D1752186

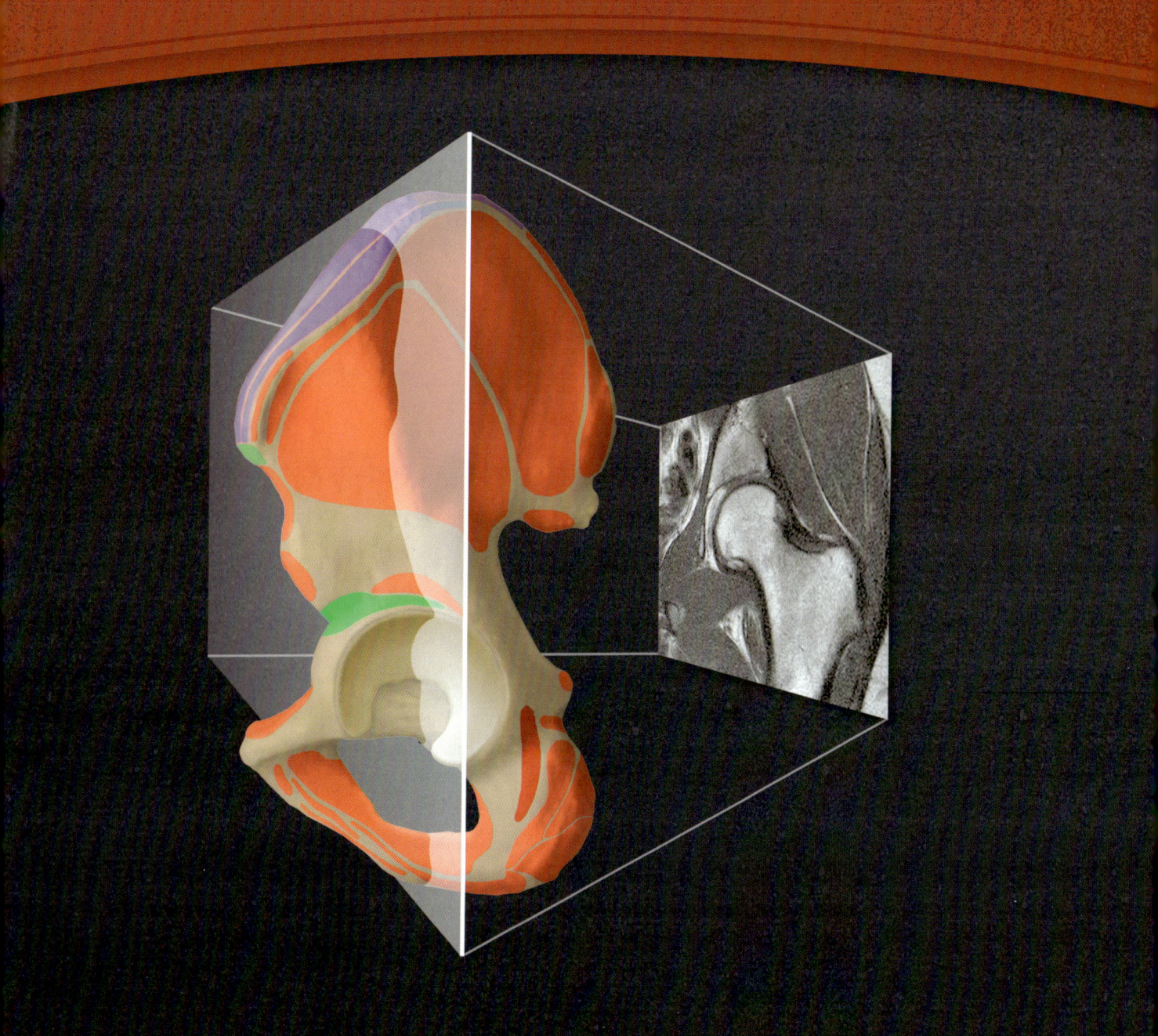

IMAGING ANATOMY
Musculoskeletal
SECOND EDITION
MANASTER | CRIM

ii

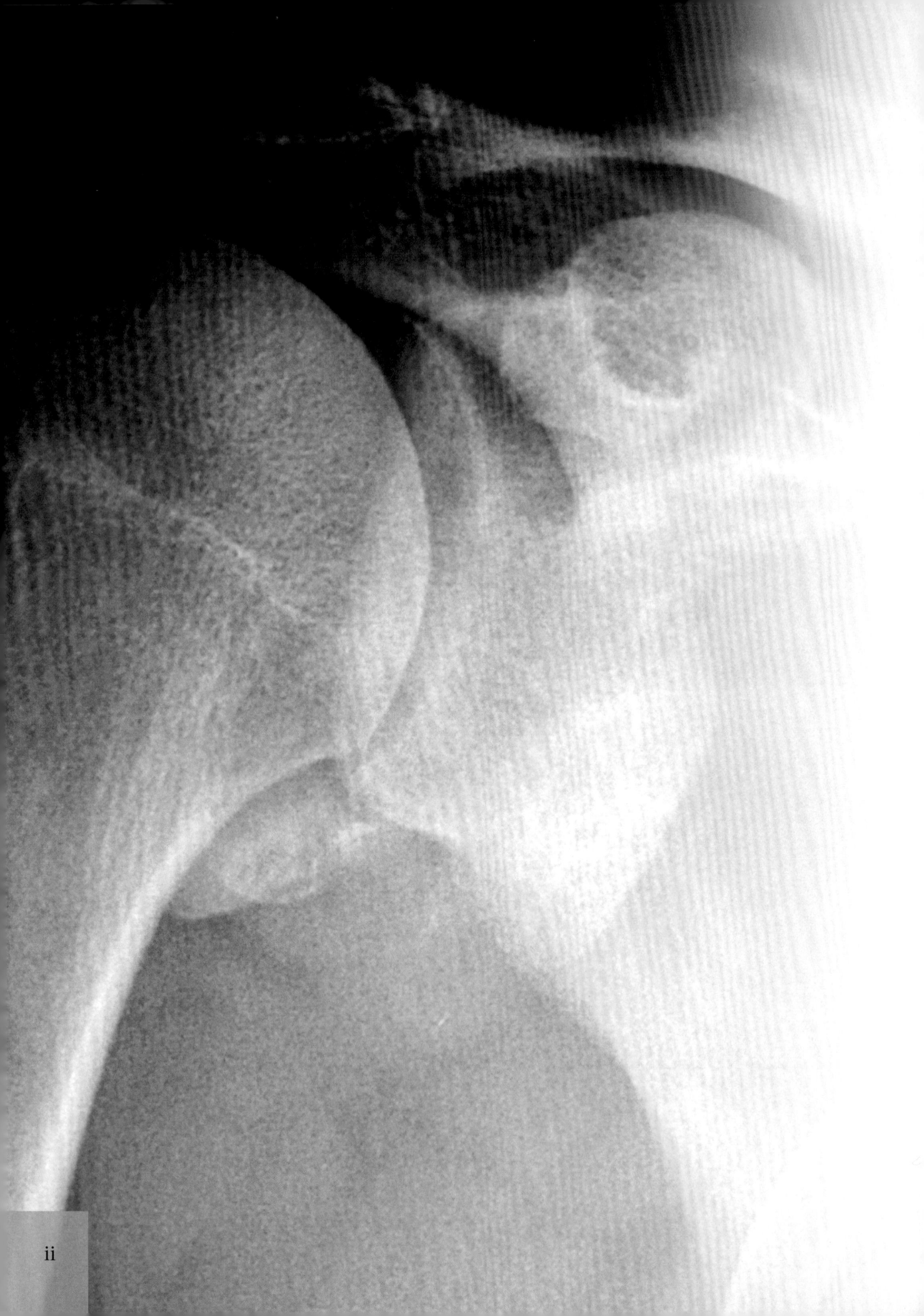

IMAGING ANATOMY
Musculoskeletal
SECOND EDITION

B.J. Manaster, MD, PhD, FACR
Emeritus Professor
Department of Radiology
University of Utah School of Medicine
Salt Lake City, Utah

Julia Crim, MD
Chief of Musculoskeletal Radiology
Department of Radiology
University of Missouri
Columbia, Missouri

ELSEVIER

1600 John F. Kennedy Blvd.
Ste 1800
Philadelphia, PA 19103-2899

IMAGING ANATOMY: MUSCULOSKELETAL, SECOND EDITION   ISBN: 978-0-323-37756-0

Copyright © 2016 by Elsevier. All rights reserved.

No part of this publication may be reproduced or transmitted in any form or by any means, electronic or mechanical, including photocopying, recording, or any information storage and retrieval system, without permission in writing from the publisher. Details on how to seek permission, further information about the Publisher's permissions policies and our arrangements with organizations such as the Copyright Clearance Center and the Copyright Licensing Agency, can be found at our website: www.elsevier.com/permissions.

This book and the individual contributions contained in it are protected under copyright by the Publisher (other than as may be noted herein).

Notices

Knowledge and best practice in this field are constantly changing. As new research and experience broaden our understanding, changes in research methods, professional practices, or medical treatment may become necessary.

Practitioners and researchers must always rely on their own experience and knowledge in evaluating and using any information, methods, compounds, or experiments described herein. In using such information or methods they should be mindful of their own safety and the safety of others, including parties for whom they have a professional responsibility.

With respect to any drug or pharmaceutical products identified, readers are advised to check the most current information provided (i) on procedures featured or (ii) by the manufacturer of each product to be administered, to verify the recommended dose or formula, the method and duration of administration, and contraindications. It is the responsibility of practitioners, relying on their own experience and knowledge of their patients, to make diagnoses, to determine dosages and the best treatment for each individual patient, and to take all appropriate safety precautions.

To the fullest extent of the law, neither the Publisher nor the authors, contributors, or editors, assume any liability for any injury and/or damage to persons or property as a matter of products liability, negligence or otherwise, or from any use or operation of any methods, products, instructions, or ideas contained in the material herein.

Publisher Cataloging-in-Publication Data

Imaging anatomy. Musculoskeletal / [edited by] B.J. Manaster and Julia Crim.
    2nd edition.
      pages ; cm
      Musculoskeletal
      Includes bibliographical references and index.
    ISBN 978-0-323-37756-0 (hardback)
    1. Musculoskeletal system--Imaging--Handbooks, manuals, etc.
    I. Manaster, B. J. II. Crim, Julia. III. Title: Musculoskeletal.
    [DNLM: 1. Musculoskeletal Diseases--diagnosis--Atlases. 2. Musculoskeletal System--injuries--Atlases. 3. Musculoskeletal System--radiography--Atlases. WE 141]
    RC925.7 .I434 2015
    616.7/0754--dc23

International Standard Book Number: 978-0-323-37756-0

Cover Designer: Tom M. Olson, BA
Cover Art: Richard Coombs, MS

Printed in Canada by Friesens, Altona, Manitoba, Canada

Last digit is the print number: 9 8 7 6 5 4 3 2 1

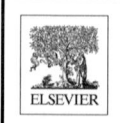

Dedications

This book is dedicated to the residents and fellows with whom we have worked over the past many years. It is a joy to have been your teachers, mentors, and friends. As we wrote the second edition of Imaging Anatomy: Musculoskeletal, we thought about you and tried to clearly answer all the anatomy questions you have asked; we hope the book is useful to you and to all scholars studying the musculoskeletal system.

BJM and JRC

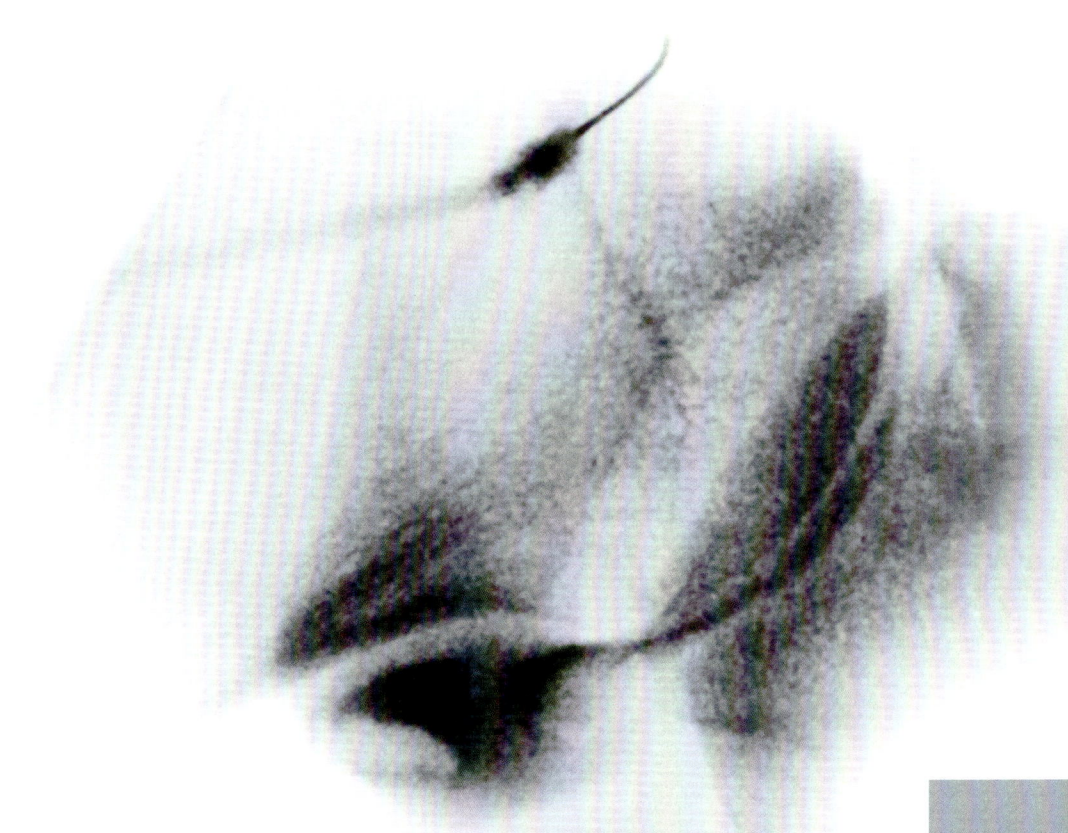

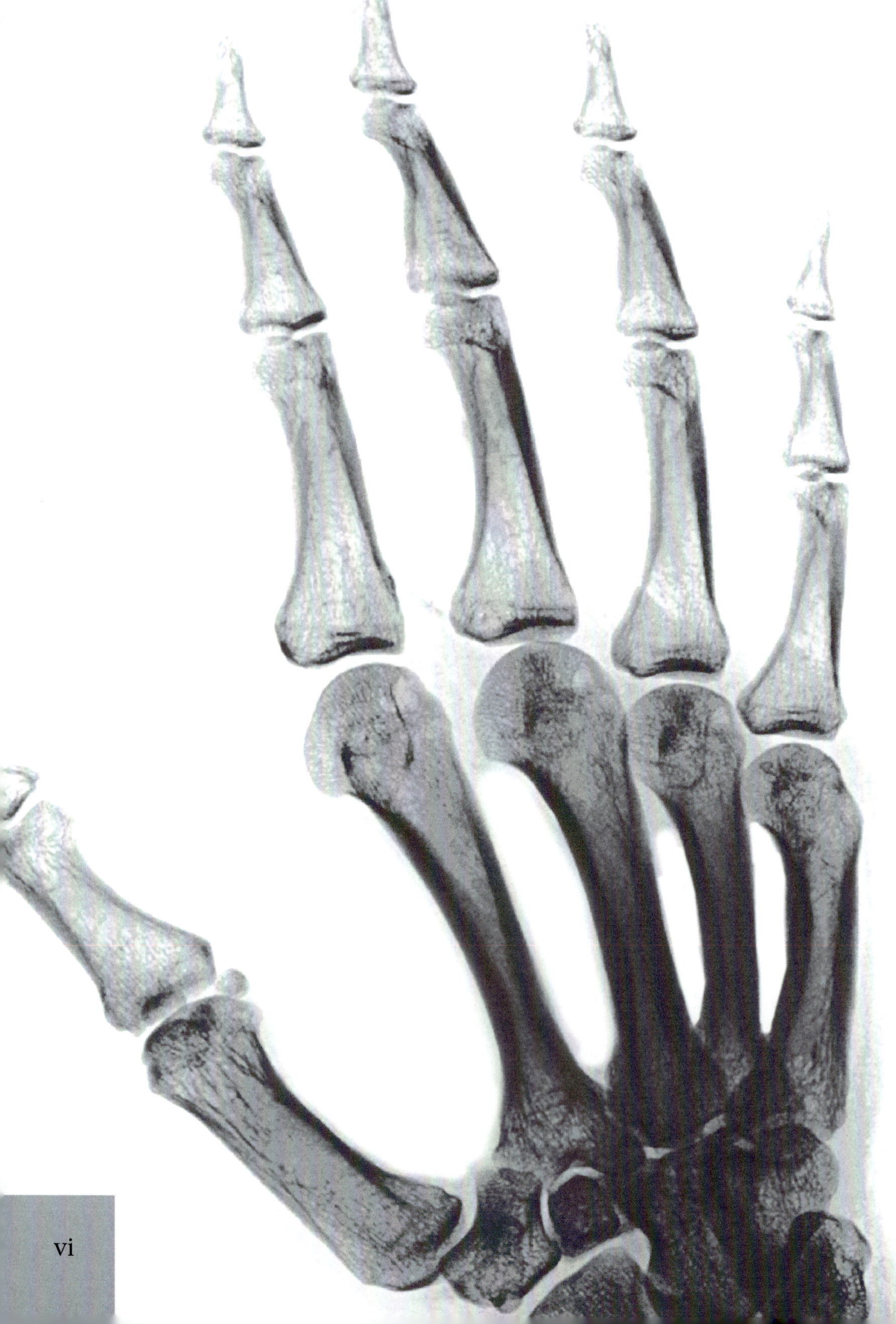

Contributing Authors

Catherine C. Roberts, MD
Professor of Radiology
Mayo Clinic
Scottsdale, Arizona

Theodore T. Miller, MD, FACR
Chief, Division of Ultrasound
Hospital for Special Surgery
Professor of Radiology
Weill Medical College of Cornell University
New York, New York

Cheryl Petersilge, MD, MBA
Clinical Professor of Radiology
Cleveland Clinic Lerner College of Medicine
Case Western Reserve University
Cleveland, Ohio

William B. Morrison, MD
Professor of Radiology
Director, Division of Musculoskeletal Imaging and Intervention
Department of Radiology
Thomas Jefferson University Hospital
Philadelphia, Pennsylvania

Carol L. Andrews, MD
Associate Professor
Division Chief, Musculoskeletal Radiology
University of Pittsburgh Medical Center
Pittsburgh, Pennsylvania

Jeffrey W. Grossman, MD
Owner/Manager
Bonehead Radiology, PLLC
Eagle, Idaho

Zehava Sadka Rosenberg, MD
Professor of Radiology and Orthopedic Surgery
NYU School of Medicine
NYU Langone Medical Center
New York, New York

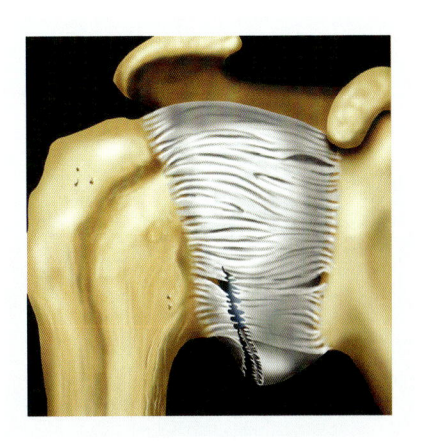

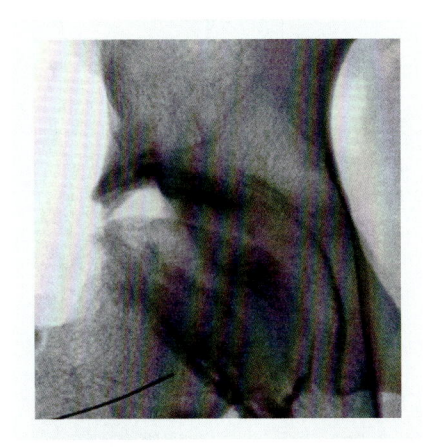

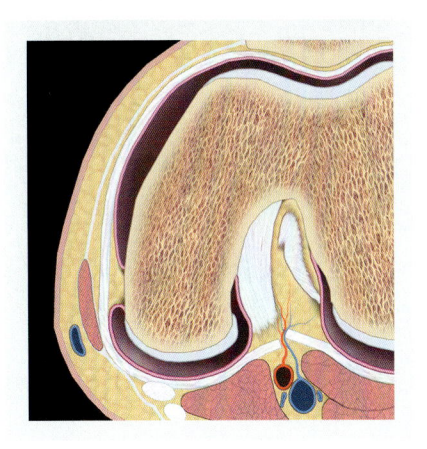

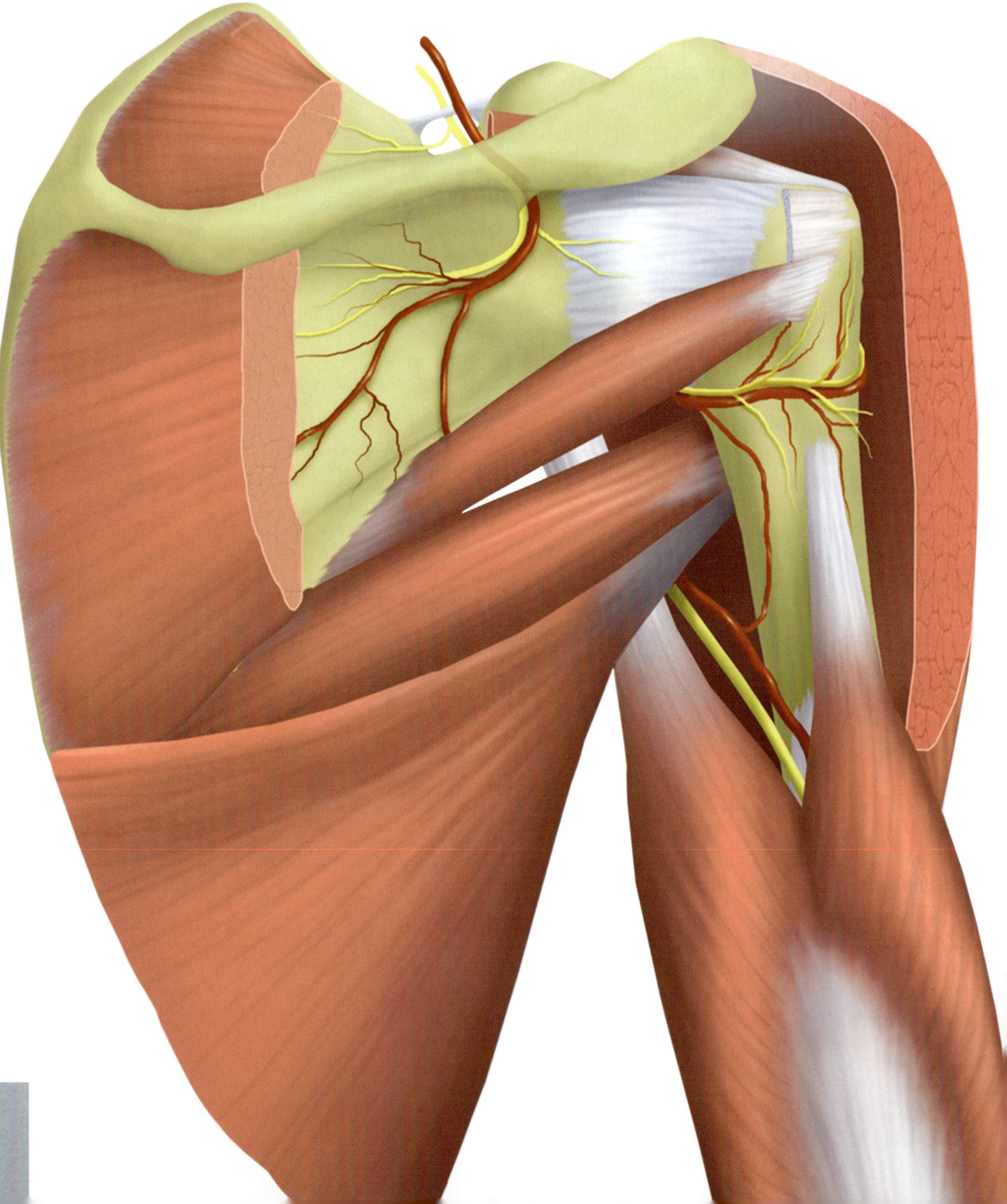

Preface

This second edition of *Imaging Anatomy: Musculoskeletal* retains features that made the first edition widely popular. Images are extensively labeled in 3 planes and include long bones as well as joints. Coronal and axial images of right and left sides are placed on facing pages. Anatomy is described with attention to issues of clinical importance. So, what is new that justifies a new edition? We have made numerous changes that we believe will make this work more complete and easier to use.

The chapter organization has been made more uniform in the second edition. The overview chapter for each anatomic region contains a written text supplemented by color anatomy illustrations. The overview is followed by a chapter describing radiographic and arthrographic anatomy, as well as an MR Atlas chapter. In the MR Atlas, the scout images are larger, making correlation easier. Additional chapters detailing uniquely difficult anatomic or functional regions follow the MR Atlas. Additional material has been added to better explicate the complex anatomy of the hip, hand, thumb, ankle, and foot.

We have standardized and expanded sections describing standard imaging lines, angles, and measurements to make it easy for radiologists to reference both methodology and normal values. In addition, chapters featuring normal variants and imaging pitfalls have been added. And last but not least, we discovered and corrected some labeling errors from the first edition.

We hope and expect the users, our colleagues, will find the improvements made in this edition to be useful in their practice.

B.J. Manaster, MD, PhD, FACR
Emeritus Professor
Department of Radiology
University of Utah School of Medicine
Salt Lake City, Utah

Julia Crim, MD
Chief of Musculoskeletal Radiology
Department of Radiology
University of Missouri
Columbia, Missouri

x

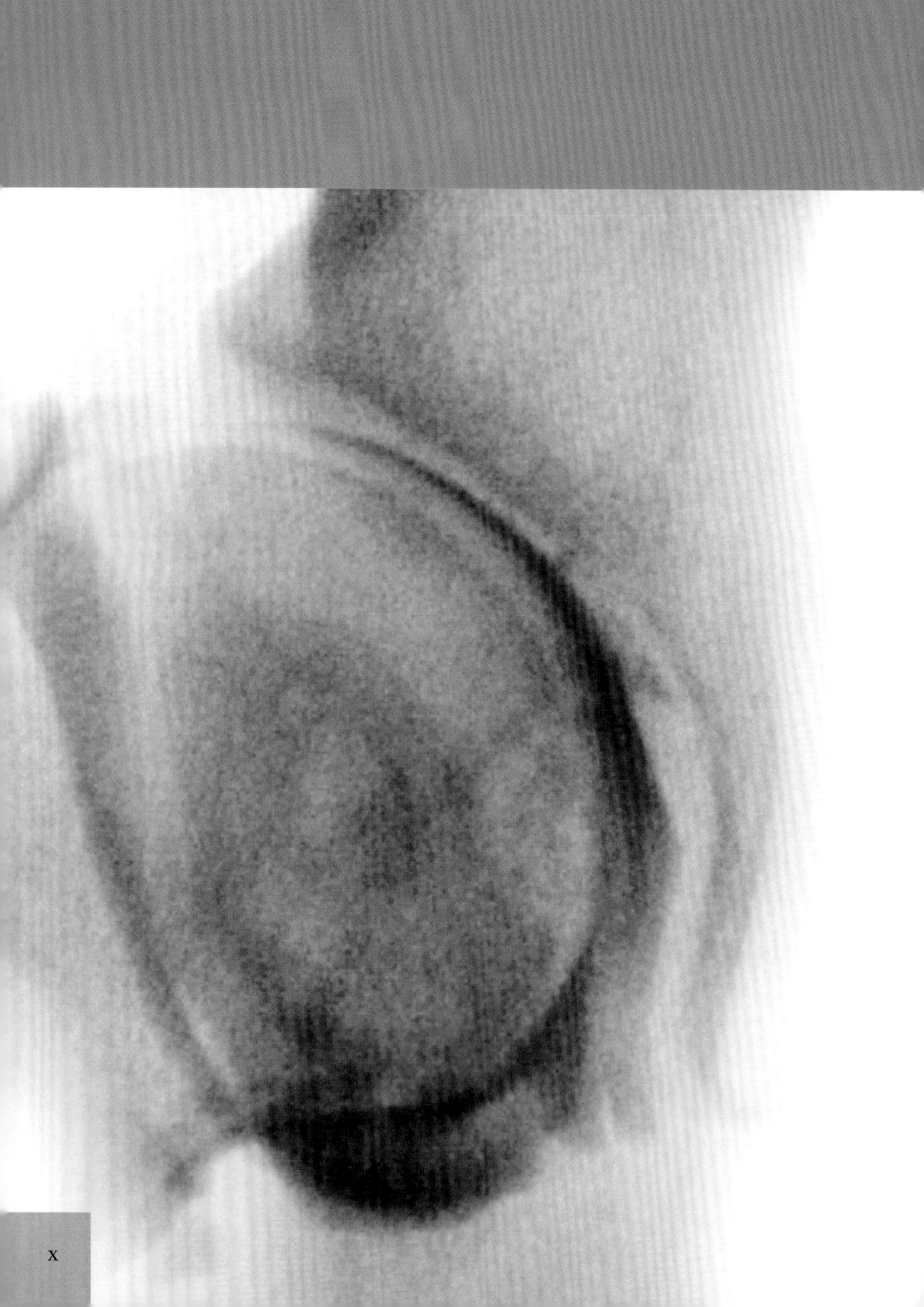

Acknowledgements

Text Editors

Dave L. Chance, MA, ELS
Arthur G. Gelsinger, MA
Nina I. Bennett, BA
Sarah J. Connor, BA
Tricia L. Cannon, BA
Terry W. Ferrell, MS

Image Editors

Jeffrey J. Marmorstone, BS
Lisa A. M. Steadman, BS

Medical Editor

Megan K. Mills, MD

Illustrations

Richard Coombs, MS
Lane R. Bennion, MS
Laura C. Sesto, MA

Art Direction and Design

Tom M. Olson, BA
Laura C. Sesto, MA

Lead Editors

Rebecca L. Hutchinson, BA
Lisa A. Gervais, BS

Production Coordinators

Angela M.G. Terry, BA
Rebecca L. Hutchinson, BA

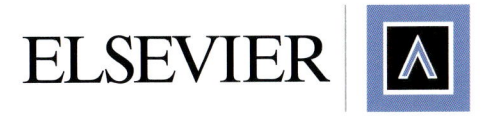

ELSEVIER

xii

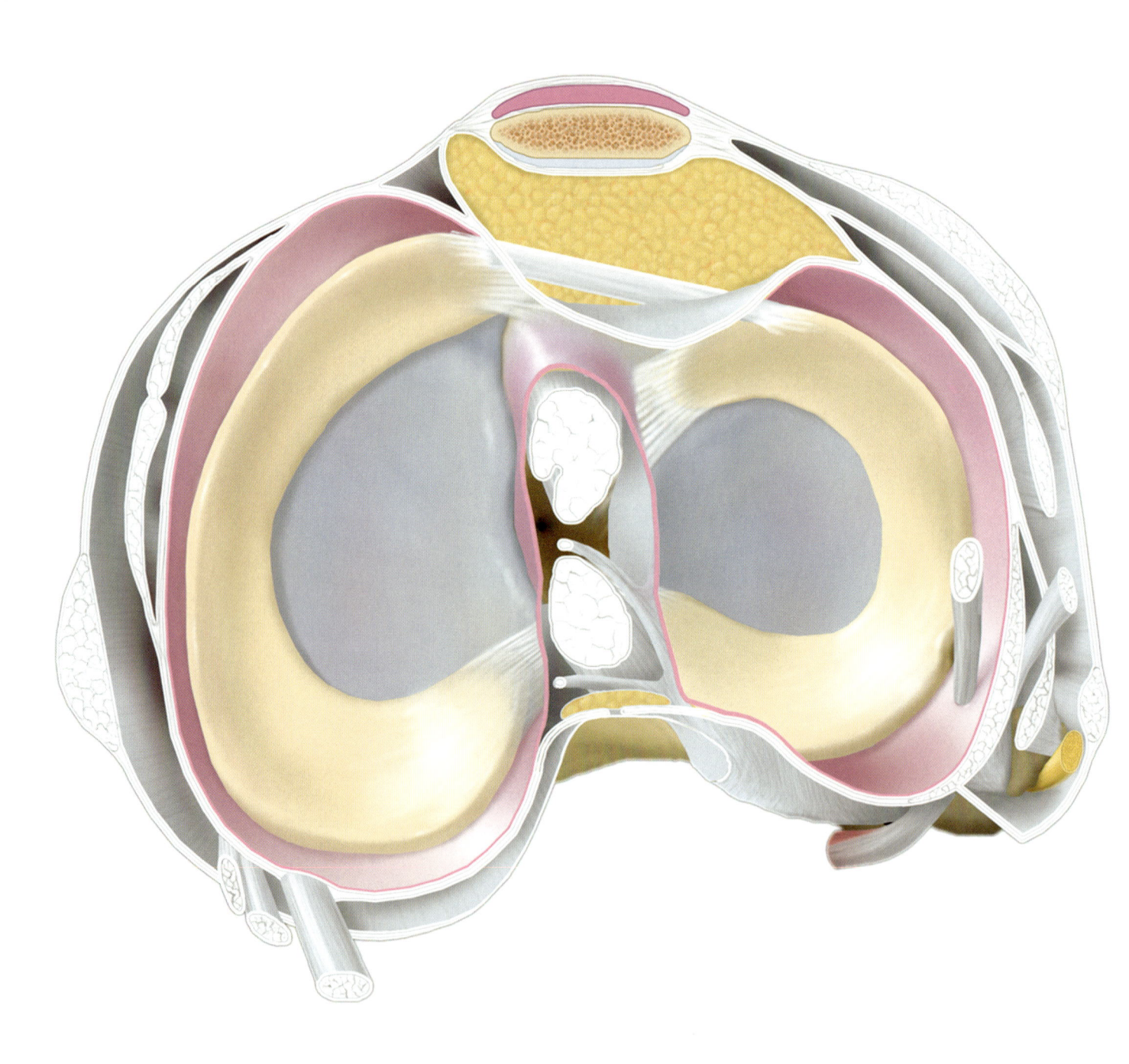

Sections

SECTION 1: SHOULDER

SECTION 2: ARM

SECTION 3: ELBOW

SECTION 4: FOREARM

SECTION 5: WRIST

SECTION 6: HAND

SECTION 7: PELVIS AND HIP

SECTION 8: THIGH

SECTION 9: KNEE

SECTION 10: LEG

SECTION 11: ANKLE

SECTION 12: FOOT

TABLE OF CONTENTS

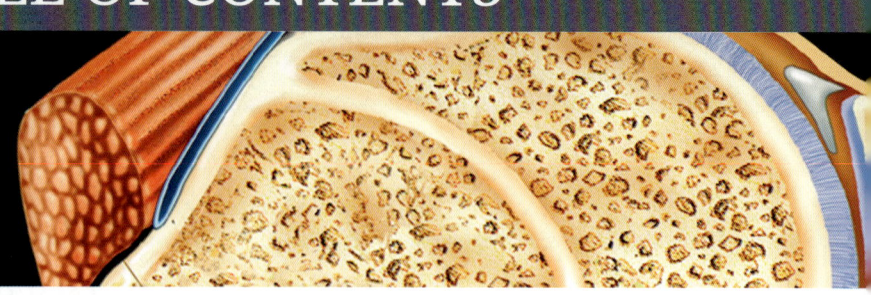

SECTION 1: SHOULDER

4 Shoulder Overview
B.J. Manaster, MD, PhD, FACR and Catherine C. Roberts, MD

14 Shoulder Radiographic and Arthrographic Anatomy
B.J. Manaster, MD, PhD, FACR and Julia Crim, MD

36 Shoulder MR Atlas
B.J. Manaster, MD, PhD, FACR and Catherine C. Roberts, MD

86 Shoulder Abduction-External Rotation (ABER) Plane
B.J. Manaster, MD, PhD, FACR and Catherine C. Roberts, MD

94 Shoulder: Rotator Cuff and Biceps Tendon
B.J. Manaster, MD, PhD, FACR and Catherine C. Roberts, MD

102 Shoulder: Rotator Interval
B.J. Manaster, MD, PhD, FACR and Catherine C. Roberts, MD

112 Shoulder Ligaments
B.J. Manaster, MD, PhD, FACR and Catherine C. Roberts, MD

126 Shoulder Labrum
B.J. Manaster, MD, PhD, FACR and Catherine C. Roberts, MD

138 Shoulder Normal Variants and Imaging Pitfalls
B.J. Manaster, MD, PhD, FACR

SECTION 2: ARM

154 Arm Radiographic Anatomy and MR Atlas
B.J. Manaster, MD, PhD, FACR and Catherine C. Roberts, MD

SECTION 3: ELBOW

194 Elbow Overview
B.J. Manaster, MD, PhD, FACR and Theodore T. Miller, MD, FACR

200 Elbow Radiographic and Arthrographic Anatomy
B.J. Manaster, MD, PhD, FACR and Julia Crim, MD

214 Elbow MR Atlas
B.J. Manaster, MD, PhD, FACR and Theodore T. Miller, MD, FACR

248 Elbow Muscles and Tendons
B.J. Manaster, MD, PhD, FACR and Theodore T. Miller, MD, FACR

270 Elbow Ligaments
B.J. Manaster, MD, PhD, FACR and Theodore T. Miller, MD, FACR

280 Elbow Normal Variants and Imaging Pitfalls
B.J. Manaster, MD, PhD, FACR

292 Elbow Measurements and Lines
B.J. Manaster, MD, PhD, FACR

SECTION 4: FOREARM

298 Forearm Radiographic Anatomy and MR Atlas
B.J. Manaster, MD, PhD, FACR and Theodore T. Miller, MD, FACR

SECTION 5: WRIST

326 Wrist Overview
Julia Crim, MD and Carol L. Andrews, MD

334 Wrist Radiographic and Arthrographic Anatomy
Julia Crim, MD

342 Wrist MR Atlas
Julia Crim, MD and Carol L. Andrews, MD

388 Wrist Ligaments
Julia Crim, MD and Carol L. Andrews, MD

398 Wrist Tendons
Julia Crim, MD and Carol L. Andrews, MD

418 Wrist and Hand Normal Variants and Imaging Pitfalls
Julia Crim, MD

428 Wrist Measurements and Lines
Julia Crim, MD and Carol L. Andrews, MD

SECTION 6: HAND

436 Hand Overview
Julia Crim, MD and Jeffrey W. Grossman, MD

444 Thumb Anatomy
Julia Crim, MD

452 Hand Radiographic Anatomy
Julia Crim, MD and Jeffrey W. Grossman, MD

456 Hand MR Atlas
Julia Crim, MD and Jeffrey W. Grossman, MD

472 Flexor and Extensor Mechanisms of Hand
Julia Crim, MD

SECTION 7: PELVIS AND HIP

486 Pelvis Overview
Julia Crim, MD and Cheryl A. Petersilge, MD, MBA

494 Pelvis MR Atlas
Julia Crim, MD and Cheryl A. Petersilge, MD, MBA

528 Anterior Pelvis
Julia Crim, MD and Cheryl A. Petersilge, MD, MBA

554 Hip Overview
Julia Crim, MD

558 Hip MR Anatomy
Julia Crim, MD and Cheryl A. Petersilge, MD, MBA

TABLE OF CONTENTS

- 574 **Pelvis and Hip Radiographic and Arthrographic Anatomy**
  Julia Crim, MD
- 590 **Pelvis and Hip Normal Variants and Imaging Pitfalls**
  Julia Crim, MD
- 598 **Pelvis and Hip Measurements and Lines**
  Julia Crim, MD and Cheryl A. Petersilge, MD, MBA

SECTION 8: THIGH

- 606 **Thigh Radiographic Anatomy and MR Atlas**
  Julia Crim, MD and Cheryl A. Petersilge, MD, MBA

SECTION 9: KNEE

- 662 **Knee Overview**
  B.J. Manaster, MD, PhD, FACR
- 670 **Knee Radiographic and Arthrographic Anatomy**
  B.J. Manaster, MD, PhD, FACR and William B. Morrison, MD
- 686 **Knee MR Atlas**
  B.J. Manaster, MD, PhD, FACR
- 734 **Knee Extensor Mechanism and Retinacula**
  B.J. Manaster, MD, PhD, FACR
- 742 **Menisci**
  B.J. Manaster, MD, PhD, FACR
- 768 **Cruciate Ligaments/Posterior Capsule**
  B.J. Manaster, MD, PhD, FACR
- 786 **Knee Medial Supporting Structures**
  B.J. Manaster, MD, PhD, FACR
- 796 **Knee Lateral Supporting Structures**
  B.J. Manaster, MD, PhD, FACR
- 812 **Knee and Leg Normal Variants and Imaging Pitfalls**
  B.J. Manaster, MD, PhD, FACR
- 858 **Knee and Leg Measurements and Lines**
  B.J. Manaster, MD, PhD, FACR

SECTION 10: LEG

- 878 **Leg Radiographic Anatomy and MR Atlas**
  B.J. Manaster, MD, PhD, FACR

SECTION 11: ANKLE

- 918 **Ankle Overview**
  Julia Crim, MD and Zehava Sadka Rosenberg, MD
- 934 **Ankle Radiographic and Arthrographic Anatomy**
  Julia Crim, MD
- 946 **Ankle MR Atlas**
  Julia Crim, MD and Zehava Sadka Rosenberg, MD
- 980 **Ankle Tendons**
  Julia Crim, MD and Zehava Sadka Rosenberg, MD
- 1004 **Ankle Ligaments**
  Julia Crim, MD and Zehava Sadka Rosenberg, MD

SECTION 12: FOOT

- 1034 **Foot Overview**
  Julia Crim, MD
- 1042 **Foot Radiographic and Arthrographic Anatomy**
  Julia Crim, MD
- 1054 **Foot MR Atlas**
  Julia Crim, MD
- 1084 **Intrinsic Muscles of Foot**
  Julia Crim, MD
- 1090 **Tarsometatarsal Joint**
  Julia Crim, MD
- 1096 **Metatarsophalangeal Joints**
  Julia Crim, MD
- 1100 **Foot and Ankle Normal Variants and Imaging Pitfalls**
  Julia Crim, MD and Zehava Sadka Rosenberg, MD
- 1128 **Foot and Ankle Measurements and Lines**
  Julia Crim, MD

IMAGING ANATOMY
Musculoskeletal
SECOND EDITION

MANASTER | CRIM

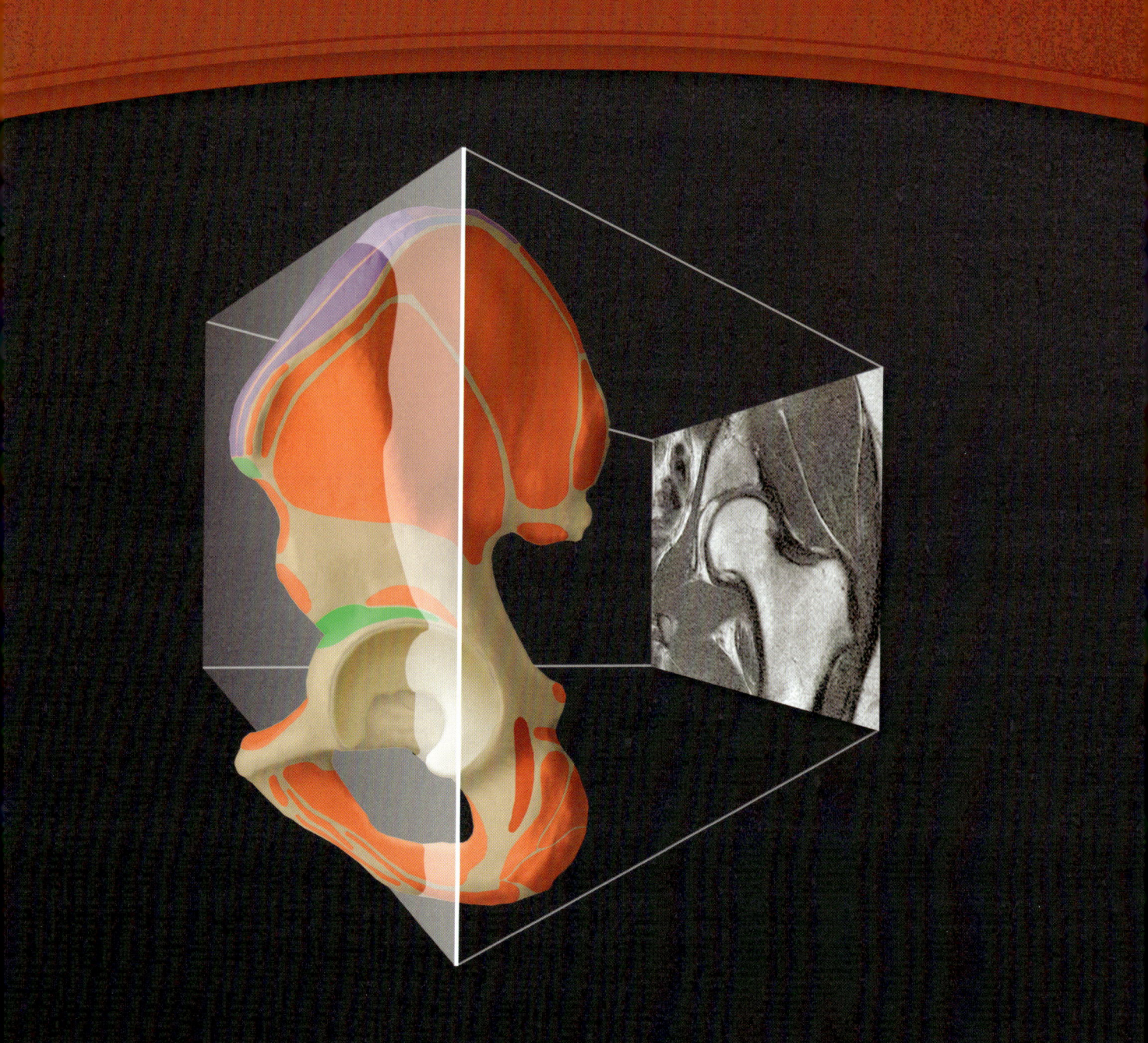

SECTION 1
Shoulder

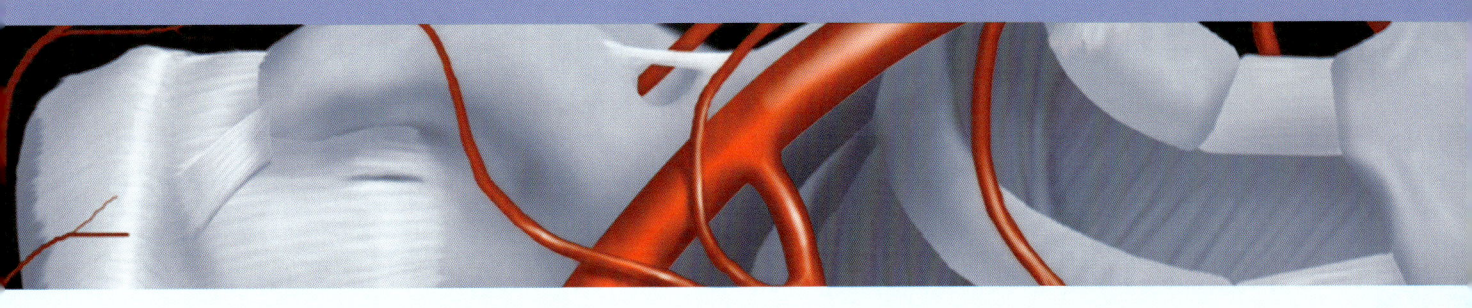

Shoulder Overview	4
Shoulder Radiographic and Arthrographic Anatomy	14
Shoulder MR Atlas	36
Shoulder Abduction-External Rotation (ABER) Plane	86
Shoulder: Rotator Cuff and Biceps Tendon	94
Shoulder: Rotator Interval	102
Shoulder Ligaments	112
Shoulder Labrum	126
Shoulder Normal Variants and Imaging Pitfalls	138

Shoulder Overview

GROSS ANATOMY

Overview
- Multiaxial ball-and-socket joint
- Hemispheric humeral head articulates with shallow pear-shaped glenoid fossa
  - Joint surrounded by synovial-lined fibrous capsule
  - Glenoid deepened by labrum, a fibrocartilage rim of tissue
  - Cartilage thins in central glenoid and in periphery of humeral head
- **Range of motion**: Flexion, extension, abduction, adduction, circumduction, medial rotation, and lateral rotation
  - **Flexion**: Pectoralis major, deltoid, coracobrachialis, & biceps muscles
  - **Extension**: Deltoid & teres major muscles
    - If against resistance, also latissimus dorsi & pectoralis major
  - **Abduction**: Deltoid & supraspinatus muscles
    - Subscapularis, infraspinatus, & teres minor exert downward traction
    - Supraspinatus contribution controversial
  - **Medial rotation**: Pectoralis major, deltoid, latissimus dorsi, & teres major muscles
    - Subscapularis when arm at side
  - **Lateral rotation**: Infraspinatus, deltoid, & teres minor muscles
- Joint stabilizers
  - Skeletally unstable joint
  - Superior support by coracoacromial arch
  - Anterior support by subscapularis tendon, anterior capsule, synovial membrane, anterior labrum and superior, middle, & inferior glenohumeral ligaments
  - Posterior support by infraspinatus and teres minor tendons, posterior capsule, synovial membrane, posterior labrum, & inferior glenohumeral ligament
- Vascular supply
  - Articular branches of anterior and posterior humeral circumflex arteries and transverse scapular artery
- Innervation
  - Axillary and suprascapular nerves

IMAGING ANATOMY

Overview
- **Humerus**
  - 8 ossification centers: Shaft, head, greater tuberosity, lesser tuberosity, capitulum, trochlea, medial, & lateral epicondyles
  - Anatomic neck located along base of articular surface, region of fused epiphyseal plate, and attachment of joint capsule
  - Surgical neck located 2 cm distal to anatomic neck, below greater and lesser tuberosities, extracapsular, most common site of fracture
  - **Greater tuberosity** anterolateral on humeral head
    - Attachment of supraspinatus, infraspinatus, & teres minor tendons
  - **Lesser tuberosity** located along proximal anterior humeral head, medial to greater tuberosity
    - Attachment of subscapularis tendon
  - Intertubercular or bicipital groove
    - Between greater and lesser tuberosities
    - Transverse ligament, an extension of subscapularis tendon, forms roof of groove
    - Contains long head of biceps tendon & anterolateral branch of anterior circumflex humeral artery and vein
- **Scapula**
  - **Acromion**
    - Acromion orientation ranges from flat to sloping, mediolaterally
    - Roughly classified into 4 types based on posterior to anterior shape
    - Type I: Flat
    - Type II: Curved, paralleling humeral head
    - Type III: Anterior hooked
    - Type IV: Convex undersurface
    - Low-lying, anterior downsloping or inferolateral tilt decreases volume of coracoacromial outlet
  - **Os acromiale**
    - Ununited acromial ossification center
    - Should fuse by 25 years of age
    - Incidence of persistent ossicle: 2-10%
    - 60% bilateral
    - Four types: Mesoacromion, metaacromion, preacromion, basiacromion
  - **Glenoid**
    - Shallow, oval recess
    - Fibrocartilage labrum increases depth
  - **Coracoid process**
    - May extend lateral to plane of glenoid
    - Normal distance between coracoid and lesser tuberosity > 11 mm with arm in internal rotation
- **Clavicle**
  - Acromioclavicular joint between distal clavicle & acromion
    - 20° range of motion
  - Synovial-lined joint capsule
  - Fibrocartilage-covered ends of bone & central fibrocartilage disk
- **Bone marrow**
  - Predominantly yellow marrow in adults with residual hematopoietic red marrow in glenoid and proximal humeral metaphysis
  - Often strikingly heterogeneous in distribution
- **Glenohumeral joint space**
  - 1-2 ml synovial fluid
  - Normal communication with biceps tendon sheath
  - Normal communication with subscapular recess
  - Posterior joint capsule typically inserts on base of labrum
  - Anterior joint capsule has variable insertion
- **Anterior joint capsule insertion**
  - Type 1: Inserts at tip or base of labrum
  - Type 2: Inserts scapular neck < 1 cm from labrum
  - Type 3: Inserts scapular neck > 1 cm from labrum
- **Subscapular recess**
  - Between scapula & subscapularis muscle and tendon
  - Joint communication via foramen of Weitbrecht: Between superior and middle glenohumeral ligaments
  - Joint communication via foramen of Rouvière: Between middle and inferior glenohumeral ligaments

Shoulder Overview

- o Normally opacified during arthrography
- **Rotator cuff**
  - o Supraspinatus, infraspinatus, subscapularis, and teres minor
  - o Tendons interdigitate forming continuous band at attachment to humerus
  - o Origins
    - – Supraspinatus: Supraspinatus fossa of scapula
    - – Infraspinatus: Infraspinatus fossa of scapula
    - – Teres minor: Lateral scapular border
    - – Subscapularis: Anterior scapular surface (subscapular fossa)
  - o Insertions
    - – Supraspinatus, infraspinatus, and teres minor insert on the greater tuberosity
    - – Supraspinatus has a direct component that inserts on anterior portion of tuberosity and posterior oblique component that undercuts the infraspinatus at posterior portion of tuberosity
    - – Subscapularis inserts on lesser tuberosity
- **Ligaments**
  - o Coracoacromial ligament
    - – Anterior 2/3 of coracoid to tip of acromion
  - o Coracoclavicular ligament
    - – Stabilizes acromioclavicular joint
    - – Base of coracoid process to clavicle
    - – Conoid (medial) & trapezoid (lateral) bands have common origin on coracoid, diverge to clavicle
  - o Coracohumeral ligament
    - – Lateral base of coracoid to lesser & greater tuberosities
    - – Blends with subscapularis tendon, supraspinatus tendon, joint capsule, & superior glenohumeral ligament
  - o Superior & inferior acromioclavicular ligaments
  - o Superior, middle, & inferior glenohumeral ligaments
    - – Superior and middle glenohumeral ligaments extend from superior glenoid region to lesser tuberosity
    - – Congenitally absent or diminutive middle glenohumeral ligament in 30% of population
    - – Inferior glenohumeral ligament (anterior band, posterior band, & axillary pouch) extends from inferior labrum to humeral anatomic neck
- **Capsulolabral complex**
  - o Labrum
    - – Oval fibrocartilage tissue along glenoid rim
    - – Hyaline cartilage may lie between labrum & bone (undercutting labrum)
    - – Varies in shape, size, and appearance
    - – Anatomic variants, most common in anterosuperior region, include sublabral foramen & Buford complex
  - o Biceps tendon
    - – Long head arises from supraglenoid tubercle or superior labrum
    - – Long head may be congenitally absent
    - – Long head may arise from intertubercular groove or joint capsule
    - – Short head originates at coracoid process as conjoined tendon with coracobrachialis
  - – Additional heads are rarely present and arise from brachialis muscle, intertubercular groove or greater tubercle
- **Bursae**
  - o Subacromial-subdeltoid bursa
    - – Normally contains a minimal amount of fluid
    - – Adherent to undersurface of acromion
    - – Lies superficial to rotator cuff
  - o Subcoracoid bursa
    - – Separate from normal subscapular recess of joint
    - – Between subscapularis tendon and coracobrachialis/short head of biceps tendon
    - – Can communicate with subacromial-subdeltoid bursa
    - – Does not normally communicate with joint
  - o Infraspinatus bursa
    - – Between infraspinatus tendon and joint capsule
    - – Can rarely communicate with joint
  - o Other less common bursae
    - – Deep to coracobrachialis muscle
    - – Between teres major & long head of triceps
    - – Anterior & posterior to latissimus dorsi tendon
    - – Superior to acromion
- **Additional muscles of upper arm**
  - o Deltoid, biceps, coracobrachialis, triceps
- **Extrinsic shoulder muscles**
  - o Trapezius, latissimus dorsi, levator scapulae, major & minor rhomboids, serratus anterior, subclavius, omohyoid, pectoralis major, pectoralis minor

Internal Contents

- **Quadrilateral or quadrangular space**
  - o Teres minor, superior border
  - o Teres major, inferior border
  - o Humerus, lateral border
  - o Long head triceps, medial border
  - o Contains axillary nerve and posterior circumflex humeral artery
- **Coracoacromial arch**
  - o Acromion, superior border
  - o Humeral head, posterior border
  - o Coracoid process and coracoacromial ligament, anterior border
  - o Contains subacromial-subdeltoid bursa, supraspinatus muscle/tendon, long head of biceps
- **Rotator interval**
  - o Triangular space between inferior border of supraspinatus muscle/tendon and superior border of subscapularis muscle/tendon
  - o Medially bordered by coracoid process
  - o Laterally bordered by transverse humeral ligament
  - o Anterior border formed by coracohumeral ligament, superior glenohumeral ligament, & joint capsule

Shoulder Overview

3D CT RECONSTRUCTION, MUSCLE ORIGINS & INSERTIONS

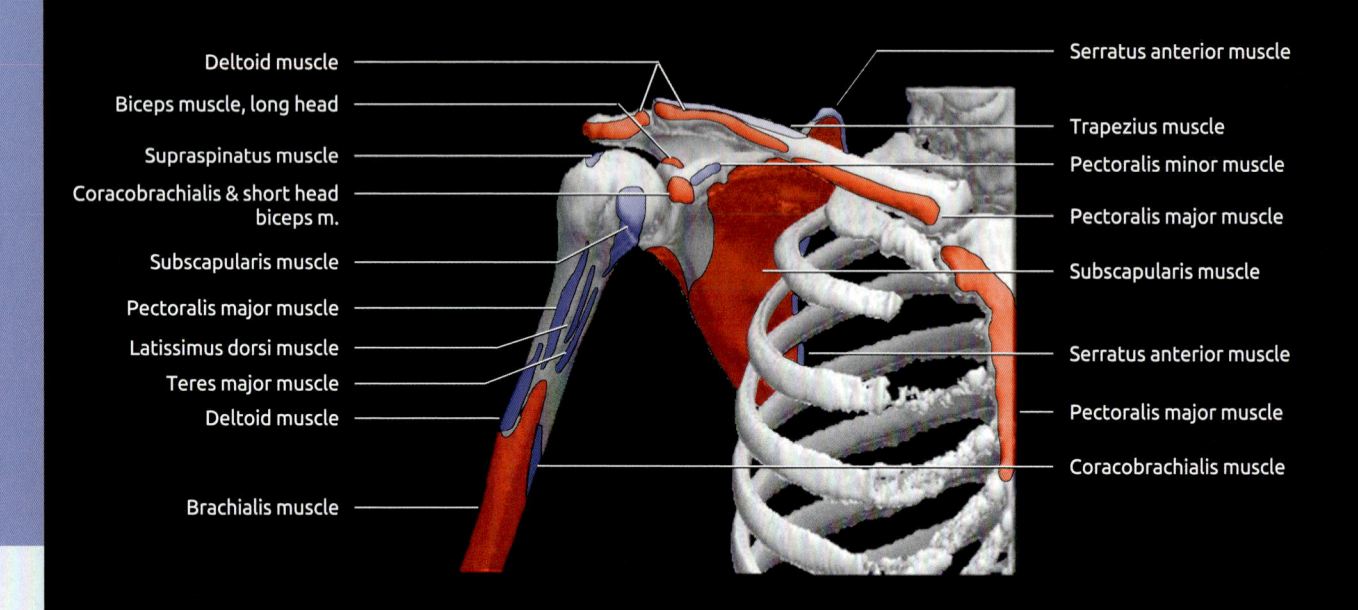

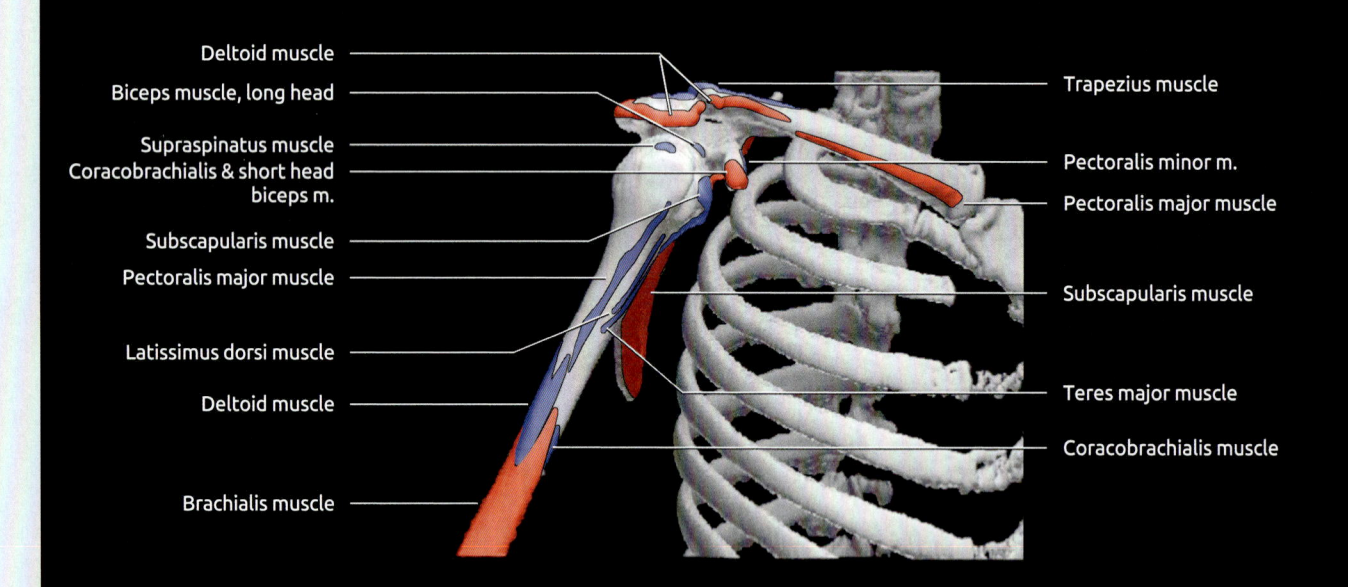

(Top) Anterior view of the right shoulder from a 3D CT reconstruction is shown. Muscle origins are shown in red. Muscle insertions are shown in blue. (Bottom) Anterior oblique view of the shoulder is shown.

Shoulder Overview

3D CT RECONSTRUCTION, MUSCLE ORIGINS & INSERTIONS

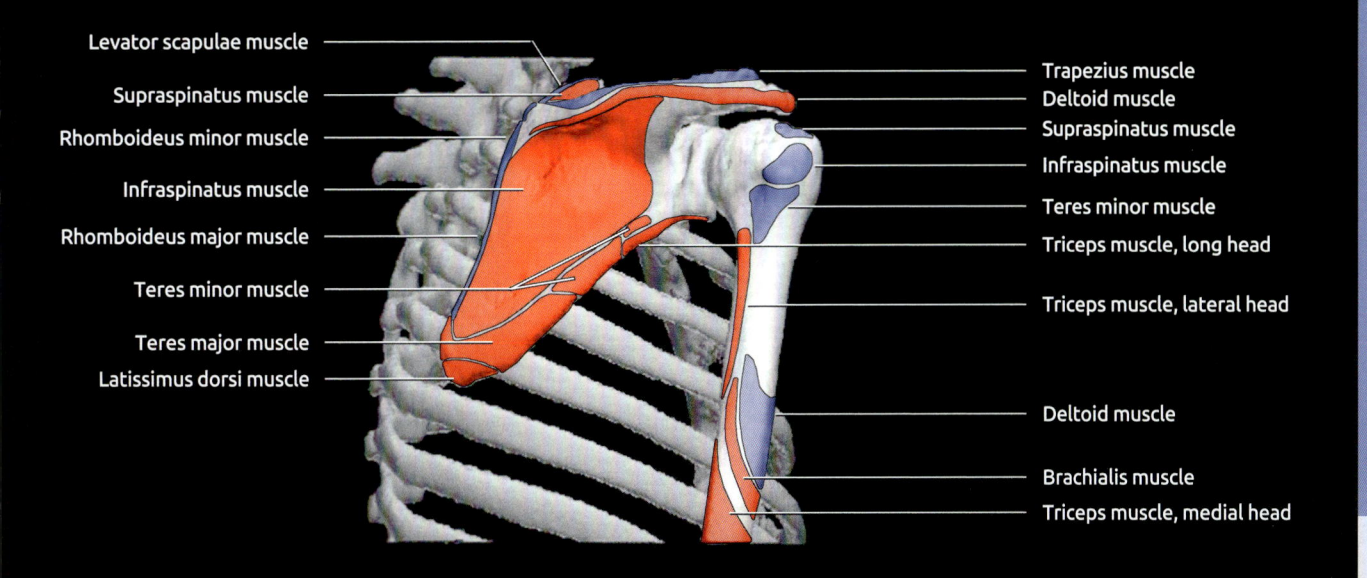

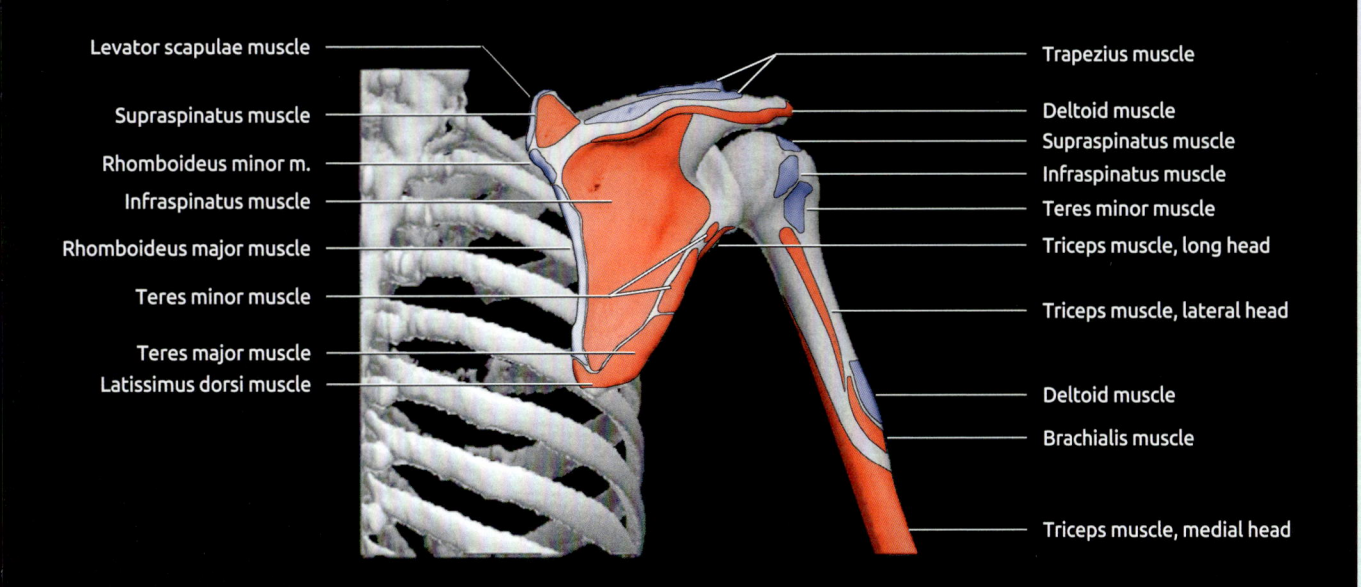

Levator scapulae muscle
Supraspinatus muscle
Rhomboideus minor muscle
Infraspinatus muscle
Rhomboideus major muscle
Teres minor muscle
Teres major muscle
Latissimus dorsi muscle

Trapezius muscle
Deltoid muscle
Supraspinatus muscle
Infraspinatus muscle
Teres minor muscle
Triceps muscle, long head
Triceps muscle, lateral head
Deltoid muscle
Brachialis muscle
Triceps muscle, medial head

Levator scapulae muscle
Supraspinatus muscle
Rhomboideus minor m.
Infraspinatus muscle
Rhomboideus major muscle
Teres minor muscle
Teres major muscle
Latissimus dorsi muscle

Trapezius muscle
Deltoid muscle
Supraspinatus muscle
Infraspinatus muscle
Teres minor muscle
Triceps muscle, long head
Triceps muscle, lateral head
Deltoid muscle
Brachialis muscle
Triceps muscle, medial head

(Top) Posterior oblique view of the shoulder from a 3D CT reconstruction is shown. Muscle origins are shown in red. Muscle insertions are shown in blue. (Bottom) Posterior view of the shoulder is shown.

Shoulder Overview

GRAPHICS: ANTERIOR, POSTERIOR SHOULDER MUSCULATURE

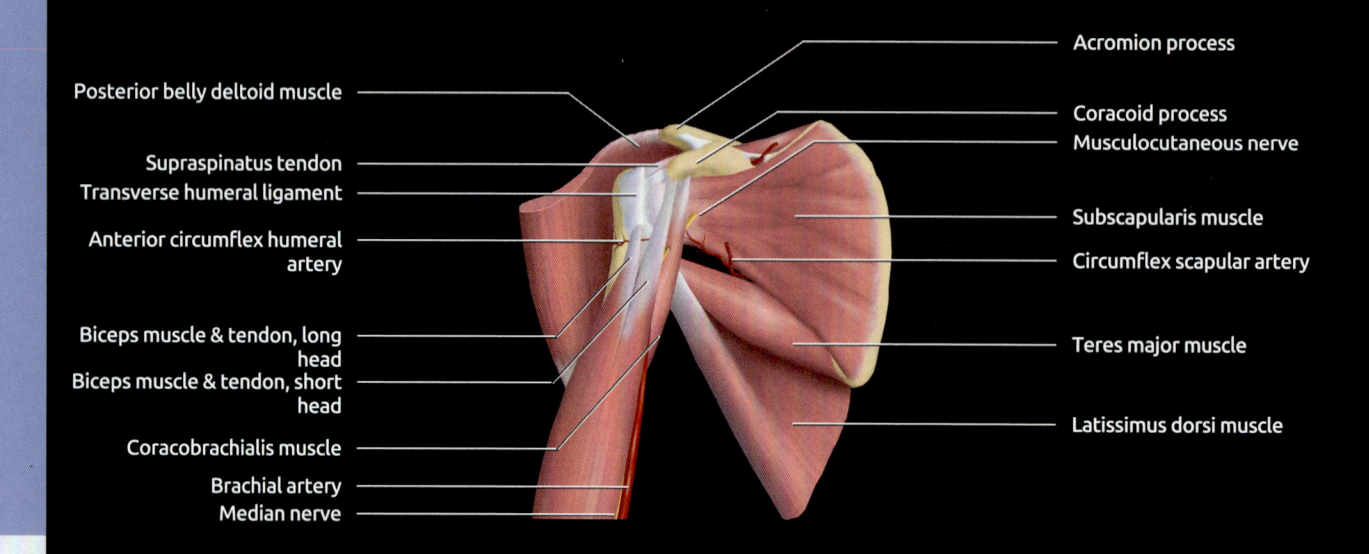

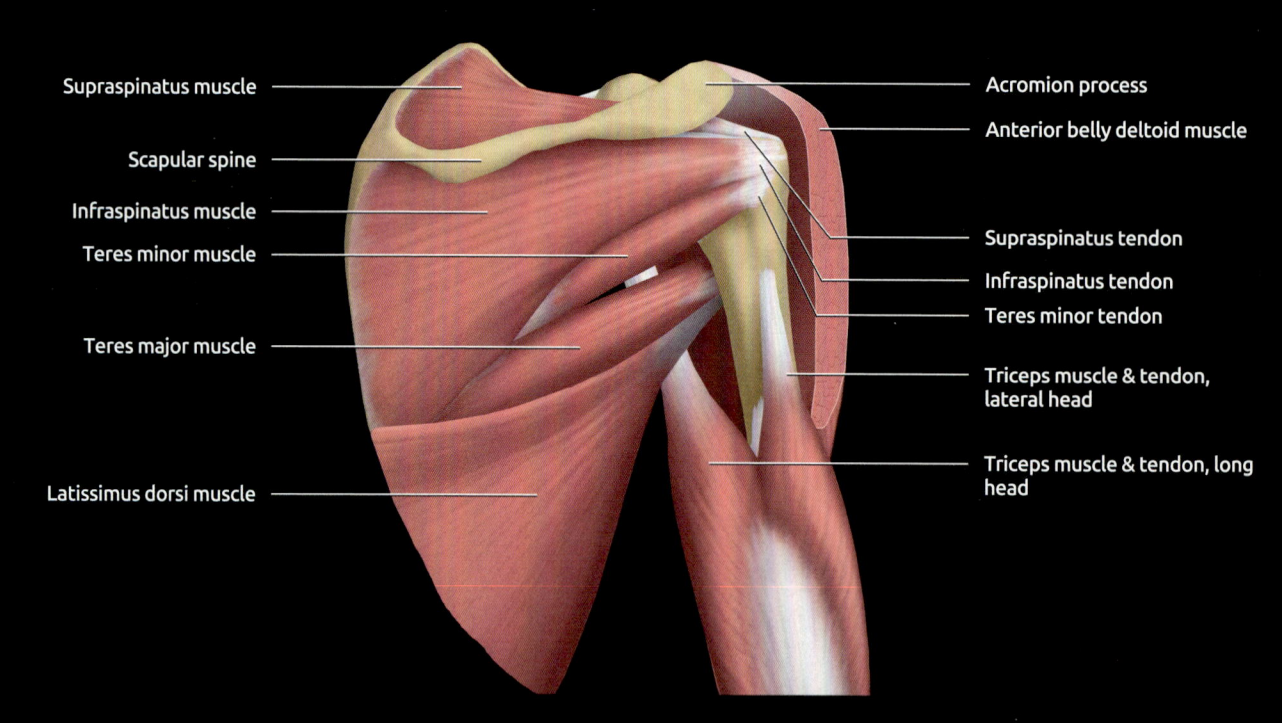

(Top) Anterior graphic of the shoulder shows a superficial scapulohumeral dissection. *(Bottom)* Posterior graphic of the shoulder shows superficial scapulohumeral dissection demonstrating the musculature.

Shoulder Overview

GRAPHICS: ROTATOR CUFF & NEUROVASCULAR STRUCTURES

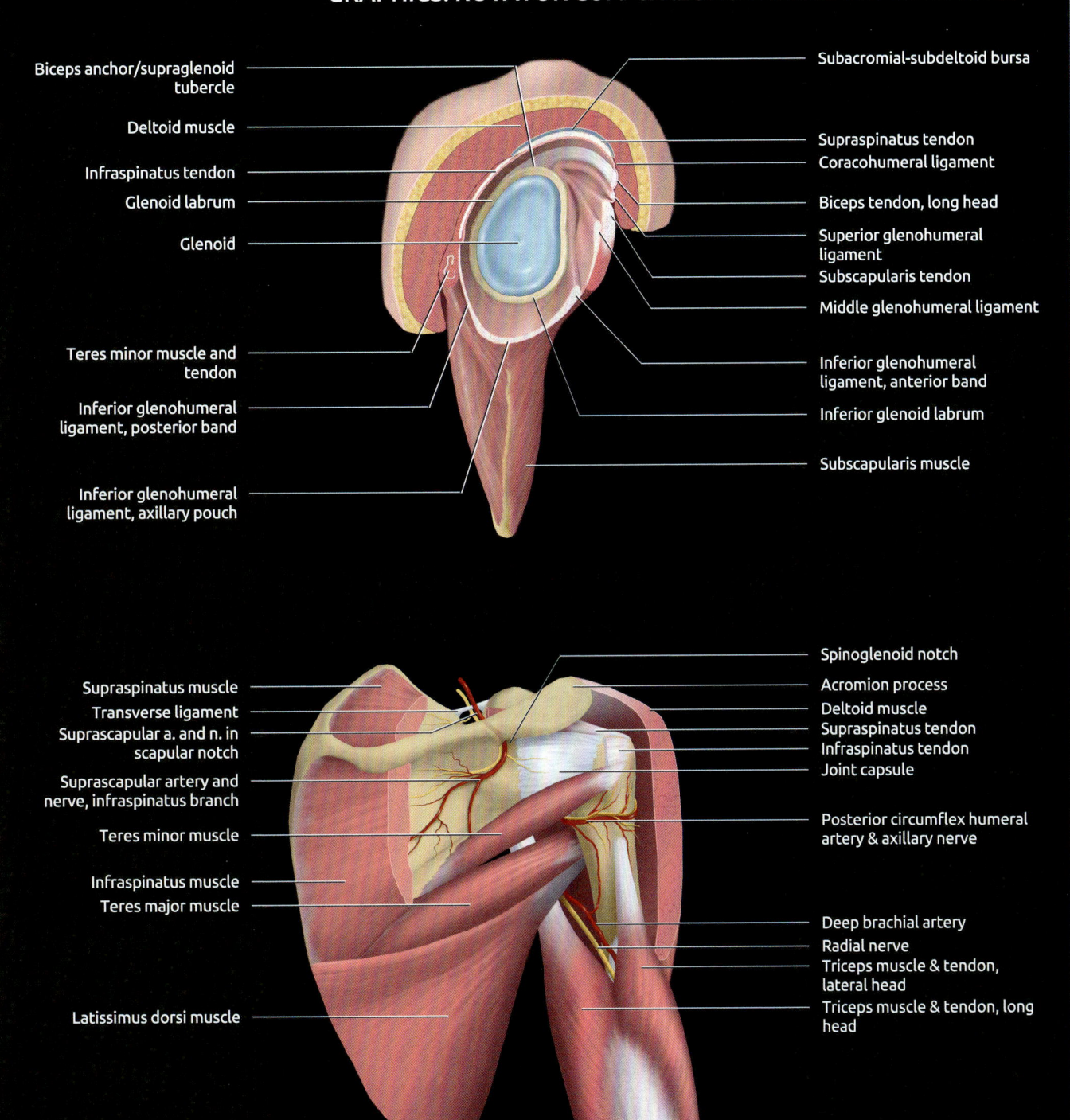

(Top) Sagittal graphic of the shoulder shows the humerus removed. (Bottom) Deep scapulohumeral dissection demonstrates the major neurovascular structures.

Shoulder Overview

GRAPHICS: VASCULAR STRUCTURES

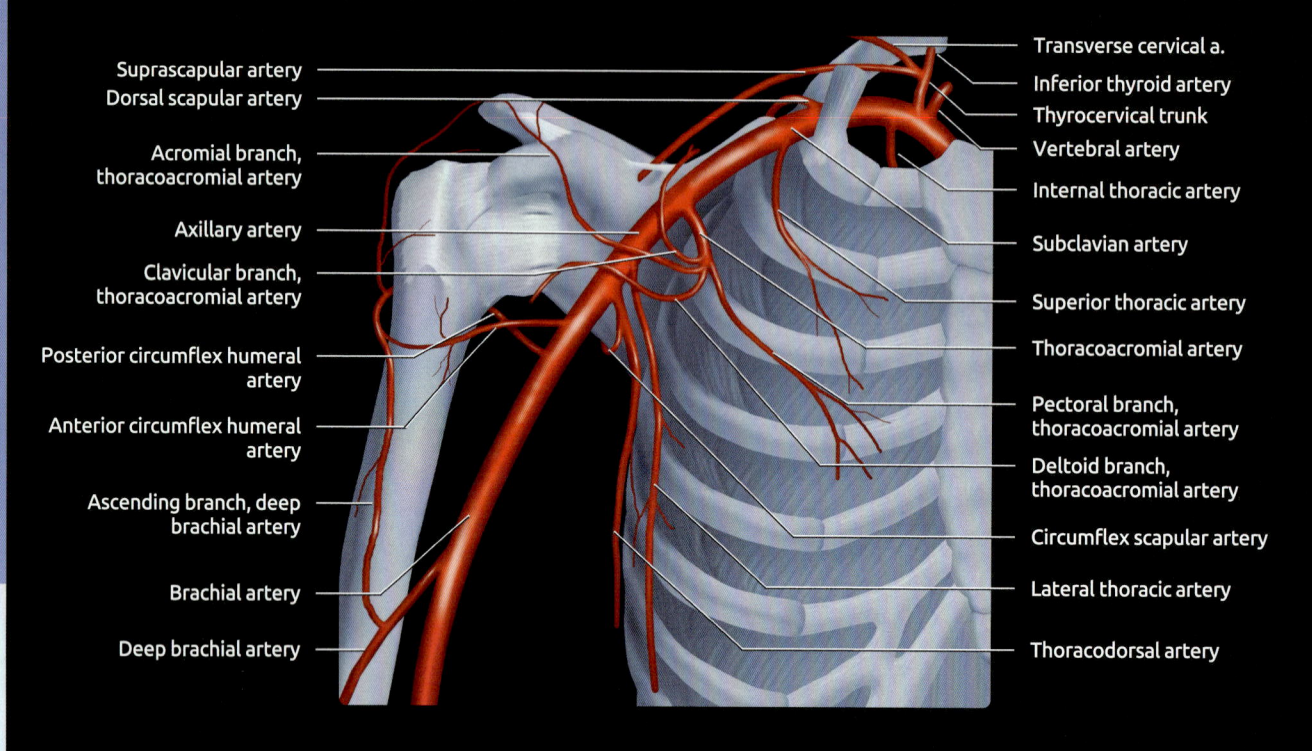

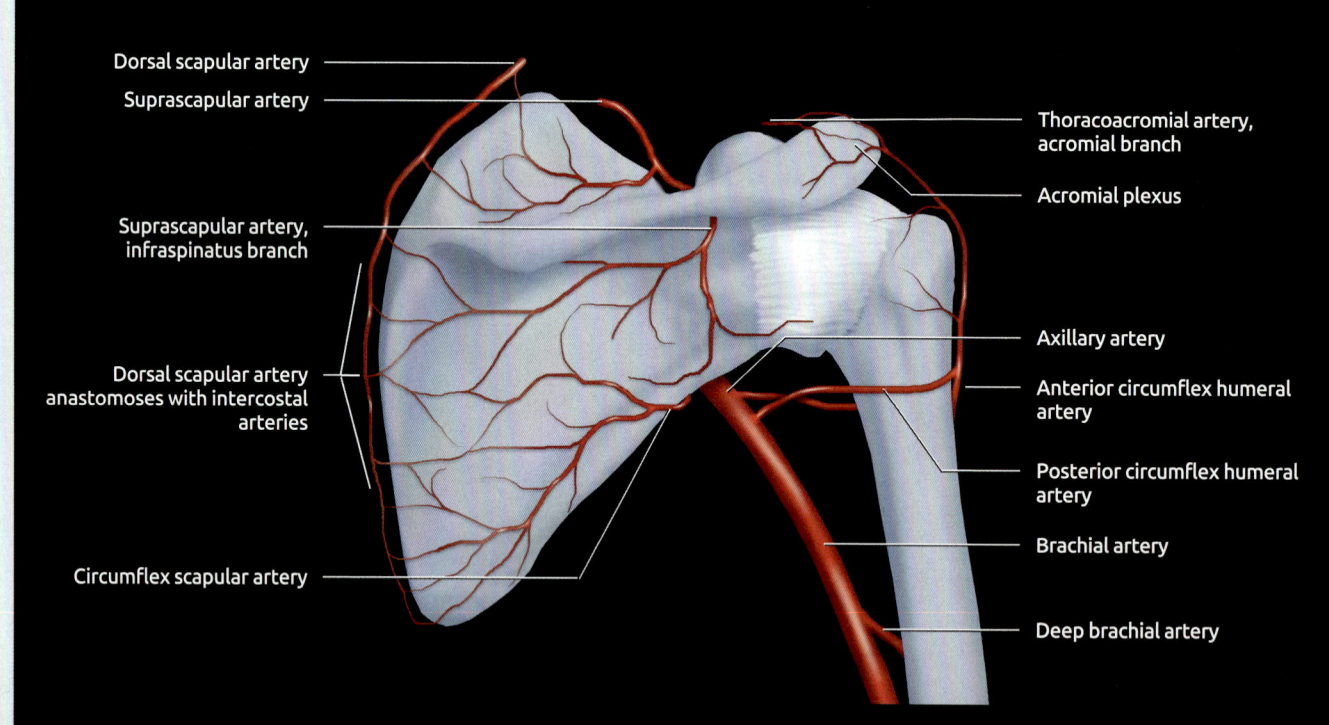

(Top) Anterior graphic of arterial supply to shoulder is shown. The shoulder is predominantly supplied by anterior and posterior circumflex humeral, suprascapular and circumflex scapular arteries. (Bottom) Posterior graphic of arterial supply to shoulder is shown. Extensive collateral blood vessels include anastomoses with intercostal arteries.

Shoulder Overview

GRAPHICS: NEURAL STRUCTURES

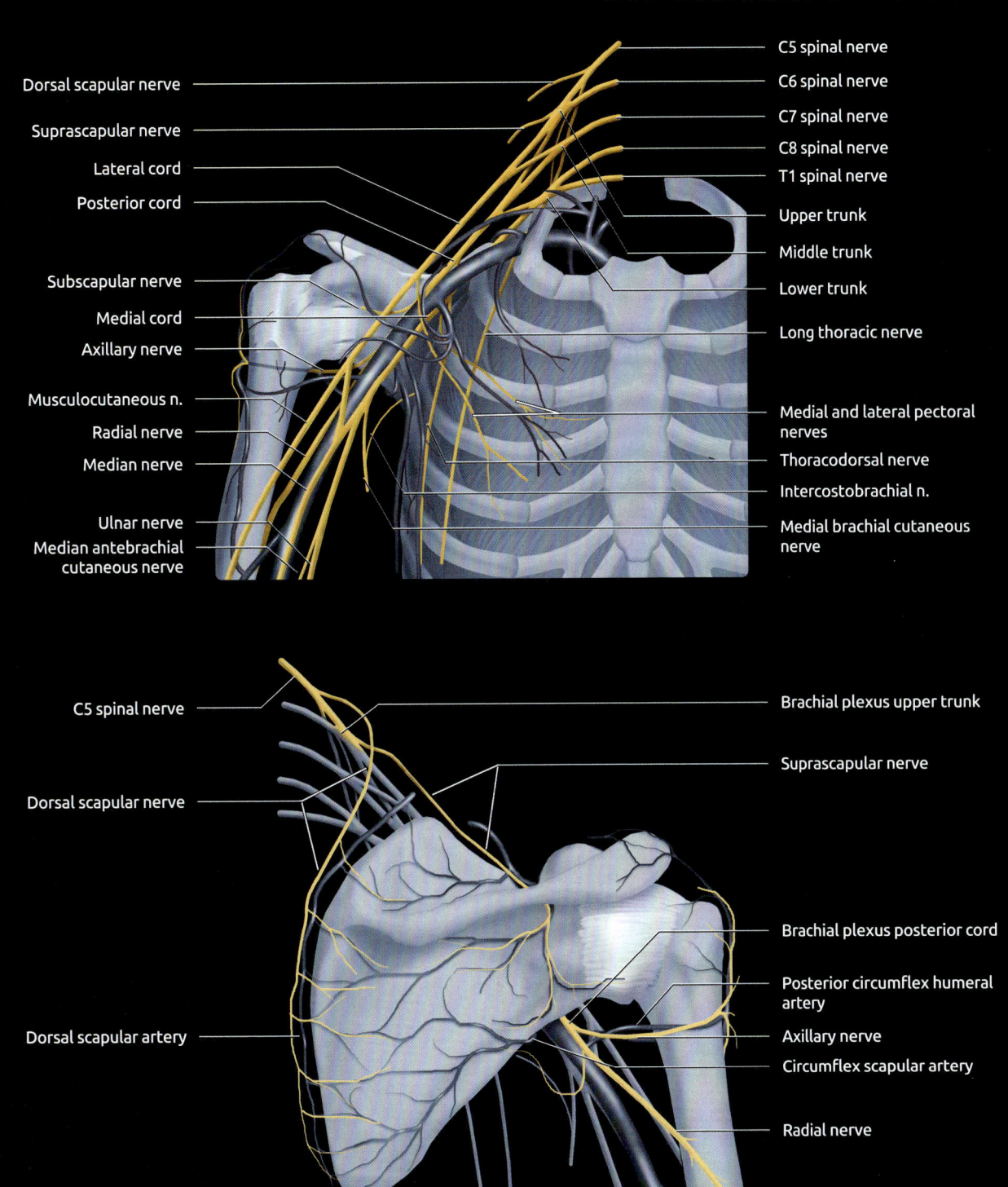

Top image labels:
- Dorsal scapular nerve
- Suprascapular nerve
- Lateral cord
- Posterior cord
- Subscapular nerve
- Medial cord
- Axillary nerve
- Musculocutaneous n.
- Radial nerve
- Median nerve
- Ulnar nerve
- Median antebrachial cutaneous nerve
- C5 spinal nerve
- C6 spinal nerve
- C7 spinal nerve
- C8 spinal nerve
- T1 spinal nerve
- Upper trunk
- Middle trunk
- Lower trunk
- Long thoracic nerve
- Medial and lateral pectoral nerves
- Thoracodorsal nerve
- Intercostobrachial n.
- Medial brachial cutaneous nerve

Bottom image labels:
- C5 spinal nerve
- Dorsal scapular nerve
- Dorsal scapular artery
- Brachial plexus upper trunk
- Suprascapular nerve
- Brachial plexus posterior cord
- Posterior circumflex humeral artery
- Axillary nerve
- Circumflex scapular artery
- Radial nerve

(Top) *Anterior graphic of the brachial plexus is shown.* (Bottom) *Posterior graphic of the brachial plexus branches innervating the shoulder is shown.*

Shoulder Overview

GRAPHICS: SUPRASCAPULAR & SPINOGLENOID NOTCH

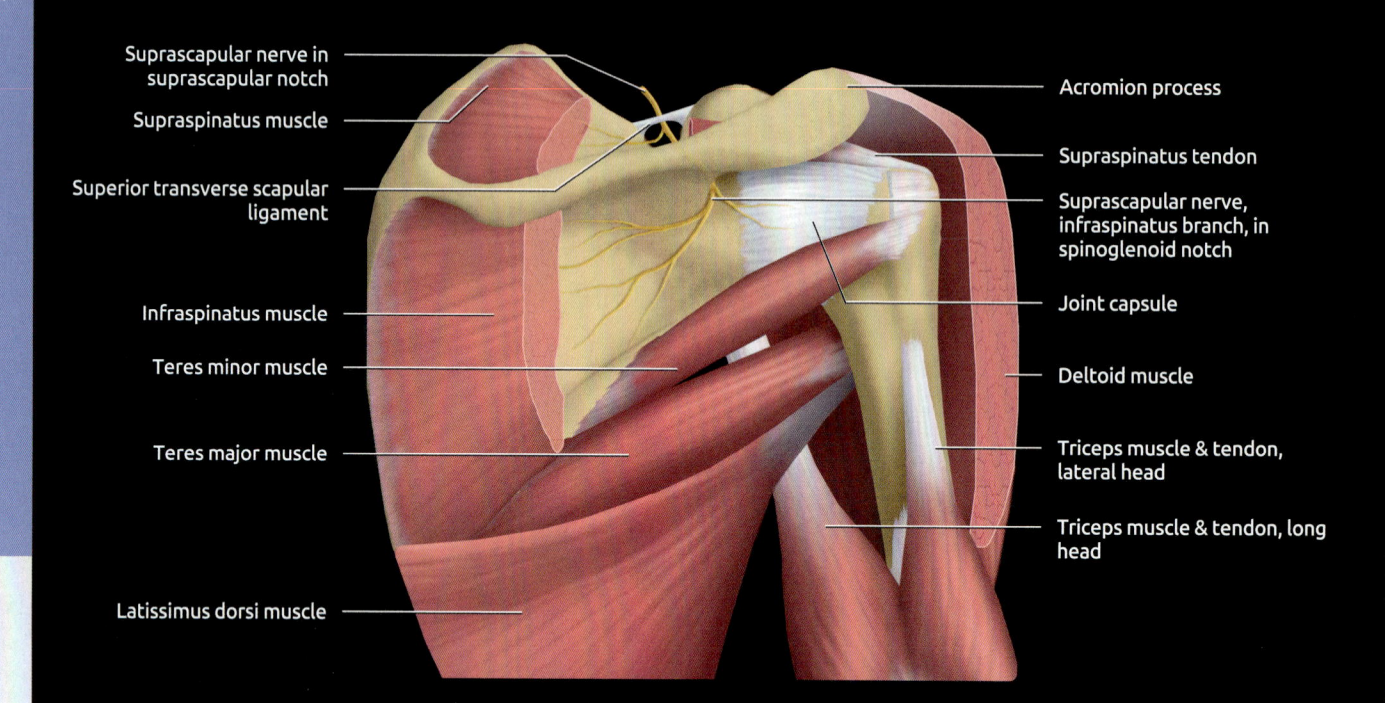

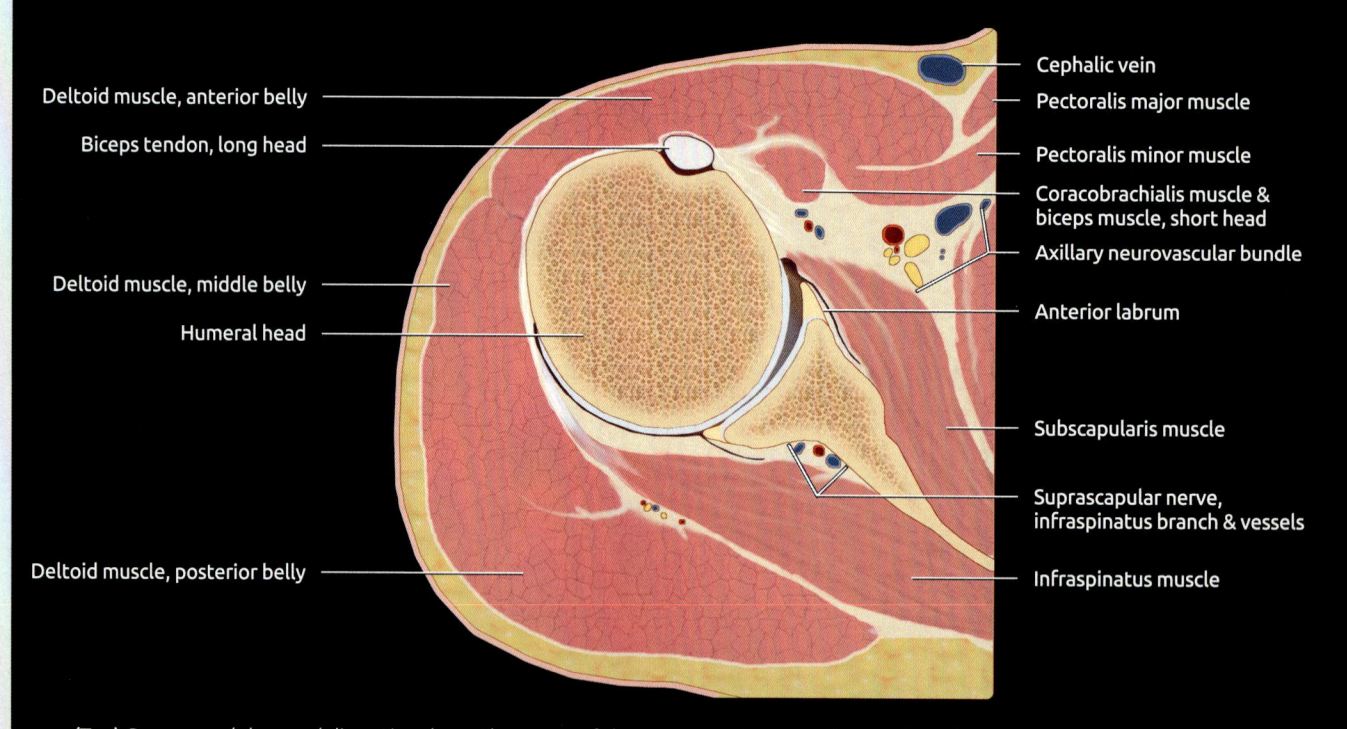

(Top) Deep scapulohumeral dissection shows the course of the suprascapular nerve. *(Bottom)* Axial graphic shows the location of the suprascapular artery, nerve and vein branches, just below the level of the spinoglenoid notch.

Shoulder Overview

GRAPHICS: QUADRILATERAL SPACE

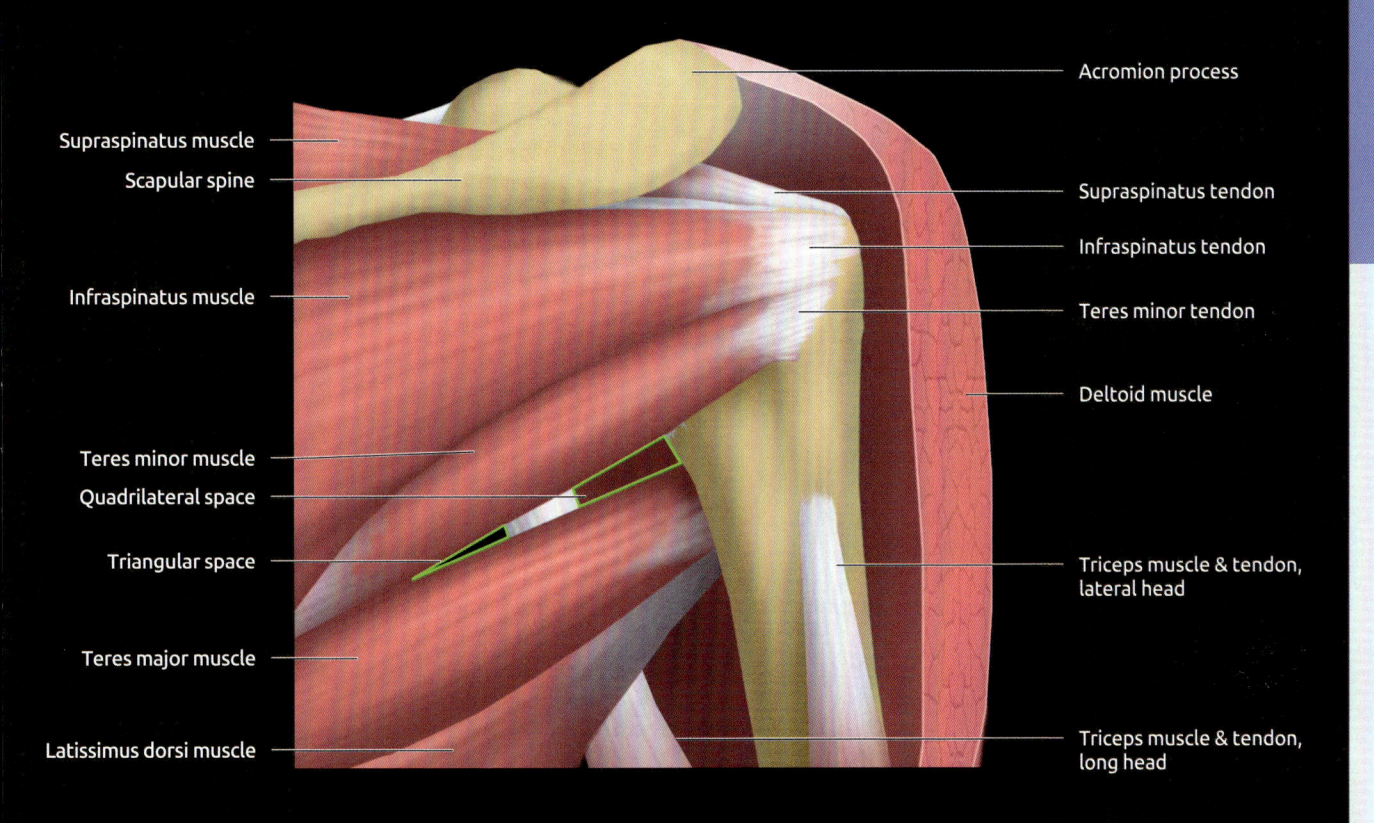

- Supraspinatus muscle
- Scapular spine
- Infraspinatus muscle
- Teres minor muscle
- Quadrilateral space
- Triangular space
- Teres major muscle
- Latissimus dorsi muscle
- Acromion process
- Supraspinatus tendon
- Infraspinatus tendon
- Teres minor tendon
- Deltoid muscle
- Triceps muscle & tendon, lateral head
- Triceps muscle & tendon, long head

Posterior graphic of the shoulder is shown. Superficial scapulohumeral dissection shows the location of the quadrilateral space and triangular space (each outlined in green).

Shoulder Radiographic and Arthrographic Anatomy

IMAGING ANATOMY

Overview

- Shoulder joint highly mobile, prone to instability
  - Rotator cuff and glenohumeral ligaments stabilize
    - Small contribution by glenoid labrum
- Joint capsule
  - Extends from glenoid margin or scapular neck to anatomic neck of humerus
  - Normal joint recesses are visualized at arthrography
    - Axillary, subscapularis, rotator interval, anterior and posterior recesses, biceps tendon sheath
- Glenoid
  - Anteverted, forms shallow cup
  - Central cartilage defect is small, smoothly marginated region that varies slightly in position
- Glenoid labrum
  - Fibrocartilaginous structure extending circumferentially around bony glenoid
  - Sits on articular surface, overlies hyaline cartilage
  - Deepens bony glenoid, improves joint congruency and stability
  - In cross section may appear triangular or rounded
  - Anterior labrum larger than posterior
- **Rotator cuff**: 4 muscles arising on scapula and inserting on humerus
  - Supraspinatus: From supraspinatus fossa of scapula to greater tuberosity
    - Abducts humerus, also depresses humeral head
  - Infraspinatus: From posterior surface of scapula to greater tuberosity
    - Externally rotates humerus
  - Teres minor: From lateral border of scapula to greater tuberosity
    - Externally rotates humerus
  - Subscapularis muscle: From anterior surface of scapula to lesser tuberosity
    - Superficial fibers extend across to anterior margin of greater tuberosity as part of transverse ligament
    - Internally rotates, adducts humerus
- **Glenohumeral ligaments**: Thickenings in joint capsule, variable morphology
  - Superior glenohumeral ligament (SGHL)
    - Stabilizes adducted shoulder against inferior subluxation
    - Thin, horizontal band at superior margin of joint
    - Originates glenoid labrum just anterior to biceps tendon
    - Inserts on lesser tuberosity
    - Merges with coracohumeral ligament
  - Middle glenohumeral ligament (MGHL)
    - Stabilizes abducted shoulder
    - Obliquely oriented from superior labrum inferolaterally
    - Originates anterior to SGHL
    - Merges with subscapularis
    - Inserts on lesser tuberosity
    - Enlarged when anterosuperior labrum absent (Buford complex)
  - Inferior glenohumeral ligament (IGHL)
    - Stabilizes abducted shoulder
    - Anterior band: Anteroinferior labrum to surgical neck of humerus
    - Posterior band: Posteroinferior labrum to surgical neck of humerus
- Coracohumeral ligament (CHL)
  - Stabilizes long head biceps, forming biceps sling together with SGHL and subscapularis tendon
  - Stabilizes against inferior and posterior subluxation
  - Originates posterior margin coracoid process, inserts greater and lesser tuberosities
  - Broad, thin ligament or capsular fold, with lateral and medial condensations (bands)
  - Lateral band merges with capsule, subscapularis tendon, transverse ligament
    - Attachments can be seen on anterior margin of subscapularis tendon
  - Medial band merges with capsule, SGHL, and distal supraspinatus tendon
- Rotator interval
  - Triangular space between supraspinatus, subscapularis tendons
    - Wide medially, narrows laterally, ends at attachments of supraspinatus and subscapularis to humerus
    - Roof formed by CHL
- Long head of biceps tendon
  - Originates superior labrum and bony glenoid
  - Extends laterally above humeral head
  - Turns to enter bicipital groove
- Biceps sling
  - Stabilizes intraarticular biceps tendon
  - Formed by CHL, SGHL, subscapularis tendon
- Transverse humeral ligament
  - Roof of bicipital groove
  - Composed of subscapularis tendon and CHL fibers
- Posterior rotator interval
  - Potential space between supraspinatus, infraspinatus tendons

ANATOMY IMAGING ISSUES

Imaging Approaches

- Radiographs
  - Standard views include AP internal rotation, AP external rotation, and axillary views
    - Often a Grashey view (true AP view of glenohumeral joint) is substituted for true AP external rotation view
  - Scapular Y-view to evaluate supraspinatus outlet and assess for dislocation
  - Rockwood view, 30 degrees caudal tilt AP, to evaluate acromion
  - Zanca view, 10-20 degrees cephalic tilt AP, to evaluate acromioclavicular joint
  - Garth apical oblique or West Point axillary view to assess anteroinferior glenoid rim
    - Garth: Patient seated, arm at side, cassette posterior lying parallel to spine of scapula, beam centered at glenohumeral joint angled 45 degrees to plane of thorax and 45 degrees caudal

Shoulder Radiographic and Arthrographic Anatomy

- West Point axillary: Patient prone, head turned away from involved side, cassette held against superior aspect of shoulder, beam centered at axilla angled 25 degrees downward from horizontal and 25 degrees medial
  - Stryker notch view to assess humeral head and base of coracoid process
    - Patient supine, cassette under involved shoulder, palm of hand on top of head with fingers toward back of head
- Arthrography
  - Conventional arthrography
    - Needle placed into glenohumeral joint under fluoroscopic guidance
    - Administer 10 to 12 ml contrast
    - Contrast should remain within joint, without extension into rotator cuff or subacromial-subdeltoid bursa
    - Opacification of subscapular recess & biceps tendon sheath is normal
  - Choice of needle placement for arthrography may depend on site of symptoms &/or patient comfort
  - Rotator interval placement: Most common choice
    - Arm must be rotated externally; patient supine
    - Needle placed high on humeral head, through rotator interval
    - Misplaced injections or partial extravasation least likely with this approach
    - Can result in extravasation into rotator interval mimicking rotator interval tear
  - Inferomedial placement on humeral head
    - Arm rotated externally; patient supine
    - Needle placed inferomedially on humeral head
    - Increased incidence of extravasation into subscapularis tendon, inferior glenohumeral ligament
    - Avoid placing too far medially, on or through labrum
    - Avoid placing in center of humeral head; external rotation compresses capsule at this site, making extravasation more likely
  - Posterior humeral head needle approach (patient in prone position)
    - May be used with anterior complaints, particularly in rotator interval region
    - Procedure: Elevate shoulder with wedge/towels, rotate arm externally
    - High entry point (superomedial humeral head) or low entry point (inferomedial aspect humeral head; has higher risk of extracapsular injection)
    - Potential problem: Posterior rotator interval injection (potential space between supraspinatus and infraspinatus tendons); inadvertent filling occurs when needle is placed superior to humeral head in a posterior approach
  - Expected flow of contrast
    - Easy injection, flowing around cartilage in joint or filling capsule
    - Extraarticular injection may flow freely and mimic filling of capsule; watch anatomy closely during intermittent fluoroscopy
    - Intracartilaginous or intraosseous injection: Puddling of contrast around needle tip
    - Injection into substance of capsule or muscle: Usually mixed injection, with contrast entering intraarticular space as well as soft tissue (watch for streaking along muscle/tendon); may mimic tear
  - CT arthrography helpful in patients with contraindication to MR
  - MR arthrography
    - Best evaluates capsulolabral complex
    - Intraarticular 12 ml dilute gadopentetate dimeglumine (2 mmol/L) mixed with iodinated contrast, Marcaine, & epinephrine according to institutional preference
    - Avoid shoulder exercise prior to imaging to minimize contrast leakage
    - Indirect method utilizes IV gadopentetate dimeglumine followed by exercise prior to imaging
    - T1 FS sequences in axial, coronal oblique, & sagittal oblique planes
    - Optional abduction-external rotation (ABER)
    - Injection of air bubbles can simulate loose bodies
    - High-field MR scanner
    - Dedicated shoulder coil centered on region of interest
    - Patient positioning: Supine, arm neutral to slight external rotation (avoid internal rotation), arm at side & slightly away from side of body

Imaging Pitfalls

- Buford complex: Absent anterosuperior labrum; thick, cord-like MGHL
- Superior labral variations: Superior labrum may have meniscoid configuration at and anterior to biceps anchor
- Injection between fibers of capsule: May mimic capsular tear

SELECTED REFERENCES

1. Hunt SA et al: The rotator interval: anatomy, pathology, and strategies for treatment. J Am Acad Orthop Surg. 15(4):218-27, 2007
2. Krief OP: MRI of the rotator interval capsule. AJR Am J Roentgenol. 184(5):1490-4, 2005
3. Morag Y et al: MR arthrography of rotator interval, long head of the biceps brachii, and biceps pulley of the shoulder. Radiology. 235(1):21-30, 2005
4. Clark JM et al: Tendons, ligaments, and capsule of the rotator cuff. Gross and microscopic anatomy. J Bone Joint Surg Am. 74(5):713-25, 1992

Shoulder Radiographic and Arthrographic Anatomy

AP EXTERNAL & INTERNAL ROTATION RADIOGRAPHS

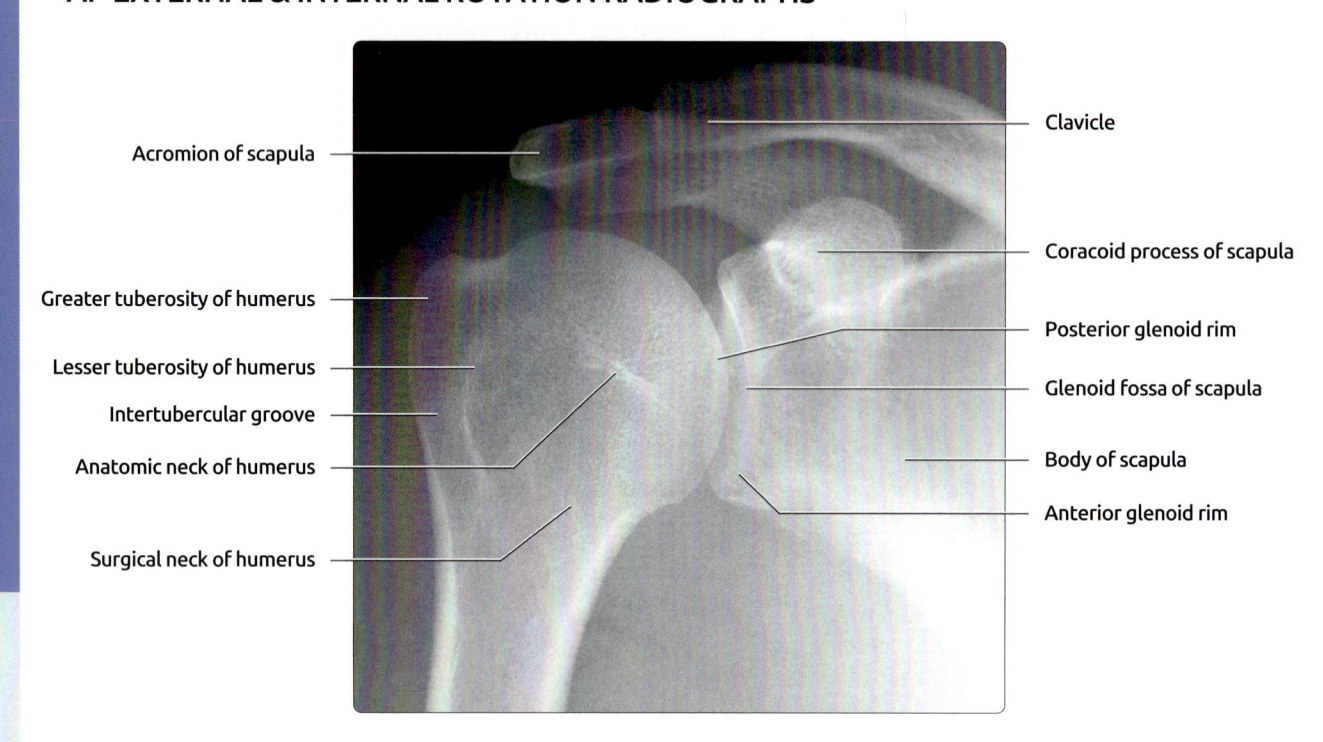

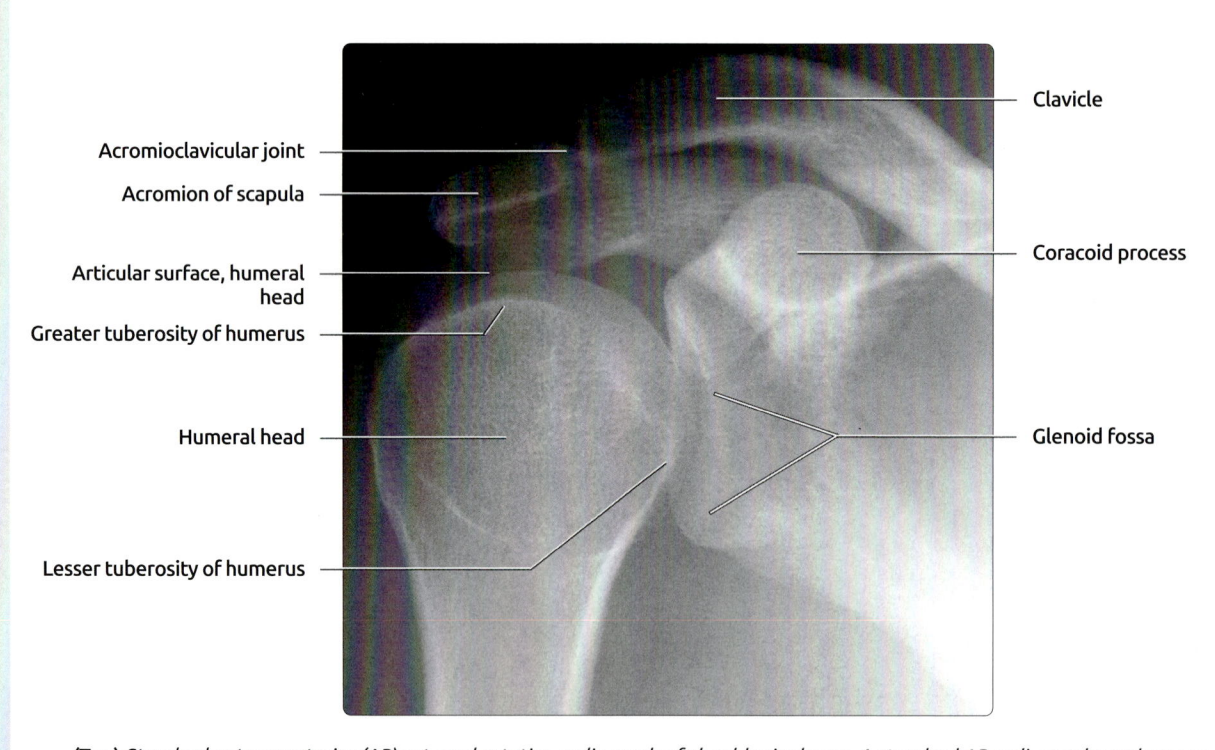

(Top) Standard anteroposterior (AP) external rotation radiograph of shoulder is shown. A standard AP radiograph produces an oblique view of the glenohumeral joint, which has a normal anterior angulation of ~ 40 degrees. The anterior glenoid rim projects medial to the posterior rim on this view. The AP view can be obtained in neutral position, internal rotation, or external rotation. With the arm in external rotation, the greater tuberosity projects at the lateral aspect of the humeral head. (Bottom) Standard AP internal rotation radiograph of the shoulder is shown. The lesser tuberosity projects at the medial aspect of the humeral head. The greater tuberosity has rotated anteriorly and its superior margin forms a dense line inferior to the articular surface. The posterolateral aspect of the humeral head projects laterally.

Shoulder Radiographic and Arthrographic Anatomy

GRASHEY & GARTH RADIOGRAPHS

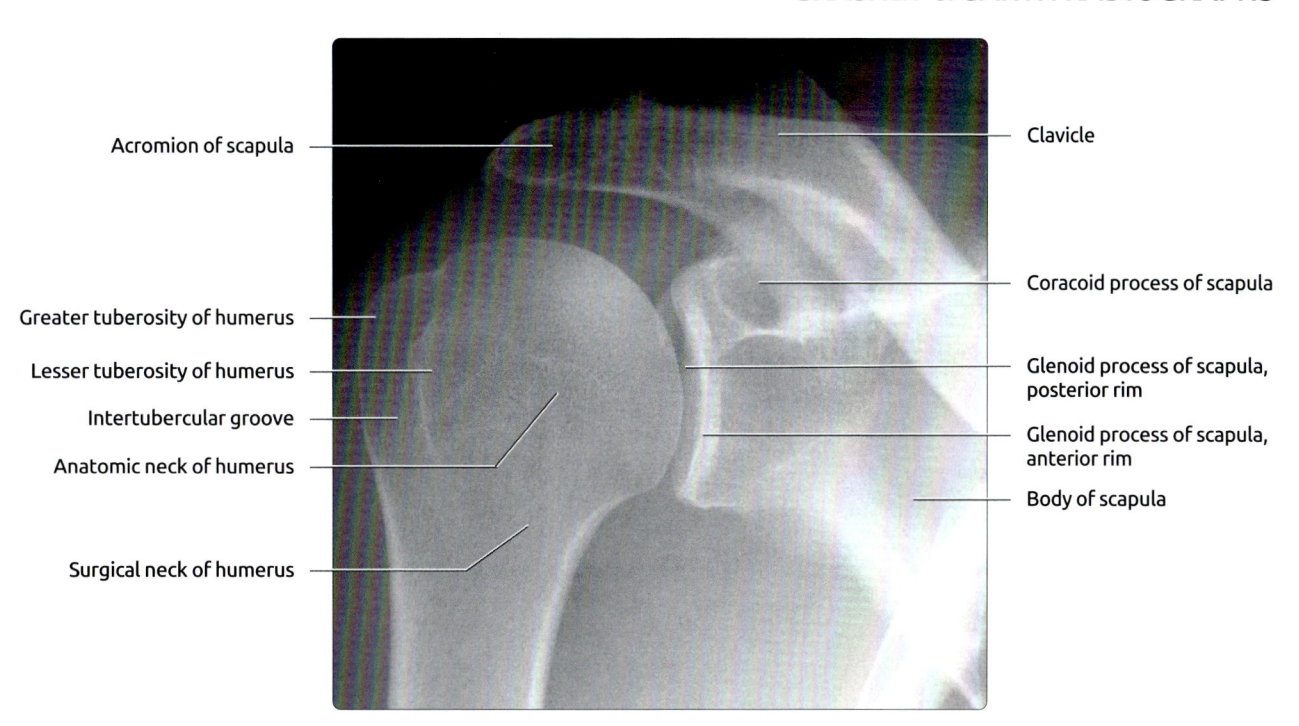

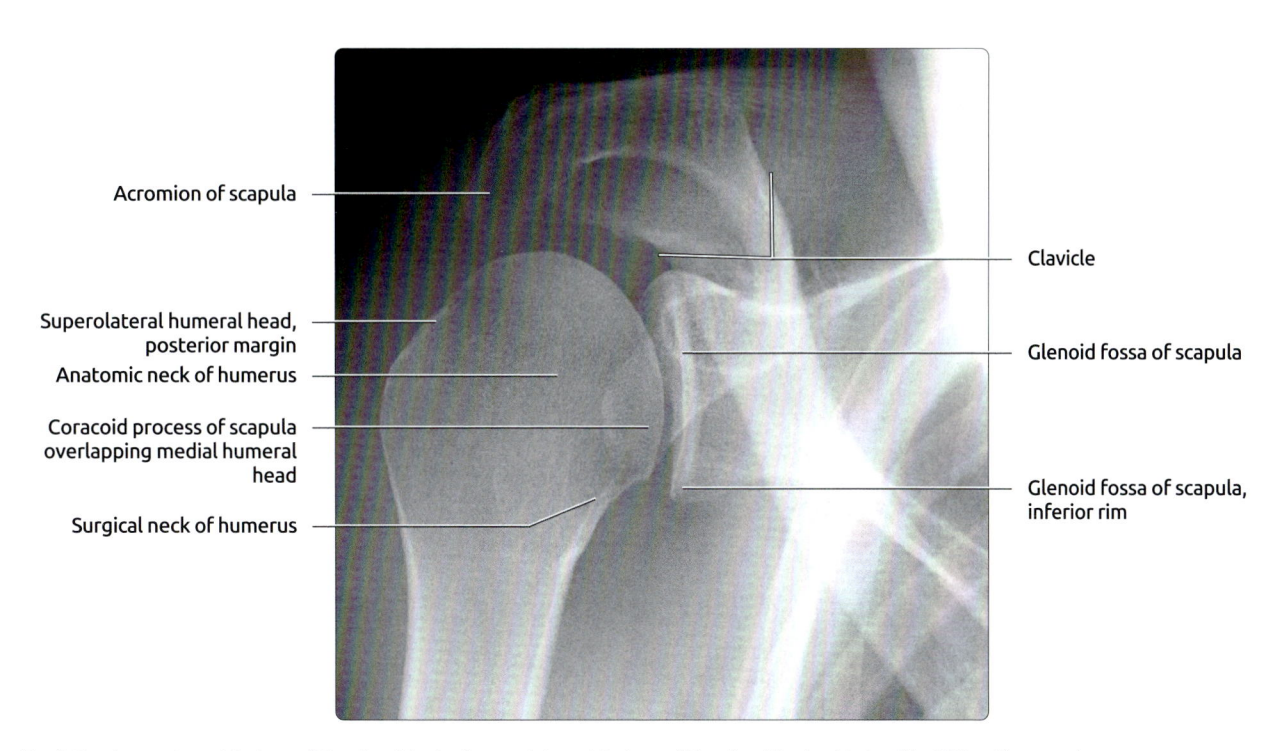

Top image labels:
- Acromion of scapula
- Greater tuberosity of humerus
- Lesser tuberosity of humerus
- Intertubercular groove
- Anatomic neck of humerus
- Surgical neck of humerus
- Clavicle
- Coracoid process of scapula
- Glenoid process of scapula, posterior rim
- Glenoid process of scapula, anterior rim
- Body of scapula

Bottom image labels:
- Acromion of scapula
- Superolateral humeral head, posterior margin
- Anatomic neck of humerus
- Coracoid process of scapula overlapping medial humeral head
- Surgical neck of humerus
- Clavicle
- Glenoid fossa of scapula
- Glenoid fossa of scapula, inferior rim

(**Top**) *Grashey or true AP view of the shoulder is shown. A true AP view of the shoulder is obtained by tilting the x-ray beam approximately 45 degrees laterally from the standard AP view. This produces a true AP view of the anteriorly angled glenohumeral joint. The anterior and posterior rims of the glenoid should nearly overlap on this view. The Grashey view is helpful for evaluating joint congruity, joint space narrowing, and humeral head subluxation.* (**Bottom**) *Garth view of shoulder is shown. The Garth view is obtained by angling the x-ray beam 45 degrees caudally from a standard AP view. The inferior glenohumeral rim and posterior margin of the superolateral humeral head are well demonstrated. In patients with acute or chronic anterior humeral head dislocations, this view may assist in detection of Bankart fractures of the inferior glenoid and Hill-Sachs deformities of the humeral head.*

Shoulder Radiographic and Arthrographic Anatomy

AXILLARY, WEST POINT, & STRYKER NOTCH RADIOGRAPHS

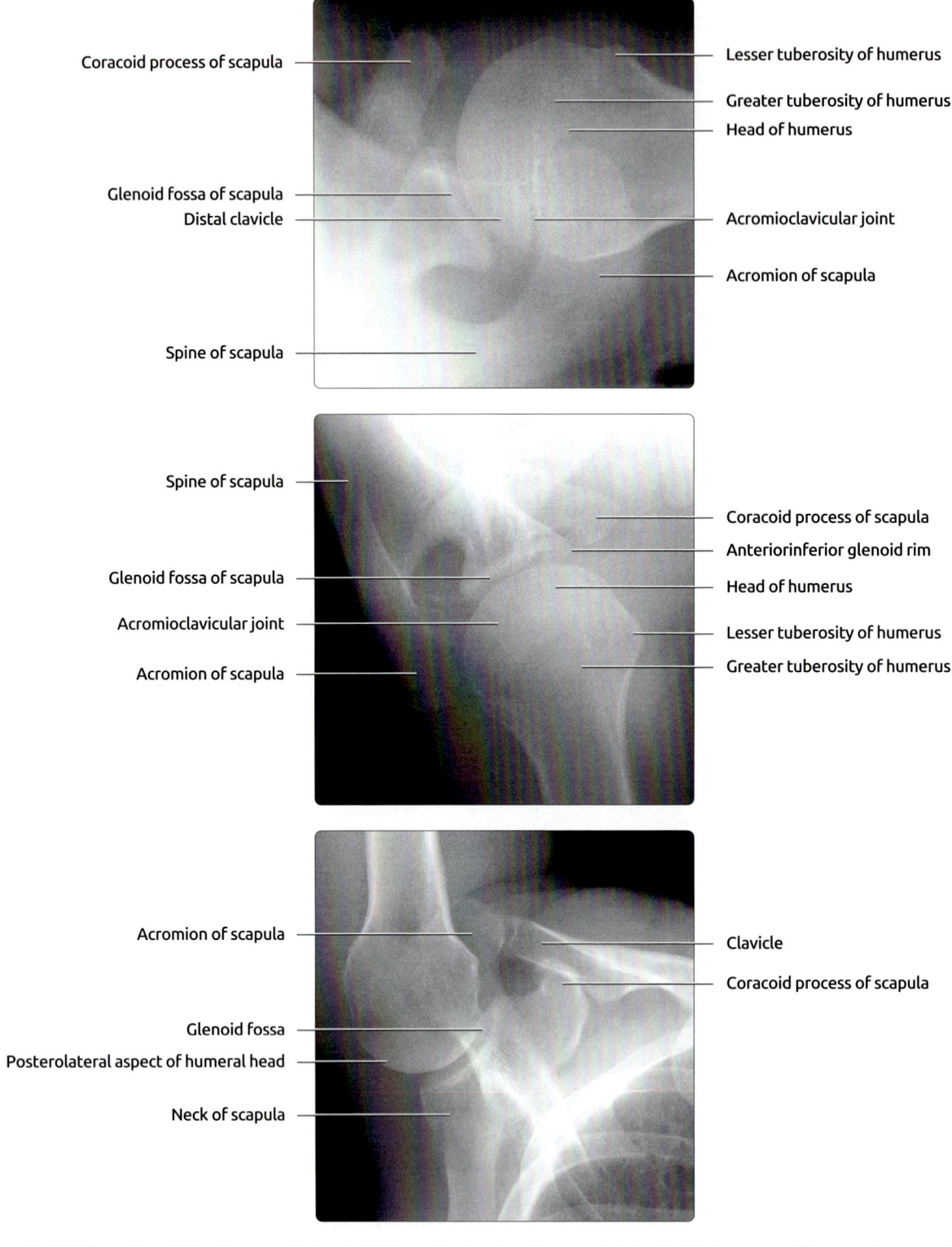

(Top) Axillary view of shoulder was obtained with the patient supine, the arm abducted to 90 degrees, and the x-ray beam angled 15 to 30 degrees medially. The resultant image is tangential to the glenohumeral joint. This view is helpful for identification of humeral head dislocation and anterior or posterior glenoid rim fractures. (Middle) West Point axillary view of the shoulder is shown. This variation on the standard axillary view is acquired with the patient prone and the abducted forearm hanging off the edge of the table. The x-ray beam is angled 25 degrees medially and anteriorly. The West Point view better demonstrates the anterior inferior glenoid, making it useful for detection of Bankart fractures. (Bottom) Stryker notch view of shoulder is shown. This view is obtained with the patient supine and the arm in an abducted and externally rotated (ABER) position. The x-ray beam is angled 10 degrees cephalic. The posterolateral aspect of the humeral head, where a Hill-Sachs deformity could be located, is well demonstrated.

Shoulder Radiographic and Arthrographic Anatomy

SUPRASPINATUS OUTLET, SCAPULAR Y, & AP SCAPULA RADIOGRAPHS

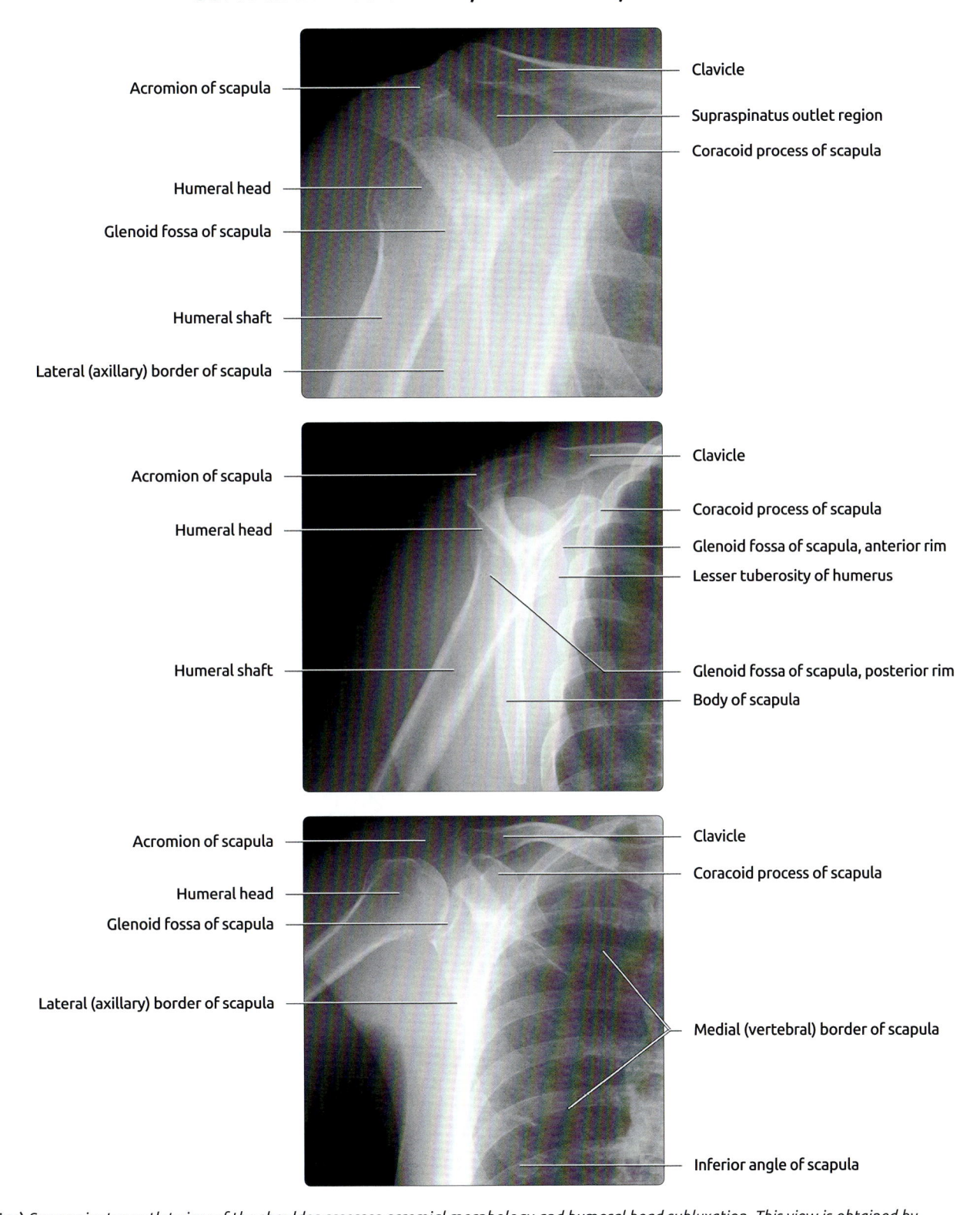

(Top) Supraspinatus outlet view of the shoulder assesses acromial morphology and humeral head subluxation. This view is obtained by placing the anterior aspect of the affected shoulder against the x-ray plate, rotating the opposite shoulder approximately 40 degrees away from the plate, then tilting the x-ray beam 5-10 degrees caudally. The acromion and subacromial space are imaged in profile. (Middle) Scapular Y view is shown. The anterior aspect of the affected shoulder is placed against the x-ray plate and the opposite shoulder rotated approximately 45-60 degrees away from the plate. The x-ray beam is directed along the scapular spine producing a true lateral view of the shoulder, with the scapula shaped like the letter Y and the humeral head located at the center of the Y. The humeral head will lie below the coracoid process in an anterior dislocation & posterior to the glenoid in posterior dislocation. (Bottom) AP view of scapula was obtained standing or supine with the arm abducted and hand supinated.

Shoulder Radiographic and Arthrographic Anatomy

CONVENTIONAL ARTHROGRAPHY: GLENOHUMERAL JOINT AND SUBDELTOID BURSA

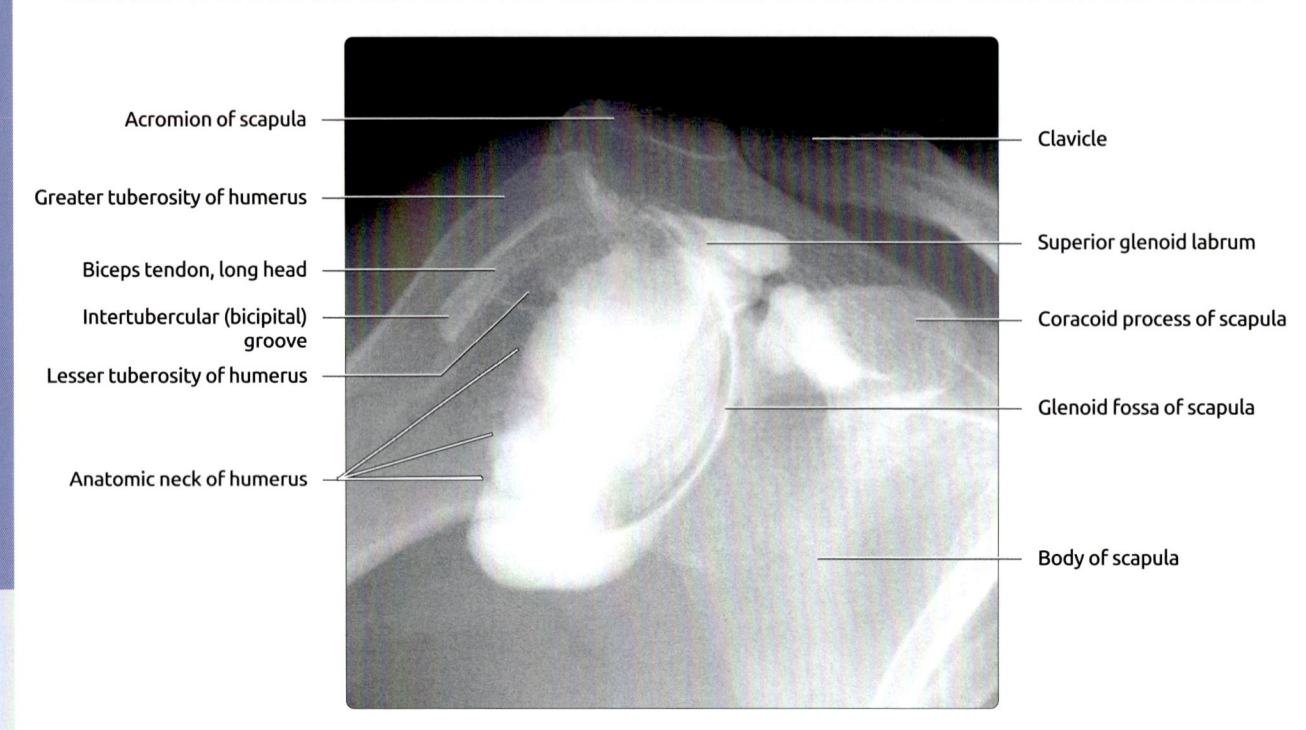

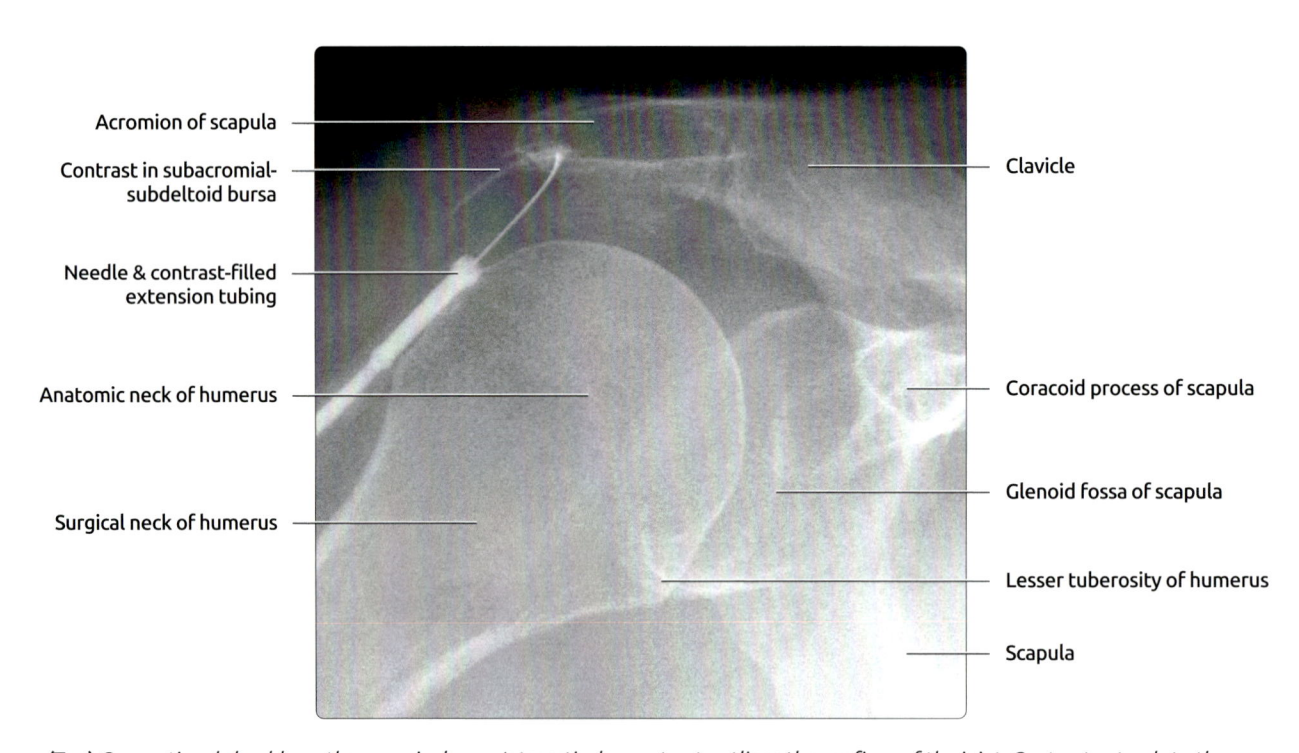

(Top) Conventional shoulder arthrogram is shown. Intraarticular contrast outlines the confines of the joint. Contrast extends to the anatomic neck of the humerus, where the joint capsule inserts. Contrast can normally extend into the biceps tendon sheath and subscapular recess. (Bottom) Subacromial-subdeltoid bursa injection is shown. A 25 g needle is placed just below the acromion process. Administered contrast will have a curvilinear configuration as it tracks within the subacromial-subdeltoid bursa. The shoulder is internally rotated on this image.

Shoulder Radiographic and Arthrographic Anatomy

NORMAL ARTHROGRAM

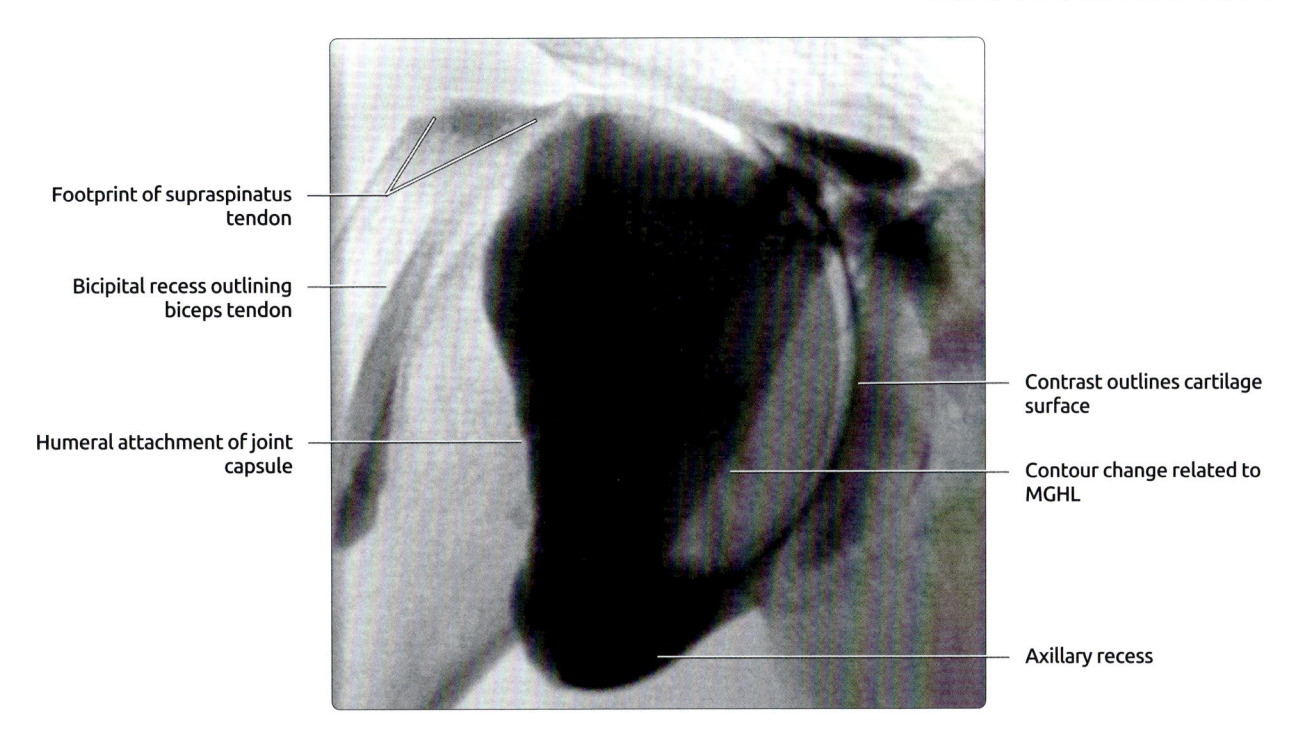

- Footprint of supraspinatus tendon
- Bicipital recess outlining biceps tendon
- Humeral attachment of joint capsule
- Contrast outlines cartilage surface
- Contour change related to MGHL
- Axillary recess

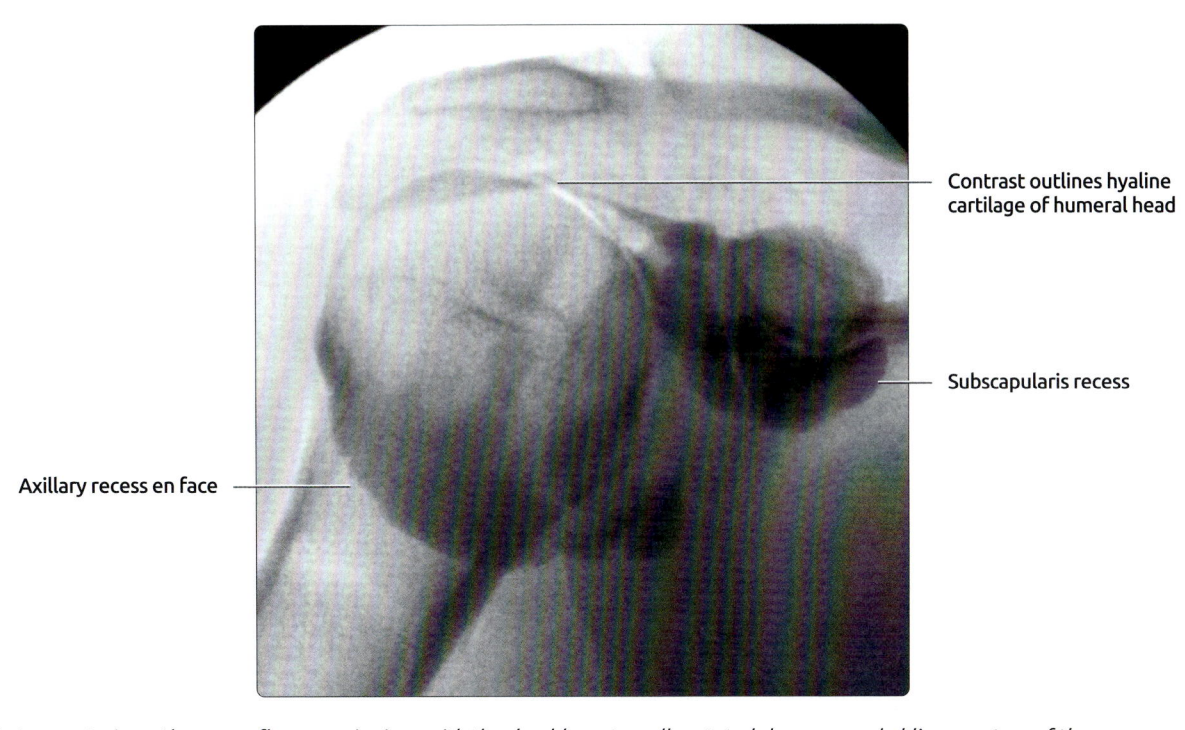

- Contrast outlines hyaline cartilage of humeral head
- Subscapularis recess
- Axillary recess en face

(Top) Anteroposterior arthrogram, fluoroscopic view, with the shoulder externally rotated shows normal oblique contour of the capsular attachment to the anatomic neck of the humerus. Contrast extension lateral to this line, &/or lateral to the greater tuberosity, indicates a rotator cuff tear. Note normal filling of the bicipital and axillary recesses of the joint. **(Bottom)** Anteroposterior arthrogram with the shoulder internally rotated shows contrast now filling the subscapularis recess.

Shoulder Radiographic and Arthrographic Anatomy

SHOULDER GRAPHICS

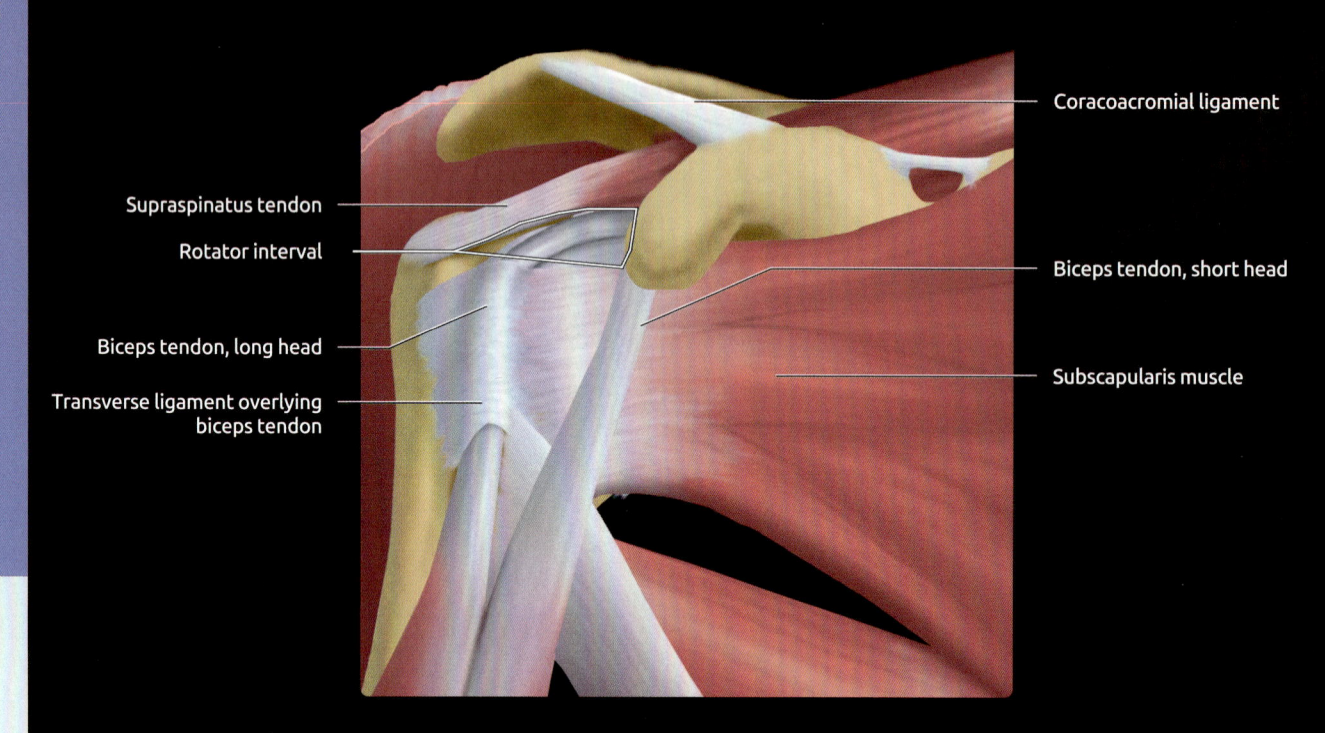

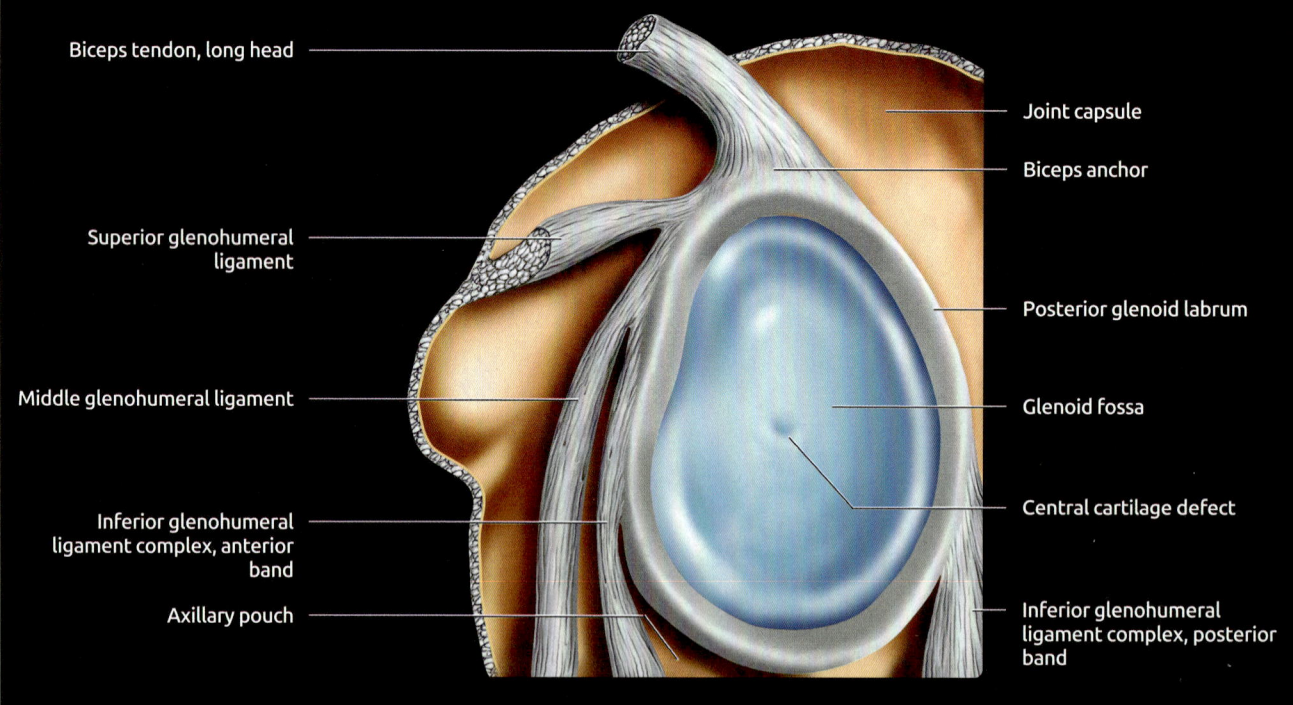

(Top) Anterior graphic shows the relationships of the rotator cuff to the rotator interval, a triangular space wide medially and narrowing laterally, with the apex at the anterior leading edge of the greater tuberosity. *(Bottom)* Sagittal graphic shows the intraarticular portion of the shoulder, humeral head removed. The superior and middle glenohumeral ligaments (SGHL & MGHL) both originate adjacent to the biceps tendon, but SGHL has a horizontal course and forms part of the biceps tendon sling. MGHL has an oblique course inferolaterally and provides anterior stability. The inferior glenohumeral ligament (IGHL) bands originate near the equator of the glenoid anteriorly & posteriorly and form anterior & posterior boundaries of the axillary recess.

Shoulder Radiographic and Arthrographic Anatomy

ROTATOR INTERVAL GRAPHIC

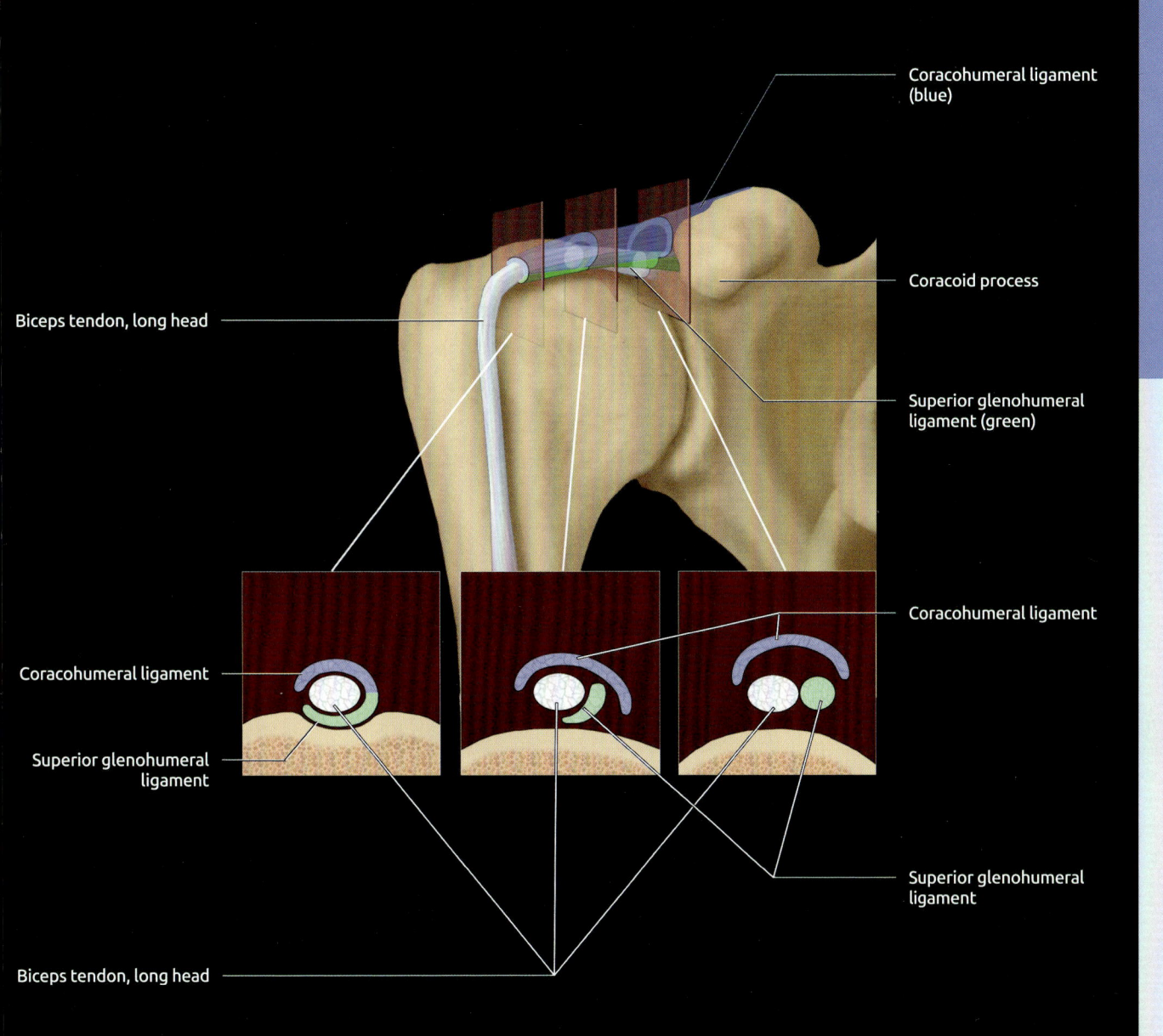

Coracohumeral ligament (blue)

Coracoid process

Biceps tendon, long head

Superior glenohumeral ligament (green)

Coracohumeral ligament

Coracohumeral ligament

Superior glenohumeral ligament

Superior glenohumeral ligament

Biceps tendon, long head

Normal rotator interval anatomy graphic is shown. Cross-section images at lateral, mid, & medial portions of rotator interval are located along bottom of image. At lateral aspect of rotator interval, just proximal to entrance to bicipital groove, medial band of coracohumeral ligament (blue) & superior glenohumeral ligament (green) form a sling around long head of the biceps tendon. At mid portion of rotator interval, coracohumeral ligament covers superior surface of biceps tendon, with superior glenohumeral ligament forming T-shaped junction with coracohumeral ligament. Near medial border of rotator interval, superior glenohumeral ligament is a round structure lying anterior to biceps tendon, & both structures are capped by U-shaped coracohumeral ligament. (Modified from Krief OP, 2005.)

Shoulder Radiographic and Arthrographic Anatomy

OBLIQUE CORONAL: POSTERIOR TO ANTERIOR

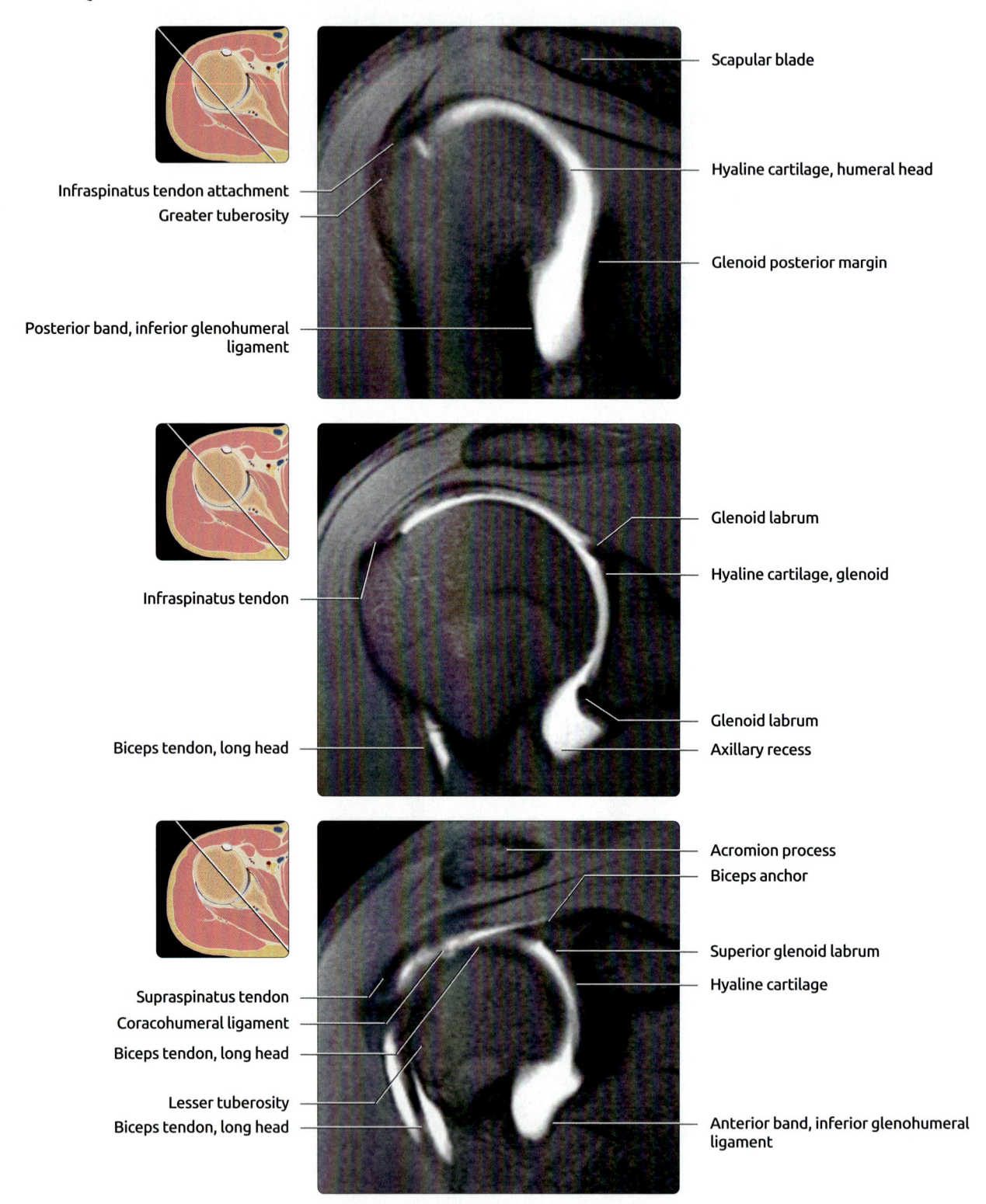

Labels (top image):
- Scapular blade
- Hyaline cartilage, humeral head
- Glenoid posterior margin
- Infraspinatus tendon attachment
- Greater tuberosity
- Posterior band, inferior glenohumeral ligament

Labels (middle image):
- Glenoid labrum
- Hyaline cartilage, glenoid
- Glenoid labrum
- Axillary recess
- Infraspinatus tendon
- Biceps tendon, long head

Labels (bottom image):
- Acromion process
- Biceps anchor
- Superior glenoid labrum
- Hyaline cartilage
- Anterior band, inferior glenohumeral ligament
- Supraspinatus tendon
- Coracohumeral ligament
- Biceps tendon, long head
- Lesser tuberosity
- Biceps tendon, long head

(**Top**) First of 6 selected coronal oblique T1WI MR arthrogram images, angled along the supraspinatus tendon axis, is shown. The posterior band of the inferior glenohumeral ligament forms a thick, distinct band at the posterior margin of the axillary pouch. (**Middle**) Posterior to the biceps anchor, the glenoid labrum is tightly adherent to the hyaline cartilage, and the sublabral sulci are never present. Because the elbow is posterior to the shoulder in a supine patient, a more anterior portion of the arm is usually seen at the inferior portion of the image than superiorly. (**Bottom**) Biceps originates from the superior bony margin of the glenoid and attaches firmly to the superior labrum. The sublabral sulcus is variably seen in this region but is absent in this patient. Intermediate signal intensity hyaline cartilage extends beneath the superior labrum. Note that the biceps tendon is seen in this mid-shoulder cut rather than more anteriorly because the shoulder is extremely externally rotated.

Shoulder Radiographic and Arthrographic Anatomy

OBLIQUE CORONAL: POSTERIOR TO ANTERIOR

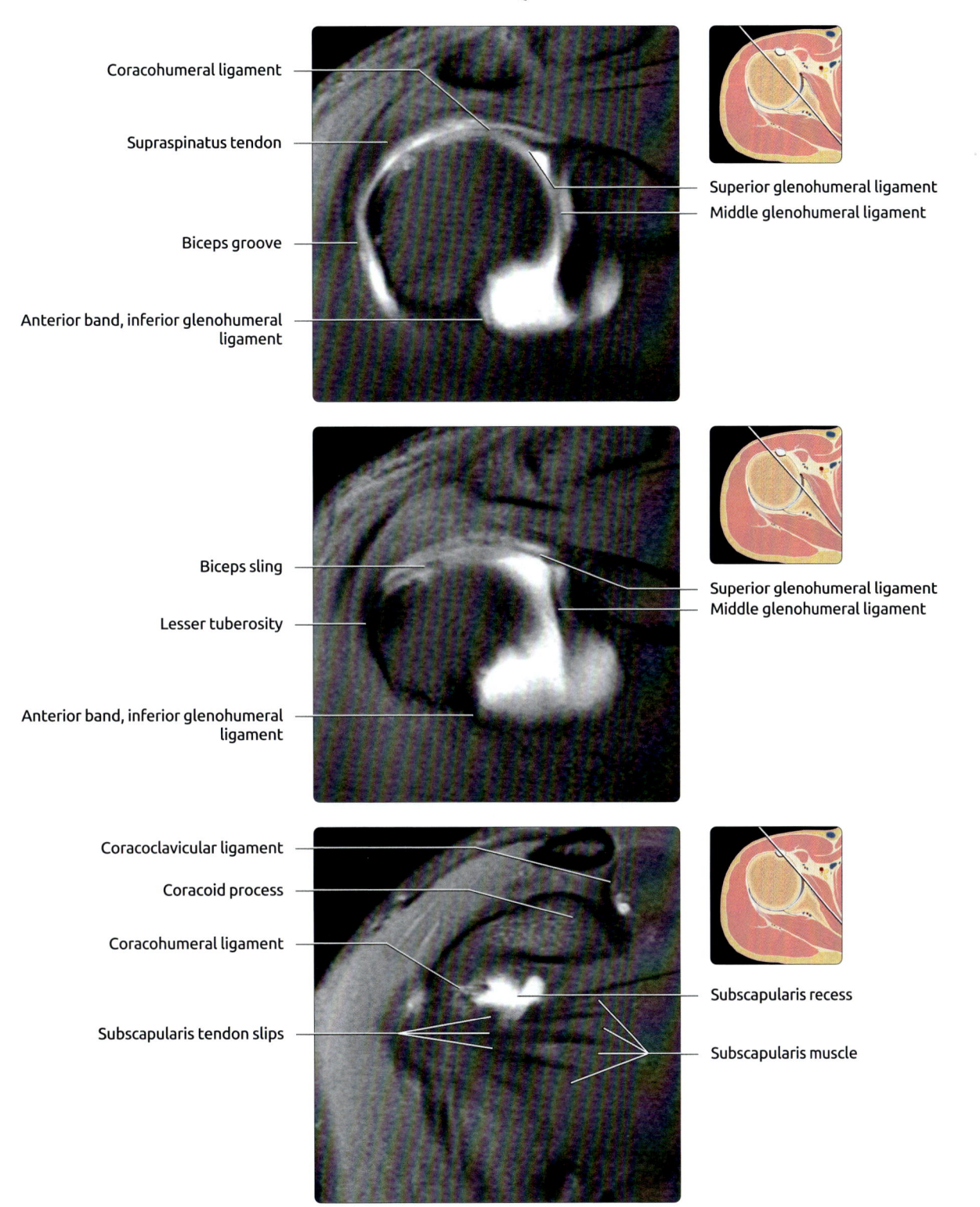

Top image labels:
- Coracohumeral ligament
- Supraspinatus tendon
- Biceps groove
- Anterior band, inferior glenohumeral ligament
- Superior glenohumeral ligament
- Middle glenohumeral ligament

Middle image labels:
- Biceps sling
- Lesser tuberosity
- Anterior band, inferior glenohumeral ligament
- Superior glenohumeral ligament
- Middle glenohumeral ligament

Bottom image labels:
- Coracoclavicular ligament
- Coracoid process
- Coracohumeral ligament
- Subscapularis tendon slips
- Subscapularis recess
- Subscapularis muscle

(Top) *Immediately anterior to horizontal portion of long head biceps tendon, superior glenohumeral ligament is seen inferior to coracohumeral ligament. Appearance on MR arthrogram varies with rotation of shoulder. Shoulder of this patient is externally rotated, so the ligaments are nearly coronal in orientation.* **(Middle)** *Additional portions of biceps sling are now visible at the anterior margin of the glenoid, spiraling to form biceps sling.* **(Bottom)** *Most anterior image through the joint shows the subscapularis recess extending over the superior margin of the subscapularis muscle. Note the normal interdigitation of the subscapularis tendon slips with muscle. Most anterior portion of coracohumeral ligament is also visible merging with the lateral subscapularis fibers.*

Shoulder Radiographic and Arthrographic Anatomy

AXIAL: SUPERIOR TO INFERIOR

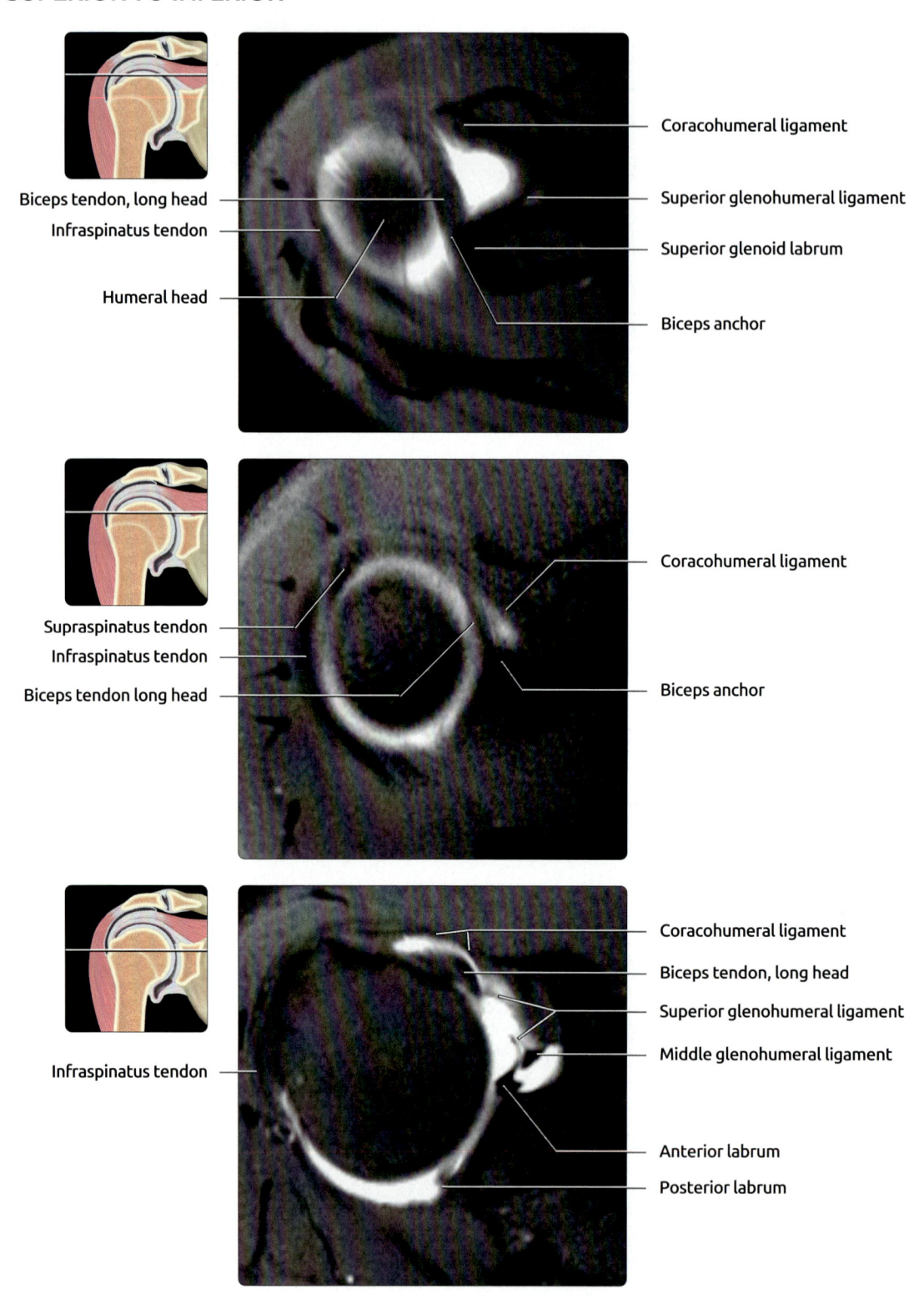

Biceps tendon, long head
Infraspinatus tendon
Humeral head

Coracohumeral ligament
Superior glenohumeral ligament
Superior glenoid labrum
Biceps anchor

Supraspinatus tendon
Infraspinatus tendon
Biceps tendon long head

Coracohumeral ligament
Biceps anchor

Infraspinatus tendon

Coracohumeral ligament
Biceps tendon, long head
Superior glenohumeral ligament
Middle glenohumeral ligament
Anterior labrum
Posterior labrum

(Top) First of 6 selected T1WI FS MR arthrogram images shows the shoulder joint from superior to inferior. Biceps anchor and horizontal portion of the long head of biceps are well seen, together with portions of the coracohumeral ligament. Superior glenohumeral ligament is deviated medially by joint distention. (Middle) Coracohumeral ligament has a medial band, which forms part of biceps sling, and a lateral band, which drapes over anterior margin of subscapularis, attaching to subscapularis and lesser and greater tuberosities. It forms part of transverse ligament. (Bottom) Coracohumeral ligament forms roof of rotator interval, as well as part of biceps sling.

Shoulder Radiographic and Arthrographic Anatomy

AXIAL: SUPERIOR TO INFERIOR

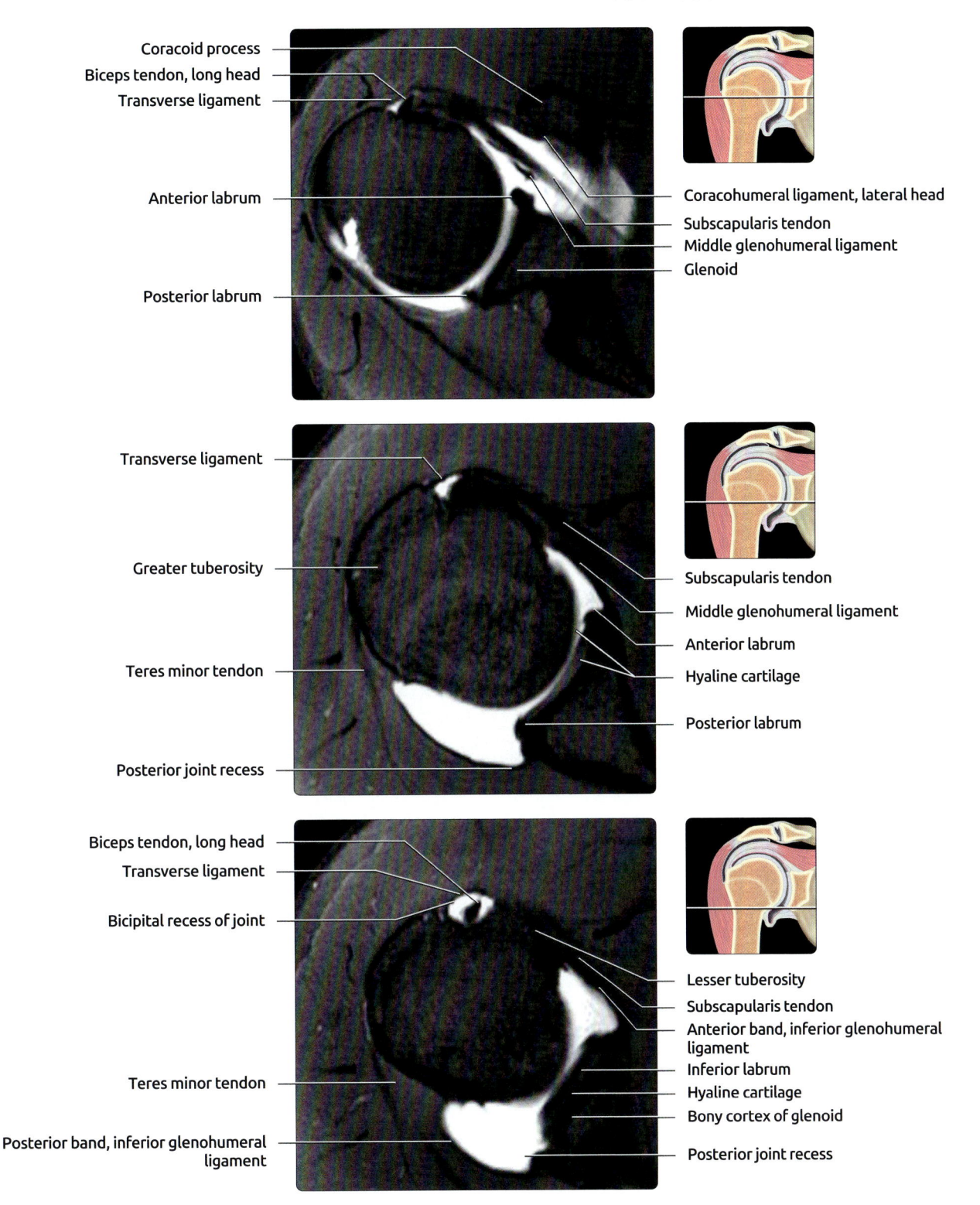

(Top) Lateral band of coracohumeral ligament (CHL) is well seen, extending anterior to subscapularis tendon and forming transverse ligament together with superficial fibers of subscapularis tendon. MGHL is adjacent to the posterior border of subscapularis tendon, with which it merges slightly more inferiorly. *(Middle)* The anterior labrum is larger than the posterior labrum. The intermediate signal intensity hyaline cartilage extends beneath the labrum both anteriorly and posteriorly. *(Bottom)* At the inferior margin of the joint, the inferior labrum is seen superficial to the hyaline cartilage. A prominent posterior joint recess adjacent to the labrum is a normal finding.

Shoulder Radiographic and Arthrographic Anatomy

SAGITTAL: LATERAL TO MEDIAL

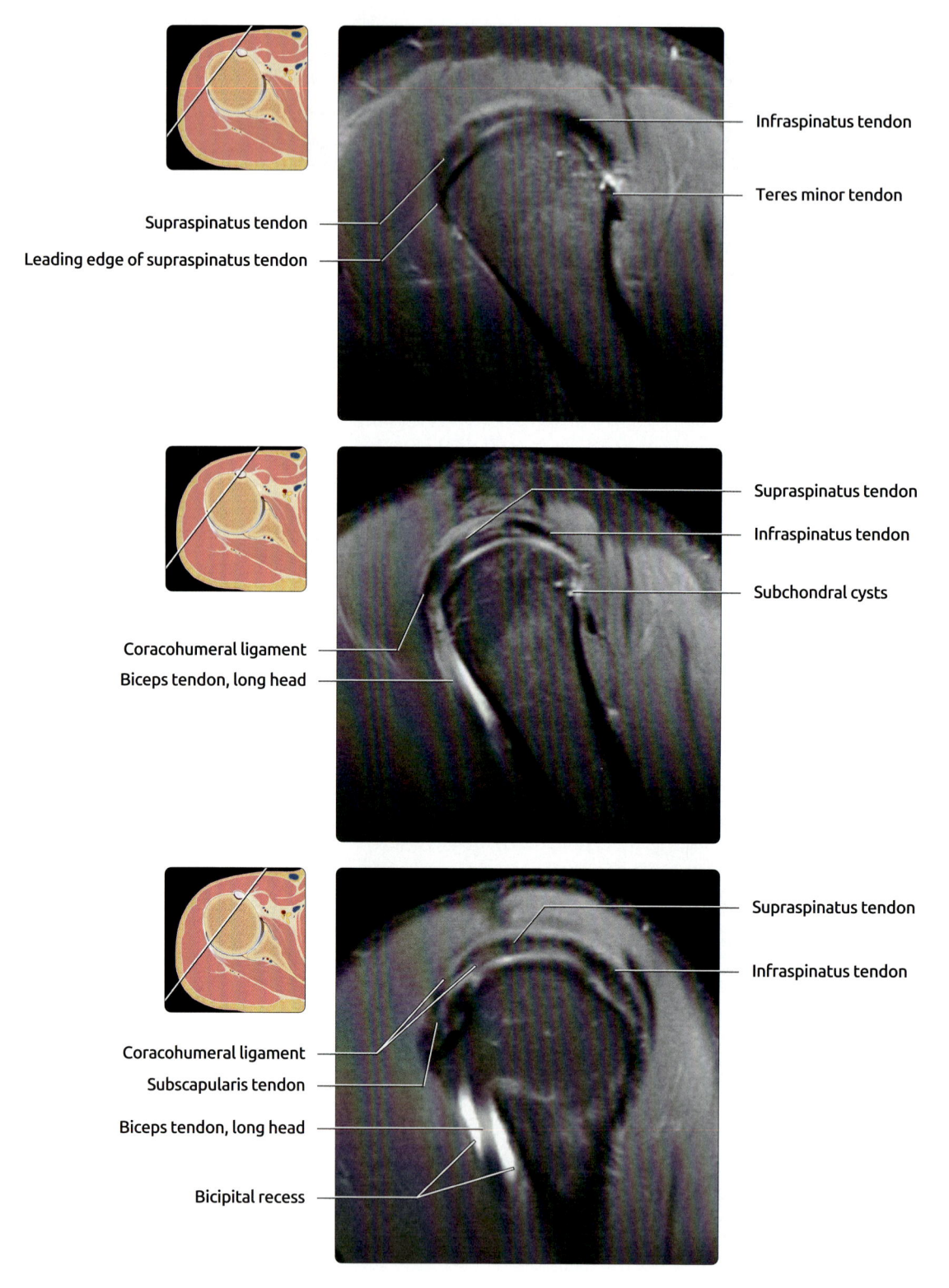

Suprapsinatus tendon — Infraspinatus tendon
Leading edge of supraspinatus tendon — Teres minor tendon

Coracohumeral ligament — Supraspinatus tendon
Biceps tendon, long head — Infraspinatus tendon
— Subchondral cysts

Coracohumeral ligament — Supraspinatus tendon
Subscapularis tendon — Infraspinatus tendon
Biceps tendon, long head
Bicipital recess

(**Top**) *First of 9 selected sagittal PD FS MR arthrogram images from lateral to medial shows normal bicycle tire rim appearance of the rotator cuff around the superior and posterior portions of the humeral head. Small tears of the supraspinatus tendon occur at the anterior margin or "leading edge." The leading edge is best seen in the sagittal oblique plane.* (**Middle**) *Just medial to the footprint of the supraspinatus and infraspinatus tendons, a thin rim of joint fluid is seen beneath the tendons. Small subchondral cysts are noted posteriorly and are an almost universal finding in patients past young adulthood.* (**Bottom**) *The coracohumeral ligament forms the roof of the rotator interval. It has a variable appearance.*

Shoulder Radiographic and Arthrographic Anatomy

SAGITTAL: LATERAL TO MEDIAL

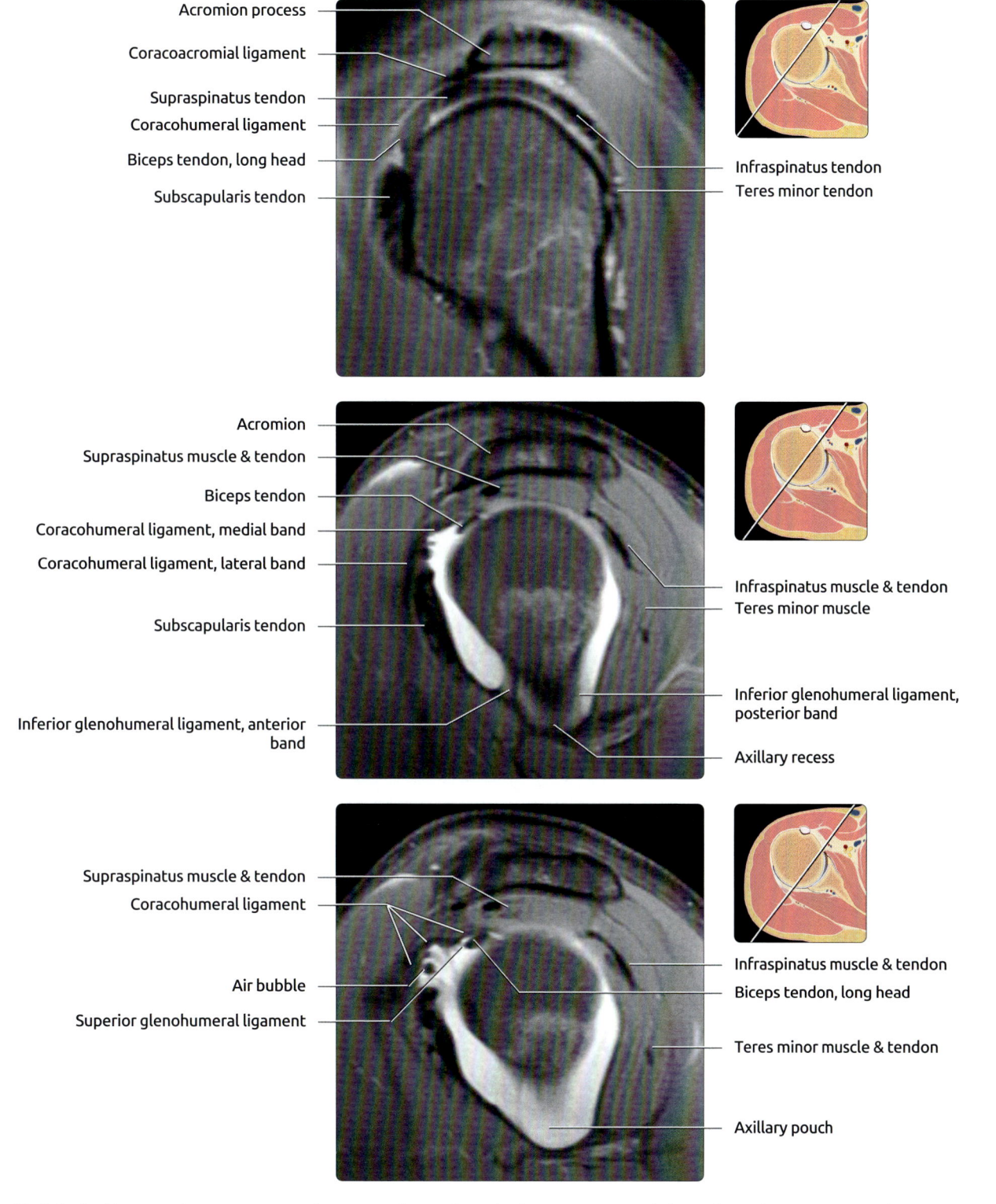

(Top) As the biceps tendon turns to enter the groove, the magic angle phenomenon can mimic tendinopathy. However, tendon subluxation and fraying in this region are common. Accurate assessment depends on careful cross-referencing of the appearance in all 3 imaging planes. **(Middle)** The anterior and posterior bands of the inferior glenohumeral ligament are seen inserting on the humeral neck. Between them lies the axillary recess. **(Bottom)** The breadth of the coracohumeral ligament is evident on this image; the ligament spans the rotator interval and arcs around the top of the biceps tendon.

Shoulder Radiographic and Arthrographic Anatomy

SAGITTAL: LATERAL TO MEDIAL

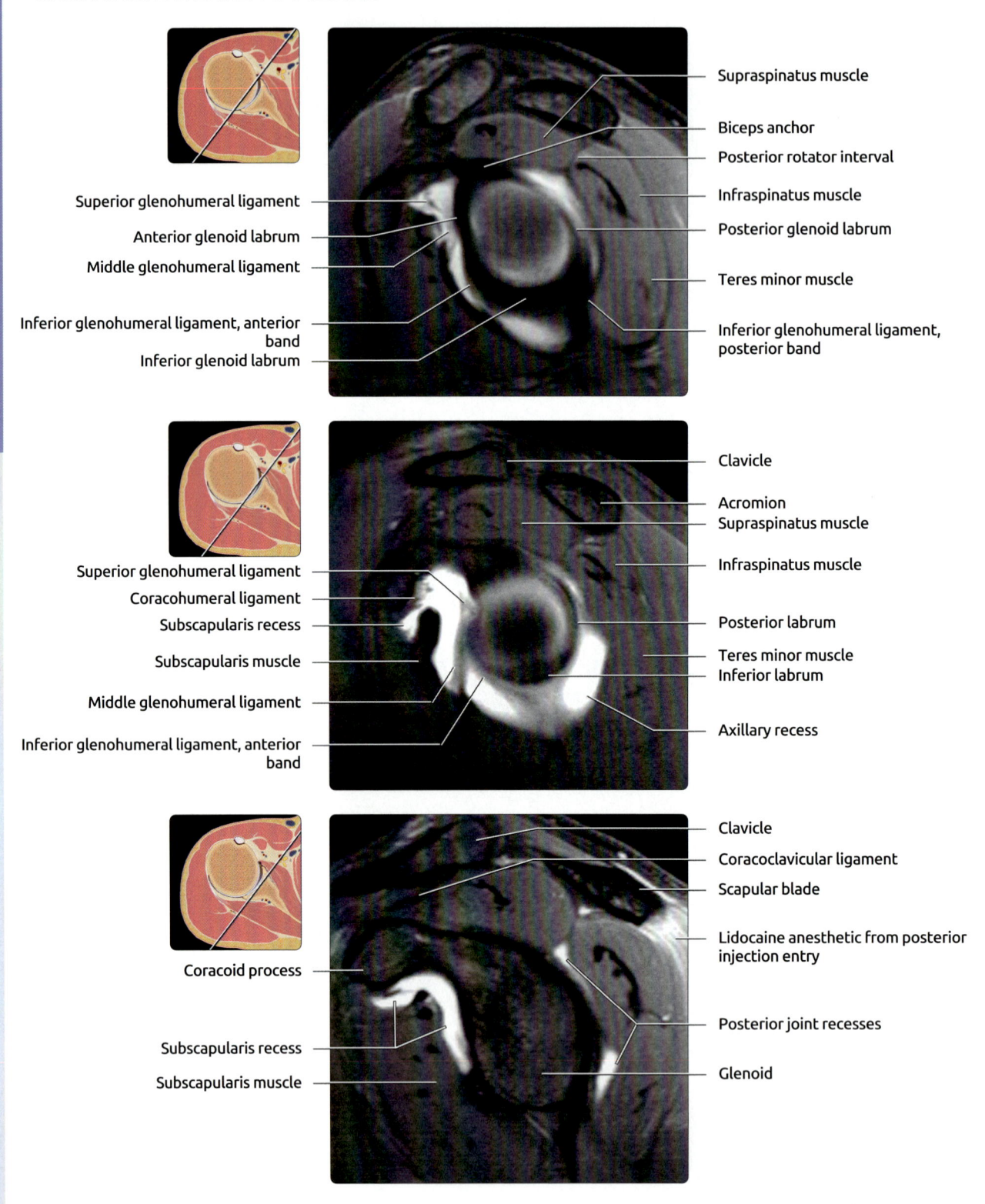

Labels (top image):
- Superior glenohumeral ligament
- Anterior glenoid labrum
- Middle glenohumeral ligament
- Inferior glenohumeral ligament, anterior band
- Inferior glenoid labrum
- Supraspinatus muscle
- Biceps anchor
- Posterior rotator interval
- Infraspinatus muscle
- Posterior glenoid labrum
- Teres minor muscle
- Inferior glenohumeral ligament, posterior band

Labels (middle image):
- Superior glenohumeral ligament
- Coracohumeral ligament
- Subscapularis recess
- Subscapularis muscle
- Middle glenohumeral ligament
- Inferior glenohumeral ligament, anterior band
- Clavicle
- Acromion
- Supraspinatus muscle
- Infraspinatus muscle
- Posterior labrum
- Teres minor muscle
- Inferior labrum
- Axillary recess

Labels (bottom image):
- Coracoid process
- Subscapularis recess
- Subscapularis muscle
- Clavicle
- Coracoclavicular ligament
- Scapular blade
- Lidocaine anesthetic from posterior injection entry
- Posterior joint recesses
- Glenoid

(Top) *The glenoid labrum is seen extending circumferentially around the bony glenoid.* **(Middle)** *This image is medial to the previous image, but in a different patient, and has improved visualization of the joint recesses and the glenohumeral ligaments due to greater joint distention.* **(Bottom)** *Medial to the articular surfaces, contrast is present in the medial joint recesses. The subscapularis recess has a saddle-bag shape draping over the superior margin of the subscapularis muscle. A subcoracoid bursa (not seen in this case) superior to the subscapularis recess does not communicate with the joint and should not fill at arthrography unless a rotator cuff tear is present, in which case it fills via the subacromial/subdeltoid bursa.*

Shoulder Radiographic and Arthrographic Anatomy

NORMAL VARIANTS: SUBLABRAL WINDOW

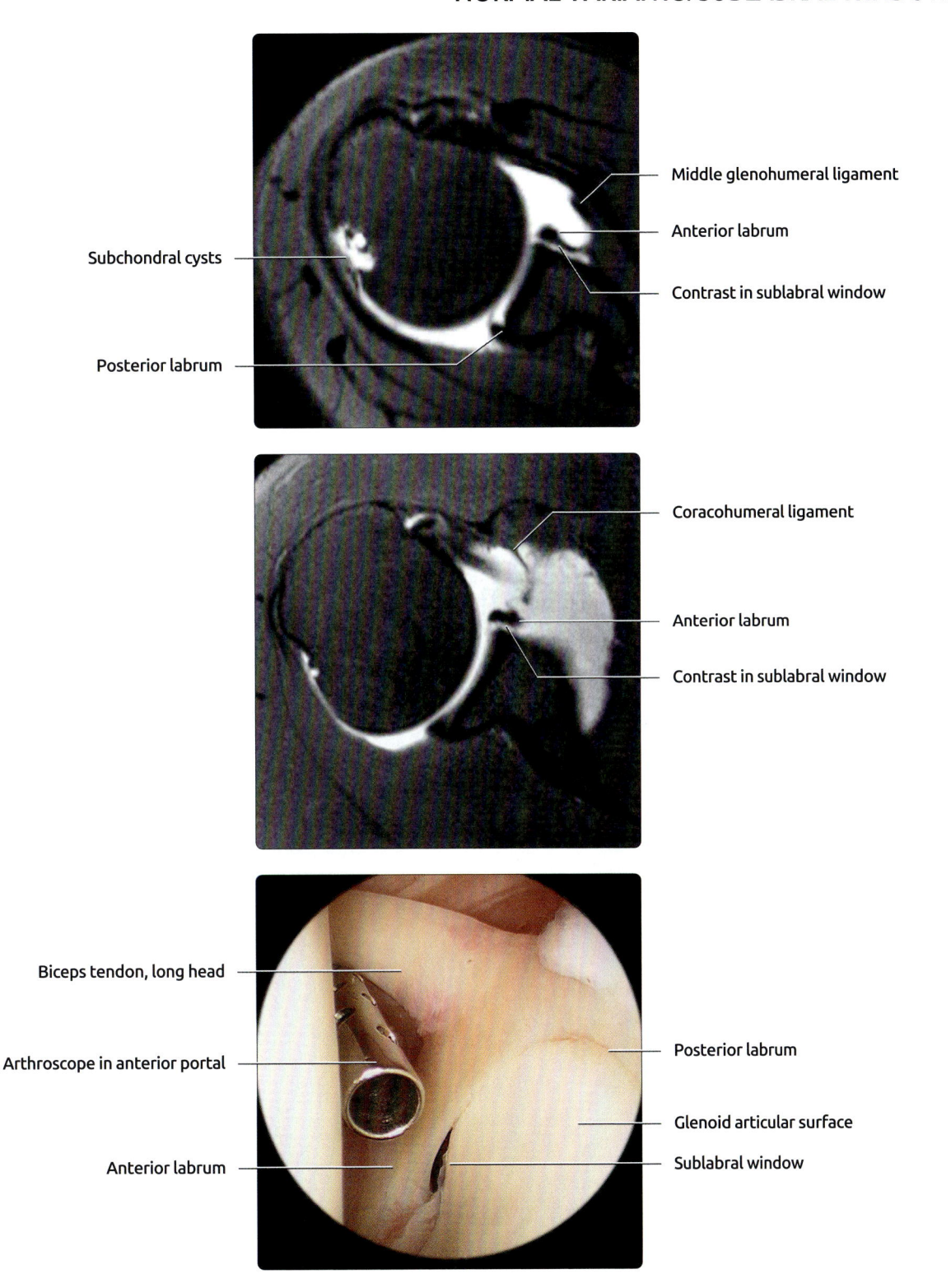

Middle glenohumeral ligament
Anterior labrum
Contrast in sublabral window
Subchondral cysts
Posterior labrum

Coracohumeral ligament
Anterior labrum
Contrast in sublabral window

Biceps tendon, long head
Arthroscope in anterior portal
Anterior labrum
Posterior labrum
Glenoid articular surface
Sublabral window

(Top) *Axial T1WI MR arthrography shows sublabral window. This normal variant occurs in the anterosuperior quadrant of the labrum, where isolated labral tears are rare. They do not extend below the level of the coracoid process. Unlike the irregular jagged line of a labral tear, the sublabral window is smoothly marginated.* (Middle) *Axial T1WI MR arthrography shows a different case of sublabral window. Images further inferiorly are used to distinguish between a labrum with sublabral window (in which case the labrum rejoins the bone more inferiorly) or a Buford complex (in which case the cord-like MGHL merges with the subscapularis and a separate labrum is present more inferiorly).* (Bottom) *Arthroscopic photograph shows different appearance of firmly attached posterior labrum compared to anterior sublabral window.*

Shoulder Radiographic and Arthrographic Anatomy

NORMAL VARIANTS: BUFORD COMPLEX

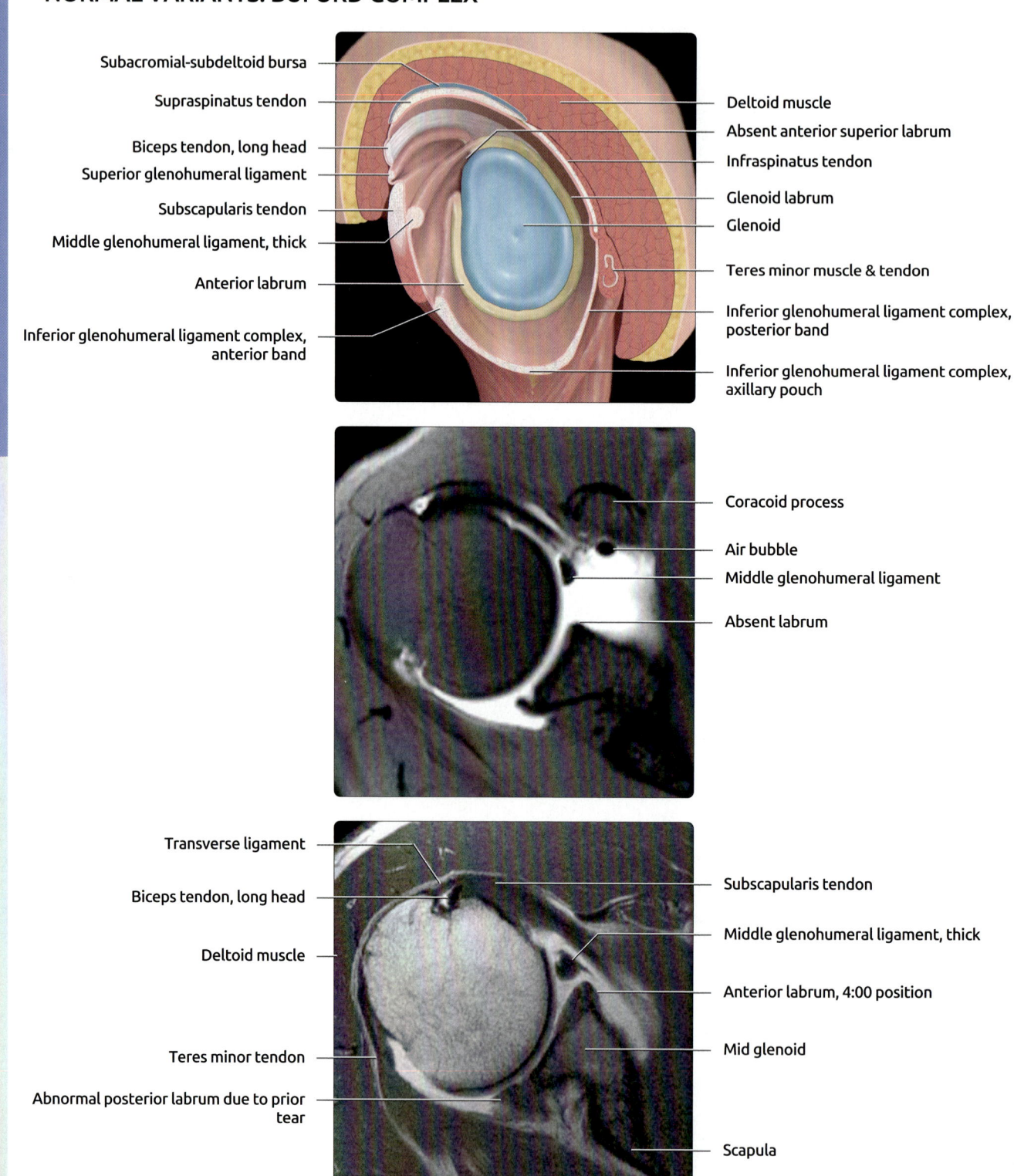

(Top) Sagittal graphic shows a Buford complex: Anterior superior glenoid labrum is absent and the middle glenohumeral ligament is enlarged and cord-like. (Middle) T1 FS MR arthrogram in axial plane shows that the middle glenohumeral ligament in the Buford complex may be as large as a normal anterior labrum. This configuration may be slightly unstable, since patients with Buford complex have an increased incidence of SLAP tears. (Bottom) Axial T2 MR below the level of coracoid shows anterior labrum separate from large middle glenohumeral ligament, a configuration expected at this inferior level in a Buford complex.

Shoulder Radiographic and Arthrographic Anatomy

NORMAL VARIANTS: BICEPS ANCHOR/LABRAL COMPLEX

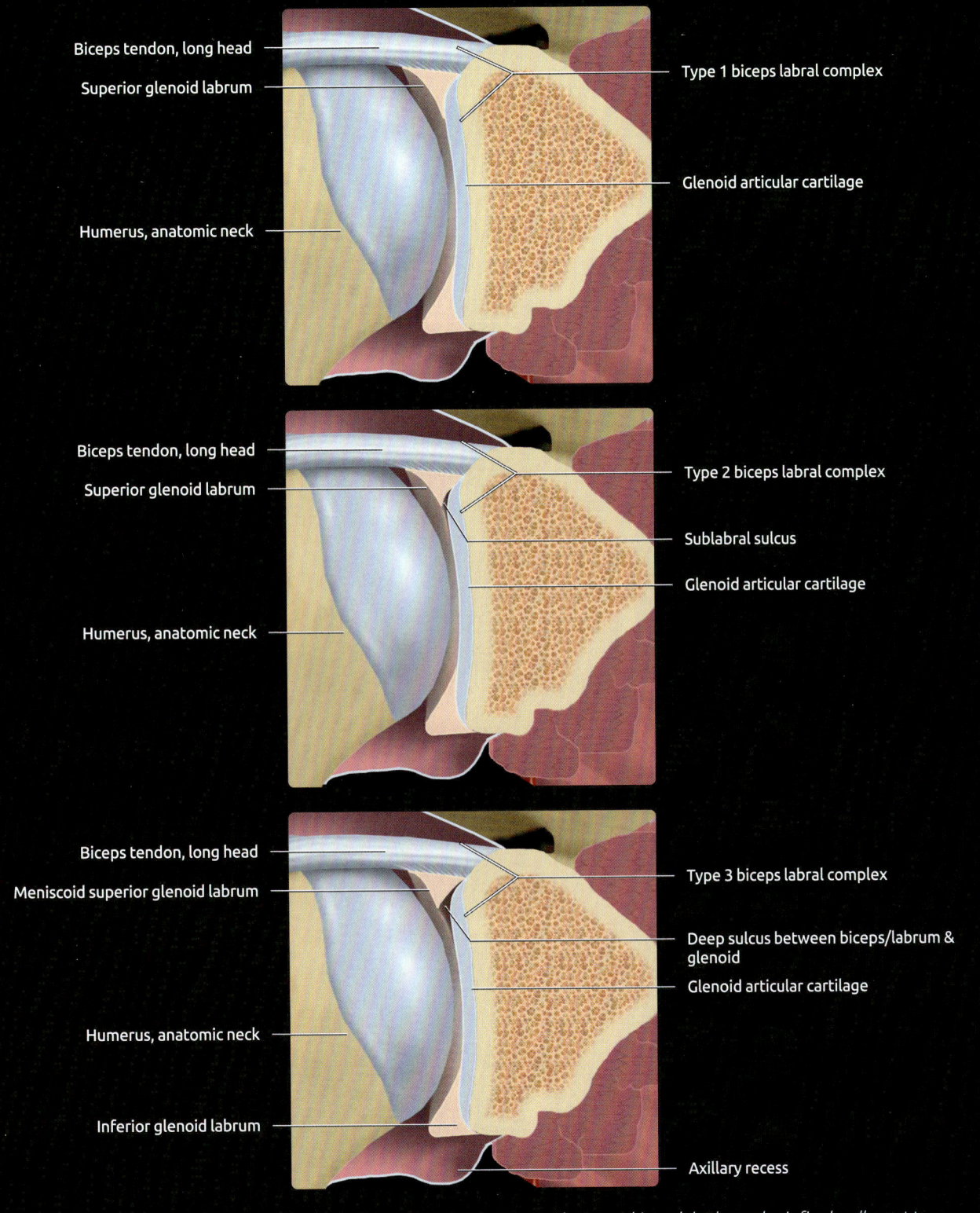

Labels (top image):
- Biceps tendon, long head
- Superior glenoid labrum
- Humerus, anatomic neck
- Type 1 biceps labral complex
- Glenoid articular cartilage

Labels (middle image):
- Biceps tendon, long head
- Superior glenoid labrum
- Humerus, anatomic neck
- Type 2 biceps labral complex
- Sublabral sulcus
- Glenoid articular cartilage

Labels (bottom image):
- Biceps tendon, long head
- Meniscoid superior glenoid labrum
- Humerus, anatomic neck
- Inferior glenoid labrum
- Type 3 biceps labral complex
- Deep sulcus between biceps/labrum & glenoid
- Glenoid articular cartilage
- Axillary recess

(**Top**) *First of 3 coronal graphics shows the biceps labral complex normal variants. The type 1 biceps labral complex is firmly adherent to the glenoid.* (**Middle**) *This shoulder shows a shallow sulcus between the glenoid and the superior labrum.* (**Bottom**) *This shoulder shows a deep sulcus between the glenoid and biceps/labrum. The superior glenoid labrum is meniscoid. The deep sulcus often continues anteriorly as a sublabral foramen.*

Shoulder Radiographic and Arthrographic Anatomy

NORMAL VARIANTS: BICEPS ANCHOR

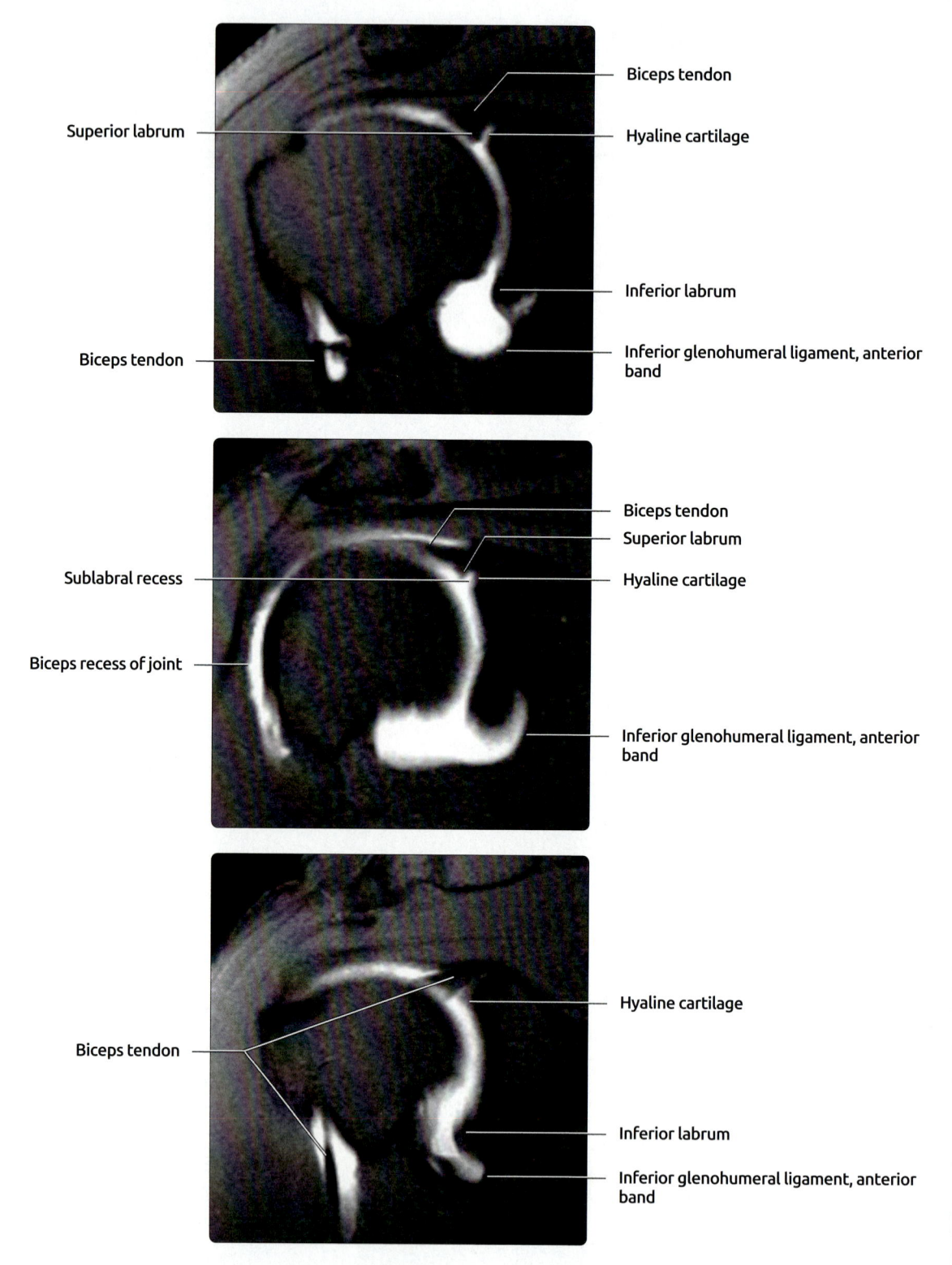

(Top) *In this patient, the superior labrum is adherent to underlying articular cartilage. Note that cartilage curves medially and extends to superior margin of bony glenoid beneath biceps anchor.* (Middle) *In a different patient, there is a sublabral recess. The apparent width of the recess varies with joint distention. Morphology is more important than quantitative measurement of width to distinguish between a recess and a SLAP tear: A recess has smooth margins, while tears tend to be more irregular and jagged.* (Bottom) *This shoulder was imaged in internal rotation. The horizontal portion of the biceps is therefore more sagittally oriented, and the anchor forms a V shape with the glenoid.*

Shoulder Radiographic and Arthrographic Anatomy

VARIABILITY DUE TO ROTATION OF ARM

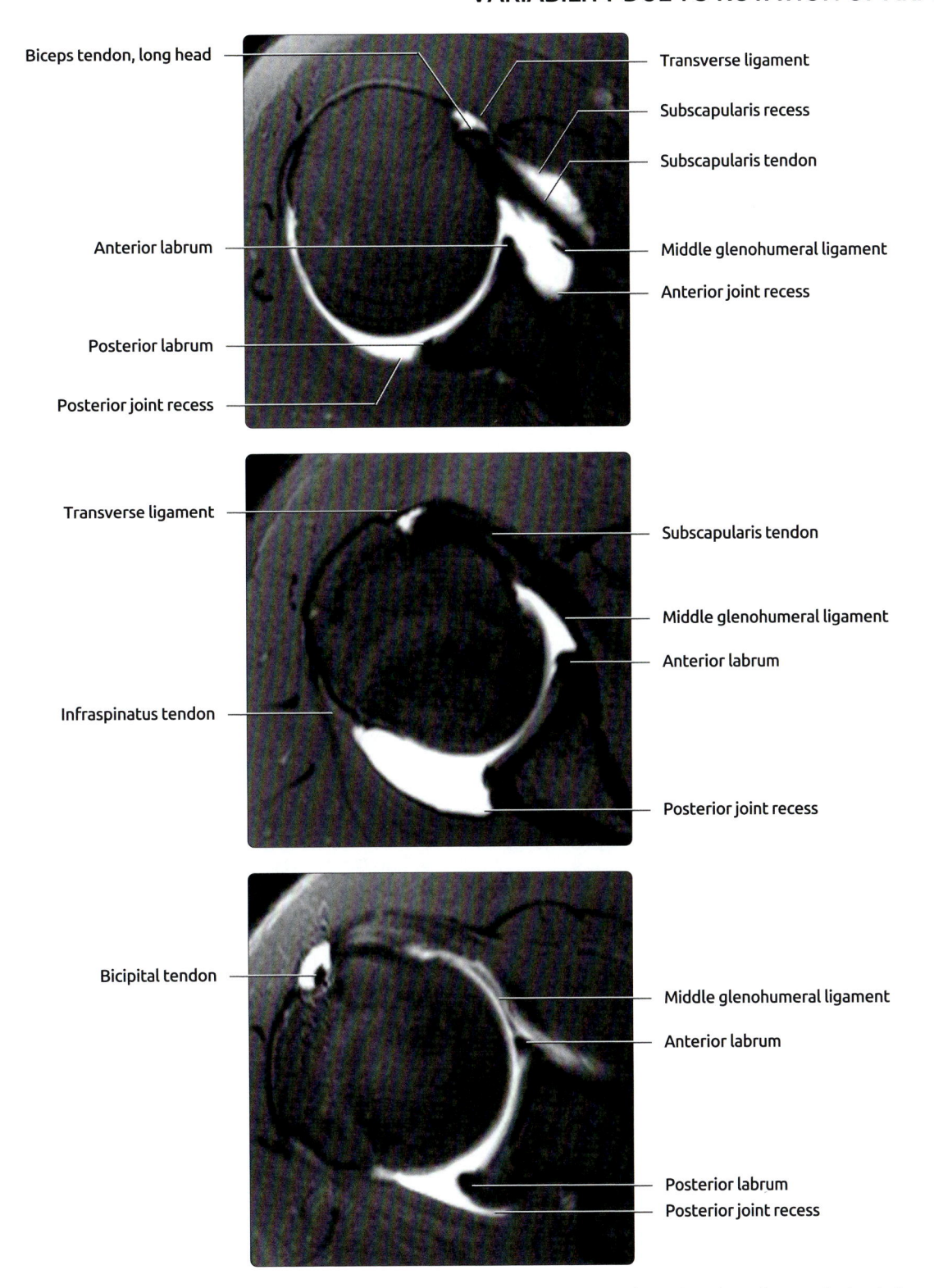

Top image labels:
- Biceps tendon, long head
- Anterior labrum
- Posterior labrum
- Posterior joint recess
- Transverse ligament
- Subscapularis recess
- Subscapularis tendon
- Middle glenohumeral ligament
- Anterior joint recess

Middle image labels:
- Transverse ligament
- Infraspinatus tendon
- Subscapularis tendon
- Middle glenohumeral ligament
- Anterior labrum
- Posterior joint recess

Bottom image labels:
- Bicipital tendon
- Middle glenohumeral ligament
- Anterior labrum
- Posterior labrum
- Posterior joint recess

(Top) The appearance of the labrum and capsule is affected significantly by arm rotation. Internal rotation, shown here at the level of the mid-glenoid, results in distention of the anterior joint recesses. The middle glenohumeral ligament is outlined by fluid. **(Middle)** External rotation at the same level empties the anterior recess and decreases the conspicuity of the middle glenohumeral ligament, which moves closer to subscapularis. Posterior recess is now filled with contrast and appears redundant. **(Bottom)** Extreme external rotation accentuates the normal posterior joint recess. The middle glenohumeral ligament is stretched and taut, paralleling the subscapularis tendon.

Shoulder MR Atlas

ANATOMY IMAGING ISSUES

Imaging Approaches

- **Magnetic resonance (MR) imaging**
  - Patient positioning
    - Supine, arm neutral to slight external rotation, avoid internal rotation
    - Arm at side and slightly away from side of body
  - Axial gradient-echo or T2 FS from acromion through inferior glenoid fossa
  - Coronal oblique T2 FS or proton density and T1 sequences oriented parallel to supraspinatus tendon
    - From subscapularis muscle anteriorly through infraspinatus muscle posteriorly
  - Sagittal oblique T2 FS oriented perpendicular to supraspinatus tendon
    - Scapular neck through lateral border of greater tuberosity

Imaging Pitfalls

- **Magic angle phenomenon on MR**
  - 55° to main magnetic field when image echo time (TE) < 30 ms
  - Increases signal intensity in otherwise normal structures
  - Most often seen in supraspinatus tendon, commonly in "critical zone," 1 cm from greater tuberosity
  - Can be seen in glenoid labrum and biceps tendon proximal to bicipital groove
  - Avoid pitfall by comparing with images acquired with longer TE
- **Interdigitation of muscle or fibrous tissue between supraspinatus and infraspinatus tendons**
  - Simulates increased T2 MR signal within supraspinatus tendon
  - Exaggerated if imaged in internal rotation
- **Volume averaging of rotator interval contents on coronal oblique images**
  - Simulates increased T2 MR signal within supraspinatus tendon
- **Normal flattening or slight concavity of posterolateral humeral head**
  - Proximal to teres minor tendon insertion
  - Can be confused with Hill-Sachs lesion, which is located more proximally, above level of coracoid process
- **Acromial pseudospurs mimicking osteophytes**
  - Fibrocartilaginous hypertrophy at insertion of coracoacromial ligament on inferior acromion
  - Superior and inferior tendon slips of deltoid muscle
- **Anterolateral branch of anterior circumflex humeral artery and vein in lateral bicipital groove**
  - Can be mistaken for biceps tendon longitudinal tear
- **Hyaline cartilage undercutting of superior labrum simulating labral tear**
- **General imaging artifacts**
  - Motion artifact can be decreased by positioning arm away from patient's body
  - Avoid superior to inferior phase encoding to decrease artifact from axillary vessels
  - Metal susceptibility artifact
    - Increase bandwidth on all sequences
    - Fast spin-echo preferred to conventional spin-echo

CLINICAL IMPLICATIONS

"Spaces" of Particular Interest Around Shoulder

- **Quadrilateral or quadrangular space**
  - Superior border: Teres minor
  - Inferior border: Teres major
  - Lateral border: Surgical neck of humerus
  - Medial border: Long head of triceps muscle
  - Contents: Axillary nerve and posterior circumflex humeral artery
    - Axillary nerve supplies teres minor muscle, deltoid muscle, posterolateral cutaneous region of shoulder and upper arm
    - Can have complications that are purely neurologic, purely vascular, or both
  - Axillary neuropathy
    - Due to abnormalities in quadrilateral space (paralabral cyst, fibrous band, glenohumeral joint dislocation, humeral fracture, extreme or prolonged abduction of arm during sleep)
    - Results in atrophy of teres minor muscle; may affect deltoid
- **Coracoacromial arch**
  - Superior border: Acromion
  - Posterior border: Humeral head
  - Anterior border: Coracoacromial ligament, coracoid process
  - Contents: Subacromial-subdeltoid bursa, supraspinatus muscle/tendon, long head of biceps
  - Space/contents affected by os acromiale
    - Normal variant anatomy (unfused acromial process) in 5%
    - Normally fused by age 25
    - May be mobile, decreasing coracoacromial space during shoulder motion, predisposing to impingement
- **Rotator interval**
  - Triangular space between inferior border of supraspinatus muscle/tendon and superior border of subscapularis muscle/tendon
  - Medially border: Coracoid process
  - Laterally border: Transverse humeral ligament
  - Anterior border: Coracohumeral ligament, superior glenohumeral ligament, and joint capsule
- **Suprascapular notch**
  - Roof of notch covered by superior transverse scapular ligament
  - Contents: Suprascapular nerve
    - Arises from brachial plexus superior trunk (4th-6th cervical nerve roots) composed of both motor and sensory fibers
    - Supplies supraspinatus and infraspinatus muscles
    - Anterior compression causes supraspinatus and infraspinatus atrophy
    - Posterior compression causes infraspinatus atrophy
- **Spinoglenoid notch**
  - Located inferior to suprascapular notch, between scapular spine and posterior surface of glenoid body
  - Contents: Infraspinatus branch of suprascapular nerve
  - Supplies infraspinatus muscle

Shoulder MR Atlas

GRAPHICS, SUPERFICIAL SHOULDER DISSECTION

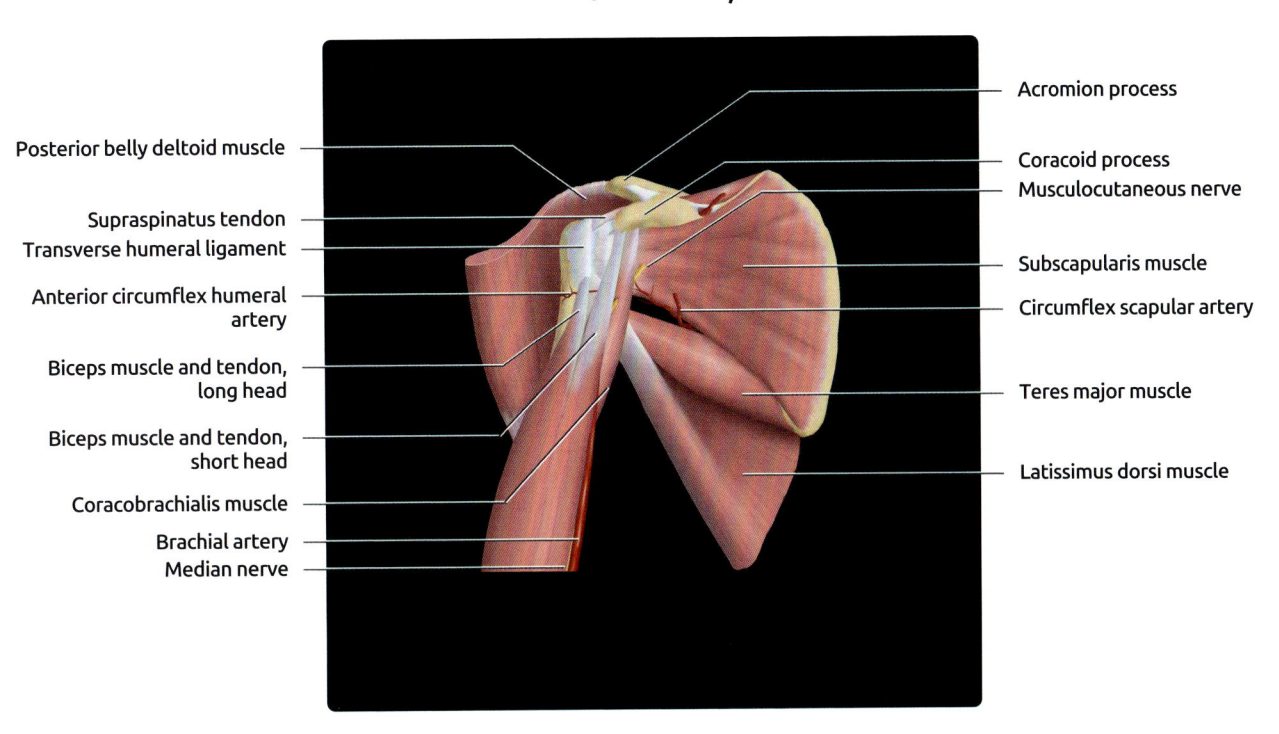

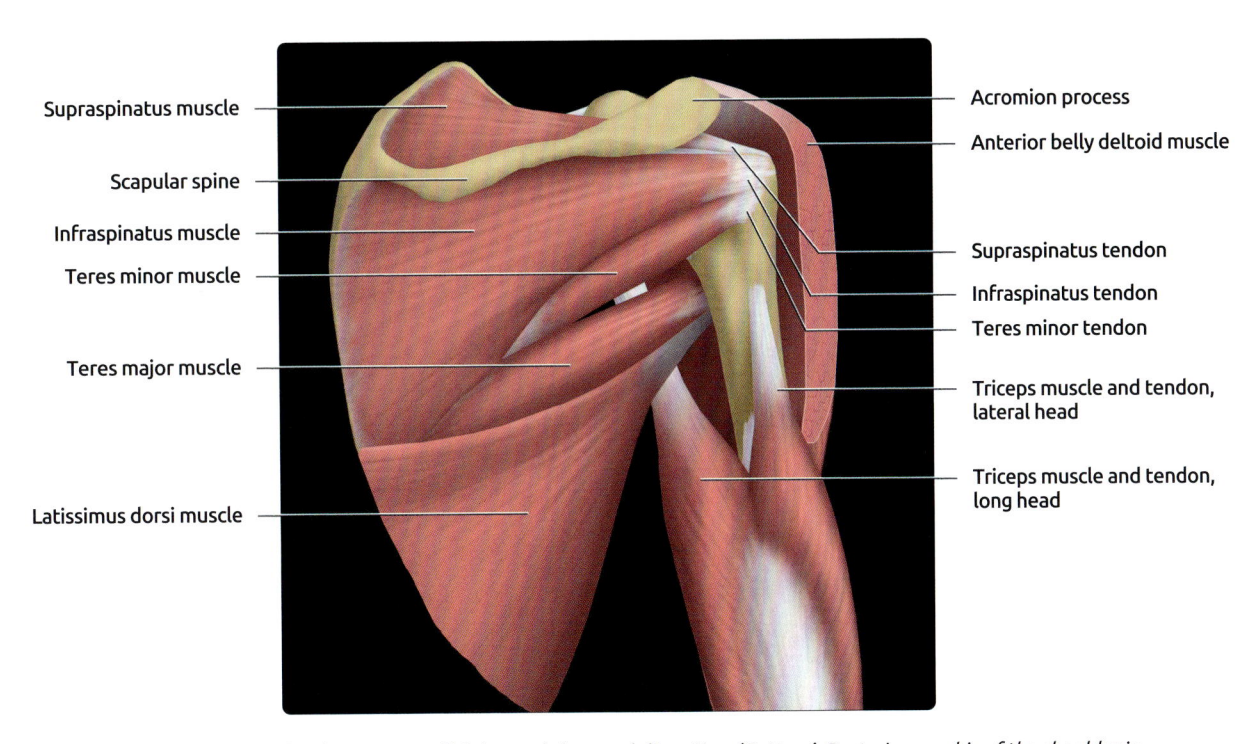

Labels (anterior view, top):
- Posterior belly deltoid muscle
- Supraspinatus tendon
- Transverse humeral ligament
- Anterior circumflex humeral artery
- Biceps muscle and tendon, long head
- Biceps muscle and tendon, short head
- Coracobrachialis muscle
- Brachial artery
- Median nerve
- Acromion process
- Coracoid process
- Musculocutaneous nerve
- Subscapularis muscle
- Circumflex scapular artery
- Teres major muscle
- Latissimus dorsi muscle

Labels (posterior view, bottom):
- Supraspinatus muscle
- Scapular spine
- Infraspinatus muscle
- Teres minor muscle
- Teres major muscle
- Latissimus dorsi muscle
- Acromion process
- Anterior belly deltoid muscle
- Supraspinatus tendon
- Infraspinatus tendon
- Teres minor tendon
- Triceps muscle and tendon, lateral head
- Triceps muscle and tendon, long head

(Top) *Anterior graphic of the shoulder shows a superficial scapulohumeral dissection.* **(Bottom)** *Posterior graphic of the shoulder is shown. Superficial scapulohumeral dissection demonstrates the musculature.*

Shoulder MR Atlas

AXIAL T1 MR, RIGHT SHOULDER

Subcutaneous fat

Skin surface

Trapezius muscle

Subcutaneous fat

Skin surface

Trapezius muscle

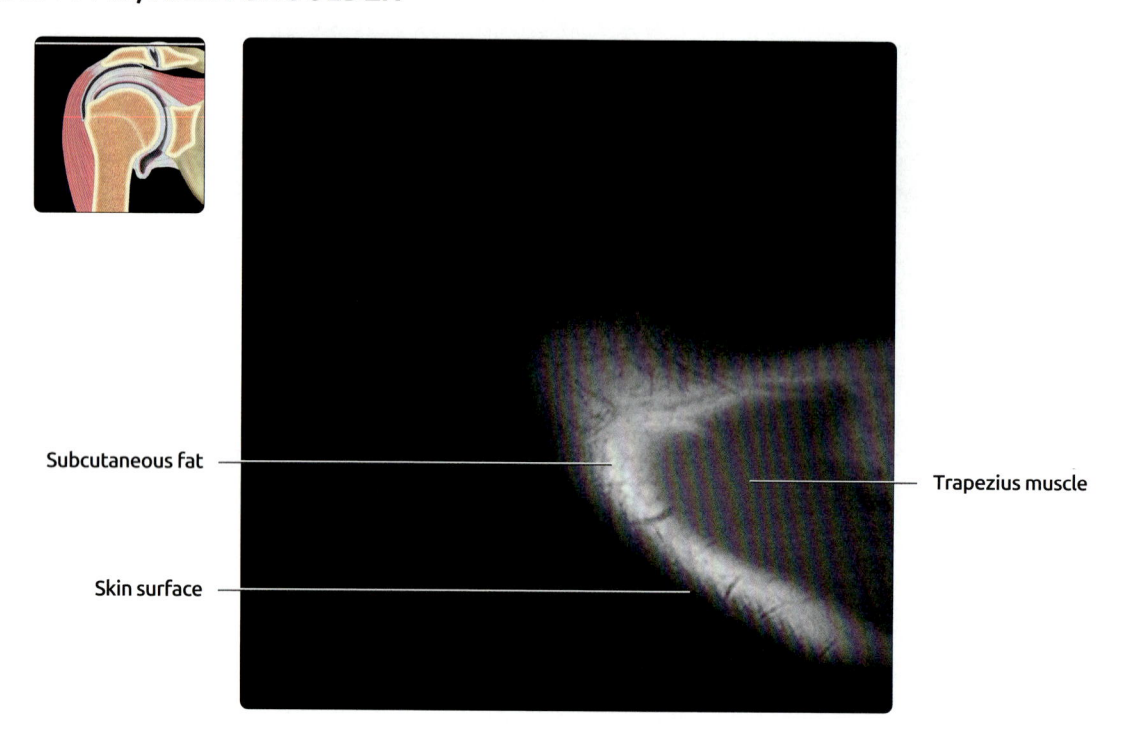

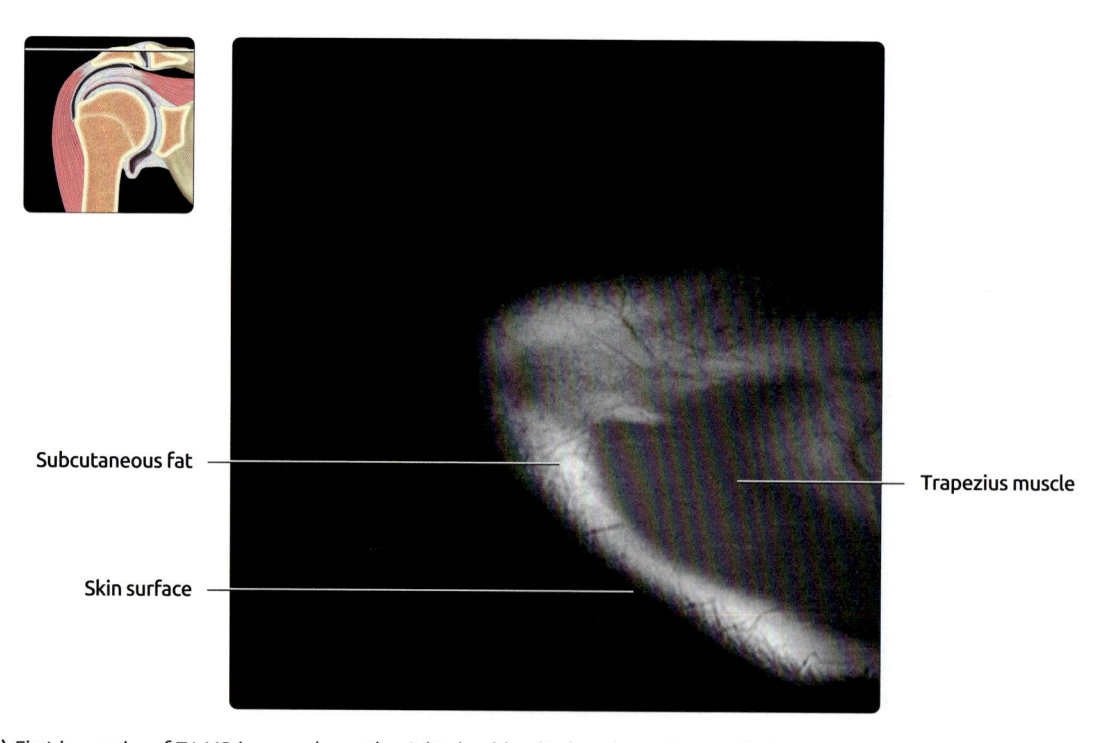

(Top) First in a series of T1 MR images shows the right shoulder displayed superior to inferior. Images were acquired using a shoulder coil on a 3T MR scanner. *(Bottom)* The trapezius muscle covers the superior and posterior aspect of the upper shoulder. It originates from the occipital bone, ligamentum nuchae, and the spinous processes of C7 to T12. It inserts on the posterior border of the lateral clavicle, the medial border of the acromion, and the spine of the scapula.

Shoulder MR Atlas

AXIAL T1 MR, LEFT SHOULDER

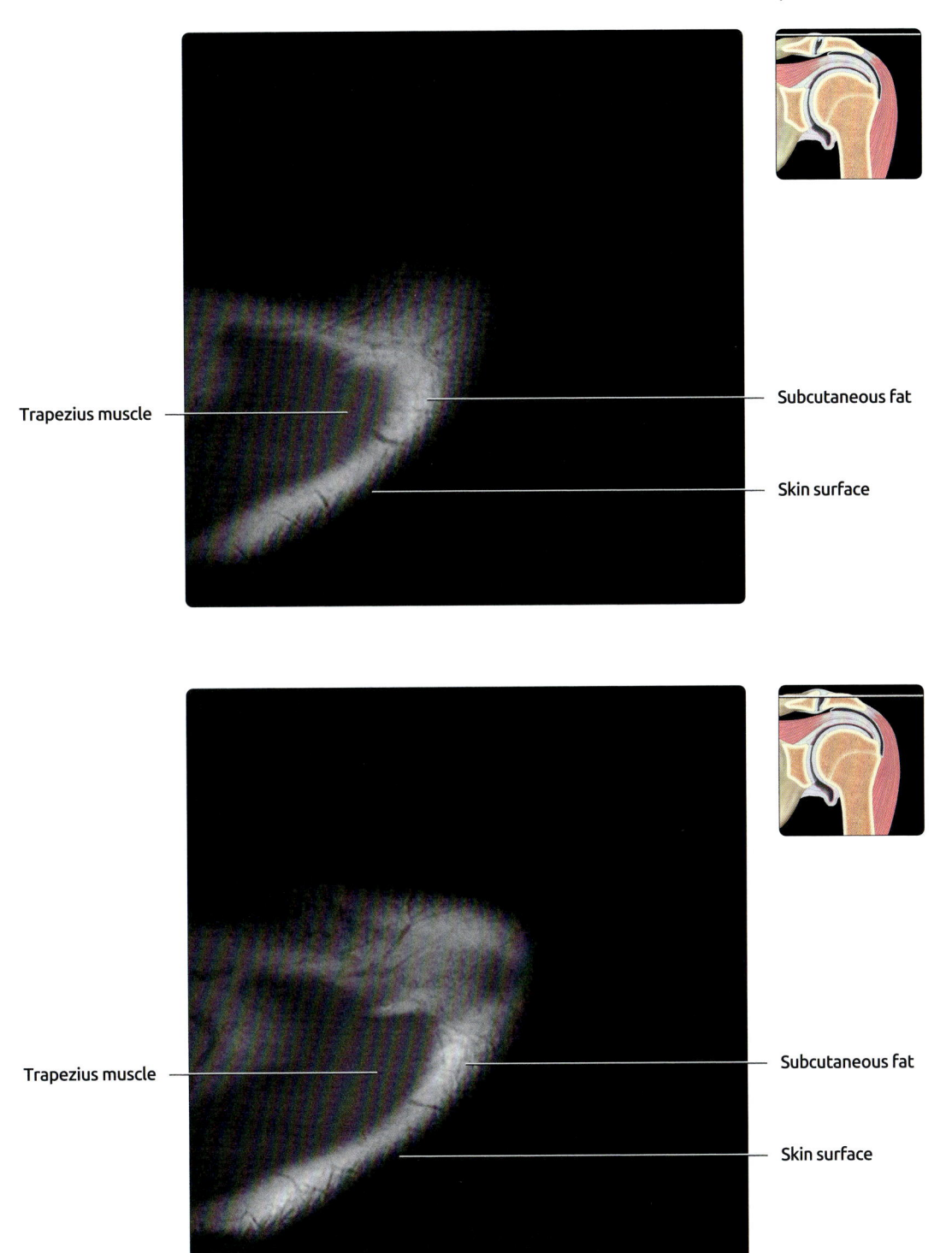

Trapezius muscle — Subcutaneous fat

Skin surface

Trapezius muscle — Subcutaneous fat

Skin surface

(Top) First in series of T1 MR images shows the left shoulder displayed superior to inferior. Images were acquired using a shoulder coil on a 3T MR scanner. **(Bottom)** The trapezius muscle covers the superior and posterior aspect of the upper shoulder. It originates from the occipital bone, ligamentum nuchae, and the spinous processes of C7 to T12. It inserts on the posterior border of the lateral clavicle, the medial border of the acromion, and the spine of the scapula.

Shoulder MR Atlas

AXIAL T1 MR, RIGHT SHOULDER

Acromioclavicular joint

Clavicle

Trapezius muscle, anterior fibers

Trapezius muscle

Acromioclavicular joint
Acromion process of scapula

Suprascapular vessels

Deltoid muscle, anterior belly

Clavicle

Supraspinatus muscle

Trapezius muscle

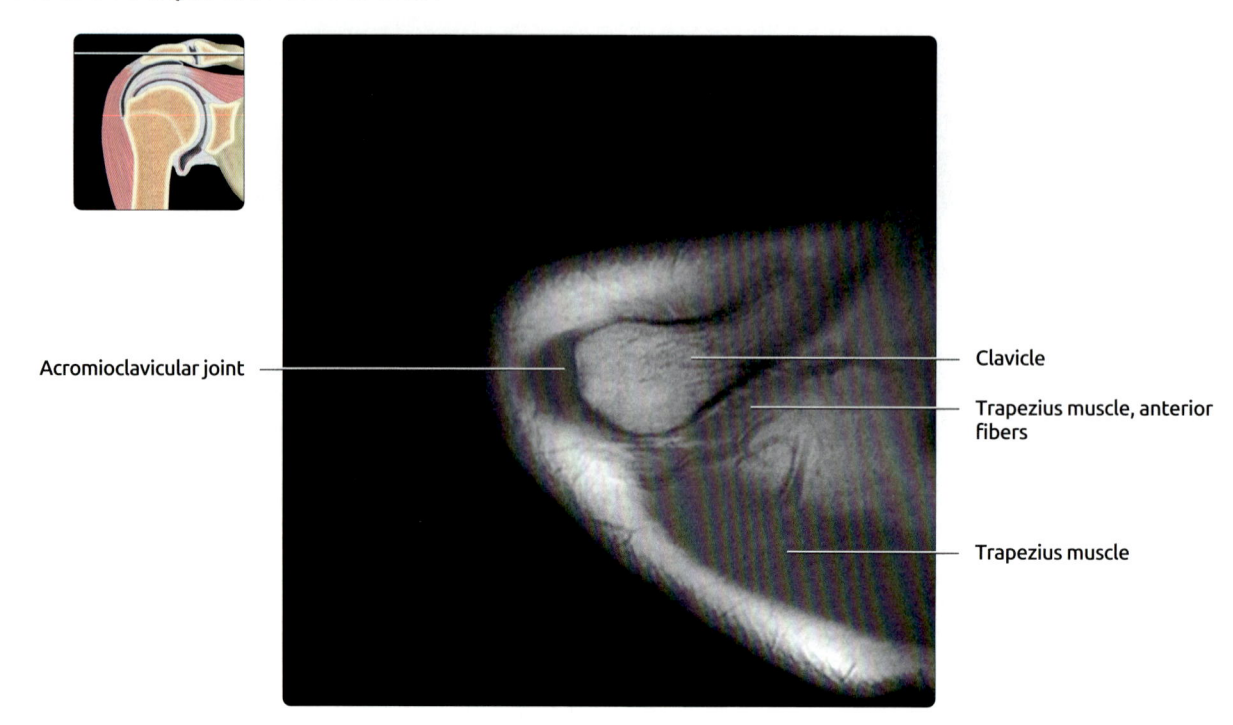

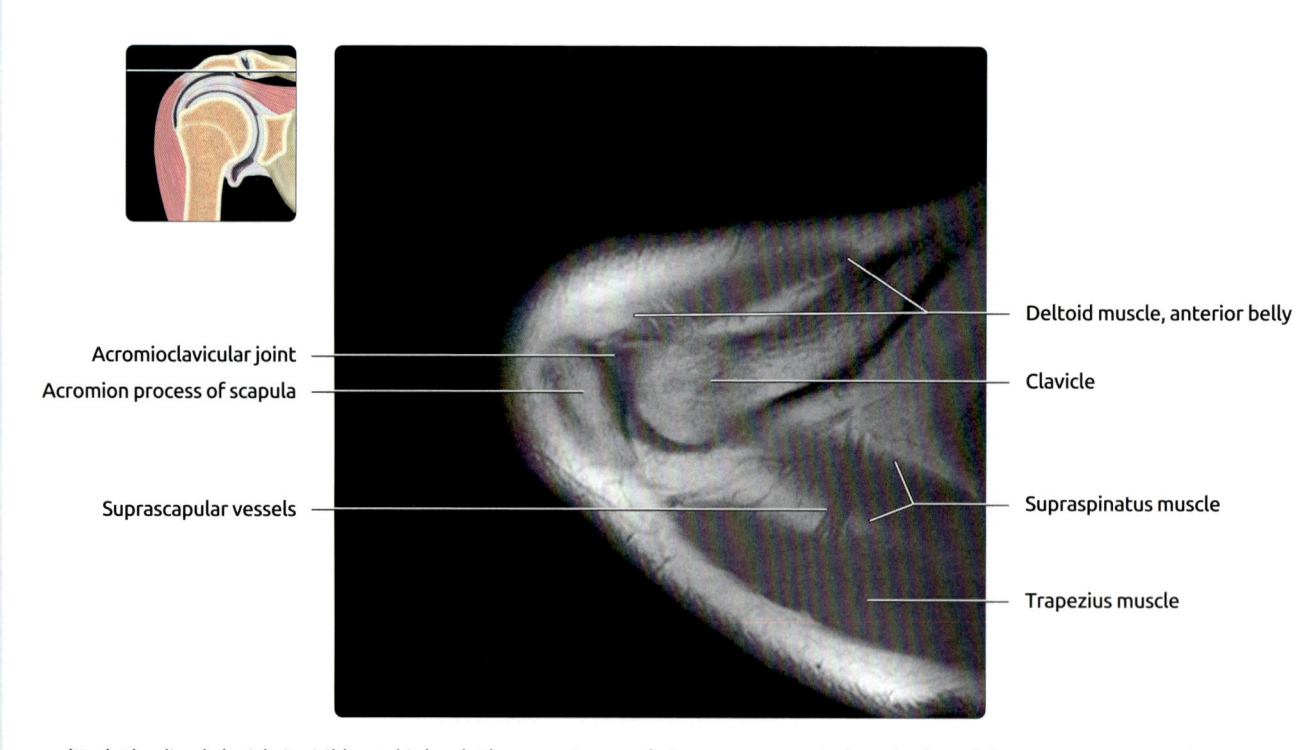

(**Top**) The distal clavicle is visible at this level. The trapezius muscle is present posteriorly and a few of the anterior trapezius fibers are inserting along the posterior border of the distal clavicle. (**Bottom**) The acromion and distal clavicle form the bony roof of the superior shoulder. The supraspinatus muscle becomes visible beneath the branches of the suprascapular vessels.

Shoulder MR Atlas

AXIAL T1 MR, LEFT SHOULDER

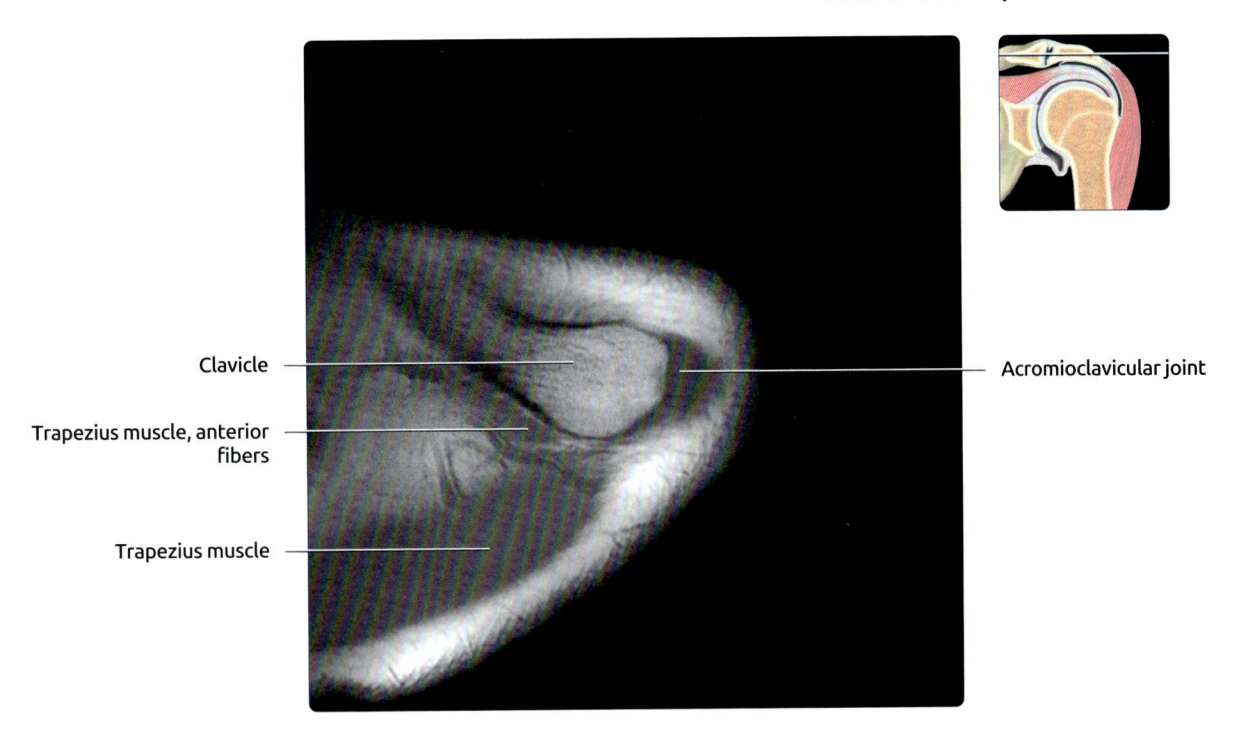

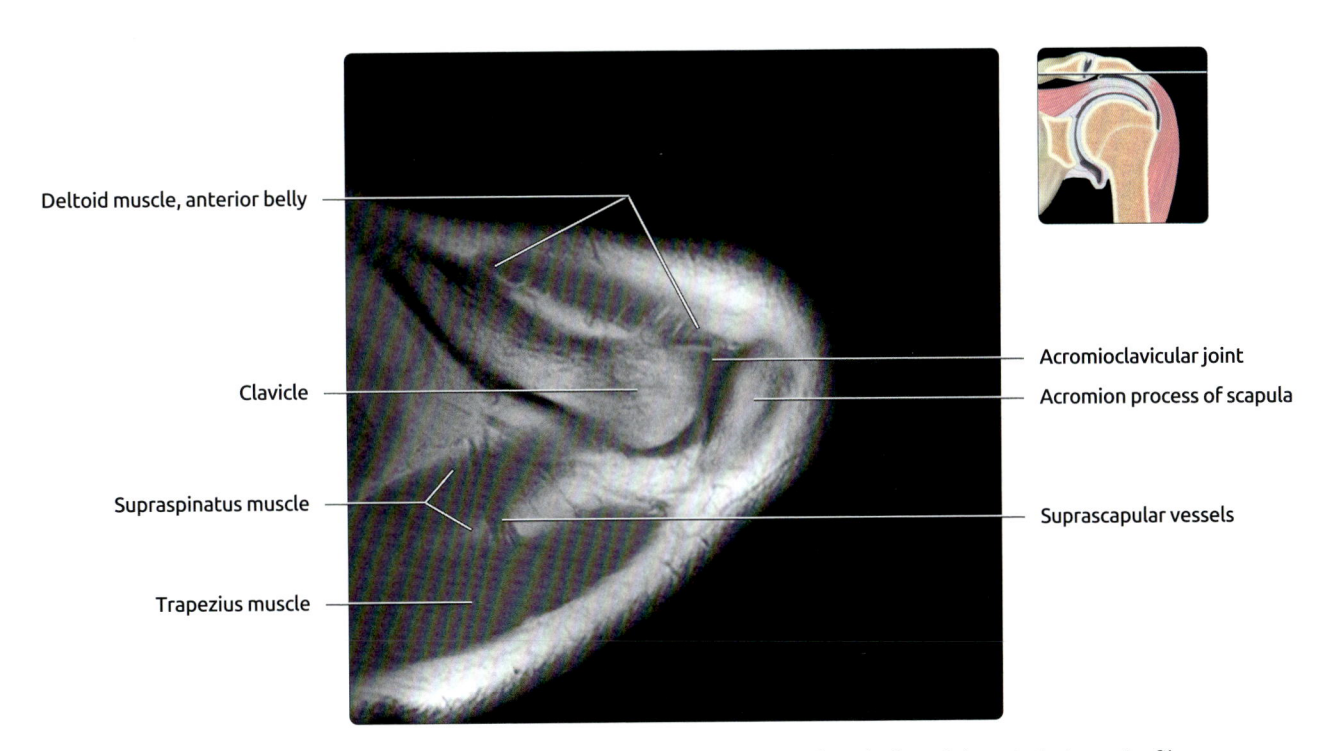

Clavicle — Acromioclavicular joint

Trapezius muscle, anterior fibers

Trapezius muscle

Deltoid muscle, anterior belly

Clavicle — Acromioclavicular joint
— Acromion process of scapula

Supraspinatus muscle — Suprascapular vessels

Trapezius muscle

(Top) The distal clavicle is visible at this level. The trapezius muscle is present posteriorly and a few of the anterior trapezius fibers are inserting along the posterior border of the distal clavicle. (Bottom) The acromion and distal clavicle form the bony roof of the superior shoulder. The supraspinatus muscle becomes visible beneath the branches of the suprascapular vessels.

Shoulder MR Atlas

AXIAL T1 MR, RIGHT SHOULDER

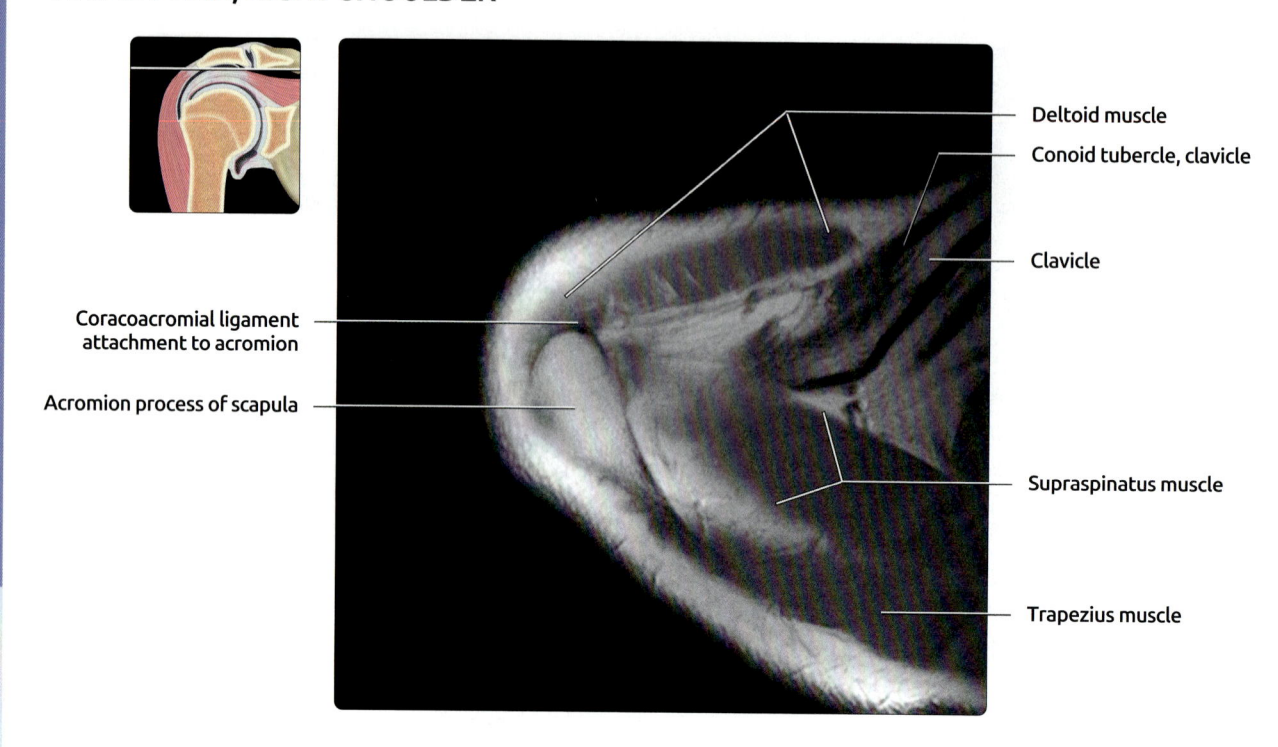

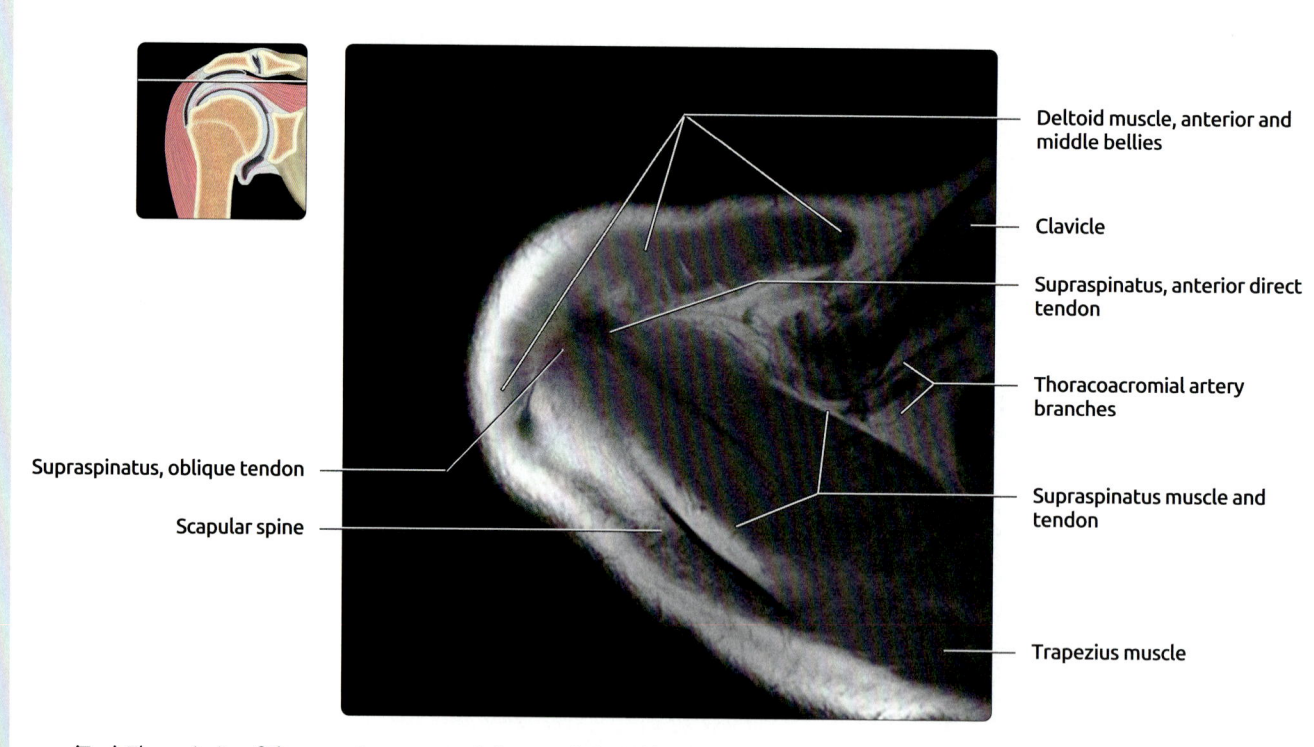

Labels (top image):
- Deltoid muscle
- Conoid tubercle, clavicle
- Clavicle
- Supraspinatus muscle
- Trapezius muscle
- Coracoacromial ligament attachment to acromion
- Acromion process of scapula

Labels (bottom image):
- Deltoid muscle, anterior and middle bellies
- Clavicle
- Supraspinatus, anterior direct tendon
- Thoracoacromial artery branches
- Supraspinatus muscle and tendon
- Trapezius muscle
- Supraspinatus, oblique tendon
- Scapular spine

(Top) *The majority of the acromion process of the scapula is visible on this axial image. This is the level to assess for the presence of an os acromiale, an unfused acromial apophysis that can be symptomatic.* **(Bottom)** *This image is just below the acromion process. The supraspinatus tendon arcs over the humeral head toward the attachment on the greater tuberosity. The deltoid muscle covers the anterior, lateral, and posterior aspect of the shoulder. It originates from the lateral 1/3 of the clavicle, lateral margin of the acromion, and posterior border of the scapular spine.*

Shoulder MR Atlas

AXIAL T1 MR, LEFT SHOULDER

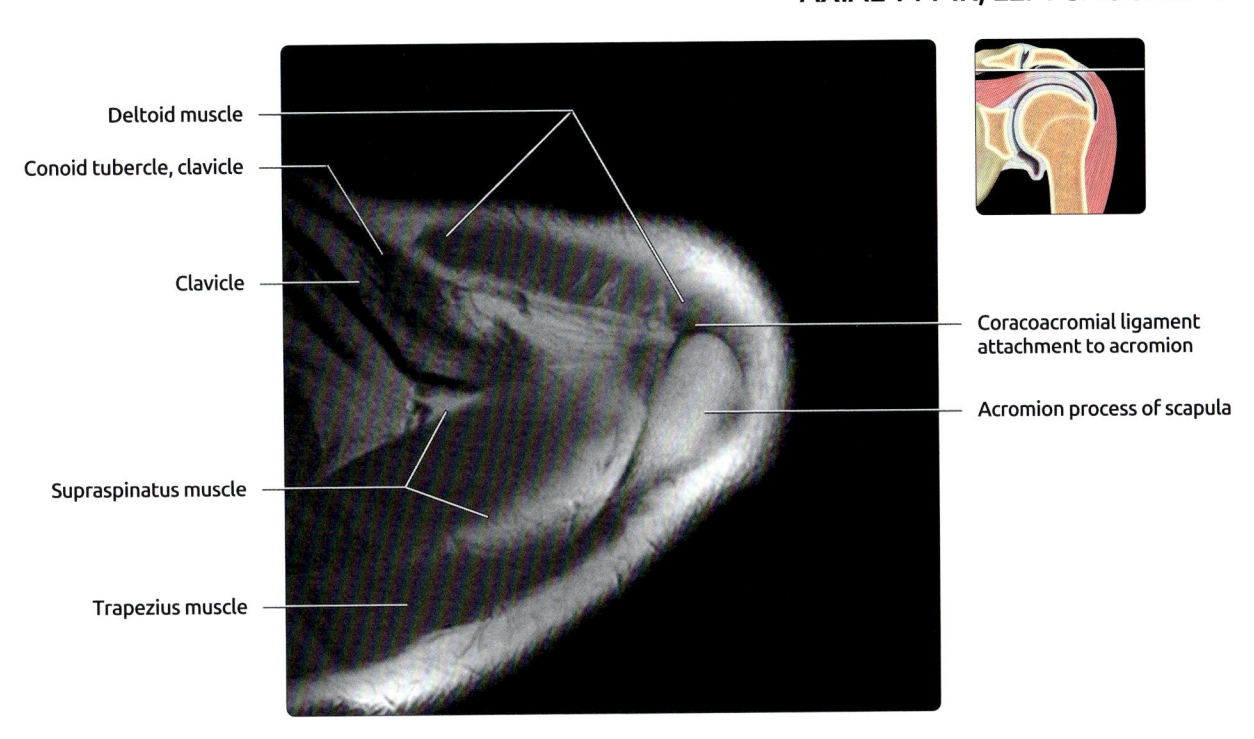

Top image labels:
- Deltoid muscle
- Conoid tubercle, clavicle
- Clavicle
- Supraspinatus muscle
- Trapezius muscle
- Coracoacromial ligament attachment to acromion
- Acromion process of scapula

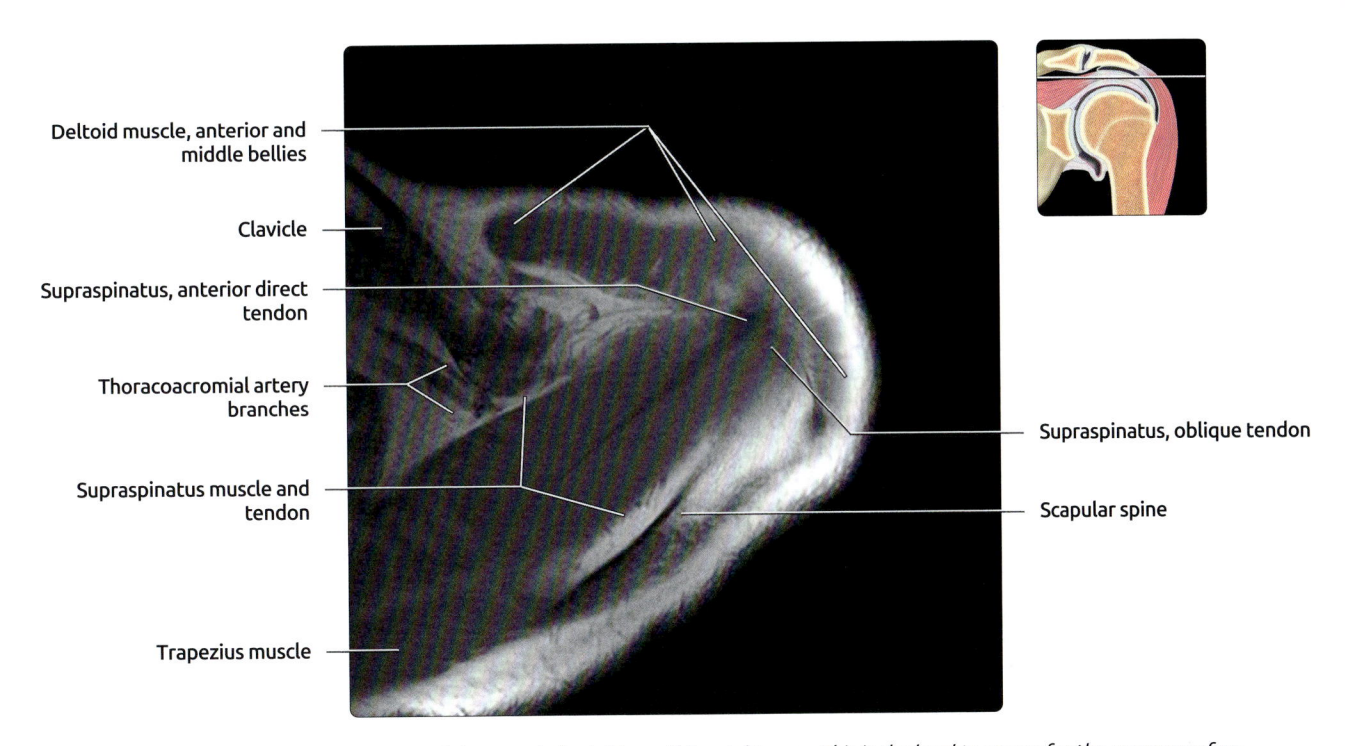

Bottom image labels:
- Deltoid muscle, anterior and middle bellies
- Clavicle
- Supraspinatus, anterior direct tendon
- Thoracoacromial artery branches
- Supraspinatus muscle and tendon
- Trapezius muscle
- Supraspinatus, oblique tendon
- Scapular spine

(Top) The majority of the acromion process of the scapula is visible on this axial image. This is the level to assess for the presence of an os acromiale, an unfused acromial apophysis that can be symptomatic. **(Bottom)** This image is just below the acromion process. The supraspinatus tendon arcs over the humeral head toward the attachment on the greater tuberosity. The deltoid muscle covers the anterior, lateral, and posterior aspect of the shoulder. It originates from the lateral 1/3 of the clavicle, lateral margin of the acromion, and posterior border of the scapular spine.

Shoulder MR Atlas

AXIAL T1 MR, RIGHT SHOULDER

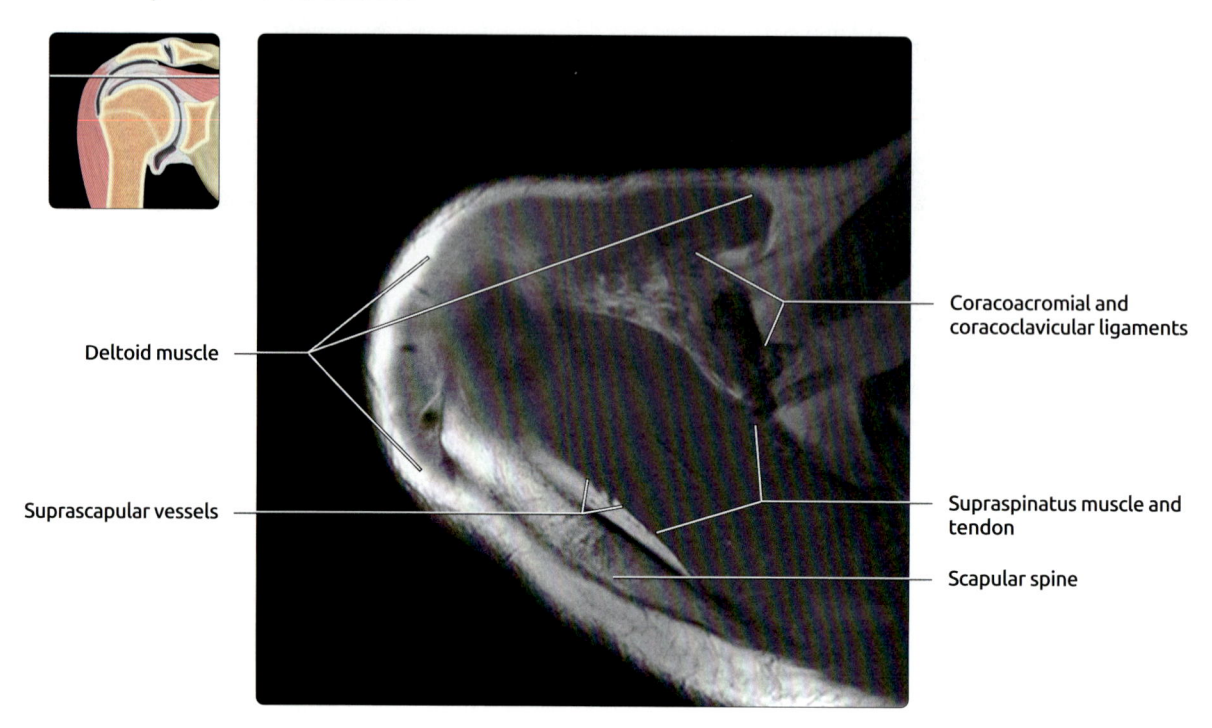

Deltoid muscle

Suprascapular vessels

Coracoacromial and coracoclavicular ligaments

Supraspinatus muscle and tendon

Scapular spine

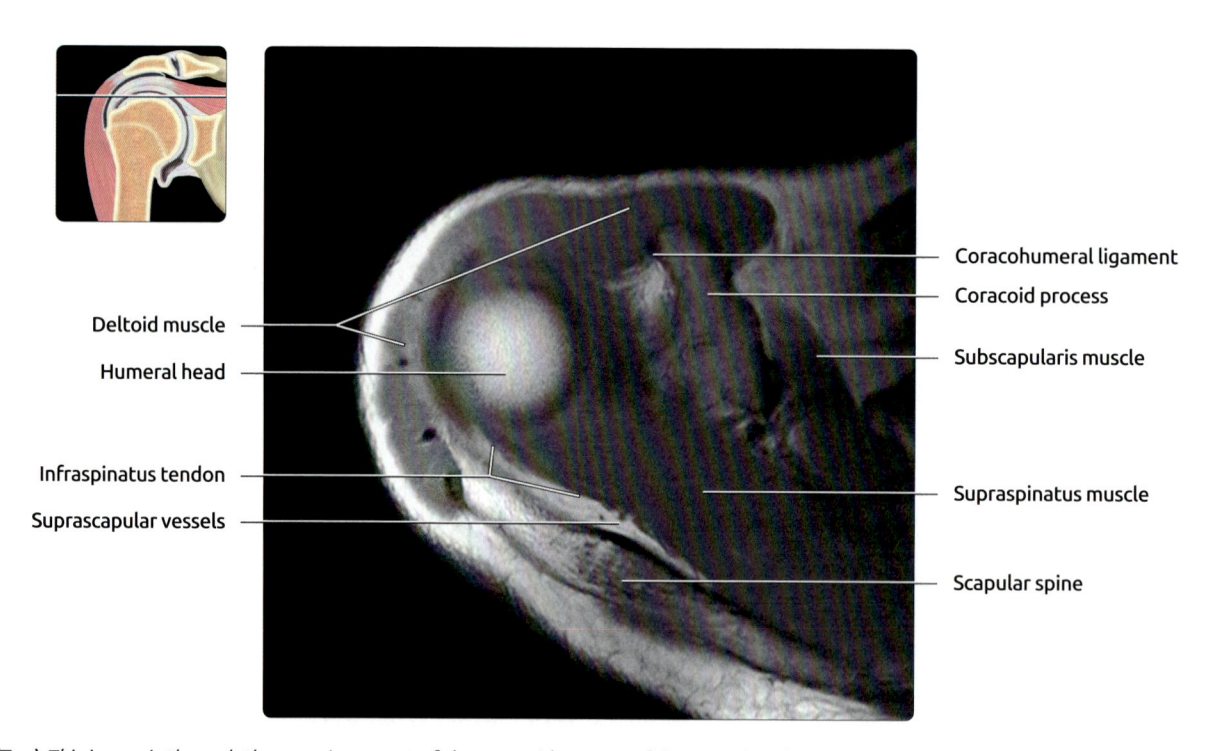

Deltoid muscle
Humeral head

Infraspinatus tendon
Suprascapular vessels

Coracohumeral ligament
Coracoid process
Subscapularis muscle

Supraspinatus muscle

Scapular spine

(Top) This image is through the superior aspect of the coracoid process of the scapula. The coracoclavicular and coracoacromial ligaments extend from the inferior border of the clavicle and acromion respectively to attach to the superior aspect of the coracoid process. **(Bottom)** The infraspinatus muscle begins to appear at the posterior aspect of the shoulder, below the level of the scapular spine. The coracohumeral ligament extends from the lateral border of the coracoid process to the anterior aspect of the greater tuberosity of the humerus. The coracohumeral ligament blends with the supraspinatus tendon at the attachment.

Shoulder MR Atlas

AXIAL T1 MR, LEFT SHOULDER

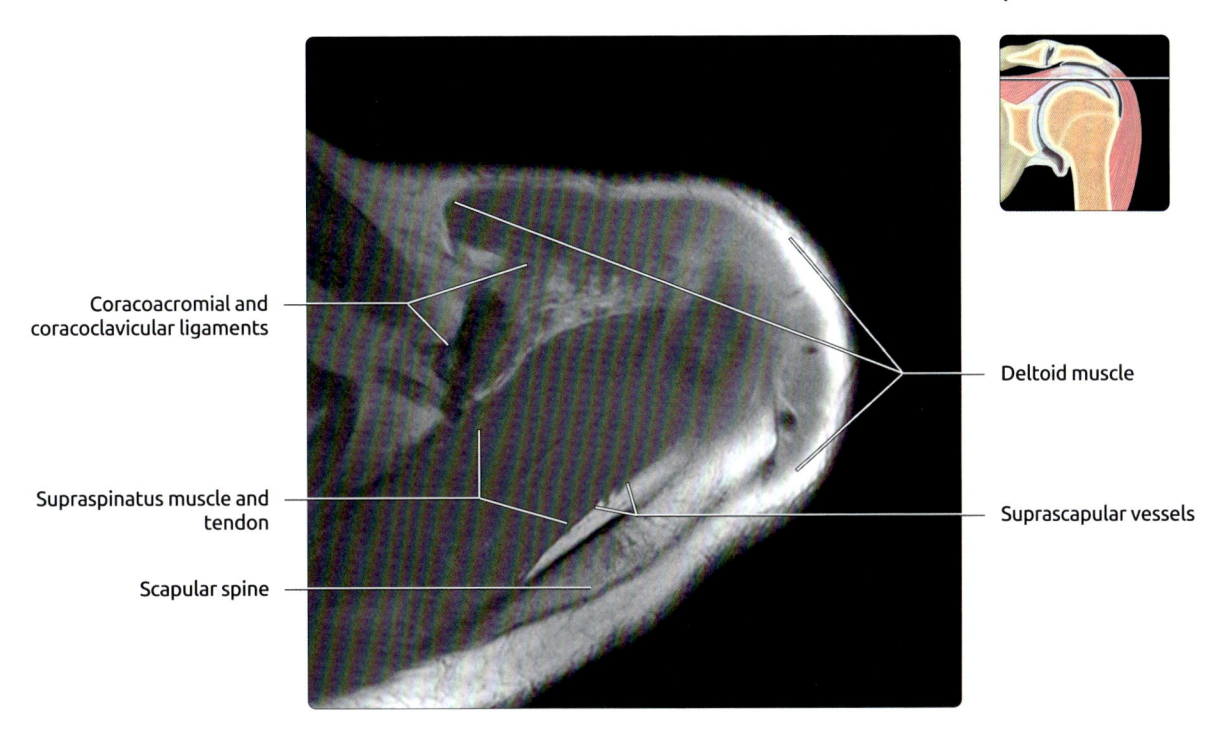

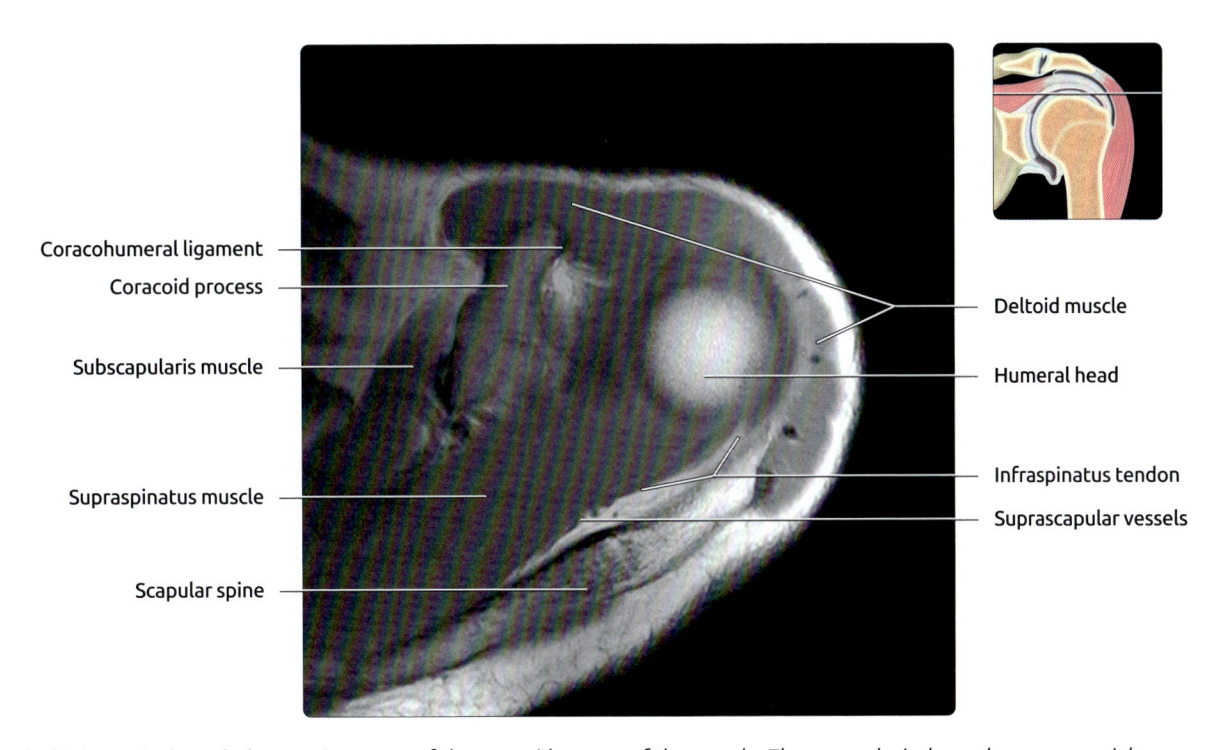

(Top) This image is through the superior aspect of the coracoid process of the scapula. The coracoclavicular and coracoacromial ligaments extend from the inferior border of the clavicle and acromion respectively to attach to the superior aspect of the coracoid process. **(Bottom)** The infraspinatus muscle begins to appear at the posterior aspect of the shoulder, below the level of the scapular spine. The coracohumeral ligament extends from the lateral border of the coracoid process to the anterior aspect of the greater tuberosity of the humerus. The coracohumeral ligament blends with the supraspinatus tendon at the attachment.

Shoulder MR Atlas

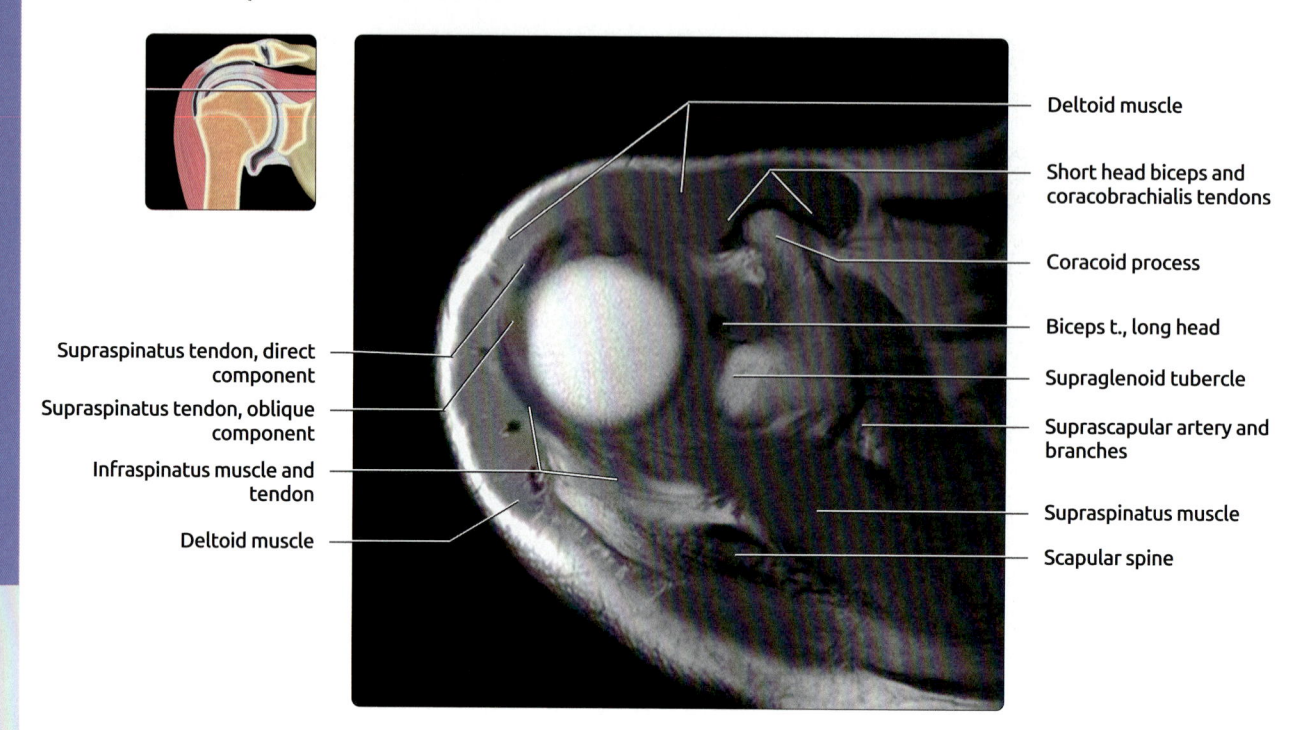

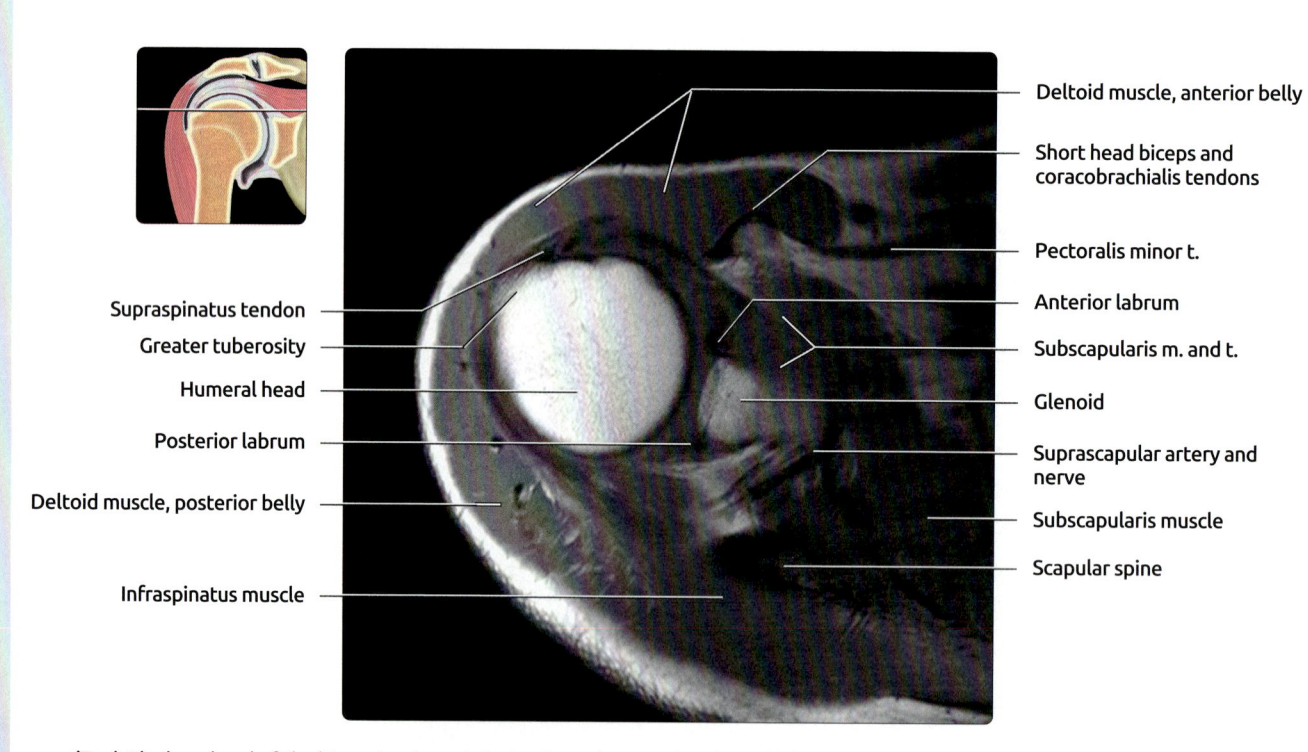

AXIAL T1 MR, RIGHT SHOULDER

Labels (top image):
- Deltoid muscle
- Short head biceps and coracobrachialis tendons
- Coracoid process
- Biceps t., long head
- Supraglenoid tubercle
- Suprascapular artery and branches
- Supraspinatus muscle
- Scapular spine
- Supraspinatus tendon, direct component
- Supraspinatus tendon, oblique component
- Infraspinatus muscle and tendon
- Deltoid muscle

Labels (bottom image):
- Deltoid muscle, anterior belly
- Short head biceps and coracobrachialis tendons
- Pectoralis minor t.
- Anterior labrum
- Subscapularis m. and t.
- Glenoid
- Suprascapular artery and nerve
- Subscapularis muscle
- Scapular spine
- Supraspinatus tendon
- Greater tuberosity
- Humeral head
- Posterior labrum
- Deltoid muscle, posterior belly
- Infraspinatus muscle

(Top) The long head of the biceps tendon originates from the superior glenoid labrum and supraglenoid tuberosity of the scapula. The short head of the biceps and coracobrachialis muscles originate from the tip of the coracoid process. **(Bottom)** The suprascapular artery and nerve branches course along the posterior glenoid fossa. The point labeled "supraspinatus tendon" represents the most lateral extent of rotator cuff interval, where the transverse ligament component of subscapularis meets the anterior edge of supraspinatus (direct tendon).

Shoulder MR Atlas

AXIAL T1 MR, LEFT SHOULDER

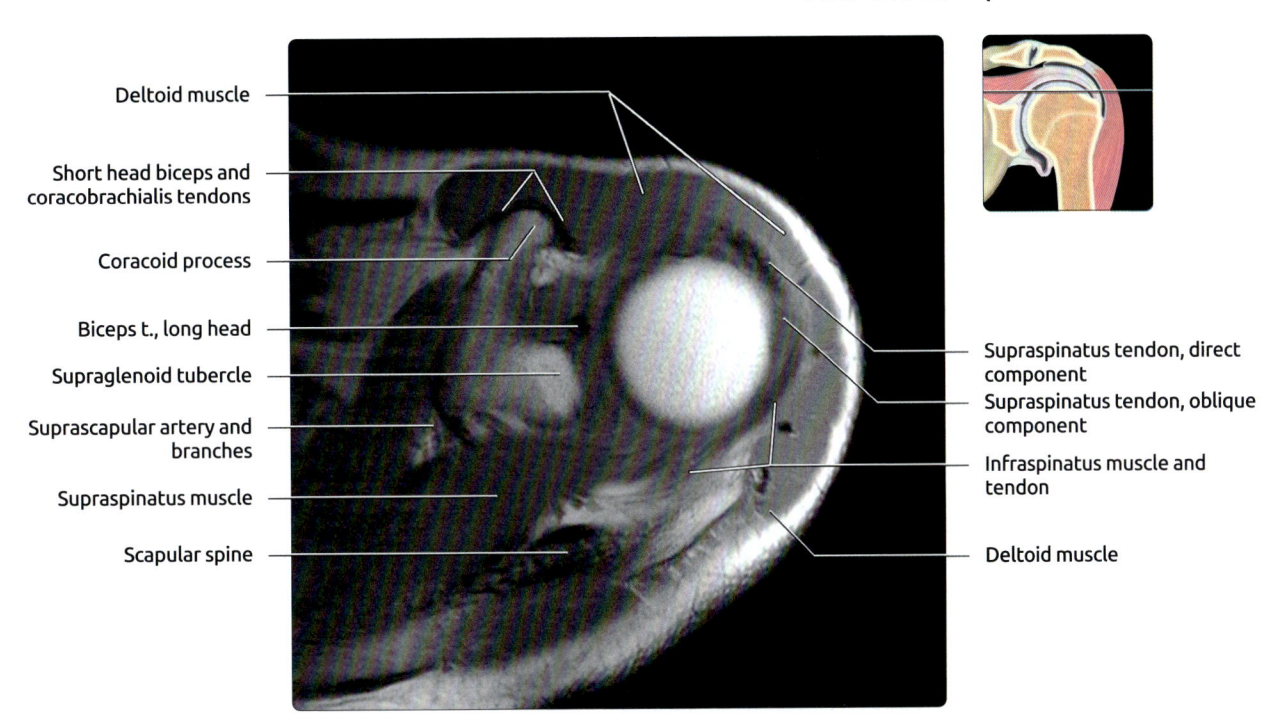

Top image labels (left):
- Deltoid muscle
- Short head biceps and coracobrachialis tendons
- Coracoid process
- Biceps t., long head
- Supraglenoid tubercle
- Suprascapular artery and branches
- Supraspinatus muscle
- Scapular spine

Top image labels (right):
- Supraspinatus tendon, direct component
- Supraspinatus tendon, oblique component
- Infraspinatus muscle and tendon
- Deltoid muscle

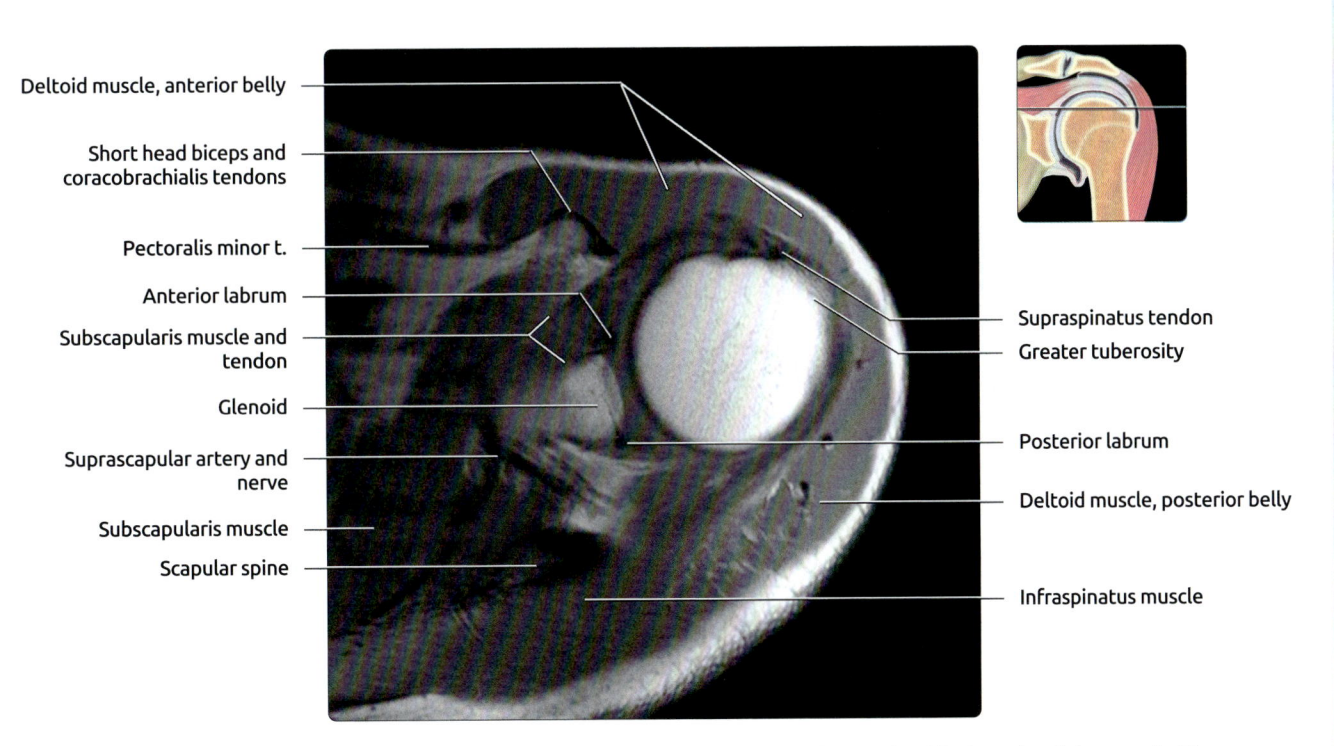

Bottom image labels (left):
- Deltoid muscle, anterior belly
- Short head biceps and coracobrachialis tendons
- Pectoralis minor t.
- Anterior labrum
- Subscapularis muscle and tendon
- Glenoid
- Suprascapular artery and nerve
- Subscapularis muscle
- Scapular spine

Bottom image labels (right):
- Supraspinatus tendon
- Greater tuberosity
- Posterior labrum
- Deltoid muscle, posterior belly
- Infraspinatus muscle

(Top) *The long head of the biceps tendon originates from the superior glenoid labrum and supraglenoid tuberosity of the scapula. The short head of the biceps and coracobrachialis muscles originate from the tip of the coracoid process.* **(Bottom)** *The suprascapular artery and nerve branches course along the posterior glenoid fossa. The point labeled "supraspinatus tendon" represents the most lateral extent of rotator cuff interval, where the transverse ligament component of subscapularis meets the anterior edge of supraspinatus (direct tendon).*

Shoulder MR Atlas

AXIAL T1 MR, RIGHT SHOULDER

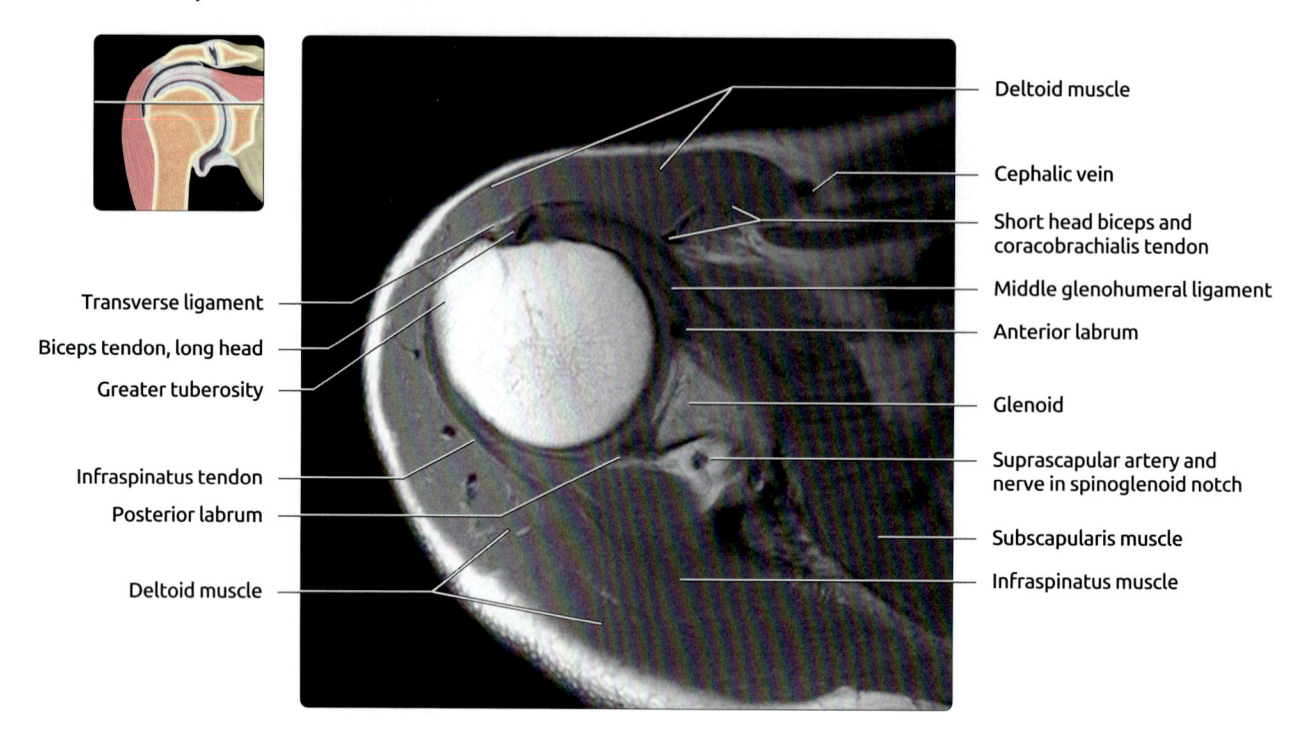

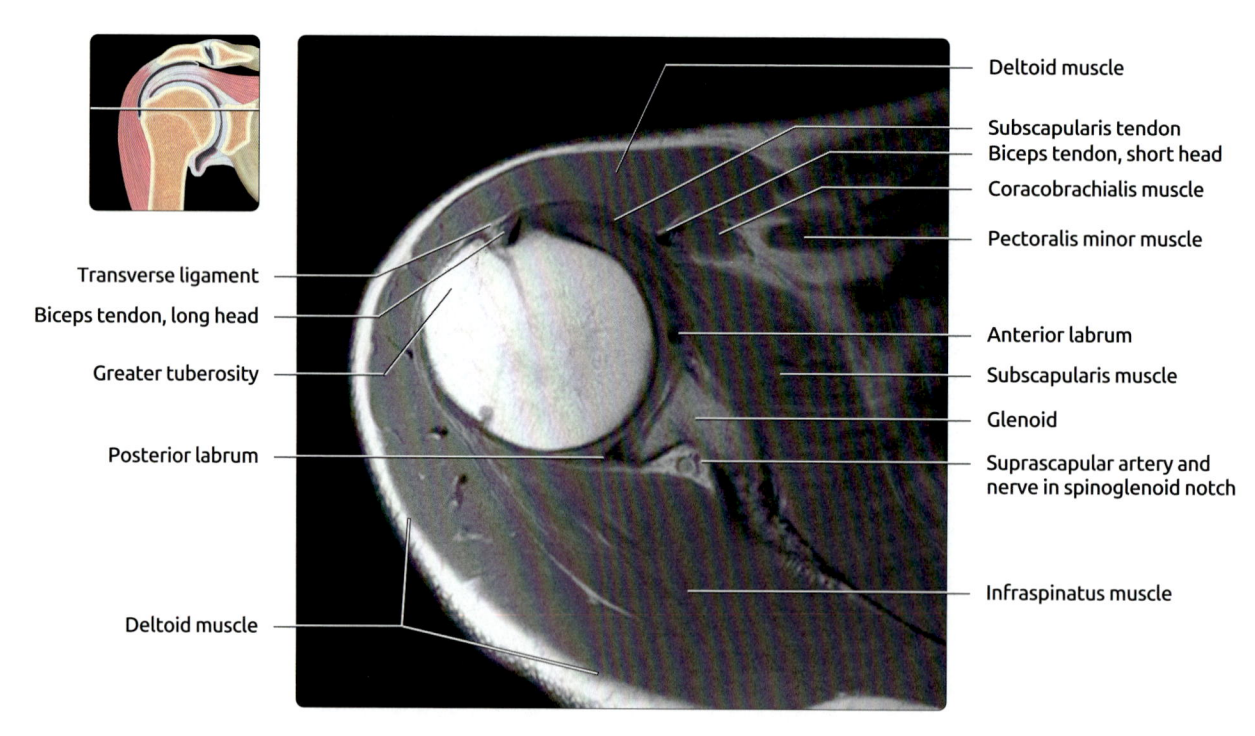

Labels (top image):
- Deltoid muscle
- Cephalic vein
- Short head biceps and coracobrachialis tendon
- Middle glenohumeral ligament
- Anterior labrum
- Glenoid
- Suprascapular artery and nerve in spinoglenoid notch
- Subscapularis muscle
- Infraspinatus muscle
- Transverse ligament
- Biceps tendon, long head
- Greater tuberosity
- Infraspinatus tendon
- Posterior labrum
- Deltoid muscle

Labels (bottom image):
- Deltoid muscle
- Subscapularis tendon
- Biceps tendon, short head
- Coracobrachialis muscle
- Pectoralis minor muscle
- Anterior labrum
- Subscapularis muscle
- Glenoid
- Suprascapular artery and nerve in spinoglenoid notch
- Infraspinatus muscle
- Transverse ligament
- Biceps tendon, long head
- Greater tuberosity
- Posterior labrum
- Deltoid muscle

(Top) *The middle glenohumeral ligament is seen as a dark band near the anterior labrum. This extends from the anterior glenoid to the lower part of the lesser tuberosity.* **(Bottom)** *The glenoid labrum is seen as low signal triangles (sometimes rounded) at the anterior and posterior rim of the glenoid.*

Shoulder MR Atlas

AXIAL T1 MR, LEFT SHOULDER

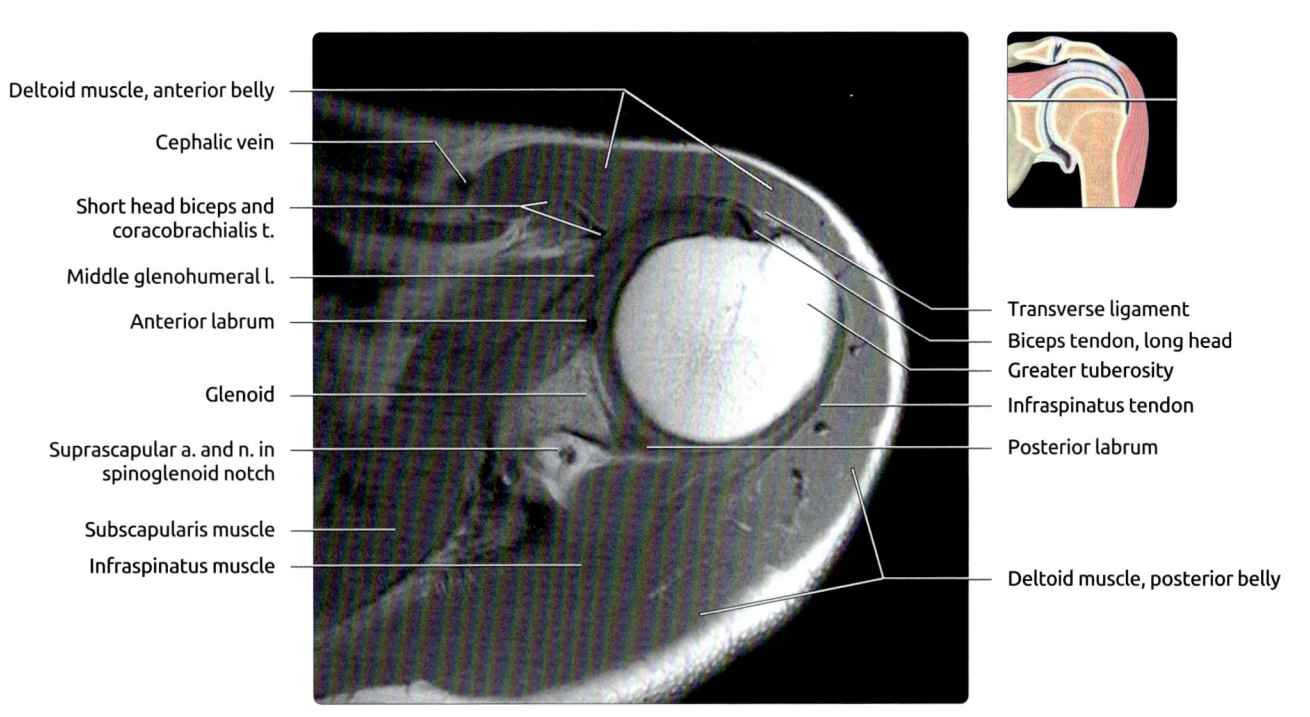

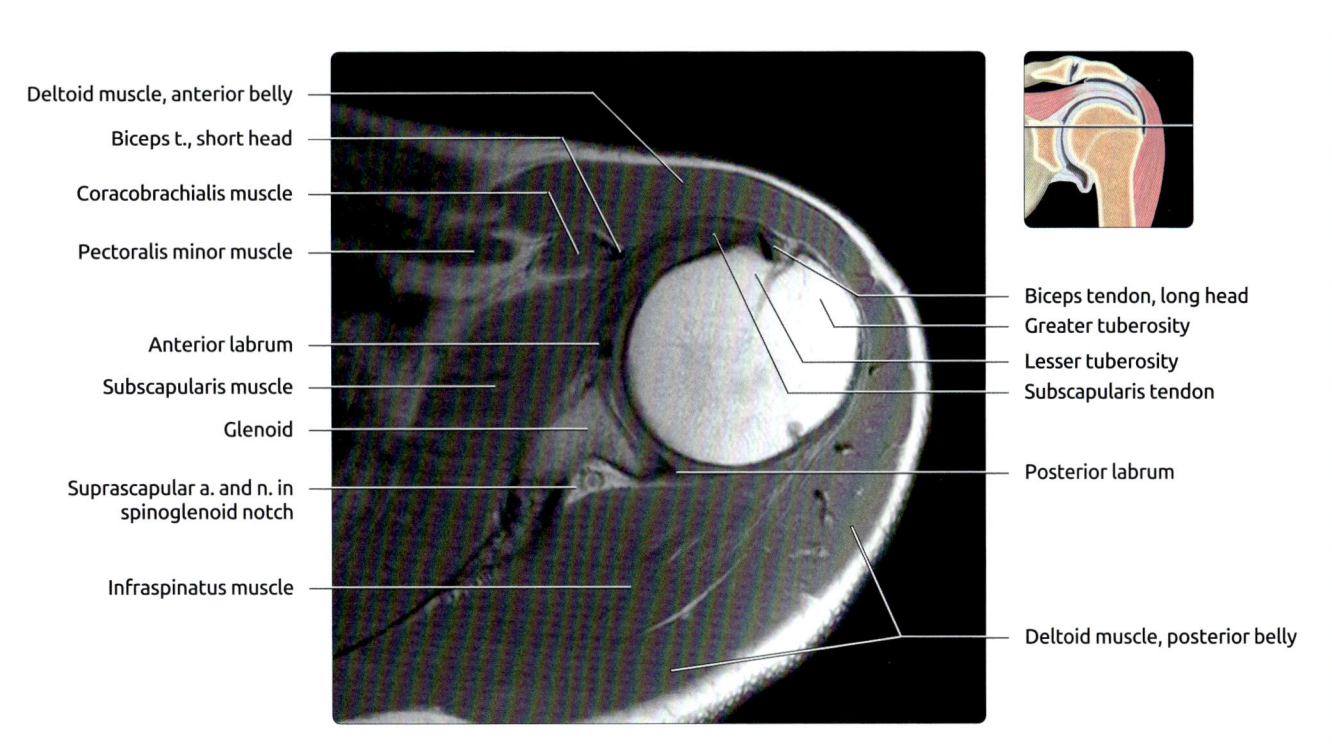

Top image labels:
- Deltoid muscle, anterior belly
- Cephalic vein
- Short head biceps and coracobrachialis t.
- Middle glenohumeral l.
- Anterior labrum
- Glenoid
- Suprascapular a. and n. in spinoglenoid notch
- Subscapularis muscle
- Infraspinatus muscle
- Transverse ligament
- Biceps tendon, long head
- Greater tuberosity
- Infraspinatus tendon
- Posterior labrum
- Deltoid muscle, posterior belly

Bottom image labels:
- Deltoid muscle, anterior belly
- Biceps t., short head
- Coracobrachialis muscle
- Pectoralis minor muscle
- Anterior labrum
- Subscapularis muscle
- Glenoid
- Suprascapular a. and n. in spinoglenoid notch
- Infraspinatus muscle
- Biceps tendon, long head
- Greater tuberosity
- Lesser tuberosity
- Subscapularis tendon
- Posterior labrum
- Deltoid muscle, posterior belly

(Top) The middle glenohumeral ligament is seen as a dark band near the anterior labrum. This extends from the anterior glenoid to the lower part of the lesser tuberosity. **(Bottom)** The glenoid labrum is seen as low signal triangles (occasionally rounded) at the anterior and posterior rim of the glenoid.

Shoulder MR Atlas

AXIAL T1 MR, RIGHT SHOULDER

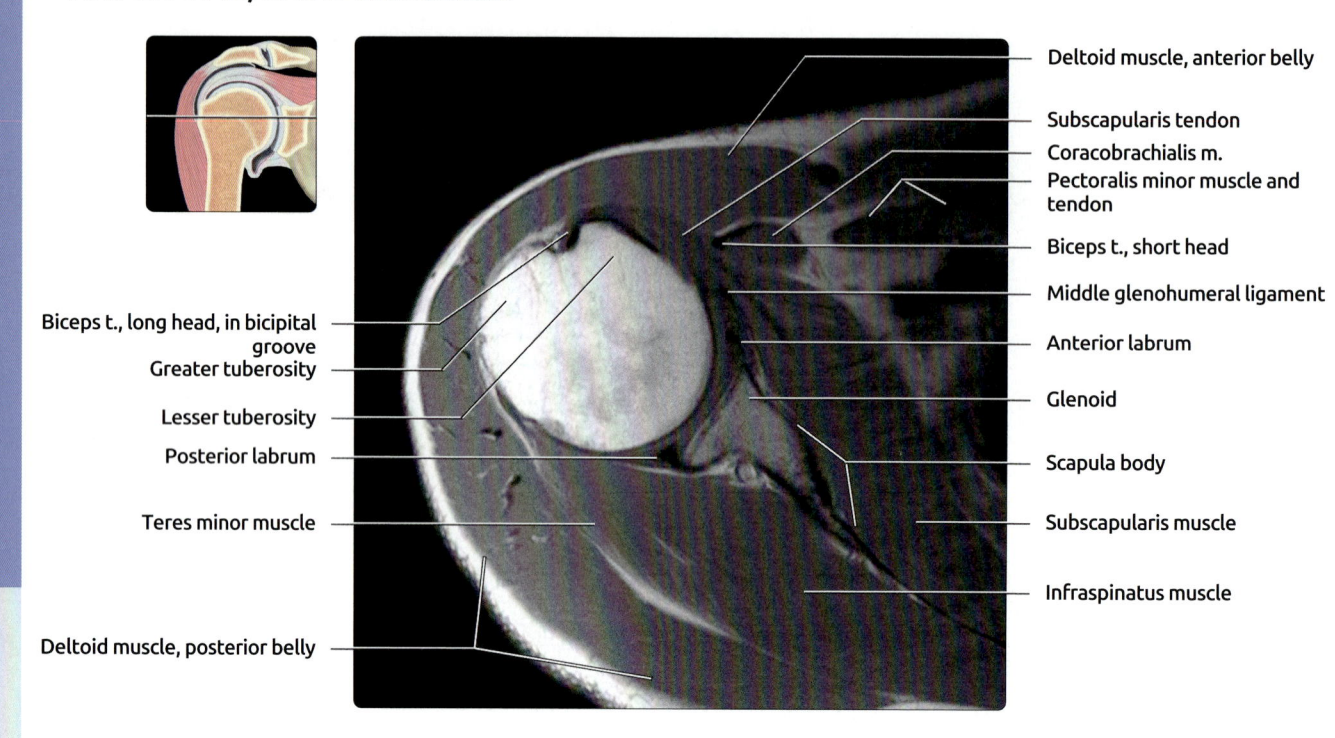

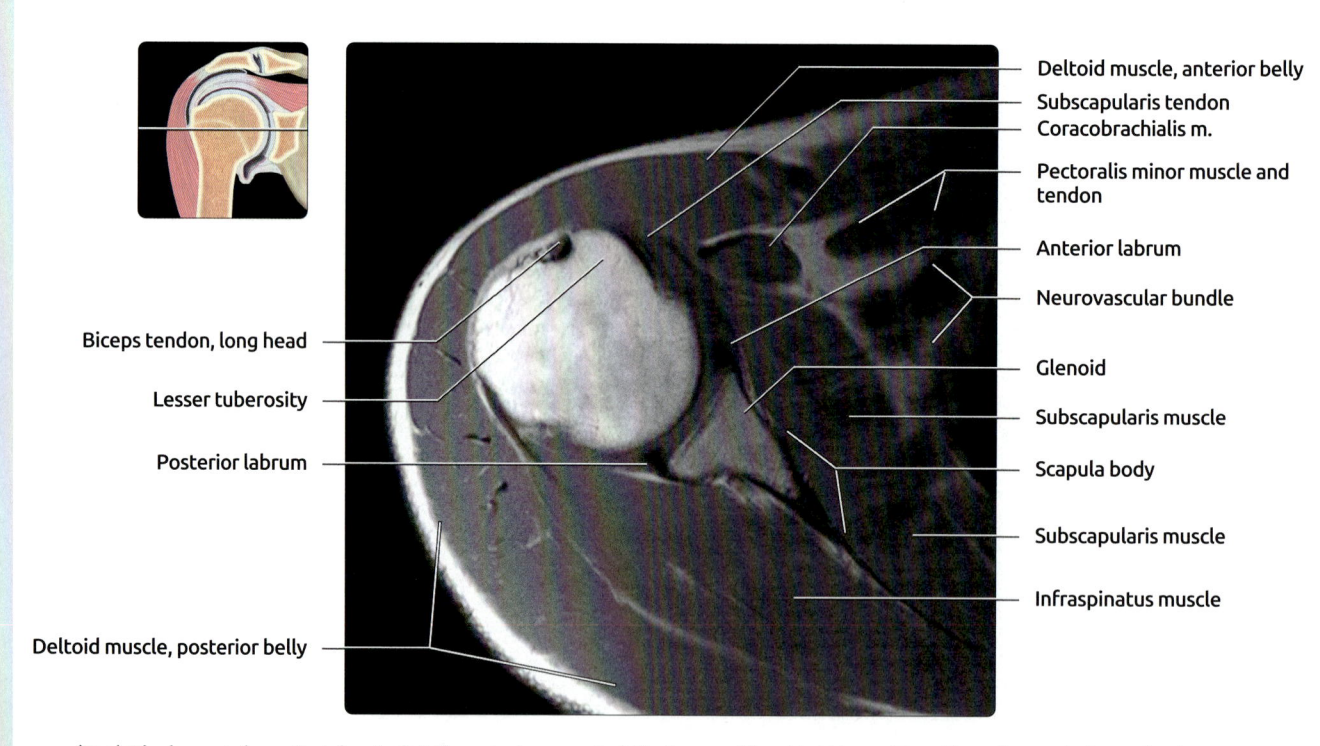

Top image labels:
- Deltoid muscle, anterior belly
- Subscapularis tendon
- Coracobrachialis m.
- Pectoralis minor muscle and tendon
- Biceps t., short head
- Middle glenohumeral ligament
- Anterior labrum
- Glenoid
- Scapula body
- Subscapularis muscle
- Infraspinatus muscle
- Biceps t., long head, in bicipital groove
- Greater tuberosity
- Lesser tuberosity
- Posterior labrum
- Teres minor muscle
- Deltoid muscle, posterior belly

Bottom image labels:
- Deltoid muscle, anterior belly
- Subscapularis tendon
- Coracobrachialis m.
- Pectoralis minor muscle and tendon
- Anterior labrum
- Neurovascular bundle
- Glenoid
- Subscapularis muscle
- Scapula body
- Subscapularis muscle
- Infraspinatus muscle
- Biceps tendon, long head
- Lesser tuberosity
- Posterior labrum
- Deltoid muscle, posterior belly

(Top) *The lesser tuberosity is located at the anterior aspect of the humeral head in this position. The subscapularis tendon is seen inserting on the lesser tuberosity. The long head of the biceps tendon is within the bicipital groove.* **(Bottom)** *The neurovascular bundle lies deep to the pectoralis minor muscle. The subclavian artery becomes the axillary artery when it extends beyond the 1st rib below the clavicle.*

Shoulder MR Atlas

AXIAL T1 MR, LEFT SHOULDER

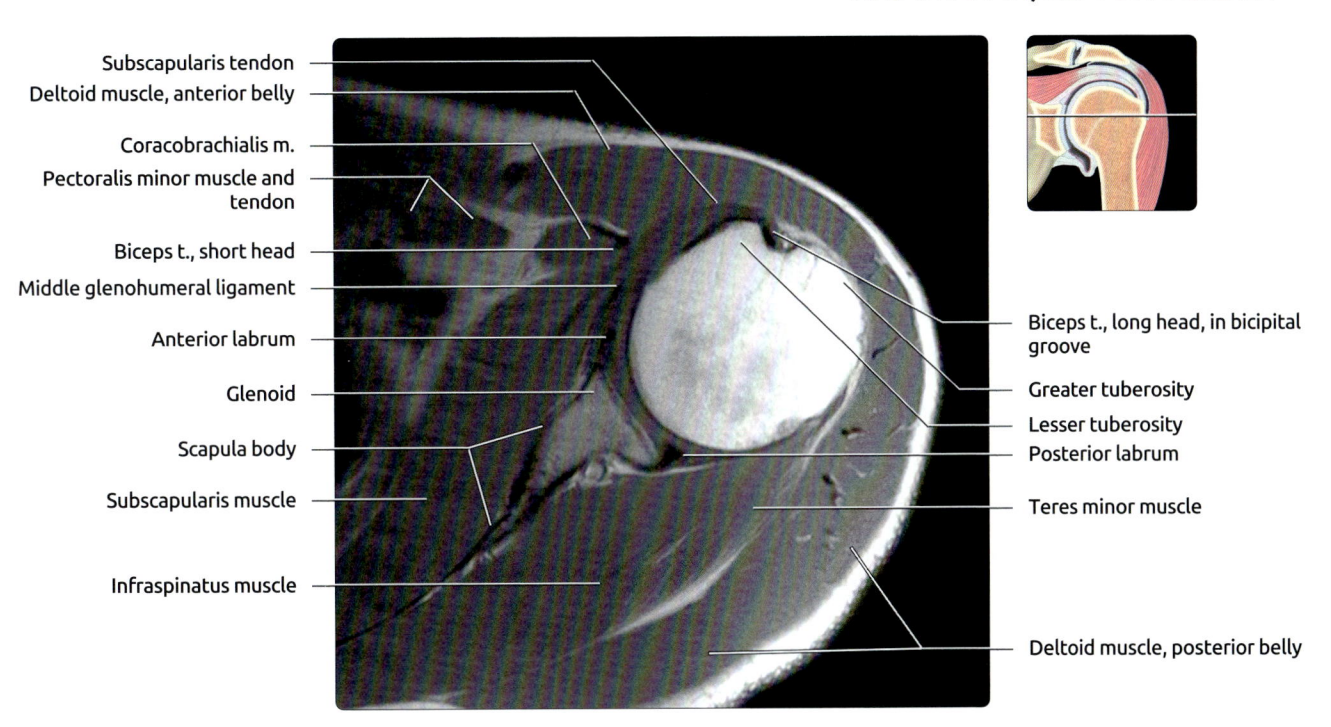

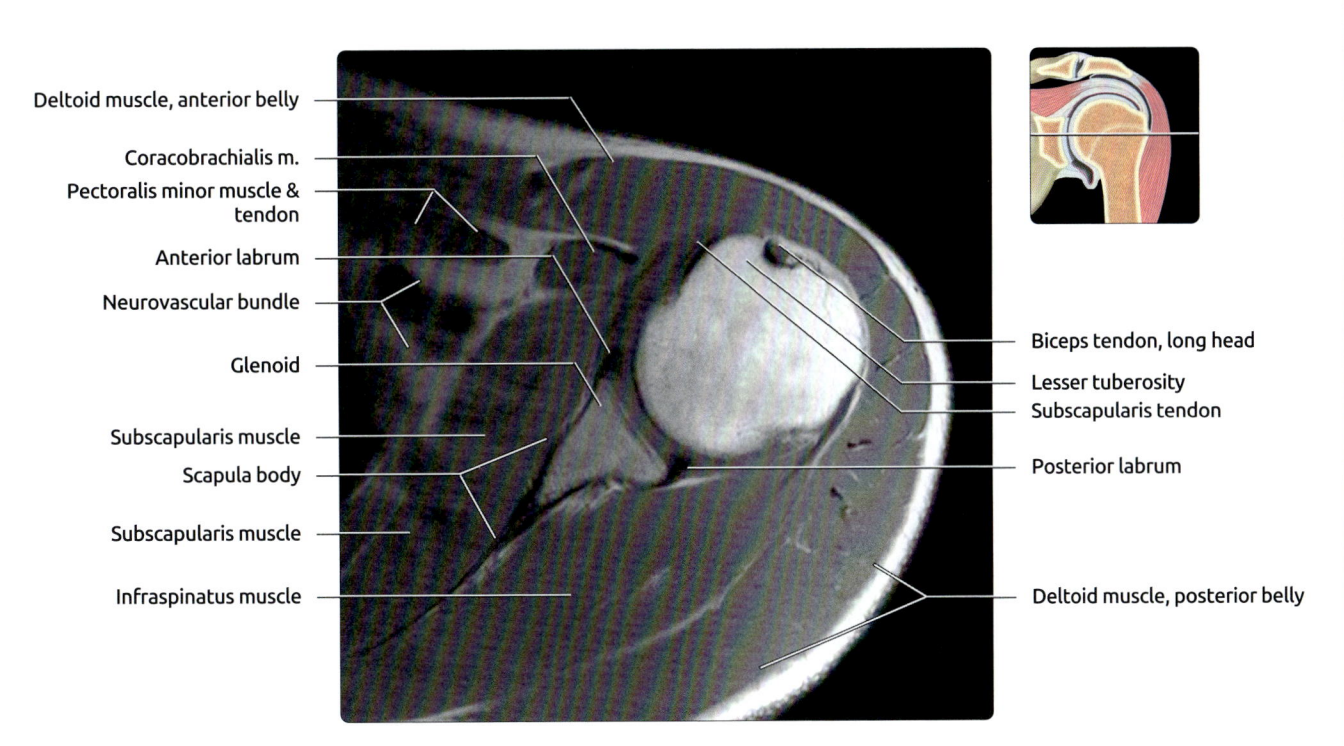

Labels (top image):
- Subscapularis tendon
- Deltoid muscle, anterior belly
- Coracobrachialis m.
- Pectoralis minor muscle and tendon
- Biceps t., short head
- Middle glenohumeral ligament
- Anterior labrum
- Glenoid
- Scapula body
- Subscapularis muscle
- Infraspinatus muscle
- Biceps t., long head, in bicipital groove
- Greater tuberosity
- Lesser tuberosity
- Posterior labrum
- Teres minor muscle
- Deltoid muscle, posterior belly

Labels (bottom image):
- Deltoid muscle, anterior belly
- Coracobrachialis m.
- Pectoralis minor muscle & tendon
- Anterior labrum
- Neurovascular bundle
- Glenoid
- Subscapularis muscle
- Scapula body
- Subscapularis muscle
- Infraspinatus muscle
- Biceps tendon, long head
- Lesser tuberosity
- Subscapularis tendon
- Posterior labrum
- Deltoid muscle, posterior belly

(Top) *The lesser tuberosity is located at the anterior aspect of the humeral head in this position. The subscapularis tendon is seen inserting on the lesser tuberosity. The long head of the biceps tendon is within the bicipital groove.* (Bottom) *The neurovascular bundle lies deep to the pectoralis minor muscle. The subclavian artery becomes the axillary artery when it extends beyond the 1st rib below the clavicle.*

Shoulder MR Atlas

AXIAL T1 MR, RIGHT SHOULDER

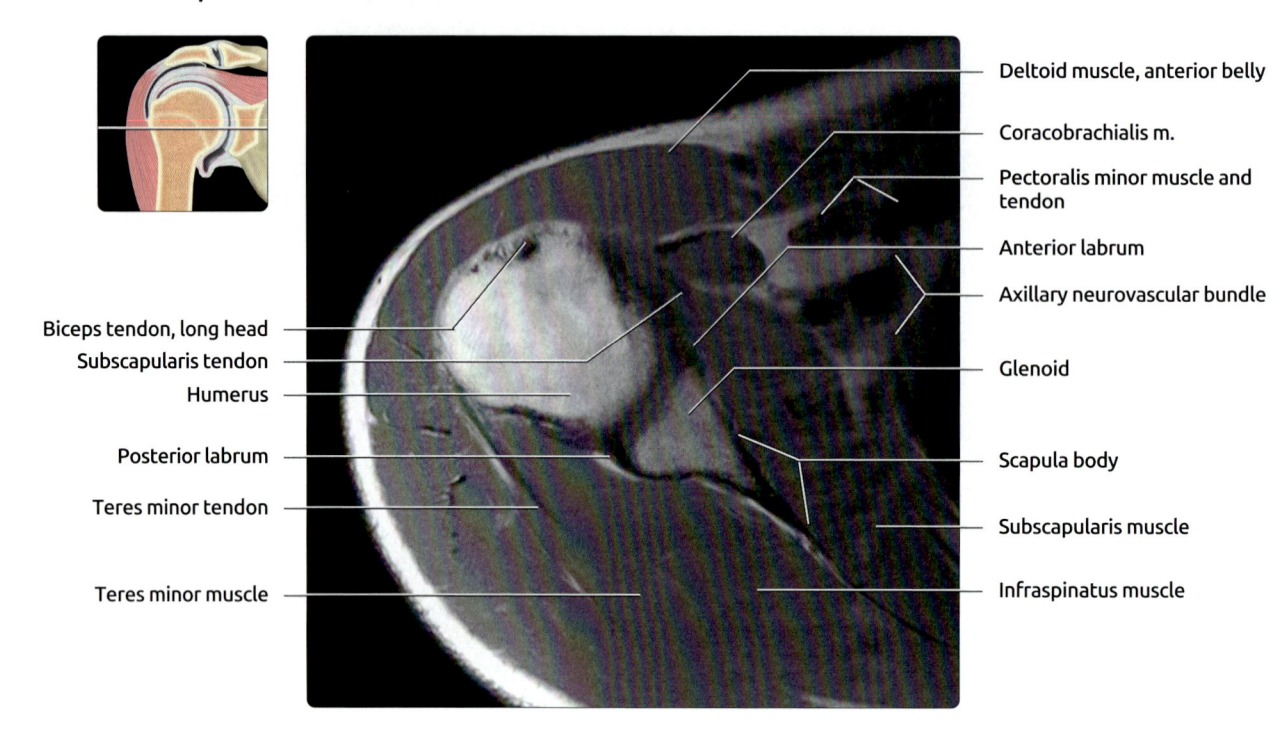

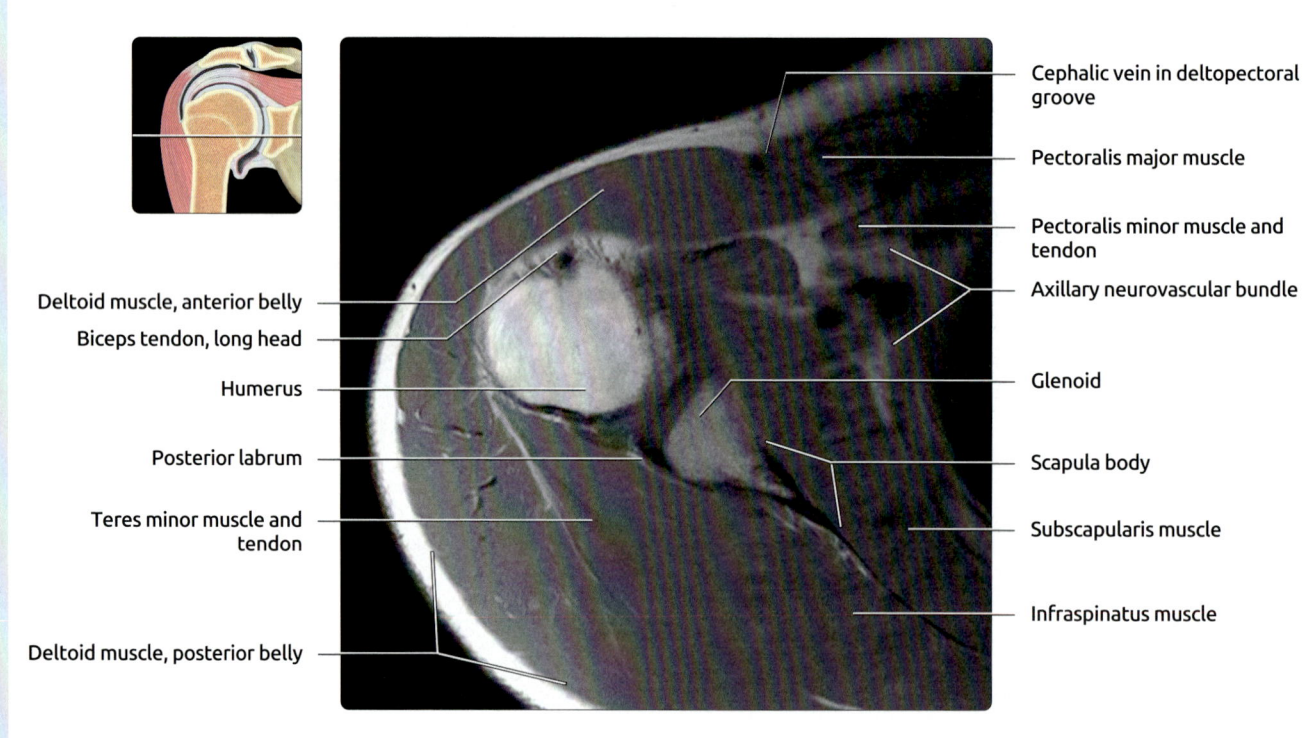

- Deltoid muscle, anterior belly
- Coracobrachialis m.
- Pectoralis minor muscle and tendon
- Anterior labrum
- Axillary neurovascular bundle
- Biceps tendon, long head
- Subscapularis tendon
- Humerus
- Glenoid
- Posterior labrum
- Scapula body
- Teres minor tendon
- Subscapularis muscle
- Teres minor muscle
- Infraspinatus muscle

- Cephalic vein in deltopectoral groove
- Pectoralis major muscle
- Pectoralis minor muscle and tendon
- Axillary neurovascular bundle
- Deltoid muscle, anterior belly
- Biceps tendon, long head
- Humerus
- Glenoid
- Posterior labrum
- Scapula body
- Teres minor muscle and tendon
- Subscapularis muscle
- Infraspinatus muscle
- Deltoid muscle, posterior belly

(Top) The teres minor and infraspinatus muscles are difficult to separate at this level. The teres minor muscle is lying more lateral than what remains of the infraspinatus muscle, lying more medial. **(Bottom)** The cephalic vein is seen anteriorly, lying within the deltopectoral groove.

Shoulder MR Atlas

AXIAL T1 MR, LEFT SHOULDER

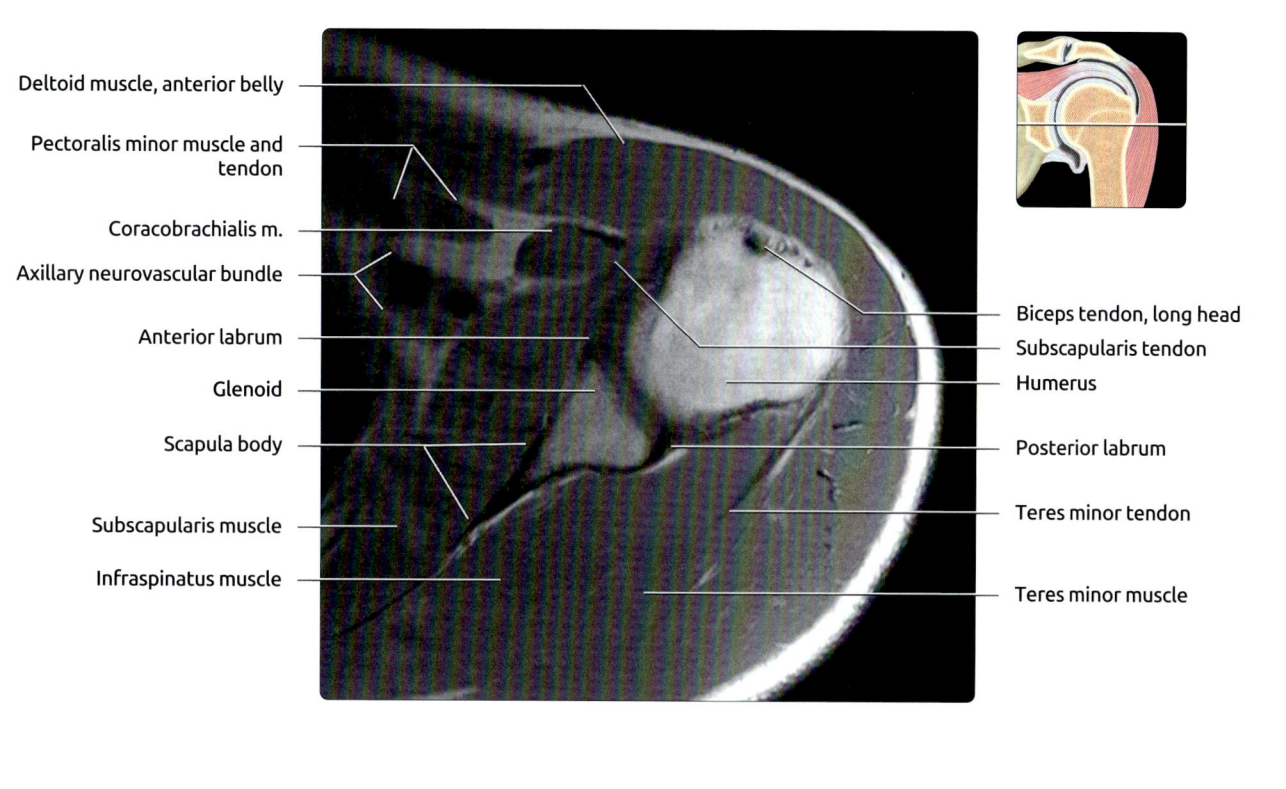

Top image labels (left):
- Deltoid muscle, anterior belly
- Pectoralis minor muscle and tendon
- Coracobrachialis m.
- Axillary neurovascular bundle
- Anterior labrum
- Glenoid
- Scapula body
- Subscapularis muscle
- Infraspinatus muscle

Top image labels (right):
- Biceps tendon, long head
- Subscapularis tendon
- Humerus
- Posterior labrum
- Teres minor tendon
- Teres minor muscle

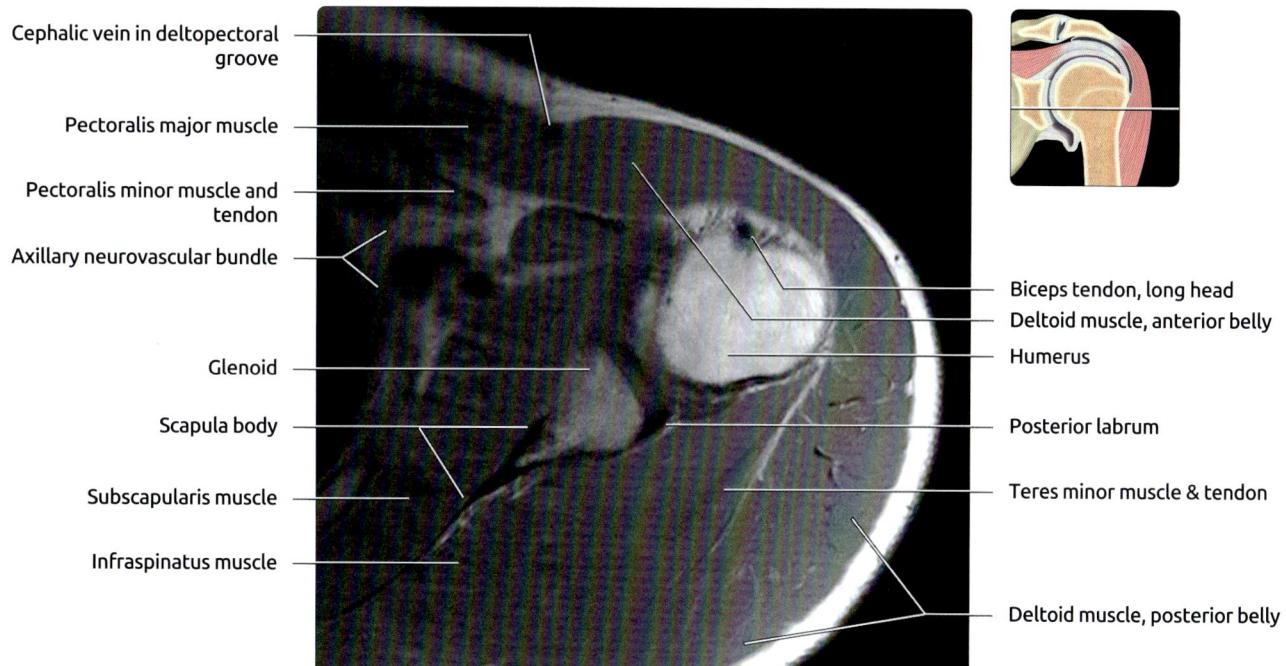

Bottom image labels (left):
- Cephalic vein in deltopectoral groove
- Pectoralis major muscle
- Pectoralis minor muscle and tendon
- Axillary neurovascular bundle
- Glenoid
- Scapula body
- Subscapularis muscle
- Infraspinatus muscle

Bottom image labels (right):
- Biceps tendon, long head
- Deltoid muscle, anterior belly
- Humerus
- Posterior labrum
- Teres minor muscle & tendon
- Deltoid muscle, posterior belly

(**Top**) The teres minor and infraspinatus muscles are difficult to separate at this level. The teres minor muscle is lying more lateral than what remains of the infraspinatus muscle, lying more medial. (**Bottom**) The cephalic vein is seen anteriorly, lying within the deltopectoral groove.

Shoulder MR Atlas

AXIAL T1 MR, RIGHT SHOULDER

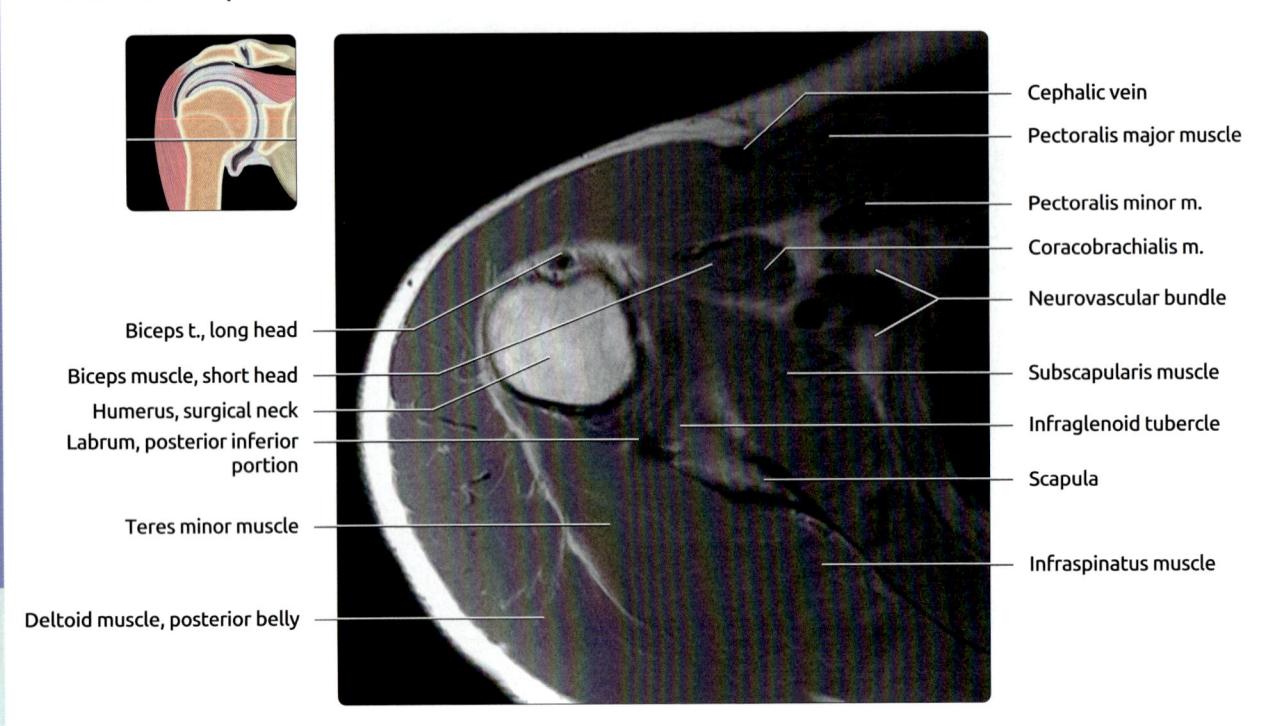

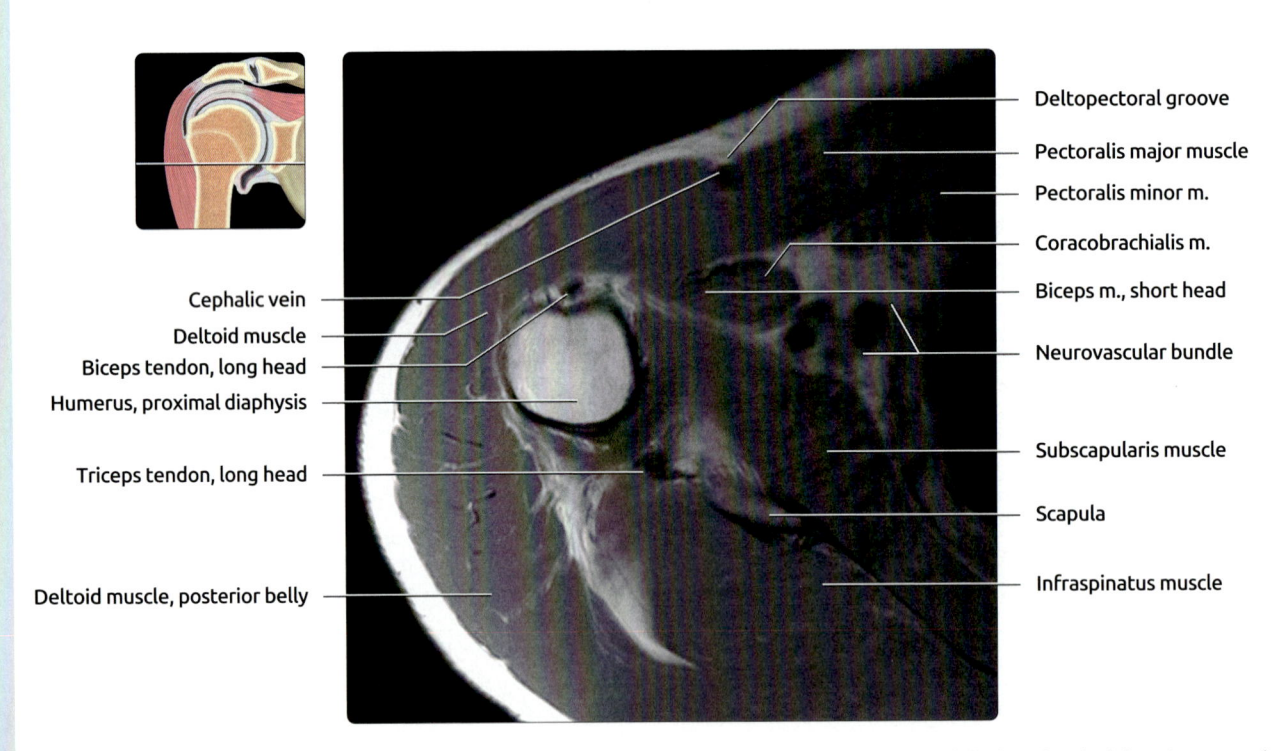

Top image labels (left side):
- Biceps t., long head
- Biceps muscle, short head
- Humerus, surgical neck
- Labrum, posterior inferior portion
- Teres minor muscle
- Deltoid muscle, posterior belly

Top image labels (right side):
- Cephalic vein
- Pectoralis major muscle
- Pectoralis minor m.
- Coracobrachialis m.
- Neurovascular bundle
- Subscapularis muscle
- Infraglenoid tubercle
- Scapula
- Infraspinatus muscle

Bottom image labels (left side):
- Cephalic vein
- Deltoid muscle
- Biceps tendon, long head
- Humerus, proximal diaphysis
- Triceps tendon, long head
- Deltoid muscle, posterior belly

Bottom image labels (right side):
- Deltopectoral groove
- Pectoralis major muscle
- Pectoralis minor m.
- Coracobrachialis m.
- Biceps m., short head
- Neurovascular bundle
- Subscapularis muscle
- Scapula
- Infraspinatus muscle

(Top) *Last image through the inferior glenoid is shown. The infraglenoid tuberosity is the origin of the long head of the triceps muscle.* **(Bottom)** *This image is just below the level of the glenoid. The long head of the triceps tendon is now visible below the infraglenoid tubercle.*

Shoulder MR Atlas

AXIAL T1 MR, LEFT SHOULDER

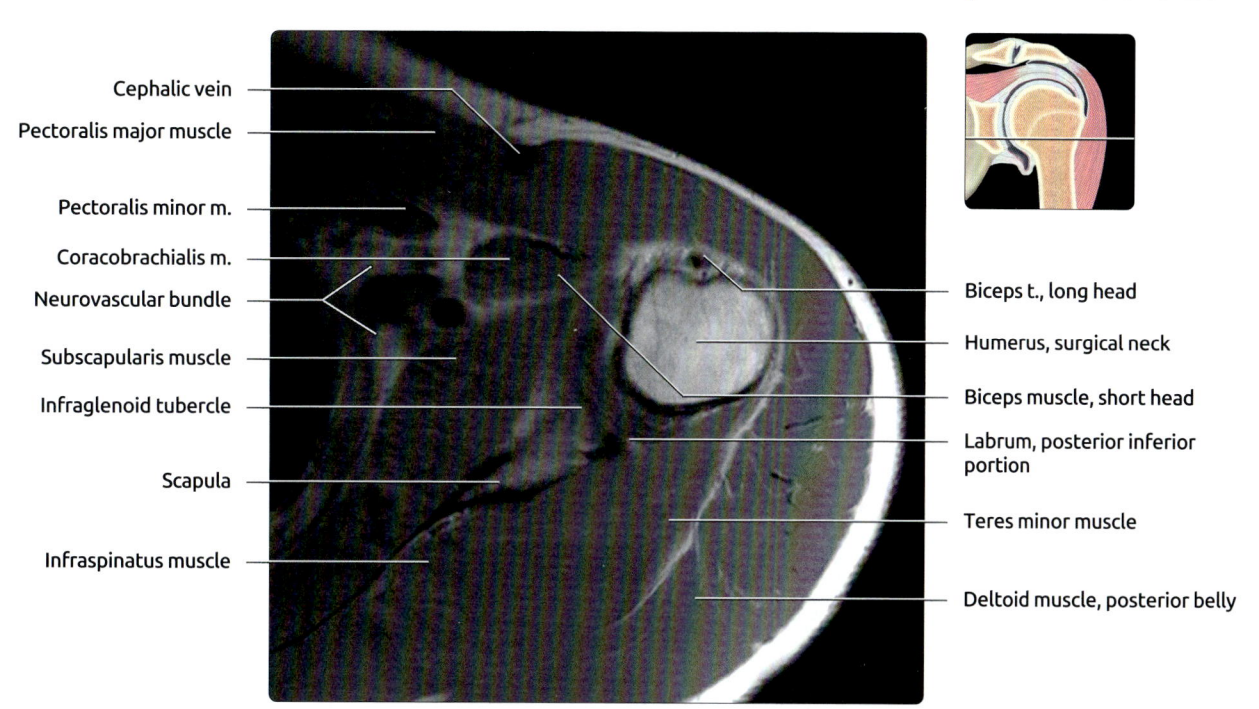

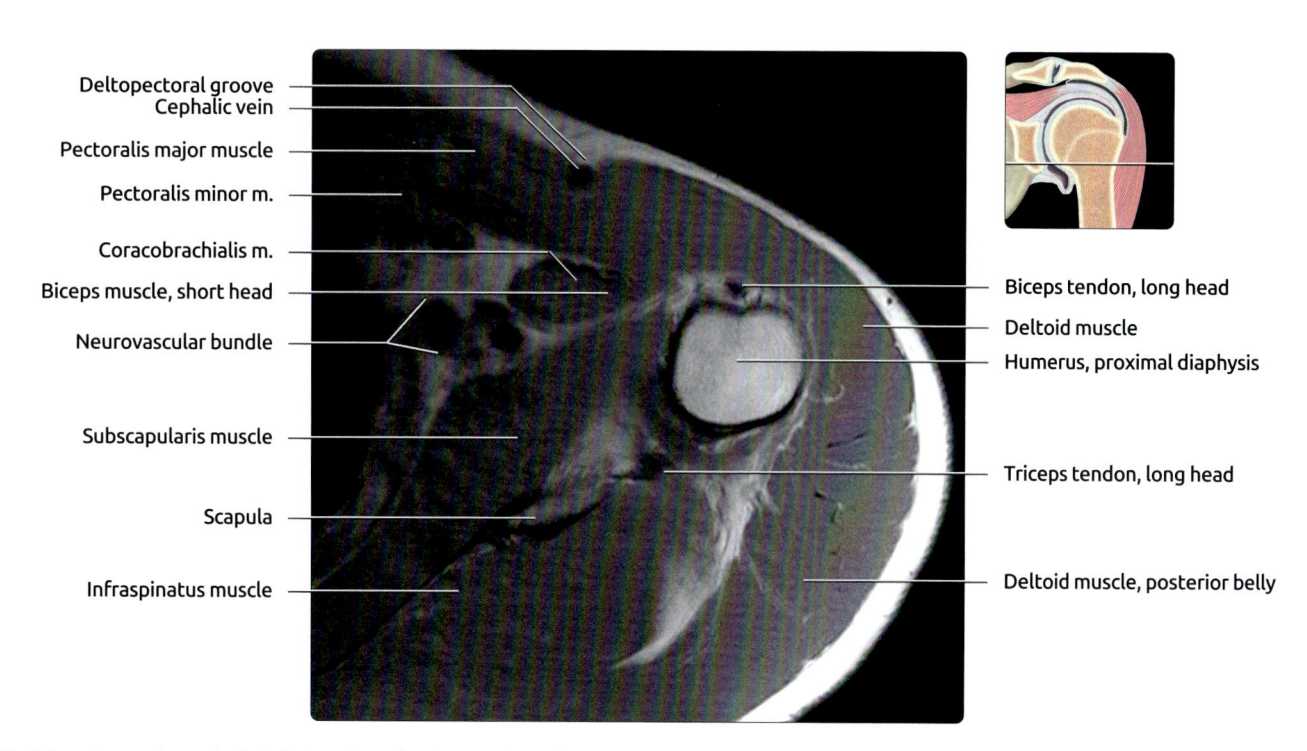

Top labels (left side):
- Cephalic vein
- Pectoralis major muscle
- Pectoralis minor m.
- Coracobrachialis m.
- Neurovascular bundle
- Subscapularis muscle
- Infraglenoid tubercle
- Scapula
- Infraspinatus muscle

Top labels (right side):
- Biceps t., long head
- Humerus, surgical neck
- Biceps muscle, short head
- Labrum, posterior inferior portion
- Teres minor muscle
- Deltoid muscle, posterior belly

Bottom labels (left side):
- Deltopectoral groove
- Cephalic vein
- Pectoralis major muscle
- Pectoralis minor m.
- Coracobrachialis m.
- Biceps muscle, short head
- Neurovascular bundle
- Subscapularis muscle
- Scapula
- Infraspinatus muscle

Bottom labels (right side):
- Biceps tendon, long head
- Deltoid muscle
- Humerus, proximal diaphysis
- Triceps tendon, long head
- Deltoid muscle, posterior belly

(*Top*) *Last image through the inferior glenoid is shown. The infraglenoid tuberosity is the origin of the long head of the triceps muscle.*
(*Bottom*) *This image is just below the level of the glenoid. The long head of the triceps tendon is now visible below the infraglenoid tubercle.*

Shoulder MR Atlas

AXIAL T1 MR, RIGHT SHOULDER

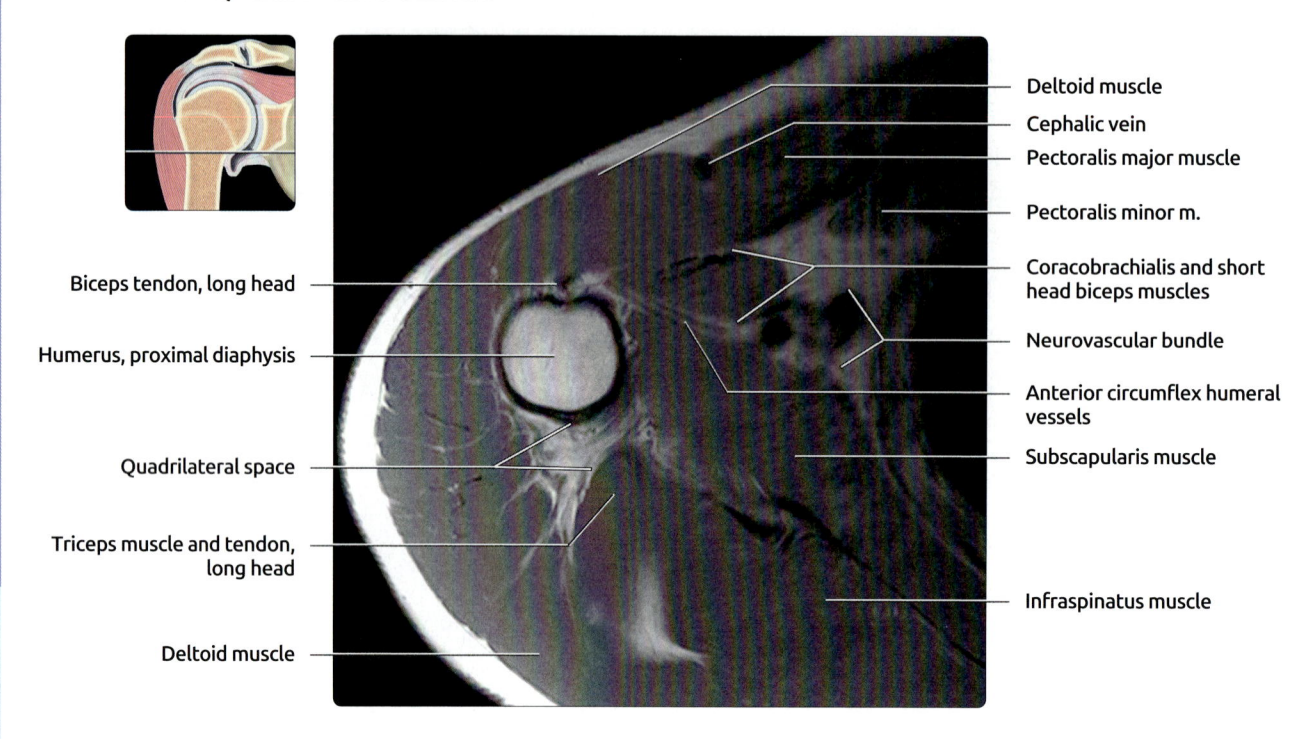

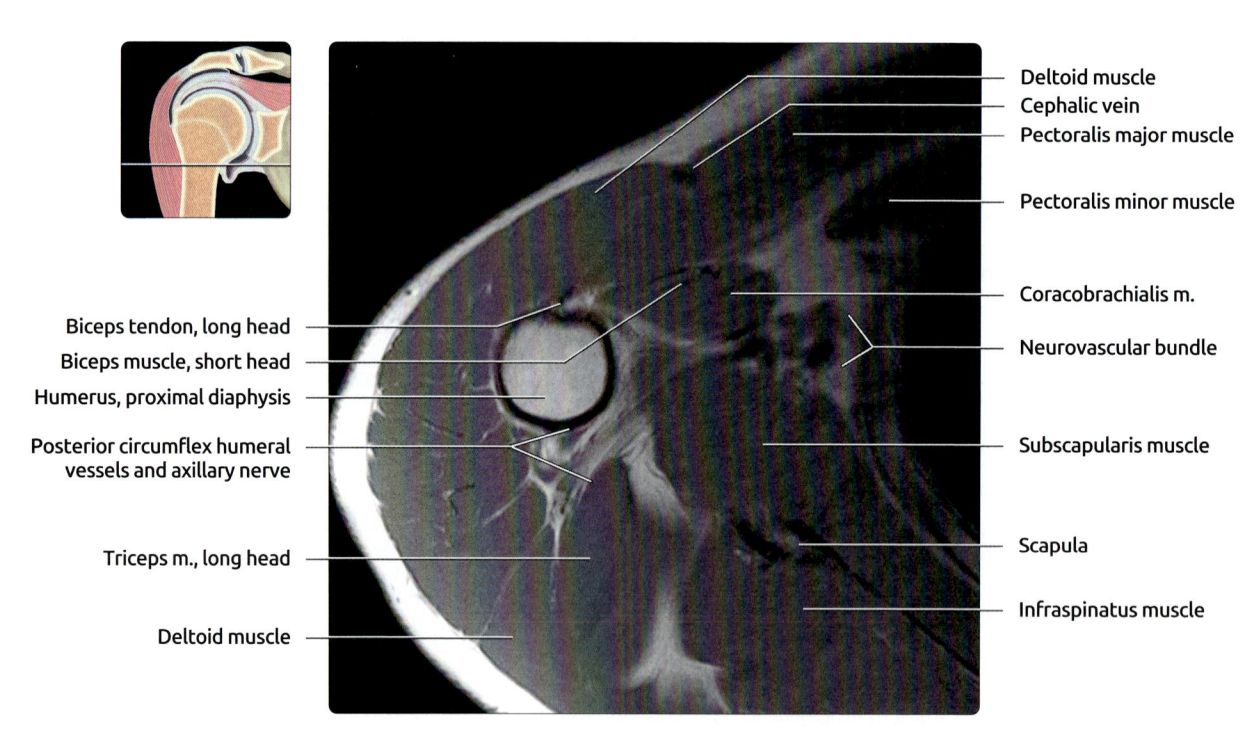

Labels (top image):
- Biceps tendon, long head
- Humerus, proximal diaphysis
- Quadrilateral space
- Triceps muscle and tendon, long head
- Deltoid muscle
- Deltoid muscle
- Cephalic vein
- Pectoralis major muscle
- Pectoralis minor m.
- Coracobrachialis and short head biceps muscles
- Neurovascular bundle
- Anterior circumflex humeral vessels
- Subscapularis muscle
- Infraspinatus muscle

Labels (bottom image):
- Biceps tendon, long head
- Biceps muscle, short head
- Humerus, proximal diaphysis
- Posterior circumflex humeral vessels and axillary nerve
- Triceps m., long head
- Deltoid muscle
- Deltoid muscle
- Cephalic vein
- Pectoralis major muscle
- Pectoralis minor muscle
- Coracobrachialis m.
- Neurovascular bundle
- Subscapularis muscle
- Scapula
- Infraspinatus muscle

(Top) The posterior circumflex humeral vessels and axillary nerve traverse the quadrilateral space. This space is formed by the subscapularis and teres minor muscles superiorly, the teres major inferiorly, the long head of the triceps medially, and the surgical neck of the humerus laterally. **(Bottom)** The short head of the biceps muscle and the coracobrachialis muscle can be difficult to distinguish as separate structures in the anterior shoulder. The coracobrachialis muscle originates from the coracoid process more laterally than the short head of the biceps muscle. The coracobrachialis muscle then swings posterior to the short head of the biceps muscle as it enters the upper arm.

Shoulder MR Atlas

AXIAL T1 MR, LEFT SHOULDER

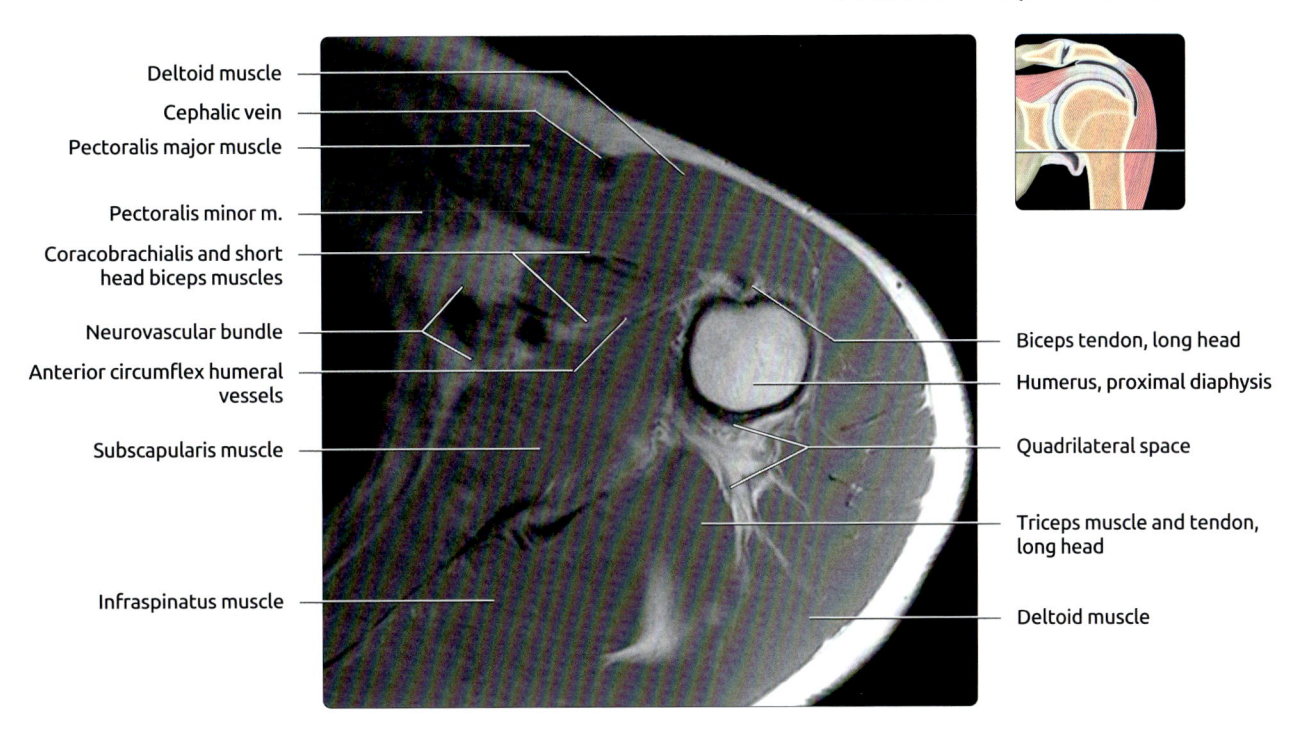

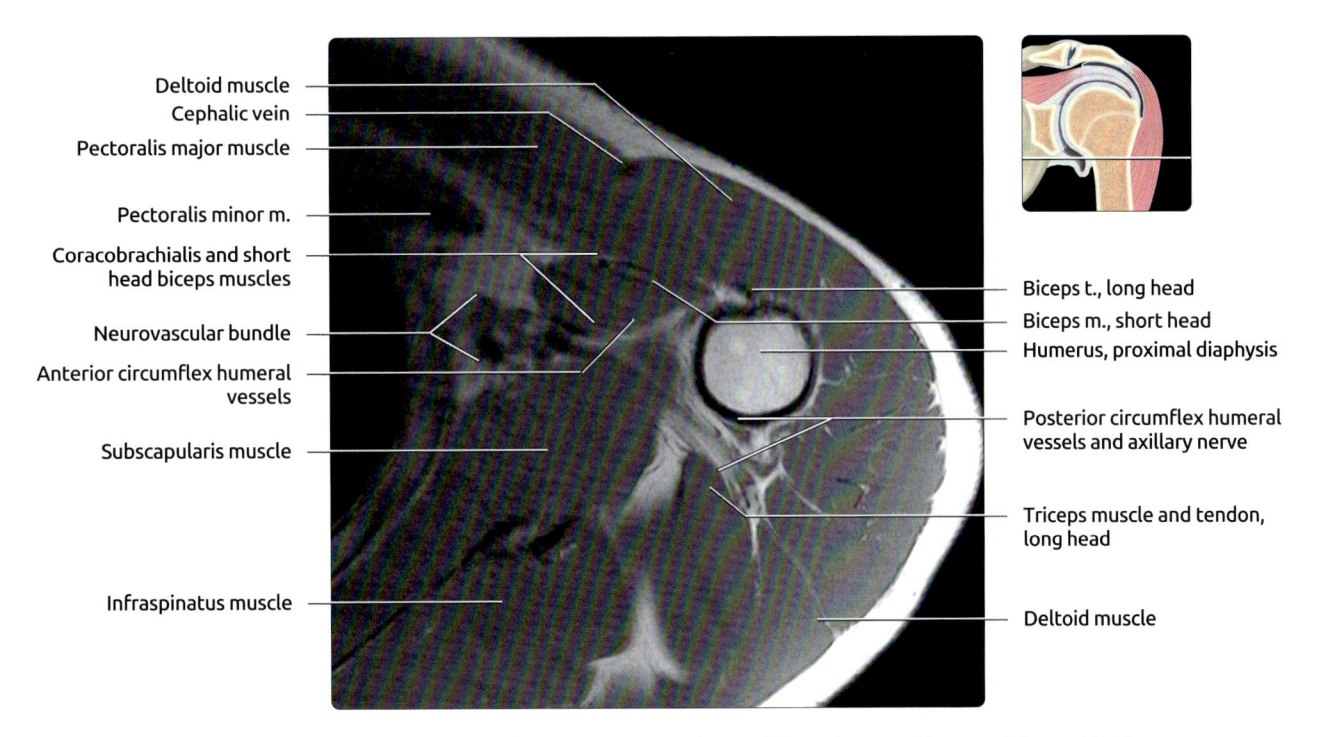

(Top) Labels:
- Deltoid muscle
- Cephalic vein
- Pectoralis major muscle
- Pectoralis minor m.
- Coracobrachialis and short head biceps muscles
- Neurovascular bundle
- Anterior circumflex humeral vessels
- Subscapularis muscle
- Infraspinatus muscle
- Biceps tendon, long head
- Humerus, proximal diaphysis
- Quadrilateral space
- Triceps muscle and tendon, long head
- Deltoid muscle

(Bottom) Labels:
- Deltoid muscle
- Cephalic vein
- Pectoralis major muscle
- Pectoralis minor m.
- Coracobrachialis and short head biceps muscles
- Neurovascular bundle
- Anterior circumflex humeral vessels
- Subscapularis muscle
- Infraspinatus muscle
- Biceps t., long head
- Biceps m., short head
- Humerus, proximal diaphysis
- Posterior circumflex humeral vessels and axillary nerve
- Triceps muscle and tendon, long head
- Deltoid muscle

(Top) The posterior circumflex humeral vessels and axillary nerve traverse the quadrilateral space. This space is formed by the subscapularis and teres minor muscles superiorly, the teres major inferiorly, the long head of the triceps medially, and the surgical neck of the humerus laterally. **(Bottom)** The short head of the biceps muscle and the coracobrachialis muscle can be difficult to distinguish as separate structures in the anterior shoulder. The coracobrachialis muscle originates from the coracoid process more laterally than the short head of the biceps muscle. The coracobrachialis muscle then swings posterior to the short head of the biceps muscle as it enters the upper arm.

Shoulder MR Atlas

AXIAL T1 MR, RIGHT SHOULDER

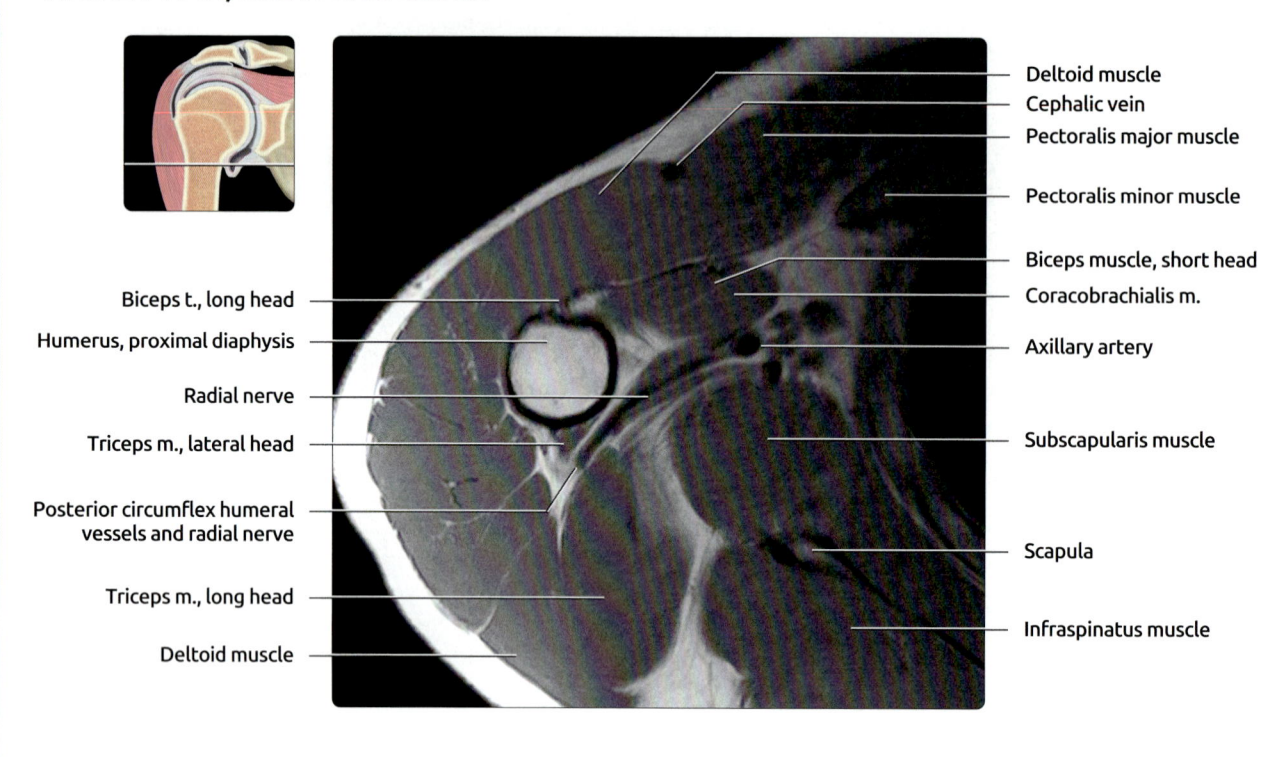

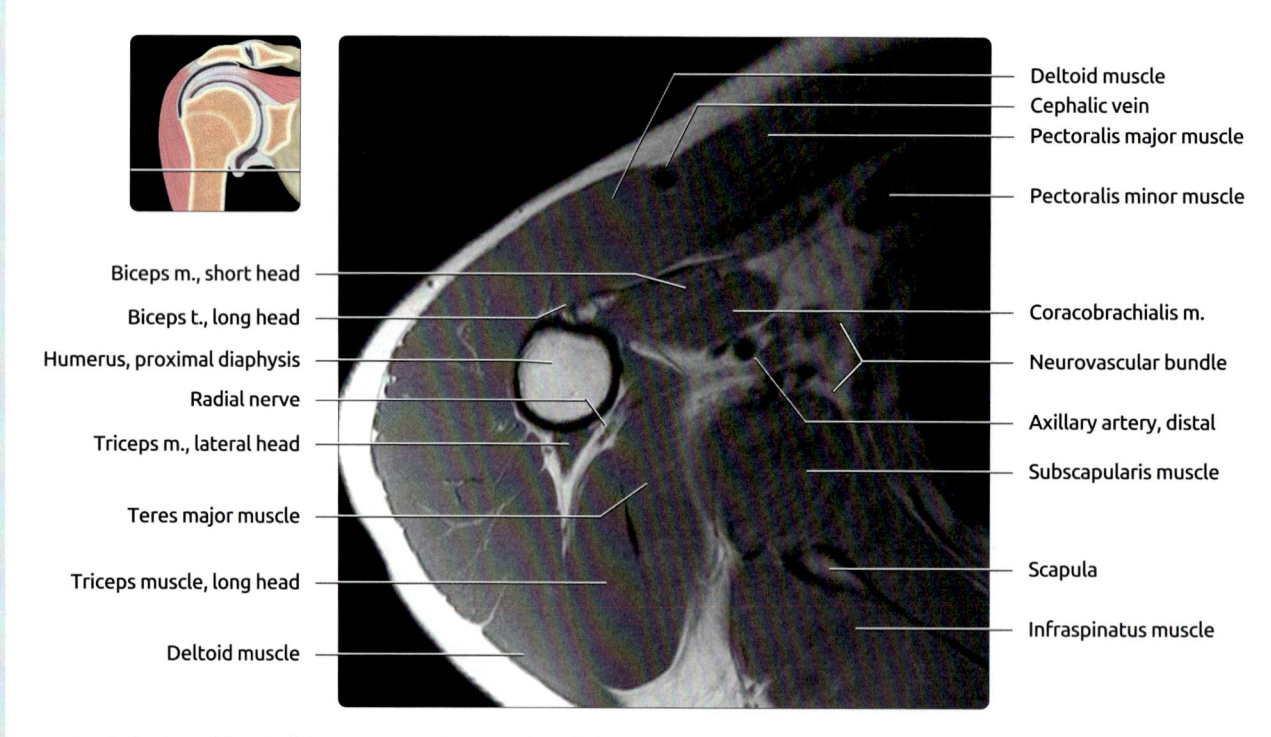

Top image labels (left):
- Biceps t., long head
- Humerus, proximal diaphysis
- Radial nerve
- Triceps m., lateral head
- Posterior circumflex humeral vessels and radial nerve
- Triceps m., long head
- Deltoid muscle

Top image labels (right):
- Deltoid muscle
- Cephalic vein
- Pectoralis major muscle
- Pectoralis minor muscle
- Biceps muscle, short head
- Coracobrachialis m.
- Axillary artery
- Subscapularis muscle
- Scapula
- Infraspinatus muscle

Bottom image labels (left):
- Biceps m., short head
- Biceps t., long head
- Humerus, proximal diaphysis
- Radial nerve
- Triceps m., lateral head
- Teres major muscle
- Triceps muscle, long head
- Deltoid muscle

Bottom image labels (right):
- Deltoid muscle
- Cephalic vein
- Pectoralis major muscle
- Pectoralis minor muscle
- Coracobrachialis m.
- Neurovascular bundle
- Axillary artery, distal
- Subscapularis muscle
- Scapula
- Infraspinatus muscle

(Top) *The lateral head of the triceps muscle arises directly from the posterior surface of the humeral shaft.* **(Bottom)** *The teres major muscle arises from the inferior angle of the scapula and inserts below the lesser tuberosity on the anteromedial humeral shaft.*

Shoulder MR Atlas

AXIAL T1 MR, LEFT SHOULDER

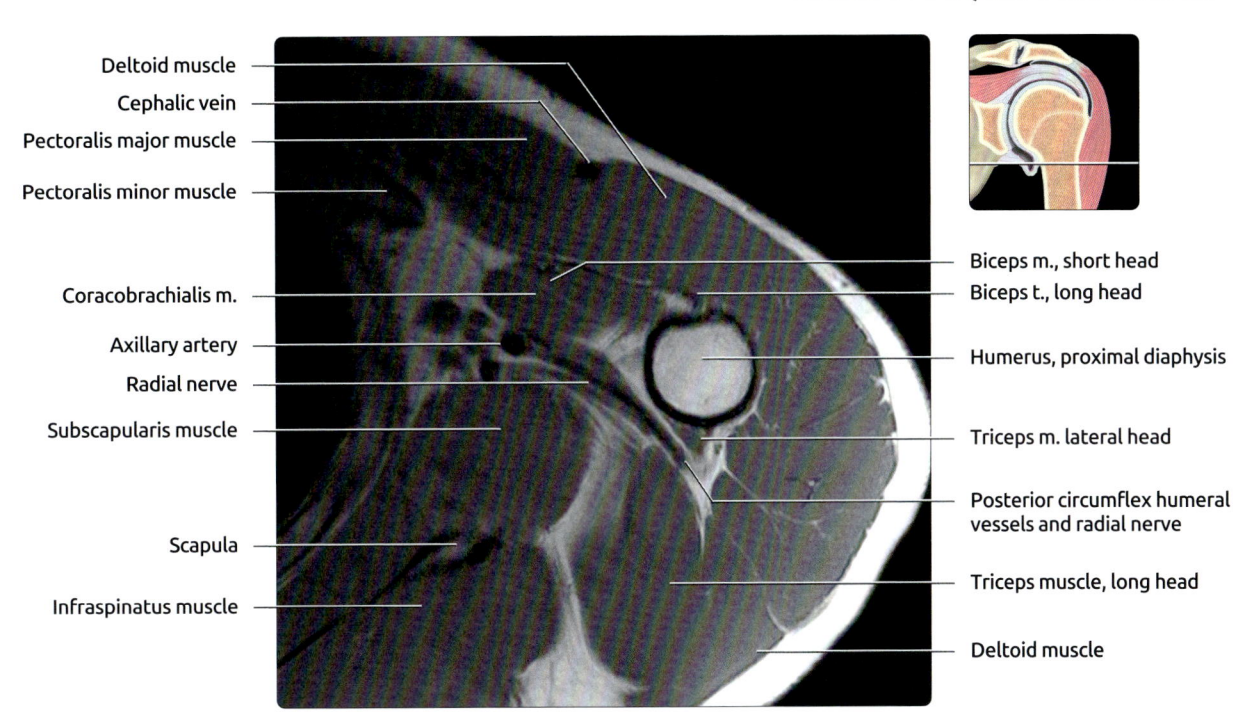

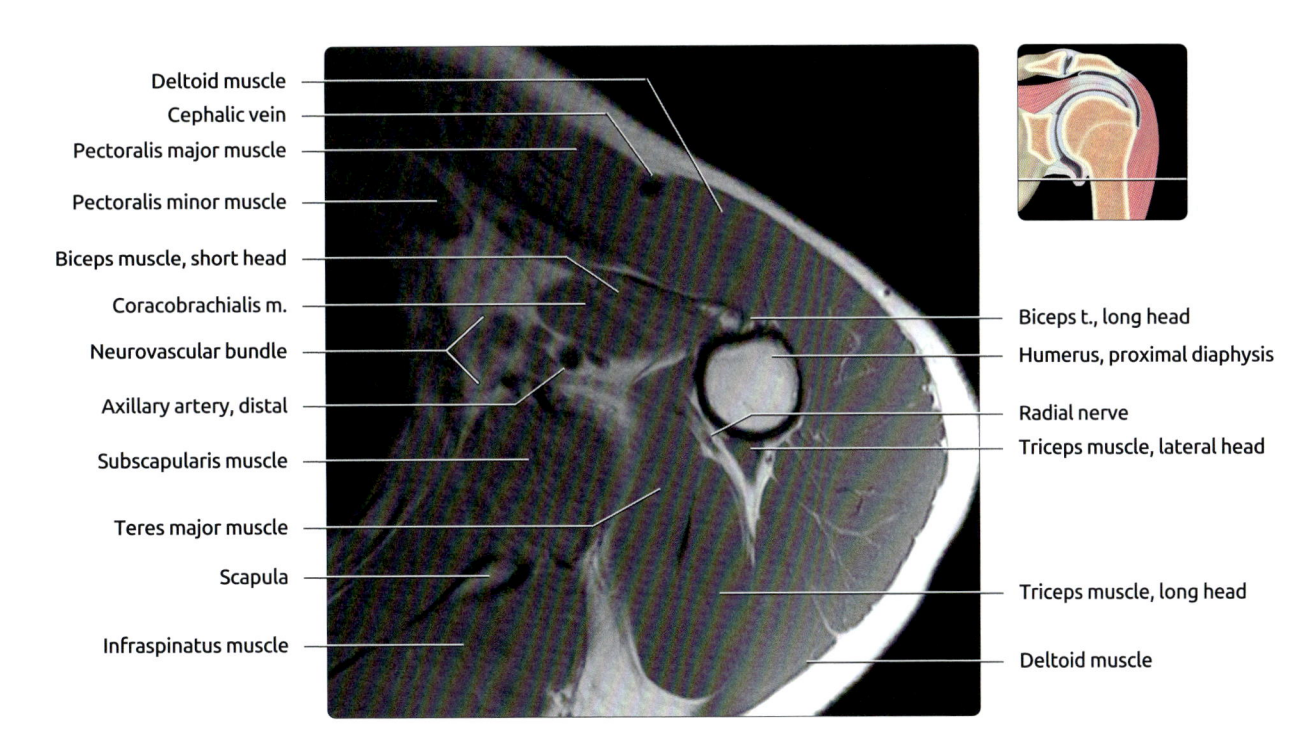

Top image labels (left): Deltoid muscle; Cephalic vein; Pectoralis major muscle; Pectoralis minor muscle; Coracobrachialis m.; Axillary artery; Radial nerve; Subscapularis muscle; Scapula; Infraspinatus muscle

Top image labels (right): Biceps m., short head; Biceps t., long head; Humerus, proximal diaphysis; Triceps m. lateral head; Posterior circumflex humeral vessels and radial nerve; Triceps muscle, long head; Deltoid muscle

Bottom image labels (left): Deltoid muscle; Cephalic vein; Pectoralis major muscle; Pectoralis minor muscle; Biceps muscle, short head; Coracobrachialis m.; Neurovascular bundle; Axillary artery, distal; Subscapularis muscle; Teres major muscle; Scapula; Infraspinatus muscle

Bottom image labels (right): Biceps t., long head; Humerus, proximal diaphysis; Radial nerve; Triceps muscle, lateral head; Triceps muscle, long head; Deltoid muscle

(Top) The lateral head of the triceps muscle arises directly from the posterior surface of the humeral shaft. (Bottom) The teres major muscle arises from the inferior angle of the scapula and inserts below the lesser tuberosity on the anteromedial humeral shaft.

Shoulder MR Atlas

AXIAL T1 MR, RIGHT SHOULDER

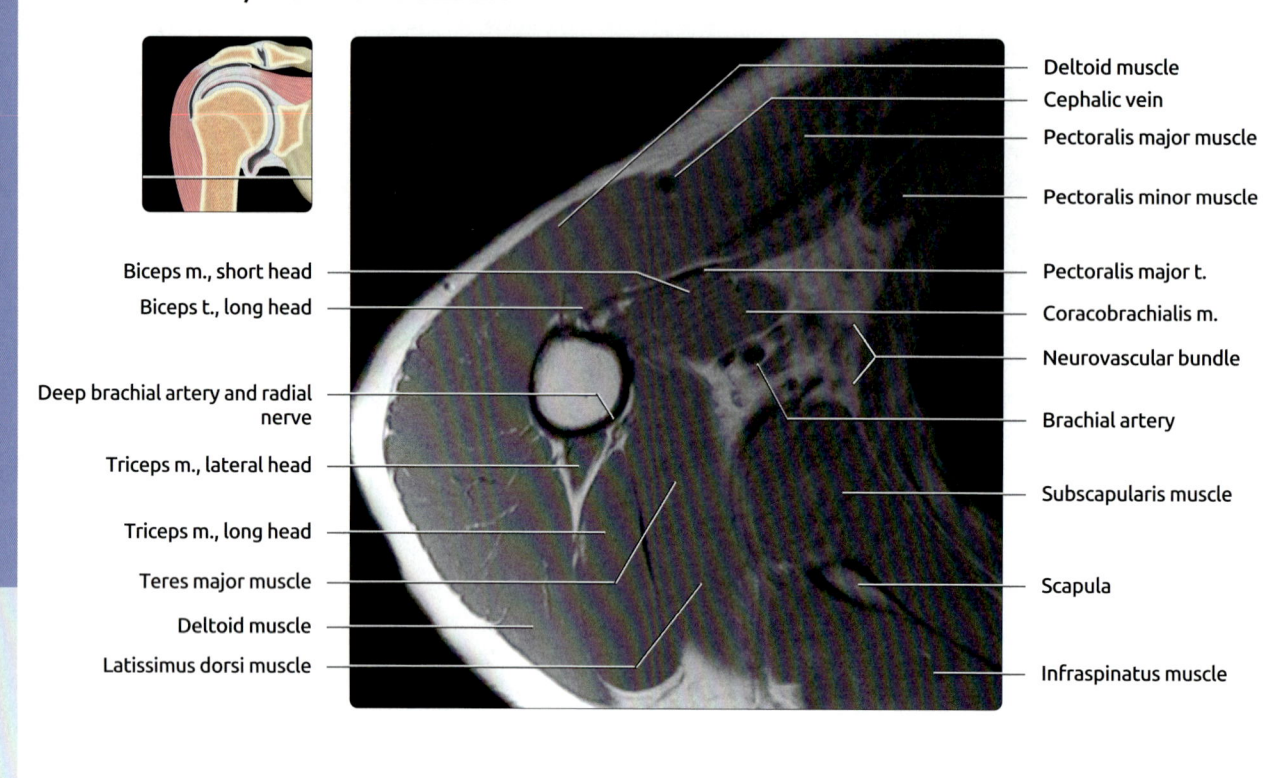

Top image labels (left side):
- Biceps m., short head
- Biceps t., long head
- Deep brachial artery and radial nerve
- Triceps m., lateral head
- Triceps m., long head
- Teres major muscle
- Deltoid muscle
- Latissimus dorsi muscle

Top image labels (right side):
- Deltoid muscle
- Cephalic vein
- Pectoralis major muscle
- Pectoralis minor muscle
- Pectoralis major t.
- Coracobrachialis m.
- Neurovascular bundle
- Brachial artery
- Subscapularis muscle
- Scapula
- Infraspinatus muscle

Bottom image labels (left side):
- Biceps muscle, short head
- Biceps muscle and tendon, long head
- Deep brachial artery and radial nerve
- Triceps m., lateral head
- Triceps m., long head
- Teres major muscle
- Deltoid muscle

Bottom image labels (right side):
- Deltoid muscle
- Cephalic vein
- Pectoralis major muscle
- Pectoralis minor muscle
- Pectoralis major t.
- Coracobrachialis m.
- Brachial artery
- Serratus anterior muscle
- Subscapularis muscle
- Scapula
- Latissimus dorsi muscle
- Infraspinatus muscle

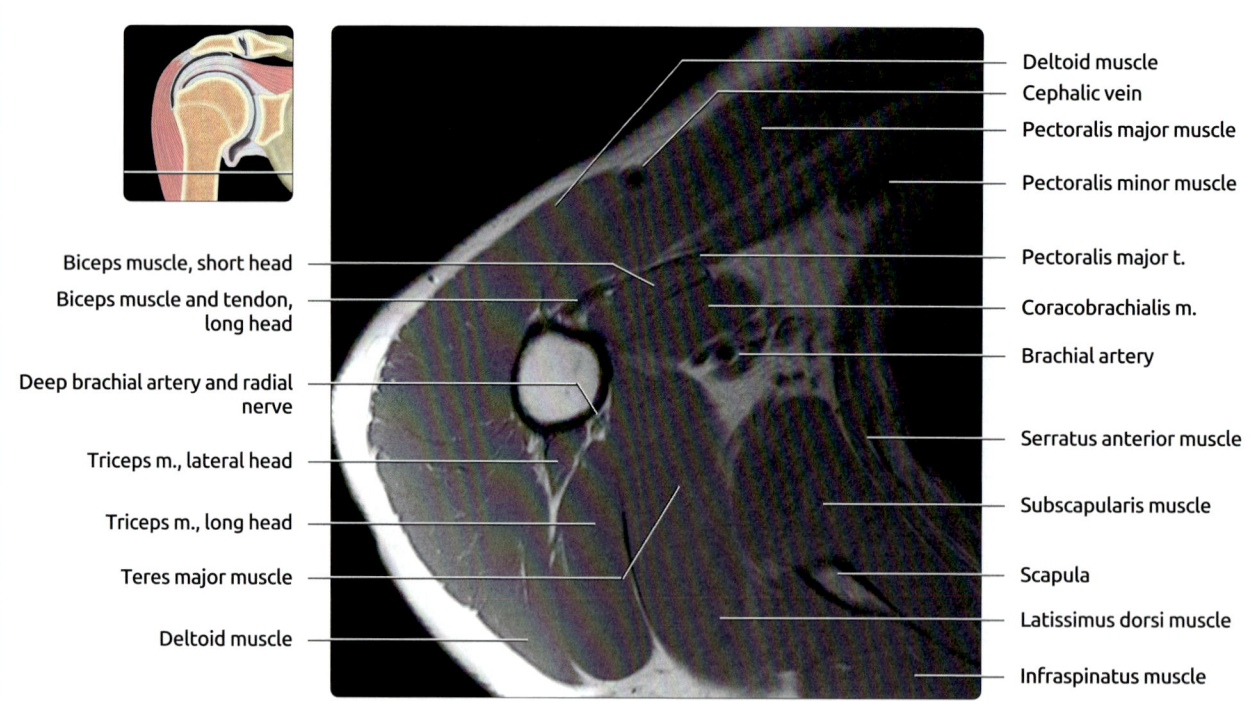

(Top) The axillary artery becomes the brachial artery at the lower margin of the teres major muscle. The brachial artery has paired brachial veins lying on each side of the artery. The pectoralis major muscle has a long insertion along the lateral aspect of the bicipital groove. In some places, it fuses with the joint capsule, deltoid tendon, and fascia of the upper arm. **(Bottom)** The deep brachial artery is the 1st branch of the brachial artery. The deep brachial artery travels with the radial nerve between the lateral and long heads of the triceps in the upper arm.

Shoulder MR Atlas

AXIAL T1 MR, LEFT SHOULDER

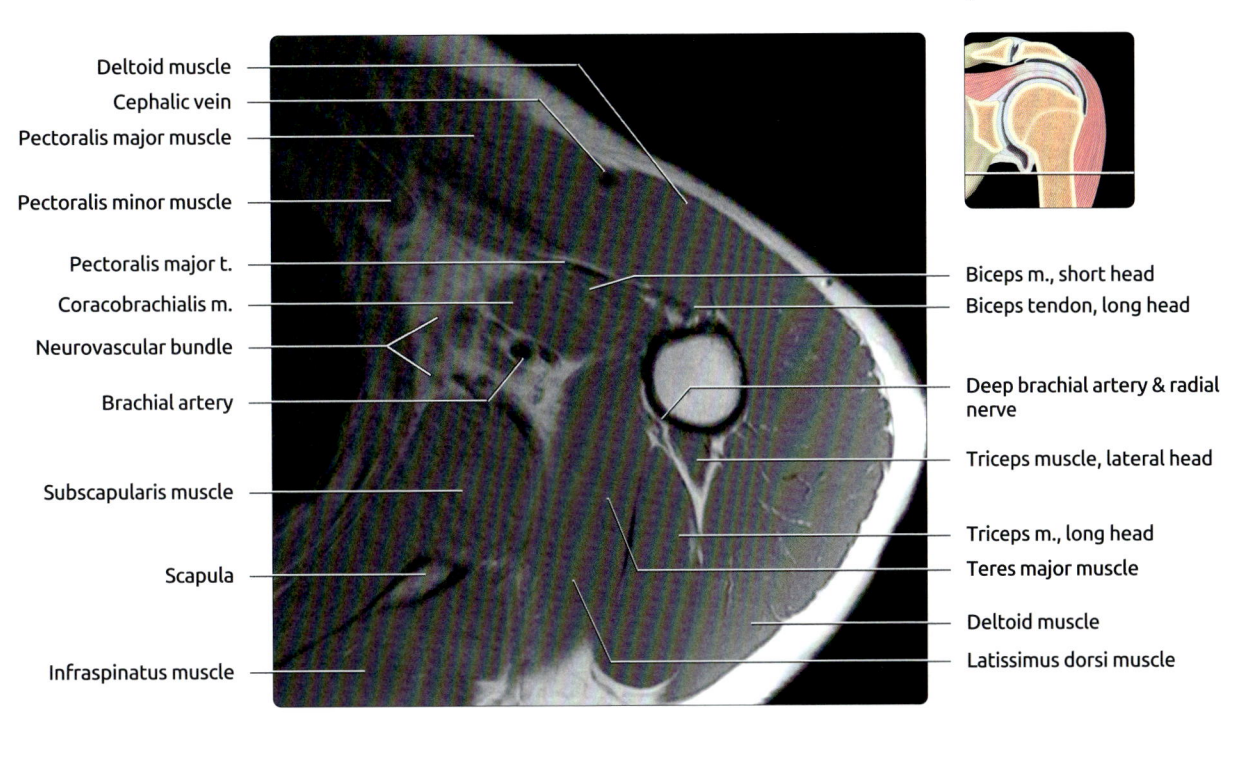

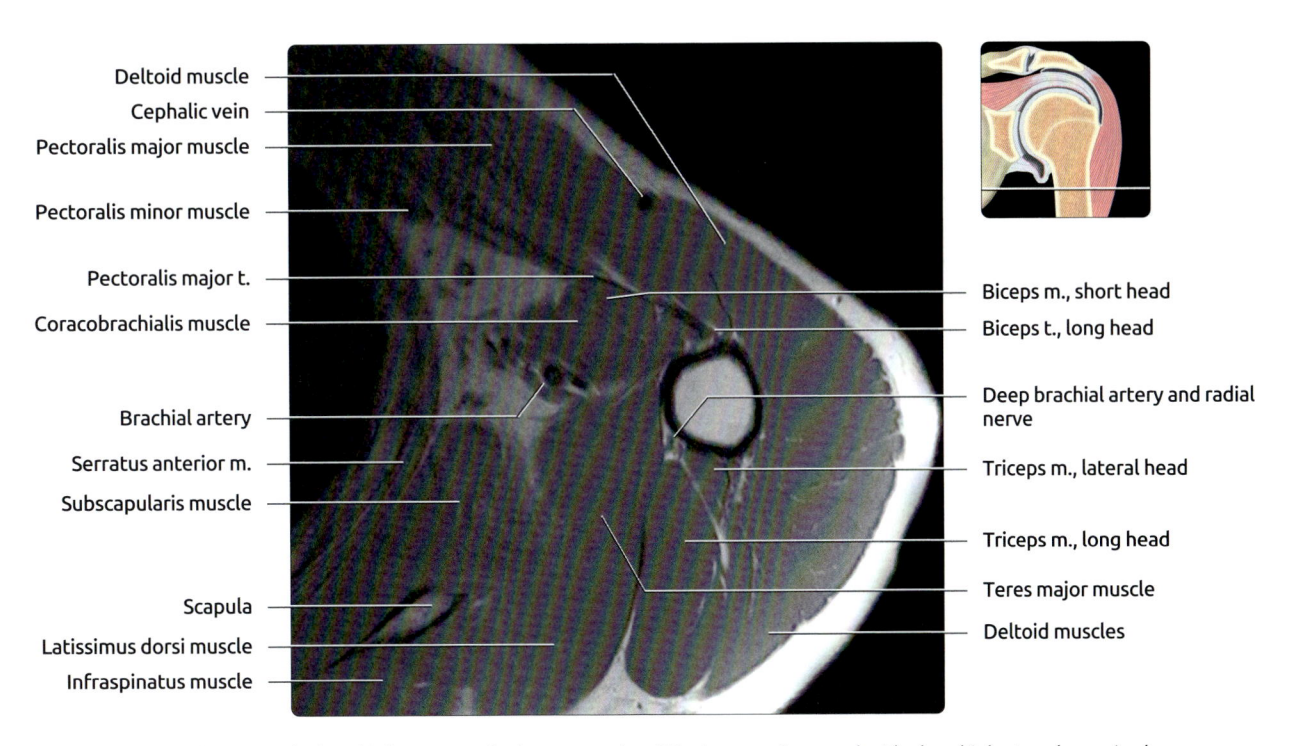

Top image labels (left): Deltoid muscle; Cephalic vein; Pectoralis major muscle; Pectoralis minor muscle; Pectoralis major t.; Coracobrachialis m.; Neurovascular bundle; Brachial artery; Subscapularis muscle; Scapula; Infraspinatus muscle.

Top image labels (right): Biceps m., short head; Biceps tendon, long head; Deep brachial artery & radial nerve; Triceps muscle, lateral head; Triceps m., long head; Teres major muscle; Deltoid muscle; Latissimus dorsi muscle.

Bottom image labels (left): Deltoid muscle; Cephalic vein; Pectoralis major muscle; Pectoralis minor muscle; Pectoralis major t.; Coracobrachialis muscle; Brachial artery; Serratus anterior m.; Subscapularis muscle; Scapula; Latissimus dorsi muscle; Infraspinatus muscle.

Bottom image labels (right): Biceps m., short head; Biceps t., long head; Deep brachial artery and radial nerve; Triceps m., lateral head; Triceps m., long head; Teres major muscle; Deltoid muscles.

(Top) The axillary artery becomes the brachial artery at the lower margin of the teres major muscle. The brachial artery has paired brachial veins lying on each side of the artery. The pectoralis major muscle has a long insertion along the lateral aspect of the bicipital groove. In some places, it fuses with the joint capsule, deltoid tendon, and fascia of the upper arm. **(Bottom)** The deep brachial artery is the 1st branch of the brachial artery. The deep brachial artery travels with the radial nerve between the lateral and long heads of the triceps in the upper arm.

Shoulder MR Atlas

AXIAL T1 MR, RIGHT SHOULDER

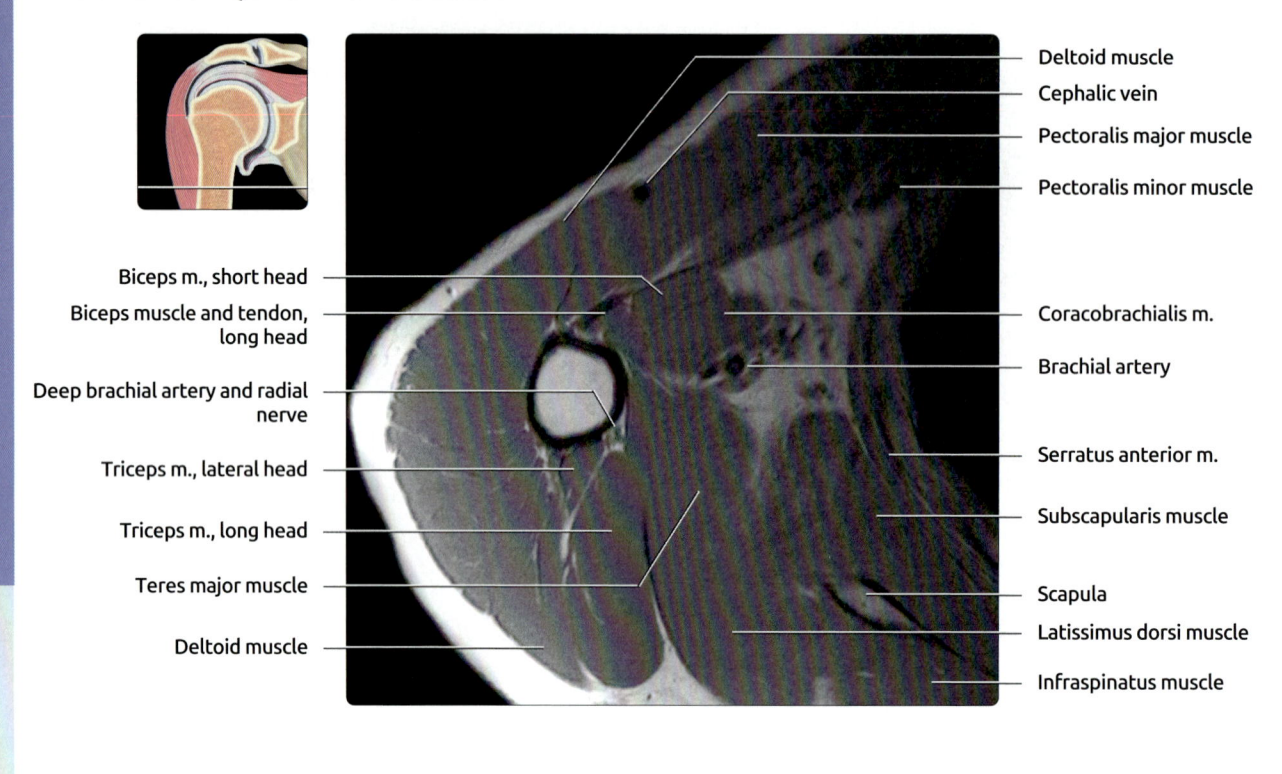

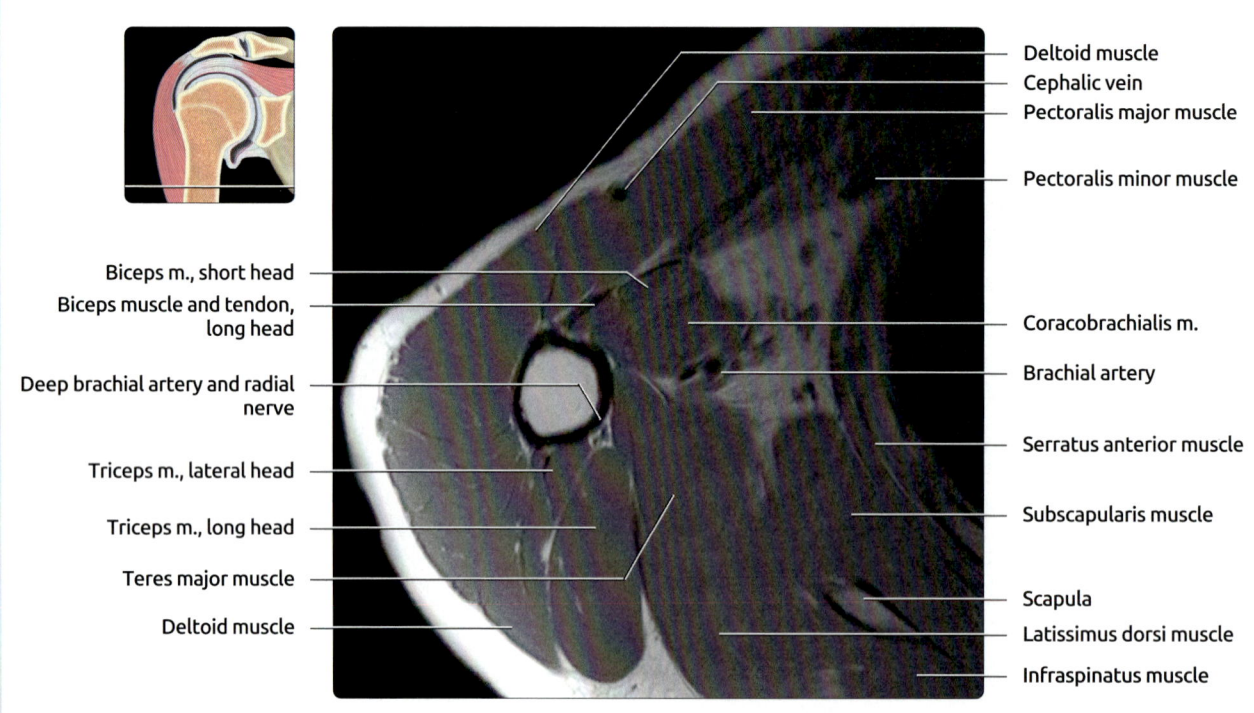

Labels (top image, left side):
- Biceps m., short head
- Biceps muscle and tendon, long head
- Deep brachial artery and radial nerve
- Triceps m., lateral head
- Triceps m., long head
- Teres major muscle
- Deltoid muscle

Labels (top image, right side):
- Deltoid muscle
- Cephalic vein
- Pectoralis major muscle
- Pectoralis minor muscle
- Coracobrachialis m.
- Brachial artery
- Serratus anterior m.
- Subscapularis muscle
- Scapula
- Latissimus dorsi muscle
- Infraspinatus muscle

Labels (bottom image, left side):
- Biceps m., short head
- Biceps muscle and tendon, long head
- Deep brachial artery and radial nerve
- Triceps m., lateral head
- Triceps m., long head
- Teres major muscle
- Deltoid muscle

Labels (bottom image, right side):
- Deltoid muscle
- Cephalic vein
- Pectoralis major muscle
- Pectoralis minor muscle
- Coracobrachialis m.
- Brachial artery
- Serratus anterior muscle
- Subscapularis muscle
- Scapula
- Latissimus dorsi muscle
- Infraspinatus muscle

(Top) *The latissimus dorsi muscle courses superiorly from the lower back, around the inferior border of the teres major muscle, to insert along the inferior aspect of the bicipital groove.* **(Bottom)** *The subscapularis muscle covers the entire ventral surface of the scapula.*

Shoulder MR Atlas

AXIAL T1 MR, LEFT SHOULDER

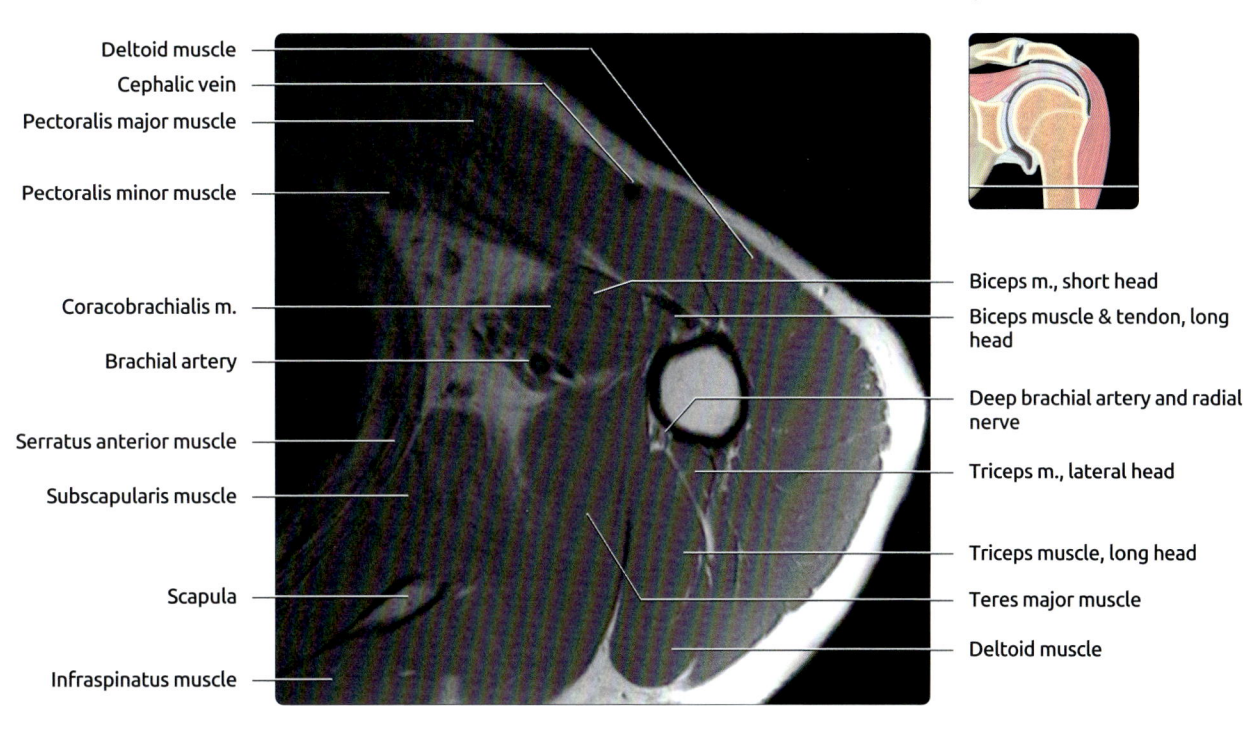

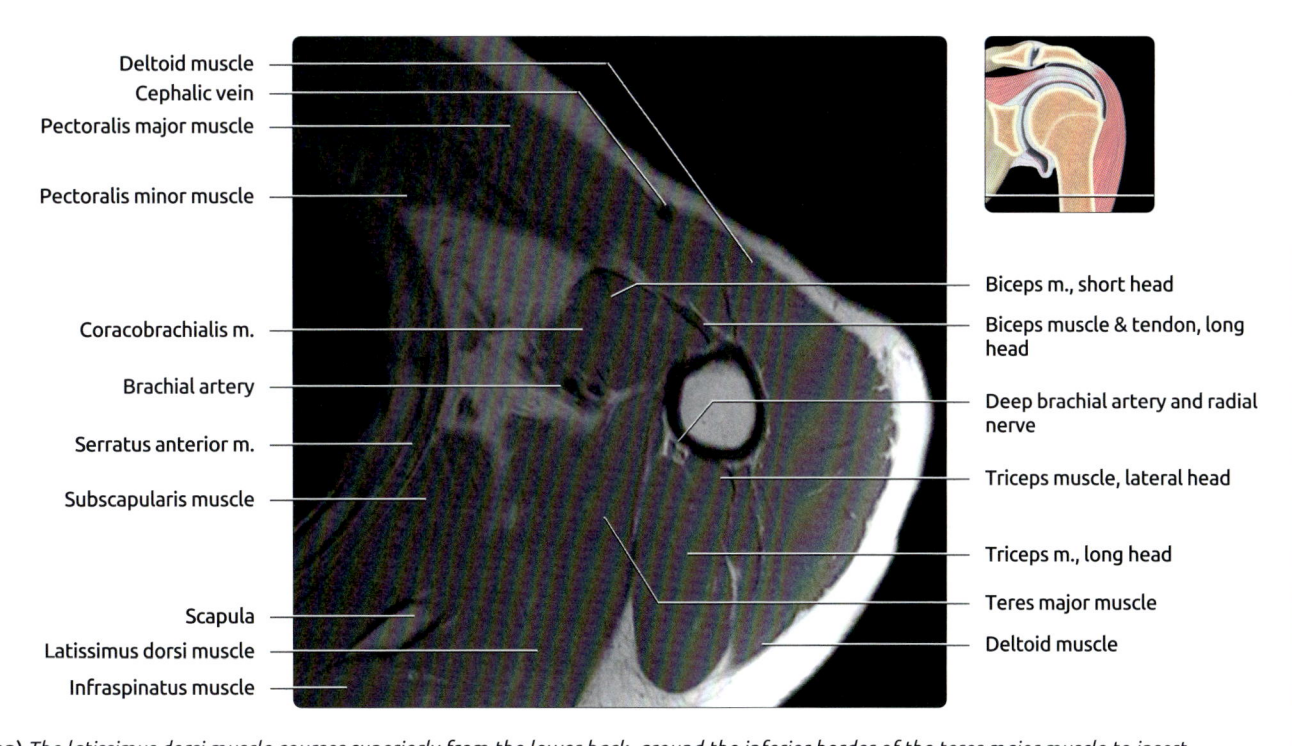

Top image labels (left):
- Deltoid muscle
- Cephalic vein
- Pectoralis major muscle
- Pectoralis minor muscle
- Coracobrachialis m.
- Brachial artery
- Serratus anterior muscle
- Subscapularis muscle
- Scapula
- Infraspinatus muscle

Top image labels (right):
- Biceps m., short head
- Biceps muscle & tendon, long head
- Deep brachial artery and radial nerve
- Triceps m., lateral head
- Triceps muscle, long head
- Teres major muscle
- Deltoid muscle

Bottom image labels (left):
- Deltoid muscle
- Cephalic vein
- Pectoralis major muscle
- Pectoralis minor muscle
- Coracobrachialis m.
- Brachial artery
- Serratus anterior m.
- Subscapularis muscle
- Scapula
- Latissimus dorsi muscle
- Infraspinatus muscle

Bottom image labels (right):
- Biceps m., short head
- Biceps muscle & tendon, long head
- Deep brachial artery and radial nerve
- Triceps muscle, lateral head
- Triceps m., long head
- Teres major muscle
- Deltoid muscle

(**Top**) *The latissimus dorsi muscle courses superiorly from the lower back, around the inferior border of the teres major muscle to insert along the inferior aspect of the bicipital groove.* (**Bottom**) *The subscapularis muscle covers the entire ventral surface of the scapula.*

Shoulder MR Atlas

AXIAL T1 MR, RIGHT SHOULDER

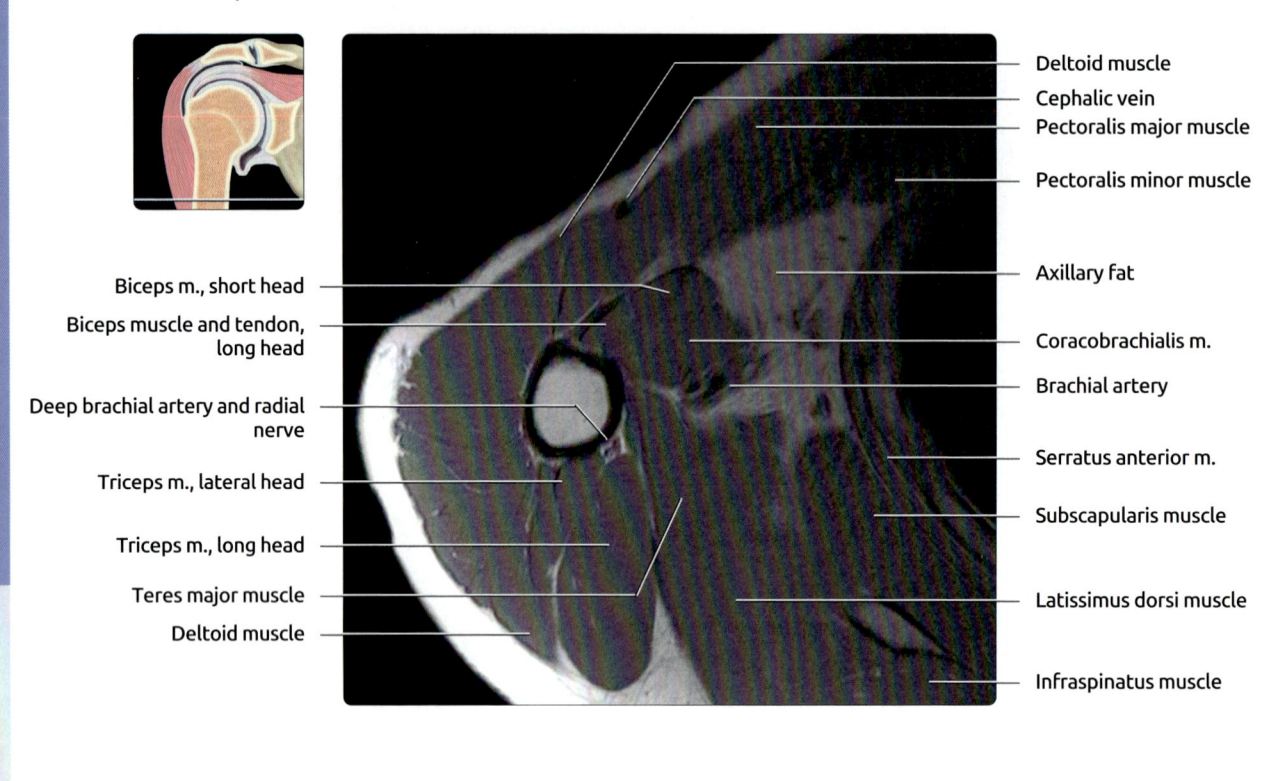

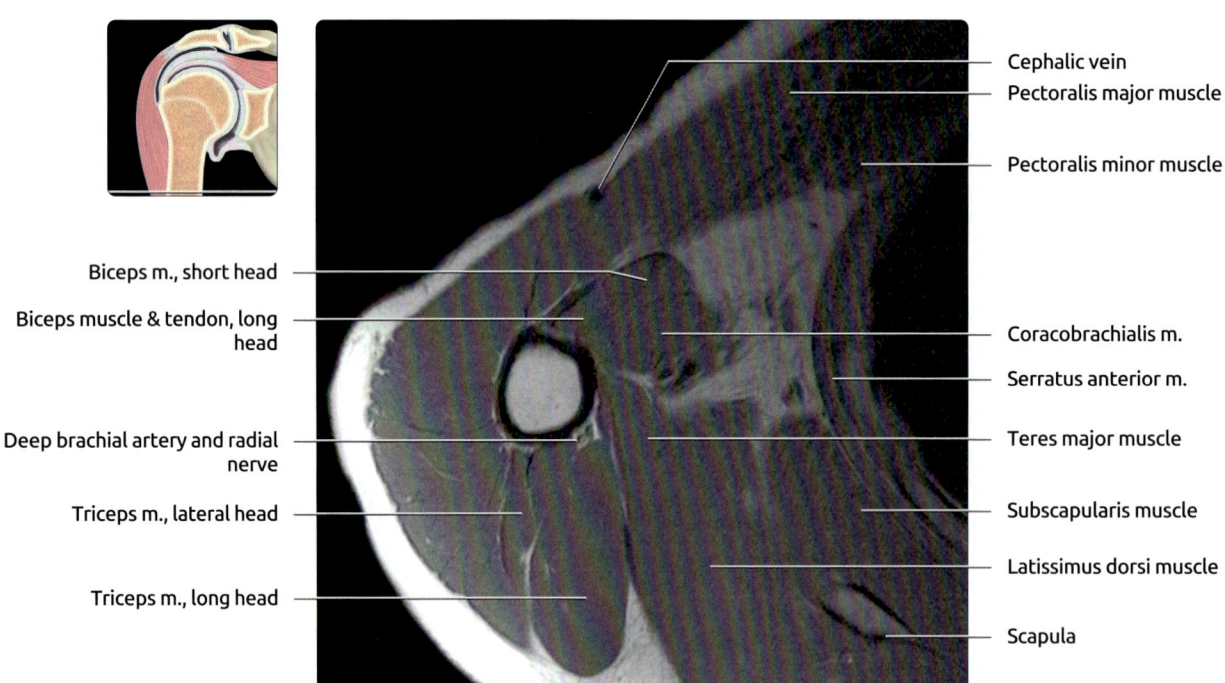

Top image labels (left side):
- Biceps m., short head
- Biceps muscle and tendon, long head
- Deep brachial artery and radial nerve
- Triceps m., lateral head
- Triceps m., long head
- Teres major muscle
- Deltoid muscle

Top image labels (right side):
- Deltoid muscle
- Cephalic vein
- Pectoralis major muscle
- Pectoralis minor muscle
- Axillary fat
- Coracobrachialis m.
- Brachial artery
- Serratus anterior m.
- Subscapularis muscle
- Latissimus dorsi muscle
- Infraspinatus muscle

Bottom image labels (left side):
- Biceps m., short head
- Biceps muscle & tendon, long head
- Deep brachial artery and radial nerve
- Triceps m., lateral head
- Triceps m., long head

Bottom image labels (right side):
- Cephalic vein
- Pectoralis major muscle
- Pectoralis minor muscle
- Coracobrachialis m.
- Serratus anterior m.
- Teres major muscle
- Subscapularis muscle
- Latissimus dorsi muscle
- Scapula

(Top) The pectoralis major and minor form the anterior wall of the axilla. **(Bottom)** The serratus anterior muscle is a thin band of muscle that lies between the ribs and scapula at the posterolateral aspect of the upper chest.

Shoulder MR Atlas

AXIAL T1 MR, LEFT SHOULDER

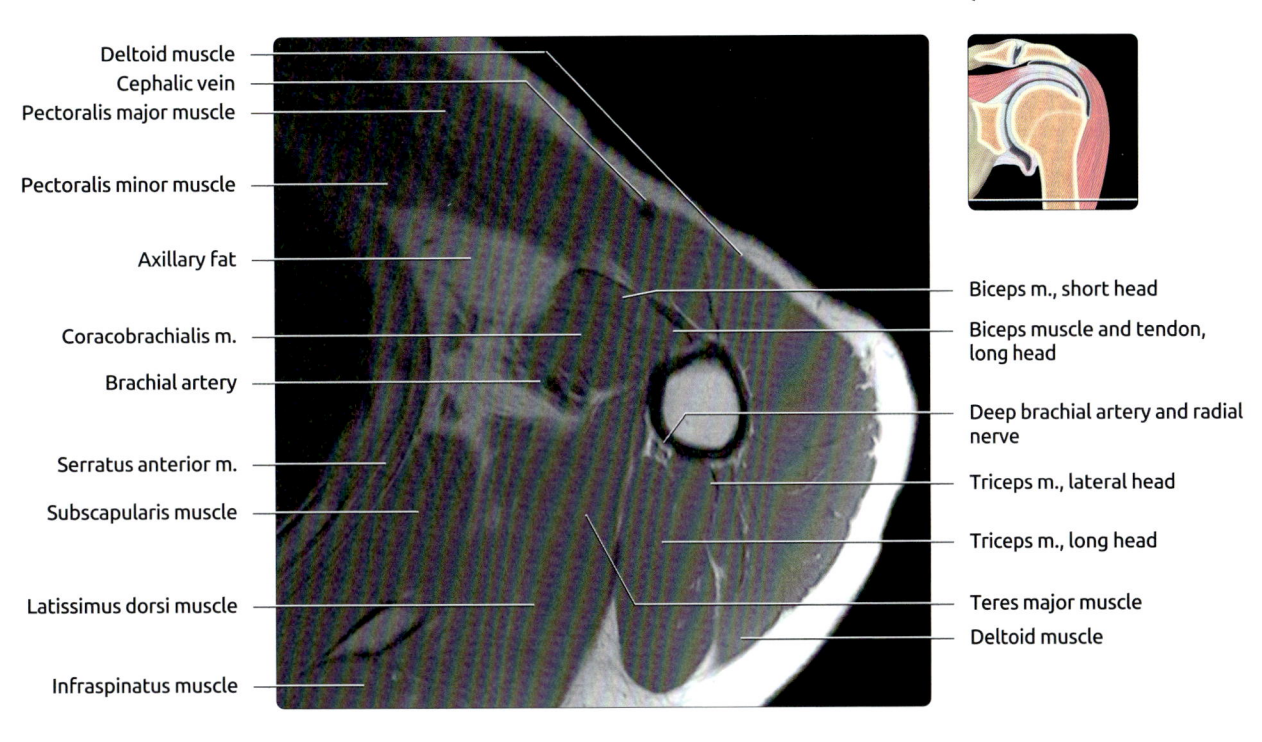

Top image labels (left): Deltoid muscle; Cephalic vein; Pectoralis major muscle; Pectoralis minor muscle; Axillary fat; Coracobrachialis m.; Brachial artery; Serratus anterior m.; Subscapularis muscle; Latissimus dorsi muscle; Infraspinatus muscle.

Top image labels (right): Biceps m., short head; Biceps muscle and tendon, long head; Deep brachial artery and radial nerve; Triceps m., lateral head; Triceps m., long head; Teres major muscle; Deltoid muscle.

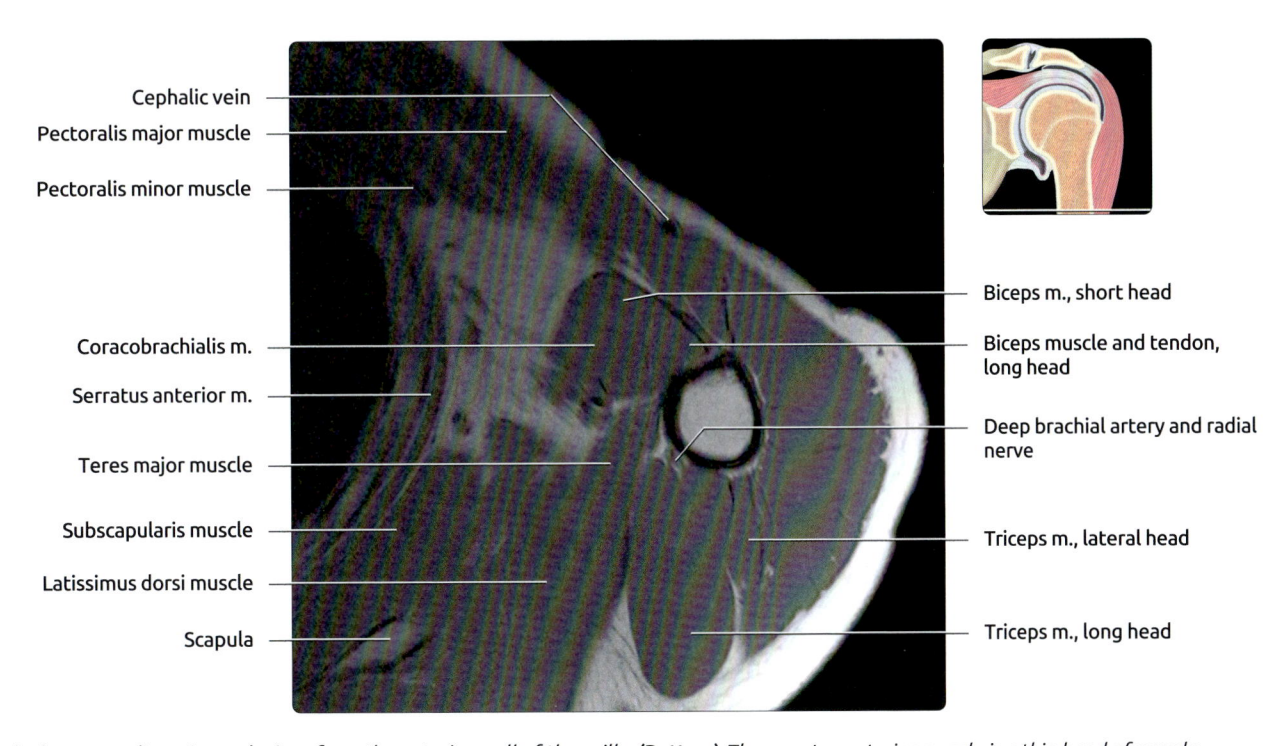

Bottom image labels (left): Cephalic vein; Pectoralis major muscle; Pectoralis minor muscle; Coracobrachialis m.; Serratus anterior m.; Teres major muscle; Subscapularis muscle; Latissimus dorsi muscle; Scapula.

Bottom image labels (right): Biceps m., short head; Biceps muscle and tendon, long head; Deep brachial artery and radial nerve; Triceps m., lateral head; Triceps m., long head.

(Top) *The pectoralis major and minor form the anterior wall of the axilla.* **(Bottom)** *The serratus anterior muscle is a thin band of muscle that lies between the ribs and scapula at the posterolateral aspect of the upper chest.*

Shoulder MR Atlas

CORONAL OBLIQUE T1 MR, RIGHT SHOULDER

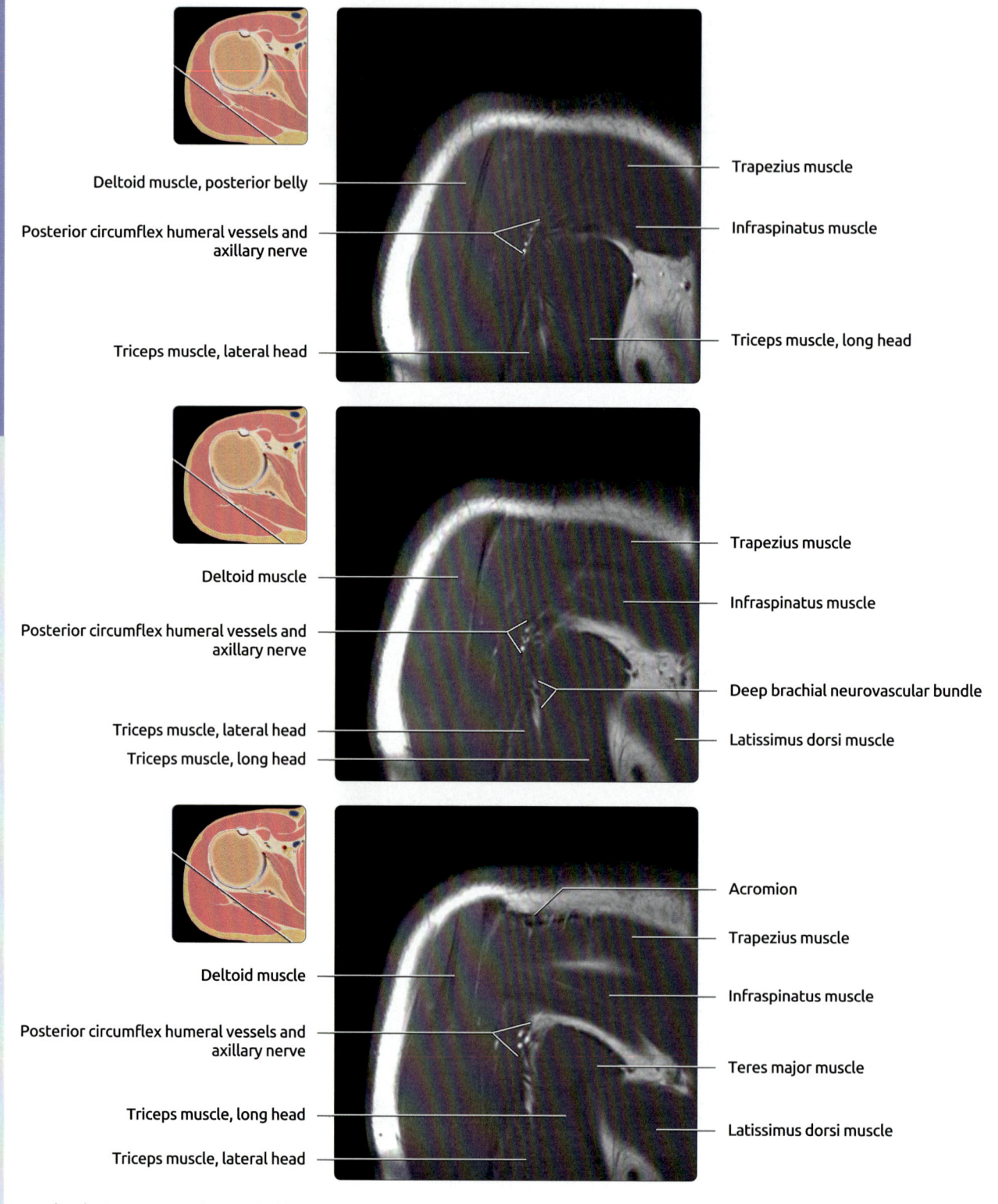

Deltoid muscle, posterior belly

Posterior circumflex humeral vessels and axillary nerve

Triceps muscle, lateral head

Trapezius muscle

Infraspinatus muscle

Triceps muscle, long head

Deltoid muscle

Posterior circumflex humeral vessels and axillary nerve

Triceps muscle, lateral head
Triceps muscle, long head

Trapezius muscle

Infraspinatus muscle

Deep brachial neurovascular bundle

Latissimus dorsi muscle

Deltoid muscle

Posterior circumflex humeral vessels and axillary nerve

Triceps muscle, long head
Triceps muscle, lateral head

Acromion

Trapezius muscle

Infraspinatus muscle

Teres major muscle

Latissimus dorsi muscle

(**Top**) *First in series of coronal oblique T1 MR images shows the right shoulder displayed posterior to anterior. Images were obtained with a shoulder coil on a 3T MR scanner. At the most posterior aspect of the shoulder, the deltoid muscle covers the majority of the shoulder joint. The trapezius muscle covers the superomedial aspect of the shoulder girdle.* (**Middle**) *The radial nerve supplies the triceps muscle. It is part of the deep brachial neurovascular bundle.* (**Bottom**) *The long head of the triceps muscle is the most medial muscle of the posterior upper arm. Axillary nerve branches supply the skin and shoulder joint.*

Shoulder MR Atlas

CORONAL OBLIQUE T1 MR, LEFT SHOULDER

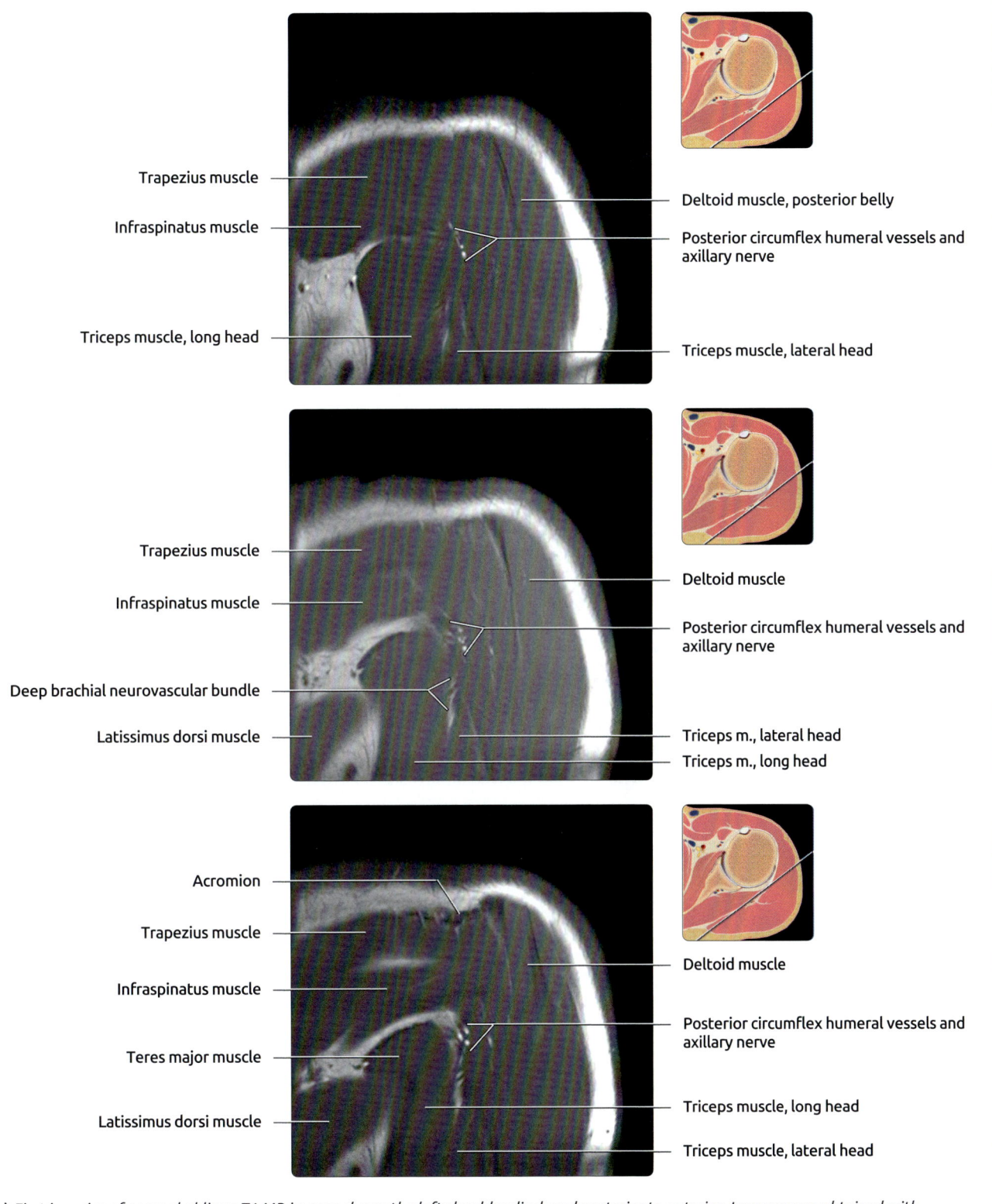

Trapezius muscle
Infraspinatus muscle
Triceps muscle, long head

Deltoid muscle, posterior belly
Posterior circumflex humeral vessels and axillary nerve
Triceps muscle, lateral head

Trapezius muscle
Infraspinatus muscle
Deep brachial neurovascular bundle
Latissimus dorsi muscle

Deltoid muscle
Posterior circumflex humeral vessels and axillary nerve
Triceps m., lateral head
Triceps m., long head

Acromion
Trapezius muscle
Infraspinatus muscle
Teres major muscle
Latissimus dorsi muscle

Deltoid muscle
Posterior circumflex humeral vessels and axillary nerve
Triceps muscle, long head
Triceps muscle, lateral head

(Top) First in series of coronal oblique T1 MR images shows the left shoulder displayed posterior to anterior. Images were obtained with a shoulder coil on a 3T MR scanner. At the most posterior aspect of the shoulder, the deltoid muscle covers the majority of the shoulder joint. The trapezius muscle covers the superomedial aspect of the shoulder girdle. (Middle) The radial nerve supplies the triceps muscle. It is part of the deep brachial neurovascular bundle. (Bottom) The long head of the triceps muscle is the most medial muscle of the posterior upper arm. Axillary nerve branches supply the skin and shoulder joint.

Shoulder MR Atlas

CORONAL OBLIQUE T1 MR, RIGHT SHOULDER

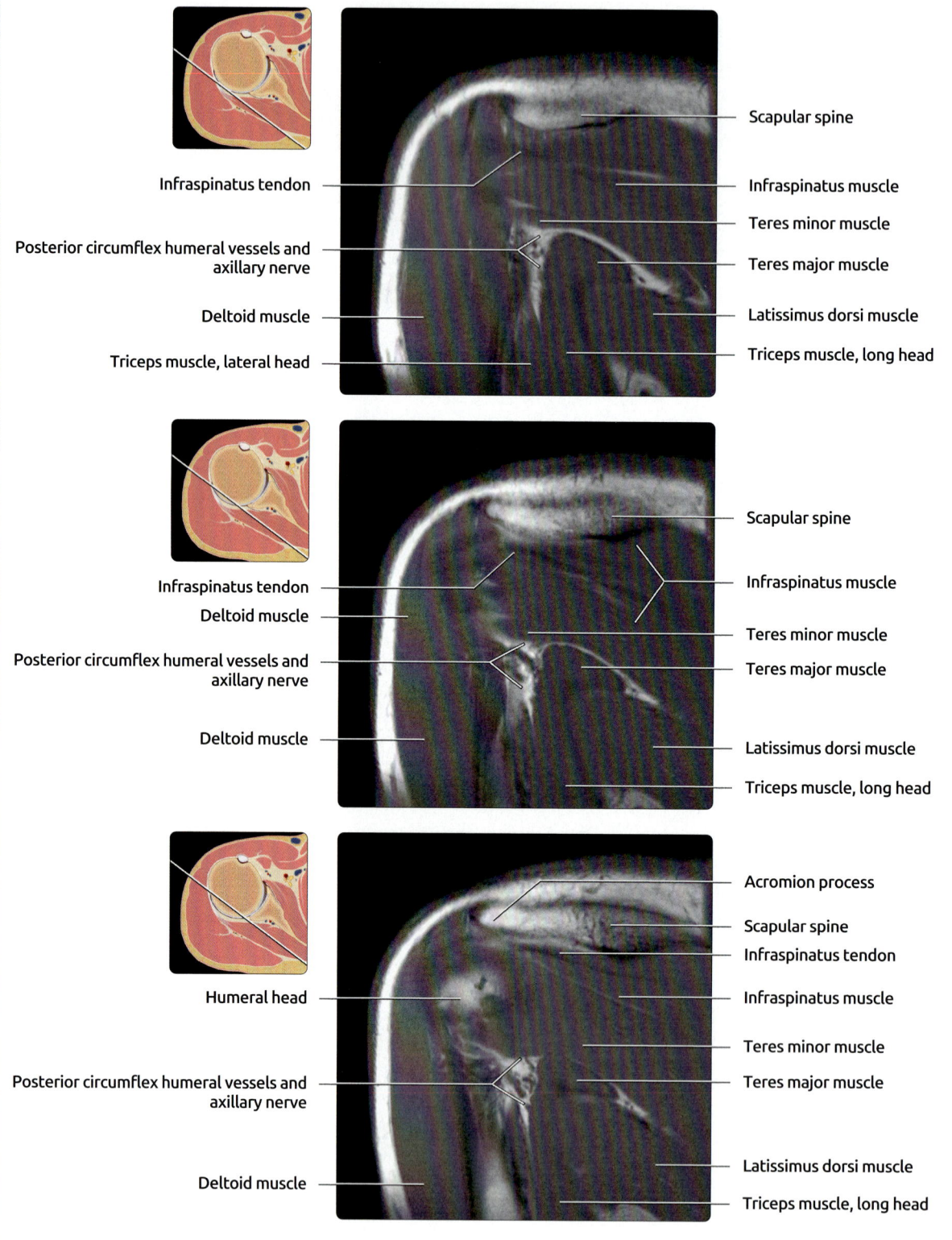

Top image labels:
- Infraspinatus tendon
- Posterior circumflex humeral vessels and axillary nerve
- Deltoid muscle
- Triceps muscle, lateral head
- Scapular spine
- Infraspinatus muscle
- Teres minor muscle
- Teres major muscle
- Latissimus dorsi muscle
- Triceps muscle, long head

Middle image labels:
- Infraspinatus tendon
- Deltoid muscle
- Posterior circumflex humeral vessels and axillary nerve
- Deltoid muscle
- Scapular spine
- Infraspinatus muscle
- Teres minor muscle
- Teres major muscle
- Latissimus dorsi muscle
- Triceps muscle, long head

Bottom image labels:
- Humeral head
- Posterior circumflex humeral vessels and axillary nerve
- Deltoid muscle
- Acromion process
- Scapular spine
- Infraspinatus tendon
- Infraspinatus muscle
- Teres minor muscle
- Teres major muscle
- Latissimus dorsi muscle
- Triceps muscle, long head

(**Top**) *The infraspinatus tendon arches over the posterosuperior aspect of the humeral head to insert on the greater tuberosity.* (**Middle**) *The teres major muscle originates from the inferolateral border of the scapula to insert on the medial aspect of the bicipital groove of the anterior humerus.* (**Bottom**) *The posterior circumflex humeral artery is a branch of the axillary artery and anastomoses with the anterior circumflex humeral artery.*

Shoulder MR Atlas

CORONAL OBLIQUE T1 MR, LEFT SHOULDER

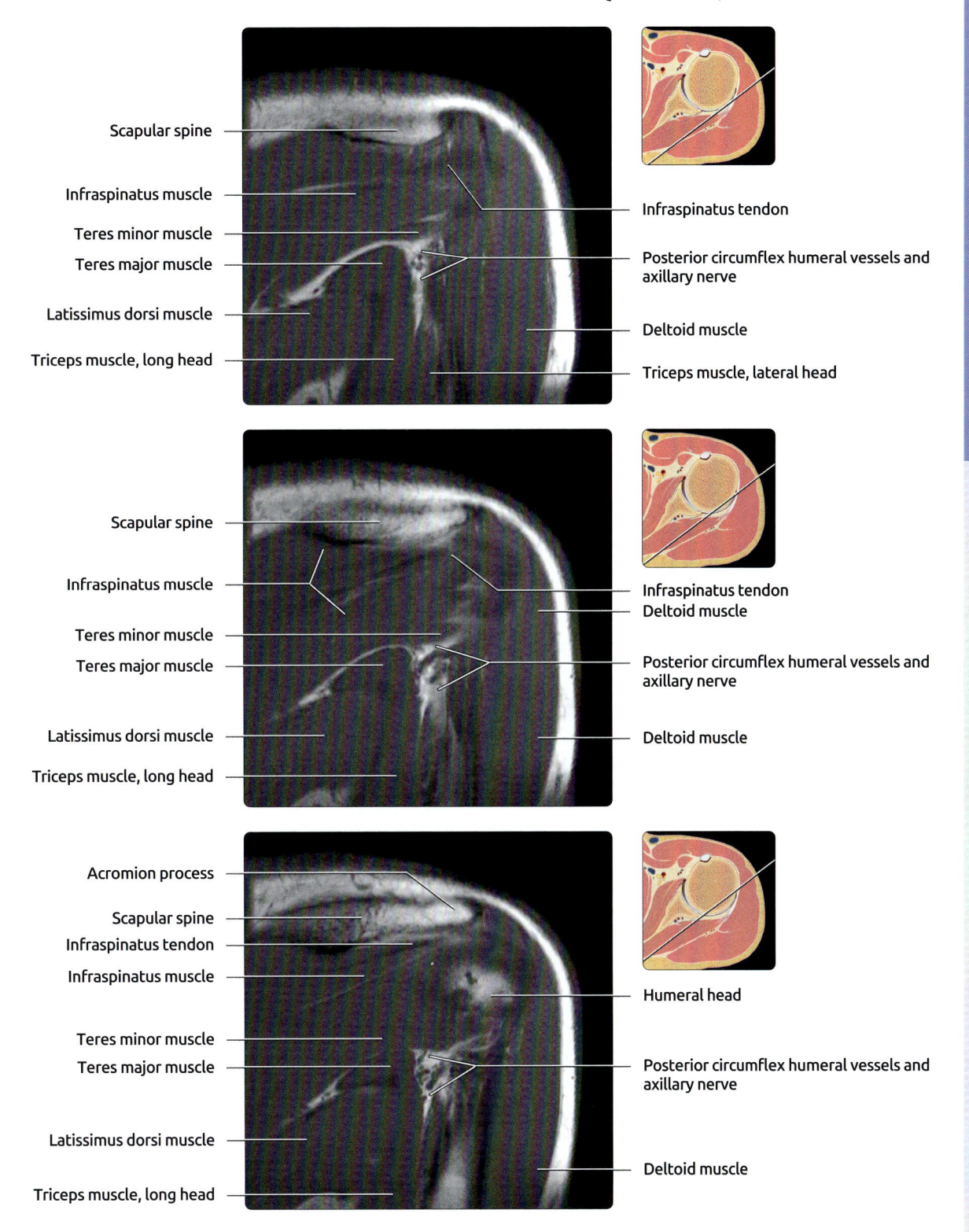

Scapular spine
Infraspinatus muscle
Teres minor muscle
Teres major muscle
Latissimus dorsi muscle
Triceps muscle, long head
Infraspinatus tendon
Posterior circumflex humeral vessels and axillary nerve
Deltoid muscle
Triceps muscle, lateral head

Scapular spine
Infraspinatus muscle
Teres minor muscle
Teres major muscle
Latissimus dorsi muscle
Triceps muscle, long head
Infraspinatus tendon
Deltoid muscle
Posterior circumflex humeral vessels and axillary nerve
Deltoid muscle

Acromion process
Scapular spine
Infraspinatus tendon
Infraspinatus muscle
Teres minor muscle
Teres major muscle
Latissimus dorsi muscle
Triceps muscle, long head
Humeral head
Posterior circumflex humeral vessels and axillary nerve
Deltoid muscle

(Top) The infraspinatus tendon arches over the posterosuperior aspect of the humeral head to insert on the greater tuberosity. (Middle) The teres major muscle originates from the inferolateral border of the scapula to insert on the medial aspect of the bicipital groove of the anterior humerus. (Bottom) The posterior circumflex humeral artery is a branch of the axillary artery and anastomoses with the anterior circumflex humeral artery.

Shoulder MR Atlas

CORONAL OBLIQUE T1 MR, RIGHT SHOULDER

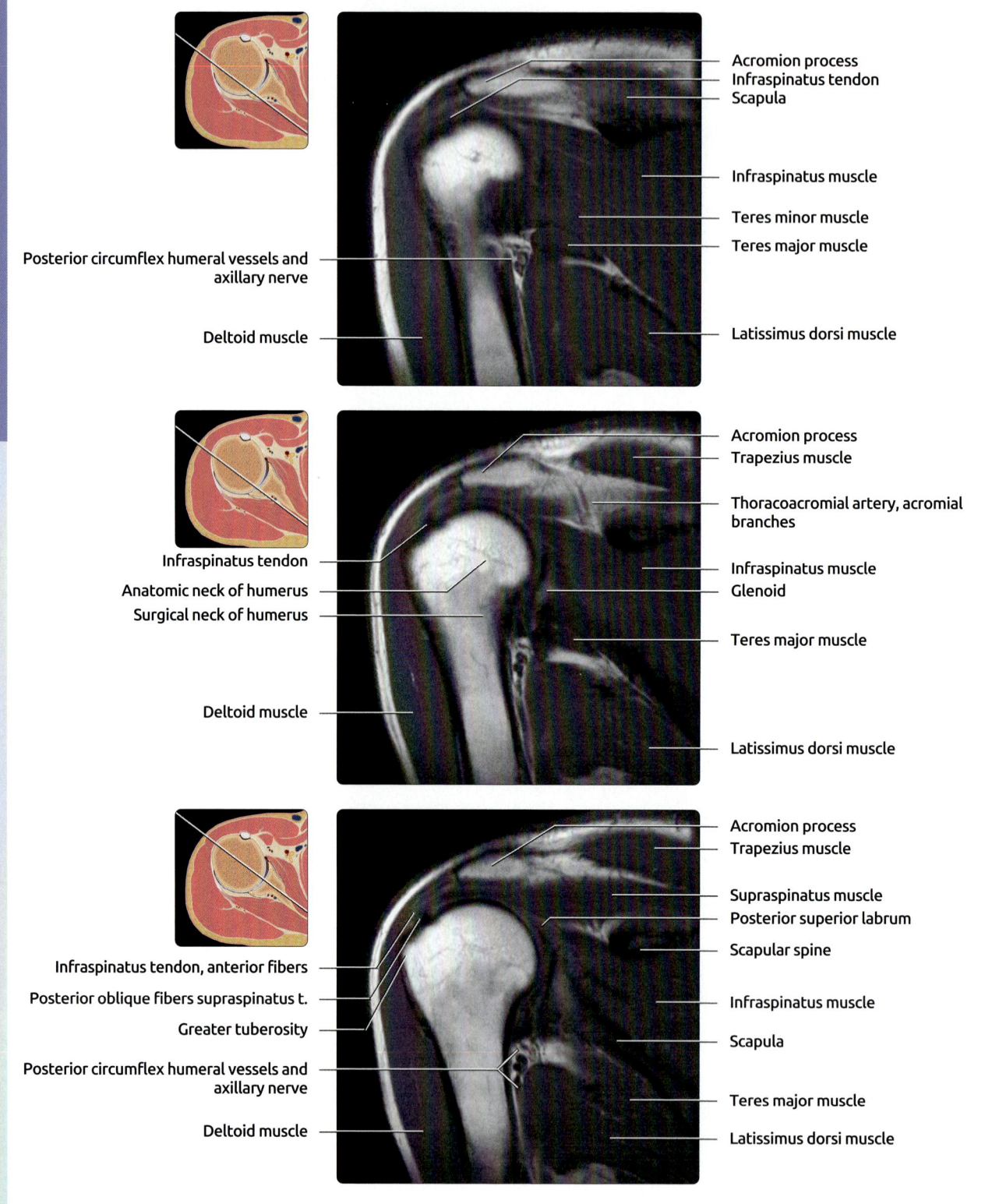

Labels (Top):
- Acromion process
- Infraspinatus tendon
- Scapula
- Infraspinatus muscle
- Teres minor muscle
- Teres major muscle
- Posterior circumflex humeral vessels and axillary nerve
- Latissimus dorsi muscle
- Deltoid muscle

Labels (Middle):
- Acromion process
- Trapezius muscle
- Thoracoacromial artery, acromial branches
- Infraspinatus muscle
- Glenoid
- Teres major muscle
- Infraspinatus tendon
- Anatomic neck of humerus
- Surgical neck of humerus
- Latissimus dorsi muscle
- Deltoid muscle

Labels (Bottom):
- Acromion process
- Trapezius muscle
- Supraspinatus muscle
- Posterior superior labrum
- Scapular spine
- Infraspinatus muscle
- Scapula
- Teres major muscle
- Latissimus dorsi muscle
- Infraspinatus tendon, anterior fibers
- Posterior oblique fibers supraspinatus t.
- Greater tuberosity
- Posterior circumflex humeral vessels and axillary nerve
- Deltoid muscle

(Top) The supraspinatus, infraspinatus, teres minor, and subscapularis muscles constitute the rotator cuff. The joint capsule fuses distally with the rotator cuff tendons. **(Middle)** The acromion process is the lateral continuation of the scapular spine. The surgical neck of the humerus is extracapsular and located distal to the anatomic neck, which is located at the attachment of the capsule, along the epiphyseal line. **(Bottom)** The scapular spine divides the posterior border of the scapula into the supraspinatus fossa and infraspinatus fossa. The supraspinatus outlet refers to the area of the lateral 1/3 of the supraspinatus muscle and tendon.

Shoulder MR Atlas

CORONAL OBLIQUE T1 MR, LEFT SHOULDER

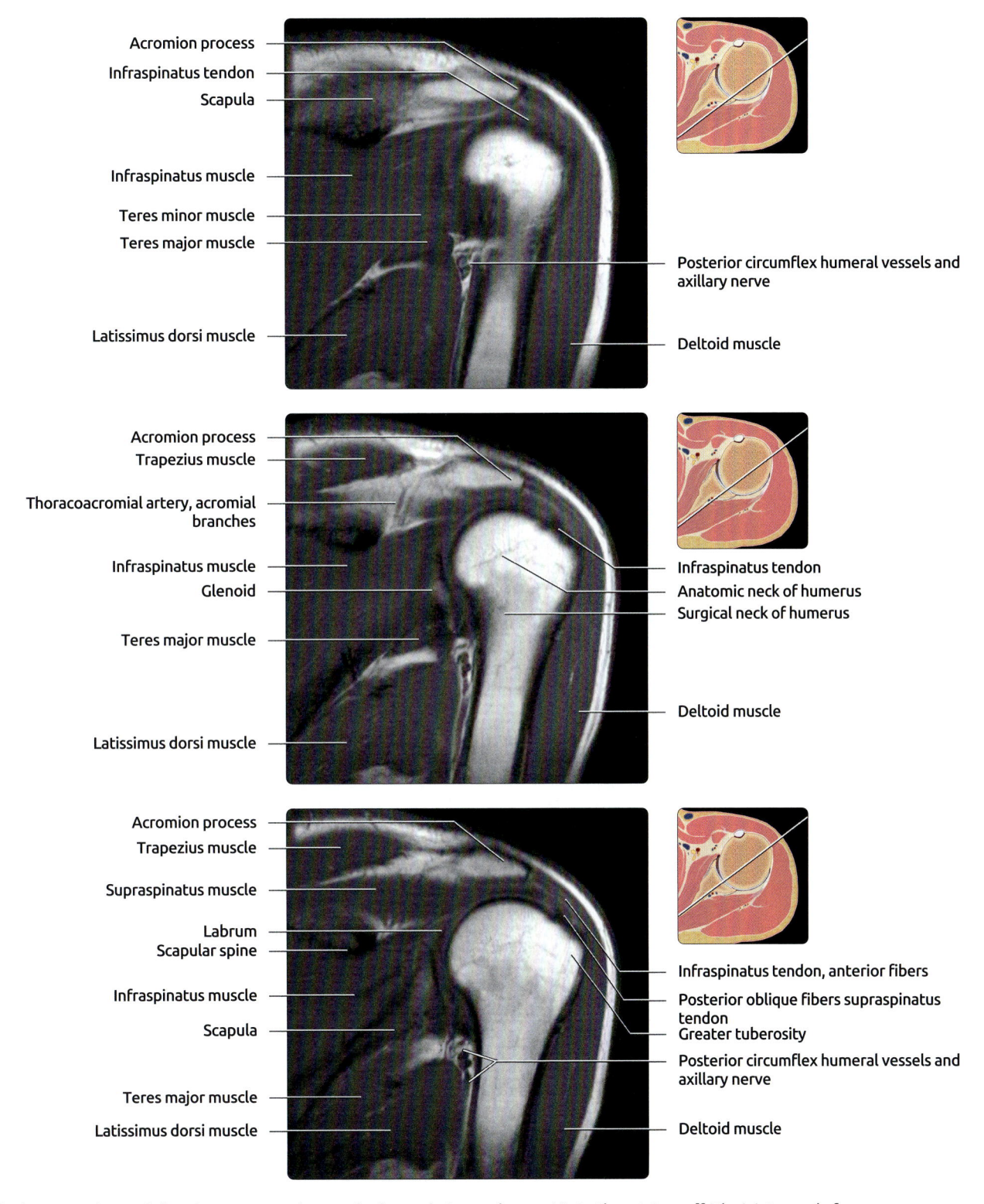

Top image labels:
- Acromion process
- Infraspinatus tendon
- Scapula
- Infraspinatus muscle
- Teres minor muscle
- Teres major muscle
- Latissimus dorsi muscle
- Posterior circumflex humeral vessels and axillary nerve
- Deltoid muscle

Middle image labels:
- Acromion process
- Trapezius muscle
- Thoracoacromial artery, acromial branches
- Infraspinatus muscle
- Glenoid
- Teres major muscle
- Latissimus dorsi muscle
- Infraspinatus tendon
- Anatomic neck of humerus
- Surgical neck of humerus
- Deltoid muscle

Bottom image labels:
- Acromion process
- Trapezius muscle
- Supraspinatus muscle
- Labrum
- Scapular spine
- Infraspinatus muscle
- Scapula
- Teres major muscle
- Latissimus dorsi muscle
- Infraspinatus tendon, anterior fibers
- Posterior oblique fibers supraspinatus tendon
- Greater tuberosity
- Posterior circumflex humeral vessels and axillary nerve
- Deltoid muscle

(**Top**) The supraspinatus, infraspinatus, teres minor, and subscapularis muscles constitute the rotator cuff. The joint capsule fuses distally with the rotator cuff tendons. (**Middle**) The acromion process is the lateral continuation of the scapular spine. The surgical neck of the humerus is extracapsular and located distal to the anatomic neck, which is located at the attachment of the capsule along the epiphyseal line. (**Bottom**) The scapular spine divides the posterior border of the scapula into the supraspinatus fossa and infraspinatus fossa. The supraspinatus outlet refers to the area of the lateral 1/3 of the supraspinatus muscle and tendon.

Shoulder MR Atlas

CORONAL OBLIQUE T1 MR, RIGHT SHOULDER

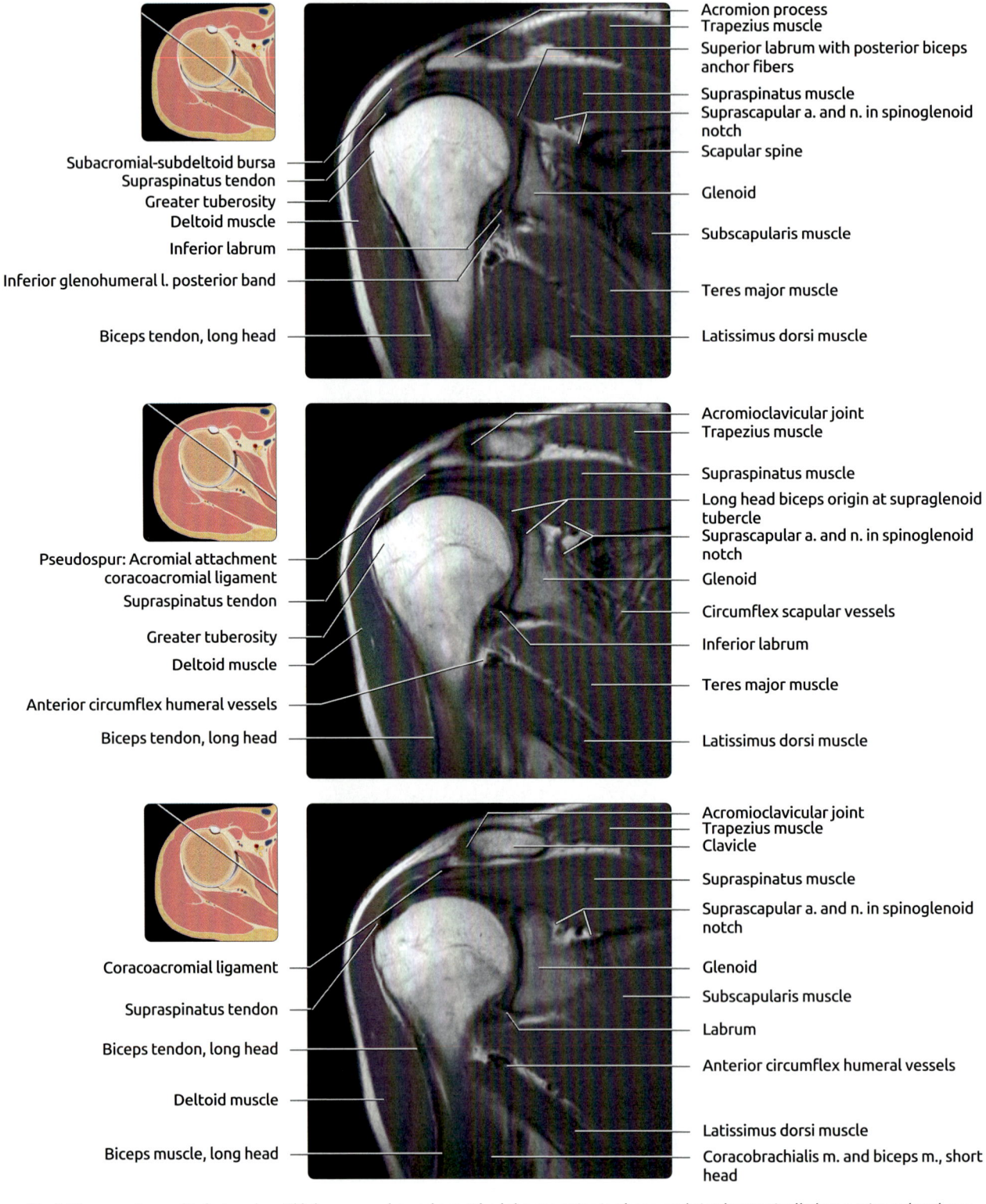

Top image labels (left):
- Subacromial-subdeltoid bursa
- Supraspinatus tendon
- Greater tuberosity
- Deltoid muscle
- Inferior labrum
- Inferior glenohumeral l. posterior band
- Biceps tendon, long head

Top image labels (right):
- Acromion process
- Trapezius muscle
- Superior labrum with posterior biceps anchor fibers
- Supraspinatus muscle
- Suprascapular a. and n. in spinoglenoid notch
- Scapular spine
- Glenoid
- Subscapularis muscle
- Teres major muscle
- Latissimus dorsi muscle

Middle image labels (left):
- Pseudospur: Acromial attachment coracoacromial ligament
- Supraspinatus tendon
- Greater tuberosity
- Deltoid muscle
- Anterior circumflex humeral vessels
- Biceps tendon, long head

Middle image labels (right):
- Acromioclavicular joint
- Trapezius muscle
- Supraspinatus muscle
- Long head biceps origin at supraglenoid tubercle
- Suprascapular a. and n. in spinoglenoid notch
- Glenoid
- Circumflex scapular vessels
- Inferior labrum
- Teres major muscle
- Latissimus dorsi muscle

Bottom image labels (left):
- Coracoacromial ligament
- Supraspinatus tendon
- Biceps tendon, long head
- Deltoid muscle
- Biceps muscle, long head

Bottom image labels (right):
- Acromioclavicular joint
- Trapezius muscle
- Clavicle
- Supraspinatus muscle
- Suprascapular a. and n. in spinoglenoid notch
- Glenoid
- Subscapularis muscle
- Labrum
- Anterior circumflex humeral vessels
- Latissimus dorsi muscle
- Coracobrachialis m. and biceps m., short head

(Top) The superior and inferior glenoid labrum are shown here. The labrum varies in shape and size but typically has a triangular shape of uniformly low signal. **(Middle)** Anterior circumflex artery is a branch of the axillary artery. **(Bottom)** The spinoglenoid notch contains fat and the suprascapular artery and nerve. A mass in this region can impinge the nerve and produce focal atrophy of the infraspinatus muscle.

Shoulder MR Atlas

CORONAL OBLIQUE T1 MR, LEFT SHOULDER

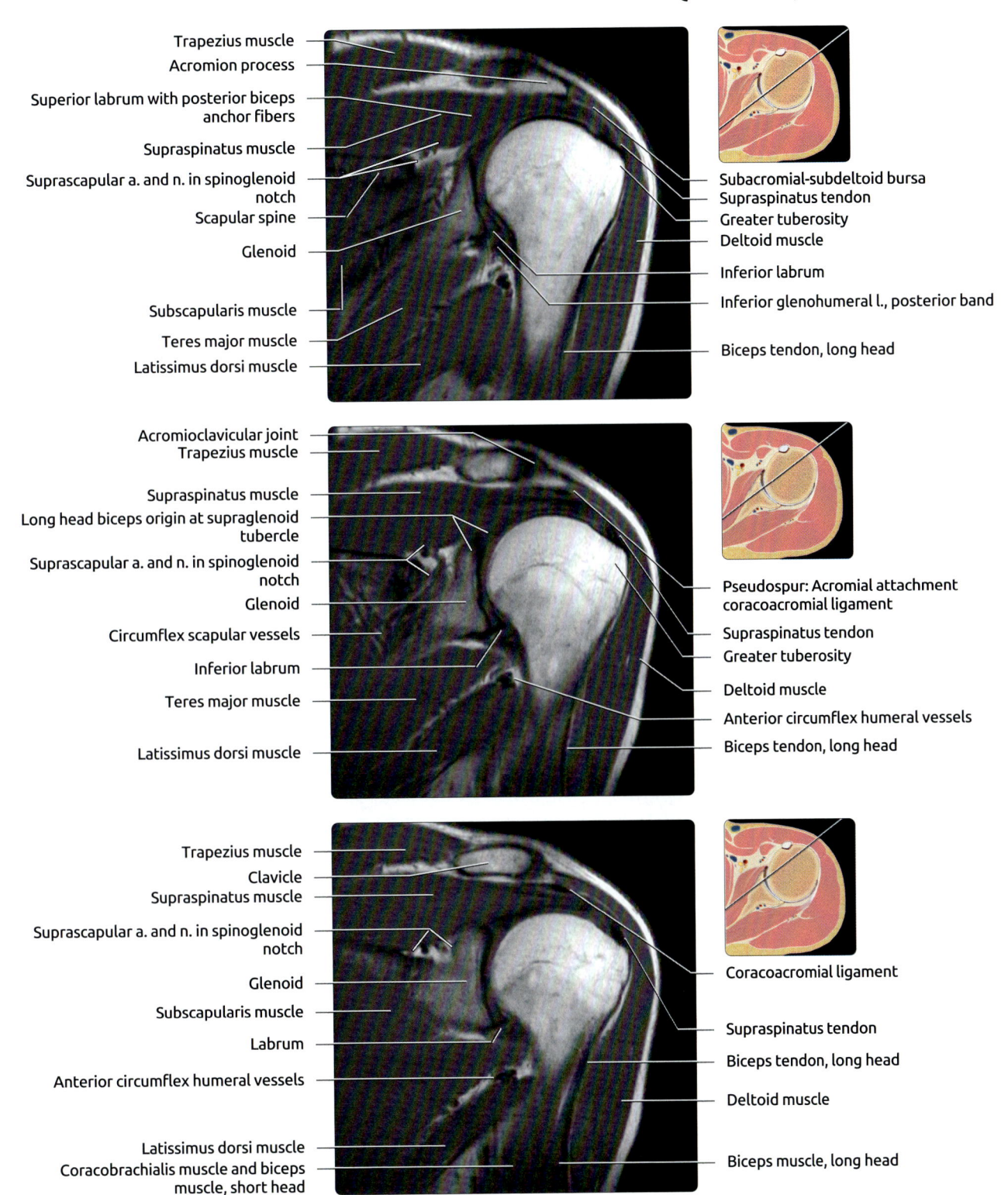

Labels (top image):
- Trapezius muscle
- Acromion process
- Superior labrum with posterior biceps anchor fibers
- Supraspinatus muscle
- Suprascapular a. and n. in spinoglenoid notch
- Scapular spine
- Glenoid
- Subscapularis muscle
- Teres major muscle
- Latissimus dorsi muscle
- Subacromial-subdeltoid bursa
- Supraspinatus tendon
- Greater tuberosity
- Deltoid muscle
- Inferior labrum
- Inferior glenohumeral l., posterior band
- Biceps tendon, long head

Labels (middle image):
- Acromioclavicular joint
- Trapezius muscle
- Supraspinatus muscle
- Long head biceps origin at supraglenoid tubercle
- Suprascapular a. and n. in spinoglenoid notch
- Glenoid
- Circumflex scapular vessels
- Inferior labrum
- Teres major muscle
- Latissimus dorsi muscle
- Pseudospur: Acromial attachment coracoacromial ligament
- Supraspinatus tendon
- Greater tuberosity
- Deltoid muscle
- Anterior circumflex humeral vessels
- Biceps tendon, long head

Labels (bottom image):
- Trapezius muscle
- Clavicle
- Supraspinatus muscle
- Suprascapular a. and n. in spinoglenoid notch
- Glenoid
- Subscapularis muscle
- Labrum
- Anterior circumflex humeral vessels
- Latissimus dorsi muscle
- Coracobrachialis muscle and biceps muscle, short head
- Coracoacromial ligament
- Supraspinatus tendon
- Biceps tendon, long head
- Deltoid muscle
- Biceps muscle, long head

(**Top**) The superior and inferior glenoid labrum are shown here. The labrum varies in shape and size but typically has a triangular shape of uniformly low signal. (**Middle**) Anterior circumflex artery is a branch of the axillary artery. (**Bottom**) The spinoglenoid notch contains fat and the suprascapular artery and nerve. A mass in this region can impinge the nerve and produce focal atrophy of the infraspinatus muscle.

Shoulder MR Atlas

CORONAL OBLIQUE T1 MR, RIGHT SHOULDER

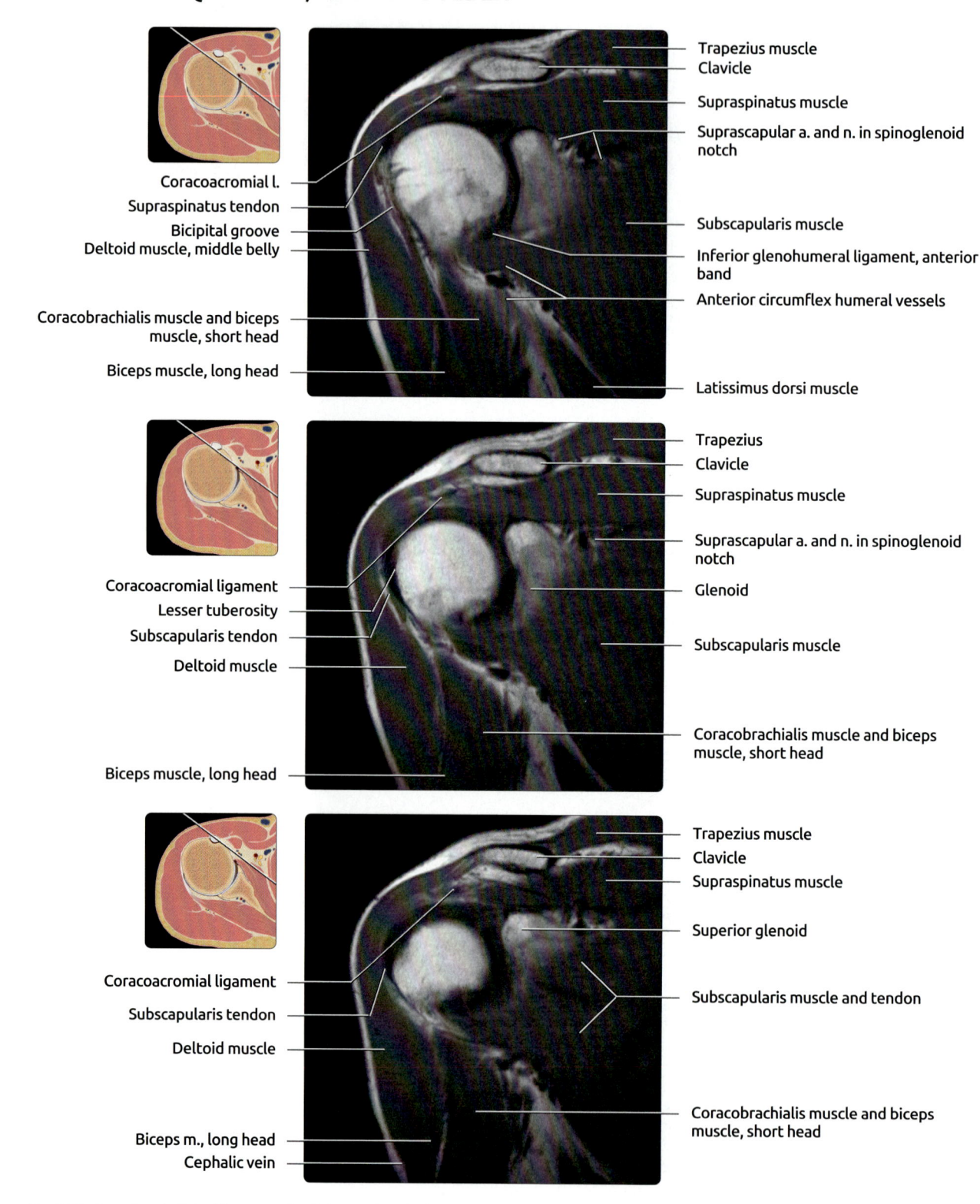

Top image labels (left): Coracoacromial l.; Supraspinatus tendon; Bicipital groove; Deltoid muscle, middle belly; Coracobrachialis muscle and biceps muscle, short head; Biceps muscle, long head

Top image labels (right): Trapezius muscle; Clavicle; Supraspinatus muscle; Suprascapular a. and n. in spinoglenoid notch; Subscapularis muscle; Inferior glenohumeral ligament, anterior band; Anterior circumflex humeral vessels; Latissimus dorsi muscle

Middle image labels (left): Coracoacromial ligament; Lesser tuberosity; Subscapularis tendon; Deltoid muscle; Biceps muscle, long head

Middle image labels (right): Trapezius; Clavicle; Supraspinatus muscle; Suprascapular a. and n. in spinoglenoid notch; Glenoid; Subscapularis muscle; Coracobrachialis muscle and biceps muscle, short head

Bottom image labels (left): Coracoacromial ligament; Subscapularis tendon; Deltoid muscle; Biceps m., long head; Cephalic vein

Bottom image labels (right): Trapezius muscle; Clavicle; Supraspinatus muscle; Superior glenoid; Subscapularis muscle and tendon; Coracobrachialis muscle and biceps muscle, short head

(Top) *The long head of the biceps tendon is located in the bicipital groove. It originates from the supraglenoid tubercle and labrum. The long head of the biceps helps prevent humeral head impingement on the acromion during deltoid contraction.* **(Middle)** *The subscapularis tendon inserts on the lesser tuberosity. The teres major and latissimus dorsi tendons insert just inferior to the subscapularis tendon.* **(Bottom)** *The deltoid and trapezius muscles attach to the scapular spine, lateral 1/3 of clavicle and acromion. Anterior compartment muscles are innervated by the musculocutaneous nerve.*

Shoulder MR Atlas

CORONAL OBLIQUE T1 MR, LEFT SHOULDER

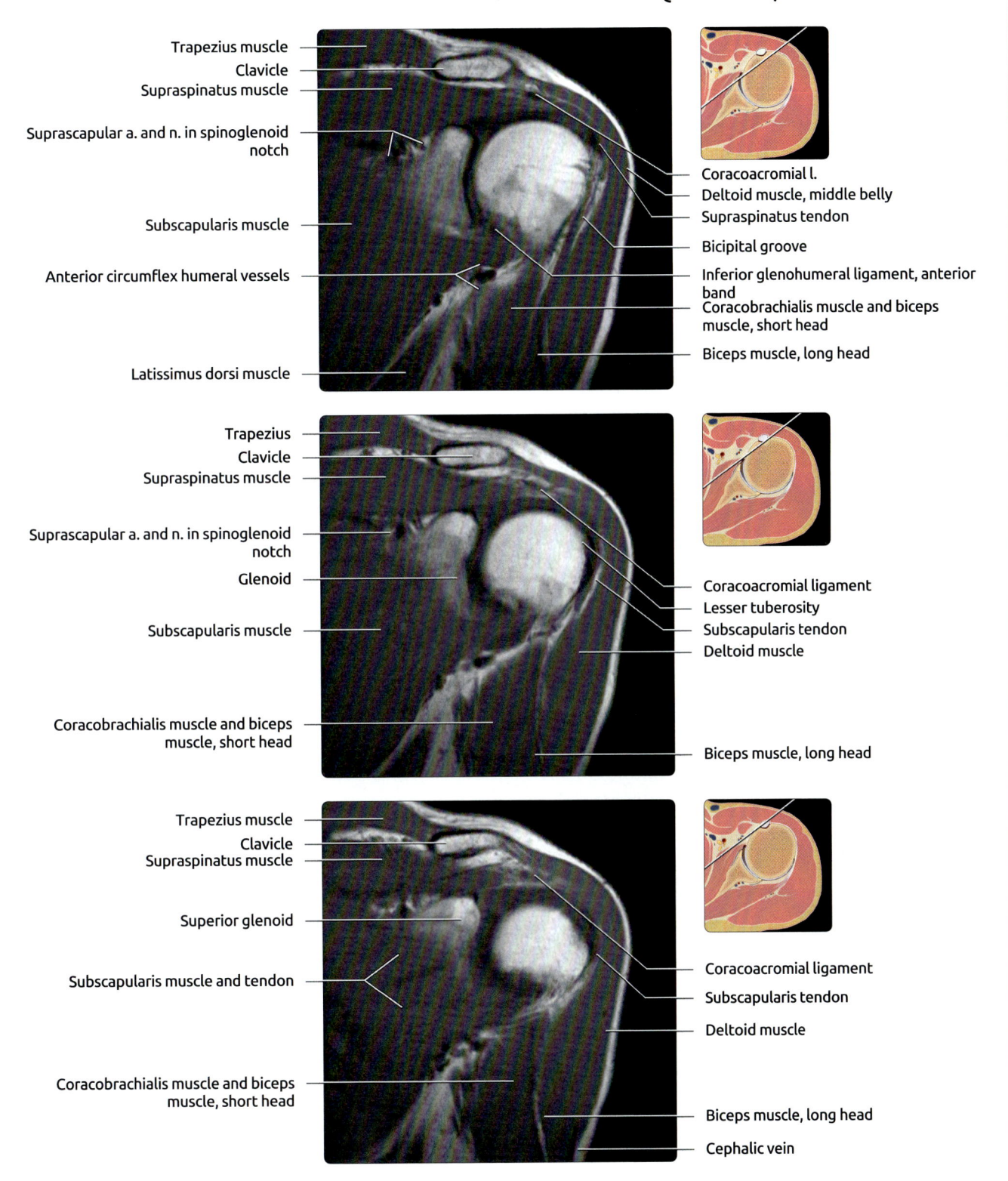

Top image labels (left): Trapezius muscle; Clavicle; Supraspinatus muscle; Suprascapular a. and n. in spinoglenoid notch; Subscapularis muscle; Anterior circumflex humeral vessels; Latissimus dorsi muscle

Top image labels (right): Coracoacromial l.; Deltoid muscle, middle belly; Supraspinatus tendon; Bicipital groove; Inferior glenohumeral ligament, anterior band; Coracobrachialis muscle and biceps muscle, short head; Biceps muscle, long head

Middle image labels (left): Trapezius; Clavicle; Supraspinatus muscle; Suprascapular a. and n. in spinoglenoid notch; Glenoid; Subscapularis muscle; Coracobrachialis muscle and biceps muscle, short head

Middle image labels (right): Coracoacromial ligament; Lesser tuberosity; Subscapularis tendon; Deltoid muscle; Biceps muscle, long head

Bottom image labels (left): Trapezius muscle; Clavicle; Supraspinatus muscle; Superior glenoid; Subscapularis muscle and tendon; Coracobrachialis muscle and biceps muscle, short head

Bottom image labels (right): Coracoacromial ligament; Subscapularis tendon; Deltoid muscle; Biceps muscle, long head; Cephalic vein

(Top) The long head of the biceps tendon is located in the bicipital groove. It originates from the supraglenoid tubercle and labrum. The long head of the biceps helps prevent humeral head impingement on the acromion during deltoid contraction. **(Middle)** The subscapularis tendon inserts on the lesser tuberosity. The teres major and latissimus dorsi tendons insert just inferior to the subscapularis tendon. **(Bottom)** The deltoid and trapezius muscles attach to the scapular spine, lateral 1/3 of clavicle and acromion. Anterior compartment muscles are innervated by the musculocutaneous nerve.

Shoulder MR Atlas

CORONAL OBLIQUE T1 MR, RIGHT SHOULDER

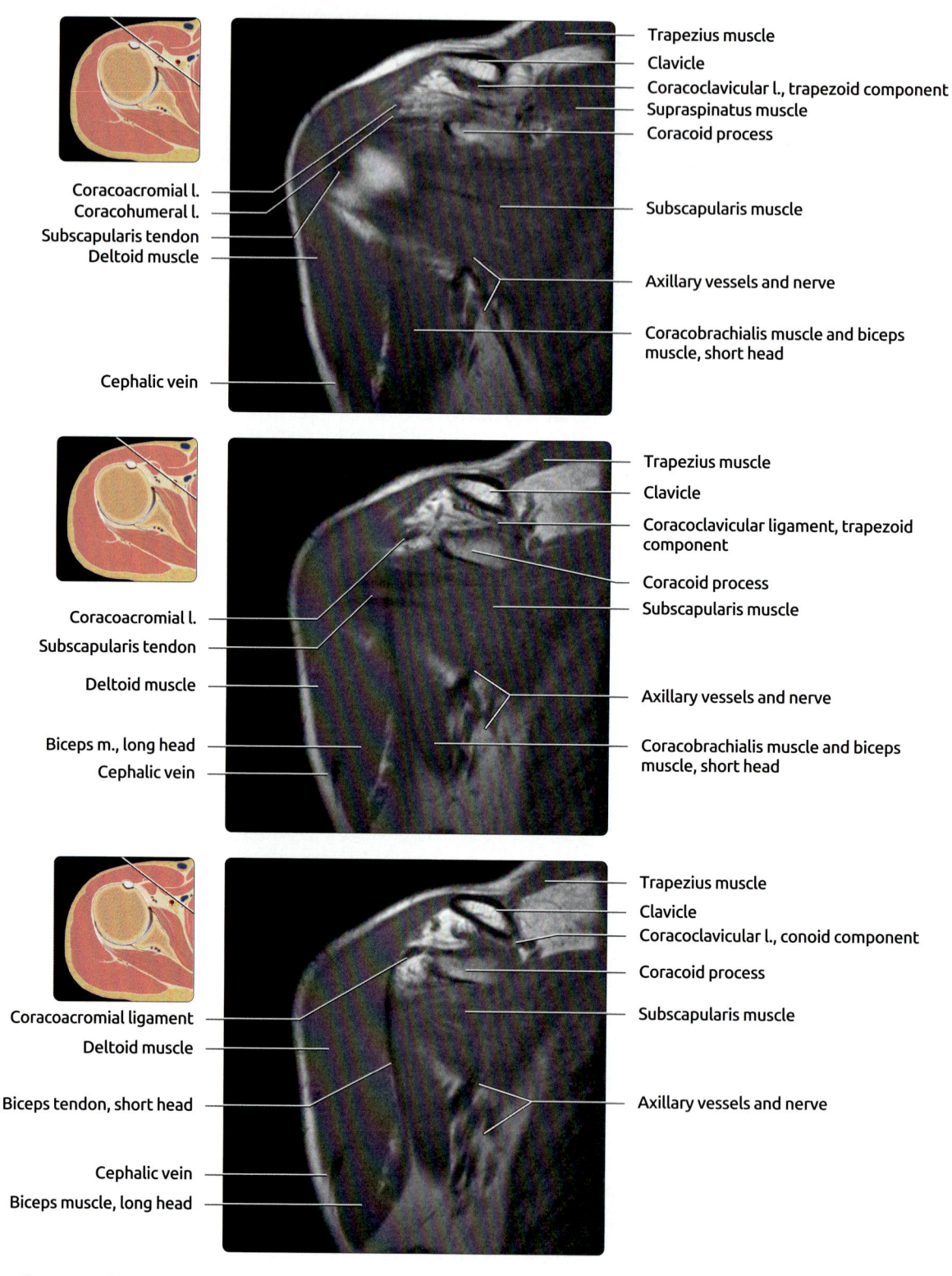

Labels (top image):
- Coracoacromial l.
- Coracohumeral l.
- Subscapularis tendon
- Deltoid muscle
- Cephalic vein
- Trapezius muscle
- Clavicle
- Coracoclavicular l., trapezoid component
- Supraspinatus muscle
- Coracoid process
- Subscapularis muscle
- Axillary vessels and nerve
- Coracobrachialis muscle and biceps muscle, short head

Labels (middle image):
- Coracoacromial l.
- Subscapularis tendon
- Deltoid muscle
- Biceps m., long head
- Cephalic vein
- Trapezius muscle
- Clavicle
- Coracoclavicular ligament, trapezoid component
- Coracoid process
- Subscapularis muscle
- Axillary vessels and nerve
- Coracobrachialis muscle and biceps muscle, short head

Labels (bottom image):
- Coracoacromial ligament
- Deltoid muscle
- Biceps tendon, short head
- Cephalic vein
- Biceps muscle, long head
- Trapezius muscle
- Clavicle
- Coracoclavicular l., conoid component
- Coracoid process
- Subscapularis muscle
- Axillary vessels and nerve

(Top) The axillary artery becomes the brachial artery below the level of the teres major muscle. On this image, the bundle still consists of the axillary neurovascular structures. The brachial artery (not shown on this image) will course along the medial border of the coracobrachialis muscle. **(Middle)** The coracoclavicular ligament helps maintain clavicular alignment with the acromion. The ligament has trapezoid and conoid portions. The trapezoid portion has an oblique lateral course from the medial horizontal coracoid process to the lateral end of the clavicle. The conoid portion has a near vertical course. **(Bottom)** The tip of the coracoid process is the site of origin for the coracobrachialis muscle, medially, and the short head of biceps muscle, laterally.

Shoulder MR Atlas

CORONAL OBLIQUE T1 MR, LEFT SHOULDER

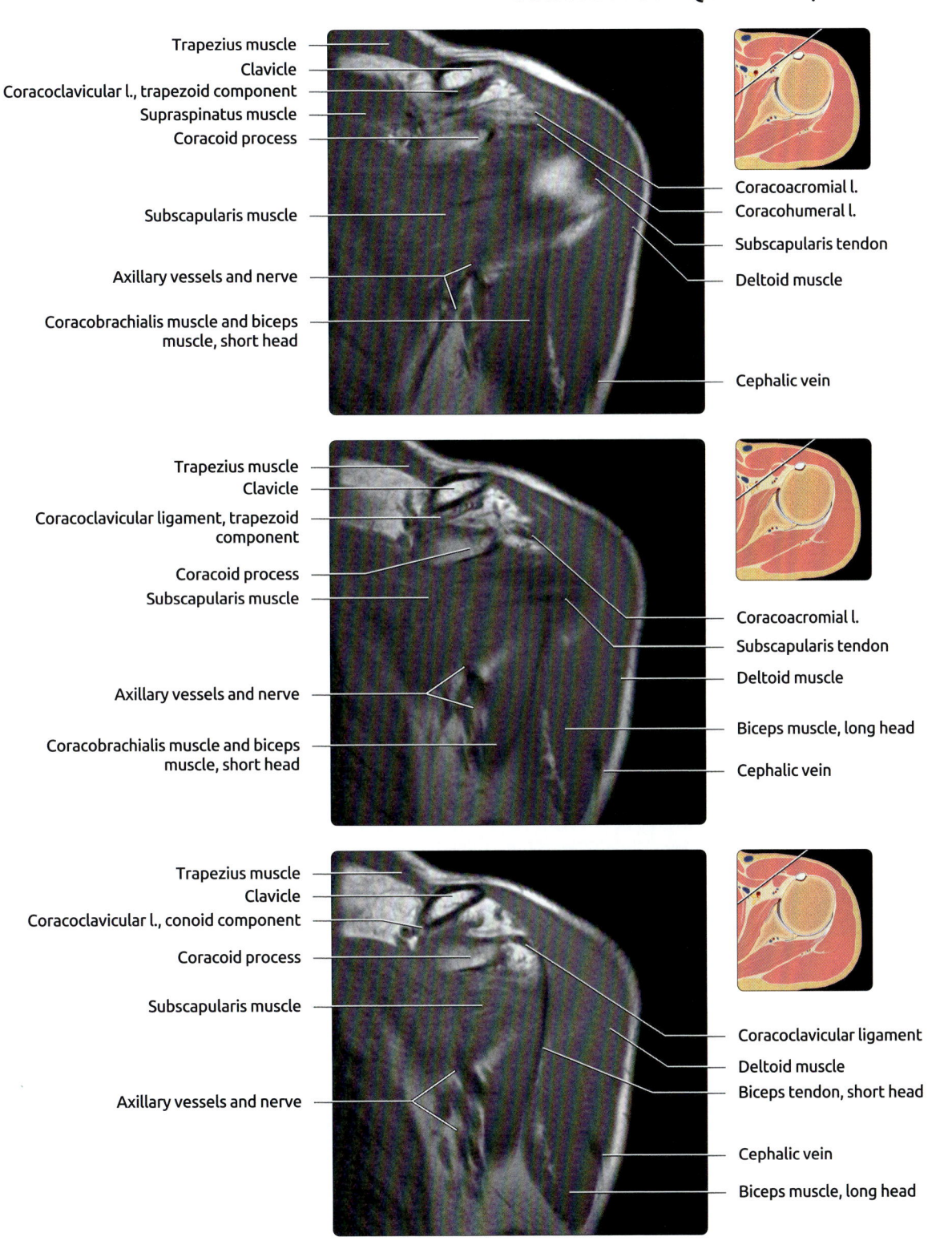

Labels (top image):
- Trapezius muscle
- Clavicle
- Coracoclavicular l., trapezoid component
- Supraspinatus muscle
- Coracoid process
- Subscapularis muscle
- Axillary vessels and nerve
- Coracobrachialis muscle and biceps muscle, short head
- Coracoacromial l.
- Coracohumeral l.
- Subscapularis tendon
- Deltoid muscle
- Cephalic vein

Labels (middle image):
- Trapezius muscle
- Clavicle
- Coracoclavicular ligament, trapezoid component
- Coracoid process
- Subscapularis muscle
- Axillary vessels and nerve
- Coracobrachialis muscle and biceps muscle, short head
- Coracoacromial l.
- Subscapularis tendon
- Deltoid muscle
- Biceps muscle, long head
- Cephalic vein

Labels (bottom image):
- Trapezius muscle
- Clavicle
- Coracoclavicular l., conoid component
- Coracoid process
- Subscapularis muscle
- Axillary vessels and nerve
- Coracoclavicular ligament
- Deltoid muscle
- Biceps tendon, short head
- Cephalic vein
- Biceps muscle, long head

(Top) The axillary artery becomes the brachial artery below the level of the teres major muscle. On this image, the bundle still consists of the axillary neurovascular structures. The brachial artery (not shown on this image) will course along the medial border of the coracobrachialis muscle. **(Middle)** The coracoclavicular ligament helps maintain clavicular alignment with the acromion. The ligament has trapezoid and conoid portions. The trapezoid portion has an oblique lateral course from the medial horizontal coracoid process to the lateral end of the clavicle. The conoid portion has a near vertical course. **(Bottom)** The tip of the coracoid process is the site of origin for the coracobrachialis muscle, medially, and the short head of biceps muscle, laterally.

Shoulder MR Atlas

SAGITTAL OBLIQUE T1 MR, RIGHT SHOULDER

Top image labels:
- Deltoid muscle
- Infraspinatus muscle
- Teres minor muscle
- Teres major muscle
- Trapezius muscle
- Scapular spine
- Supraspinatus muscle
- Serratus anterior muscle
- Subscapularis muscle
- Lung
- Latissimus dorsi muscle

Middle image labels:
- Deltoid muscle
- Infraspinatus muscle
- Teres minor muscle
- Teres major muscle
- Trapezius muscle
- Scapular spine
- Supraspinatus muscle
- Serratus anterior muscle
- Subscapularis muscle
- Lung
- Latissimus dorsi muscle

Bottom image labels:
- Scapular spine
- Deltoid muscle
- Infraspinatus muscle
- Teres minor muscle
- Teres major muscle
- Triceps muscle, long head
- Trapezius muscle
- Supraspinatus muscle
- Suprascapular vessels
- Serratus anterior muscle
- Subscapularis muscle
- Lung
- Latissimus dorsi muscle

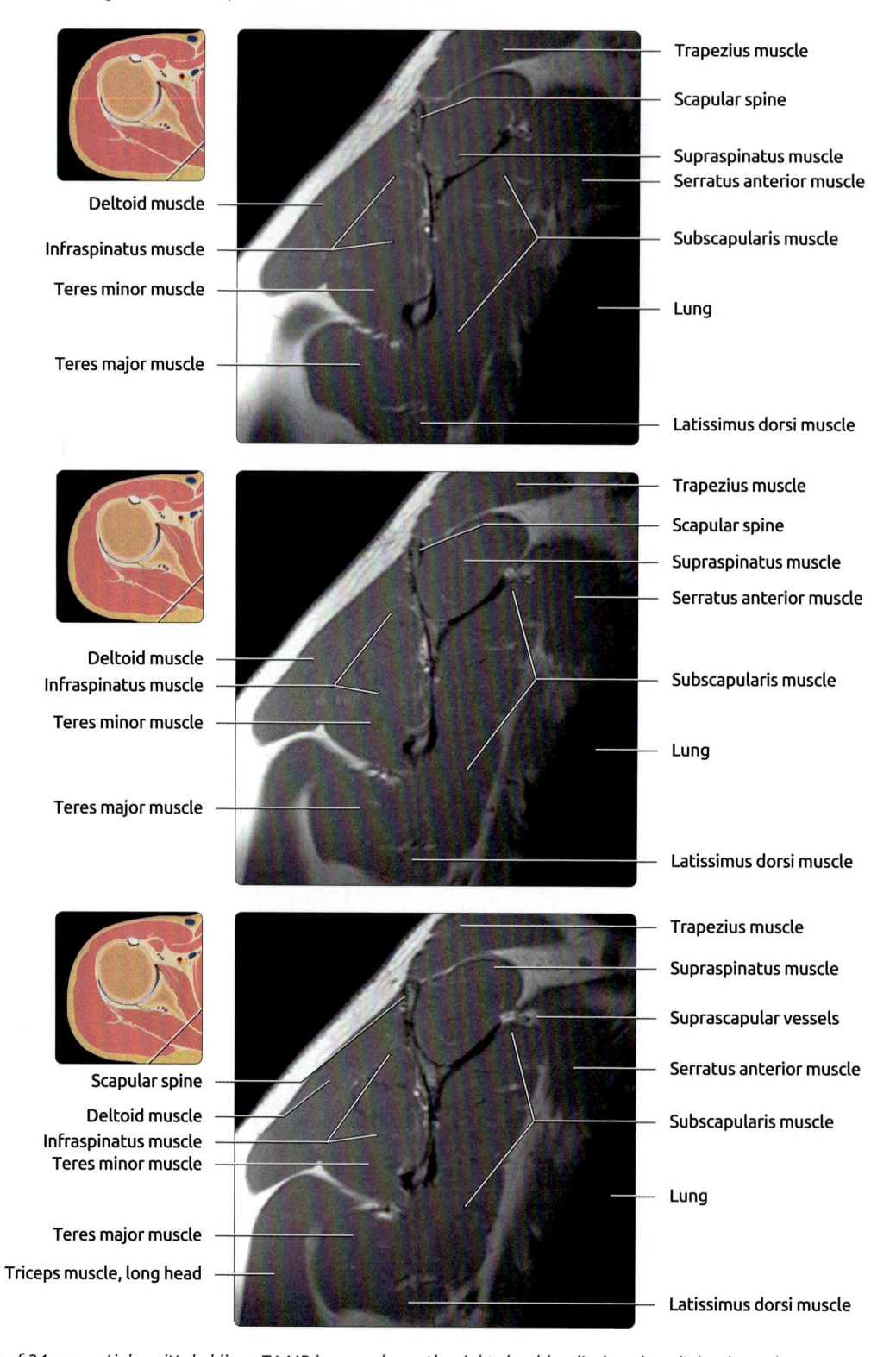

(**Top**) *First of 24 sequential sagittal oblique T1 MR images shows the right shoulder displayed medial to lateral. Images were obtained with a shoulder coil on a 3T MR scanner. Image is far medial, including a portion of the lateral lung and chest wall.* (**Middle**) *The latissimus dorsi muscle wraps around the inferior aspect of the teres major muscle. These 2 muscles can be difficult to differentiate as separate structures. Each courses superiorly and laterally to insert on the crest of the lesser tuberosity.* (**Bottom**) *The rotator cuff muscles consist of the supraspinatus, infraspinatus, teres minor, and subscapularis. All of the rotator cuff muscles originate from the scapula.*

Shoulder MR Atlas

SAGITTAL OBLIQUE T1 MR, RIGHT SHOULDER

Top image labels (left): Trapezius muscle; Supraspinatus muscle; Omohyoid muscle; Scapular spine; Deltoid muscle; Infraspinatus muscle; Teres minor muscle; Teres major muscle; Triceps muscle, long head

Top image labels (right): Serratus anterior muscle; Subscapularis muscle; Lung; Latissimus dorsi muscle

Middle image labels (left): Trapezius muscle; Scapular spine; Supraspinatus muscle; Supraspinous fossa; Suprascapular branch vessels; Infraspinatus muscle; Deltoid muscle; Teres minor muscle; Triceps muscle, long head; Teres major muscle; Latissimus dorsi muscle

Middle image labels (right): Subscapularis muscle; Scapula; Rib; Lung

Bottom image labels (left): Scapular spine; Supraspinatus muscle; Infraspinatus muscle; Deltoid muscle, posterior belly; Teres minor muscle; Teres major muscle; Triceps muscle, long head

Bottom image labels (right): Brachial plexus; Axillary artery and vein; Subscapularis muscle; Lymph node; Latissimus dorsi muscle; Lung

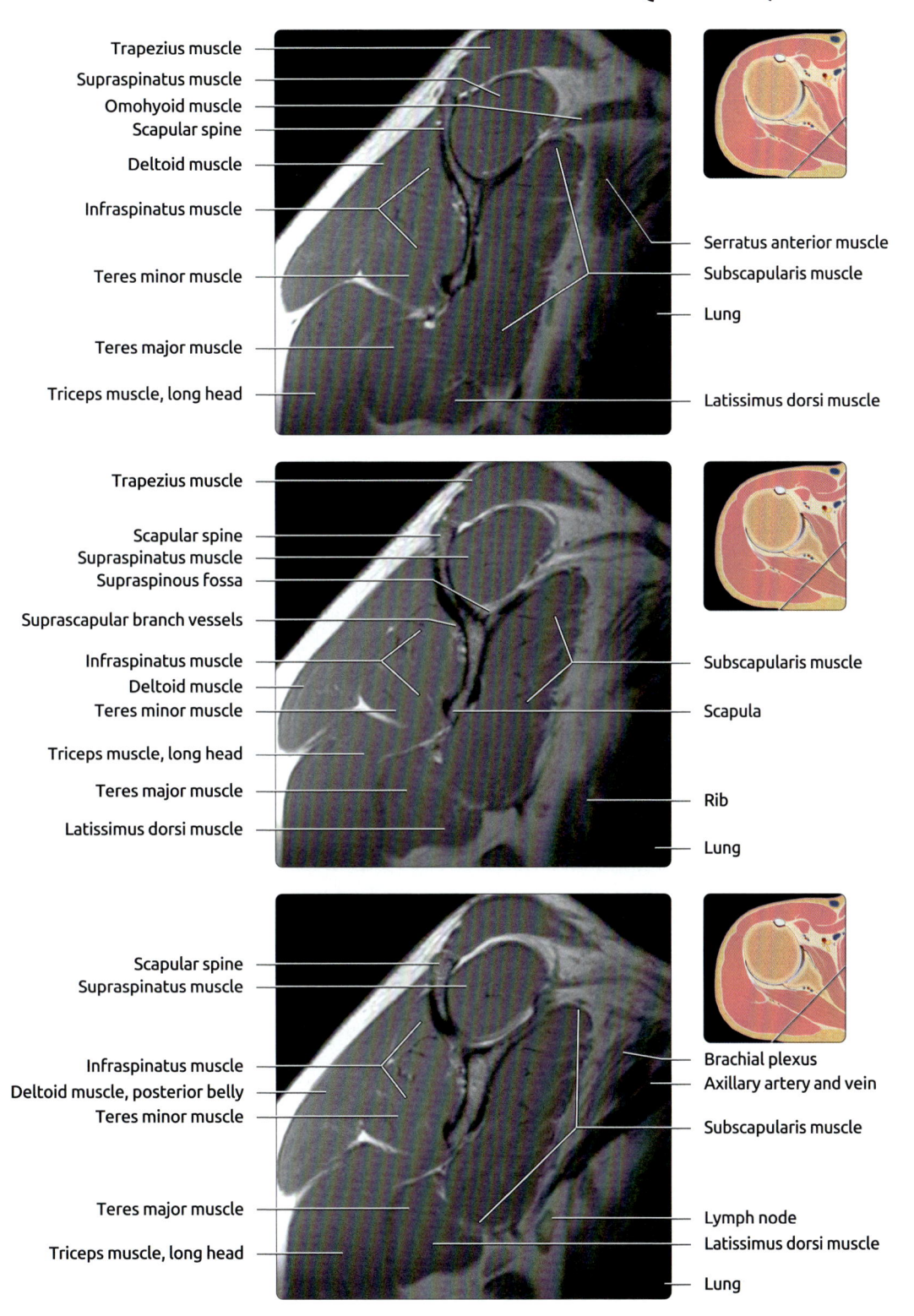

(Top) The omohyoid muscle originates from the superior border of the scapula. It has an inferior belly and a superior belly. The superior portion inserts on the lower border of the hyoid bone. **(Middle)** The scapula has a Y-shaped configuration due to the posterior extent of the scapular spine. The supraspinatus muscle is contained entirely within the crux of the Y and should roughly fill this area unless the muscle is atrophied. **(Bottom)** A portion of the trapezius muscle is seen at the superior aspect of the shoulder. The trapezius inserts on the superior border of the lateral clavicle, the medial border of the acromion, and the superior border of the scapular spine. The deltoid muscle originates at the same osseous sites, adjacent to the trapezius, but on the opposite border of each of the bones (inferior border of lateral clavicle, lateral border of acromion, inferior border of scapular spine).

SAGITTAL OBLIQUE T1 MR, RIGHT SHOULDER

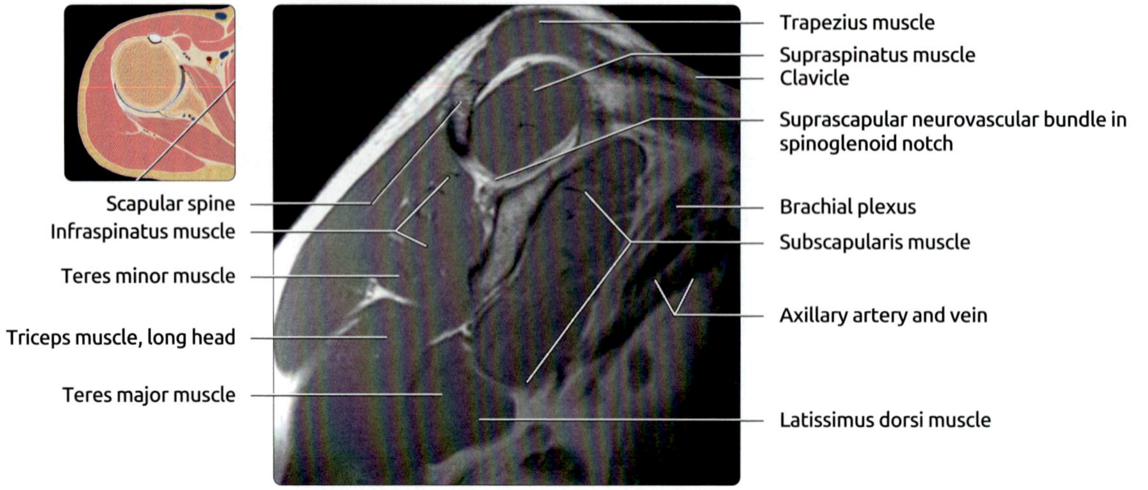
Trapezius muscle
Supraspinatus muscle
Clavicle
Suprascapular neurovascular bundle in spinoglenoid notch
Brachial plexus
Subscapularis muscle
Axillary artery and vein
Latissimus dorsi muscle
Scapular spine
Infraspinatus muscle
Teres minor muscle
Triceps muscle, long head
Teres major muscle

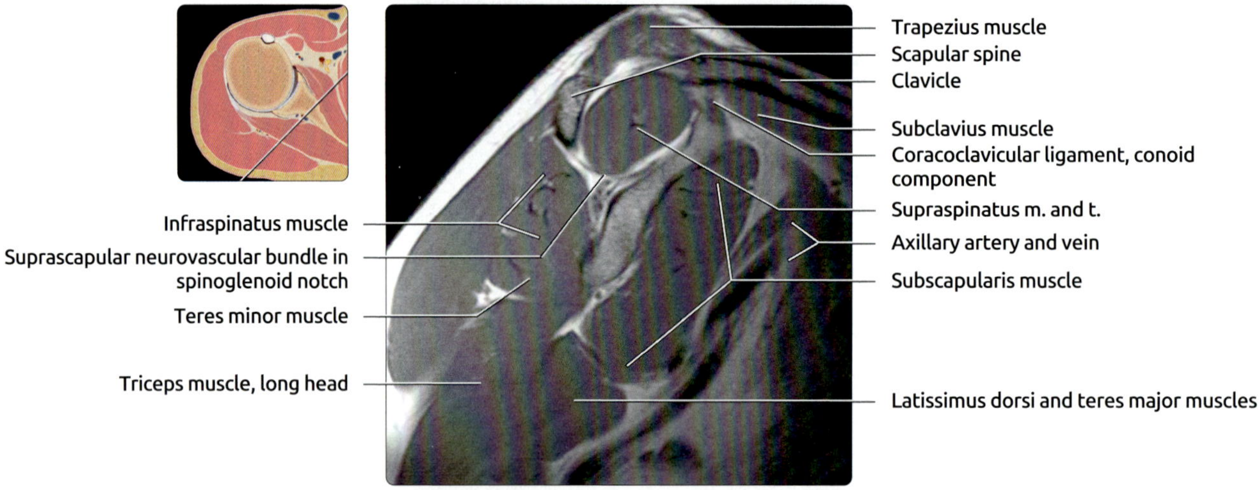
Trapezius muscle
Scapular spine
Clavicle
Subclavius muscle
Coracoclavicular ligament, conoid component
Supraspinatus m. and t.
Axillary artery and vein
Subscapularis muscle
Latissimus dorsi and teres major muscles
Infraspinatus muscle
Suprascapular neurovascular bundle in spinoglenoid notch
Teres minor muscle
Triceps muscle, long head

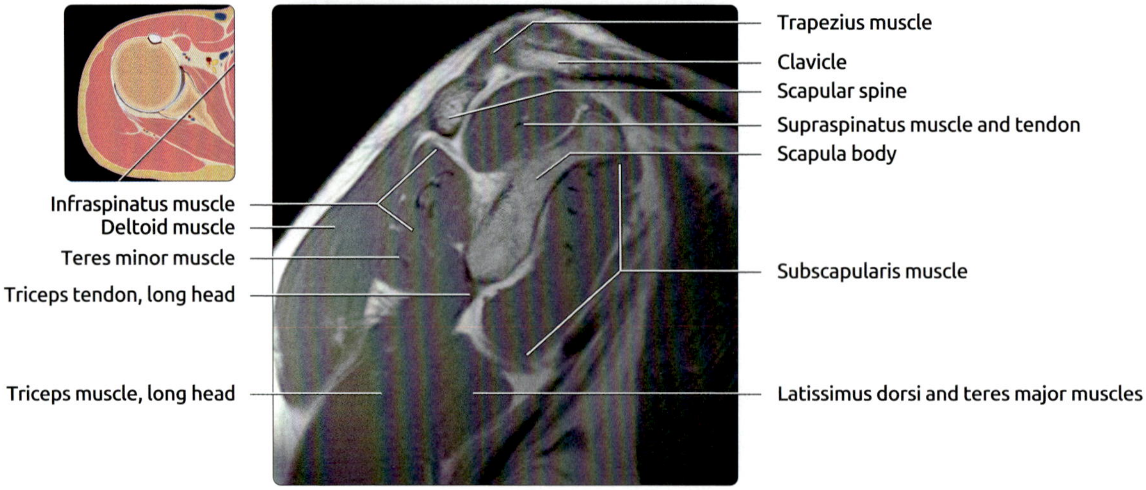
Trapezius muscle
Clavicle
Scapular spine
Supraspinatus muscle and tendon
Scapula body
Subscapularis muscle
Latissimus dorsi and teres major muscles
Infraspinatus muscle
Deltoid muscle
Teres minor muscle
Triceps tendon, long head
Triceps muscle, long head

(Top) *The subscapularis muscle fills the subscapular fossa of the scapula.* **(Middle)** *The infraspinatus and teres minor muscles are located below the scapular spine. The infraspinatus muscle is the larger and is located more superiorly than teres minor.* **(Bottom)** *The supraspinatus, subscapularis, teres minor, and infraspinatus (clockwise) continue to course laterally. The tendons of the supraspinatus and infraspinatus will conjoin as they reach the lateral aspect of the humeral head.*

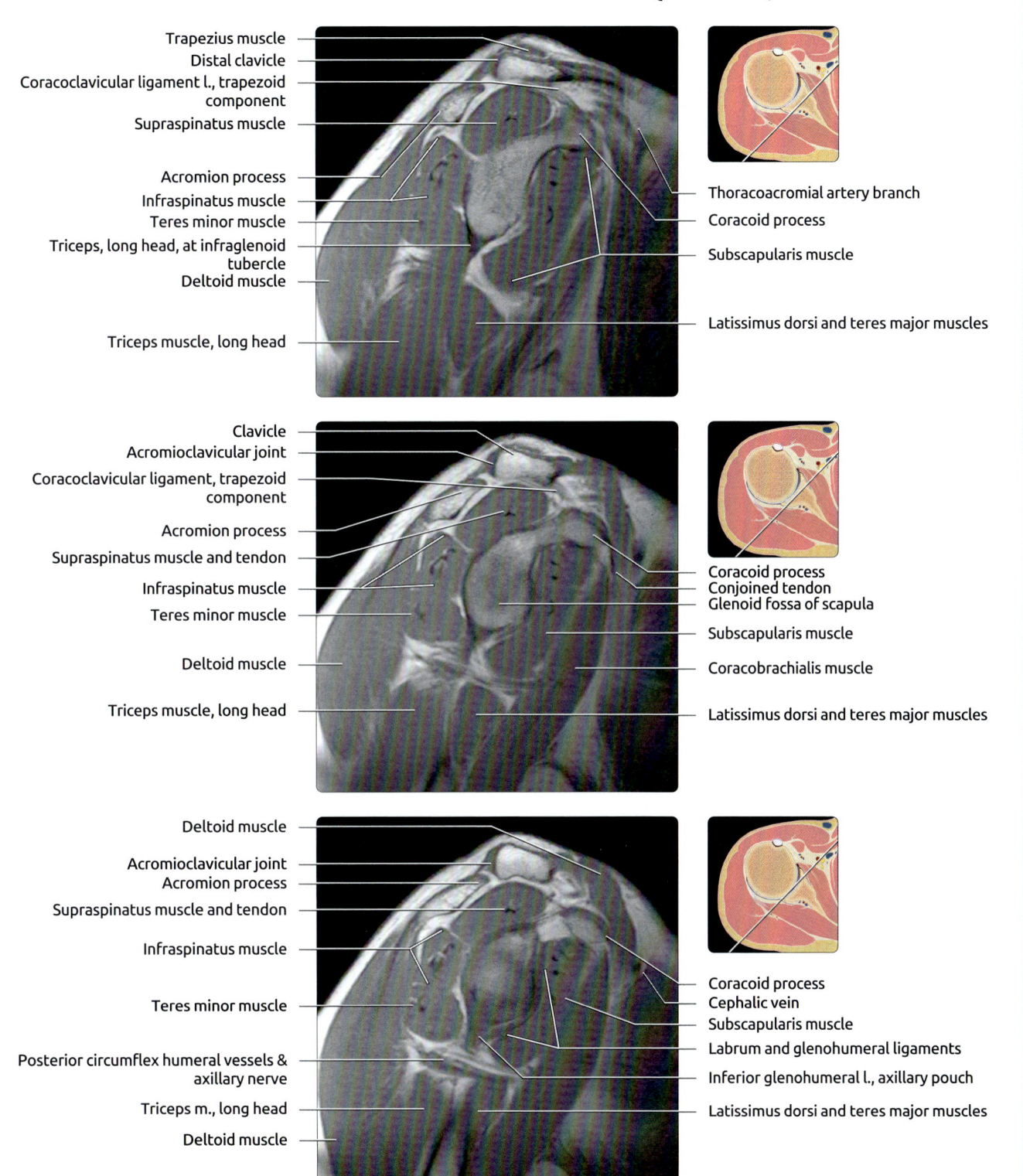

Shoulder MR Atlas

SAGITTAL OBLIQUE T1 MR, RIGHT SHOULDER

Top image labels:
- Trapezius muscle
- Distal clavicle
- Coracoclavicular ligament l., trapezoid component
- Supraspinatus muscle
- Acromion process
- Infraspinatus muscle
- Teres minor muscle
- Triceps, long head, at infraglenoid tubercle
- Deltoid muscle
- Triceps muscle, long head
- Thoracoacromial artery branch
- Coracoid process
- Subscapularis muscle
- Latissimus dorsi and teres major muscles

Middle image labels:
- Clavicle
- Acromioclavicular joint
- Coracoclavicular ligament, trapezoid component
- Acromion process
- Supraspinatus muscle and tendon
- Infraspinatus muscle
- Teres minor muscle
- Deltoid muscle
- Triceps muscle, long head
- Coracoid process
- Conjoined tendon
- Glenoid fossa of scapula
- Subscapularis muscle
- Coracobrachialis muscle
- Latissimus dorsi and teres major muscles

Bottom image labels:
- Deltoid muscle
- Acromioclavicular joint
- Acromion process
- Supraspinatus muscle and tendon
- Infraspinatus muscle
- Teres minor muscle
- Posterior circumflex humeral vessels & axillary nerve
- Triceps m., long head
- Deltoid muscle
- Coracoid process
- Cephalic vein
- Subscapularis muscle
- Labrum and glenohumeral ligaments
- Inferior glenohumeral l., axillary pouch
- Latissimus dorsi and teres major muscles

(Top) The scapular spine ends at the acromion process. The acromioclavicular joint is becoming visible. The neurovascular bundle lies along the anterior surface of the subscapularis muscle. *(Middle)* Image is at the level of the glenoid fossa of the scapula. The dark surrounding rim of the glenoid labrum is becoming visible. The coracoid process is the origin of the coracobrachialis and short head of the biceps tendon. *(Bottom)* The glenohumeral ligaments are seen as low signal bands of tissue surrounding the anterior, inferior, and posteroinferior aspects of the shoulder joint. The glenohumeral ligaments strengthen the joint capsule.

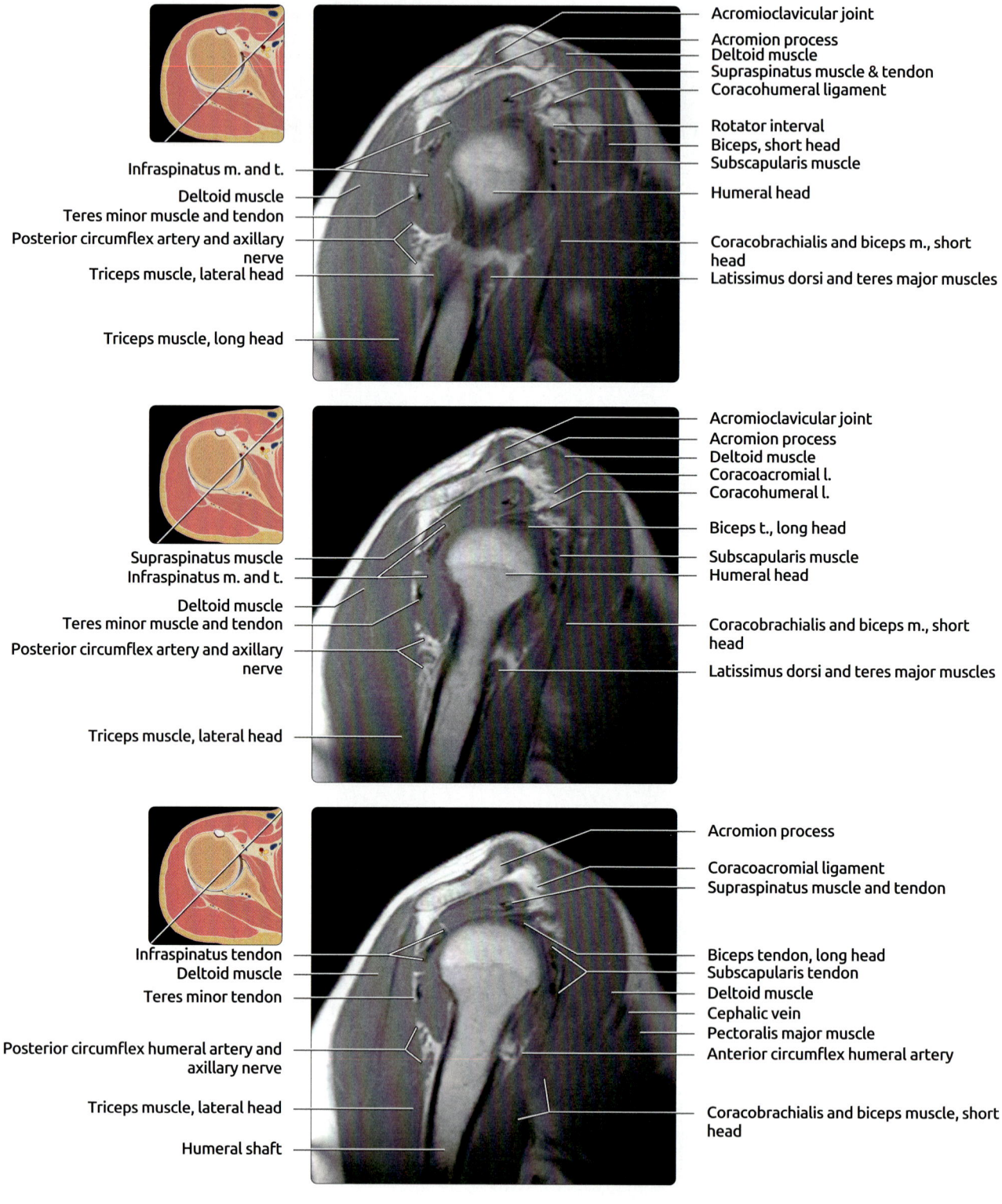

Shoulder MR Atlas

SAGITTAL OBLIQUE T1 MR, RIGHT SHOULDER

Top image labels (left):
- Infraspinatus m. and t.
- Deltoid muscle
- Teres minor muscle and tendon
- Posterior circumflex artery and axillary nerve
- Triceps muscle, lateral head
- Triceps muscle, long head

Top image labels (right):
- Acromioclavicular joint
- Acromion process
- Deltoid muscle
- Supraspinatus muscle & tendon
- Coracohumeral ligament
- Rotator interval
- Biceps, short head
- Subscapularis muscle
- Humeral head
- Coracobrachialis and biceps m., short head
- Latissimus dorsi and teres major muscles

Middle image labels (left):
- Supraspinatus muscle
- Infraspinatus m. and t.
- Deltoid muscle
- Teres minor muscle and tendon
- Posterior circumflex artery and axillary nerve
- Triceps muscle, lateral head

Middle image labels (right):
- Acromioclavicular joint
- Acromion process
- Deltoid muscle
- Coracoacromial l.
- Coracohumeral l.
- Biceps t., long head
- Subscapularis muscle
- Humeral head
- Coracobrachialis and biceps m., short head
- Latissimus dorsi and teres major muscles

Bottom image labels (left):
- Infraspinatus tendon
- Deltoid muscle
- Teres minor tendon
- Posterior circumflex humeral artery and axillary nerve
- Triceps muscle, lateral head
- Humeral shaft

Bottom image labels (right):
- Acromion process
- Coracoacromial ligament
- Supraspinatus muscle and tendon
- Biceps tendon, long head
- Subscapularis tendon
- Deltoid muscle
- Cephalic vein
- Pectoralis major muscle
- Anterior circumflex humeral artery
- Coracobrachialis and biceps muscle, short head

(**Top**) *Image is at the medial border of the humeral head. The posterior circumflex humeral artery winds around the neck of the humerus to anastomose with the anterior circumflex humeral artery.* (**Middle**) *The rotator interval is a triangular space bordered superiorly by the supraspinatus tendon anterior margin, inferiorly by the subscapularis tendon superior border, medially by the coracoid base, and laterally by the long head of the biceps tendon bicipital groove.* (**Bottom**) *The long head of the biceps tendon arises from the supraglenoid tuberosity at the upper margin of the glenoid cavity. On this image, it is seen coursing distally over the humeral head, surrounded by a synovial membrane sheath. The tendon traverses the capsule through an opening near the intertubercular groove.*

Shoulder MR Atlas

SAGITTAL OBLIQUE T1 MR, RIGHT SHOULDER

Top image labels:
- Acromion process
- Coracoacromial ligament
- Supraspinatus anterior direct tendon
- Supraspinatus posterior oblique tendon
- Infraspinatus tendon
- Deltoid muscle
- Teres minor tendon
- Posterior circumflex humeral artery and axillary nerve
- Triceps muscle, lateral head
- Biceps t., long head
- Subscapularis tendon
- Deltoid muscle
- Anterior circumflex humeral vessels
- Pectoralis major muscle

Middle image labels:
- Acromion process
- Coracoacromial ligament
- Supraspinatus tendon, direct component
- Supraspinatus tendon, posterior oblique component
- Infraspinatus tendon
- Deltoid muscle
- Teres minor tendon
- Posterior circumflex humeral artery and axillary nerve
- Triceps muscle, lateral head
- Subscapularis tendon
- Deltoid muscle
- Anterior circumflex humeral artery
- Pectoralis major muscle

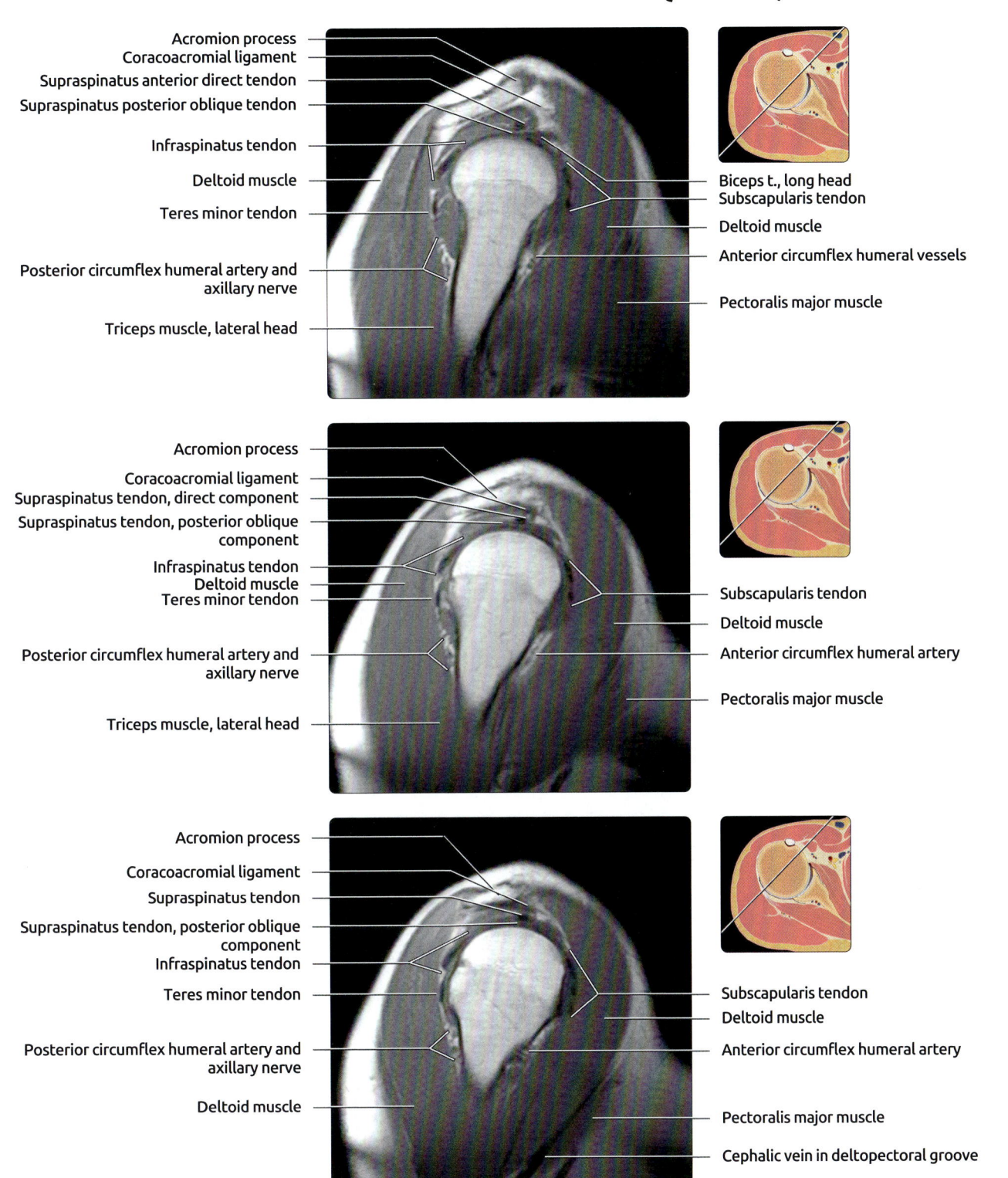

Bottom image labels:
- Acromion process
- Coracoacromial ligament
- Supraspinatus tendon
- Supraspinatus tendon, posterior oblique component
- Infraspinatus tendon
- Teres minor tendon
- Posterior circumflex humeral artery and axillary nerve
- Deltoid muscle
- Subscapularis tendon
- Deltoid muscle
- Anterior circumflex humeral artery
- Pectoralis major muscle
- Cephalic vein in deltopectoral groove

(Top) At the level of the midhumeral head, the deltoid muscle covers the superficial aspect of the shoulder. **(Middle)** Evaluation of the morphologic type of acromion is best done on the 1st image lateral to the acromioclavicular joint. **(Bottom)** The rotator cuff is predominantly tendinous as it passes toward the lateral aspect of the humeral head. The tendons are beginning to fuse with each other and the joint capsule.

Shoulder MR Atlas

SAGITTAL OBLIQUE T1 MR, RIGHT SHOULDER

Supraspinatus tendon and joint capsule

Infraspinatus tendon

Teres minor tendon

Posterior circumflex artery and axillary nerve

Deltoid muscle

Subscapularis tendon

Anterior circumflex humeral artery

Supraspinatus tendon and joint capsule

Infraspinatus tendon

Teres minor tendon

Posterior circumflex artery and axillary nerve

Deltoid muscle

Subscapularis tendon

Lesser tuberosity

Supraspinatus tendon

Infraspinatus tendon

Teres minor tendon

Subscapularis tendon

Biceps tendon, long head

Deltoid muscle

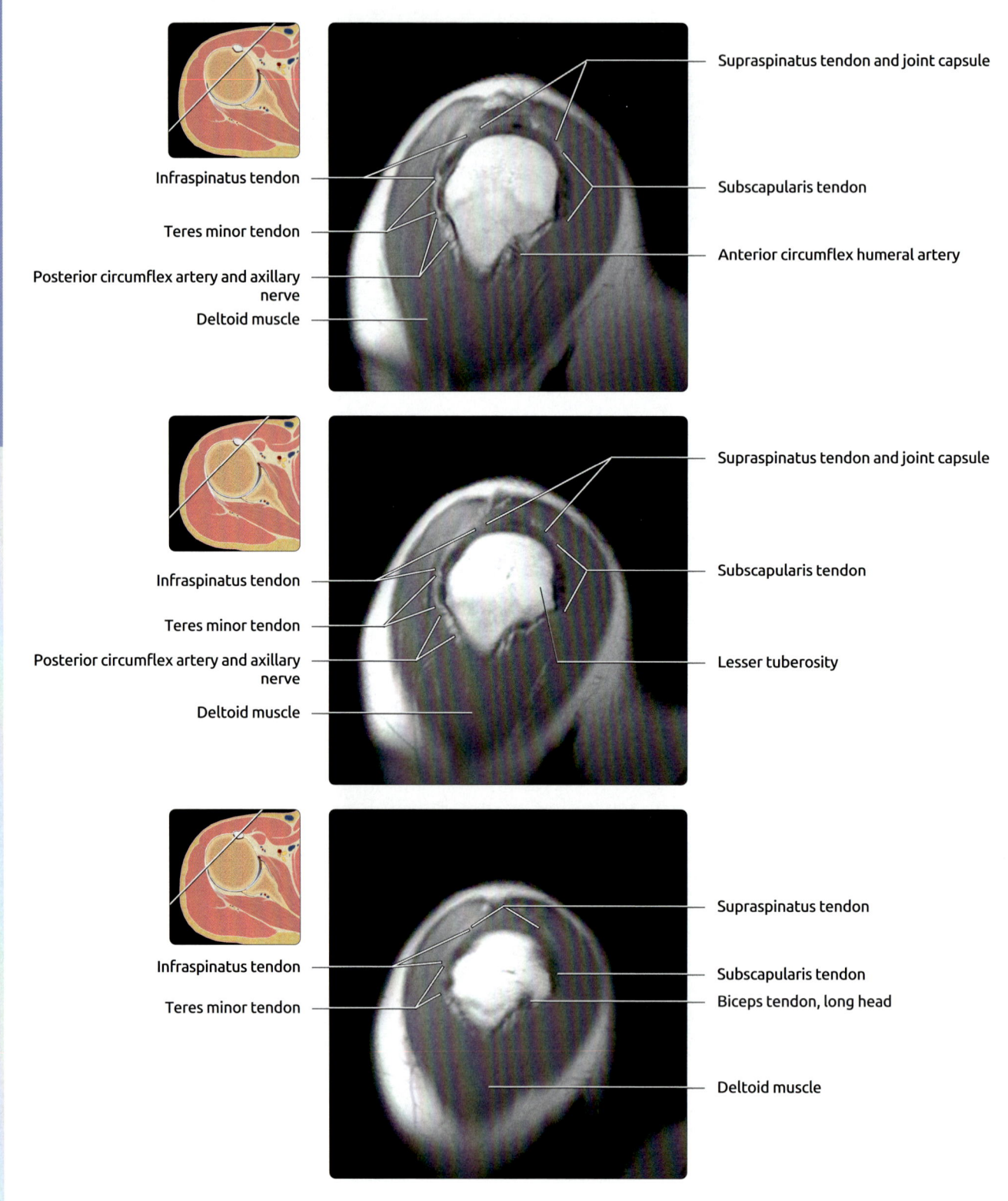

(Top) *Image is nearing the lateral aspect of the humeral head. The rotator cuff tendons are forming a solid arc of tissue over the humeral head as they continue to course laterally. On this T1-weighted sequence, the rotator cuff tendons have higher signal than the normally very low tendon signal due to magic angle artifact. Normal tendon signal can be confirmed with sequences acquired using intermediate or long TE.* **(Middle)** *The rotator cuff tendons are approaching their insertions on the greater and lesser tuberosities.* **(Bottom)** *The subscapularis tendon inserts on the lesser tuberosity and forms the roof of the bicipital groove.*

Shoulder MR Atlas

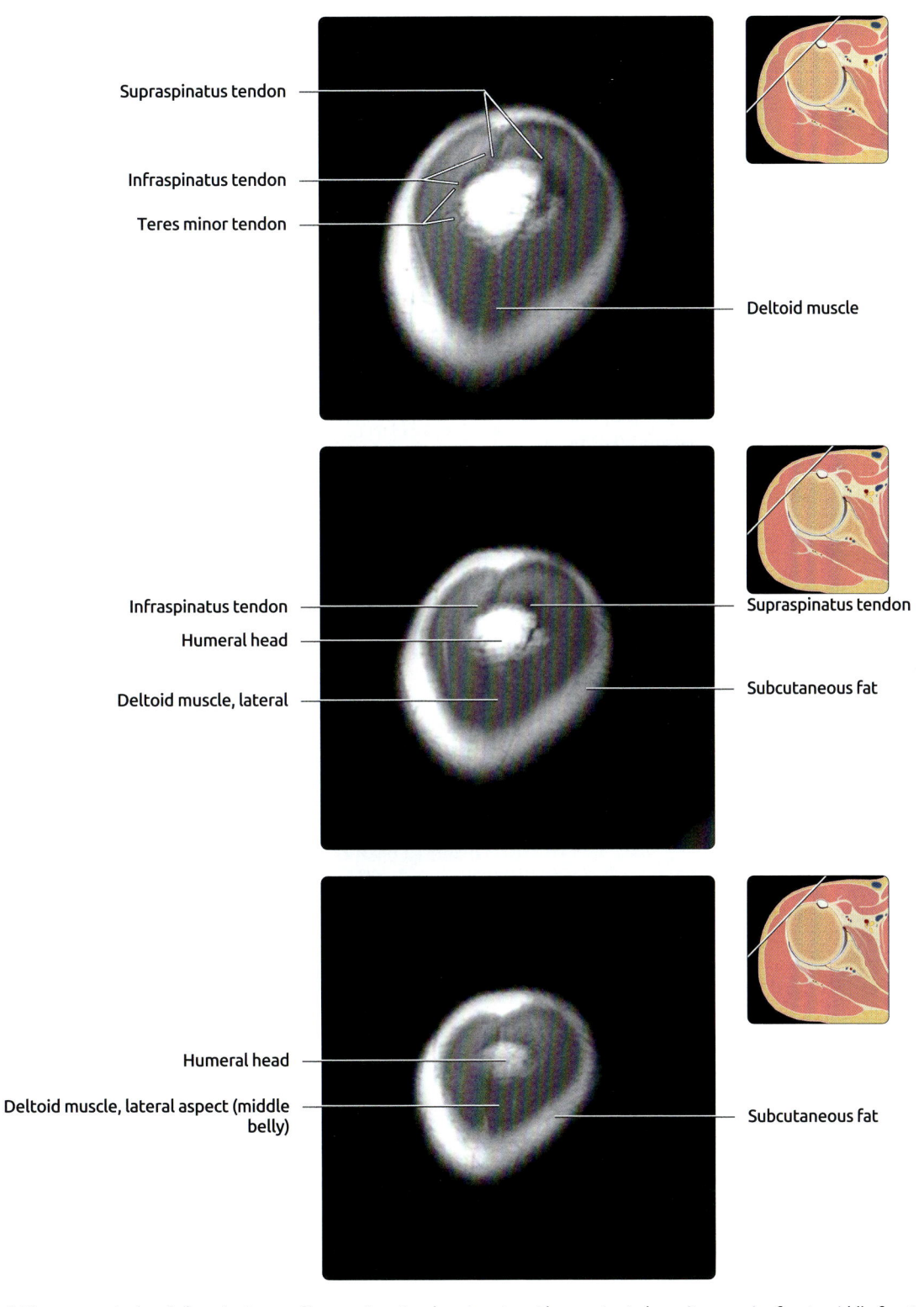

SAGITTAL OBLIQUE T1 MR, RIGHT SHOULDER

(Top) The supraspinatus, infraspinatus, and teres minor tendons insert on the greater tuberosity superior facet, middle facet, and inferior facet, respectively. **(Middle)** Small portions of the supraspinatus and infraspinatus tendons are still visible inserting on the greater tuberosity. **(Bottom)** The far lateral, superficial aspect of the shoulder is entirely covered by the middle belly of deltoid muscle.

Shoulder Abduction-External Rotation (ABER) Plane

TERMINOLOGY

Abbreviations
- Abduction external rotation (ABER)

IMAGING ANATOMY

Overview
- Optional patient position for MR arthrography

Anatomy Relationships
- **Bicipital groove rotated to lie at superior aspect of humeral head**
  - Externally rotated and elevated
  - Above spinoglenoid notch
- **Inferior glenohumeral ligament is pulled taut**
  - Exerts traction on anterior labral ligamentous complex
  - Allows intraarticular contrast to flow into labral tears that may be obscured by compression in normal externally rotated position
- **Coracoid process tip indicates approximately 2:00-3:00 position of anterior labrum**
- Inferior images show the 5:00-7:00 position of labrum, depending on alignment

Internal Contents
- **Articular surface of rotator cuff and rotator cuff "footprint"**
  - Relieved of tension, may kink slightly
  - **Undersurface tears and fraying fill with contrast**
    - Subtle tears/fraying of supraspinatus, infraspinatus, teres minor tendons may be seen with ABER when not visualized in standard adducted external rotation view
- **Labrum**
  - **Anterior labrum under tension**
  - Posterior labrum in contact with articular surface of rotator cuff
- Osteochondral surfaces, particularly of posterosuperior humeral head and inferior glenoid may be seen to better advantage

ANATOMY IMAGING ISSUES

Imaging Recommendations
- High field strength MR scanner
- Flexible shoulder coil or phased array coil

Imaging Approaches
- Standard MR arthrogram injection performed
  - 12 ml dilute gadopentetate dimeglumine (2 mmol/L) mixed with iodinated contrast, Marcaine, & epinephrine according to institutional preference
- Indirect MR arthrogram IV injection also useful when direct injection not performed
- **Arm abducted greater than 90°**, unless imaging with open MR system
- **Hand placed on top of head, over head, or behind neck**
  - Elbow flexed
- Scout view obtained in coronal plane
- **Images aligned with shaft of humerus**
  - Humerus long axis images
  - Results on oblique axial images through joint
  - (Oblique sagittal images with respect to body)

Imaging Pitfalls
- **Improper positioning**
  - Patients unwilling or unable to hold this position due to pain or apprehension
  - Unfamiliar position for technologists
    - Requires extra time positioning patient and coil
- **Improper alignment of axial images**
  - **Images need to be prescribed along shaft of humerus from orthogonal coronal plane scout**
  - This nonstandard alignment may be difficult to achieve when not part of routine study
- **Wrap artifact**
  - Saturation band can be placed over medial chest wall
- **Inadequate signal**
  - Clamshell coil vs. multi-element array
  - Malposition of array elements
- **Meniscoid (type 3) labrum**
  - Contrast extends into normal gap between meniscoid labrum and cartilage

CLINICAL IMPLICATIONS

Clinical Importance
- **ABER position for MR imaging improves visualization of several regions**
  - **Anterior and posterior labrum**
    - Especially nondetached tears of anterior labrum
  - **Anterior capsular attachment**
  - **Inferior glenohumeral ligament**
  - **Undersurface of rotator cuff**
    - When differentiation between tendinosis and partial thickness tear is clinically important
    - Throwing athletes
  - **Intrasubstance or horizontal component tears of rotator cuff**
  - **Coracohumeral ligament**

SELECTED REFERENCES

1. Herold T et al: Indirect MR arthrography of the shoulder: use of abduction and external rotation to detect full- and partial-thickness tears of the supraspinatus tendon. Radiology. 2006
2. Lee SY et al: Horizontal component of partial-thickness tears of rotator cuff: imaging characteristics and comparison of ABER view with oblique coronal view at MR arthrography initial results. Radiology. 224(2):470-6, 2002
3. Choi JA et al: Comparison between conventional MR arthrography and abduction and external rotation MR arthrography in revealing tears of the antero-inferior glenoid labrum. Korean J Radiol. 2(4):216-21, 2001
4. Kwak SM et al: Glenohumeral joint: comparison of shoulder positions at MR arthrography. Radiology. 208(2):375-80, 1998
5. Wintzell G et al: Indirect MR arthrography of anterior shoulder instability in the ABER and the apprehension test positions: a prospective comparative study of two different shoulder positions during MRI using intravenous gadodiamide contrast for enhancement of the joint fluid. Skeletal Radiol. 27(9):488-94, 1998
6. Cvitanic O et al: Using abduction and external rotation of the shoulder to increase the sensitivity of MR arthrography in revealing tears of the anterior glenoid labrum. AJR Am J Roentgenol. 169(3):837-44, 1997
7. Tirman PF et al: MR arthrographic depiction of tears of the rotator cuff: benefit of abduction and external rotation of the arm. Radiology. 192(3):851-6, 1994

Shoulder Abduction-External Rotation (ABER) Plane

GRAPHICS: ANTERIOR AND SUPERIOR VIEWS

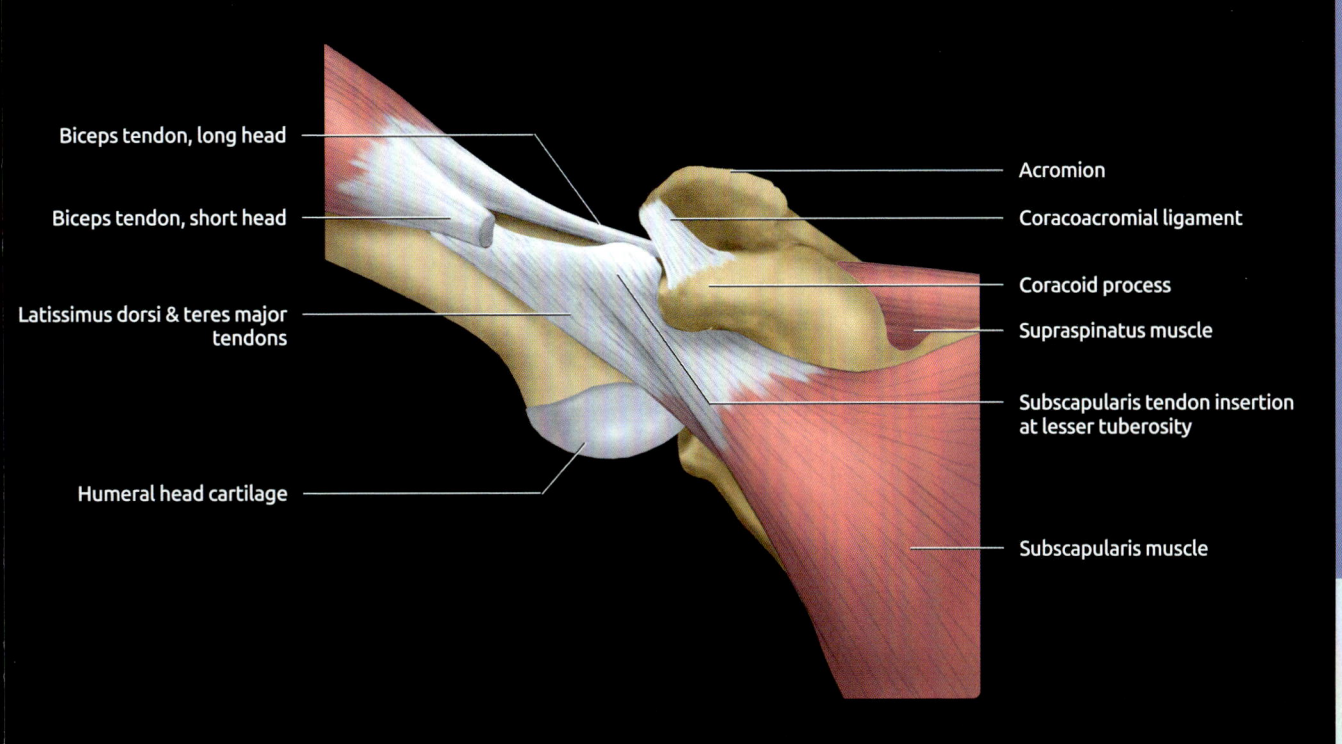

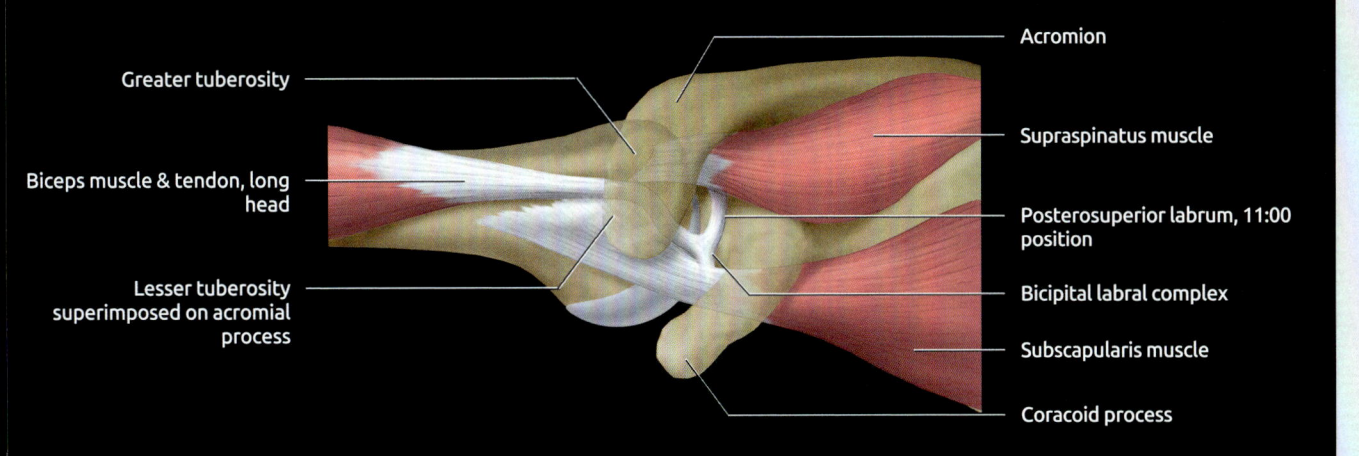

Labels (top image):
- Biceps tendon, long head
- Biceps tendon, short head
- Latissimus dorsi & teres major tendons
- Humeral head cartilage
- Acromion
- Coracoacromial ligament
- Coracoid process
- Supraspinatus muscle
- Subscapularis tendon insertion at lesser tuberosity
- Subscapularis muscle

Labels (bottom image):
- Greater tuberosity
- Biceps muscle & tendon, long head
- Lesser tuberosity superimposed on acromial process
- Acromion
- Supraspinatus muscle
- Posterosuperior labrum, 11:00 position
- Bicipital labral complex
- Subscapularis muscle
- Coracoid process

(**Top**) *Anterior graphic shows the shoulder in the ABER position. The coronal scout image of this position is used to prescribe oblique axial images of the glenohumeral joint, with cuts paralleling the shaft of the humerus.* (**Bottom**) *Graphic shows the shoulder in the ABER position, as seen from the superior aspect of the shoulder. The tip of the coracoid process corresponds to the 2:00 or 3:00 position of anterior labrum (variability relates to patient positioning).*

Shoulder Abduction-External Rotation (ABER) Plane

ABER T1 FS MR ARTHROGRAM

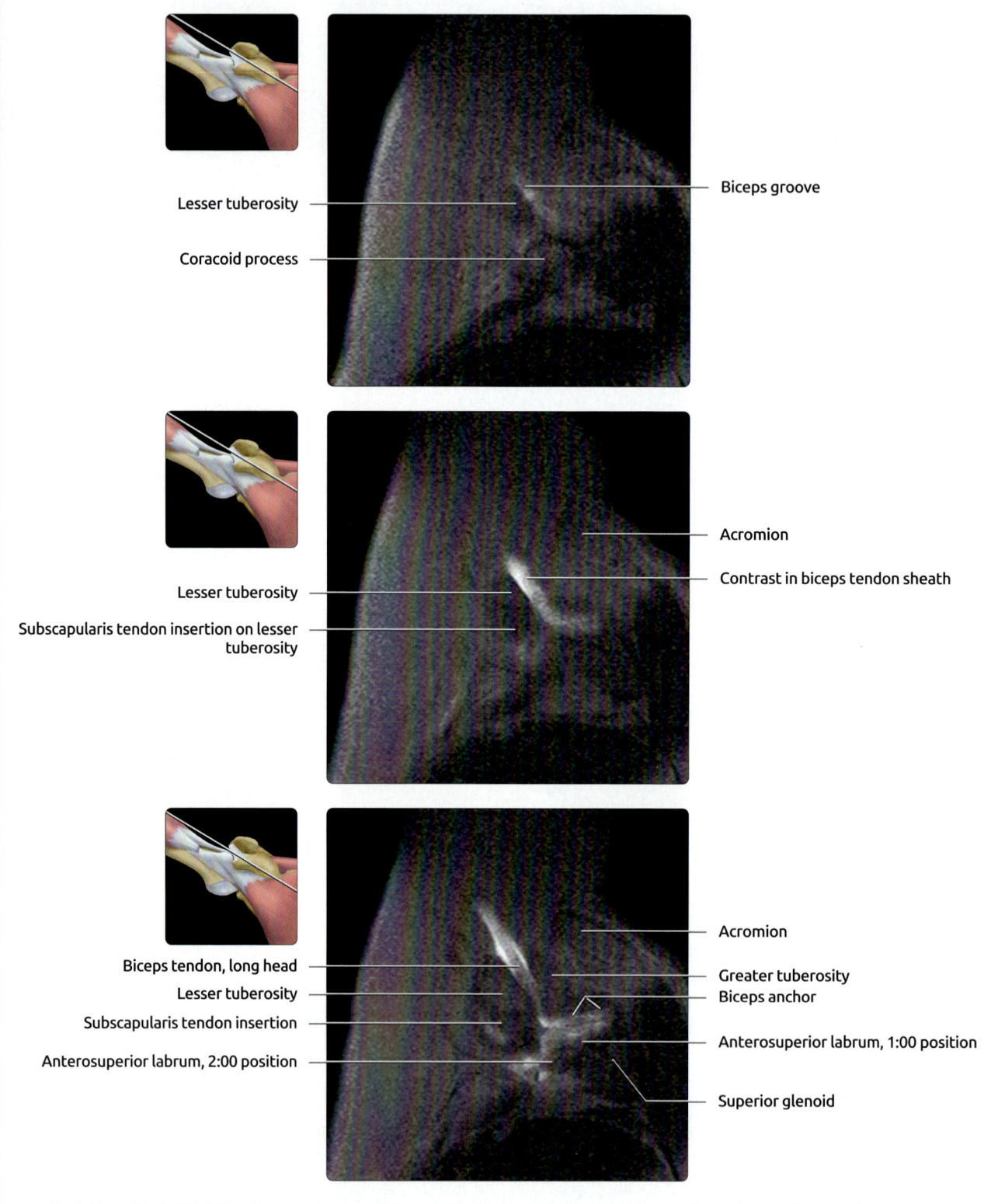

Lesser tuberosity

Coracoid process

Biceps groove

Lesser tuberosity

Subscapularis tendon insertion on lesser tuberosity

Acromion

Contrast in biceps tendon sheath

Biceps tendon, long head

Lesser tuberosity

Subscapularis tendon insertion

Anterosuperior labrum, 2:00 position

Acromion

Greater tuberosity

Biceps anchor

Anterosuperior labrum, 1:00 position

Superior glenoid

(Top) *First of 18 T1 FS MR arthrogram images of the shoulder in the ABER position presented superior to inferior is shown. This superior cut is outside the glenohumeral joint and includes portions of both the acromion and coracoid processes. The patient is positioned with the arm held behind the neck or head. An orthogonal coronal scout image is obtained and axial oblique images are prescribed along the long axis of the humeral shaft.* **(Middle)** *The subscapularis tendon insertion on the lesser tuberosity is shown on this image. Intra-articular contrast can normally extend into the biceps tendon sheath.* **(Bottom)** *The long head of the biceps tendon is shown along the length of the proximal bicipital groove.*

Shoulder Abduction-External Rotation (ABER) Plane

ABER T1 FS MR ARTHROGRAM

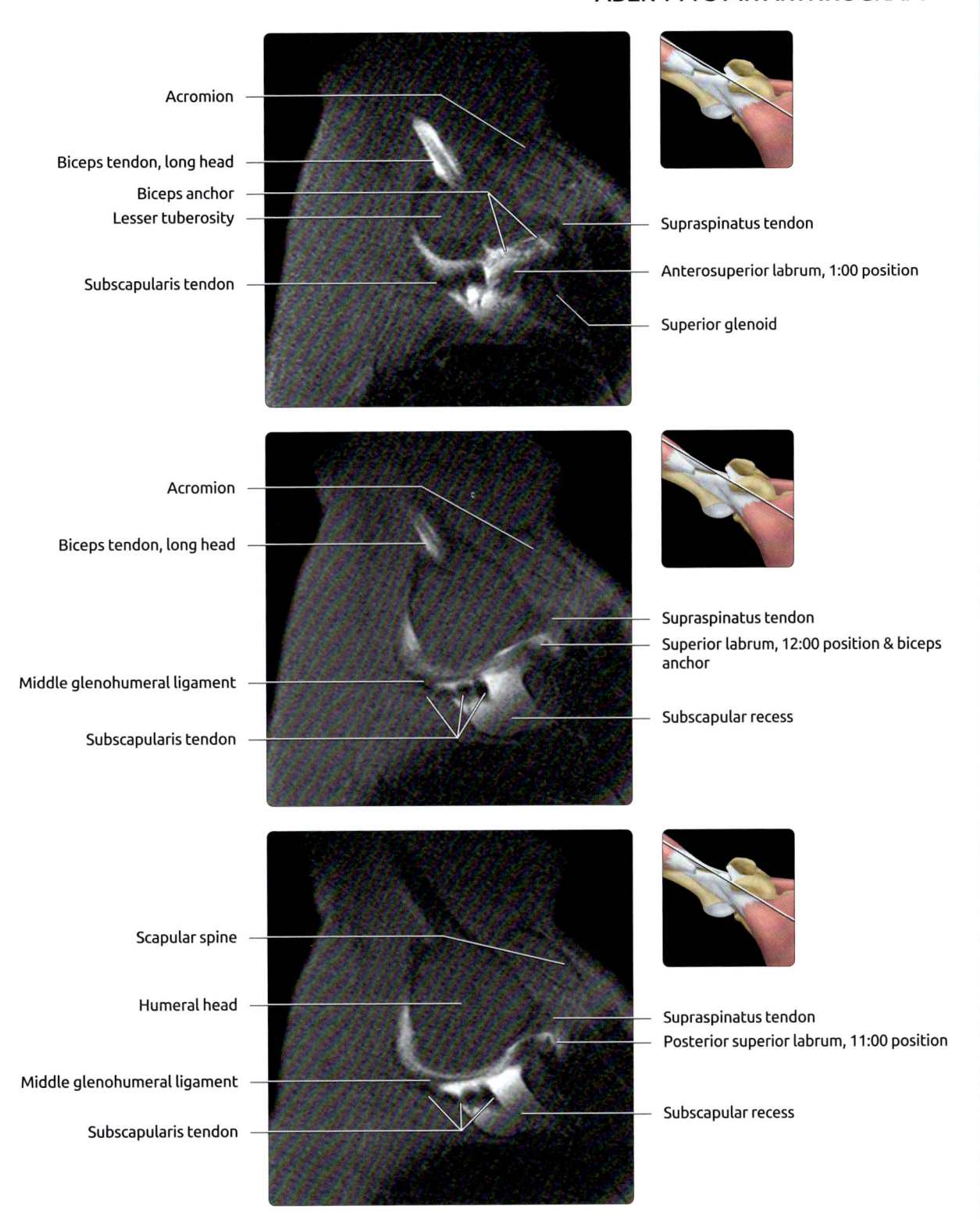

(Top) The most superior images through the shoulder joint show the long head of the biceps tendon. The biceps anchor to the labrum is also demonstrated. This position is relatively insensitive for the detection of superior labral anterior to posterior (SLAP) tears. (Middle) The biceps tendon, just proximal to the labral attachment, can be kinked due to positioning. Kinking of the biceps tendon can sometimes be associated with a SLAP tear. (Bottom) The posterosuperior labrum is partially visualized at this level. The ABER position best shows the 2:00-10:00 position of the labrum.

Shoulder Abduction-External Rotation (ABER) Plane

ABER T1 FS MR ARTHROGRAM

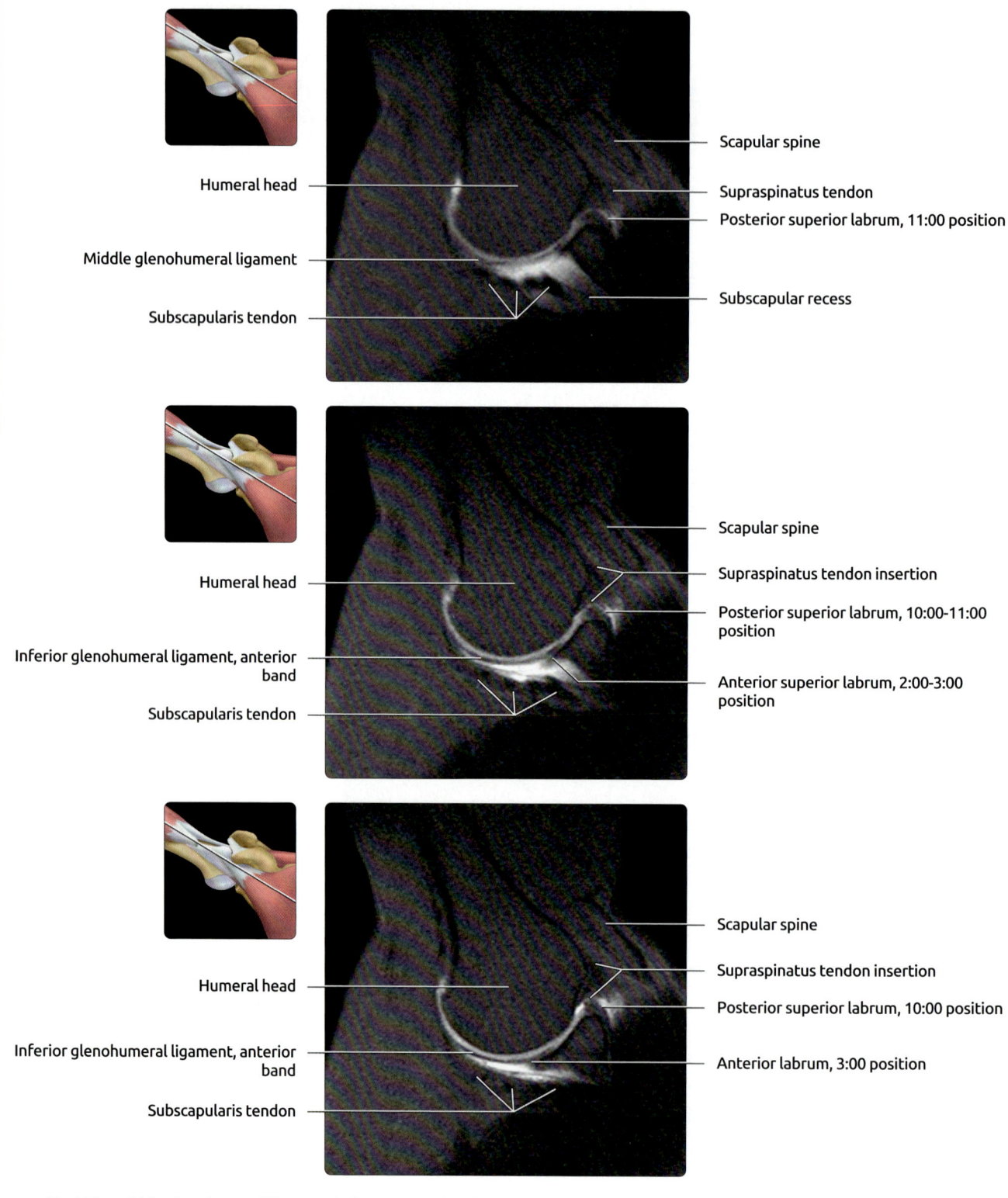

Labels (top image):
- Humeral head
- Middle glenohumeral ligament
- Subscapularis tendon
- Scapular spine
- Supraspinatus tendon
- Posterior superior labrum, 11:00 position
- Subscapular recess

Labels (middle image):
- Humeral head
- Inferior glenohumeral ligament, anterior band
- Subscapularis tendon
- Scapular spine
- Supraspinatus tendon insertion
- Posterior superior labrum, 10:00-11:00 position
- Anterior superior labrum, 2:00-3:00 position

Labels (bottom image):
- Humeral head
- Inferior glenohumeral ligament, anterior band
- Subscapularis tendon
- Scapular spine
- Supraspinatus tendon insertion
- Posterior superior labrum, 10:00 position
- Anterior labrum, 3:00 position

(Top) The middle glenohumeral ligament is demonstrated at the attachment to the subscapularis tendon. The presence of true glenohumeral ligaments is debated. The glenohumeral ligaments may represent folds of the joint capsule. (Middle) The anterior band of the inferior glenohumeral ligament is under traction and is seen curving around the anterior border of the humeral head. The traction force is transmitted to the anterior labrum, increasing the likelihood of contrast entering and making a small tear visible. (Bottom) If posterosuperior subglenoid impingement of the humeral head were present, it may be seen at this level. Contact between the rotator cuff undersurface and labrum can be seen in asymptomatic patients.

Shoulder Abduction-External Rotation (ABER) Plane

ABER T1 FS MR ARTHROGRAM

Top image labels:
- Scapular spine
- Humeral head
- Inferior glenohumeral ligament, anterior band
- Subscapularis muscle
- Transition between supraspinatus & infraspinatus tendons
- Posterior labrum, 9:00-10:00 position
- Anterior labrum, 3:00 position

Middle image labels:
- Scapular spine
- Humeral head
- Axillary recess
- Axillary vein
- Subscapularis muscle
- Transition between supraspinatus & infraspinatus tendons
- Posterior labrum, 9:00 position
- Anterior labrum, 3:00-4:00 position

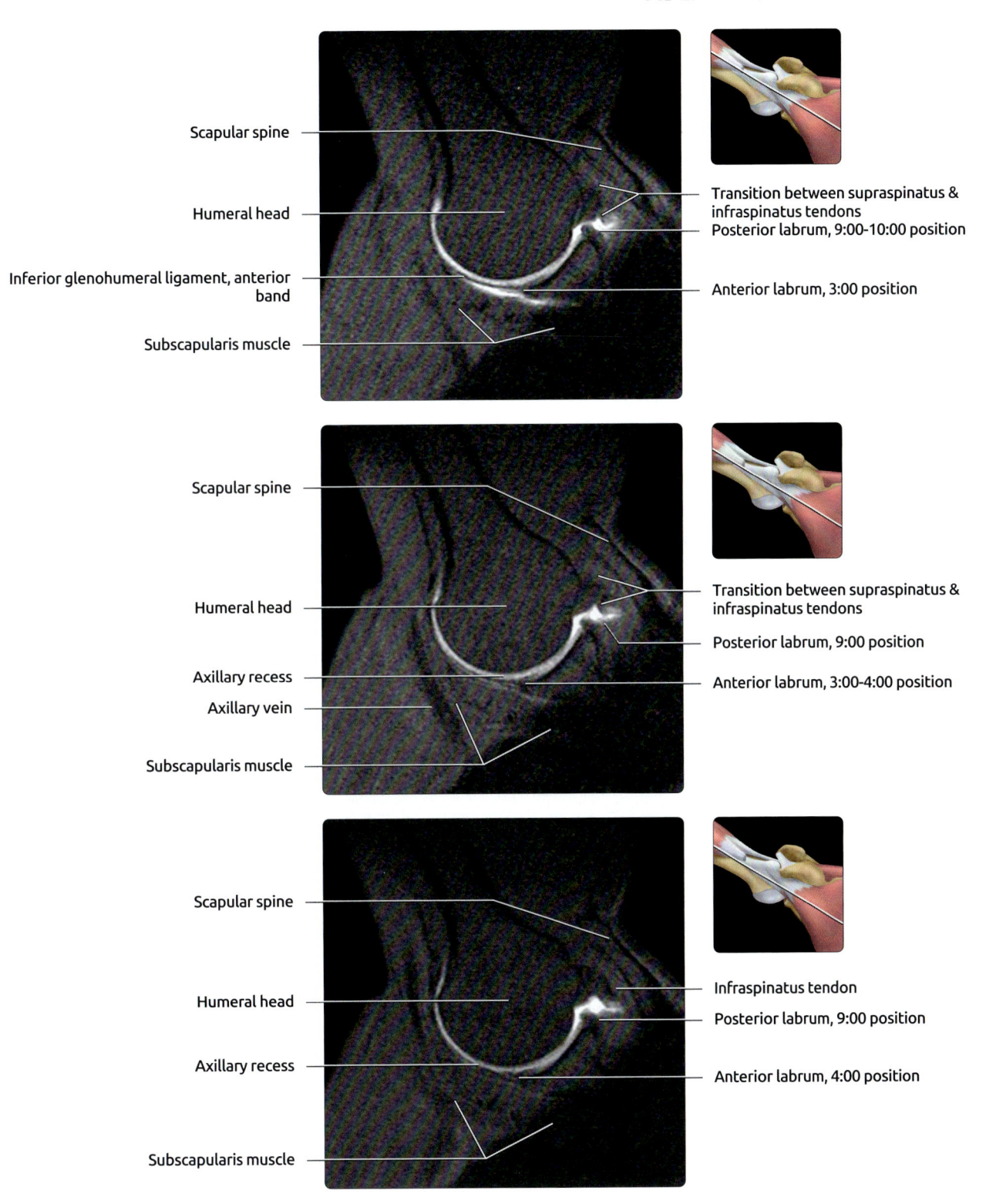

Bottom image labels:
- Scapular spine
- Humeral head
- Axillary recess
- Subscapularis muscle
- Infraspinatus tendon
- Posterior labrum, 9:00 position
- Anterior labrum, 4:00 position

(Top) *The traction of the anterior band of the inferior glenohumeral ligament also increases visualization of labral tears at the 3:00 to 5:00 position that have partially healed or have been resynovialized.* **(Middle)** *The ABER position allows the anteroinferior labrum to be imaged without a magic angle artifact that can be present with standard, adducted positioning.* **(Bottom)** *Osteochondral injuries of the posterosuperior humeral head, not present in this case, are accentuated in the ABER position.*

Shoulder Abduction-External Rotation (ABER) Plane

ABER T1 FS MR ARTHROGRAM

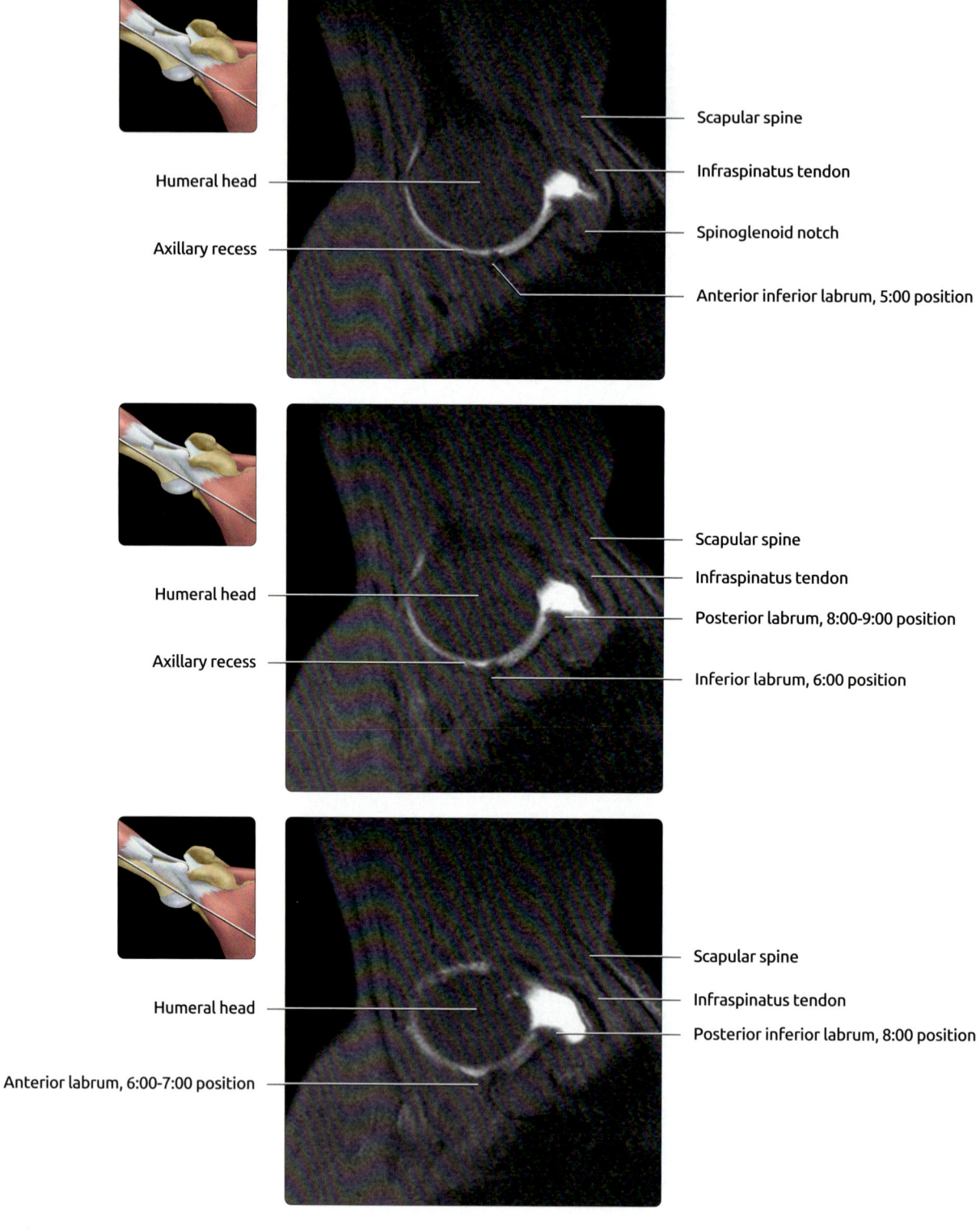

Top image labels:
- Humeral head
- Axillary recess
- Scapular spine
- Infraspinatus tendon
- Spinoglenoid notch
- Anterior inferior labrum, 5:00 position

Middle image labels:
- Humeral head
- Axillary recess
- Scapular spine
- Infraspinatus tendon
- Posterior labrum, 8:00-9:00 position
- Inferior labrum, 6:00 position

Bottom image labels:
- Humeral head
- Anterior labrum, 6:00-7:00 position
- Scapular spine
- Infraspinatus tendon
- Posterior inferior labrum, 8:00 position

(Top) *Detection of anteroinferior labral tears is improved in the ABER position.* **(Middle)** *The smooth undersurface of the infraspinatus tendon is shown.* **(Bottom)** *The ABER position allows the supraspinatus, infraspinatus, and teres minor tendons to kink. This would potentially allow contrast to fill small undersurface tears. The ABER position is very helpful for detection of delaminated rotator cuff tears.*

Shoulder Abduction-External Rotation (ABER) Plane

ABER T1 FS MR ARTHROGRAM

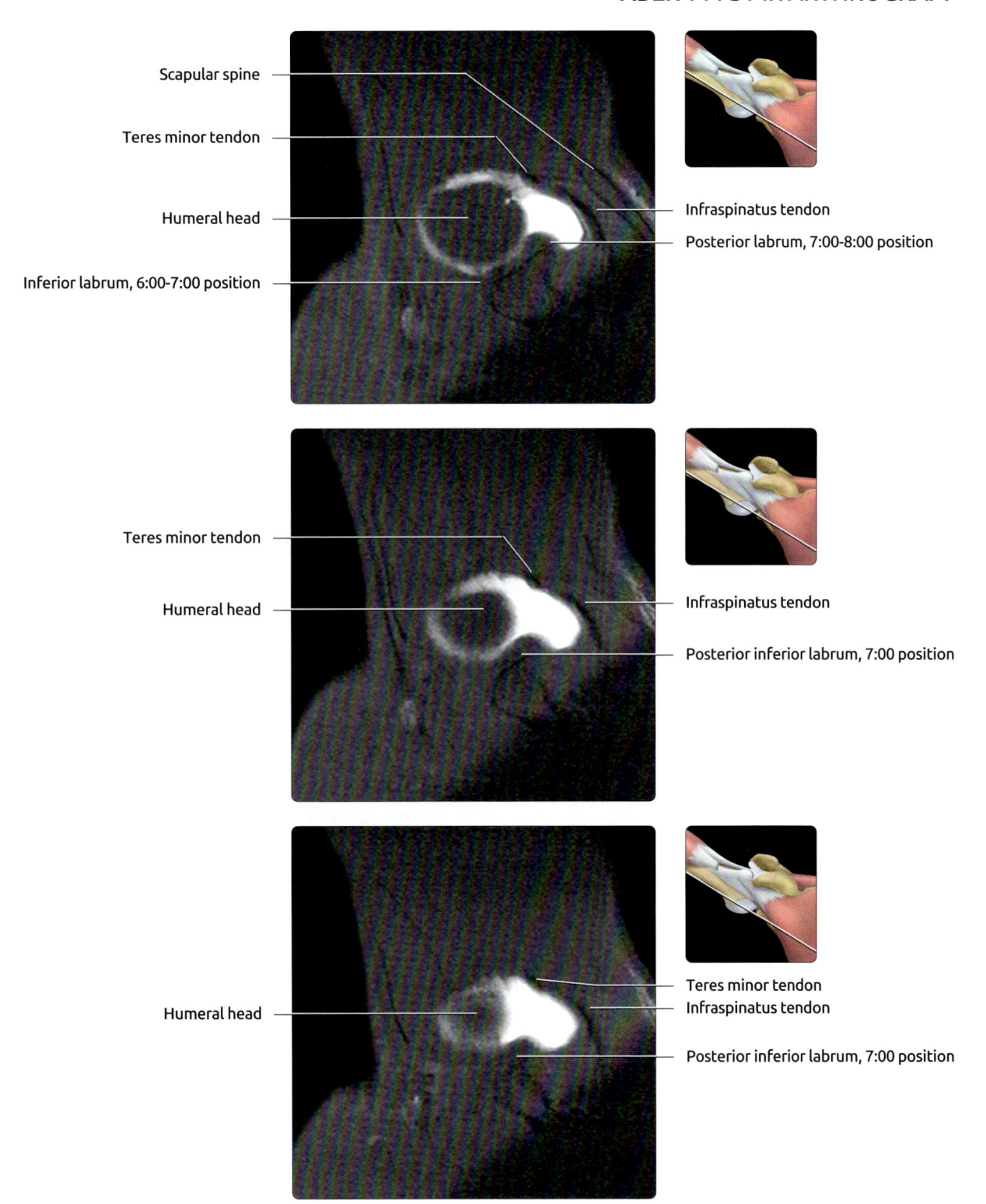

(Top image labels) Scapular spine; Teres minor tendon; Humeral head; Inferior labrum, 6:00-7:00 position; Infraspinatus tendon; Posterior labrum, 7:00-8:00 position

(Middle image labels) Teres minor tendon; Humeral head; Infraspinatus tendon; Posterior inferior labrum, 7:00 position

(Bottom image labels) Humeral head; Teres minor tendon; Infraspinatus tendon; Posterior inferior labrum, 7:00 position

(Top) Undersurface tears of the teres minor can be accentuated in this position, when compared with standard adducted MR images. (Middle) The most inferior image through the glenoid labrum ranges from the 5:00-7:00 position. The exact location depends on patient positioning and image alignment. (Bottom) Although ABER positioning may improve visualization of some anatomic structures and abnormalities in the shoulder, there are limitations. The most significant limitation is that many patients with shoulder pain will not be able to tolerate this position. Additionally, proper placement of the shoulder coil and alignment of the images can be challenging for technologist unfamiliar with this technique.

Shoulder: Rotator Cuff and Biceps Tendon

IMAGING ANATOMY

Overview

- **Rotator cuff**
  - Consists of supraspinatus, infraspinatus, teres minor and subscapularis muscles, and tendons
  - Uniform, hypointense tendons on all sequences
  - Cuff tendons blend with shoulder joint capsule
- **Supraspinatus muscle**
  - Origin: Supraspinatus fossa of scapula
  - Insertion: Superior facet (horizontal orientation) and portion of middle facet of greater tuberosity
  - Nerve supply: Suprascapular nerve
  - Blood supply: Suprascapular artery and circumflex scapular branches of subscapular artery
  - Action: Abduction of humerus
  - Anterior and posterior muscle bellies
    - Anterior belly is larger, has central tendon and is more likely to tear
    - Posterior belly is strap-like & has terminal tendon
  - Most commonly injured rotator cuff muscle
- **Infraspinatus muscle**
  - Origin: Infraspinatus fossa of scapula
  - Insertion: Middle facet greater tuberosity
  - Nerve supply: Suprascapular nerve, distal fibers
  - Blood supply: Suprascapular artery and circumflex scapular branches of subscapular artery
  - Action: External rotation of humerus and resists posterior subluxation
- **Teres minor muscle**
  - Origin: Lateral (axillary) scapular border, middle half
  - Insertion: Inferior facet (vertical orientation) of humerus greater tuberosity
  - Nerve supply: Axillary nerve
  - Blood supply: Posterior circumflex humeral artery & circumflex scapular branches of subscapular artery
  - Action: External rotation of humerus
  - Least commonly injured rotator cuff muscle
- **Subscapularis muscle**
  - Origin: Subscapular fossa of scapula
  - Insertion: Lesser tuberosity and up to 40% may insert at surgical neck
  - Nerve supply: Subscapular nerve, upper and lower
  - Blood supply: Subscapularis artery
  - Action: Internal rotation of humerus, also adduction, depression, and flexion
  - 4-6 tendon slips converge into main tendon; multipennate morphology increases strength
- **Rotator cuff tendon blood supply**
  - Derived from adjacent muscle, bone, and bursae
  - Normal hypovascular regions in tendons, particularly musculotendinous junction
    - Termed "critical zone"
    - Vulnerable to degeneration
    - However, not the most common region of tearing
- **Biceps tendon, long head**
  - Low signal intensity on all sequences
  - Origin: Superior glenoid labrum
    - Portions may attach to supraglenoid tubercle, anterosuperior labrum, posterosuperior labrum, and coracoid base
  - Courses through superior shoulder joint to intertubercular or bicipital groove
  - Action: Stabilizes and depresses humeral head
  - Anatomic variants
    - Anomalous intraarticular and extraarticular origins from rotator cuff and joint capsule
    - May be bifid or absent
  - **Tendon sheath** communicates with joint and normally contains small amount of fluid

ANATOMY IMAGING ISSUES

Imaging Recommendations

- **Radiographs**: AP and supraspinatus outlet views to assess humeral head position and thus indirectly assess supraspinatus tendon
- **MR**: Fluid sensitive MR sequences best study for rotator cuff
  - T1 sequences without fat suppression are helpful for evaluating muscle mass
- **MR arthrography**: Improves evaluation of rotator cuff and capsulolabral complex

Imaging Pitfalls

- **Increased signal in supraspinatus tendon approximately 1 cm from insertion**
  - Present in asymptomatic patients
  - Attributed to magic angle artifact, tendon degeneration, partial volume effect, and positioning artifacts
- **Magic angle artifact**
  - Increased signal in collagen fibers oriented 55° to main magnetic field on short TE images
  - Can occur in rotator cuff and biceps tendon
  - Recognize by comparing with long TE images
- **Partial volume averaging**
  - Anterior supraspinatus may volume average with fluid in subscapularis bursa or biceps tendon sheath simulating tear
  - Posterior oblique fibers of supraspinatus attach deep to overlapping anterior fibers of infraspinatus; cuff may appear thin in this zone, sometimes with increased linear signal
  - Mid supraspinatus may average with thickened region of humeral head cartilage
  - Tendons may average with normal variant muscle slips extending above or below tendon
- **Dilated veins in supraspinatus muscle**
  - Usually in periphery of muscle
  - May simulate intramuscular ganglion cysts
- **Interruption of subacromial-subdeltoid fat plane**
  - Fat plane is superficial to bursa
  - Can be interrupted or absent in normal patients
  - Not a reliable sign of rotator cuff abnormality
- **Increased signal in lateral bicipital groove**
  - Due to anterolateral branch of anterior circumflex humeral artery and vein
  - Do not confuse with fluid from tenosynovitis or tear

Shoulder: Rotator Cuff and Biceps Tendon

GRAPHICS: ROTATOR CUFF

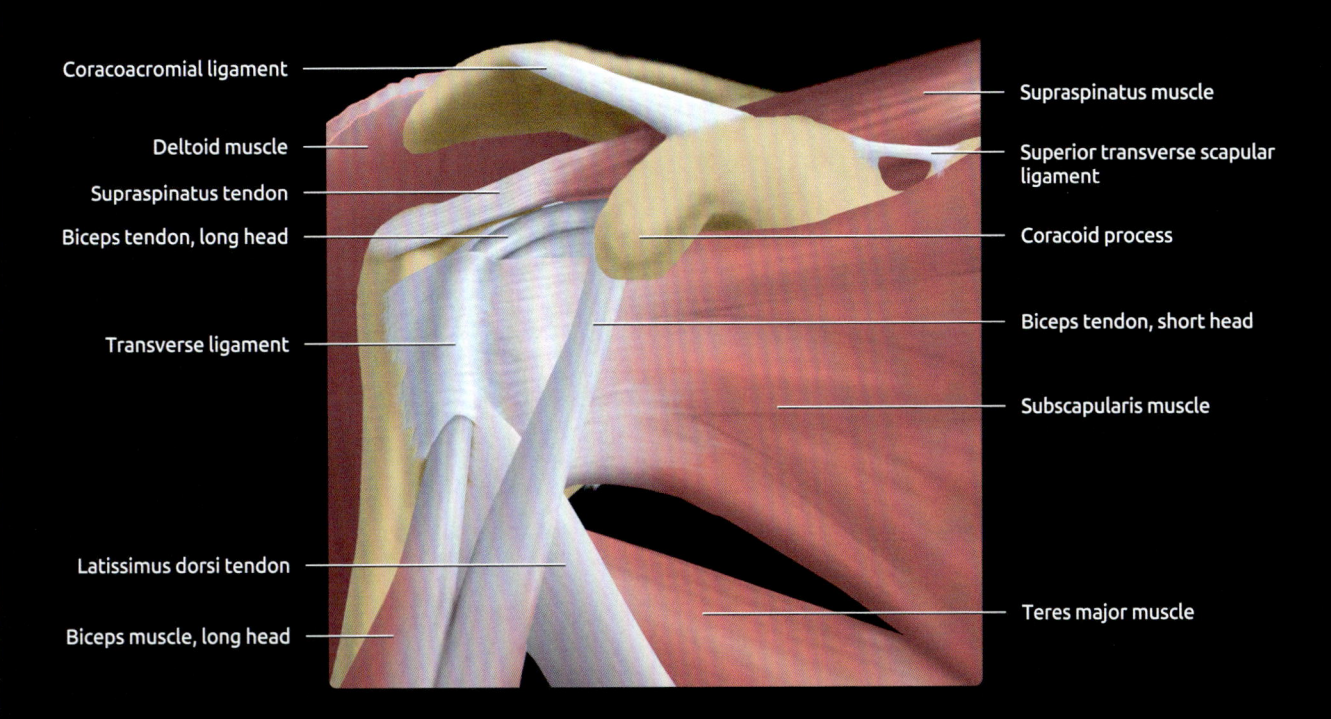

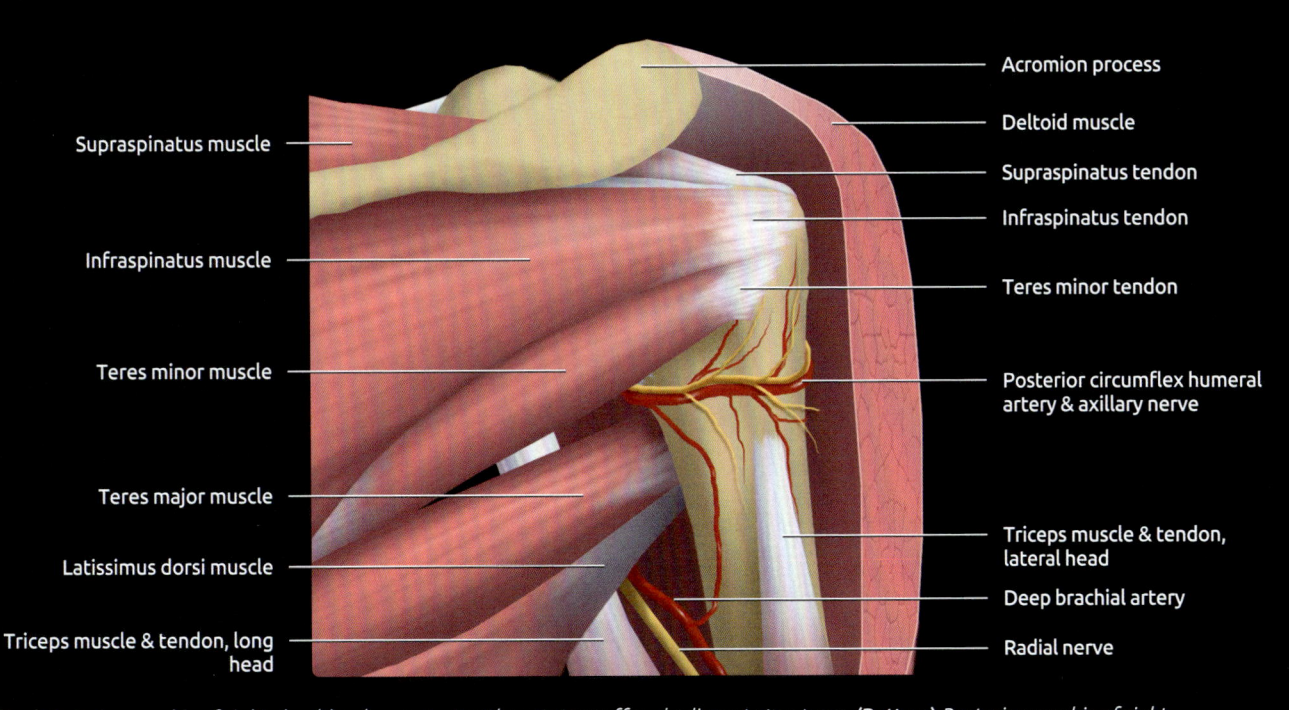

(Top) Anterior graphic of right shoulder demonstrates the rotator cuff and adjacent structures. (Bottom) Posterior graphic of right shoulder demonstrates the rotator cuff and adjacent structures.

Shoulder: Rotator Cuff and Biceps Tendon

SAGITTAL T2 FS MR, RIGHT SHOULDER

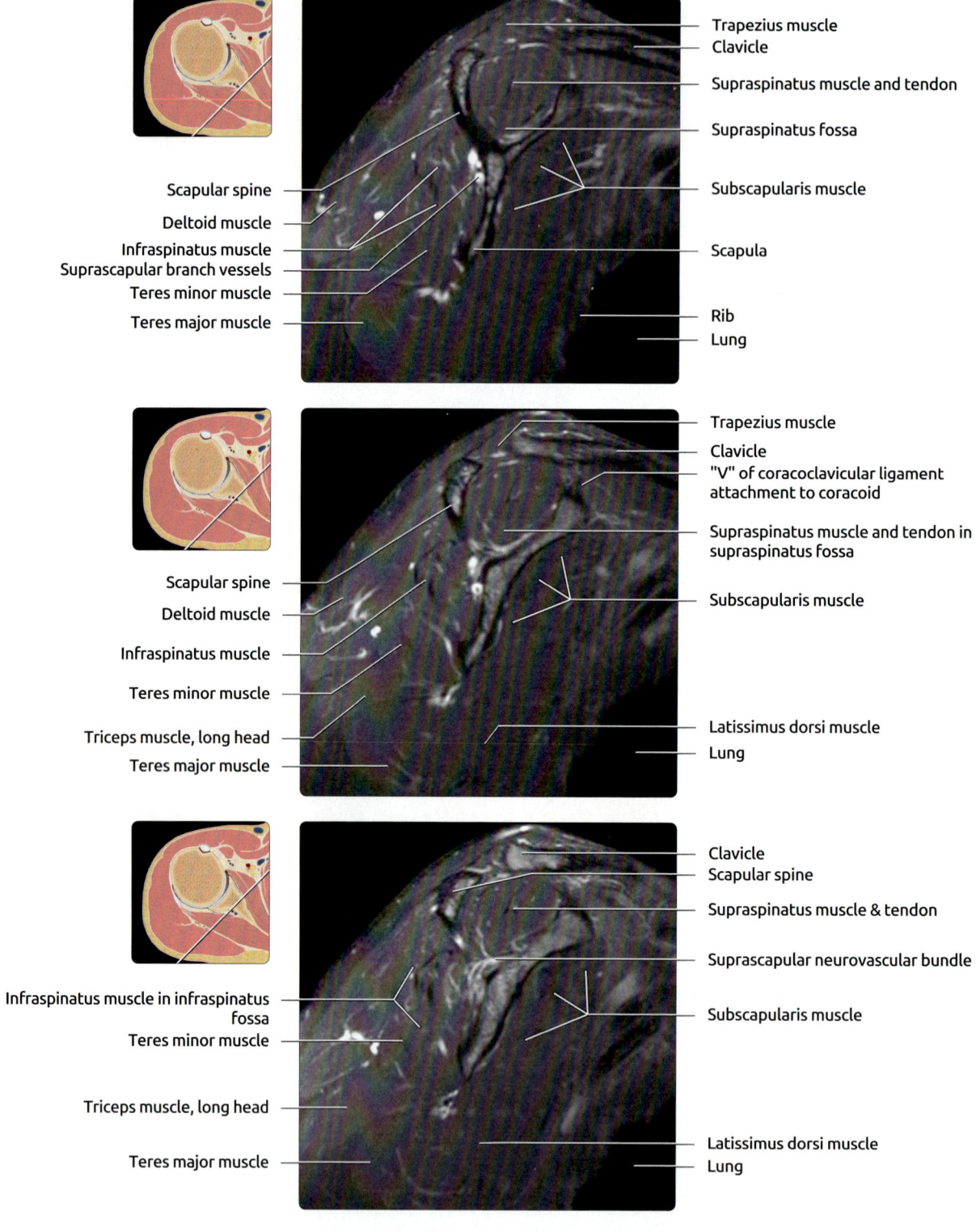

(Top) First of 18 sequential sagittal oblique T2 FS MR images of the right shoulder displayed medial to lateral is shown. Images were acquired at 1.5 T with a shoulder coil. *(Middle)* The supraspinatus muscle fills the supraspinatus fossa of the scapula. The normal muscle should fill or extend slightly above a line drawn along the top border of the "Y" of the scapula. When the muscle atrophies, the muscle will be replaced by fat. With atrophy, the supraspinatus tendon may become eccentric in location, approaching the superior border of the muscle. *(Bottom)* The infraspinatus muscle fills the infraspinatus fossa of the scapula. A normal infraspinatus muscle should fill the fossa and extend posterior to a line drawn from the posterior aspect of the scapular spine to the inferior border of the scapula. Infraspinatus muscle atrophy may occur in the absence of tendon abnormality.

Shoulder: Rotator Cuff and Biceps Tendon

SAGITTAL T2 FS MR, RIGHT SHOULDER

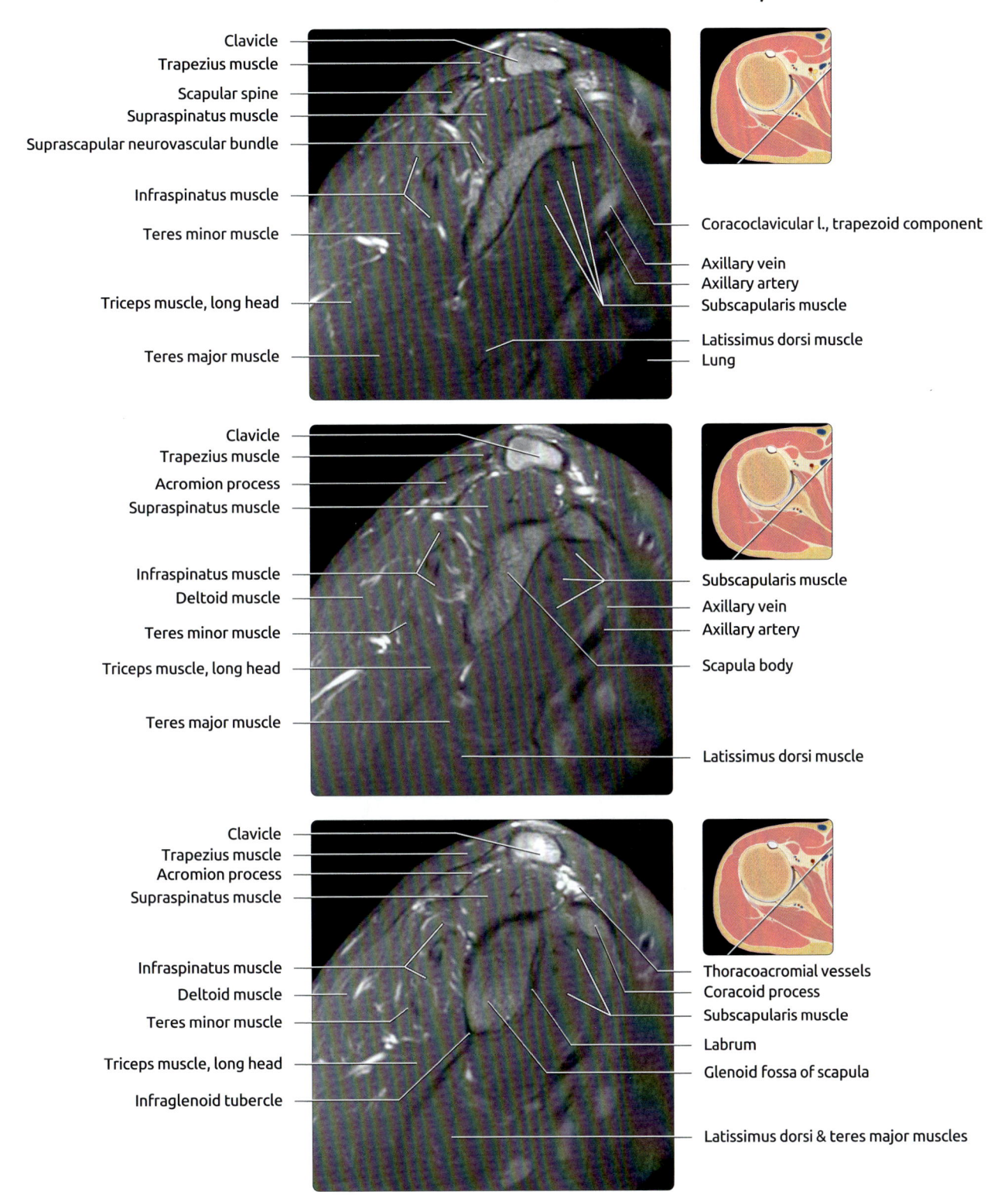

(Top) The normal subscapularis muscle should fill the subscapular fossa. The muscle should have a convex anterior border. **(Middle)** The teres muscle lies inferior to the infraspinatus muscle. It assists in external rotation of the humerus. The teres minor also resists posterior subluxation of the humeral head. **(Bottom)** All of the rotator cuff muscles originate from the scapula and insert on the humeral head.

Shoulder: Rotator Cuff and Biceps Tendon

SAGITTAL T2 FS MR, RIGHT SHOULDER

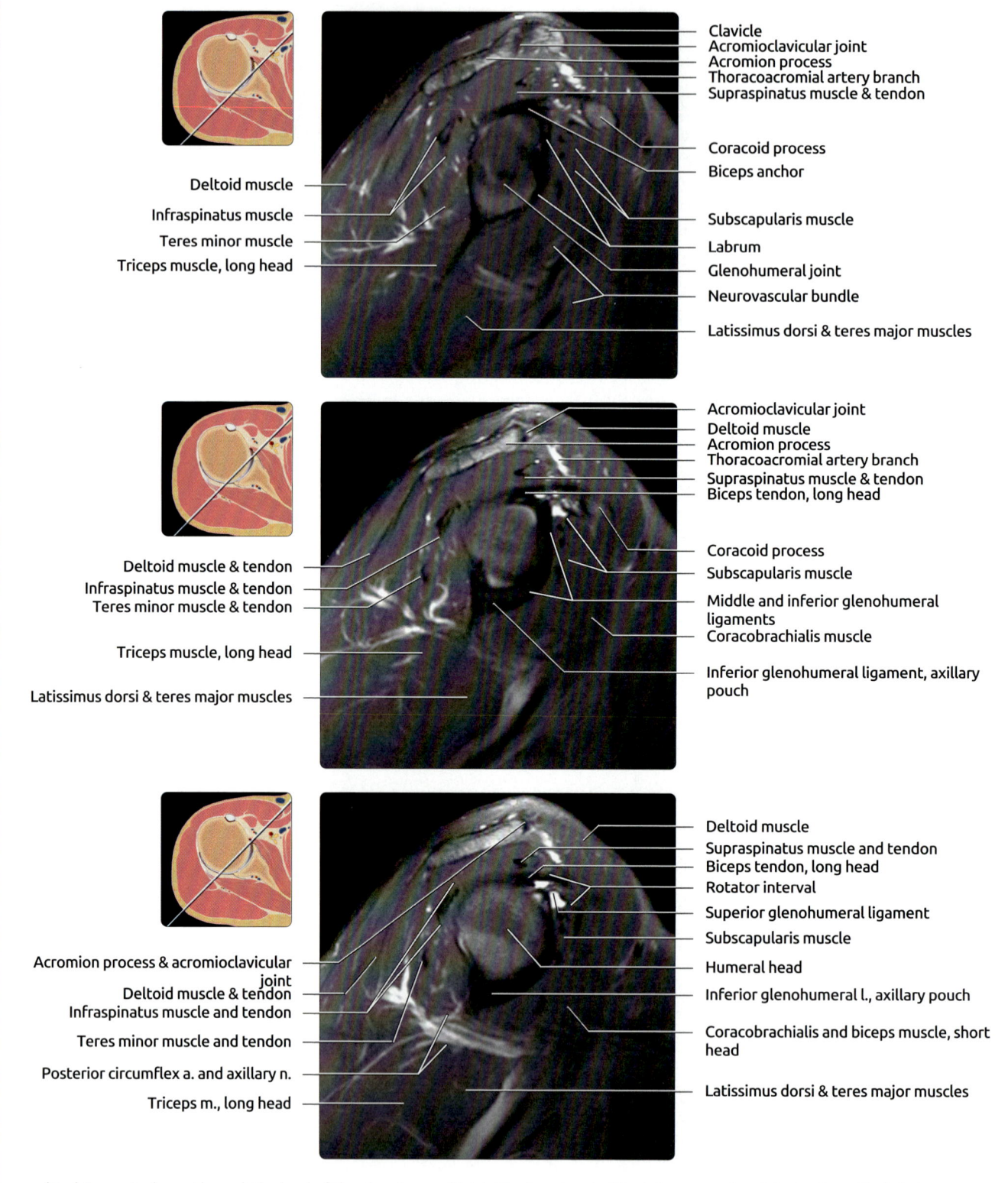

Top image labels:
- Deltoid muscle
- Infraspinatus muscle
- Teres minor muscle
- Triceps muscle, long head
- Clavicle
- Acromioclavicular joint
- Acromion process
- Thoracoacromial artery branch
- Supraspinatus muscle & tendon
- Coracoid process
- Biceps anchor
- Subscapularis muscle
- Labrum
- Glenohumeral joint
- Neurovascular bundle
- Latissimus dorsi & teres major muscles

Middle image labels:
- Deltoid muscle & tendon
- Infraspinatus muscle & tendon
- Teres minor muscle & tendon
- Triceps muscle, long head
- Latissimus dorsi & teres major muscles
- Acromioclavicular joint
- Deltoid muscle
- Acromion process
- Thoracoacromial artery branch
- Supraspinatus muscle & tendon
- Biceps tendon, long head
- Coracoid process
- Subscapularis muscle
- Middle and inferior glenohumeral ligaments
- Coracobrachialis muscle
- Inferior glenohumeral ligament, axillary pouch

Bottom image labels:
- Acromion process & acromioclavicular joint
- Deltoid muscle & tendon
- Infraspinatus muscle and tendon
- Teres minor muscle and tendon
- Posterior circumflex a. and axillary n.
- Triceps m., long head
- Deltoid muscle
- Supraspinatus muscle and tendon
- Biceps tendon, long head
- Rotator interval
- Superior glenohumeral ligament
- Subscapularis muscle
- Humeral head
- Inferior glenohumeral l., axillary pouch
- Coracobrachialis and biceps muscle, short head
- Latissimus dorsi & teres major muscles

(Top) Image is shown through the level of the glenohumeral joint. The long head of the triceps muscle originates from the inferior border of the glenoid. **(Middle)** The glenoid labrum and glenohumeral ligaments provide support for the humeral head in the somewhat shallow bony glenoid fossa. **(Bottom)** The rotator interval is a triangular space between the supraspinatus and subscapularis tendons. The long head of the biceps traverses the rotator interval. The coracohumeral ligament and superior glenohumeral ligament provide support for the long head of the biceps tendon in the rotator interval.

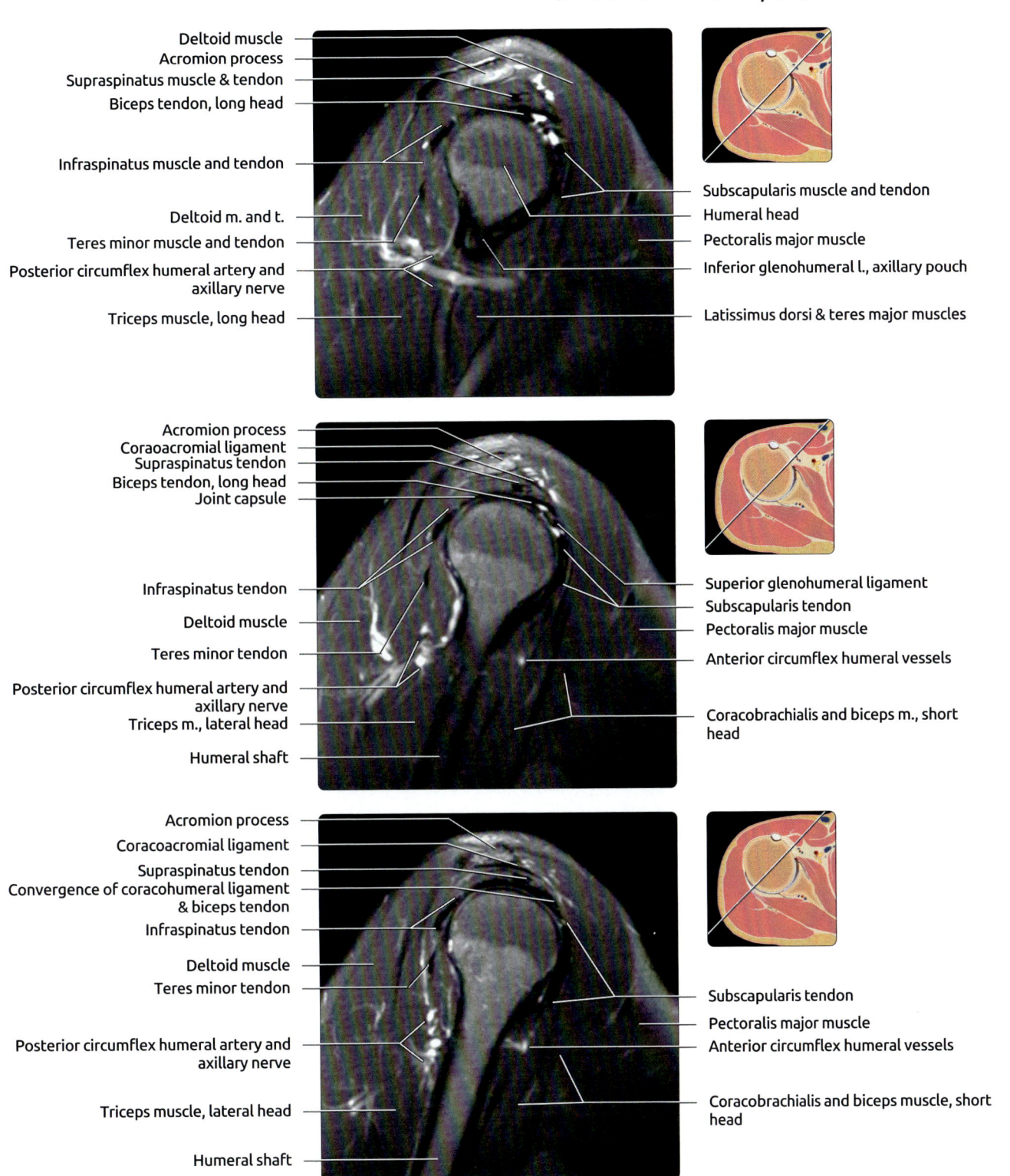

Shoulder: Rotator Cuff and Biceps Tendon

SAGITTAL T2 FS MR, RIGHT SHOULDER

Top image labels:
- Deltoid muscle
- Acromion process
- Supraspinatus muscle & tendon
- Biceps tendon, long head
- Infraspinatus muscle and tendon
- Deltoid m. and t.
- Teres minor muscle and tendon
- Posterior circumflex humeral artery and axillary nerve
- Triceps muscle, long head
- Subscapularis muscle and tendon
- Humeral head
- Pectoralis major muscle
- Inferior glenohumeral l., axillary pouch
- Latissimus dorsi & teres major muscles

Middle image labels:
- Acromion process
- Coracoacromial ligament
- Supraspinatus tendon
- Biceps tendon, long head
- Joint capsule
- Infraspinatus tendon
- Deltoid muscle
- Teres minor tendon
- Posterior circumflex humeral artery and axillary nerve
- Triceps m., lateral head
- Humeral shaft
- Superior glenohumeral ligament
- Subscapularis tendon
- Pectoralis major muscle
- Anterior circumflex humeral vessels
- Coracobrachialis and biceps m., short head

Bottom image labels:
- Acromion process
- Coracoacromial ligament
- Supraspinatus tendon
- Convergence of coracohumeral ligament & biceps tendon
- Infraspinatus tendon
- Deltoid muscle
- Teres minor tendon
- Posterior circumflex humeral artery and axillary nerve
- Triceps muscle, lateral head
- Humeral shaft
- Subscapularis tendon
- Pectoralis major muscle
- Anterior circumflex humeral vessels
- Coracobrachialis and biceps muscle, short head

(Top) *The long head of the biceps in this region is intraarticular but extrasynovial.* **(Middle)** *As the images move laterally, the superior glenohumeral ligament will form an anterior sling around the long head of the biceps tendon, along with the coracohumeral ligament.* **(Bottom)** *The rotator cuff is becoming progressively tendinous.*

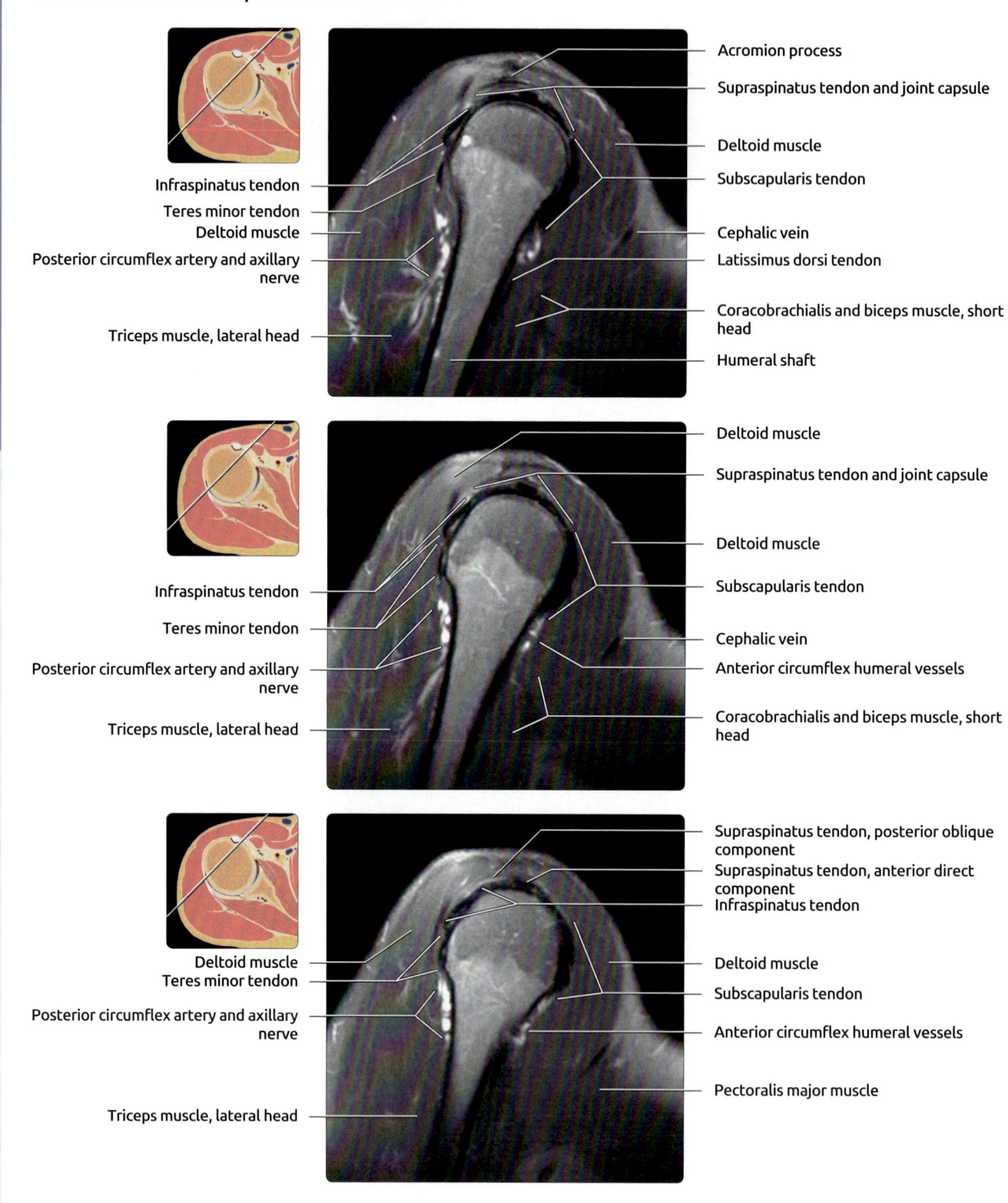

Shoulder: Rotator Cuff and Biceps Tendon

SAGITTAL T2 FS MR, RIGHT SHOULDER

Labels (top image):
- Acromion process
- Supraspinatus tendon and joint capsule
- Deltoid muscle
- Subscapularis tendon
- Cephalic vein
- Latissimus dorsi tendon
- Coracobrachialis and biceps muscle, short head
- Humeral shaft
- Infraspinatus tendon
- Teres minor tendon
- Deltoid muscle
- Posterior circumflex artery and axillary nerve
- Triceps muscle, lateral head

Labels (middle image):
- Deltoid muscle
- Supraspinatus tendon and joint capsule
- Deltoid muscle
- Subscapularis tendon
- Cephalic vein
- Anterior circumflex humeral vessels
- Coracobrachialis and biceps muscle, short head
- Infraspinatus tendon
- Teres minor tendon
- Posterior circumflex artery and axillary nerve
- Triceps muscle, lateral head

Labels (bottom image):
- Supraspinatus tendon, posterior oblique component
- Supraspinatus tendon, anterior direct component
- Infraspinatus tendon
- Deltoid muscle
- Subscapularis tendon
- Anterior circumflex humeral vessels
- Pectoralis major muscle
- Deltoid muscle
- Teres minor tendon
- Posterior circumflex artery and axillary nerve
- Triceps muscle, lateral head

(**Top**) The rotator cuff tendons fuse with the joint capsule. The coracohumeral ligament fuses with the supraspinatus and subscapularis tendons, spanning the gap between the 2 tendons. (**Middle**) Anterior and posterior circumflex humeral vessels anastomose at the lateral aspect of the humeral neck. (**Bottom**) The rotator cuff is entirely tendinous at this level. Individual tendons have fused together. The supraspinatus, infraspinatus, teres minor, and subscapularis tendons can be inferred by their location and insertion on the humeral head.

Shoulder: Rotator Cuff and Biceps Tendon

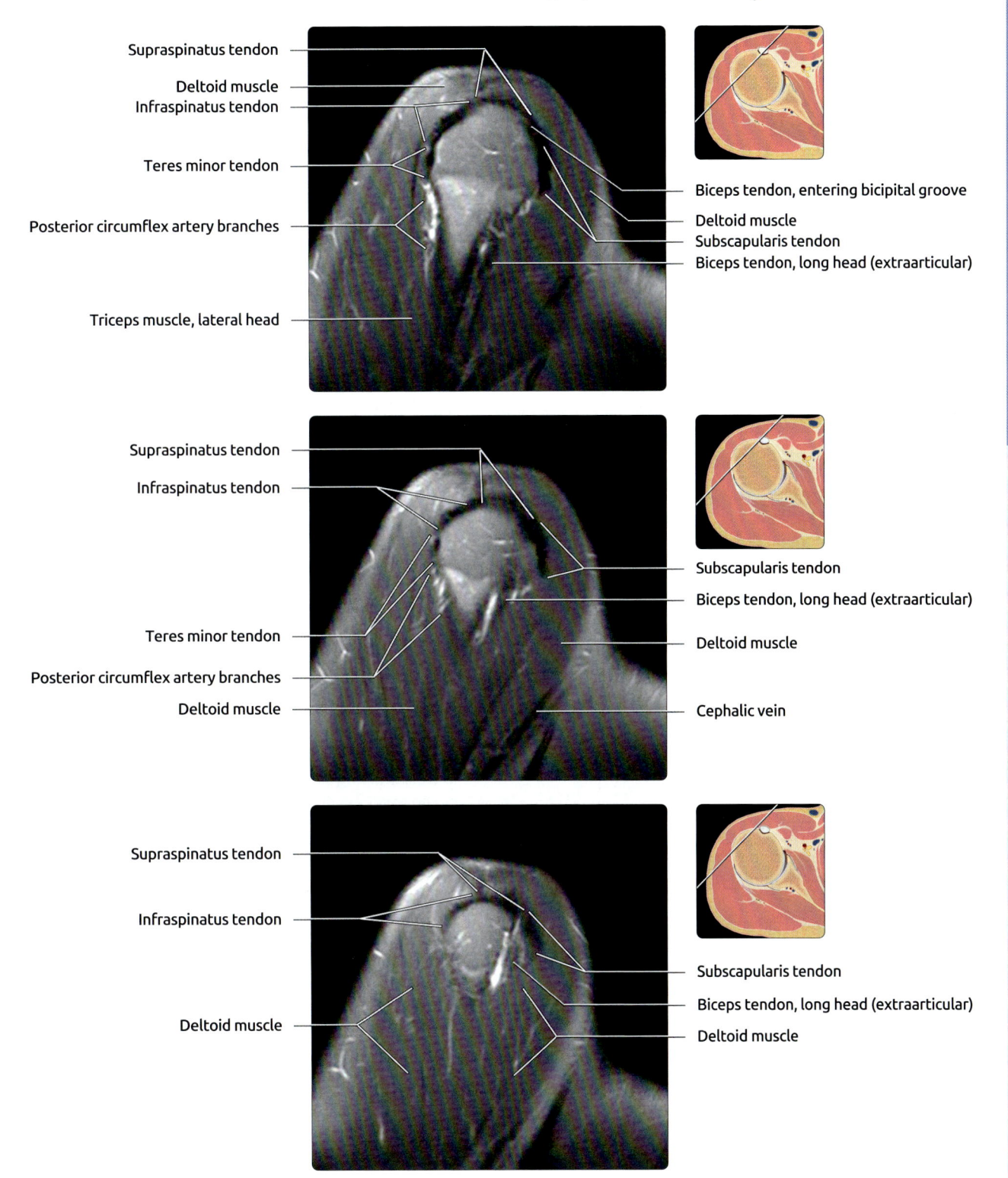

SAGITTAL T2 FS MR, RIGHT SHOULDER

(Top) The deltoid muscle covers the superficial aspect of the shoulder anteriorly, laterally, and posteriorly. *(Middle)* There are 3 facets of the greater tuberosity. The superior facet is horizontally oriented. The middle facet is obliquely oriented. The inferior facet is vertically oriented. The supraspinatus, infraspinatus, and teres minor tendons insert on the superior, middle, and inferior facets of the greater tuberosity respectively. The supraspinatus partially inserts on the middle facet, as as well as on the superior facet. *(Bottom)* The subscapularis tendon inserts primarily on the lesser tuberosity.

Shoulder: Rotator Interval

TERMINOLOGY

Abbreviations
- Coracohumeral ligament (CHL)
- Superior glenohumeral ligament (SGHL)
- Long head, biceps tendon (LBT)

IMAGING ANATOMY

Overview
- **Triangular space between supraspinatus and subscapularis tendons**
  - Base of triangle at coracoid process
  - Tip of triangle at transverse ligament
- **Borders of rotator interval**
  - Medial extent: Coracoid base
  - Lateral extent: Entrance to bicipital groove, transverse ligament
  - Floor: Humeral head cartilage
  - Roof: Joint capsule
    - Coracohumeral ligament on bursal surface
    - Fasciculus obliquus on articular surface
    - Synovial lining
- **Contents of rotator interval**
  - Coracohumeral ligament
  - Superior glenohumeral ligament
  - Biceps tendon, long head
- Coracohumeral ligament and superior glenohumeral ligament stabilize long head of biceps tendon as it enters bicipital groove

Internal Contents
- **Coracohumeral ligament**
  - Origin: Base of coracoid process
  - Insertion: Lesser and greater tuberosities, humerus
    - Forms 2 bands laterally
    - Larger inserts on greater tuberosity and supraspinatus anterior border
    - Smaller band inserts on lesser tuberosity, transverse ligament, and superior subscapularis tendon
  - Histologically more similar to a capsule than a true ligament
  - Blends with superficial and deep layers of rotator cuff tendons and joint capsule
  - Forms solid layer of tissue between supraspinatus and subscapularis tendons
  - Covers intraarticular portion of LBT
  - Optimal imaging plane: Sagittal oblique but should be visible in all planes
  - Homogeneous low signal on all sequences
  - Cannot be differentiated from supraspinatus and subscapularis tendons where it is fused
- **Superior glenohumeral ligament (SGHL)**
  - Origin: Superior tubercle of glenoid, anterior to biceps
  - Insertion: Superolateral lesser tuberosity, deep to superior border of subscapularis tendon
  - May not be possible to differentiate from coracohumeral ligament in absence of intraarticular contrast or joint effusion
  - Changes configuration through course of interval
    - Medial: Tubular, anterior to LBT
    - Mid portion: Flattened anterior band with T-shaped connection to CHL
    - Lateral: Fuses with CHL to form sling around LBT
  - **On axial images, may be seen as band anterior to biceps tendon**
    - Forms a "Y" on high axial images, with one arm being SGHL and other LBT
  - Optimal imaging plane: Sagittal oblique MR arthrogram or MR with joint effusion
- **Biceps tendon, long head**
  - Origin: Superior glenoid labrum
    - May also have origin from supraglenoid tubercle, rotator cuff, joint capsule and coracoid base
  - Courses through superior shoulder joint to intertubercular or bicipital groove
    - Traction zone: Intraarticular, extrasynovial, tendon histology
    - Sliding zone: Contacts humerus, fibrocartilage histology
  - Action: Stabilizes and depresses humeral head
  - Uniform low signal intensity on all sequences

Other
- **Lower rotator interval**
  - Separate entity from classic rotator interval described above
  - Located between teres minor and subscapularis tendons
  - Instability may disrupt this region
  - Encompasses axillary sling

ANATOMY IMAGING ISSUES

Imaging Recommendations
- MR: Sagittal oblique T2 FS images to accentuate fluid in rotator interval
- MR arthrography (direct)
  - **Best imaging study for rotator interval**
  - Sagittal oblique arthrogram, T1 with fat saturation
- CT arthrography: May be useful for patients with contraindication to MR

Imaging Pitfalls
- **Synovium and capsule may herniate into interval**
  - Present in asymptomatic shoulders
  - Causes focal fluid signal intensity
  - May simulate tear
- **Iatrogenic disruption of rotator interval**
  - Arthroscopic surgery with probe placed through rotator interval
  - Arthrography using a rotator interval approach

CLINICAL IMPLICATIONS

Clinical Importance
- Provides passive shoulder stability
- Injury to one structure often associated with injuries to other structures within rotator interval
- Rotator interval injury predisposes to additional injuries due to humeral head instability

Shoulder: Rotator Interval

CORACOHUMERAL LIGAMENT

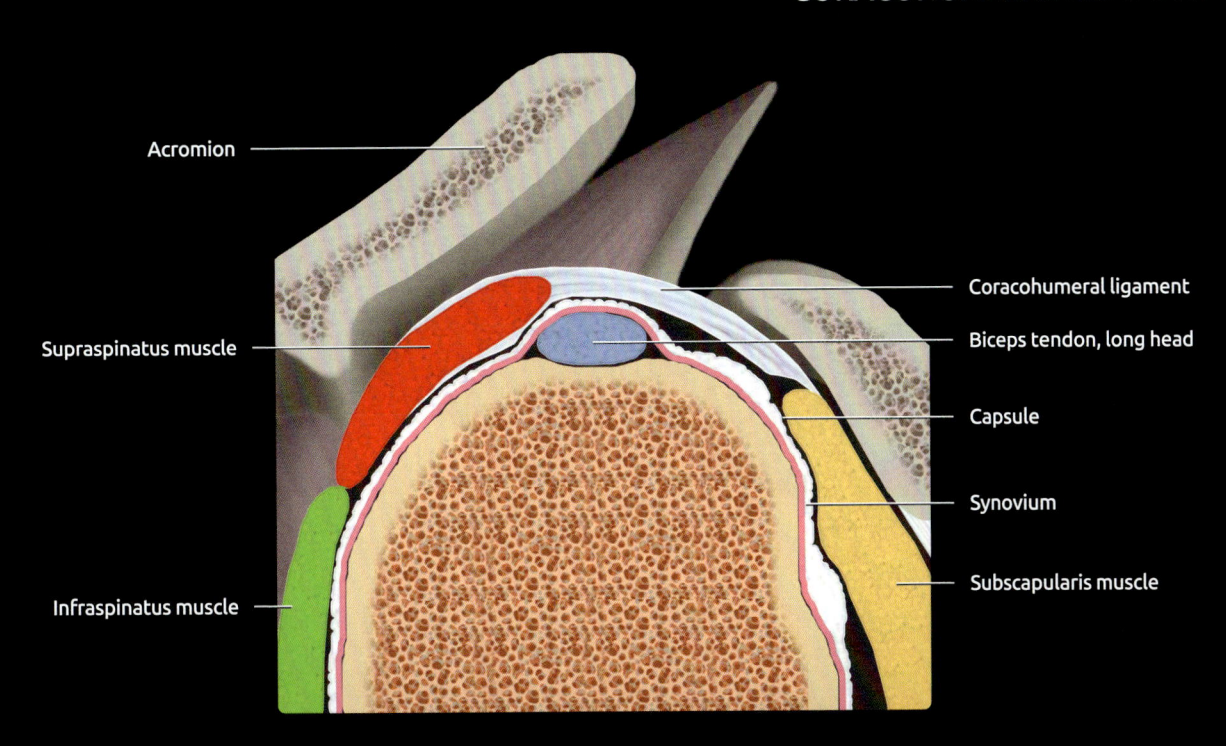

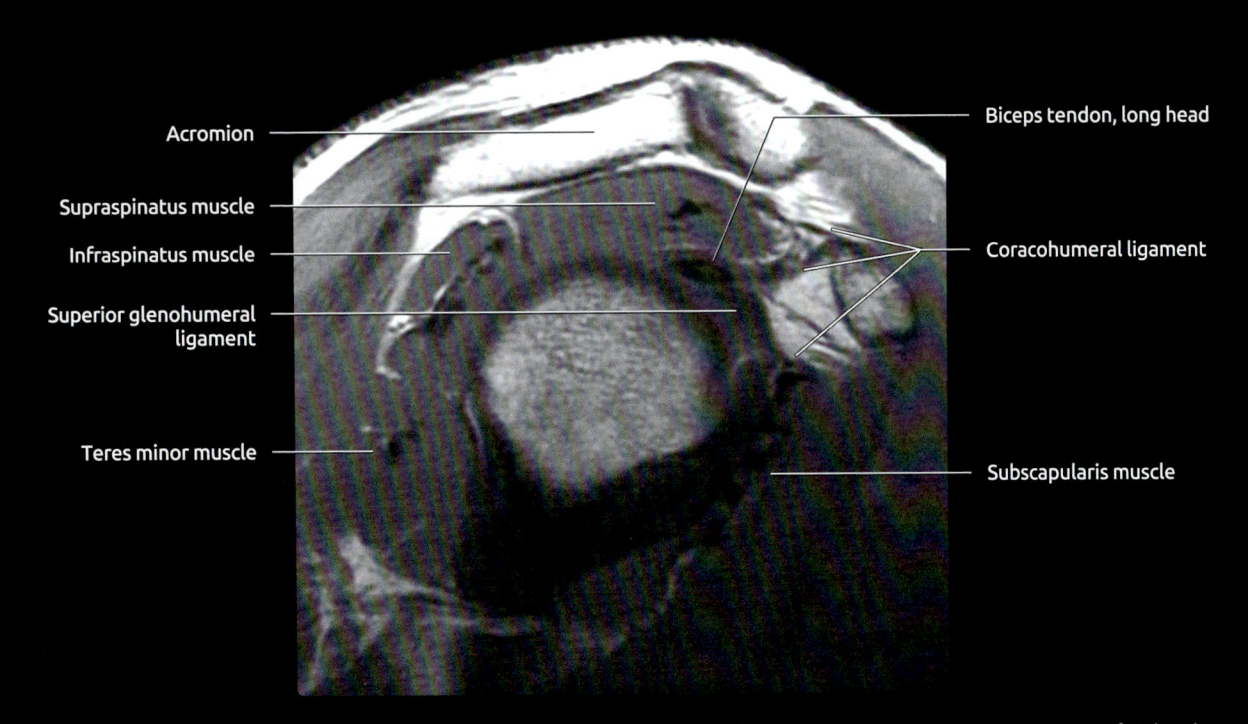

(Top) Graphic shows the relationship of coracohumeral ligament with the rotator cuff muscles. Portions of the CHL pass superficial and deep to the supraspinatus muscle. The CHL attaches to the superior border of the subscapularis muscle. (Bottom) Sagittal oblique T1 MR image is shown through the rotator interval of the right shoulder. Portions of the coracohumeral ligament blend with the superficial and deep aspects of the supraspinatus. A portion also blends with the superficial subscapularis. The superior glenohumeral ligament is seen as globular low signal anterior to the long head of the biceps tendon. Without fluid in the joint, the superior glenohumeral ligament can be difficult to differentiate as a separate structure from the coracohumeral ligament.

Shoulder: Rotator Interval

ROTATOR INTERVAL ANATOMY

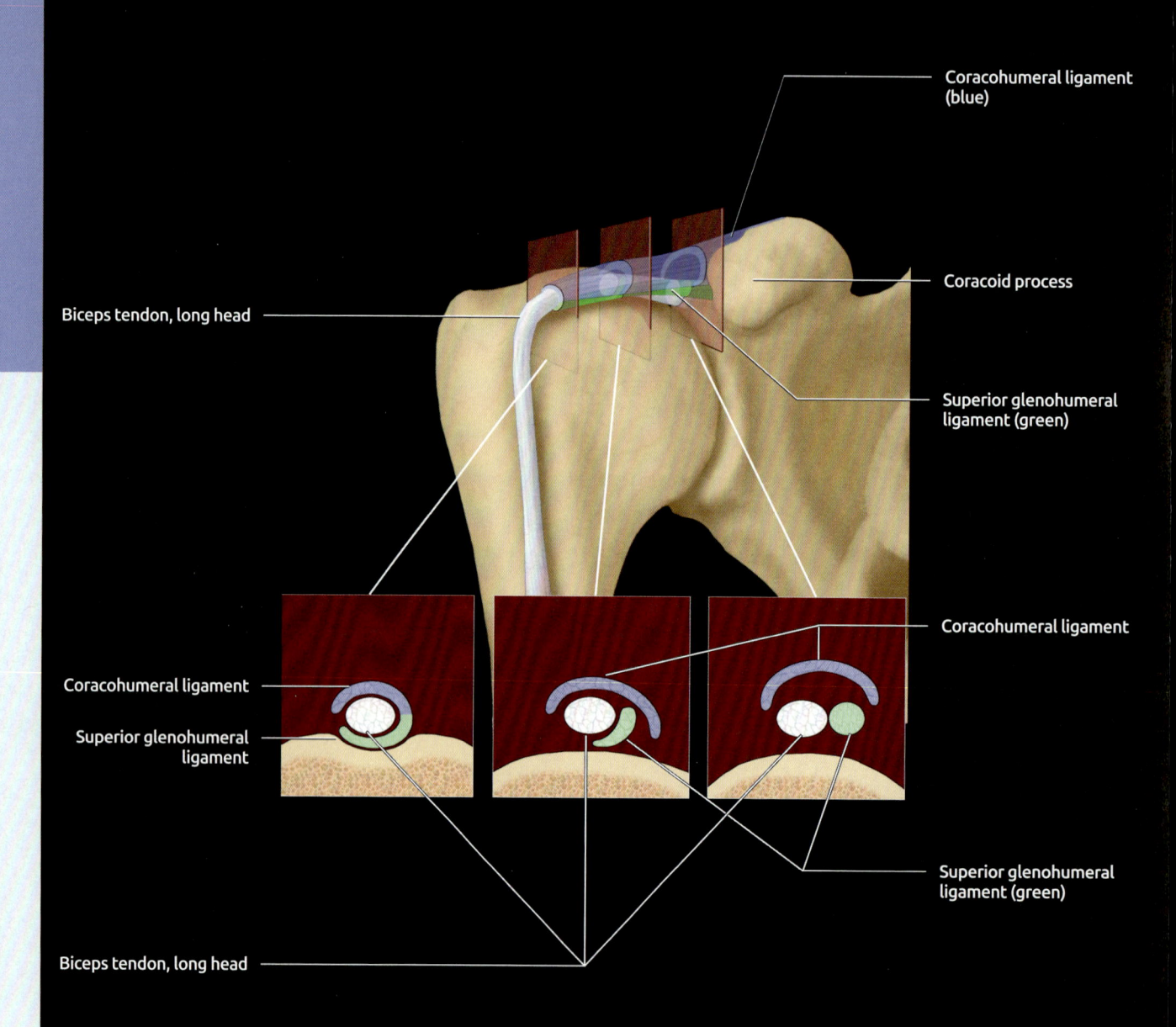

A normal rotator interval anatomy graphic is shown. Cross section images at the lateral, mid, and medial portions of the rotator interval are located along the bottom of the image. At the lateral aspect of the rotator interval, just proximal to the entrance to the bicipital groove, the coracohumeral ligament (blue) and superior glenohumeral ligament (green) form a sling around the long head of the biceps tendon. At the mid portion of the rotator interval, the CHL covers the superior aspect of the LBT, with the SGHL forming a T-shaped junction with the CHL. Near the medial border of the rotator interval, the SGHL is a round structure lying anterior to the LBT. The CHL forms a U-shaped roof over the LBT and SGHL. (Modified from Krief OP, 2005.)

Shoulder: Rotator Interval

SAGITTAL PD FS ARTHROGRAM, ROTATOR INTERVAL

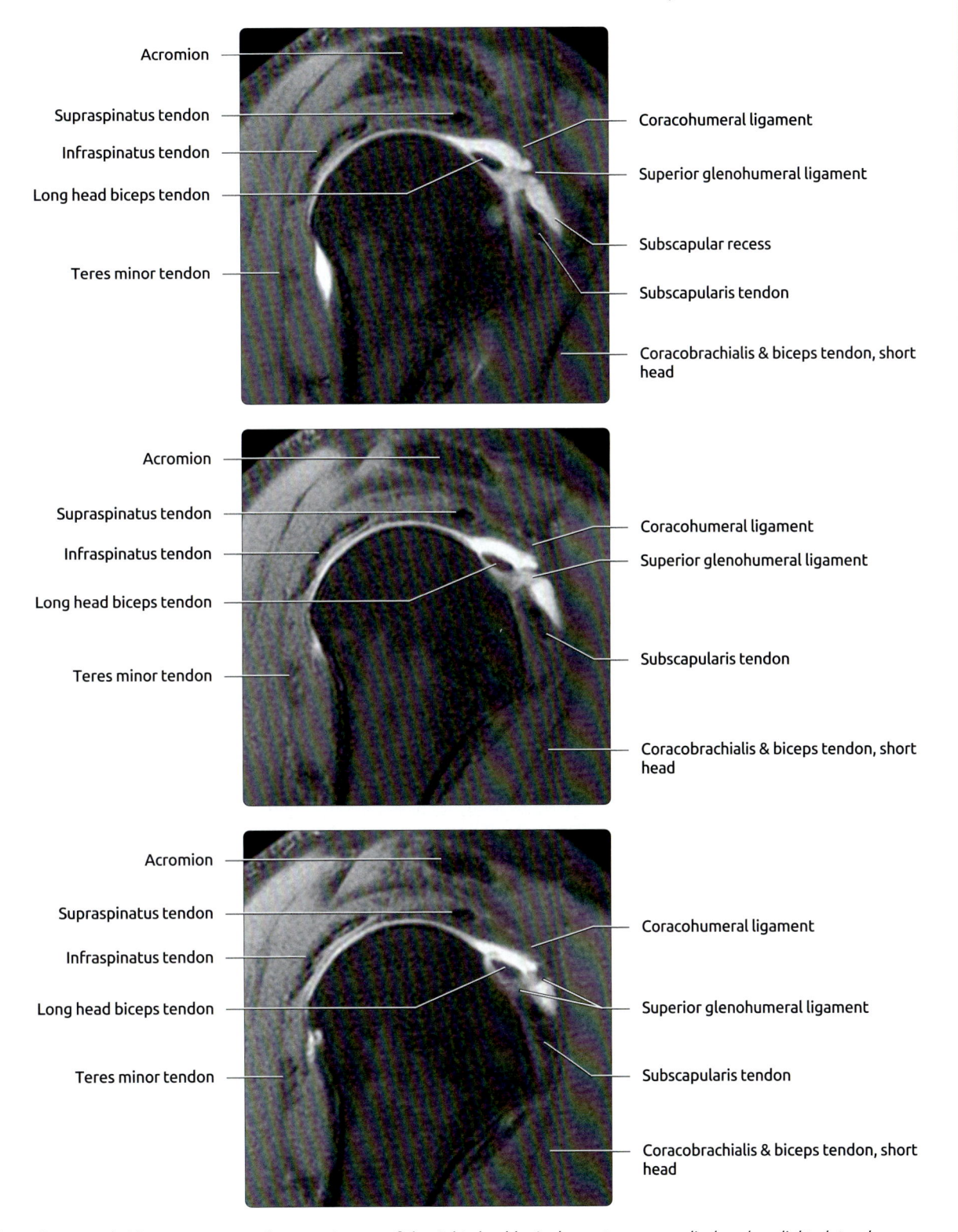

(Top) The first of 3 sagittal oblique T1 FS MR arthrogram images of the right shoulder is shown. Images are displayed medial to lateral. The sagittal oblique plane is the optimal plane for evaluating the rotator interval. These images were chosen to match the cross section graphics on the prior page. The coracohumeral ligament forms the roof of the rotator interval on all 3 images. (Middle) The superior glenohumeral ligament has a T-shaped junction with the coracohumeral ligament at the mid portion of the rotator interval. (Bottom) At the lateral aspect of the rotator interval, the superior glenohumeral ligament forms the inferior portion of the sling around the long head of the biceps tendon.

Shoulder: Rotator Interval

AXIAL T2 MR ARTHROGRAM, ROTATOR INTERVAL

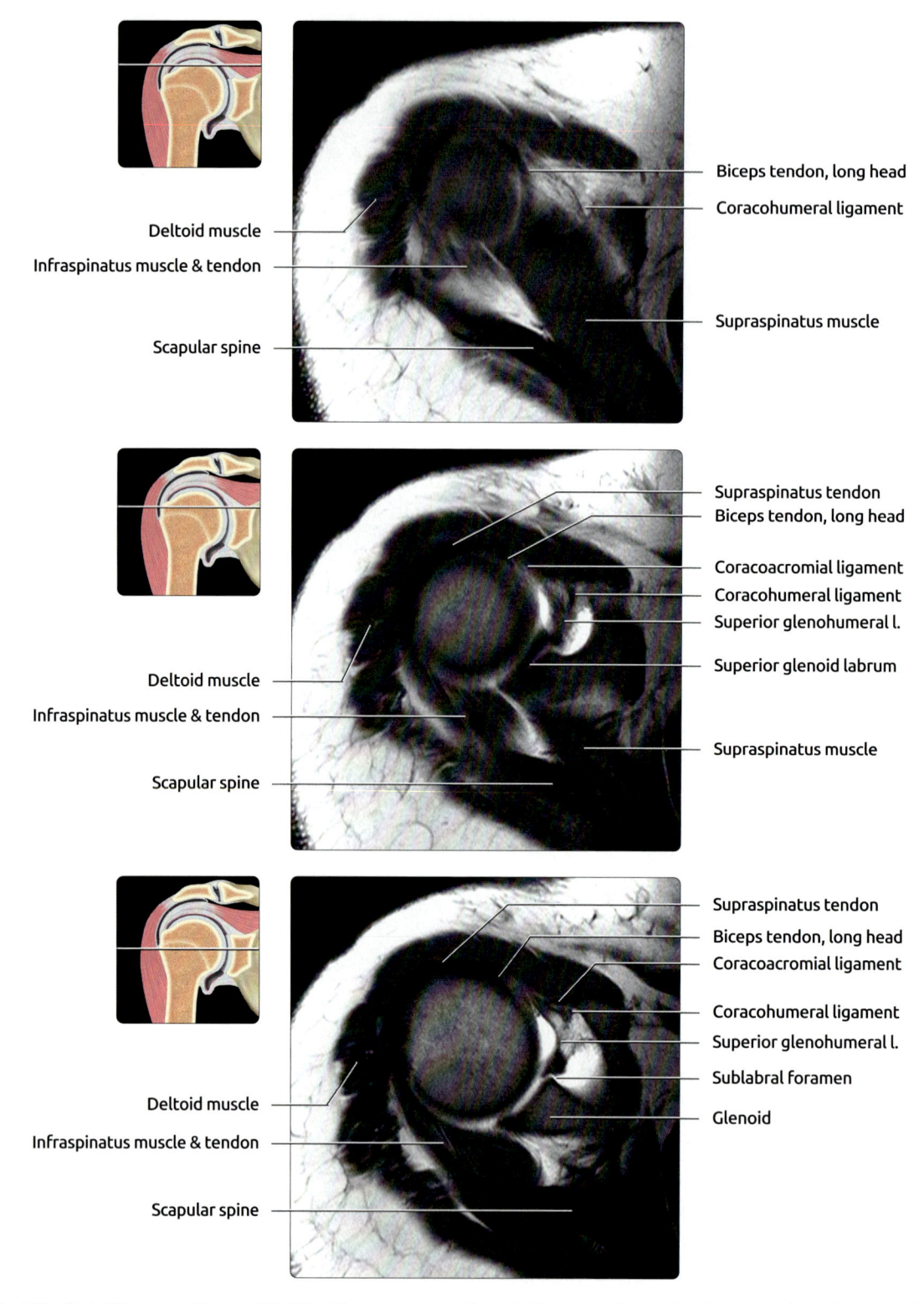

Labels (Top image): Deltoid muscle; Infraspinatus muscle & tendon; Scapular spine; Biceps tendon, long head; Coracohumeral ligament; Supraspinatus muscle

Labels (Middle image): Deltoid muscle; Infraspinatus muscle & tendon; Scapular spine; Supraspinatus tendon; Biceps tendon, long head; Coracoacromial ligament; Coracohumeral ligament; Superior glenohumeral l.; Superior glenoid labrum; Supraspinatus muscle

Labels (Bottom image): Deltoid muscle; Infraspinatus muscle & tendon; Scapular spine; Supraspinatus tendon; Biceps tendon, long head; Coracoacromial ligament; Coracohumeral ligament; Superior glenohumeral l.; Sublabral foramen; Glenoid

(Top) The first of 3 consecutive axial T2 MR arthrogram images through the rotator interval is shown. Axial imaging is not the optimal plane for evaluating the rotator interval, but can be useful. The long head of the biceps tendon is seen traversing the superomedial humeral head. (Middle) The superior glenohumeral ligament has a roughly parallel course to the long head of the biceps tendon on axial images but diverges slightly, forming a "Y." (Bottom) The superior glenohumeral ligament fuses with the coracohumeral ligament. These in turn will fuse with the joint capsule and rotator cuff tendons. These images are T2WI and have intraarticular contrast. The fat and bone marrow are near the intensity of a T1WI study due to a relatively short TE.

Shoulder: Rotator Interval

CORONAL T2 MR ARTHROGRAM, ROTATOR INTERVAL

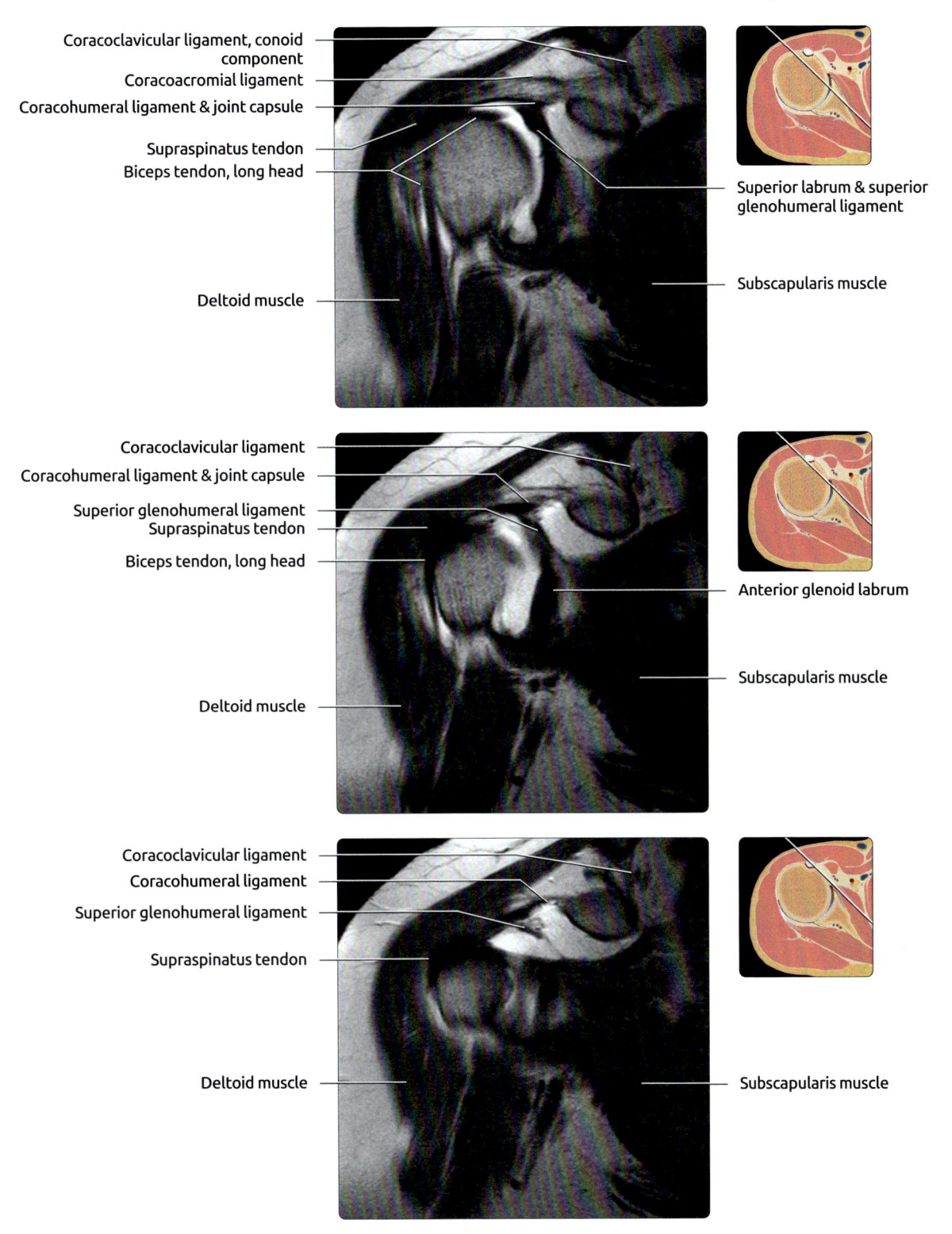

Top image labels:
- Coracoclavicular ligament, conoid component
- Coracoacromial ligament
- Coracohumeral ligament & joint capsule
- Supraspinatus tendon
- Biceps tendon, long head
- Deltoid muscle
- Superior labrum & superior glenohumeral ligament
- Subscapularis muscle

Middle image labels:
- Coracoclavicular ligament
- Coracohumeral ligament & joint capsule
- Superior glenohumeral ligament
- Supraspinatus tendon
- Biceps tendon, long head
- Deltoid muscle
- Anterior glenoid labrum
- Subscapularis muscle

Bottom image labels:
- Coracoclavicular ligament
- Coracohumeral ligament
- Superior glenohumeral ligament
- Supraspinatus tendon
- Deltoid muscle
- Subscapularis muscle

(Top) The first of 3 consecutive coronal oblique T2 MR images through the rotator interval is shown. Images are displayed posterior to anterior. The rotator interval is best evaluated in the sagittal oblique plane but the coronal plane may be additive to the evaluation of the region. (Middle) The long head of the biceps tendon is exiting the rotator interval as it enters the bicipital groove. (Bottom) In any plane, it may be difficult to separate the superior glenohumeral ligament, coracohumeral ligament, joint capsule, and rotator cuff tendons, especially at the anterolateral aspect of the rotator interval.

Shoulder: Rotator Interval

SAGITTAL T1 FS MR ARTHROGRAM

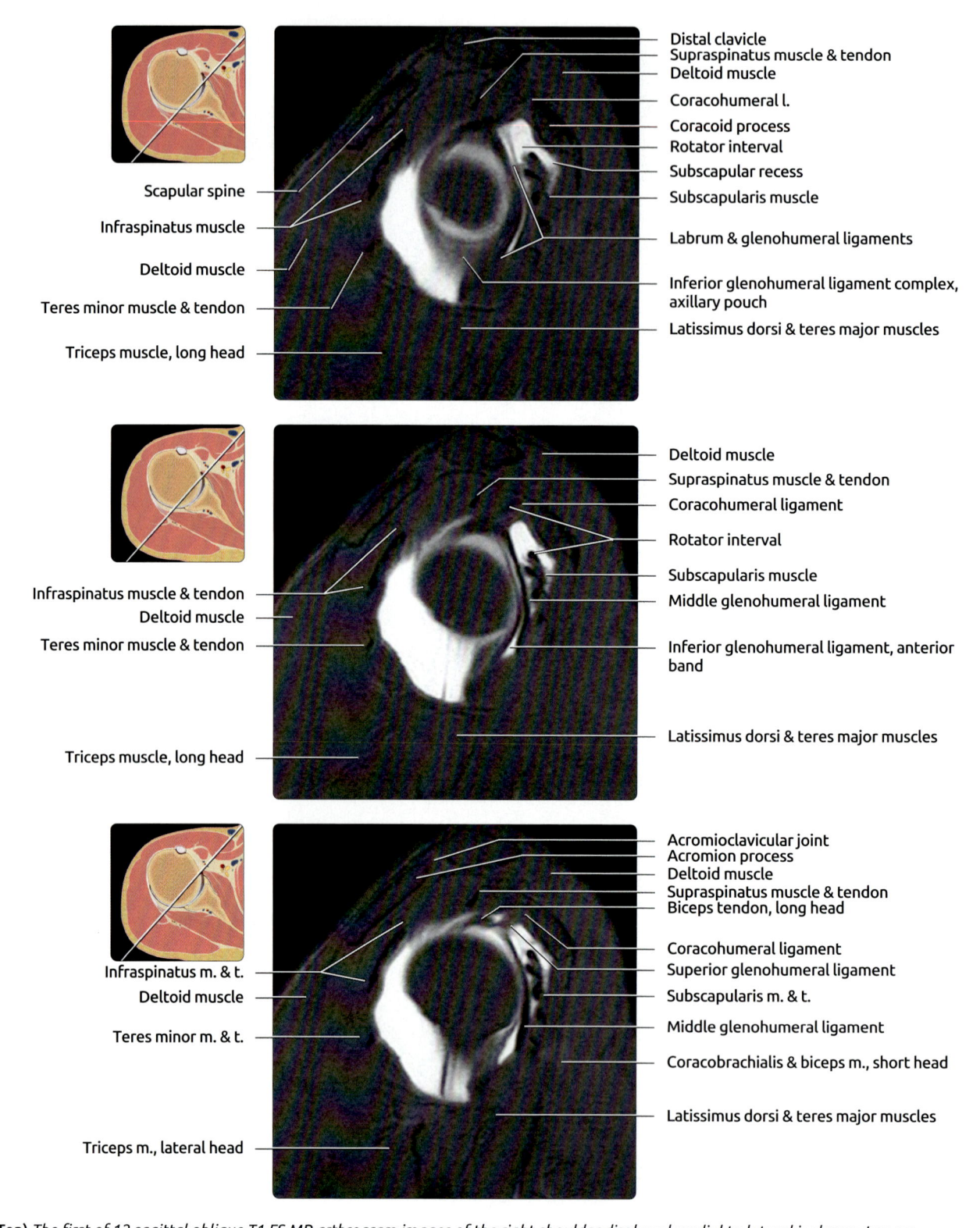

Labels (top image):
- Distal clavicle
- Supraspinatus muscle & tendon
- Deltoid muscle
- Coracohumeral l.
- Coracoid process
- Rotator interval
- Subscapular recess
- Subscapularis muscle
- Labrum & glenohumeral ligaments
- Inferior glenohumeral ligament complex, axillary pouch
- Latissimus dorsi & teres major muscles
- Scapular spine
- Infraspinatus muscle
- Deltoid muscle
- Teres minor muscle & tendon
- Triceps muscle, long head

Labels (middle image):
- Deltoid muscle
- Supraspinatus muscle & tendon
- Coracohumeral ligament
- Rotator interval
- Subscapularis muscle
- Middle glenohumeral ligament
- Inferior glenohumeral ligament, anterior band
- Latissimus dorsi & teres major muscles
- Infraspinatus muscle & tendon
- Deltoid muscle
- Teres minor muscle & tendon
- Triceps muscle, long head

Labels (bottom image):
- Acromioclavicular joint
- Acromion process
- Deltoid muscle
- Supraspinatus muscle & tendon
- Biceps tendon, long head
- Coracohumeral ligament
- Superior glenohumeral ligament
- Subscapularis m. & t.
- Middle glenohumeral ligament
- Coracobrachialis & biceps m., short head
- Latissimus dorsi & teres major muscles
- Infraspinatus m. & t.
- Deltoid muscle
- Teres minor m. & t.
- Triceps m., lateral head

(Top) The first of 12 sagittal oblique T1 FS MR arthrogram images of the right shoulder displayed medial to lateral is shown. Images were acquired at 1.5 T with a shoulder coil. This image is through the level of the glenohumeral joint. The glenoid labrum forms an oval low-signal band around the medial aspect of the humeral head. **(Middle)** The rotator interval is the space between the supraspinatus and subscapularis tendons. The medial extent is the coracoid process. **(Bottom)** The superior glenohumeral ligament has a T-shaped connection with the coracohumeral ligament at this level.

Shoulder: Rotator Interval

SAGITTAL T1 FS MR ARTHROGRAM

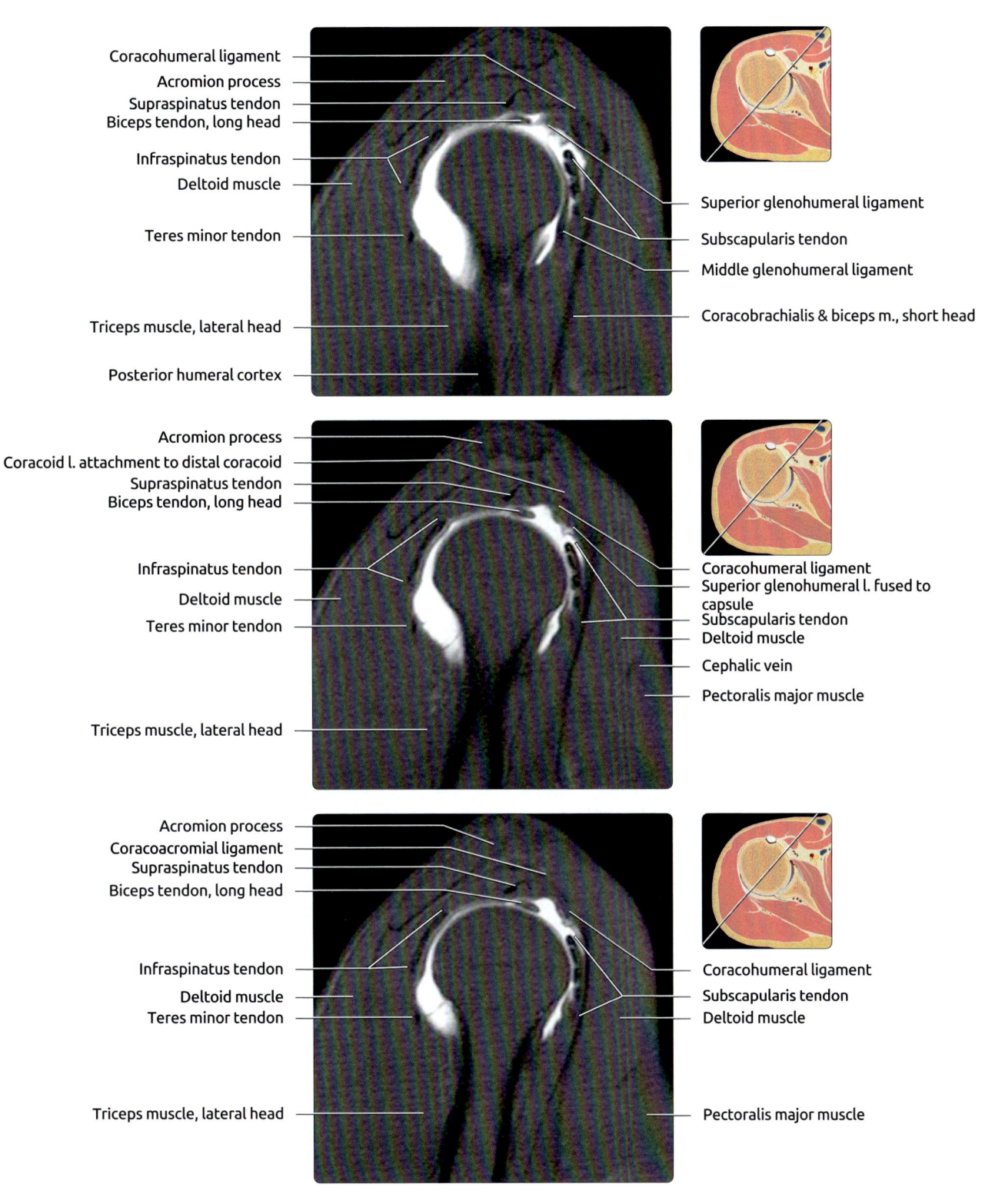

(Top) The coracohumeral ligament forms the roof of the rotator interval. Portions of the coracohumeral ligament fuse with the joint capsule, supraspinatus tendon, and subscapularis tendons. Note that at this level the coracohumeral ligament extends to the articular surface of supraspinatus and is medial to the origin of the more superficial coracoacromial ligament (shown on the next lateral image). (Middle) The long head of the biceps tendon courses over the top of the humeral head. (Bottom) The floor of the rotator interval is the humeral head cartilage.

Shoulder: Rotator Interval

SAGITTAL T1 FS MR ARTHROGRAM

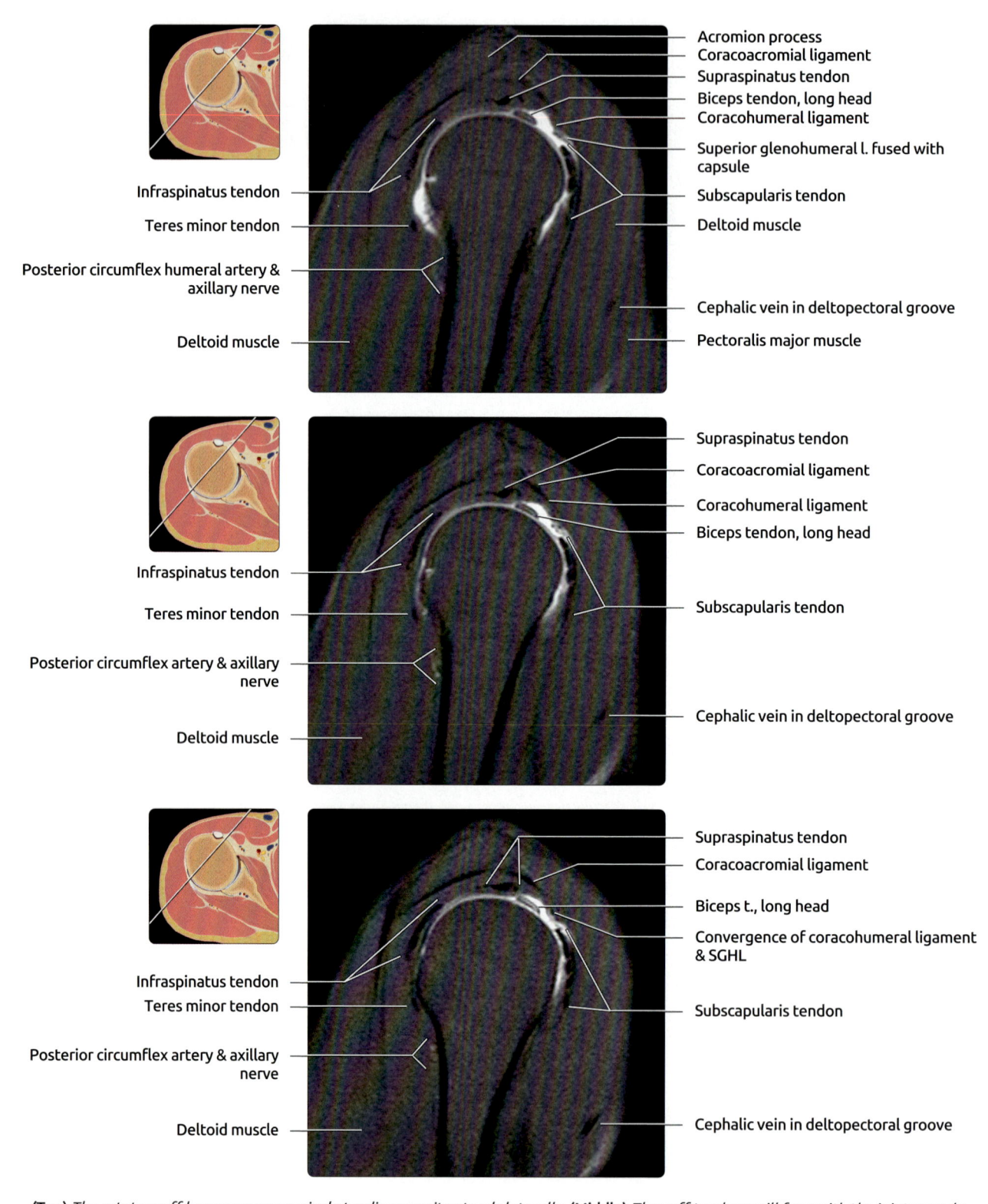

(Top) The rotator cuff becomes progressively tendinous as it extends laterally. *(Middle)* The cuff tendons will fuse with the joint capsule, as will the coracohumeral ligament. The coracohumeral ligament will span the rotator interval roof to fill the space between the supraspinatus and subscapularis tendons. The coracohumeral ligament will not be distinguishable from the rotator cuff tendons or joint capsule when it fuses. *(Bottom)* The long head of the biceps tendon is nearing the entrance into the bicipital groove. The coracohumeral ligament and superior glenohumeral ligament can be difficult to appreciate but are within the globular soft tissue anterior to the biceps tendon.

Shoulder: Rotator Interval

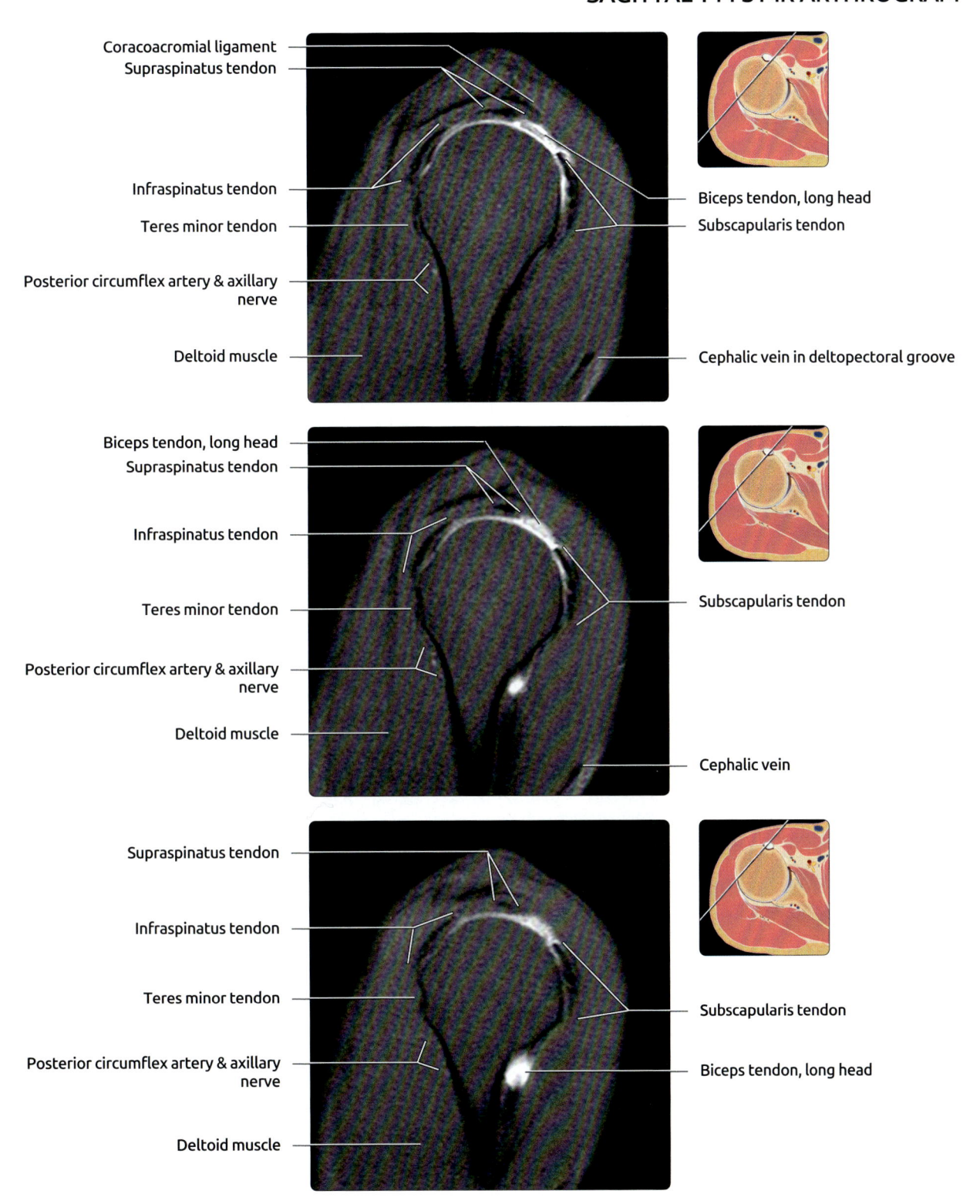

SAGITTAL T1 FS MR ARTHROGRAM

(Top) The coracohumeral ligament and superior glenohumeral ligament provide support to the long head of the biceps tendon. **(Middle)** The long head of the biceps tendon is entering the bicipital groove. The rotator interval ends at this level. **(Bottom)** This is one image beyond the lateral extent of the rotator interval. The long head of the biceps tendon has exited the joint and is now traversing the bicipital groove.

Shoulder Ligaments

TERMINOLOGY

Abbreviations
- Acromioclavicular (AC)
- Coracohumeral (CH)
- Superior glenohumeral ligament (SGHL)
- Middle glenohumeral ligament (MGHL)
- Inferior glenohumeral ligament (IGHL)

IMAGING ANATOMY

Anatomy Relationships
- **Glenohumeral ligaments**
  - Strengthen and fuse with joint capsule
  - **Presence of true ligaments debated**
    - May represent folds in joint capsule
    - Termed glenolabral periarticular fiber complex
  - **Vary in number and size**
    - Type I: Classic 3 ligaments (SGHL, MGHL, IGHL)
    - Type II: MGHL cord, pseudo-Buford
    - Type III: Combined MGHL/IGHL cord, pseudo-Buford
    - Type IV: No ligaments
  - **Superior glenohumeral ligament**
    - Stabilizes shoulder in adduction
    - May originate from biceps tendon, anterior labrum, or in common with MGHL
    - Extends to lesser tuberosity
    - Fuses with coracohumeral ligament
    - Transverse orientation
    - Gentle curving shape on axial images at level of superior coracoid process
    - Almost always anatomically present
    - Visible on 30% conventional MR, 85% MR arthrograms
  - **Middle glenohumeral ligament**
    - Stabilizes shoulder in abduction
    - Originates from anterior labrum or scapular neck
    - Extends along deep surface of subscapularis to lesser tuberosity
    - Oblique orientation
    - Blends with joint capsule and labrum anteriorly
    - Absent or small MGHL in 30%
    - May be enlarged and cord-like
    - Buford complex: Thick or cord-like MGHL and absent anterosuperior labrum
    - Can fuse with anterior band of IGHL
  - **Inferior glenohumeral ligament**
    - Resists anterior dislocation and stabilizes in abduction
    - More accurately termed IGHL complex
    - Anterior band, fascicles of axillary pouch and posterior band
    - Extends from inferior glenoid labrum to inferior humeral anatomic neck
    - Vertical orientation of anterior & posterior bands
    - Anterior band is usually larger than posterior band
- **Coracohumeral ligament**
  - Coracoid process base to greater & lesser tuberosities
  - Horizontal orientation
  - **Forms roof of rotator interval**
  - Stabilizes long head of biceps tendon from subluxing medially into subscapularis
  - Strengthens transverse ligament covering bicipital groove
  - Fuses with supraspinatus tendon, subscapularis tendon, joint capsule, and SGHL
- **Coracoacromial ligament**
  - Forms coracoacromial arch along with acromion and coracoid process
  - Reinforces inferior aspect of acromioclavicular joint
  - Extends from distal 2/3 of coracoid to acromion tip
  - 2 conjoined or closely associated bands
  - May have a broad acromial insertion
- **Coracoclavicular ligament**
  - Major stabilizer of acromioclavicular joint
  - Extends from base of coracoid process to undersurface of clavicle
  - Fan-shaped complex with 2 fasciculi
    - Conoid ligament: Posteromedial, vertical
    - Trapezoid ligament: Anterolateral, oblique
- **Acromioclavicular ligaments**
  - Superior and inferior AC ligaments
  - Reinforce acromioclavicular joint capsule
- **Transverse humeral ligament**
  - Extends between greater and lesser tuberosities
  - Contains fibers from subscapularis tendon
  - Covers bicipital groove
- **Superior transverse scapular ligament**
  - Converts suprascapular notch into foramen
  - Suprascapular nerve passes below ligament
    - Potential for suprascapular nerve entrapment
  - Suprascapular vessels pass above ligament
- **Inferior transverse scapular ligament**
  - Extends from scapular spine to glenoid rim
  - Lateral to spinoglenoid notch
  - Subscapular nerve passes beneath ligament
  - Inconsistently present

ANATOMY IMAGING ISSUES

Imaging Recommendations
- MR: Ligaments have low signal intensity on all sequences
- MR arthrography
  - **Best imaging study for glenohumeral ligaments**
    - Sagittal oblique for MGHL and IGHL
    - Axial for SGHL and MGHL

Imaging Pitfalls
- **Subacromial pseudospur**
  - **Coracoacromial ligament hypertrophy**
    - Located at insertion on acromion
  - **Hypertrophied deltoid muscle inferior tendon slip**
  - Can simulate a subacromial enthesophyte
  - On T1 MR, mature osteophytes should demonstrate fatty bone marrow
  - Sclerotic or immature osteophytes may not have marrow fat, so compare with radiographs
- **MGHL origin from scapular neck** (uncommon)
  - May simulate stripping of anterior capsule

Shoulder Ligaments

ANTERIOR GRAPHIC

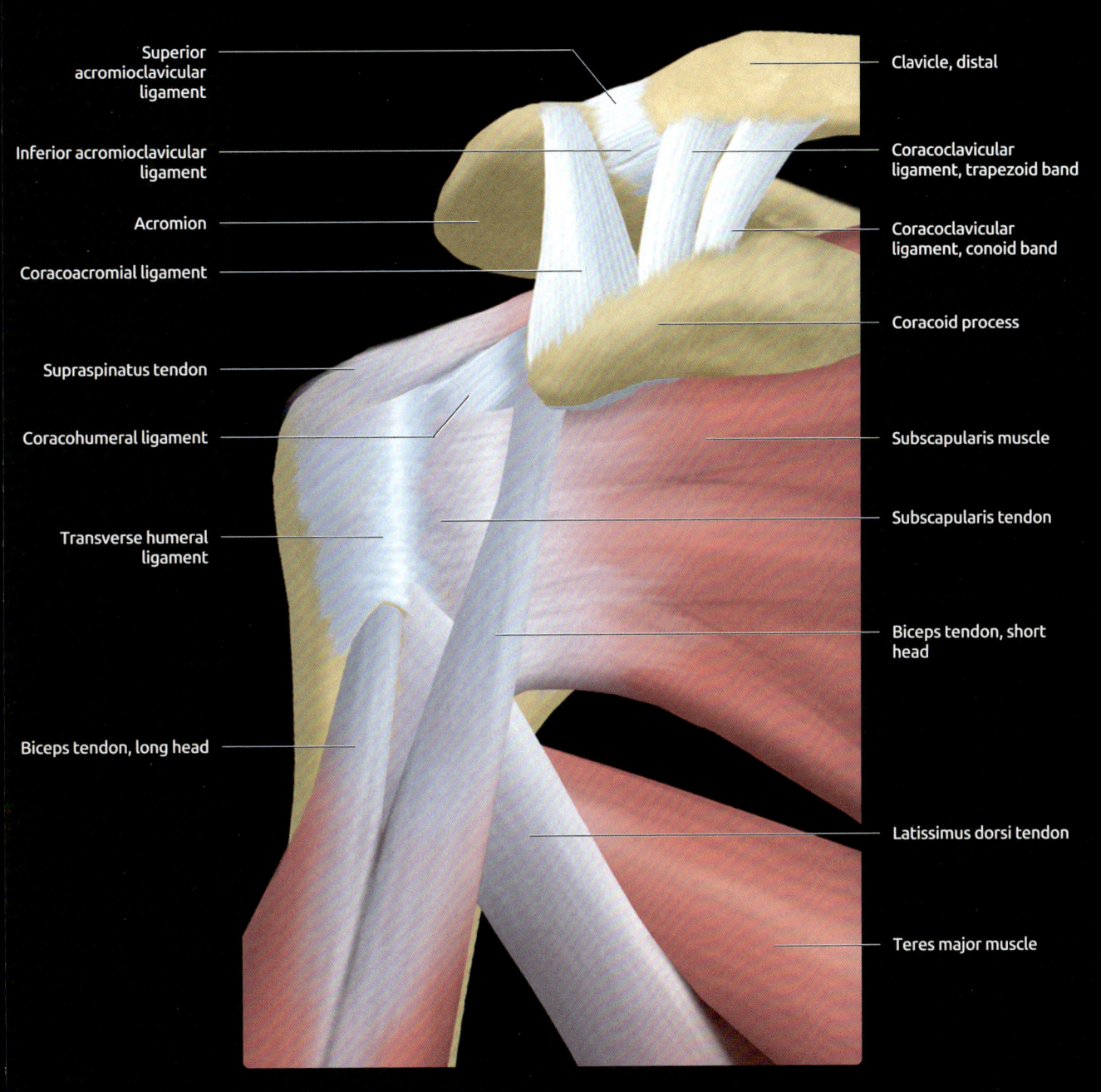

- Superior acromioclavicular ligament
- Inferior acromioclavicular ligament
- Acromion
- Coracoacromial ligament
- Supraspinatus tendon
- Coracohumeral ligament
- Transverse humeral ligament
- Biceps tendon, long head
- Clavicle, distal
- Coracoclavicular ligament, trapezoid band
- Coracoclavicular ligament, conoid band
- Coracoid process
- Subscapularis muscle
- Subscapularis tendon
- Biceps tendon, short head
- Latissimus dorsi tendon
- Teres major muscle

This anterior lordotic graphic of the shoulder shows superficial dissection.

Shoulder Ligaments

ANTERIOR AND SAGITTAL GRAPHICS

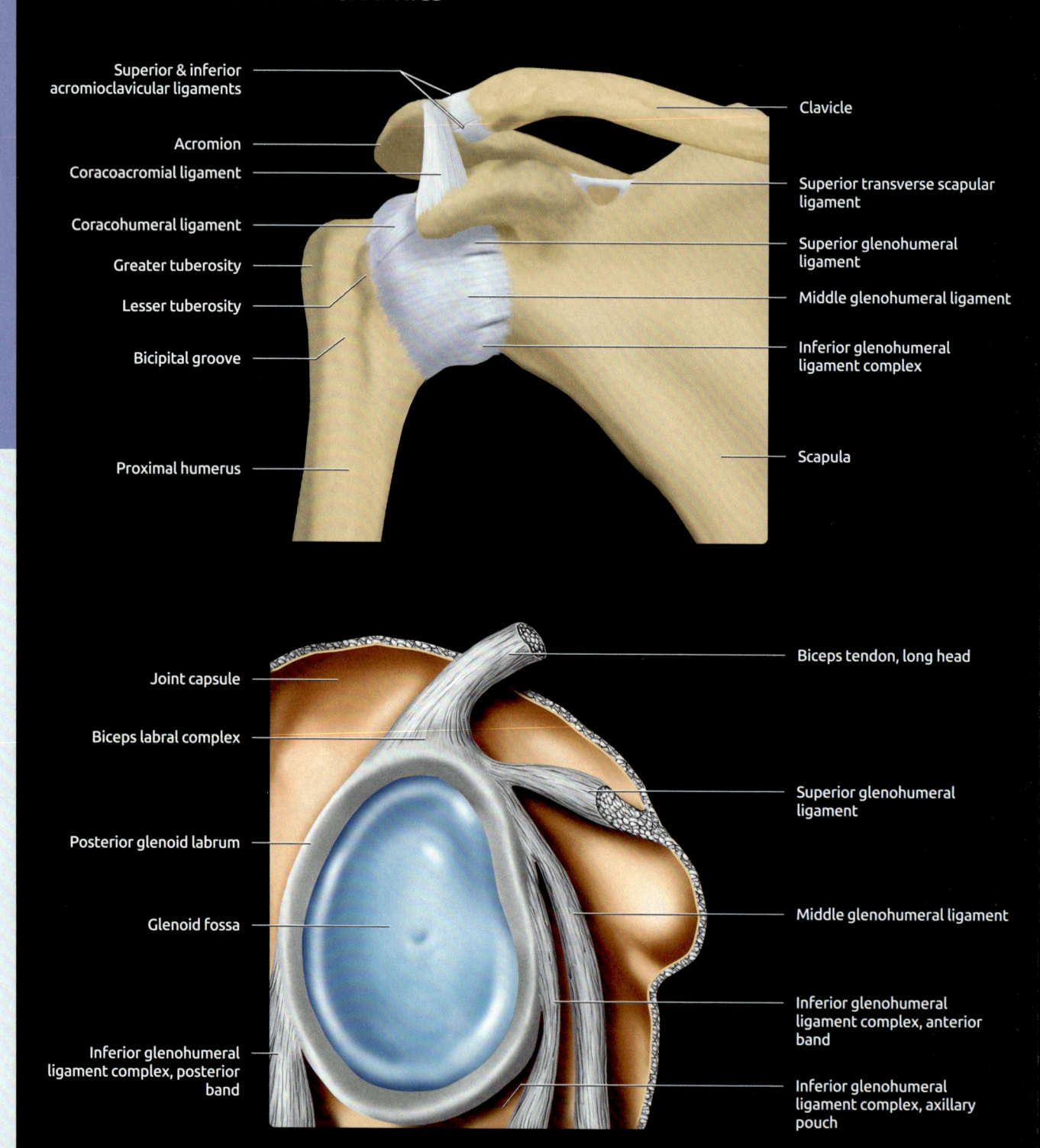

(Top) This anterior graphic of the right shoulder shows deep dissection. The muscles have been removed. *(Bottom)* Shown is a sagittal graphic of the intraarticular portion of the shoulder. The humeral head has been removed.

Shoulder Ligaments

ARTHROGRAM, GLENOHUMERAL LIGAMENTS

Top image labels (left): Supraspinatus tendon; Biceps labral complex; Infraspinatus tendon; Teres minor tendon.
Top image labels (right): Coracohumeral l.; Superior glenohumeral ligament; Middle glenohumeral ligament; Subscapularis tendon; Inferior glenohumeral ligament complex, anterior band.

Bottom image labels (left): Supraspinatus tendon; Biceps tendon, long head; Infraspinatus tendon; Teres minor tendon.
Bottom image labels (right): Superior glenohumeral ligament; Coracohumeral l.; Middle glenohumeral ligament; Subscapularis tendon; Inferior glenohumeral ligament complex, anterior band.

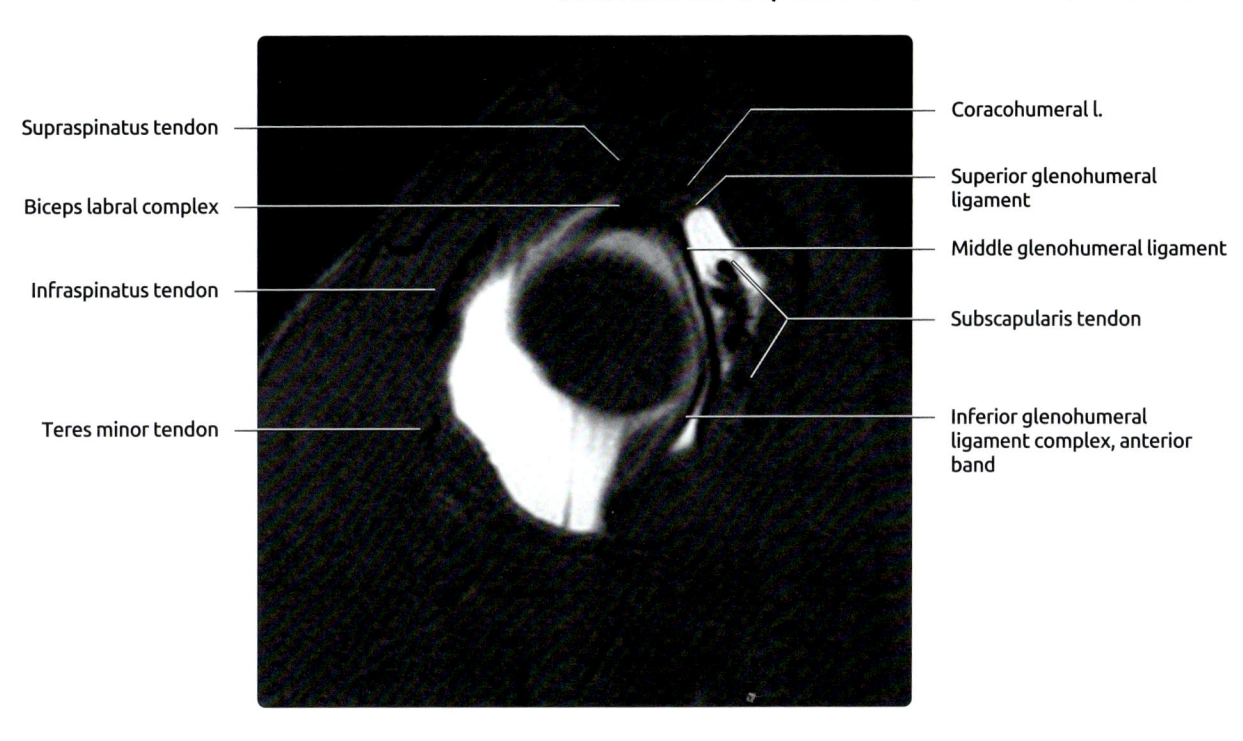

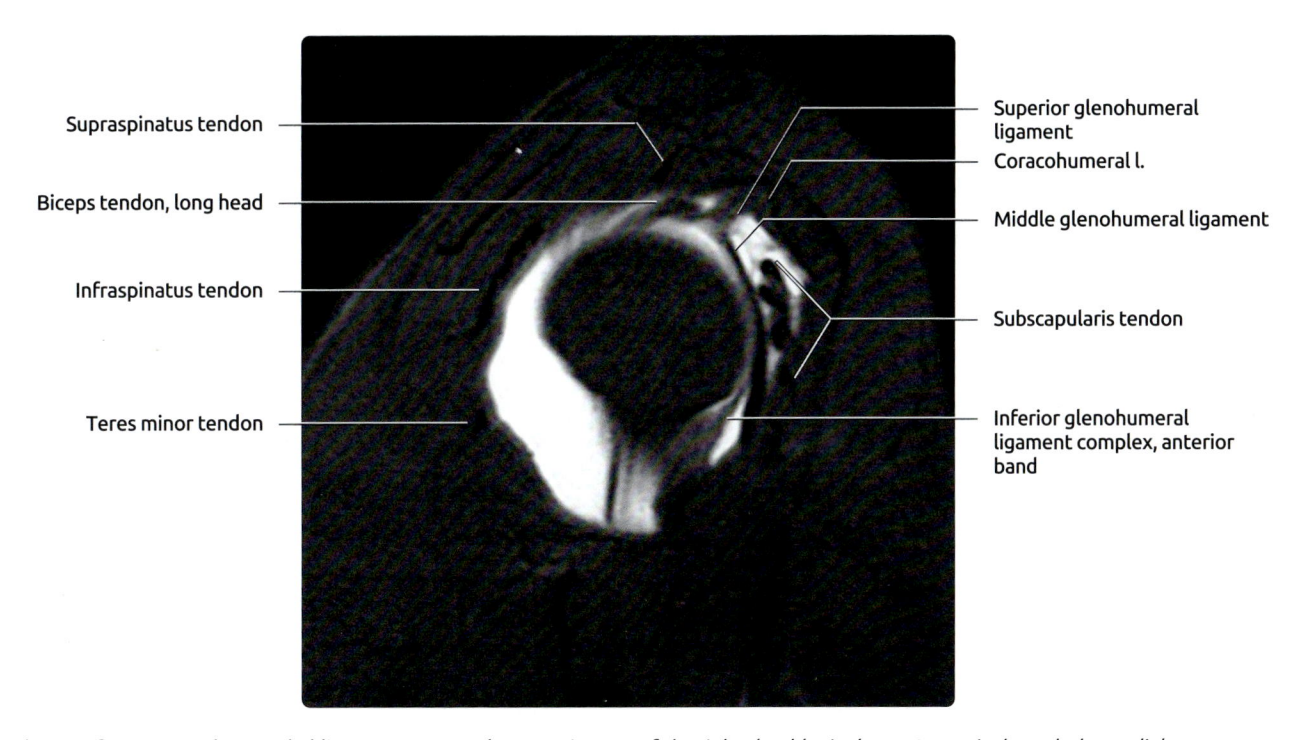

(**Top**) *First of 2 sequential sagittal oblique T1 FS MR arthrogram images of the right shoulder is shown. Image is through the medial aspect of the humeral head. The middle and inferior glenohumeral ligaments have an oblique to vertical course.* (**Bottom**) *This image is located just lateral to the previous image. The superior glenohumeral ligament is the rounded soft tissue density located anterior to the long head of the biceps tendon.*

ARTHROGRAM, SUPERIOR GLENOHUMERAL LIGAMENT

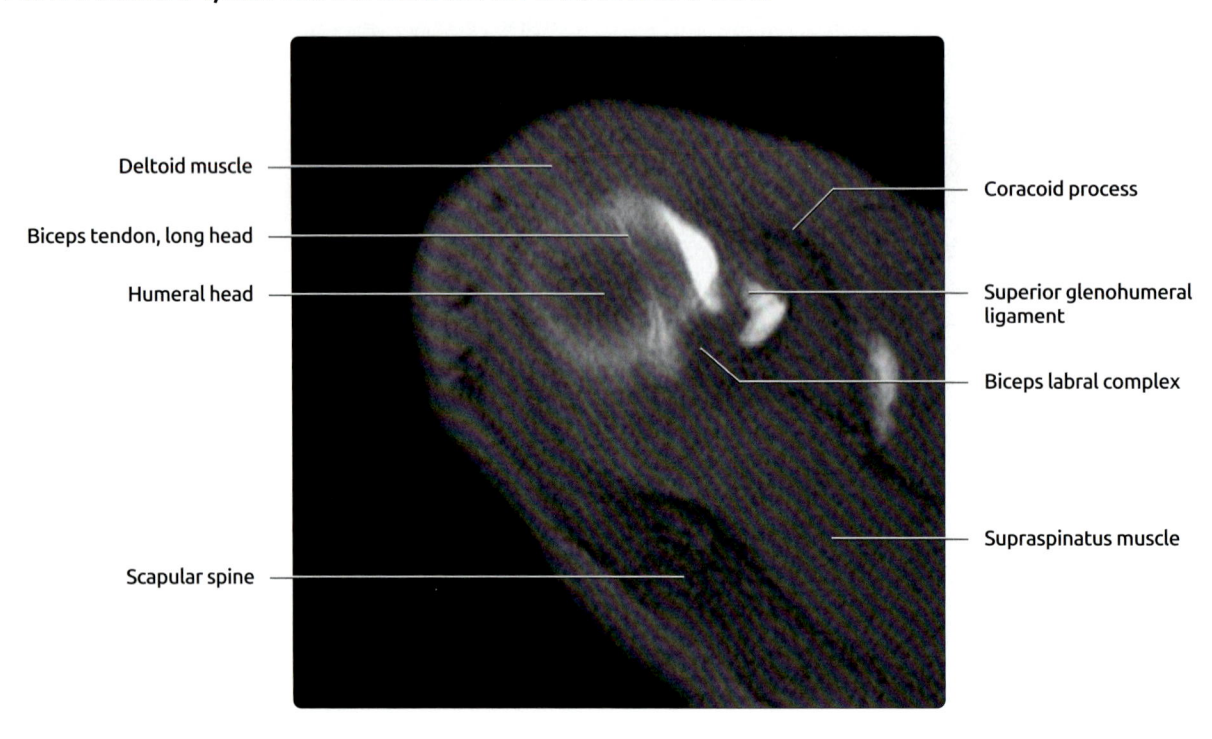

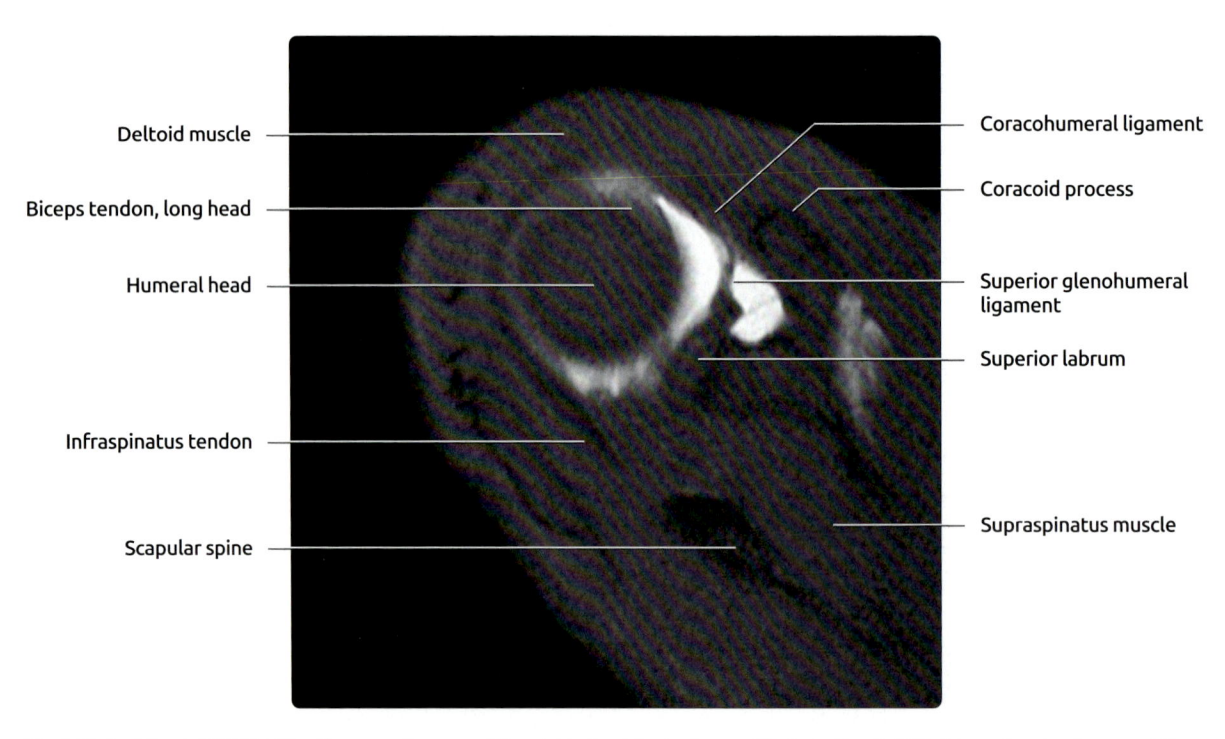

(Top) First of 2 axial T1 FS MR arthrogram images of the right shoulder is shown. The long head of the biceps tendon has an oblique course across the top of the humeral head. The superior glenohumeral ligament is located medial to the long head of the biceps and has a roughly parallel but slightly oblique course on axial images, forming a "V" or "Y" with the biceps tendon. **(Bottom)** This image is located below the previous image. The biceps tendon is curving along the anterior humeral head toward the bicipital groove. The superior glenohumeral ligament fuses with the coracohumeral ligament anteriorly. These structures in turn fuse with the joint capsule, supraspinatus tendon and subscapularis tendon to form the rotator interval.

Shoulder Ligaments

ARTHROGRAM, MIDDLE GLENOHUMERAL LIGAMENT

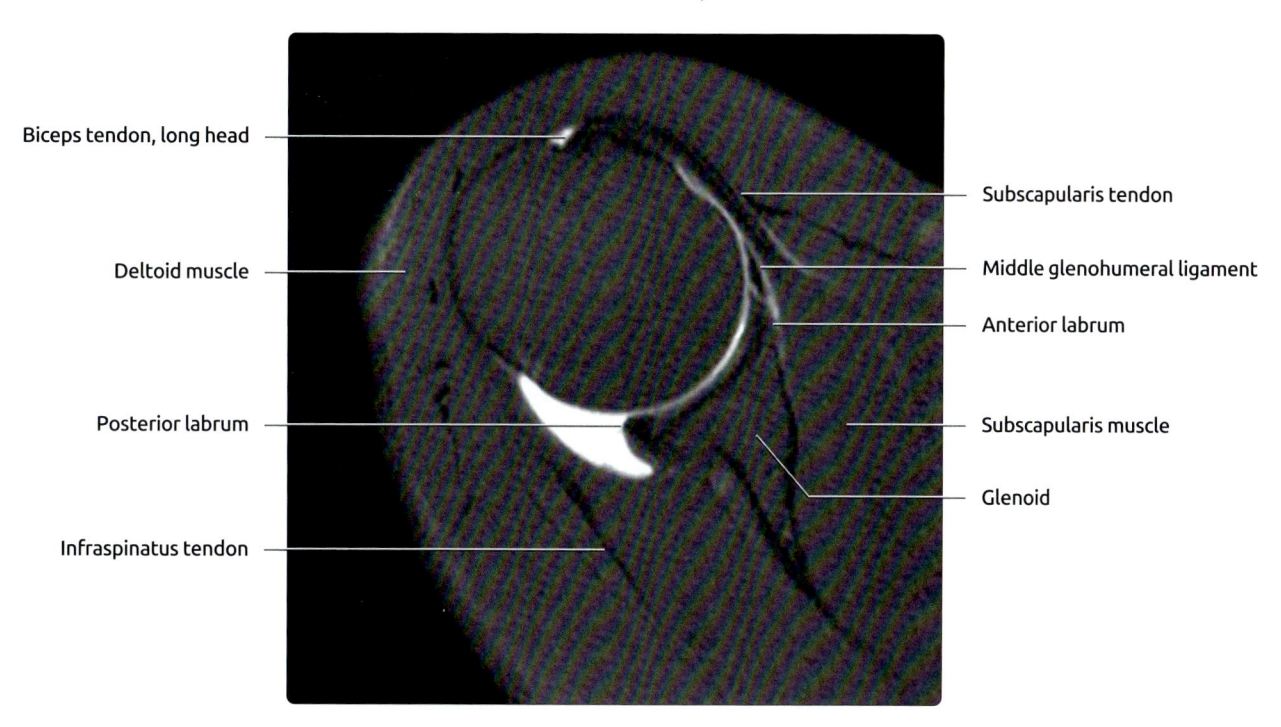

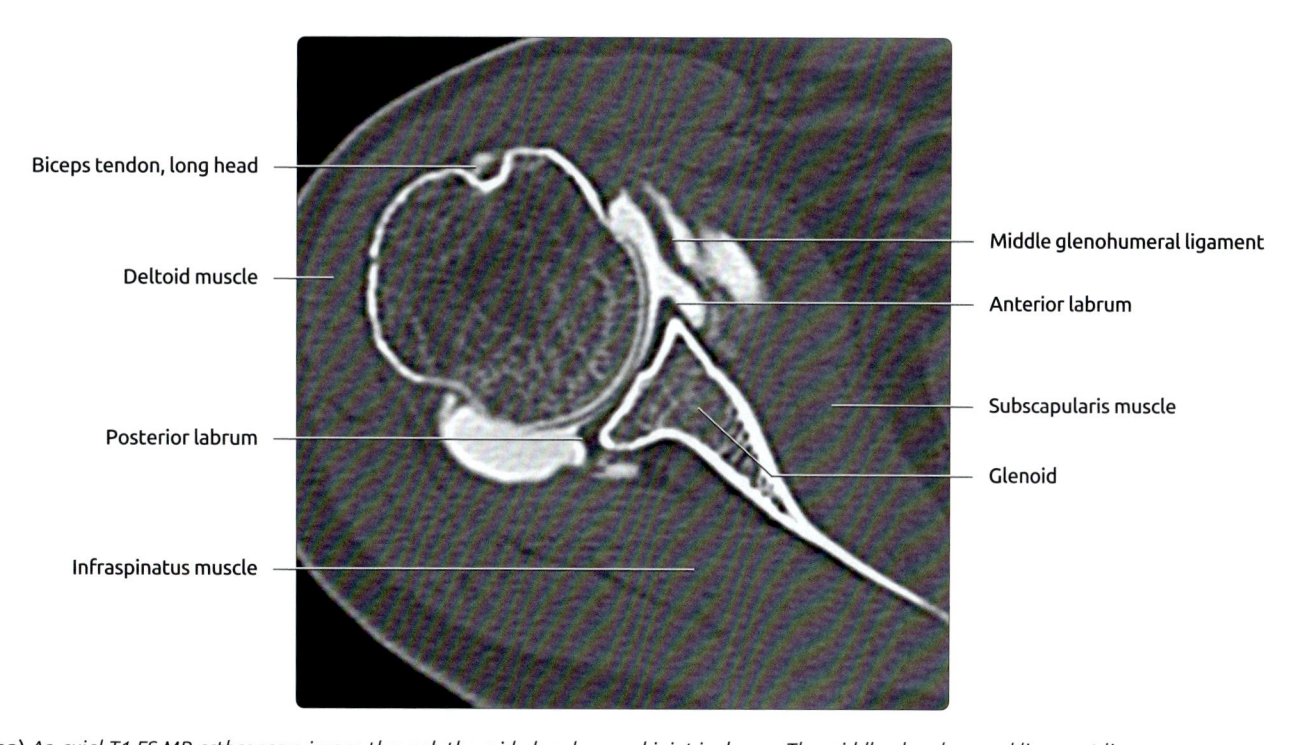

(Top) An axial T1 FS MR arthrogram image through the mid glenohumeral joint is shown. The middle glenohumeral ligament lies anterior to the anterior labrum and roughly parallels the subscapularis tendon. *(Bottom)* An axial CT arthrogram image is shown. The middle glenohumeral ligament is displaced further from the anterior labrum due to better distension of the joint compared with the prior image.

Shoulder Ligaments

GLENOHUMERAL LIGAMENT MR PITFALL: BUFORD COMPLEX

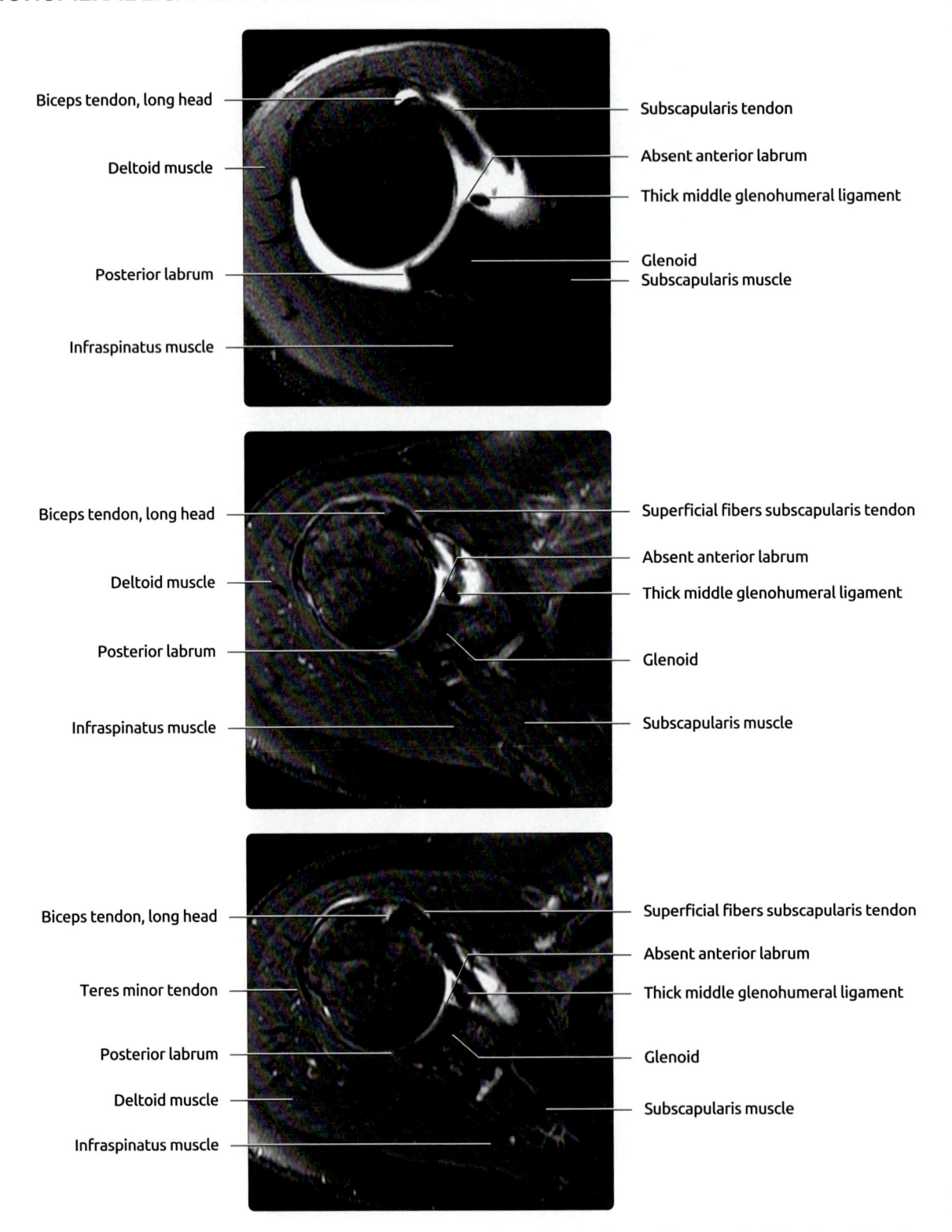

Top image labels:
- Biceps tendon, long head
- Deltoid muscle
- Posterior labrum
- Infraspinatus muscle
- Subscapularis tendon
- Absent anterior labrum
- Thick middle glenohumeral ligament
- Glenoid
- Subscapularis muscle

Middle image labels:
- Biceps tendon, long head
- Deltoid muscle
- Posterior labrum
- Infraspinatus muscle
- Superficial fibers subscapularis tendon
- Absent anterior labrum
- Thick middle glenohumeral ligament
- Glenoid
- Subscapularis muscle

Bottom image labels:
- Biceps tendon, long head
- Teres minor tendon
- Posterior labrum
- Deltoid muscle
- Infraspinatus muscle
- Superficial fibers subscapularis tendon
- Absent anterior labrum
- Thick middle glenohumeral ligament
- Glenoid
- Subscapularis muscle

(Top) An axial T1 FS MR arthrogram image of a Buford complex is shown. The middle glenohumeral ligament is thick and cord-like. The anterior glenoid labrum is absent. **(Middle)** First of 2 sequential axial T1 FS MR arthrogram images of a Buford complex is shown. **(Bottom)** This image is located distal to the previous image. A thick middle glenohumeral ligament is a relatively common normal variant and must not be mistaken for a torn or displaced labrum.

Shoulder Ligaments

INFERIOR GLENOHUMERAL LIGAMENT COMPLEX

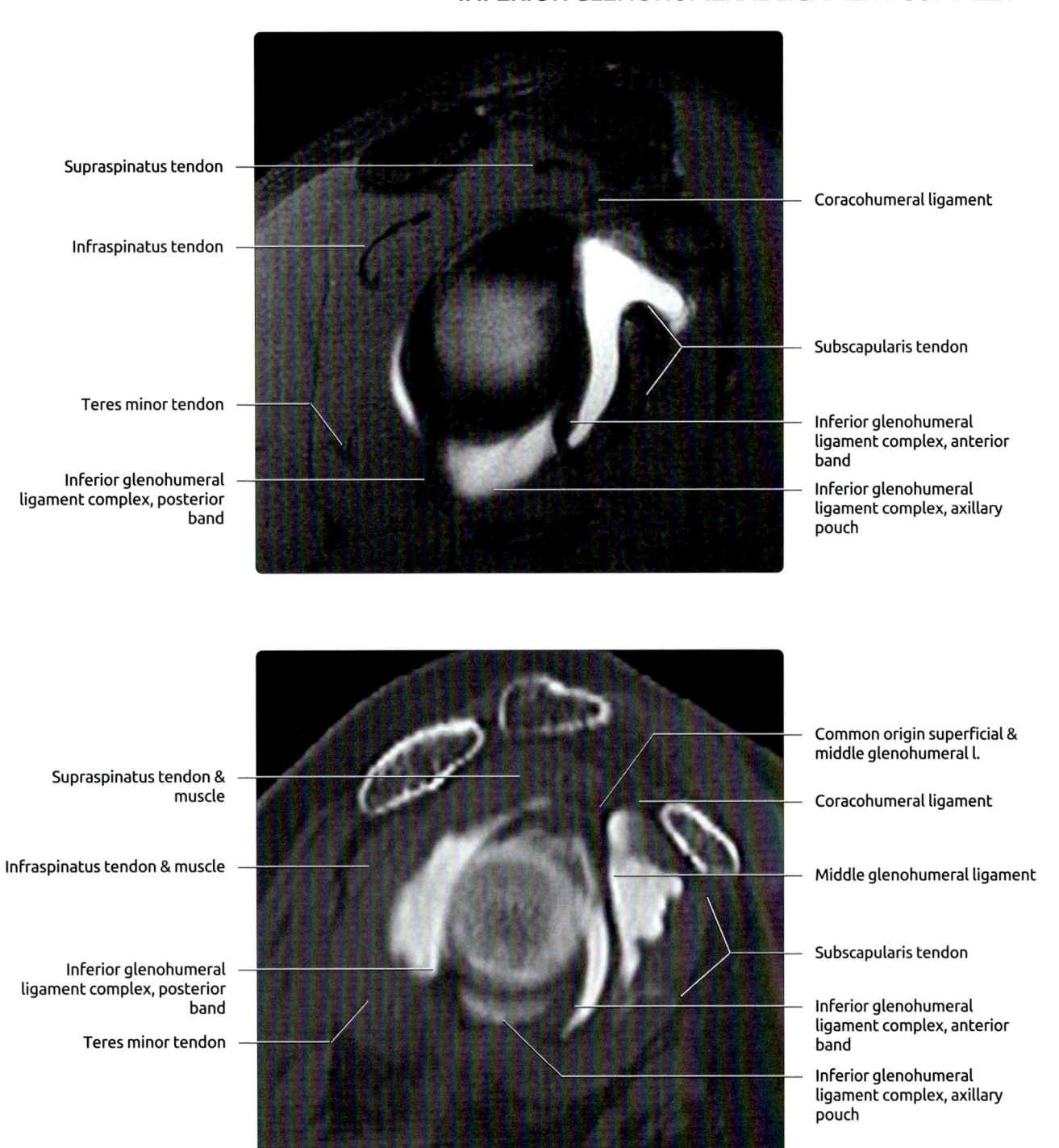

(Top) A sagittal oblique T1 FS MR arthrogram image of the right shoulder shows the inferior glenohumeral ligament complex is shown.
(Bottom) A sagittal oblique CT arthrogram image of the right shoulder shows the inferior glenohumeral ligament complex and middle glenohumeral ligament.

Shoulder Ligaments

CORACOHUMERAL LIGAMENT, SAGITTAL OBLIQUE

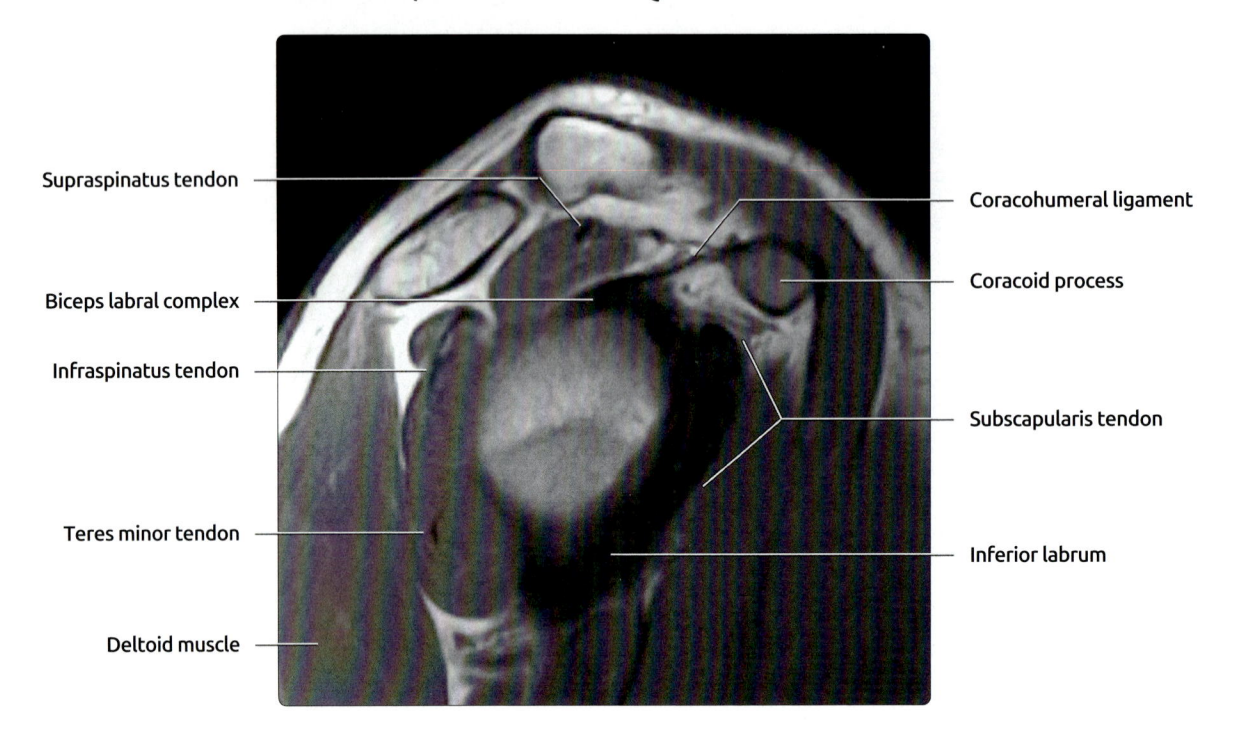

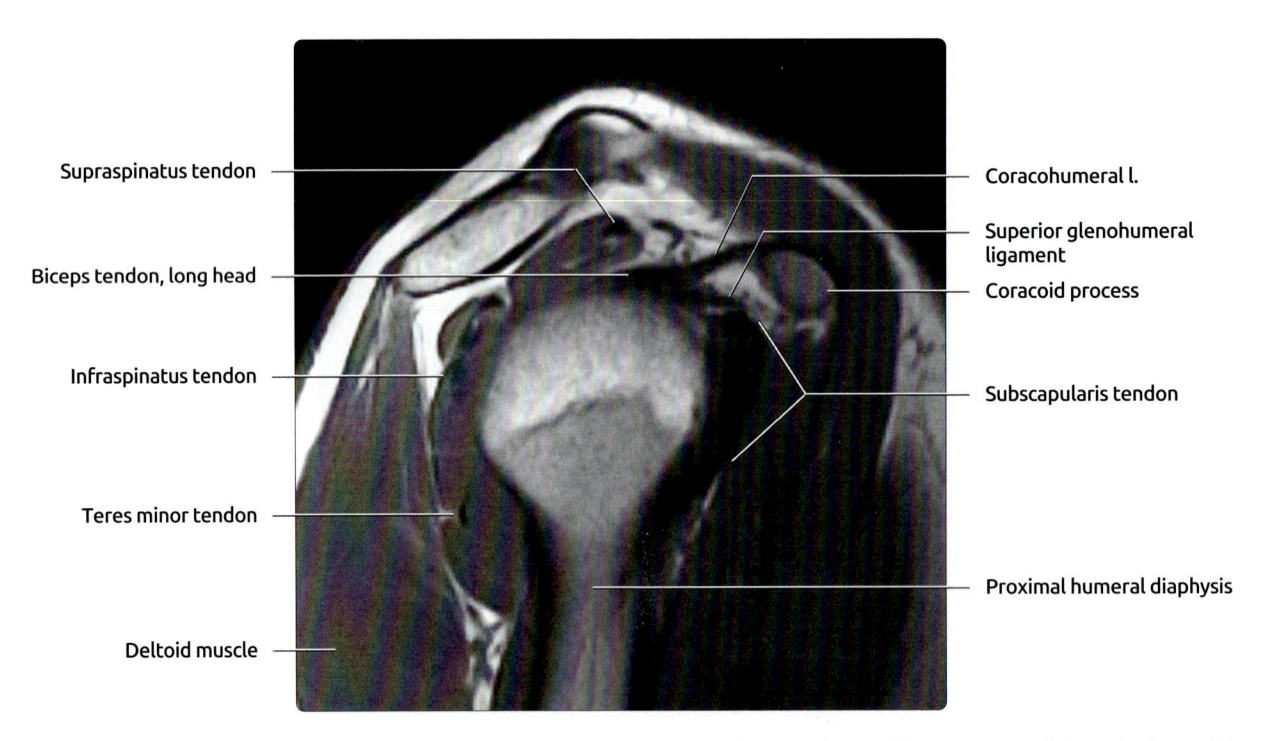

(Top) First of 2 sagittal oblique PD MR images of the right shoulder is shown. The coracohumeral ligament extends from the base of the coracoid process to the greater and lesser tuberosities. *(Bottom)* Image is of the right shoulder located lateral to the previous image. The coracohumeral ligament forms the roof of the rotator interval. It fuses with several structures including the supraspinatus tendon, subscapularis tendon, joint capsule, and superior glenohumeral ligament.

Shoulder Ligaments

CORACOHUMERAL LIGAMENT, AXIAL

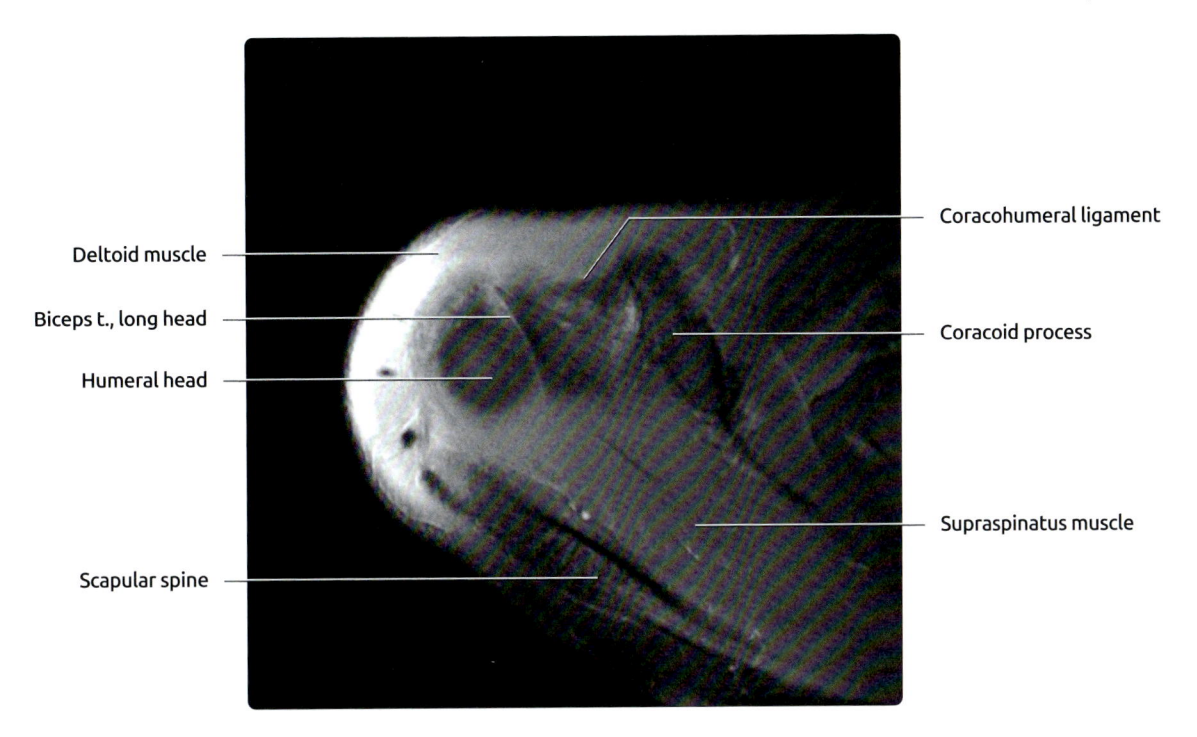

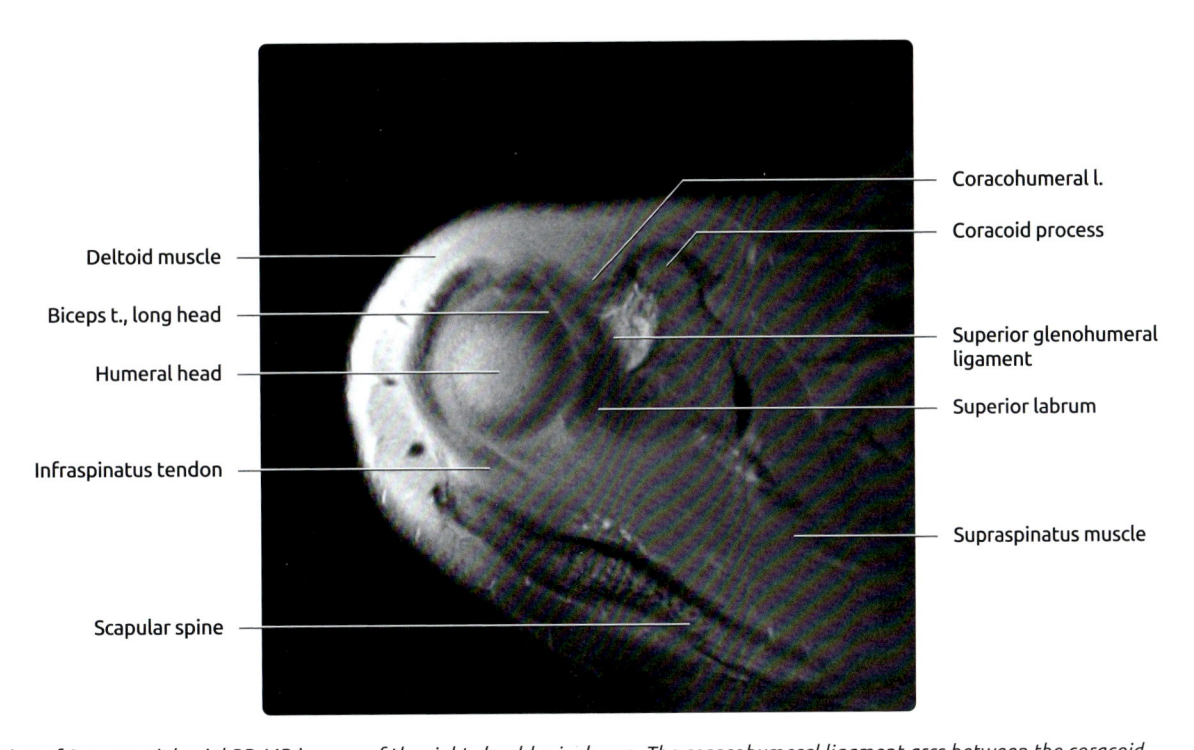

(Top) First of 2 sequential axial PD MR images of the right shoulder is shown. The coracohumeral ligament arcs between the coracoid process and anterior humeral head. (Bottom) This image is located below the previous image. The coracohumeral ligament is fusing with the superior glenohumeral ligament and joint capsule.

Shoulder Ligaments

CORACOHUMERAL LIGAMENT, CORONAL OBLIQUE

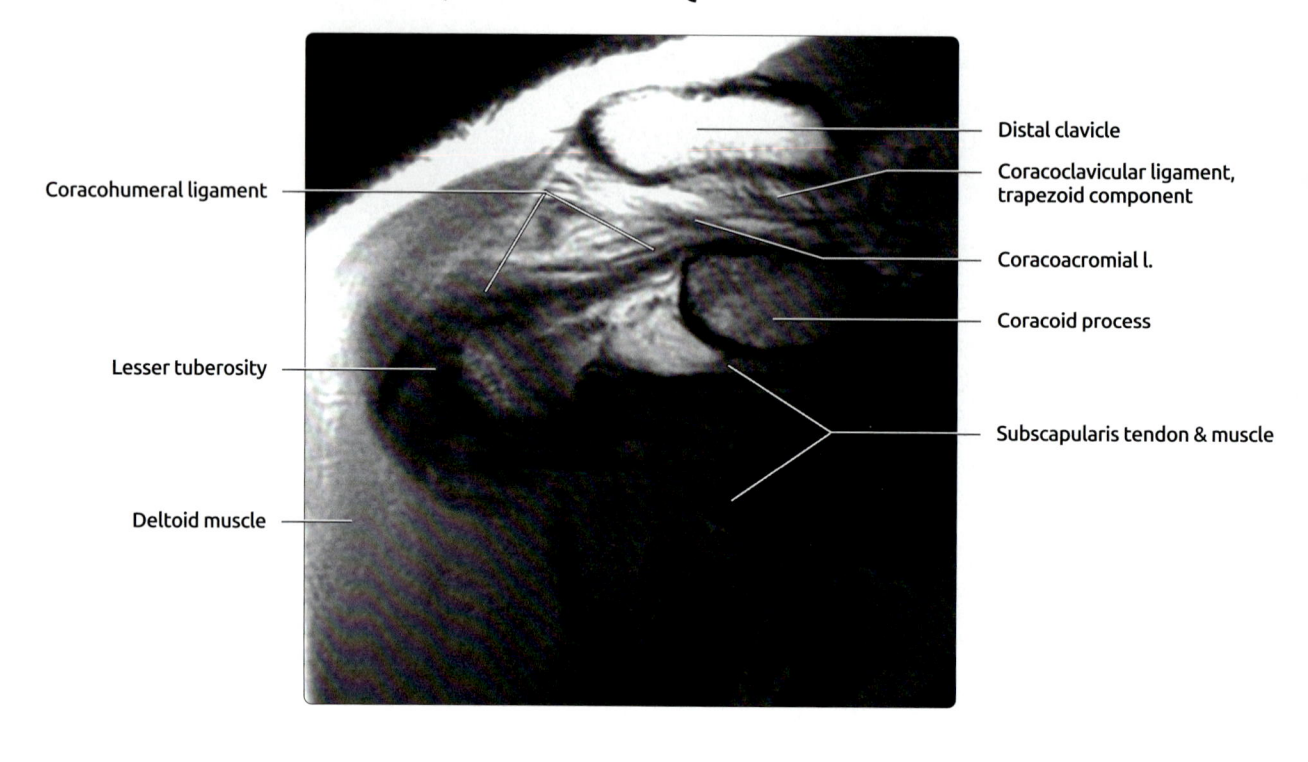

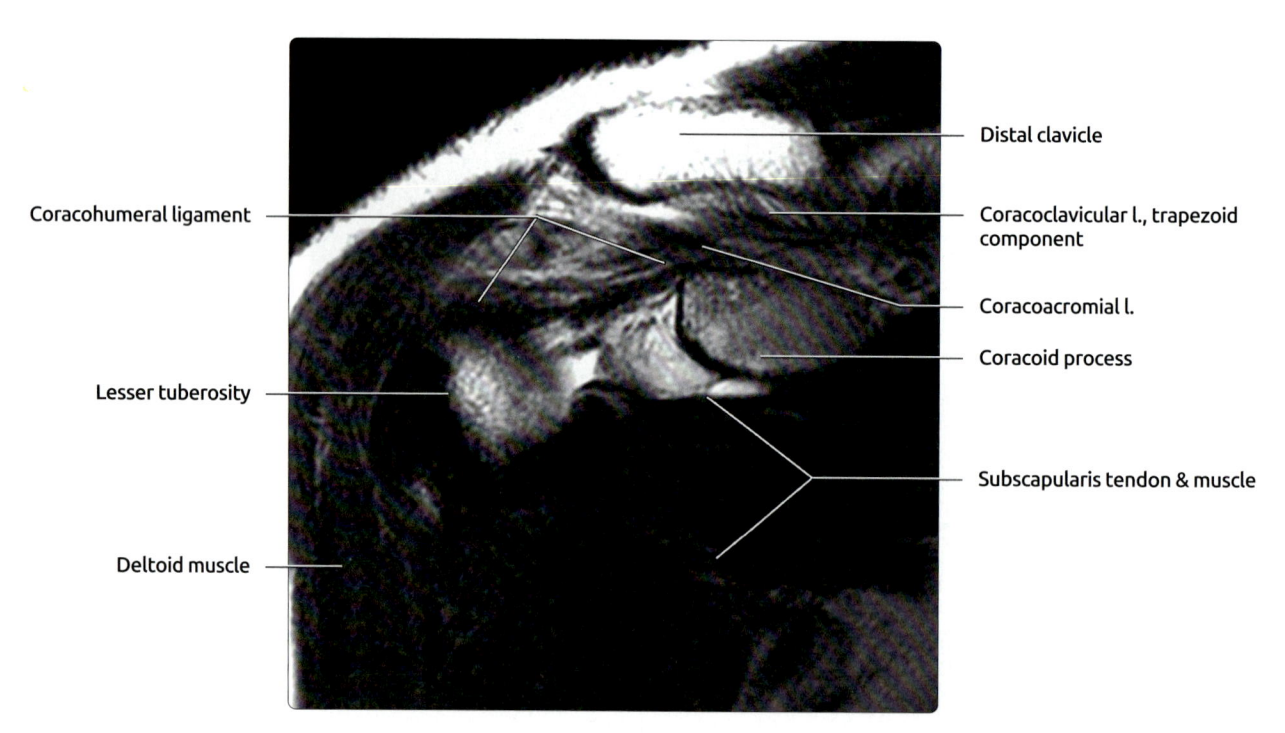

(Top) The first of 2 coronal oblique images through the same level is shown. The coracohumeral ligament has a roughly transverse course on coronal oblique images. **(Bottom)** A coronal T2 MR in a different patient is through the same level as the previous image is shown. Surrounding fat outlines the coracohumeral ligament. When this ligament fuses with the supraspinatus tendon, subscapularis tendon and joint capsule, the structures cannot be differentiated from each other.

Shoulder Ligaments

CORACOCLAVICULAR LIGAMENT

Top image labels:
- Distal clavicle
- Coracohumeral ligament
- Humeral head
- Deltoid muscle
- Coracoclavicular ligament, conoid
- Coracoclavicular ligament, trapezoid
- Coracoid process
- Subscapularis tendon & muscle

Bottom image labels:
- Distal clavicle
- Coracohumeral ligament
- Humeral head
- Deltoid muscle
- Coracoclavicular ligament, conoid
- Coracoclavicular ligament, trapezoid
- Coracoid process
- Subscapularis tendon & muscle

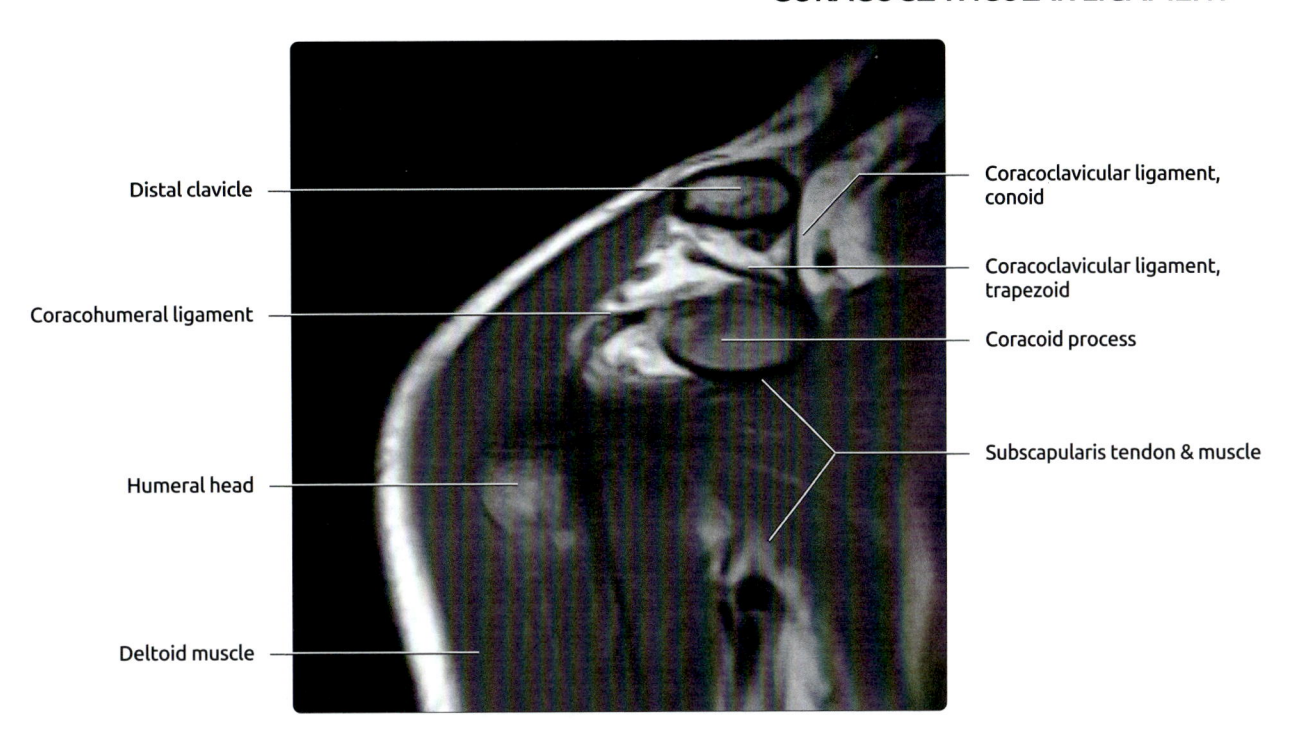

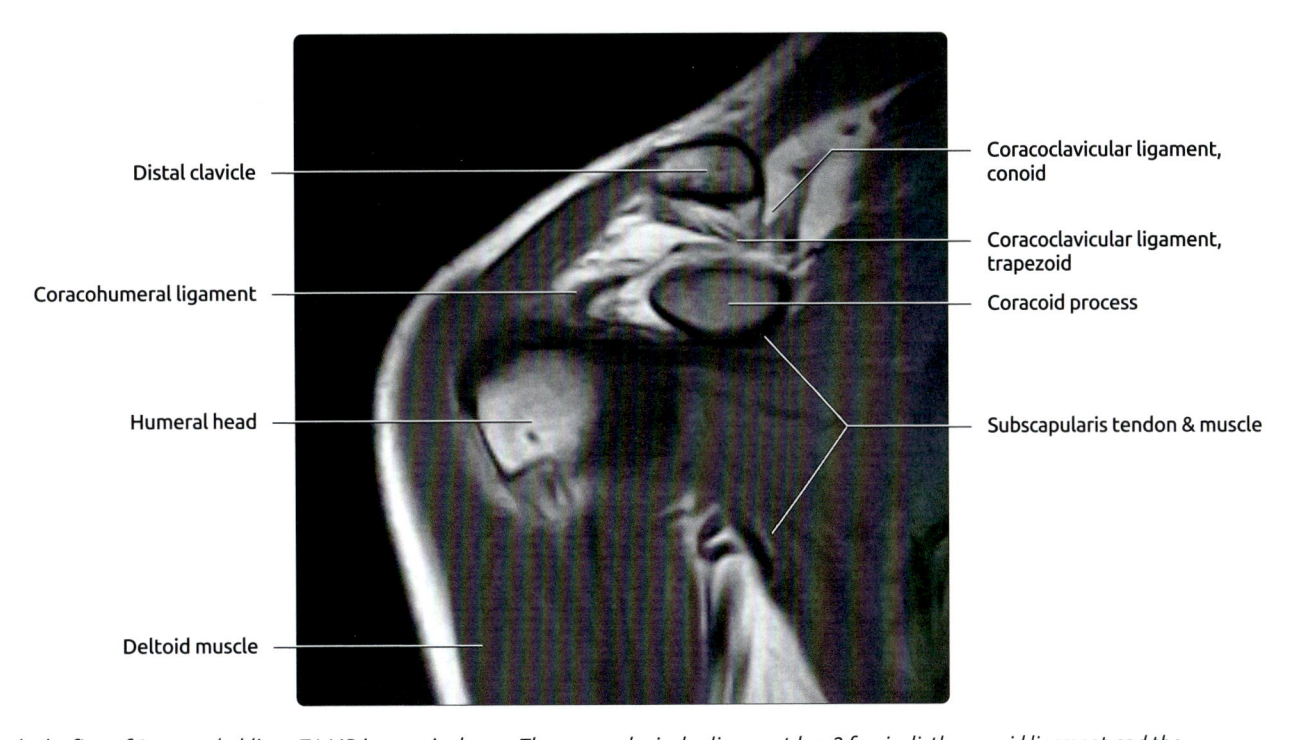

(**Top**) *The first of 2 coronal oblique T1 MR images is shown. The coracoclavicular ligament has 2 fasciculi, the conoid ligament and the trapezoid ligament. The conoid ligament is located medially and is more vertical in orientation. The trapezoid ligament is more laterally located and has an oblique course.* (**Bottom**) *The coracoclavicular ligament extends from the base of the coracoid process to the undersurface of the clavicle. It acts to stabilize the acromioclavicular joint.*

Shoulder Ligaments

CORACOACROMIAL LIGAMENT

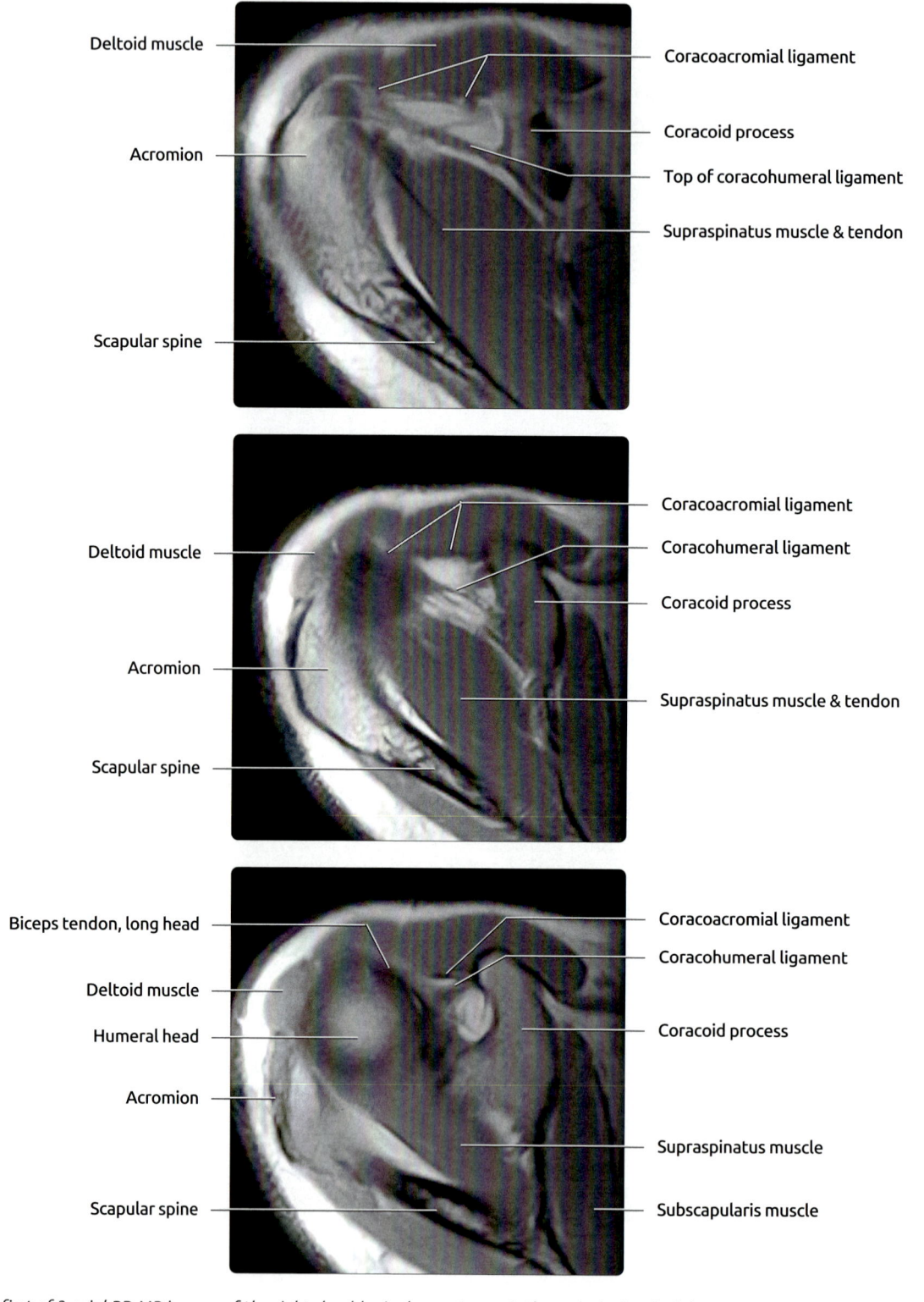

(Top) The first of 3 axial PD MR images of the right shoulder is shown. Image is through the level of the acromion. The coracoacromial ligament extends from the coracoid process to the anterior aspect of the acromion. *(Middle)* Strands of the coracoacromial ligament are visible in this obliquely oriented structure. *(Bottom)* The image shown is below the level of the acromial process, at the base of the acromion. The origins of the coracoacromial and coracohumeral ligaments from the coracoid are seen.

Shoulder Ligaments

ACROMIOCLAVICULAR LIGAMENTS

Top image labels:
- Superior acromioclavicular ligament
- Inferior acromioclavicular ligament
- Deltoid muscle
- Supraspinatus tendon
- Distal clavicle
- Supraspinatus tendon & muscle
- Superior labrum
- Biceps tendon, long head
- Glenoid

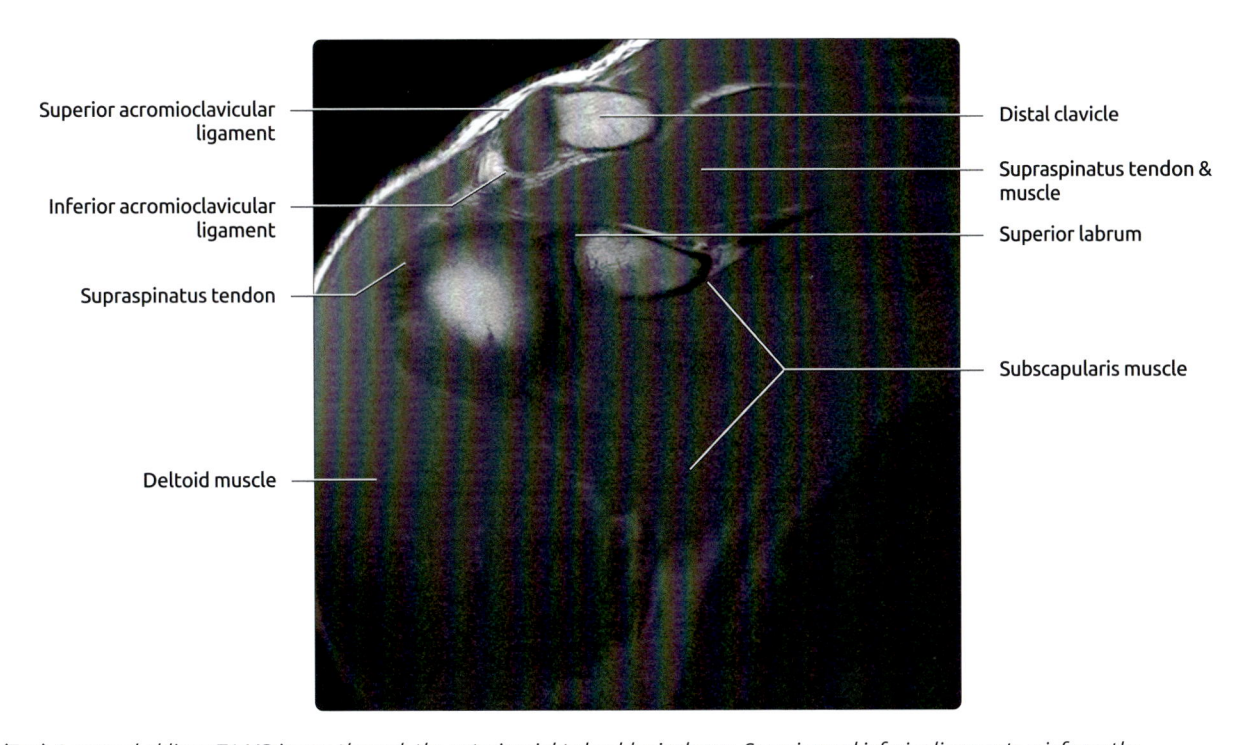

Bottom image labels:
- Superior acromioclavicular ligament
- Inferior acromioclavicular ligament
- Supraspinatus tendon
- Deltoid muscle
- Distal clavicle
- Supraspinatus tendon & muscle
- Superior labrum
- Subscapularis muscle

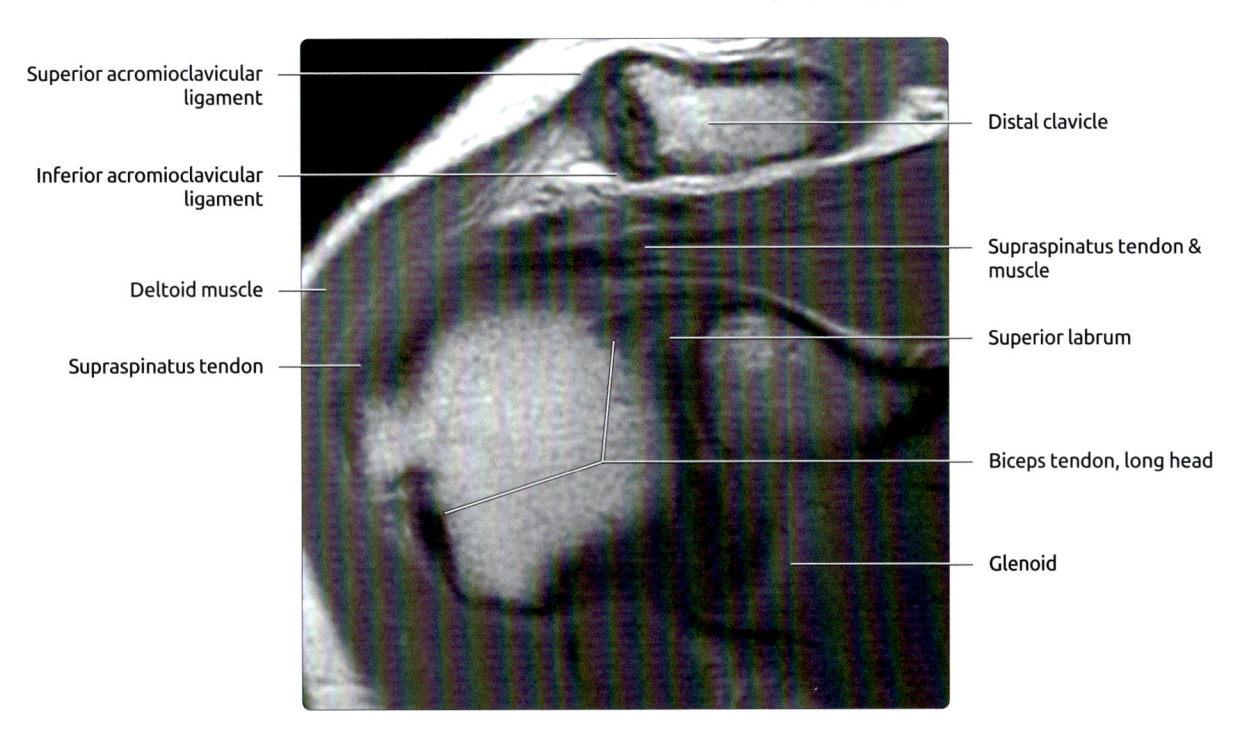

(Top) *A coronal oblique T1 MR image through the anterior right shoulder is shown. Superior and inferior ligaments reinforce the acromioclavicular joint.* (Bottom) *A coronal oblique T1 MR image in a different patient from previous image shows the superior and inferior acromioclavicular ligaments.*

Shoulder Labrum

TERMINOLOGY

Abbreviations
- Biceps labral complex (BLC)

IMAGING ANATOMY

Overview
- **Glenoid labrum consists of hyaline cartilage, fibrocartilage, and fibrous tissue**
  - Increases joint circumference and depth
  - Increases surface area and surface contact
  - Approximately 4 mm wide
  - Provides increased rotational stability
- **Variable size, shape, and signal intensity**
  - Classic triangle or wedge shape on axial imaging is present in less than 50% of normal anterior labra and less than 80% of posterior labra
  - Normal shapes include round, blunted, crescentic, flat, notched, and cleaved
  - May be small or absent anteriorly
  - Not always symmetric anterior to posterior
  - Can vary in signal intensity due to mucinous and myxoid contents
- **Portions of labrum described as positions on face of clock** (either shoulder)
  - 12:00: Superior
  - 3:00: Anterior
  - 6:00: Inferior
  - 9:00: Posterior

Anatomy Relationships
- **Labral attachment types**
  - Type A: Detached free edge overlying glenoid articular cartilage (meniscoid)
  - Type B: Adherent to glenoid articular cartilage
- **Biceps labral complex**
  - Biceps tendon attachment to labrum
  - Type 1 BLC: Firmly adherent to glenoid and superior labrum, slab type
  - Type 2 BLC: Small sulcus between biceps/labrum and glenoid, may be continuous with sublabral foramen, intermediate type
  - Type 3 BLC: Large sulcus between biceps/labrum and glenoid, labrum often continues as sublabral foramen, meniscoid type
- **Buford complex**
  - Diminutive or absent anterosuperior labrum
  - Thick or cord-like middle glenohumeral ligament
  - Present in 1-6.5% of population
  - Pseudo-Buford appearance can occur when middle and inferior glenohumeral ligaments are combined
- **Superior sublabral recess (sulcus)**
  - Located along superior labrum
    - 1-2 mm in thickness along full anterior to posterior extent
    - Does not extend posterior to biceps tendon
  - Fluid may extend into recess simulating tear
    - Medial or vertical orientation of fluid between base of labrum & cartilaginous margin of glenoid rim suggests recess
    - Laterally angulated, irregular fluid cleft distal to glenolabral attachment suggests tear
  - May be continuous with sublabral foramen
- **Sublabral foramen (hole)**
  - Present in 8-18% of population
  - Anterosuperior quadrant of labrum only
  - Can mimic tear if filled with fluid or contrast
  - Foramen is smooth and tapered
  - Tears are irregular and displace labrum away from glenoid when filled with fluid
- **Sublabral foramen with sulcus between biceps tendon and superior labrum**
  - "Double Oreo cookie" sign on coronal oblique MR
  - Glenoid cortex (black) + sublabral recess (white) + labrum (black) + biceps/superior labrum sulcus (white) + biceps tendon (black)
  - Similar appearance can be seen with superior labral tear instead of biceps/superior labrum sulcus

ANATOMY IMAGING ISSUES

Imaging Recommendations
- **MR arthrography (direct)**
  - Coronal oblique plane best demonstrates BLC
  - Fibrocartilaginous labrum outlined by contrast

Imaging Pitfalls
- **Variant anatomy**
  - Many normal variants of labral anatomy can be confused with pathology
  - Most normal variants occur at 11:00-3:00 position
- **Magic angle artifact**
  - Anteroinferior and posterosuperior labrum
- **Intraarticular biceps tendon dislocation**
  - Dislocated tendon lies adjacent to labrum
  - May simulate displaced tear
- **Hyaline cartilage undercutting**
  - Cartilage lying beneath labrum may simulate tear
  - Cartilage signal intensity is higher than fibrous labrum
  - Differentiate by smooth, even character of cartilage
    - Tears tend to be irregular
  - Cartilage does not extend through to opposite labral surface
- **Confusion with middle glenohumeral ligament**
  - On axial images, middle glenohumeral ligament lies adjacent to anterior labrum
    - May appear to be fragment of anterior labrum
  - Crescent of fluid between labrum and middle glenohumeral ligament can simulate tear
  - "Pseudo-sublabral foramen" appearance may occur when oblique sagittal images are improperly oriented
  - Follow oblique course of middle glenohumeral ligament on consecutive images to confirm that it is a separate structure from labrum
  - Confirm normal signal in underlying labrum
- **Volume averaging with contrast in sublabral foramen on MR arthrogram may simulate tear**

Shoulder Labrum

SAGITTAL GRAPHIC, LABRUM & BICEPS LABRAL COMPLEX

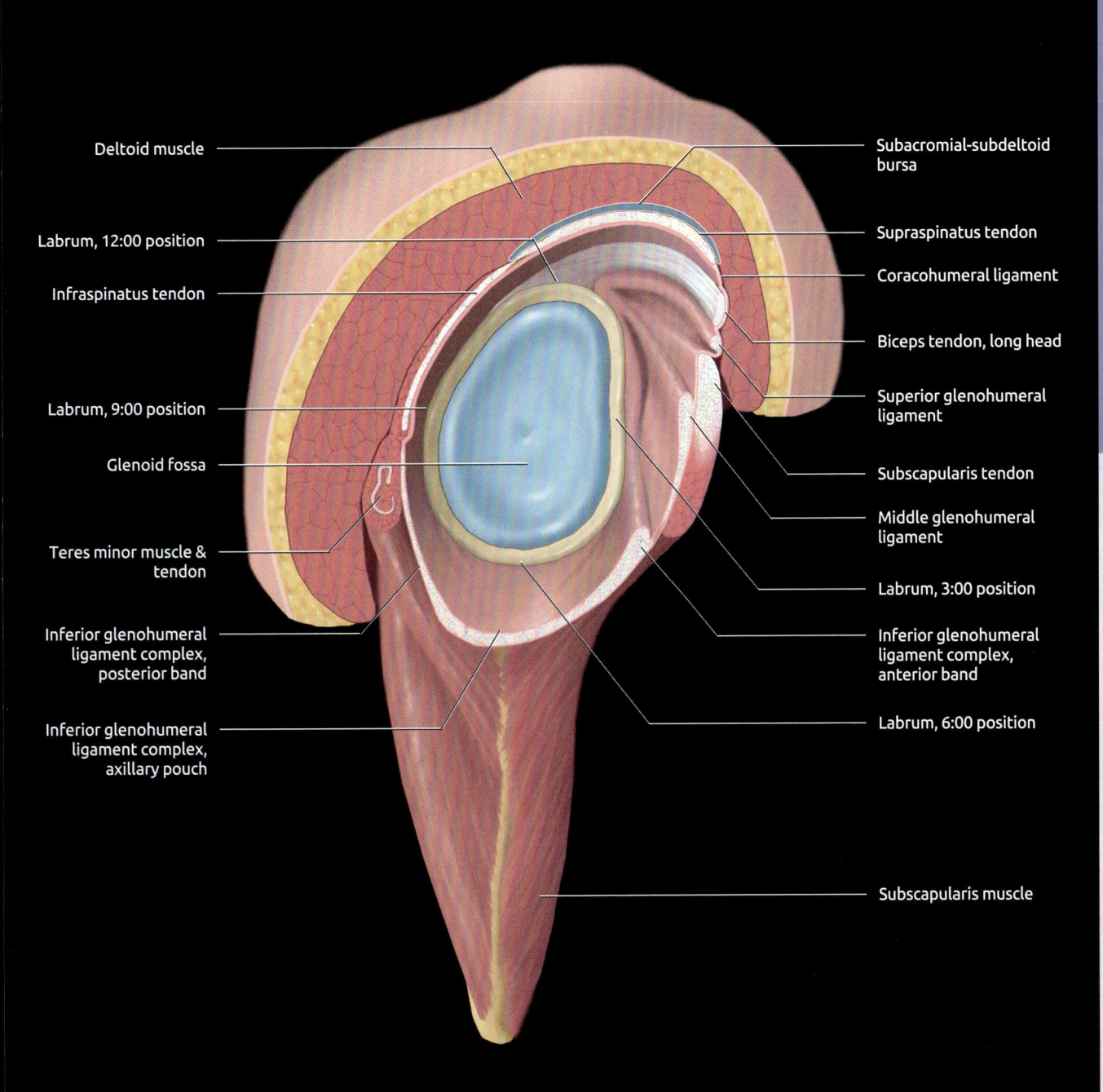

Sagittal graphic of the glenoid fossa is shown. The labrum lines the edge of the glenoid, increasing the circumference and depth of the shoulder joint.

Shoulder Labrum

NORMAL LABRUM, SAGITTAL

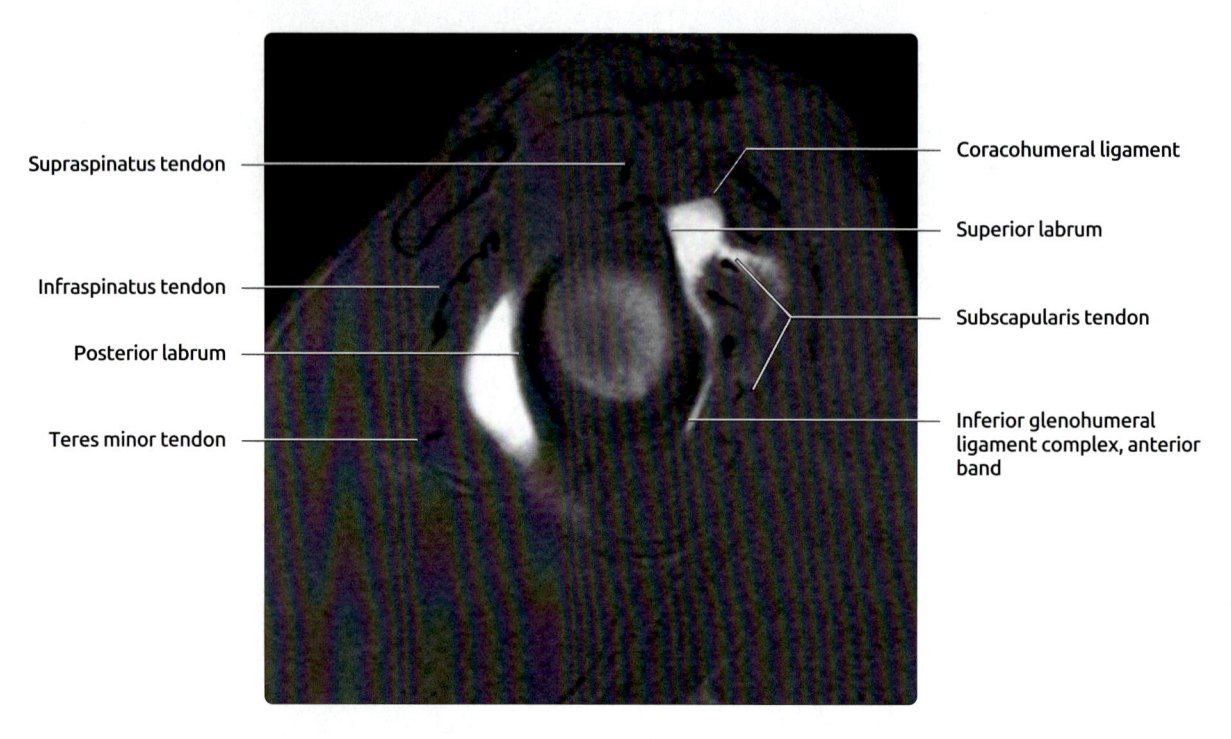

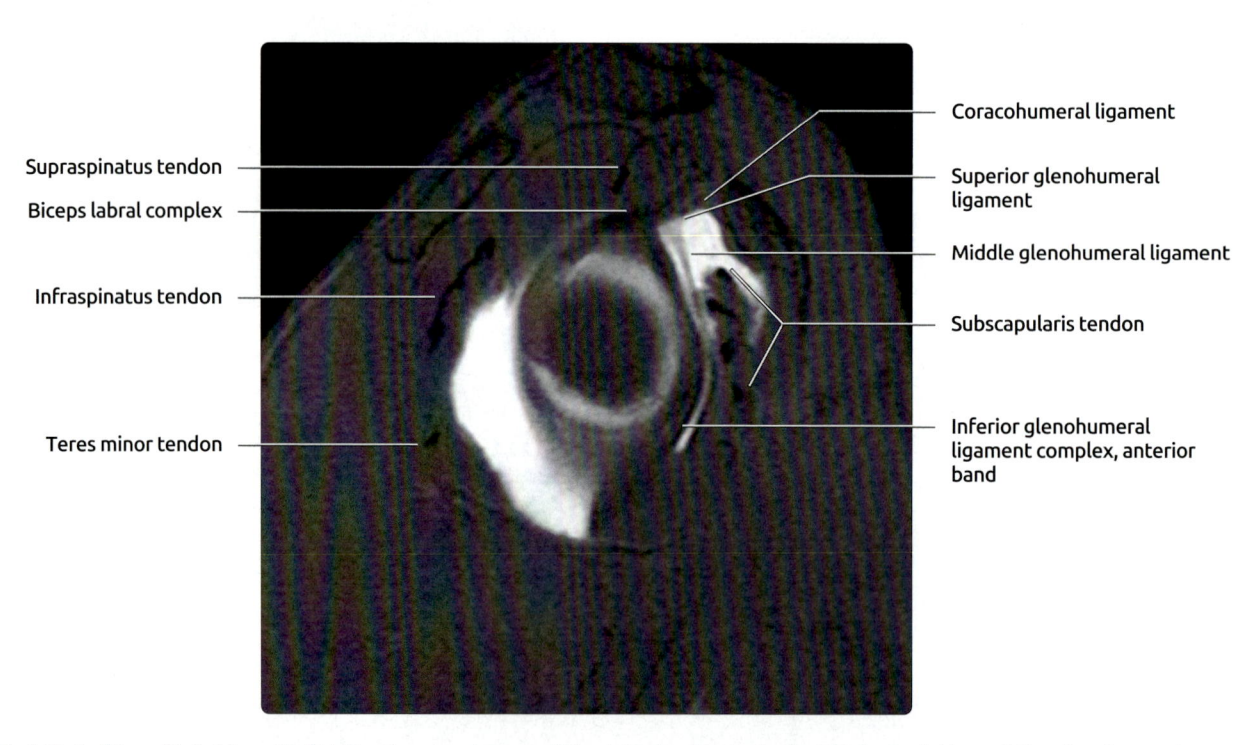

Top image labels:
- Supraspinatus tendon
- Infraspinatus tendon
- Posterior labrum
- Teres minor tendon
- Coracohumeral ligament
- Superior labrum
- Subscapularis tendon
- Inferior glenohumeral ligament complex, anterior band

Bottom image labels:
- Supraspinatus tendon
- Biceps labral complex
- Infraspinatus tendon
- Teres minor tendon
- Coracohumeral ligament
- Superior glenohumeral ligament
- Middle glenohumeral ligament
- Subscapularis tendon
- Inferior glenohumeral ligament complex, anterior band

(**Top**) *First of 2 sagittal oblique T1 FS MR arthrogram images of the right shoulder is shown. This image is through the glenohumeral joint. The labrum is a low signal, pear-shaped structure lining the edge of the glenoid fossa.* (**Bottom**) *Just lateral to the previous image, the medial aspect of the humeral head is coming into view. The long head of the biceps tendon fuses with the superior labrum to form the biceps labral complex.*

Shoulder Labrum

AXIAL PD FS MR, NORMAL LABRUM

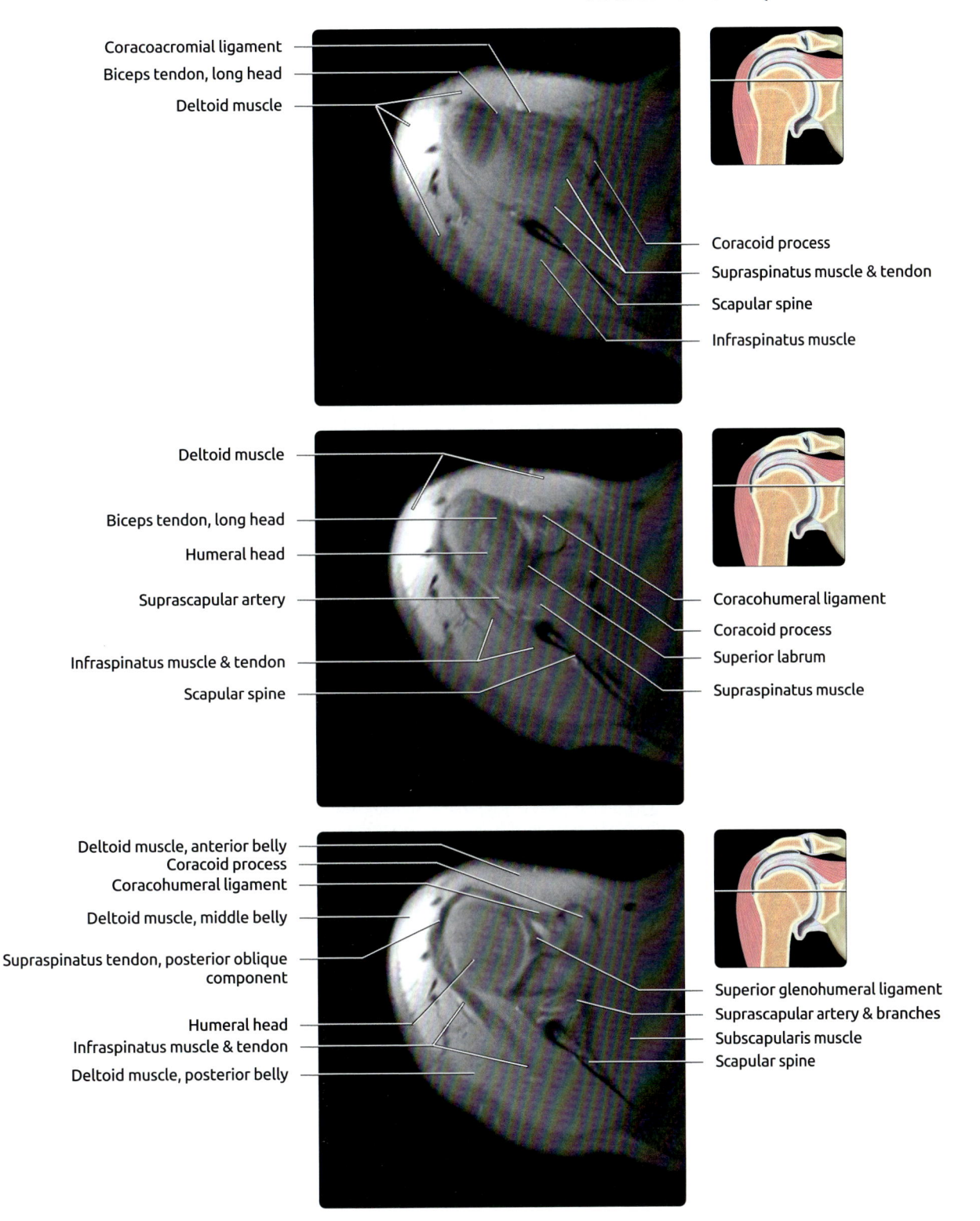

(Top) First of 12 axial PD FS MR images of the right shoulder presented from proximal to distal is shown. Image is above the level of the glenoid labrum. The fibrous labrum increases the stability of the glenohumeral joint and is an important attachment site for the glenohumeral ligaments and long head of the biceps tendon. (Middle) The superior glenoid labrum comes into view on this image. It has normal low signal. The long head of the biceps tendon attaches to the superior labrum, forming the biceps labral complex. Note that the coracohumeral ligament is unusually taut and well demonstrated in this hyper-externally rotated shoulder. (Bottom) The superior glenohumeral ligament attachment to the anterior superior labrum is shown on this image. The glenohumeral ligaments may actually represent folds of the joint capsule, as opposed to true ligaments. The superior glenohumeral ligament will fuse with the coracohumeral ligament to form a supportive sling around the long head of the biceps tendon.

Shoulder Labrum

AXIAL PD FS MR, NORMAL LABRUM

Supraspinatus tendon
Greater tuberosity
Infraspinatus tendon
Posterior labrum
Deltoid muscle
Infraspinatus muscle

Deltoid muscle, anterior belly
Conjoined tendon of short head biceps & coracobrachialis t.
Coracoid process
Middle glenohumeral l.
Subscapularis m. & t.
Glenoid
Suprascapular artery & nerve
Scapula

Greater tuberosity
Posterior labrum
Deltoid muscle, posterior belly

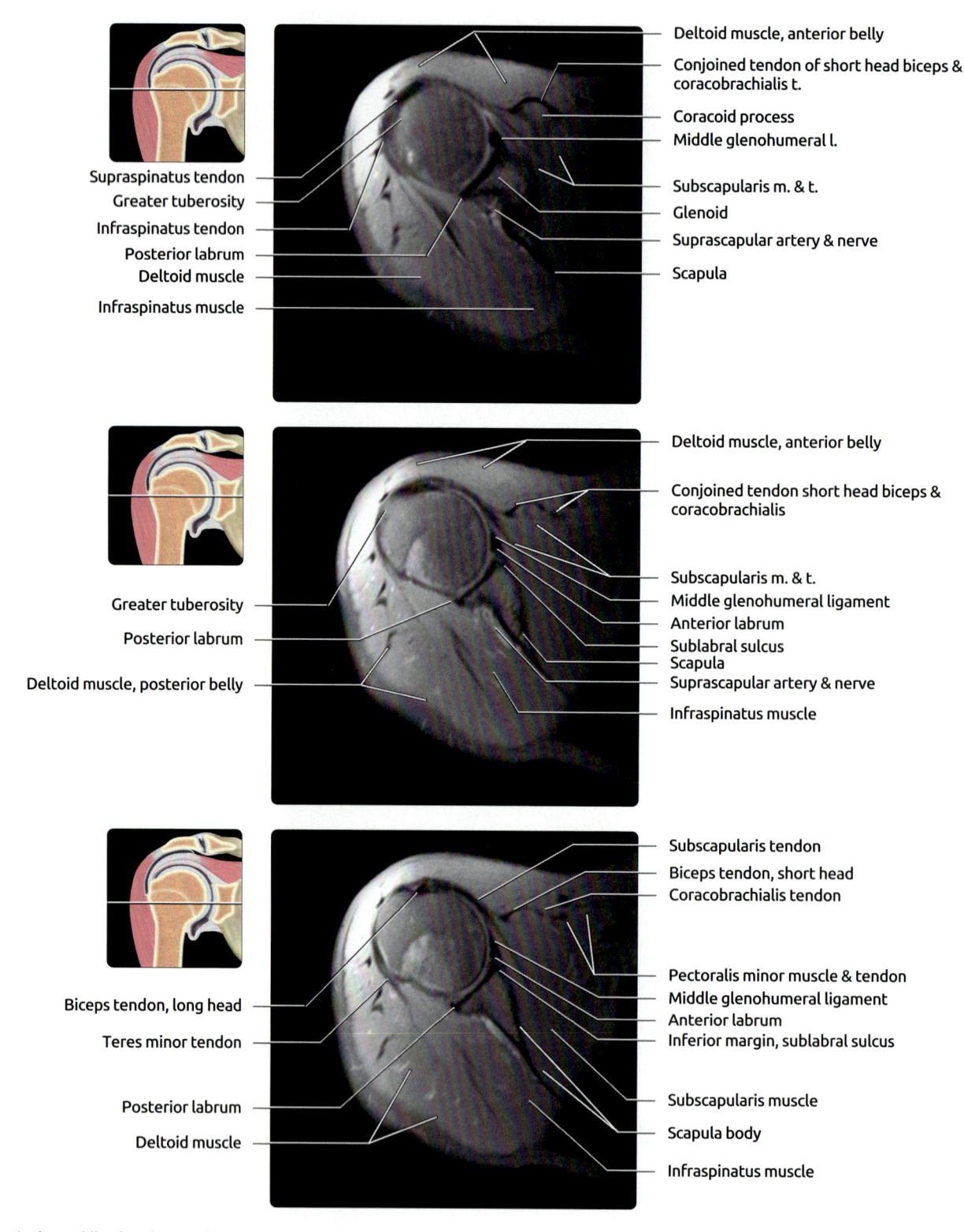

Deltoid muscle, anterior belly
Conjoined tendon short head biceps & coracobrachialis
Subscapularis m. & t.
Middle glenohumeral ligament
Anterior labrum
Sublabral sulcus
Scapula
Suprascapular artery & nerve
Infraspinatus muscle

Biceps tendon, long head
Teres minor tendon
Posterior labrum
Deltoid muscle

Subscapularis tendon
Biceps tendon, short head
Coracobrachialis tendon
Pectoralis minor muscle & tendon
Middle glenohumeral ligament
Anterior labrum
Inferior margin, sublabral sulcus
Subscapularis muscle
Scapula body
Infraspinatus muscle

(**Top**) The middle glenohumeral ligament also arises anteriorly. It is larger than the superior glenohumeral ligament and can be confused for a torn fragment of labrum if it is not followed along its oblique course. (**Middle**) The glenoid labrum has a wide range of normal appearances. The typical appearance of the labrum on axial images is a low signal triangle or wedge adjacent to the anterior and posterior rim of the glenoid. (**Bottom**) The labrum in asymptomatic patients can be round, blunted, notched, crescentic, cleaved, flat, or absent.

Shoulder Labrum

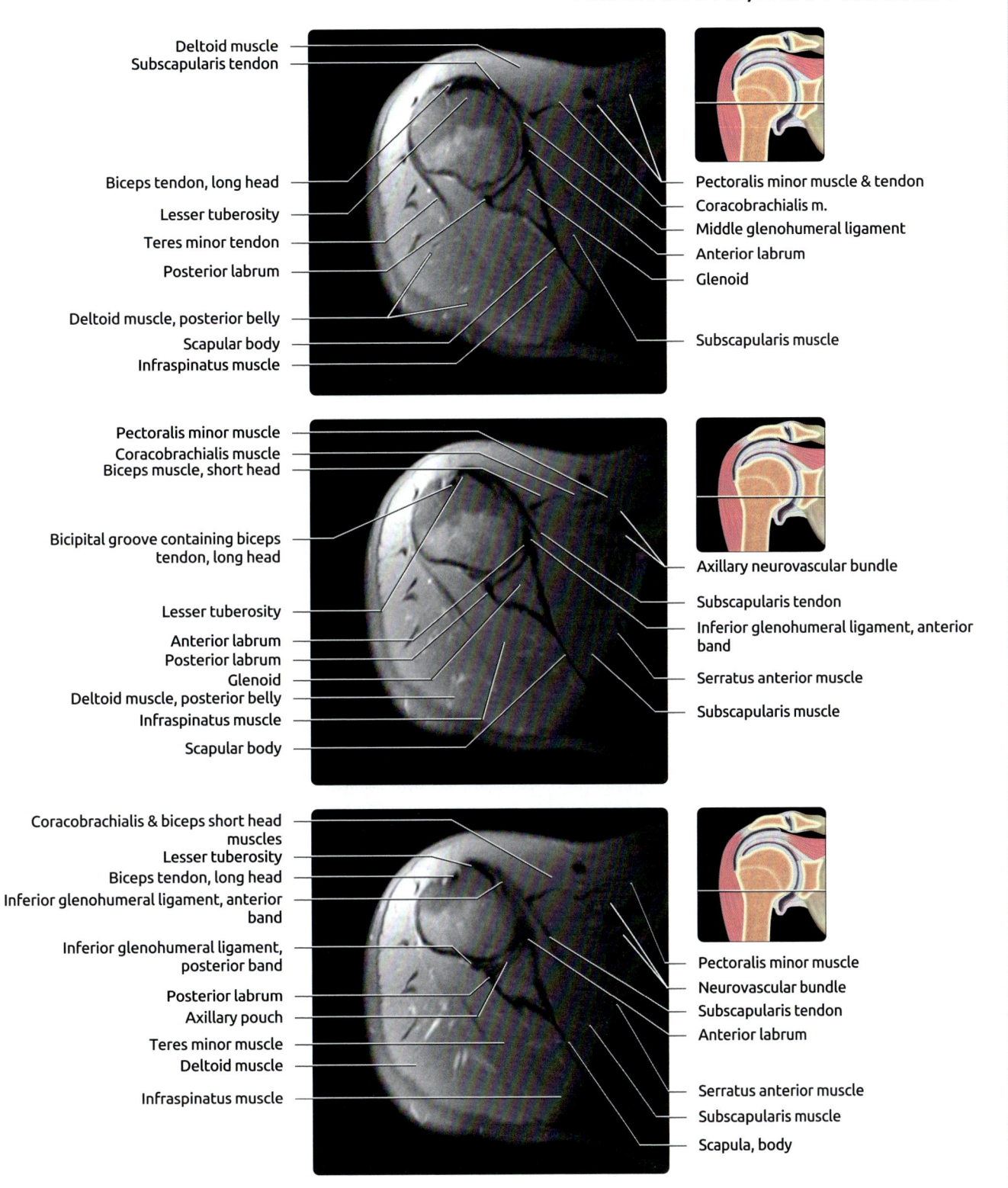

AXIAL PD FS MR, NORMAL LABRUM

Top image labels:
- Deltoid muscle
- Subscapularis tendon
- Biceps tendon, long head
- Lesser tuberosity
- Teres minor tendon
- Posterior labrum
- Deltoid muscle, posterior belly
- Scapular body
- Infraspinatus muscle
- Pectoralis minor muscle & tendon
- Coracobrachialis m.
- Middle glenohumeral ligament
- Anterior labrum
- Glenoid
- Subscapularis muscle

Middle image labels:
- Pectoralis minor muscle
- Coracobrachialis muscle
- Biceps muscle, short head
- Bicipital groove containing biceps tendon, long head
- Lesser tuberosity
- Anterior labrum
- Posterior labrum
- Glenoid
- Deltoid muscle, posterior belly
- Infraspinatus muscle
- Scapular body
- Axillary neurovascular bundle
- Subscapularis tendon
- Inferior glenohumeral ligament, anterior band
- Serratus anterior muscle
- Subscapularis muscle

Bottom image labels:
- Coracobrachialis & biceps short head muscles
- Lesser tuberosity
- Biceps tendon, long head
- Inferior glenohumeral ligament, anterior band
- Inferior glenohumeral ligament, posterior band
- Posterior labrum
- Axillary pouch
- Teres minor muscle
- Deltoid muscle
- Infraspinatus muscle
- Pectoralis minor muscle
- Neurovascular bundle
- Subscapularis tendon
- Anterior labrum
- Serratus anterior muscle
- Subscapularis muscle
- Scapula, body

(**Top**) *The inferior glenohumeral ligament complex consists of an anterior band, axillary pouch, and posterior band. This complex represents the thickest portion of the joint capsule. A distinct site of origin of this triangular-shaped complex is more difficult to identify than the superior and middle glenohumeral ligament origins.* (**Middle**) *The anterior and posterior labrum can normally have asymmetric shapes. Hyaline cartilage undercutting of the labrum, seen anteriorly in this case, can simulate a tear due to the relatively increased signal of cartilage compared with the fibrous labrum.* (**Bottom**) *Near the inferior aspect of the glenohumeral joint, the axillary pouch normally contains a small amount of joint fluid. The joint capsule may become redundant in this area, simulating loose bodies.*

Shoulder Labrum

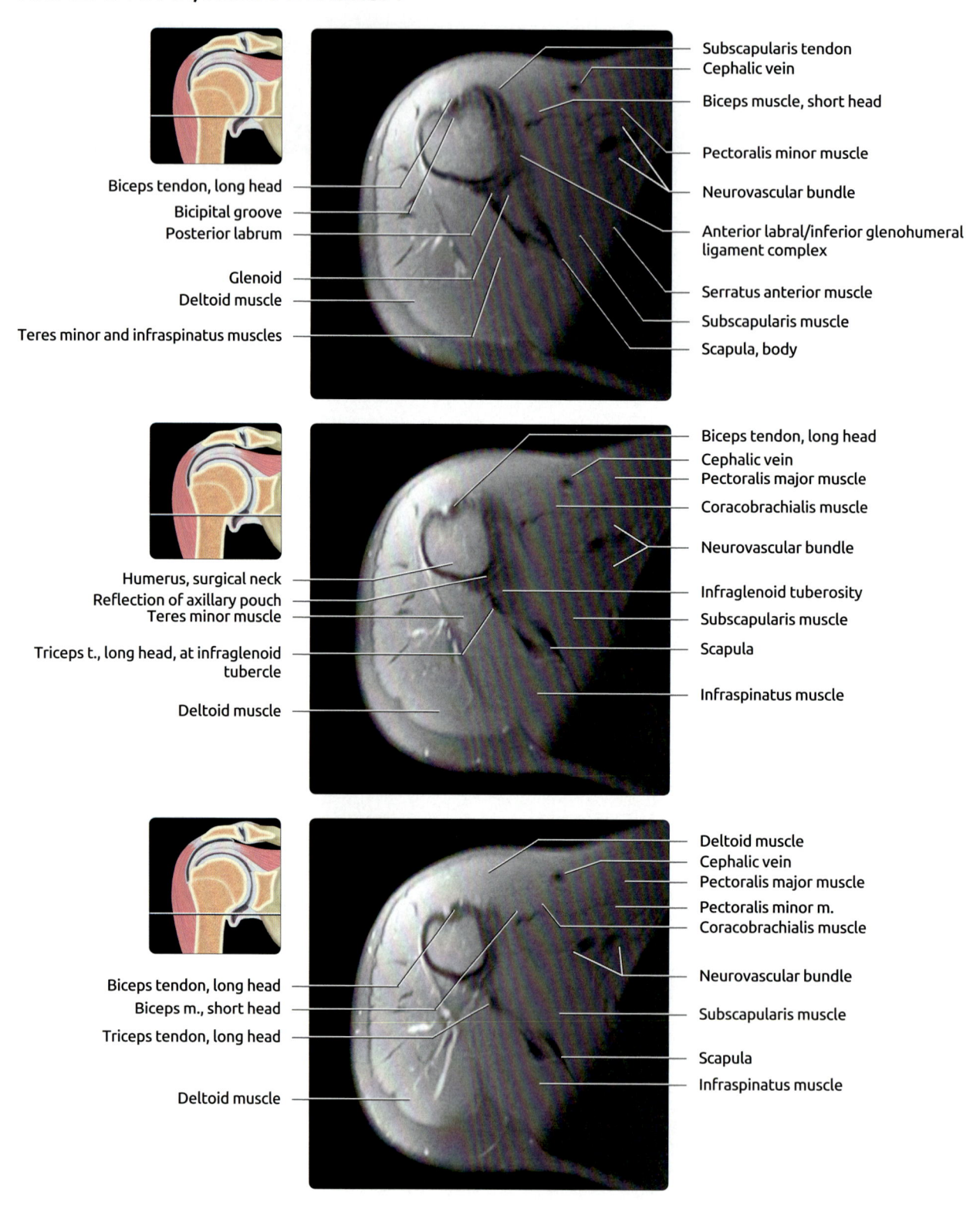

AXIAL PD FS MR, NORMAL LABRUM

Top image labels (left): Biceps tendon, long head; Bicipital groove; Posterior labrum; Glenoid; Deltoid muscle; Teres minor and infraspinatus muscles

Top image labels (right): Subscapularis tendon; Cephalic vein; Biceps muscle, short head; Pectoralis minor muscle; Neurovascular bundle; Anterior labral/inferior glenohumeral ligament complex; Serratus anterior muscle; Subscapularis muscle; Scapula, body

Middle image labels (left): Humerus, surgical neck; Reflection of axillary pouch; Teres minor muscle; Triceps t., long head, at infraglenoid tubercle; Deltoid muscle

Middle image labels (right): Biceps tendon, long head; Cephalic vein; Pectoralis major muscle; Coracobrachialis muscle; Neurovascular bundle; Infraglenoid tuberosity; Subscapularis muscle; Scapula; Infraspinatus muscle

Bottom image labels (left): Biceps tendon, long head; Biceps m., short head; Triceps tendon, long head; Deltoid muscle

Bottom image labels (right): Deltoid muscle; Cephalic vein; Pectoralis major muscle; Pectoralis minor m.; Coracobrachialis muscle; Neurovascular bundle; Subscapularis muscle; Scapula; Infraspinatus muscle

(**Top**) Magic angle artifact can cause increased signal in the labrum. This is most commonly seen in the superior and inferior aspects of both the anterior and posterior labrum on short TE images. Any abnormal labral signal should be confirmed on T2 sequences. (**Middle**) Image is shown through the labrum, representing the 6:00 position. (**Bottom**) Just below the level of the glenoid, there is no labral tissue visible. The long head of the triceps muscle has its origin from the infraglenoid tubercle.

Shoulder Labrum

LABRAL VARIANTS

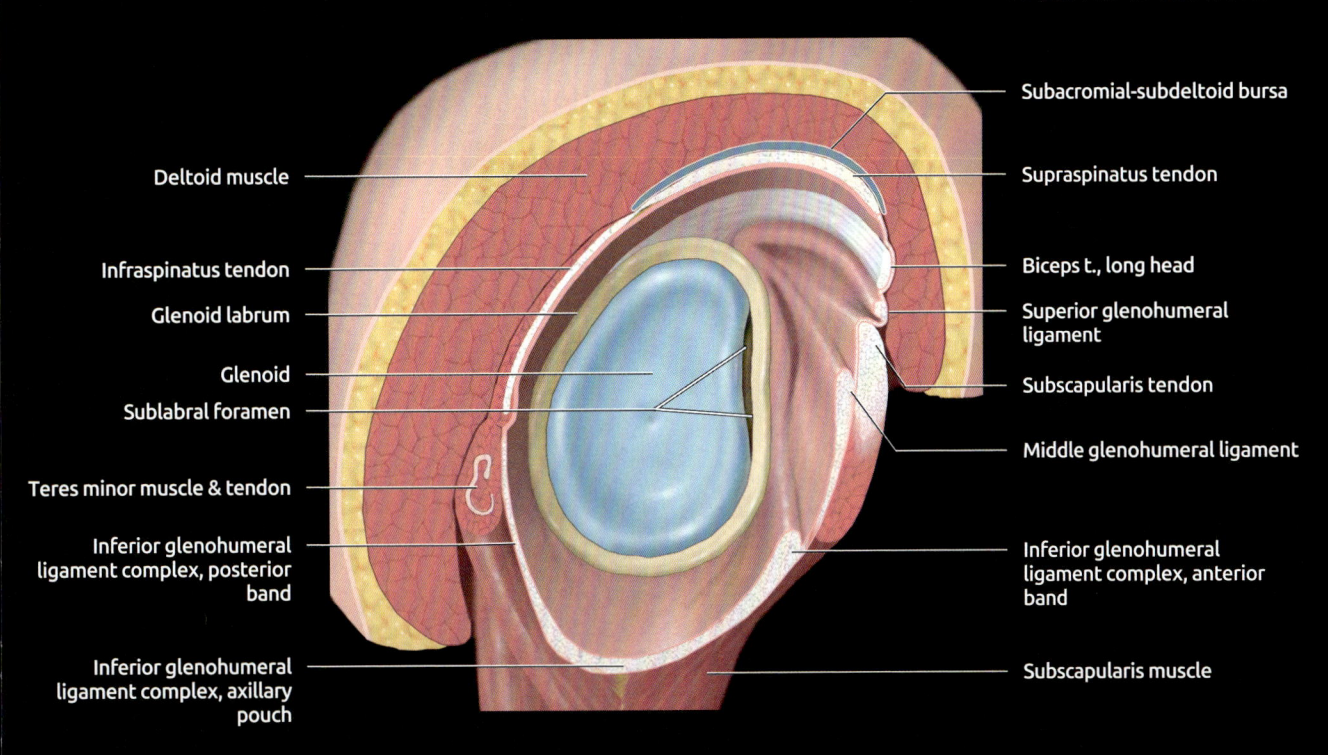

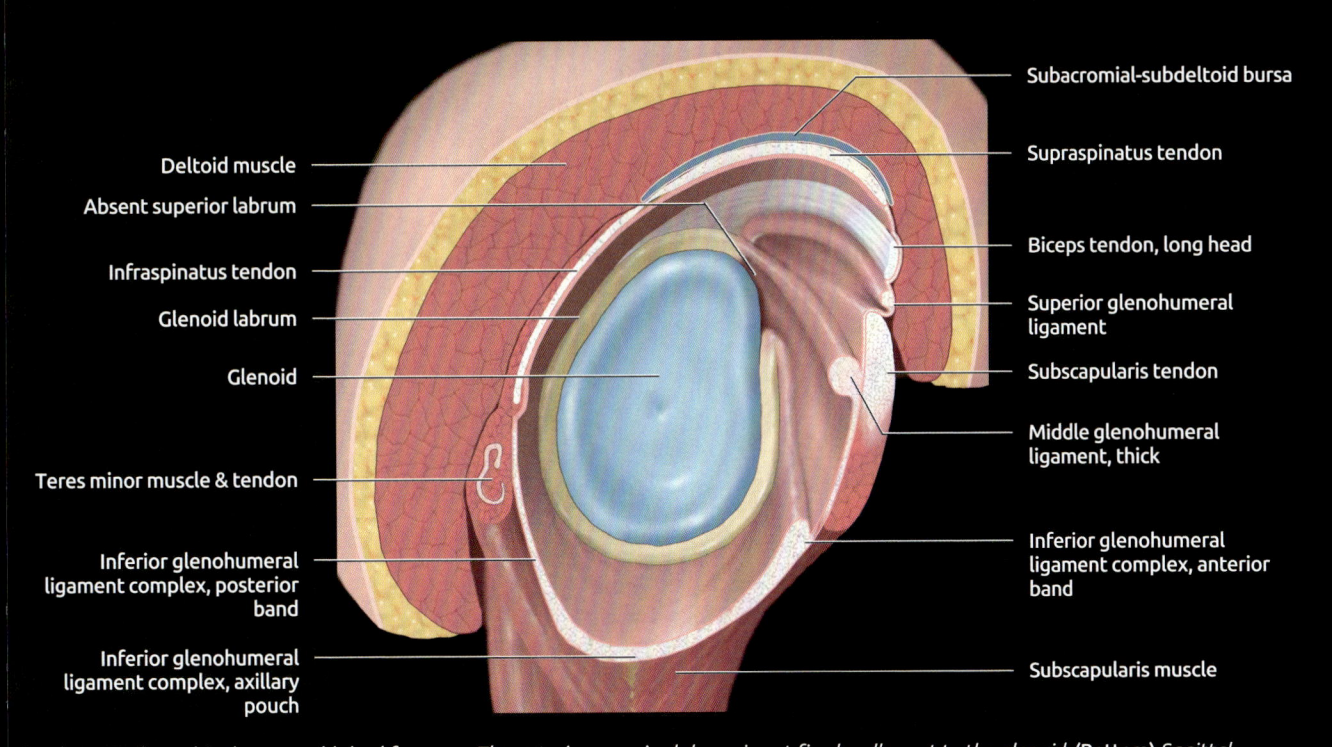

(Top) Sagittal graphic shows a sublabral foramen. The anterior superior labrum is not firmly adherent to the glenoid. **(Bottom)** Sagittal graphic shows a Buford complex. The anterior superior glenoid labrum is absent. The middle glenohumeral ligament is enlarged and cord-like.

Shoulder Labrum

LABRAL VARIANT: BUFORD COMPLEX

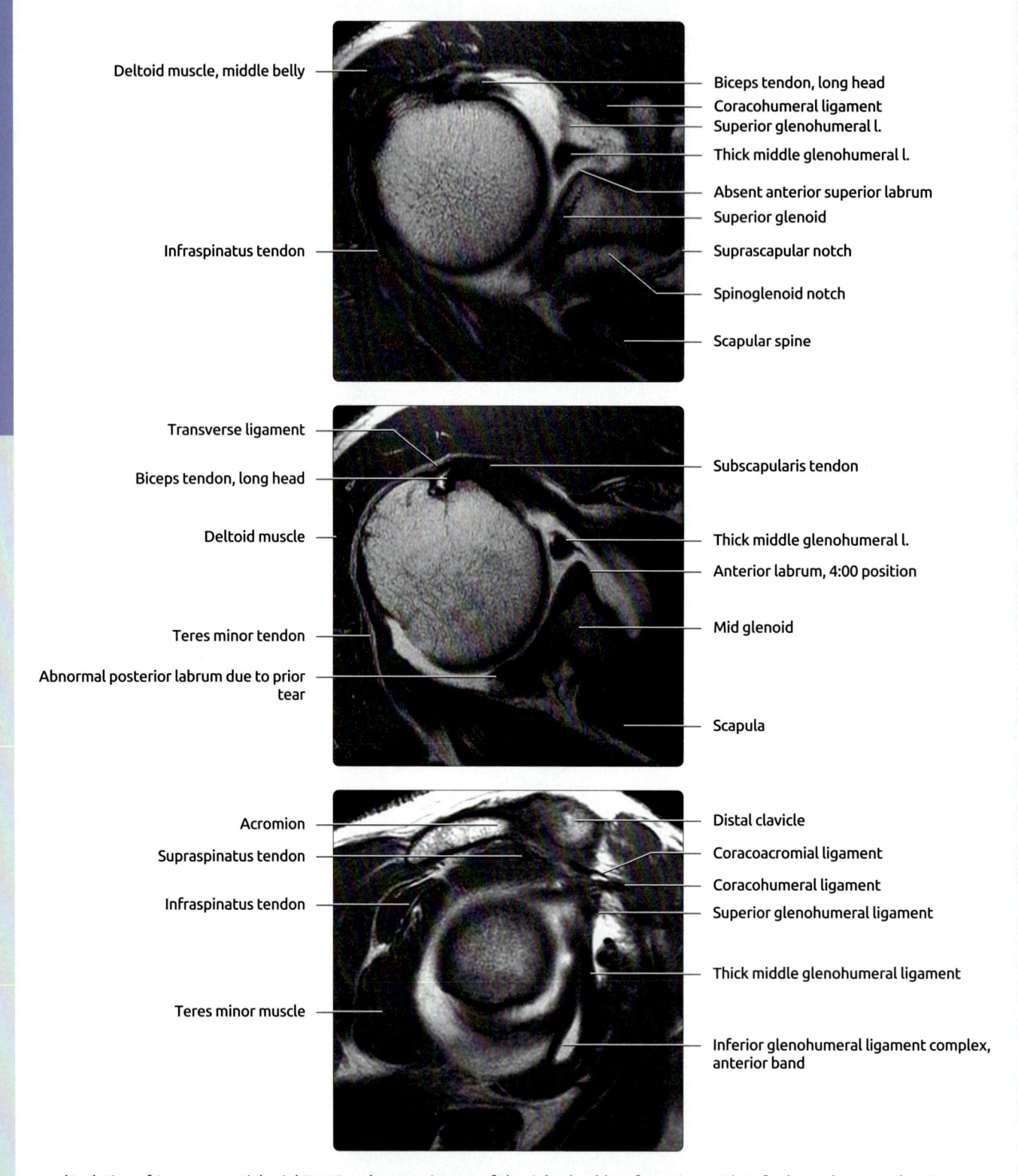

(Top) First of 2 nonsequential axial T1 MR arthrogram images of the right shoulder of a patient with Buford complex normal variant. The anterior superior glenoid labrum is absent. The middle glenohumeral ligament is thickened. The posterior labrum has abnormal size and shape due to a tear. This is unrelated to the Buford complex. *(Middle)* Image at the mid-glenoid level is shown. The middle glenohumeral ligament is still thick and cord-like. Labral tissue has reappeared anteriorly. *(Bottom)* Sagittal oblique T1 MR arthrogram image of the same patient is shown. The middle glenohumeral ligament is enlarged.

Shoulder Labrum

LABRAL ATTACHMENT VARIANTS

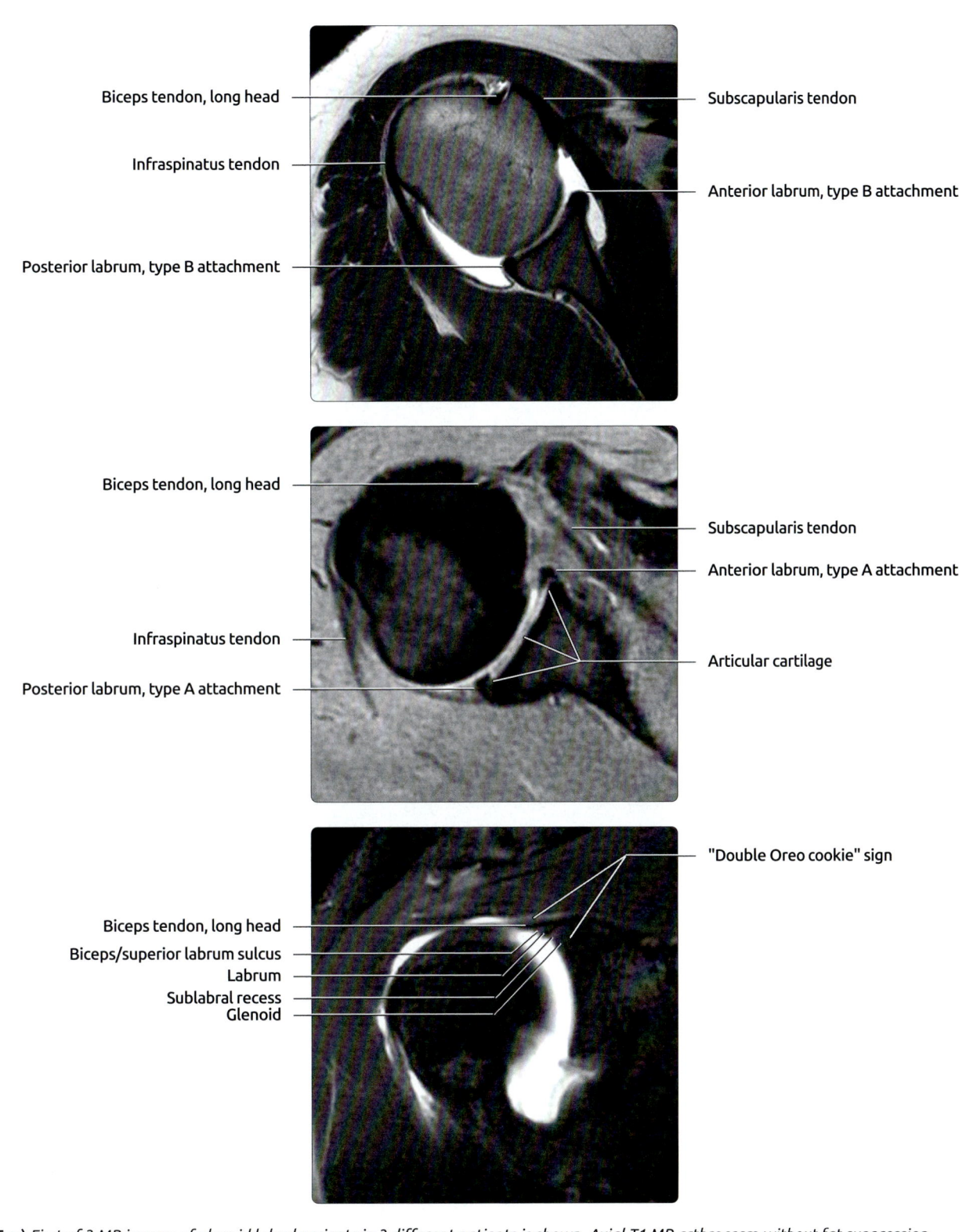

Top image labels:
- Biceps tendon, long head
- Infraspinatus tendon
- Posterior labrum, type B attachment
- Subscapularis tendon
- Anterior labrum, type B attachment

Middle image labels:
- Biceps tendon, long head
- Infraspinatus tendon
- Posterior labrum, type A attachment
- Subscapularis tendon
- Anterior labrum, type A attachment
- Articular cartilage

Bottom image labels:
- Biceps tendon, long head
- Biceps/superior labrum sulcus
- Labrum
- Sublabral recess
- Glenoid
- "Double Oreo cookie" sign

(Top) *First of 3 MR images of glenoid labral variants in 3 different patients is shown. Axial T1 MR arthrogram without fat suppression. The anterior and posterior labrum are firmly adherent to the articular cartilage. This is referred to as a type B attachment.* **(Middle)** *Axial PD MR of the anterior and posterior labrum overlie the articular cartilage, giving the appearance of the cartilage "undercutting" the labrum. This is referred to as a type A attachment.* **(Bottom)** *The "double Oreo cookie" sign on coronal T2 FS arthrogram is shown. From medial to lateral, the layers of the cookie correspond to the glenoid cortex (black) + sublabral recess (white) + labrum (black) + biceps/superior labrum sulcus (white) + biceps tendon (black). This sign can also be seen when a superior labral tear is present in place of the biceps/superior labrum sulcus.*

Shoulder Labrum

BICEPS LABRAL COMPLEX, NORMAL VARIANTS

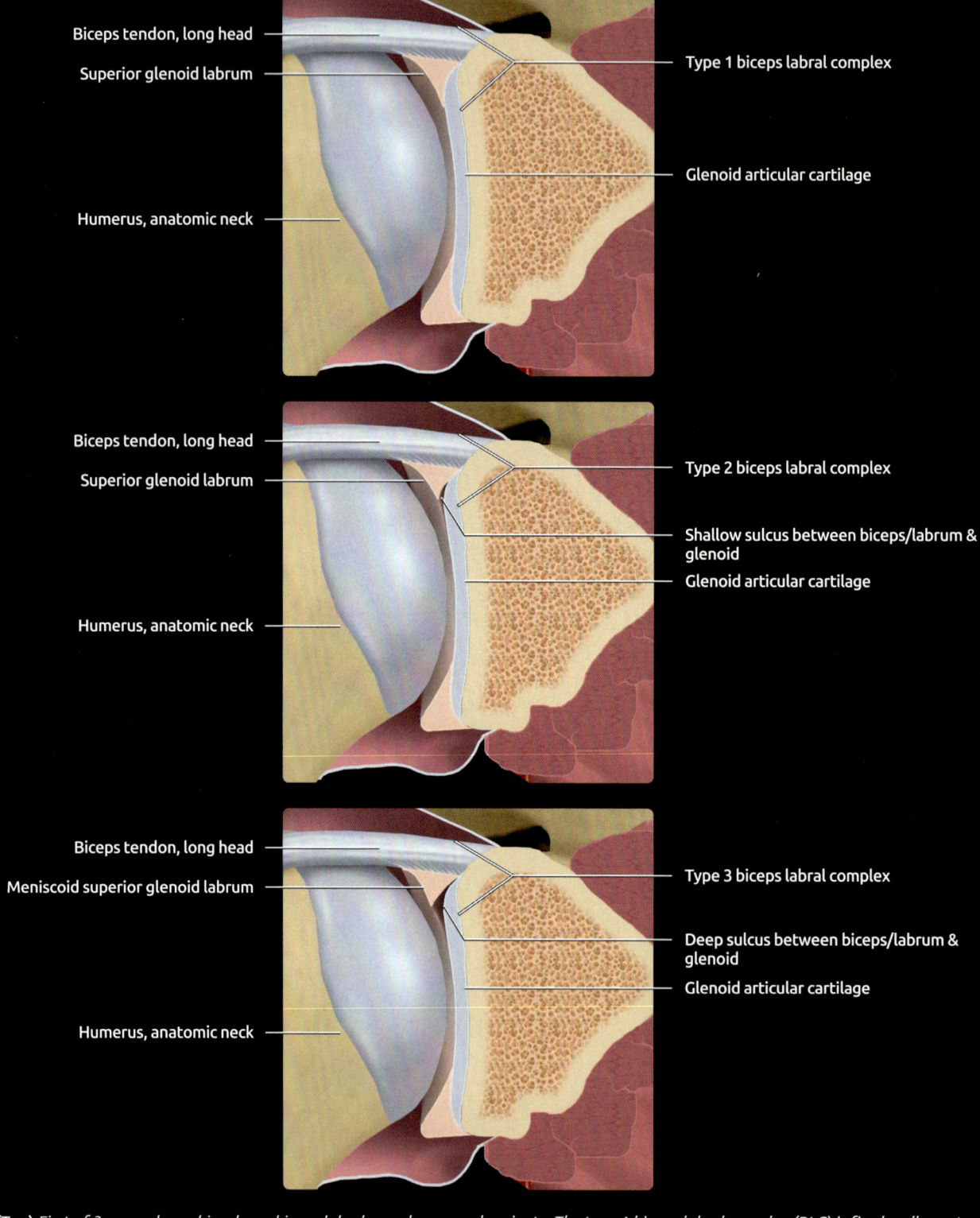

(Top) First of 3 coronal graphics shows biceps labral complex normal variants. The type 1 biceps labral complex (BLC) is firmly adherent to the glenoid. This is also referred to as the slab-type BLC. **(Middle)** The type 2 BLC has a shallow sulcus between the glenoid and biceps/labrum. This morphology is also referred to as intermediate type BLC. **(Bottom)** The type 3 BLC has a deep sulcus between the glenoid and biceps/labrum. The superior glenoid labrum is meniscoid, thus this normal variant is also called the meniscoid type BLC. This deep sulcus often continues anteriorly as a sublabral foramen.

Shoulder Labrum

BICEPS LABRAL COMPLEX, NORMAL VARIANTS

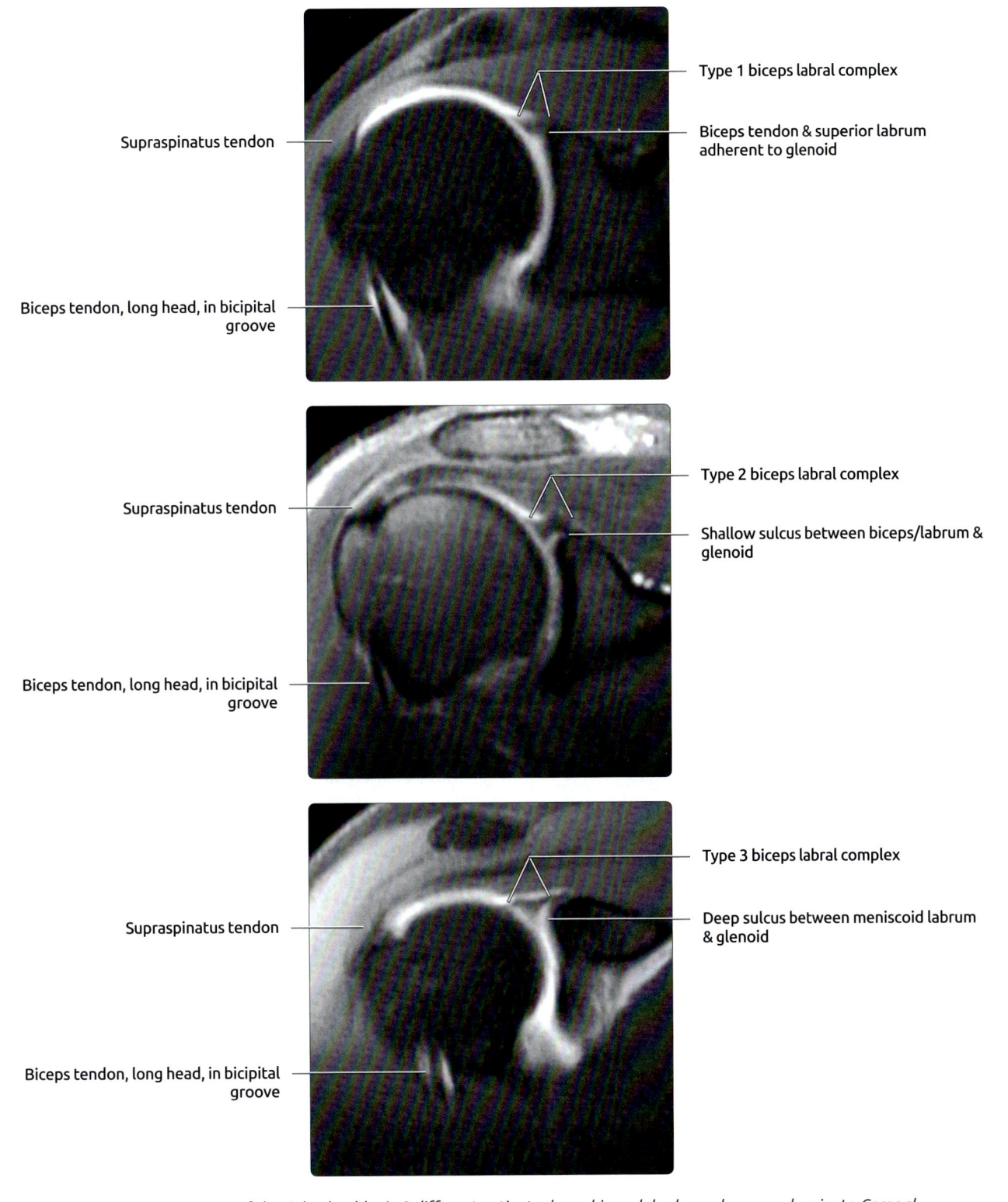

Suprapinatus tendon — Type 1 biceps labral complex — Biceps tendon & superior labrum adherent to glenoid — Biceps tendon, long head, in bicipital groove

Supraspinatus tendon — Type 2 biceps labral complex — Shallow sulcus between biceps/labrum & glenoid — Biceps tendon, long head, in bicipital groove

Supraspinatus tendon — Type 3 biceps labral complex — Deep sulcus between meniscoid labrum & glenoid — Biceps tendon, long head, in bicipital groove

(Top) First of 3 coronal MR images of the right shoulder in 3 different patients shows biceps labral complex normal variants. Coronal oblique T1 FS MR arthrogram is shown. The biceps tendon is firmly adherent to the labrum and superior glenoid. This is a type 1 or slab type BLC. (Middle) Coronal oblique T1 MR shows a relatively shallow sulcus that lies between the biceps/labrum and glenoid. This is a type 2 or intermediate-type BLC. (Bottom) Coronal oblique T1 FS MR arthrogram shows a deep sulcus that lies between the biceps/labrum and glenoid. This is a type 3 or meniscoid type BLC.

Shoulder Normal Variants and Imaging Pitfalls

IMAGING PITFALLS

Magic Angle Phenomenon on MR
- 55° to main magnetic field when image TE < 30 ms
- Increases signal intensity in otherwise normal structures
- Most often seen in supraspinatus tendon, commonly in "critical zone," 1 cm from greater tuberosity
- Can be seen in glenoid labrum and biceps tendon proximal to bicipital groove
- Avoid pitfall by comparing with images acquired with longer TE

Interdigitation of Muscle or Fibrous Tissue Between Supraspinatus and Infraspinatus Tendons
- Simulates increased T2 MR signal within supraspinatus tendon
- Exaggerated if imaged in internal rotation

Volume Averaging of Rotator Interval Contents on Coronal Oblique Images
- Simulates increased T2 MR signal within supraspinatus tendon

Normal Flattening or Slight Concavity of Posterolateral Humeral Head
- Proximal to teres minor tendon insertion
- Can be confused with Hill-Sachs lesion, which is located more proximally, above level of coracoid process

Acromial Pseudospurs Mimicking Osteophytes
- Fibrocartilaginous hypertrophy at insertion of coracoacromial ligament on inferior acromion
- Superior and inferior tendon slips of deltoid muscle

Normal Residual Red Bone Marrow in Glenoid and Proximal Humeral Metaphysis Can Mimic Neoplastic Process
- Red marrow has higher T1 signal than adjacent muscle
- Red marrow typically decreases in signal on out-of-phase images, compared with in-phase images

Anterolateral Branch of Anterior Circumflex Humeral Artery & Vein in Lateral Bicipital Groove
- Can be mistaken for biceps tendon longitudinal tear

Hyaline Cartilage Undercutting of Superior Labrum Simulating Labral Tear
- Distinguish between signal of cartilage vs. true tear

Vacuum Effect Simulating Loose Bodies or Chondrocalcinosis
- Round or curvilinear intraarticular low signal
- Exaggerated on gradient-echo MR sequences & with external rotation positioning

General Imaging Artifacts
- Motion artifact can be decreased by positioning arm away from patient's body
- Avoid superior to inferior phase encoding to decrease artifact from axillary vessels
- Metal susceptibility artifact
  - Increase bandwidth on all sequences
- Use fast spin-echo rather than conventional spin-echo sequences

NORMAL VARIANTS

Osseous
- **Os acromiale**
  - Unfused acromial apophysis (normally fuses by age 25)
  - Occurs in 5% of population
  - May be mobile & decrease coracoacromial space during motion
  - Predisposes to impingement & rotator cuff tear; therefore is a clinically important normal variant
- **Hypoplastic glenoid**
  - Congenital anomaly resulting in hypoplasia of posterior & inferior glenoid
  - Associated hyperplasia of posterior & inferior glenoid with associated tear &/or detachment
  - Associated findings of shoulder instability

Labrum
- **Sublabral cleft and foramen**
  - Sublabral recess (sulcus or cleft) restricted to anterosuperior labrum (does not extend posterior to biceps tendon origin)
  - Recess 1-2 mm thick; fluid may enter recess, simulating tear
  - Recess may be continuous with sublabral foramen
  - Foramen found in 8-18% of population
  - Foramen restricted to anterosuperior labral quadrant
  - Recess or foramen smooth & tapered; morphology may help differentiate from tear
- **Labral attachment types**
  - Type A: Detached free edge overlying glenoid articular cartilage (meniscoid)
  - Type B: Adherent to glenoid articular cartilage
- **Biceps labral complex (BLC)**
  - Biceps attachment to labrum
  - Type 1 BLC: Biceps firmly adherent to glenoid and superior labrum, slab type
  - Type 2 BLC: Small sulcus between biceps/labrum and glenoid, may be continuous with sublabral foramen, intermediate type
  - Type 3 BLC: Large sulcus between biceps/labrum and glenoid, labrum often continues as sublabral foramen, meniscoid type
- **Variability in size (or absence) of glenohumeral ligaments**
  - Most common variant is absent (or very small middle glenohumeral ligament
- **Buford complex**
  - Diminutive or absent anterosuperior labrum
  - Thick cord-like middle glenohumeral ligament
  - Present in 1-6.5% of population
  - Must not be misinterpreted as glenoid labral detachment

SELECTED REFERENCES
1. Wilson WR et al: Variability of the capsular anatomy in the rotator interval region of the shoulder. J Shoulder Elbow Surg. 22(6):856-61, 2013

Shoulder Normal Variants and Imaging Pitfalls

NORMAL VARIANT: HYPERINTENSITY DISTAL SUPRASPINATUS TENDON

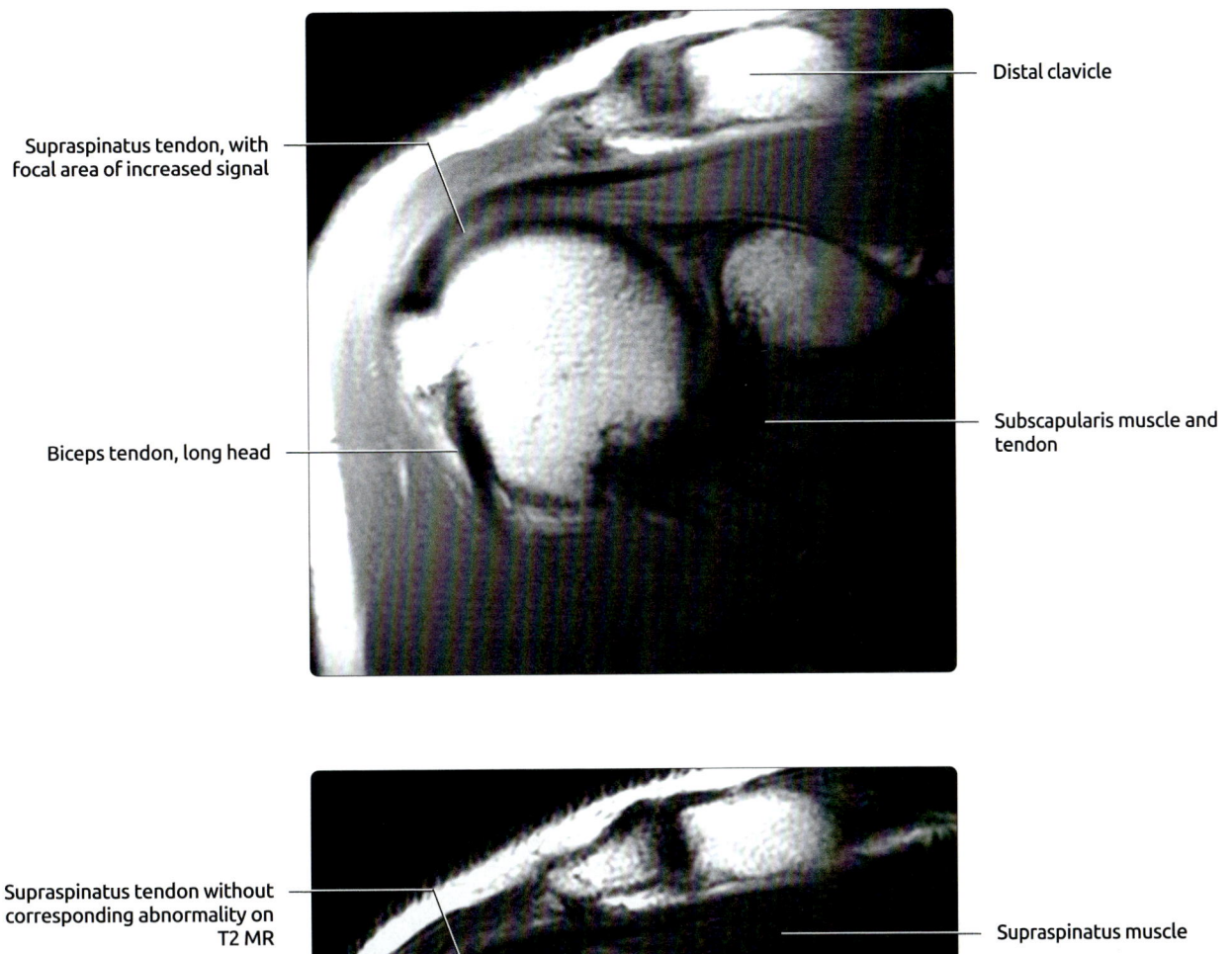

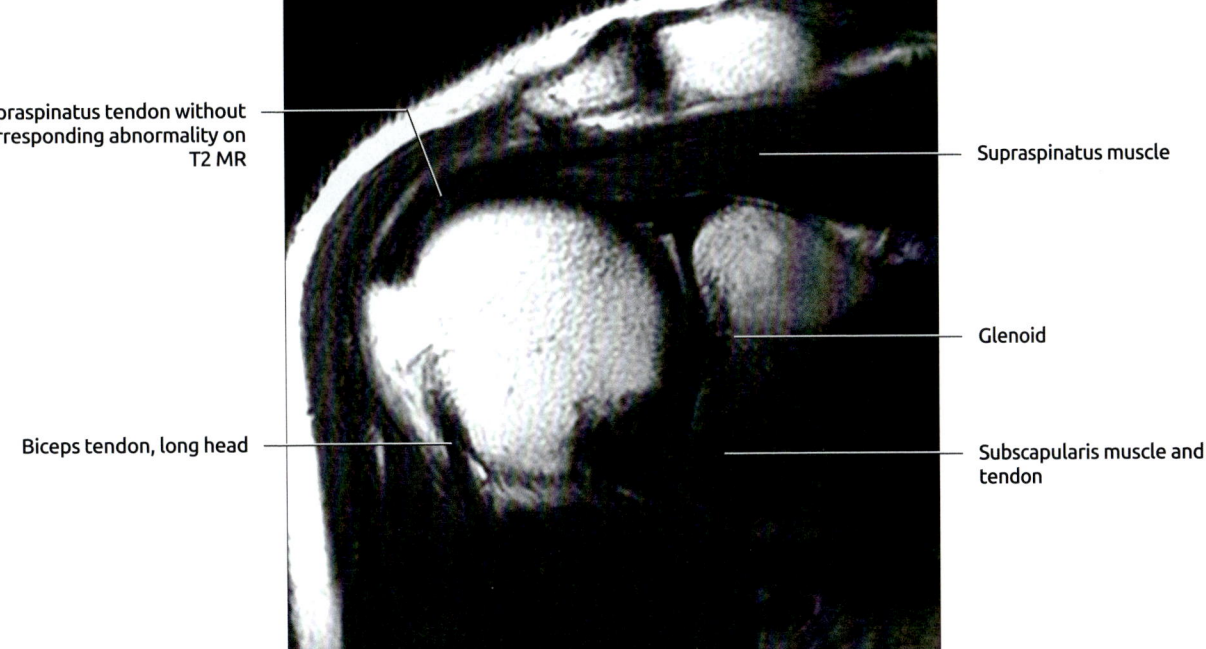

(Top) First of 2 coronal oblique images through the same level in the same patient is shown. Image is proton density weighted with a TE of 11. A focal area of increased signal in the supraspinatus tendon is located approximately 1 cm from the insertion on the greater tuberosity. *(Bottom)* Image is T2 weighted with a TE of 93. There is no corresponding abnormal signal on this sequence. Abnormal signal in this area of the supraspinatus tendon has been attributed to many different entities including magic angle artifact, tendon degeneration, and partial volume effect. The resolution of the abnormal signal when the TE of the sequence was increased favors magic angle artifact.

Shoulder Normal Variants and Imaging Pitfalls

NORMAL VARIANT: VESSELS LATERAL ASPECT BICIPITAL GROOVE

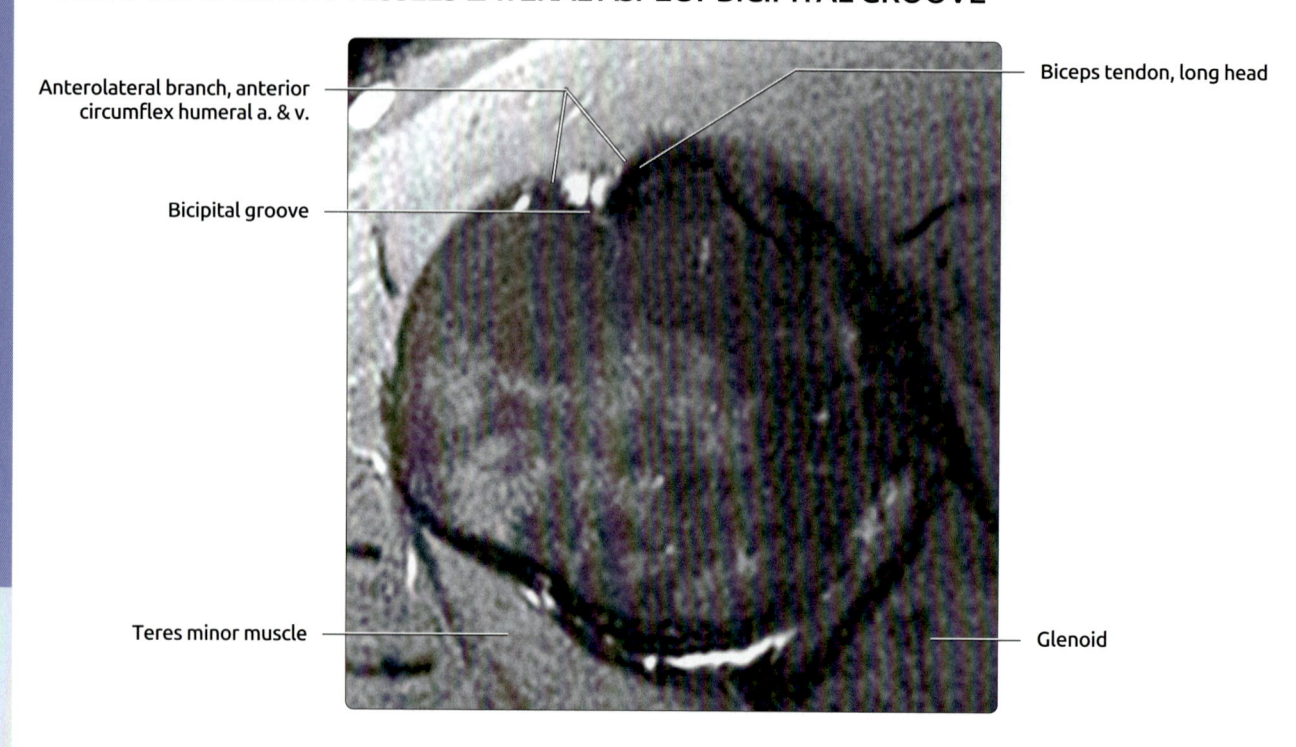

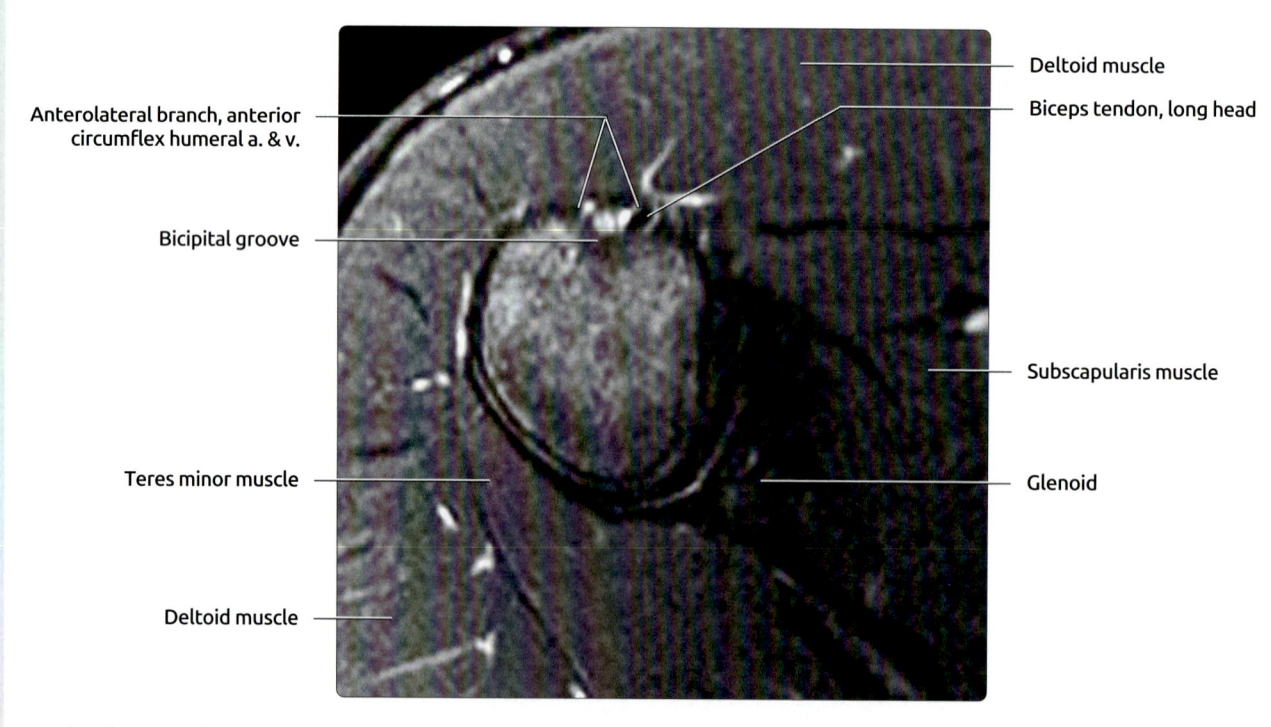

(Top) Increased signal within the lateral aspect of bicipital groove on axial T2 FS MR image is shown. The anterolateral branch of the anterior circumflex humeral artery and vein lie within the groove. These vessels should not be confused with fluid from tenosynovitis or a tear of the biceps tendon. (Bottom) Companion case shows the anterolateral branch of the anterior circumflex humeral artery and vein within lateral aspect of bicipital groove on axial T2 FS MR image.

Shoulder Normal Variants and Imaging Pitfalls

MR PITFALLS: ACROMION PSEUDOSPUR

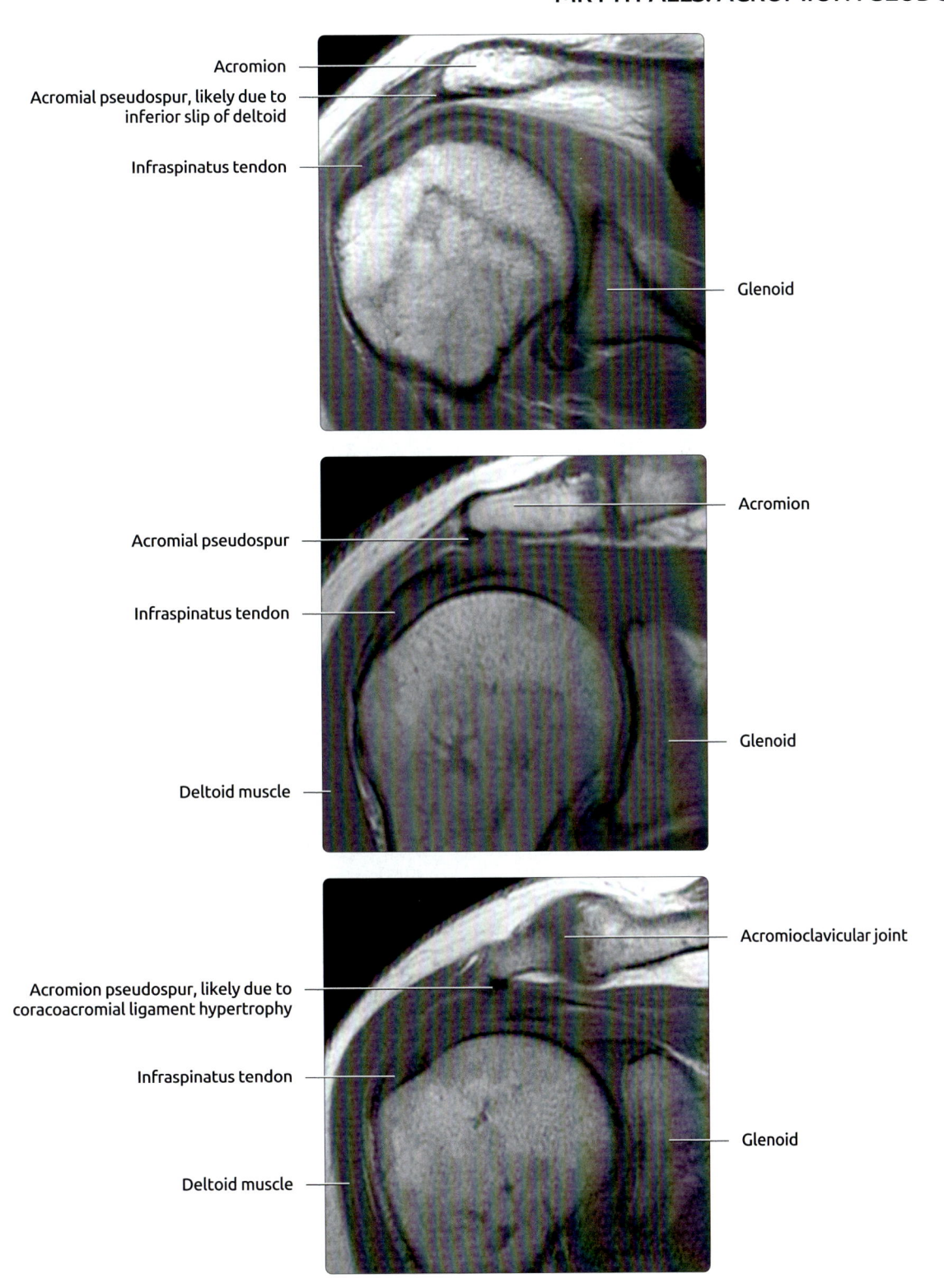

(Top) First of 3 coronal oblique T1 MR images of the right shoulder in 3 different patients with subacromial pseudospurs is shown. None of the patients had a bony spur on radiographs. The low signal subacromial pseudospur in this patient is oriented laterally and likely represents the inferior tendon slip of the deltoid muscle. *(Middle)* In this patient, the low signal subacromial pseudospur is globular. It could be due to hypertrophy of the inferior tendon slip of the deltoid muscle or the coracoacromial ligament. *(Bottom)* In this patient, the low signal subacromial pseudospur is oriented medially. It is likely due to coracoacromial ligament hypertrophy.

Shoulder Normal Variants and Imaging Pitfalls

RADIOGRAPHIC PITFALL: NORMAL FLATTENING OF POSTERIOR HUMERAL HEAD

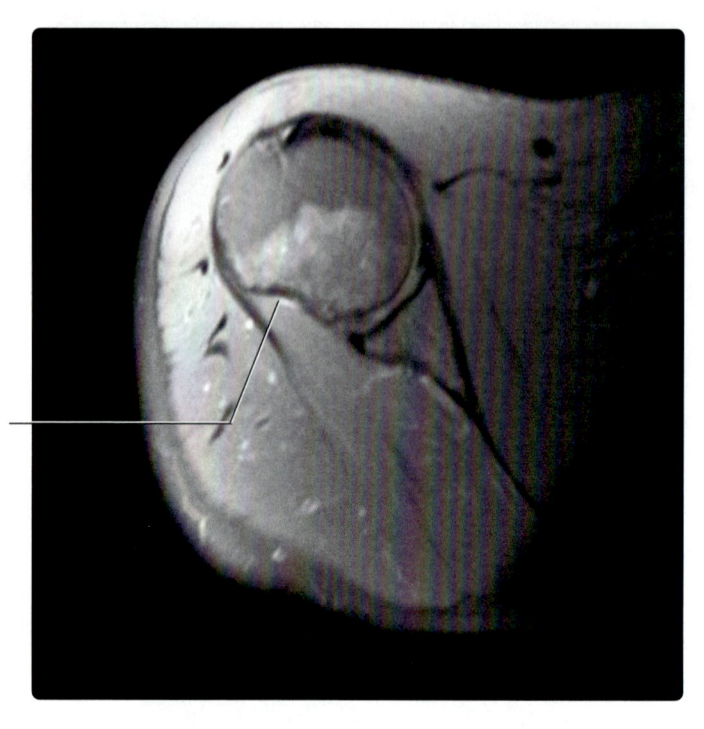

Normal flattening humeral head

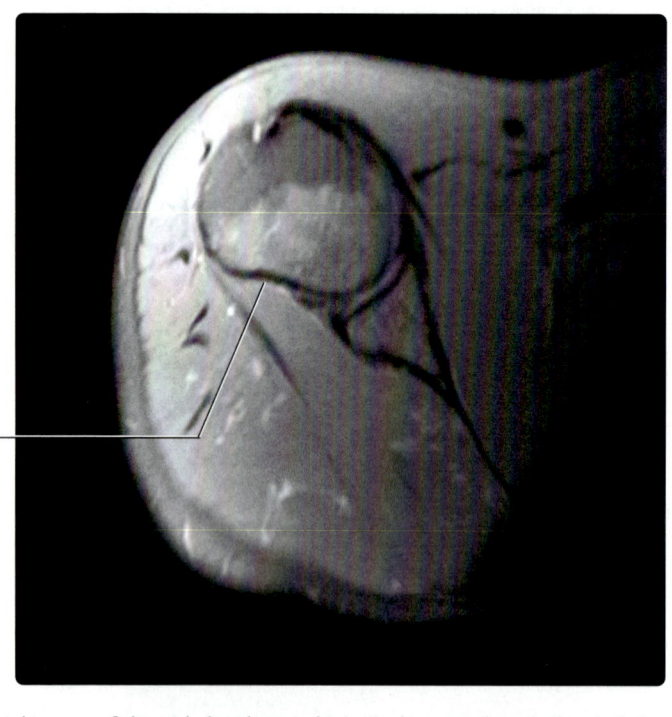

Normal flat contour posterior humeral head, approaching surgical neck of humerus

(Top) First of 2 sequential axial images of the mid-glenohumeral joint is shown. Below the level of the coracoid process (at or below the level of mid-glenohumeral joint), the posterior aspect of the humeral head loses its normal round contour, becoming flattened. (Bottom) Adjacent axial image, same patient, shows the normal flattening posteriorly on the humeral head. It is important that the posterior flattening, which may appear abrupt in the 1st image, not be misinterpreted as a Hill-Sachs impaction fracture. These fractures occur posterolaterally, not directly posteriorly, and more superiorly (superior portion of humeral head).

Shoulder Normal Variants and Imaging Pitfalls

OS ACROMIALE, RADIOGRAPHS

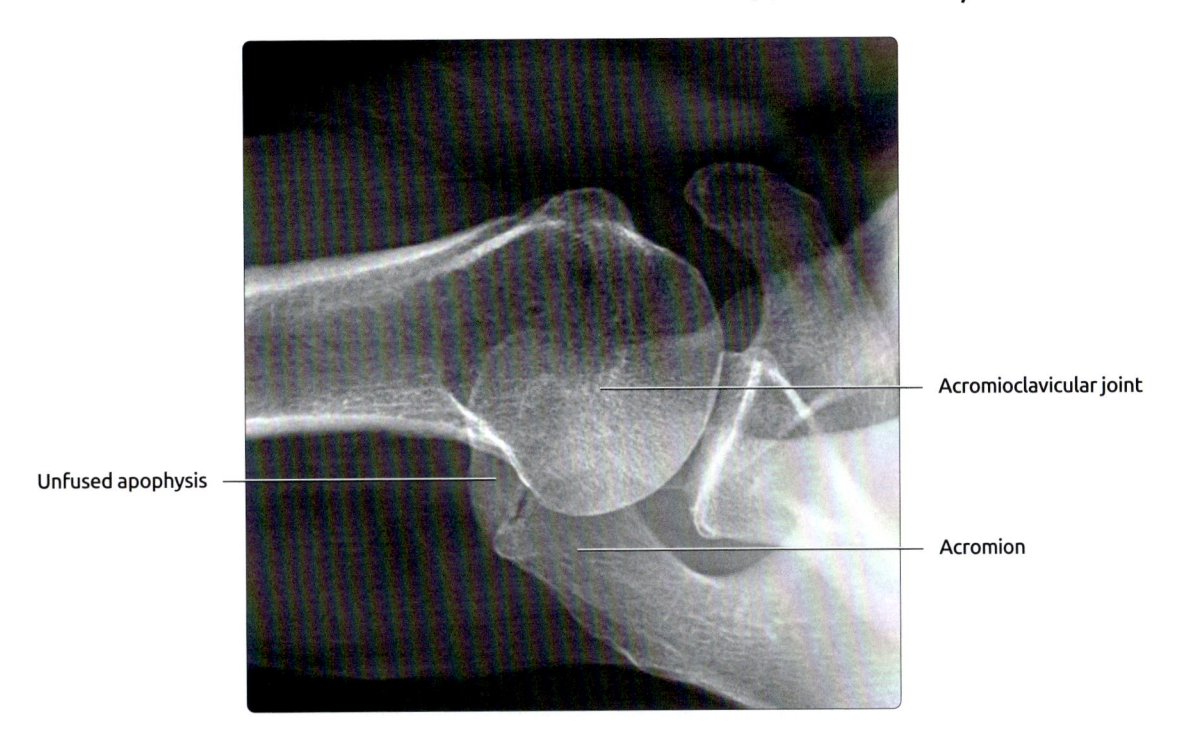

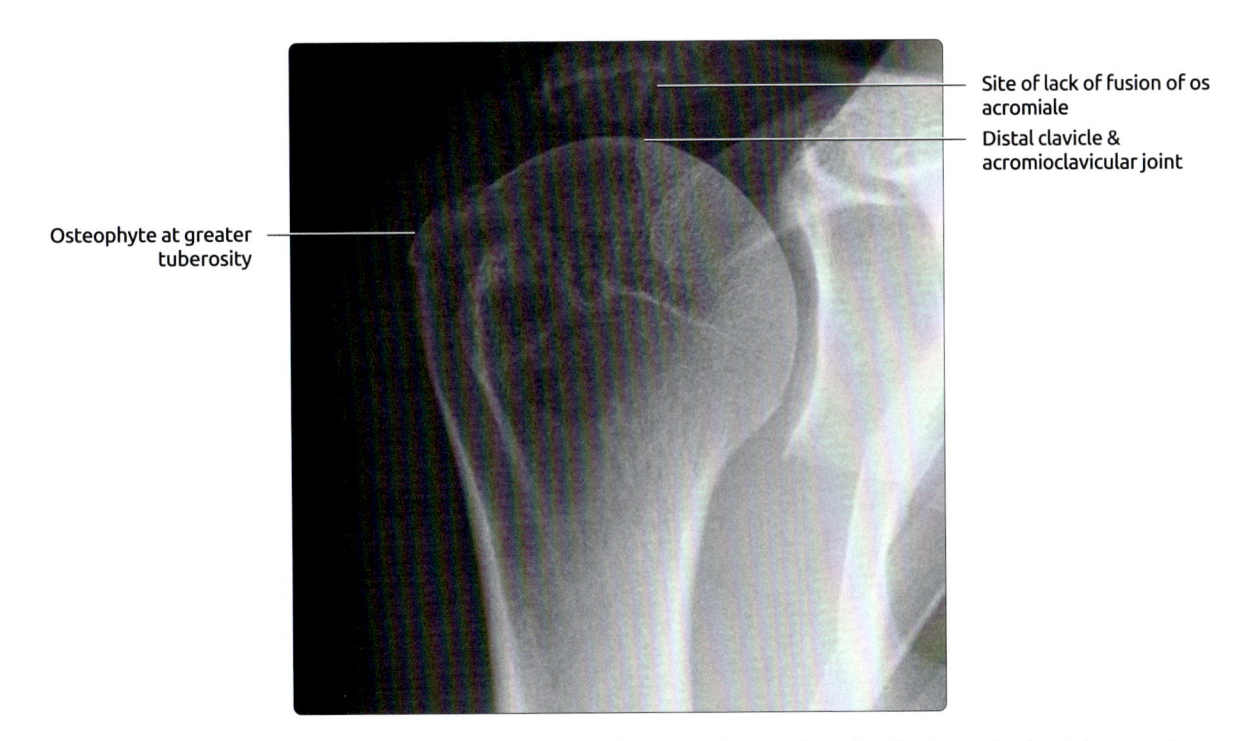

Acromioclavicular joint

Unfused apophysis

Acromion

Site of lack of fusion of os acromiale

Distal clavicle & acromioclavicular joint

Osteophyte at greater tuberosity

(Top) Os acromiale is seen best on axillary lateral radiographs. In a well-positioned image, the unfused os is seen to clearly be separate from the acromioclavicular joint, which is correctly positioned superimposed over the center of the humeral head. (Bottom) An os acromiale may be more subtle to identify on AP view of the shoulder joint. With care, the unfused portion of the acromion is seen to be separate from the acromioclavicular joint. In this case, long-term motion of the os has restricted the space in the coracoacromial arch, resulting in rotator cuff pathology and secondary degenerative disease, seen as an osteophyte on the greater tuberosity.

Shoulder Normal Variants and Imaging Pitfalls

OS ACROMIALE, RADIOGRAPH AND MR

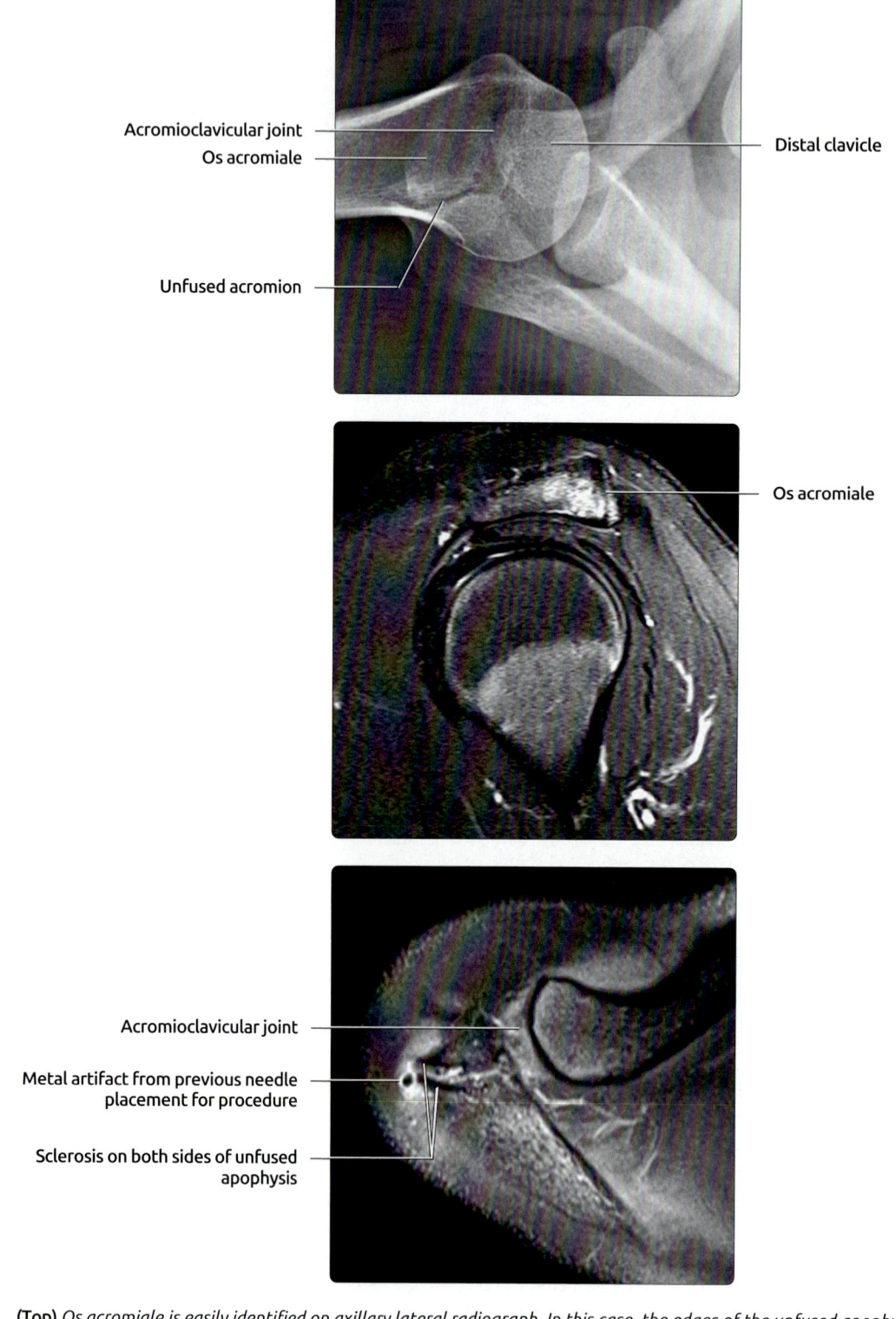

(Top) Os acromiale is easily identified on axillary lateral radiograph. In this case, the edges of the unfused apophysis are sclerotic, suggestive of chronic motion at the site. *(Middle)* Oblique sagittal T2 FS MR in the same patient demonstrates the site of lack of fusion of the os, as well as high signal edema on either side of the mobile segment. In this section, no associated rotator cuff injury is noted. *(Bottom)* Axial PD FS MR in the same patient shows sclerosis and adjacent high signal edema at the os acromiale, indicating chronic motion at the site.

Shoulder Normal Variants and Imaging Pitfalls

OS ACROMIALE, 3D CT AND MR

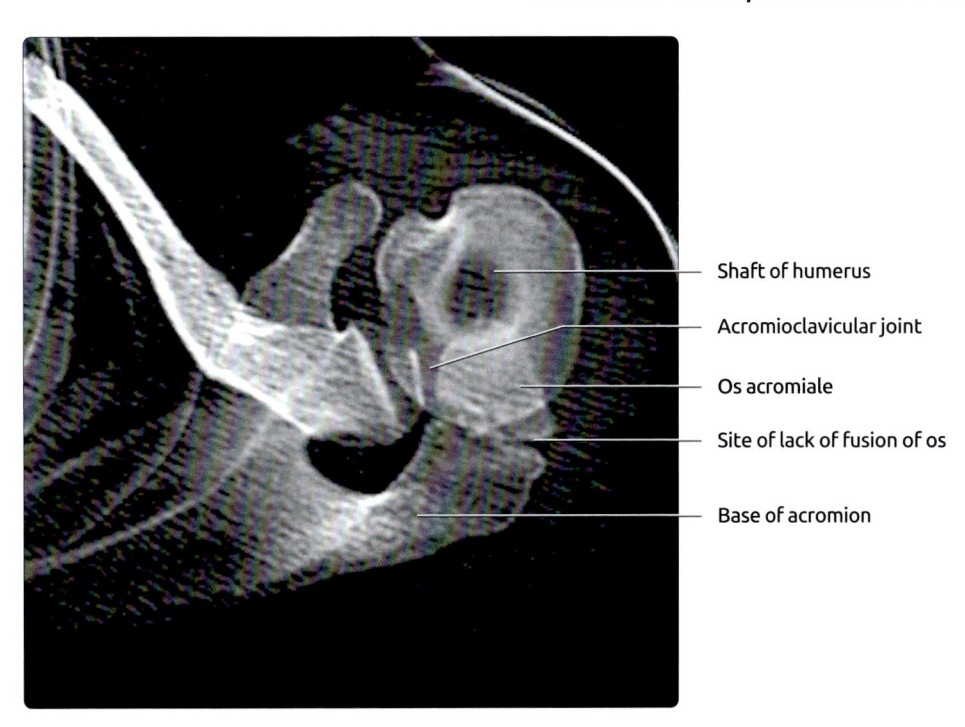

Shaft of humerus
Acromioclavicular joint
Os acromiale
Site of lack of fusion of os
Base of acromion

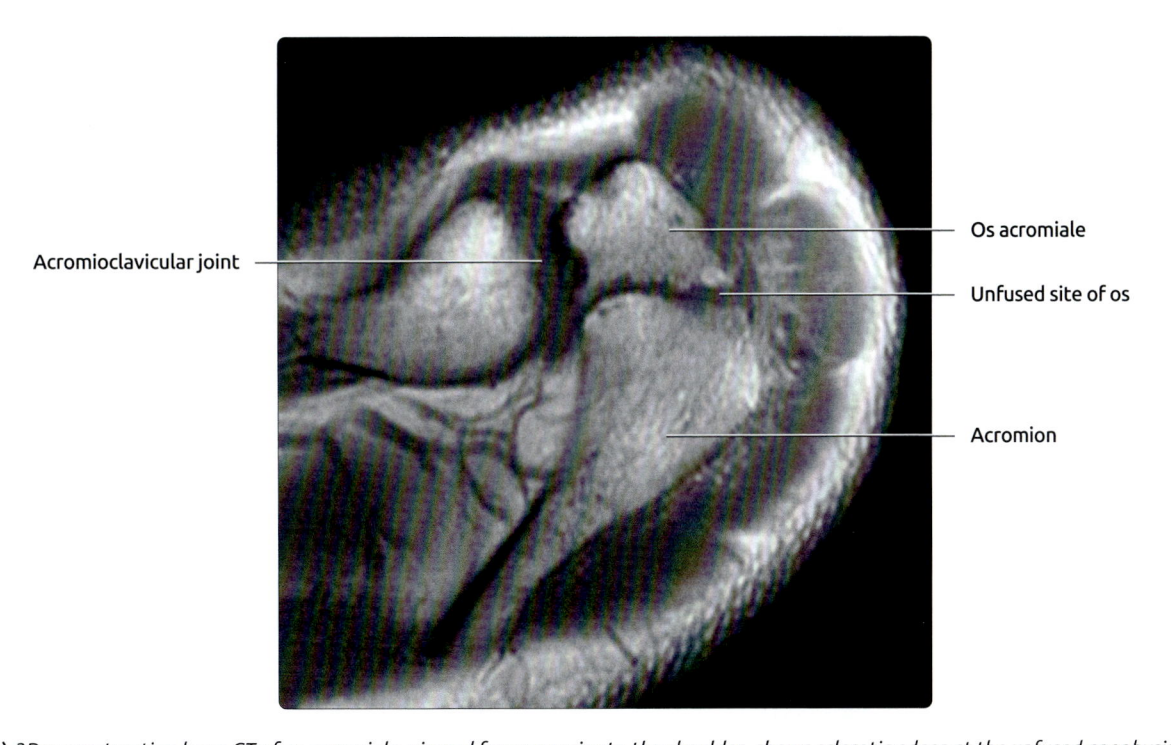

Acromioclavicular joint
Os acromiale
Unfused site of os
Acromion

(Top) *3D reconstruction bone CT of os acromiale, viewed from superior to the shoulder, shows sclerotic edges at the unfused apophysis.*
(Bottom) *Axial T1-weighted MR shows sclerotic edges of an os acromiale.*

Shoulder Normal Variants and Imaging Pitfalls

VARIANT: HYPOPLASTIC GLENOID

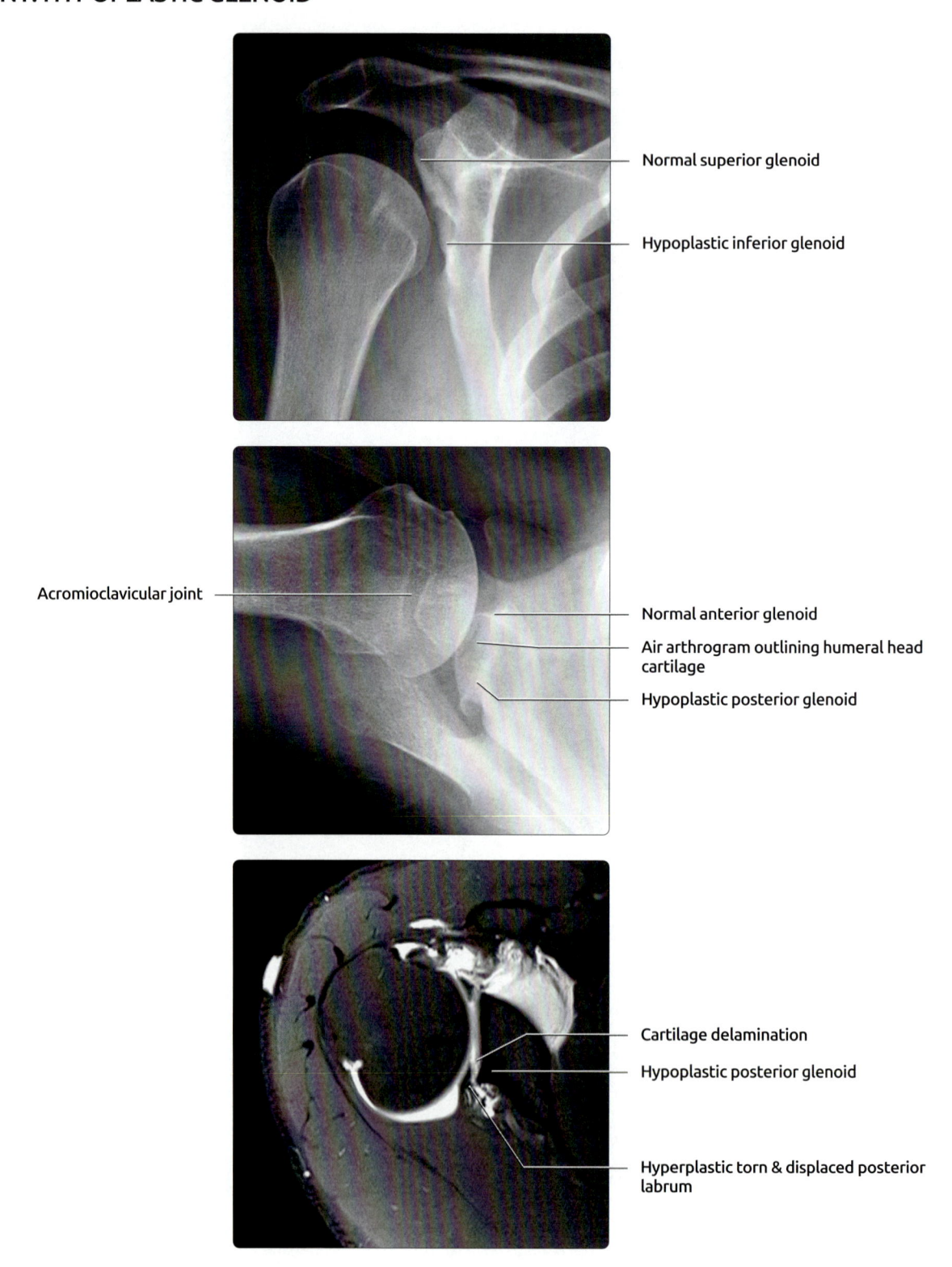

Normal superior glenoid

Hypoplastic inferior glenoid

Acromioclavicular joint

Normal anterior glenoid

Air arthrogram outlining humeral head cartilage

Hypoplastic posterior glenoid

Cartilage delamination

Hypoplastic posterior glenoid

Hyperplastic torn & displaced posterior labrum

(Top) *AP internal rotation radiograph demonstrates a hypoplastic glenoid. This congenital anomaly almost exclusively involves the inferior and posterior aspects of the glenoid, leaving the superior glenoid with a normal morphology.* **(Middle)** *Axillary lateral radiograph demonstrates a hypoplastic glenoid, with deficient bone in the posterior aspect of the glenoid. The anterior glenoid has normal morphology. One might initially try to fault the patient positioning for this appearance; however, the acromioclavicular joint is superimposed on the center of the humeral head, as is expected for an appropriately positioned axillary lateral radiograph.* **(Bottom)** *T1FS MR arthrogram in the same patient demonstrates the deficient osseous glenoid posteriorly, along with associated glenoid labral cartilage defect and torn/displaced posterior labrum. The posterior labrum is mildly hyperplastic relative to the normal anterior labrum.*

Shoulder Normal Variants and Imaging Pitfalls

VARIANT: HYPOPLASTIC GLENOID

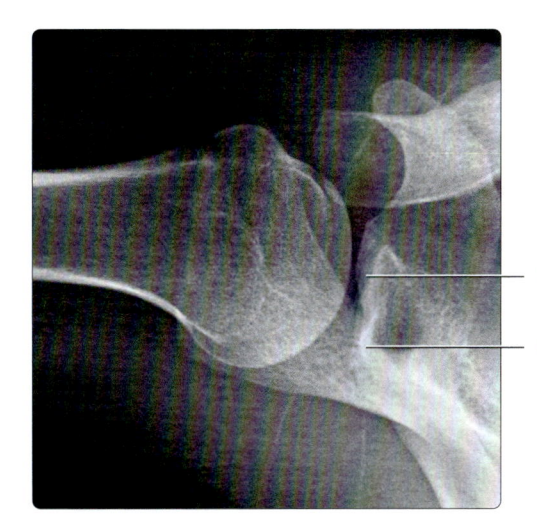

- Normal anterior glenoid
- Hypoplastic posterior glenoid

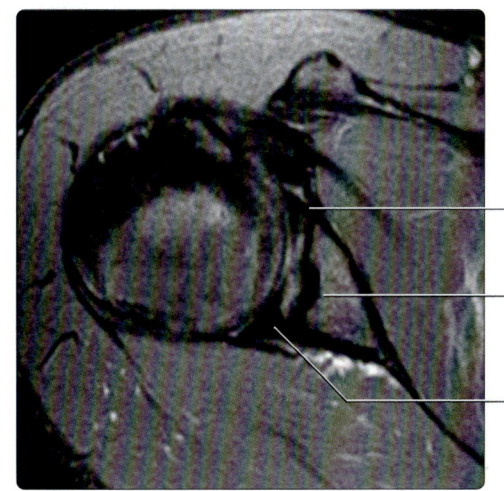

- Normal anterior glenoid & labrum
- Hypoplastic posterior glenoid
- Hyperplastic posterior labrum with detachment from underlying abnormal bony glenoid

- Normal anterior glenoid
- Hypoplastic posterior glenoid
- Detached posterior labrum

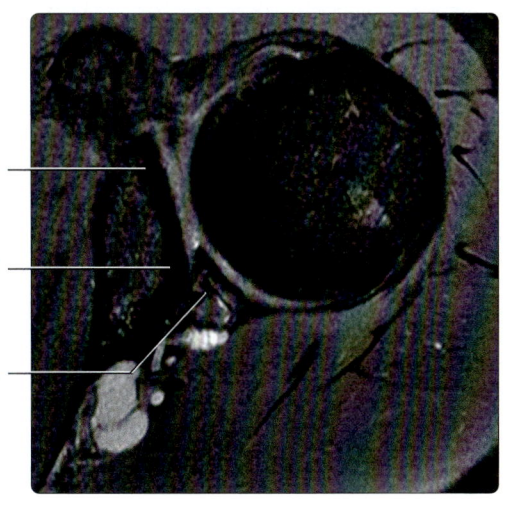

(Top) Axillary lateral radiograph is not perfectly positioned, but demonstrates the posterior glenoid to be hypoplastic relative to the normal anterior glenoid. (Middle) Axial PD FS MR of the same patient confirms the posterior glenoid to be hypoplastic relative to the normal anterior glenoid. Note that the posterior labrum is significantly hyperplastic relative to the normal anterior labrum; the posterior labrum undergoes shear stress in this situation and has become detached. (Bottom) Axial T2 FS image in another patient shows hypoplastic posterior glenoid, with hyperplastic and detached posterior labrum.

Shoulder Normal Variants and Imaging Pitfalls

MR VARIANT: SIZE/PRESENCE OF GLENOHUMERAL LIGAMENTS

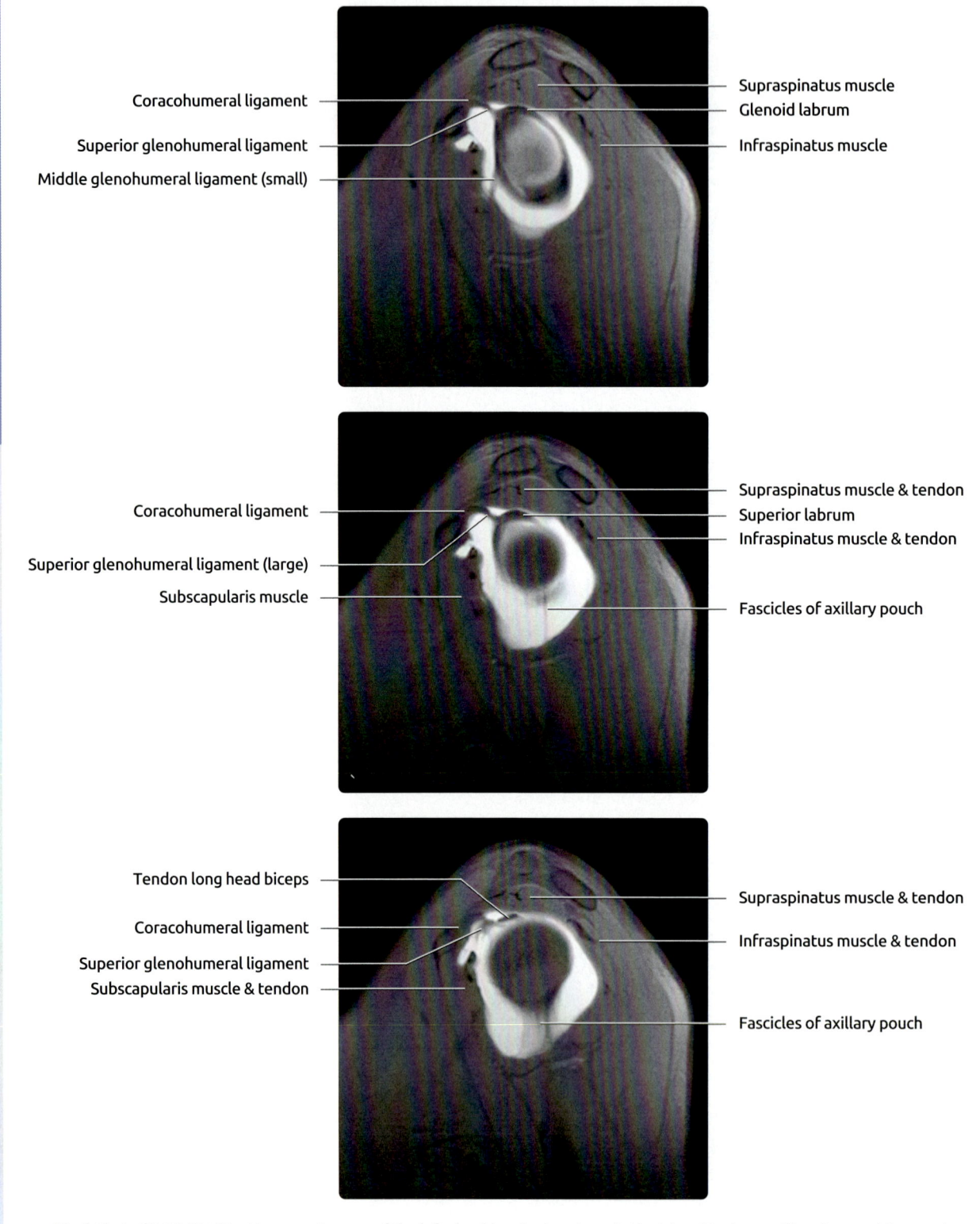

Coracohumeral ligament
Superior glenohumeral ligament
Middle glenohumeral ligament (small)

Supraspinatus muscle
Glenoid labrum
Infraspinatus muscle

Coracohumeral ligament
Superior glenohumeral ligament (large)
Subscapularis muscle

Supraspinatus muscle & tendon
Superior labrum
Infraspinatus muscle & tendon
Fascicles of axillary pouch

Tendon long head biceps
Coracohumeral ligament
Superior glenohumeral ligament
Subscapularis muscle & tendon

Supraspinatus muscle & tendon
Infraspinatus muscle & tendon
Fascicles of axillary pouch

(Top) First of 3 T1 FS MR arthrogram images of the left shoulder displayed medial to lateral is shown. Glenohumeral ligaments can normally vary in size and presence. The superior and middle glenohumeral ligaments are outlined by contrast in this image. The middle glenohumeral ligament is smaller than is typically seen. (Middle) The superior glenohumeral ligament is larger than usual and blends with the coracohumeral ligament and joint capsule in this image. These structures will also fuse with the supraspinatus and subscapularis tendons as they extend laterally. (Bottom) Anterior and posterior bands of the inferior glenohumeral ligament complex are absent. Fascicles of the axillary pouch are present.

Shoulder Normal Variants and Imaging Pitfalls

NORMAL VARIANT: SUBLABRAL FORAMEN

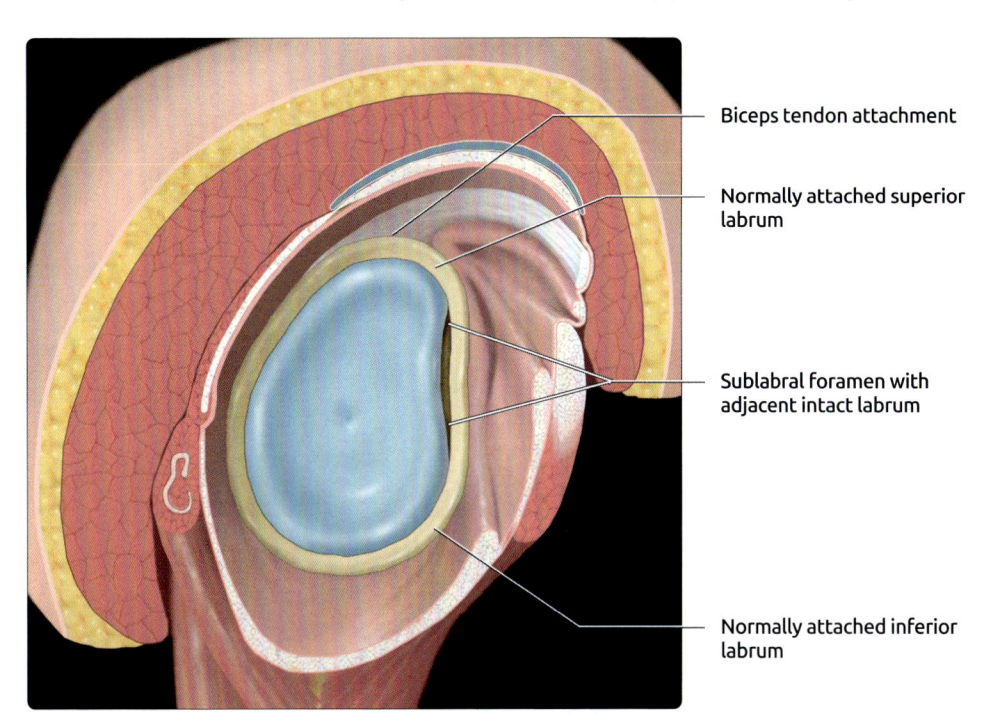

- Biceps tendon attachment
- Normally attached superior labrum
- Sublabral foramen with adjacent intact labrum
- Normally attached inferior labrum

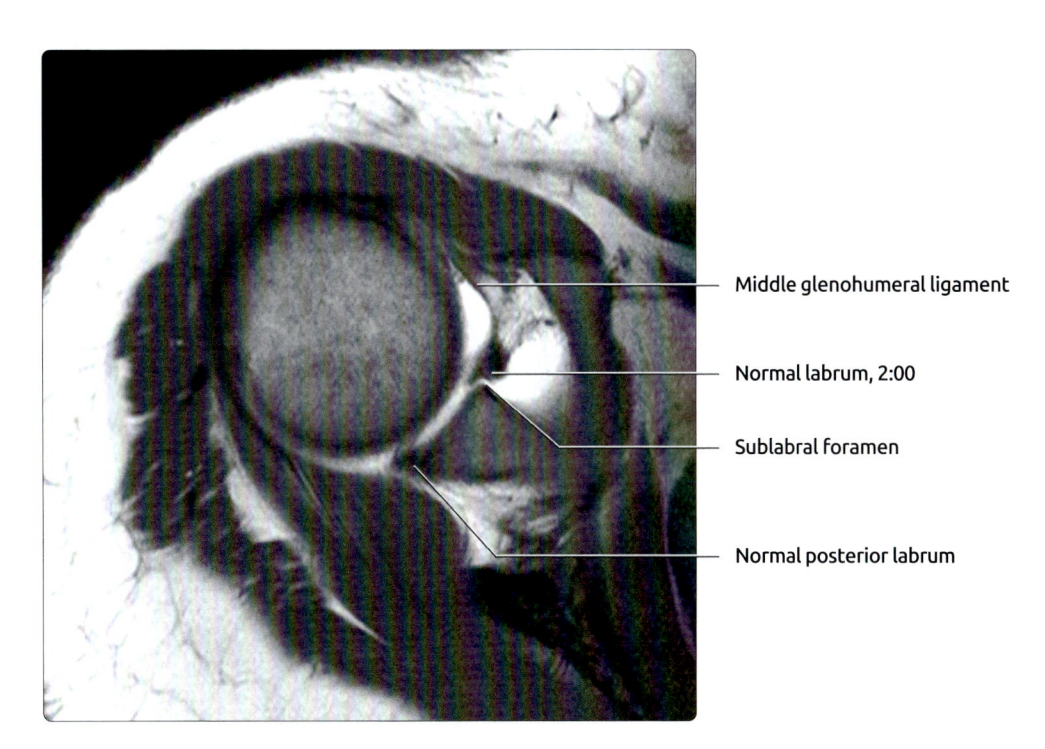

- Middle glenohumeral ligament
- Normal labrum, 2:00
- Sublabral foramen
- Normal posterior labrum

(Top) *A normal sublabral foramen may be found, restricted to the anterosuperior labrum. The foramen does not extend posterior to the biceps tendon attachment* **(Bottom)** *T1WI MR arthrogram, in the axial plane at the 2:00 level, shows a sublabral foramen between the normal anterosuperior labrum and the underlying bony glenoid. Note that the fluid extending through the foramen outlines smooth surfaces, helping to differentiate from a labral tear or detachment.*

Shoulder Normal Variants and Imaging Pitfalls

NORMAL VARIANT: BUFORD COMPLEX

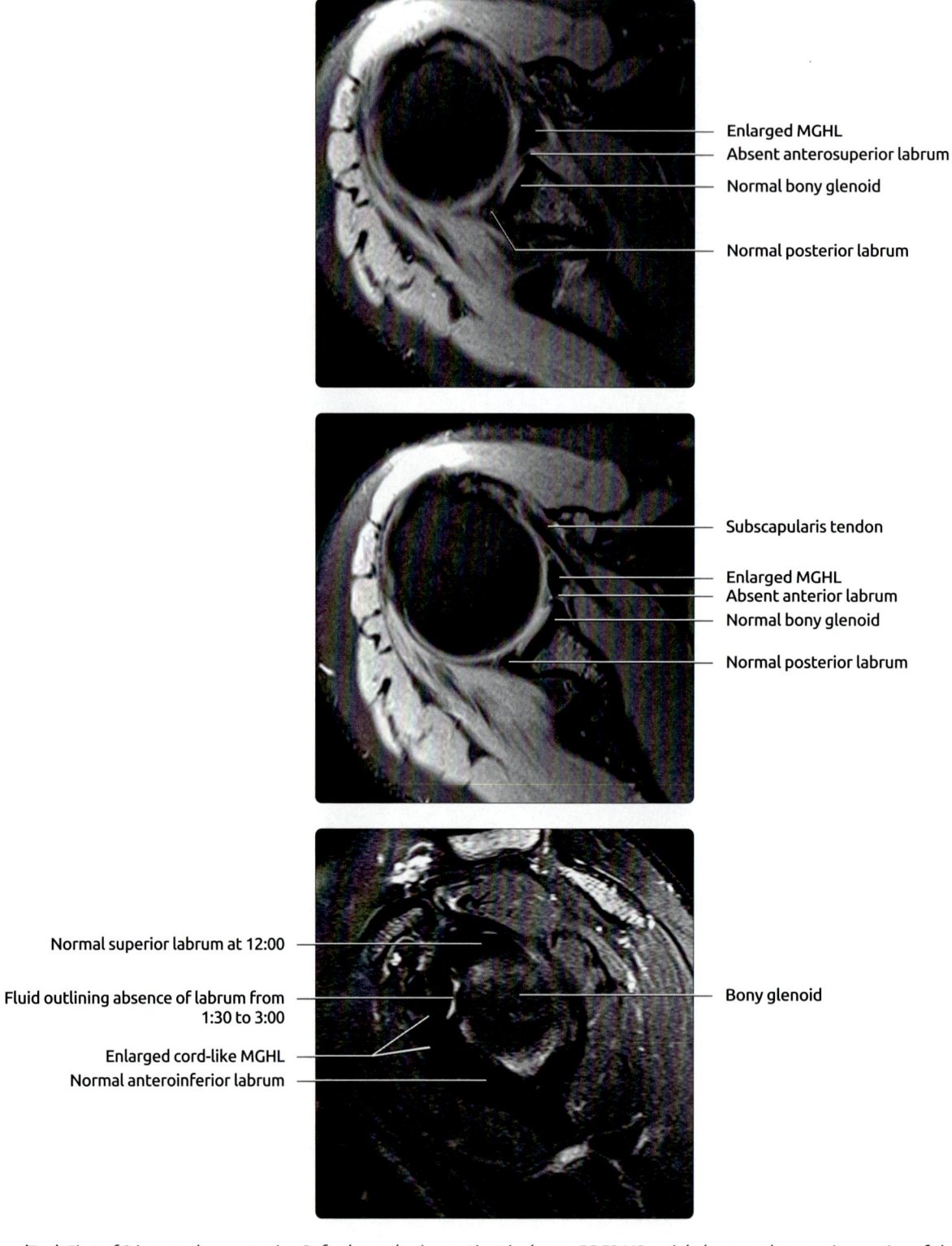

Enlarged MGHL
Absent anterosuperior labrum
Normal bony glenoid
Normal posterior labrum

Subscapularis tendon
Enlarged MGHL
Absent anterior labrum
Normal bony glenoid
Normal posterior labrum

Normal superior labrum at 12:00
Fluid outlining absence of labrum from 1:30 to 3:00
Enlarged cord-like MGHL
Normal anteroinferior labrum
Bony glenoid

(Top) *First of 3 images demonstrating Buford complex in a patient is shown. PDFS MR, axial plane, at the superior portion of the glenohumeral joint (~ 1:30 on the clock face) is shown. There is an extremely large middle glenohumeral ligament (MGHL). This is associated with an absent anterior labrum. The posterior labrum is normal.* **(Middle)** *Second axial PDFS MR shows the significantly enlarged MGHL to continue in its course toward the subscapularis tendon as a cord-like structure. There is continued absence of the anterior glenoid. This image is at about the 3:00 level.* **(Bottom)** *Oblique sagittal T2 FS MR in the same patient shows fluid outlining the bony glenoid, delineating the absence of the anterosuperior labrum from approximately 1:30 to 3:00. The anterior labrum "reconstitutes" to a normal attachment from 3:00 to 12:00. The absent portion of anterosuperior labrum is associated with a thick, cord-like MGHL; this latter structure can often be seen well on sagittal images in the Buford complex.*

Shoulder Normal Variants and Imaging Pitfalls

NORMAL VARIANT: BUFORD COMPLEX

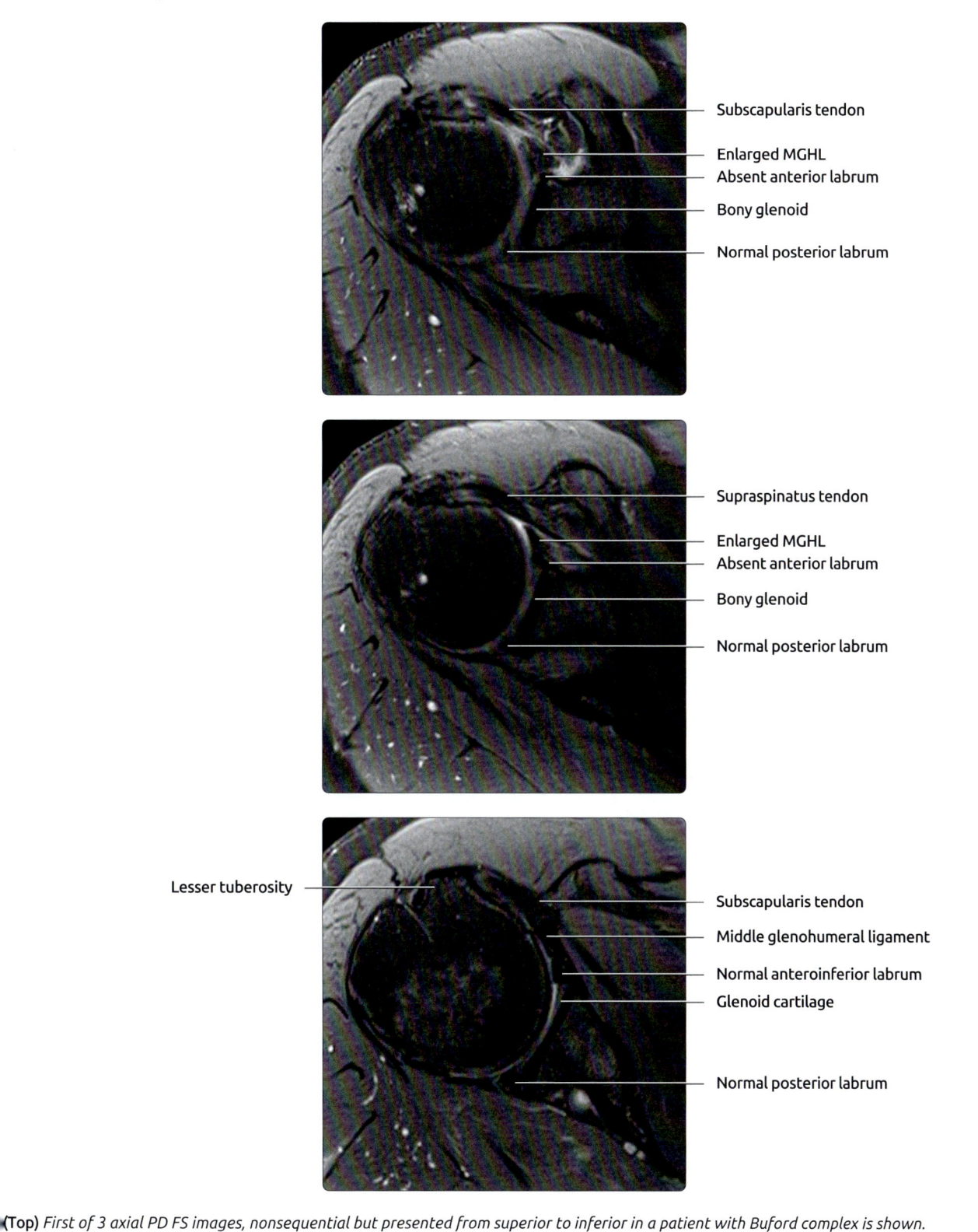

Top image labels: Subscapularis tendon; Enlarged MGHL; Absent anterior labrum; Bony glenoid; Normal posterior labrum

Middle image labels: Supraspinatus tendon; Enlarged MGHL; Absent anterior labrum; Bony glenoid; Normal posterior labrum

Bottom image labels: Lesser tuberosity; Subscapularis tendon; Middle glenohumeral ligament; Normal anteroinferior labrum; Glenoid cartilage; Normal posterior labrum

(**Top**) First of 3 axial PD FS images, nonsequential but presented from superior to inferior in a patient with Buford complex is shown. This image is obtained at approximately 2:00 and shows an absent anterior labrum with associated enlarged middle glenohumeral ligament (MGHL). (**Middle**) Second image in series of axial PD FS images, at approximately 3:00, shows continuation of the enlarged cord-like MGHL and continued absence of anterior labrum. (**Bottom**) Third axial PD FS image in the series, at approximately 4:00, shows "reconstituted" normal anterior inferior labrum and the MGHL merging with the subscapularis tendon as it approaches its insertion on the lesser tuberosity. This is the expected appearance of a Buford complex in the anteroinferior aspect of the shoulder.

SECTION 2
Arm

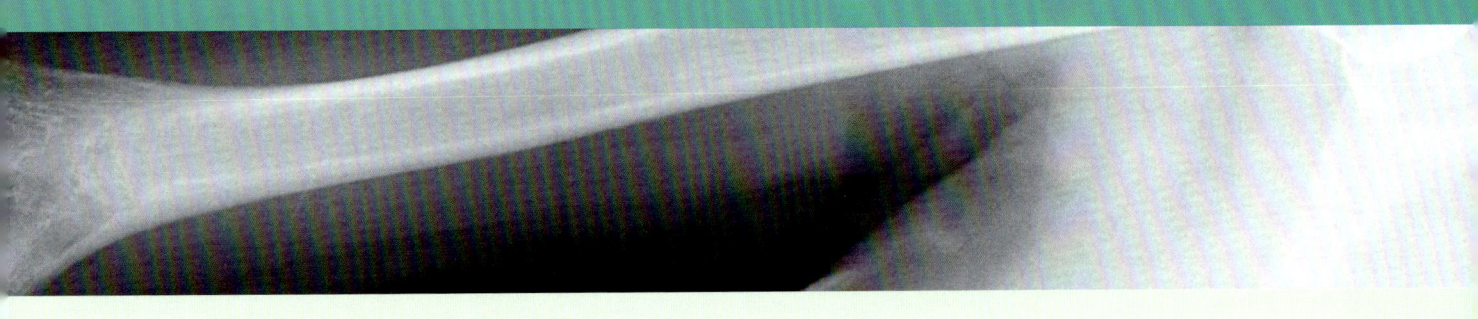

Arm Radiographic Anatomy and MR Atlas   **154**

Arm Radiographic Anatomy and MR Atlas

IMAGING ANATOMY

Anatomy Relationships
- Proximal muscle insertions
  - Deltoid muscle
    - Origin: Anterior, middle, and posterior bellies arise from clavicle, acromion process, and spine of scapula, respectively
    - Insertion: Muscle bellies merge and insert on deltoid tuberosity of humerus, located laterally at approximate midpoint of humeral length, over distance of nearly 5 cm
    - Innervation: Axillary nerve (C5 & C6)
    - Blood supply: Deltoid branch of thoracoacromial artery
    - Action: Anterior belly flexes and medially rotates shoulder, middle belly abducts shoulder, posterior belly extends and laterally rotates shoulder
  - Teres major muscle
    - Origin: Dorsal surface of inferior angle of scapula
    - Insertion: Medial lip of intertubercular groove of humerus (below subscapularis insertion)
    - Innervation: Lower subscapular nerve (C6 & C7)
    - Blood supply: Subscapular and circumflex scapular arteries
    - Action: Adducts and medially rotates arm
  - Pectoralis major muscle
    - Origin: Clavicular head arises from anterior surface of medial half of clavicle; sternocostal head arises from anterior surface of sternum, superior 6 costal cartilages, and aponeurosis of external oblique muscle
    - Insertion: Lateral lip of intertubercular groove of humerus (immediately lateral to teres major insertion)
    - Innervation: C5, C6, C7, C8, T1
    - Blood supply: Pectoral branch of thoracoacromial trunk
    - Action: Adducts and medially rotates humerus, draws scapula anteriorly and inferiorly
  - Latissimus dorsi muscle
    - Origin: Spinous process of inferior 6 thoracic vertebrae, thoracolumbar fascia, iliac crest, and inferior 3 or 4 ribs
    - Insertion: Floor of intertubercular groove of humerus (between pectoralis major and teres major)
    - Innervation: Thoracodorsal nerve (C6, C7, C8)
    - Blood supply: Thoracodorsal artery
    - Action: Extends, adducts, and medially rotates humerus; raises body towards arms when climbing
- Anterior compartment of arm
  - Coracobrachialis muscle
    - Origin: Coracoid process tip, in common with and medial to short head biceps tendon
    - Insertion: Medial surface of humeral mid shaft, between brachialis and triceps muscle origins
    - Nerve supply: Musculocutaneous nerve, perforates muscle
    - Blood supply: Brachial artery, muscular branches
    - Action: Flexes and adducts shoulder, supports humeral head in glenoid
    - Variants: Bony head extending to medial epicondyle, short head extending to lesser tuberosity
  - Biceps muscle, short head
    - Origin: Coracoid process tip, in common with and lateral to coracobrachialis tendon
    - Insertion: Radial tuberosity after joining long head
    - Nerve supply: Musculocutaneous nerve
    - Blood supply: Brachial artery, muscular branches
    - Action: Flexes elbow and shoulder, supinates forearm
  - Biceps muscle, long head
    - Origin: Predominantly supraglenoid tubercle; also superior glenoid labrum and coracoid base
    - Insertion: Radial tuberosity after joining with short head
    - Nerve supply: Musculocutaneous nerve
    - Blood supply: Brachial artery, muscular branches
    - Action: Flexes elbow and shoulder, supinates forearm
    - Lacertus fibrosus (distal bicipital fascia/aponeurosis) provides traction on deep fascia of forearm
    - Variants, biceps muscle: 3rd head in 10% arising at upper medial aspect of brachialis muscle, 4th head can arise from lateral humerus, bicipital groove, or greater tuberosity
  - Brachialis muscle
    - Origin: Distal half of anterior humeral shaft and 2 intermuscular septa
    - Insertion: Tuberosity of ulna and anterior surface of coronoid process
    - Nerve supply: Musculocutaneous nerve plus branch of radial nerve
    - Blood supply: Brachial artery, muscular branches, and recurrent radial artery
    - Action: Flexes elbow
    - Covers anterior aspect of elbow joint
    - Variants: Doubled; slips to supinator, pronator teres, biceps, lacertus fibrosus, or radius
- Posterior compartment of arm
  - Triceps muscle, long head
    - Origin: Infraglenoid tubercle of scapula
    - Insertion: Proximal olecranon and deep fascia of arm after joining with lateral and medial heads
    - Nerve supply: Radial nerve
    - Blood supply: Deep brachial artery branches
    - Action: Elbow extension, adducts humerus when arm is extended
  - Triceps muscle, lateral head
    - Origin: Posterior and lateral humeral shaft, lateral intermuscular septum
    - Insertion: Proximal olecranon and deep fascia of arm after joining with long and medial heads
    - Nerve supply: Radial nerve
    - Blood supply: Deep brachial artery branches
    - Action: Elbow extension
  - Triceps muscle, medial head
    - Origin: Posterior humeral shaft from teres major insertion to near trochlea, medial intermuscular septum
    - Insertion: Proximal olecranon and deep fascia of arm after joining with lateral and long heads
    - Nerve supply: Radial and branches of ulnar nerve
    - Blood supply: Deep brachial artery branches
    - Action: Elbow extension

Arm Radiographic Anatomy and MR Atlas

- Variants, triceps muscle: 4th head from medial humerus, slip termed dorso-epitrochlearis extending between triceps and latissimus dorsi
  - Anconeus muscle
    - Origin: Lateral epicondyle of humerus
    - Insertion: Lateral olecranon and posterior 1/4 of ulna
    - Nerve supply: Radial nerve
    - Blood supply: Deep brachial artery, middle collateral branch
    - Action: Assists elbow extension, abducts ulna
- Fascia
  - Brachial fascia
    - Continuous with fascia covering deltoid and pectoralis major
    - Varies in thickness being thin over biceps and thick over triceps muscles
    - Lateral intermuscular septum from lower aspect of greater tuberosity to lateral epicondyle
    - Medial intermuscular septum from lower aspect of lesser tuberosity to medial epicondyle
    - Perforated by ulnar nerve, superior ulnar collateral artery, and posterior branch of inferior ulnar collateral artery
  - Bicipital fascia
    - Also known as lacertus fibrosus
    - Arises from medial side of distal biceps tendon at level of elbow joint
    - Passes superficial to brachial artery
    - Continuous with deep fascia of forearm
- Neurovascular structures
  - Brachial artery
    - Continuation of axillary artery at inferior border of teres major muscle
    - Brachial artery runs medial to median nerve in upper part of arm and lateral to median nerve in lower part of arm
    - Deep brachial (profunda brachii) branch wraps around posterior surface of humerus, descending branch becomes radial collateral artery and runs in radial groove with radial nerve, and supplies posterior compartment of arm
    - Superior ulnar collateral branch runs with ulnar nerve and passes posterior to medial epicondyle
    - Distally, brachial artery passes deep to bicipital aponeurosis lateral to median nerve and medial to bicipital tendon, then branches into radial and ulnar arteries
  - Radial nerve
    - Continuation of posterior cord of brachial plexus (C5-C8, T1)
    - Passes under teres major muscle, winding around medial side of neck of humerus to enter substance of triceps muscle
    - Continues through spiral groove of posterior humerus to lateral side of arm
    - Pierces lateral intermuscular septum just proximal to level of lateral humeral condyle
    - Divides into superficial cutaneous sensory branch and deep motor branch
  - Median nerve
    - Arises from lateral and medial cords of brachial plexus (C6-T1)
    - Follows course of axillary artery, then enters upper arm deep in relation to fascia of biceps muscle and superficial to brachialis muscle
  - Ulnar nerve
    - Arises from medial cord of brachial plexus (C8 & T1)
    - Runs along medial border of axillary-brachial artery to mid humeral level where it angles dorsally, piercing medial intermuscular septum
    - Follows medial head of triceps to cubital tunnel

ANATOMY IMAGING ISSUES

Imaging Recommendations

- **Radiographs and CT**: Evaluation of bone cortex and matrix of any identified bone lesion
- **MR**: Axial plane most helpful to delineate borders of anterior and posterior compartments and relationship to neurovascular structures

CLINICAL IMPLICATIONS

Traumatic Pathology Related to Anatomy

- **Radial nerve palsy**
  - Nerve at risk in fracture of distal half of humeral shaft due to its close association to bone, running posteriorly in spiral groove between lateral and medial heads of triceps muscle
  - 16% of midshaft fractures develop radial nerve palsy
  - Denervation changes seen on MR
    - Brachioradialis
    - Extensor carpi radialis longus
    - Extensor carpi radialis brevis
    - May also involve muscles innervated by posterior interosseous nerve if injury is at proximal margin of supinator muscle due to entrapment by fibrous bands (arcade of Frohse)
- **Displacement/angulation following humeral shaft fracture**
  - Midshaft humeral fracture usually significantly displaced and angulated
    - Varus angulation due to abduction of proximal fragment by deltoid muscle
    - Proximal displacement of distal fragment due to contraction of biceps and brachialis muscles

SELECTED REFERENCES

1. Kim SJ et al: MR imaging mapping of skeletal muscle denervation in entrapment and compressive neuropathies. Radiographics. 31(2):319-32, 2011
2. Sallomi D et al: Muscle denervation patterns in upper limb nerve injuries: MR imaging findings and anatomic basis. AJR Am J Roentgenol. 171(3):779-84, 1998

Arm Radiographic Anatomy and MR Atlas

RADIOGRAPHS

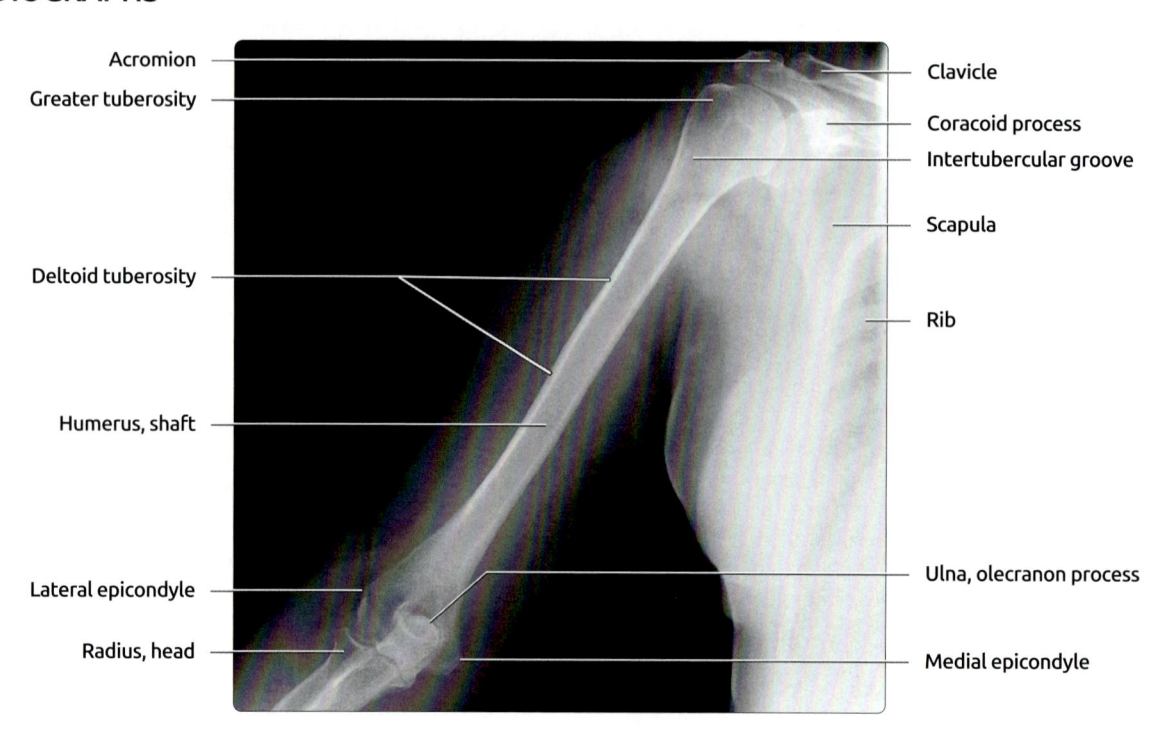

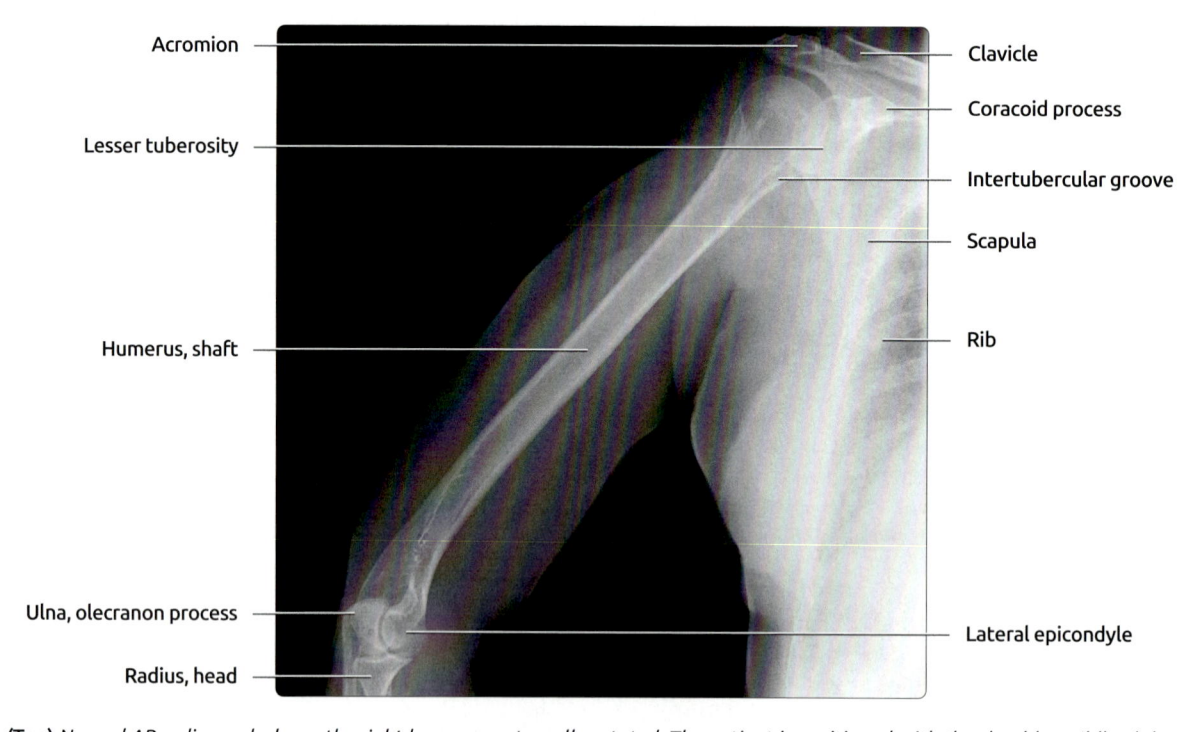

(Top) *Normal AP radiograph shows the right humerus, externally rotated. The patient is positioned with the shoulder mildly abducted, the elbow extended, and the hand supinated. Both the shoulder and elbow joints should be visible on the radiograph.* (Bottom) *This image is of a normal lateral radiograph of right humerus. The patient is positioned with the shoulder internally rotated and mildly abducted. If obtained lateromedial, as in this case, the elbow is partially flexed. If obtained mediolateral, then the elbow would be flexed 90 degrees.*

Arm Radiographic Anatomy and MR Atlas

GRAPHICS, ANTERIOR ARM

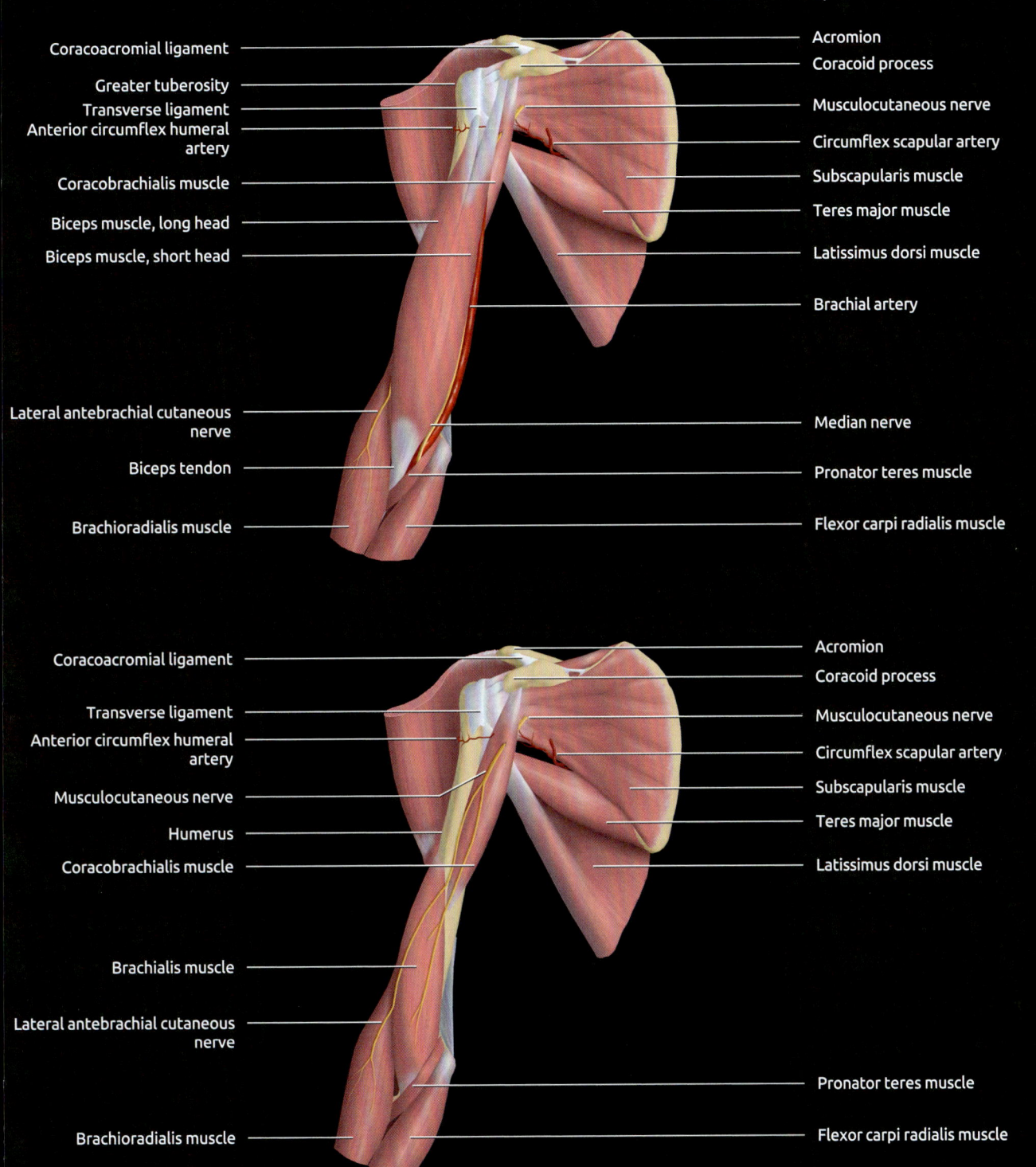

Labels (top, superficial dissection):
- Coracoacromial ligament
- Greater tuberosity
- Transverse ligament
- Anterior circumflex humeral artery
- Coracobrachialis muscle
- Biceps muscle, long head
- Biceps muscle, short head
- Lateral antebrachial cutaneous nerve
- Biceps tendon
- Brachioradialis muscle
- Acromion
- Coracoid process
- Musculocutaneous nerve
- Circumflex scapular artery
- Subscapularis muscle
- Teres major muscle
- Latissimus dorsi muscle
- Brachial artery
- Median nerve
- Pronator teres muscle
- Flexor carpi radialis muscle

Labels (bottom, deep dissection):
- Coracoacromial ligament
- Transverse ligament
- Anterior circumflex humeral artery
- Musculocutaneous nerve
- Humerus
- Coracobrachialis muscle
- Brachialis muscle
- Lateral antebrachial cutaneous nerve
- Brachioradialis muscle
- Acromion
- Coracoid process
- Musculocutaneous nerve
- Circumflex scapular artery
- Subscapularis muscle
- Teres major muscle
- Latissimus dorsi muscle
- Pronator teres muscle
- Flexor carpi radialis muscle

(**Top**) *First of 2 anterior graphics of the right arm shows a superficial dissection.* (**Bottom**) *Anterior graphic of the arm shows a deep dissection.*

Arm Radiographic Anatomy and MR Atlas

GRAPHICS, POSTERIOR ARM

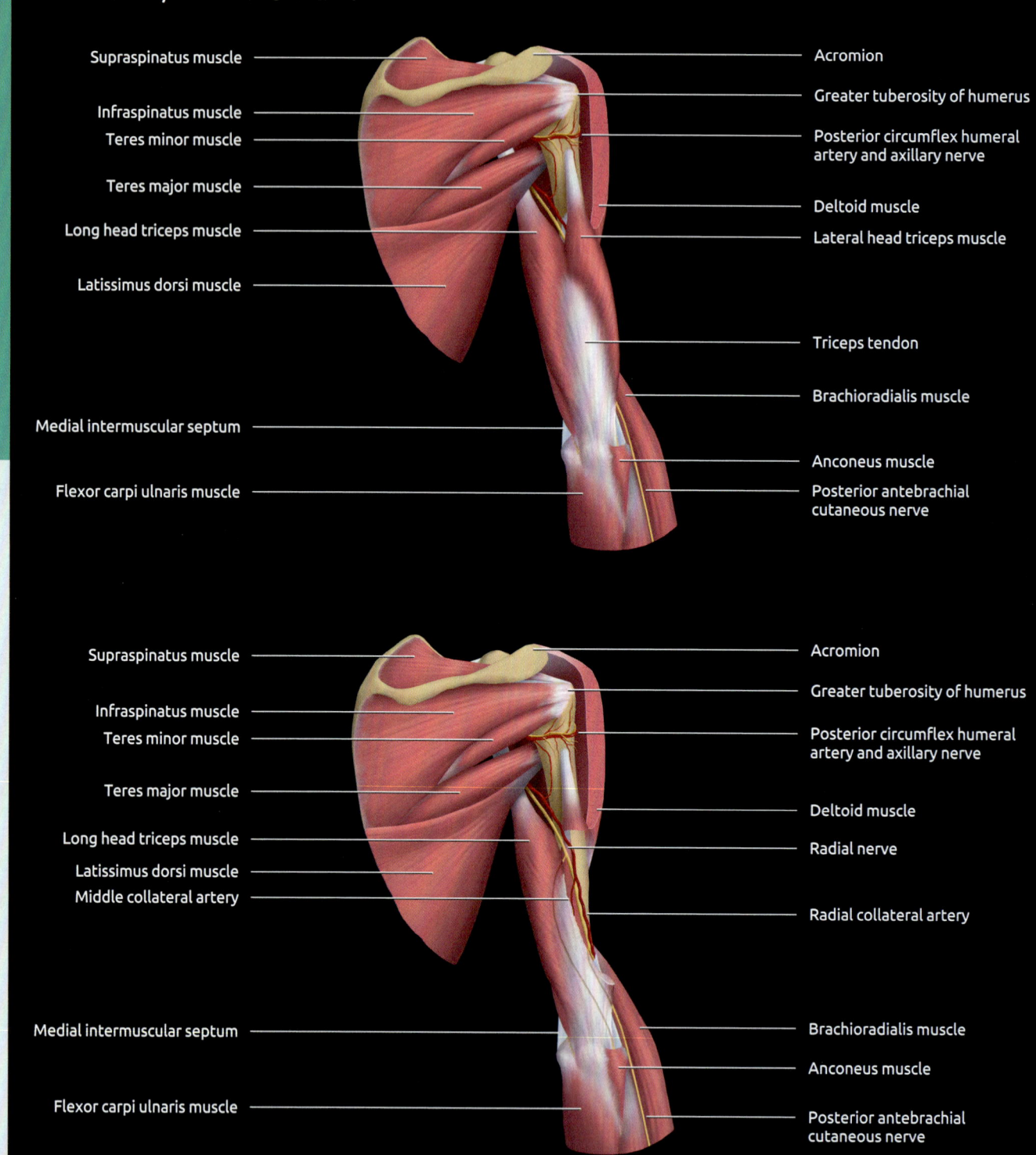

(Top) First of 2 posterior graphics of the right arm shows a superficial dissection. (Bottom) Posterior graphic of the arm shows a deep dissection.

Arm Radiographic Anatomy and MR Atlas

AXIAL GRAPHICS, ARM

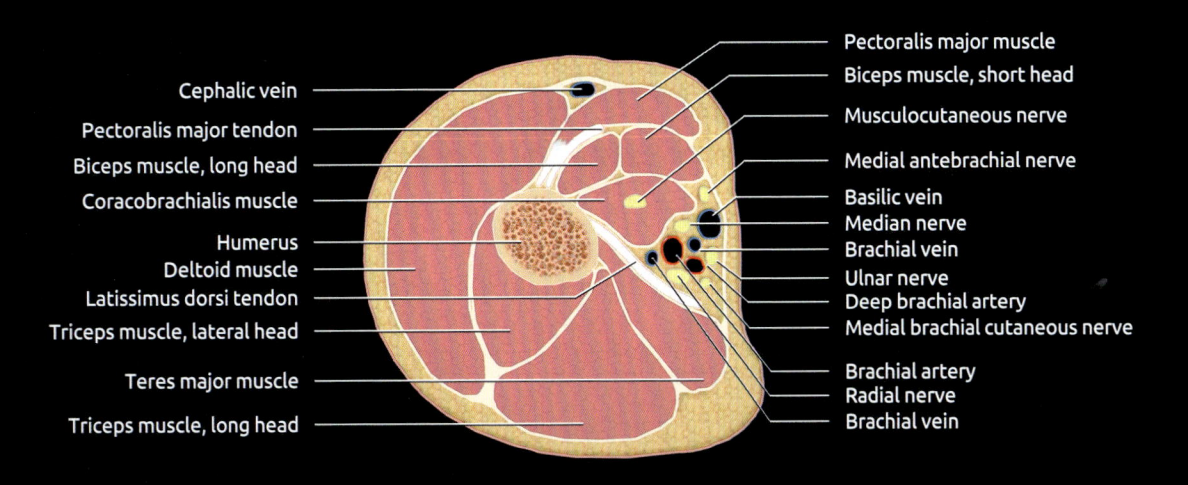

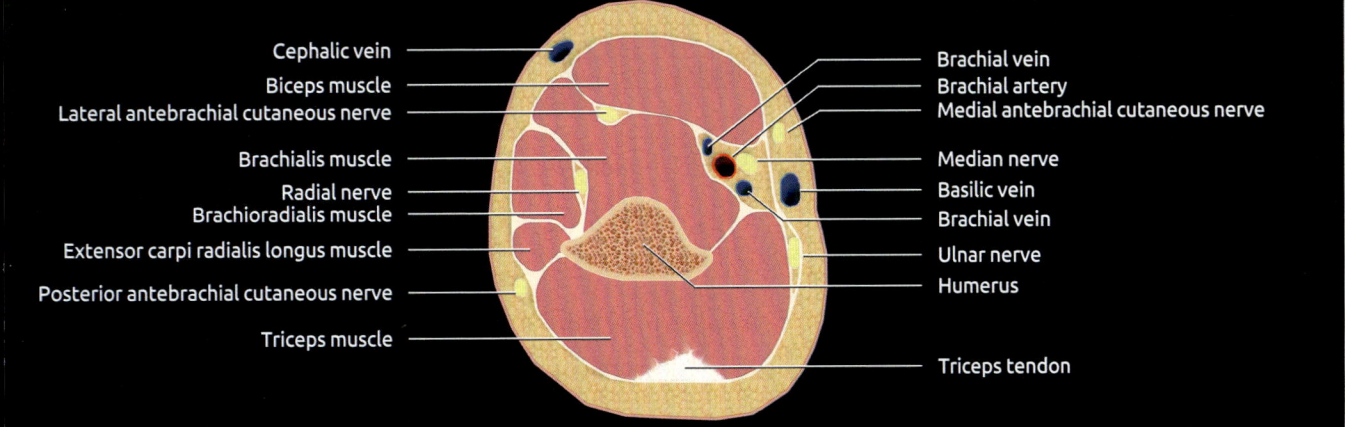

Top image labels:
- Cephalic vein
- Pectoralis major tendon
- Biceps muscle, long head
- Coracobrachialis muscle
- Humerus
- Deltoid muscle
- Latissimus dorsi tendon
- Triceps muscle, lateral head
- Teres major muscle
- Triceps muscle, long head
- Pectoralis major muscle
- Biceps muscle, short head
- Musculocutaneous nerve
- Medial antebrachial nerve
- Basilic vein
- Median nerve
- Brachial vein
- Ulnar nerve
- Deep brachial artery
- Medial brachial cutaneous nerve
- Brachial artery
- Radial nerve
- Brachial vein

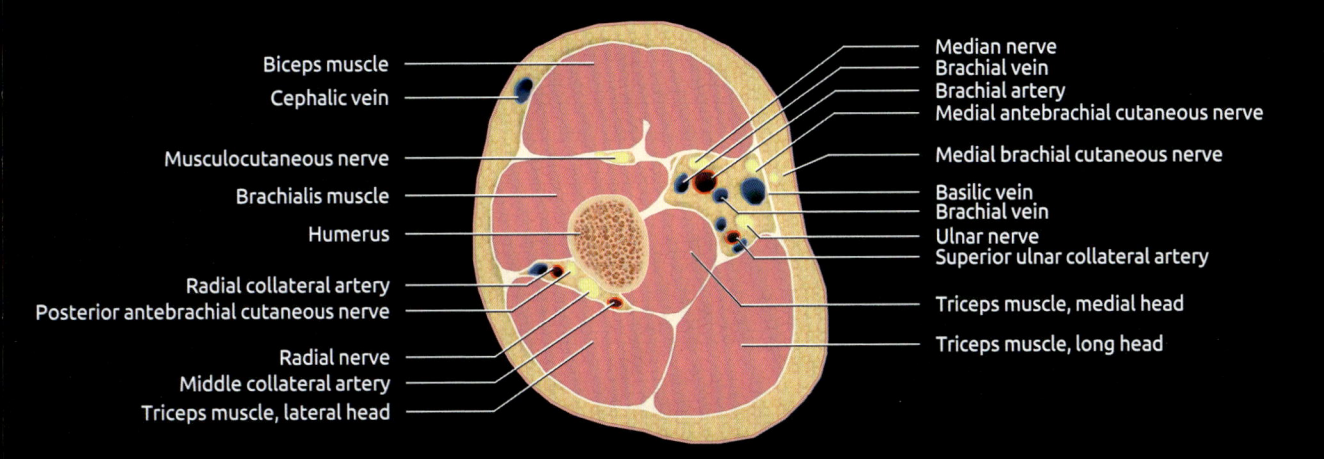

Middle image labels:
- Biceps muscle
- Cephalic vein
- Musculocutaneous nerve
- Brachialis muscle
- Humerus
- Radial collateral artery
- Posterior antebrachial cutaneous nerve
- Radial nerve
- Middle collateral artery
- Triceps muscle, lateral head
- Median nerve
- Brachial vein
- Brachial artery
- Medial antebrachial cutaneous nerve
- Medial brachial cutaneous nerve
- Basilic vein
- Brachial vein
- Ulnar nerve
- Superior ulnar collateral artery
- Triceps muscle, medial head
- Triceps muscle, long head

Bottom image labels:
- Cephalic vein
- Biceps muscle
- Lateral antebrachial cutaneous nerve
- Brachialis muscle
- Radial nerve
- Brachioradialis muscle
- Extensor carpi radialis longus muscle
- Posterior antebrachial cutaneous nerve
- Triceps muscle
- Brachial vein
- Brachial artery
- Medial antebrachial cutaneous nerve
- Median nerve
- Basilic vein
- Brachial vein
- Ulnar nerve
- Humerus
- Triceps tendon

(Top) Axial graphic shows the structures at the level of the upper humeral shaft. (Middle) Axial graphic of the right arm shows the mid humeral level. (Bottom) Axial graphic of the right arm shows the distal humeral level.

Arm Radiographic Anatomy and MR Atlas

AXIAL T1 MR, RIGHT ARM

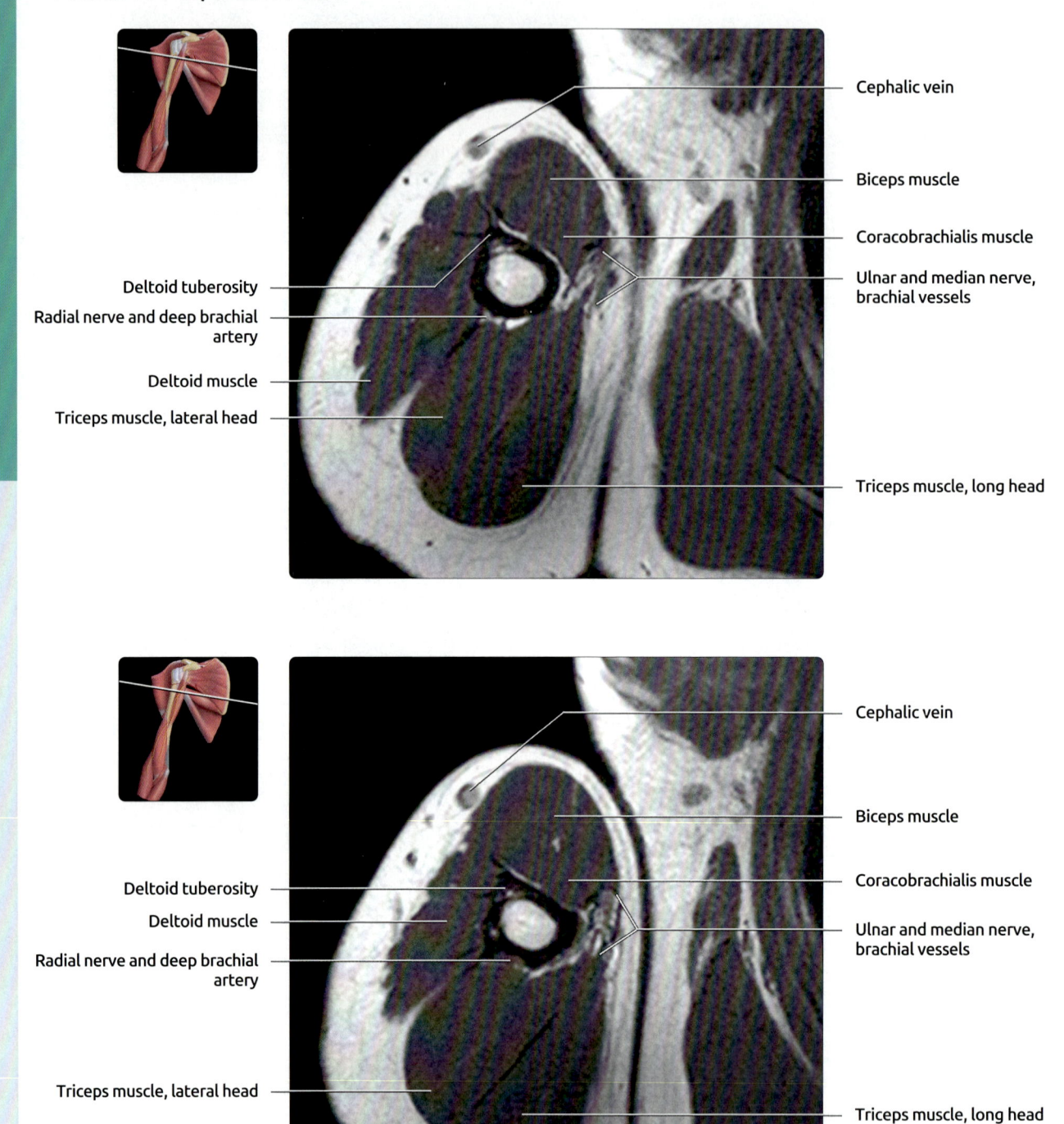

Top image labels:
- Cephalic vein
- Biceps muscle
- Coracobrachialis muscle
- Ulnar and median nerve, brachial vessels
- Deltoid tuberosity
- Radial nerve and deep brachial artery
- Deltoid muscle
- Triceps muscle, lateral head
- Triceps muscle, long head

Bottom image labels:
- Cephalic vein
- Biceps muscle
- Coracobrachialis muscle
- Ulnar and median nerve, brachial vessels
- Deltoid tuberosity
- Deltoid muscle
- Radial nerve and deep brachial artery
- Triceps muscle, lateral head
- Triceps muscle, long head

(Top) This is the first in a series of axial T1 MR images of the right arm, displayed proximal to distal. Images were acquired at 3T. This image is located just distal to the axilla. (Bottom) The deltoid muscle inserts on the deltoid tuberosity.

Arm Radiographic Anatomy and MR Atlas

AXIAL T1 MR, LEFT ARM

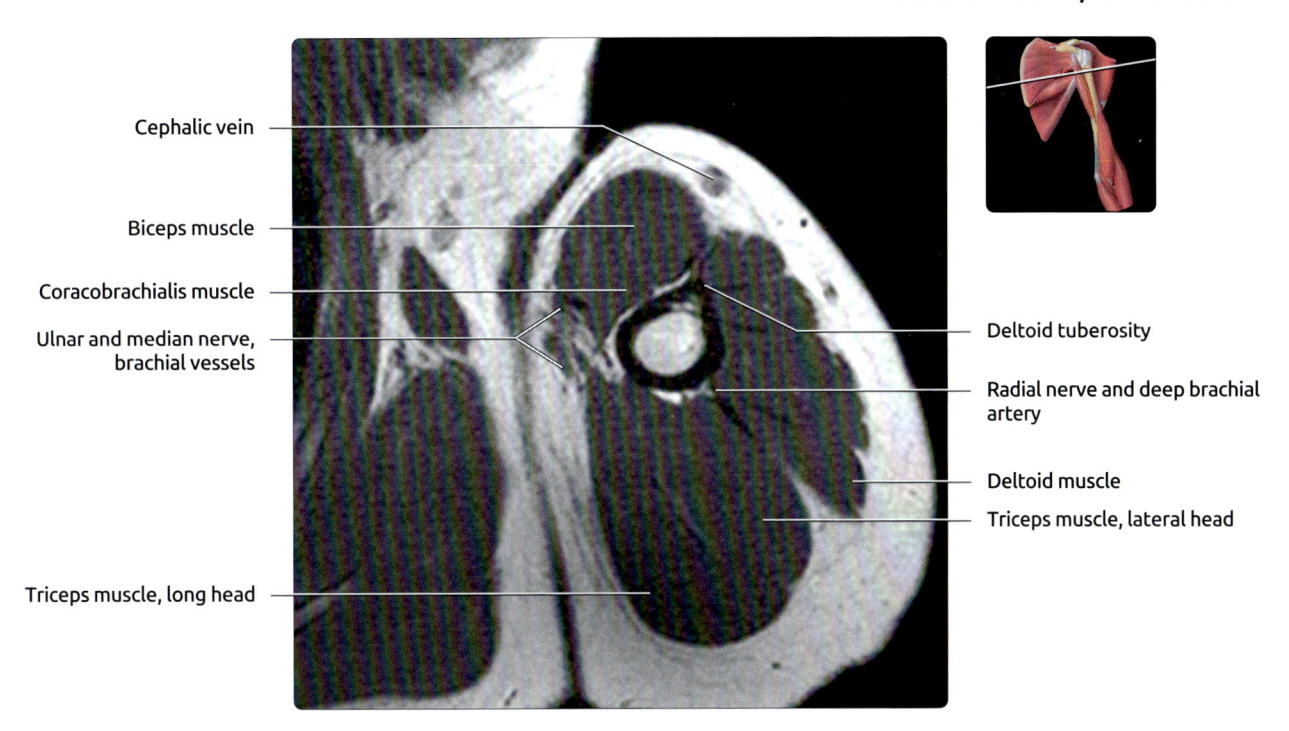

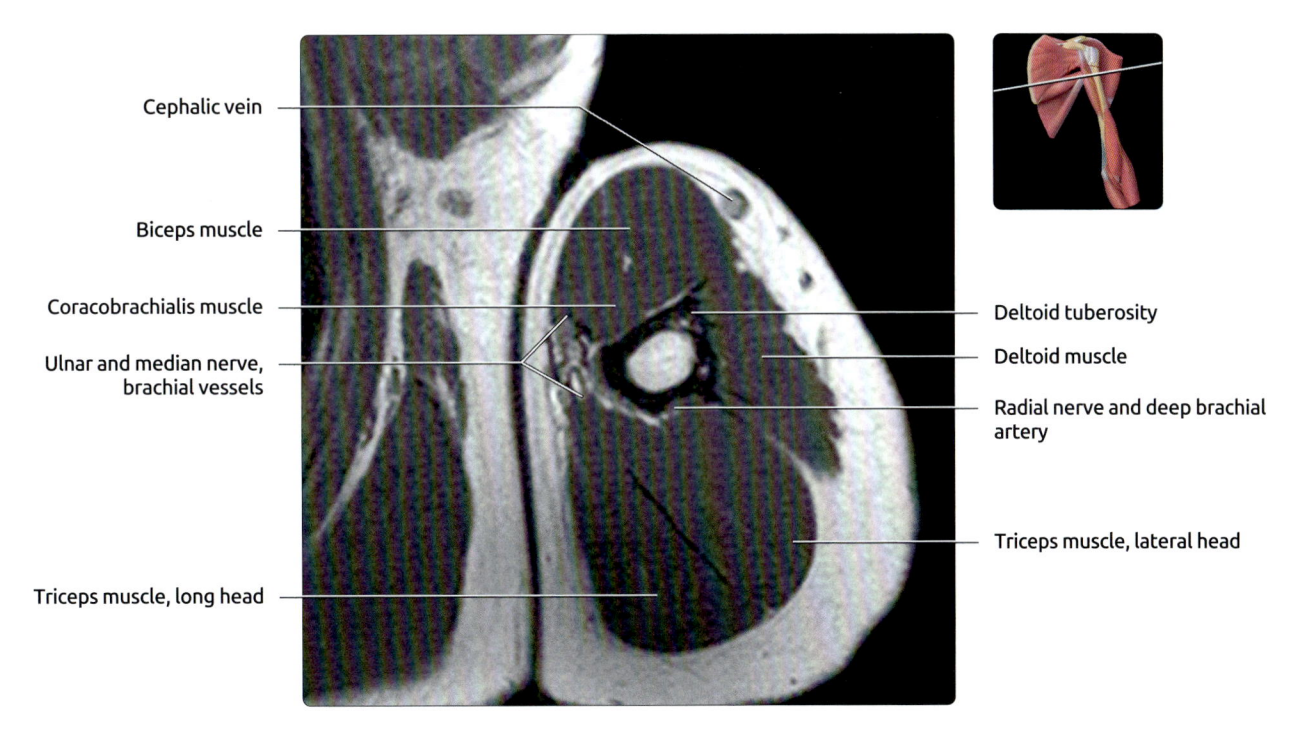

Top labels:
- Cephalic vein
- Biceps muscle
- Coracobrachialis muscle
- Ulnar and median nerve, brachial vessels
- Triceps muscle, long head
- Deltoid tuberosity
- Radial nerve and deep brachial artery
- Deltoid muscle
- Triceps muscle, lateral head

Bottom labels:
- Cephalic vein
- Biceps muscle
- Coracobrachialis muscle
- Ulnar and median nerve, brachial vessels
- Triceps muscle, long head
- Deltoid tuberosity
- Deltoid muscle
- Radial nerve and deep brachial artery
- Triceps muscle, lateral head

(**Top**) *First in a series of axial T1 MR images of the left arm displayed proximal to distal is shown. Images were acquired at 3T. This image is located just distal to the axilla.* (**Bottom**) *The deltoid muscle inserts on the deltoid tuberosity.*

Arm Radiographic Anatomy and MR Atlas

AXIAL T1 MR, RIGHT ARM

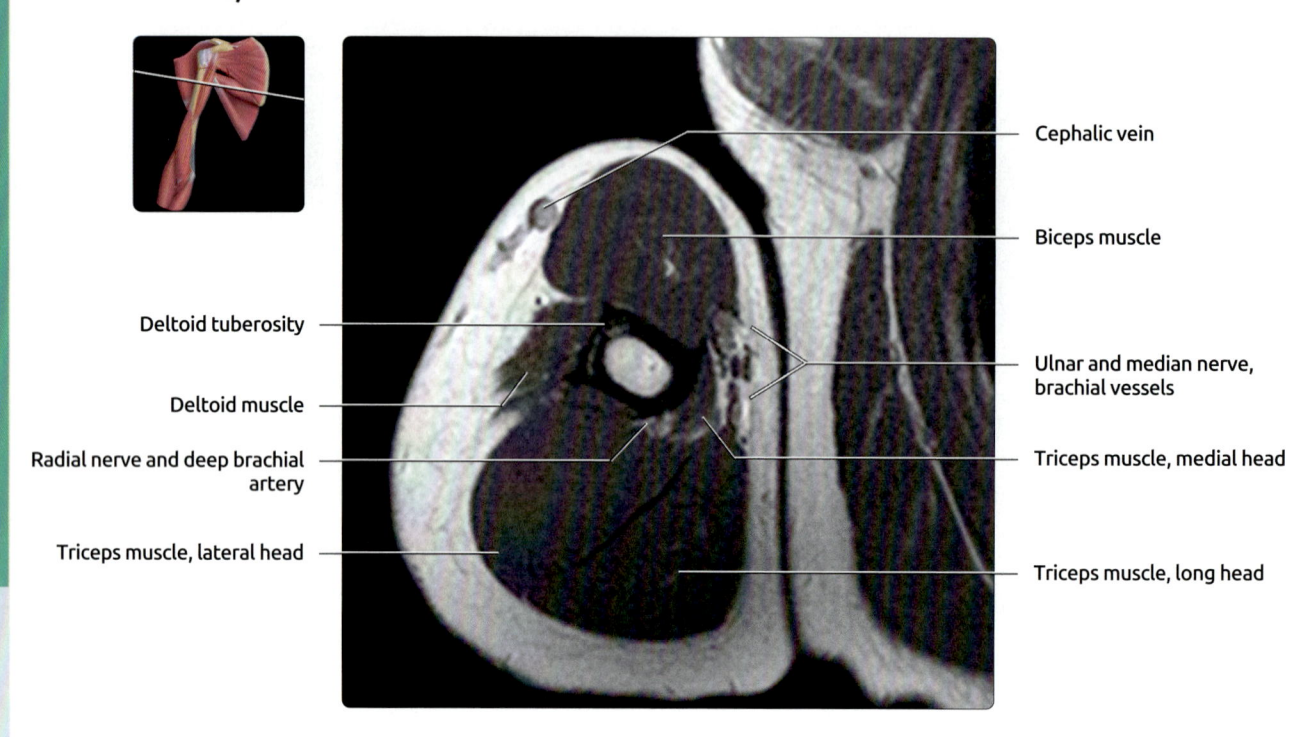

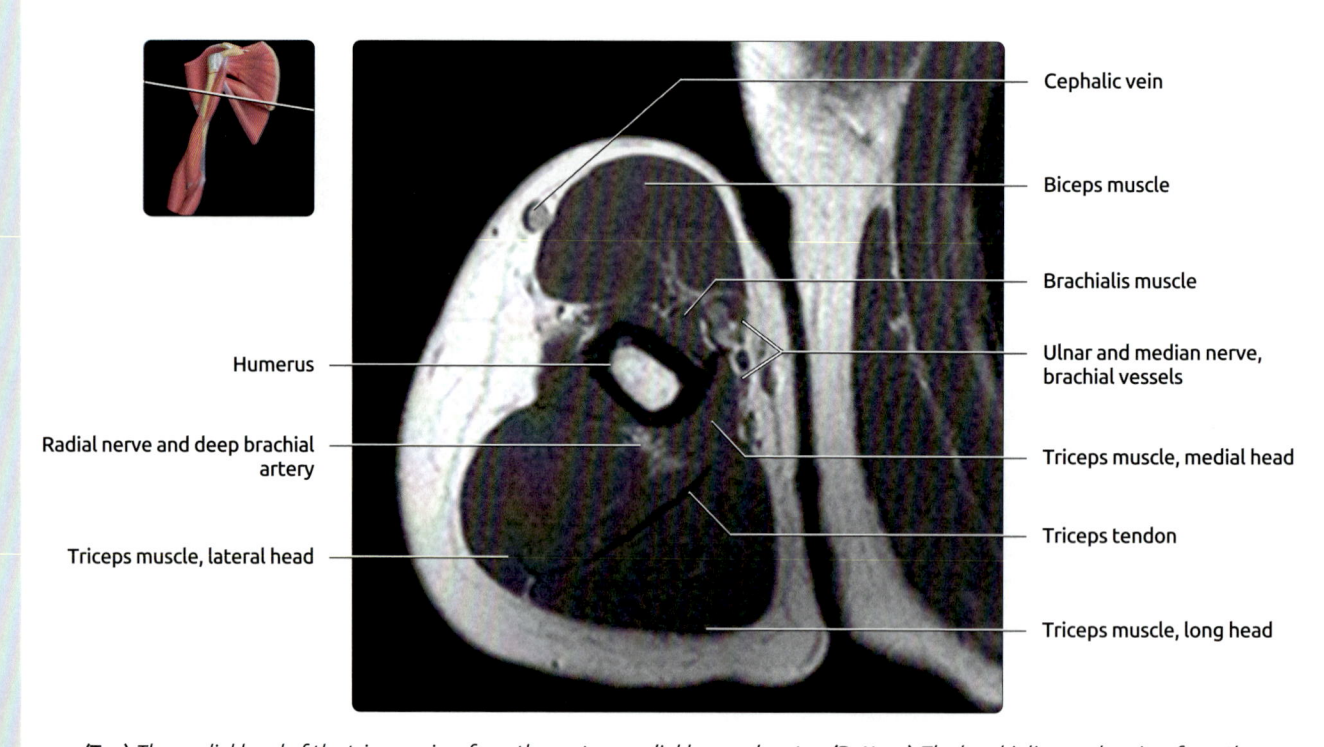

- Cephalic vein
- Biceps muscle
- Deltoid tuberosity
- Ulnar and median nerve, brachial vessels
- Deltoid muscle
- Radial nerve and deep brachial artery
- Triceps muscle, medial head
- Triceps muscle, lateral head
- Triceps muscle, long head

- Cephalic vein
- Biceps muscle
- Brachialis muscle
- Humerus
- Ulnar and median nerve, brachial vessels
- Radial nerve and deep brachial artery
- Triceps muscle, medial head
- Triceps tendon
- Triceps muscle, lateral head
- Triceps muscle, long head

(**Top**) *The medial head of the triceps arises from the posteromedial humeral cortex.* (**Bottom**) *The brachialis muscle arises from the anterior humeral cortex.*

Arm Radiographic Anatomy and MR Atlas

AXIAL T1 MR, LEFT ARM

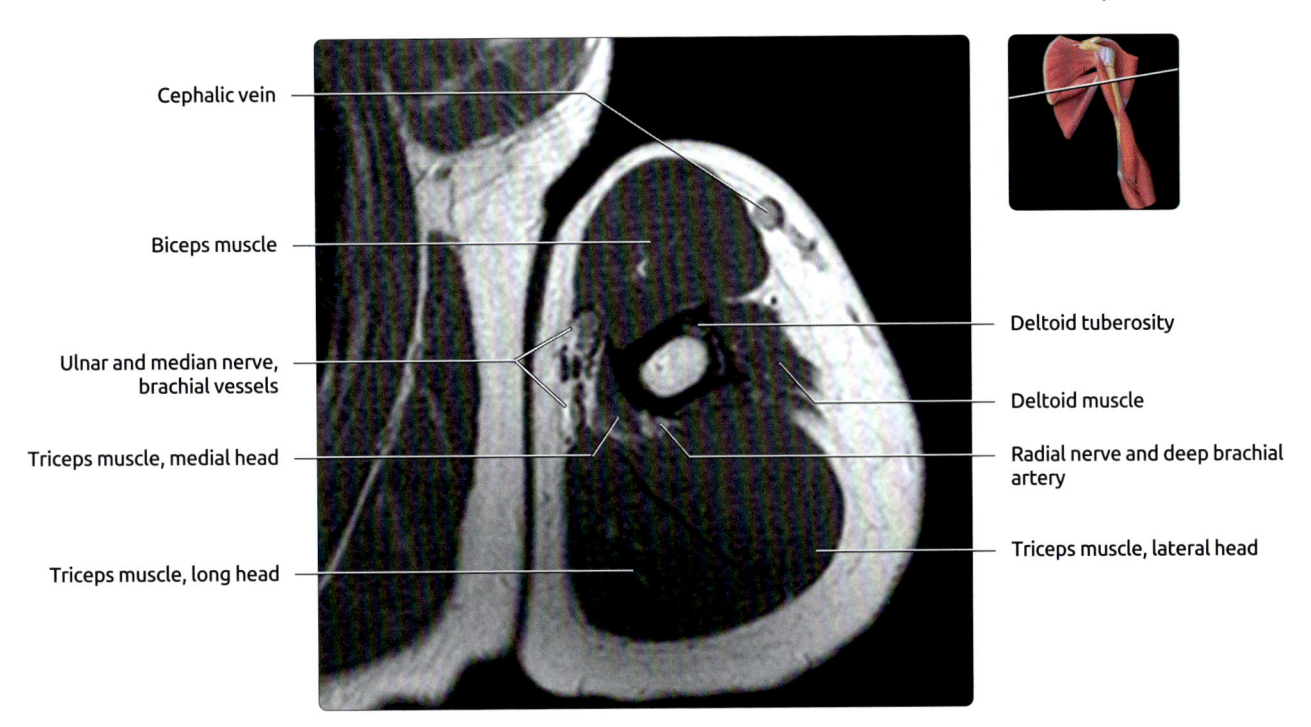

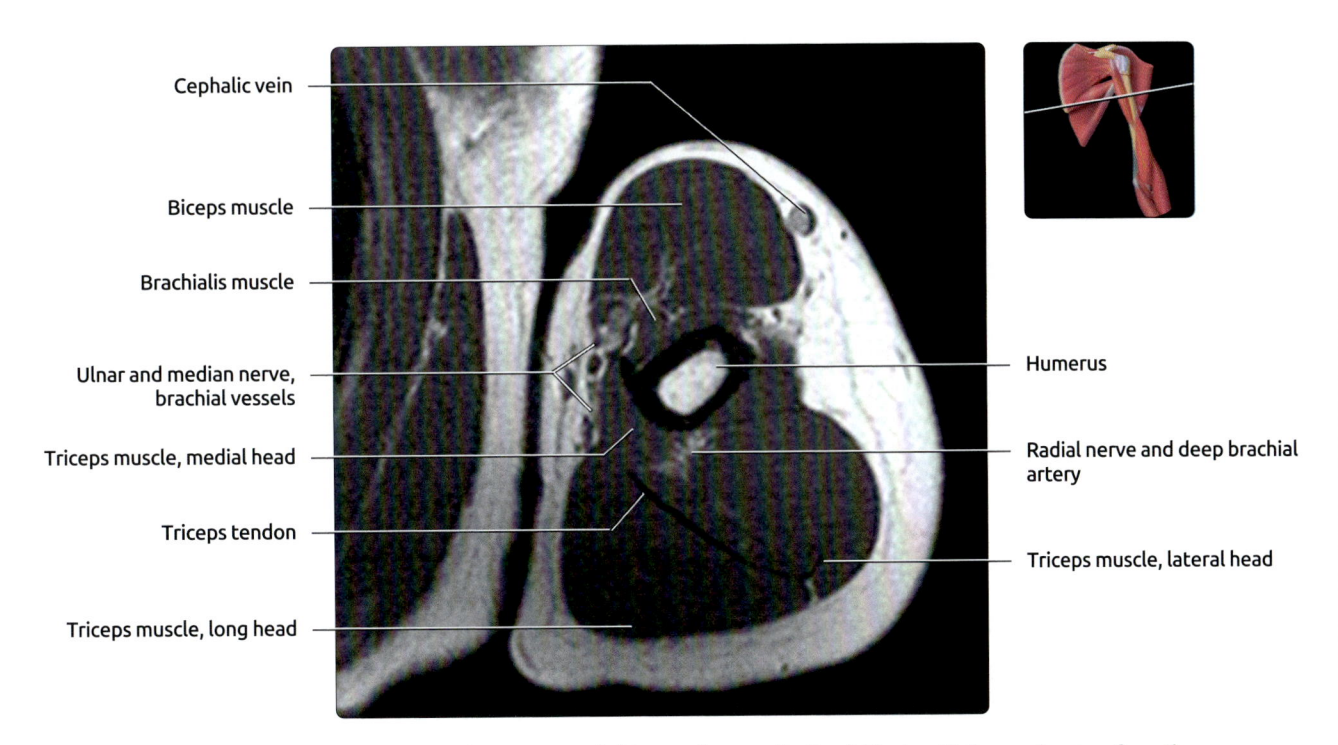

Top image labels:
- Cephalic vein
- Biceps muscle
- Ulnar and median nerve, brachial vessels
- Triceps muscle, medial head
- Triceps muscle, long head
- Deltoid tuberosity
- Deltoid muscle
- Radial nerve and deep brachial artery
- Triceps muscle, lateral head

Bottom image labels:
- Cephalic vein
- Biceps muscle
- Brachialis muscle
- Ulnar and median nerve, brachial vessels
- Triceps muscle, medial head
- Triceps tendon
- Triceps muscle, long head
- Humerus
- Radial nerve and deep brachial artery
- Triceps muscle, lateral head

(**Top**) The medial head of the triceps arises from the posteromedial humeral cortex. (**Bottom**) The brachialis muscle arises from the anterior humeral cortex.

Arm Radiographic Anatomy and MR Atlas

AXIAL T1 MR, RIGHT ARM

Labels (top image):
- Cephalic vein
- Biceps muscle
- Ulnar and median nerve, brachial vessels
- Triceps muscle, medial head
- Triceps tendon
- Triceps muscle, long head
- Brachialis muscle
- Radial nerve and deep brachial artery
- Triceps muscle, lateral head

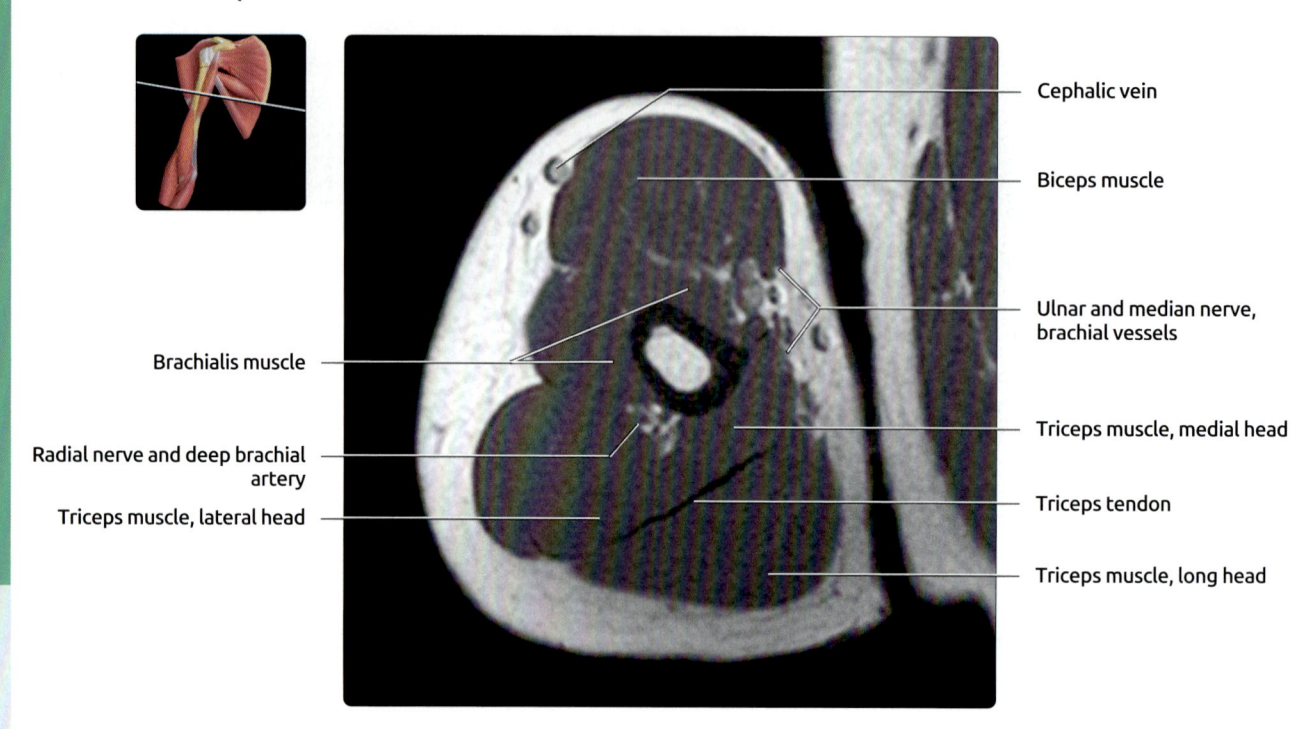

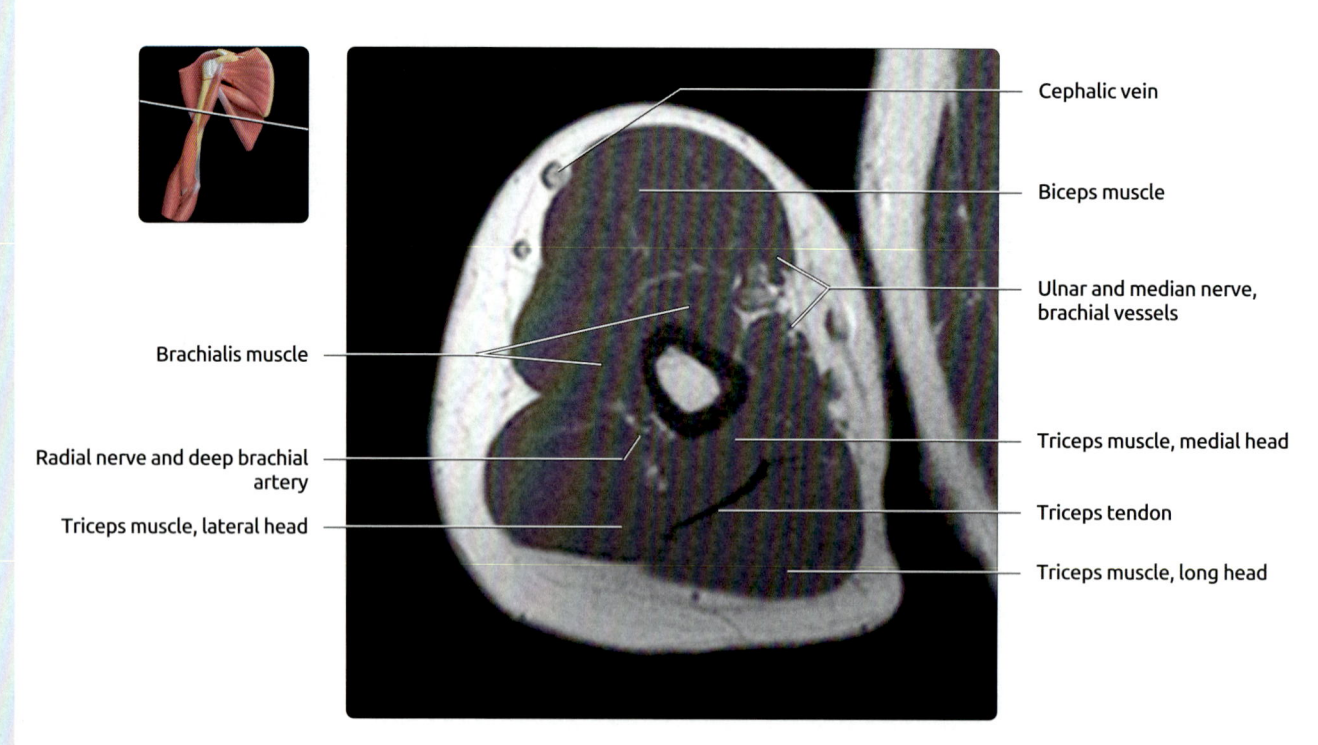

Labels (bottom image):
- Cephalic vein
- Biceps muscle
- Ulnar and median nerve, brachial vessels
- Triceps muscle, medial head
- Triceps tendon
- Triceps muscle, long head
- Brachialis muscle
- Radial nerve and deep brachial artery
- Triceps muscle, lateral head

(Top) The posterior compartment of the arm consists of the 3 heads of the triceps muscle. **(Bottom)** The deep brachial artery and radial nerve course along the posterolateral humerus.

Arm Radiographic Anatomy and MR Atlas

AXIAL T1 MR, LEFT ARM

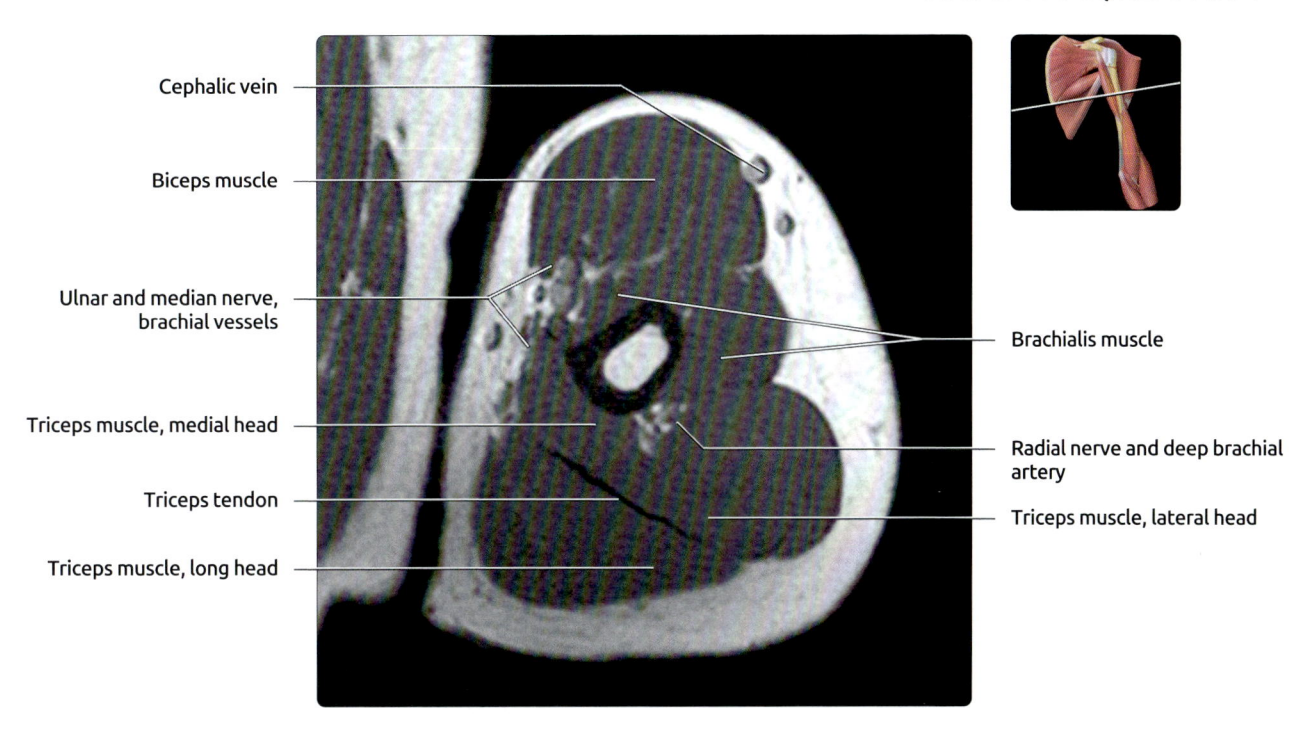

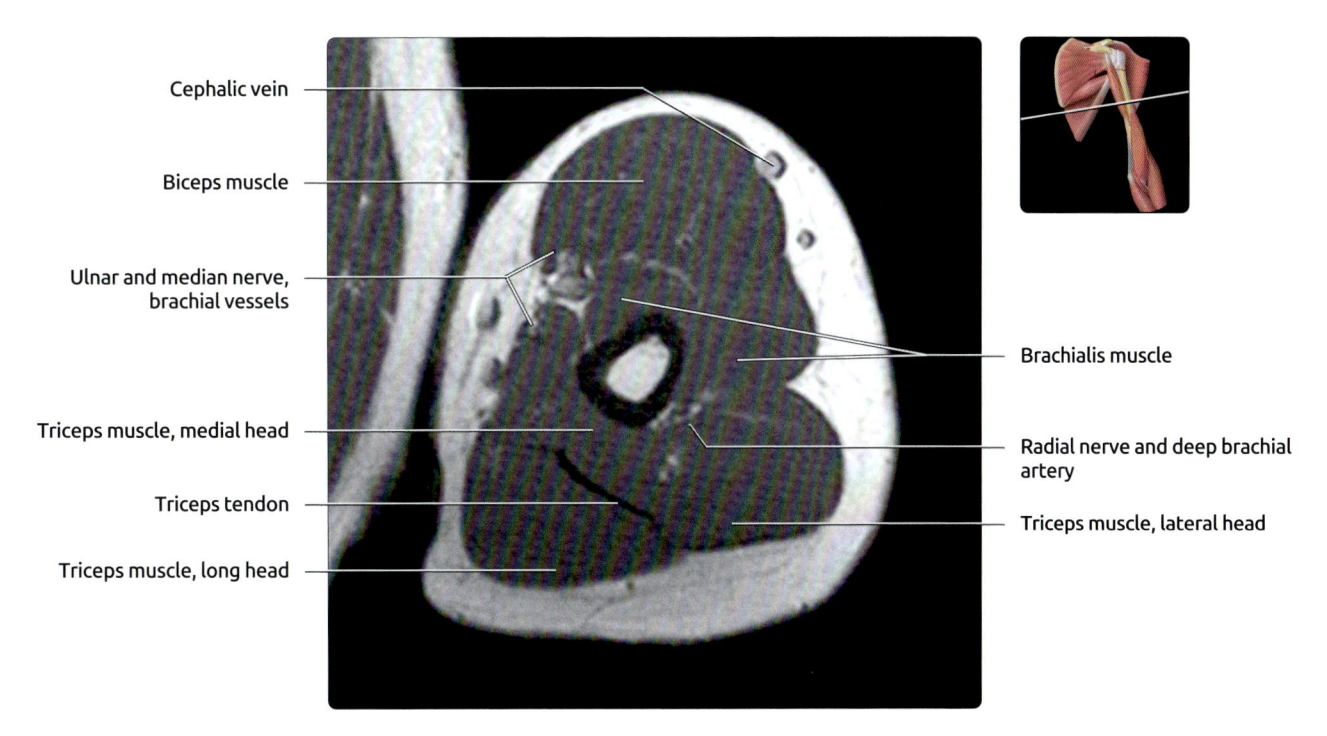

(Top) The posterior compartment of the arm consists of the 3 heads of the triceps muscle. *(Bottom)* The deep brachial artery and radial nerve course along the posterolateral humerus.

Arm Radiographic Anatomy and MR Atlas

AXIAL T1 MR, RIGHT ARM

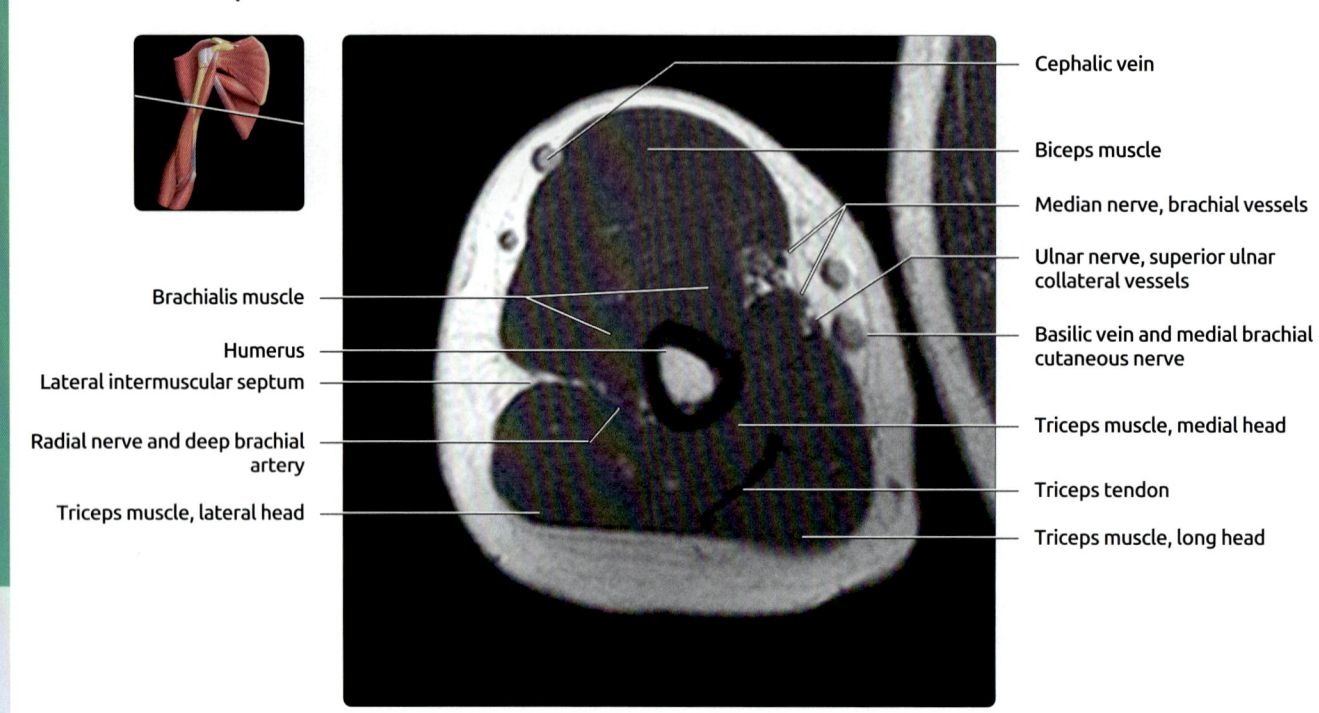

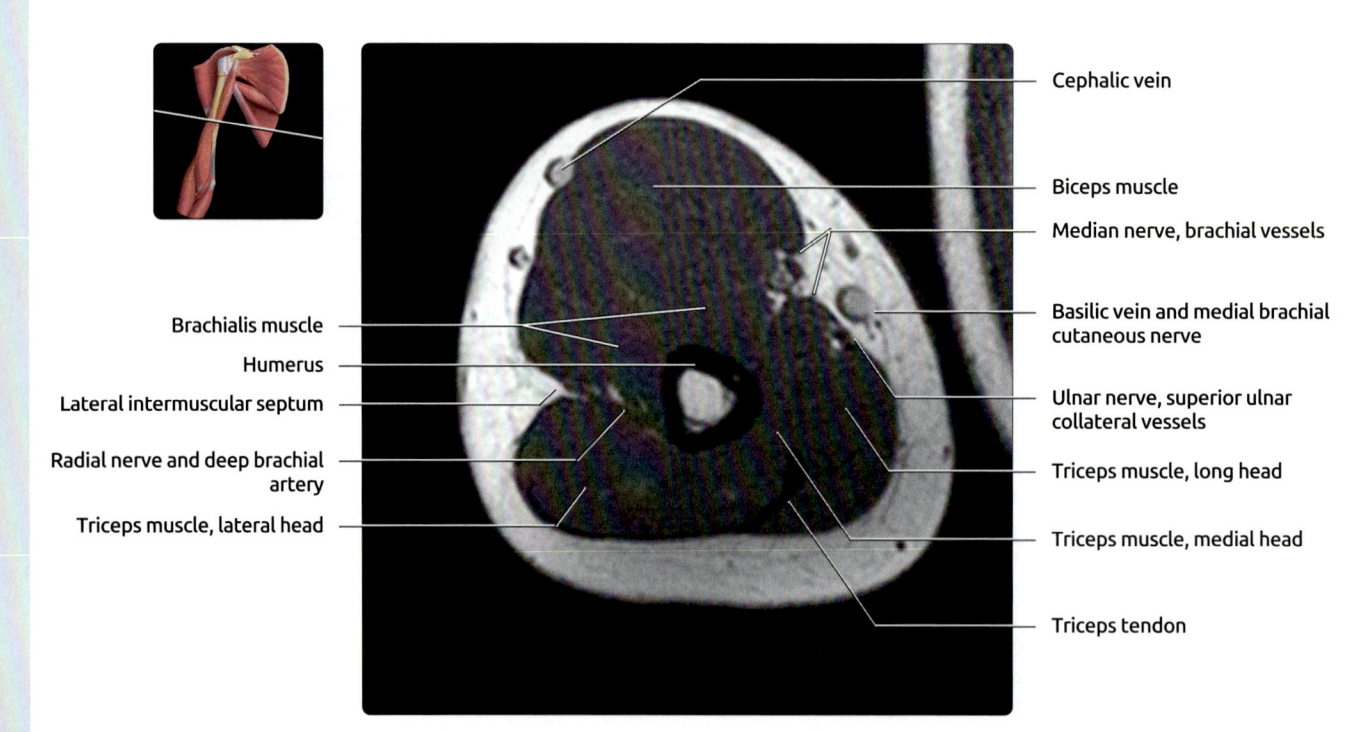

Labels (top image):
- Cephalic vein
- Biceps muscle
- Median nerve, brachial vessels
- Ulnar nerve, superior ulnar collateral vessels
- Basilic vein and medial brachial cutaneous nerve
- Triceps muscle, medial head
- Triceps tendon
- Triceps muscle, long head
- Brachialis muscle
- Humerus
- Lateral intermuscular septum
- Radial nerve and deep brachial artery
- Triceps muscle, lateral head

Labels (bottom image):
- Cephalic vein
- Biceps muscle
- Median nerve, brachial vessels
- Basilic vein and medial brachial cutaneous nerve
- Ulnar nerve, superior ulnar collateral vessels
- Triceps muscle, long head
- Triceps muscle, medial head
- Triceps tendon
- Brachialis muscle
- Humerus
- Lateral intermuscular septum
- Radial nerve and deep brachial artery
- Triceps muscle, lateral head

(Top) Branches of the radial nerve innervate the lateral, long, and medial heads of the triceps muscle. *(Bottom)* The neurovascular bundle containing the median nerve and brachial vessels denotes the location of the medial intermuscular septum.

Arm Radiographic Anatomy and MR Atlas

AXIAL T1 MR, LEFT ARM

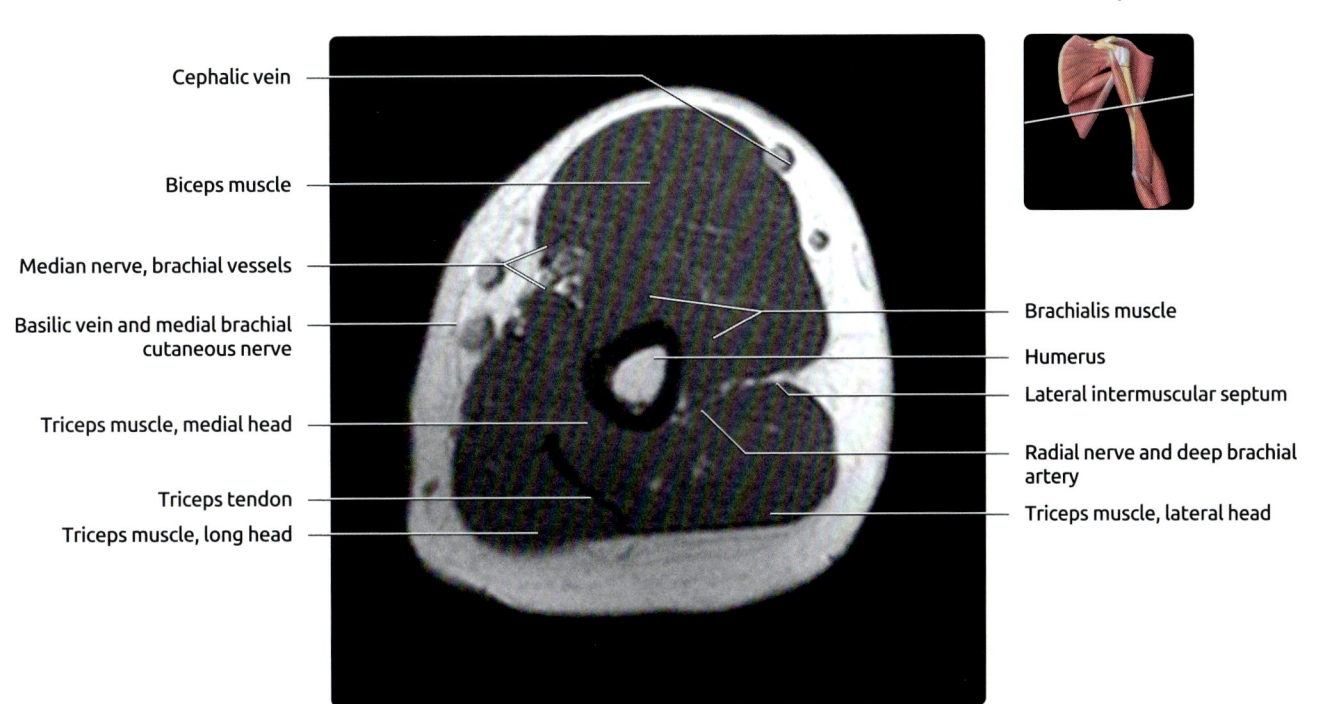

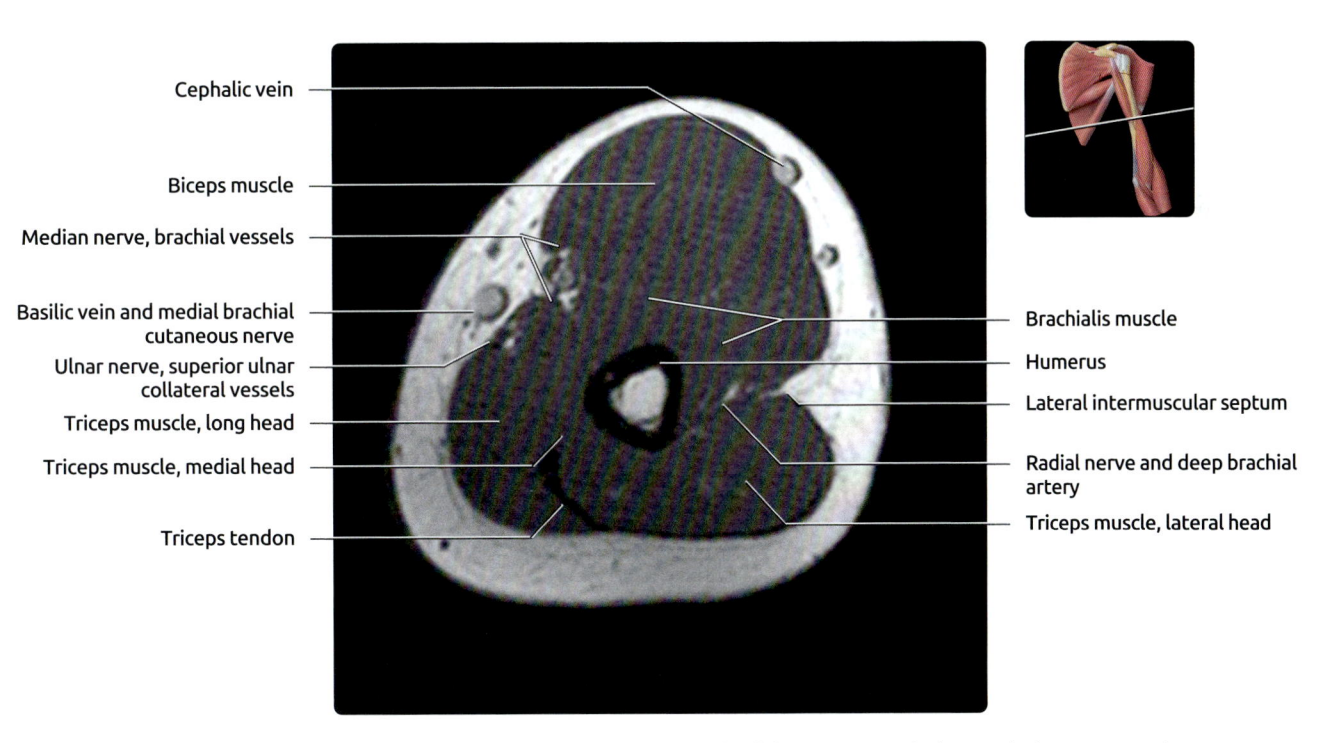

Top image labels:
- Cephalic vein
- Biceps muscle
- Median nerve, brachial vessels
- Basilic vein and medial brachial cutaneous nerve
- Triceps muscle, medial head
- Triceps tendon
- Triceps muscle, long head
- Brachialis muscle
- Humerus
- Lateral intermuscular septum
- Radial nerve and deep brachial artery
- Triceps muscle, lateral head

Bottom image labels:
- Cephalic vein
- Biceps muscle
- Median nerve, brachial vessels
- Basilic vein and medial brachial cutaneous nerve
- Ulnar nerve, superior ulnar collateral vessels
- Triceps muscle, long head
- Triceps muscle, medial head
- Triceps tendon
- Brachialis muscle
- Humerus
- Lateral intermuscular septum
- Radial nerve and deep brachial artery
- Triceps muscle, lateral head

(**Top**) *Branches of the radial nerve innervate the lateral, long, and medial heads of the triceps muscle.* (**Bottom**) *The neurovascular bundle containing the ulnar nerve, median nerve, and brachial vessels denotes the location of the medial intermuscular septum.*

Arm Radiographic Anatomy and MR Atlas

AXIAL T1 MR, RIGHT ARM

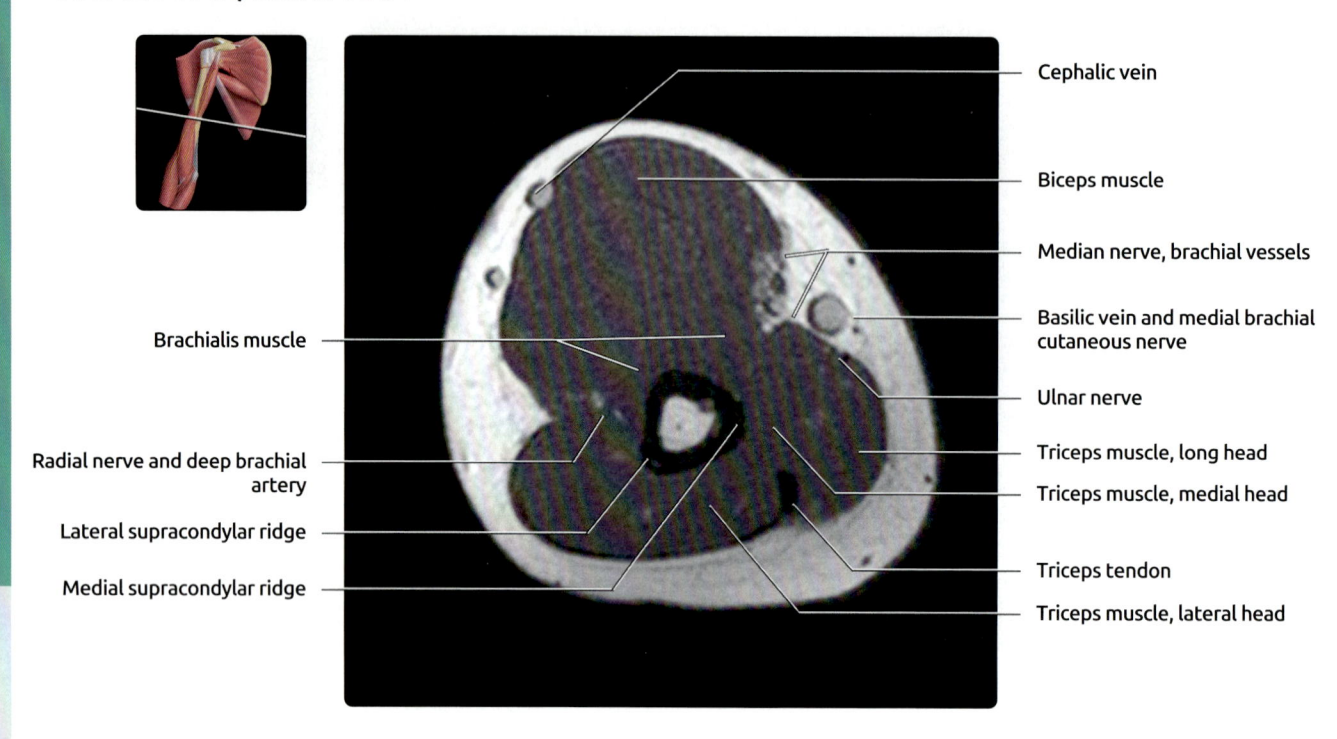

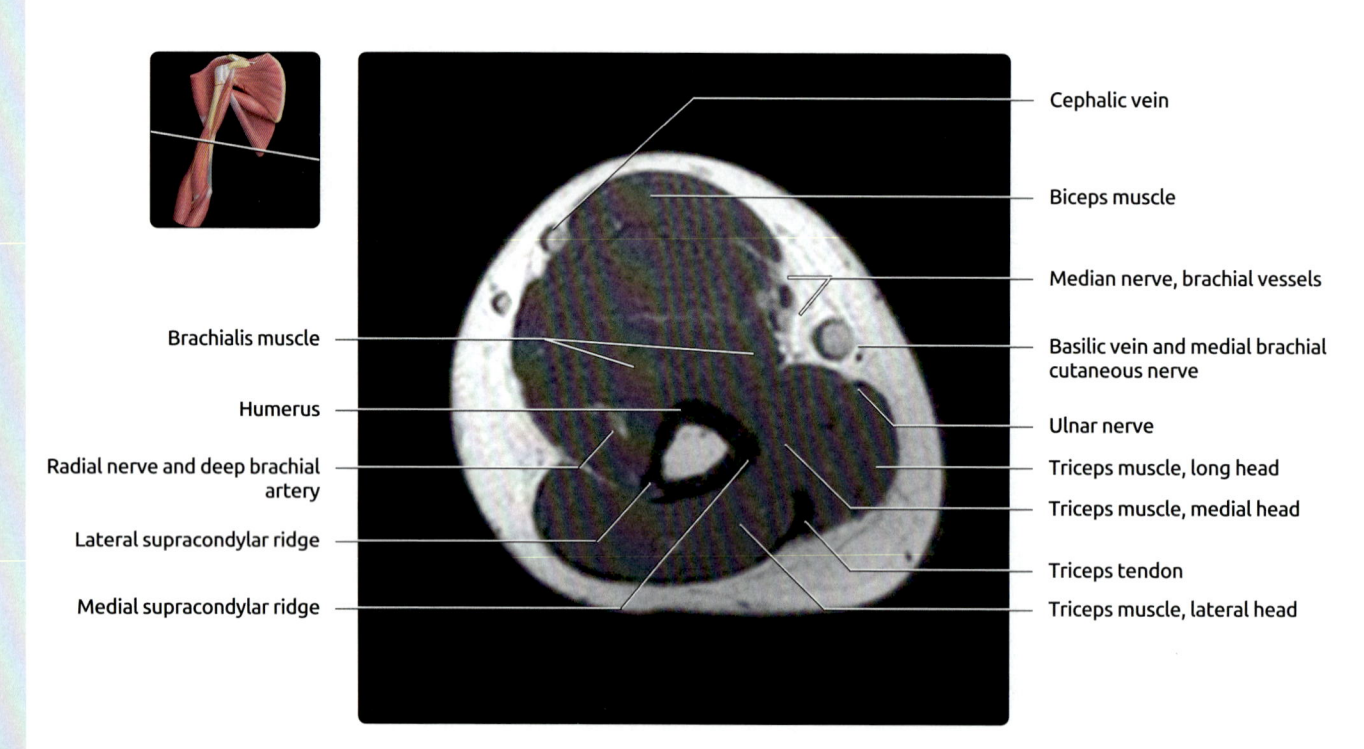

Top image labels:
- Cephalic vein
- Biceps muscle
- Median nerve, brachial vessels
- Basilic vein and medial brachial cutaneous nerve
- Ulnar nerve
- Triceps muscle, long head
- Triceps muscle, medial head
- Triceps tendon
- Triceps muscle, lateral head
- Brachialis muscle
- Radial nerve and deep brachial artery
- Lateral supracondylar ridge
- Medial supracondylar ridge

Bottom image labels:
- Cephalic vein
- Biceps muscle
- Median nerve, brachial vessels
- Basilic vein and medial brachial cutaneous nerve
- Ulnar nerve
- Triceps muscle, long head
- Triceps muscle, medial head
- Triceps tendon
- Triceps muscle, lateral head
- Brachialis muscle
- Humerus
- Radial nerve and deep brachial artery
- Lateral supracondylar ridge
- Medial supracondylar ridge

(Top) The thick triceps tendon lies between the triceps lateral and long heads. **(Bottom)** The biceps muscle is thinning anteriorly.

Arm Radiographic Anatomy and MR Atlas

AXIAL T1 MR, LEFT ARM

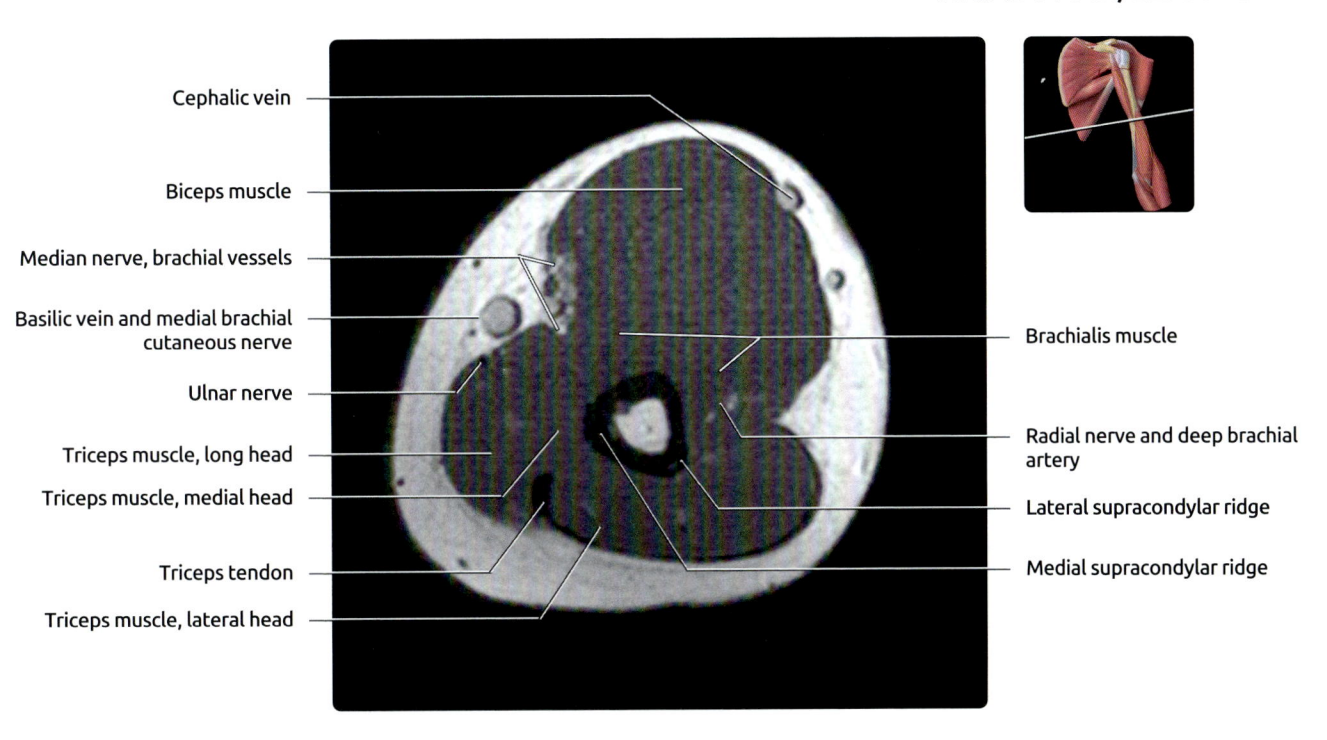

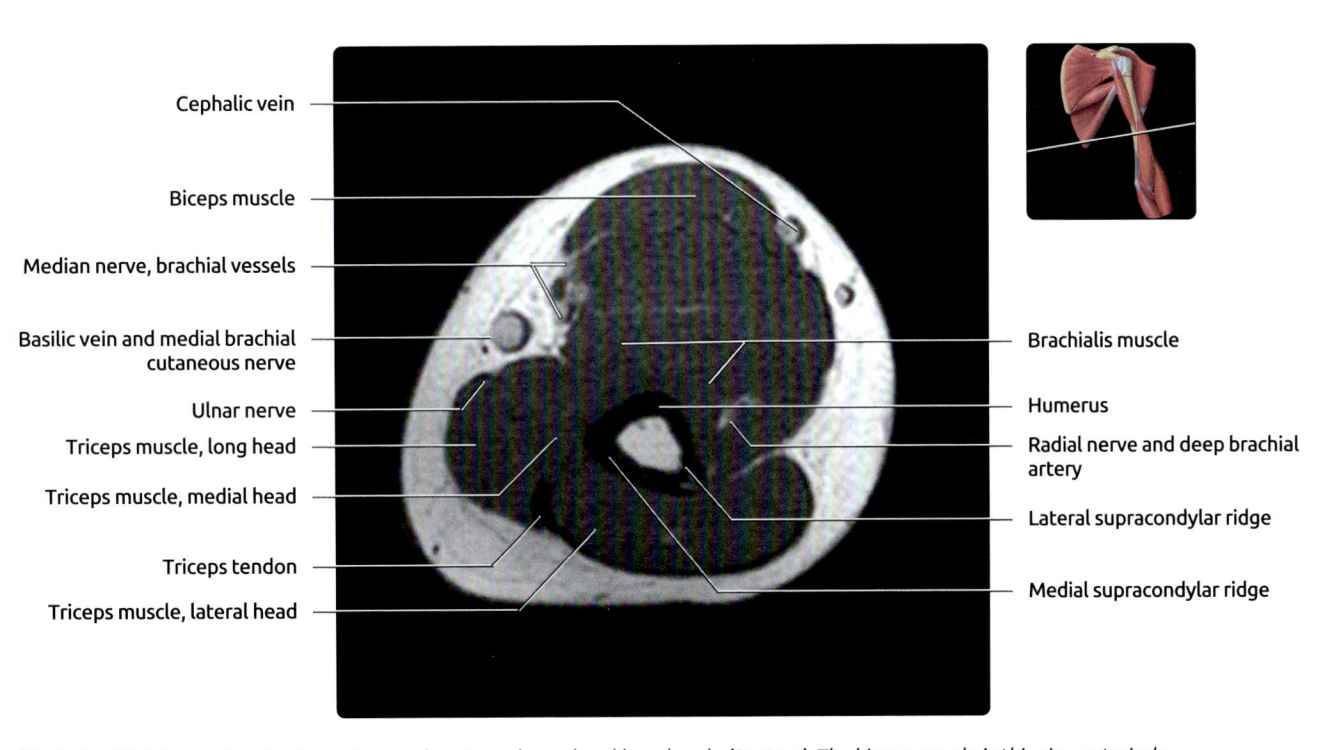

Top image labels:
- Cephalic vein
- Biceps muscle
- Median nerve, brachial vessels
- Basilic vein and medial brachial cutaneous nerve
- Ulnar nerve
- Triceps muscle, long head
- Triceps muscle, medial head
- Triceps tendon
- Triceps muscle, lateral head
- Brachialis muscle
- Radial nerve and deep brachial artery
- Lateral supracondylar ridge
- Medial supracondylar ridge

Bottom image labels:
- Cephalic vein
- Biceps muscle
- Median nerve, brachial vessels
- Basilic vein and medial brachial cutaneous nerve
- Ulnar nerve
- Triceps muscle, long head
- Triceps muscle, medial head
- Triceps tendon
- Triceps muscle, lateral head
- Brachialis muscle
- Humerus
- Radial nerve and deep brachial artery
- Lateral supracondylar ridge
- Medial supracondylar ridge

(Top) *The thick triceps tendon lies between the triceps lateral and long heads.* **(Bottom)** *The biceps muscle is thinning anteriorly.*

Arm Radiographic Anatomy and MR Atlas

AXIAL T1 MR, RIGHT ARM

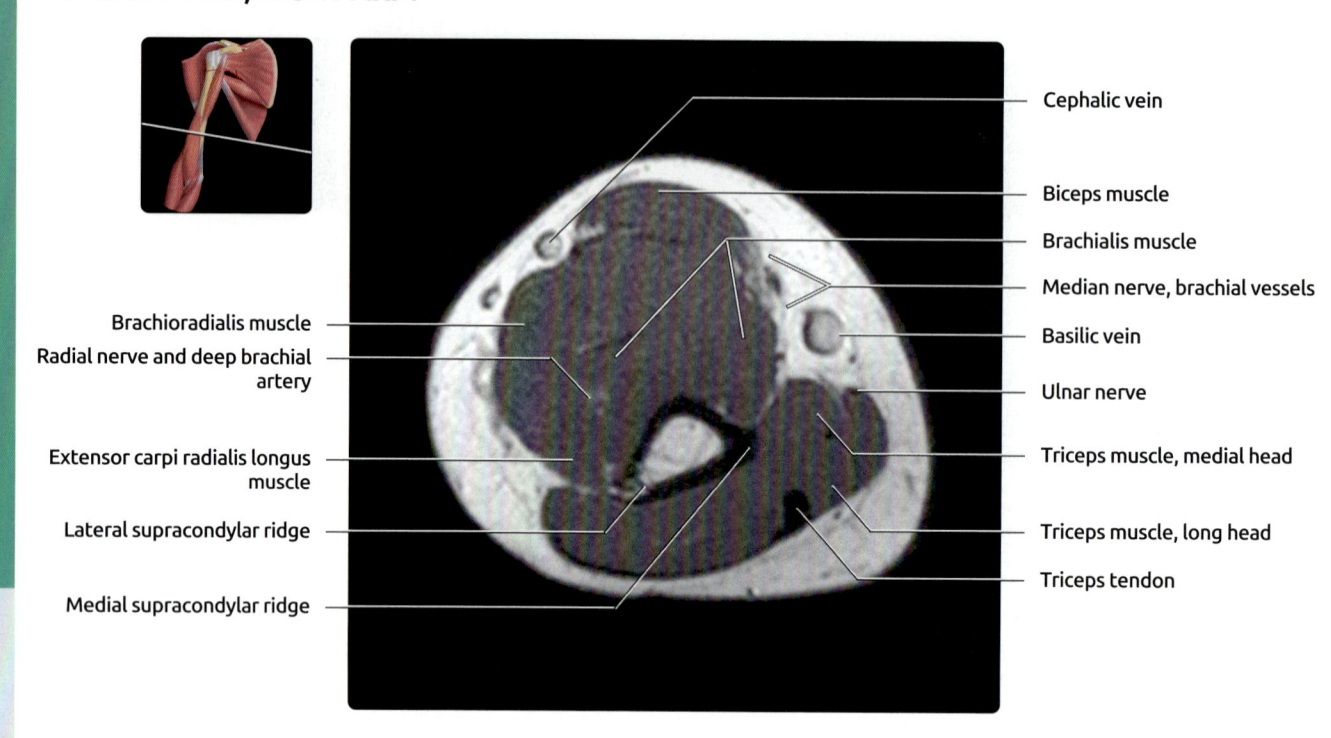

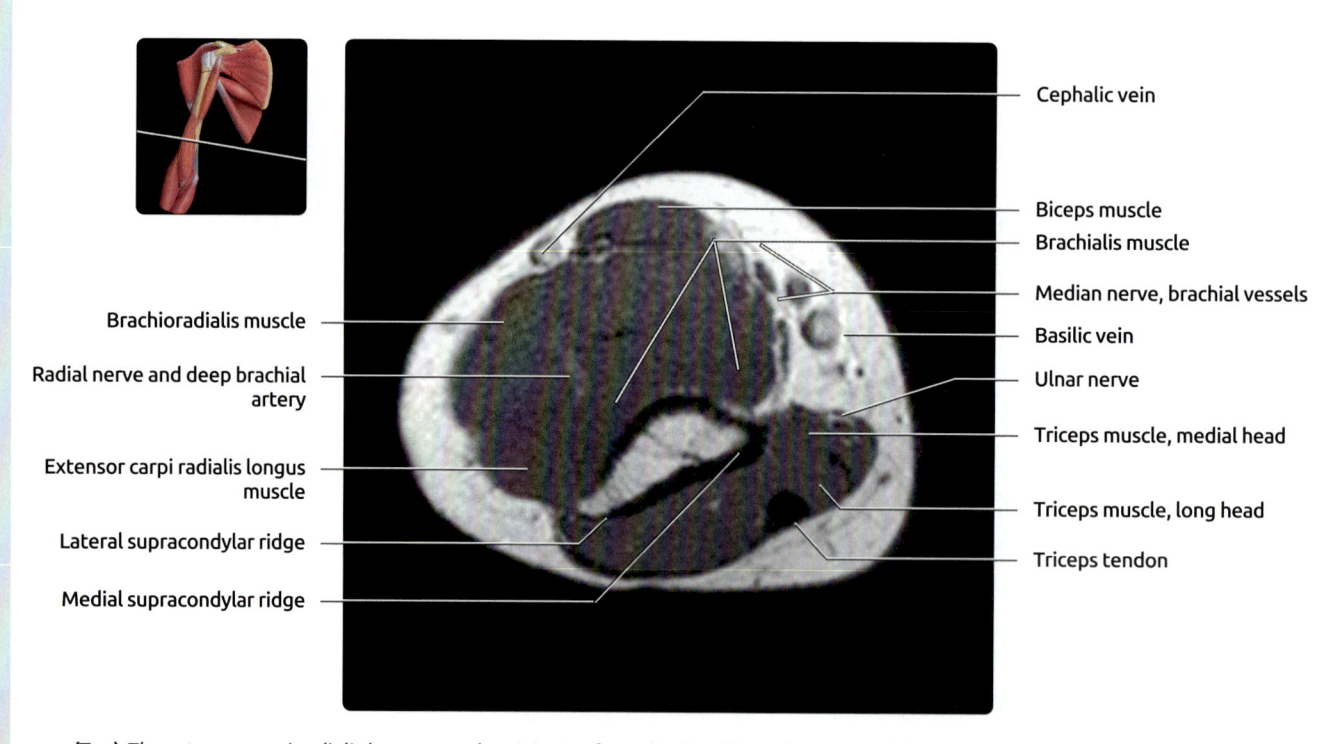

Labels (top image):
- Cephalic vein
- Biceps muscle
- Brachialis muscle
- Median nerve, brachial vessels
- Basilic vein
- Ulnar nerve
- Triceps muscle, medial head
- Triceps muscle, long head
- Triceps tendon
- Brachioradialis muscle
- Radial nerve and deep brachial artery
- Extensor carpi radialis longus muscle
- Lateral supracondylar ridge
- Medial supracondylar ridge

Labels (bottom image):
- Cephalic vein
- Biceps muscle
- Brachialis muscle
- Median nerve, brachial vessels
- Basilic vein
- Ulnar nerve
- Triceps muscle, medial head
- Triceps muscle, long head
- Triceps tendon
- Brachioradialis muscle
- Radial nerve and deep brachial artery
- Extensor carpi radialis longus muscle
- Lateral supracondylar ridge
- Medial supracondylar ridge

(Top) The extensor carpi radialis longus muscle originates from the distal lateral supracondylar ridge. **(Bottom)** The brachioradialis has become the largest muscle in the anterior compartment.

Arm Radiographic Anatomy and MR Atlas

AXIAL T1 MR, LEFT ARM

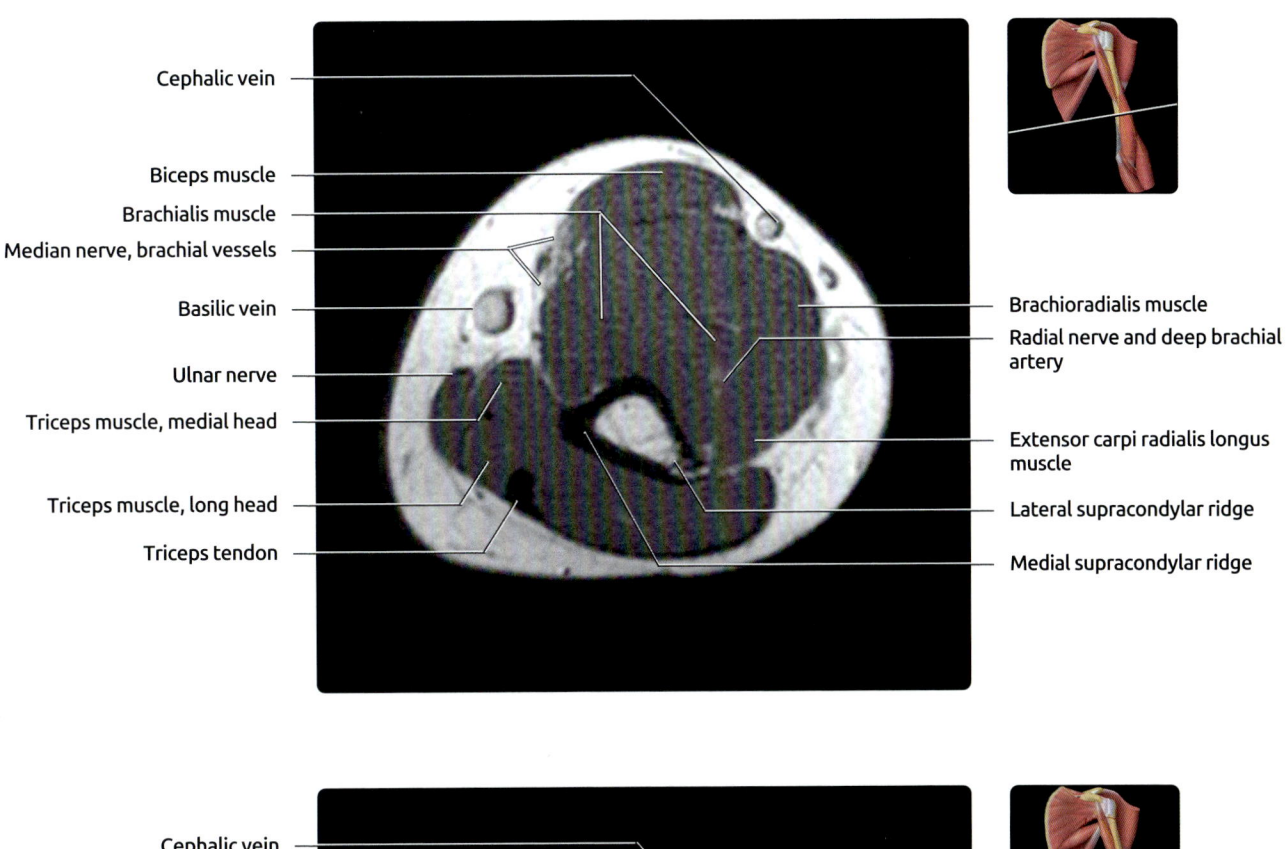

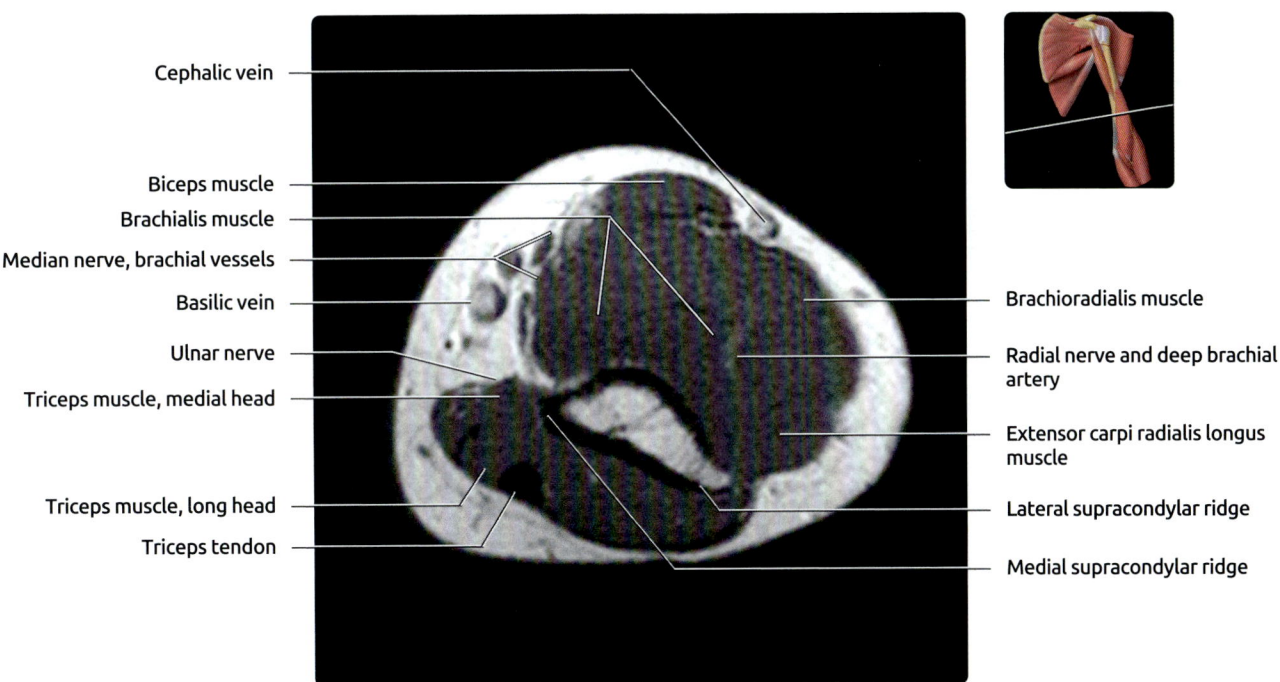

Cephalic vein

Biceps muscle
Brachialis muscle
Median nerve, brachial vessels

Basilic vein

Ulnar nerve
Triceps muscle, medial head

Triceps muscle, long head
Triceps tendon

Brachioradialis muscle
Radial nerve and deep brachial artery
Extensor carpi radialis longus muscle
Lateral supracondylar ridge
Medial supracondylar ridge

Cephalic vein

Biceps muscle
Brachialis muscle
Median nerve, brachial vessels
Basilic vein
Ulnar nerve
Triceps muscle, medial head

Triceps muscle, long head
Triceps tendon

Brachioradialis muscle
Radial nerve and deep brachial artery
Extensor carpi radialis longus muscle
Lateral supracondylar ridge
Medial supracondylar ridge

(Top) The extensor carpi radialis longus muscle originates from the distal lateral supracondylar ridge. *(Bottom)* The brachioradialis has become the largest muscle in the anterior compartment.

Arm Radiographic Anatomy and MR Atlas

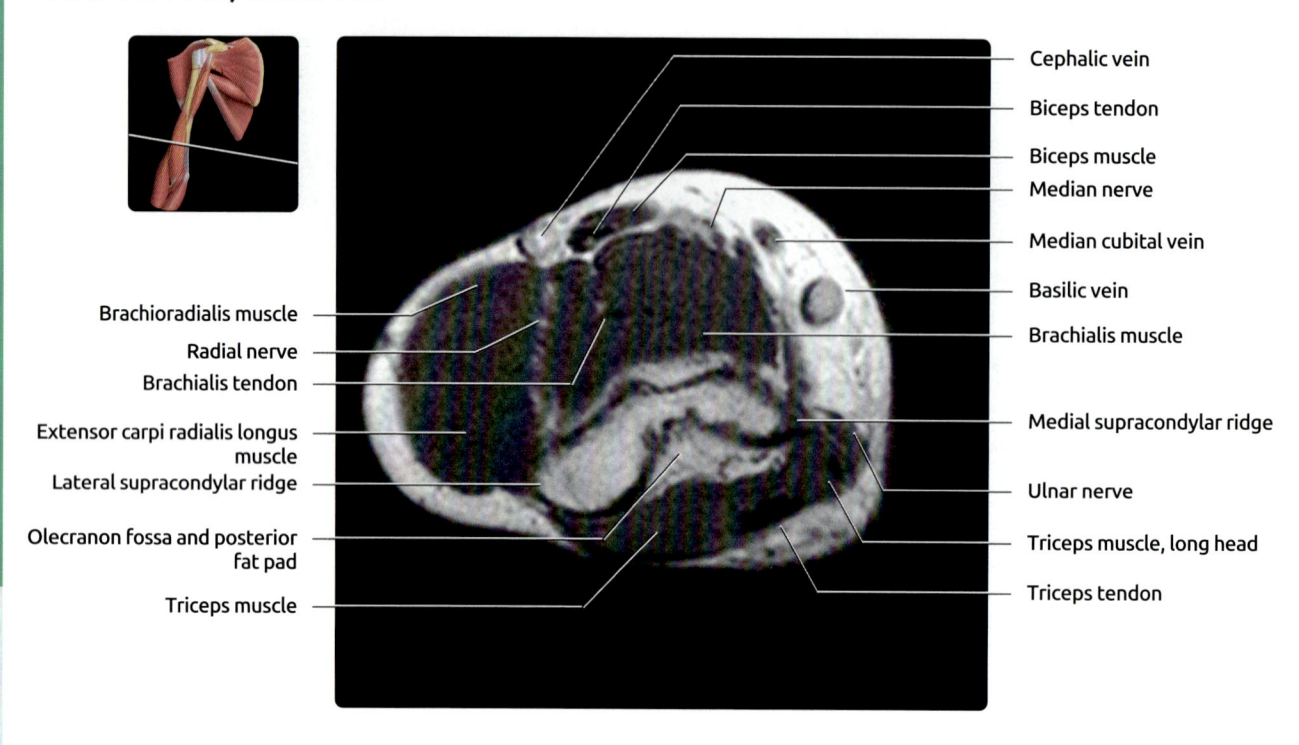

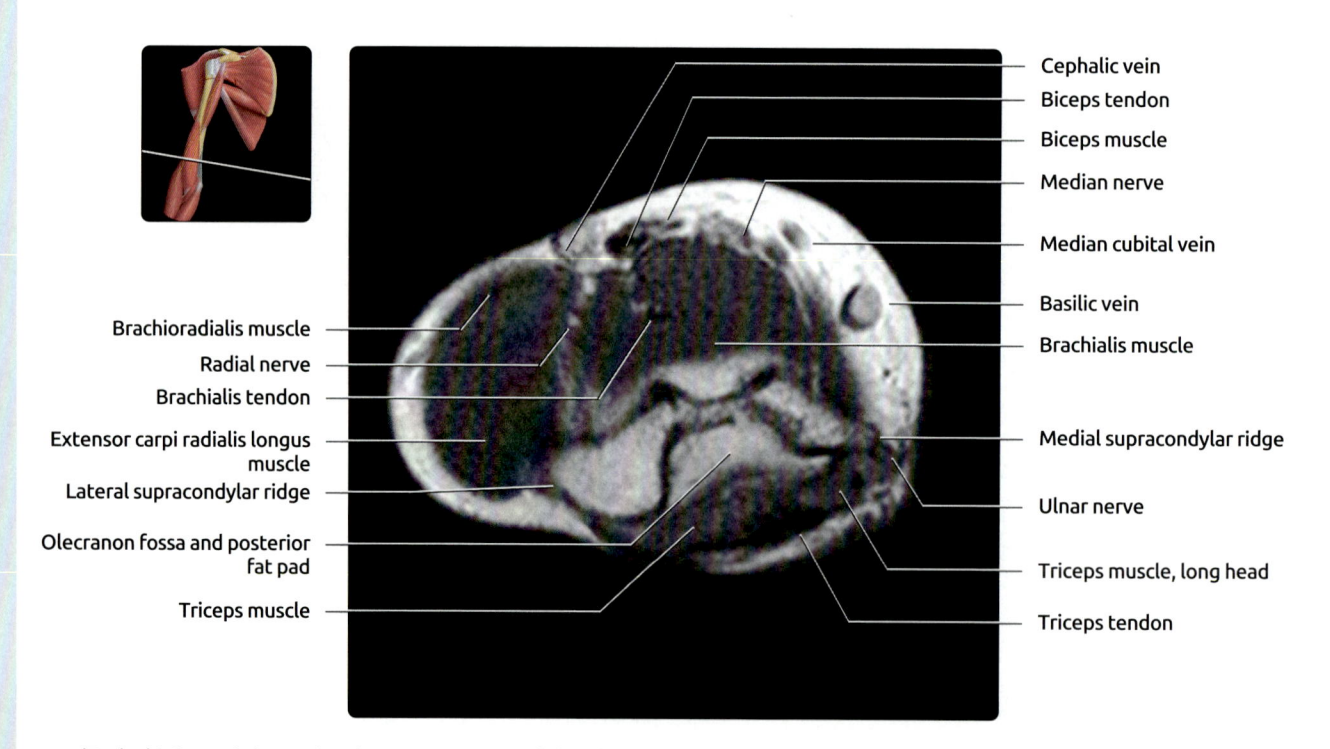

AXIAL T1 MR, RIGHT ARM

Top image labels:
- Cephalic vein
- Biceps tendon
- Biceps muscle
- Median nerve
- Median cubital vein
- Basilic vein
- Brachialis muscle
- Medial supracondylar ridge
- Ulnar nerve
- Triceps muscle, long head
- Triceps tendon
- Brachioradialis muscle
- Radial nerve
- Brachialis tendon
- Extensor carpi radialis longus muscle
- Lateral supracondylar ridge
- Olecranon fossa and posterior fat pad
- Triceps muscle

Bottom image labels:
- Cephalic vein
- Biceps tendon
- Biceps muscle
- Median nerve
- Median cubital vein
- Basilic vein
- Brachialis muscle
- Medial supracondylar ridge
- Ulnar nerve
- Triceps muscle, long head
- Triceps tendon
- Brachioradialis muscle
- Radial nerve
- Brachialis tendon
- Extensor carpi radialis longus muscle
- Lateral supracondylar ridge
- Olecranon fossa and posterior fat pad
- Triceps muscle

(Top) *This image is located at the superior aspect of the elbow. The olecranon fossa contains the posterior fat pad.* **(Bottom)** *The biceps is now almost entirely tendinous.*

Arm Radiographic Anatomy and MR Atlas

AXIAL T1 MR, LEFT ARM

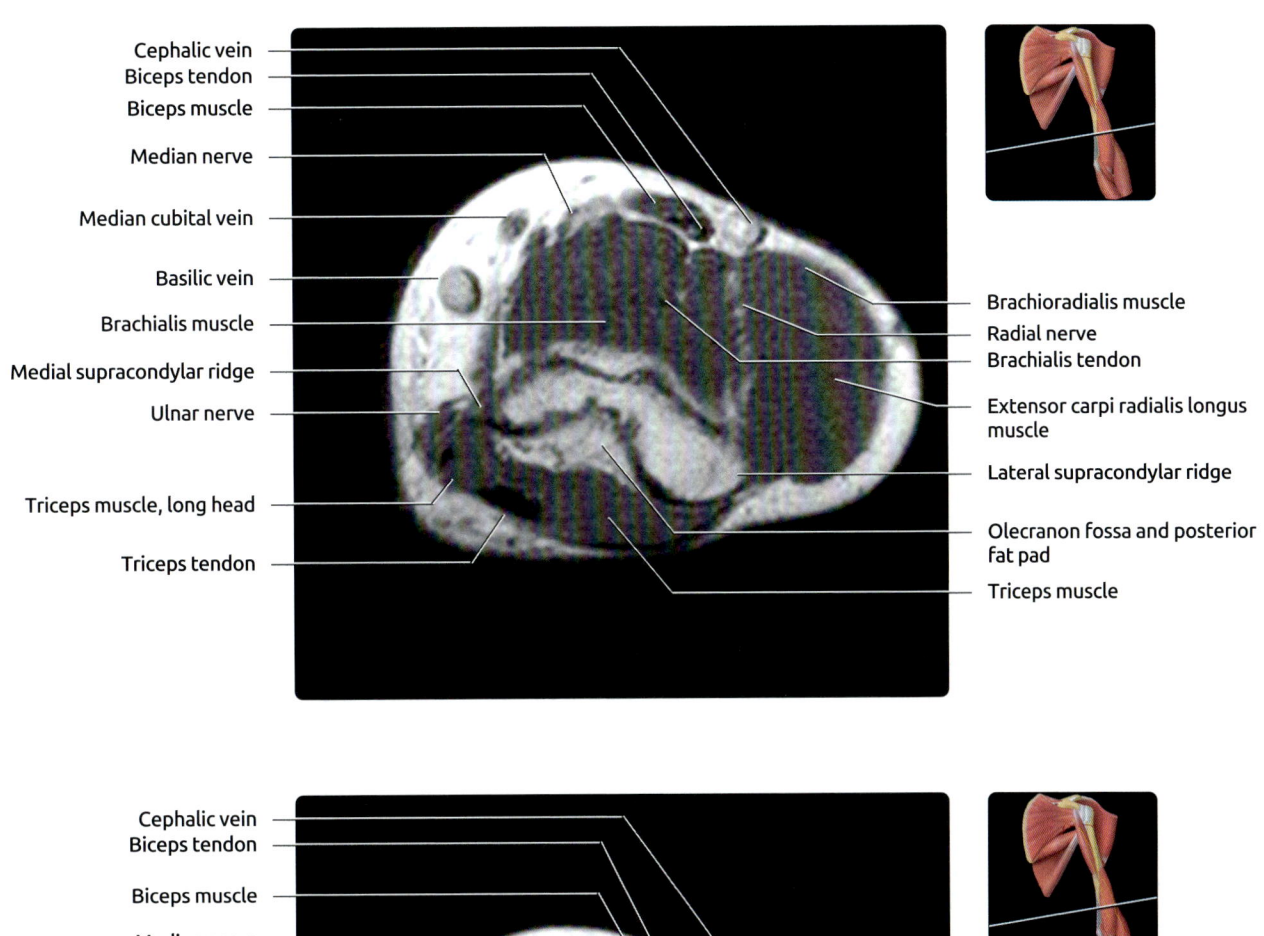

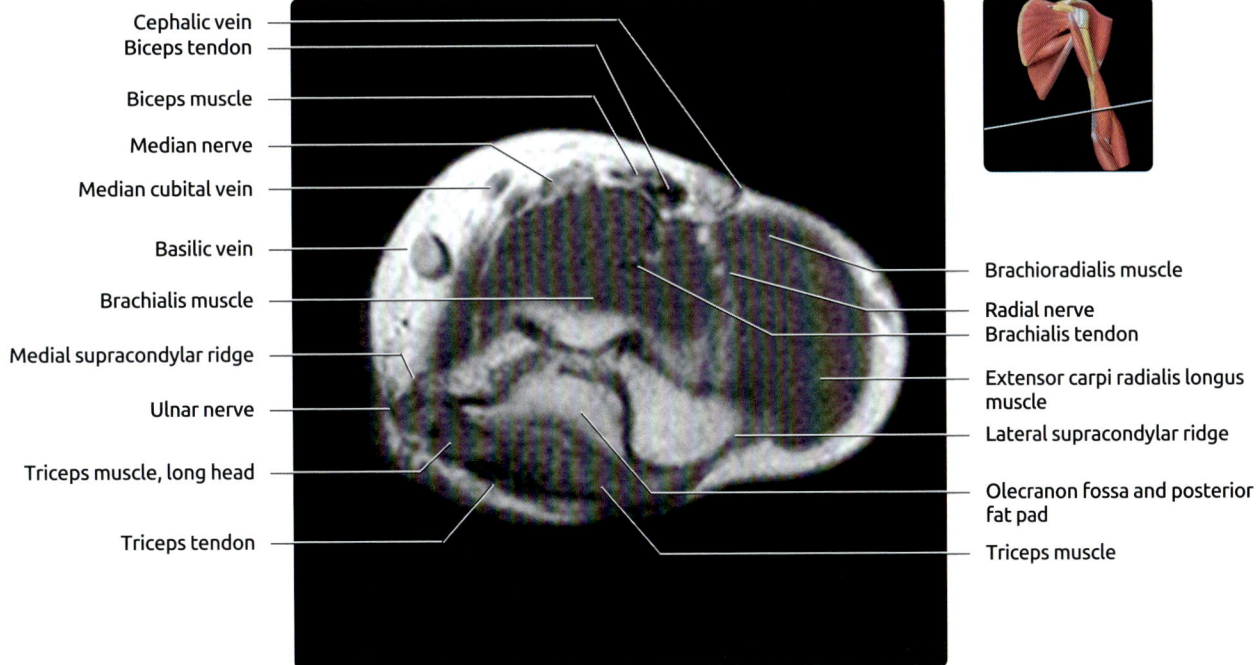

(Top) *This image is located at the superior aspect of the elbow. The olecranon fossa contains the posterior fat pad.* (Bottom) *The biceps is now almost entirely tendinous.*

Arm Radiographic Anatomy and MR Atlas

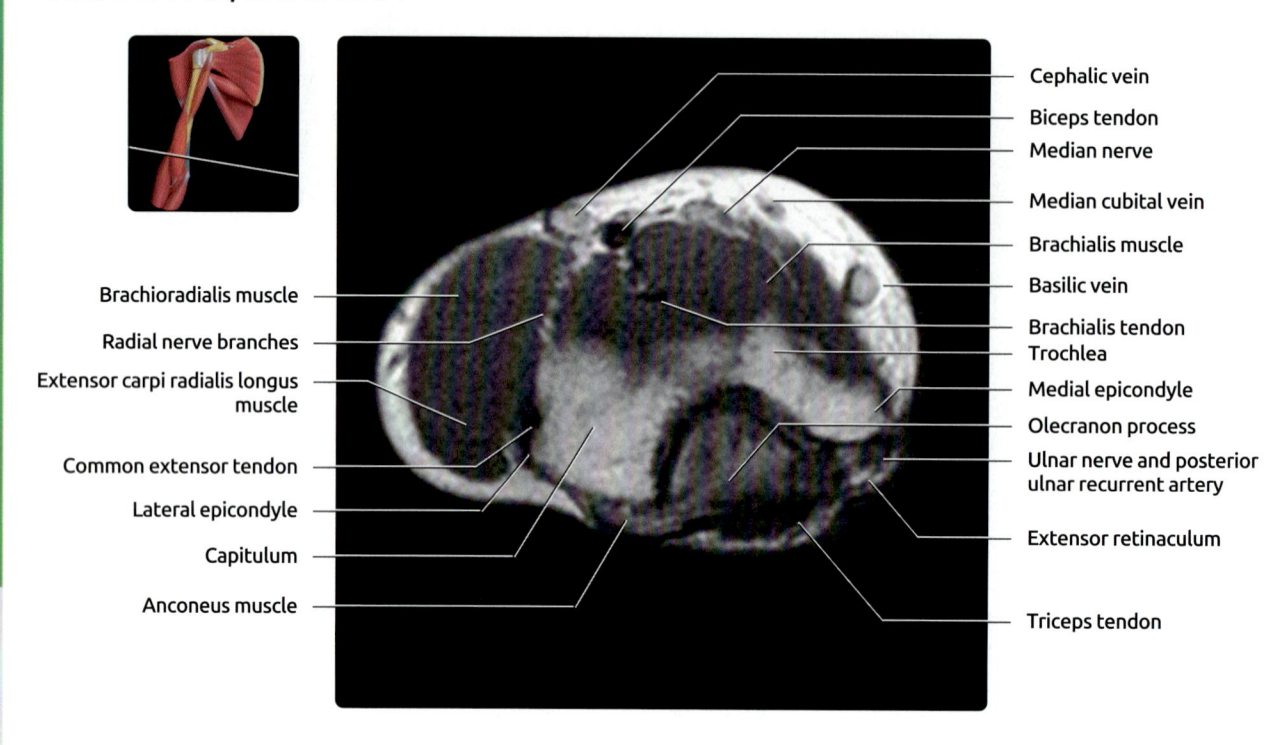

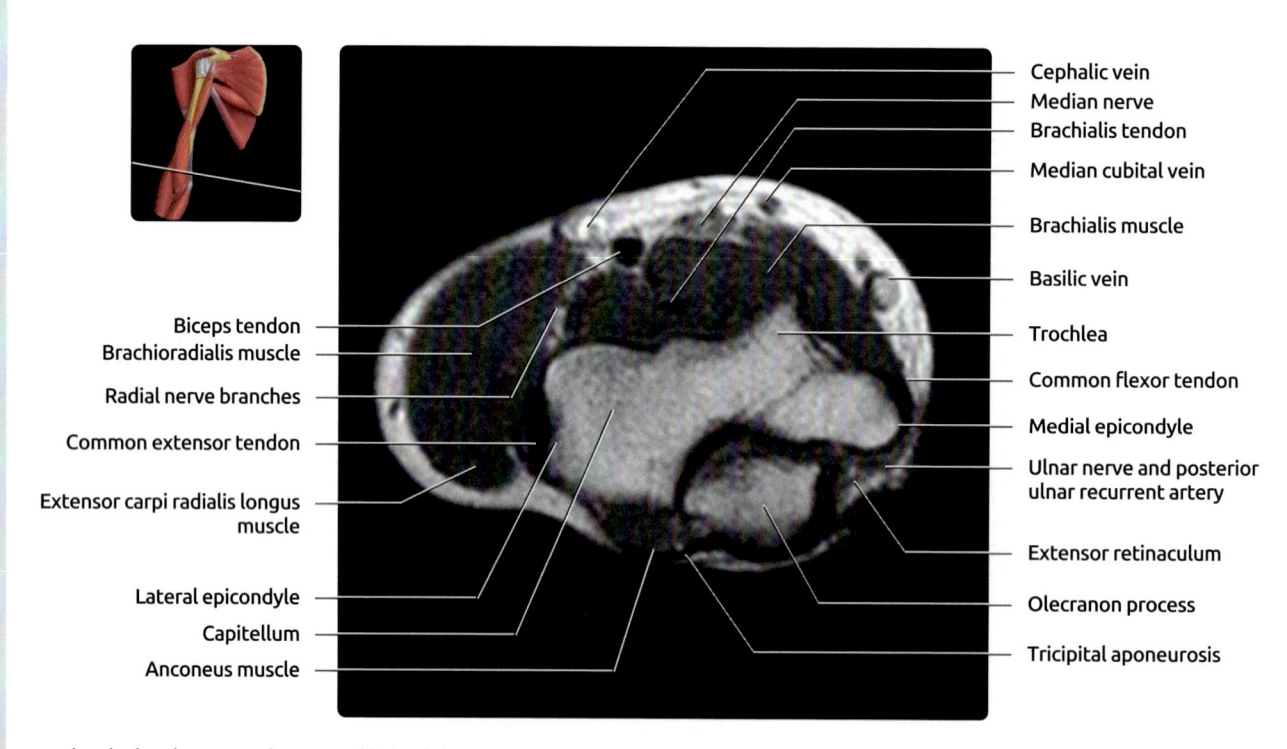

AXIAL T1 MR, RIGHT ARM

Labels (top image):
- Cephalic vein
- Biceps tendon
- Median nerve
- Median cubital vein
- Brachialis muscle
- Basilic vein
- Brachialis tendon
- Trochlea
- Medial epicondyle
- Olecranon process
- Ulnar nerve and posterior ulnar recurrent artery
- Extensor retinaculum
- Triceps tendon
- Brachioradialis muscle
- Radial nerve branches
- Extensor carpi radialis longus muscle
- Common extensor tendon
- Lateral epicondyle
- Capitulum
- Anconeus muscle

Labels (bottom image):
- Cephalic vein
- Median nerve
- Brachialis tendon
- Median cubital vein
- Brachialis muscle
- Basilic vein
- Trochlea
- Common flexor tendon
- Medial epicondyle
- Ulnar nerve and posterior ulnar recurrent artery
- Extensor retinaculum
- Olecranon process
- Tricipital aponeurosis
- Biceps tendon
- Brachioradialis muscle
- Radial nerve branches
- Common extensor tendon
- Extensor carpi radialis longus muscle
- Lateral epicondyle
- Capitellum
- Anconeus muscle

(Top) *The ulnar nerve has passed behind the medial epicondyle.* **(Bottom)** *The anconeus muscle arises from the lateral epicondyle.*

Arm Radiographic Anatomy and MR Atlas

AXIAL T1 MR, LEFT ARM

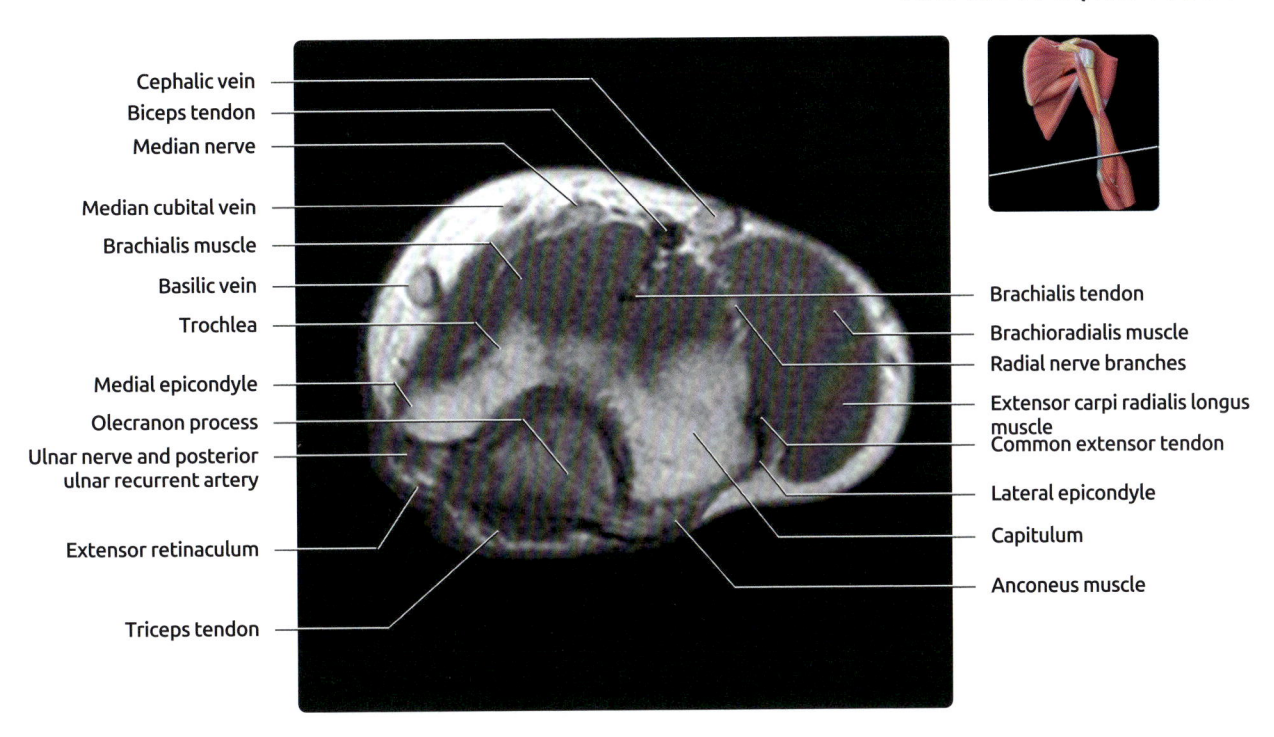

Top image labels (left side): Cephalic vein; Biceps tendon; Median nerve; Median cubital vein; Brachialis muscle; Basilic vein; Trochlea; Medial epicondyle; Olecranon process; Ulnar nerve and posterior ulnar recurrent artery; Extensor retinaculum; Triceps tendon

Top image labels (right side): Brachialis tendon; Brachioradialis muscle; Radial nerve branches; Extensor carpi radialis longus muscle; Common extensor tendon; Lateral epicondyle; Capitulum; Anconeus muscle

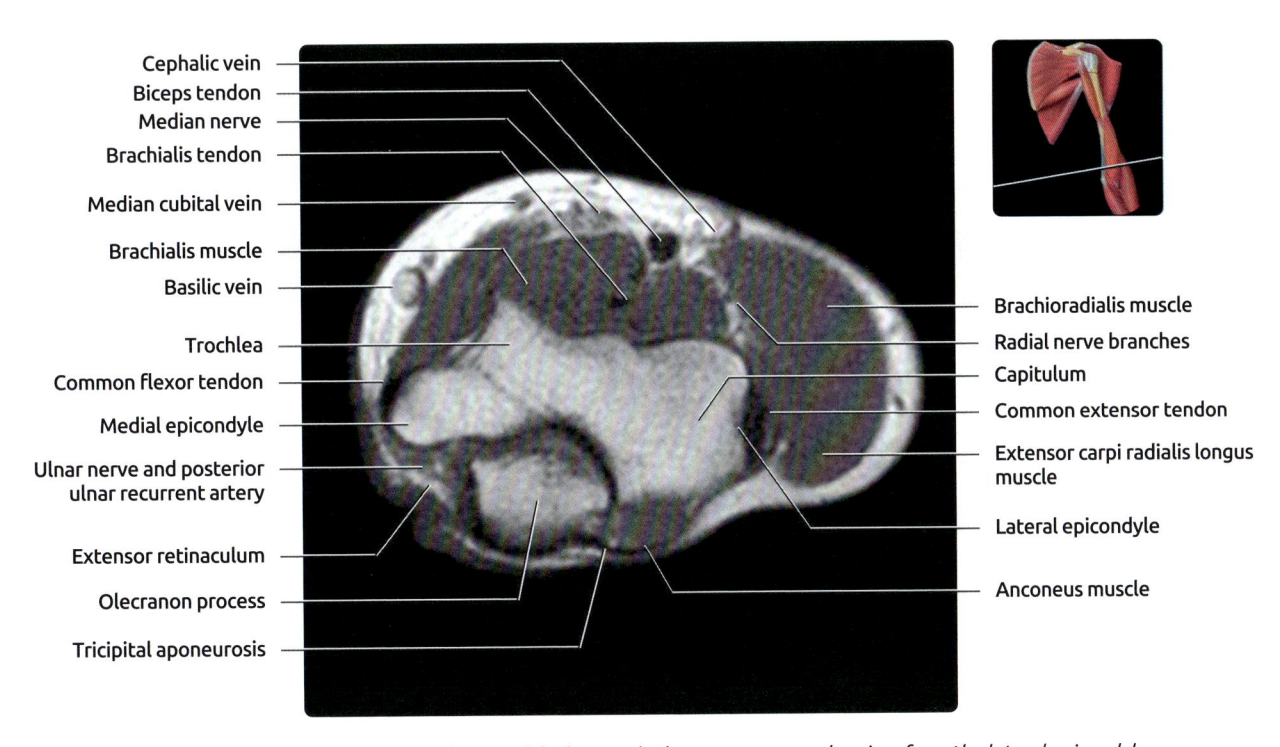

Bottom image labels (left side): Cephalic vein; Biceps tendon; Median nerve; Brachialis tendon; Median cubital vein; Brachialis muscle; Basilic vein; Trochlea; Common flexor tendon; Medial epicondyle; Ulnar nerve and posterior ulnar recurrent artery; Extensor retinaculum; Olecranon process; Tricipital aponeurosis

Bottom image labels (right side): Brachioradialis muscle; Radial nerve branches; Capitulum; Common extensor tendon; Extensor carpi radialis longus muscle; Lateral epicondyle; Anconeus muscle

(Top) The ulnar nerve has passed behind the medial epicondyle. **(Bottom)** The anconeus muscle arises from the lateral epicondyle.

Arm Radiographic Anatomy and MR Atlas

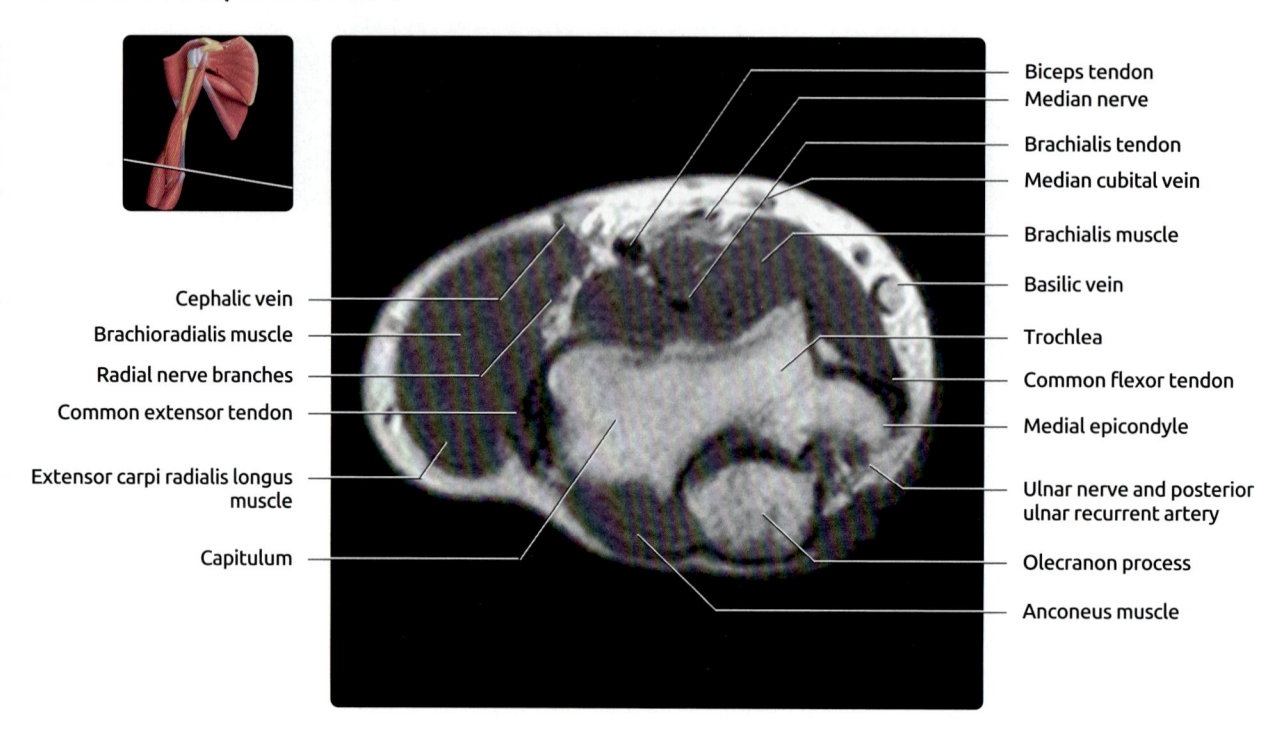

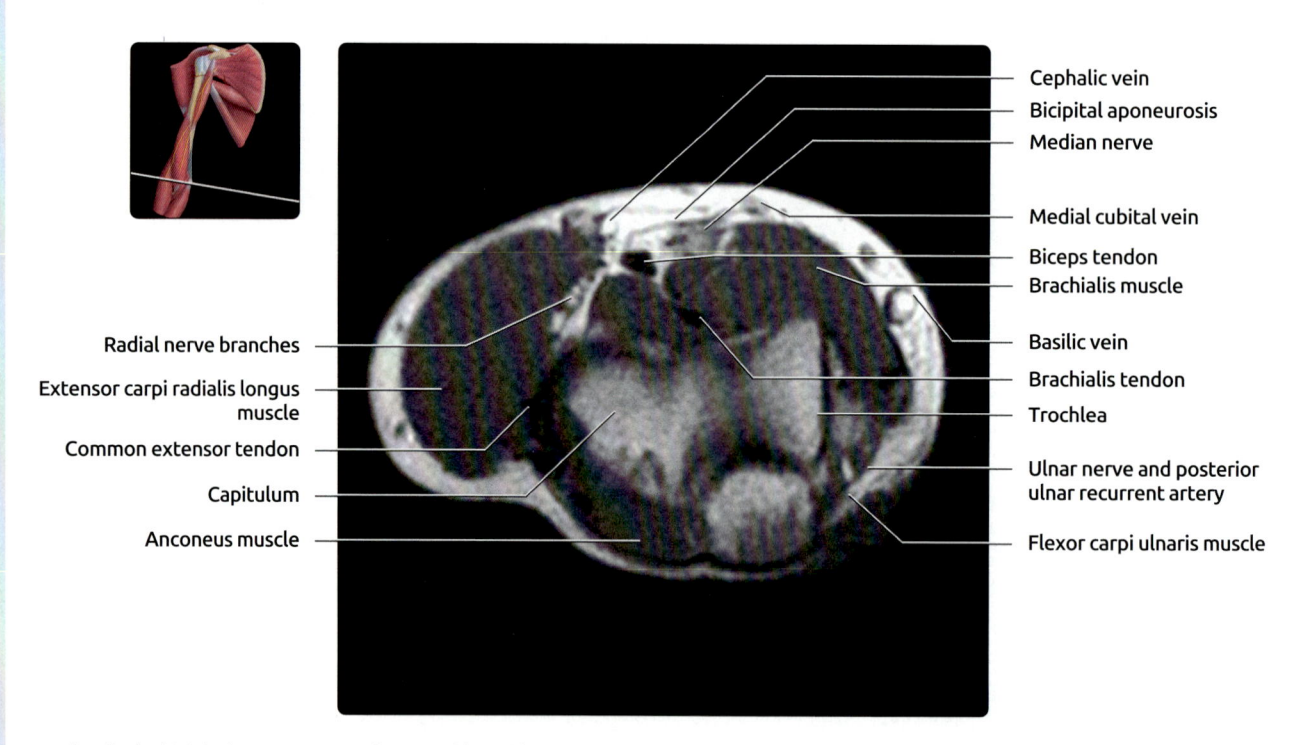

AXIAL T1 MR, RIGHT ARM

Labels (top image):
- Biceps tendon
- Median nerve
- Brachialis tendon
- Median cubital vein
- Brachialis muscle
- Basilic vein
- Trochlea
- Common flexor tendon
- Medial epicondyle
- Ulnar nerve and posterior ulnar recurrent artery
- Olecranon process
- Anconeus muscle
- Cephalic vein
- Brachioradialis muscle
- Radial nerve branches
- Common extensor tendon
- Extensor carpi radialis longus muscle
- Capitulum

Labels (bottom image):
- Cephalic vein
- Bicipital aponeurosis
- Median nerve
- Medial cubital vein
- Biceps tendon
- Brachialis muscle
- Basilic vein
- Brachialis tendon
- Trochlea
- Ulnar nerve and posterior ulnar recurrent artery
- Flexor carpi ulnaris muscle
- Radial nerve branches
- Extensor carpi radialis longus muscle
- Common extensor tendon
- Capitulum
- Anconeus muscle

(Top) *The bicipital aponeurosis or lacertus fibrosis has originated from the medial side of the biceps tendon.* **(Bottom)** *The brachialis tendon is nearing the insertion on the ulnar tuberosity.*

Arm Radiographic Anatomy and MR Atlas

AXIAL T1 MR, LEFT ARM

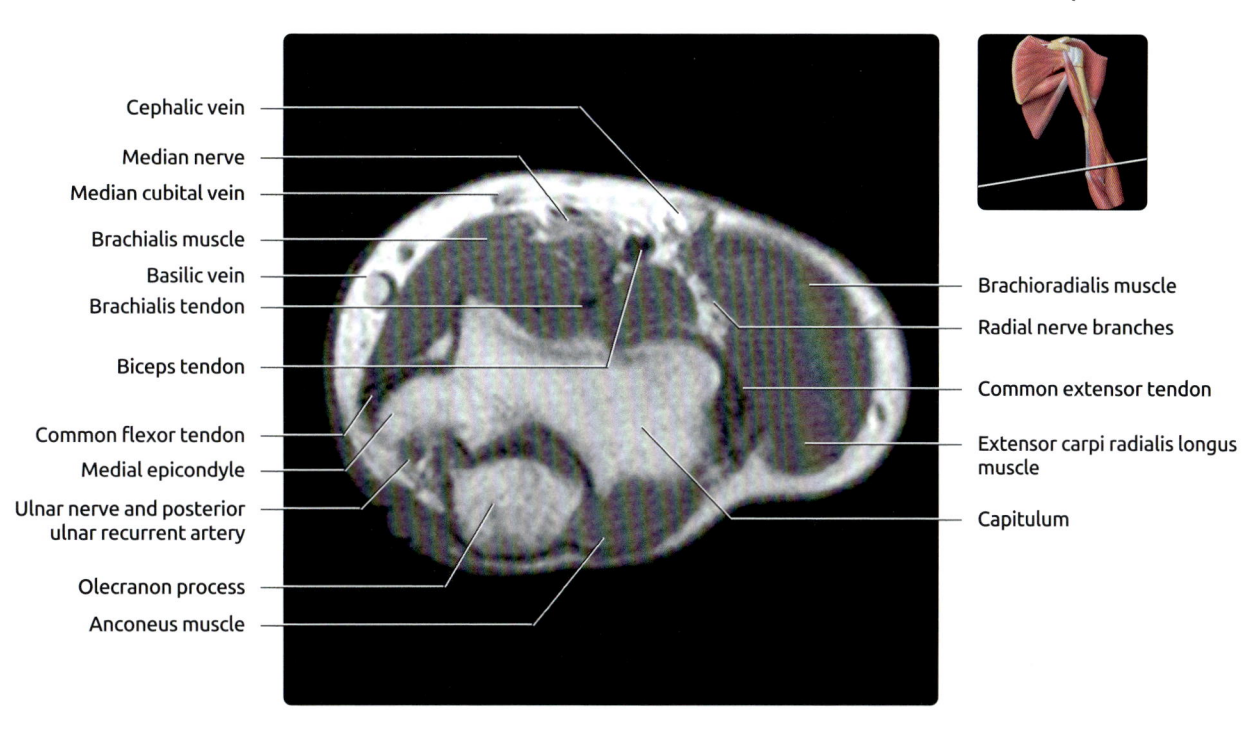

Top image labels:
- Cephalic vein
- Median nerve
- Median cubital vein
- Brachialis muscle
- Basilic vein
- Brachialis tendon
- Biceps tendon
- Common flexor tendon
- Medial epicondyle
- Ulnar nerve and posterior ulnar recurrent artery
- Olecranon process
- Anconeus muscle
- Brachioradialis muscle
- Radial nerve branches
- Common extensor tendon
- Extensor carpi radialis longus muscle
- Capitulum

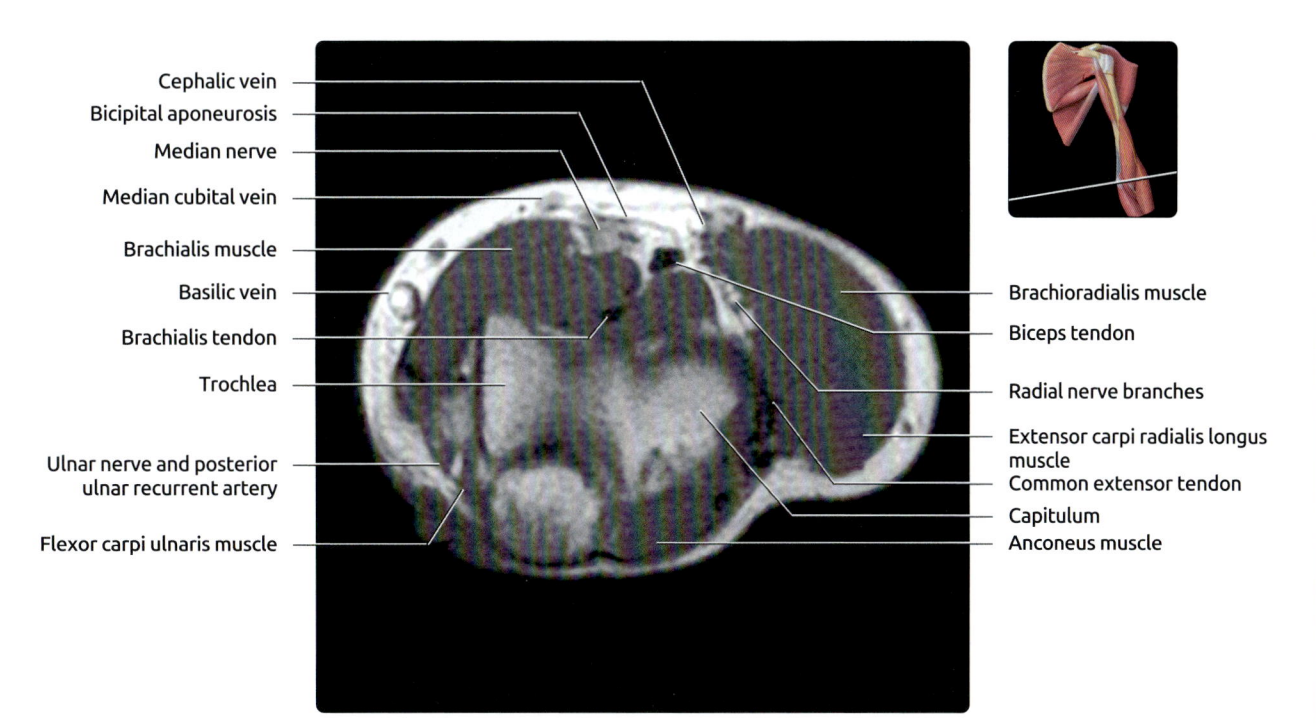

Bottom image labels:
- Cephalic vein
- Bicipital aponeurosis
- Median nerve
- Median cubital vein
- Brachialis muscle
- Basilic vein
- Brachialis tendon
- Trochlea
- Ulnar nerve and posterior ulnar recurrent artery
- Flexor carpi ulnaris muscle
- Brachioradialis muscle
- Biceps tendon
- Radial nerve branches
- Extensor carpi radialis longus muscle
- Common extensor tendon
- Capitulum
- Anconeus muscle

(Top) The bicipital aponeurosis or lacertus fibrosis has originated from the medial side of the biceps tendon. **(Bottom)** The brachialis tendon is nearing the insertion on the ulnar tuberosity.

Arm Radiographic Anatomy and MR Atlas

AXIAL T1 MR, RIGHT ARM

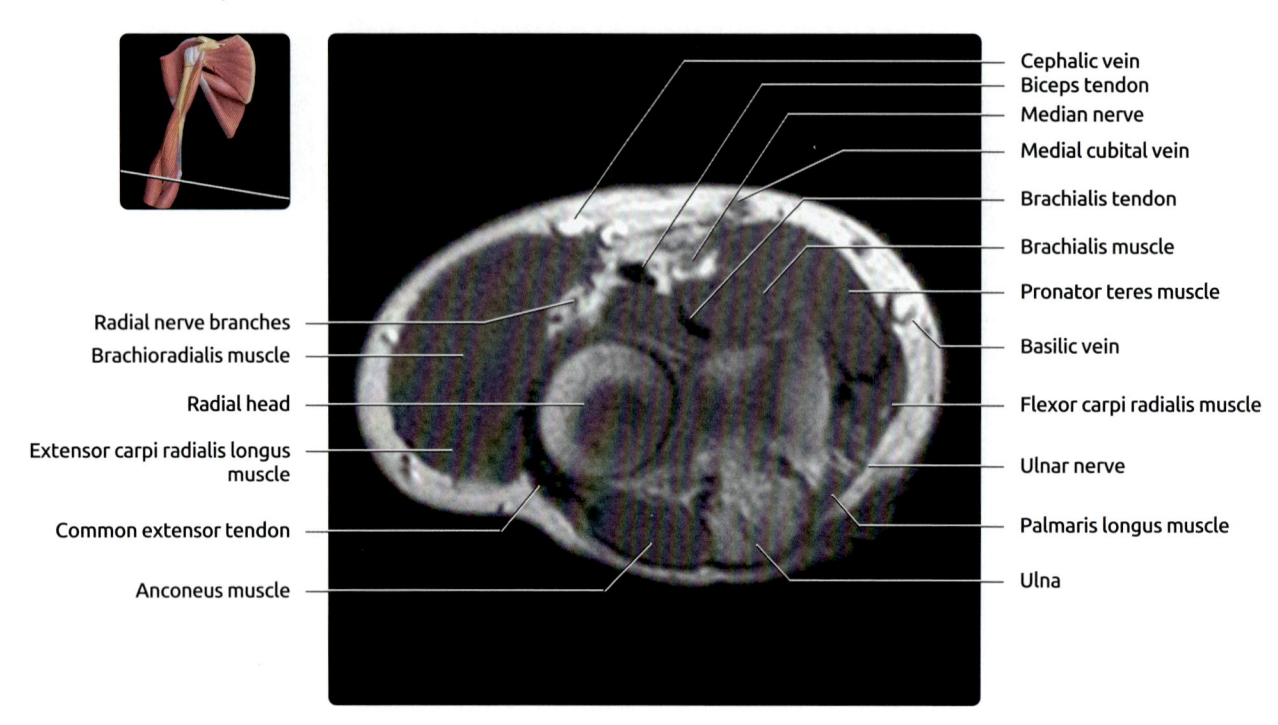

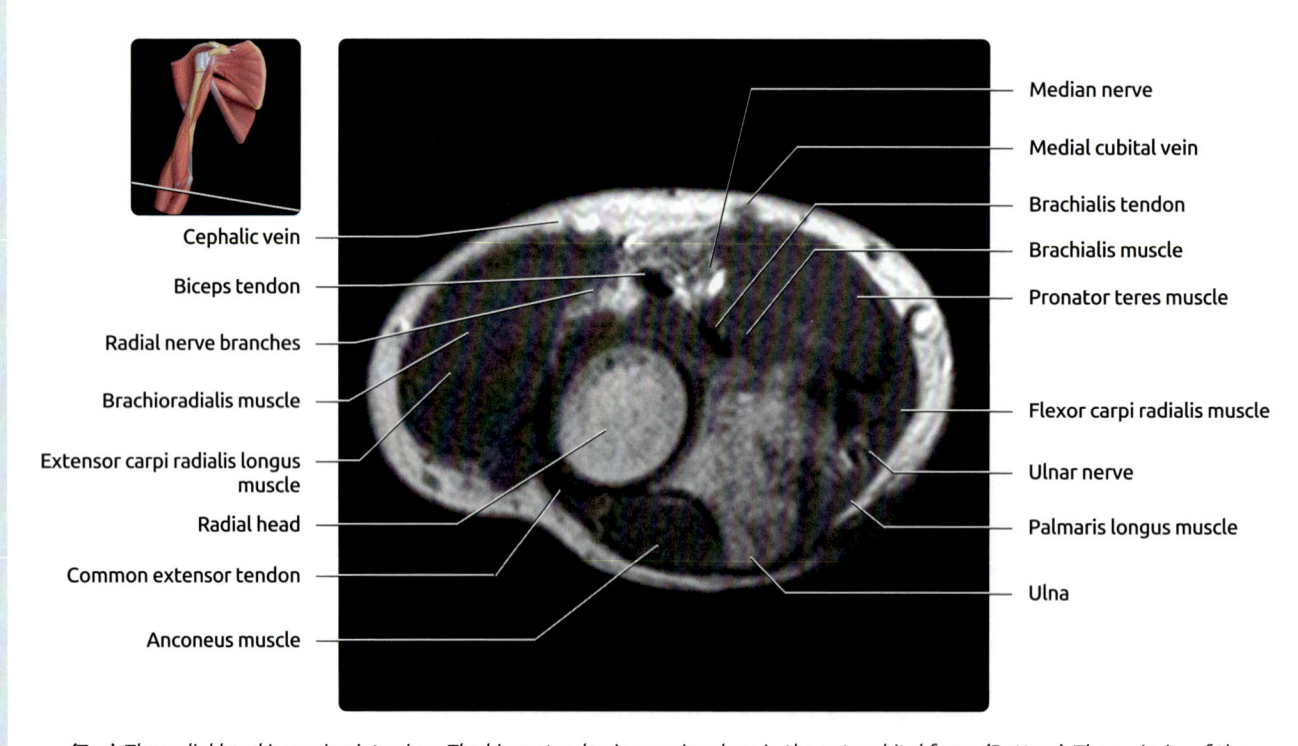

Top image labels (right side):
- Cephalic vein
- Biceps tendon
- Median nerve
- Medial cubital vein
- Brachialis tendon
- Brachialis muscle
- Pronator teres muscle
- Basilic vein
- Flexor carpi radialis muscle
- Ulnar nerve
- Palmaris longus muscle
- Ulna

Top image labels (left side):
- Radial nerve branches
- Brachioradialis muscle
- Radial head
- Extensor carpi radialis longus muscle
- Common extensor tendon
- Anconeus muscle

Bottom image labels (right side):
- Median nerve
- Medial cubital vein
- Brachialis tendon
- Brachialis muscle
- Pronator teres muscle
- Flexor carpi radialis muscle
- Ulnar nerve
- Palmaris longus muscle
- Ulna

Bottom image labels (left side):
- Cephalic vein
- Biceps tendon
- Radial nerve branches
- Brachioradialis muscle
- Extensor carpi radialis longus muscle
- Radial head
- Common extensor tendon
- Anconeus muscle

(Top) The radial head is coming into view. The biceps tendon is coursing deep in the antecubital fossa. **(Bottom)** The majority of the muscle mass at the lateral aspect of the elbow consists of the brachioradialis and extensor carpi radialis longus muscles.

Arm Radiographic Anatomy and MR Atlas

AXIAL T1 MR, LEFT ARM

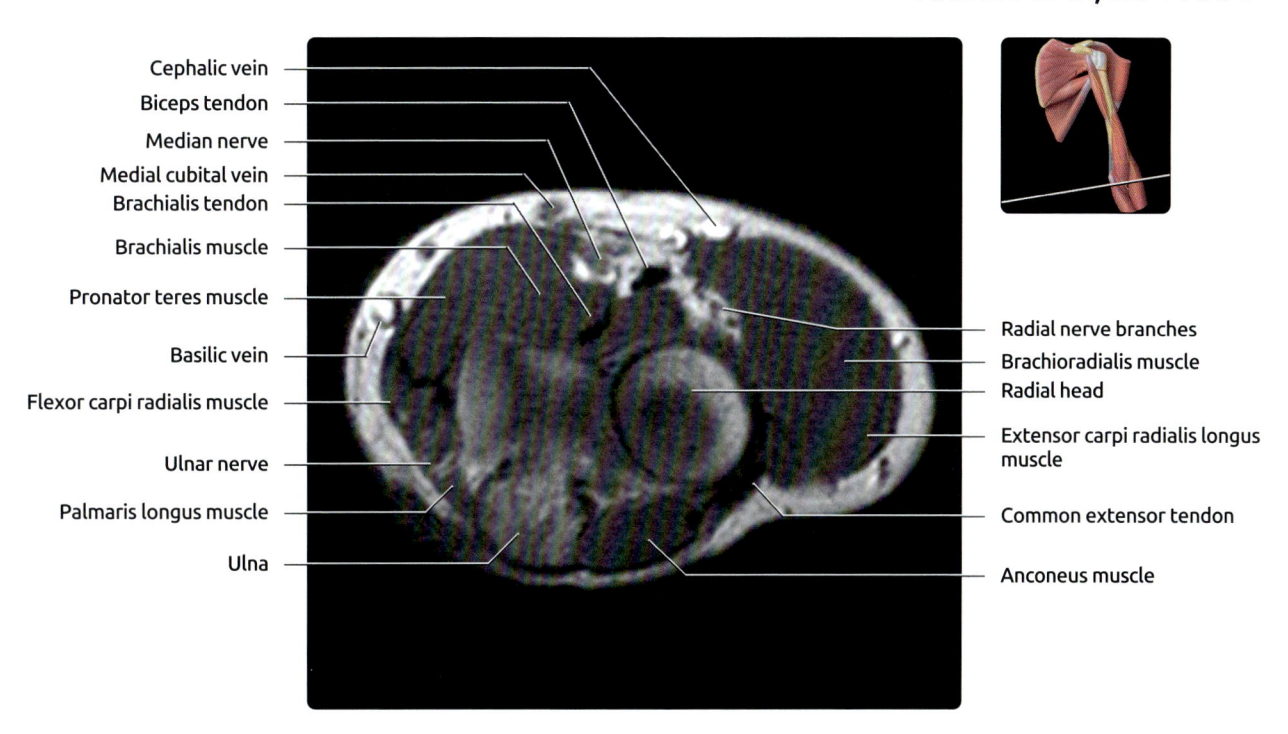

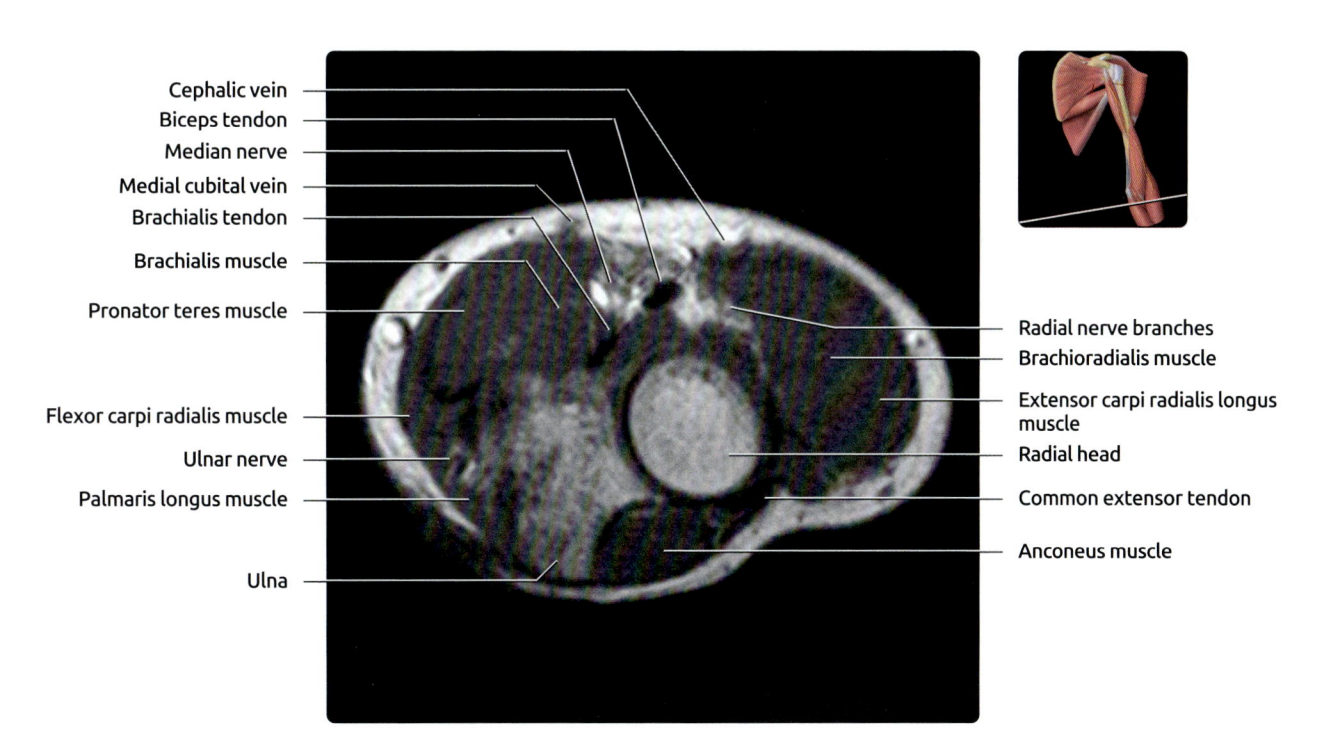

(Top) The radial head is coming into view. The biceps tendon is coursing deep in the antecubital fossa. (Bottom) The majority of the muscle mass at the lateral aspect of the elbow consists of the brachioradialis and extensor carpi radialis longus muscles.

Arm Radiographic Anatomy and MR Atlas

CORONAL T1 MR, RIGHT ARM

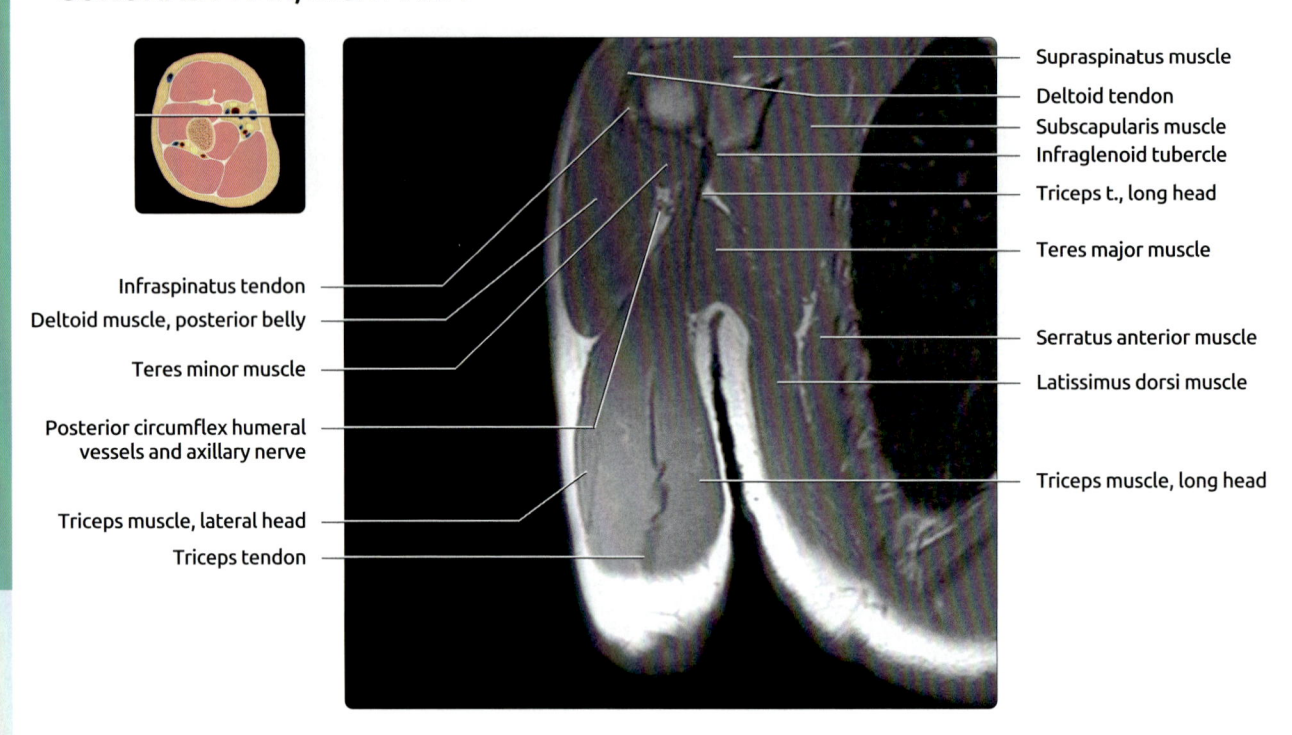

Labels (top image, left): Infraspinatus tendon; Deltoid muscle, posterior belly; Teres minor muscle; Posterior circumflex humeral vessels and axillary nerve; Triceps muscle, lateral head; Triceps tendon

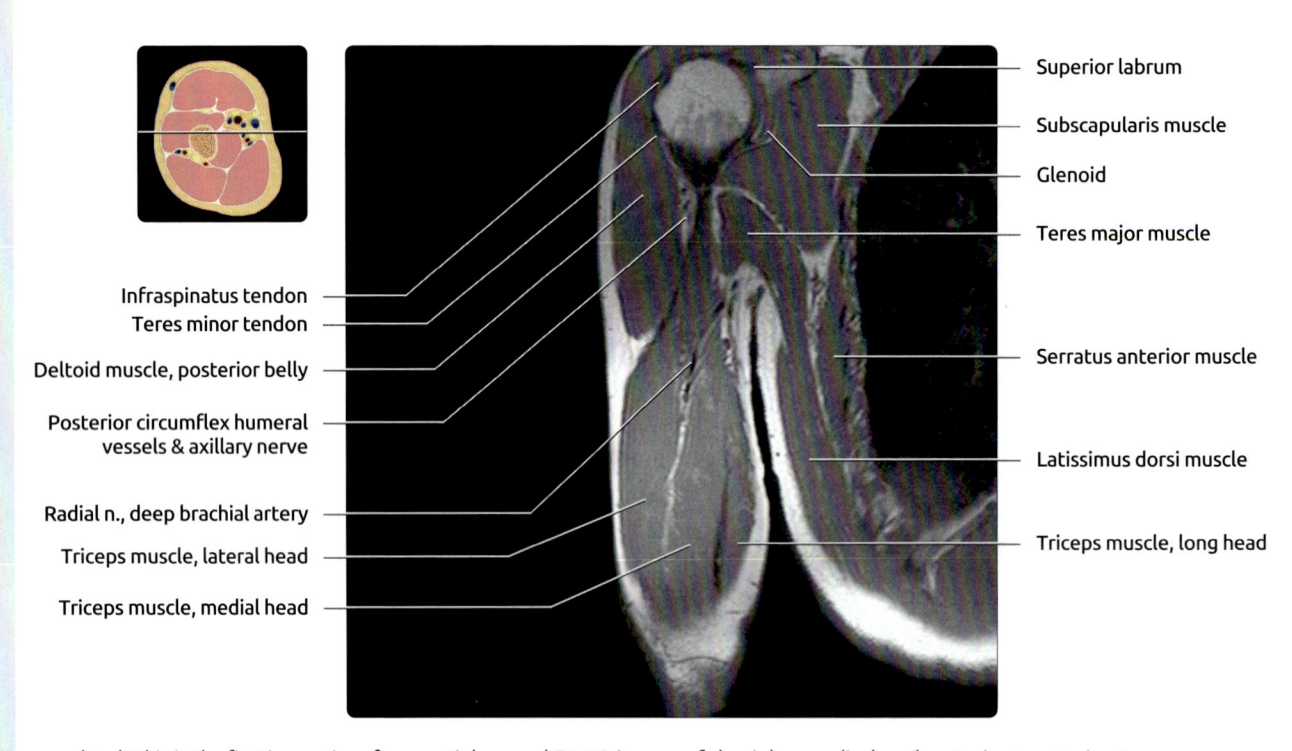

Labels (top image, right): Supraspinatus muscle; Deltoid tendon; Subscapularis muscle; Infraglenoid tubercle; Triceps t., long head; Teres major muscle; Serratus anterior muscle; Latissimus dorsi muscle; Triceps muscle, long head

Labels (bottom image, left): Infraspinatus tendon; Teres minor tendon; Deltoid muscle, posterior belly; Posterior circumflex humeral vessels & axillary nerve; Radial n., deep brachial artery; Triceps muscle, lateral head; Triceps muscle, medial head

Labels (bottom image, right): Superior labrum; Subscapularis muscle; Glenoid; Teres major muscle; Serratus anterior muscle; Latissimus dorsi muscle; Triceps muscle, long head

(Top) This is the first in a series of sequential coronal T1 MR images of the right arm displayed posterior to anterior. Images were acquired at 3T. The long head of the triceps originates from the infraglenoid tubercle of the scapula. **(Bottom)** The muscle mass of the posterior arm consists of the 3 heads of the triceps muscle.

Arm Radiographic Anatomy and MR Atlas

CORONAL T1 MR, LEFT ARM

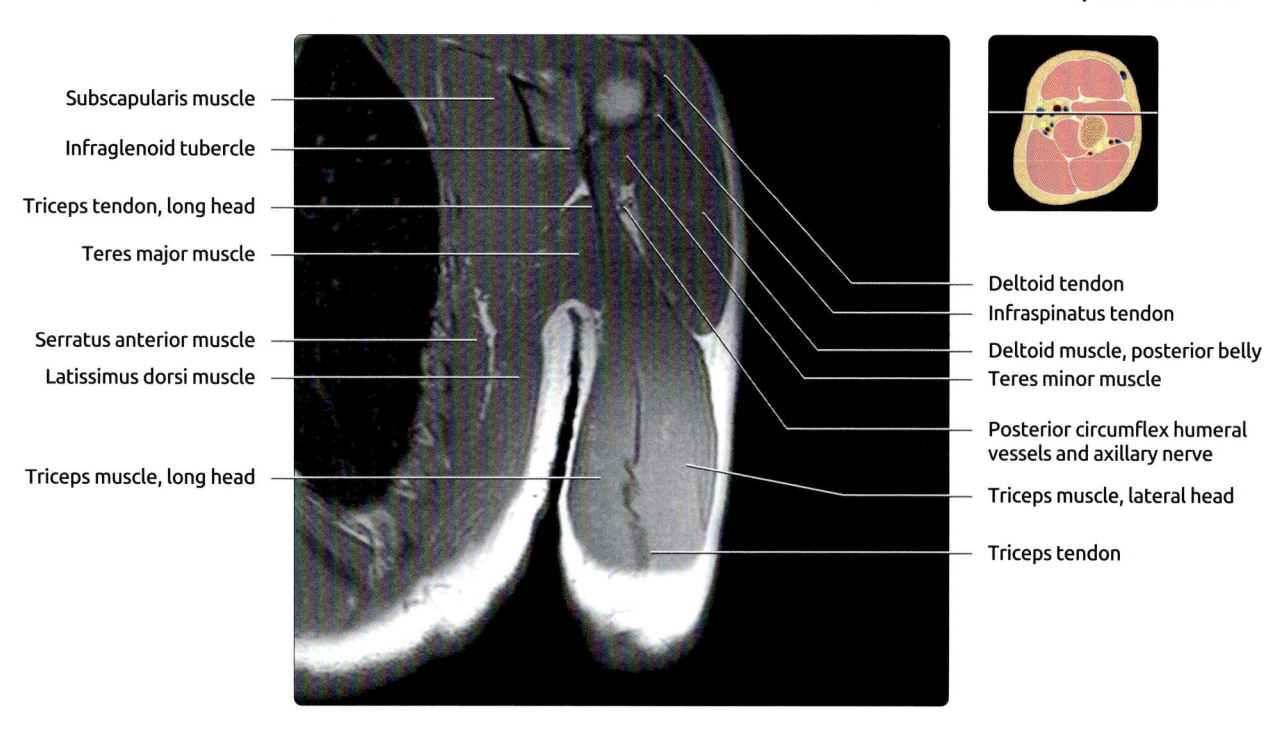

Labels (top image):
- Subscapularis muscle
- Infraglenoid tubercle
- Triceps tendon, long head
- Teres major muscle
- Serratus anterior muscle
- Latissimus dorsi muscle
- Triceps muscle, long head
- Deltoid tendon
- Infraspinatus tendon
- Deltoid muscle, posterior belly
- Teres minor muscle
- Posterior circumflex humeral vessels and axillary nerve
- Triceps muscle, lateral head
- Triceps tendon

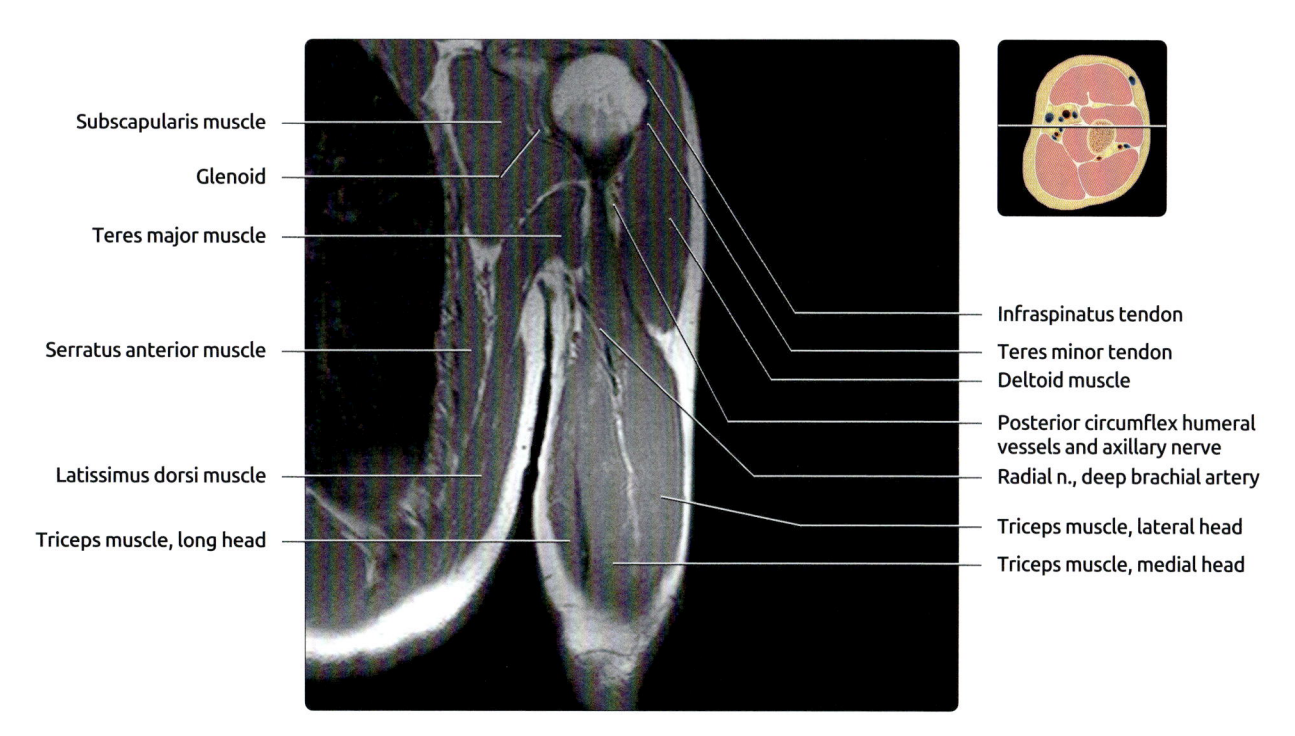

Labels (bottom image):
- Subscapularis muscle
- Glenoid
- Teres major muscle
- Serratus anterior muscle
- Latissimus dorsi muscle
- Triceps muscle, long head
- Infraspinatus tendon
- Teres minor tendon
- Deltoid muscle
- Posterior circumflex humeral vessels and axillary nerve
- Radial n., deep brachial artery
- Triceps muscle, lateral head
- Triceps muscle, medial head

(Top) This is the first in a series of sequential coronal T1 MR images of the left arm displayed posterior to anterior. Images were acquired at 3T. The long head of the triceps originates from the infraglenoid tubercle of the scapula. **(Bottom)** The muscle mass of the posterior arm consists of the 3 heads of the triceps muscle.

Arm Radiographic Anatomy and MR Atlas

CORONAL T1 MR, RIGHT ARM

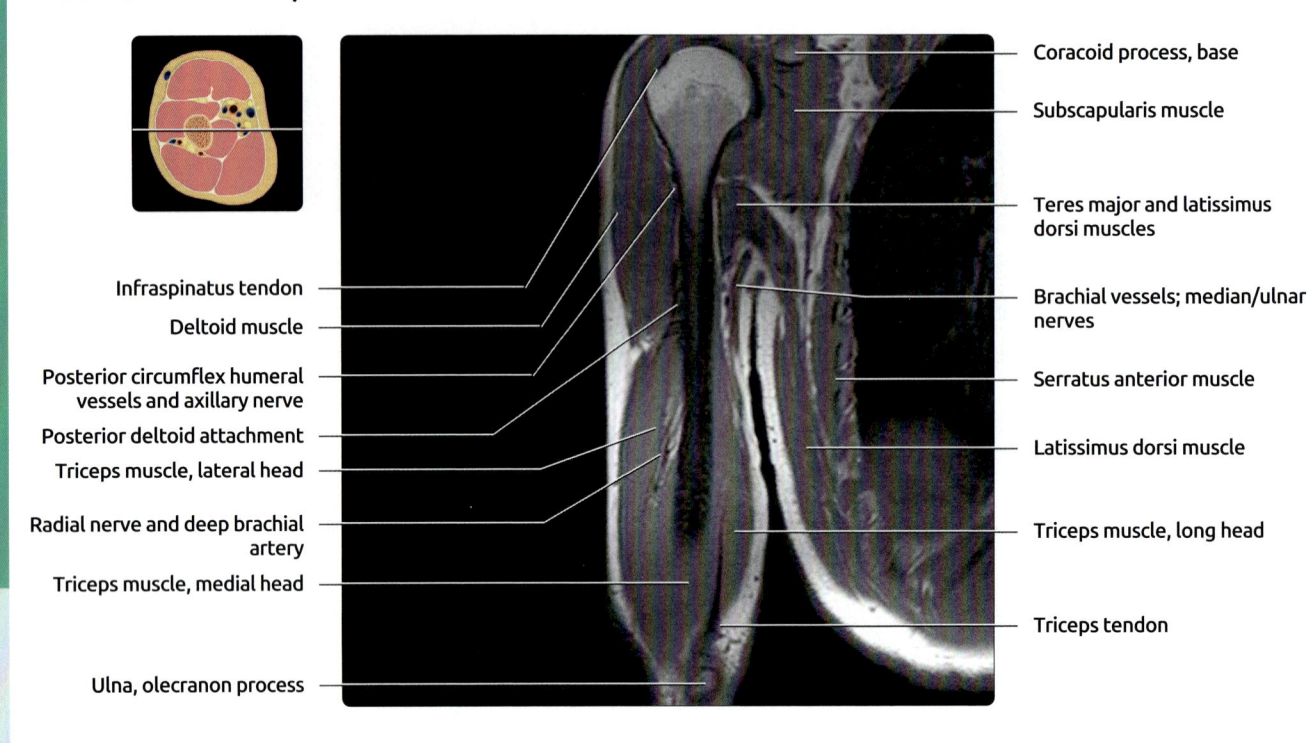

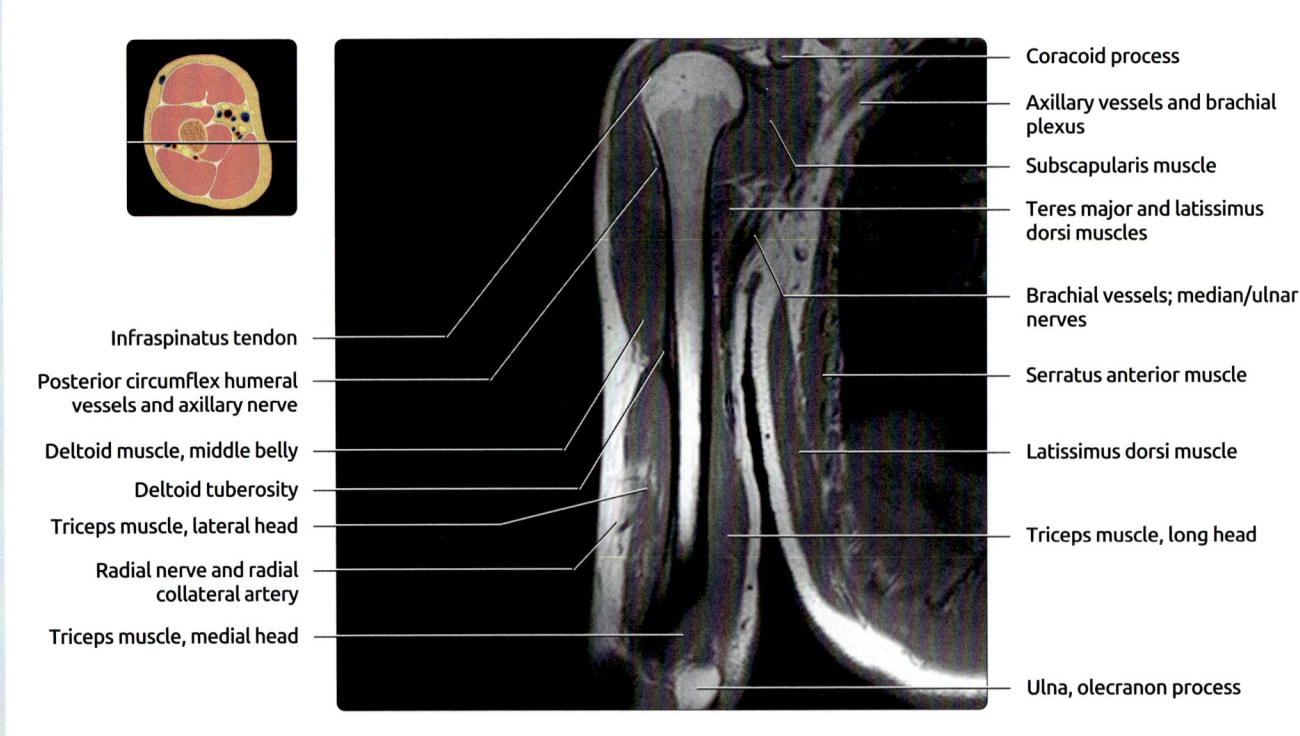

Labels (top image):
- Coracoid process, base
- Subscapularis muscle
- Teres major and latissimus dorsi muscles
- Brachial vessels; median/ulnar nerves
- Serratus anterior muscle
- Latissimus dorsi muscle
- Triceps muscle, long head
- Triceps tendon
- Infraspinatus tendon
- Deltoid muscle
- Posterior circumflex humeral vessels and axillary nerve
- Posterior deltoid attachment
- Triceps muscle, lateral head
- Radial nerve and deep brachial artery
- Triceps muscle, medial head
- Ulna, olecranon process

Labels (bottom image):
- Coracoid process
- Axillary vessels and brachial plexus
- Subscapularis muscle
- Teres major and latissimus dorsi muscles
- Brachial vessels; median/ulnar nerves
- Serratus anterior muscle
- Latissimus dorsi muscle
- Triceps muscle, long head
- Ulna, olecranon process
- Infraspinatus tendon
- Posterior circumflex humeral vessels and axillary nerve
- Deltoid muscle, middle belly
- Deltoid tuberosity
- Triceps muscle, lateral head
- Radial nerve and radial collateral artery
- Triceps muscle, medial head

(Top) *The teres major and latissimus dorsi muscles course anteriorly to insert on the anterior humeral cortex.* (Bottom) *The deltoid muscle tapers distally at the attachment to the deltoid tuberosity.*

Arm Radiographic Anatomy and MR Atlas

CORONAL T1 MR, LEFT ARM

Top image labels:
- Coracoid process, base
- Subscapularis muscle
- Teres major and latissimus dorsi muscles
- Brachial vessels; median/ulnar nerves
- Serratus anterior muscle
- Latissimus dorsi muscle
- Triceps muscle, long head
- Triceps tendon
- Infraspinatus tendon
- Posterior circumflex humeral vessels and axillary nerve
- Deltoid muscle
- Posterior deltoid attachment
- Triceps muscle, lateral head
- Radial nerve and deep brachial artery
- Triceps muscle, medial head
- Ulna, olecranon process

Bottom image labels:
- Coracoid process
- Axillary vessels and brachial plexus
- Subscapularis muscle
- Teres major and latissimus dorsi muscles
- Brachial vessels; median/ulnar nerves
- Serratus anterior muscle
- Latissimus dorsi muscle
- Triceps muscle, long head
- Ulna, olecranon process
- Infraspinatus tendon
- Posterior circumflex humeral vessels and axillary nerve
- Deltoid muscle
- Deltoid tuberosity
- Triceps muscle, lateral head
- Radial nerve and radial collateral artery
- Triceps muscle, medial head

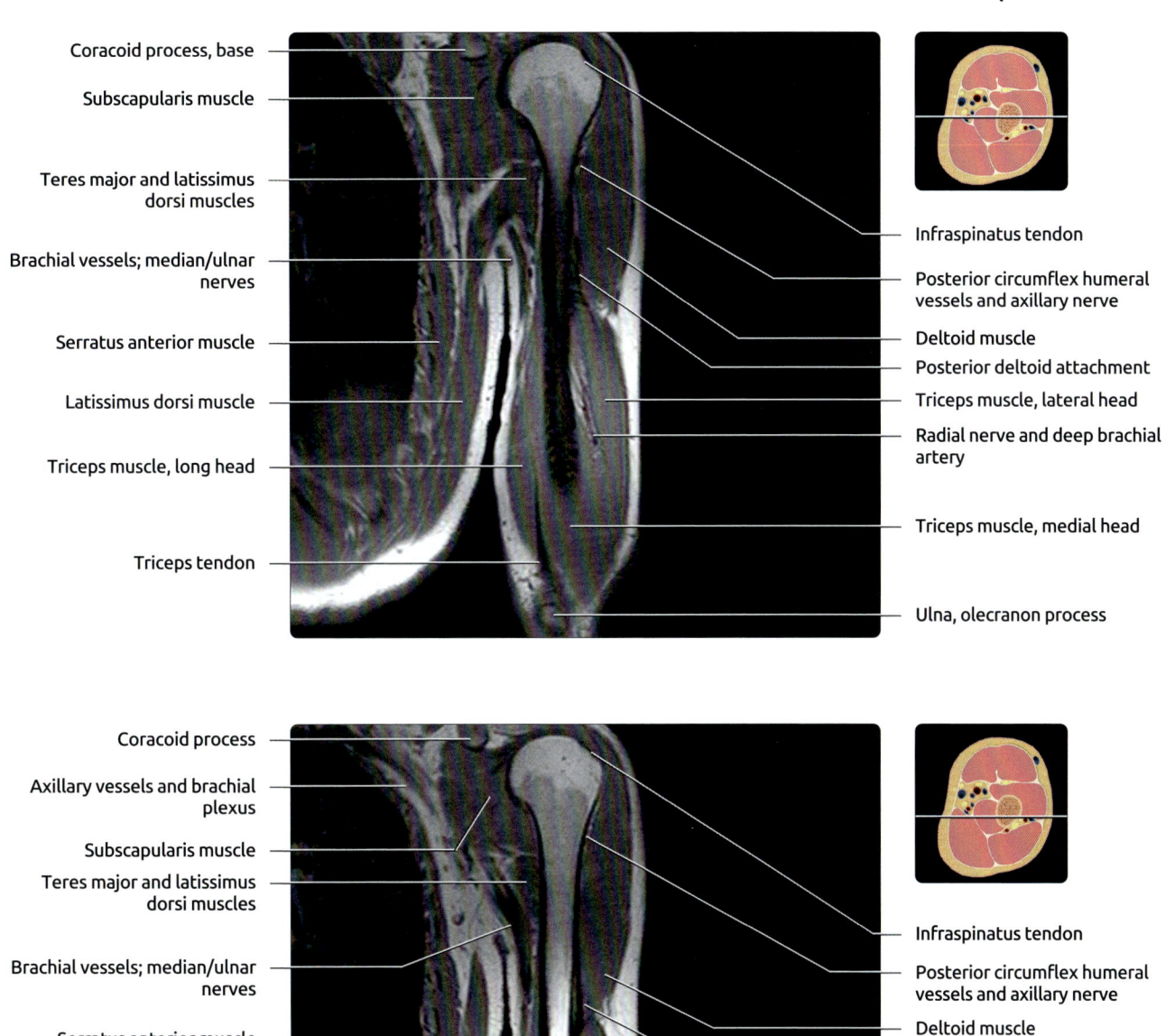

(Top) *The teres major and latissimus dorsi muscles course anteriorly to insert on the anterior humeral cortex.* **(Bottom)** *The deltoid muscle tapers distally at the attachment to the deltoid tuberosity.*

Arm Radiographic Anatomy and MR Atlas

CORONAL T1 MR, RIGHT ARM

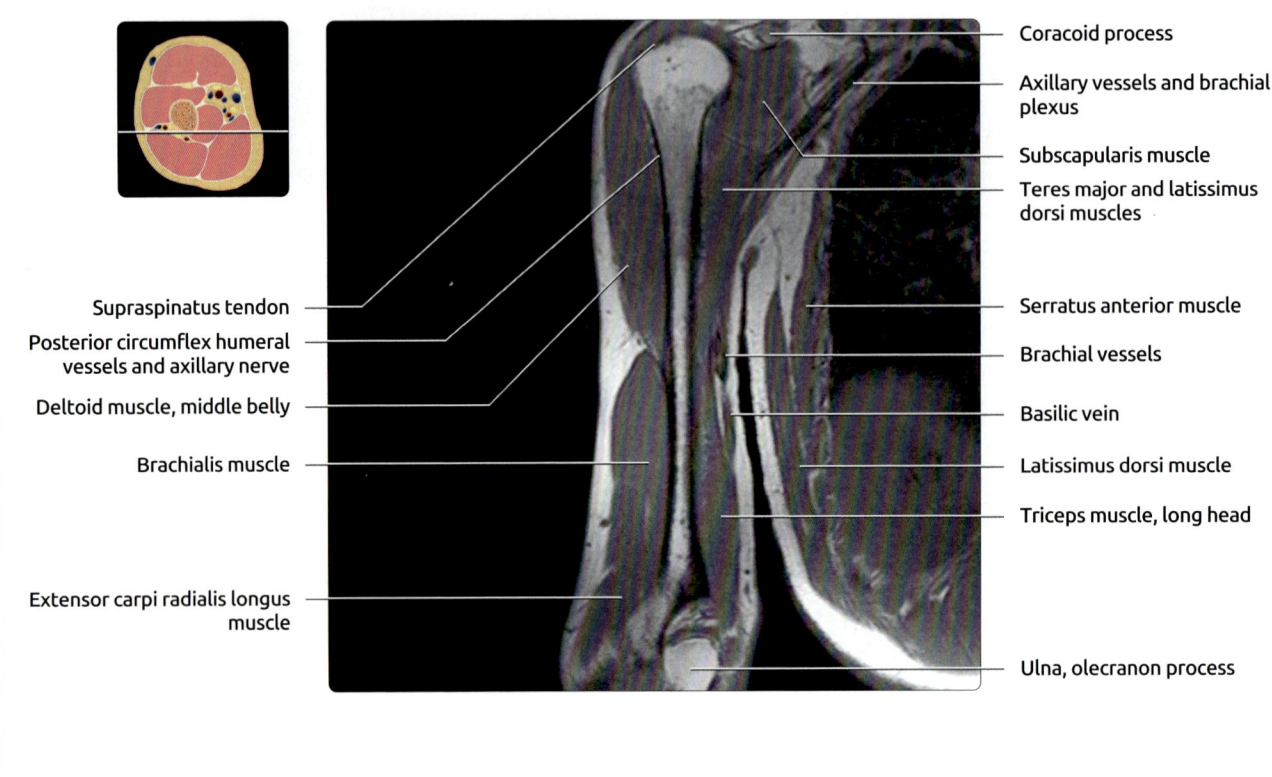

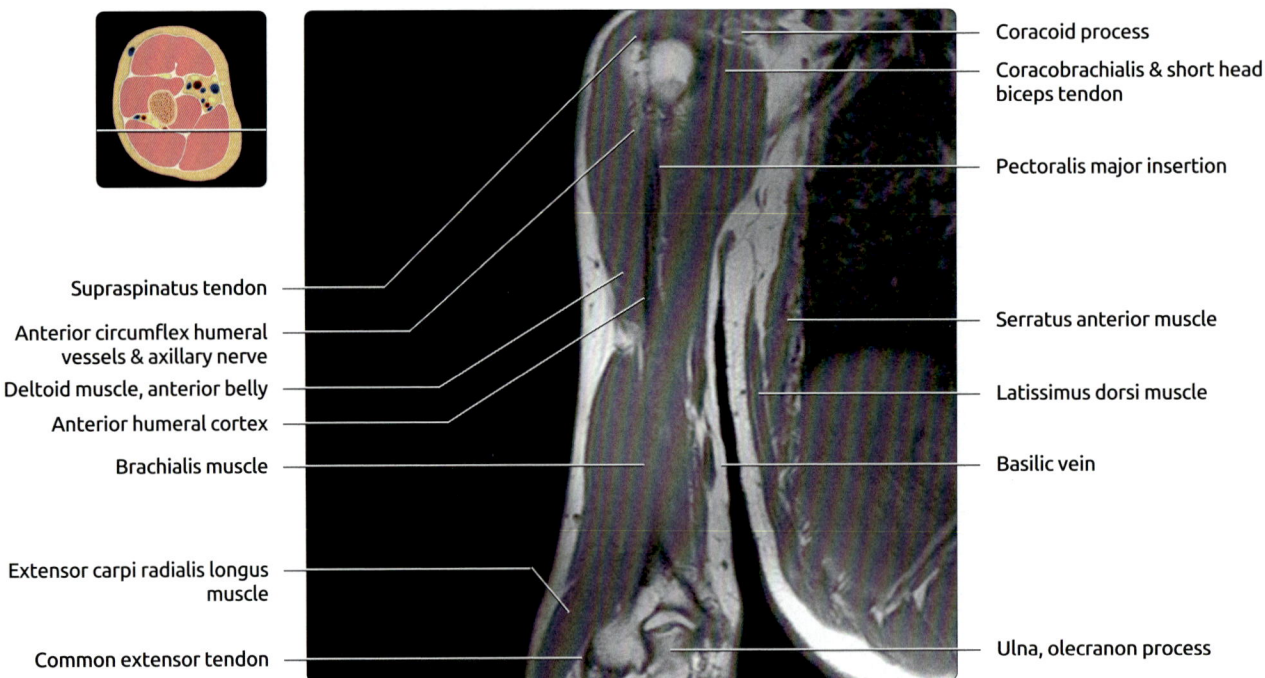

Labels (top image):
- Coracoid process
- Axillary vessels and brachial plexus
- Subscapularis muscle
- Teres major and latissimus dorsi muscles
- Serratus anterior muscle
- Brachial vessels
- Basilic vein
- Latissimus dorsi muscle
- Triceps muscle, long head
- Ulna, olecranon process
- Supraspinatus tendon
- Posterior circumflex humeral vessels and axillary nerve
- Deltoid muscle, middle belly
- Brachialis muscle
- Extensor carpi radialis longus muscle

Labels (bottom image):
- Coracoid process
- Coracobrachialis & short head biceps tendon
- Pectoralis major insertion
- Serratus anterior muscle
- Latissimus dorsi muscle
- Basilic vein
- Ulna, olecranon process
- Supraspinatus tendon
- Anterior circumflex humeral vessels & axillary nerve
- Deltoid muscle, anterior belly
- Anterior humeral cortex
- Brachialis muscle
- Extensor carpi radialis longus muscle
- Common extensor tendon

(Top) *The brachialis muscle originates from the distal half of the anterior humeral cortex.* **(Bottom)** *The coracobrachialis and biceps short head originate from the coracoid process.*

Arm Radiographic Anatomy and MR Atlas

CORONAL T1 MR, LEFT ARM

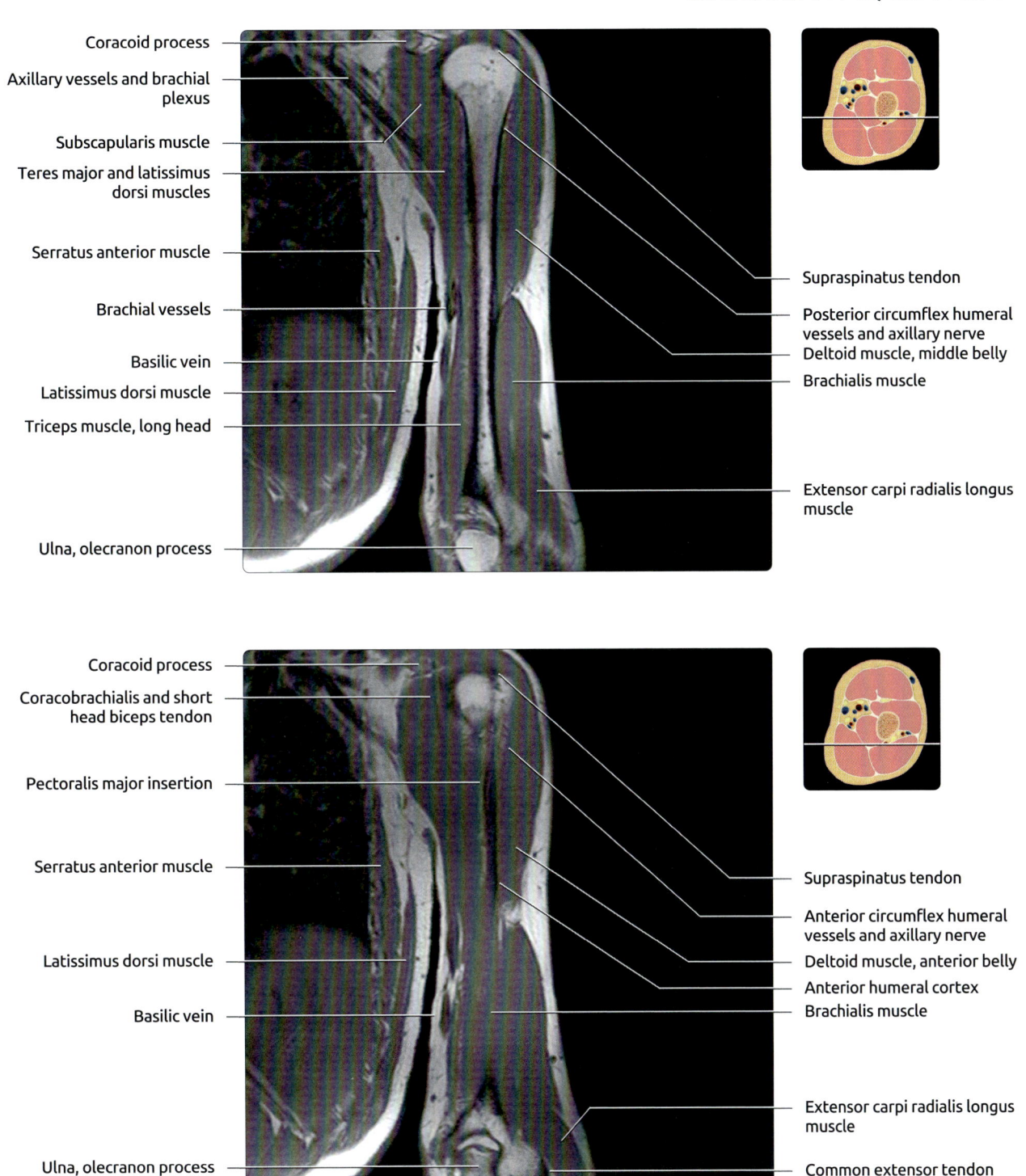

Top image labels:
- Coracoid process
- Axillary vessels and brachial plexus
- Subscapularis muscle
- Teres major and latissimus dorsi muscles
- Serratus anterior muscle
- Brachial vessels
- Basilic vein
- Latissimus dorsi muscle
- Triceps muscle, long head
- Ulna, olecranon process
- Supraspinatus tendon
- Posterior circumflex humeral vessels and axillary nerve
- Deltoid muscle, middle belly
- Brachialis muscle
- Extensor carpi radialis longus muscle

Bottom image labels:
- Coracoid process
- Coracobrachialis and short head biceps tendon
- Pectoralis major insertion
- Serratus anterior muscle
- Latissimus dorsi muscle
- Basilic vein
- Ulna, olecranon process
- Supraspinatus tendon
- Anterior circumflex humeral vessels and axillary nerve
- Deltoid muscle, anterior belly
- Anterior humeral cortex
- Brachialis muscle
- Extensor carpi radialis longus muscle
- Common extensor tendon

(Top) The brachialis muscle originates from the distal half of the anterior humeral cortex. *(Bottom)* The coracobrachialis and biceps short head originate from the coracoid process.

Arm Radiographic Anatomy and MR Atlas

CORONAL T1 MR, RIGHT ARM

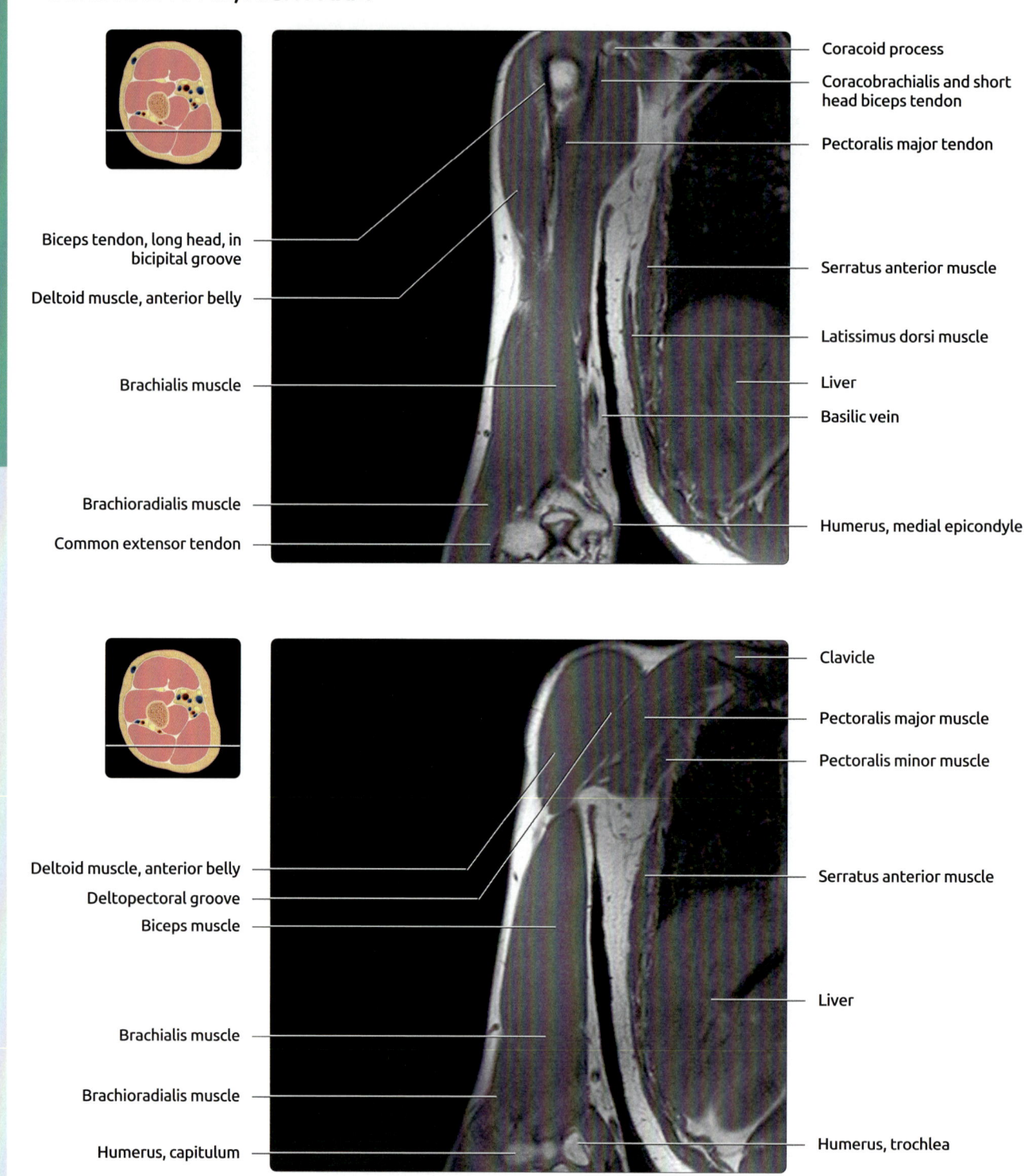

Labels (top image):
- Coracoid process
- Coracobrachialis and short head biceps tendon
- Pectoralis major tendon
- Biceps tendon, long head, in bicipital groove
- Deltoid muscle, anterior belly
- Serratus anterior muscle
- Latissimus dorsi muscle
- Brachialis muscle
- Liver
- Basilic vein
- Brachioradialis muscle
- Common extensor tendon
- Humerus, medial epicondyle

Labels (bottom image):
- Clavicle
- Pectoralis major muscle
- Pectoralis minor muscle
- Deltoid muscle, anterior belly
- Deltopectoral groove
- Biceps muscle
- Serratus anterior muscle
- Liver
- Brachialis muscle
- Brachioradialis muscle
- Humerus, capitulum
- Humerus, trochlea

(**Top**) The long head of the biceps tendon traverses the bicipital groove. The biceps long head and short head fuse at the upper humeral level. (**Bottom**) The most anterior image shows the deltoid muscle at the shoulder level and the biceps muscle along the length of the upper arm.

Arm Radiographic Anatomy and MR Atlas

CORONAL T1 MR, LEFT ARM

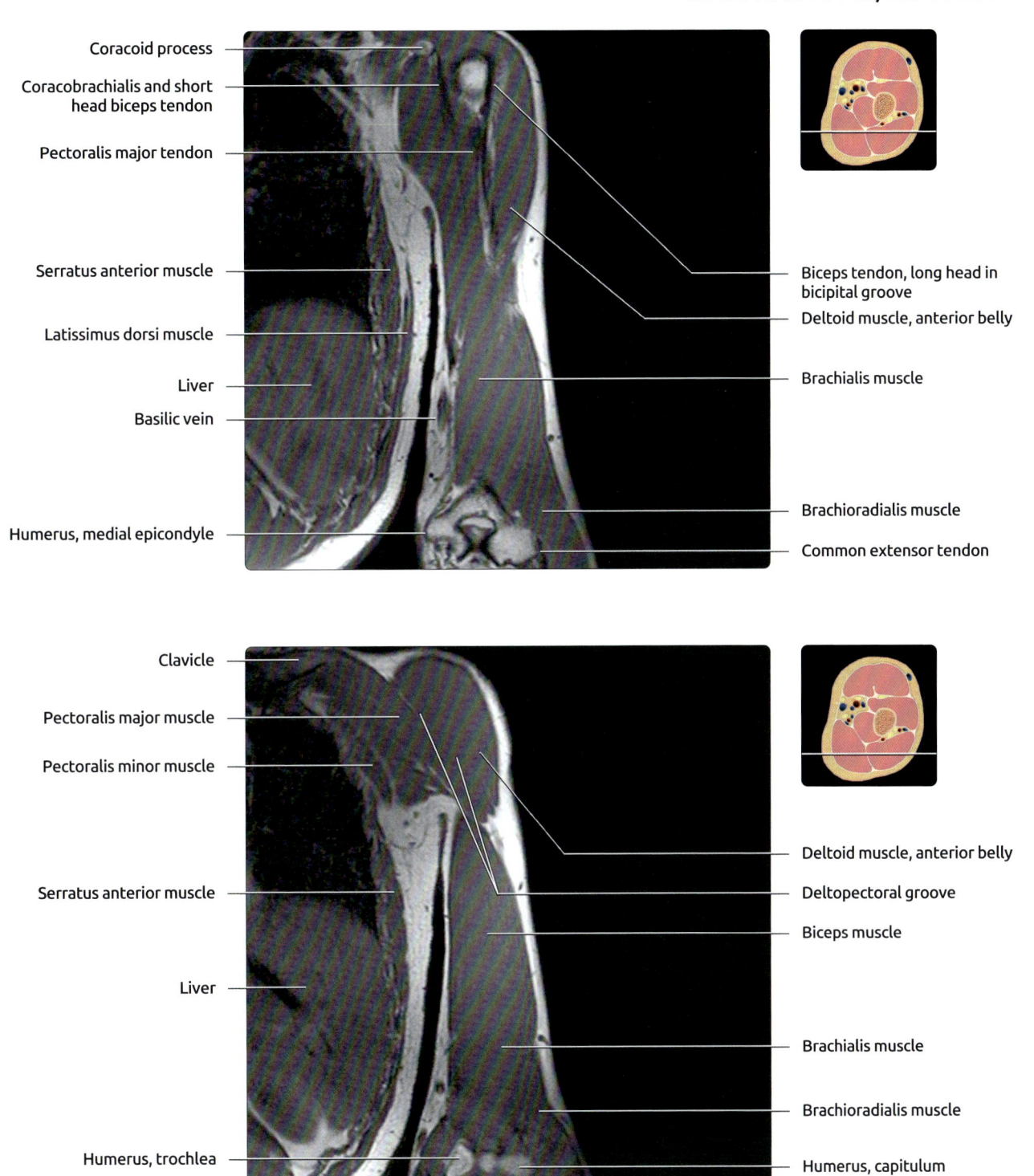

(Top) *The long head of the biceps tendon traverses the bicipital groove. The biceps long head and short head fuse at the upper humeral level.* (Bottom) *The most anterior image shows the deltoid muscle at the shoulder level and the biceps muscle along the length of the upper arm.*

Arm Radiographic Anatomy and MR Atlas

SAGITTAL T1 MR, RIGHT ARM

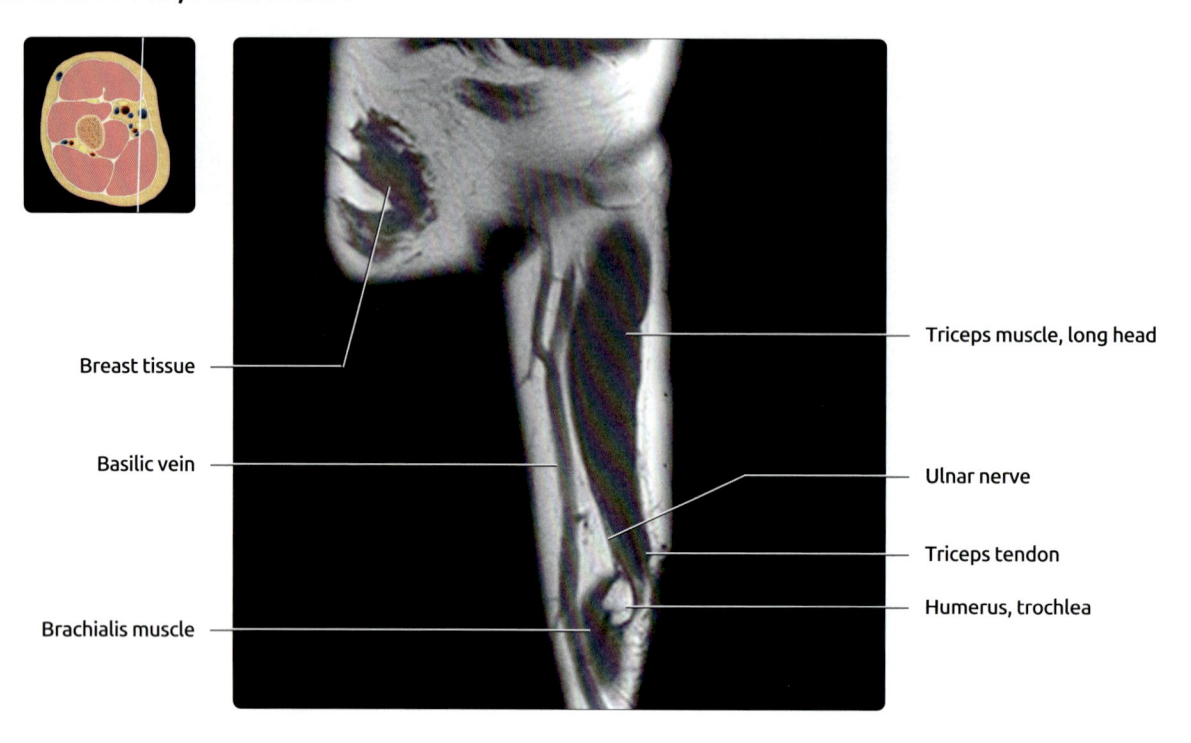

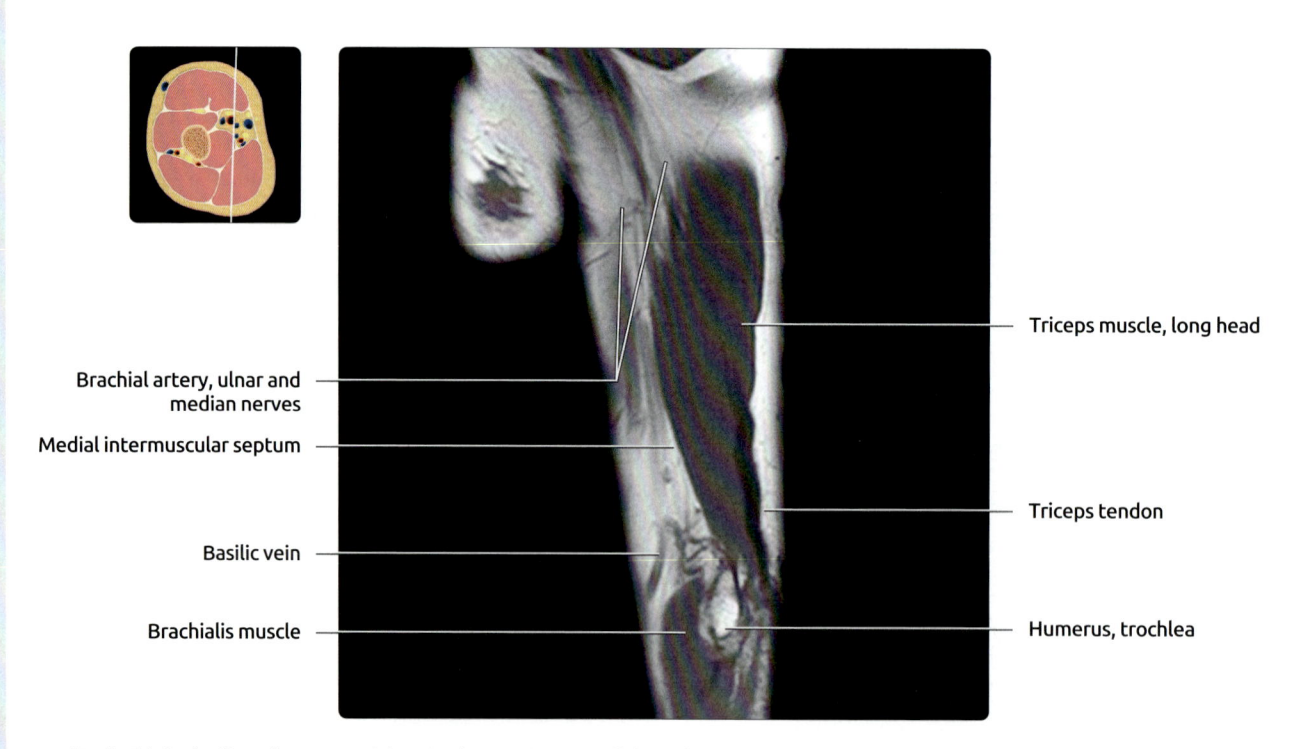

Top image labels:
- Breast tissue
- Basilic vein
- Brachialis muscle
- Triceps muscle, long head
- Ulnar nerve
- Triceps tendon
- Humerus, trochlea

Bottom image labels:
- Brachial artery, ulnar and median nerves
- Medial intermuscular septum
- Basilic vein
- Brachialis muscle
- Triceps muscle, long head
- Triceps tendon
- Humerus, trochlea

(Top) This is the first of 8 sequential sagittal T1 MR images of the right arm displayed medial to lateral. Images were acquired at 3T. The basilic vein courses distally down the medial arm. **(Bottom)** The medial intermuscular septum separates the anterior compartment from the triceps muscle in the posterior compartment.

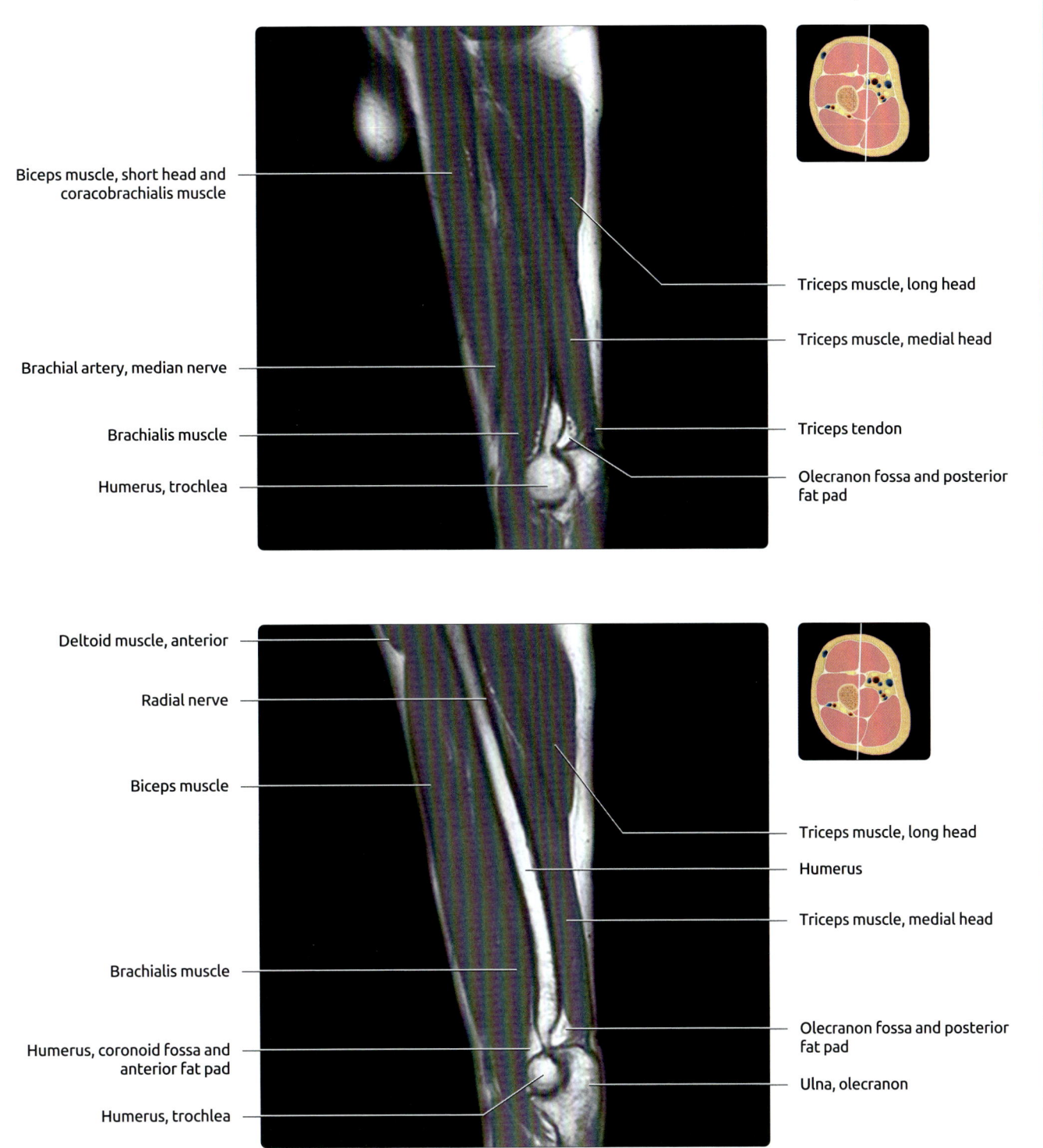

Arm Radiographic Anatomy and MR Atlas

SAGITTAL T1 MR, RIGHT ARM

- Biceps muscle, short head and coracobrachialis muscle
- Brachial artery, median nerve
- Brachialis muscle
- Humerus, trochlea
- Triceps muscle, long head
- Triceps muscle, medial head
- Triceps tendon
- Olecranon fossa and posterior fat pad

- Deltoid muscle, anterior
- Radial nerve
- Biceps muscle
- Brachialis muscle
- Humerus, coronoid fossa and anterior fat pad
- Humerus, trochlea
- Triceps muscle, long head
- Humerus
- Triceps muscle, medial head
- Olecranon fossa and posterior fat pad
- Ulna, olecranon

(**Top**) *The triceps medial head lies deep to the long and lateral heads.* (**Bottom**) *The brachialis muscle originates from the anterior humeral cortex and inserts on the ulnar tuberosity.*

Arm Radiographic Anatomy and MR Atlas

SAGITTAL T1 MR, RIGHT ARM

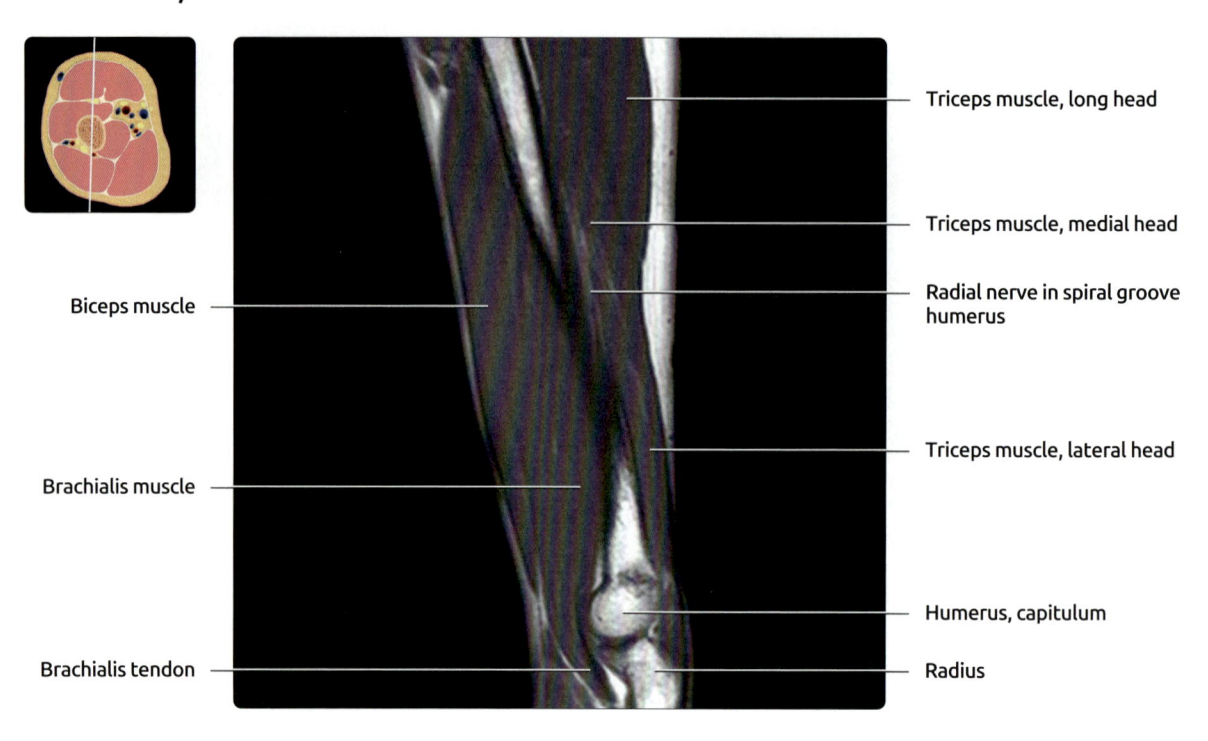

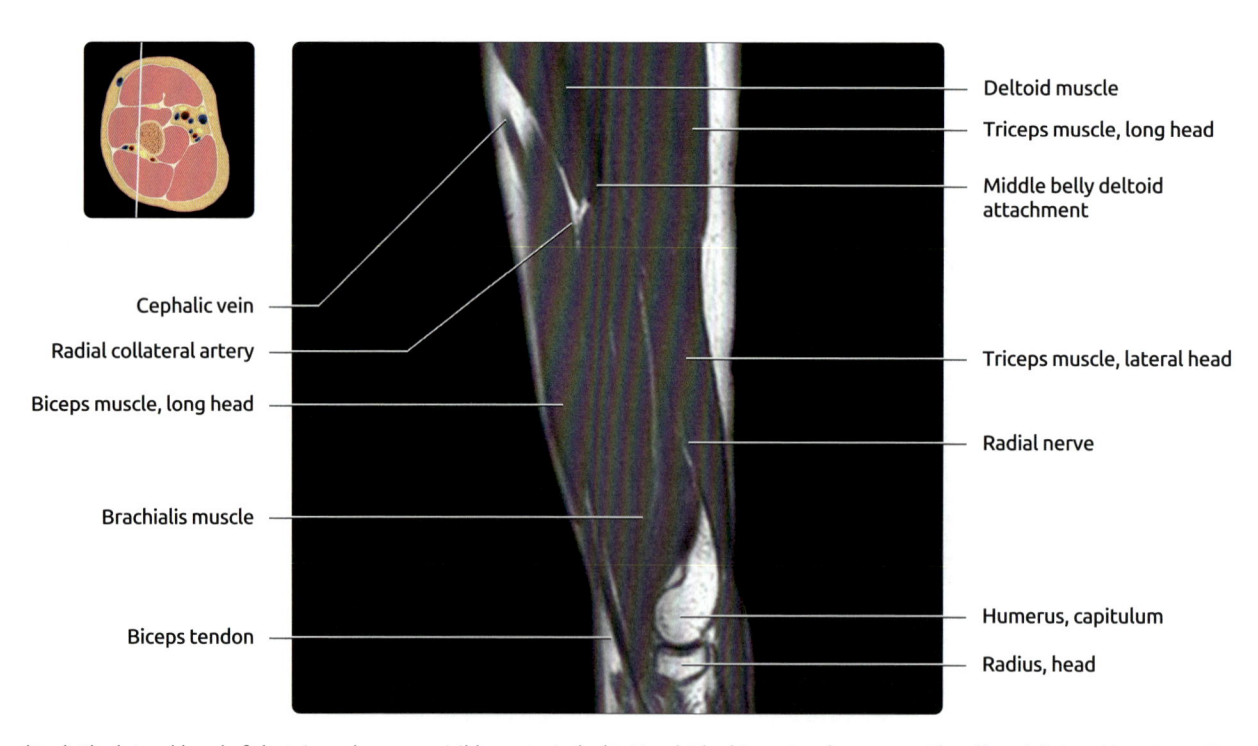

Top image labels:
- Triceps muscle, long head
- Triceps muscle, medial head
- Radial nerve in spiral groove humerus
- Triceps muscle, lateral head
- Humerus, capitulum
- Radius
- Biceps muscle
- Brachialis muscle
- Brachialis tendon

Bottom image labels:
- Deltoid muscle
- Triceps muscle, long head
- Middle belly deltoid attachment
- Triceps muscle, lateral head
- Radial nerve
- Humerus, capitulum
- Radius, head
- Cephalic vein
- Radial collateral artery
- Biceps muscle, long head
- Brachialis muscle
- Biceps tendon

(**Top**) *The lateral head of the triceps becomes visible posteriorly.* (**Bottom**) *The biceps tendon crosses the elbow joint and inserts on the radial tuberosity.*

Arm Radiographic Anatomy and MR Atlas

SAGITTAL T1 MR, RIGHT ARM

Top image labels:
- Deltoid muscle, middle belly
- Cephalic vein
- Triceps muscle, lateral head
- Lateral intermuscular septum
- Brachialis muscle
- Humerus, lateral epicondyle
- Radius, head

Bottom image labels:
- Deltoid muscle
- Cephalic vein
- Brachialis muscle
- Triceps muscle, lateral head
- Median cephalic vein
- Brachioradialis muscle
- Extensor carpi radialis longus

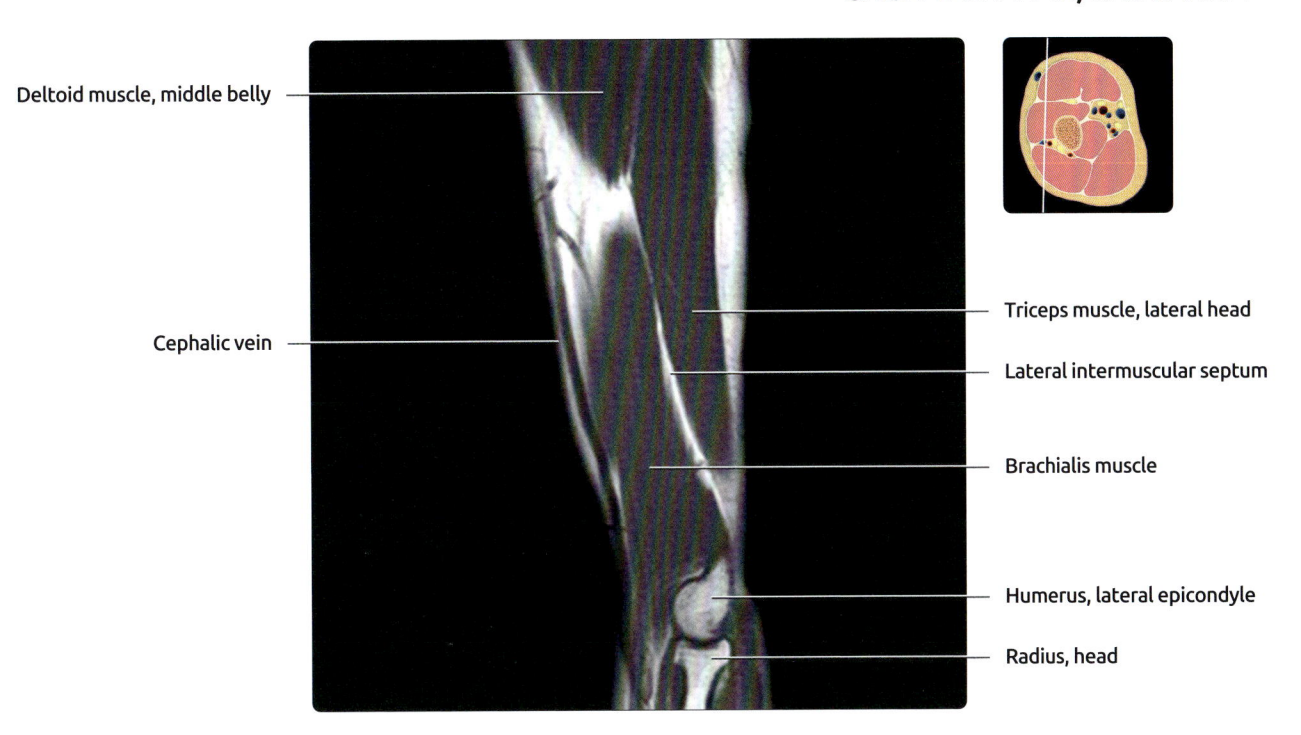

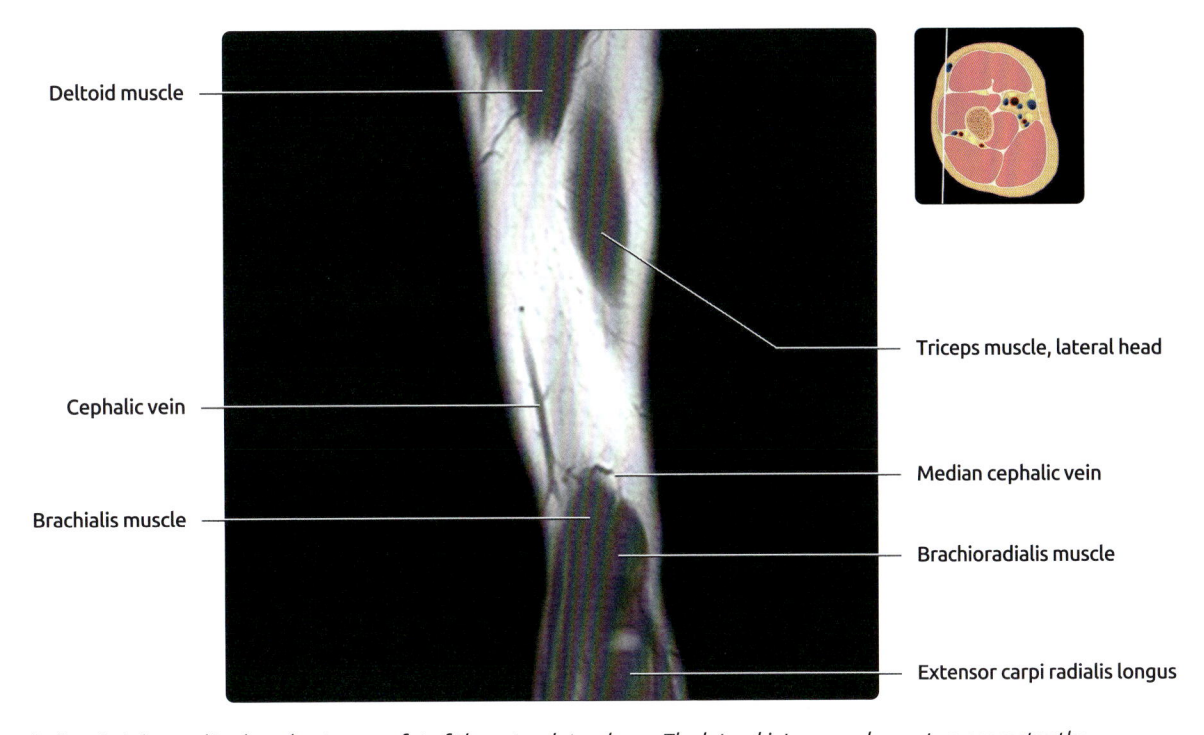

(Top) The cephalic vein is located in the subcutaneous fat of the anterolateral arm. The lateral intermuscular septum separates the anterior from posterior compartment. (Bottom) The extensor carpi radialis longus originates from the lateral epicondyle of the humerus.

SECTION 3
Elbow

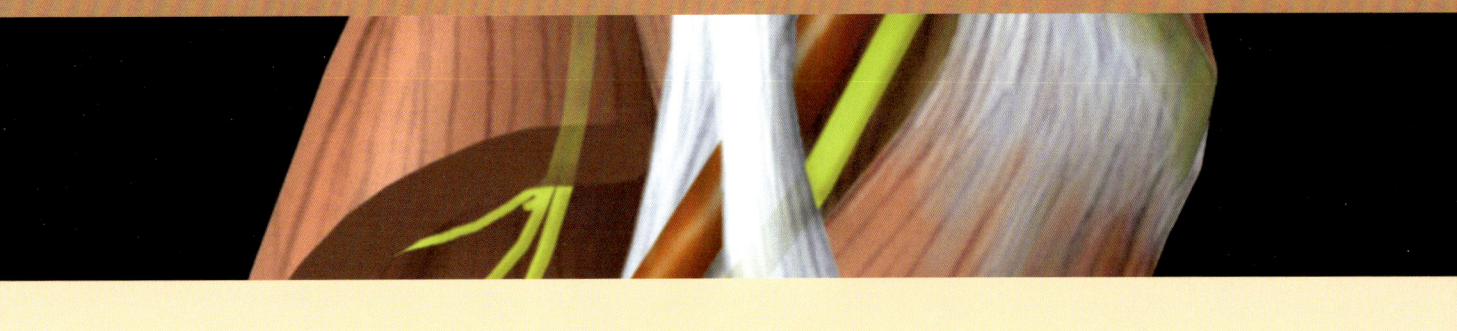

Elbow Overview	**194**
Elbow Radiographic and Arthrographic Anatomy	**200**
Elbow MR Atlas	**214**
Elbow Muscles and Tendons	**248**
Elbow Ligaments	**270**
Elbow Normal Variants and Imaging Pitfalls	**280**
Elbow Measurements and Lines	**292**

Elbow Overview

GROSS ANATOMY

Joint
- Complex joint composed of humerus, ulna, and radius
- Has 3 articulations
  - **Humeroulnar articulation**
    - Composed of trochlea of humerus and trochlear notch of ulna
    - Hinge joint, allowing flexion and extension
    - Osseous configuration provides medial-lateral stability between 0° and 30° flexion
  - **Humeroradial articulation**
    - Composed of capitellum and radial head
    - Allows both hinge and pivot motion
    - No inherent osseous stability
  - **Proximal radioulnar joint**
    - Composed of radial head and sigmoid notch of proximal ulna
    - Pivot joint, allowing radial head to rotate as forearm supinates and pronates
    - Stability is provided by annular ligament, holding head within notch
  - Congruity of articulating surfaces varies with position of both elbow and forearm: Greatest congruity when elbow flexed 90° and forearm midway between supination and pronation
- **Joint capsule**
  - Encloses all 3 articulations
  - Posterior attachments: Humerus proximal to olecranon fossa and capitellum, olecranon process anterior to triceps tendon
  - Anterior attachments: Humerus proximal to coronoid and radial fossae, coronoid process, annular ligament
  - Anterior and posterior fat pads are intracapsular but extrasynovial
- **Motion of elbow joint**
  - **Flexion**
    - Brachialis muscle: Originates at anterior surface of humerus and inserts on anterior tuberosity of ulna
    - Biceps brachii muscle: Originates at shoulder and inserts on radial tuberosity
    - Brachioradialis muscle: Originates from lateral supracondylar ridge of humerus and inserts on lateral side of distal radius
    - Pronator teres muscle: Originates from medial epicondyle and coronoid process of ulna and inserts on lateral side of midshaft of radius
  - **Extension**
    - Triceps muscle: Originates from shoulder and proximal humerus and inserts on olecranon
    - Anconeus muscle: Originates from posterior aspect of lateral epicondyle and inserts on lateral aspect of ulna and olecranon (also abducts ulna during pronation)
- **Motion of proximal radioulnar joint**
  - **Supination**
    - Biceps brachii muscle (see "flexion" bullet)
    - Supinator muscle: Originates from lateral epicondyle and supinator crest of ulna and inserts anteriorly & on lateral side of proximal shaft of radius
  - **Pronation**
    - Pronator teres muscle (see "flexion" bullet)
    - Pronator quadratus muscle: Located in distal forearm, originates on distal ulna and inserts on distal radius

Ligaments
- Lateral
  - **Radial collateral ligament**
    - Restrains against varus stress
    - Originates on lateral epicondyle and distally blends with annular ligament
  - **Lateral ulnar collateral ligament**
    - Restrains against posterolateral instability
    - Originates on lateral epicondyle, just posterior to radial collateral ligament
    - Courses posteromedially behind radial neck to insert on supinator crest on radial side of proximal ulna
- Medial
  - **Medial (also called ulnar) collateral ligament**
    - Restrains against valgus stress
    - Fan-shaped, extending from medial epicondyle to ulna
    - Has 3 components: Anterior band (functionally most important), posterior band, transverse band
- Ligaments of proximal radioulnar joint
  - **Annular ligament**: Attached to anterior and posterior aspects of radial notch of ulna, forming collar around radial head
  - **Quadrate ligament**: Thin fibrous band extending from radial neck to ulna, distal to annular ligament

Tendons
- Several flexor and extensor muscles of forearm arise from medial and lateral epicondyles of humerus
  - **Common flexor tendon**
    - Arises from medial epicondyle
    - Superficial to medial collateral ligament
    - Composed of flexor/pronator group: Flexor carpi radialis, flexor carpi ulnaris, flexor digitorum superficialis, pronator teres, palmaris longus
  - **Common extensor tendon**
    - Arises from lateral epicondyle
    - Superficial to radial collateral ligament
    - Composed of extensor/supinator group: Extensor carpi radialis brevis, extensor carpi radialis longus, extensor digiti minimi, extensor digitorum communis

Bursae
- Posterior
  - **Subcutaneous olecranon bursa**: Located subcutaneously, superficial to olecranon process
  - **Subtendinous olecranon bursa**: Located between triceps tendon and olecranon
- Anterior
  - **Bicipitoradial bursa**: Located between biceps tendon and radial tuberosity
- Lateral
  - **Radioulnar bursa**: Located between extensor digitorum and radiohumeral joint

Vessels
- Brachial artery
  - Continuation of axillary artery

Elbow Overview

- Located in cubital fossa, medial to biceps tendon and deep to biceps aponeurosis
- Accompanies median nerve
- Has several branches in arm
  - Deep brachial: Descends posterolaterally with radial nerve, has branches anterior and posterior to lateral condyle forming anastomosis
  - Superior ulnar collateral: Arises medially and descends with ulnar nerve posterior to medial condyle, forms anastomosis with branches of ulnar artery
  - Inferior ulnar collateral: Arises distal to superior ulnar collateral artery, descends anterior to medial condyle, forming anastomosis with branches of ulnar artery
- Divides into radial artery and ulnar artery at level of radial neck
- **Cephalic vein**
  - Lies lateral to biceps
- **Basilic vein**
  - Lies medial to biceps

Nerves

- **Radial nerve**
  - Arises from posterior cord of brachial plexus (C5-C8, T1)
  - Spirals posterolaterally around humerus with deep brachial artery
    - Gives off posterior cutaneous nerve of forearm, which passes posterior to lateral condyle and supplies posterior forearm
  - Located anterolateral, between brachialis and brachioradialis
  - Supplies triceps, anconeus, brachioradialis, and lateral portion of brachialis
  - Gives articular branches to elbow joint
  - Divides into deep and superficial branches at lateral epicondyle
  - **Deep branch**
    - Purely motor
    - Supplies extensor carpi radialis brevis and supinator muscles
    - Pierces supinator muscle and winds around lateral aspect of radial neck
    - Exits supinator muscle in posterior compartment of forearm as posterior interosseous nerve
    - Posterior interosseous nerve supplies extensor muscles of posterior compartment of forearm
    - Posterior interosseous nerve syndrome: Compression of deep branch by arcade of Frohse (superficial proximal margin of supinator)
  - **Superficial branch**
    - Purely sensory
    - Located in anterolateral aspect of forearm superficial to supinator and pronator teres muscles
- **Median nerve**
  - Arises from both medial and lateral cords of brachial plexus (C5-C8, T1)
  - Located in cubital fossa, deep to biceps aponeurosis
  - Gives articular branches to elbow joint
  - Enters forearm by passing between heads of pronator teres and located in forearm between flexor digitorum superficialis and profundus muscles
  - May get compressed by biceps aponeurosis or by either head of pronator teres (pronator teres syndrome)
  - Supplies pronator teres, pronator quadratus, and flexors of anterior compartment of forearm (except flexor carpi ulnaris and medial half of flexor digitorum profundus, supplied by ulnar nerve)
  - **Anterior interosseous nerve**
    - Arises from median nerve at level of pronator teres
    - Located in forearm, anterior to interosseous membrane, between flexor pollicis longus and flexor digitorum profundus
    - Supplies flexor pollicis longus, pronator quadratus, and lateral half of flexor digitorum profundus
    - Kiloh-Nevin syndrome: Compression of anterior interosseous nerve by ulnar head of pronator teres
- **Ulnar nerve**
  - Arises from medial cord of brachial plexus (C8, T1)
  - Located posteromedially, deep to triceps muscles in distal arm
  - Passes posterior to medial epicondyle in cubital tunnel
    - **Cubital tunnel**: Fibroosseous tunnel formed by medial epicondyle and cubital retinaculum (arcuate ligament of Osborne)
    - Cubital tunnel syndrome: Pain and weakness of 4th and 5th fingers due to compression of ulnar nerve in cubital tunnel
  - May sublux anterior to medial epicondyle in about 15% of people, usually during flexion
  - Gives articular branches to elbow joint
  - Continues into forearm by dividing into superficial and deep heads of flexor carpi ulnaris
  - Supplies flexor carpi ulnaris and medial half of flexor digitorum profundus
- **Musculocutaneous nerve**
  - Arises from lateral cord of brachial plexus (C5, C6, C7)
  - Lies between brachialis and biceps brachii muscles and supplies both
  - Gives articular branches to elbow joint
  - Becomes superficial at elbow joint, continuing laterally as lateral cutaneous nerve of forearm, which innervates skin of lateral side of forearm
- **Medial cutaneous nerve of forearm**
  - Accompanies basilic vein in arm
  - Located superficially at elbow, anterior to medial epicondyle
  - Supplies sensation to posteromedial forearm

SELECTED REFERENCES

1. Rosenberg ZS et al: MR features of nerve disorders at the elbow. Magn Reson Imaging Clin N Am. 5(3):545-65, 1997
2. Rosenberg ZS et al: MR imaging of normal variants and interpretation pitfalls of the elbow. Magn Reson Imaging Clin N Am. 5(3):481-99, 1997

GRAPHIC: JOINT CAPSULE, LATERAL VIEW

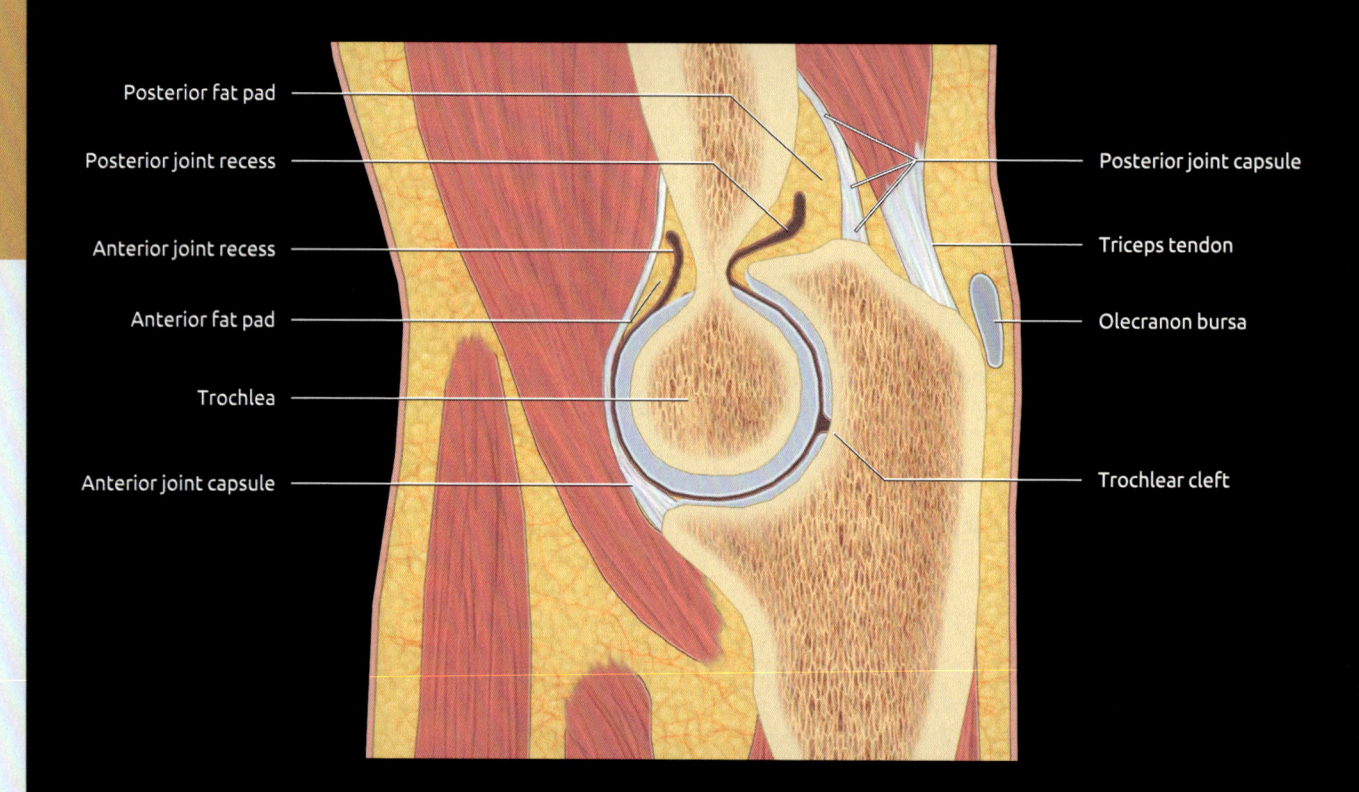

- Posterior fat pad
- Posterior joint recess
- Anterior joint recess
- Anterior fat pad
- Trochlea
- Anterior joint capsule
- Posterior joint capsule
- Triceps tendon
- Olecranon bursa
- Trochlear cleft

The anterior and posterior fat pads are intracapsular but extrasynovial. They may be pushed outward by a joint effusion. Note the trochlear cleft, which is the border of the olecranon and coronoid and is not covered by articular cartilage; it may mimic a loose body or be seen as a pseudodefect.

Elbow Overview

GRAPHICS: AXIAL ELBOW

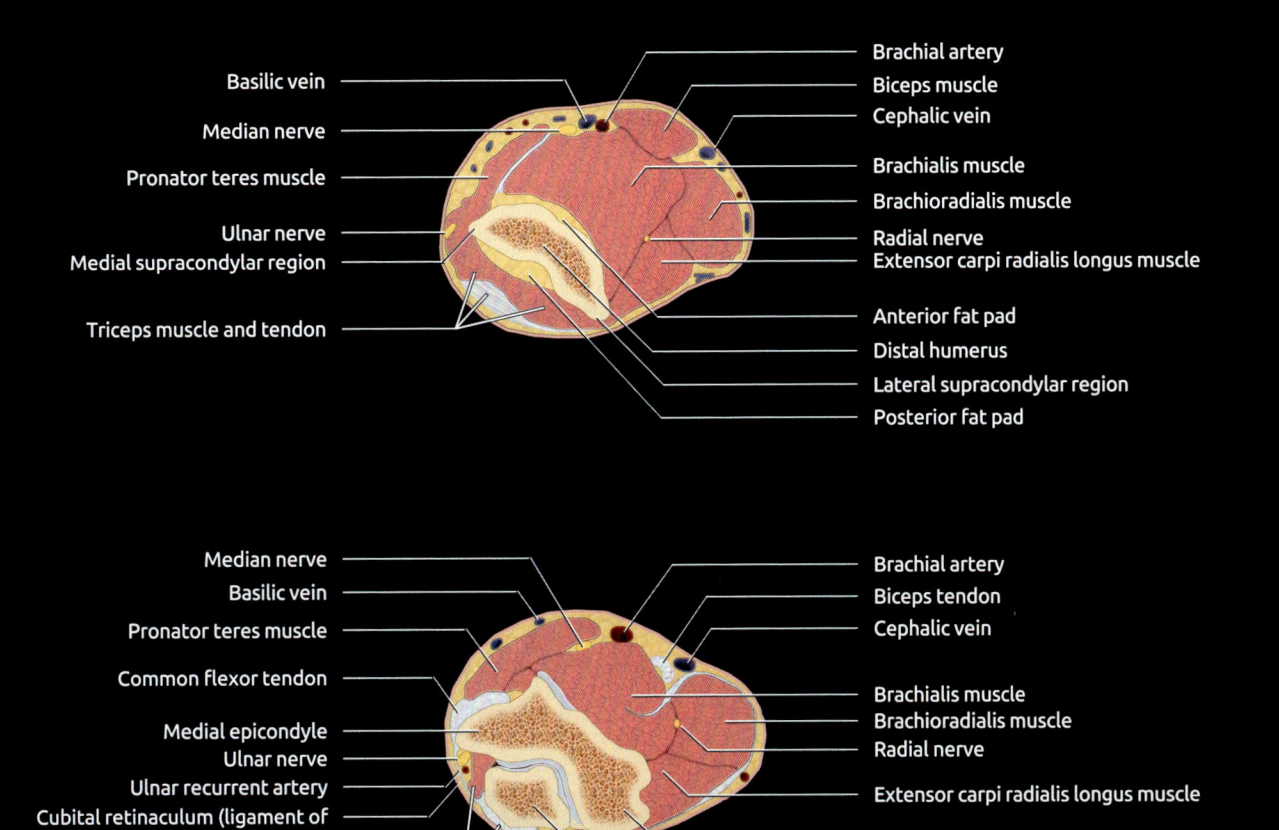

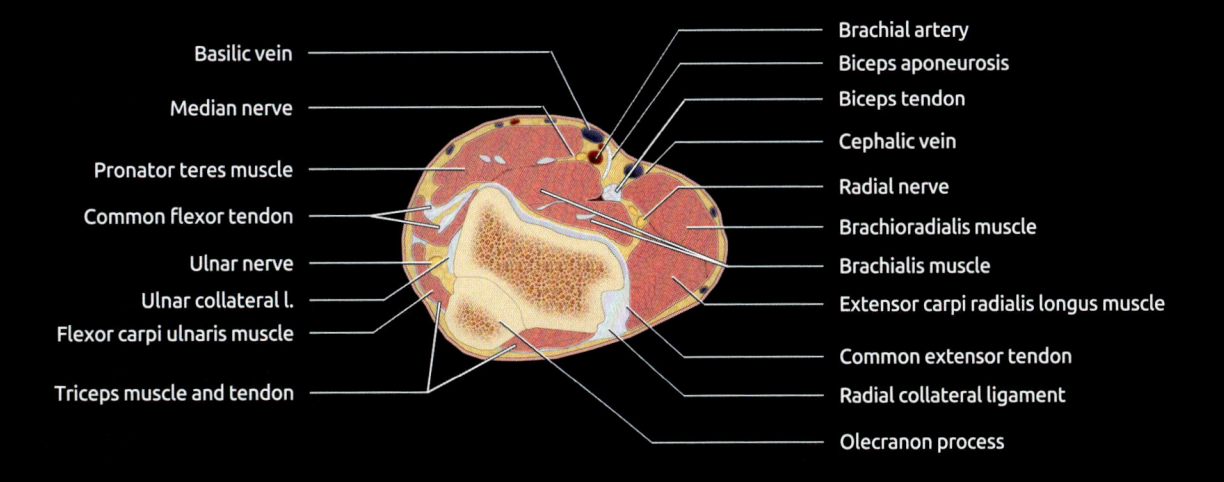

(Top) Axial graphic shows the supracondylar region of the humerus. The anterior and posterior fat pads are seen in the coronoid and olecranon fossae, respectively. The brachialis muscle accounts for the bulk of the anterior compartment of the distal arm. (Middle) Axial graphic shows the epicondylar region of the distal humerus. The triceps muscle thins as its tendon attaches to the olecranon. The ulnar nerve and posterior ulnar recurrent artery are held in the cubital tunnel by the cubital retinaculum (the ligament of Osborne). (Bottom) Axial graphic immediately proximal to the elbow joint, below the level of the epicondyles is shown. The common extensor tendon overlies the radial collateral ligament and may be difficult to distinguish at this level. The ulnar nerve has exited the cubital tunnel and is entering the flexor carpi ulnaris.

Elbow Overview

GRAPHICS: AXIAL ELBOW

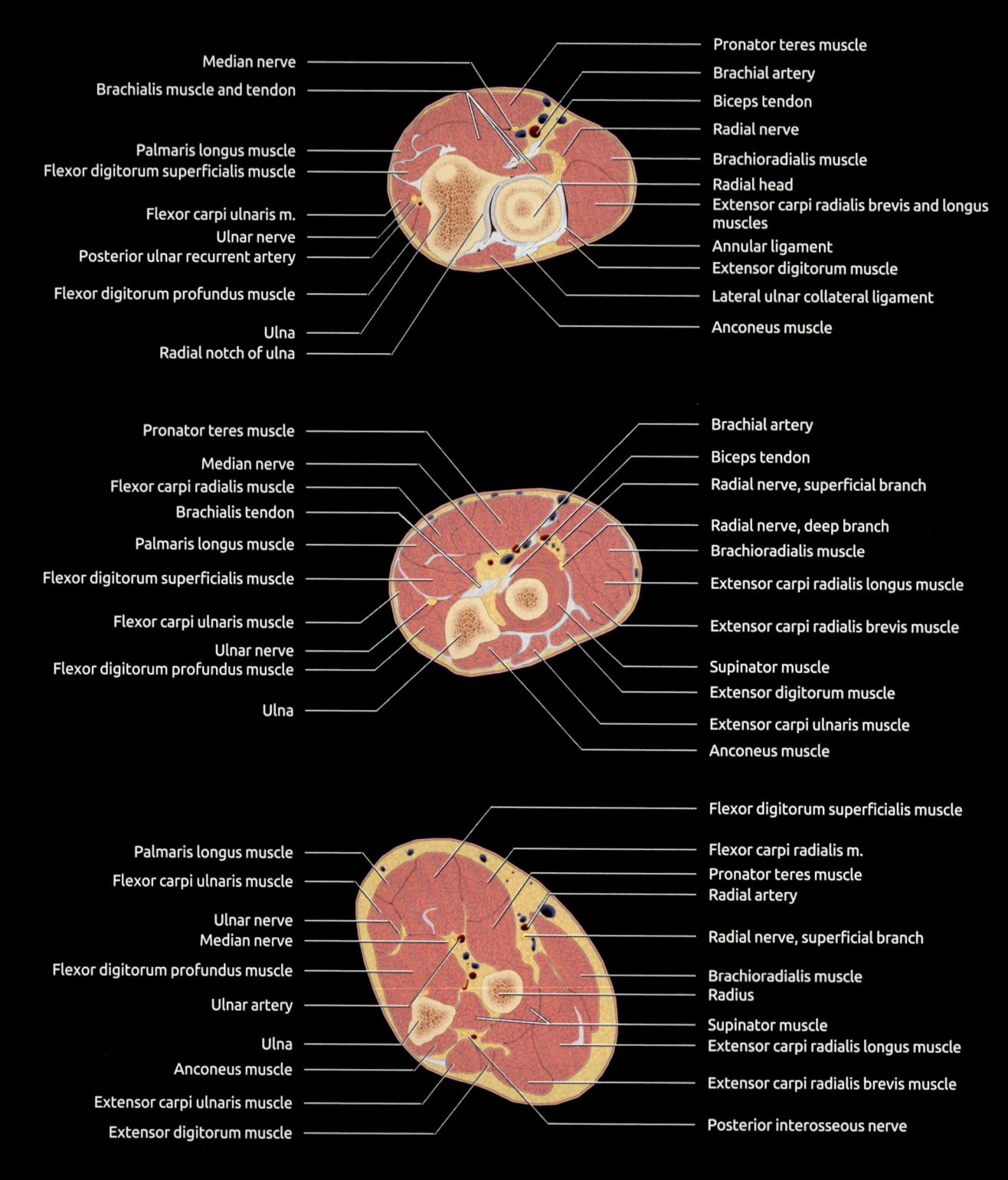

(Top) Axial graphic at the level of the proximal radioulnar joint. The articulating surfaces of the proximal radioulnar joint are well seen as the radial head is held in the radial notch of the ulna by the annular ligament. The lateral ulnar collateral ligament blends with the posterior aspect of the annular ligament before inserting on the ulna. **(Middle)** This graphic shows the axial elbow at a level immediately above the radial tuberosity. The brachialis tendon is inserting on the ulnar tuberosity and the biceps tendon is approaching its insertion on the radial tuberosity, which is more distal than the brachialis insertion. **(Bottom)** At the level of the proximal forearm, the muscles are starting to align themselves into the anterior (flexor) compartment and the posterior (extensor) compartment.

Elbow Overview

GRAPHICS: ARTERIES AND NERVES AROUND ELBOW

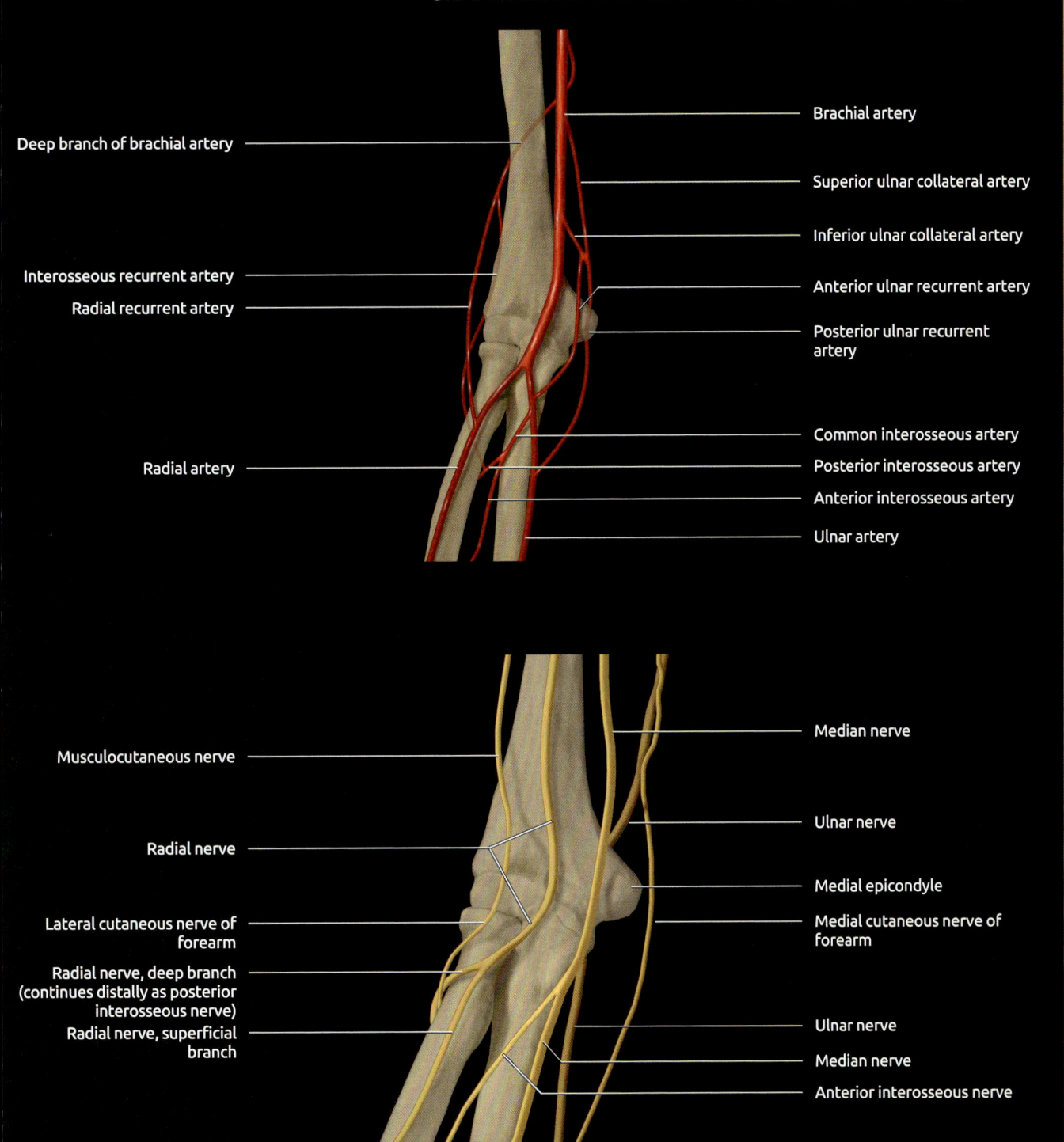

Labels (top image):
- Deep branch of brachial artery
- Interosseous recurrent artery
- Radial recurrent artery
- Radial artery
- Brachial artery
- Superior ulnar collateral artery
- Inferior ulnar collateral artery
- Anterior ulnar recurrent artery
- Posterior ulnar recurrent artery
- Common interosseous artery
- Posterior interosseous artery
- Anterior interosseous artery
- Ulnar artery

Labels (bottom image):
- Musculocutaneous nerve
- Radial nerve
- Lateral cutaneous nerve of forearm
- Radial nerve, deep branch (continues distally as posterior interosseous nerve)
- Radial nerve, superficial branch
- Median nerve
- Ulnar nerve
- Medial epicondyle
- Medial cutaneous nerve of forearm
- Ulnar nerve
- Median nerve
- Anterior interosseous nerve

(Top) The brachial artery, the major artery of the arm, is a direct continuation of the axillary artery. It gives off several branches in the arm that form anastomoses medially and laterally with branches from the ulnar and radial arteries, respectively, which are themselves terminal branches of the brachial artery. *(Bottom)* The nerves of the elbow region and their major branches are shown. The lateral cutaneous nerve of the forearm is a continuation of the musculocutaneous nerve of the arm. The deep branch of the radial nerve winds around the radial neck through the supinator muscle to become the posterior interosseous nerve of the forearm. The ulnar nerve is located posterior to the medial epicondyle and enters the forearm by passing between the superficial and deep heads of the flexor carpi ulnaris muscle. The anterior interosseous nerve is a branch of the median nerve, originating between the pronator teres muscle proximally and the biceps aponeurosis distally.

Elbow Radiographic and Arthrographic Anatomy

IMAGING ANATOMY

Overview

- Distal humerus has 2 articular surfaces
  - Trochlea located medially, articulates with ulna
    - Continuous posteriorly with olecranon fossa
    - Olecranon fossa articulates with olecranon process of ulna
  - Capitellum located laterally, articulates with radius
  - Trochlea and capitellum separated by intercondylar ridge
  - Hyaline cartilage continuous across trochlea and capitellum
- Proximal radius
  - Round, slightly concave articular surface (fovea) articulates with capitellum
- Proximal ulna
  - Olecranon process articulates with trochlea and olecranon fossa
    - Articular surface called trochlear notch
  - Coronoid process: Triangular tip of anterior articular margin
  - Sublime tubercle: Discrete projection medial margin
    - Insertion of ulnar collateral ligament
- Ulna-humeral joint is a pure hinge joint
  - Flexion and extension only
- Radiocapitellar joint allows more complex motions
  - Flexion, extension, pronation, supination
- Proximal radioulnar joint
  - Hyaline cartilage surfaces on apposing surfaces of radius and ulna
  - Allows pronation, supination

Internal Contents

- **Joint capsule**
  - Capsule redundant anteriorly and posteriorly to allow flexion/extension
  - Capsule tight medially and laterally, prohibiting varus/valgus motion
    - Reinforced by medial and lateral collateral ligaments
  - Superior extent: Slightly above olecranon fossa both anteriorly and posteriorly
  - Inferior extent: Metaphysis of radius, coronoid process of ulna
    - Joint recesses distal to annular ligament consistently fill at arthrography
  - Medially and laterally: Capsule tightly parallels underlying bones, reinforced by collateral ligaments
- **Ulnar collateral ligament (UCL)**
  - Also called medial collateral ligament
  - Stabilizes to valgus stress
  - Has 3 components: Anterior, posterior, and transverse bands
  - Anterior band
    - Functionally most important
    - Arises on inferior surface of medial epicondyle
    - Inserts on sublime tubercle of ulna
    - Deep to flexor tendon origin
  - Posterior band
    - Arises on medial epicondyle
    - Inserts on olecranon process
  - Transverse band
    - Functionally not important
    - Extends from posterior to anterior on olecranon process
- **Radial collateral ligament (RCL)**
  - Also called lateral collateral ligament (LCL)
  - Stabilizes to varus stress
  - Thinner than ulnar collateral ligament
  - Extends from lateral epicondyle to annular ligament
- **Lateral ulnar collateral ligament (LUCL)**
  - Also called radial ulnar collateral ligament
  - Provides posterolateral rotational stability
  - Arises posterior to radial collateral ligament on lateral epicondyle
  - Extends obliquely posteriorly and inferiorly, around radial head and neck
  - Blends with annular ligament posteriorly
  - Inserts distally on supinator crest of ulna
- **Annular ligament**
  - Forms collar around radial head
  - Attaches to radial notch of ulnar anteriorly and posteriorly
  - Blends with radial collateral and lateral ulnar collateral ligaments
  - Superficial head of supinator muscle arises from it
- **Accessory radial collateral ligament**
  - Variably present
  - Arises from anterior portion annular ligament
  - Inserts on supinator crest of ulna
  - Stabilizes annular ligament during varus stress
- **Synovial fringe or fold**
  - Meniscus-like structure variably present between capitellum and radial head
  - Infolding of synovium
  - May cause locking (snapping if enlarged) but no definite criteria accepted

ANATOMY IMAGING ISSUES

Imaging Approaches

- **Radiographs**
  - Standard views: AP, lateral, external oblique
  - AP view
    - Full extension, in full supination
    - Medial condyle is larger than lateral
    - Lucency in distal humerus due to olecranon & coronoid fossae
  - Lateral view
    - 90° flexion
    - Lucent anterior fat pad is normally visible as straight, slightly oblique line anterior to distal humerus
    - Posterior fat pad not visible unless there is effusion
    - Supinator line: Thin lucency of fat superficial to supinator muscle, parallels proximal radial shaft, displaced by radial head fracture or joint effusion
  - External oblique view
    - Useful to visualize radial head without overlap
  - Radial head view
    - Lateral, in 90° flexion, with x-ray beam angled transversely 45° to profile radial head & neck

Elbow Radiographic and Arthrographic Anatomy

- Flexed "ulnar sulcus" view
  - Elbow flexed with hand on shoulder, shoulder & elbow in same plane, x-ray beam straight down
  - Demonstrates olecranon process en face, medial & lateral epicondyles, and ulnar sulcus
- Arthrography
  - Best approach for procedure: Lateral
    - Patient prone, face turned away from procedure
    - Elbow flexed near 90° with arm over head
    - Thumb turned up
    - Position profiles radiocapitellar joint for needle placement at this site
    - May obtain same elbow position for lateral approach with patient seated next to fluoroscopy table, but experience shows this position more likely to result in vasovagal response to needle placement
  - Alternate approach for procedure: Posterior
    - Patient supine, elbow flexed, & elevated on pillow
    - Concavity posterior to capitellum is palpated, needle is placed at this dorsolateral side of joint and directed between olecranon and capitellum toward radial head
    - Position may be used with ultrasonic guidance
  - Avoid medial approach because of medial location of ulnar nerve
- MR arthrography
  - Preferred over routine MR for evaluation of stability of osteochondral fracture
  - May be preferred over routine MR for evaluation of integrity of medial collateral ligament
- MR protocol
  - In supine position, elbow may be scanned at patient's side
    - Imaging challenging in large patients because elbow is at periphery of magnet bore
  - "Superman" position
    - Patient prone, arm straight out over head
    - Bend head to side to avoid wraparound artifact
    - Motion may be a problem, especially in older patients who also have limited shoulder mobility
  - Use 3T magnet if possible
  - High-quality send-receive coil essential
    - Wrap coil
    - Wrist coil often works in children
    - If arm above head, can use combination of spine coil under elbow, flex coil on top of elbow (may provide increased signal compared to flex coil alone)
  - Axial, coronal, sagittal planes
  - For MR arthrogram, T1 FS MR weighting in 3 planes, plus T1 MR &/or T2 MR in most useful plane for individual clinical question
  - For nonarthrographic MR, PD FS weighted imaging in all 3 planes plus T1 MR in most useful plane for individual clinical question
- CT protocol
  - CT arthrography useful if MR contraindicated for patient
  - Positioning
    - Patient prone, arm above head
    - Patient on side, arm above head
    - Bend head to side to avoid beam-hardening artifact
    - Avoid imaging with arm to side if possible because of beam-hardening artifact

Imaging Pitfalls
- **Radiographic pitfalls**
  - Thin flange at medial & lateral distal humeral metaphysis
    - May mimic periosteal reaction
  - Lucency when radial tuberosity viewed en face
    - May mimic lytic lesion
  - Irregular ossification of epiphyses/apophyses in skeletally immature patients
    - Lateral epicondyle, trochlea, capitellum
    - May mimic osteochondral fracture or osteonecrosis
  - Notch at annular ligament insertion
    - May mimic incomplete fracture or erosion
- **MR arthrogram pitfalls**
  - Capitellar pseudodefect
    - Posterior aspect of articular surface of capitellum
    - Bony indentation with absent overlying cartilage
    - Osteochondral injuries may occur in this region; evaluate on T2WI to differentiate
  - Trochlear notch cartilage defect
    - Small, bowl-shaped
    - Centrally located in articular surface
  - Ulnar & radial collateral ligaments are thin
    - Be sure to visualize on MR arthrography as separate structure from adjacent flexor tendons

SELECTED REFERENCES

1. Magee T: Accuracy of 3-T MR arthrography versus conventional 3-T MRI of elbow tendons and ligaments compared with surgery. AJR Am J Roentgenol. 204(1):W70-5, 2015
2. van Wagenberg JM et al: The posterior transtriceps approach for intra-articular elbow diagnostics, definitely not forgotten. Skeletal Radiol. 42(1):55-9, 2013
3. Delport AG et al: MR and CT arthrography of the elbow. Semin Musculoskelet Radiol. 16(1):15-26, 2012
4. Munshi M et al: Anterior bundle of ulnar collateral ligament: evaluation of anatomic relationships by using MR imaging, MR arthrography, and gross anatomic and histologic analysis. Radiology. 231(3):797-803, 2004
5. Cotten A et al: Normal Anatomy of the Elbow on Conventional MR Imaging and MR Arthrography. Semin Musculoskelet Radiol. 2(2):133-140, 1998

Elbow Radiographic and Arthrographic Anatomy

RADIOGRAPHS: AP AND LATERAL

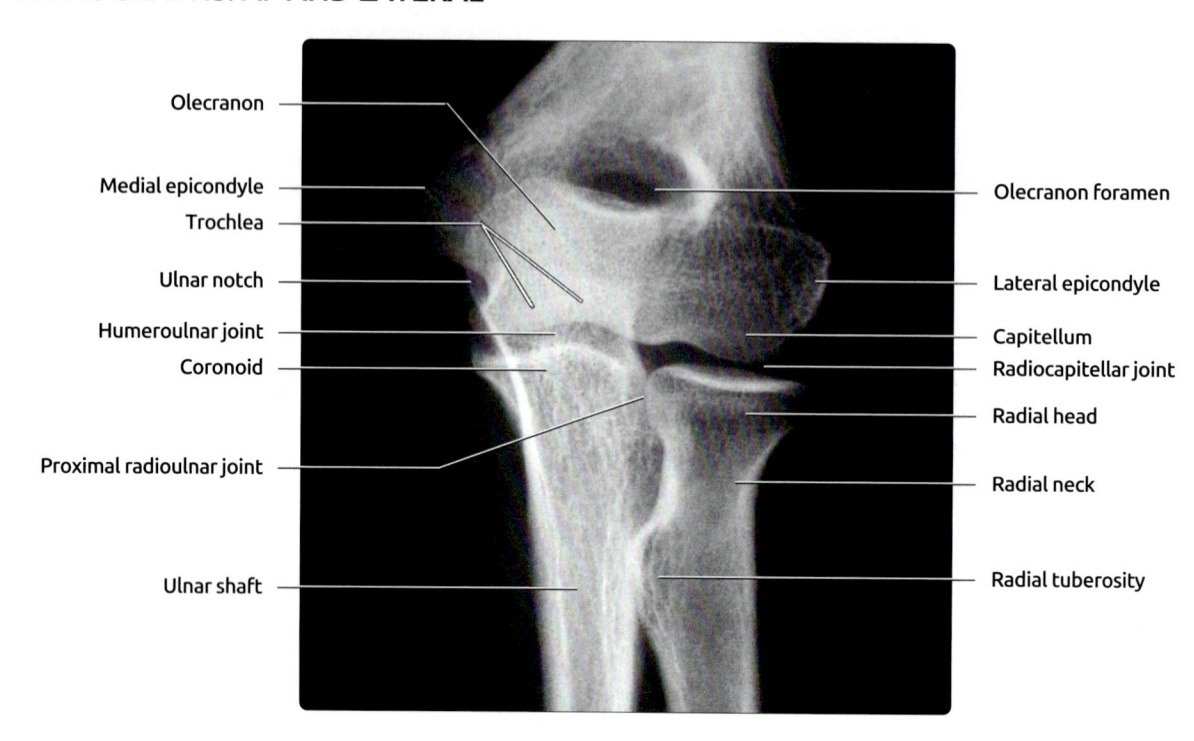

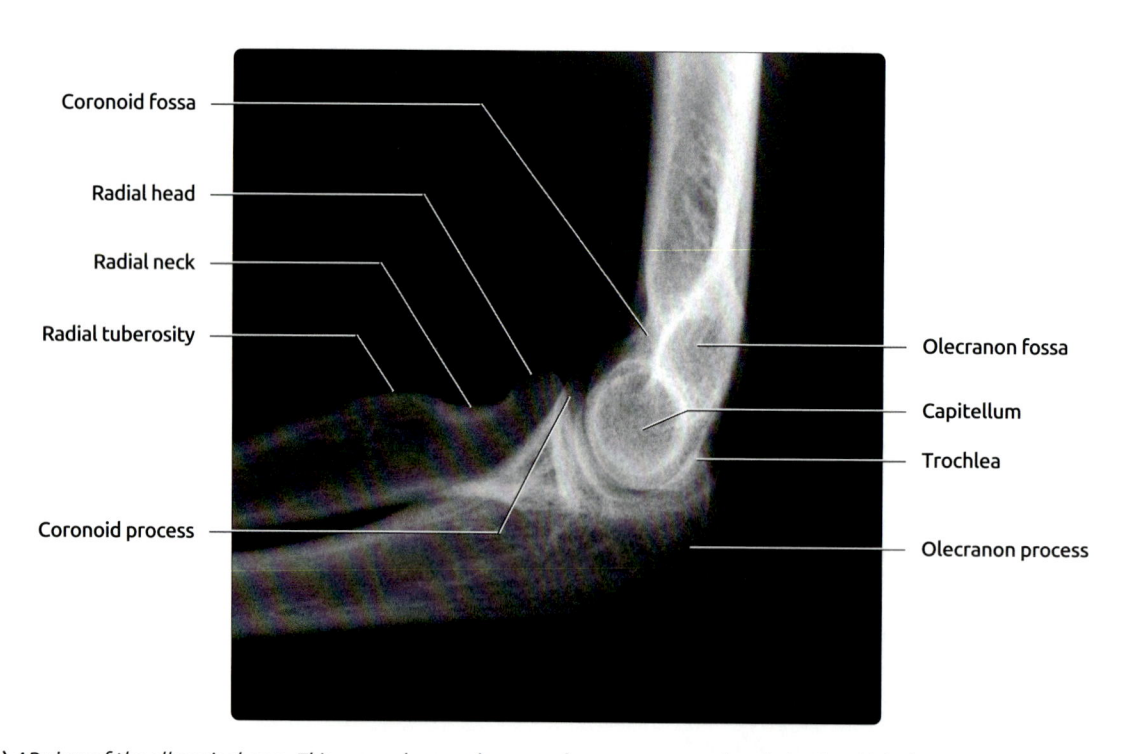

Labels (top, AP view): Olecranon; Medial epicondyle; Trochlea; Ulnar notch; Humeroulnar joint; Coronoid; Proximal radioulnar joint; Ulnar shaft; Olecranon foramen; Lateral epicondyle; Capitellum; Radiocapitellar joint; Radial head; Radial neck; Radial tuberosity.

Labels (bottom, lateral view): Coronoid fossa; Radial head; Radial neck; Radial tuberosity; Coronoid process; Olecranon fossa; Capitellum; Trochlea; Olecranon process.

(Top) *AP view of the elbow is shown. This person has an olecranon foramen, a normal variation in which there is a hole in the cortex between the olecranon fossa and coronoid fossa.* **(Bottom)** *A lateral radiograph is shown. The capitellum and trochlea are superimposed on each other. The head of the radius should always intersect the capitellum (radiocapitellar line) and a line drawn along the anterior cortex of the humerus should always intersect the middle of the capitellum (anterior humeral line).*

Elbow Radiographic and Arthrographic Anatomy

RADIOGRAPHS: EXTERNAL OBLIQUE AND RADIAL HEAD VIEWS

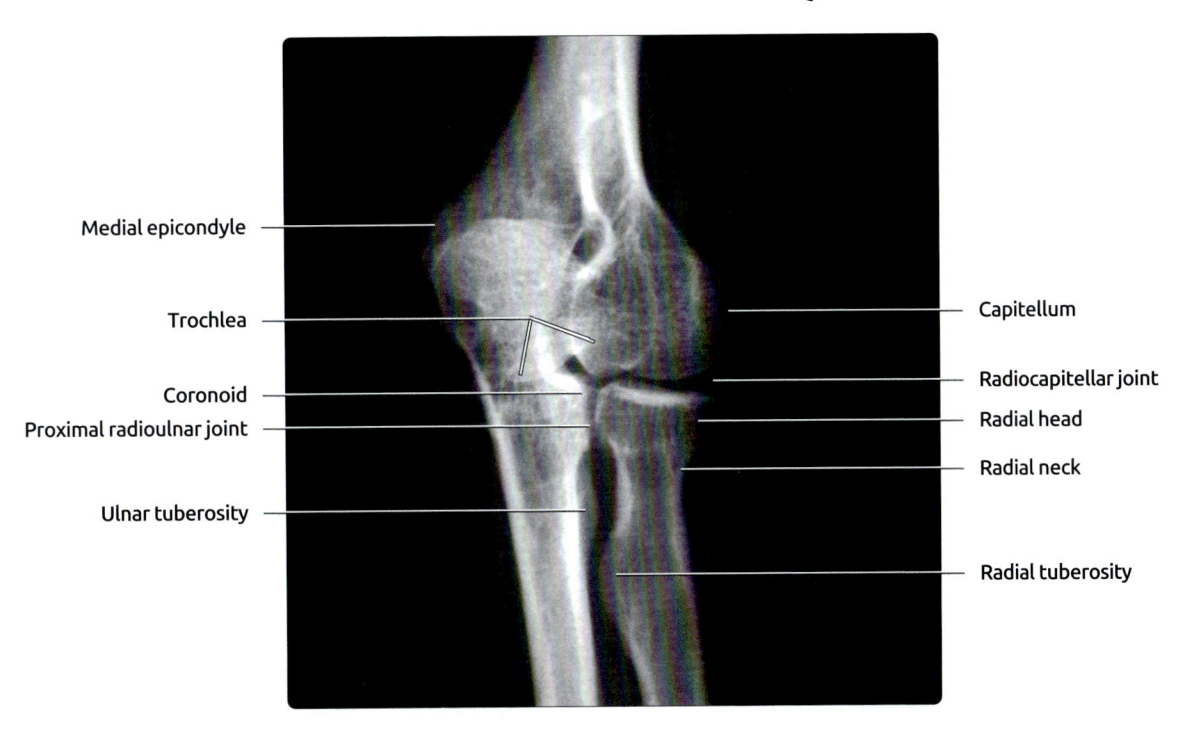

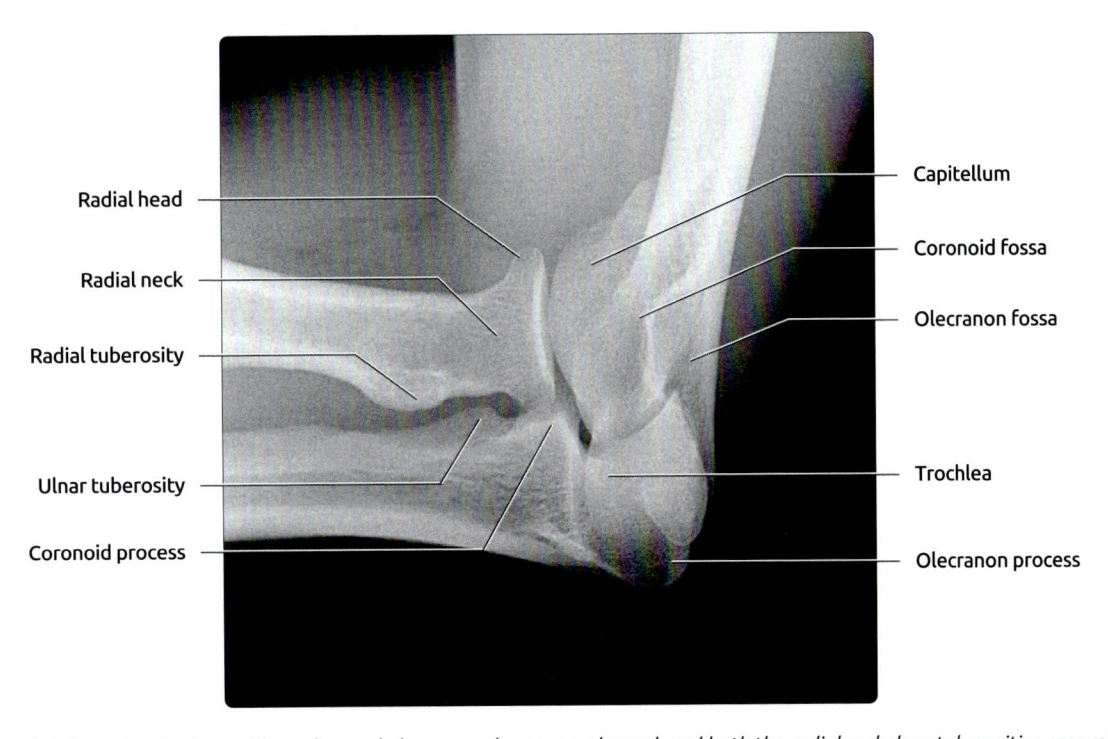

Top image labels:
- Medial epicondyle
- Trochlea
- Coronoid
- Proximal radioulnar joint
- Ulnar tuberosity
- Capitellum
- Radiocapitellar joint
- Radial head
- Radial neck
- Radial tuberosity

Bottom image labels:
- Radial head
- Radial neck
- Radial tuberosity
- Ulnar tuberosity
- Coronoid process
- Capitellum
- Coronoid fossa
- Olecranon fossa
- Trochlea
- Olecranon process

(Top) *External oblique view is shown. The radius and ulna are no longer overlapped, and both the radial and ulnar tuberosities are well seen. The internal oblique view is rarely obtained.* **(Bottom)** *Radial head view is shown. A lateral view with the x-ray beam angled transversely is demonstrated. The radial head is better seen than on a conventional lateral because the head is not overlapping the coronoid. This view is useful for the evaluation of a suspected radial head fracture.*

Elbow Radiographic and Arthrographic Anatomy

GRAPHIC: JOINT CAPSULE AND CORONAL CROSS SECTION

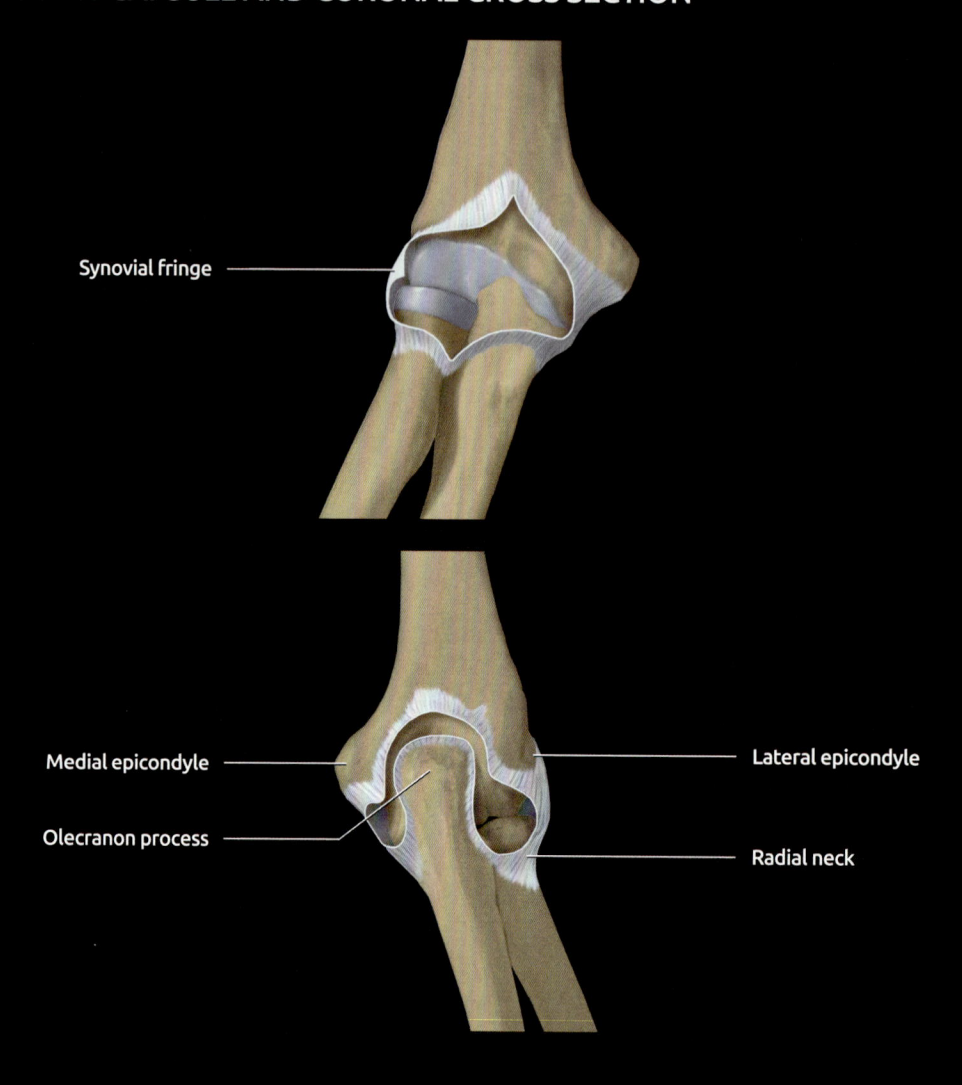

Synovial fringe

Medial epicondyle
Olecranon process

Lateral epicondyle
Radial neck

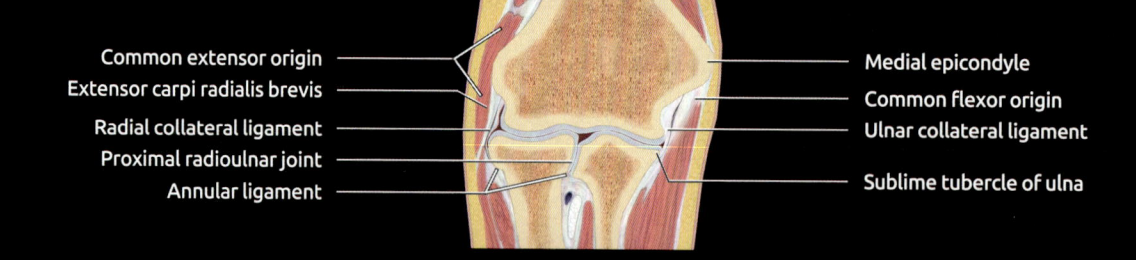

Common extensor origin
Extensor carpi radialis brevis
Radial collateral ligament
Proximal radioulnar joint
Annular ligament

Medial epicondyle
Common flexor origin
Ulnar collateral ligament
Sublime tubercle of ulna

(**Top**) The anterior aspect of the joint capsule has been removed, showing the outline of its osseous attachments. Notice the focal meniscus-like thickening of the capsule at the radiocapitellar joint, called the synovial fringe. (**Middle**) The posterior aspect of the joint capsule has been removed to show the outline of its posterior osseous attachment. (**Bottom**) The radial collateral ligament is deep to the extensor carpi radialis brevis tendon, which originates deep and distal to the common extensor tendon origin. The ulnar collateral ligament is deep to the common flexor tendon origin.

Elbow Radiographic and Arthrographic Anatomy

GRAPHICS: LIGAMENTOUS ANATOMY

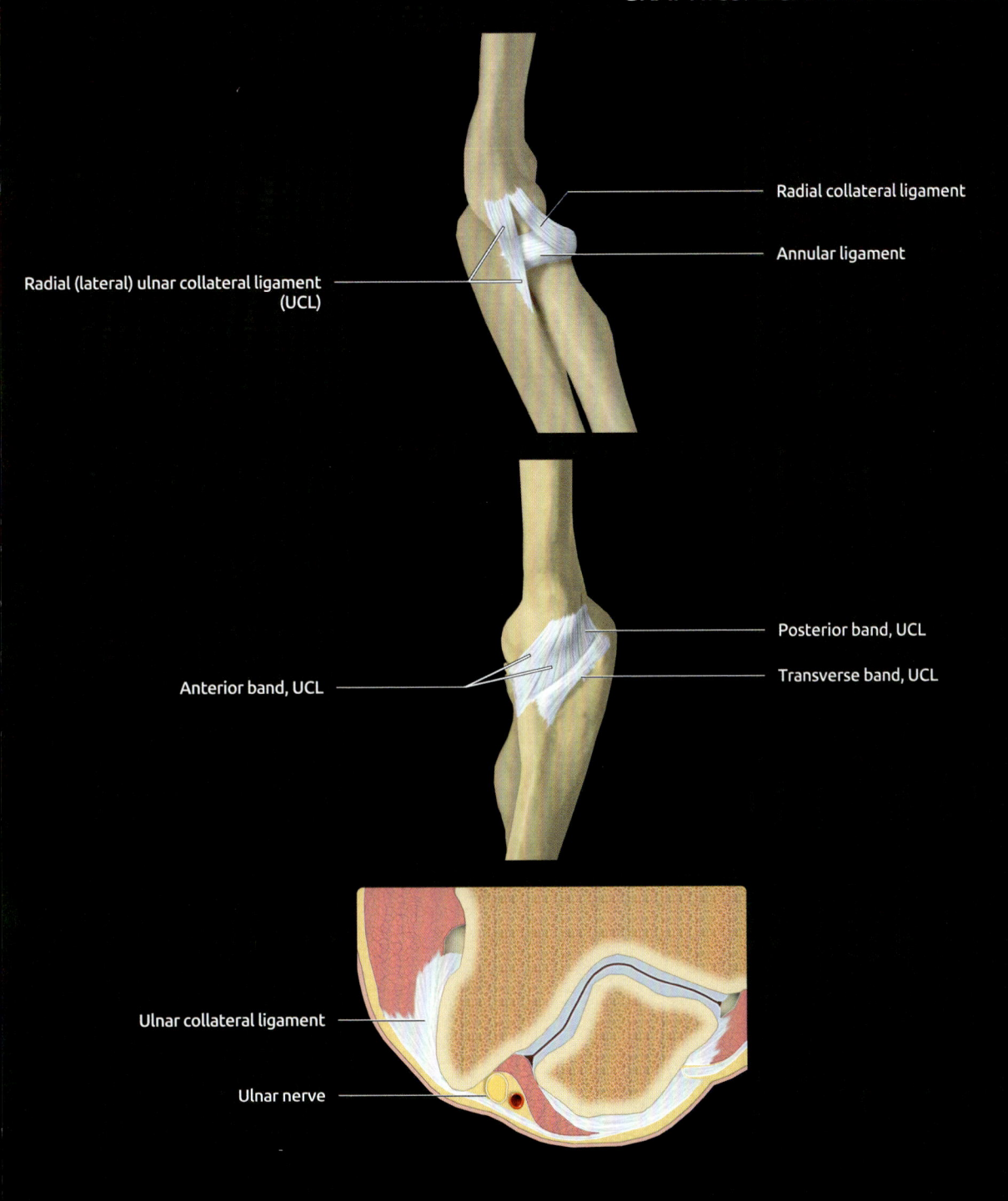

- Radial collateral ligament
- Annular ligament
- Radial (lateral) ulnar collateral ligament (UCL)
- Posterior band, UCL
- Transverse band, UCL
- Anterior band, UCL
- Ulnar collateral ligament
- Ulnar nerve

(Top) *Lateral view shows the radial collateral ligament extending from the lateral epicondyle to the radial neck. The radial ulnar collateral ligament has a diagonal course from the posterior margin of the lateral epicondyle behind the radial head (where it blends with the annular ligament) to the lateral ridge of the ulna.* **(Middle)** *Side view of the medial aspect of the elbow shows the 3 components of the ulnar collateral ligament. The anterior band is functionally most important and extends from the medial epicondyle to the sublime tubercle of the ulna.* **(Bottom)** *Position of the ulnar nerve in the cubital tunnel, immediately adjacent to the ulnar collateral ligament, explains why ulnar collateral ligament tears are often associated with ulnar neuropathy.*

Elbow Radiographic and Arthrographic Anatomy

ARTHROGRAM IMAGES: NEEDLE PLACEMENT

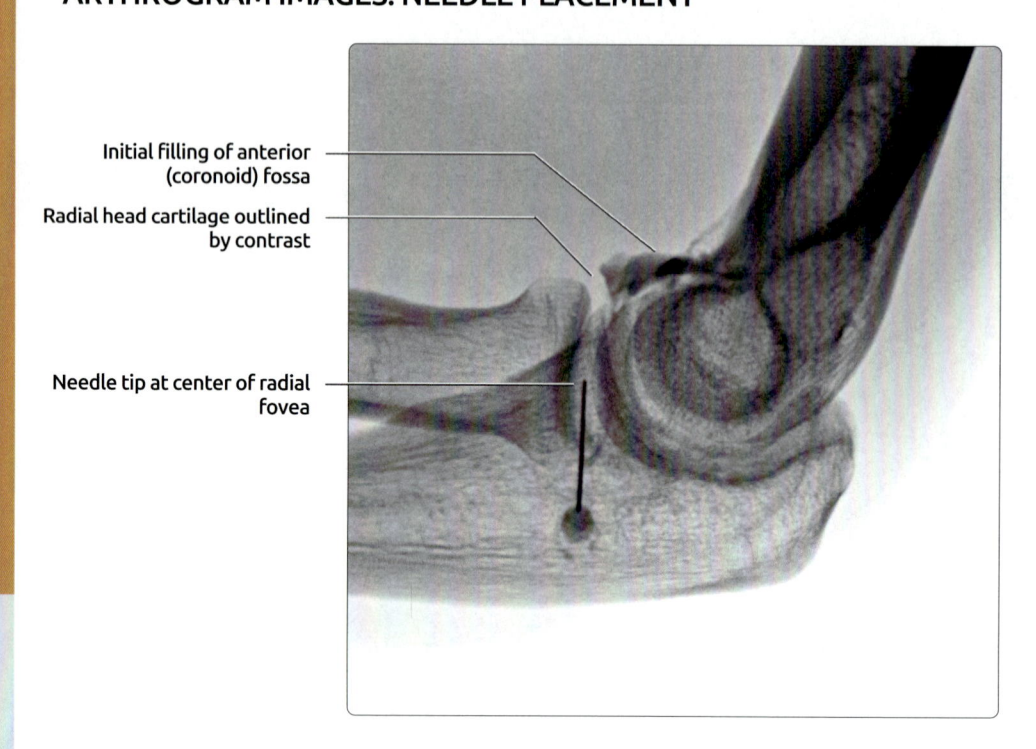

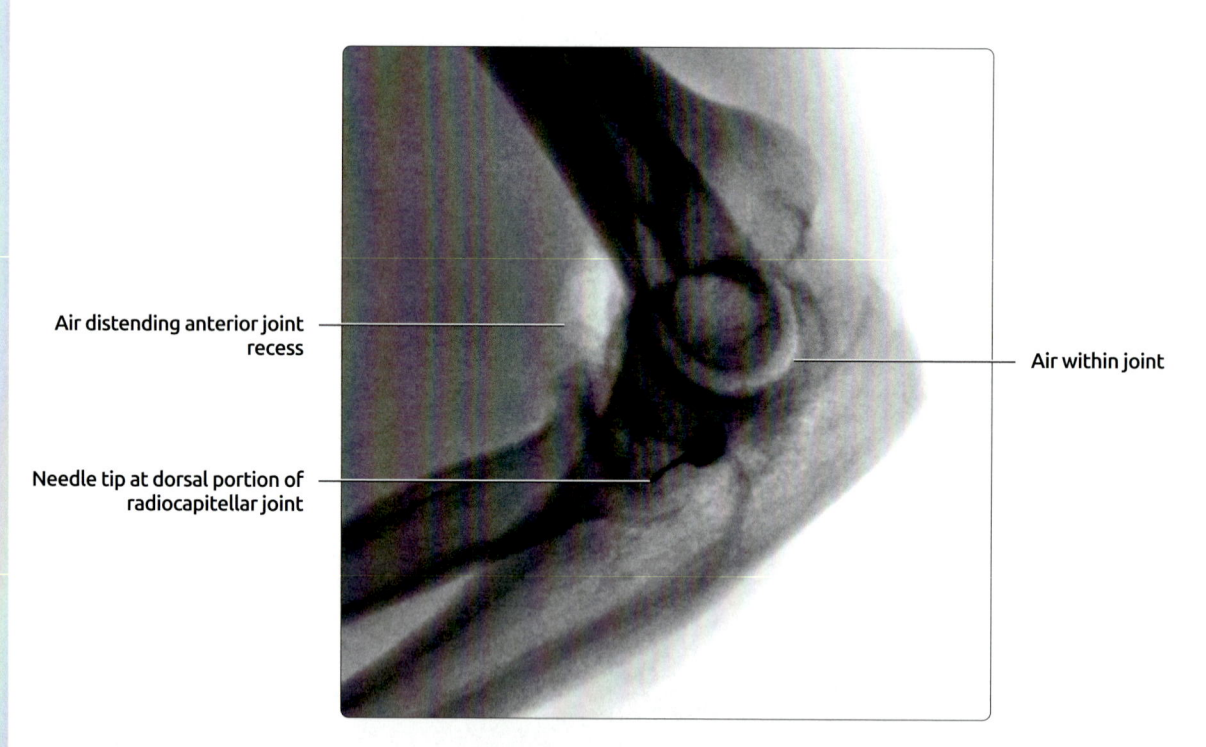

- Initial filling of anterior (coronoid) fossa
- Radial head cartilage outlined by contrast
- Needle tip at center of radial fovea

- Air distending anterior joint recess
- Needle tip at dorsal portion of radiocapitellar joint
- Air within joint

(Top) Lateral elbow arthrogram shows the ideal position of the needle tip, adjacent to the center of the radial fovea. Contrast typically fills the coronoid fossa prior to filling posteriorly. If the posterior recesses fail to fill, the joint should be exercised after the needle is removed in order to establish if scarring is preventing normal joint filling. Note that the joint capsule is quite tight and it is difficult to see contrast outlining the hyaline cartilage except at the volar-most portion of the radial head. **(Bottom)** Lateral arthrogram shows the air technique used for injection of corticosteroid in a patient allergic to iodine. Air fills the normal anterior joint recess.

Elbow Radiographic and Arthrographic Anatomy

ARTHROGRAPHIC ANATOMY

- Anterior joint recess
- Inferior joint recess
- Radial and capitellar articular cartilage
- Olecranon recess
- Olecranon articular cartilage
- Posterior joint recess

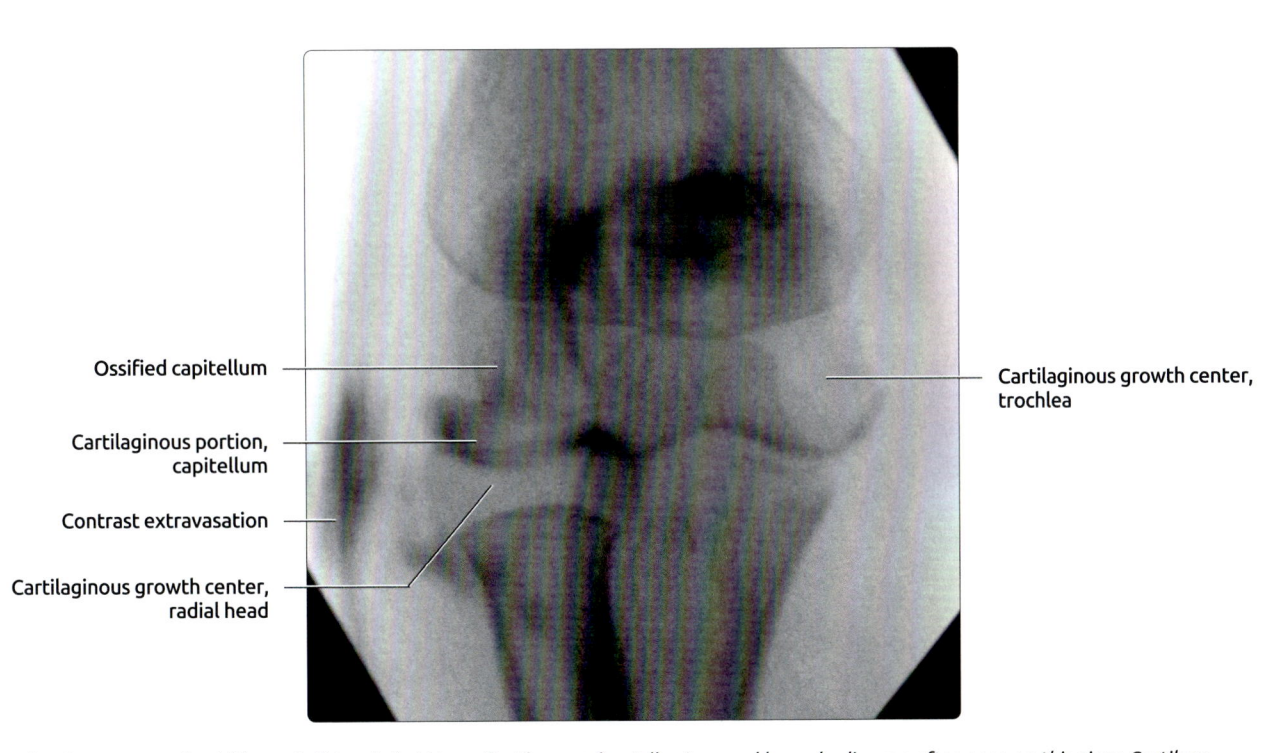

- Ossified capitellum
- Cartilaginous portion, capitellum
- Contrast extravasation
- Cartilaginous growth center, radial head
- Cartilaginous growth center, trochlea

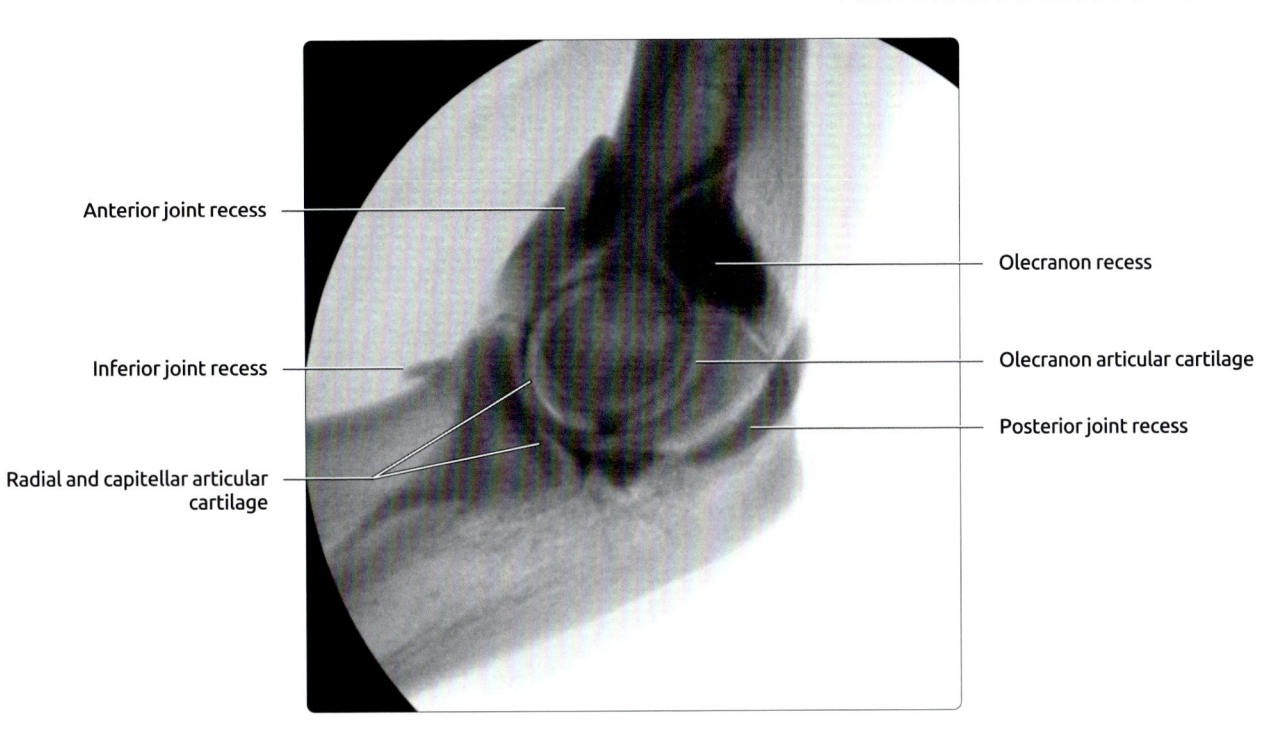

(Top) *Joint recesses should be well distended at time of arthrography. Adhesions and loose bodies are often seen on this view. Cartilage visualization is limited.* (Bottom) *Anteroposterior arthrogram in a 4 year old, performed to evaluate for cartilage injury, shows normal cartilaginous ossification centers outlined by contrast. Ossification centers appear in the following order: Capitellum, radial head, medial epicondyle, trochlea, olecranon process, lateral epicondyle.*

Elbow Radiographic and Arthrographic Anatomy

CORONAL MR ARTHROGRAM

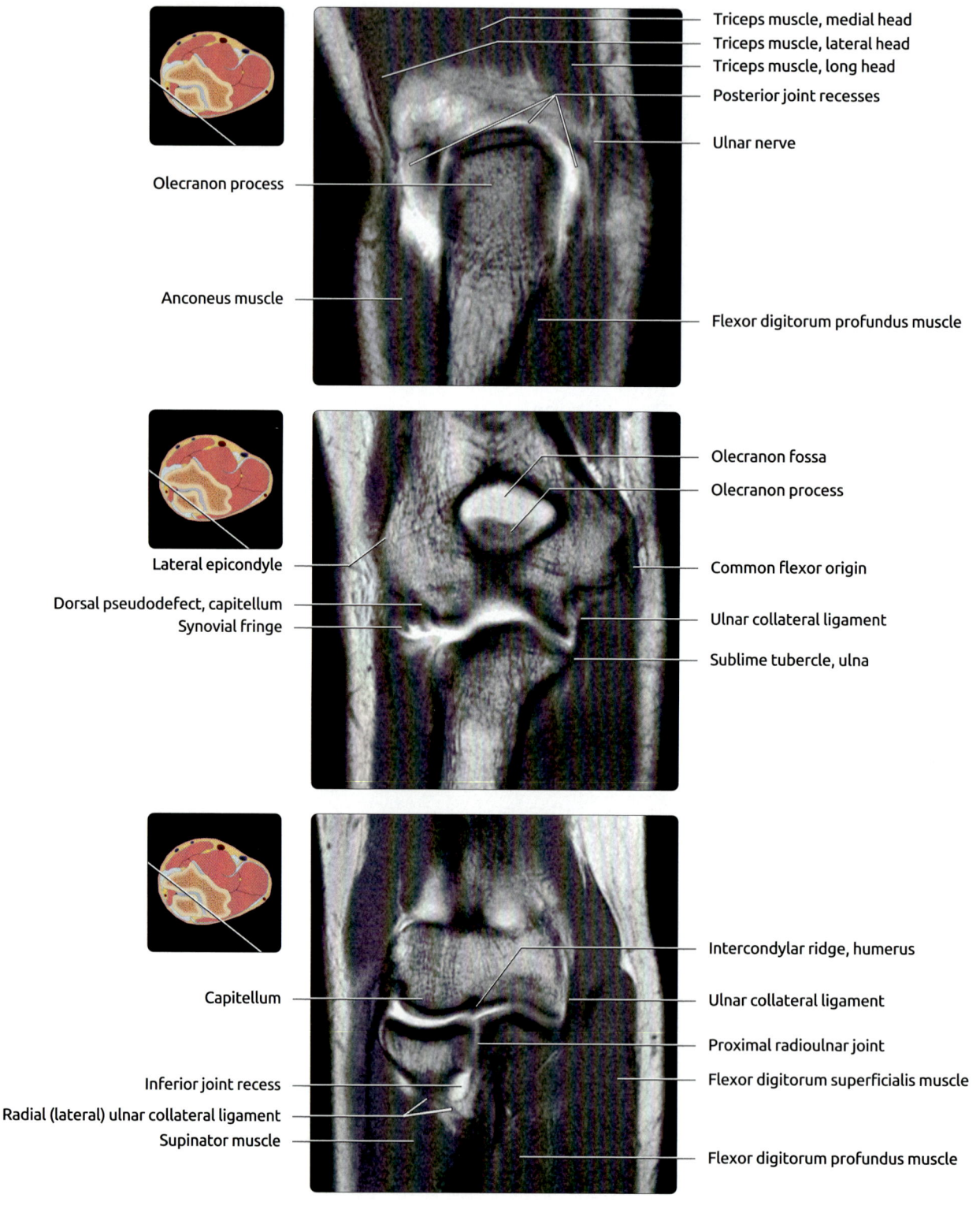

Labels (top image): Triceps muscle, medial head; Triceps muscle, lateral head; Triceps muscle, long head; Posterior joint recesses; Ulnar nerve; Olecranon process; Anconeus muscle; Flexor digitorum profundus muscle

Labels (middle image): Olecranon fossa; Olecranon process; Common flexor origin; Ulnar collateral ligament; Sublime tubercle, ulna; Lateral epicondyle; Dorsal pseudodefect, capitellum; Synovial fringe

Labels (bottom image): Intercondylar ridge, humerus; Ulnar collateral ligament; Proximal radioulnar joint; Flexor digitorum superficialis muscle; Flexor digitorum profundus muscle; Capitellum; Inferior joint recess; Radial (lateral) ulnar collateral ligament; Supinator muscle

(**Top**) *The 1st of 6 selected MR arthrogram coronal T1 images from posterior to anterior in the same patient is shown. On this most posterior image, the posterior joint recesses form a horseshoe shape around the olecranon process. The joint capsule is normally redundant both anteriorly and posteriorly.* (**Middle**) *The anterior margin of the olecranon process is seen at the inferior margin of the olecranon fossa. The ulnar collateral ligament extends from the medial epicondyle to the sublime tubercle of the ulna. Note the normal notch in the posterior aspect of the capitellum, called a pseudodefect.* (**Bottom**) *The radial (lateral) ulnar collateral ligament forms a sling posterior to the radius, providing posterolateral stability.*

Elbow Radiographic and Arthrographic Anatomy

CORONAL MR ARTHROGRAM

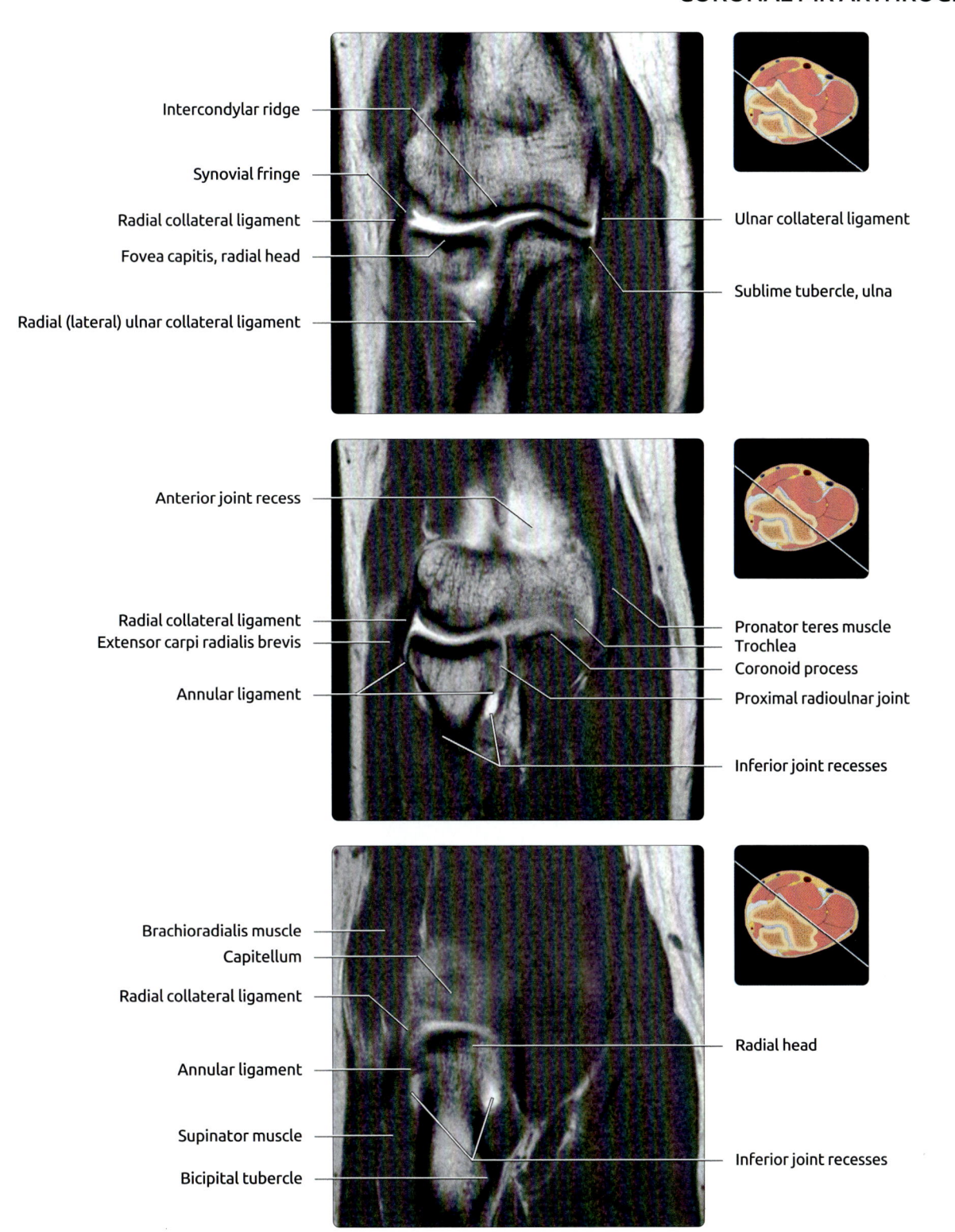

Labels (top image):
- Intercondylar ridge
- Synovial fringe
- Radial collateral ligament
- Fovea capitis, radial head
- Radial (lateral) ulnar collateral ligament
- Ulnar collateral ligament
- Sublime tubercle, ulna

Labels (middle image):
- Anterior joint recess
- Radial collateral ligament
- Extensor carpi radialis brevis
- Annular ligament
- Pronator teres muscle
- Trochlea
- Coronoid process
- Proximal radioulnar joint
- Inferior joint recesses

Labels (bottom image):
- Brachioradialis muscle
- Capitellum
- Radial collateral ligament
- Annular ligament
- Supinator muscle
- Bicipital tubercle
- Radial head
- Inferior joint recesses

(Top) Cartilage in the central portion of the fovea capitis of the radius is normally thin. The synovial fringe forms the meniscoid structure between the radius and capitellum. The capitellar and trochlear articular surfaces of the humerus are separated by the intercondylar ridge. (Middle) The radial collateral ligament is tightly apposed to the lateral margin of the humerus and radius. Distally, it merges with the annular ligament. (Bottom) Radiohumeral articulation extends anterior to ulnohumeral articulation.

Elbow Radiographic and Arthrographic Anatomy

SAGITTAL MR ARTHROGRAM

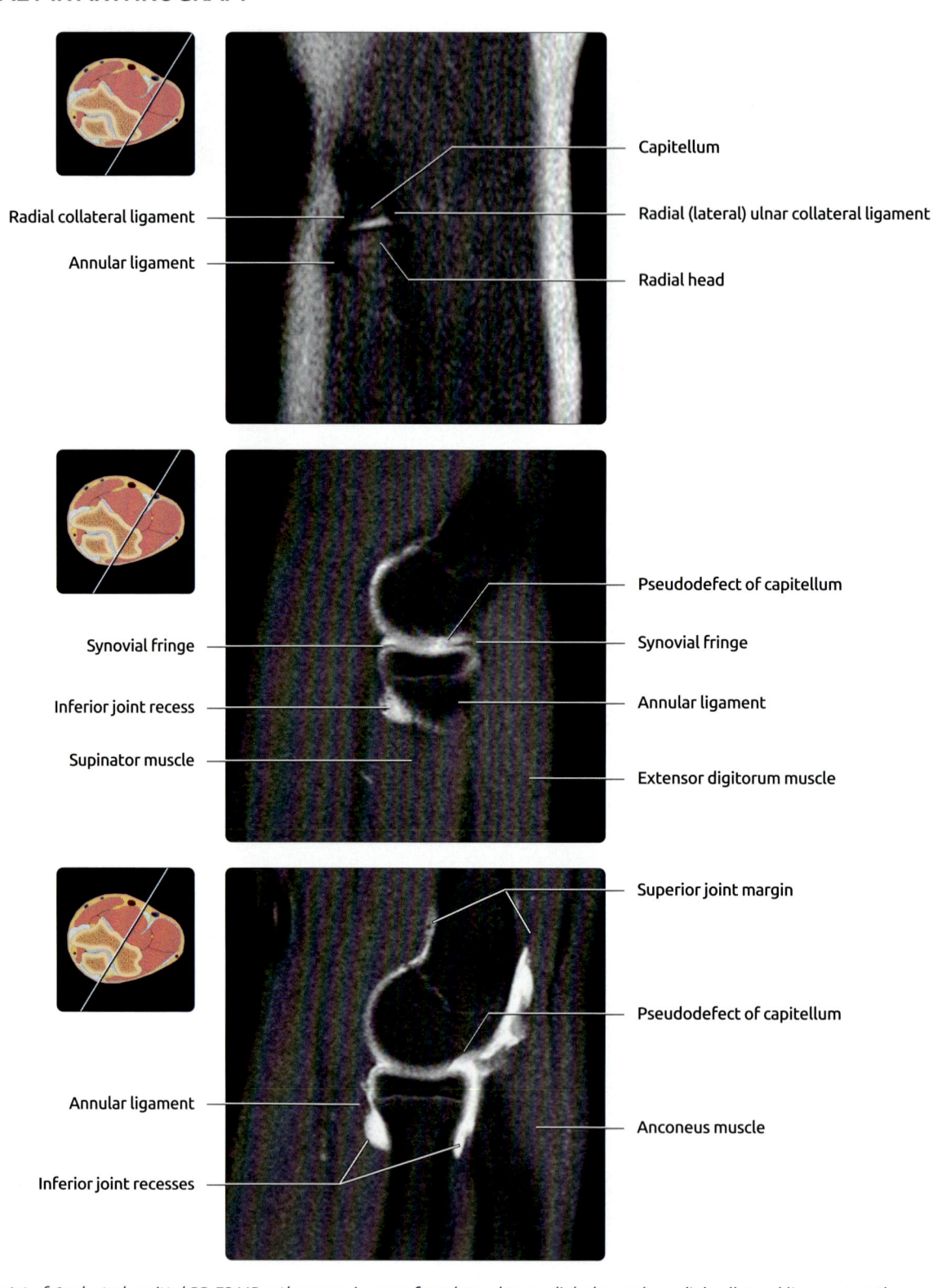

Top image labels:
- Radial collateral ligament
- Annular ligament
- Capitellum
- Radial (lateral) ulnar collateral ligament
- Radial head

Middle image labels:
- Synovial fringe
- Inferior joint recess
- Supinator muscle
- Pseudodefect of capitellum
- Synovial fringe
- Annular ligament
- Extensor digitorum muscle

Bottom image labels:
- Annular ligament
- Inferior joint recesses
- Superior joint margin
- Pseudodefect of capitellum
- Anconeus muscle

(**Top**) *The 1st of 6 selected sagittal PD FS MR arthrogram images, from lateral to medial, shows the radial collateral ligament at the anterior portion of the elbow joint and the radial (lateral) ulnar collateral ligament posteriorly.* (**Middle**) *Note the normal bony concavity and absent cartilage at the dorsal portion of the capitellum (pseudodefect) in this 12-year-old patient with normal cartilage proven at arthroscopy.* (**Bottom**) *This image through the center of the capitellum in the same patient again shows a pseudodefect. There are normal outpouchings of the joint distal to the annular ligament, forming inferior joint recesses.*

Elbow Radiographic and Arthrographic Anatomy

SAGITTAL MR ARTHROGRAM

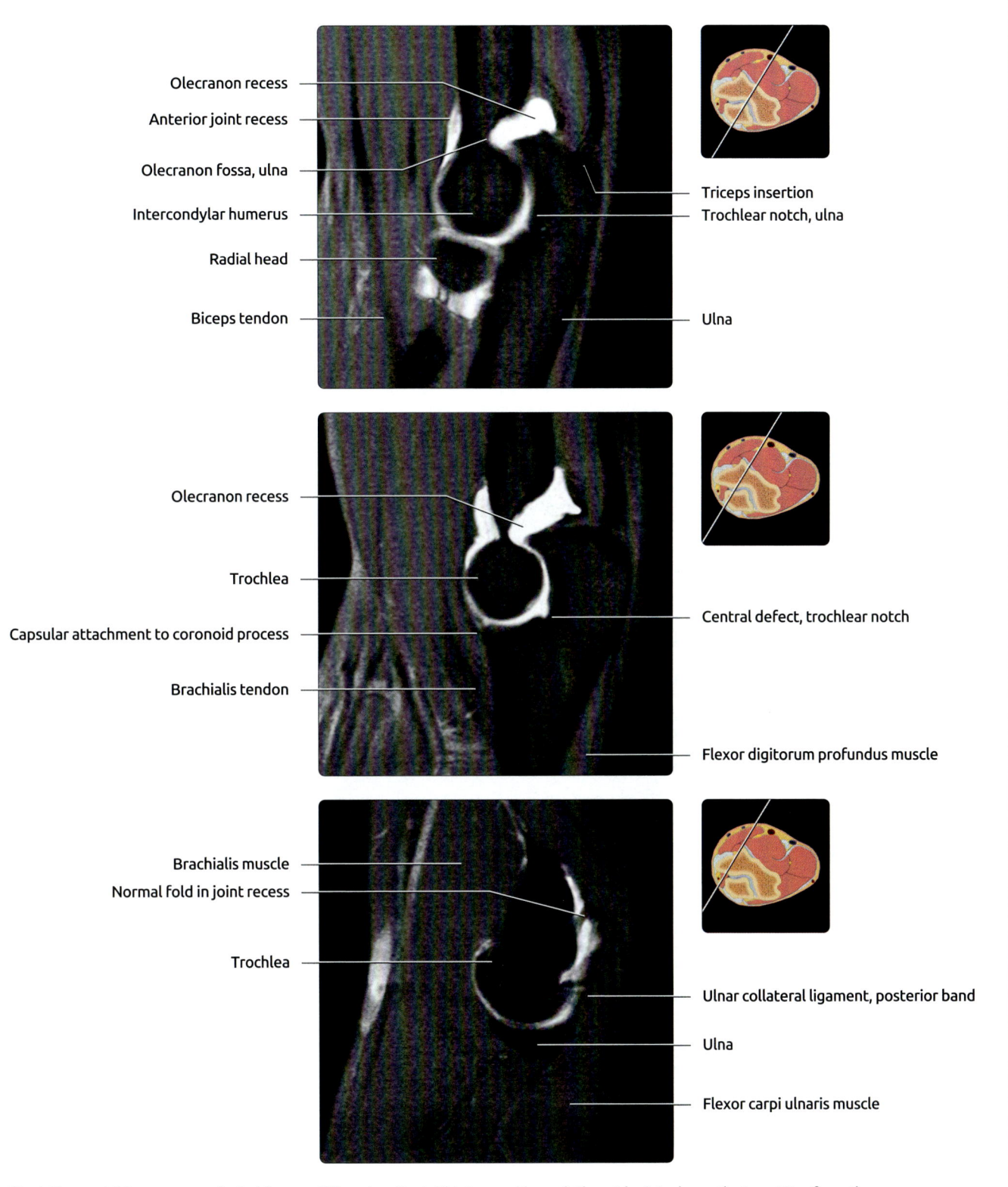

Labels (top image): Olecranon recess; Anterior joint recess; Olecranon fossa, ulna; Intercondylar humerus; Radial head; Biceps tendon; Triceps insertion; Trochlear notch, ulna; Ulna

Labels (middle image): Olecranon recess; Trochlea; Capsular attachment to coronoid process; Brachialis tendon; Central defect, trochlear notch; Flexor digitorum profundus muscle

Labels (bottom image): Brachialis muscle; Normal fold in joint recess; Trochlea; Ulnar collateral ligament, posterior band; Ulna; Flexor carpi ulnaris muscle

(Top) The next 3 images are selected from a different patient. This image, through the midpoint, shows the transition from the radiocapitellar to ulnohumeral surfaces. (Middle) The joint capsule extends superior to the olecranon fossa both anteriorly and posteriorly. The trochlea is more spherical in the sagittal section than the capitellum. The olecranon process has a normal bowl-shaped defect in the articular cartilage midway between the coronoid process and the tip of the olecranon process. (Bottom) On this image through the far medial portion of the joint, the horizontally oriented posterior band of the ulnar collateral ligament is visible.

Elbow Radiographic and Arthrographic Anatomy

AXIAL MR ARTHROGRAM

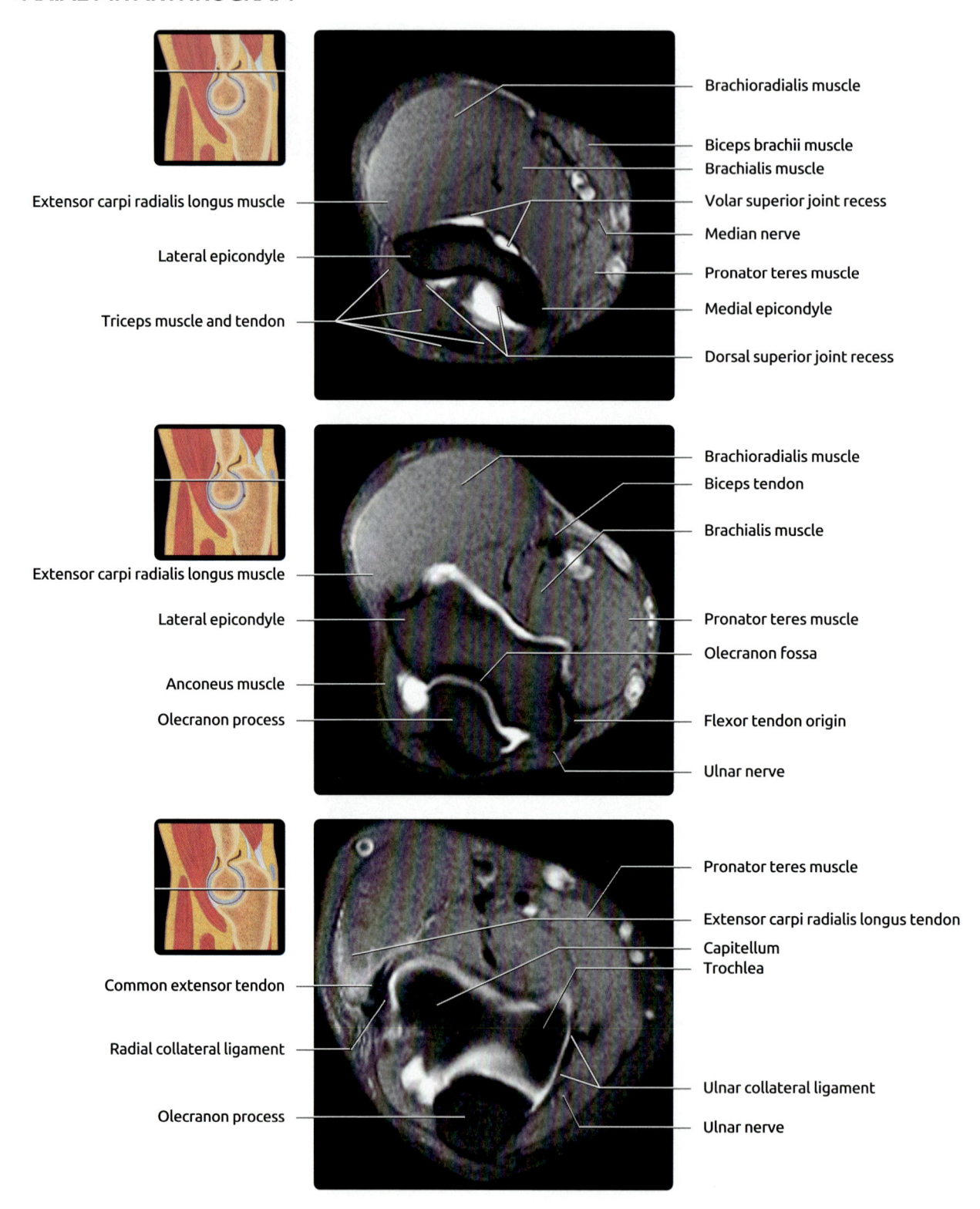

Labels (top image):
- Brachioradialis muscle
- Biceps brachii muscle
- Brachialis muscle
- Volar superior joint recess
- Median nerve
- Pronator teres muscle
- Medial epicondyle
- Dorsal superior joint recess
- Extensor carpi radialis longus muscle
- Lateral epicondyle
- Triceps muscle and tendon

Labels (middle image):
- Brachioradialis muscle
- Biceps tendon
- Brachialis muscle
- Pronator teres muscle
- Olecranon fossa
- Flexor tendon origin
- Ulnar nerve
- Extensor carpi radialis longus muscle
- Lateral epicondyle
- Anconeus muscle
- Olecranon process

Labels (bottom image):
- Pronator teres muscle
- Extensor carpi radialis longus tendon
- Capitellum
- Trochlea
- Ulnar collateral ligament
- Ulnar nerve
- Common extensor tendon
- Radial collateral ligament
- Olecranon process

(**Top**) *The 1st of 6 selected axial PD FS MR arthrogram images, from superior to inferior (different patients), shows broad attachments of the joint capsule. There is a normal fold in the dorsal superior joint recess.* (**Middle**) *Medial epicondyle has a horizontal undersurface, from which the flexor tendons and ulnar collateral ligament originate. The lateral epicondyle is more vertically oriented, and the tendons and radial collateral ligament originate from its lateral margin.* (**Bottom**) *Note the proximity of the ulnar nerve to the ulnar collateral ligament. This close anatomic relationship requires careful attention to the ulnar nerve at the time of ulnar collateral ligament repair.*

Elbow Radiographic and Arthrographic Anatomy

AXIAL MR ARTHROGRAM

Pronator teres muscle
Annular ligament
Radial collateral ligament
Fovea capitis, radial head
Olecranon process
Flexor digitorum profundus muscle
Palmaris longus muscle
Ulnar collateral ligament
Flexor carpi ulnaris muscle

Biceps tendon
Brachioradialis muscle
Annular ligament
Common extensor tendon
Annular ligament
Proximal radioulnar joint
Anconeus muscle
Pronator teres muscle
Flexors

Biceps tendon
Supinator muscle
Inferior joint recesses
Ulna
Brachialis muscle
Ulnar nerve

(Top) *Portions of the annular ligament encircling the radial head are visible deep to the radial collateral ligament. The ulnar collateral ligament is not clearly separable from the adjacent flexor muscles.* (Middle) *The proximal radioulnar joint is now visible. The ulnar joint capsule ends cephalad to this image.* (Bottom) *The inferior joint recess extends nearly circumferentially around the radial neck, deep to the supinator muscle.*

Elbow MR Atlas

ANATOMY IMAGING ISSUES

MR Imaging Recommendations

- Elbow may be scanned at patient's side or **"superman" position** (patient prone, arm straight out over head)
- Axial, sagittal, coronal planes
  - Sagittal images unreliable for differentiating distal biceps tendon from vascular structures; rely on axial imaging for biceps evaluation
  - Note: Axial imaging MUST extend to distal aspect of radial tuberosity in order to adequately evaluate biceps insertion
- T1-weighted and proton density ± fat suppression
- Supplemental imaging
  - Coronal plane with 20° posteroinferior tilt: Better demonstrates medial collateral and lateral ulnar collateral ligaments
  - **FABS**: **F**lexed (elbow), **AB**ducted (arm), **S**upinated (forearm); superman position with elbow flexed, excellent demonstration of distal biceps tendon and insertion
  - MR arthrography: Useful for evaluation of stability of capitellar osteochondral fracture and integrity of ulnar collateral ligament

CLINICAL IMPLICATIONS

Denervation Syndromes Related to Elbow Anatomy

- Radial nerve
  - Posterior interosseous nerve denervation
  - 2 clinical syndromes: May be variations of 1 condition
    - Radial tunnel syndrome: Pain ± mild motor weakness; MR denervation pattern in 52%
    - Posterior interosseous nerve syndrome: Pure motor weakness with muscle denervation pattern; no pain
  - Radial tunnel anatomy
    - Posterior: Capitellum
    - Medial: Brachialis muscle
    - Anterolaterally: Brachioradialis and extensor carpi radialis muscles
  - Common sites of compression in radial tunnel
    - Under arcade of Frohse (fibrous adhesion between brachialis and brachioradialis muscles; found in 30-50% of population) at proximal edge of supinator muscle (most common site of compression)
    - Fibrous bands of anterior capsule of radiocapitellar joint at entrance to tunnel
    - Radial recurrent artery (leash of Henry)
    - Fibrous edge of extensor carpi radialis brevis
    - Below fascial arcade at distal margin of supinator muscle
  - Most common denervation pattern
    - Denervation of supinator, extensor digitorum, extensor carpi ulnaris, extensor digiti minimi, abductor pollicis longus, extensor pollicis longus, extensor indicis
    - Extensor carpi radialis longus and brevis commonly spared because branches arise proximal to radial tunnel
    - Supinator occasionally spared if branches to it arise proximal to radial tunnel
- Median nerve
  - Proximal median nerve denervation: Pronator syndrome has several potential sites of entrapment of median nerve
    - Between humeral (superficial) and ulnar (deep) heads of pronator teres muscle
    - At bicipital aponeurosis (lacertus fibrosus)
    - At arch (sublimis bridge) of origin of flexor digitorum superficialis
    - Hypertrophy of muscles or congenital abnormalities of muscle belly/tendons
    - Clinically have pain and numbness in volar aspect of elbow/forearm/hand; generally no muscle weakness
    - Occasional denervation signs in pronator teres, flexor carpi radialis, flexor digitorum superficialis
  - Proximal median nerve denervation: Supracondylar process syndrome
    - Rare ligament of Struthers connecting supracondylar process to medial epicondyle may compress median nerve
    - Clinical findings of paresthesias and numbness of hand; occasional weakness
  - Anterior interosseous nerve syndrome (Kiloh-Nevin): Compression of nerve in proximal forearm
    - Most lesions have a location distal to those that cause pronator syndrome
    - Usually due to direct trauma or external compression (as from cast, soft tissue mass, anomalous muscle, or fibrous bands)
    - Clinically have volar forearm pain and acute muscle weakness of thumb, index, and occasionally middle finger
    - Muscles involved: Flexor digitorum profundus, flexor pollicis longus, pronator quadratus
- Ulnar nerve: Cubital tunnel syndrome
  - Within cubital tunnel at posterior medial epicondyle, ulnar nerve passes beneath cubital tunnel retinaculum (ligament of Osborne)
  - Causes of ulnar neuropathy at cubital tunnel
    - Subluxation secondary to trauma or fibrous tissue laxity
    - Loose bodies, fracture callus, or osteophyte
    - Soft tissue mass
    - Synovitis or hemorrhage in joint
    - Thickened retinaculum of flexor carpi ulnaris
    - Anomalous muscle: Anconeus epitrochlearis
    - Direct trauma
  - Clinical findings: Pain involving 4th and 5th digits and claw-like hand position
  - Muscles involved: Flexor carpi ulnaris and ulnar half of flexor digitorum profundus

SELECTED REFERENCES

1. Kim SJ et al: MR imaging mapping of skeletal muscle denervation in entrapment and compressive neuropathies. Radiographics. 31(2):319-32, 2011
2. Husarik DB et al: Elbow nerves: MR findings in 60 asymptomatic subjects– normal anatomy, variants, and pitfalls. Radiology. 252(1):148-56, 2009

Elbow MR Atlas

AXIAL ANATOMY

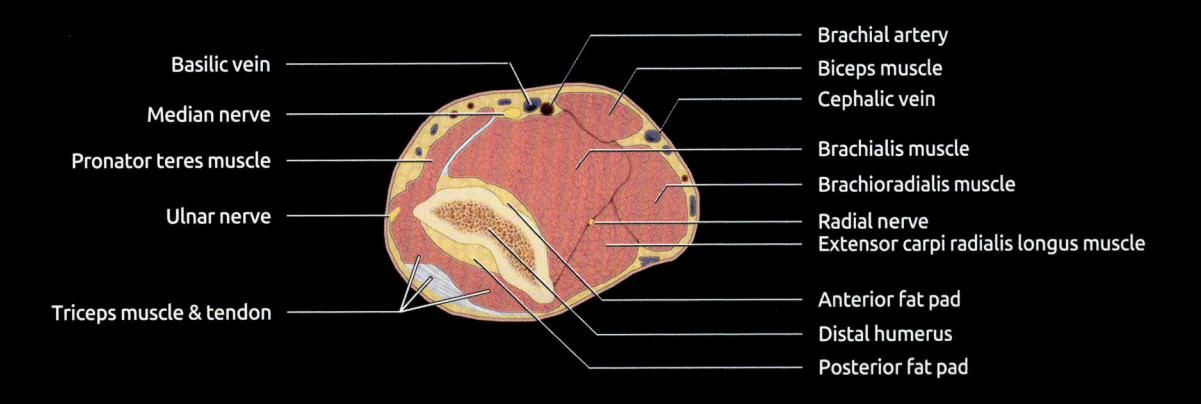

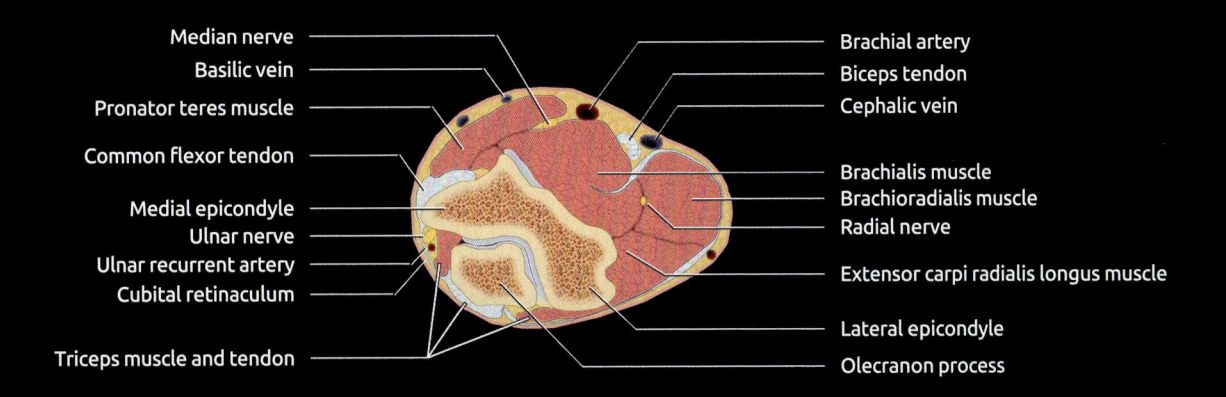

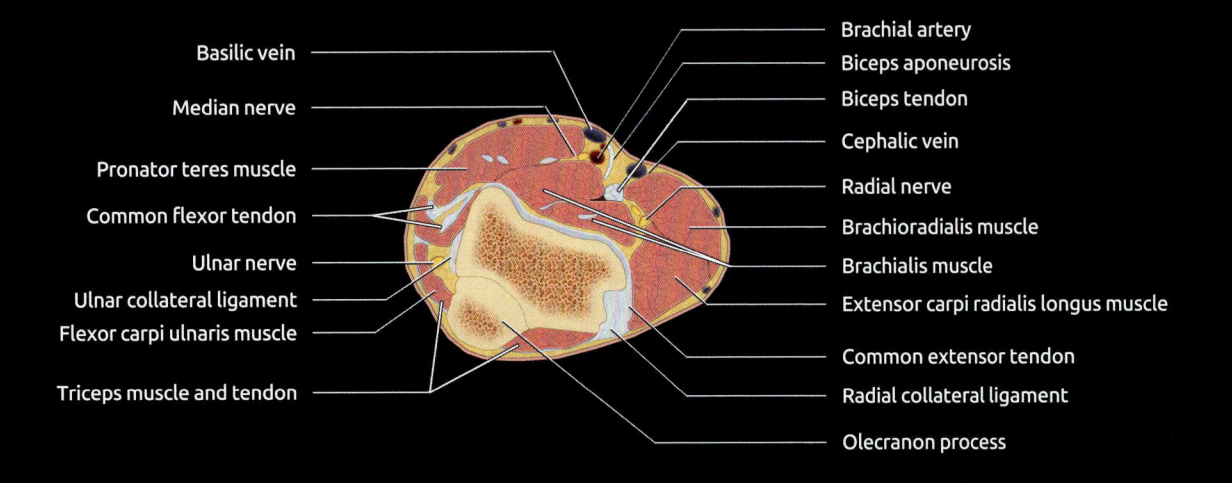

(Top) Labels: Basilic vein, Median nerve, Pronator teres muscle, Ulnar nerve, Triceps muscle & tendon, Brachial artery, Biceps muscle, Cephalic vein, Brachialis muscle, Brachioradialis muscle, Radial nerve, Extensor carpi radialis longus muscle, Anterior fat pad, Distal humerus, Posterior fat pad.

(Middle) Labels: Median nerve, Basilic vein, Pronator teres muscle, Common flexor tendon, Medial epicondyle, Ulnar nerve, Ulnar recurrent artery, Cubital retinaculum, Triceps muscle and tendon, Brachial artery, Biceps tendon, Cephalic vein, Brachialis muscle, Brachioradialis muscle, Radial nerve, Extensor carpi radialis longus muscle, Lateral epicondyle, Olecranon process.

(Bottom) Labels: Basilic vein, Median nerve, Pronator teres muscle, Common flexor tendon, Ulnar nerve, Ulnar collateral ligament, Flexor carpi ulnaris muscle, Triceps muscle and tendon, Brachial artery, Biceps aponeurosis, Biceps tendon, Cephalic vein, Radial nerve, Brachioradialis muscle, Brachialis muscle, Extensor carpi radialis longus muscle, Common extensor tendon, Radial collateral ligament, Olecranon process.

(Top) *Axial graphic shows the supracondylar region of the humerus. The anterior and posterior fat pads are seen in the coronoid and olecranon fossae, respectively. The brachialis muscle accounts for the bulk of the anterior compartment of the distal arm.* **(Middle)** *Axial graphic shows the epicondylar region of the distal humerus. The triceps muscle thins as its tendon attaches to the olecranon. The ulnar nerve and posterior ulnar recurrent artery are held in the cubital tunnel by the cubital retinaculum (the ligament of Osborne).* **(Bottom)** *Axial graphic immediately proximal to the elbow joint is shown. The common extensor tendon overlies the radial collateral ligament and may be difficult to distinguish at this level. The ulnar nerve has exited the cubital tunnel and is entering the flexor carpi ulnaris.*

Elbow MR Atlas

AXIAL ANATOMY

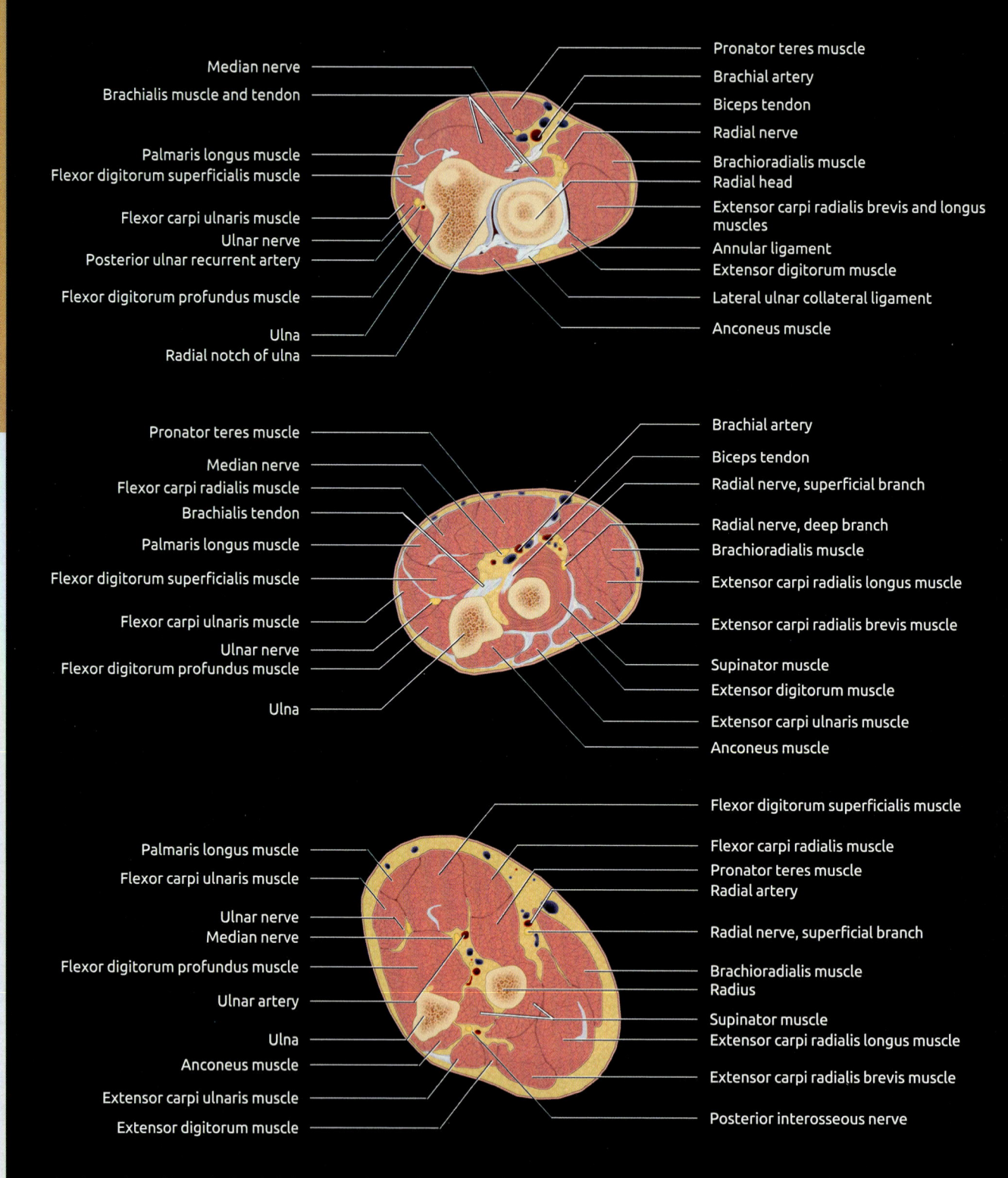

Top image labels:
- Median nerve
- Brachialis muscle and tendon
- Palmaris longus muscle
- Flexor digitorum superficialis muscle
- Flexor carpi ulnaris muscle
- Ulnar nerve
- Posterior ulnar recurrent artery
- Flexor digitorum profundus muscle
- Ulna
- Radial notch of ulna
- Pronator teres muscle
- Brachial artery
- Biceps tendon
- Radial nerve
- Brachioradialis muscle
- Radial head
- Extensor carpi radialis brevis and longus muscles
- Annular ligament
- Extensor digitorum muscle
- Lateral ulnar collateral ligament
- Anconeus muscle

Middle image labels:
- Pronator teres muscle
- Median nerve
- Flexor carpi radialis muscle
- Brachialis tendon
- Palmaris longus muscle
- Flexor digitorum superficialis muscle
- Flexor carpi ulnaris muscle
- Ulnar nerve
- Flexor digitorum profundus muscle
- Ulna
- Brachial artery
- Biceps tendon
- Radial nerve, superficial branch
- Radial nerve, deep branch
- Brachioradialis muscle
- Extensor carpi radialis longus muscle
- Extensor carpi radialis brevis muscle
- Supinator muscle
- Extensor digitorum muscle
- Extensor carpi ulnaris muscle
- Anconeus muscle

Bottom image labels:
- Palmaris longus muscle
- Flexor carpi ulnaris muscle
- Ulnar nerve
- Median nerve
- Flexor digitorum profundus muscle
- Ulnar artery
- Ulna
- Anconeus muscle
- Extensor carpi ulnaris muscle
- Extensor digitorum muscle
- Flexor digitorum superficialis muscle
- Flexor carpi radialis muscle
- Pronator teres muscle
- Radial artery
- Radial nerve, superficial branch
- Brachioradialis muscle
- Radius
- Supinator muscle
- Extensor carpi radialis longus muscle
- Extensor carpi radialis brevis muscle
- Posterior interosseous nerve

(Top) Axial graphic at the level of the proximal radioulnar joint is shown. The articulating surfaces of the proximal radioulnar joint are well seen as the radial head is held in the radial notch of the ulna by the annular ligament. The lateral ulnar collateral ligament blends with the posterior aspect of the annular ligament. (Middle) This graphic shows the axial elbow at a level immediately above the radial tuberosity. The brachialis tendon is inserting on the ulnar tuberosity and the biceps tendon is approaching its insertion on the radial tuberosity, which is more distal than the brachialis insertion. (Bottom) At the level of the proximal forearm, the muscles are starting to align themselves into the anterior (flexor) compartment, and the posterior (extensor) compartment.

Elbow MR Atlas

CUBITAL FOSSA, RADIAL & MEDIAN NERVE RELATIONSHIPS

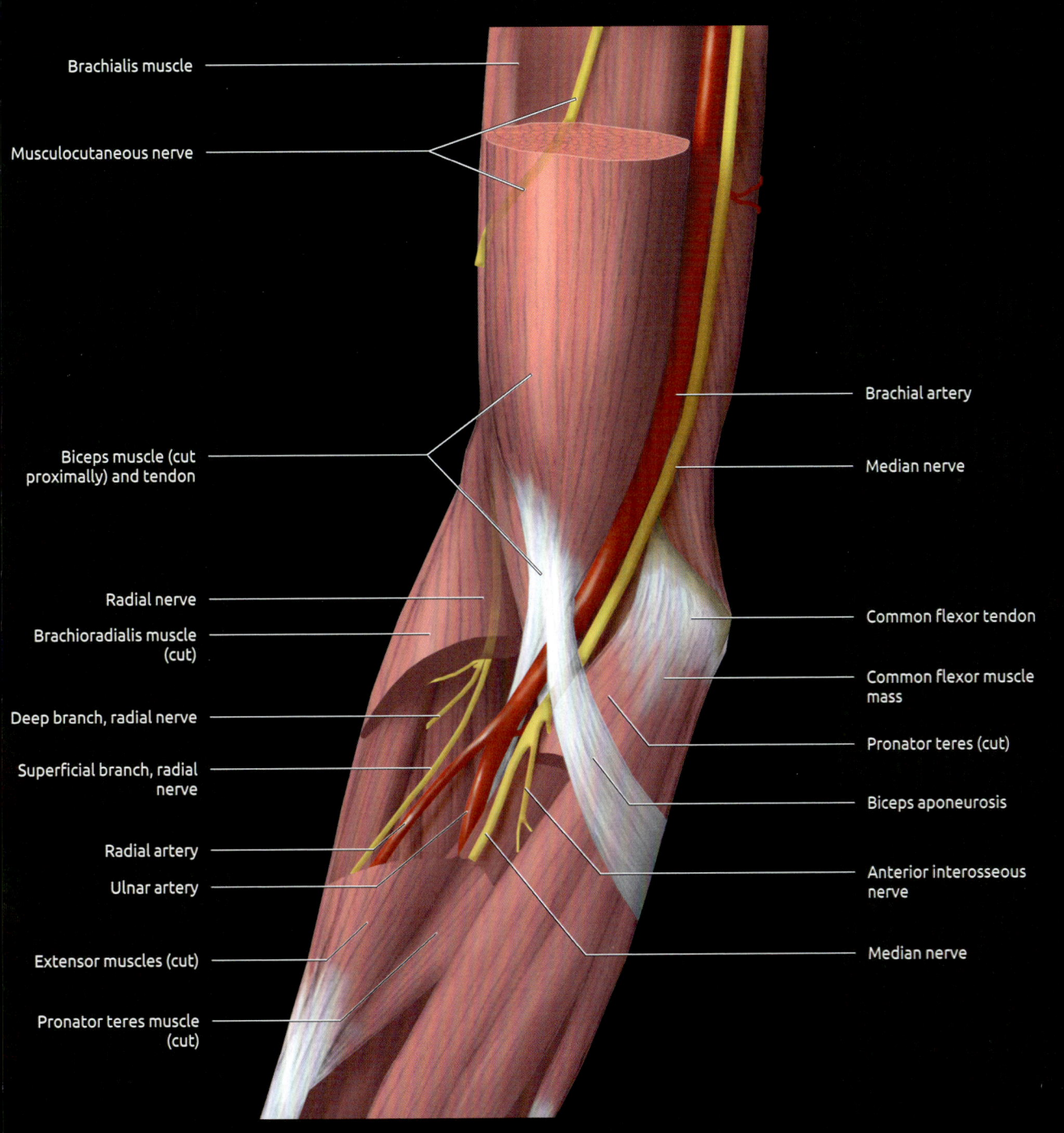

- Brachialis muscle
- Musculocutaneous nerve
- Biceps muscle (cut proximally) and tendon
- Radial nerve
- Brachioradialis muscle (cut)
- Deep branch, radial nerve
- Superficial branch, radial nerve
- Radial artery
- Ulnar artery
- Extensor muscles (cut)
- Pronator teres muscle (cut)
- Brachial artery
- Median nerve
- Common flexor tendon
- Common flexor muscle mass
- Pronator teres (cut)
- Biceps aponeurosis
- Anterior interosseous nerve
- Median nerve

Anterior view of the cubital fossa shows the median nerve and brachial artery passing underneath the the biceps aponeurosis. The anterior interosseous nerve arises from the median nerve as the median nerve passes between the 2 heads of the pronator teres muscle. The radial nerve, deep to the brachioradialis muscle, is seen dividing into superficial and deep branches.

Elbow MR Atlas

RADIAL & MEDIAN NERVE ENTRAPMENT

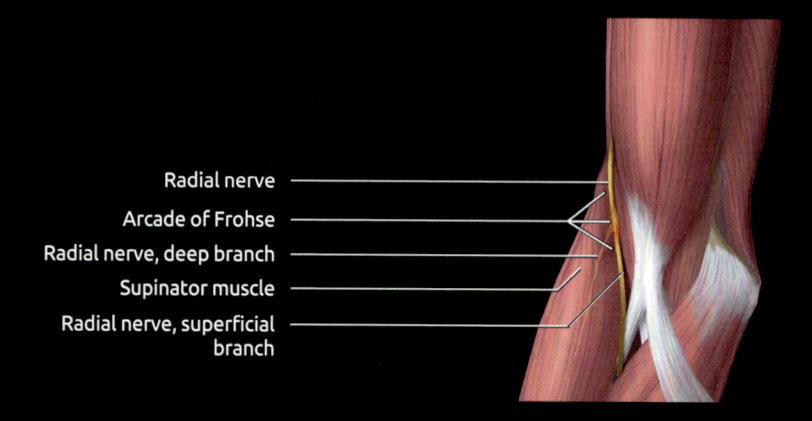

Radial nerve
Arcade of Frohse
Radial nerve, deep branch
Supinator muscle
Radial nerve, superficial branch

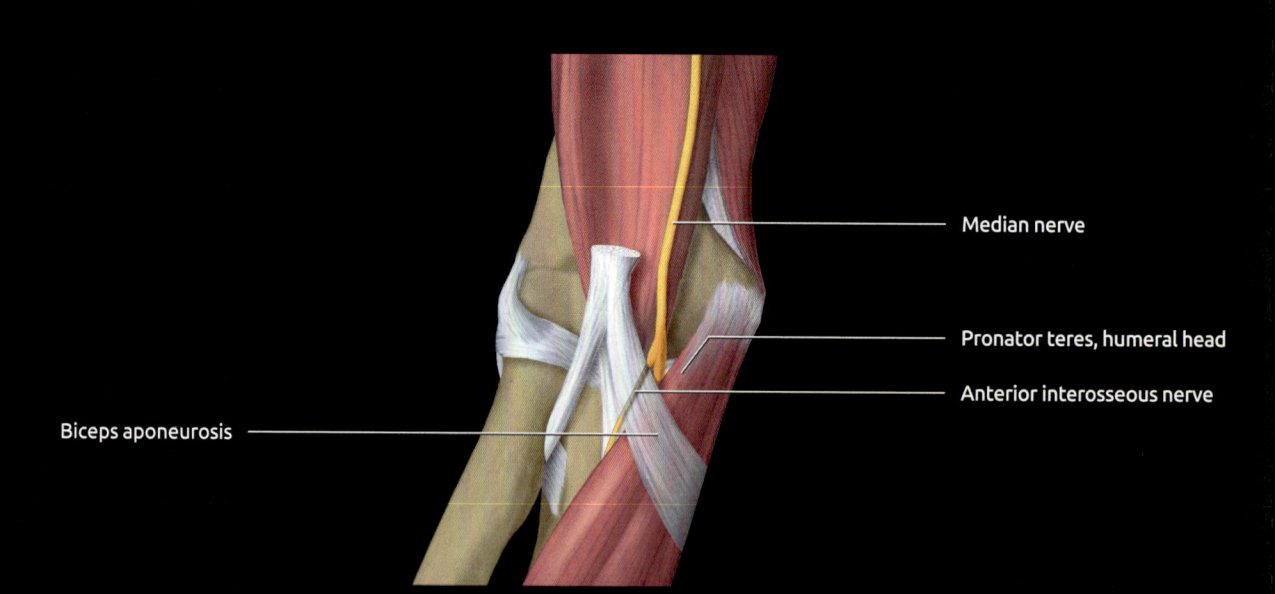

Median nerve
Pronator teres, humeral head
Anterior interosseous nerve
Biceps aponeurosis

(Top) The radial nerve &/or its deep branch may be impinged by the arcade of Frohse, the superior edge of the supinator muscle. (Bottom) The median nerve may be entrapped between the 2 heads of the pronator teres muscle or by the overlying biceps aponeurosis. The anterior interosseous branch of the median nerve may also be compressed by the overlying bicipital aponeurosis.

Elbow MR Atlas

ULNAR NERVE ENTRAPMENT

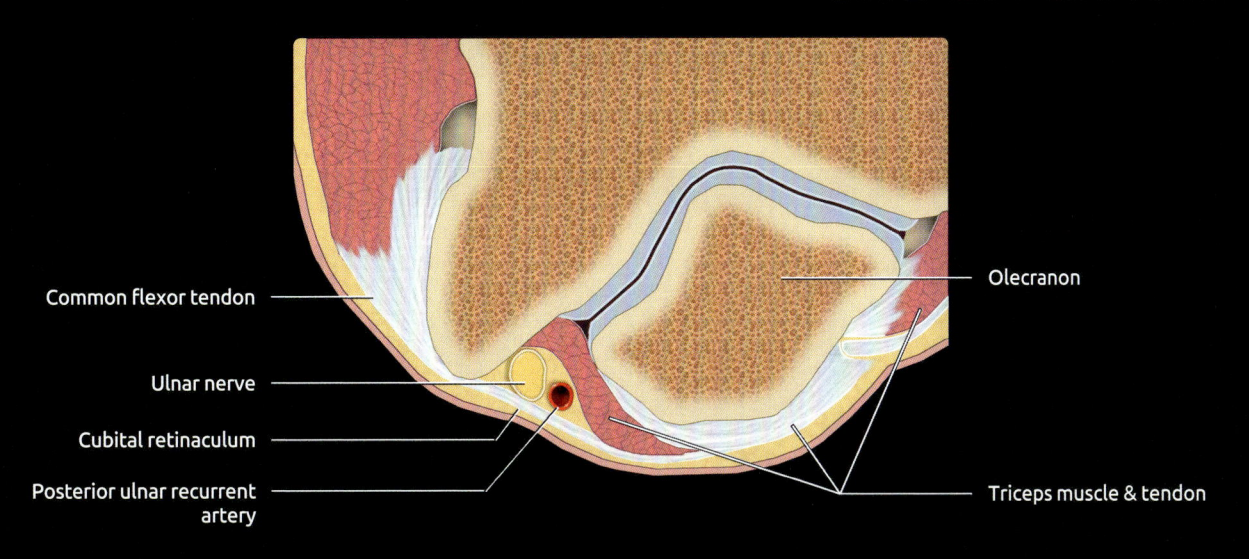

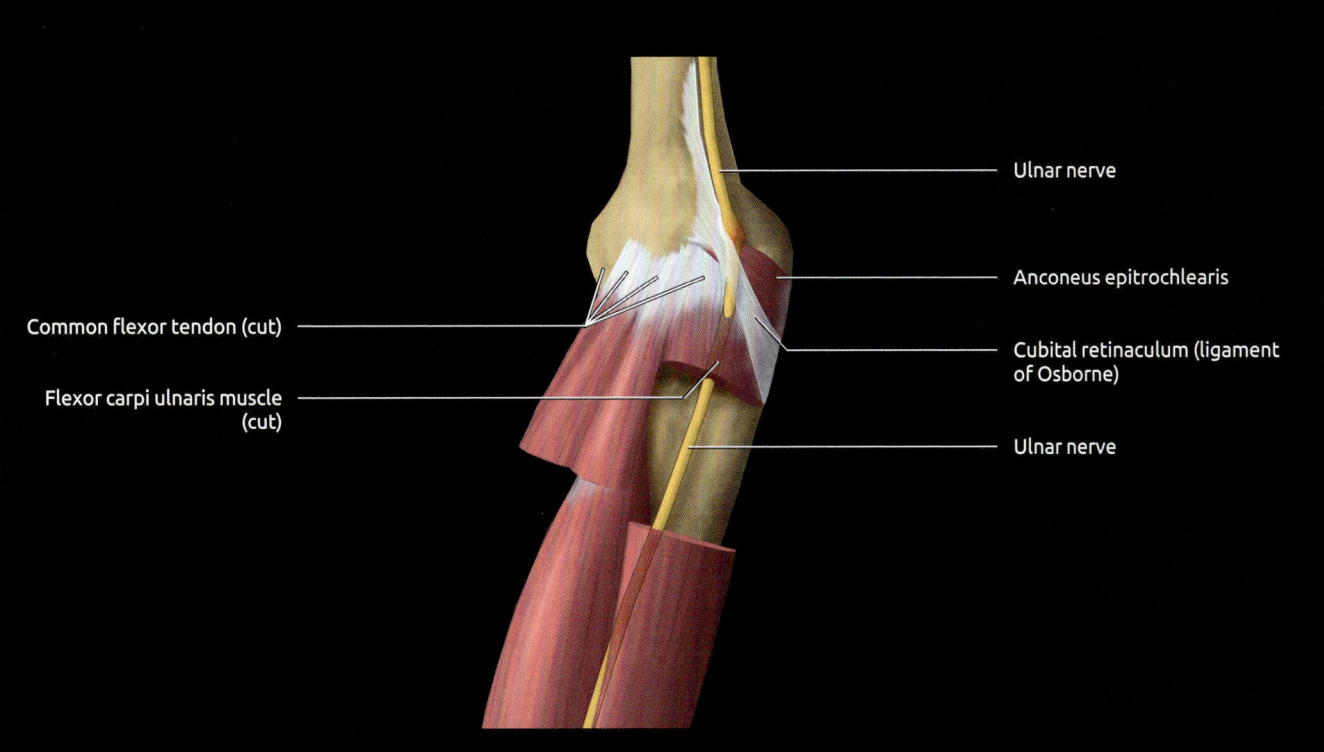

Common flexor tendon

Ulnar nerve

Cubital retinaculum

Posterior ulnar recurrent artery

Olecranon

Triceps muscle & tendon

Common flexor tendon (cut)

Flexor carpi ulnaris muscle (cut)

Ulnar nerve

Anconeus epitrochlearis

Cubital retinaculum (ligament of Osborne)

Ulnar nerve

(Top) *Axial graphic shows the cubital tunnel. The ulnar nerve may be compressed within the cubital tunnel (cubital tunnel syndrome) by a mass, post-traumatic osseous deformity, or aneurysm of the recurrent ulnar artery. The ulnar nerve may also be subluxed out of the cubital tunnel by the adjacent medial head of the triceps.* **(Bottom)** *Medial graphic shows the cubital tunnel. The anconeus epitrochlearis is an inconstant accessory muscle that is posterior to the ulnar nerve and may compress the nerve against the cubital retinaculum and medial epicondyle.*

Elbow MR Atlas

AXIAL T1 MR, RIGHT ELBOW

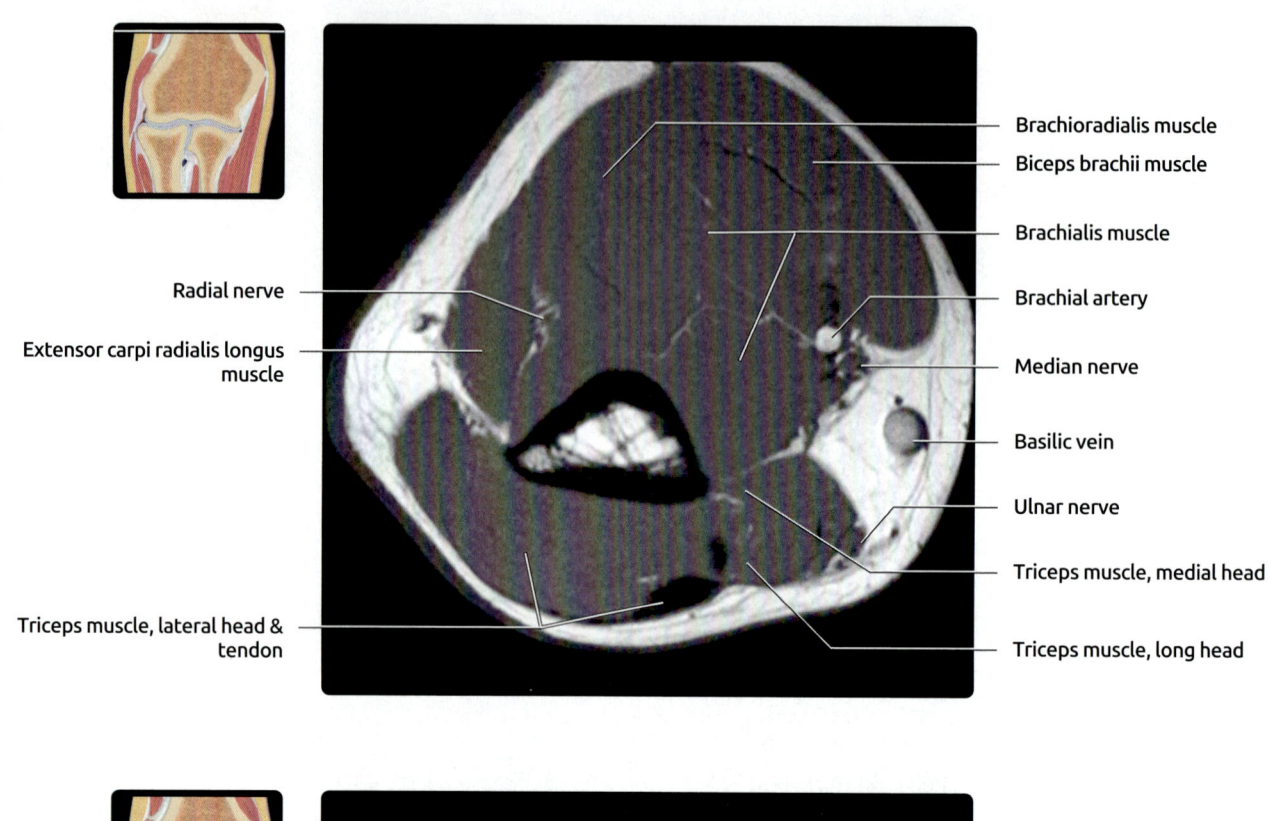

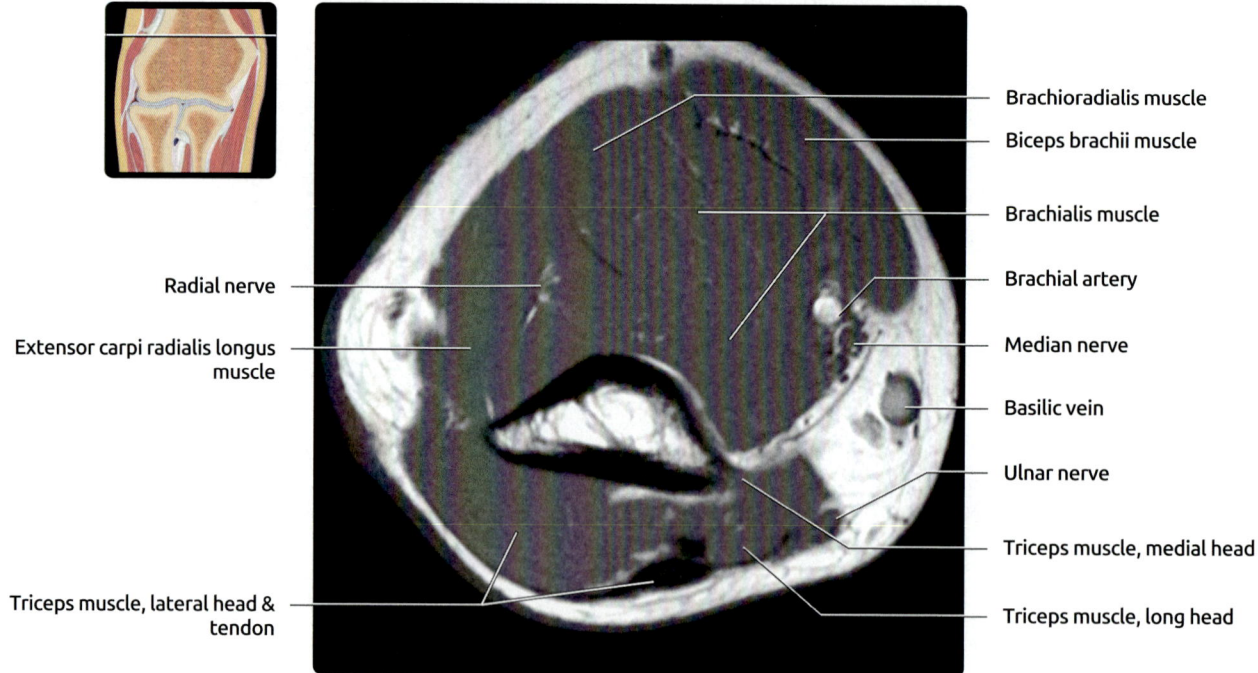

Labels (top image):
- Brachioradialis muscle
- Biceps brachii muscle
- Brachialis muscle
- Brachial artery
- Median nerve
- Basilic vein
- Ulnar nerve
- Triceps muscle, medial head
- Triceps muscle, long head
- Triceps muscle, lateral head & tendon
- Extensor carpi radialis longus muscle
- Radial nerve

Labels (bottom image):
- Brachioradialis muscle
- Biceps brachii muscle
- Brachialis muscle
- Brachial artery
- Median nerve
- Basilic vein
- Ulnar nerve
- Triceps muscle, medial head
- Triceps muscle, long head
- Triceps muscle, lateral head & tendon
- Extensor carpi radialis longus muscle
- Radial nerve

(Top) Axial T1 MR series through the elbow, proximal to distal, is shown. In this proximal image, the radial, ulnar, and median nerves are visibile. The 3 heads of the triceps occupy the entire posterior compartment. **(Bottom)** The brachialis muscle accounts for most of the bulk in the anterior compartment.

Elbow MR Atlas

AXIAL T1 MR, LEFT ELBOW

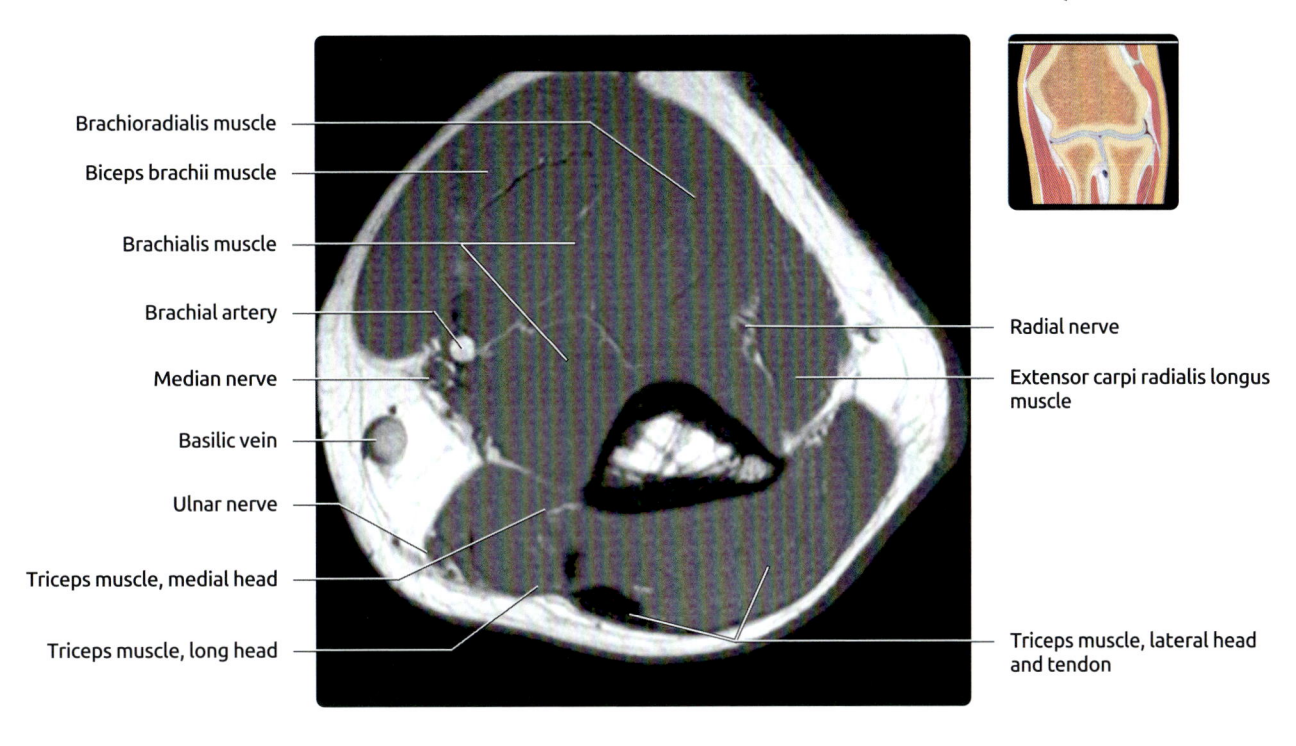

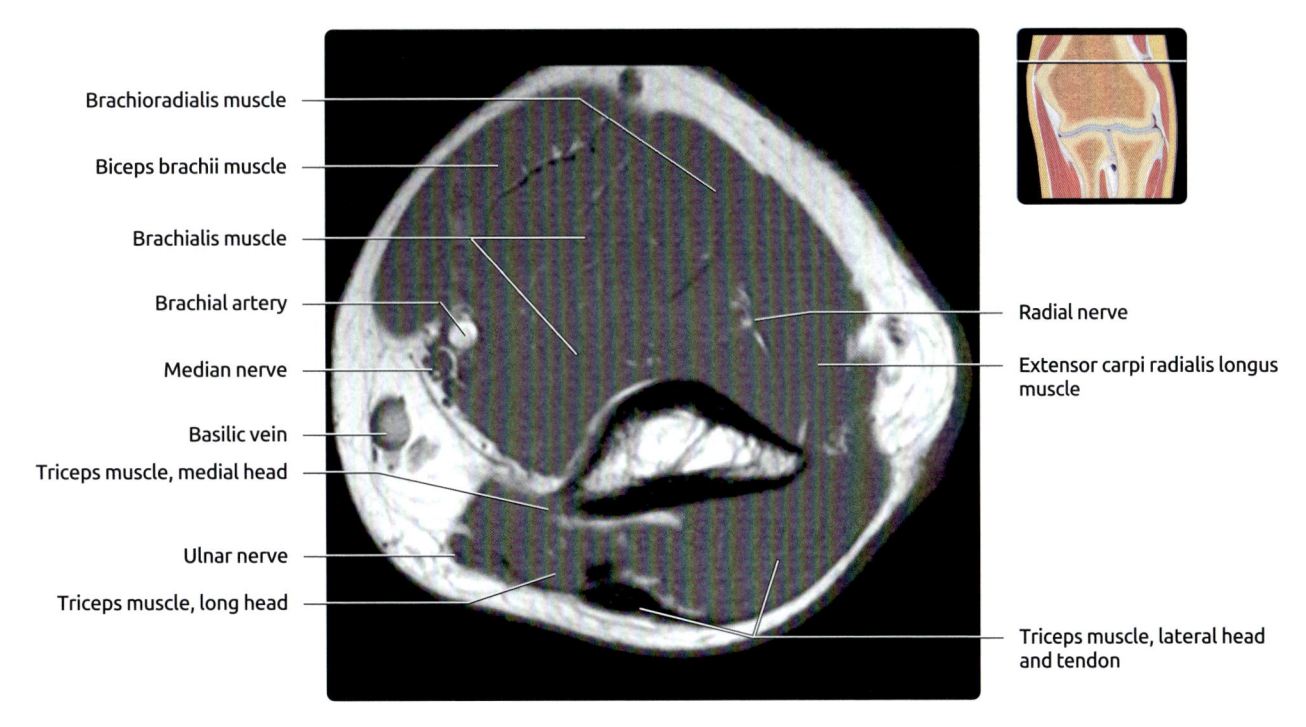

(Top) Axial T1 MR series through the elbow, proximal to distal, is shown. In this proximal image, the radial, ulnar, and median nerves are visibile. The 3 heads of the triceps occupy the entire posterior compartment. *(Bottom)* The brachialis muscle accounts for most of the bulk in the anterior compartment.

Elbow MR Atlas

AXIAL T1 MR, RIGHT ELBOW

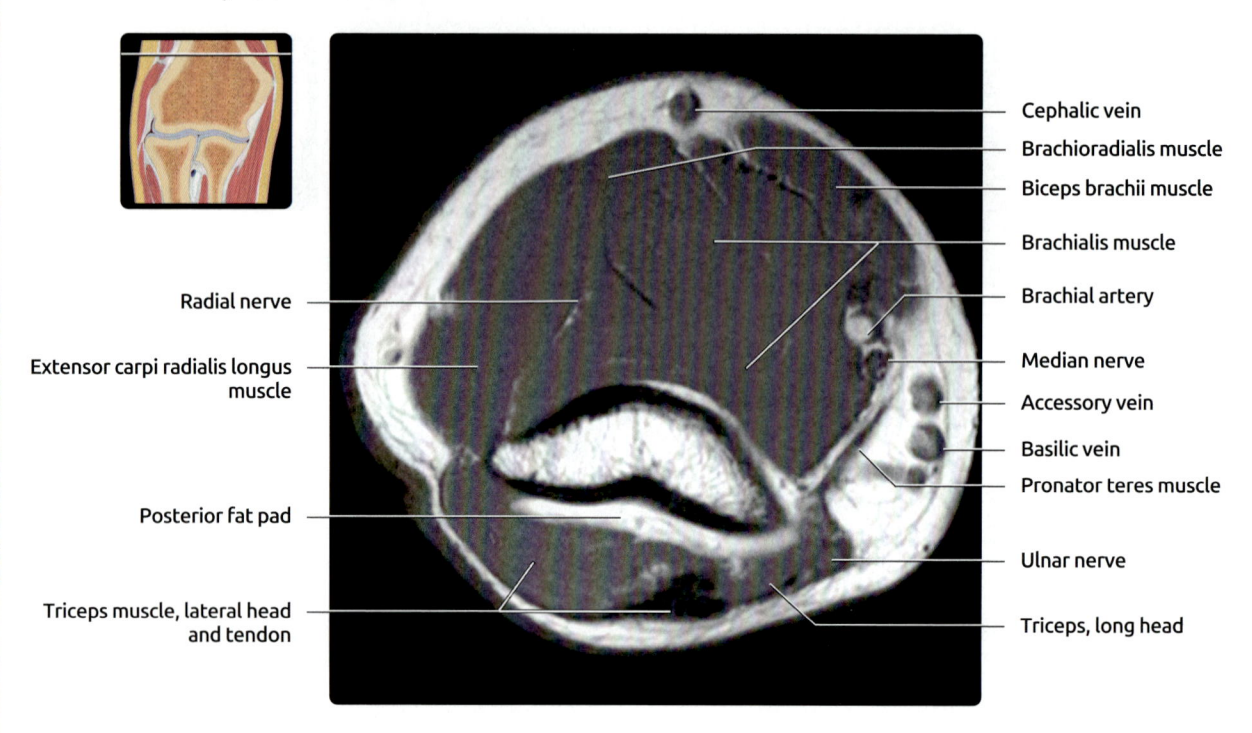

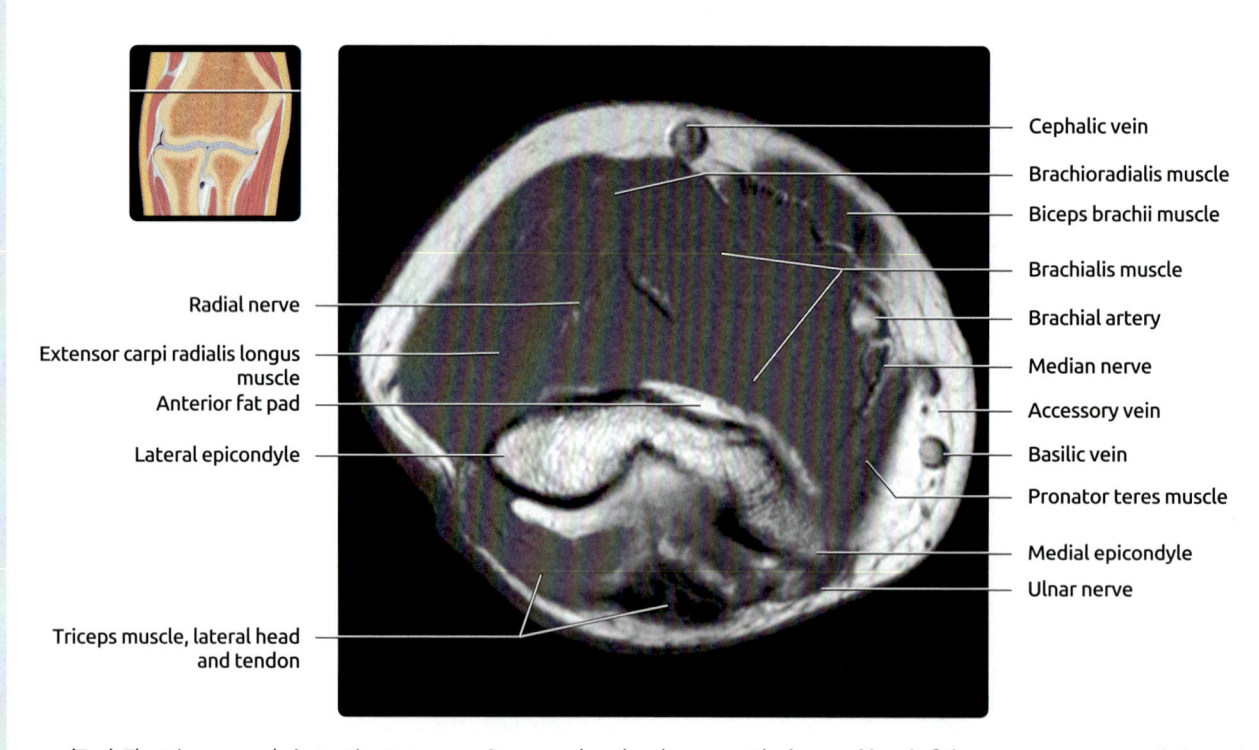

Labels (top image):
- Cephalic vein
- Brachioradialis muscle
- Biceps brachii muscle
- Brachialis muscle
- Brachial artery
- Median nerve
- Accessory vein
- Basilic vein
- Pronator teres muscle
- Ulnar nerve
- Triceps, long head
- Radial nerve
- Extensor carpi radialis longus muscle
- Posterior fat pad
- Triceps muscle, lateral head and tendon

Labels (bottom image):
- Cephalic vein
- Brachioradialis muscle
- Biceps brachii muscle
- Brachialis muscle
- Brachial artery
- Median nerve
- Accessory vein
- Basilic vein
- Pronator teres muscle
- Medial epicondyle
- Ulnar nerve
- Radial nerve
- Extensor carpi radialis longus muscle
- Anterior fat pad
- Lateral epicondyle
- Triceps muscle, lateral head and tendon

(Top) *The triceps muscle is starting to taper as it approaches the olecranon. The humeral head of the pronator teres muscle is coming into view. This is the most proximal tendon to arise from the medial epicondyle.* **(Bottom)** *The medial and lateral epicondyles are now in view. The ulnar nerve is entering the cubital tunnel.*

Elbow MR Atlas

AXIAL T1 MR, LEFT ELBOW

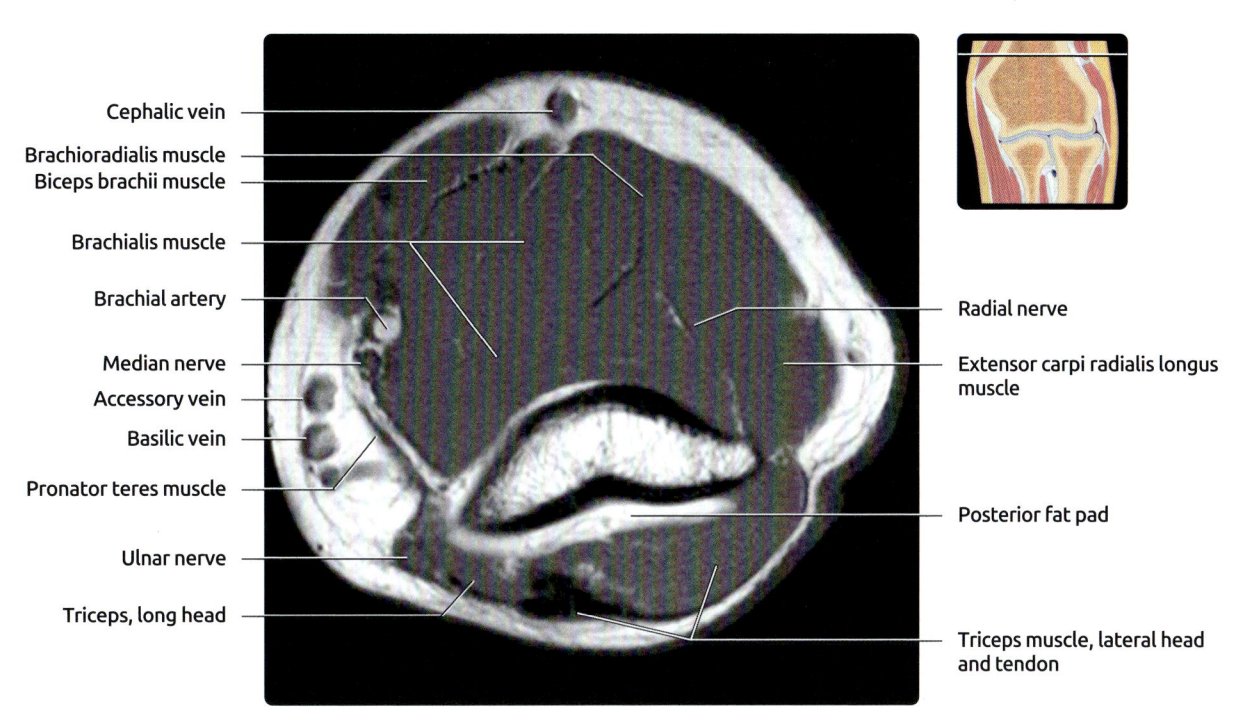

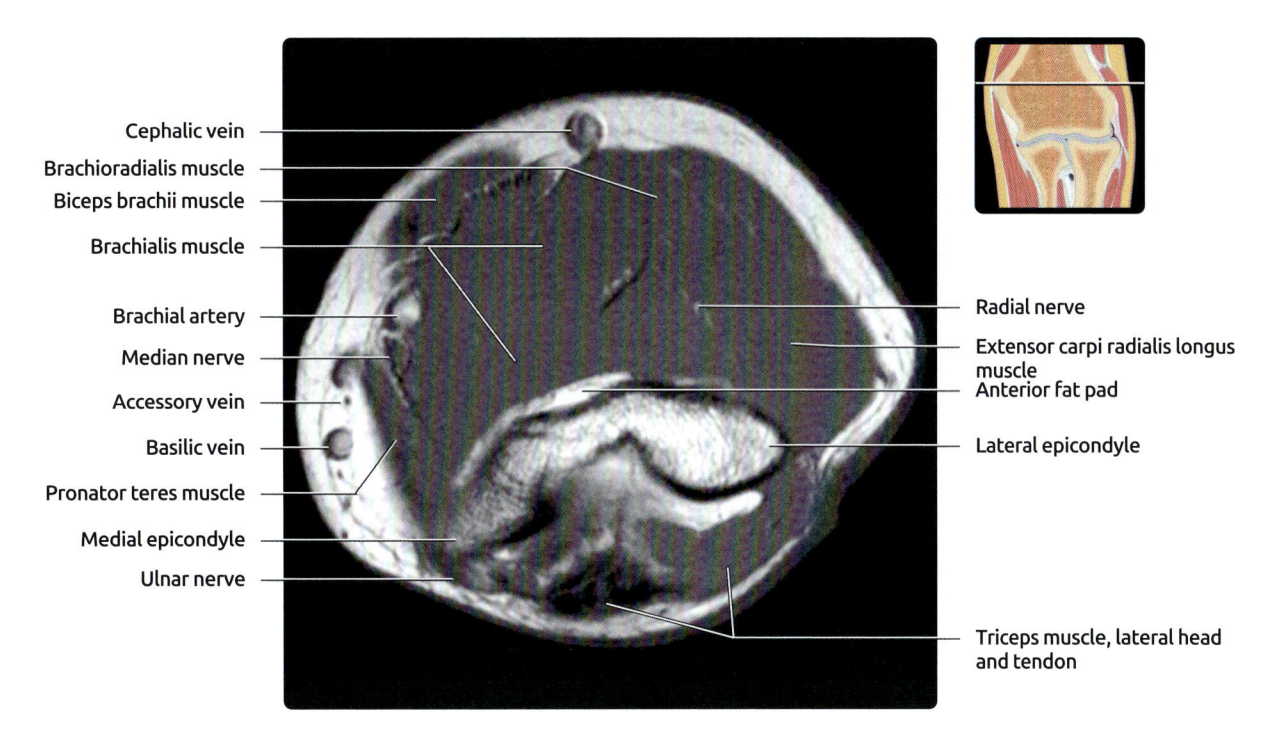

(Top) The triceps muscle is starting to taper as it approaches the olecranon. The humeral head of the pronator teres muscle is coming into view. This is the most proximal tendon to arise from the medial epicondyle. **(Bottom)** The medial and lateral epicondyles are now in view. The ulnar nerve is entering the cubital tunnel.

Elbow MR Atlas

AXIAL T1 MR, RIGHT ELBOW

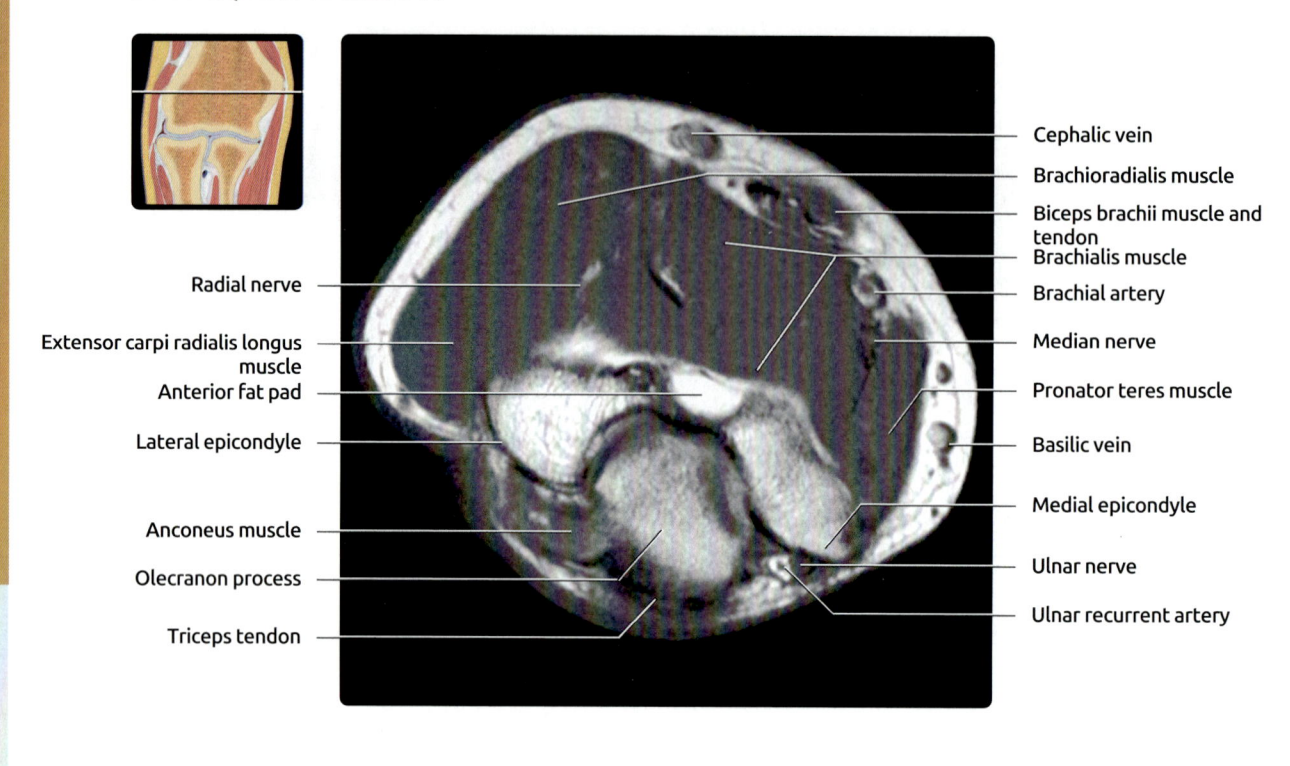

Top image labels:
- Cephalic vein
- Brachioradialis muscle
- Biceps brachii muscle and tendon
- Brachialis muscle
- Brachial artery
- Median nerve
- Pronator teres muscle
- Basilic vein
- Medial epicondyle
- Ulnar nerve
- Ulnar recurrent artery
- Radial nerve
- Extensor carpi radialis longus muscle
- Anterior fat pad
- Lateral epicondyle
- Anconeus muscle
- Olecranon process
- Triceps tendon

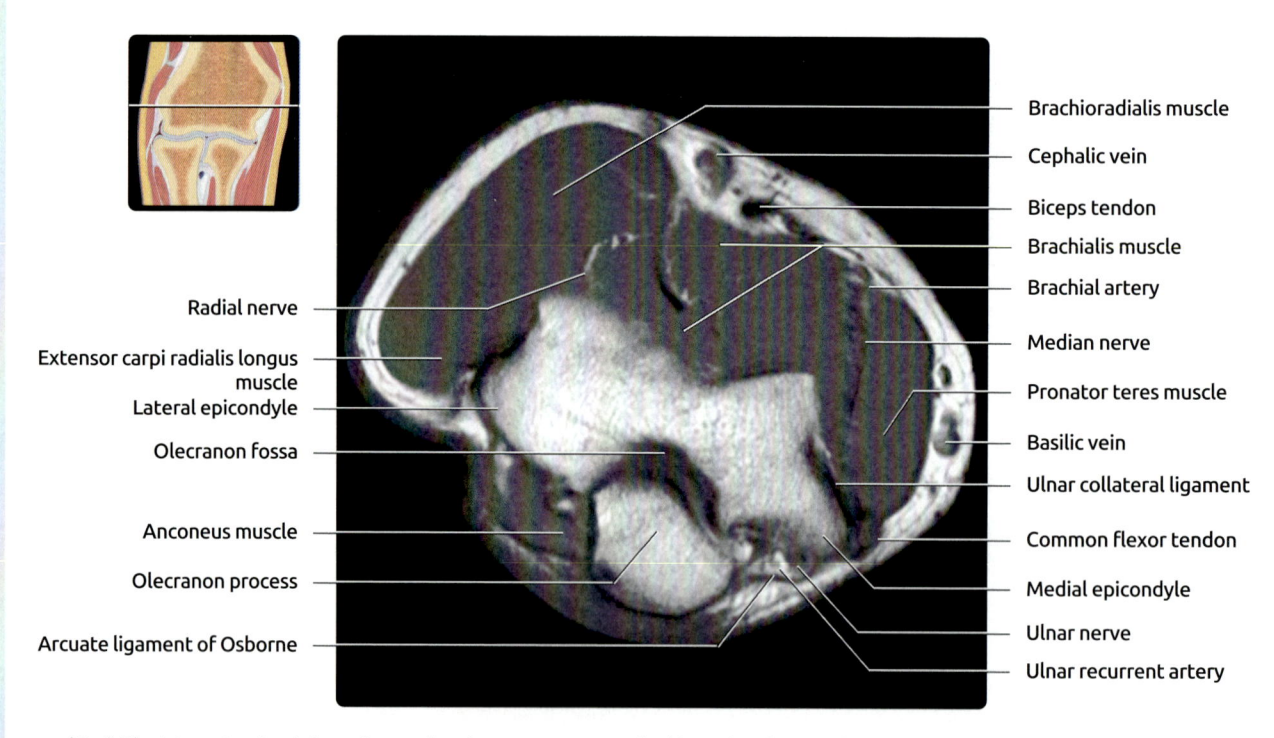

Bottom image labels:
- Brachioradialis muscle
- Cephalic vein
- Biceps tendon
- Brachialis muscle
- Brachial artery
- Median nerve
- Pronator teres muscle
- Basilic vein
- Ulnar collateral ligament
- Common flexor tendon
- Medial epicondyle
- Ulnar nerve
- Ulnar recurrent artery
- Radial nerve
- Extensor carpi radialis longus muscle
- Lateral epicondyle
- Olecranon fossa
- Anconeus muscle
- Olecranon process
- Arcuate ligament of Osborne

(Top) The triceps tendon is inserting on the olecranon process. The biceps brachii muscle is tapering to its distal tendon. **(Bottom)** The ulnar nerve is in the cubital tunnel, accompanied by the posterior ulnar recurrent artery.

Elbow MR Atlas

AXIAL T1 MR, LEFT ELBOW

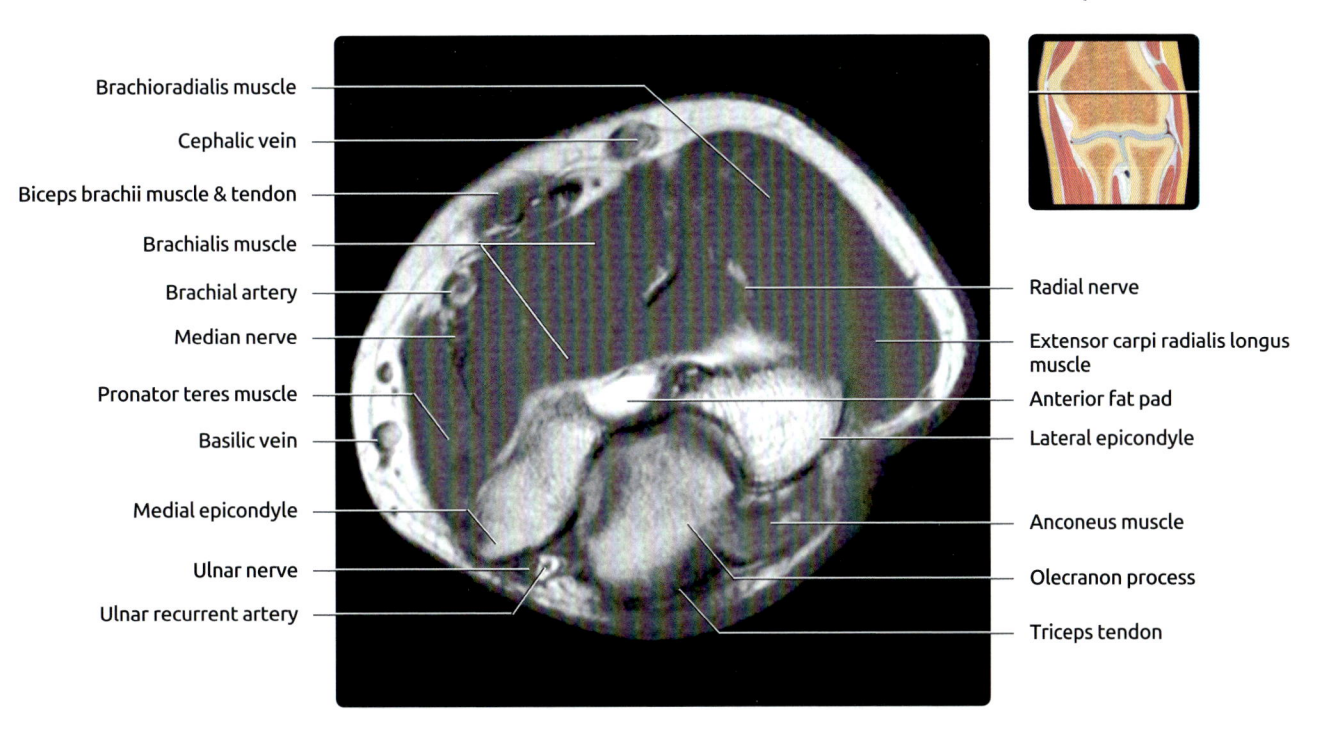

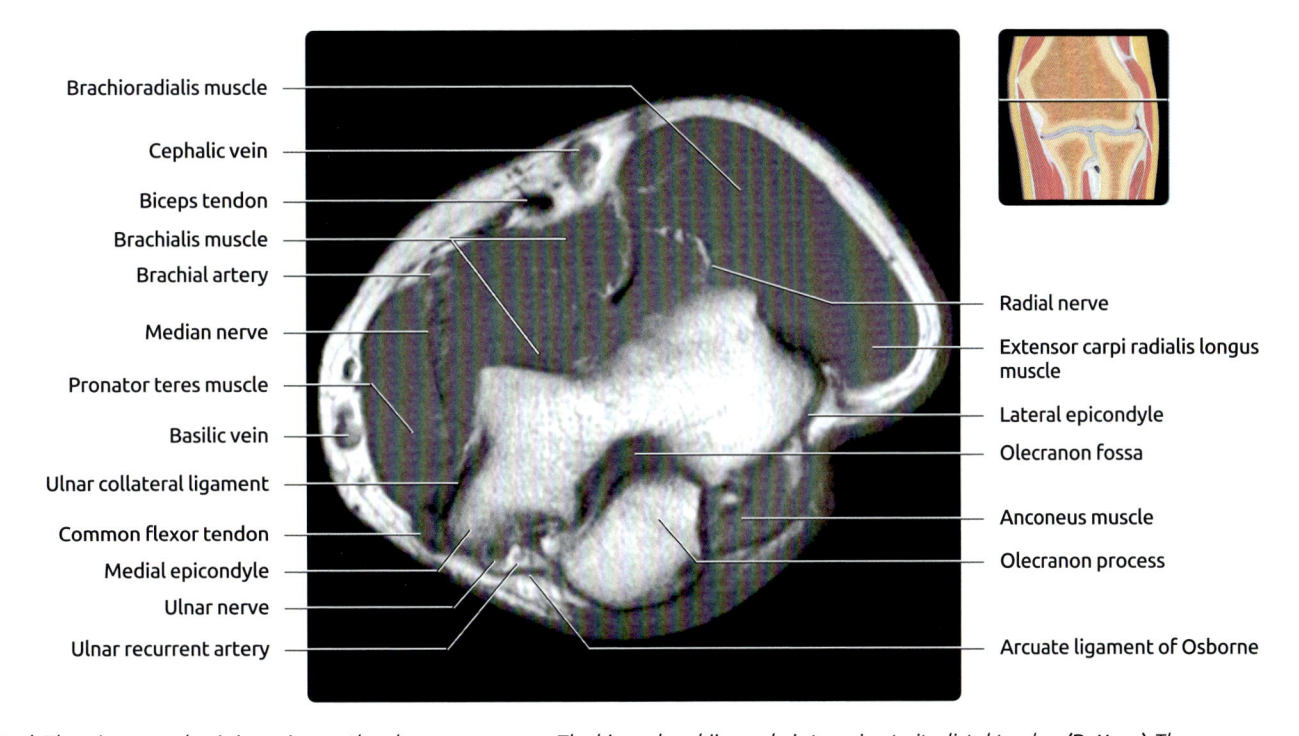

(Top) The triceps tendon is inserting on the olecranon process. The biceps brachii muscle is tapering to its distal tendon. (Bottom) The ulnar nerve is in the cubital tunnel, accompanied by the posterior ulnar recurrent artery.

Elbow MR Atlas

AXIAL T1 MR, RIGHT ELBOW

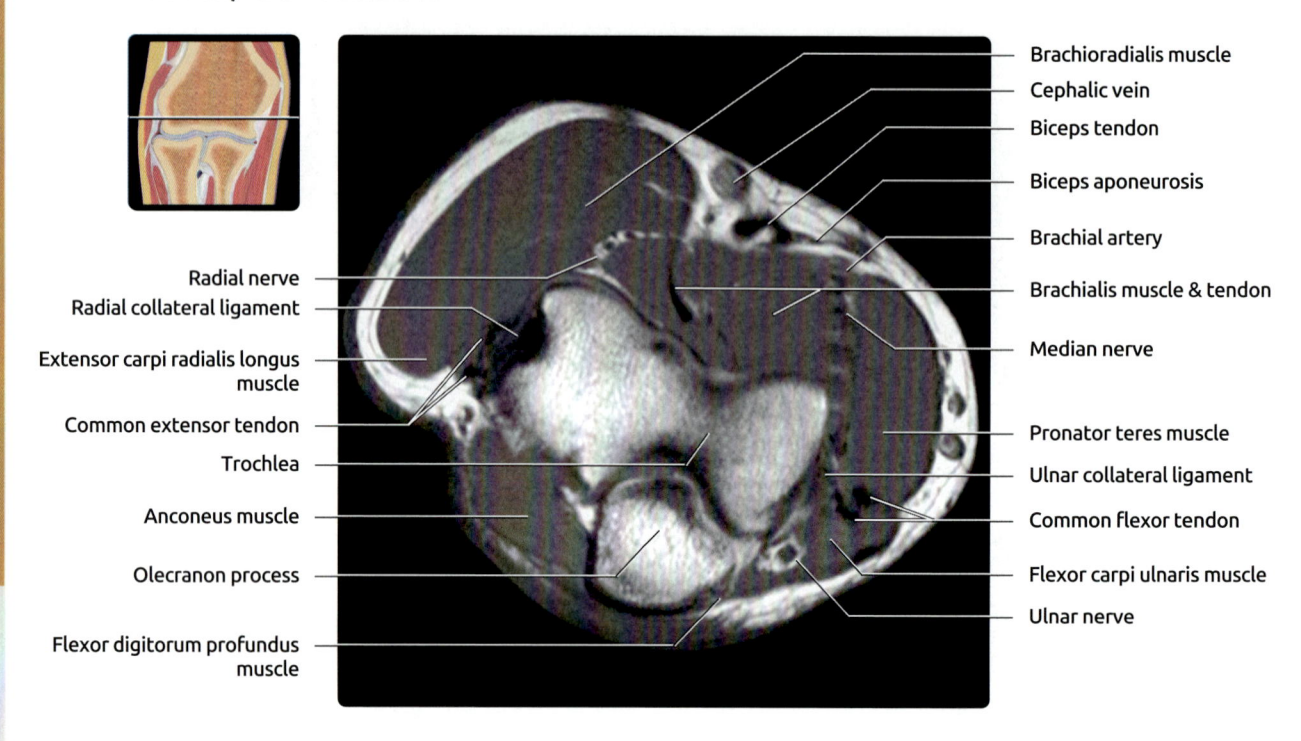

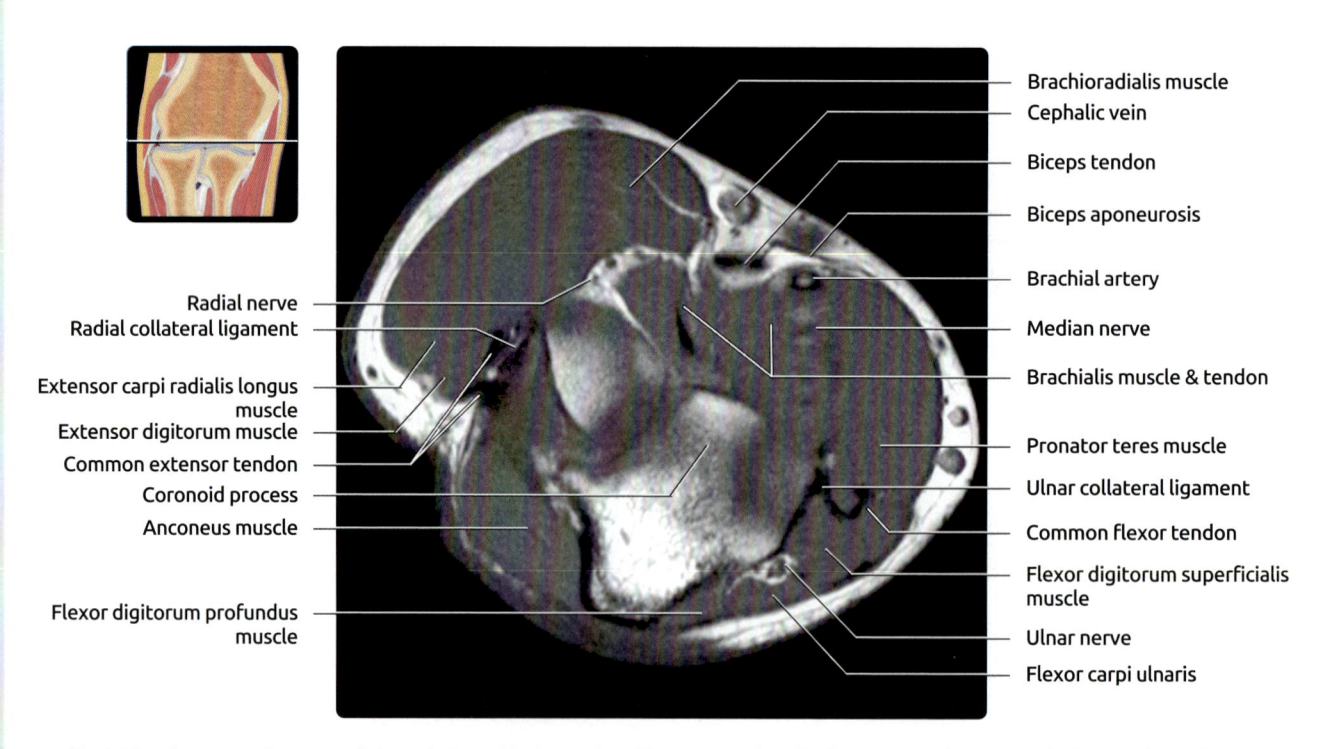

Top image labels (left side):
- Radial nerve
- Radial collateral ligament
- Extensor carpi radialis longus muscle
- Common extensor tendon
- Trochlea
- Anconeus muscle
- Olecranon process
- Flexor digitorum profundus muscle

Top image labels (right side):
- Brachioradialis muscle
- Cephalic vein
- Biceps tendon
- Biceps aponeurosis
- Brachial artery
- Brachialis muscle & tendon
- Median nerve
- Pronator teres muscle
- Ulnar collateral ligament
- Common flexor tendon
- Flexor carpi ulnaris muscle
- Ulnar nerve

Bottom image labels (left side):
- Radial nerve
- Radial collateral ligament
- Extensor carpi radialis longus muscle
- Extensor digitorum muscle
- Common extensor tendon
- Coronoid process
- Anconeus muscle
- Flexor digitorum profundus muscle

Bottom image labels (right side):
- Brachioradialis muscle
- Cephalic vein
- Biceps tendon
- Biceps aponeurosis
- Brachial artery
- Median nerve
- Brachialis muscle & tendon
- Pronator teres muscle
- Ulnar collateral ligament
- Common flexor tendon
- Flexor digitorum superficialis muscle
- Ulnar nerve
- Flexor carpi ulnaris

(**Top**) The ulnar nerve has passed through the cubital tunnel and is now entering the flexor carpi ulnaris muscle. (**Bottom**) The flexor digitorum profundus muscle is now visible, arising from the medial side of the olecranon. The biceps aponeurosis extends from the biceps tendon to the superficial surface of the common flexor mass.

Elbow MR Atlas

AXIAL T1 MR, LEFT ELBOW

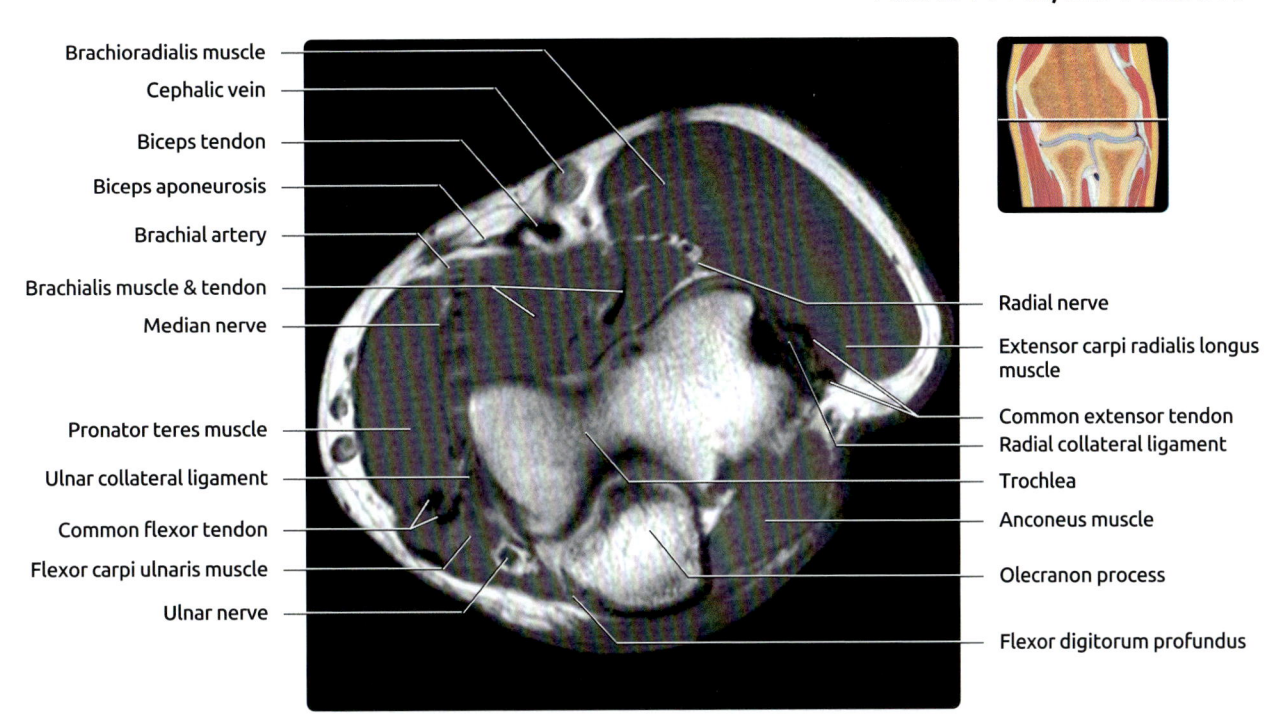

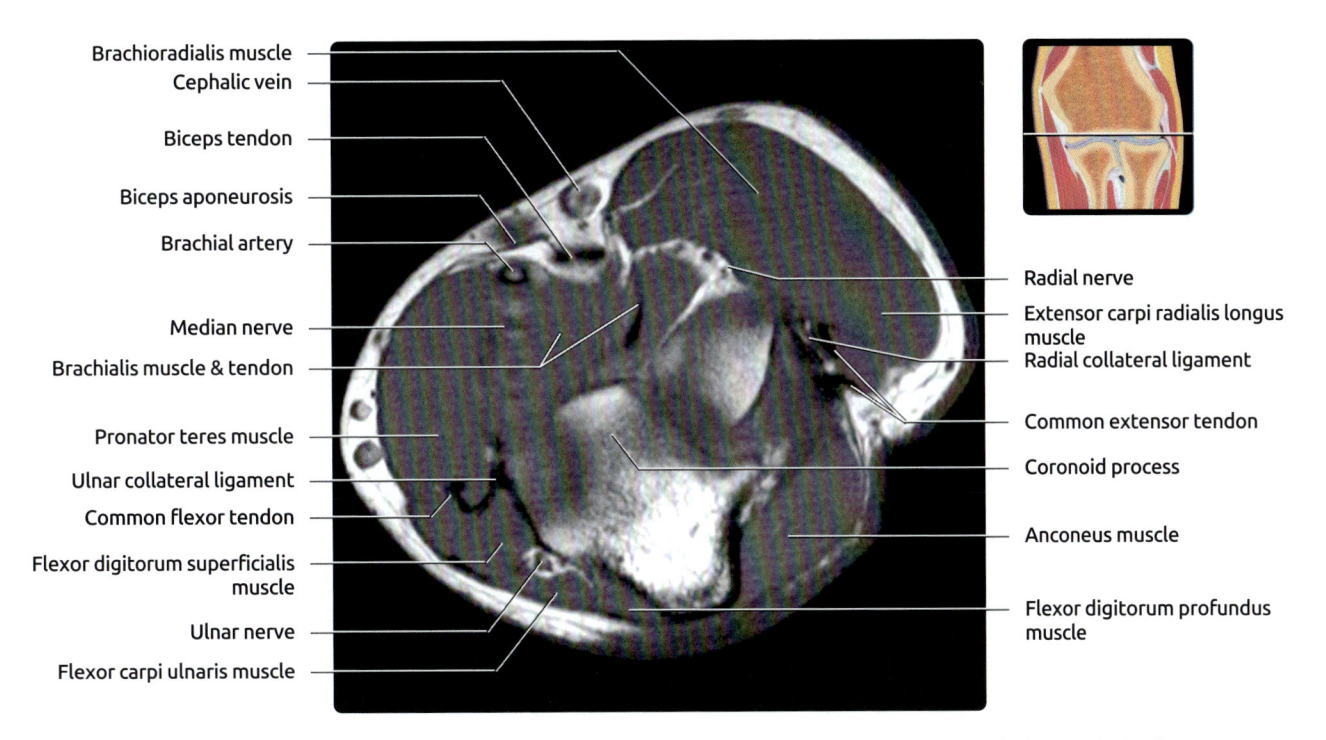

Labels (top image):
- Brachioradialis muscle
- Cephalic vein
- Biceps tendon
- Biceps aponeurosis
- Brachial artery
- Brachialis muscle & tendon
- Median nerve
- Pronator teres muscle
- Ulnar collateral ligament
- Common flexor tendon
- Flexor carpi ulnaris muscle
- Ulnar nerve
- Radial nerve
- Extensor carpi radialis longus muscle
- Common extensor tendon
- Radial collateral ligament
- Trochlea
- Anconeus muscle
- Olecranon process
- Flexor digitorum profundus

Labels (bottom image):
- Brachioradialis muscle
- Cephalic vein
- Biceps tendon
- Biceps aponeurosis
- Brachial artery
- Median nerve
- Brachialis muscle & tendon
- Pronator teres muscle
- Ulnar collateral ligament
- Common flexor tendon
- Flexor digitorum superficialis muscle
- Ulnar nerve
- Flexor carpi ulnaris muscle
- Radial nerve
- Extensor carpi radialis longus muscle
- Radial collateral ligament
- Common extensor tendon
- Coronoid process
- Anconeus muscle
- Flexor digitorum profundus muscle

(Top) *The ulnar nerve has passed through the cubital tunnel and is now entering the flexor carpi ulnaris muscle.* (Bottom) *The flexor digitorum profundus muscle is now visible, arising from the medial side of the olecranon. The biceps aponeurosis extends from the biceps tendon to the superficial surface of the common flexor mass.*

Elbow MR Atlas

AXIAL T1 MR, RIGHT ELBOW

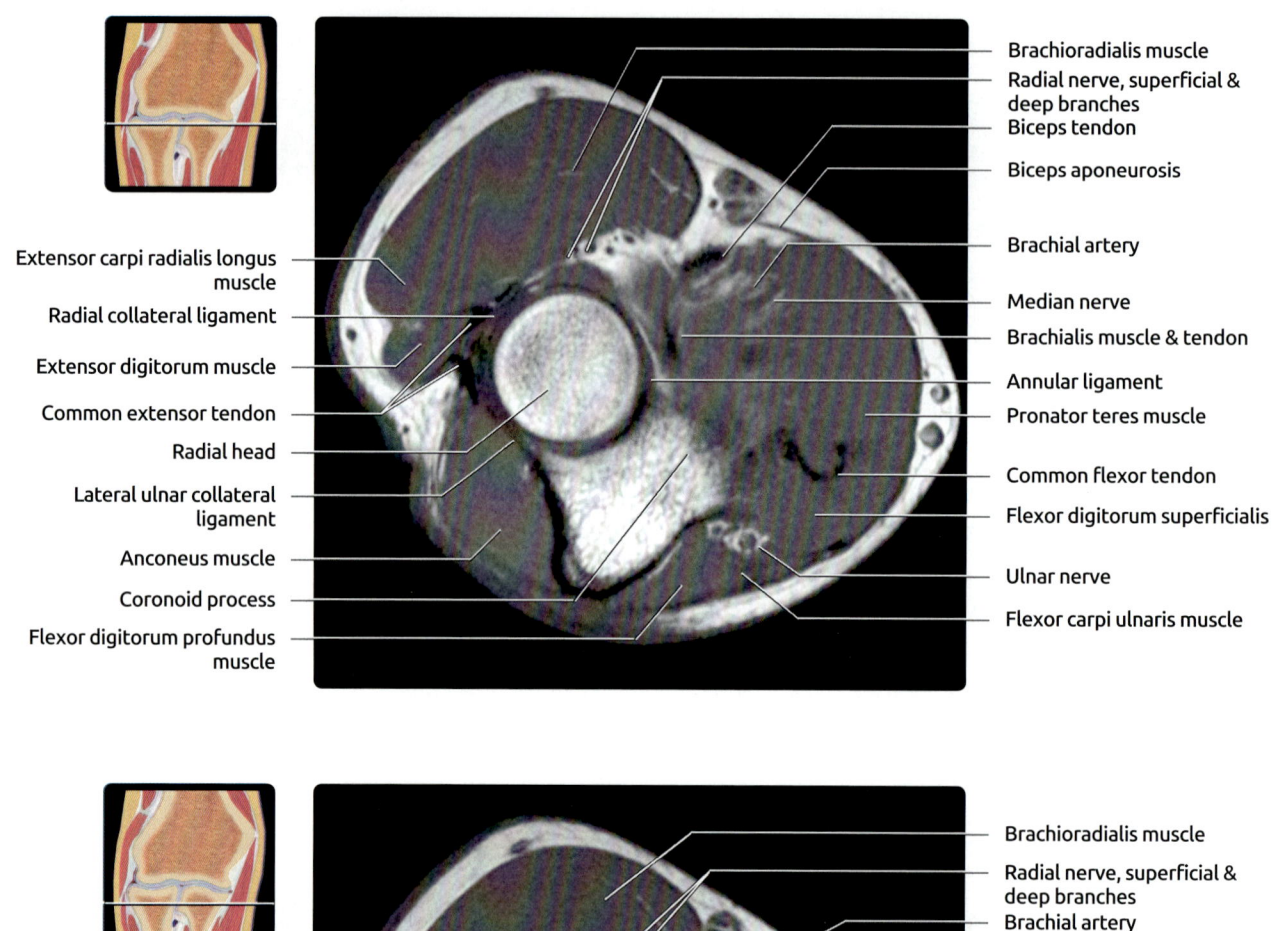

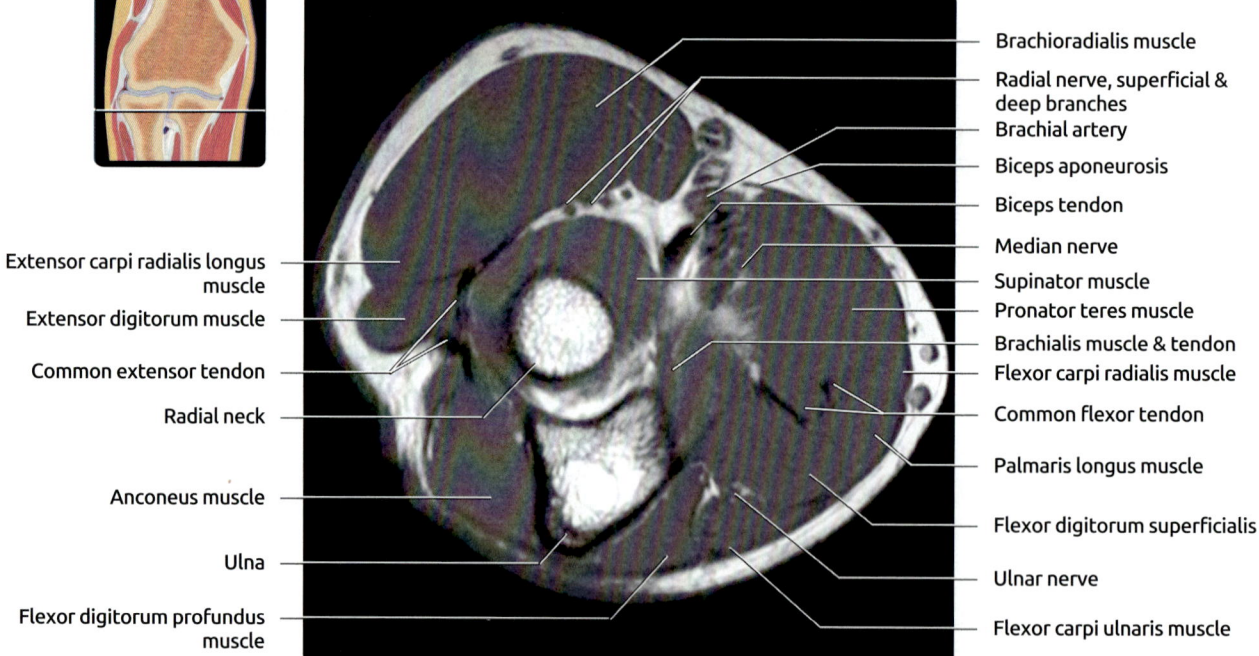

Top image labels:
- Brachioradialis muscle
- Radial nerve, superficial & deep branches
- Biceps tendon
- Biceps aponeurosis
- Brachial artery
- Median nerve
- Brachialis muscle & tendon
- Annular ligament
- Pronator teres muscle
- Common flexor tendon
- Flexor digitorum superficialis
- Ulnar nerve
- Flexor carpi ulnaris muscle
- Extensor carpi radialis longus muscle
- Radial collateral ligament
- Extensor digitorum muscle
- Common extensor tendon
- Radial head
- Lateral ulnar collateral ligament
- Anconeus muscle
- Coronoid process
- Flexor digitorum profundus muscle

Bottom image labels:
- Brachioradialis muscle
- Radial nerve, superficial & deep branches
- Brachial artery
- Biceps aponeurosis
- Biceps tendon
- Median nerve
- Supinator muscle
- Pronator teres muscle
- Brachialis muscle & tendon
- Flexor carpi radialis muscle
- Common flexor tendon
- Palmaris longus muscle
- Flexor digitorum superficialis
- Ulnar nerve
- Flexor carpi ulnaris muscle
- Extensor carpi radialis longus muscle
- Extensor digitorum muscle
- Common extensor tendon
- Radial neck
- Anconeus muscle
- Ulna
- Flexor digitorum profundus muscle

(Top) The annular ligament wraps around the radial head. The radial collateral ligament is seen inserting on the lateral aspect of the annular ligament. The radial nerve has branched into superficial and deep components. *(Bottom)* The supinator muscle wraps around the neck of the radius.

Elbow MR Atlas

AXIAL T1 MR, LEFT ELBOW

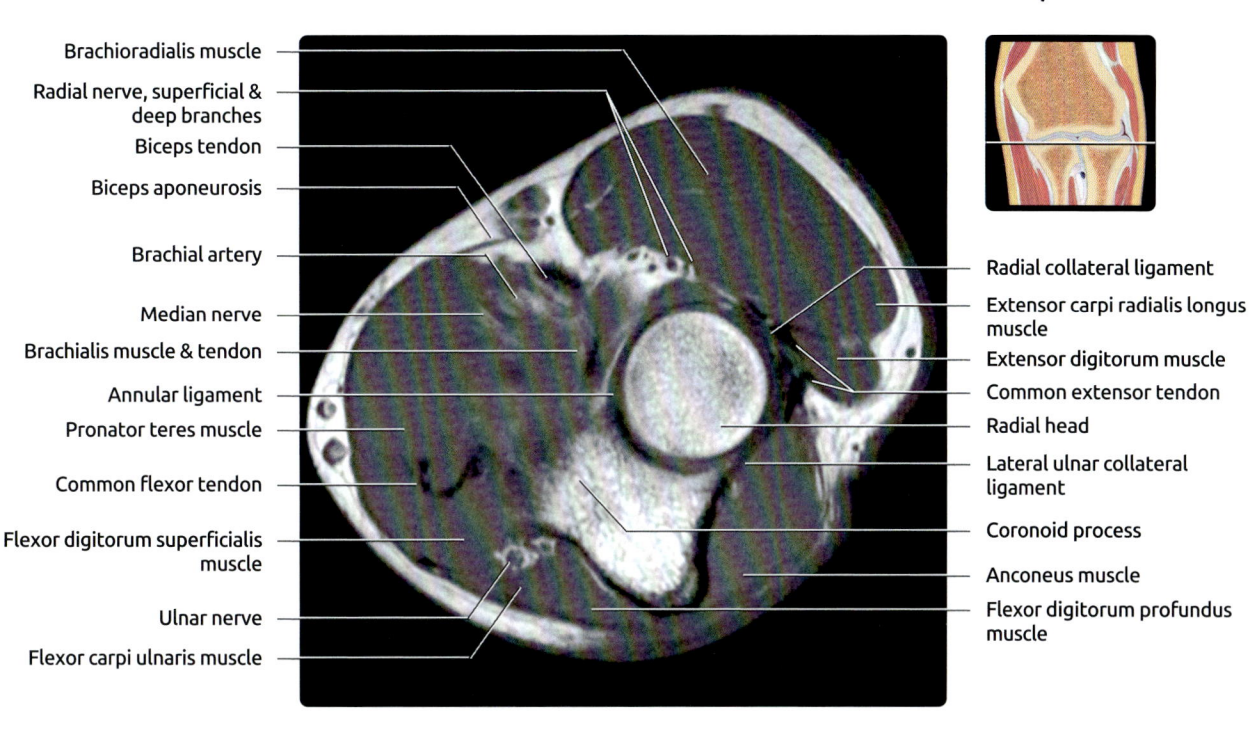

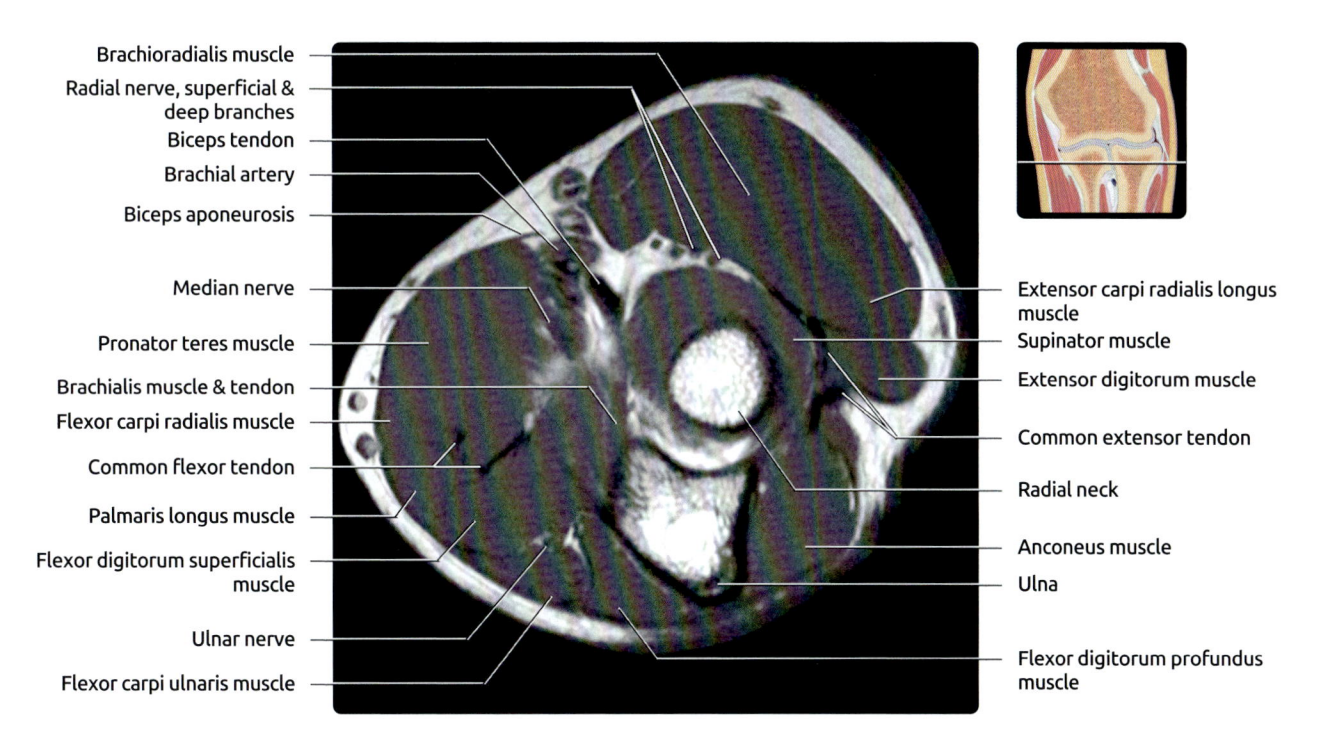

Top image labels (left side): Brachioradialis muscle; Radial nerve, superficial & deep branches; Biceps tendon; Biceps aponeurosis; Brachial artery; Median nerve; Brachialis muscle & tendon; Annular ligament; Pronator teres muscle; Common flexor tendon; Flexor digitorum superficialis muscle; Ulnar nerve; Flexor carpi ulnaris muscle

Top image labels (right side): Radial collateral ligament; Extensor carpi radialis longus muscle; Extensor digitorum muscle; Common extensor tendon; Radial head; Lateral ulnar collateral ligament; Coronoid process; Anconeus muscle; Flexor digitorum profundus muscle

Bottom image labels (left side): Brachioradialis muscle; Radial nerve, superficial & deep branches; Biceps tendon; Brachial artery; Biceps aponeurosis; Median nerve; Pronator teres muscle; Brachialis muscle & tendon; Flexor carpi radialis muscle; Common flexor tendon; Palmaris longus muscle; Flexor digitorum superficialis muscle; Ulnar nerve; Flexor carpi ulnaris muscle

Bottom image labels (right side): Extensor carpi radialis longus muscle; Supinator muscle; Extensor digitorum muscle; Common extensor tendon; Radial neck; Anconeus muscle; Ulna; Flexor digitorum profundus muscle

(Top) *The annular ligament wraps around the radial head. The radial collateral ligament is seen inserting on the lateral aspect of the annular ligament. The radial nerve has branched into superficial and deep components.* **(Bottom)** *The supinator muscle wraps around the neck of the radius.*

Elbow MR Atlas

AXIAL T1 MR, RIGHT ELBOW

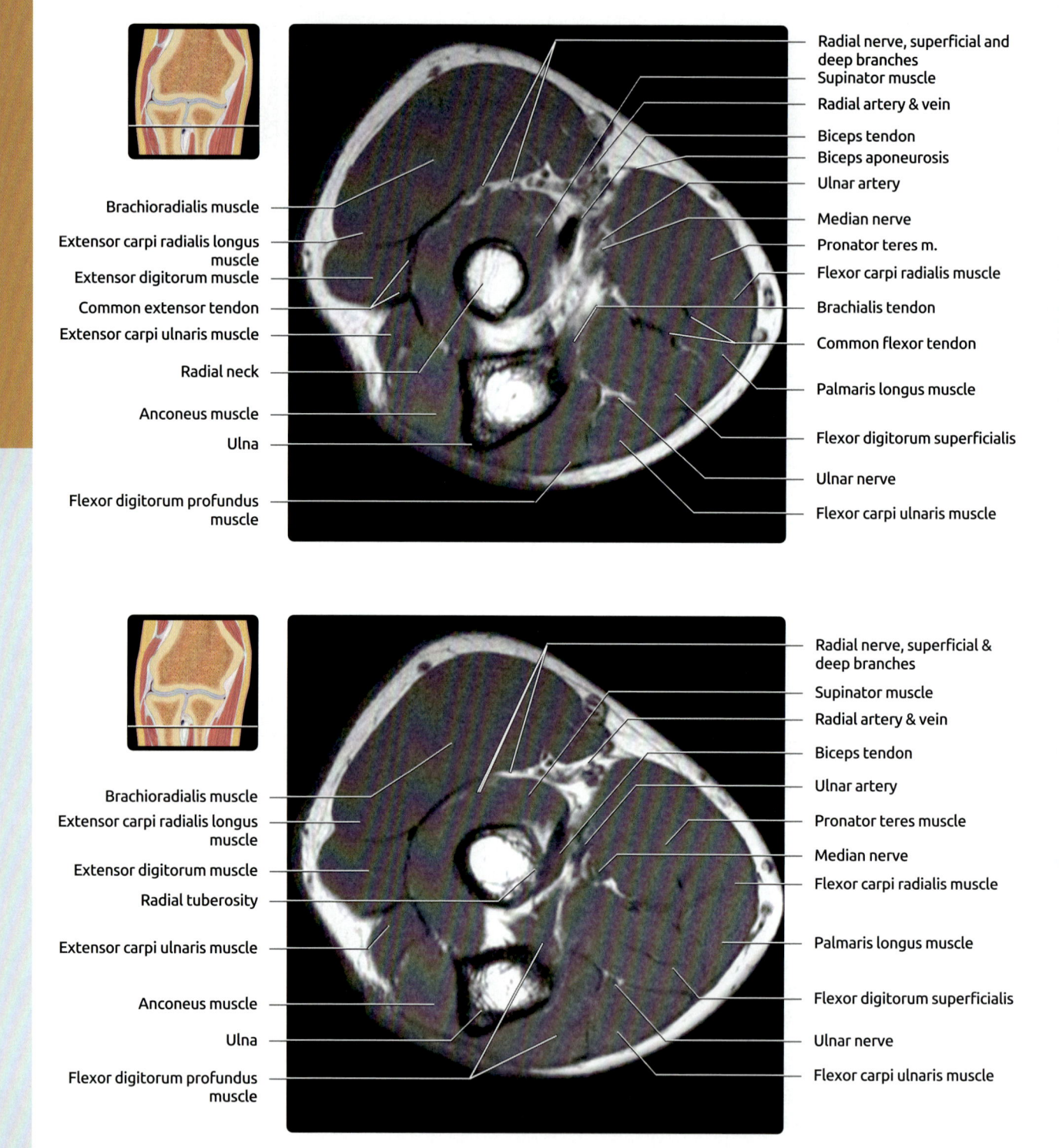

Labels (top image):
- Radial nerve, superficial and deep branches
- Supinator muscle
- Radial artery & vein
- Biceps tendon
- Biceps aponeurosis
- Ulnar artery
- Median nerve
- Pronator teres m.
- Flexor carpi radialis muscle
- Brachialis tendon
- Common flexor tendon
- Palmaris longus muscle
- Flexor digitorum superficialis
- Ulnar nerve
- Flexor carpi ulnaris muscle
- Brachioradialis muscle
- Extensor carpi radialis longus muscle
- Extensor digitorum muscle
- Common extensor tendon
- Extensor carpi ulnaris muscle
- Radial neck
- Anconeus muscle
- Ulna
- Flexor digitorum profundus muscle

Labels (bottom image):
- Radial nerve, superficial & deep branches
- Supinator muscle
- Radial artery & vein
- Biceps tendon
- Ulnar artery
- Pronator teres muscle
- Median nerve
- Flexor carpi radialis muscle
- Palmaris longus muscle
- Flexor digitorum superficialis
- Ulnar nerve
- Flexor carpi ulnaris muscle
- Brachioradialis muscle
- Extensor carpi radialis longus muscle
- Extensor digitorum muscle
- Radial tuberosity
- Extensor carpi ulnaris muscle
- Anconeus muscle
- Ulna
- Flexor digitorum profundus muscle

(Top) The brachialis tendon is seen inserting on the ulnar tuberosity. The brachial artery has divided into radial and ulnar branches. **(Bottom)** The biceps tendon is seen inserting on the radial tuberosity. The deep branch of the radial nerve is starting to enter the supinator muscle on its way to the posterior compartment of the forearm to become the posterior interosseous nerve.

AXIAL T1 MR, LEFT ELBOW

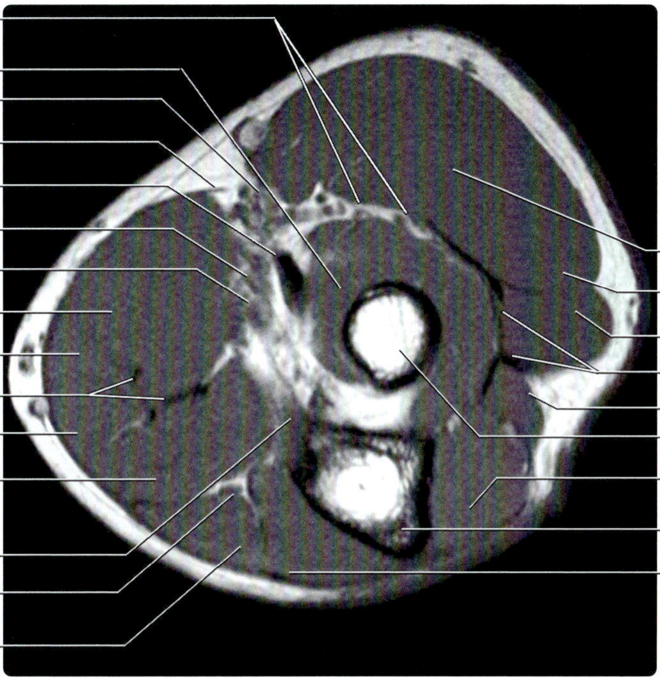
Radial nerve, superficial & deep branches
Supinator muscle
Radial artery & vein
Biceps aponeurosis
Biceps tendon
Ulnar artery
Median nerve
Pronator teres muscle
Flexor carpi radialis muscle
Common flexor tendon
Palmaris longus muscle
Flexor digitorum superficialis muscle
Brachialis tendon
Ulnar nerve
Flexor carpi ulnaris muscle
Brachioradialis muscle
Extensor carpi radialis longus muscle
Extensor digitorum muscle
Common extensor tendon
Extensor carpi ulnaris muscle
Radial neck
Anconeus muscle
Ulna
Flexor digitorum profundus muscle

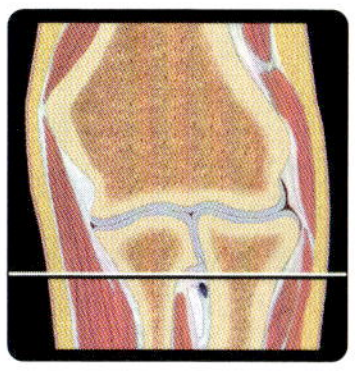

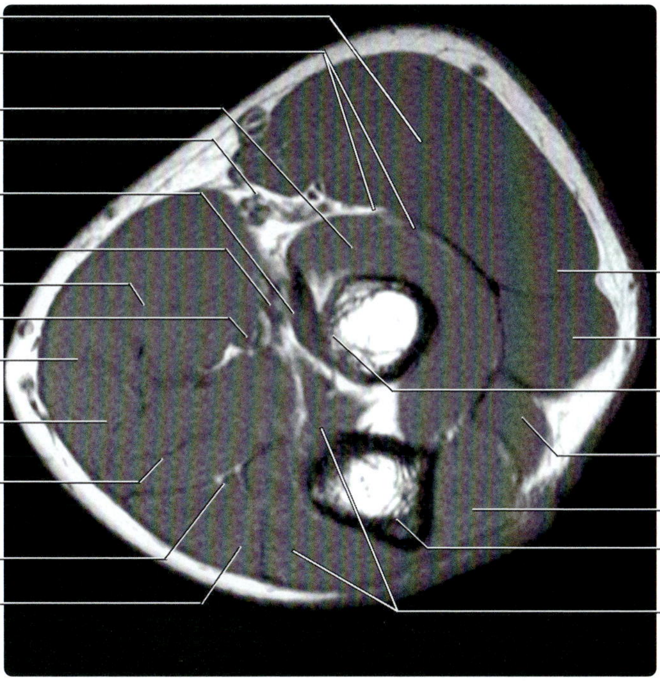
Brachioradialis muscle
Radial nerve, superficial & deep branches
Supinator muscle
Radial artery & vein
Biceps tendon
Ulnar artery
Pronator teres muscle
Median nerve
Flexor carpi radialis muscle
Palmaris longus muscle
Flexor digitorum superficialis muscle
Ulnar nerve
Flexor carpi ulnaris muscle
Extensor carpi radialis longus muscle
Extensor digitorum muscle
Radial tuberosity
Extensor carpi ulnaris muscle
Anconeus muscle
Ulna
Flexor digitorum profundus muscle

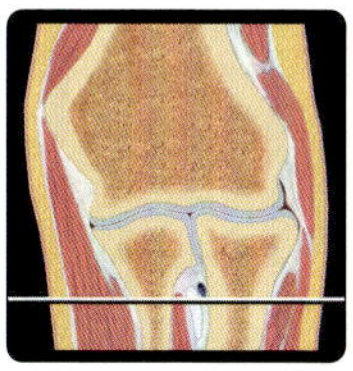

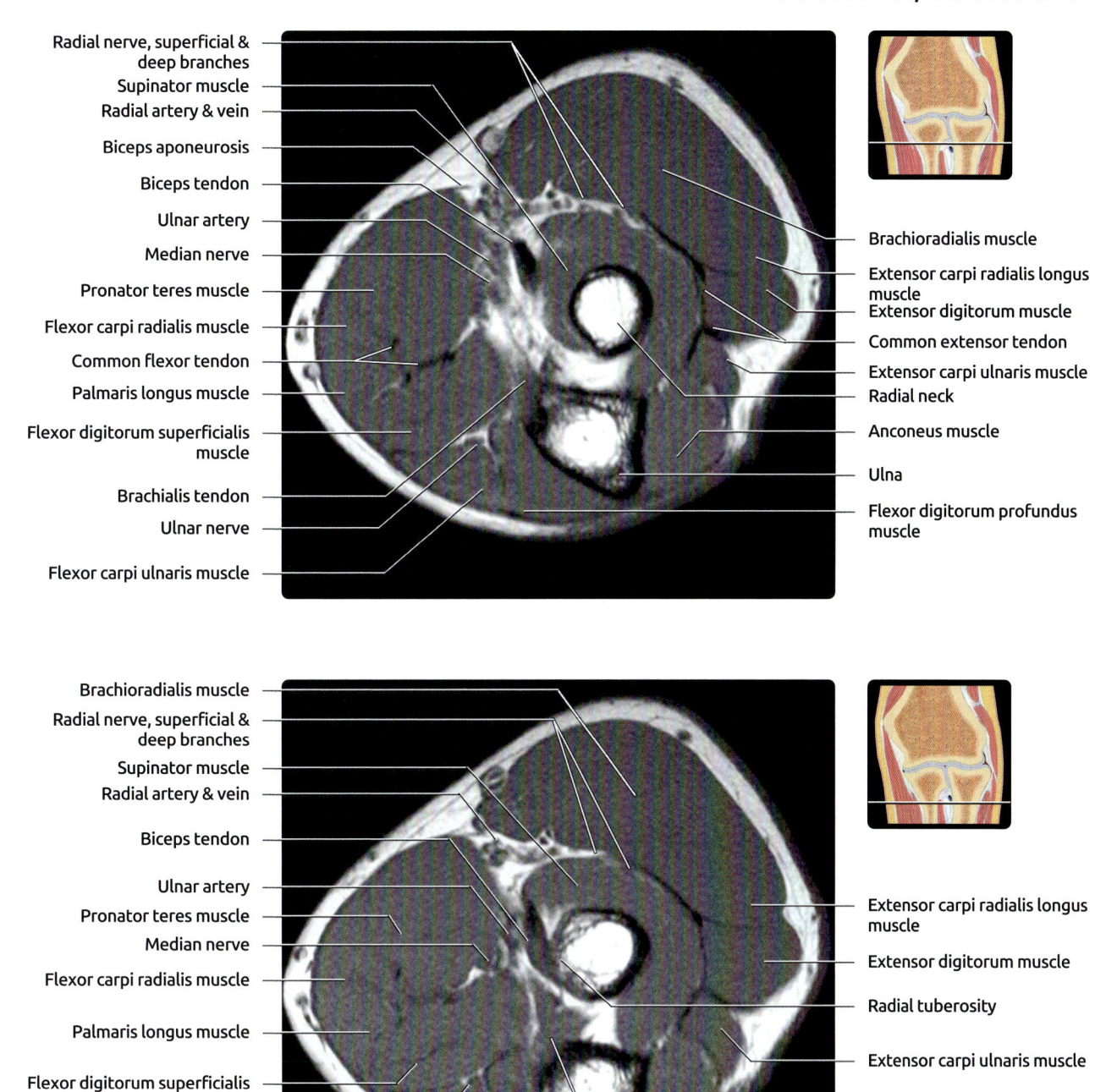

(Top) *The brachialis tendon is seen inserting on the ulnar tuberosity.* **(Bottom)** *The biceps tendon is seen inserting on the radial tuberosity. The deep branch of the radial nerve is starting to enter the supinator muscle on its way to the posterior compartment of the forearm to become the posterior interosseous nerve.*

Elbow MR Atlas

AXIAL T1 MR, RIGHT ELBOW

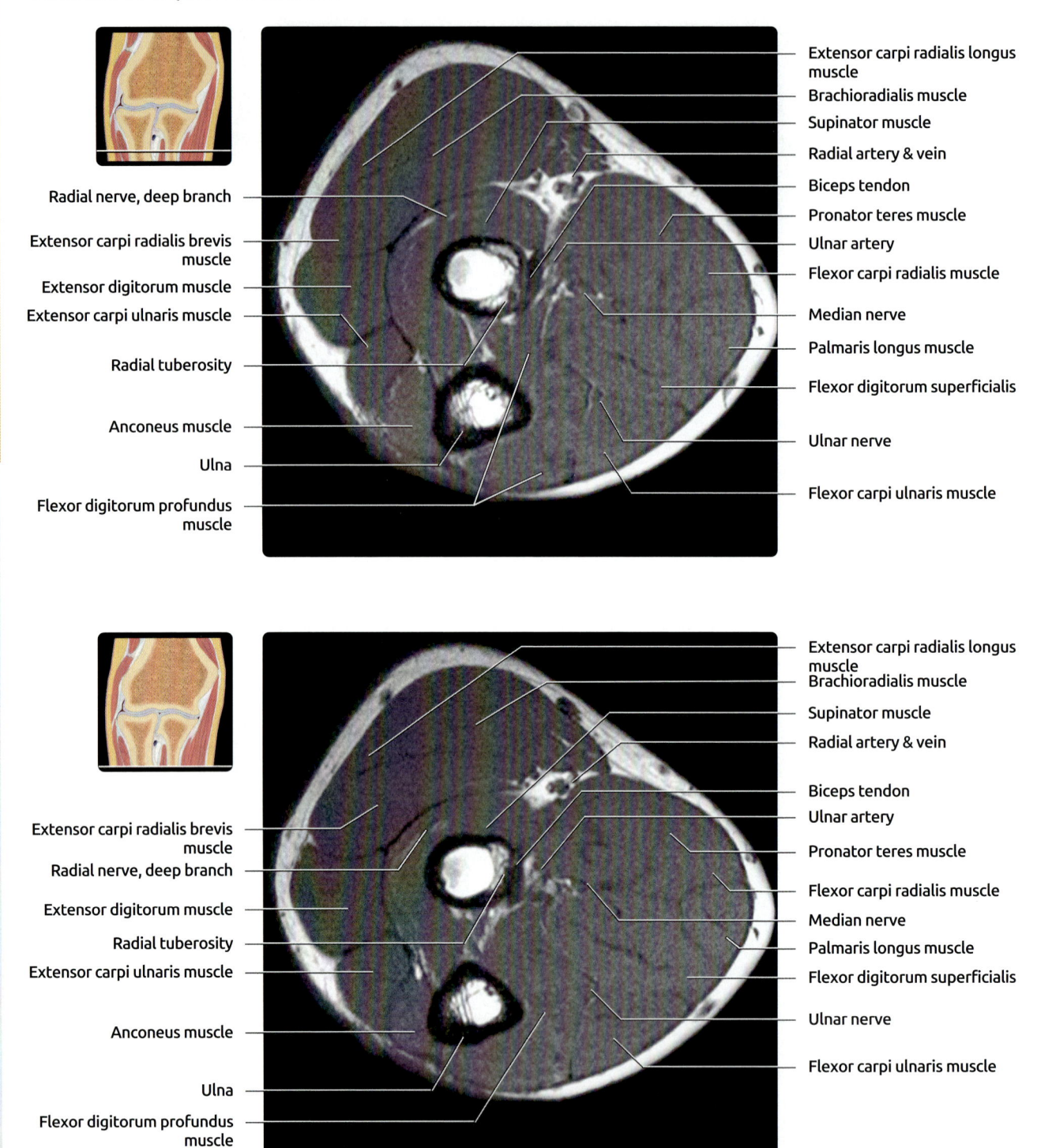

(Top) The deep branch of the radial nerve has entered the supinator muscle. The biceps tendon is attaching to the radial tuberosity.
(Bottom) The muscles of the flexor-pronator group are becoming well defined. Note how far distally one must image in order to see the full extent of the biceps tendon insertion on the radial tuberosity.

Elbow MR Atlas

AXIAL T1 MR, LEFT ELBOW

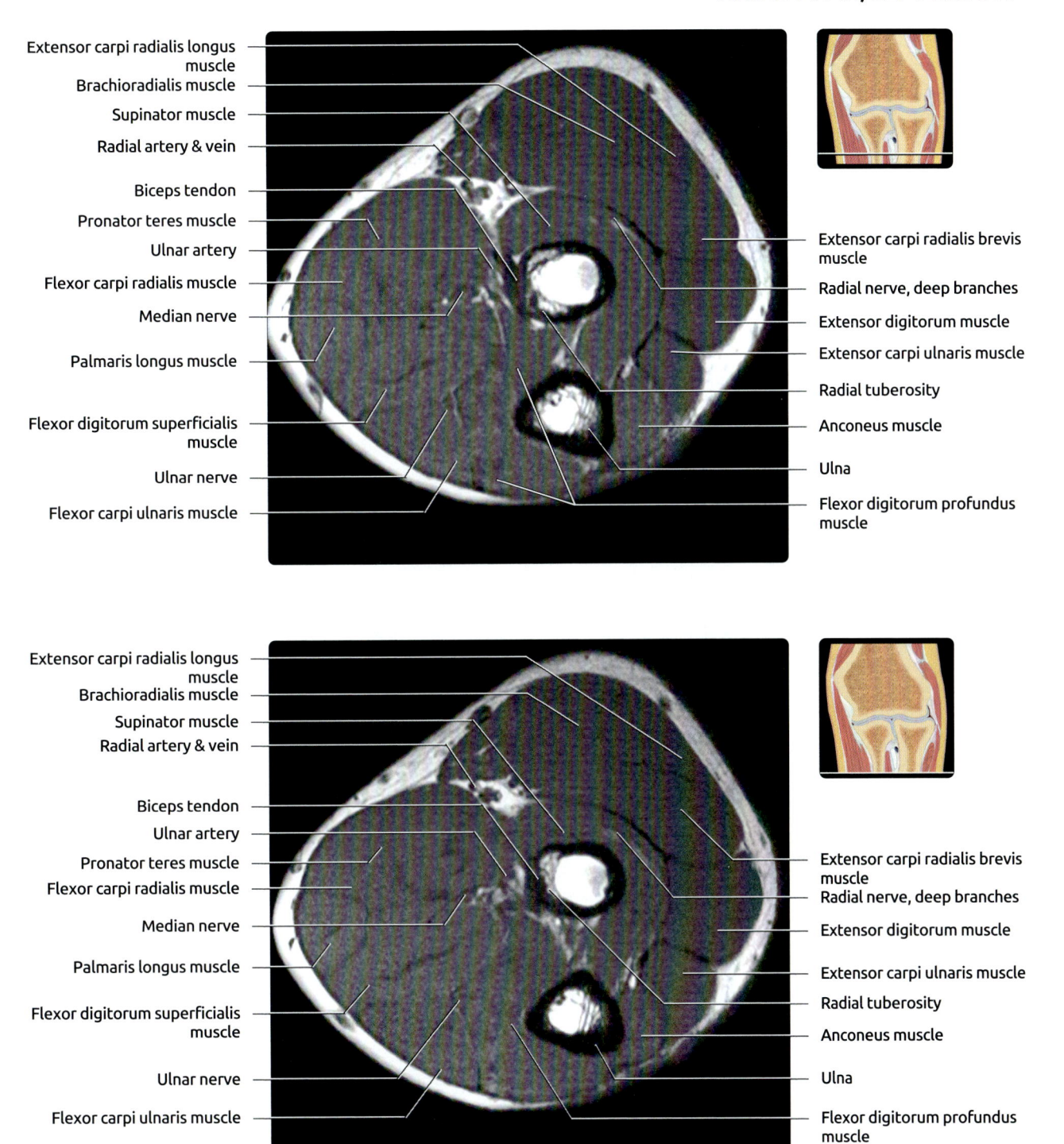

(Top) The deep branch of the radial nerve has entered the supinator muscle. The biceps tendon is attaching to the radial tuberosity.
(Bottom) The muscles of the flexor-pronator group are becoming well defined. Note how far distally one must image in order to see the full extent of the biceps tendon insertion on the radial tuberosity.

CORONAL T1 MR, RIGHT ELBOW

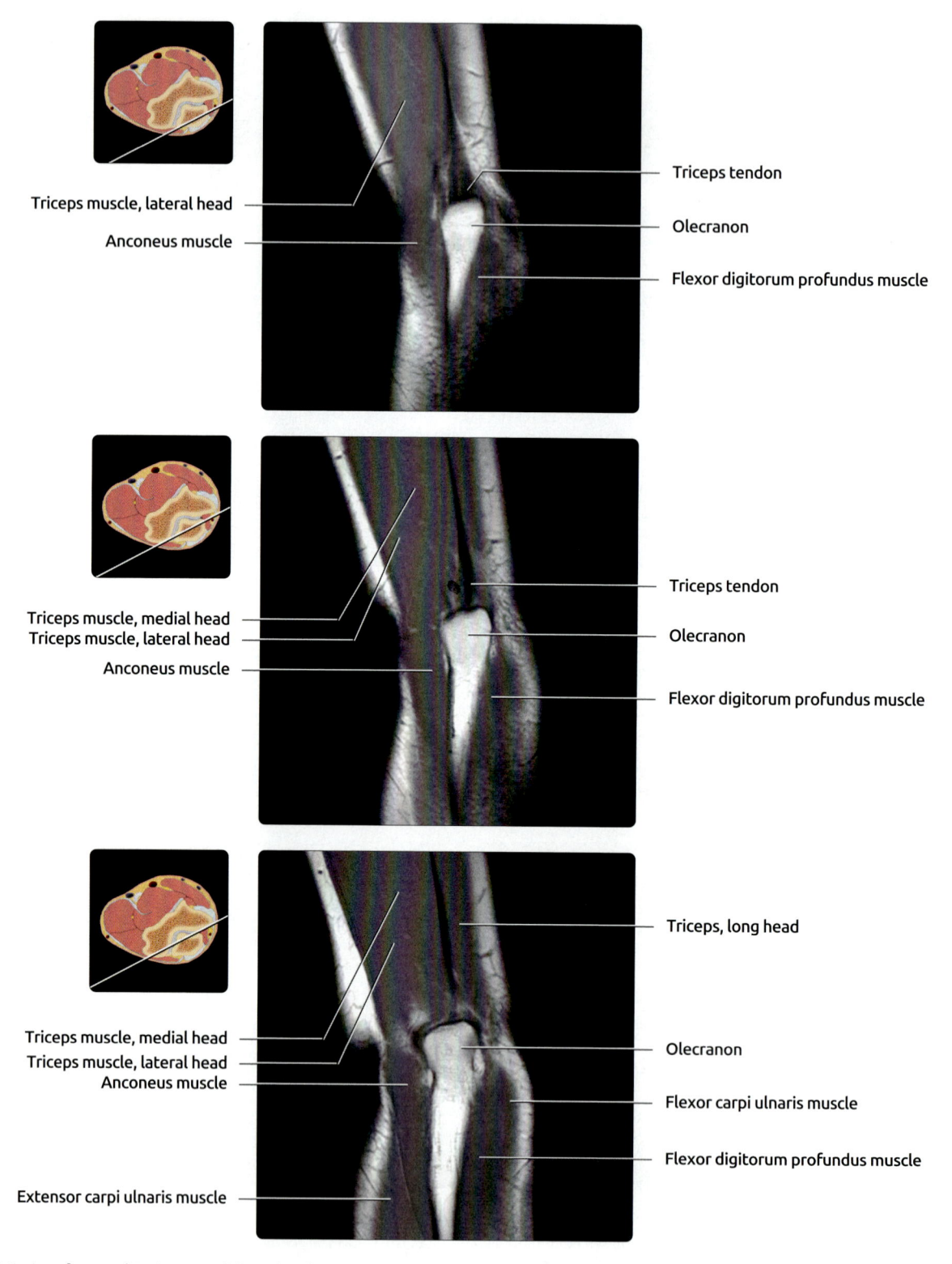

Triceps muscle, lateral head
Anconeus muscle
Triceps tendon
Olecranon
Flexor digitorum profundus muscle

Triceps muscle, medial head
Triceps muscle, lateral head
Anconeus muscle
Triceps tendon
Olecranon
Flexor digitorum profundus muscle

Triceps muscle, medial head
Triceps muscle, lateral head
Anconeus muscle
Extensor carpi ulnaris muscle
Triceps, long head
Olecranon
Flexor carpi ulnaris muscle
Flexor digitorum profundus muscle

(Top) Series of coronal T1 images of the right elbow, posterior to anterior, is shown. The triceps tendon is inserting on the olecranon. (Middle) The anconeus and flexor digitorum profundus muscles are now better seen. (Bottom) The flexor carpi ulnaris and extensor carpi ulnaris tendons are now coming into view.

Elbow MR Atlas

CORONAL T1 MR, LEFT ELBOW

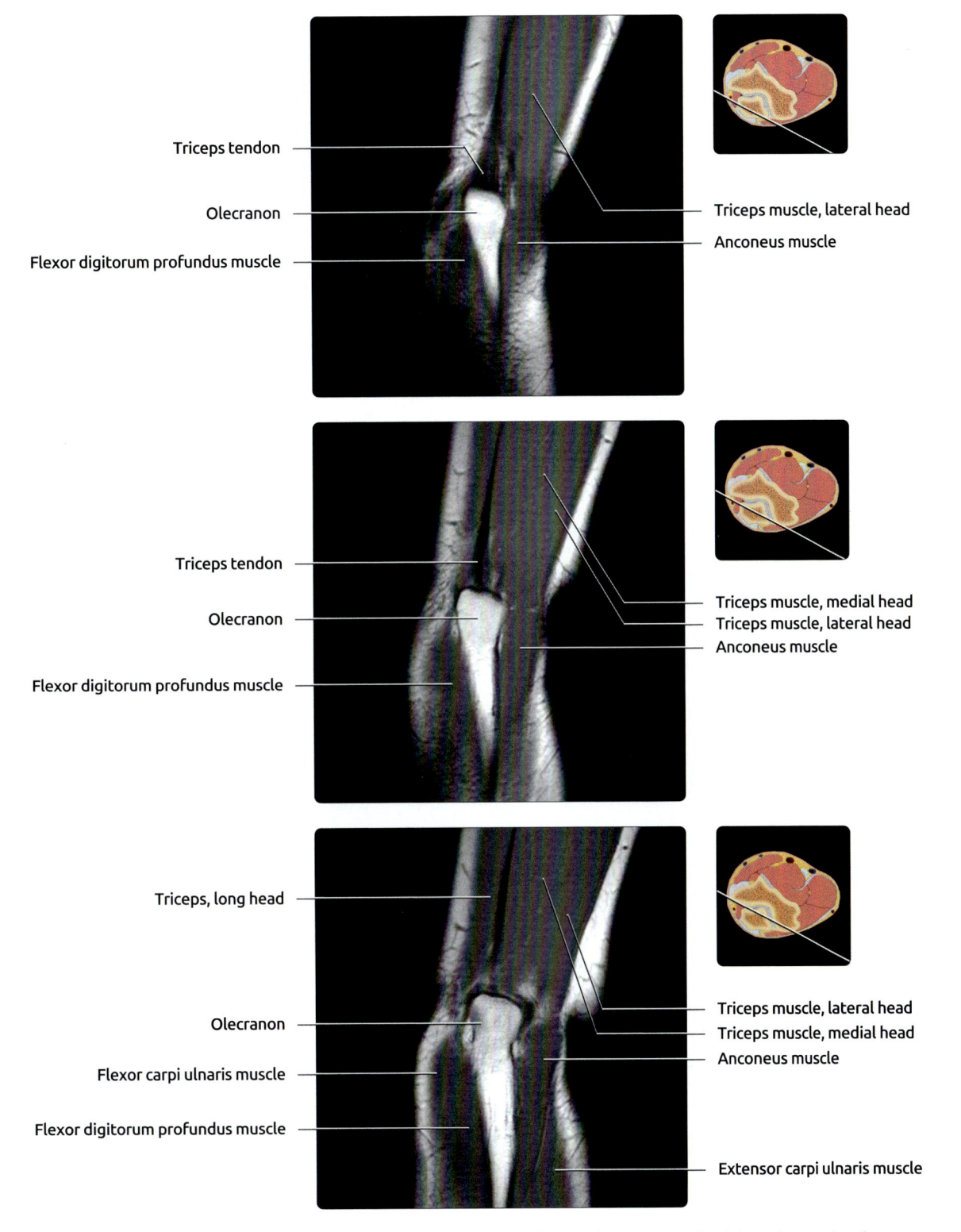

Triceps tendon
Olecranon
Flexor digitorum profundus muscle
Triceps muscle, lateral head
Anconeus muscle

Triceps tendon
Olecranon
Flexor digitorum profundus muscle
Triceps muscle, medial head
Triceps muscle, lateral head
Anconeus muscle

Triceps, long head
Olecranon
Flexor carpi ulnaris muscle
Flexor digitorum profundus muscle
Triceps muscle, lateral head
Triceps muscle, medial head
Anconeus muscle
Extensor carpi ulnaris muscle

(Top) Series of coronal T1 images of the left elbow, posterior to anterior, is shown. The triceps tendon is inserting on the olecranon. (Middle) The anconeus and flexor digitorum profundus muscles are now better seen. (Bottom) The flexor carpi ulnaris and extensor carpi ulnaris tendons are now coming into view.

Elbow MR Atlas

CORONAL T1 MR, RIGHT ELBOW

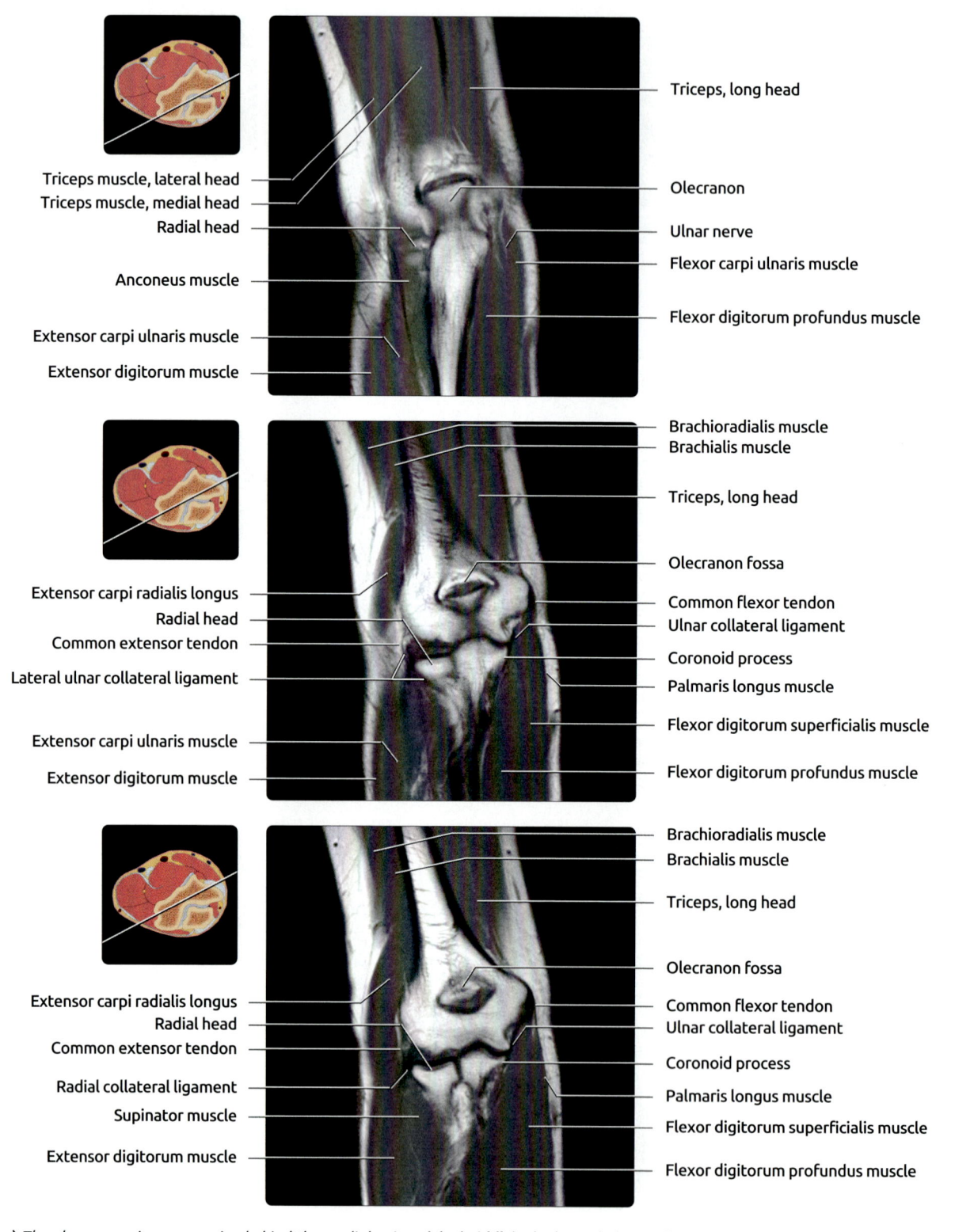

Triceps muscle, lateral head
Triceps muscle, medial head
Radial head
Anconeus muscle
Extensor carpi ulnaris muscle
Extensor digitorum muscle

Triceps, long head
Olecranon
Ulnar nerve
Flexor carpi ulnaris muscle
Flexor digitorum profundus muscle

Extensor carpi radialis longus
Radial head
Common extensor tendon
Lateral ulnar collateral ligament
Extensor carpi ulnaris muscle
Extensor digitorum muscle

Brachioradialis muscle
Brachialis muscle
Triceps, long head
Olecranon fossa
Common flexor tendon
Ulnar collateral ligament
Coronoid process
Palmaris longus muscle
Flexor digitorum superficialis muscle
Flexor digitorum profundus muscle

Extensor carpi radialis longus
Radial head
Common extensor tendon
Radial collateral ligament
Supinator muscle
Extensor digitorum muscle

Brachioradialis muscle
Brachialis muscle
Triceps, long head
Olecranon fossa
Common flexor tendon
Ulnar collateral ligament
Coronoid process
Palmaris longus muscle
Flexor digitorum superficialis muscle
Flexor digitorum profundus muscle

(Top) *The ulnar nerve is seen passing behind the medial epicondyle.* **(Middle)** *The lateral ulnar collateral ligament runs like a sling behind the radial neck to prevent posterolateral instability.* **(Bottom)** *The common extensor tendon is long and thin, while the common flexor tendon is short and broad.*

Elbow MR Atlas

CORONAL T1 MR, LEFT ELBOW

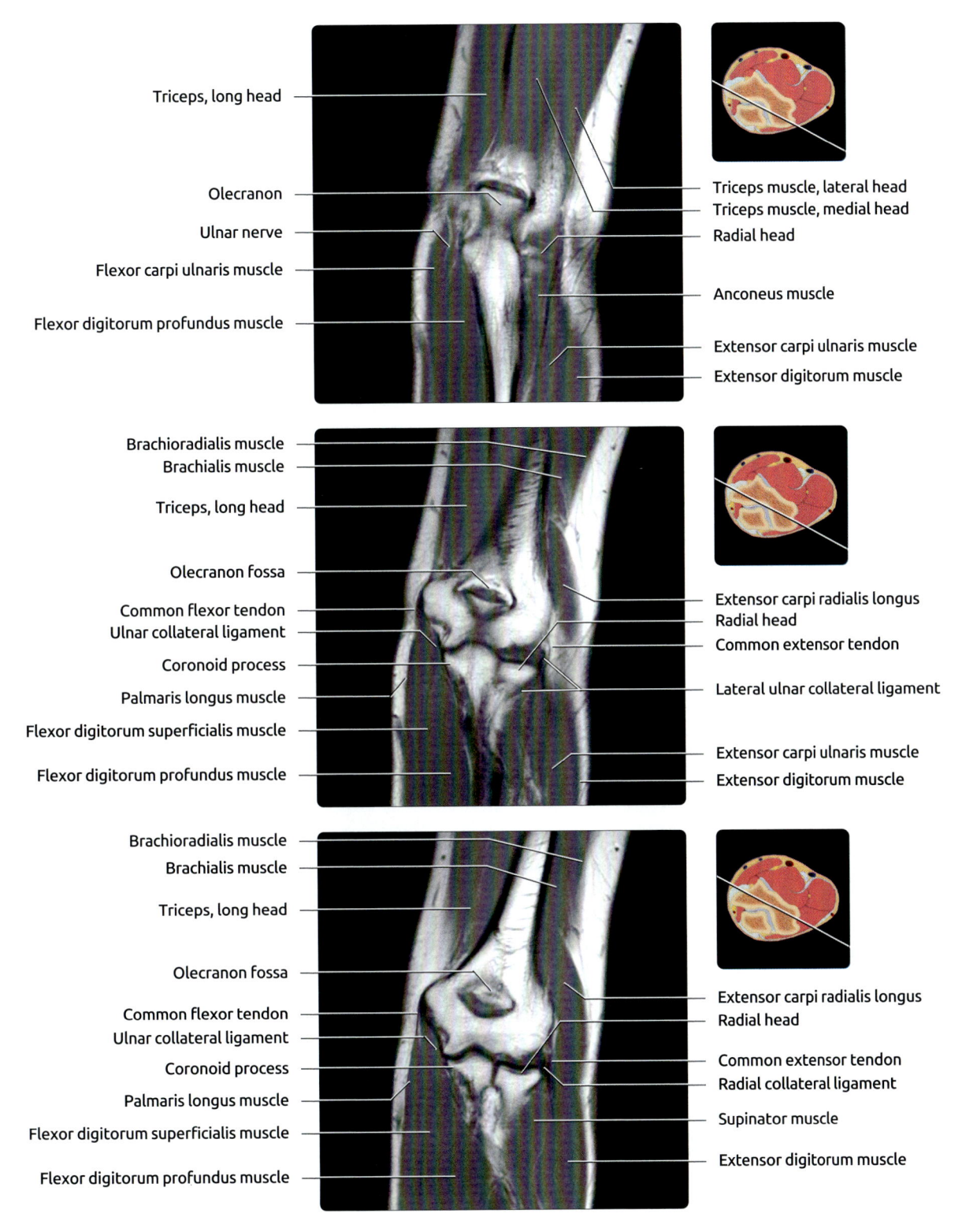

(Top) The ulnar nerve is seen passing behind the medial epicondyle. **(Middle)** The lateral ulnar collateral ligament runs like a sling behind the radial neck to prevent posterolateral instability. **(Bottom)** The common extensor tendon is long and thin, while the common flexor tendon is short and broad.

Elbow MR Atlas

CORONAL T1 MR, RIGHT ELBOW

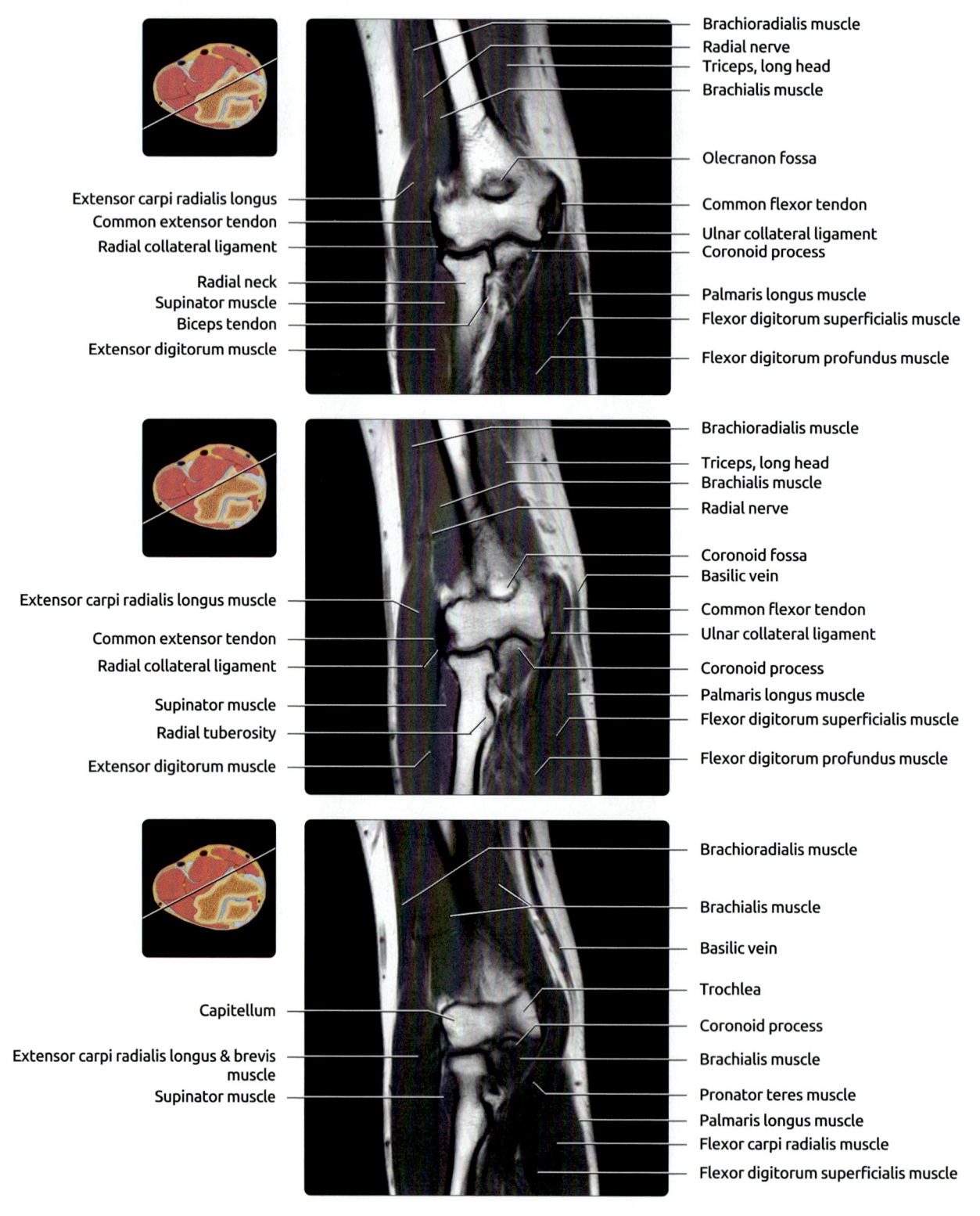

Labels (Top image):
- Brachioradialis muscle
- Radial nerve
- Triceps, long head
- Brachialis muscle
- Olecranon fossa
- Common flexor tendon
- Ulnar collateral ligament
- Coronoid process
- Palmaris longus muscle
- Flexor digitorum superficialis muscle
- Flexor digitorum profundus muscle
- Extensor carpi radialis longus
- Common extensor tendon
- Radial collateral ligament
- Radial neck
- Supinator muscle
- Biceps tendon
- Extensor digitorum muscle

Labels (Middle image):
- Brachioradialis muscle
- Triceps, long head
- Brachialis muscle
- Radial nerve
- Coronoid fossa
- Basilic vein
- Common flexor tendon
- Ulnar collateral ligament
- Coronoid process
- Palmaris longus muscle
- Flexor digitorum superficialis muscle
- Flexor digitorum profundus muscle
- Extensor carpi radialis longus muscle
- Common extensor tendon
- Radial collateral ligament
- Supinator muscle
- Radial tuberosity
- Extensor digitorum muscle

Labels (Bottom image):
- Brachioradialis muscle
- Brachialis muscle
- Basilic vein
- Trochlea
- Coronoid process
- Brachialis muscle
- Pronator teres muscle
- Palmaris longus muscle
- Flexor carpi radialis muscle
- Flexor digitorum superficialis muscle
- Capitellum
- Extensor carpi radialis longus & brevis muscle
- Supinator muscle

(Top) The radial nerve courses between the brachialis and brachioradialis muscles. The distal biceps tendon is approaching its insertion on the radial tuberosity. **(Middle)** The profile of the radial tuberosity is well seen. **(Bottom)** The brachialis muscle is draping over the anterior aspect of the humeral shaft.

Elbow MR Atlas

CORONAL T1 MR, LEFT ELBOW

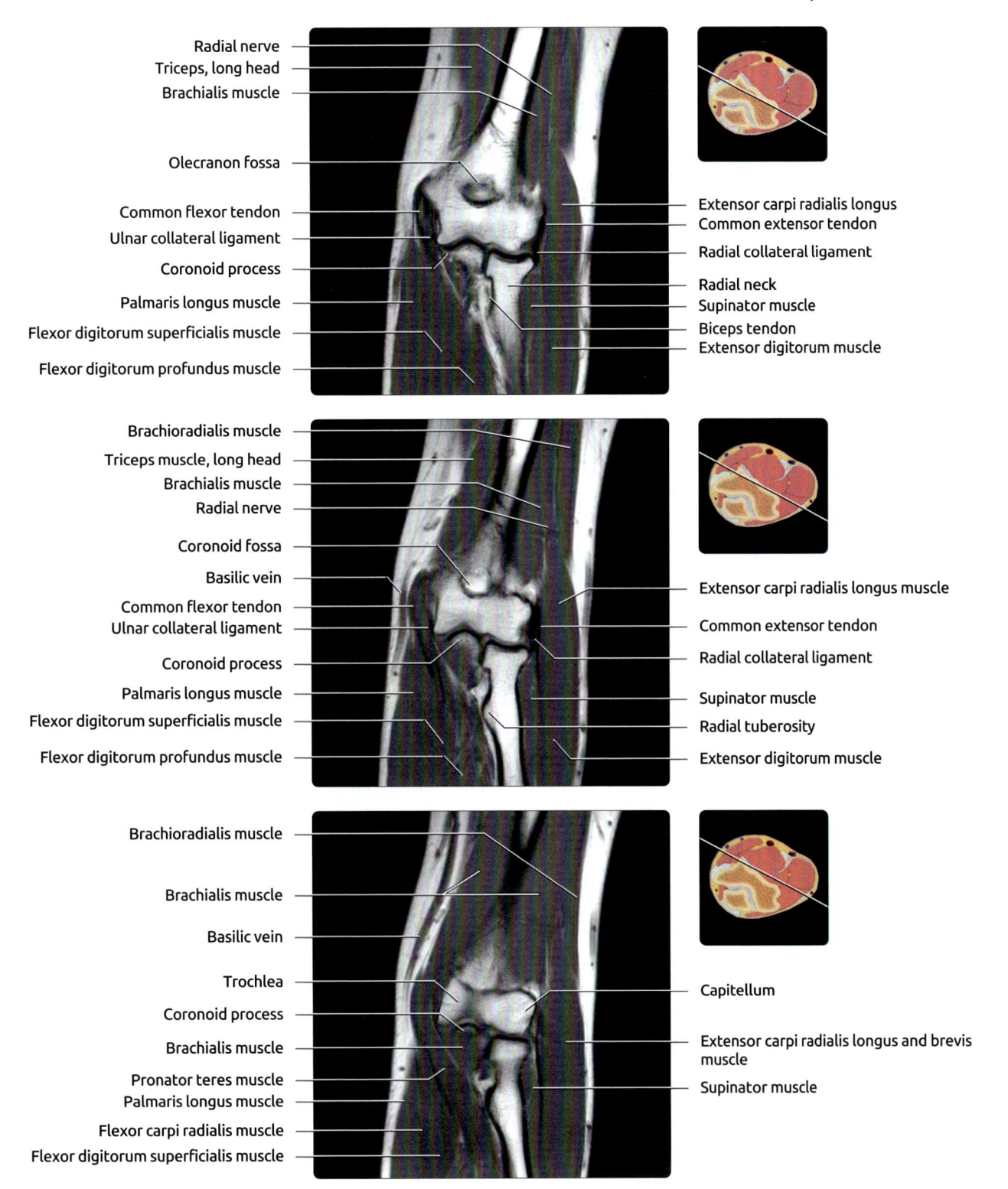

Top image labels:
- Radial nerve
- Triceps, long head
- Brachialis muscle
- Olecranon fossa
- Common flexor tendon
- Ulnar collateral ligament
- Coronoid process
- Palmaris longus muscle
- Flexor digitorum superficialis muscle
- Flexor digitorum profundus muscle
- Extensor carpi radialis longus
- Common extensor tendon
- Radial collateral ligament
- Radial neck
- Supinator muscle
- Biceps tendon
- Extensor digitorum muscle

Middle image labels:
- Brachioradialis muscle
- Triceps muscle, long head
- Brachialis muscle
- Radial nerve
- Coronoid fossa
- Basilic vein
- Common flexor tendon
- Ulnar collateral ligament
- Coronoid process
- Palmaris longus muscle
- Flexor digitorum superficialis muscle
- Flexor digitorum profundus muscle
- Extensor carpi radialis longus muscle
- Common extensor tendon
- Radial collateral ligament
- Supinator muscle
- Radial tuberosity
- Extensor digitorum muscle

Bottom image labels:
- Brachioradialis muscle
- Brachialis muscle
- Basilic vein
- Trochlea
- Coronoid process
- Brachialis muscle
- Pronator teres muscle
- Palmaris longus muscle
- Flexor carpi radialis muscle
- Flexor digitorum superficialis muscle
- Capitellum
- Extensor carpi radialis longus and brevis muscle
- Supinator muscle

(**Top**) The radial nerve courses between the brachialis and brachioradialis muscles. The distal biceps tendon is approaching its insertion on the radial tuberosity. (**Middle**) The profile of the radial tuberosity is well seen. (**Bottom**) The brachialis muscle is draping over the anterior aspect of the humeral shaft.

Elbow MR Atlas

CORONAL T1 MR, RIGHT ELBOW

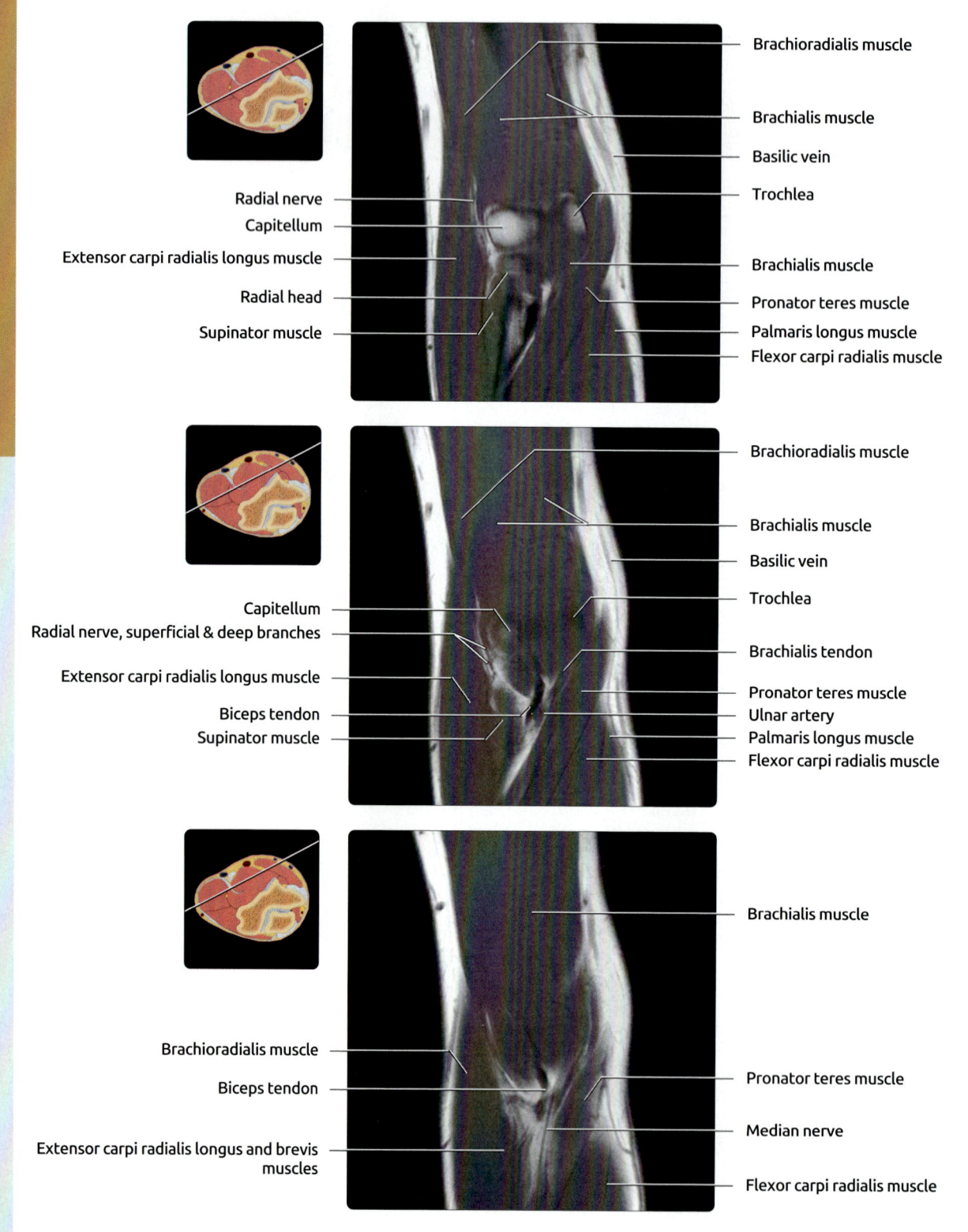

- Brachioradialis muscle
- Brachialis muscle
- Basilic vein
- Trochlea
- Brachialis muscle
- Pronator teres muscle
- Palmaris longus muscle
- Flexor carpi radialis muscle

- Radial nerve
- Capitellum
- Extensor carpi radialis longus muscle
- Radial head
- Supinator muscle

- Brachioradialis muscle
- Brachialis muscle
- Basilic vein
- Trochlea
- Brachialis tendon
- Pronator teres muscle
- Ulnar artery
- Palmaris longus muscle
- Flexor carpi radialis muscle

- Capitellum
- Radial nerve, superficial & deep branches
- Extensor carpi radialis longus muscle
- Biceps tendon
- Supinator muscle

- Brachialis muscle
- Pronator teres muscle
- Median nerve
- Flexor carpi radialis muscle

- Brachioradialis muscle
- Biceps tendon
- Extensor carpi radialis longus and brevis muscles

(Top) The pronator teres muscle wraps around the anterior aspect of the forearm. **(Middle)** The biceps and brachialis tendons are visualized as they dive toward their insertions. The radial nerve has split into its superficial and deep branches. **(Bottom)** The median nerve courses lateral to the pronator teres muscle.

Elbow MR Atlas

CORONAL T1 MR, LEFT ELBOW

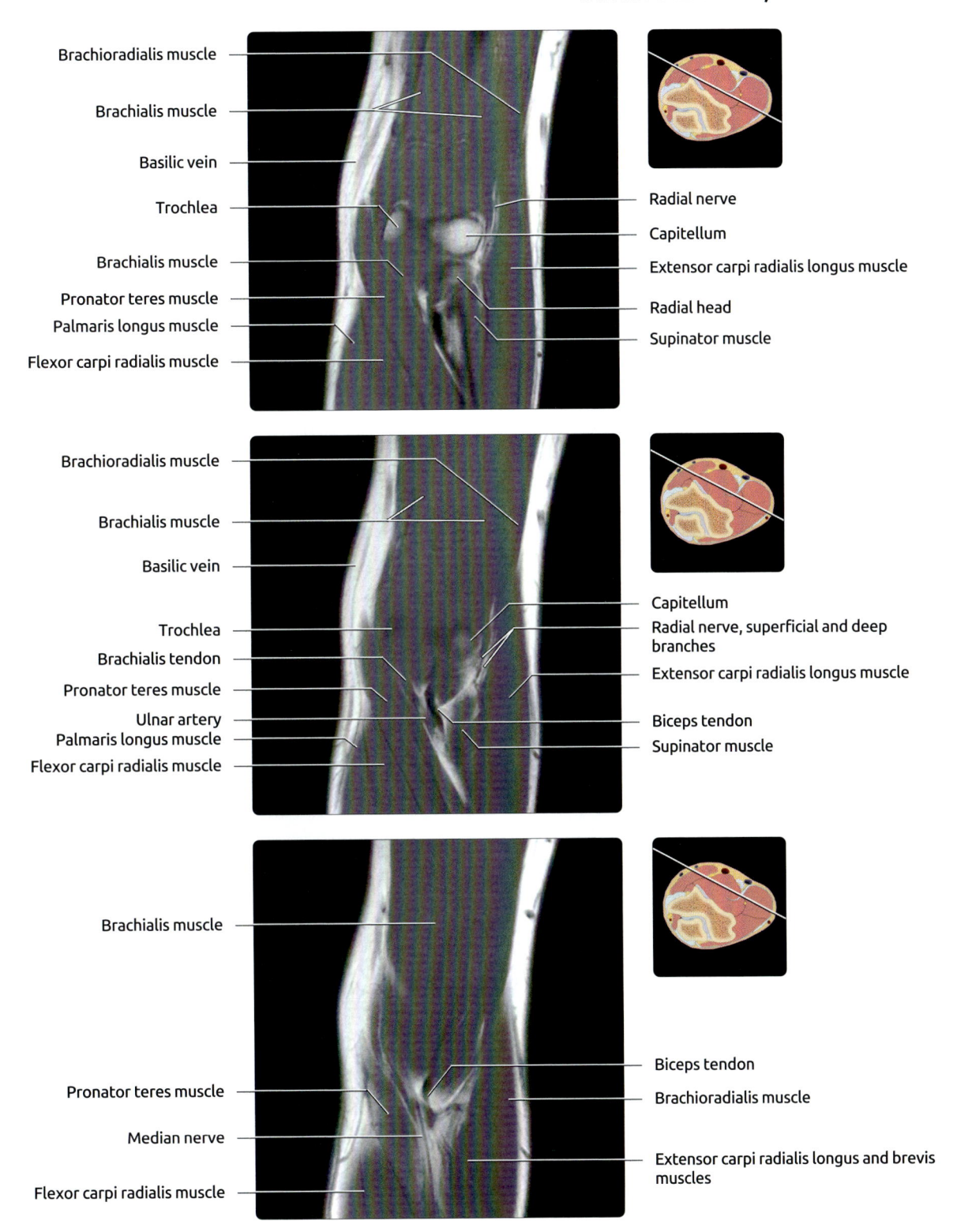

(Top) The pronator teres muscle wraps around the anterior aspect of the forearm. (Middle) The biceps and brachialis tendons are visualized as they dive toward their insertions. The radial nerve has split into its superficial and deep branches. (Bottom) The median nerve courses lateral to the pronator teres muscle.

CORONAL T1 MR, RIGHT ELBOW

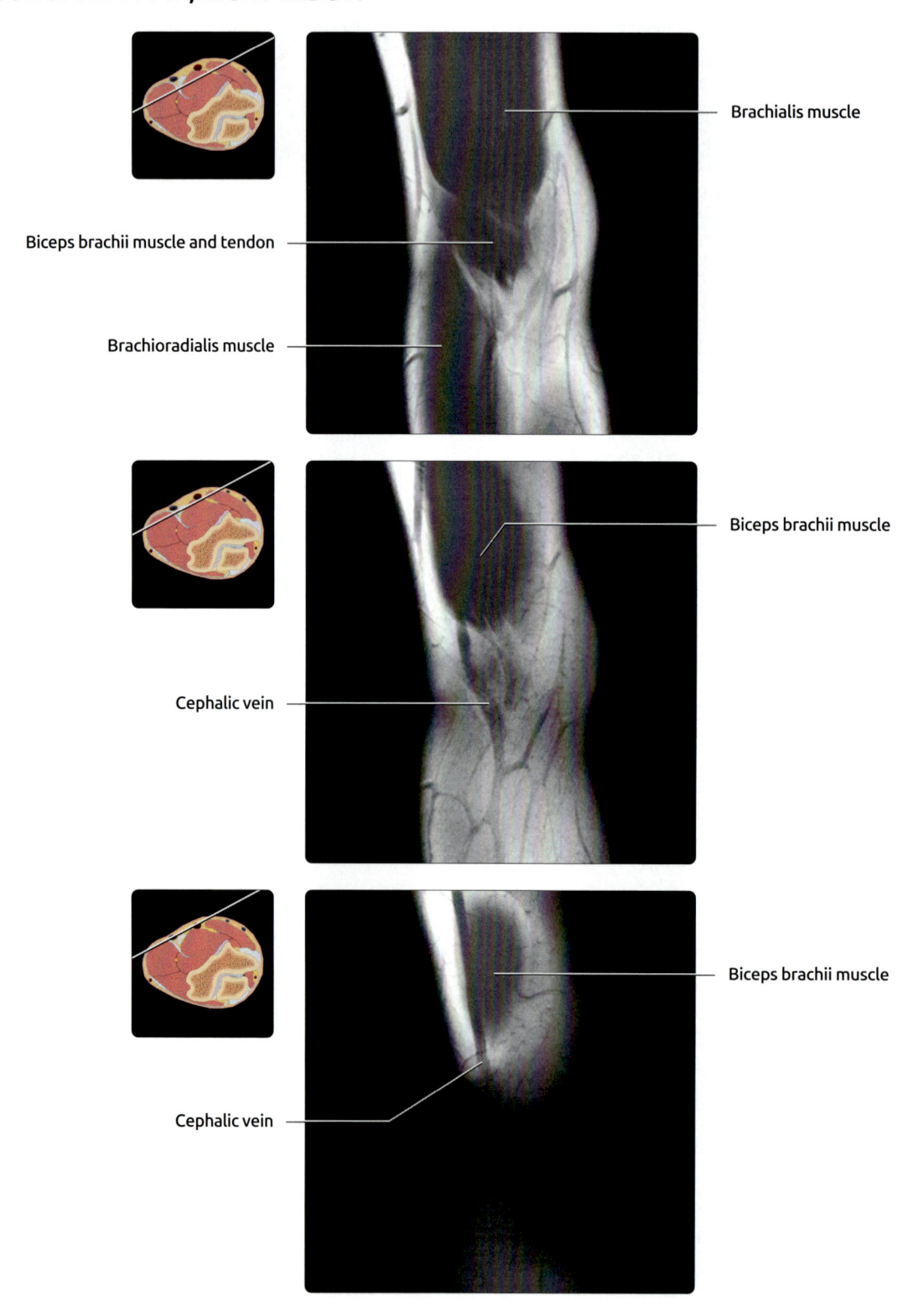

Brachialis muscle

Biceps brachii muscle and tendon

Brachioradialis muscle

Biceps brachii muscle

Cephalic vein

Biceps brachii muscle

Cephalic vein

(Top) *The brachioradialis muscle is the only muscle in the forearm still visualized.* **(Middle)** *The biceps brachii muscle is the only muscle still visualized.* **(Bottom)** *Just below the subcutaneous fat, the cephalic vein and biceps muscle are still seen.*

Elbow MR Atlas

CORONAL T1 MR, LEFT ELBOW

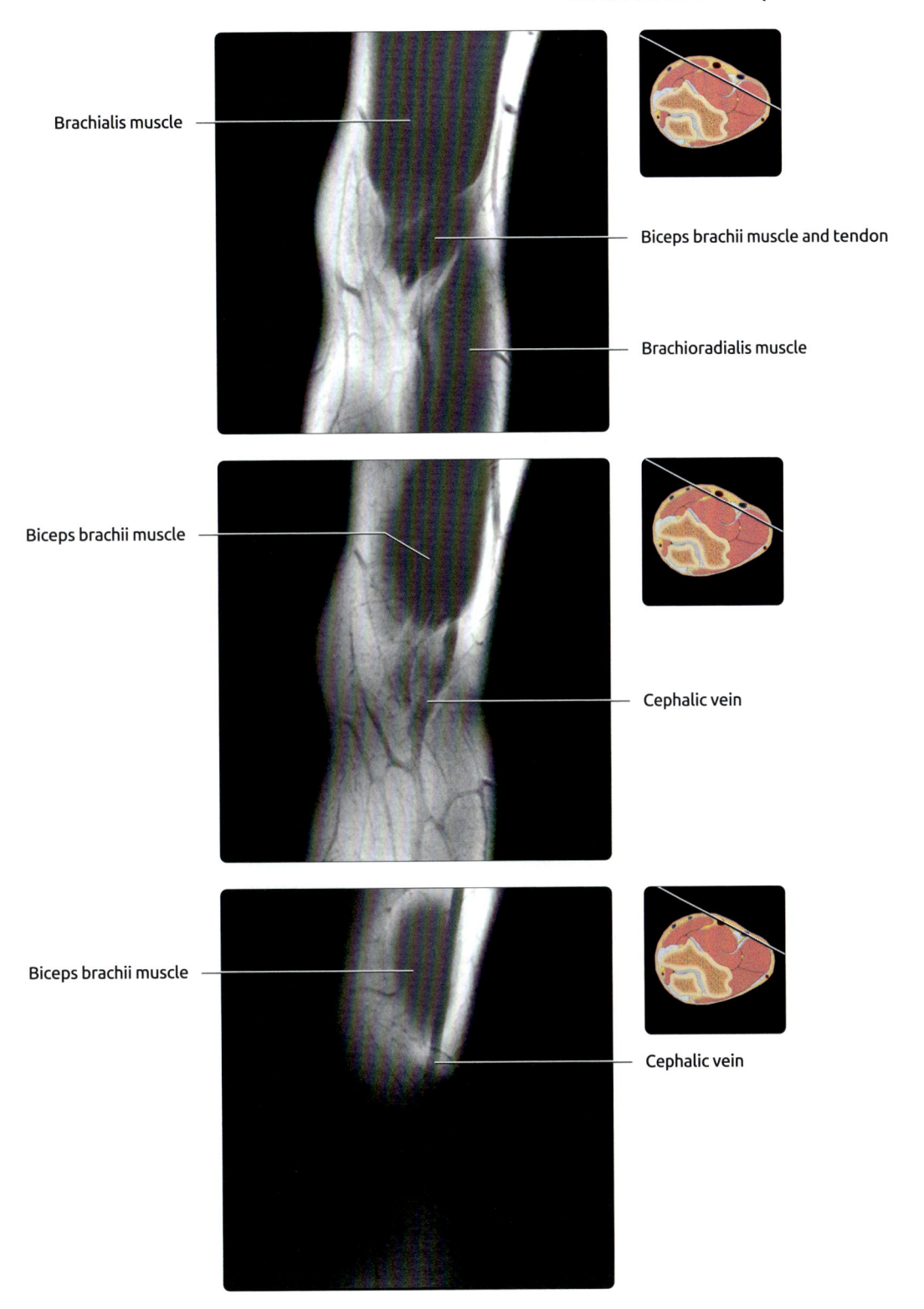

Brachialis muscle

Biceps brachii muscle and tendon

Brachioradialis muscle

Biceps brachii muscle

Cephalic vein

Biceps brachii muscle

Cephalic vein

(Top) *The brachioradialis muscle is the only muscle in the forearm still visualized.* (Middle) *The biceps brachii muscle is the only muscle still visualized.* (Bottom) *Just below the subcutaneous fat, the cephalic vein and biceps muscle are still seen.*

Elbow MR Atlas

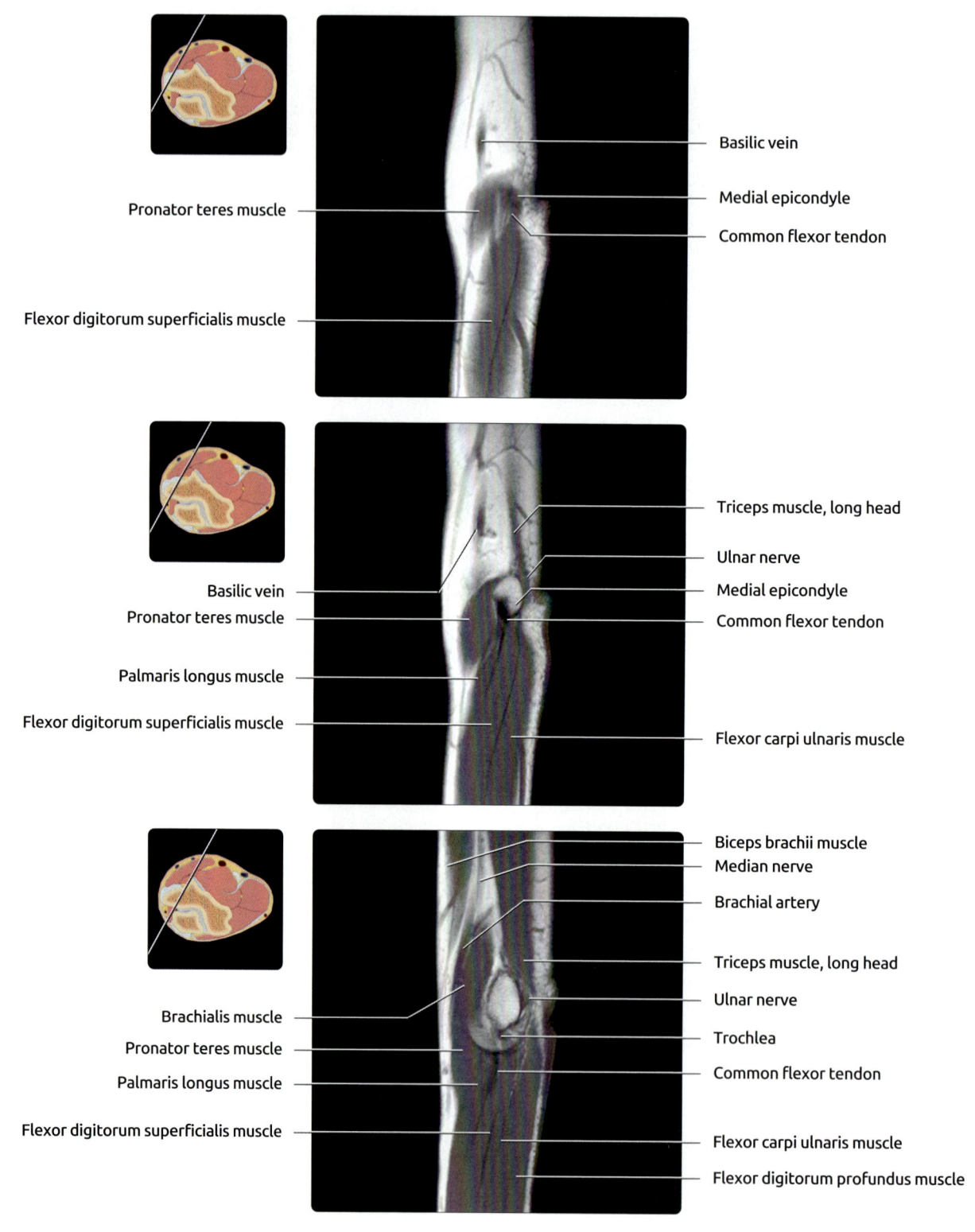

SAGITTAL T1 MR, LEFT ELBOW

Pronator teres muscle

Flexor digitorum superficialis muscle

Basilic vein
Medial epicondyle
Common flexor tendon

Basilic vein
Pronator teres muscle
Palmaris longus muscle
Flexor digitorum superficialis muscle

Triceps muscle, long head
Ulnar nerve
Medial epicondyle
Common flexor tendon

Flexor carpi ulnaris muscle

Brachialis muscle
Pronator teres muscle
Palmaris longus muscle
Flexor digitorum superficialis muscle

Biceps brachii muscle
Median nerve
Brachial artery
Triceps muscle, long head
Ulnar nerve
Trochlea
Common flexor tendon
Flexor carpi ulnaris muscle
Flexor digitorum profundus muscle

(Top) *This sagittal series starts far medially in the elbow, where the basilic vein is seen in the subcutaneous fat. The tip of the medial epicondyle is visualized, as are the most medial muscles.* **(Middle)** *The common flexor tendon and the muscles of the flexor-pronator group are seen.* **(Bottom)** *The structures of the anterior compartment of the arm are now coming into view.*

Elbow MR Atlas

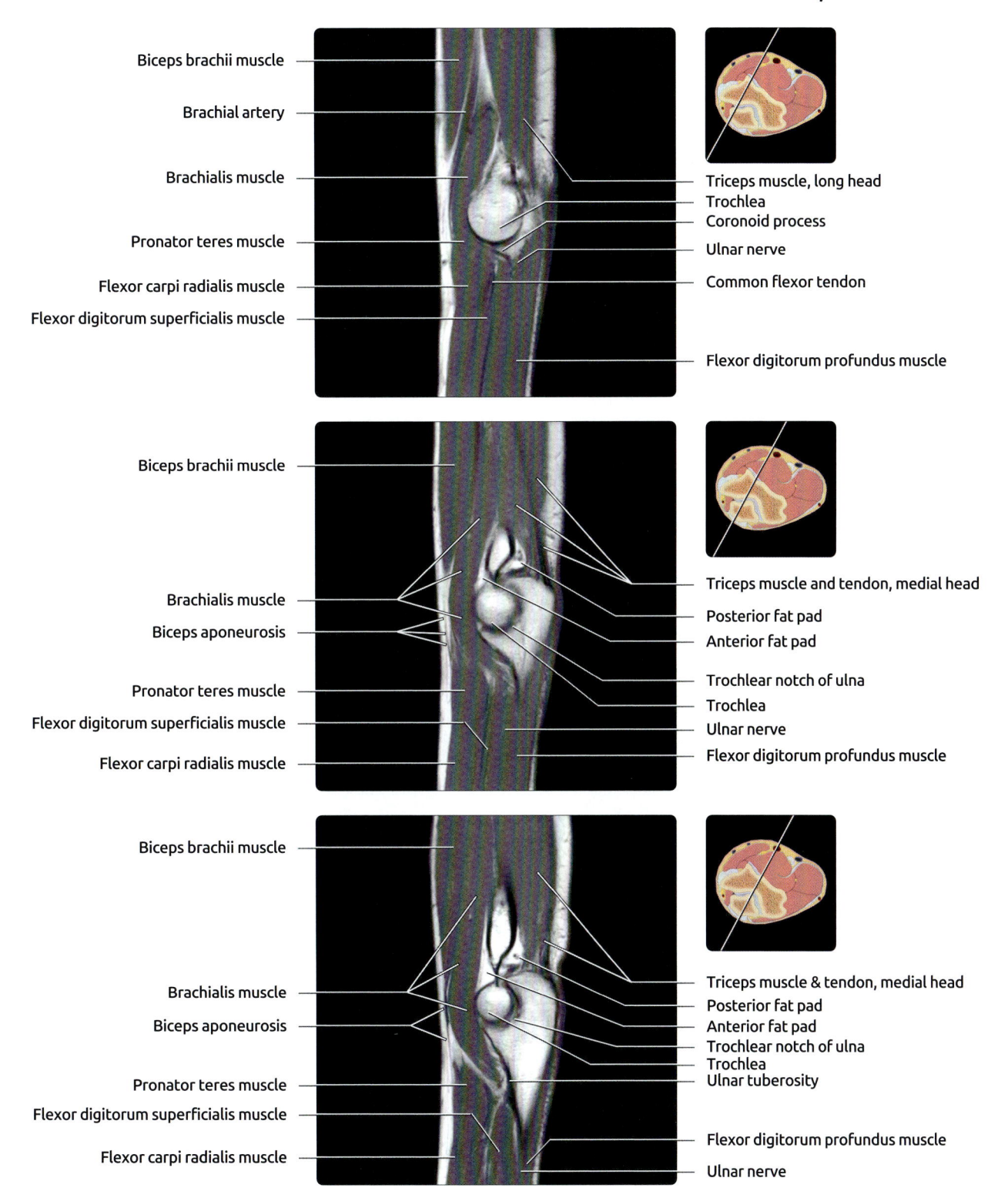

SAGITTAL T1 MR, LEFT ELBOW

Top image labels:
- Biceps brachii muscle
- Brachial artery
- Brachialis muscle
- Pronator teres muscle
- Flexor carpi radialis muscle
- Flexor digitorum superficialis muscle
- Triceps muscle, long head
- Trochlea
- Coronoid process
- Ulnar nerve
- Common flexor tendon
- Flexor digitorum profundus muscle

Middle image labels:
- Biceps brachii muscle
- Brachialis muscle
- Biceps aponeurosis
- Pronator teres muscle
- Flexor digitorum superficialis muscle
- Flexor carpi radialis muscle
- Triceps muscle and tendon, medial head
- Posterior fat pad
- Anterior fat pad
- Trochlear notch of ulna
- Trochlea
- Ulnar nerve
- Flexor digitorum profundus muscle

Bottom image labels:
- Biceps brachii muscle
- Brachialis muscle
- Biceps aponeurosis
- Pronator teres muscle
- Flexor digitorum superficialis muscle
- Flexor carpi radialis muscle
- Triceps muscle & tendon, medial head
- Posterior fat pad
- Anterior fat pad
- Trochlear notch of ulna
- Trochlea
- Ulnar tuberosity
- Flexor digitorum profundus muscle
- Ulnar nerve

(**Top**) The coronoid process of the ulna is coming into view. The biceps brachii muscle is seen anteriorly in the arm. (**Middle**) The triceps tendon is seen inserting on the olecranon process of the ulna. Notice that the triceps muscle itself also inserts on the olecranon. (**Bottom**) The distal aspect of the brachialis muscle is seen diving toward its insertion on the ulnar tuberosity. The biceps aponeurosis is seen in cross section, anterior to the brachialis.

Elbow MR Atlas

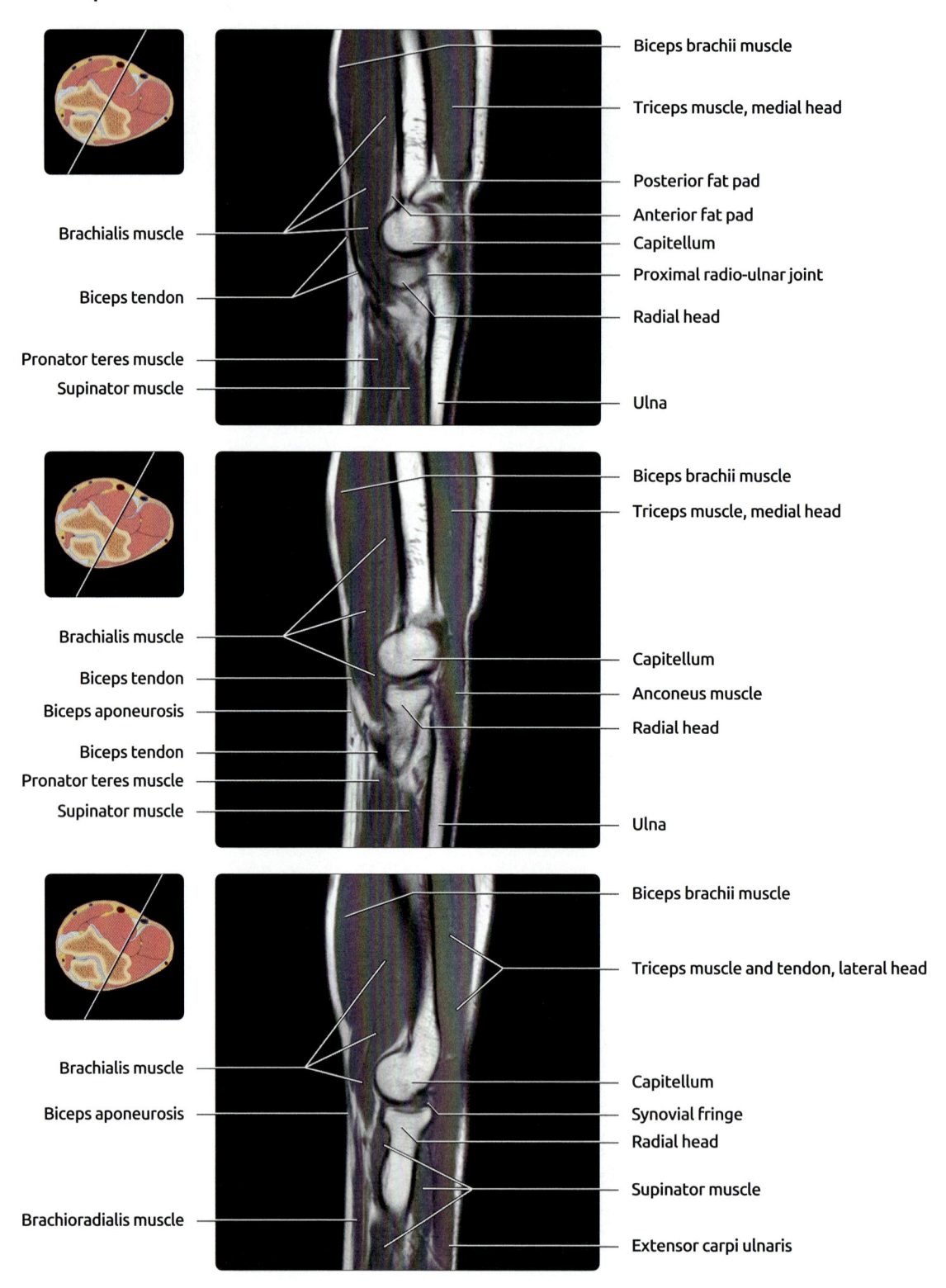

SAGITTAL T1 MR, LEFT ELBOW

Top image labels:
- Biceps brachii muscle
- Triceps muscle, medial head
- Posterior fat pad
- Anterior fat pad
- Capitellum
- Proximal radio-ulnar joint
- Radial head
- Ulna
- Brachialis muscle
- Biceps tendon
- Pronator teres muscle
- Supinator muscle

Middle image labels:
- Biceps brachii muscle
- Triceps muscle, medial head
- Capitellum
- Anconeus muscle
- Radial head
- Ulna
- Brachialis muscle
- Biceps tendon
- Biceps aponeurosis
- Biceps tendon
- Pronator teres muscle
- Supinator muscle

Bottom image labels:
- Biceps brachii muscle
- Triceps muscle and tendon, lateral head
- Capitellum
- Synovial fringe
- Radial head
- Supinator muscle
- Extensor carpi ulnaris
- Brachialis muscle
- Biceps aponeurosis
- Brachioradialis muscle

(Top) The biceps tendon is now seen, diving toward the insertion on the radial tuberosity. **(Middle)** The anconeus muscle is now visible as the cut passes lateral to the olecranon. **(Bottom)** The brachioradialis muscle is seen anteriorly. A fold of synovium, called the synovial fringe or plica, projects into the radiocapitellar joint.

Elbow MR Atlas

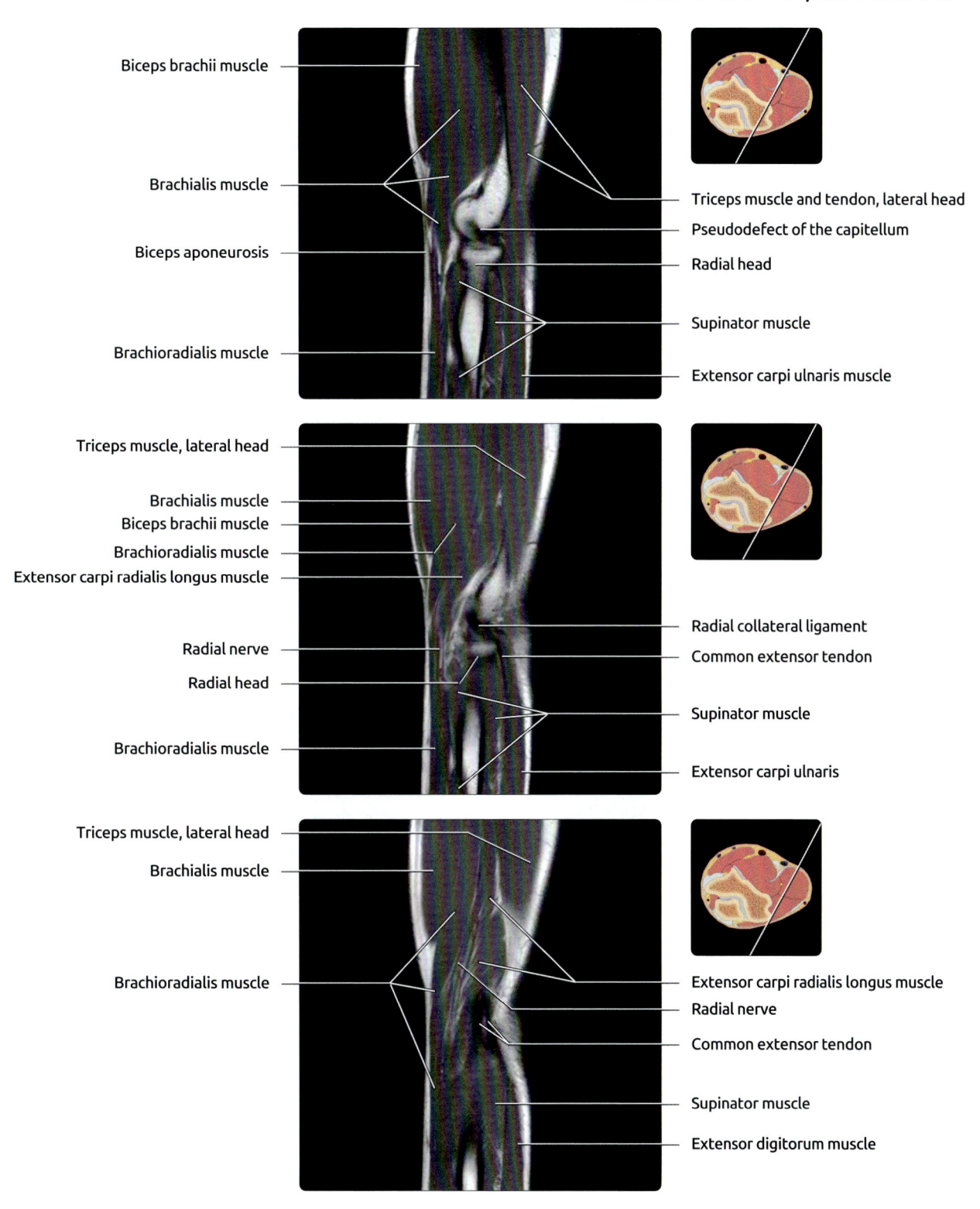

SAGITTAL T1 MR, LEFT ELBOW

(Top) The pseudodefect of the capitellum, located in the posterior aspect of the capitellum, is a groove between the capitellum and lateral epicondyle, mimicking an osteochondral defect. **(Middle)** The common extensor tendon is coming into view, along with the radial collateral ligament. **(Bottom)** The common extensor tendon is now well seen. The brachioradialis muscle sweeps forward and becomes the most lateral muscle of the forearm.

Elbow Muscles and Tendons

GROSS ANATOMY

Overview
- Elbow is divided into 4 compartments: Anterior, posterior, medial, lateral

Compartments
- Anterior
  - Contains elbow flexors
  - **Biceps brachii**
    - Origin: Supraglenoid tubercle (long head), coracoid process (short head)
    - Insertion: Radial tuberosity
    - Innervation: Musculocutaneous nerve
    - Blood supply: Muscular branches brachial artery
    - Action: Elbow flexion, forearm supination
  - **Lacertus fibrosus (biceps aponeurosis)**: Connects distal biceps tendon to fascia overlying common flexor mass
    - Lacertus fibrosus may compress underlying median nerve
    - Lacertus fibrosus can prevent retraction of ruptured biceps tendon
  - **Brachialis**
    - Origin: Anterior surface of humerus
    - Insertion: Ulnar tuberosity
    - Innervation: Musculocutaneous nerve
    - Blood supply: Muscular branches brachial artery, recurrent radial artery
    - Action: Elbow flexion
    - Lies deep to biceps brachii
- Posterior
  - Contains elbow extensors
  - **Triceps**
    - Origin: Infraglenoid tubercle (long head), posterior humerus proximal to radial groove (lateral head), posterior humerus distal to radial groove (medial head)
    - Insertion: Olecranon process
    - Innervation: Radial nerve
    - Blood supply: Branches of deep brachial artery
    - Action: Elbow extension
  - **Anconeus**
    - Origin: Lateral epicondyle
    - Insertion: Lateral portion of olecranon, posterior aspect of ulna
    - Innervation: Radial nerve
    - Blood supply: Middle collateral branch of deep brachial artery, recurrent interosseous artery
    - Action: Elbow extension, abduction of ulna during pronation
  - **Anconeus epitrochlearis**
    - Accessory muscle present in 3-28% of population
    - Anatomically inconstant
    - Origin: Medial epicondyle
    - Insertion: Medial portion of olecranon
    - Innervation: Radial nerve
    - Blood supply: Middle collateral branch of deep brachial artery
    - Action: Elbow extension
    - Courses through cubital tunnel, posteromedial to ulnar nerve
    - May protect ulnar nerve from direct trauma, but may also compress nerve, resulting in cubital tunnel syndrome
- Lateral
  - Contains the extensor-supinator group and one elbow flexor
  - **Brachioradialis**
    - Origin: Proximal 2/3 of lateral supracondylar ridge
    - Insertion: Lateral side of distal radius
    - Innervation: Radial nerve (otherwise only supplies extensors)
    - Blood supply: Radial recurrent artery
    - Action: Elbow flexion
    - Only elbow flexor in lateral compartment
  - **Extensor carpi radialis longus**
    - Origin: Inferior aspect of lateral supracondylar ridge (may blend with origin of brachioradialis)
    - Insertion: Dorsum of base of second metacarpal
    - Innervation: Radial nerve
    - Blood supply: Brachial artery
    - Action: Extends and abducts wrist
  - **Common extensor tendon**
    - Conjoined tendon of extensor carpi radialis brevis, extensor digitorum, extensor digiti minimi, extensor carpi ulnaris
    - Origin: Anterior aspect of lateral epicondyle and lateral supracondylar ridge
    - Insertion: See following individual muscles listed
  - **Extensor carpi radialis brevis**
    - Origin: Common extensor tendon and radial collateral ligament
    - Insertion: Dorsum of base of third metacarpal
    - Innervation: Deep branch of radial nerve
    - Blood supply: Radial artery
    - Action: Extends and abducts wrist
  - **Extensor digitorum**
    - Origin: Common extensor tendon, intermuscular septum
    - Insertion: Dorsum of 2nd-5th fingers
    - Innervation: Posterior interosseous branch of radial nerve
    - Blood supply: Interosseous recurrent and posterior interosseous arteries
    - Action: Extends fingers at metacarpophalangeal and interphalangeal joints, extends wrist
  - **Extensor digiti minimi**
    - Origin: Common extensor tendon
    - Insertion: Dorsum of 5th finger
    - Innervation: Posterior interosseous branch of radial nerve
    - Blood supply: Interosseous recurrent artery
    - Action: Extends 5th finger
  - **Extensor carpi ulnaris**
    - Origin: Common extensor tendon and posterior aspect of ulna
    - Insertion: Dorsum of 5th metacarpal
    - Innervation: Posterior interosseous branch of radial nerve

Elbow Muscles and Tendons

- Blood supply: Ulnar artery
- Action: Extends and adducts wrist
- **Supinator**
  - Has 2 heads of origin
  - Origin of humeral head: Lateral epicondyle, radial collateral ligament, annular ligament
  - Origin of ulnar head: Supinator fossa of ulna (anterior) and supinator crest of ulna (posterior)
  - Insertion: Lateral side of proximal radial shaft
  - Innervation: Deep branch of radial nerve
  - Blood supply: Recurrent interosseous artery
  - Action: Supinates forearm
- Medial
  - Contains the flexor-pronator group
  - **Common flexor tendon**
    - Conjoined tendon of flexor carpi radialis, flexor carpi ulnaris, flexor digitorum superficialis (also called sublimis), palmaris longus, pronator teres
    - Origin: Medial epicondyle and medial supracondylar ridge
    - Insertion: See individual muscles listed below
  - **Flexor carpi radialis**
    - Origin: Common flexor tendon
    - Insertion: Volar aspect of base of 2nd metacarpal
    - Innervation: Median nerve
    - Blood supply: Ulnar artery
    - Action: Flexes and abducts wrist, weak flexor of elbow
  - **Flexor carpi ulnaris**
    - Has 2 heads
    - Origin of humeral head: Common flexor tendon
    - Origin of ulnar head: Medial aspect of olecranon and posterior aspect of ulna
    - Insertion: Pisiform, hook of hamate, base of 5th metacarpal
    - Innervation: Ulnar nerve
    - Blood supply: Ulnar artery
    - Action: Flexes and adducts wrist
  - **Flexor digitorum superficialis**
    - Has 2 heads
    - Origin of humeroulnar head: Common flexor tendon, ulnar collateral ligament, coronoid process
    - Origin of radial head: Anterior aspect of proximal radius
    - Insertion: Volar aspect of middle phalanges of 2nd-5th fingers
    - Innervation: Median nerve
    - Blood supply: Ulnar artery
    - Action: Flexes the proximal interphalangeal joints, weak flexor of metacarpophalangeal and wrist joints
  - **Palmaris longus**
    - Origin: Common flexor tendon
    - Insertion: Palmar aponeurosis of hand
    - Innervation: Median nerve
    - Blood supply: Ulnar artery
    - Action: Flexes wrist
  - **Pronator teres**
    - Has 2 heads
    - Origin of humeral head: Common flexor tendon
    - Origin of ulnar head: Coronoid process
    - Insertion: Lateral aspect of mid shaft of radius
    - Innervation: Median nerve
    - Blood supply: Ulnar artery, anterior recurrent ulnar artery
    - Action: Pronates forearm, flexes elbow

IMAGING ANATOMY

Overview
- Common extensor tendon
  - Longer and thinner than common flexor tendon
  - May be hard to distinguish from underlying radial collateral ligament
- Triceps tendon
  - May look wavy on sagittal images with full elbow extension
- Bicipitoradial bursa
  - Located between distal biceps tendon and radial tuberosity
  - Reduces friction on biceps tendon during pronation
  - Has inverted tear-drop shape

ANATOMY IMAGING ISSUES

Imaging Recommendations
- Distal biceps tendon
  - Hard to visualize longitudinally in standard sagittal plane
    - Difficult to differentiate biceps tendon from adjacent vascular structures
    - Lacertus fibrosus may prevent retraction of ruptured biceps tendon, so do not depend on seeing retracted muscle mass to diagnosis biceps tendon rupture
    - If using 3 standard planes, rely on axial, but **must** image distally through entire radial tuberosity
  - FABS view
    - **F**lexed (elbow), **ab**ducted (arm), **s**upinated (forearm)
    - Patient in superman position with arm flexed
    - Allows full longitudinal visualization of biceps tendon and insertion on radial tuberosity
    - Obtain scout images in plane coronal to patient's body (will be sagittal to flexed elbow)
    - Plot images perpendicular to radius (coronal to humerus)
    - Also shows longitudinal extent of brachialis tendon
- Snapping triceps tendon
  - Medial head snaps over medial epicondyle during elbow flexion
  - May cause ulnar nerve to dislocate anteriorly during flexion
  - Must image in axial plane in both extension and flexion
  - Dynamic scanning can be performed sonographically as elbow flexes and extends

SELECTED REFERENCES

1. Giuffre BM et al: Optimal positioning for MRI of the distal biceps brachii tendon: flexed abducted supinated view. AJR Am J Roentgenol. 182(4):944-6, 2004

Elbow Muscles and Tendons

GRAPHIC: BICEPS TENDON AND APONEUROSIS (LACERTUS FIBROSUS)

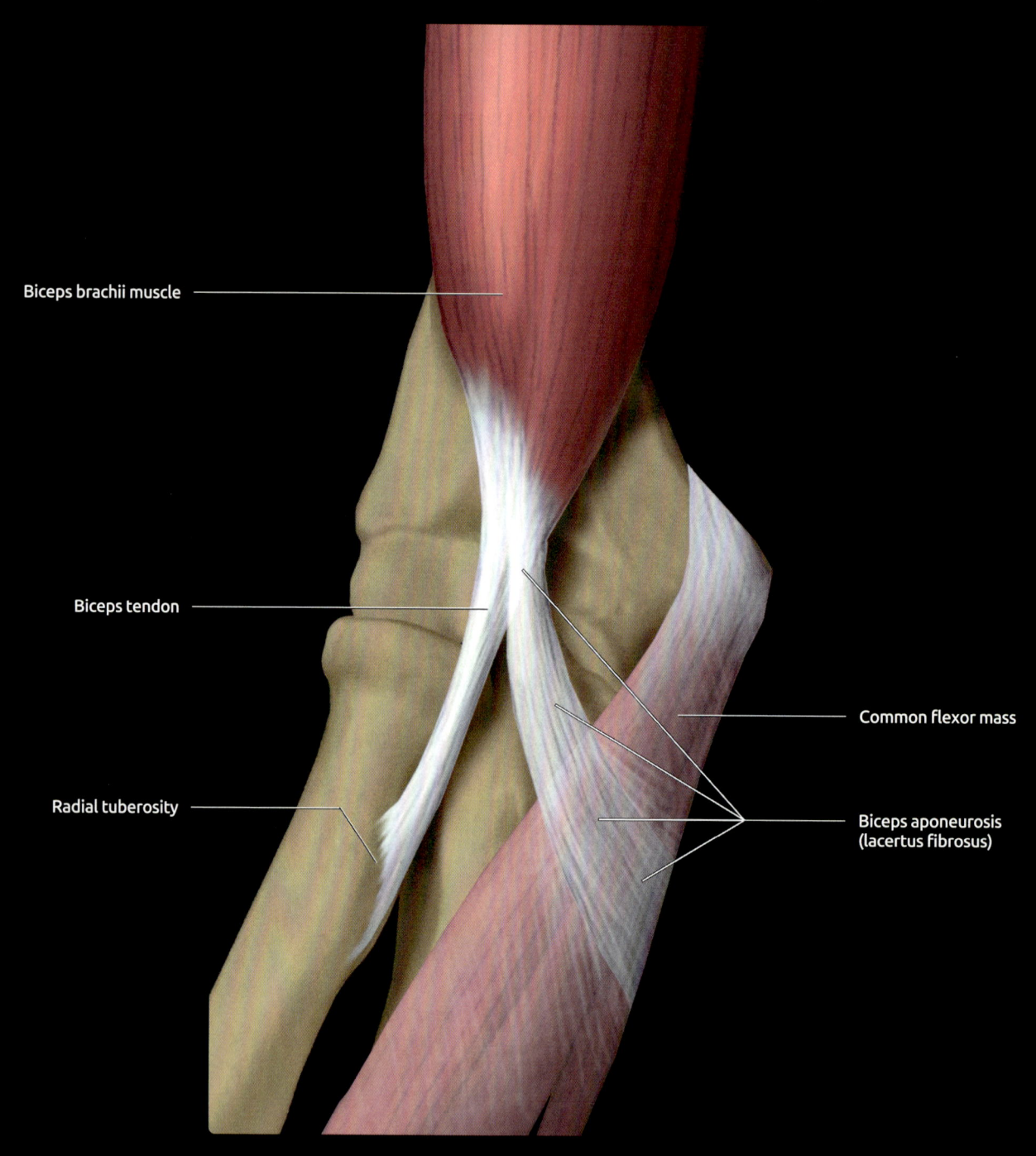

- Biceps brachii muscle
- Biceps tendon
- Radial tuberosity
- Common flexor mass
- Biceps aponeurosis (lacertus fibrosus)

The biceps aponeurosis, also called the lacertus fibrosus, is a thin sheet of fascia that connects the biceps tendon to the superficial fascia of the common flexor mass. It may prevent a ruptured biceps tendon from retracting proximally.

Elbow Muscles and Tendons

GRAPHICS: COMMON EXTENSOR AND COMMON FLEXOR TENDONS

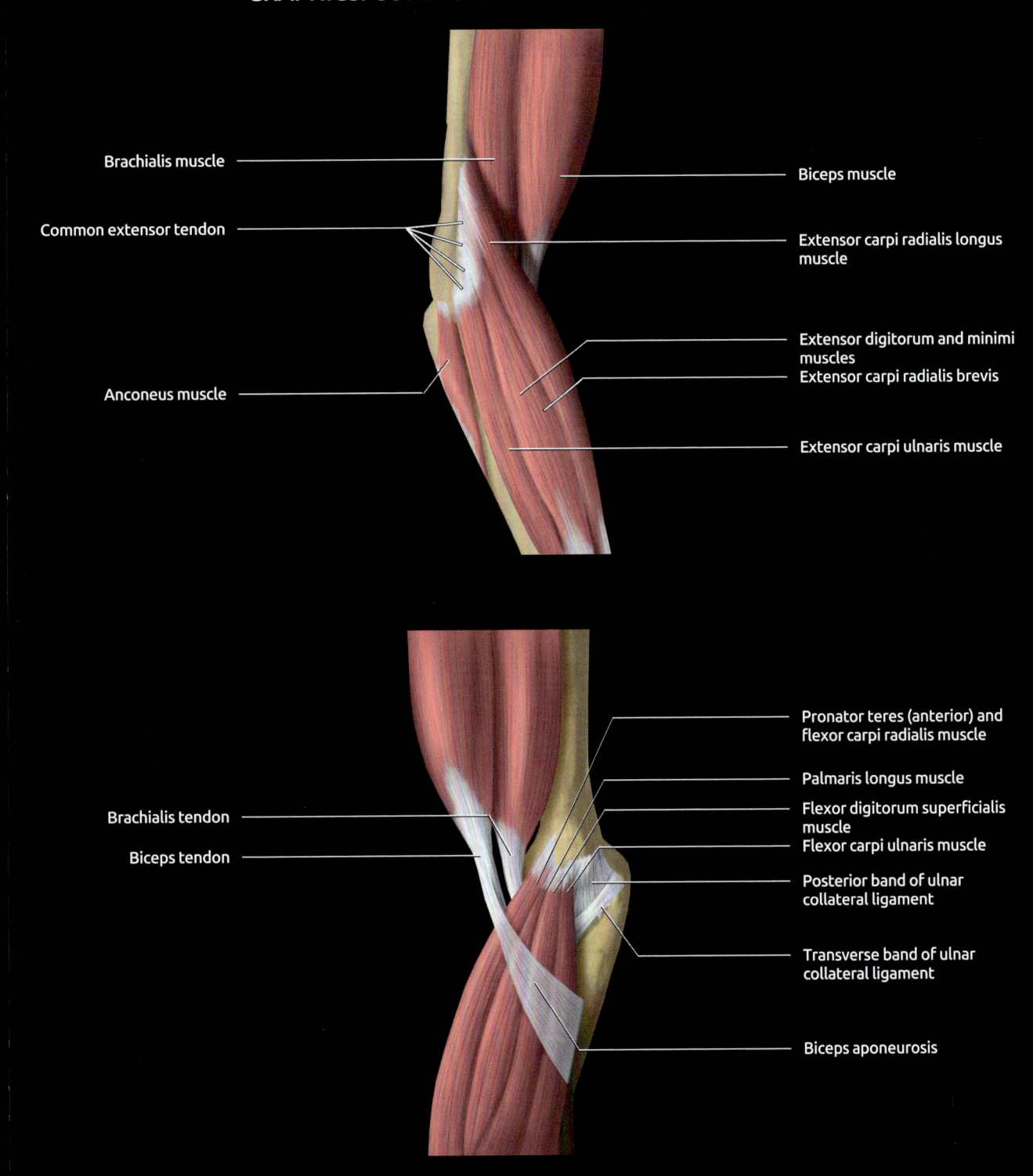

(Top) A side view of the lateral aspect of the elbow shows the extensor-supinator group and its common extensor tendon, attaching to the lateral epicondyle and supracondylar aspect of the humerus. The tendon of the extensor carpi radialis longus originates just superior to the common extensor tendon. The common extensor tendon is comprised of the extensor carpi radialis brevis, extensor digitorum, extensor digiti minimi, and extensor carpi ulnaris. The brachioradialis, which originates at the most superior aspect of the lateral supracondylar ridge, is not shown in this graphic. (Bottom) A side view of the medial aspect of the elbow shows the flexor-pronator group and its common flexor tendon attaching to the medial epicondyle. The anterior band of the ulnar collateral ligament is deep to the common tendon.

Elbow Muscles and Tendons

AXIAL T1 MR, RIGHT ELBOW

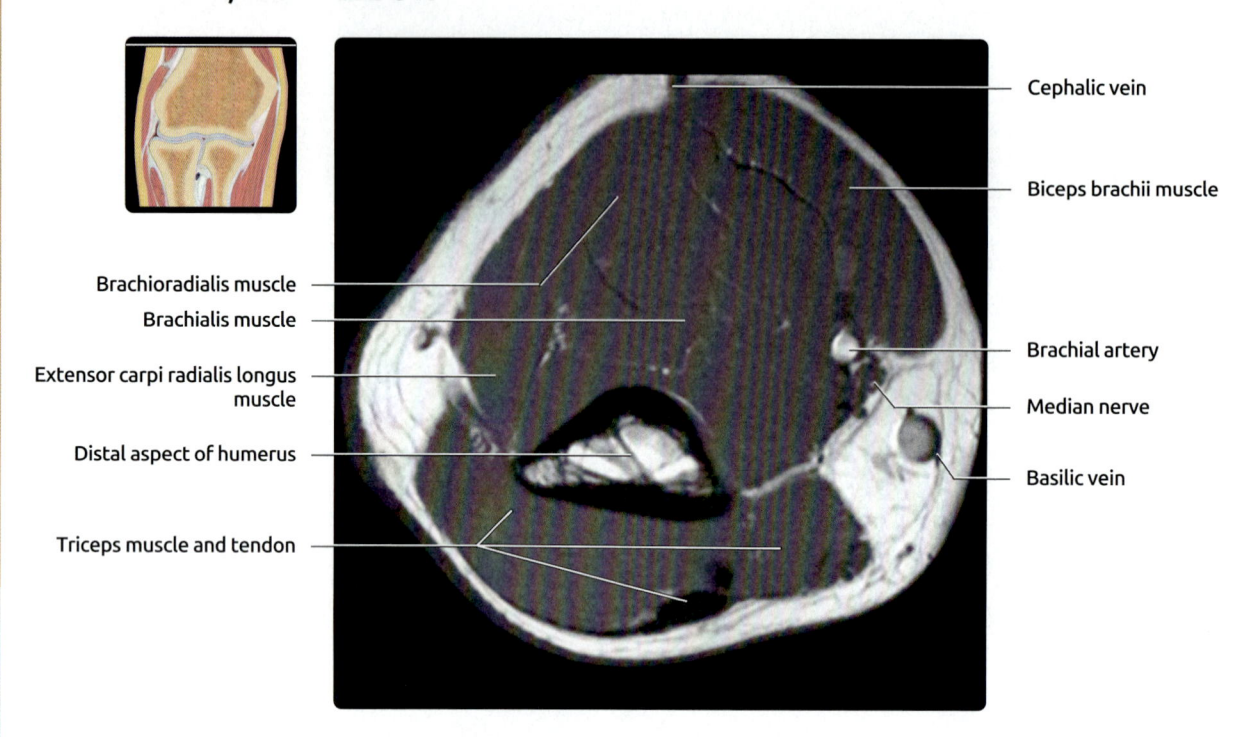

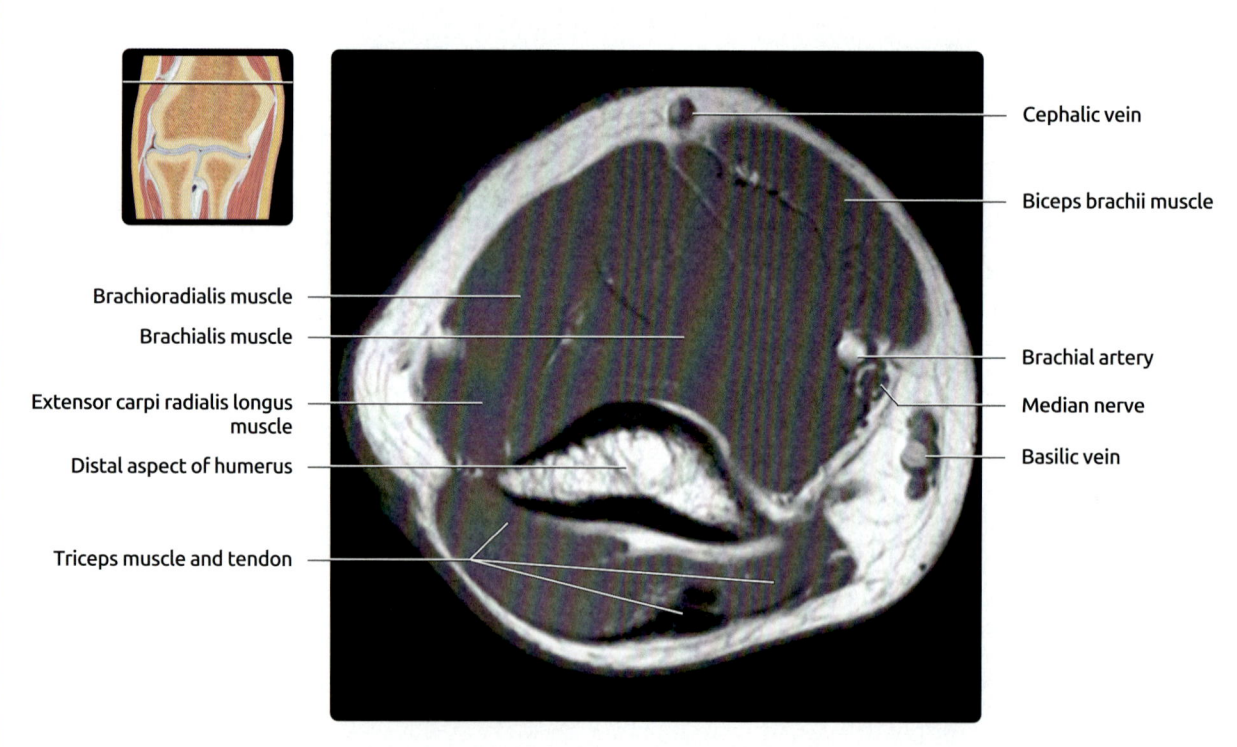

Labels (top image):
- Cephalic vein
- Biceps brachii muscle
- Brachioradialis muscle
- Brachialis muscle
- Extensor carpi radialis longus muscle
- Distal aspect of humerus
- Triceps muscle and tendon
- Brachial artery
- Median nerve
- Basilic vein

Labels (bottom image):
- Cephalic vein
- Biceps brachii muscle
- Brachioradialis muscle
- Brachialis muscle
- Extensor carpi radialis longus muscle
- Distal aspect of humerus
- Triceps muscle and tendon
- Brachial artery
- Median nerve
- Basilic vein

(Top) First of 14 axial images in the distal aspect of the arm is shown. The triceps muscle accounts for the entire posterior compartment, and the brachialis muscle accounts for most of the anterior compartment. **(Bottom)** At the supracondylar level of the humerus, the triceps muscle is starting to thin out.

Elbow Muscles and Tendons

AXIAL T1 MR, RIGHT ELBOW

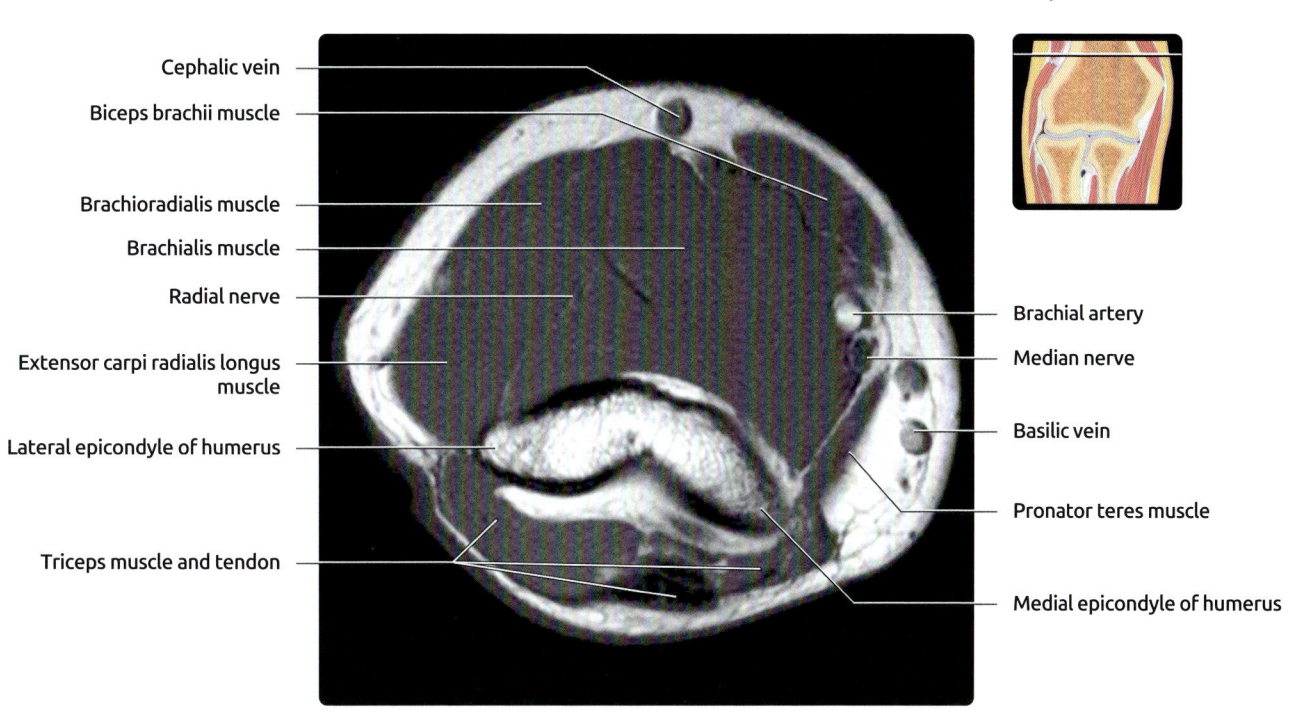

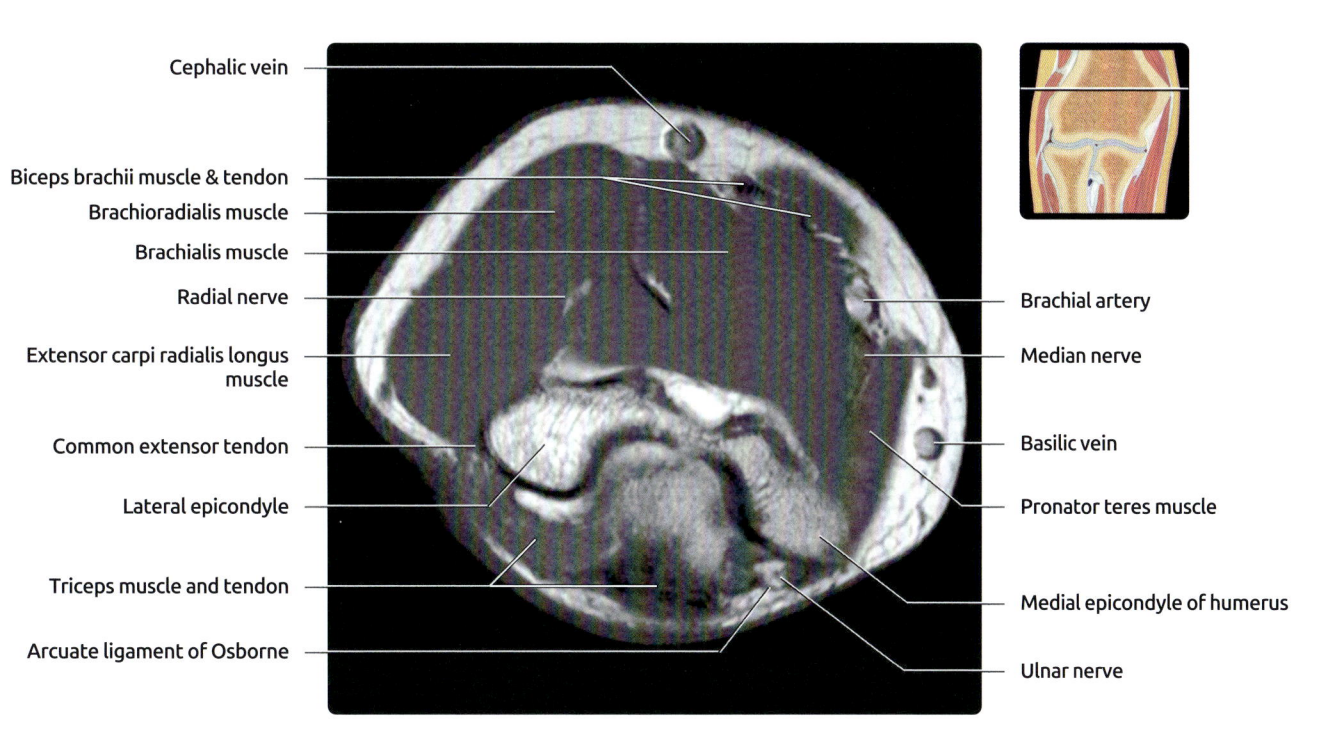

Top image labels:
- Cephalic vein
- Biceps brachii muscle
- Brachioradialis muscle
- Brachialis muscle
- Radial nerve
- Extensor carpi radialis longus muscle
- Lateral epicondyle of humerus
- Triceps muscle and tendon
- Brachial artery
- Median nerve
- Basilic vein
- Pronator teres muscle
- Medial epicondyle of humerus

Bottom image labels:
- Cephalic vein
- Biceps brachii muscle & tendon
- Brachioradialis muscle
- Brachialis muscle
- Radial nerve
- Extensor carpi radialis longus muscle
- Common extensor tendon
- Lateral epicondyle
- Triceps muscle and tendon
- Arcuate ligament of Osborne
- Brachial artery
- Median nerve
- Basilic vein
- Pronator teres muscle
- Medial epicondyle of humerus
- Ulnar nerve

(**Top**) *At the level of the superior aspect of the epicondyles, the humeral head of the pronator teres muscle origin is now visualized. Pronator teres is the most proximal tendon to arise from the medial epicondyle.* (**Bottom**) *The lateral head of the triceps is still present, adjacent to the olecranon process, but the remainder of the triceps is tendinous. The ulnar nerve is well seen in the cubital tunnel, surrounded by high signal intensity fat and enclosed by the arcuate ligament.*

Elbow Muscles and Tendons

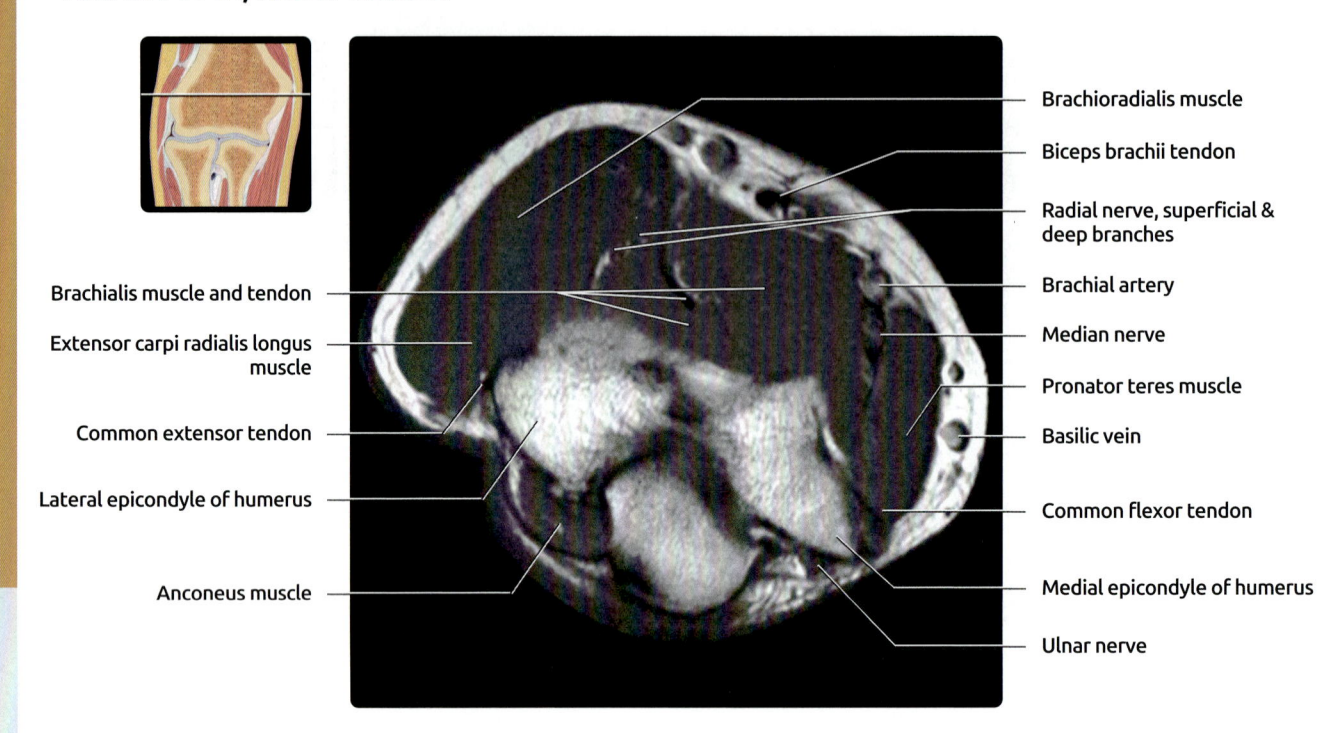

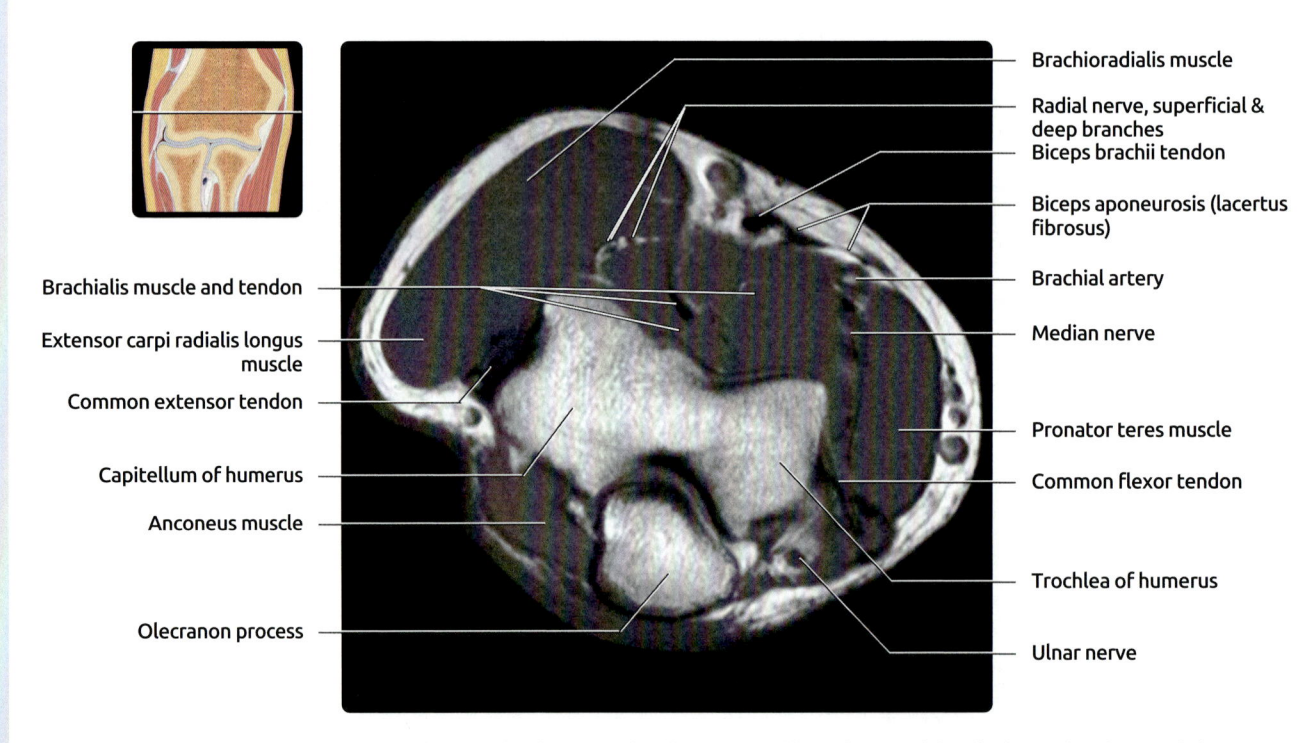

AXIAL T1 MR, RIGHT ELBOW

(Top) The anconeus muscle is now visible extending between the olecranon and lateral epicondyle. The biceps brachii muscle has tapered to its distal tendon, and the common extensor and flexor tendons are visible at their attachments to the condyles. The radial nerve has split into its superficial and deep branches. **(Bottom)** The thin biceps aponeurosis ("lacertus fibrosus") can be seen arising from the distal biceps tendon and heading medially toward the pronator teres of the common flexor muscle group.

Elbow Muscles and Tendons

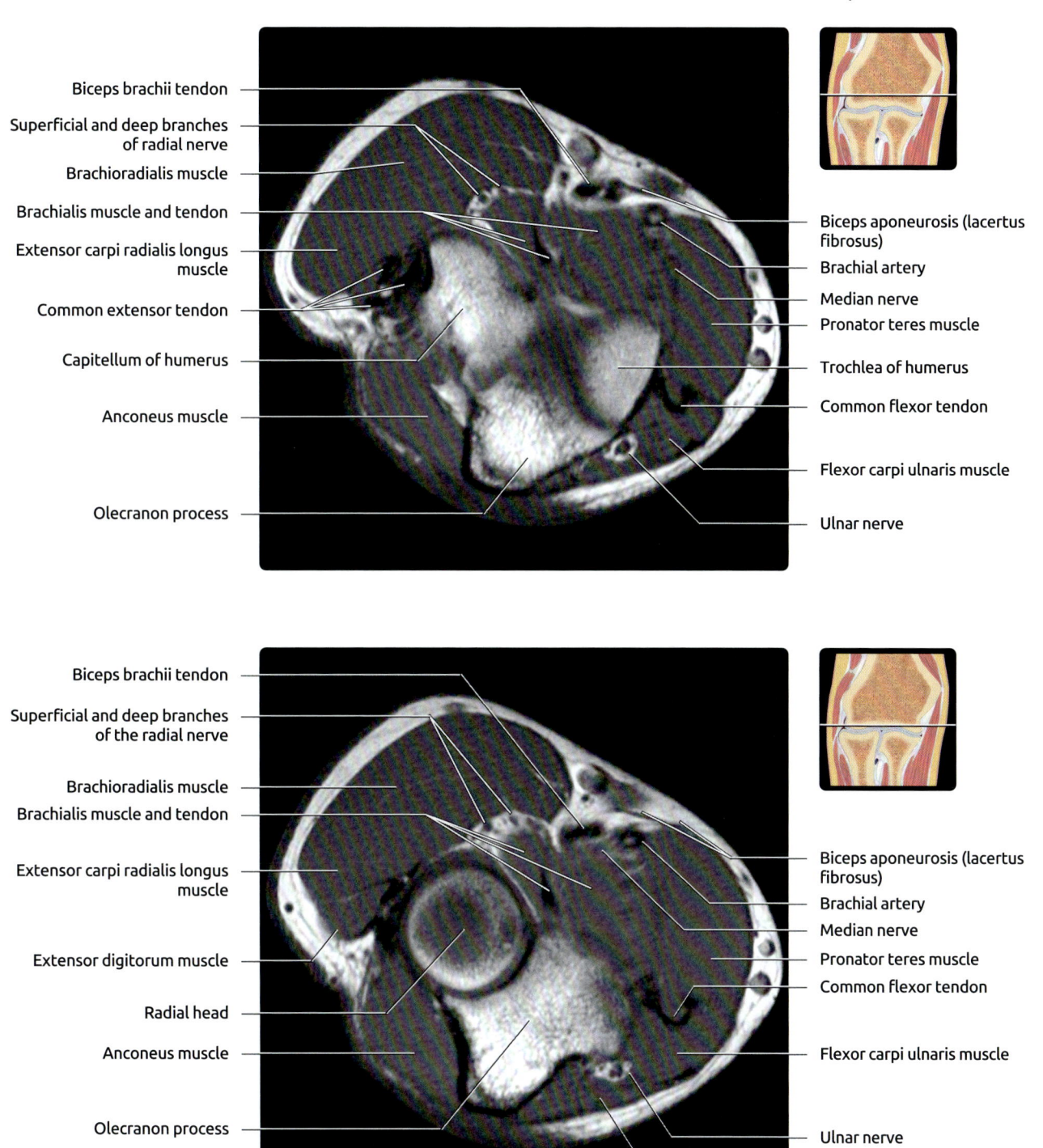

AXIAL T1 MR, RIGHT ELBOW

Top image labels:
- Biceps brachii tendon
- Superficial and deep branches of radial nerve
- Brachioradialis muscle
- Brachialis muscle and tendon
- Extensor carpi radialis longus muscle
- Common extensor tendon
- Capitellum of humerus
- Anconeus muscle
- Olecranon process
- Biceps aponeurosis (lacertus fibrosus)
- Brachial artery
- Median nerve
- Pronator teres muscle
- Trochlea of humerus
- Common flexor tendon
- Flexor carpi ulnaris muscle
- Ulnar nerve

Bottom image labels:
- Biceps brachii tendon
- Superficial and deep branches of the radial nerve
- Brachioradialis muscle
- Brachialis muscle and tendon
- Extensor carpi radialis longus muscle
- Extensor digitorum muscle
- Radial head
- Anconeus muscle
- Olecranon process
- Biceps aponeurosis (lacertus fibrosus)
- Brachial artery
- Median nerve
- Pronator teres muscle
- Common flexor tendon
- Flexor carpi ulnaris muscle
- Ulnar nerve
- Flexor digitorum profundus

(**Top**) The ulnar nerve has passed through the cubital tunnel and is now entering the forearm between the 2 heads of the flexor carpi ulnaris muscle. The common extensor tendon is starting to divide into its individual components. (**Bottom**) The brachialis muscle is tapering as its tendon heads toward its insertion on the ulnar tuberosity.

Elbow Muscles and Tendons

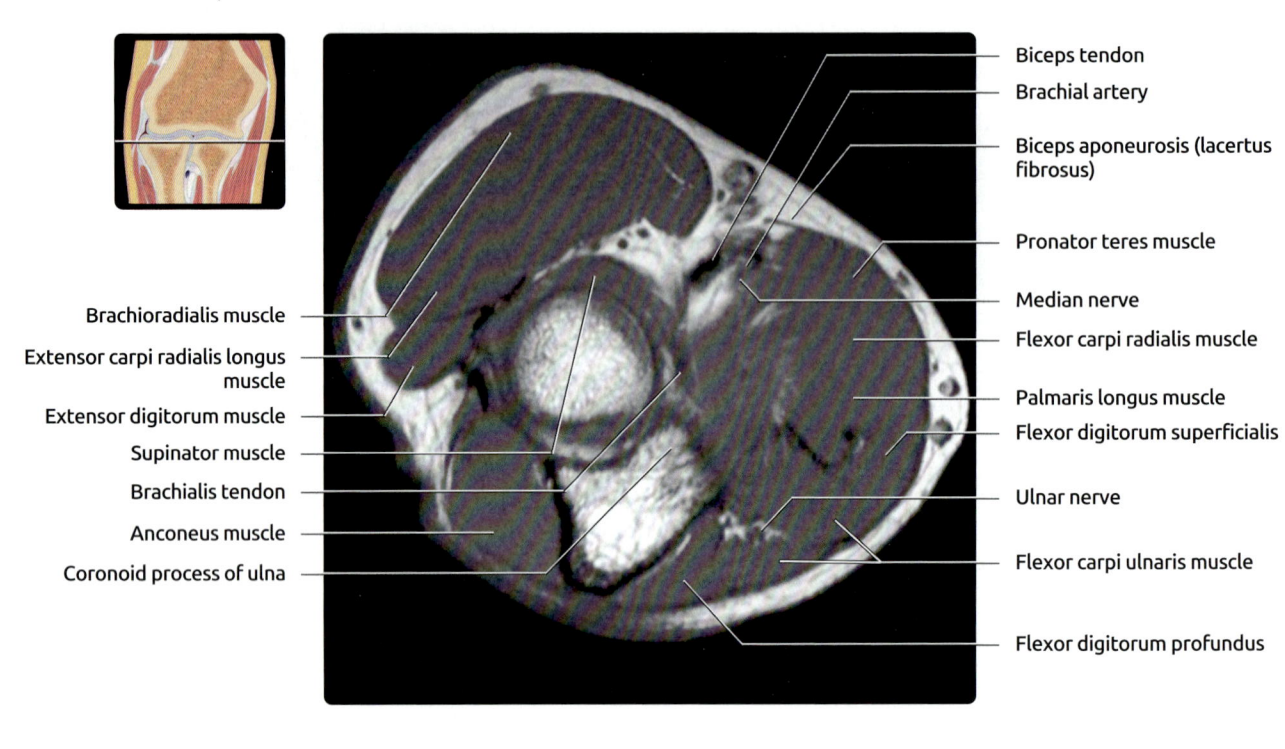

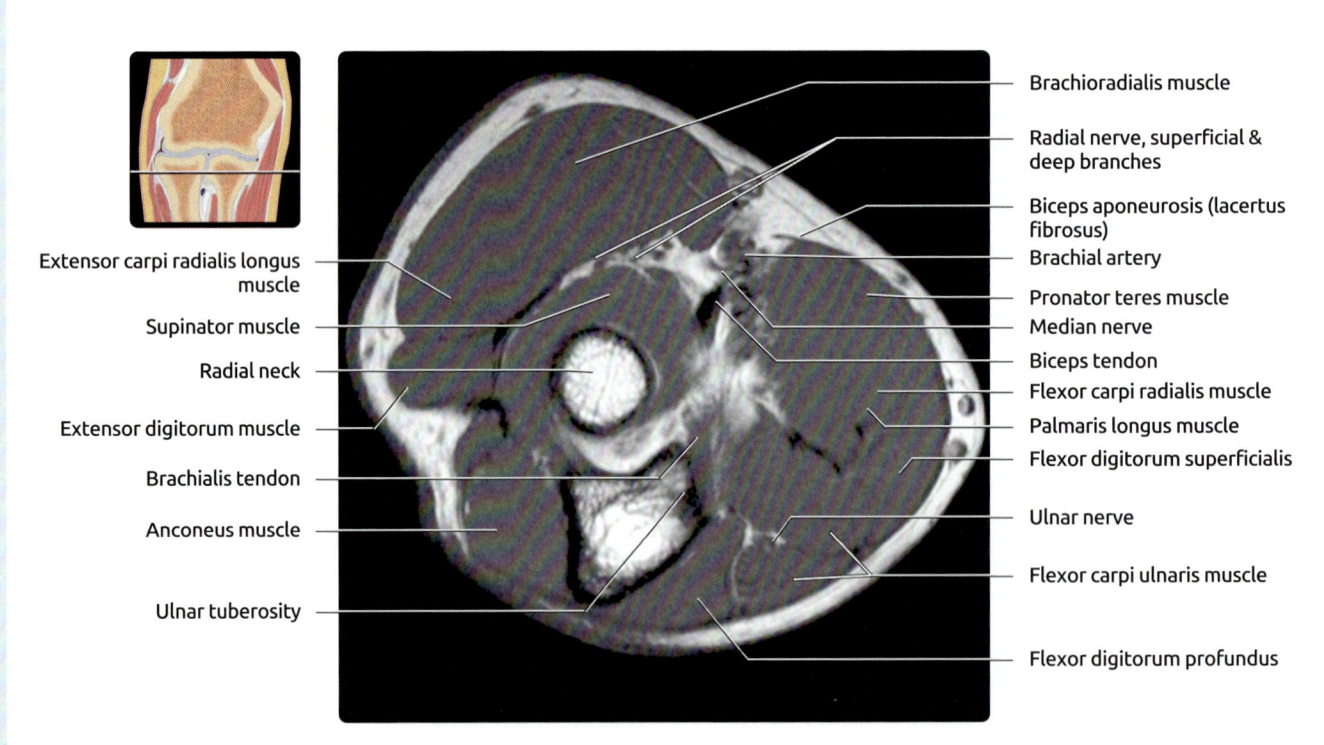

AXIAL T1 MR, RIGHT ELBOW

(Top) The components of the common flexor mass are becoming visible, as the biceps aponeurosis blends with the anterior surface. The proximal aspect of the supinator muscle is also becoming visible around the radial head and neck. (Bottom) The brachialis tendon inserts on the ulnar tuberosity. The supinator muscle is now well seen extending around the radial neck, with the superficial and deep branches of the radial nerve on its anterior aspect. The ulnar nerve lies between the superficial and deep heads of the flexor carpi ulnaris muscle.

Elbow Muscles and Tendons

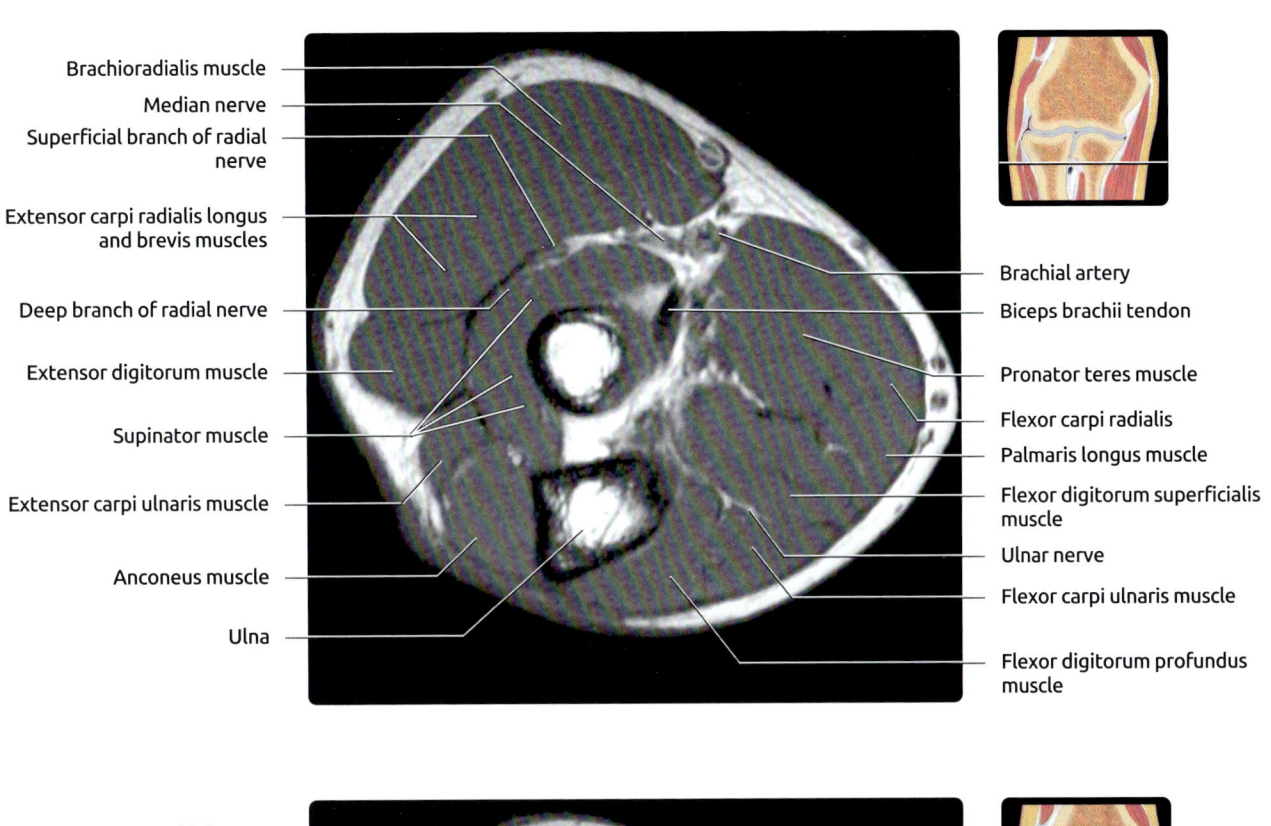

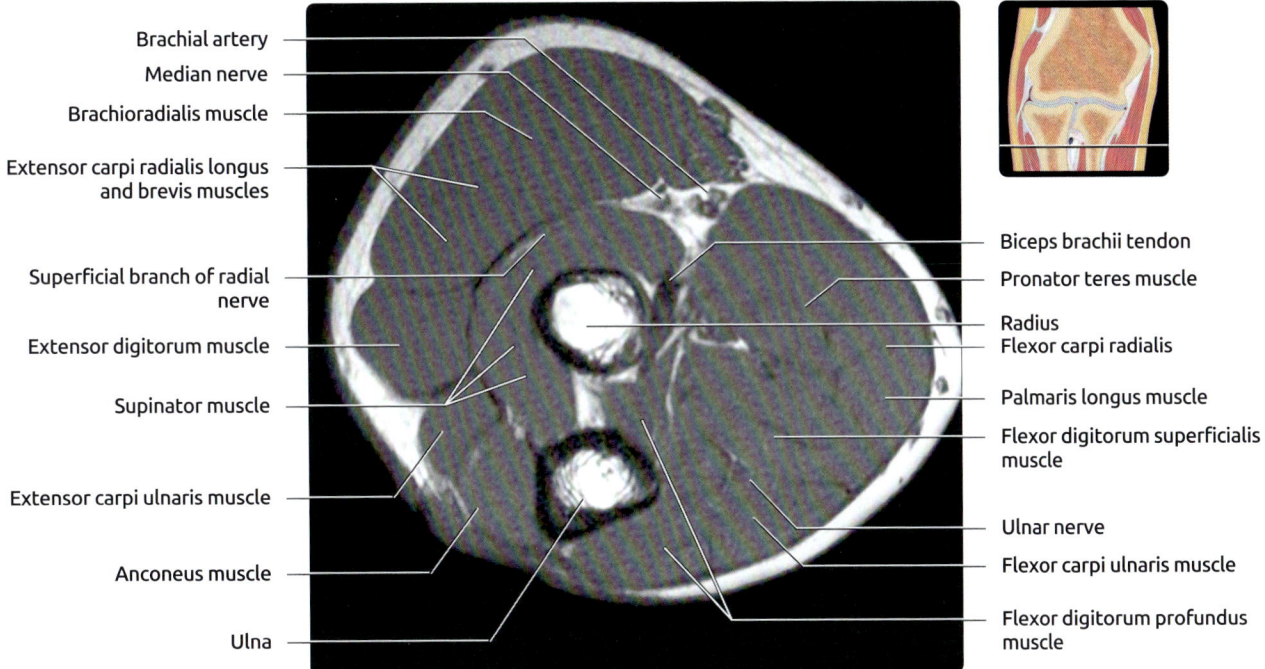

AXIAL T1 MR, RIGHT ELBOW

(**Top**) The deep branch of the radial nerve starts to enter the anterior aspect of the supinator muscle, where it will exit posteriorly as the posterior interosseous nerve. The distal biceps tendon nears its insertion on the radial tuberosity. (**Bottom**) The biceps tendon inserts on the radial tuberosity. The deep branch of the radial nerve is not well appreciated on this image but is passing through the supinator muscle.

Elbow Muscles and Tendons

AXIAL T1 MR, RIGHT ELBOW

Labels (top image):
- Brachioradialis muscle
- Radius
- Radial artery
- Median nerve
- Ulnar artery
- Pronator teres muscle
- Flexor carpi radialis
- Palmaris longus muscle
- Flexor digitorum superficialis muscle
- Ulnar nerve
- Flexor carpi ulnaris muscle
- Flexor digitorum profundus muscle
- Extensor carpi radialis longus muscle
- Extensor carpi radialis brevis muscle
- Deep branch of radial nerve
- Extensor digitorum muscle
- Supinator muscle
- Extensor carpi ulnaris muscle
- Anconeus muscle
- Ulna

Labels (bottom image):
- Extensor carpi radialis longus m.
- Brachioradialis muscle
- Radius
- Radial artery
- Ulnar artery
- Median nerve
- Pronator teres muscle
- Flexor carpi radialis
- Palmaris longus muscle
- Flexor digitorum superficialis muscle
- Ulnar nerve
- Flexor carpi ulnaris muscle
- Flexor digitorum profundus muscle
- Extensor carpi radialis brevis muscle
- Radial nerve, deep branch
- Extensor digitorum muscle
- Supinator muscle
- Extensor carpi ulnaris muscle
- Anconeus muscle
- Ulna

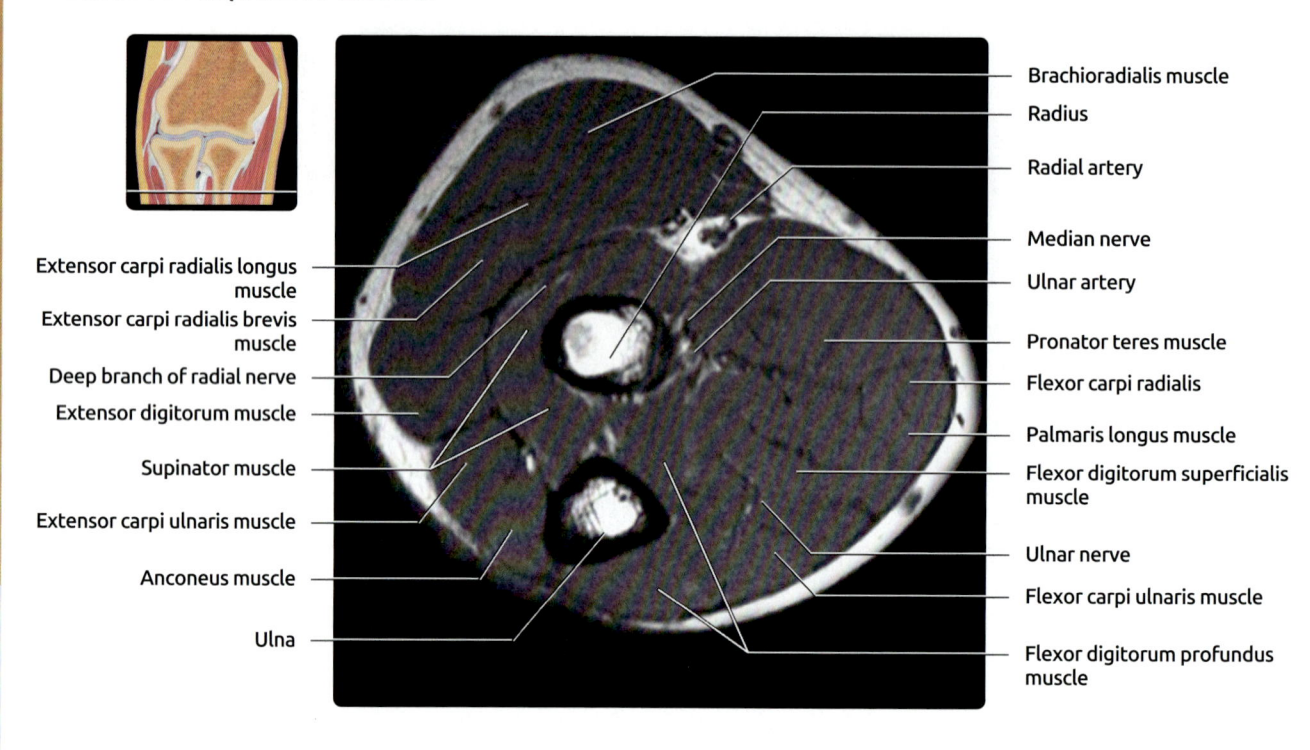

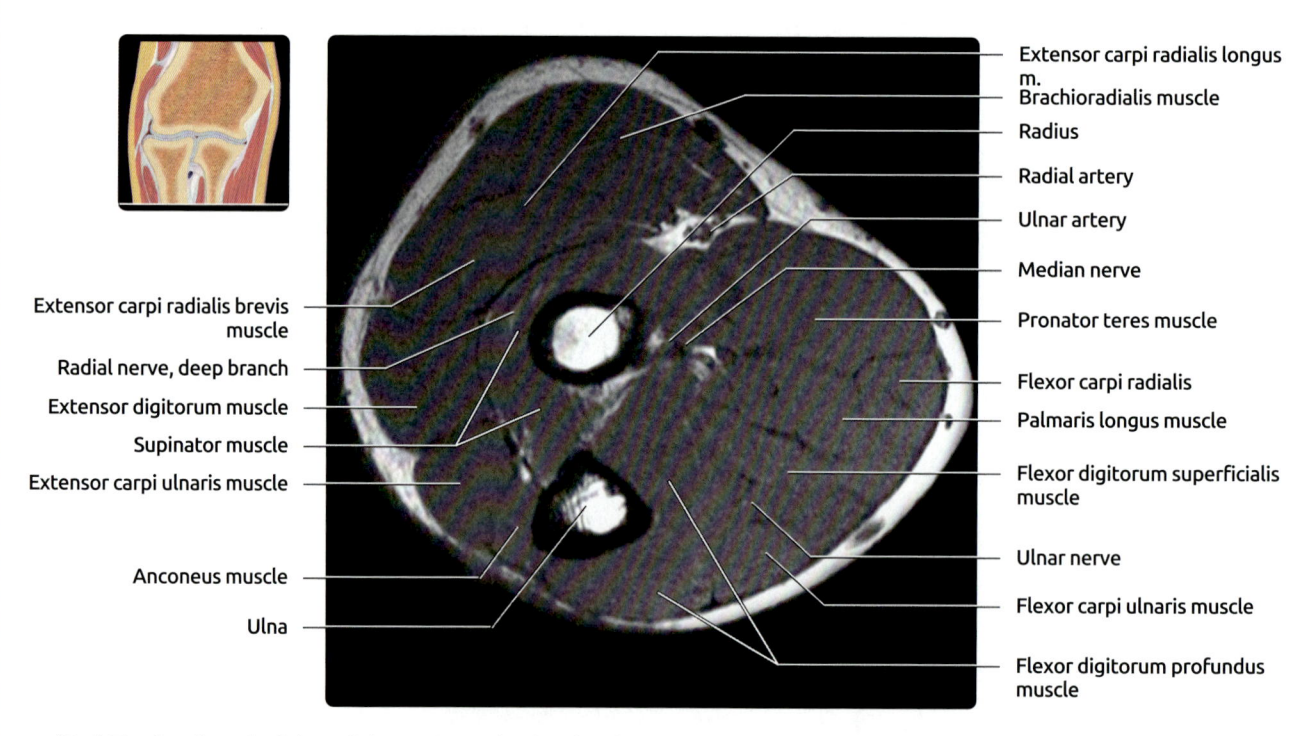

(**Top**) The deep branch of the radial nerve is visualized within the supinator muscle, but the superficial branch is not well seen on this image. The individual components of the flexor-pronator group are now well delineated. (**Bottom**) The components of the extensor group are now starting to be delineated.

Elbow Muscles and Tendons

CORONAL T1 MR, LEFT ELBOW

Triceps muscle

Olecranon process

Triceps muscle & tendon

Olecranon process

Flexor digitorum profundus muscle

Anconeus muscle

Triceps muscle and tendon

Olecranon process

Flexor carpi ulnaris muscle

Flexor digitorum profundus muscle

Anconeus muscle

Extensor carpi ulnaris

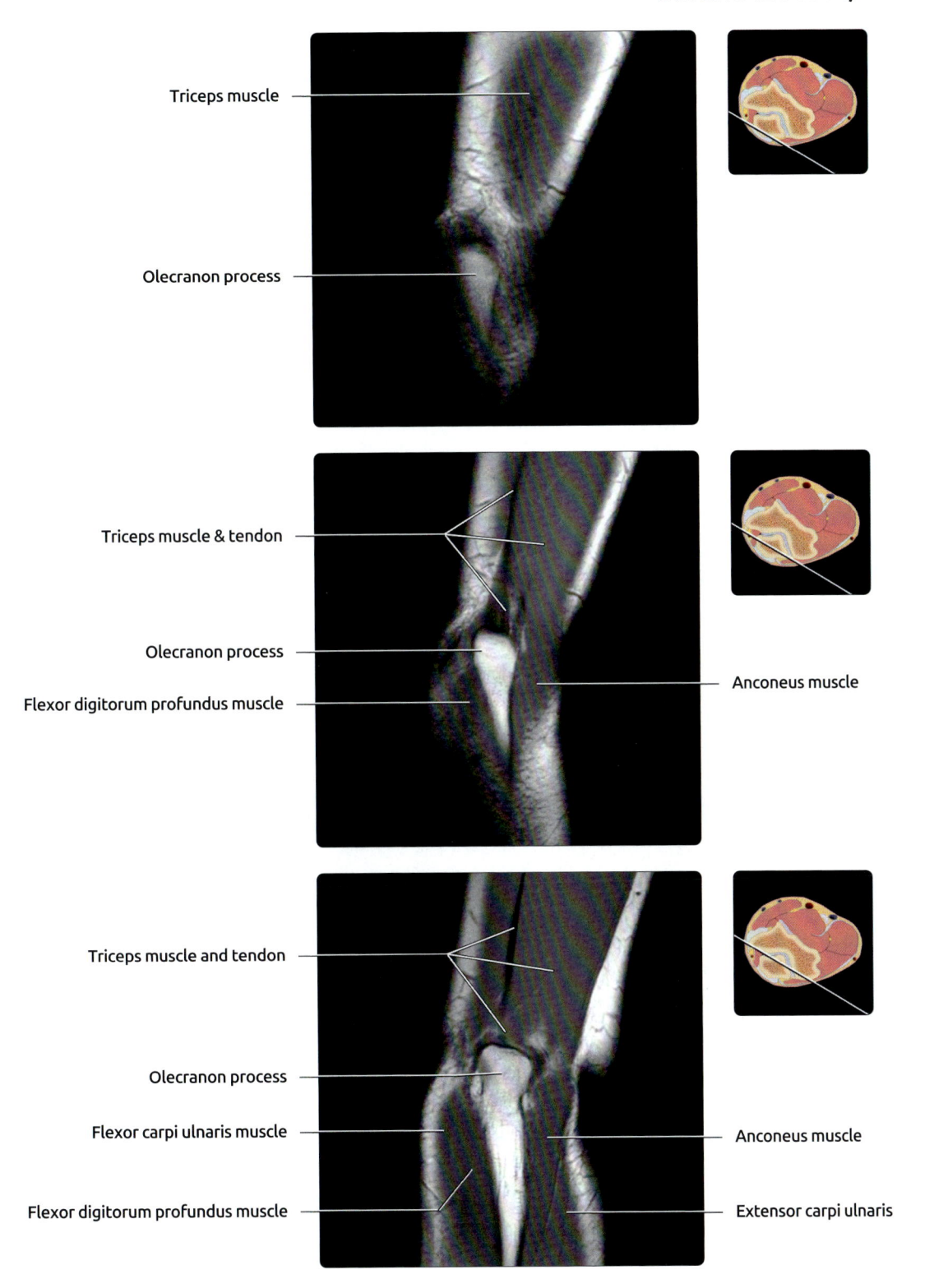

(Top) First of 12 coronal images at the posterior aspect of the elbow, the triceps muscle, and olecranon process are seen. The triceps tendon is not yet visualized. (Middle) The triceps tendon is now seen attaching to the olecranon. The posterior aspects of the anconeus on the lateral side and flexor digitorum profundus on the medial side are also now coming into view. (Bottom) The flexor carpi ulnaris and extensor carpi ulnaris muscles are now becoming visible.

259

Elbow Muscles and Tendons

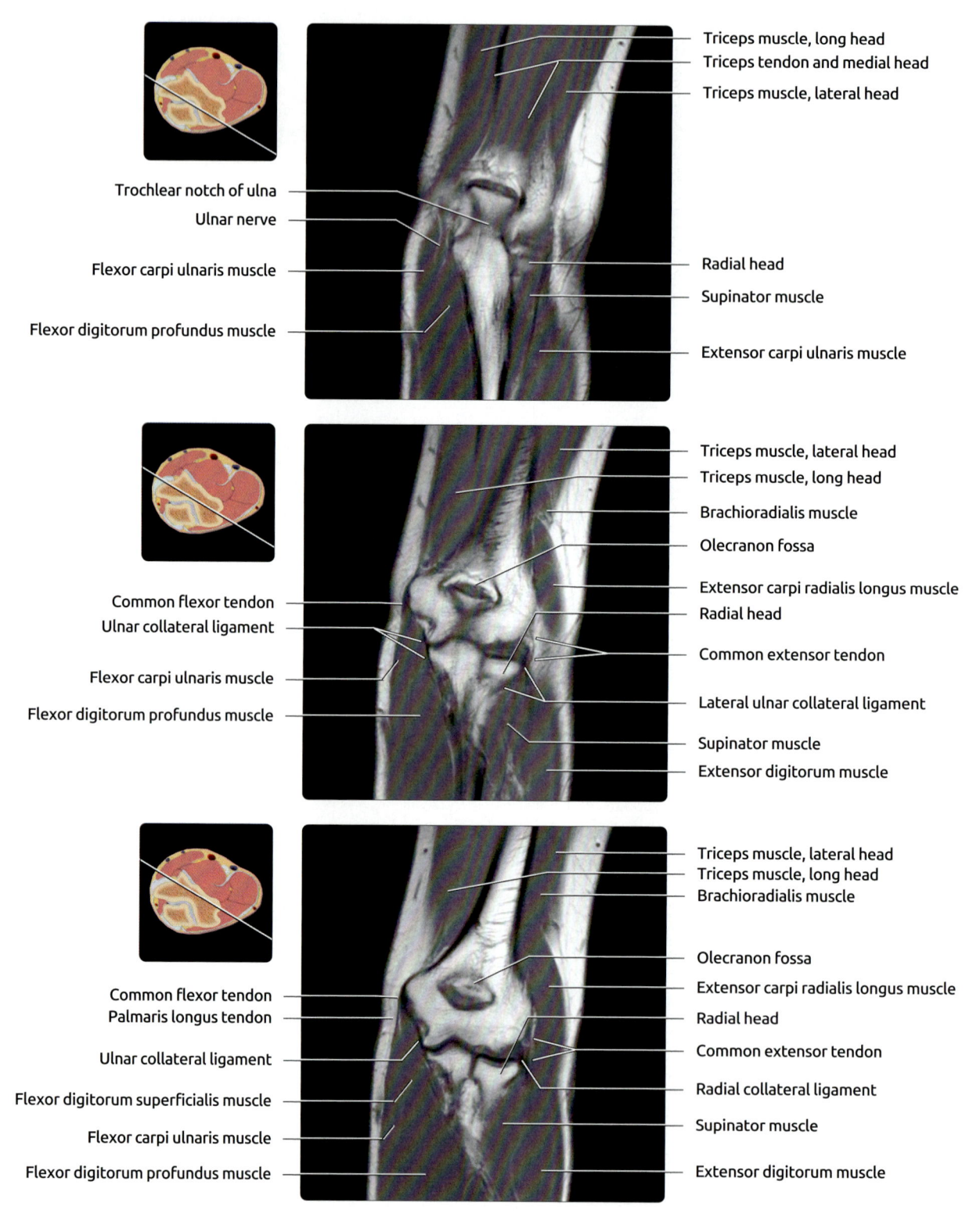

CORONAL T1 MR, LEFT ELBOW

(Top) Just behind the medial epicondyle (epicondyle not seen on this image), the ulnar nerve passes through the cubital tunnel and passes between the 2 heads of the flexor carpi ulnaris muscle. The posterior aspect of the radial head is just coming into view, with the surrounding supinator muscle. (Middle) The posterior aspect of the common extensor tendon is seen superficial to the lateral ulnar collateral ligament. The lateral ulnar collateral ligament is seen winding posterior to the radius toward its attachment on the ulna. The common flexor tendon is shorter and broader than the common extensor tendon and is seen attaching to the medial epicondyle. (Bottom) The common extensor tendon is now better visualized, superficial to the radial collateral ligament. The palmaris longus component of the common flexor tendon is also seen, with the ulnar collateral ligament deep to the common flexor muscle group.

Elbow Muscles and Tendons

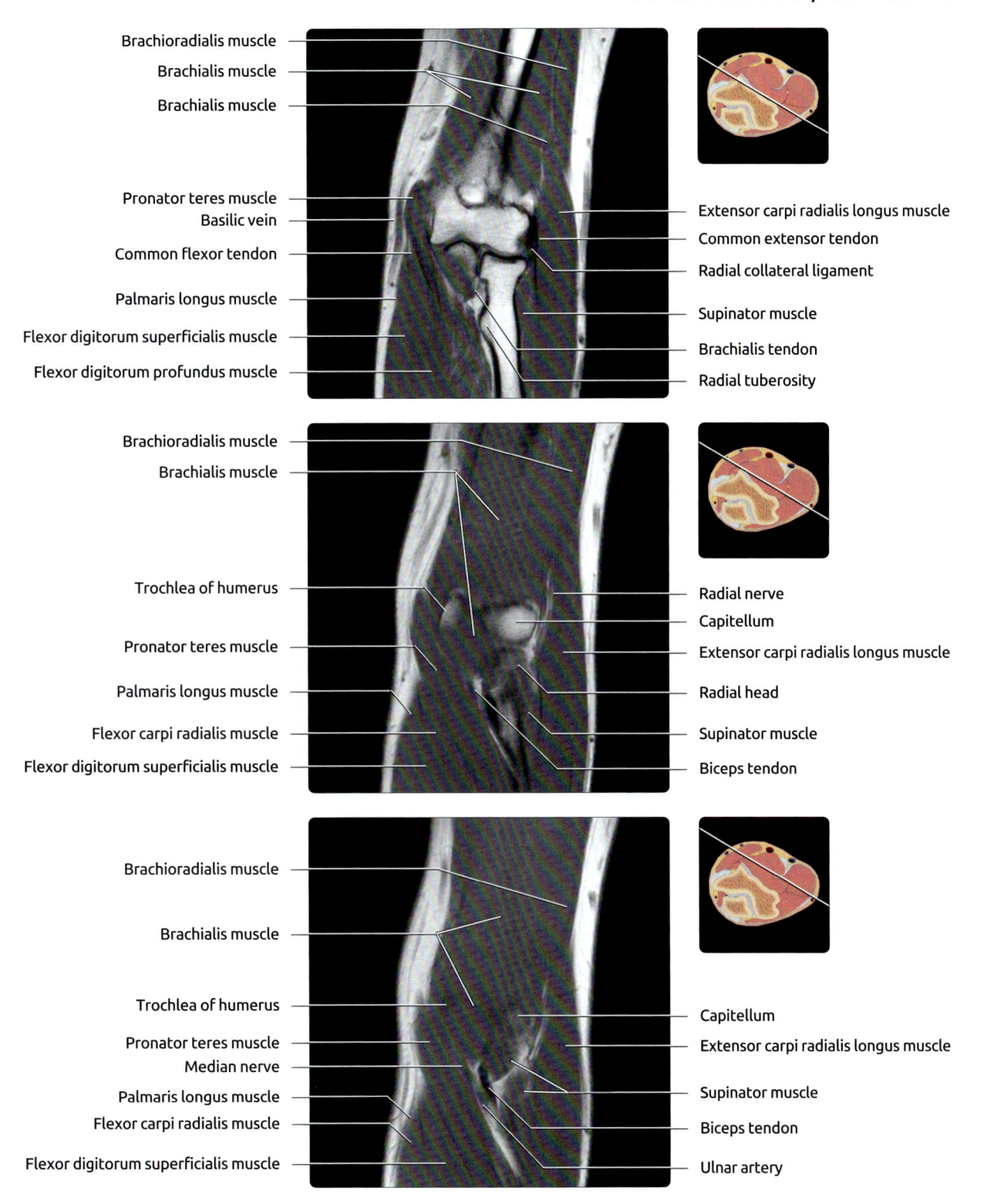

CORONAL T1 MR, LEFT ELBOW

Labels (top image):
- Brachioradialis muscle
- Brachialis muscle
- Brachialis muscle
- Pronator teres muscle
- Basilic vein
- Common flexor tendon
- Palmaris longus muscle
- Flexor digitorum superficialis muscle
- Flexor digitorum profundus muscle
- Extensor carpi radialis longus muscle
- Common extensor tendon
- Radial collateral ligament
- Supinator muscle
- Brachialis tendon
- Radial tuberosity

Labels (middle image):
- Brachioradialis muscle
- Brachialis muscle
- Trochlea of humerus
- Pronator teres muscle
- Palmaris longus muscle
- Flexor carpi radialis muscle
- Flexor digitorum superficialis muscle
- Radial nerve
- Capitellum
- Extensor carpi radialis longus muscle
- Radial head
- Supinator muscle
- Biceps tendon

Labels (bottom image):
- Brachioradialis muscle
- Brachialis muscle
- Trochlea of humerus
- Pronator teres muscle
- Median nerve
- Palmaris longus muscle
- Flexor carpi radialis muscle
- Flexor digitorum superficialis muscle
- Capitellum
- Extensor carpi radialis longus muscle
- Supinator muscle
- Biceps tendon
- Ulnar artery

(Top) The radial nerve can be seen running between the brachioradialis and brachialis muscles. The brachialis tendon approaches its insertion on the ulnar tuberosity. (Middle) The distal biceps tendon is visualized, proximal to its insertion on the radial tuberosity. The course of the pronator teres muscle is well seen, extending from the medial side of the humerus to the proximal shaft of the radius. (Bottom) The median nerve and ulnar artery are coming into view, adjacent to the biceps tendon.

Elbow Muscles and Tendons

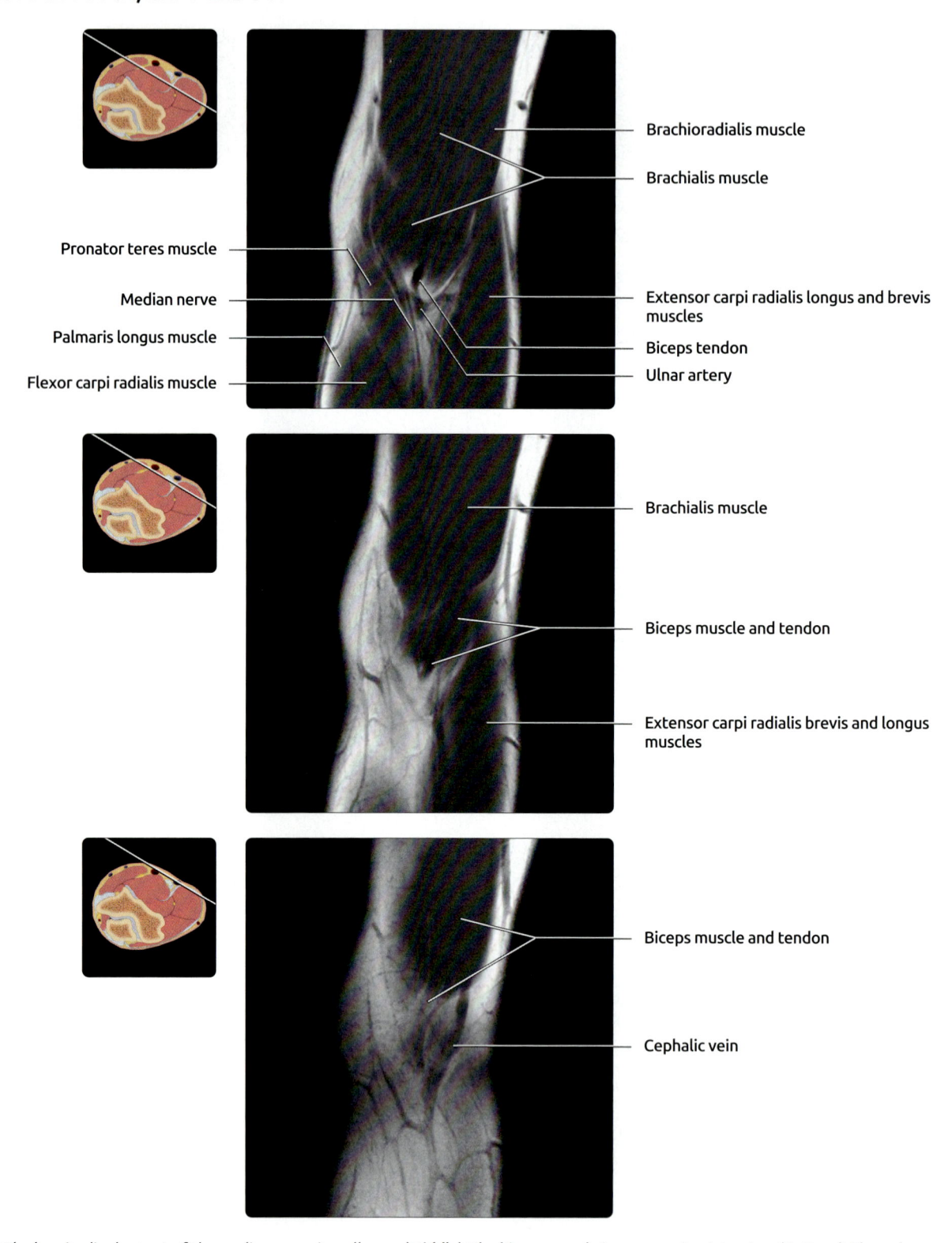

CORONAL T1 MR, LEFT ELBOW

- Brachioradialis muscle
- Brachialis muscle
- Pronator teres muscle
- Median nerve
- Palmaris longus muscle
- Flexor carpi radialis muscle
- Extensor carpi radialis longus and brevis muscles
- Biceps tendon
- Ulnar artery

- Brachialis muscle
- Biceps muscle and tendon
- Extensor carpi radialis brevis and longus muscles

- Biceps muscle and tendon
- Cephalic vein

(Top) The longitudinal extent of the median nerve is well seen. (Middle) The biceps muscle is now coming into view. (Bottom) The only muscle seen at the most extreme anterior of the elbow is the biceps.

Elbow Muscles and Tendons

SAGITTAL T1 MR, LEFT ELBOW

Top image labels:
- Basilic vein
- Pronator teres muscle
- Palmaris longus muscle
- Medial epicondyle

Middle image labels:
- Triceps muscle, long head
- Ulnar collateral ligament
- Pronator teres muscle
- Palmaris longus muscle
- Medial epicondyle
- Common flexor tendon
- Flexor digitorum superficialis muscle
- Flexor carpi ulnaris muscle

Bottom image labels:
- Triceps muscle, long head
- Brachialis muscle
- Ulnar collateral ligament
- Pronator teres muscle
- Palmaris longus muscle
- Medial epicondyle
- Common flexor tendon
- Flexor digitorum superficialis muscle
- Flexor carpi ulnaris muscle

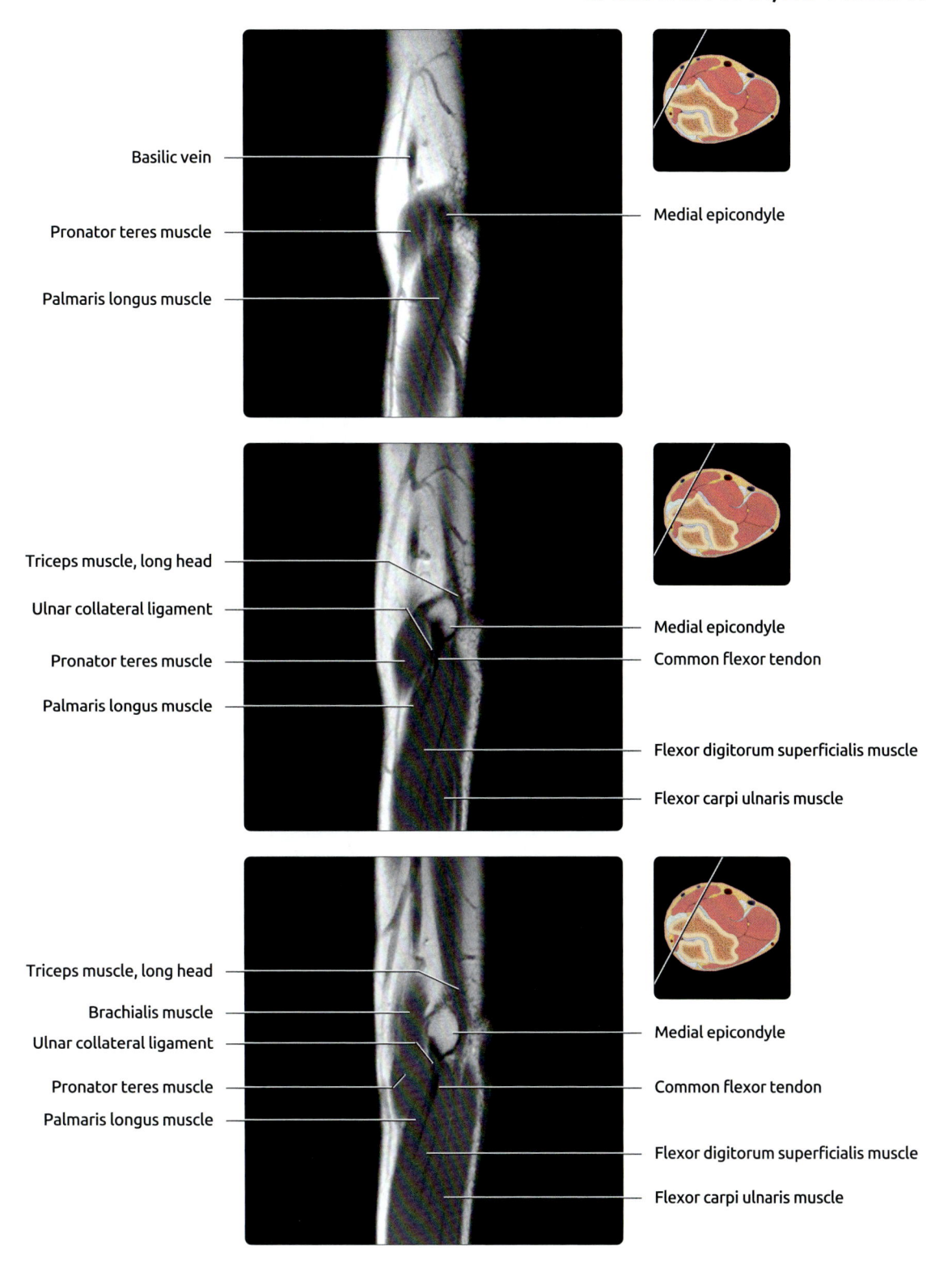

(Top) This is the 1st of 12 sagittal images, shown from medial to lateral. Only the extreme tip of the medial epicondyle is visible in this section. The pronator teres and palmaris longus muscles are the most medially located and are just coming into view. **(Middle)** The medial epicondyle is now better seen, with the attachments of the ulnar collateral ligament and common flexor tendon. **(Bottom)** The brachialis muscle is now coming into view.

Elbow Muscles and Tendons

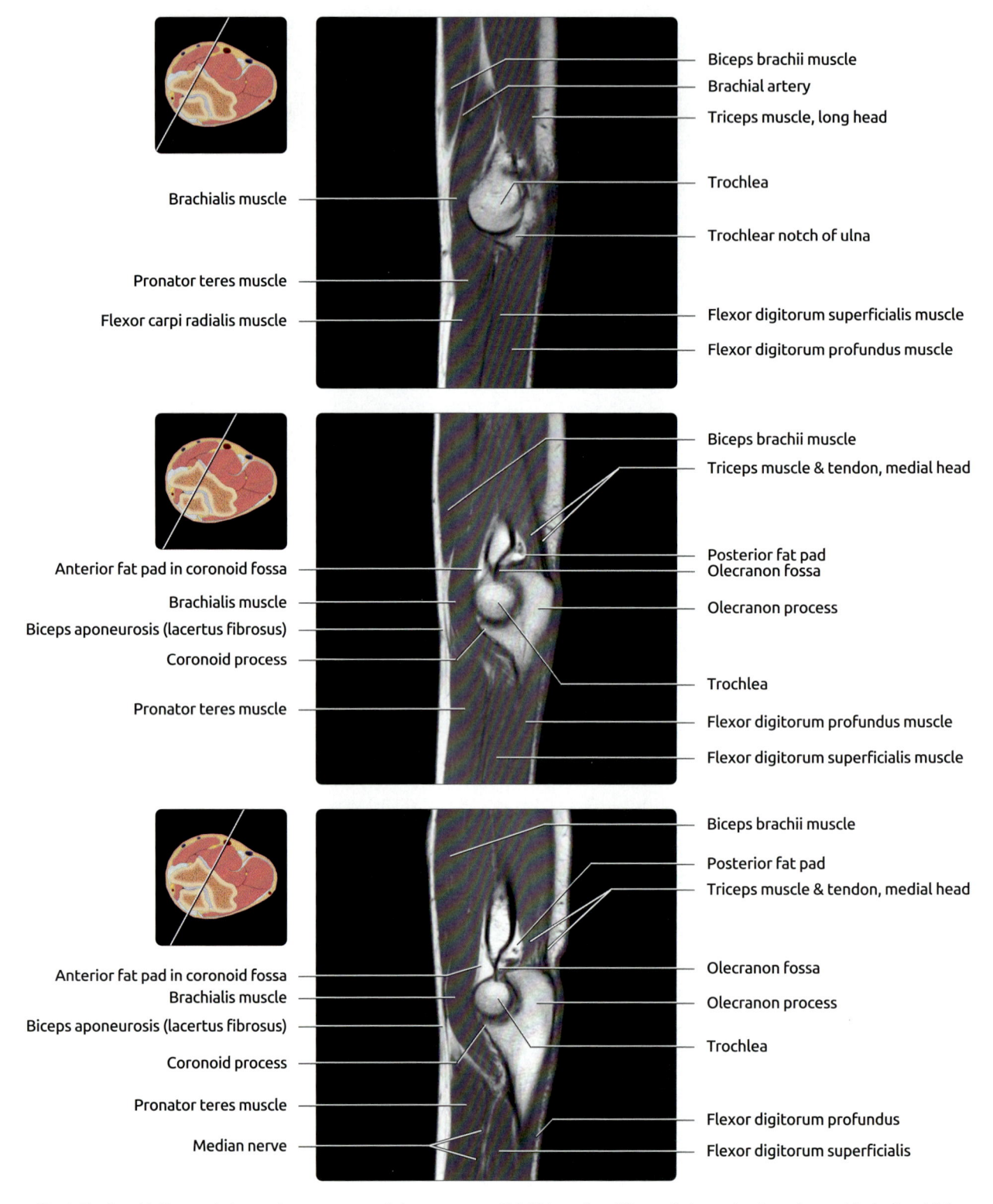

SAGITTAL T1 MR, LEFT ELBOW

Top image labels (left): Brachialis muscle; Pronator teres muscle; Flexor carpi radialis muscle
Top image labels (right): Biceps brachii muscle; Brachial artery; Triceps muscle, long head; Trochlea; Trochlear notch of ulna; Flexor digitorum superficialis muscle; Flexor digitorum profundus muscle

Middle image labels (left): Anterior fat pad in coronoid fossa; Brachialis muscle; Biceps aponeurosis (lacertus fibrosus); Coronoid process; Pronator teres muscle
Middle image labels (right): Biceps brachii muscle; Triceps muscle & tendon, medial head; Posterior fat pad; Olecranon fossa; Olecranon process; Trochlea; Flexor digitorum profundus muscle; Flexor digitorum superficialis muscle

Bottom image labels (left): Anterior fat pad in coronoid fossa; Brachialis muscle; Biceps aponeurosis (lacertus fibrosus); Coronoid process; Pronator teres muscle; Median nerve
Bottom image labels (right): Biceps brachii muscle; Posterior fat pad; Triceps muscle & tendon, medial head; Olecranon fossa; Olecranon process; Trochlea; Flexor digitorum profundus; Flexor digitorum superficialis

(**Top**) The brachialis muscle is now better seen, and the more superficial biceps brachii muscle is coming into view, with the brachial artery running between these 2 muscles. (**Middle**) Part of the triceps muscle itself is seen inserting on the olecranon process. The biceps aponeurosis is now visible. (**Bottom**) The brachialis muscle is nearing its insertion on the ulnar tuberosity. The median nerve is now visible between the pronator teres and flexor digitorum superficialis muscles.

Elbow Muscles and Tendons

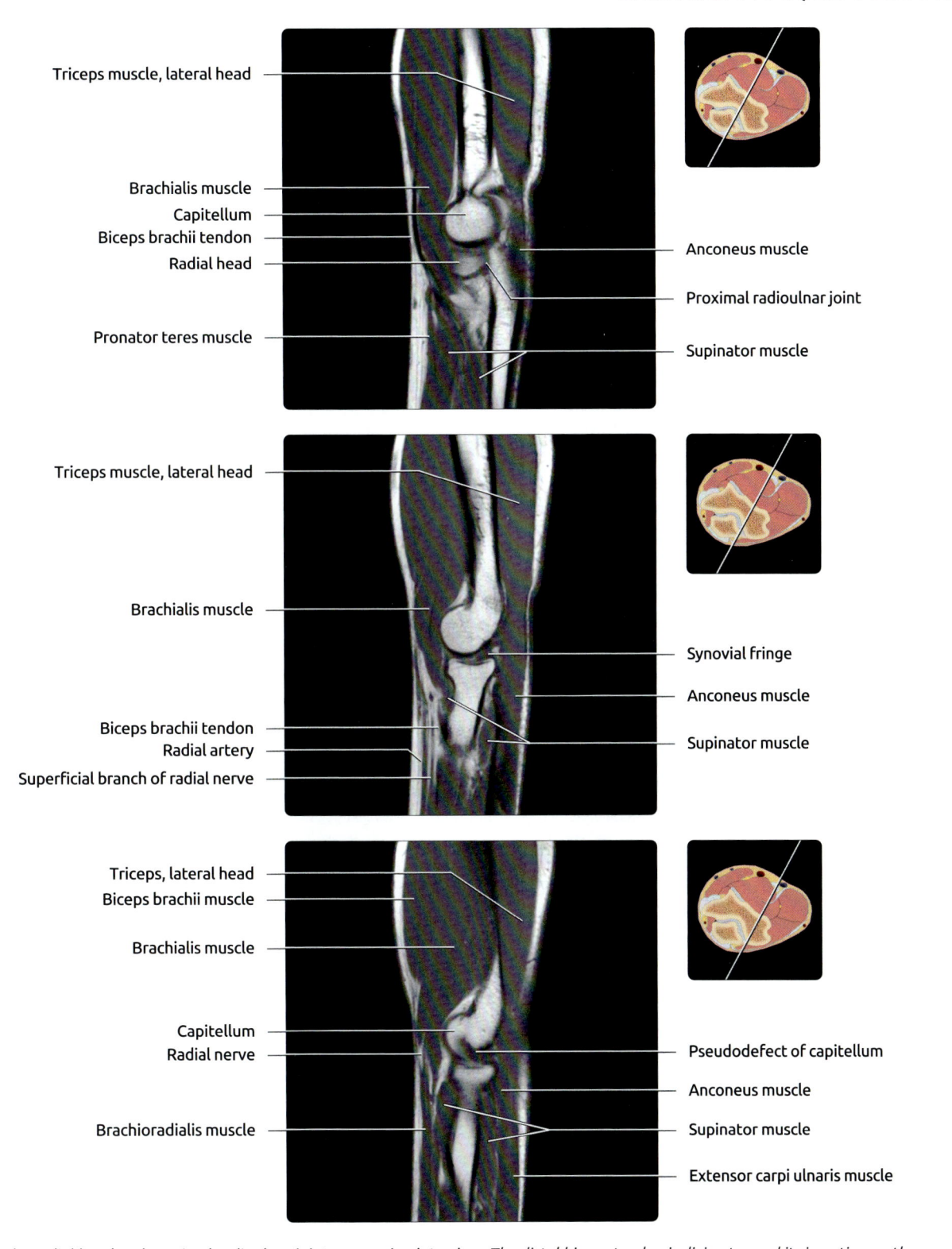

SAGITTAL T1 MR, LEFT ELBOW

Labels (Top image):
- Triceps muscle, lateral head
- Brachialis muscle
- Capitellum
- Biceps brachii tendon
- Radial head
- Pronator teres muscle
- Anconeus muscle
- Proximal radioulnar joint
- Supinator muscle

Labels (Middle image):
- Triceps muscle, lateral head
- Brachialis muscle
- Biceps brachii tendon
- Radial artery
- Superficial branch of radial nerve
- Synovial fringe
- Anconeus muscle
- Supinator muscle

Labels (Bottom image):
- Triceps, lateral head
- Biceps brachii muscle
- Brachialis muscle
- Capitellum
- Radial nerve
- Brachioradialis muscle
- Pseudodefect of capitellum
- Anconeus muscle
- Supinator muscle
- Extensor carpi ulnaris muscle

(Top) The radial head and proximal radioulnar joint are coming into view. The distal biceps tendon is diving toward its insertion on the radial tuberosity. (Middle) The biceps tendon is seen attaching to the radial tuberosity. A synovial fringe, also called a synovial plica, is a meniscus-shaped in-folding of the joint capsule. (Bottom) The pseudodefect of the capitellum is seen at the posterior aspect of the capitellum, representing a normal groove between the round capitellum and lateral condyle.

Elbow Muscles and Tendons

SAGITTAL T1 MR, LEFT ELBOW

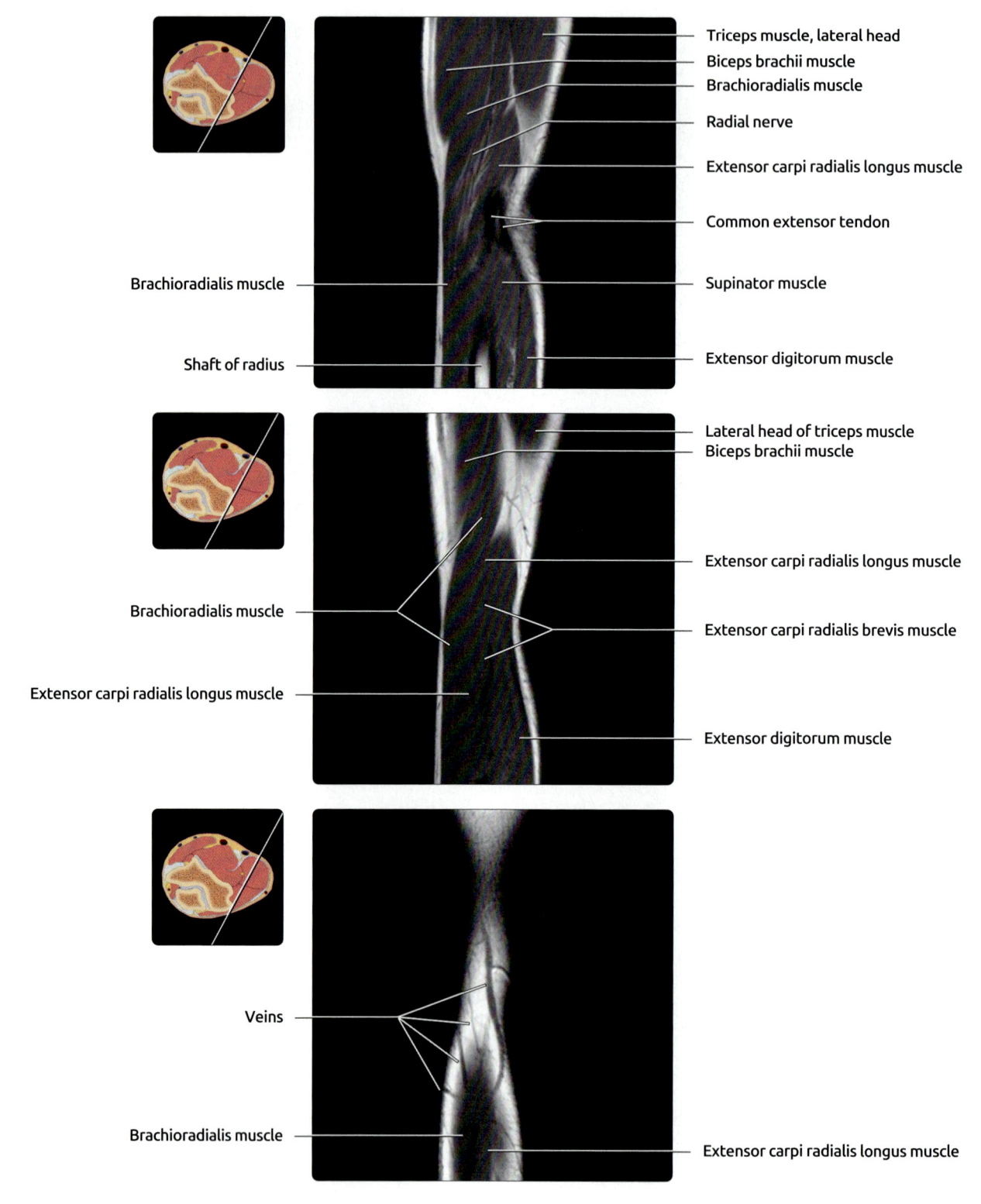

Labels (top image):
- Triceps muscle, lateral head
- Biceps brachii muscle
- Brachioradialis muscle
- Radial nerve
- Extensor carpi radialis longus muscle
- Common extensor tendon
- Supinator muscle
- Extensor digitorum muscle
- Brachioradialis muscle
- Shaft of radius

Labels (middle image):
- Lateral head of triceps muscle
- Biceps brachii muscle
- Extensor carpi radialis longus muscle
- Extensor carpi radialis brevis muscle
- Extensor digitorum muscle
- Brachioradialis muscle
- Extensor carpi radialis longus muscle

Labels (bottom image):
- Veins
- Brachioradialis muscle
- Extensor carpi radialis longus muscle

(**Top**) The common extensor tendon is arising at the tip of the lateral epicondyle. (**Middle**) Along the far lateral aspect of the elbow, the muscles of the extensor group are visualized, forming the fleshy lateral aspect of the forearm. (**Bottom**) Coming out of the lateral muscles into the subcutaneous fat, numerous veins are seen.

Elbow Muscles and Tendons

AXIAL T2 FS MR, BICIPITORADIAL BURSA

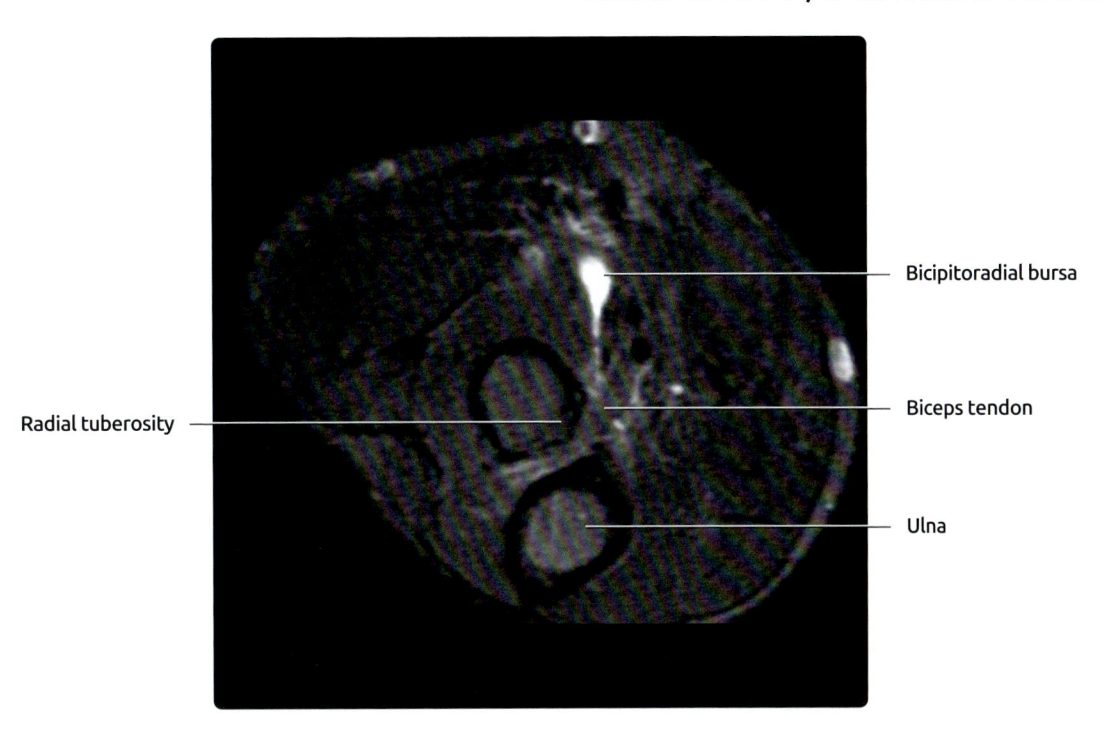

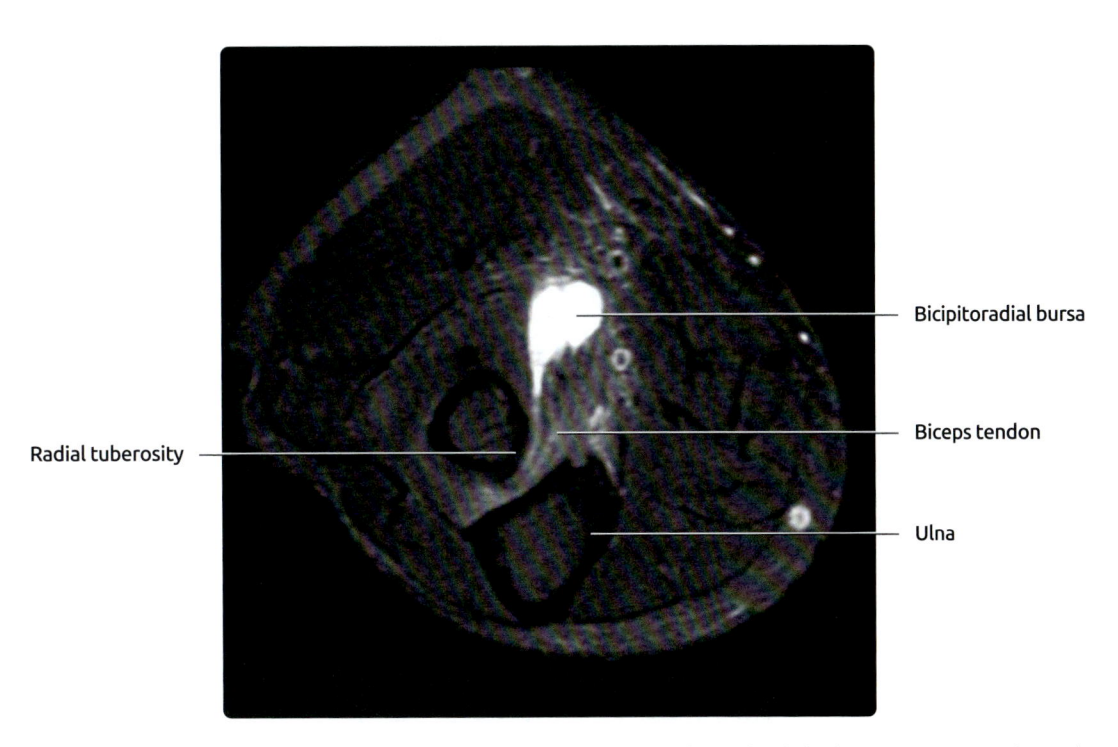

(Top) The bicipitoradial bursa is tear-drop shaped and located between the biceps tendon and radial tuberosity to protect the tendon during pronation. (Bottom) In a different patient, the bicipitoradial bursa is more distended but still tear-drop shaped. The biceps tendon is mildly tendinotic, manifest by swelling and signal alteration.

Elbow Muscles and Tendons

FABS POSITIONING AND IMAGE

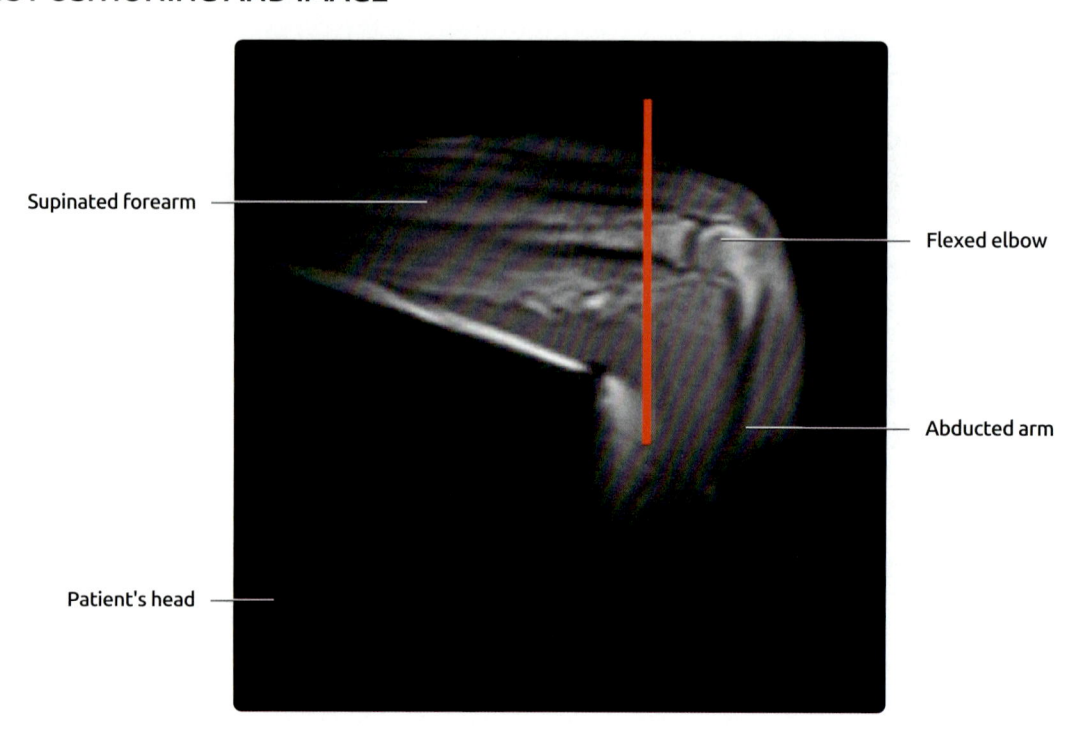

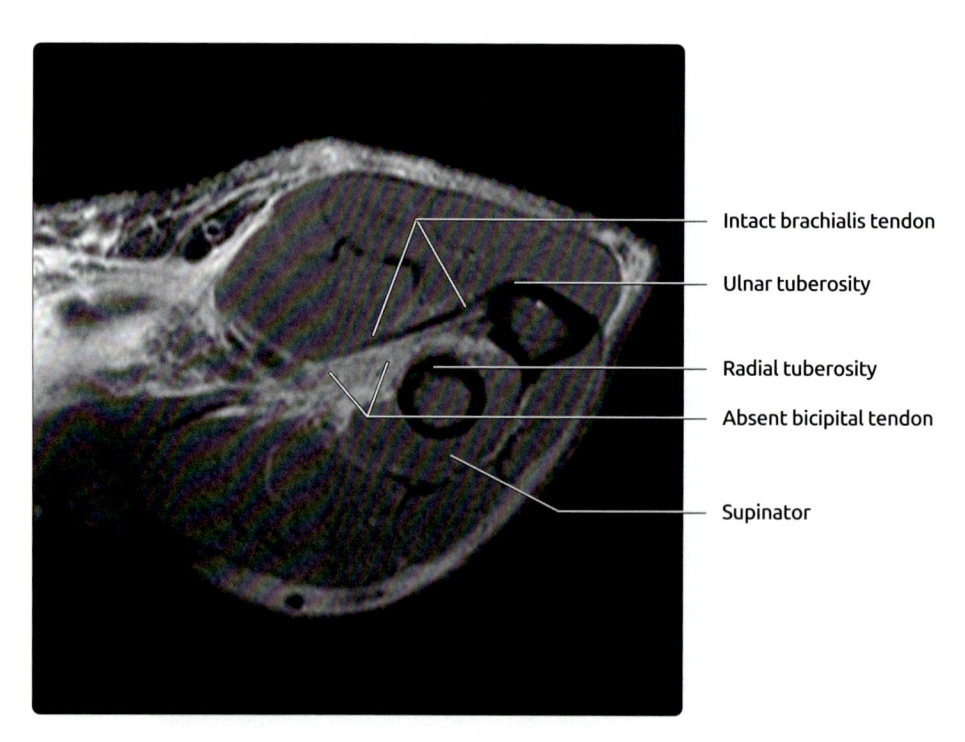

(Top) Scout image shows coronal plane for FABS view. The elbow is flexed, arm is abducted, and forearm is supinated. The red line shows the cut (perpendicular to the radius and coronal to the humerus) used to obtain the subsequent image. *(Bottom)* T2 MR obtained at the cut shown on the prior scout image shows intact brachialis tendon attaching to the ulnar tuberosity but disrupted biceps tendon at the site of its insertion on the radial tuberosity.

Elbow Muscles and Tendons

FABS VIEW: T1 MR, LEFT ELBOW

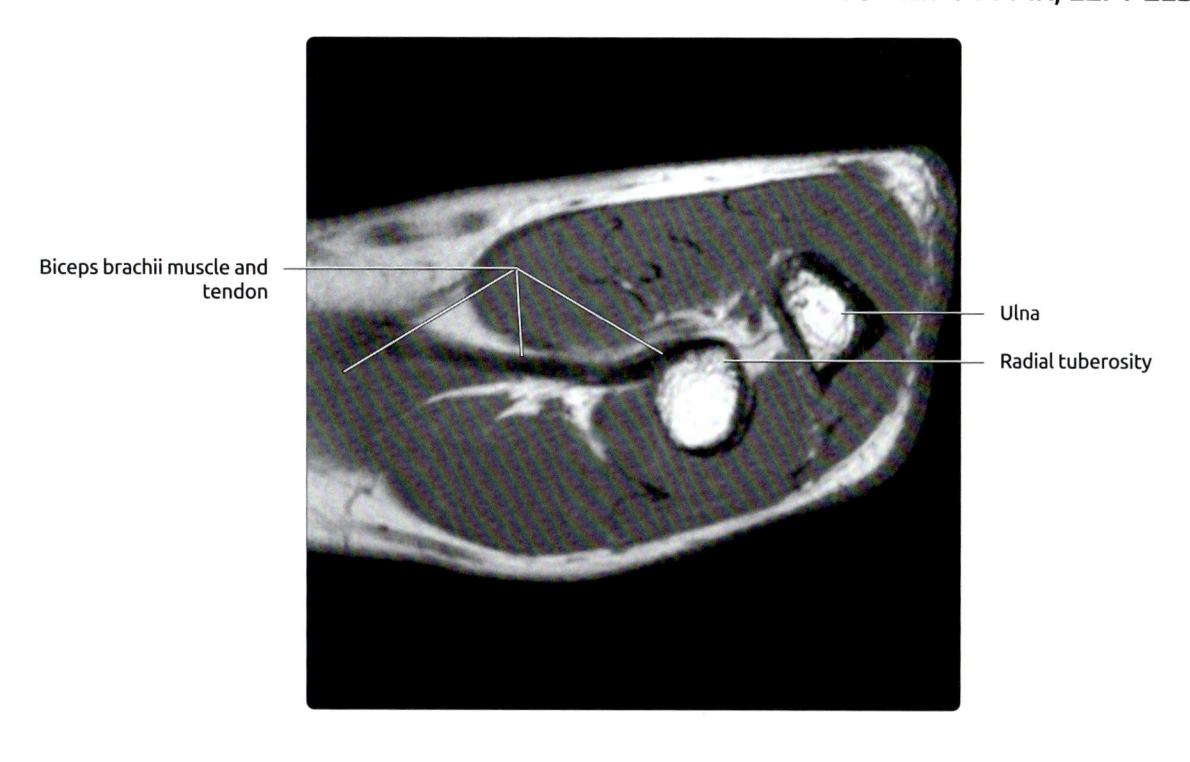

Biceps brachii muscle and tendon — Ulna — Radial tuberosity

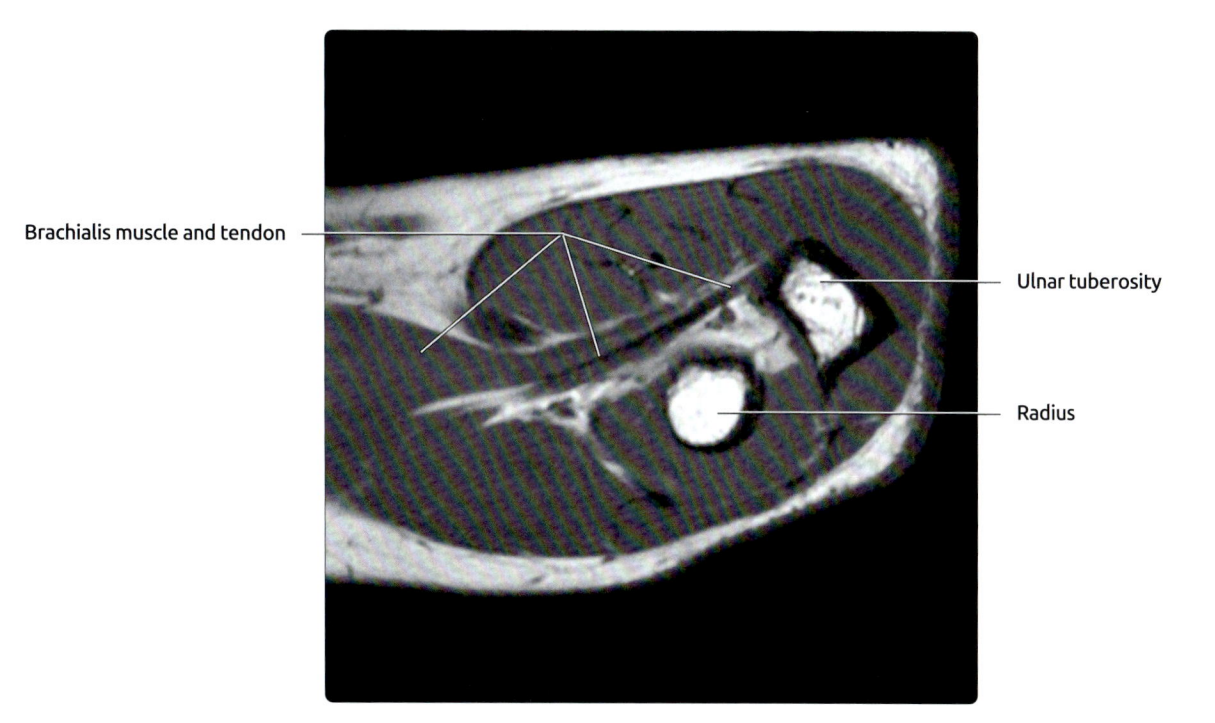

Brachialis muscle and tendon — Ulnar tuberosity — Radius

(**Top**) *Normal patient: Imaging transverse to the forearm in the FABS position shows the full longitudinal extent of the normal distal biceps tendon inserting on the radial tuberosity. The image is slightly out of plane to demonstrate the brachialis tendon.* (**Bottom**) *Adjacent image transverse to the forearm in the FABS position also shows the full longitudinal extent of the brachialis tendon inserting on the ulnar tuberosity.*

Elbow Ligaments

TERMINOLOGY

Abbreviations
- Ulnar collateral ligament (UCL)
- Radial collateral ligament (RCL)

Definitions
- Elbow ligaments are intrinsic ligaments: Thickening of joint capsule

IMAGING ANATOMY

Lateral Side of Elbow Joint
- Lateral collateral ligament complex
  - Radial collateral ligament
    - Triangular shaped with apex on lateral epicondyle, broader base at radial attachments
    - Origin: Lateral epicondyle, immediately anterior to lateral ulnar collateral ligament
    - Insertion: Base blends with annular ligament around radial head
    - Lies deep to extensor carpi radialis brevis tendon
    - Provides origin for the superficial head of supinator muscle
    - Primary restraint to varus stress
  - Lateral UCL (also termed radial UCL)
    - Thin ligament
    - Origin: Lateral epicondyle, posterior to and blending with posterior aspect of origin of RCL
    - Insertion: Supinator crest of lateral side of proximal ulna
    - Courses posterior to radial head, with its mid portion partially blending with annular ligament
    - Provides restraint to posterolateral instability of radial head
  - Annular ligament
    - Attached to anterior and posterior aspects of radial notch of ulna
    - Forms a ring or collar around radial head
    - Anterior attachment becomes taut in supination
    - Posterior attachment becomes taut in extreme pronation
    - Provides origin for superficial head of supinator muscle
  - Accessory lateral collateral ligament
    - Anatomically inconstant
    - Origin: Anterior inferior aspect of annular ligament
    - Insertion: Supinator crest of ulna, blending with insertion of lateral UCL
    - Stabilizes annular ligament during varus stress

Medial Side of Elbow Joint
- Ulnar (medial) collateral ligament
  - Triangular shaped with apex on inferior surface of medial epicondyle
  - Insertion: Coronoid and olecranon portions of ulna
  - Composed of 3 bands
    - Anterior: Functionally most important, extends from medial epicondyle of humerus to sublime tubercle of coronoid process
    - Posterior: Functionally less important but maintains reciprocal tautness with anterior band, extends from medial epicondyle to olecranon
    - Transverse: Functionally unimportant, forms base of triangle between anterior and posterior bands
  - Lies deep to common flexor tendon
  - Restraint against valgus stress

Proximal Radioulnar Joint
- Annular ligament: See discussion on lateral side of elbow joint
- Quadrate ligament
  - Thin fibrous band
  - Origin: Lateral side of ulna, distal to radial notch
  - Insertion: Medial side of radial neck, distal to annular ligament
  - Stabilizes proximal radio-ulnar joint in full supination
- Oblique cord
  - Anatomically inconstant
  - Origin: Lateral side of ulna, distal to tuberosity
  - Insertion: Medial side of radius, distal to tuberosity

ANATOMY IMAGING ISSUES

Radial Collateral Ligament
- Seen best on coronal images; visible throughout course in all patients
- Low signal intensity structure, may be difficult to distinguish from overlying extensor carpi radialis brevis tendon
- Meniscus-like synovial fold (synovial fringe) may project from its deep surface into the radiocapitellar joint

Lateral UCL
- Difficult to visualize because of thin size and oblique course
  - Visible in 85% using multiple cuts
  - Improved visualization with
    - Thin section coronal plane
    - Oblique coronal plane

Ulnar Collateral Ligament
- Anterior band is routinely visualized (100%) on coronal images, other bands are not
- Coronal images: Inverted triangle appearance
  - Broad proximal aspect attaching to undersurface of medial condyle
    - May have intermediate signal intensity
  - Thin distal aspect attaching to sublime tubercle of coronoid process, flush with edge of coronoid
    - Uniformly low signal intensity
- Usually separated from overlying common flexor tendon by deep fascial fat
- Improved visualization with oblique coronal plane
- May require MR-arthrography to visualize partial tear of deep distal aspect (T sign)

Annular Ligament
- Best visualized on axial images at level of radial head

SELECTED REFERENCES

1. Husarik DB et al: Ligaments and plicae of the elbow: normal MR imaging variability in 60 asymptomatic subjects. Radiology. 257(1):185-94, 2010

Elbow Ligaments

GRAPHICS, RADIAL COLLATERAL LIGAMENT COMPLEX

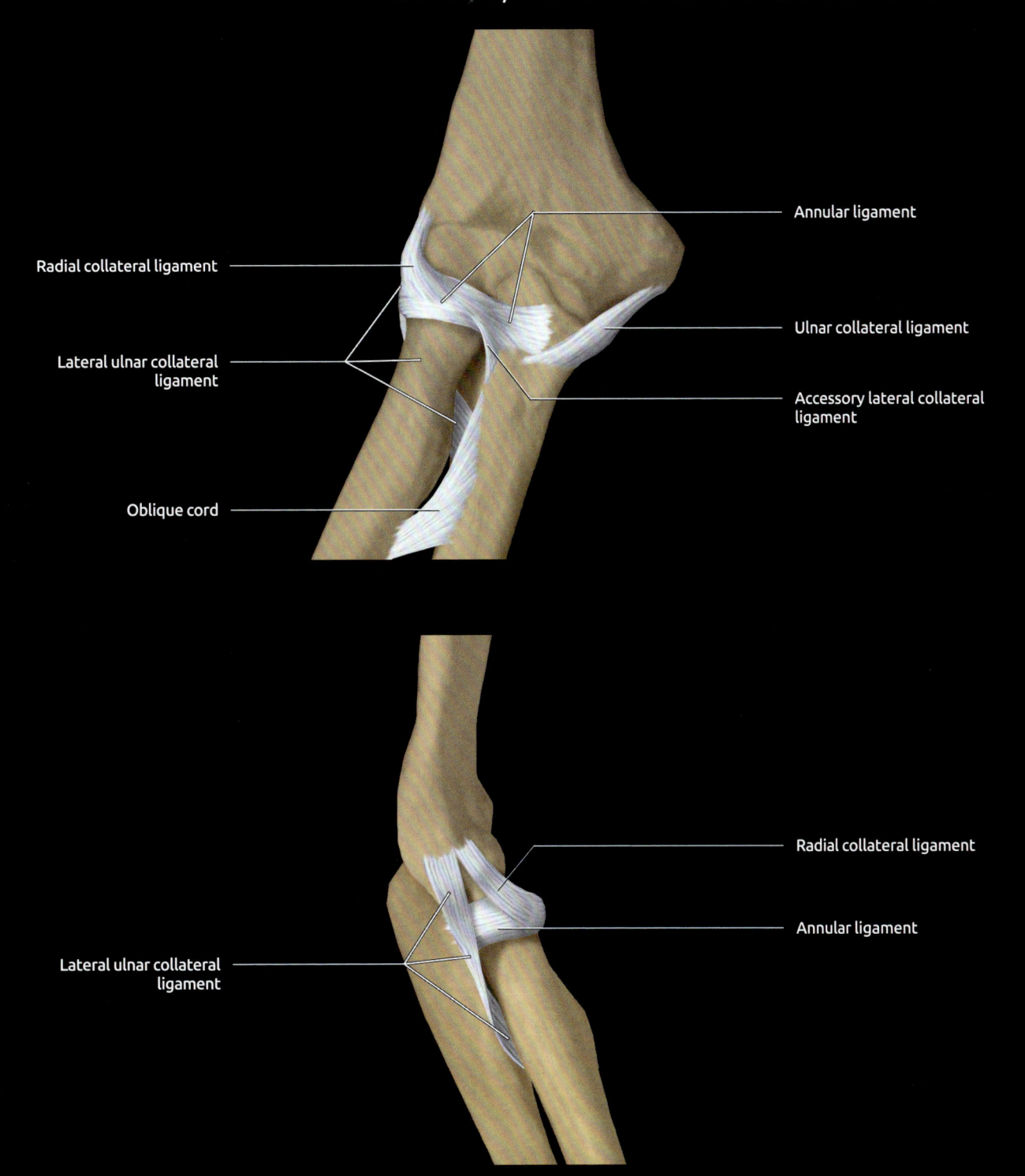

(Top) *Anterior view of the elbow shows the radial collateral ligament complex, which is composed of the radial collateral ligament (provides varus stability), the lateral ulnar collateral ligament (provides posterolateral stability), the annular ligament (holds the radial head against the radial notch of the ulna), and the accessory lateral collateral ligament (reinforces the annular ligament). The oblique cord is part of the proximal radioulnar joint.* **(Bottom)** *Lateral view shows the posterior course of the lateral ulnar collateral ligament. It blends with the annular ligament as it passes behind the radial head.*

Elbow Ligaments

GRAPHICS, ELBOW COLLATERAL LIGAMENTS

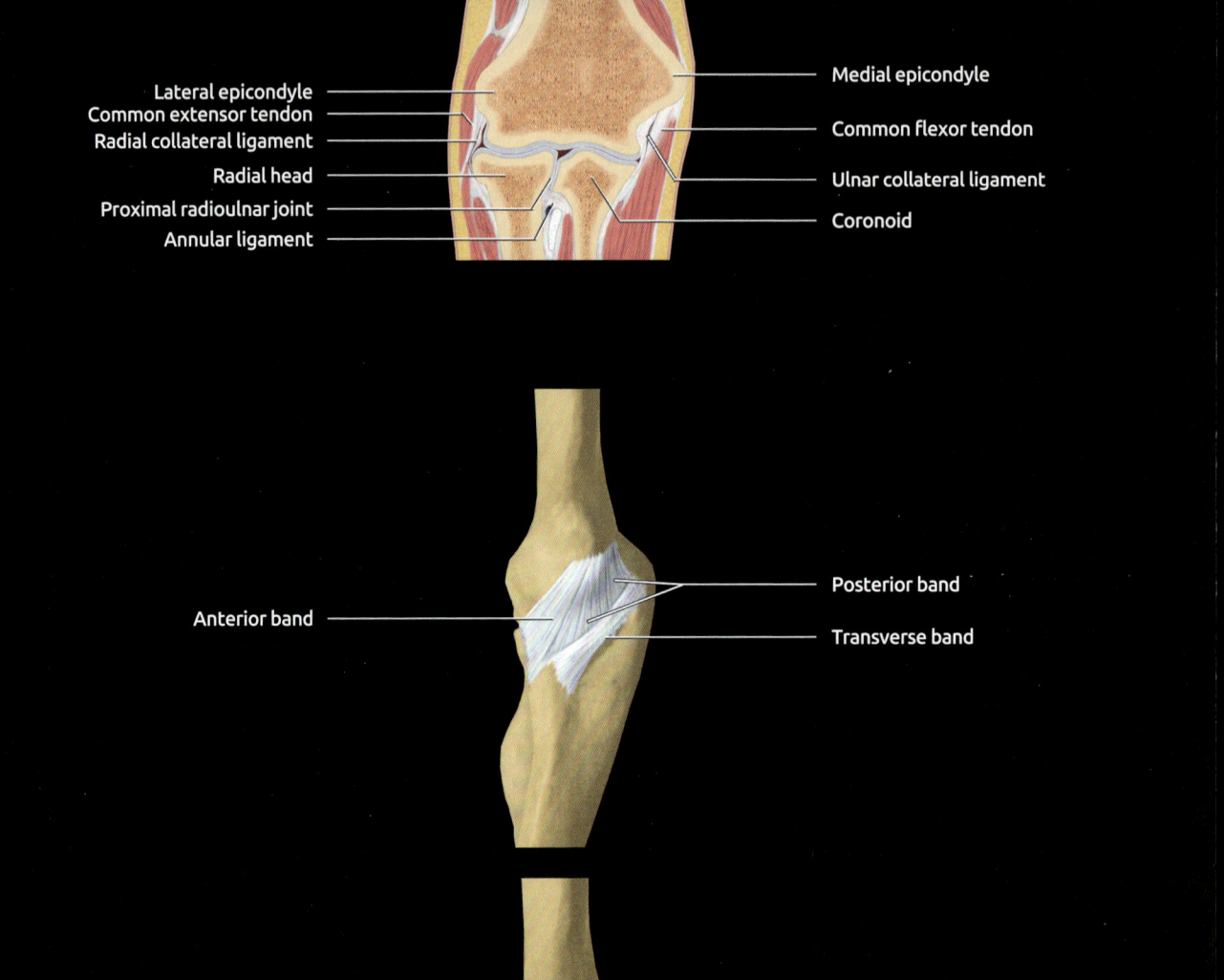

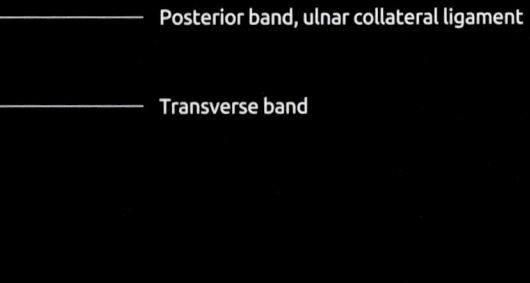

(Top) Coronal section through the level of the epicondyles shows the collateral ligaments deep to the common tendon groups. Although the radial collateral ligament is shown, the section is too anterior to show the ulnar lateral collateral ligament, which originates just posterior to the radial collateral. *(Middle)* Side view of the medial aspect of the elbow shows the 3 components of the ulnar collateral ligament: Anterior band, posterior band, and transverse band. *(Bottom)* The common flexor tendon overlies the anterior band of the ulnar collateral ligament.

Elbow Ligaments

RADIAL COLLATERAL LIGAMENT COMPLEX

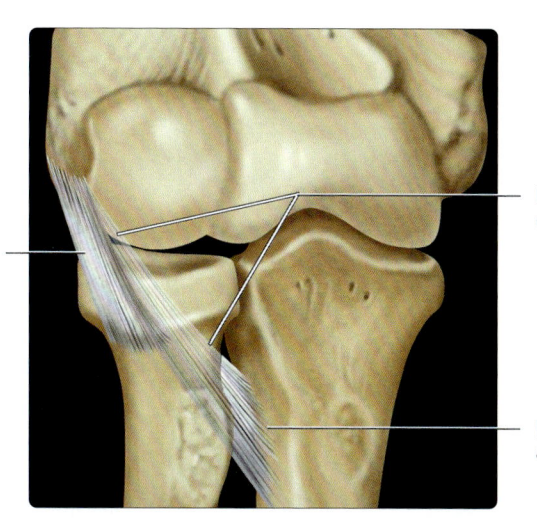

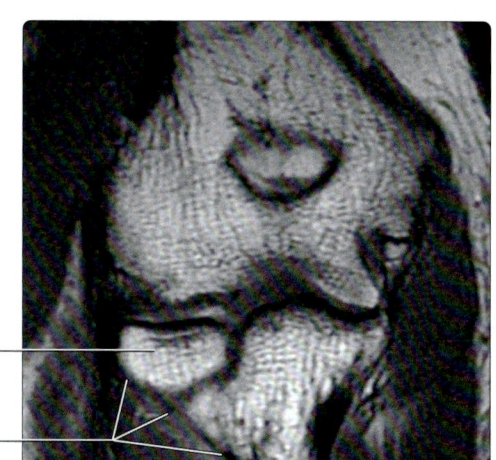

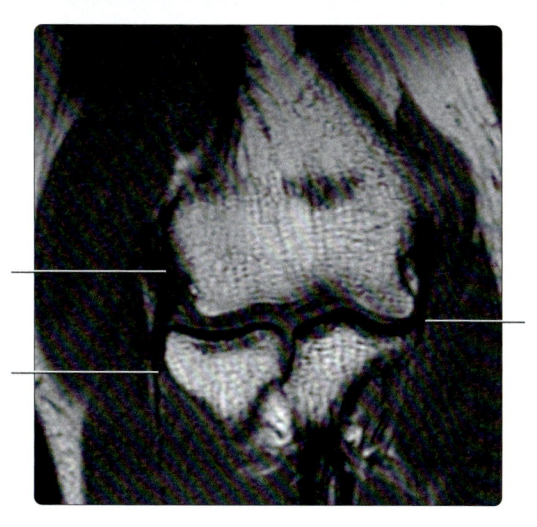

Radial collateral ligament

Lateral (radial) ulnar collateral ligament extending posterior to radial head & neck

Lateral (radial) ulnar collateral ligament at its insertion on supinator crest of ulna

Posterior (dorsal) aspect of radial head

Lateral (radial) ulnar collateral ligament

Supinator crest of ulna

Origin radial collateral ligament

Insertion radial collateral ligament

Ulnar collateral ligament at insertion on sublime tubercle

(Top) Graphic shows the radial collateral ligament extending from its origin at the lateral epicondyle to its insertion (fibers blend into annular ligament, not shown). Graphic depicts the full extent of the lateral (radial) ulnar collateral ligament, originating on the lateral epicondyle posterior to the RCL, sweeping posterior to the radial head and neck, and inserting on the lateral ulna at the supinator crest. **(Middle)** First of 2 coronal T2 MR images at mid-elbow, immediately dorsal (posterior) to the radial neck, showing the lateral (radial) ulnar collateral ligament sweeping posterior to the radial head and neck to insert on the supinator crest of the ulna. **(Bottom)** Second T2 MR image, immediately anterior (volar) to the previous image, shows the radial collateral ligament origin and insertion to be more anteriorly located relatively to the lateral (radial) ulnar collateral ligament (latter ligament not seen on this image).

CORONAL MR ARTHROGRAPHY OF ELBOW LIGAMENTS

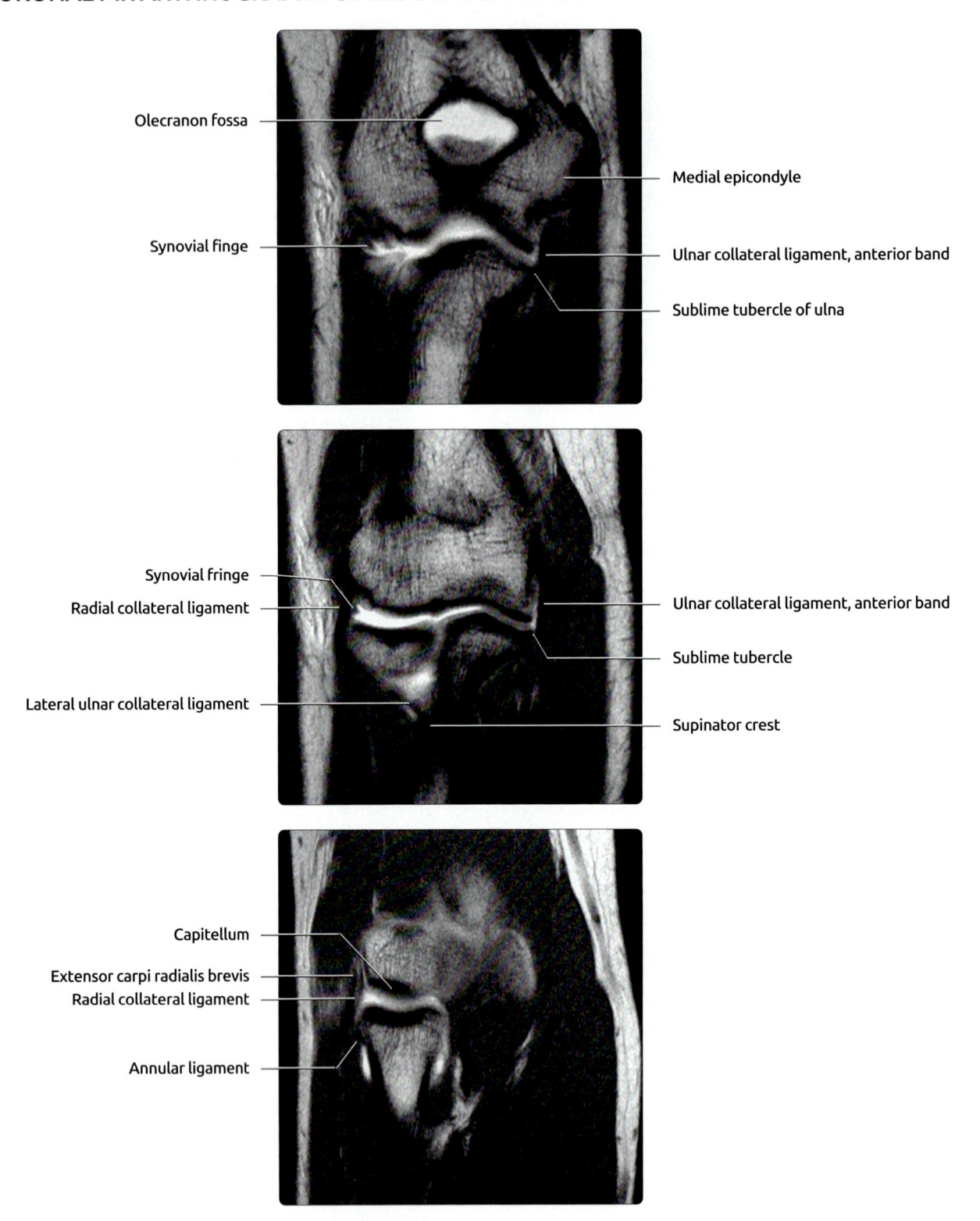

(Top) Three selected coronal MR arthrography T1 images through the right elbow show the main portions of the collateral ligaments. On this posterior image, the anterior band of the ulnar collateral ligament is seen extending from the inferior surface of the medial epicondyle to the sublime tubercle of the ulna. (Middle) Slightly more anteriorly, the lateral ulnar collateral ligament is seen inserting on the supinator crest of the ulna. It courses posterior to the radial head and neck, and provides rotational stability to the radius. Proximally, it merges with the fibers of the radial collateral ligament. (Bottom) More anteriorly, the radial collateral ligament is seen extending from the lateral condyle towards its insertion on the annular ligament. Annular ligament is not well seen on coronal images. Radial collateral ligament lies deep to the extensor carpi radialis brevis muscle.

Elbow Ligaments

AXIAL T1 MR, RIGHT ELBOW

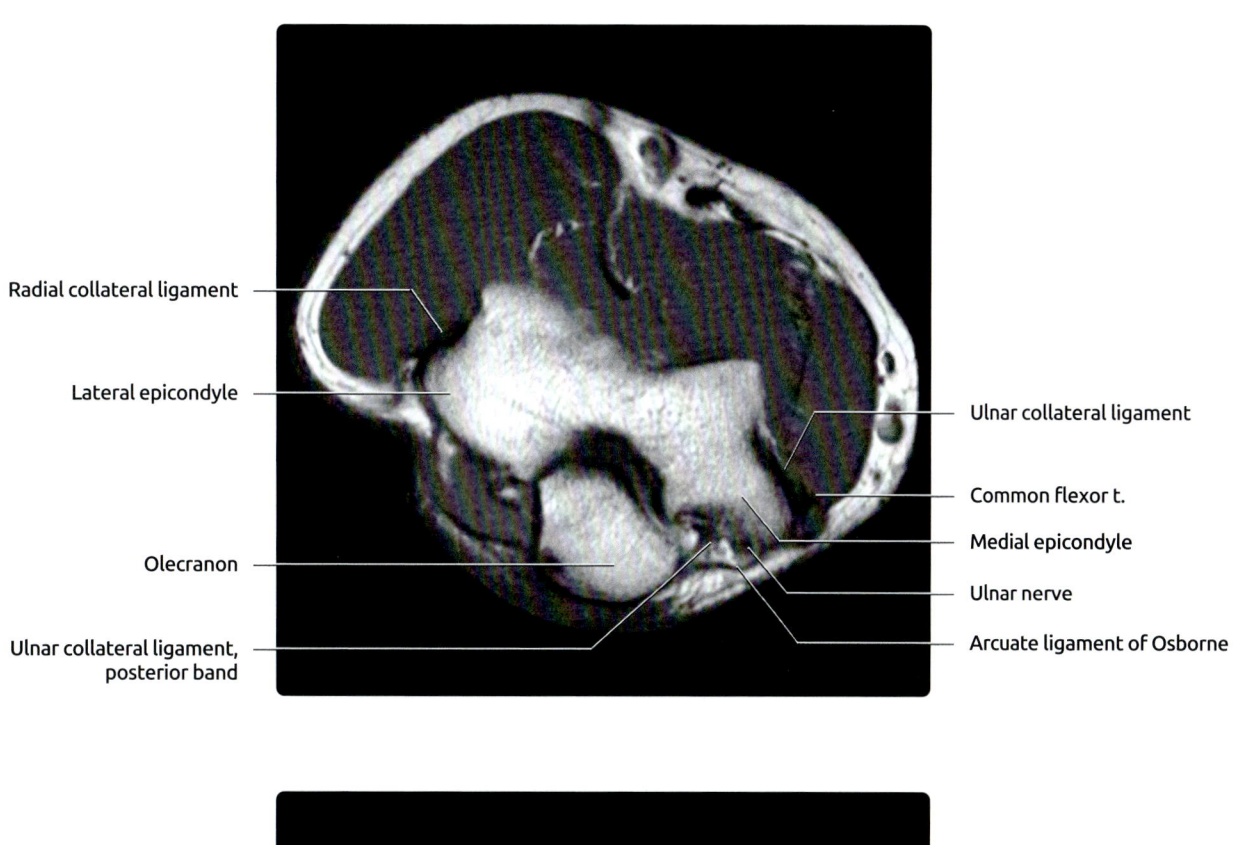

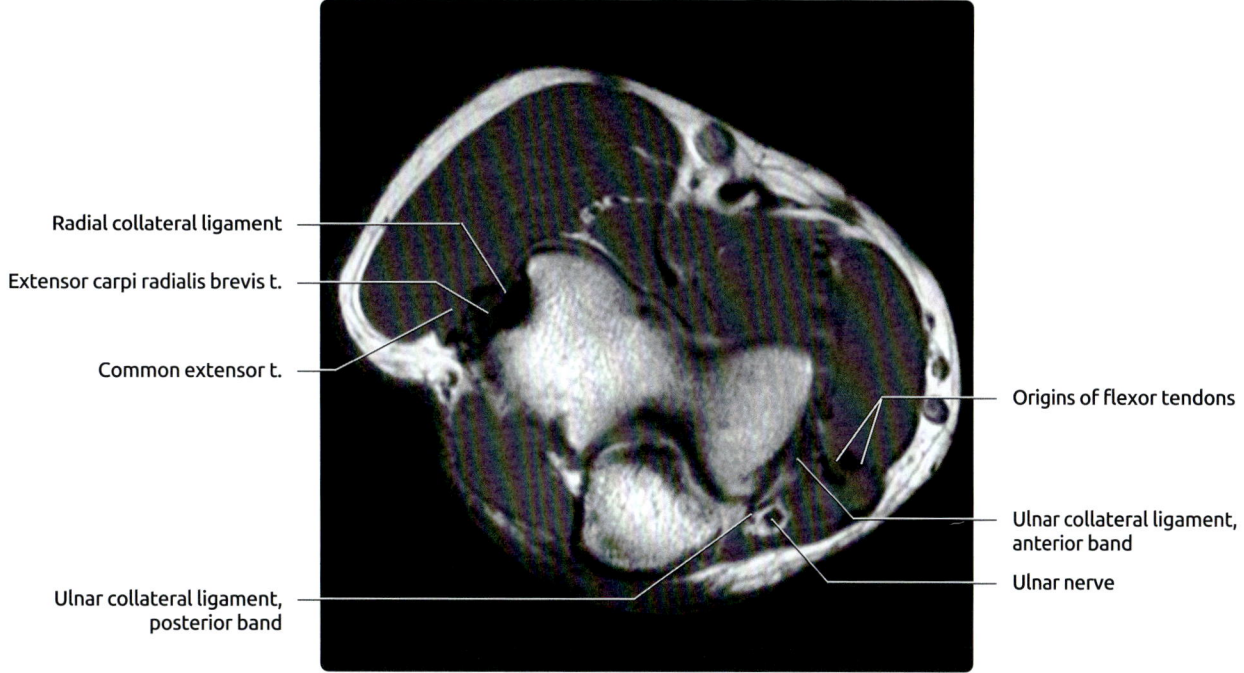

Top image labels:
- Radial collateral ligament
- Lateral epicondyle
- Olecranon
- Ulnar collateral ligament, posterior band
- Ulnar collateral ligament
- Common flexor t.
- Medial epicondyle
- Ulnar nerve
- Arcuate ligament of Osborne

Bottom image labels:
- Radial collateral ligament
- Extensor carpi radialis brevis t.
- Common extensor t.
- Ulnar collateral ligament, posterior band
- Origins of flexor tendons
- Ulnar collateral ligament, anterior band
- Ulnar nerve

(Top) This is the 1st of 6 axial images at the level of the epicondyles; the attachments of the radial and ulnar collateral ligaments are seen. The arcuate ligament of Osborne holds the ulnar nerve in the cubital tunnel. The ulnar nerve is well seen because it is surrounded by fat. **(Bottom)** Distal to their attachments to the epicondyles, the collateral ligaments and overlying common tendons are more visibly separated.

Elbow Ligaments

AXIAL T1 MR, RIGHT ELBOW

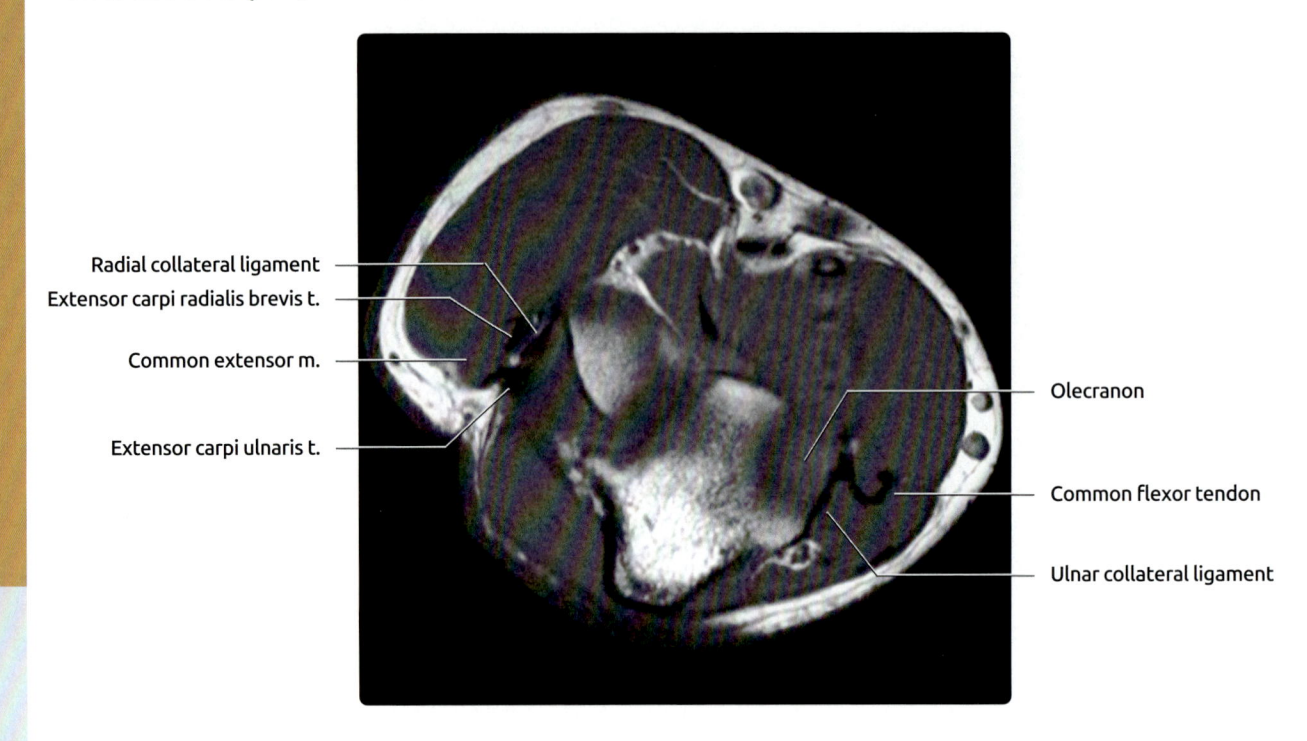

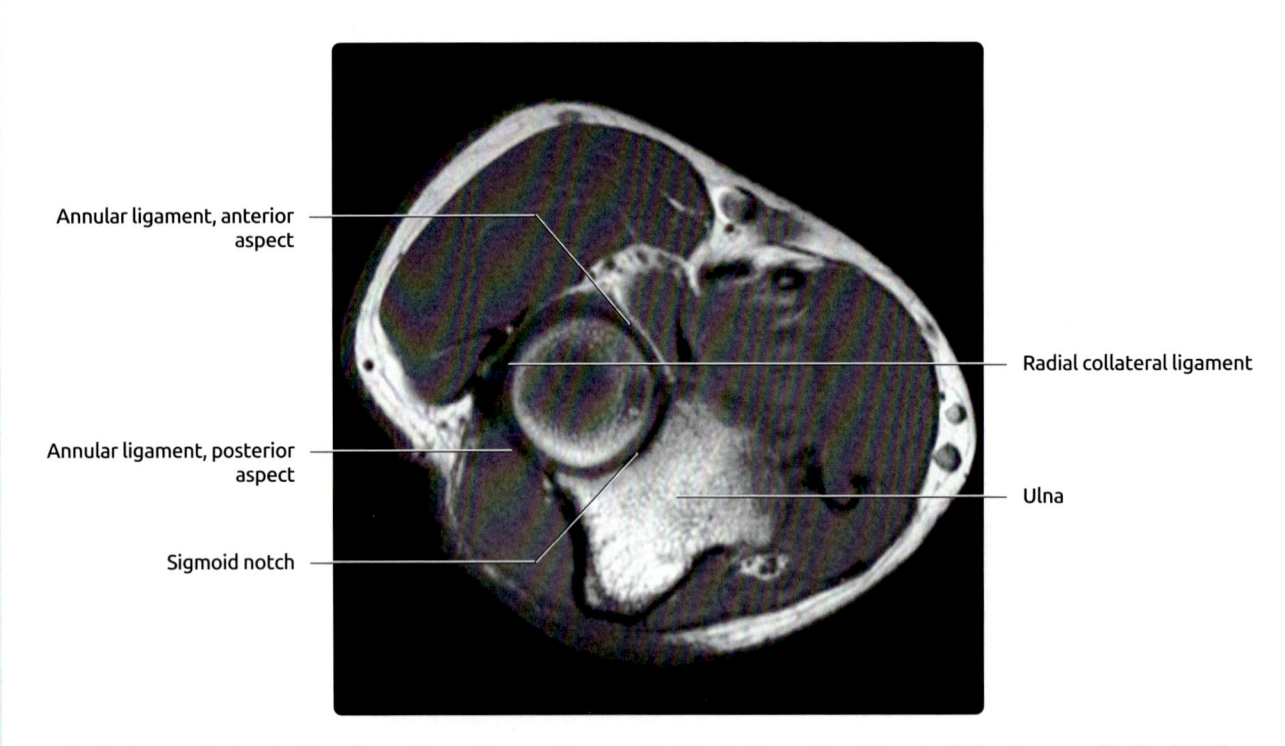

(Top) The anterior band of the ulnar collateral ligament is seen attaching to the sublime tubercle of the olecranon. *(Bottom)* At the level of the radial head, the radial collateral ligament inserts on the annular ligament.

Elbow Ligaments

AXIAL T1 MR, RIGHT ELBOW

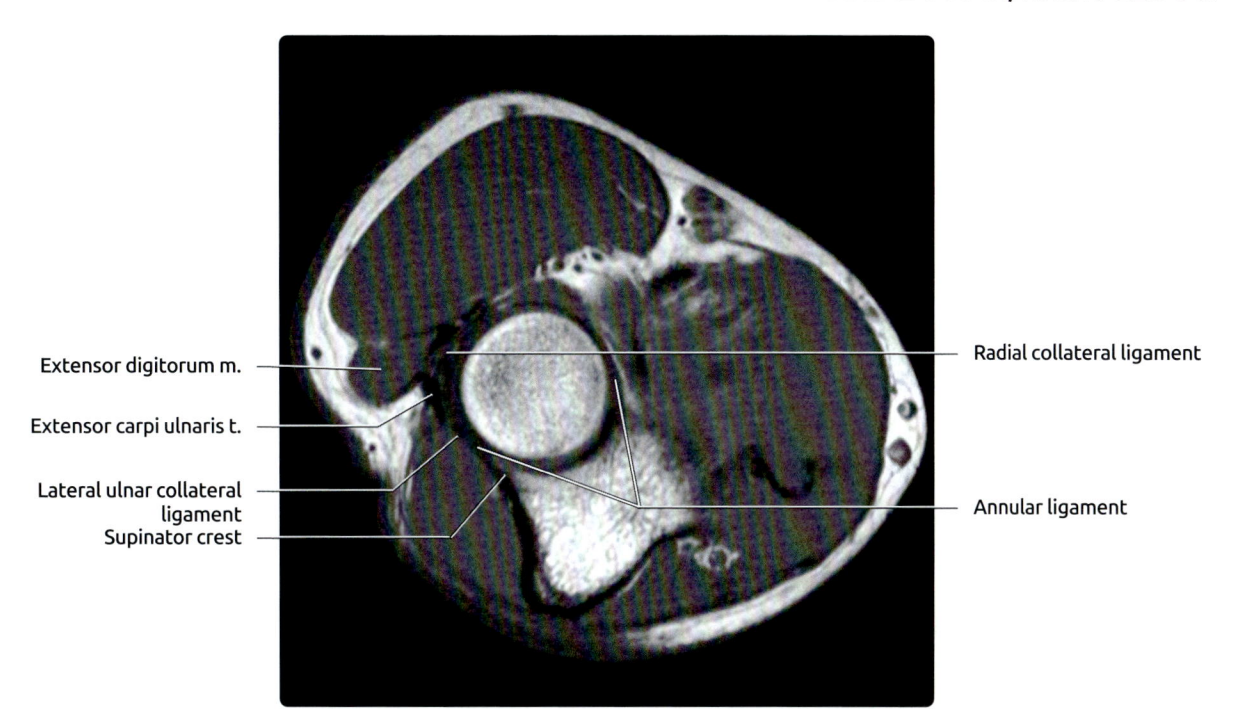

Labels (top image):
- Extensor digitorum m.
- Extensor carpi ulnaris t.
- Lateral ulnar collateral ligament
- Supinator crest
- Radial collateral ligament
- Annular ligament

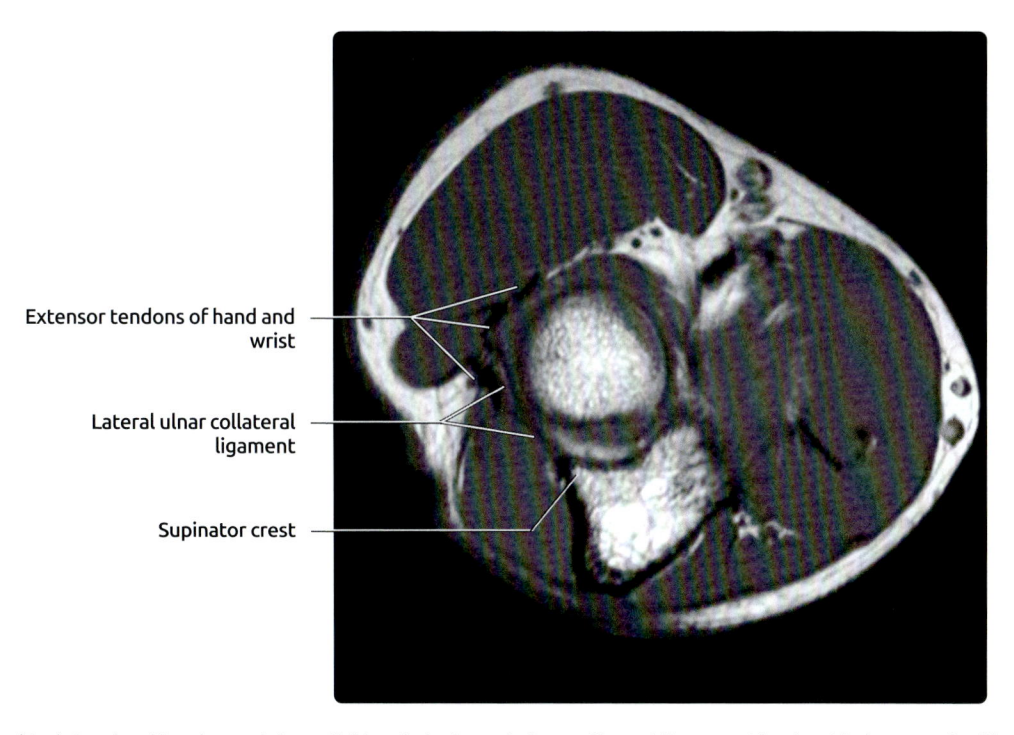

Labels (bottom image):
- Extensor tendons of hand and wrist
- Lateral ulnar collateral ligament
- Supinator crest

(Top) At a level just beyond the radial head, the lateral ulnar collateral ligament blends with the posterior fibers of the annular ligament on its way to attach to the supinator crest of the ulna. (Bottom) At the level of the radial neck, the lateral ulnar collateral ligament can be seen attaching to the supinator crest of the ulna. This is below the level of the radial collateral and annular ligaments.

Elbow Ligaments

CORONAL T1 MR, LEFT ELBOW

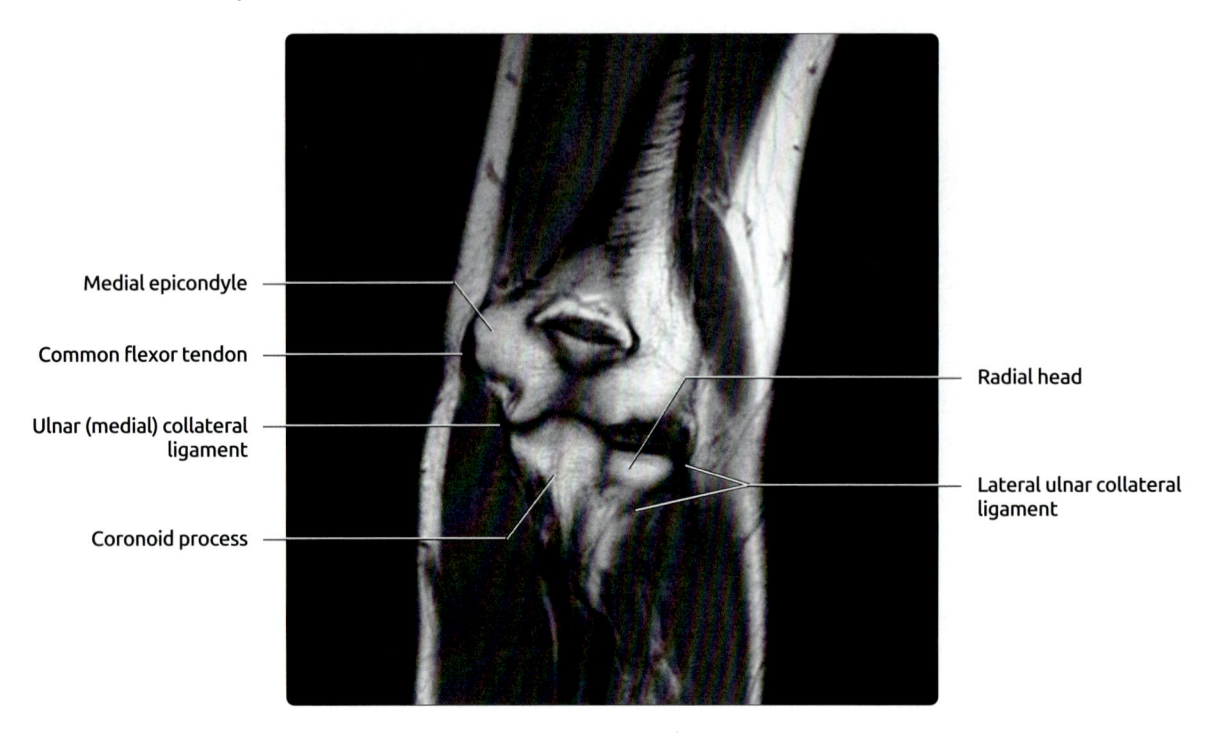

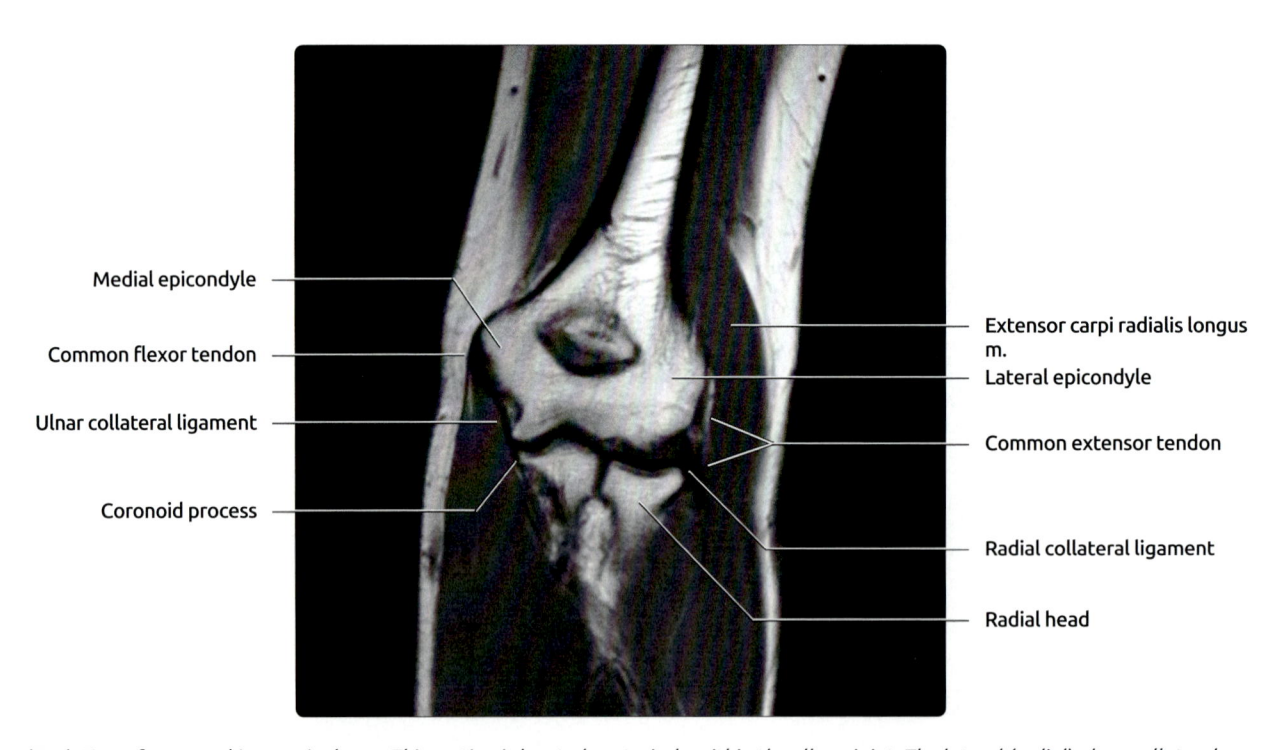

(Top) First of 4 coronal images is shown. This section is located posteriorly within the elbow joint. The lateral (radial) ulnar collateral ligament is a thin band, seen at the level of the posterior aspect of the radial head. It extends posteriorly from its origin to the origin of the radial collateral ligament, and extends posterior to the radial head & neck to insert on the supinator crest of the ulna. **(Bottom)** At a coronal image midway through the radial head (anterior to the prior image), the radial collateral ligament is seen, deep to the common extensor tendon. The ulnar collateral ligament extends from the undersurface of the medial epicondyle to the coronoid process of the ulna, also well seen at this level.

Elbow Ligaments

CORONAL T1 MR, LEFT ELBOW

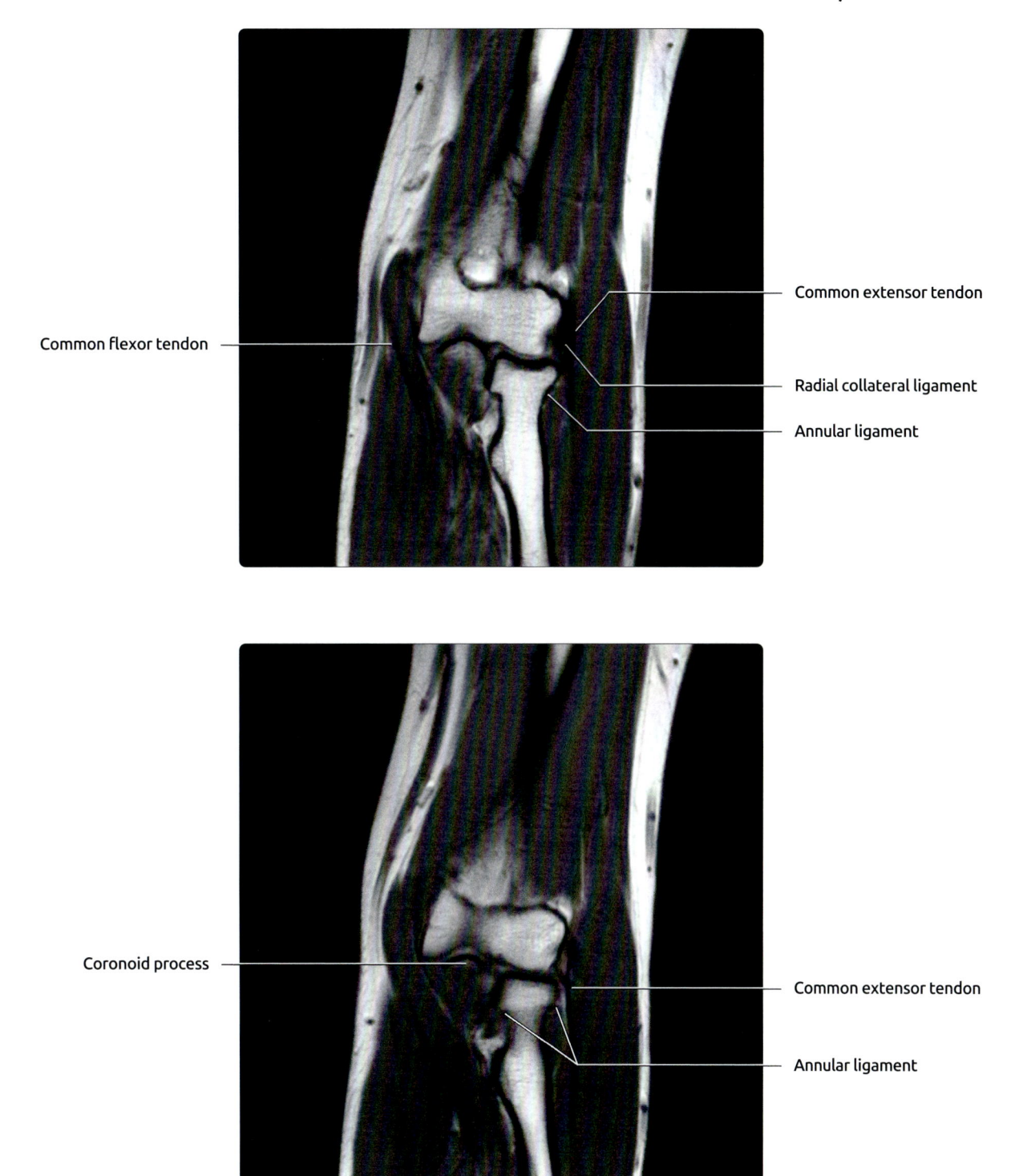

Common flexor tendon

Common extensor tendon

Radial collateral ligament

Annular ligament

Coronoid process

Common extensor tendon

Annular ligament

(Top) At a level through the extreme anterior aspect of the coronoid, the ulnar collateral ligament is no longer seen. The radial collateral ligament is seen deep to the common extensor tendon. *(Bottom)* Further anteriorly, the collateral ligaments are no longer seen.

Elbow Normal Variants and Imaging Pitfalls

IMAGING PITFALLS

Radiographs

- Metaphyseal notch
  - "Notch" at radial head metaphysis in young children
  - Fills in normally as bone matures and physis closes
- Annular ligament insertion
  - Notch at ulnar metaphysis where annular ligament inserts
  - Inconsistently seen
- Radial tuberosity lucency
  - Normal tuberosity, when seen en face, appears as oval lucency
  - Mimics osseous lesion
- Incomplete union of ossification centers
  - Mimics incomplete fracture

MR

- Pseudodefect of capitellum
  - Normal osseous groove or slight concavity between capitellum and lateral condyle
    - No articular cartilage over this 2-3 mm region
  - Reproducibly located on posterolateral aspect of capitellum
  - Mimics osteochondral fracture on coronal & sagittal images
    - However, osteochondral injury may occur at this site due to subluxation or dislocation
    - Use T2 MR to evaluate for marrow edema, differentiating injury from normal morphology
- Central pseudodefect of articular cartilage in olecranon
  - Olecranon process has normal bowl-shaped defect in articular cartilage midway between coronoid process and tip of olecranon process
  - Mimics osteochondral injury, but no marrow edema to support such a diagnosis
- Pseudodefect of trochlear groove
  - Normal notch on both medial & lateral sides of trochlear notch of ulna, at junction of olecranon and coronoid
  - Mimics fracture on sagittal images through medial or lateral side of ulna
  - Not present on midline sagittal images and no marrow edema, differentiating normal morphology from fracture
- Transverse trochlear ridge
  - Normal bony ridge running transversely across trochlear notch of ulna, at junction of olecranon and coronoid
  - May be incomplete
  - Has no overlying articular cartilage
  - Mimics intraarticular osteophyte or post-traumatic deformity on sagittal images

NORMAL VARIANTS

Osseous

- Avian (supracondylar) spur
  - Bony spur about 5 cm proximal to medial epicondyle, seen on lateral view
  - 1-3% of population
  - Usually asymptomatic
- Irregular ossification of trochlear epiphysis
  - Trochlear epiphysis may normally appear fragmented early in its ossification, mimicking osteonecrosis or osteochondral fracture
  - Ossification proceeds normally with skeletal maturation, without consequence
- Irregular ossification of lateral epicondyle apophysis
  - Lateral epicondylar apophysis may normally appear fragmented early in its ossification, mimicking osteonecrosis or osteochondral fracture
  - Ossification proceeds normally with skeletal maturation, without consequence
- Irregular ossification of capitellar epiphysis
  - May appear analogous to irregular ossification in other elbow epiphyses/apophysis
  - However, has been termed "Panner disease" since it may be caused by insufficient blood supply to capitellum
  - Capitellum initially appears normal but develops fragmented appearance at ~ ages 5-12 years
  - Overlying cartilage usually intact
  - Usually resolves over time with rest
- Os supratrochlear
  - Accessory ossicle in olecranon fossa
  - May mimic loose body
- Patella cubiti
  - Sesamoid in distal triceps muscle
  - May mimic loose body

MR

- Ligament of Struthers
  - Accessory origin of pronator teres arising from supracondylar spur
  - Extends from supracondylar (avian) spur to medial epicondyle
  - May compress median nerve & brachial artery
- Hyperplastic synovial fringe
  - Synovial fold normally seen at posterolateral aspect of radiocapitellar joint
  - Fold may become hyperplastic & unstable
    - No definite established measurement criteria for hyperplasia of synovial fringe
    - Synovial fold thickness of > 2.6 mm suggestive of hyperplasia: Seen in 67% of patients with synovial fringe syndrome in small series
  - Anecdotally related to painful snapping of elbow
- Anconeus epitrochlearis
  - Accessory muscle (do not confuse with normal anconeus)
  - Originates from olecranon, inserts on medial epicondyle
  - When present, forms roof of cubital tunnel
  - May be asymptomatic
  - May result in cubital tunnel syndrome & ulnar neuritis

SELECTED REFERENCES

1. Opanova MI et al: Supracondylar process syndrome: case report and literature review. J Hand Surg Am. 39(6):1130-5, 2014
2. Ruiz de Luzuriaga BC et al: Elbow MR imaging findings in patients with synovial fringe syndrome. Skeletal Radiol. 42(5):675-80, 2013
3. Husarik DB et al: Ligaments and plicae of the elbow: normal MR imaging variability in 60 asymptomatic subjects. Radiology. 257(1):185-94, 2010

Elbow Normal Variants and Imaging Pitfalls

METAPHYSEAL NOTCH & ANNULAR LIGAMENT NOTCH

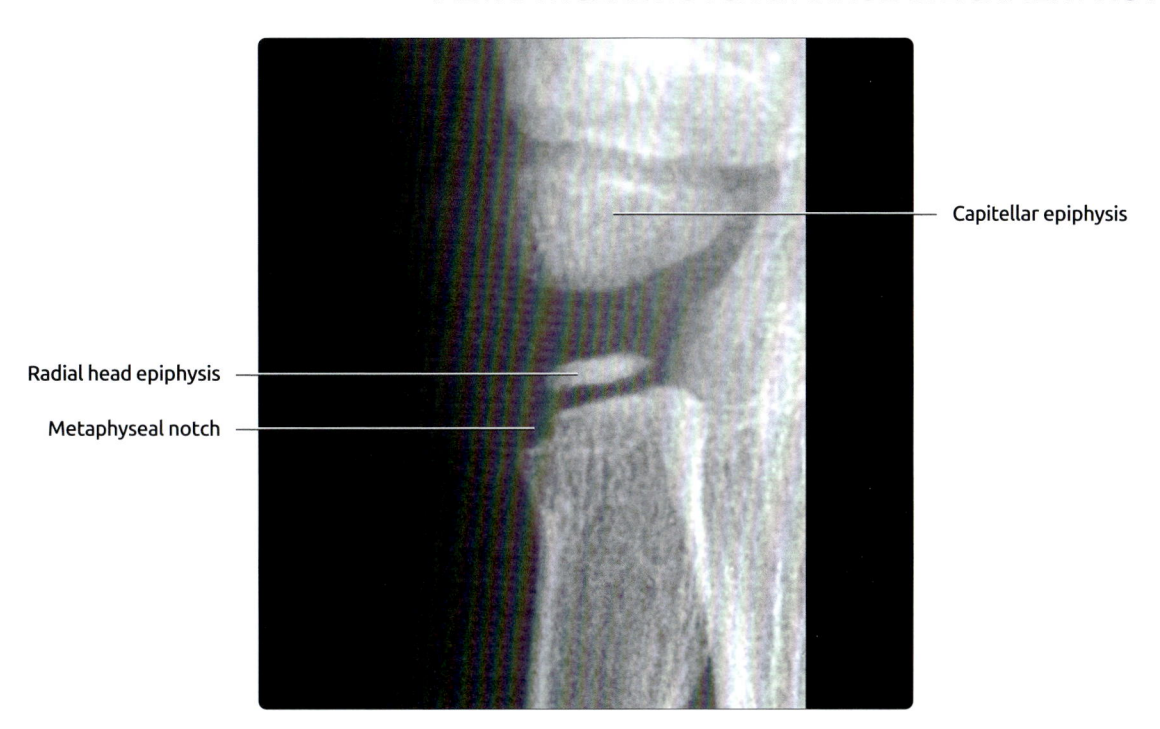

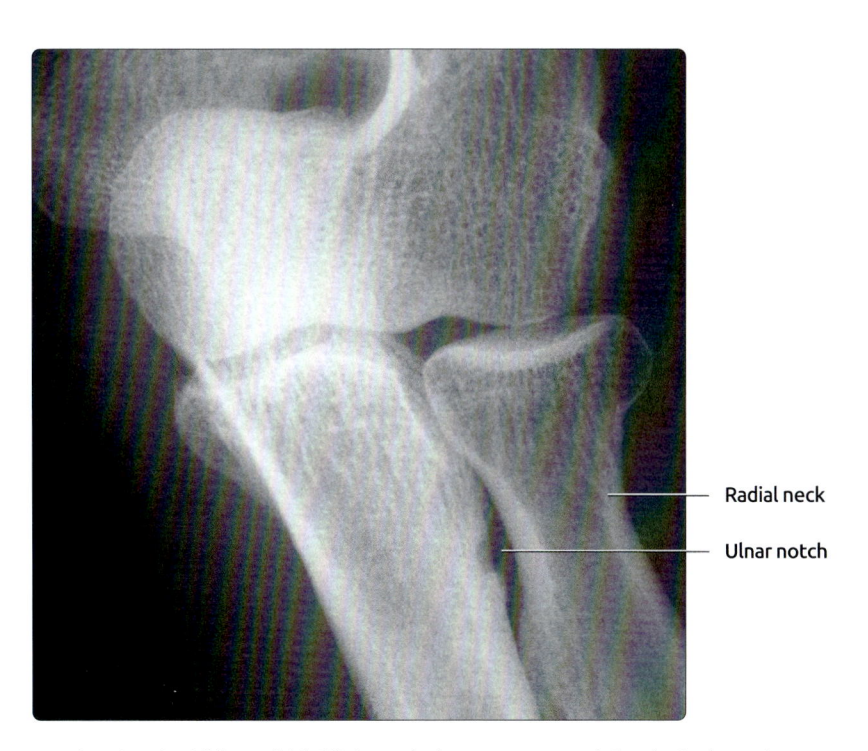

(Top) The metaphyseal notch is a normal variant in children which fills in as the bone matures and the physis closes. (Courtesy R. Shore, MD.) (Bottom) The annular ligament notch occurs as a normal variant at the site of insertion of the annular ligament on the ulnar metaphysis.

Elbow Normal Variants and Imaging Pitfalls

RADIAL TUBEROSITY LUCENCY MIMICKING LESION

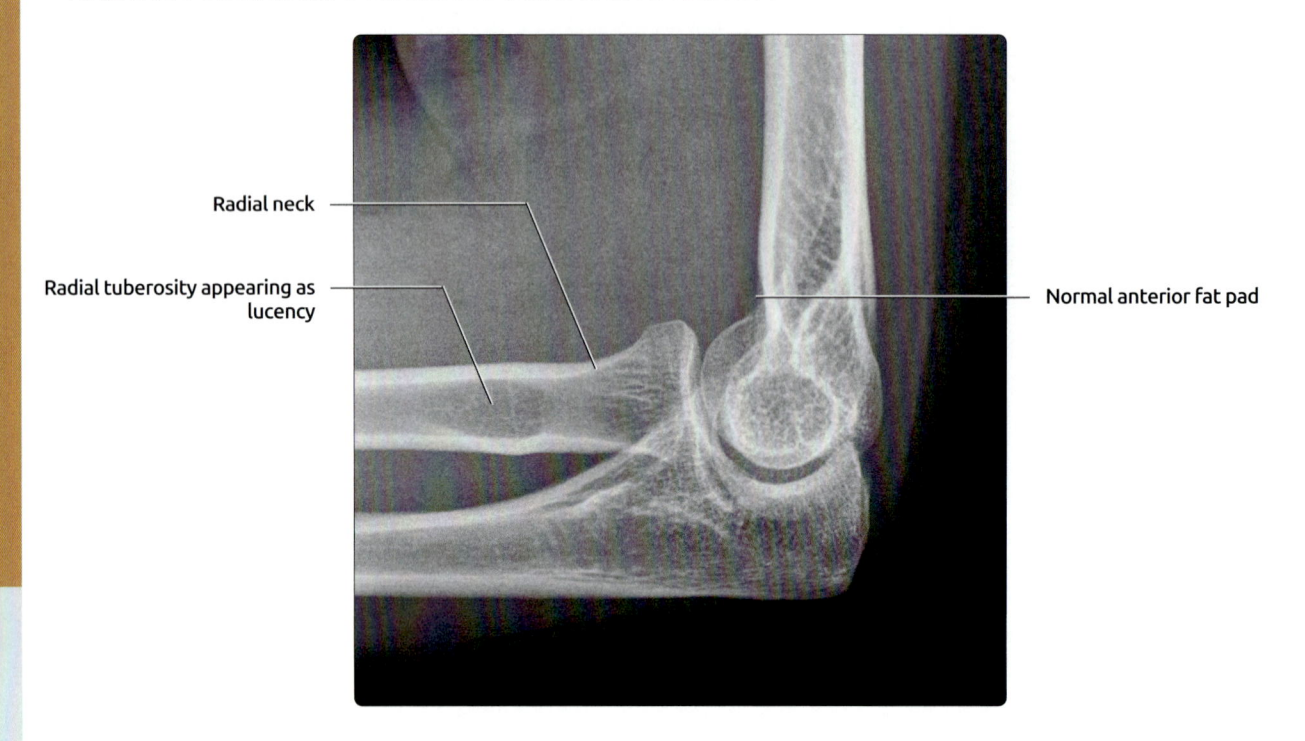

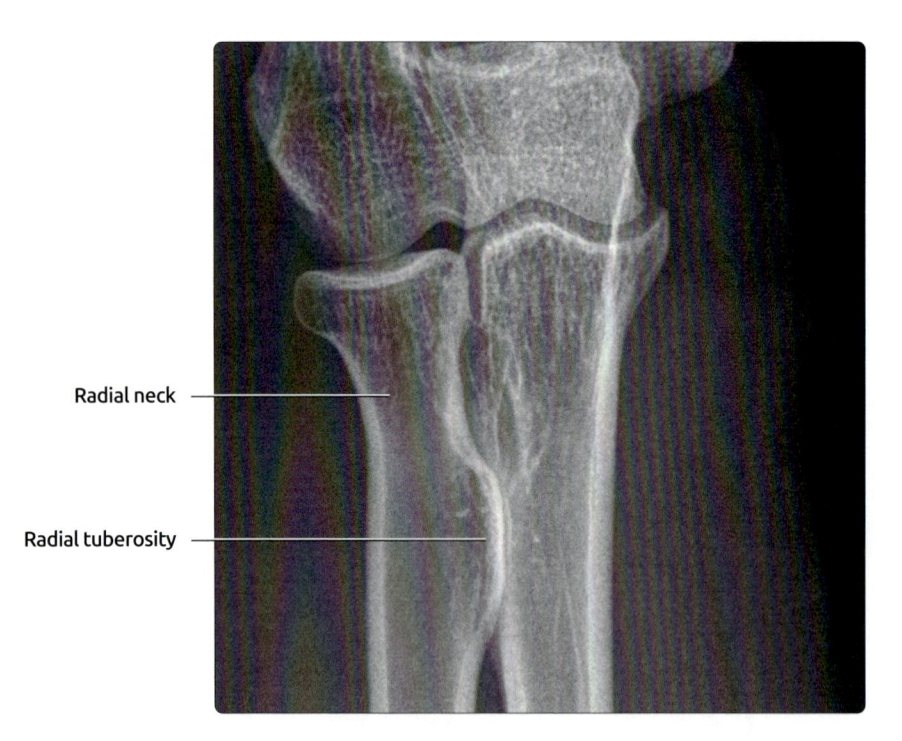

(Top) This lateral radiograph shows an oval lucency representing the radial tuberosity seen en face. *(Bottom)* AP radiograph in same patient shows the normal radial tuberosity in profile, at the same location as the "lucency" noted on the lateral image.

Elbow Normal Variants and Imaging Pitfalls

PSEUDODEFECT OF CAPITELLUM

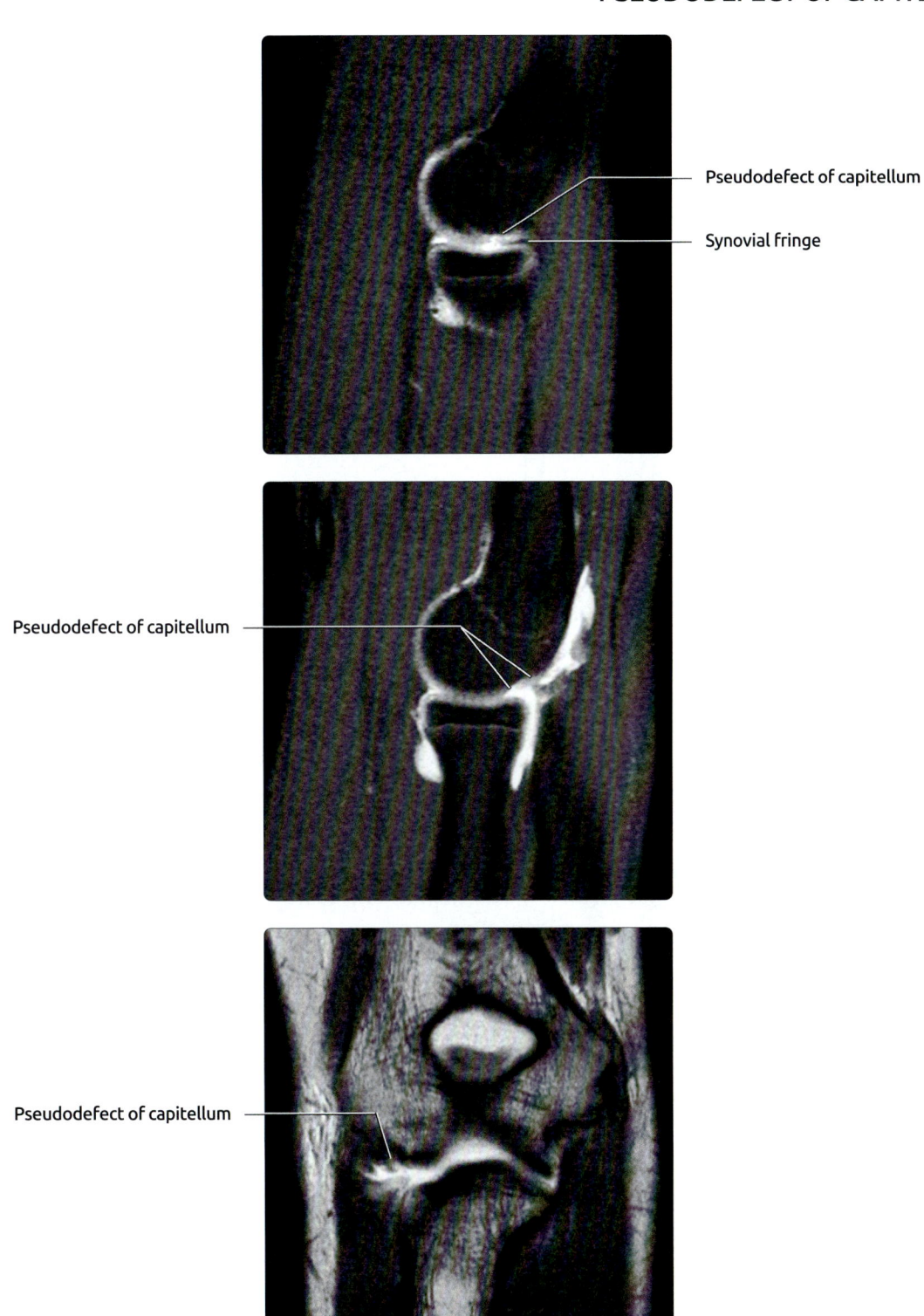

(Top) The capitellar pseudodefect is located reproducibly at the posterior aspect of the articular surface of the capitellum. This sagittal PD FS MR arthrographic image is located at the far radial side of the joint, and the capitellar pseudodefect is just coming into view. (Middle) Sagittal PD FS MR arthrographic image immediately adjacent to the prior image shows the capitellar pseudodefect more fully. There is a slight bony concavity and absence of overlying cartilage in this normal morphology. In the absence of marrow edema, it should not be mistaken for an osteochondral defect. (Bottom) Dorsal coronal image of same patient, T1 MR arthrogram, shows the capitellar pseudodefect.

PSEUDODEFECT OF CAPITELLUM

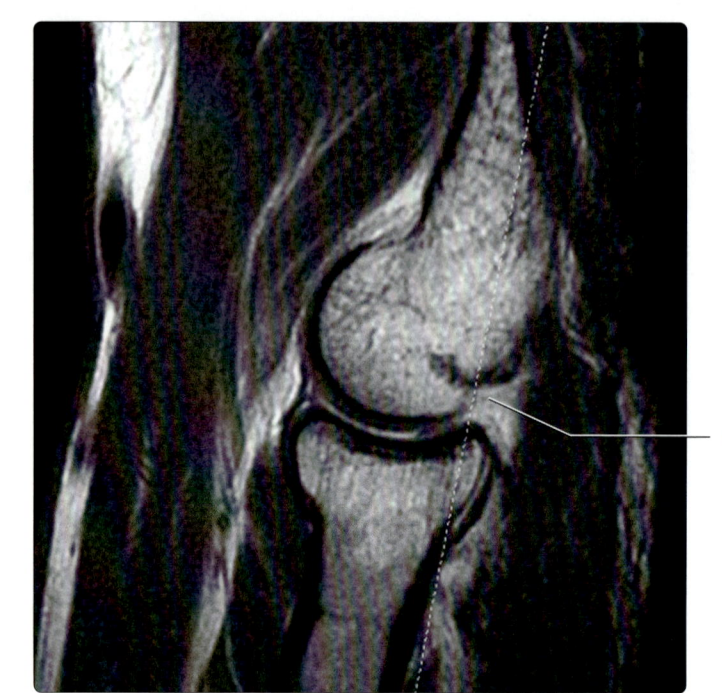

Pseudodefect of capitellum

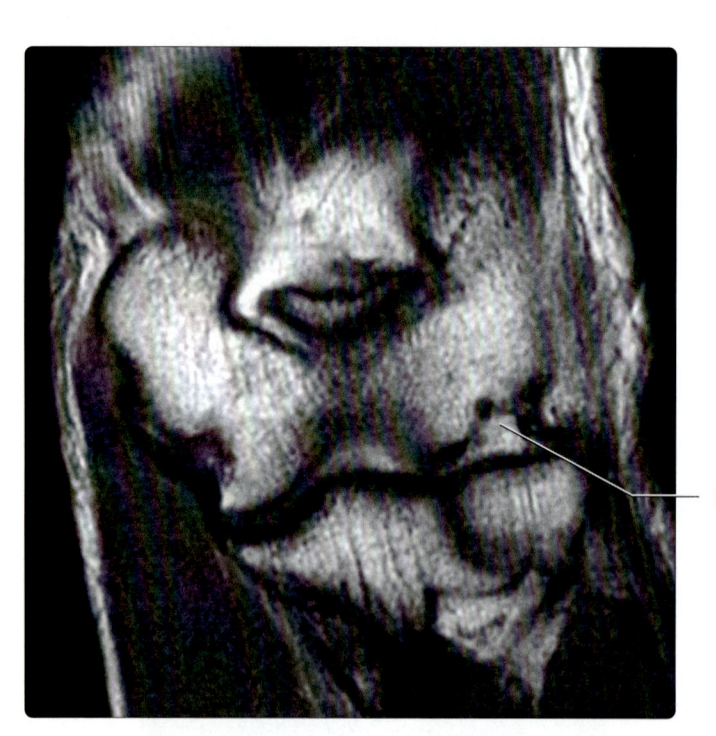

Pseudodefect of capitellum

(Top) Sagittal T2 MR shows the normal location and morphology of the pseudodefect of capitellum. The dotted line represents the plane of the oblique coronal image shown next. (Bottom) An oblique coronal T2 MR in the same patient, obtained through the plane indicated on the prior image, shows the dorsally located pseudodefect of the capitellum to good advantage.

Elbow Normal Variants and Imaging Pitfalls

OLECRANON PSEUDODEFECT AND AVIAN SPUR

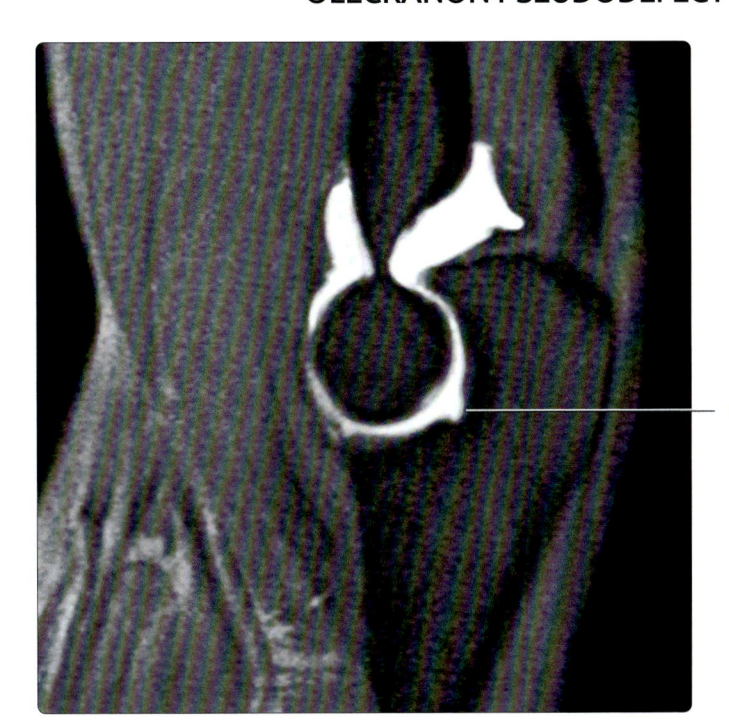

Central defect, trochlear notch

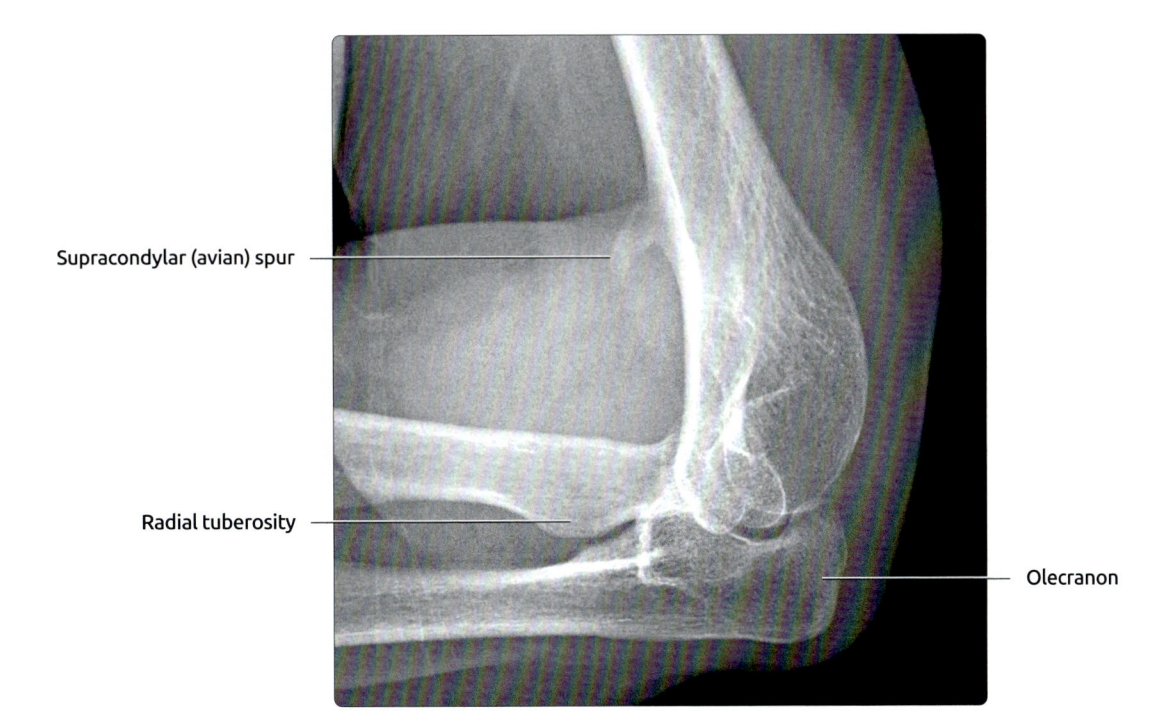

Supracondylar (avian) spur

Radial tuberosity

Olecranon

(Top) Sagittal PD FS MR arthrographic image through the center of the olecranon demonstrates the normal central defect within the trochlear notch. The osseous defect is bowl-shaped and regular, measures 2-3 mm in diameter, and has no overlying articular cartilage. It is located midway between the coronoid process and olecranon process tips. With no marrow edema and this normal morphology, it should not be mistaken for an osteochondral injury. **(Bottom)** The supracondylar (avian) spur is a normal variation that may become symptomatic if the ligament of Struthers, which connects it to the medial epicondyle, compresses the median nerve.

2 NORMAL VARIANTS: AVIAN SPUR & IRREGULAR OSSIFICATION OF TROCHLEA

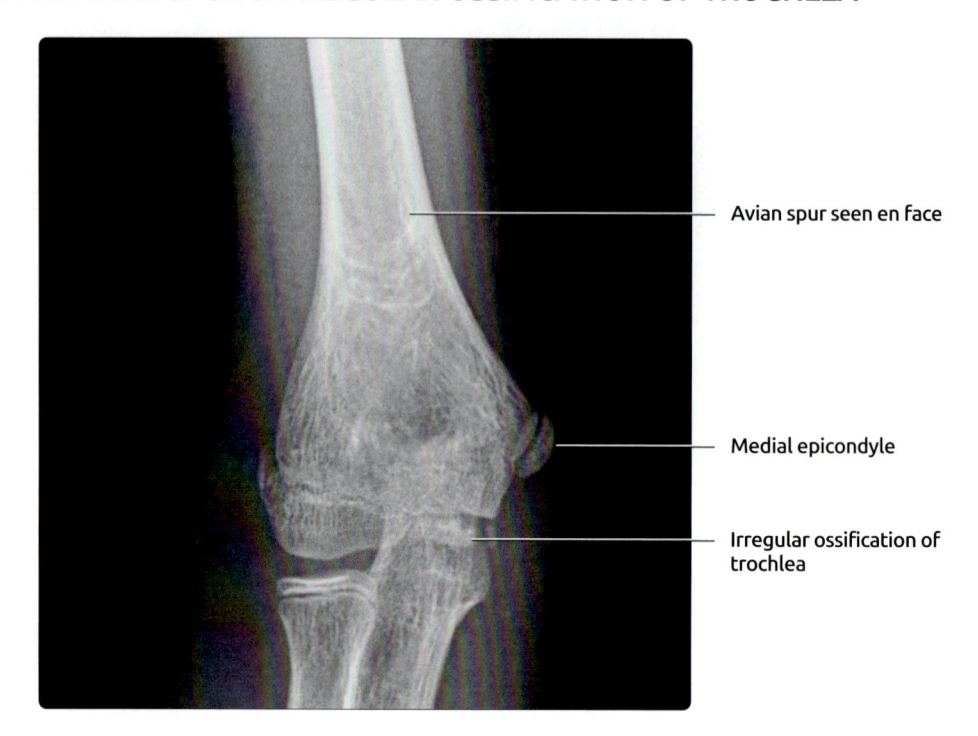

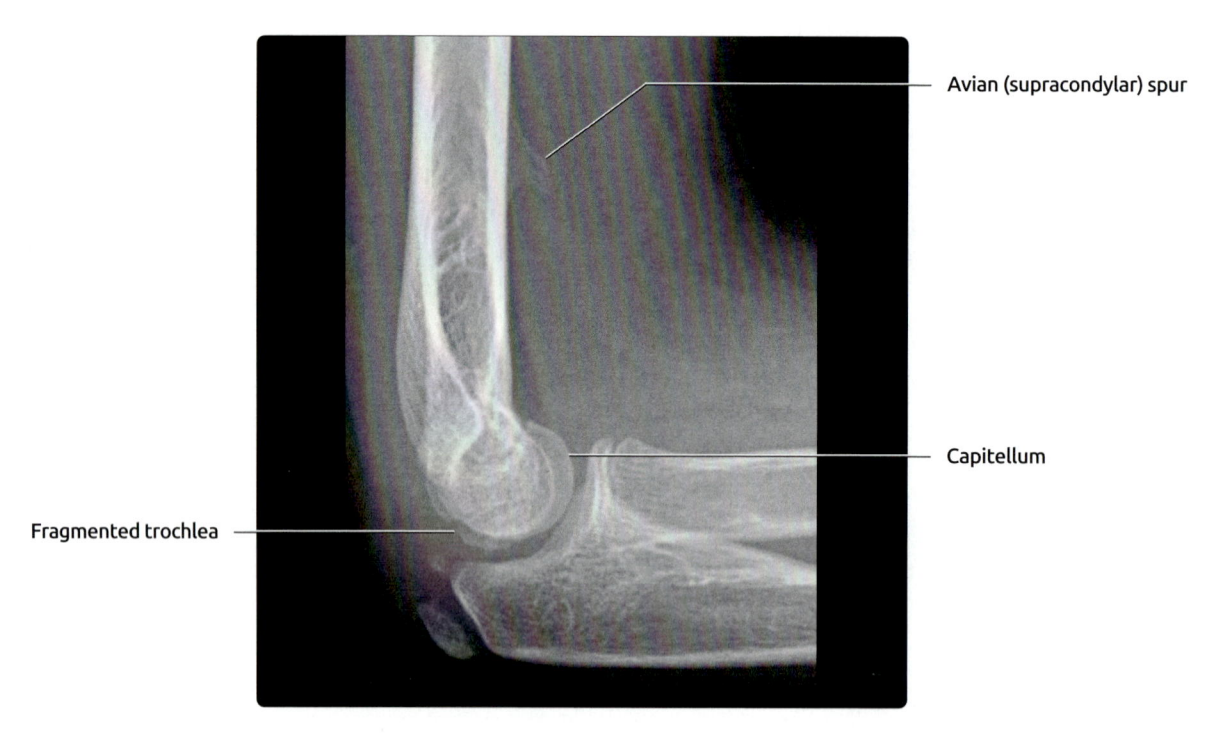

(Top) AP radiograph shows fragmentation of the trochlea, a normal variant that is expected to resolve with progressive skeletal maturation. A subtle linear sclerosis in the metadiaphysis represents the avian spur seen en face. *(Bottom)* Lateral radiograph in the same patient shows the avian spur. The fragmented trochlea is seen superimposed on the normal capitellum.

Elbow Normal Variants and Imaging Pitfalls

IRREGULAR OSSIFICATION OF TROCHLEA AND LATERAL EPICONDYLE

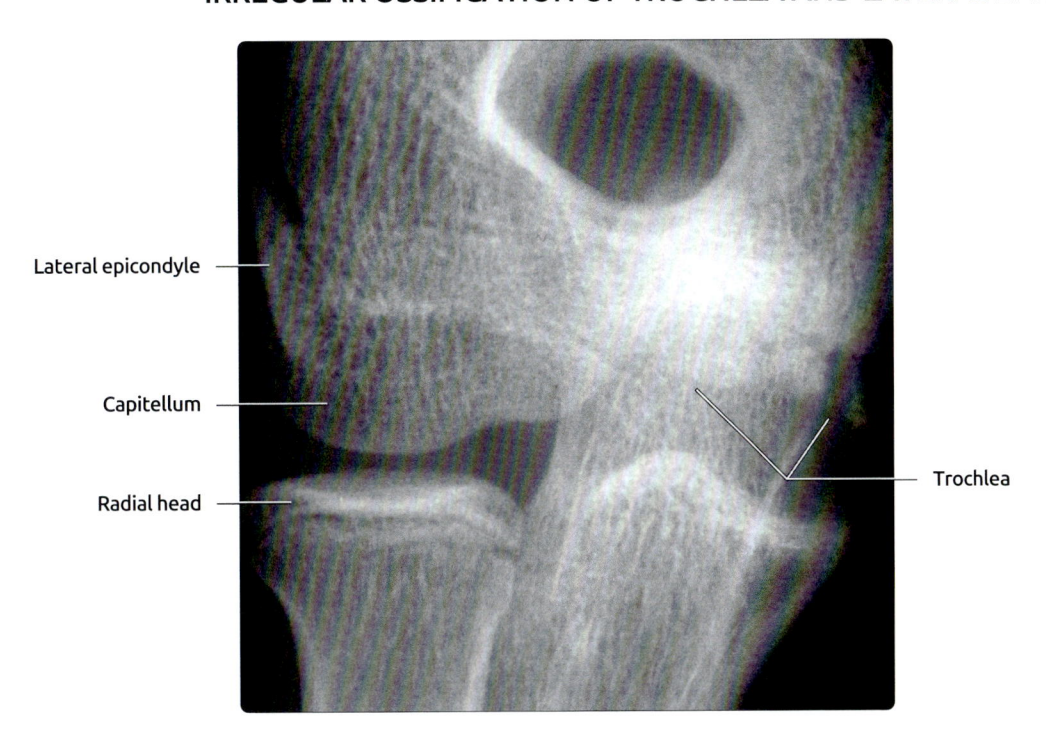

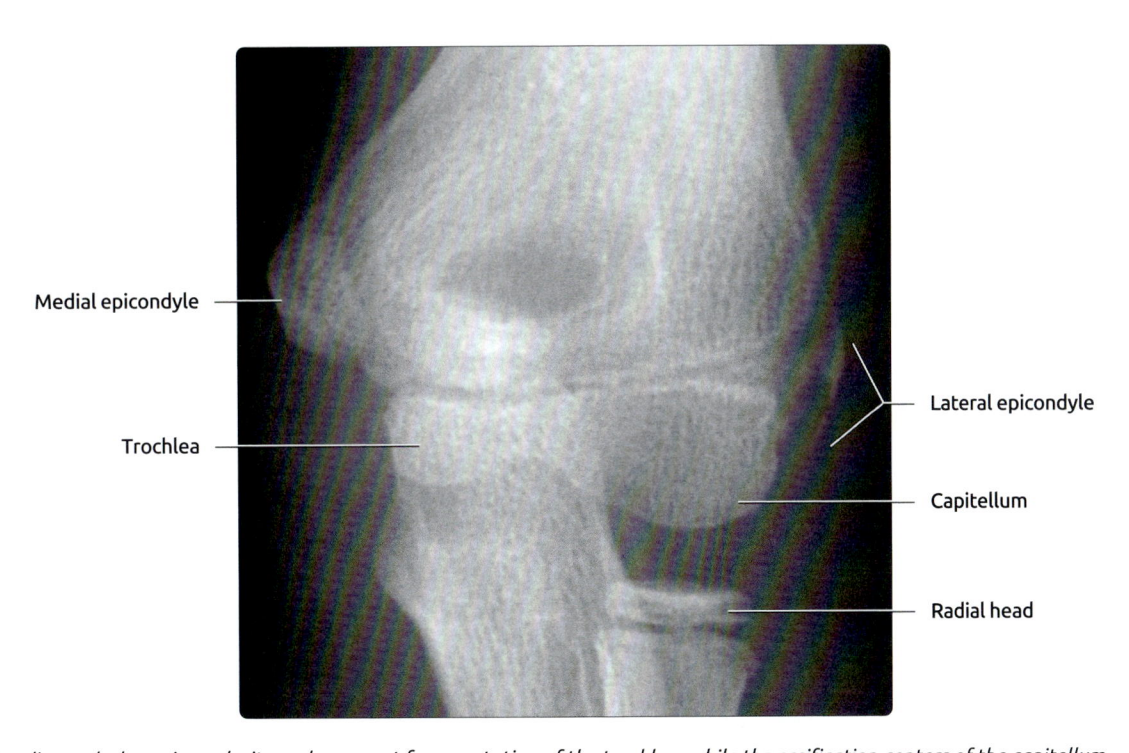

(Top) *AP radiograph shows irregularity and apparent fragmentation of the trochlea, while the ossification centers of the capitellum, radial head, and lateral epicondyle appear normal. This appearance of the trochlea, while potentially alarming, is in fact normal. Although it is not needed, MR would show the overlying cartilage to be normal. With skeletal maturation, the ossification of the trochlea proceeds normally and the mature trochlea will have a normal contour.* (Bottom) *AP radiograph shows fragmentation and apparent displacement of the lateral epicondylar apophysis. This is a normal variant; with skeletal maturation, the apophysis will demonstrate normal morphology. No treatment or change in athletic behavior is indicated for this patient.*

Elbow Normal Variants and Imaging Pitfalls

IRREGULAR OSSIFICATION CAPITELLAR EPIPHYSIS: PANNER DISEASE

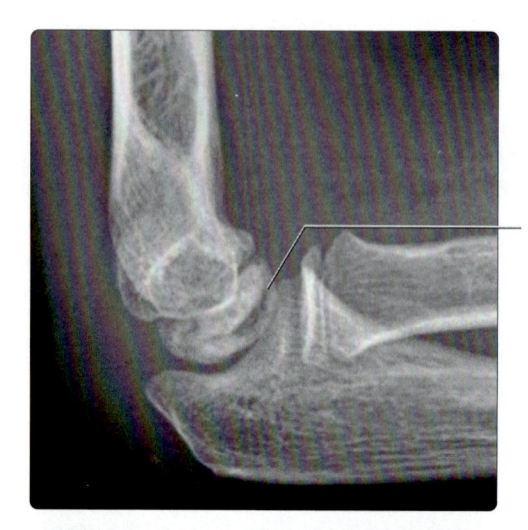

Fragmentation of capitellum

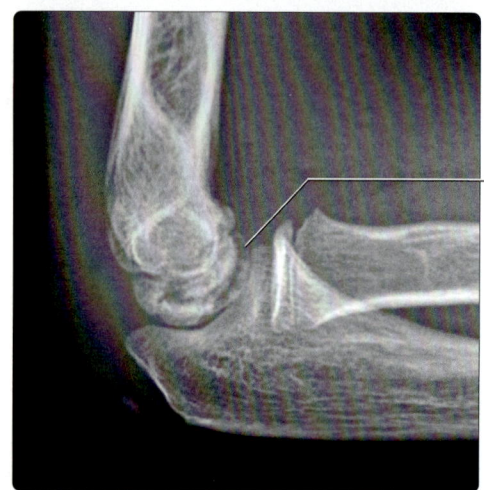

Worsening fragmentation capitellum

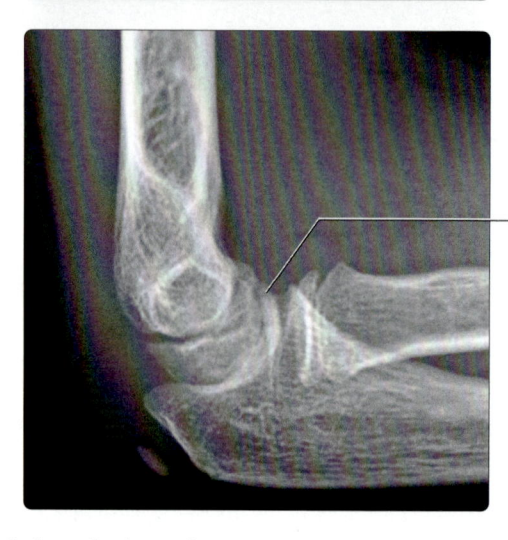

Reconstituted capitellum

(Top) This is the 1st image in a series of 3 lateral radiographs in a 9-year-old gymnast. The initial radiograph demonstrates early fragmentation of the capitellum. The remainder of the epiphyses are normal, as was the contralateral elbow. The appearance is typical of Panner disease, and the patient was treated with rest. (Middle) Second lateral radiograph, obtained 3 months later, shows worsening of the capitellar fragmentation. (Bottom) Final lateral radiograph, obtained 1 year following diagnosis, shows complete reconstitution of the capitellum. The patient was asymptomatic at this time. This is the usual natural history of this process. Although Panner disease of the capitellum has a similar appearance to the normal fragmentation of the trochlea or lateral epicondyle, it is treated with more concern; rest and physical therapy are usually offered to a patient with Panners rather than the presumption of a normal outcome as is found with trochlear and lateral epicondylar fragmentation.

Elbow Normal Variants and Imaging Pitfalls

AVIAN SPUR WITH LIGAMENT OF STRUTHERS

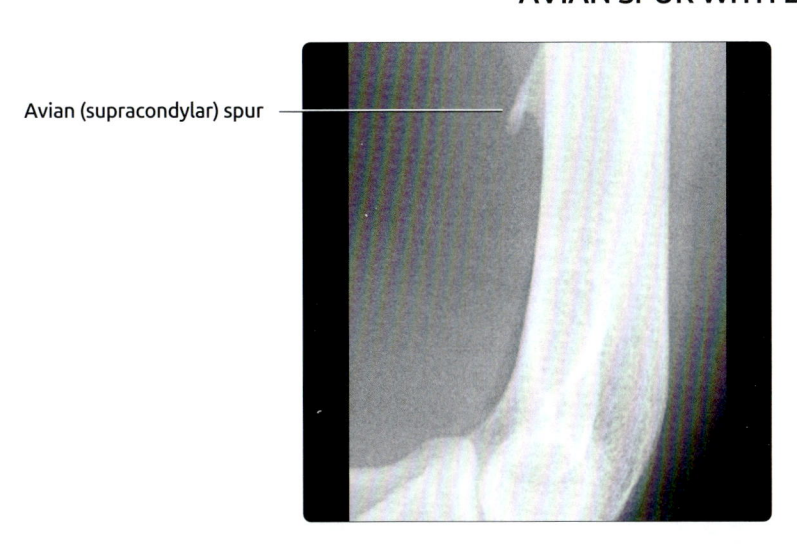

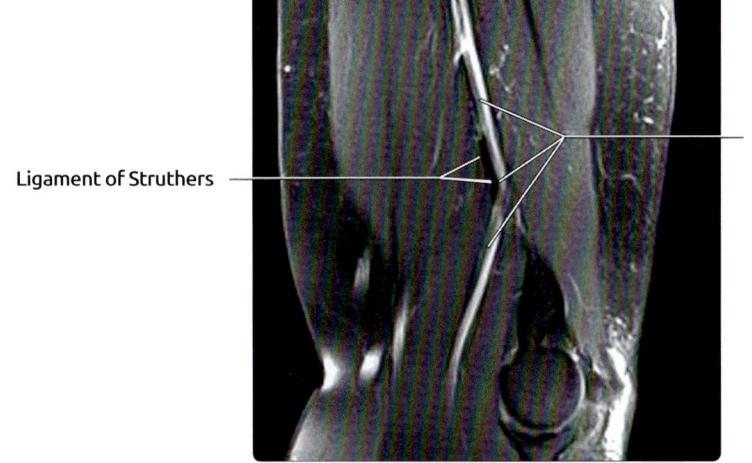

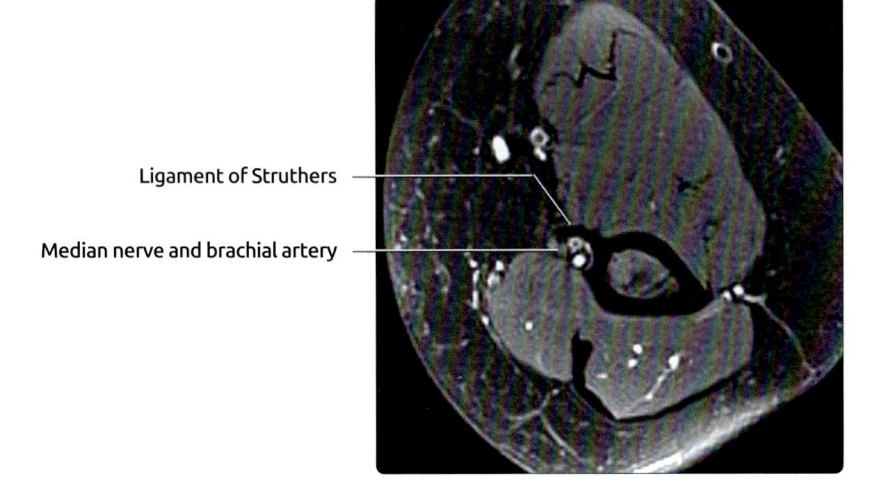

(Top) Lateral radiograph in a middle-aged woman who presents with arm/forearm pain is shown. There is a large avian (supracondylar) spur present. (Middle) Sagittal T2 FS MR in the same patient shows the thick ligament of Struthers arising from the avian spur, extending towards the medial epicondyle. The ligament tethers and compresses the median nerve and brachial artery. (Bottom) Axial PD FS MR in the same patient obtained just distal to the level of the avian spur, showing the thick ligament of Struthers compressing the neurovascular structures.

Elbow Normal Variants and Imaging Pitfalls

HYPERPLASTIC SYNOVIAL FRINGE

Capitellum

Hyperplastic synovial fringe

Radial head

Capitellum

Hyperplastic synovial fringe

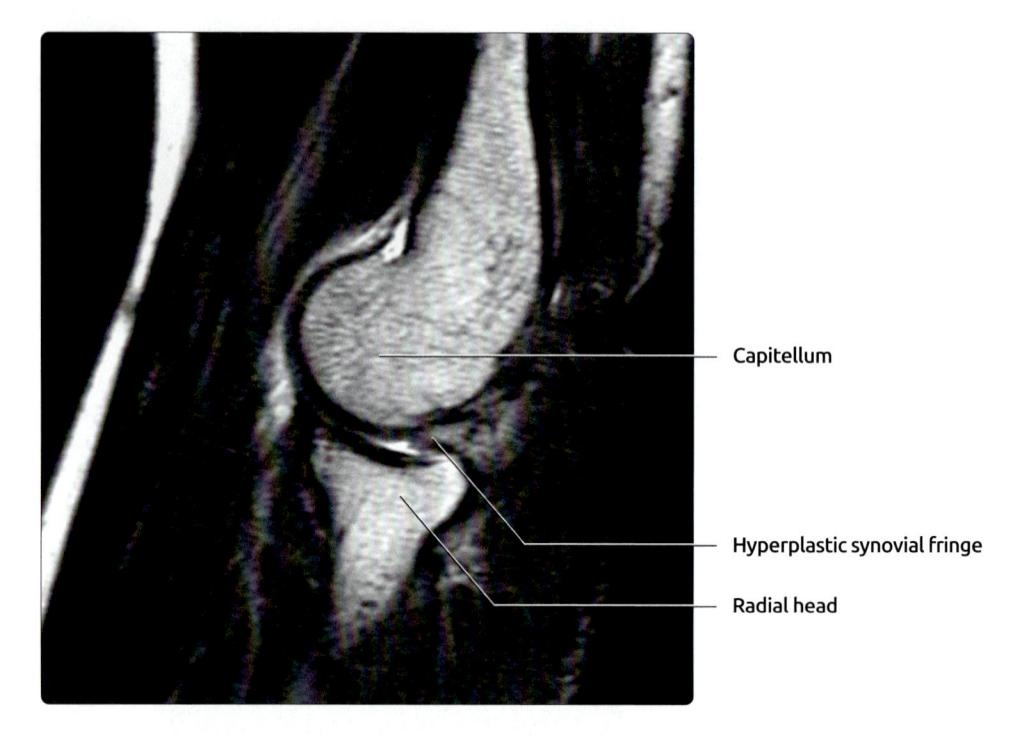

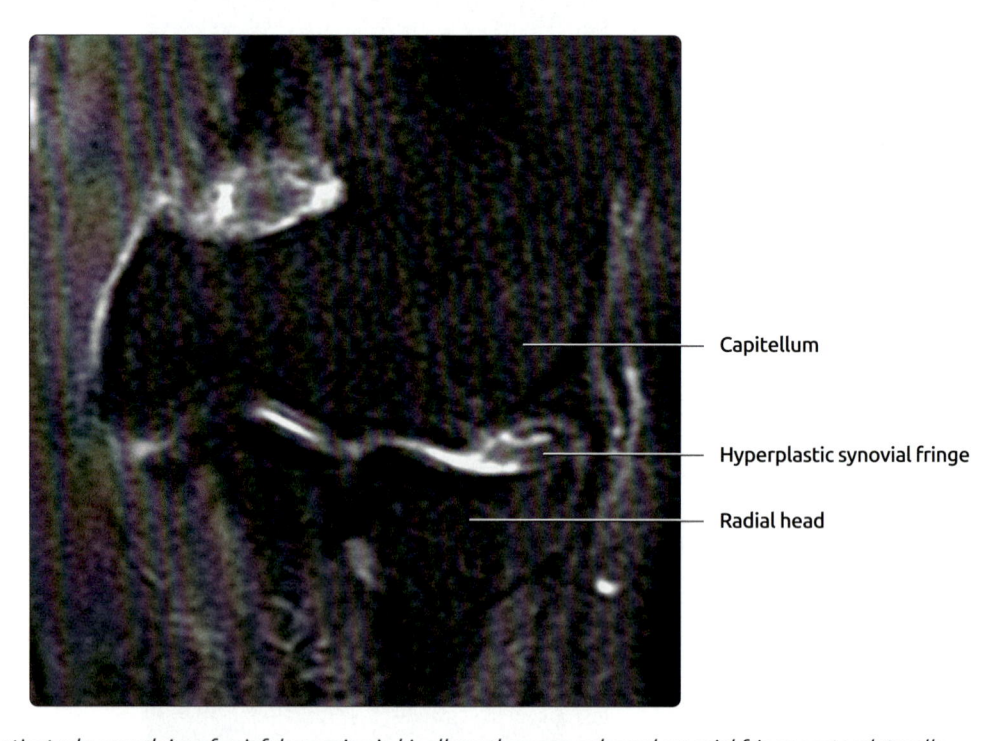

Radial head

(Top) Sagittal T2 MR in a patient who complains of painful snapping in his elbow shows an enlarged synovial fringe posterolaterally within the radiocapitellar joint space. **(Bottom)** Coronal T2 FS MR in the same patient confirms the hyperplastic tissue at the synovial fringe. Although there is no established diagnostic criterion for the "normal" size of this synovial fold, in this case it appears significantly outsized. Resection of the synovial fringe cured the patient's complaints.

Elbow Normal Variants and Imaging Pitfalls

ANCONEUS EPITROCHLEARIS

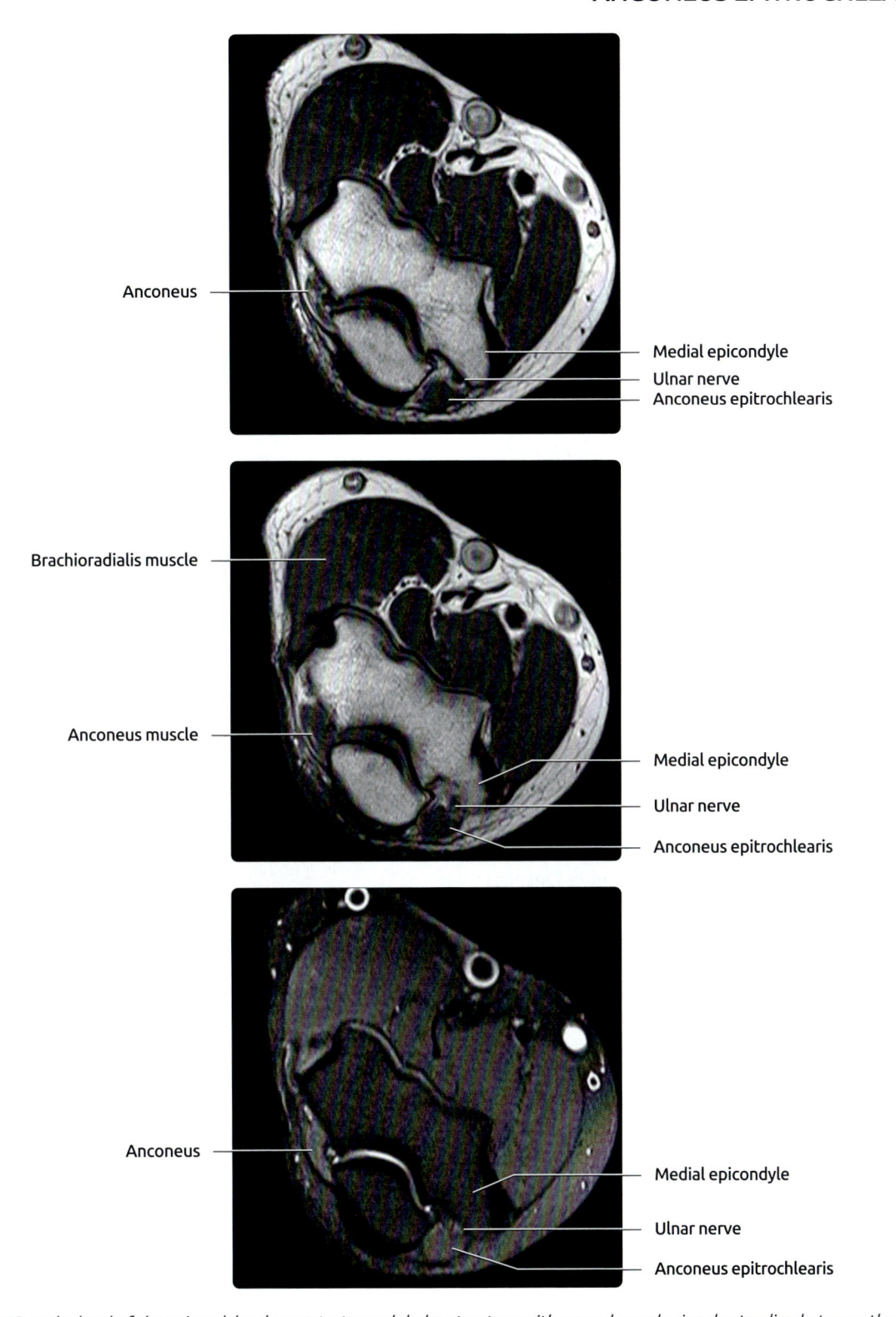

(Top) Axial T1 MR at the level of the epicondyles demonstrates a globular structure with normal muscle signal extending between the olecranon process and posterior aspect of the medial epicondyle. This is an accessory muscle, termed anconeus epitrochlearis (note the normal anconeus muscle on the lateral side of the olecranon). The ulnar nerve is potentially compressed against the posterior aspect of the medial epicondyle by the anconeus epitrochlearis. (Middle) Axial T1 MR, slightly distal to the prior image, shows the anconeus epitrochlearis to be slightly more bulky. There is a fascial plane between the muscle and the ulnar nerve; the latter structure does not appear to be compressed against the medial epicondyle. (Bottom) Axial PD FS MR in the same patient confirms the normal variant anconeus epitrochlearis to have normal muscle signal. It also shows normal signal and caliber of the ulnar nerve. This patient was asymptomatic with regard to ulnar nerve symptoms.

Elbow Measurements and Lines

MEASUREMENTS DEFINING NORMAL ANGULATION AT THE ELBOW

Carrying Angle of Elbow

- Imaging technique
  - Evaluated on AP radiograph with arm fully extended, with epicondyles flat with respect to film
  - Central ray perpendicular to plane of film
- Measurement
  - Intersection of longitudinal axes of humerus and ulna
  - Normal for males: 154-178°
  - Normal for females: 158-178°

Humeral Angle

- Imaging technique
  - Evaluated on AP radiograph with arm fully extended, with epicondyles flat with respect to film
  - Central ray perpendicular to plane of film
- Measurement
  - Intersection of longitudinal axis of humerus and line tangential to articular surfaces of trochlea and capitellum
  - Normal for males: 77-95°
  - Normal for females: 72-91°

Ulnar Angle

- Imaging technique
  - Evaluated on AP radiograph with arm fully extended, with epicondyles flat with respect to film
  - Central ray perpendicular to plane of film
- Measurement
  - Intersection of longitudinal axis of ulna and line tangential to articular surfaces of trochlea and capitellum
  - Normal for males: 74-99°
  - Normal for females: 72-93°

Significance: Any of These Measurements Detect Abnormal Carrying Angle of Elbow

- Elbow is normally in mild valgus, allowing normal back-and-forth movement of upper extremity while striding
- Following shaft fracture or physeal injury at elbow, varus deformity may result, resulting in "gunstock" deformity

USEFUL LINES FOR DETECTION OF SUBTLE TRAUMA

Radiocapitellar Line

- On any view of elbow, line extending along axis of proximal radius should intersect capitellum at ~ its center
- Significance: Detection of radial head dislocation
  - Particularly useful in children in whom epiphyseal ossification centers have not yet appeared and relationships between radius and humerus may be difficult to determine

Anterior Humeral Line

- Position: True lateral of elbow, with central x-ray perpendicular to plane of film
- Line drawn along anterior cortex of humerus and extended through its condyles will intersect middle 1/3 of capitellum
- Significance: Detection of supracondylar fracture of distal humerus
  - Supracondylar fracture in child may be subtle, without displacement
  - Results from fall on outstretched hand, resulting in slight posterior angulation of distal fracture fragment
  - Since distal fracture fragment includes capitellum, posterior displacement of this structure results in anterior humeral line falling either anterior to capitellum (if angulation is large) or within anterior 1/3 of capitellum (if angulation is slight)

ORDER OF OSSIFICATION OF ELBOW EPIPHYSES/APOPHYSES

Ossification Occurs in Reproducible Order

- Capitellum: 1 year of age
- Radial head: 3 years of age
- Medial epicondyle: 5 years of age
- Trochlea: 7 years of age
- Olecranon: 9 years of age
- Lateral epicondyle: 11 years of age

Mnemonic: CRITOE

- Each letter represents 1st letter of ossification center (with I standing for internal or medial epicondyle and E standing for lateral epicondyle), demonstrating order of ossification
- Useful since it is more important (and easier to remember) to know the **order** of ossification than to memorize actual expected age of ossification for each center

Significance: Detection of Avulsion Fracture of Medial Epicondyle

- Greatest significance falls in age range of 5-7 years
- Common elbow injury at this age is avulsion of medial epicondyle
  - Medial epicondyle is origin of common flexor tendon
  - With avulsion, common flexor tendon tends to pull medial epicondylar ossification center distally, often trapping it in joint
  - Trapped position of medial epicondyle may mimic normal trochlea within medial portion of joint, particularly if there is no ossified trochlea
- **Therefore**, since medial epicondyle ossifies before trochlea, if "trochlea" is seen in absence of medial epicondyle, that ossification center must in fact be displaced medial epicondyle, representing avulsion fracture

SELECTED REFERENCES

1. Keats TE et al: Normal axial relationships of the major joints. Radiology. 87(5):904-7, 1966

Elbow Measurements and Lines

ELBOW CARRYING ANGLE

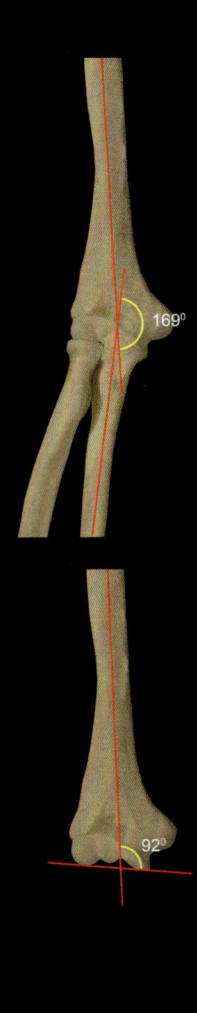

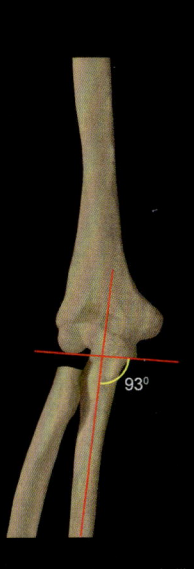

169°

92°

93°

(Top) There are 3 methods to evaluate for the normal valgus (or "carrying angle") expected at the elbow. The carrying angle is measured by the longitudinal axes of the humerus and ulna. (Middle) The humeral angle is measured by the lines formed by the longitudinal axis of the humerus and the line intersecting the bottoms of the capitellum and trochlea. (Bottom) The ulnar angle is measured by the lines formed by the longitudinal axis of the ulna and the line intersecting the bottoms of the capitellum and trochlea.

ELBOW RADIOCAPITELLAR LINE

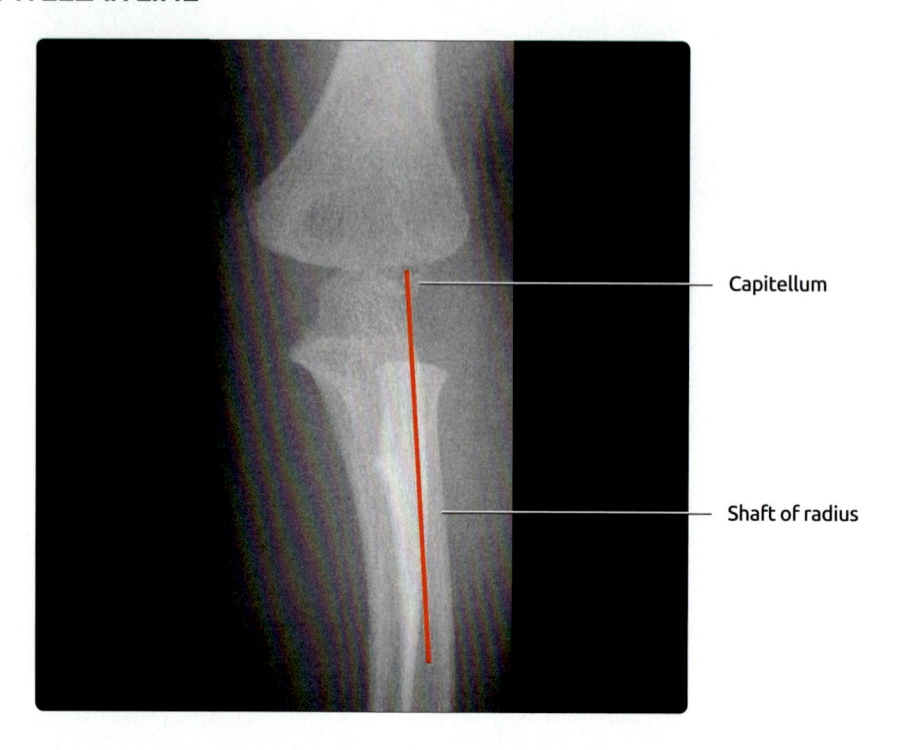

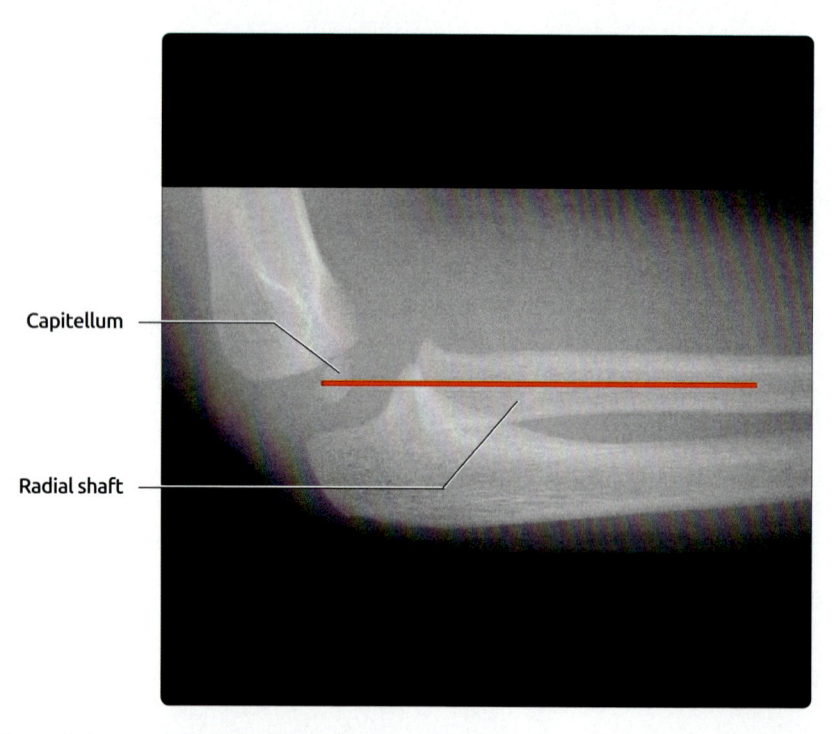

Capitellum

Shaft of radius

Capitellum

Radial shaft

(Top) *AP radiograph shows a skeletally immature patient with the radiocapitellar line drawn along the axis of the radius intersecting the capitellum.* **(Bottom)** *Lateral radiograph in the same patient shows the normal radiocapitellar line again intersecting the capitellum, indicating there is no radial head dislocation.*

Elbow Measurements and Lines

ELBOW ANTERIOR HUMERAL LINE AND ORDER OF OSSIFICATION

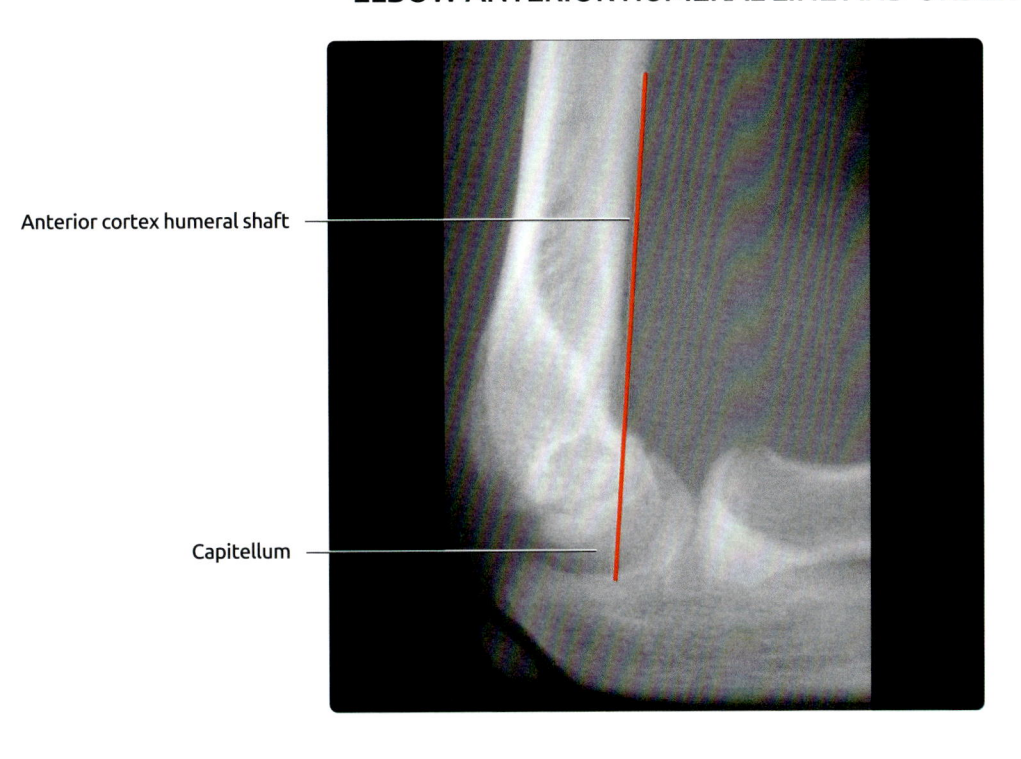

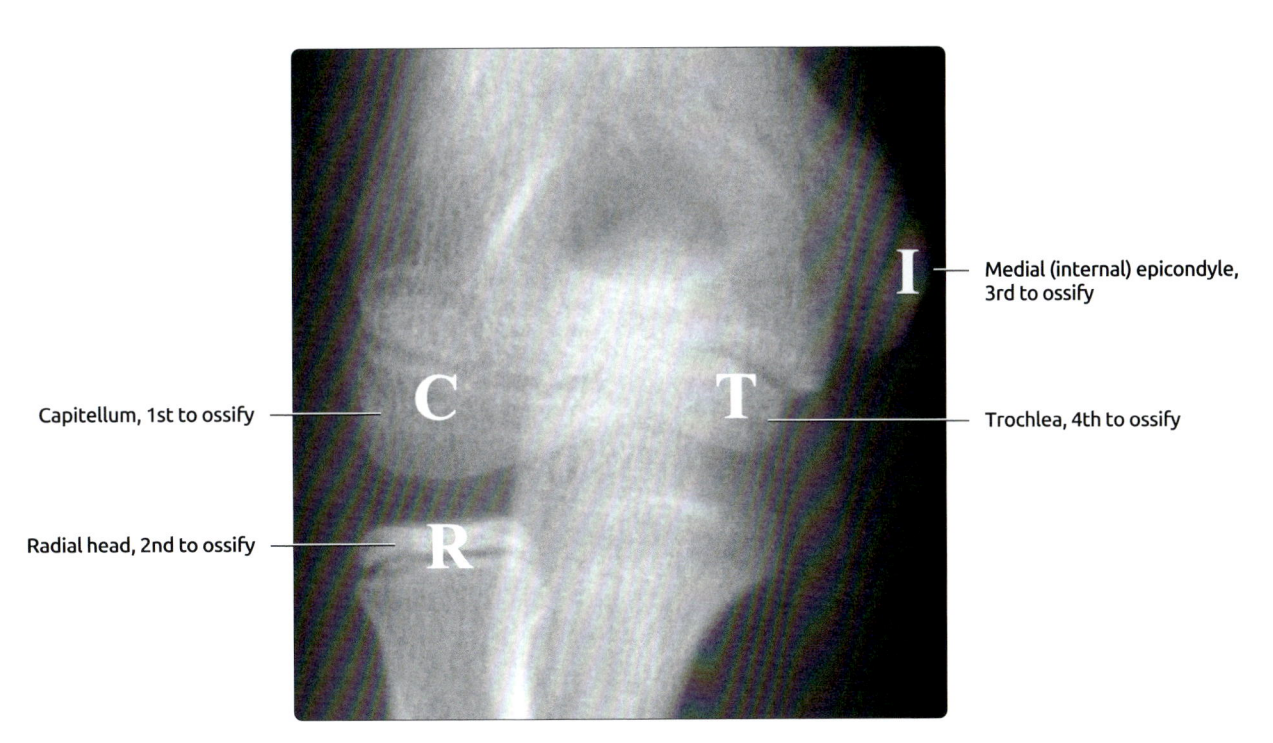

Anterior cortex humeral shaft

Capitellum

Capitellum, 1st to ossify

Radial head, 2nd to ossify

Medial (internal) epicondyle, 3rd to ossify

Trochlea, 4th to ossify

(Top) Lateral radiograph shows the anterior humeral line extending down the anterior cortex of the humeral shaft, extending to intersect the middle 1/3 of the capitellum. If the line extends into the anterior rather than middle 1/3 of the capitellum, it indicates a subtle supracondylar fracture with posterior angulation of the distal fragment. (Bottom) Understanding the order of ossification of the epiphyses/apophyses of the elbow is important. If there is an ossified body located in the position of the trochlea, but no ossified medial epicondyle is seen in its expected position. This indicates avulsion of the medial epicondyle with the fragment pulled into the joint, mimicking a trochlea.

SECTION 4
Forearm

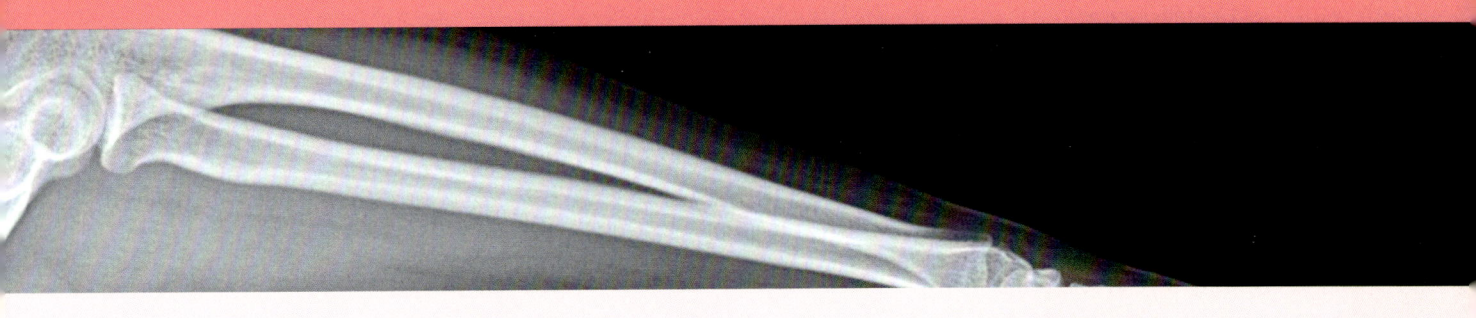

Forearm Radiographic Anatomy and MR Atlas 298

Forearm Radiographic Anatomy and MR Atlas

GROSS ANATOMY

Osseous Anatomy

- **Radius**
  - Laterally located
  - Shorter than ulna
  - Wider distally
  - Head
    - Disc shaped
    - Covered with articular cartilage along superior surface and circumference
    - Articulates with capitellum of elbow joint and ulnar notch of proximal radioulnar joint
  - Neck
    - Attachment of joint capsule
    - Angled 15° with shaft of radius
  - Radial tuberosity
    - At junction of neck and shaft
    - Insertion of biceps brachii tendon
  - Shaft
    - Medial surface: Sharp and straight, attachment site of interosseous membrane
    - Lateral surface: Rounded and convex lateral, with pronator tubercle at apex
    - **Anterior oblique line**: Ridge on anterior surface extending from radial tuberosity (proximal medial) to pronator tubercle (distal lateral)
    - Proximal 75% of shaft is concave anteriorly
    - Distal 25% of shaft is flat and wide
    - Styloid process: Most distal extent of radius
    - **Dorsal ("Lister") tubercle**: On dorsum of distal aspect, separates 2nd and 3rd extensor compartments and is origin of some extrinsic ligaments of wrist
    - **Ulnar notch**: Medial distal aspect, articulates with distal ulna
    - Distal articular surface articulates with carpus via scaphoid fossa and lunate fossa
- **Ulna**
  - Located medially
  - Longer than radius
  - Wider proximally
  - Olecranon process: Most proximal extent
  - **Coronoid process**
    - Anterior projection of proximal shaft
    - **Ulnar tuberosity**: Anterior inferior aspect of coronoid, proximal ulna, insertion of brachialis tendon
  - **Trochlear notch**
    - Formed by coronoid and olecranon processes
    - Articulates with trochlea of humerus
    - Transverse trochlear ridge: Demarcates junction of olecranon and coronoid
    - Trochlear grooves: Normal grooves on either side of trochlear notch
  - **Radial notch**
    - Lateral aspect of coronoid process
    - Articulates with radial head
  - **Supinator fossa**
    - Depression on lateral side of shaft, just below radial notch
    - Gives clearance to radial tuberosity during pronation/supination
    - Origin of ulnar head of supinator muscle
  - **Supinator crest**
    - Posterior aspect of supinator fossa
    - Origin of ulnar head of supinator muscle
    - Insertion of lateral ulnar collateral ligament
  - Shaft: Has 3 surfaces
    - Lateral: Flat and sharp, attachment site of interosseous membrane
    - Posterior: Rounded ridge, dividing line between extensors (lateral) and flexors (medial)
    - Anterior: Rounded, covered by flexor digitorum profundus origin
  - Distal
    - Small styloid process medially
    - Small round head: Articulates with ulnar notch of distal radius
    - Does not articulate with carpus

Articulations

- **Proximal radioulnar joint**
  - Pivot joint
  - Disc-shaped radial head articulates with radial notch of ulna
  - Held in place by annular ligament
  - Enclosed within elbow joint capsule
  - Communicates with elbow joint
- **Distal radioulnar joint**
  - Pivot joint
  - Ulnar head and ulnar notch of radius
  - Held in place by the triangular fibrocartilage (articular disc)
  - Synovial joint with its own capsule
  - Does not normally communicate with radiocarpal joint
- Motions
  - Supination
    - Principal muscles: Biceps brachii, supinator
  - Pronation
    - Principal muscles: Pronator teres, pronator quadratus

Interosseous Fibrous Attachments

- **Annular ligament**: Holds radial head in radial notch of proximal radioulnar joint
- **Quadrate ligament**: Thin fibrous band connecting radial neck to ulna, distal to annular ligament
- **Oblique cord**
  - Anatomically inconstant
  - Unknown functional significance, if any
  - Extends from inferior aspect of ulnar tuberosity to inferior aspect of radial tuberosity
- **Interosseous membrane**
  - Thin, broad sheet of fibrous tissue
  - Connects medial side of radius to lateral side of ulna
  - Begins 2-3 cm distal to radial tuberosity
  - Provides attachment for deep muscles of forearm
  - Fibers course inferomedially (though variable)
    - Transfers load from distal radius to ulna, and from there up to humerus and shoulder
    - Fibers are taut in midprone position (usual position of function)

Forearm Radiographic Anatomy and MR Atlas

- **Triangular fibrocartilage** (articular disc): Holds ulnar head in ulna notch of distal radioulnar joint
- **Extensor retinaculum**
  - Dorsum of distal forearm and wrist
  - Origin: Distal radius
  - Insertion: Ulnar styloid, triquetrum, pisiform
  - Has deep slips that form 6 extensor tendon compartments of distal forearm and wrist
    - 1st extensor compartment: Abductor pollicis longus, extensor pollicis brevis
    - 2nd extensor compartment: Extensor carpi radialis longus and brevis
    - 3rd extensor compartment: Extensor pollicis longus
    - 4th extensor compartment: Extensor digitorum, extensor indicis
    - 5th extensor compartment: Extensor digiti minimi
    - 6th extensor compartment: Extensor carpi ulnaris
  - Prevents bowstringing of extensor tendons

Muscles

- **Anterior compartment**
  - Has 8 flexor muscles, in 3 groups
- Anterior compartment: **Superficial group**
  - Flexor carpi radialis, flexor carpi ulnaris, pronator teres, palmaris longus
  - Originate from common flexor tendon of elbow
- Anterior compartment: **Intermediate group**
  - Flexor digitorum superficialis
  - Originates from common flexor tendon of elbow
- Anterior compartment: **Deep group**
  - Flexor digitorum profundus
    - Origin: Proximal 75% of anterior and medial surfaces of ulna and adjacent interosseous membrane
    - Insertion: Base of 2nd-5th distal phalanges
    - Innervation: Ulnar nerve for 4th and 5th fingers, anterior interosseous branch of median nerve for 2nd and 3rd fingers
    - Actions: Flexion of distal and proximal interphalangeal joints, metacarpophalangeal joints, wrist joint
  - Flexor pollicis longus
    - Lies lateral to flexor digitorum profundus
    - Origin: Anterior surface of radius (distal to anterior oblique line), lateral aspect of interosseous membrane
    - Insertion: Palmar aspect of base of distal phalanx of thumb
    - Innervation: Anterior interosseous branch of median nerve
    - Action: Flexion of interphalangeal joint of thumb, 1st metacarpophalangeal joint, carpometacarpal joint, and wrist joint
  - Pronator quadratus
    - Deepest muscle of anterior forearm
    - Origin: Distal 25% of anterior surface of ulna
    - Insertion: Distal 25% of anterior surface of radius
    - Innervation: Anterior interosseous branch of median nerve
    - Action: Pronation of forearm, holds distal radius and ulna together
- **Posterior compartment**
  - Has 9 extensor muscles, in 2 groups
- Posterior compartment: **Superficial group**
  - Extensor carpi radialis brevis, extensor carpi ulnaris, extensor digitorum, extensor digiti minimi
    - Originate from common extensor tendon of elbow
  - Extensor carpi radialis longus
    - Arises from lateral supracondylar ridge humerus
- Posterior compartment: **Deep group**
  - Abductor pollicis longus
    - Origin: Posterior surfaces of radius, ulna, and interosseous membrane
    - Insertion: Posterior surface of base of 1st metacarpal
    - Innervation: Posterior interosseous nerve
    - Action: Abducts and extends thumb at metacarpophalangeal joint
    - Distal tendon forms anterior (volar) aspect of anatomic snuff box of wrist
  - Extensor pollicis brevis
    - Origin: Posterior surface of radius and interosseous membrane
    - Insertion: Posterior surface of base of 1st proximal phalanx
    - Innervation: Posterior interosseous nerve
    - Action: Extends thumb at carpometacarpal and metacarpophalangeal joints
    - Distal tendon forms anterior (volar) aspect of anatomic snuff box of wrist
  - Extensor pollicis longus
    - Origin: Posterior surface of ulna and interosseous membrane
    - Insertion: Posterior surface of base of 1st distal phalanx
    - Innervation: Posterior interosseous nerve
    - Action: Extends interphalangeal joint of thumb and 1st metacarpophalangeal joint
    - Distal tendon forms posterior (dorsal) aspect of anatomic snuff box of wrist
  - Extensor indicis
    - Origin: Posterior surface of ulna and interosseous membrane
    - Insertion: Extensor hood expansion of 2nd finger
    - Innervation: Posterior interosseous nerve
    - Action: Extends 2nd metacarpophalangeal joint

Arteries

- **Brachial artery** divides into radial artery and ulnar artery in cubital fossa
- **Radial artery**
  - Medial to distal biceps tendon
  - Covered by brachioradialis muscle
  - Distally, leaves forearm and moves laterally, crossing floor of anatomical snuff box
  - Terminates in deep palmar arch of hand
  - Radial recurrent artery
    - Runs proximally along lateral side of elbow to form anastomosis with branches of deep brachial artery
  - Muscular branches to lateral side of forearm
  - Distal anastomotic branches: Palmar carpal arch, superficial palmar arch, dorsal carpal arch
- **Ulnar artery**
  - Proximally, deep to pronator teres
  - Distally, lies on flexor digitorum profundus and is lateral to ulnar nerve

Forearm Radiographic Anatomy and MR Atlas

- Anterior and posterior ulnar recurrent arteries: Form anastomosis around medial side of elbow with branches of brachial artery
- Common interosseous artery: Arises in distal aspect of cubital fossa
  - Anterior interosseous artery: Runs distally on interosseous membrane and ends in dorsal carpal arch
  - Posterior interosseous artery: Enters posterior compartment proximal to interosseous membrane, between supinator and abductor pollicis longus, supplies posterior muscles
- Muscular branches to medial side of forearm
- Distal anastomotic branches: Palmar carpal arch, dorsal carpal arch

Nerves

- **Anterior compartment**
  - **Median nerve**
    - Principal nerve of anterior compartment
    - Supplies: Pronator teres, flexor carpi radialis, palmaris longus, flexor digitorum superficialis
    - Enters forearm from cubital fossa by passing between the humeral and ulnar heads of pronator teres
    - Courses distally, attached to deep surface of flexor digitorum superficialis muscle by a fascial sheath
    - Pronator syndrome: Compression of median nerve as it passes between pronator heads and under flexor digitorum superficialis
    - At wrist, emerges from lateral side of flexor digitorum superficialis and is deep to palmaris longus tendon and flexor retinaculum
  - **Anterior interosseous nerve**
    - Arises from median nerve at level of pronator teres
    - Courses distally along anterior surface of interosseous membrane
    - Accompanied by interosseous branch of ulnar artery
    - Lies between flexor digitorum profundus and flexor pollicis longus
    - Ends at pronator quadratus muscle, giving articular branches to wrist joint and the palmar cutaneous branch (superficial to flexor retinaculum)
    - Supplies: Flexor pollicis longus, pronator quadratus, lateral 1/2 of flexor digitorum profundus
    - Kiloh-Nevin syndrome: Compression of anterior interoseus nerve, most often due to fibrous bands
  - **Ulnar nerve**
    - After passing behind medial epicondyle, enters forearm by passing between humeral and ulnar heads of flexor carpi ulnaris
    - Courses distally between flexor carpi ulnaris and flexor digitorum profundus
    - Distally, becomes superficial and passes into wrist superficial to flexor retinaculum
    - Supplies: Flexor carpi ulnaris, medial 1/2 of flexor digitorum profundus
    - Palmer cutaneous branch: Arises in middle of forearm and supplies skin over medial side of palm
    - Dorsal cutaneous branch: Arises distally between ulna and flexor carpi ulnaris to supply dorsal surface of medial side of hand
  - **Superficial branch of radial nerve**
    - Direct continuation of radial nerve after deep branch has split off at level of lateral epicondyle
    - Courses distally, deep to brachioradialis
    - In distal forearm passes into posterior compartment
    - Gives terminal branches to supply skin of lateral 2/3 of dorsum of wrist, hand, and lateral 2.5 fingers
  - **Lateral cutaneous nerve**
    - Continuation of musculocutaneous nerve of elbow
    - Supplies skin of lateral aspect of forearm
  - **Medial cutaneous nerve**
    - Arises from medial cord of brachial plexus (C8, T1)
    - Accompanies basilic vein in arm
    - Anterior to medial epicondyle
    - Supplies skin of posteromedial forearm
- **Posterior compartment**
  - **Posterior interosseous nerve**
    - Purely motor
    - Continuation of deep branch of radial nerve after deep branch passes through supinator muscle to reach posterior compartment
    - Lies on posterior surface of interosseous membrane, deep to extensor pollicis longus
    - Accompanied by posterior interosseous artery
    - Supplies: Extensor digitorum, extensor digiti minimi, extensor indicis, extensor carpi ulnaris, abductor pollicis longus, extensor pollicis brevis, extensor pollicis longus
    - Terminates in articular branches to wrist joint
    - Posterior osseous nerve syndrome: Compression of deep branch of radial nerve as it enters supinator muscle

ANATOMY IMAGING ISSUES

Anomalous Muscles

- Duplicate muscles, accessory muscles, anomalous origins and insertions
  - Commonly involve palmaris longus, flexor carpi ulnaris, abductor digiti minimi, flexor digiti minimi
    - May present clinically as mass: Has signal characteristics and appearance of muscle
    - May present clinically due to compression of adjacent nerve

SELECTED REFERENCES

1. Hodler J et al: Magnetic resonance imaging of the forearm: cross-sectional anatomy in a cadaveric model. Invest Radiol. 33(1):6-11, 1998
2. Skahen JR 3rd et al: The interosseous membrane of the forearm: anatomy and function. J Hand Surg Am. 22(6):981-5, 1997

Forearm Radiographic Anatomy and MR Atlas

AP AND LATERAL RADIOGRAPHS OF FOREARM

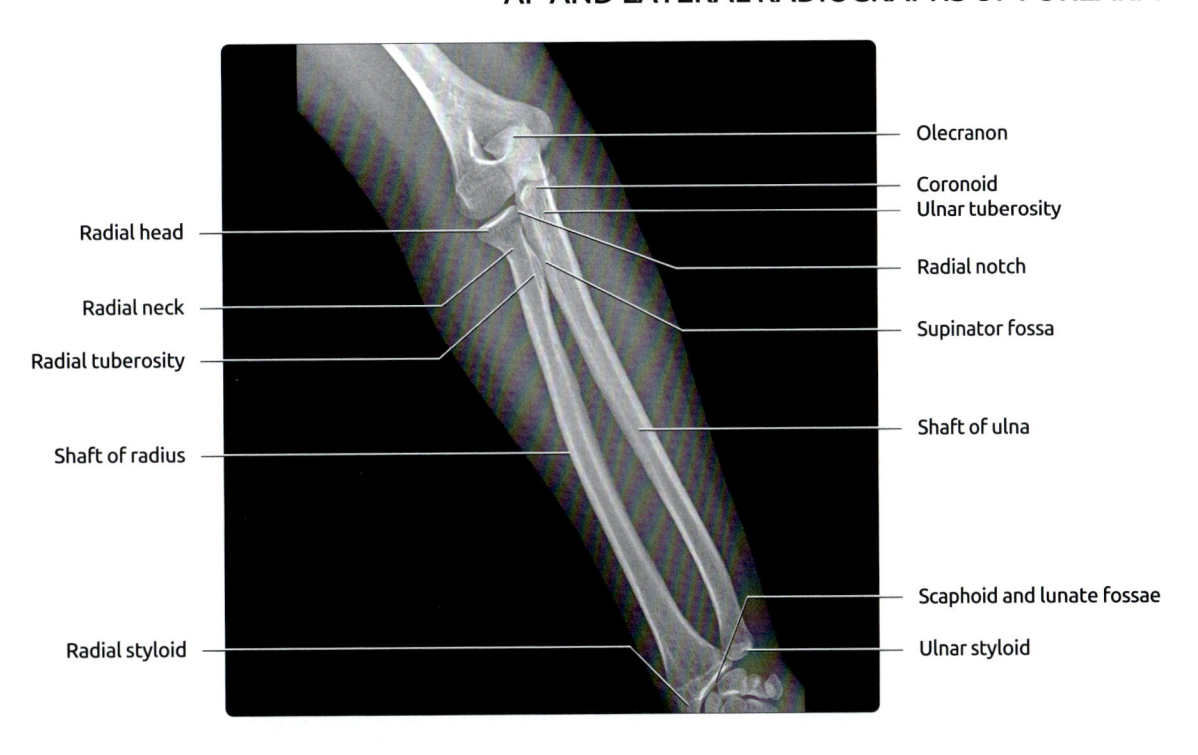

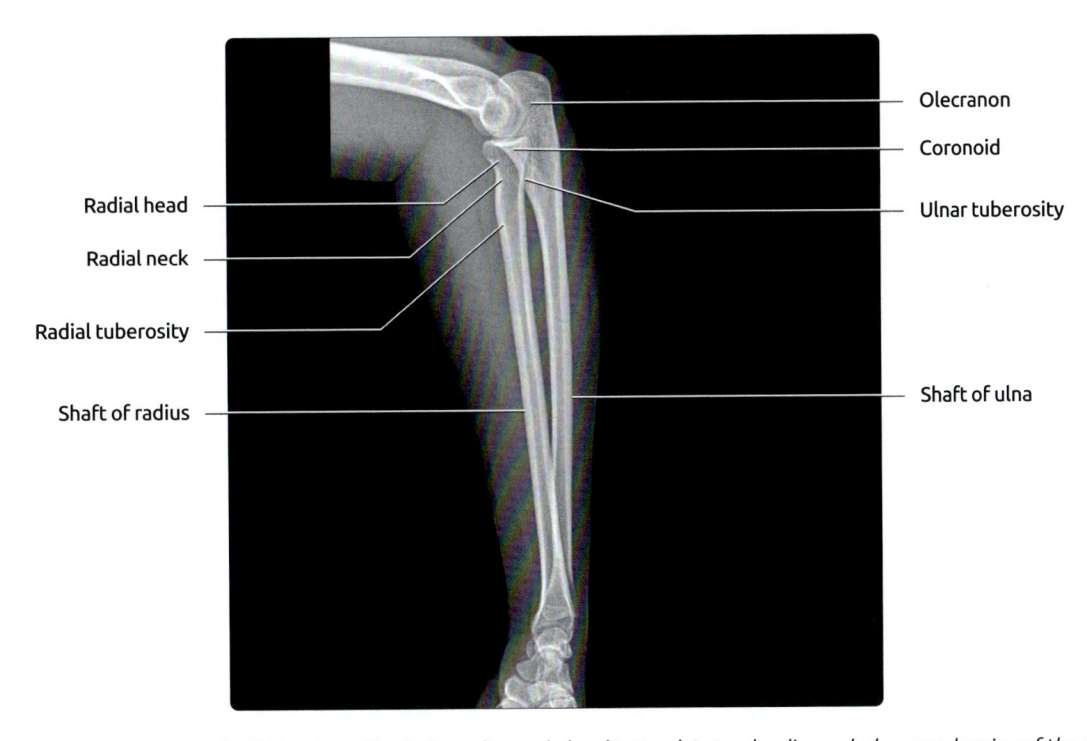

(Top) AP radiograph shows normal mild bowing of both the radius and ulna. **(Bottom)** Lateral radiograph shows no bowing of the radius and ulna. The distal aspects of the radius and ulna should overlap at the distal radioulnar joint.

Forearm Radiographic Anatomy and MR Atlas

GRAPHIC, ANTERIOR AND POSTERIOR VIEWS OF FOREARM: ORIGINS AND INSERTIONS

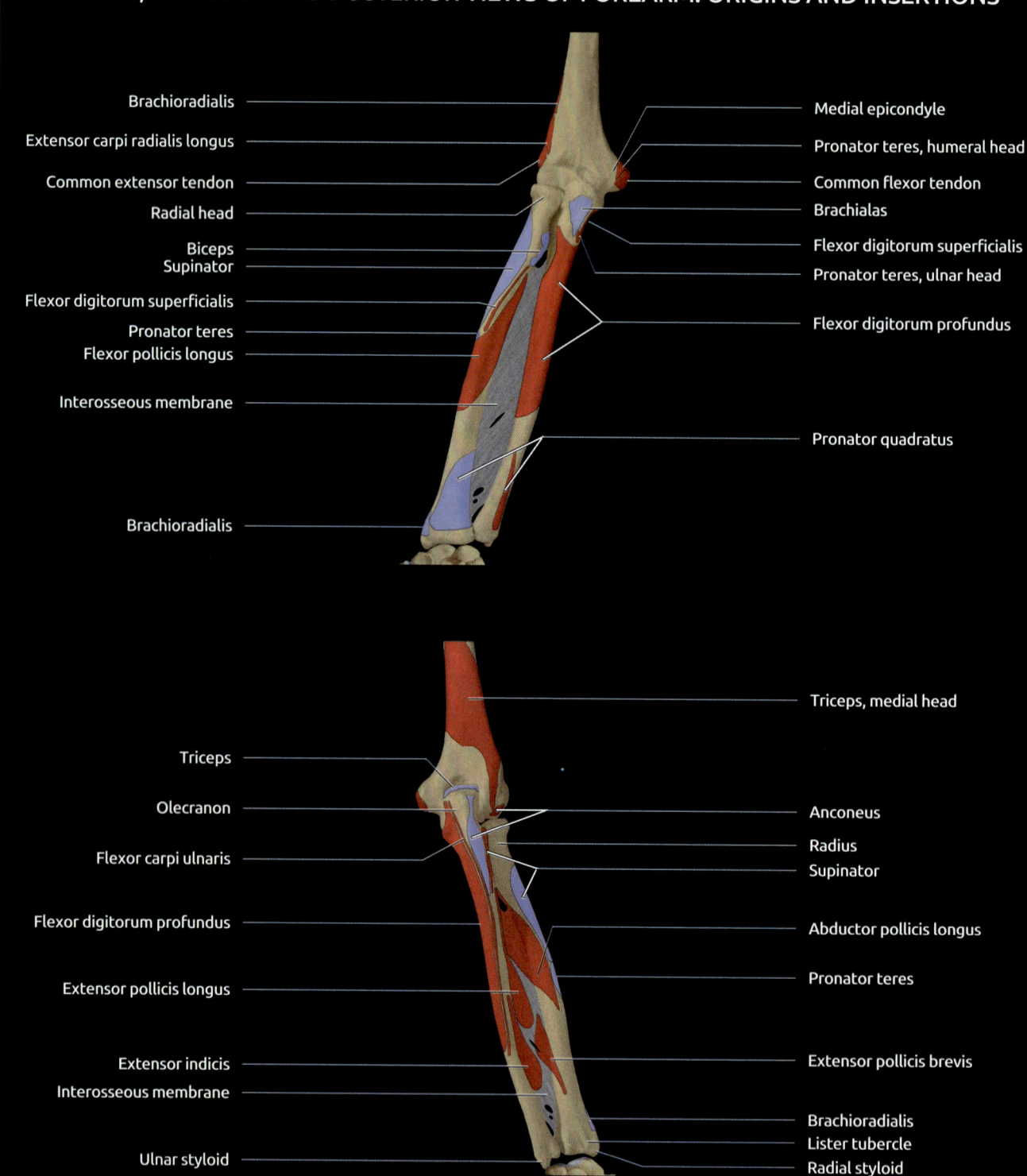

Brachioradialis — Medial epicondyle
Extensor carpi radialis longus — Pronator teres, humeral head
Common extensor tendon — Common flexor tendon
Radial head — Brachialas
Biceps — Flexor digitorum superficialis
Supinator — Pronator teres, ulnar head
Flexor digitorum superficialis — Flexor digitorum profundus
Pronator teres
Flexor pollicis longus
Interosseous membrane — Pronator quadratus
Brachioradialis

Triceps, medial head
Triceps
Olecranon — Anconeus
Flexor carpi ulnaris — Radius
— Supinator
Flexor digitorum profundus — Abductor pollicis longus
Extensor pollicis longus — Pronator teres
Extensor indicis — Extensor pollicis brevis
Interosseous membrane — Brachioradialis
— Lister tubercle
Ulnar styloid — Radial styloid

(Top) *The origins are in red, and the insertions are in blue. Note that no muscles originate from the anterior surface of the interosseous membrane.* **(Bottom)** *The origins are in red, and the insertions are in blue. Notice that several muscles take origin partially from the posterior surface of the interosseous membrane.*

Forearm Radiographic Anatomy and MR Atlas

GRAPHICS, AXIAL VIEW OF THE FOREARM AND NEUROVASCULAR STRUCTURES

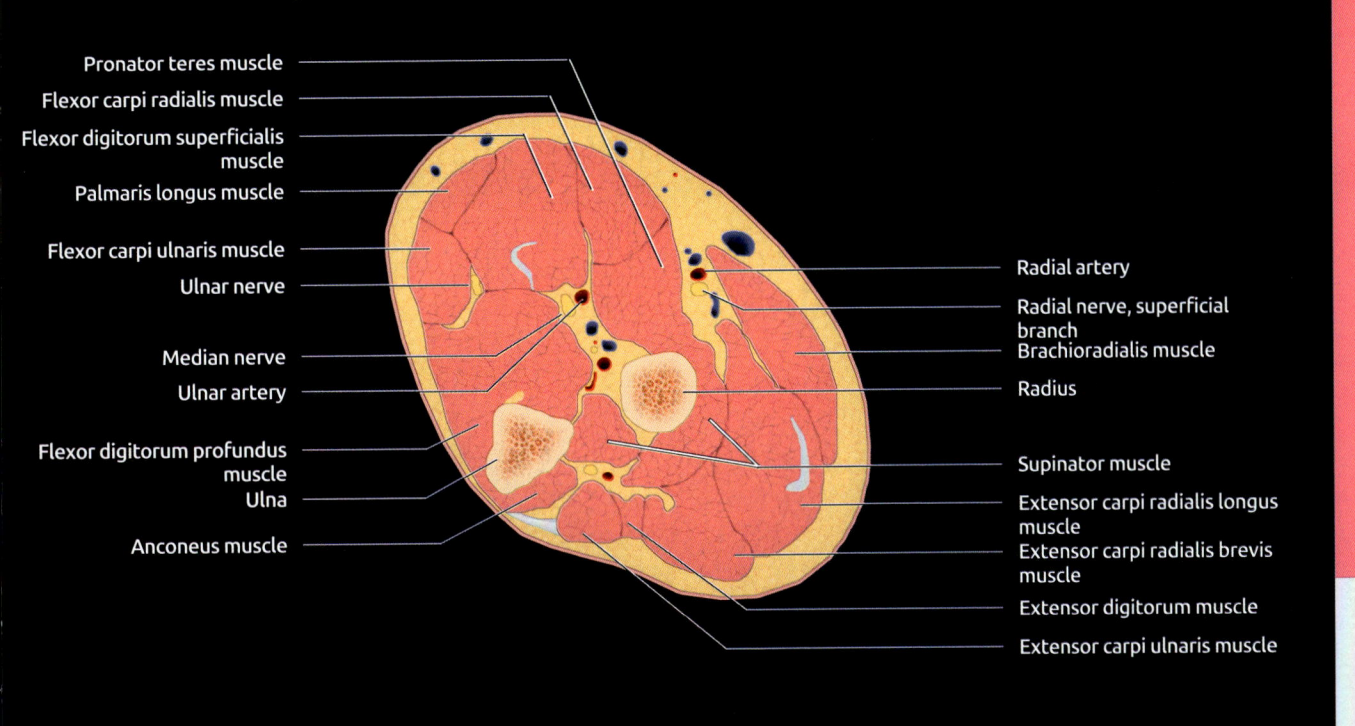

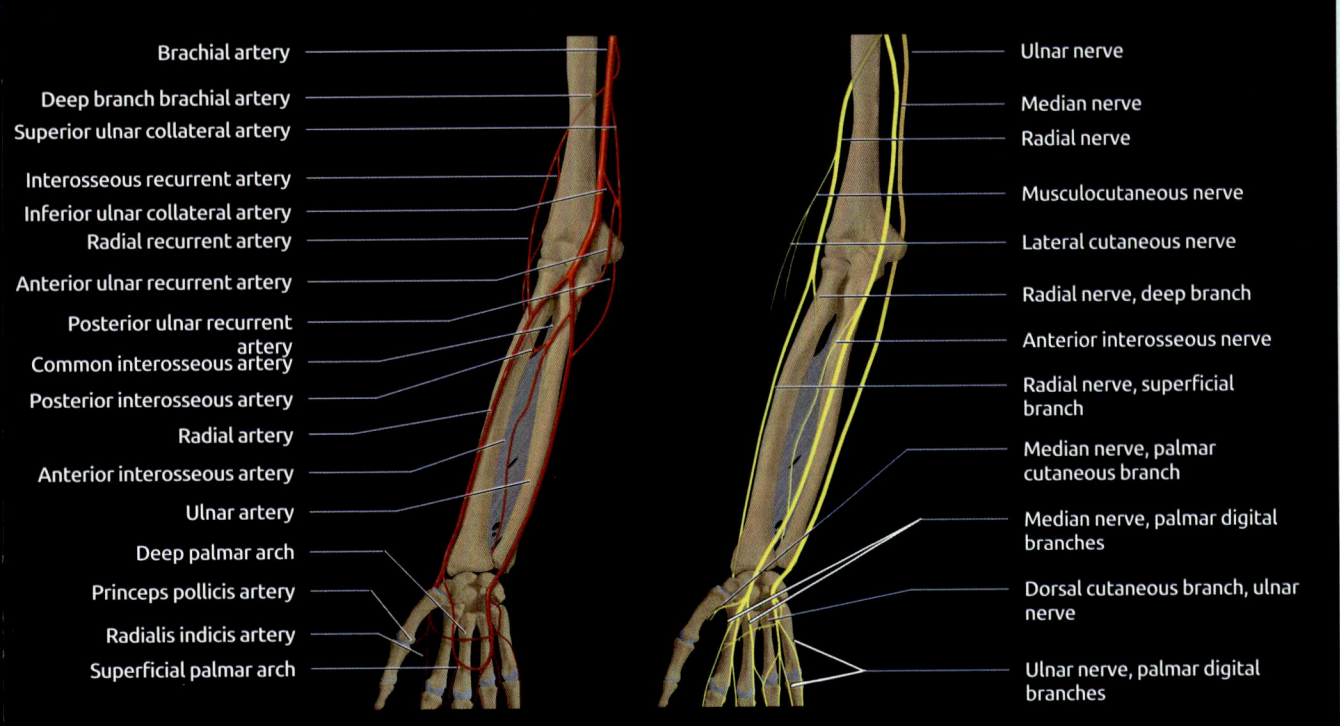

Labels (top, axial graphic):
- Pronator teres muscle
- Flexor carpi radialis muscle
- Flexor digitorum superficialis muscle
- Palmaris longus muscle
- Flexor carpi ulnaris muscle
- Ulnar nerve
- Median nerve
- Ulnar artery
- Flexor digitorum profundus muscle
- Ulna
- Anconeus muscle
- Radial artery
- Radial nerve, superficial branch
- Brachioradialis muscle
- Radius
- Supinator muscle
- Extensor carpi radialis longus muscle
- Extensor carpi radialis brevis muscle
- Extensor digitorum muscle
- Extensor carpi ulnaris muscle

Labels (bottom, vascular and neural):
- Brachial artery
- Deep branch brachial artery
- Superior ulnar collateral artery
- Interosseous recurrent artery
- Inferior ulnar collateral artery
- Radial recurrent artery
- Anterior ulnar recurrent artery
- Posterior ulnar recurrent artery
- Common interosseous artery
- Posterior interosseous artery
- Radial artery
- Anterior interosseous artery
- Ulnar artery
- Deep palmar arch
- Princeps pollicis artery
- Radialis indicis artery
- Superficial palmar arch
- Ulnar nerve
- Median nerve
- Radial nerve
- Musculocutaneous nerve
- Lateral cutaneous nerve
- Radial nerve, deep branch
- Anterior interosseous nerve
- Radial nerve, superficial branch
- Median nerve, palmar cutaneous branch
- Median nerve, palmar digital branches
- Dorsal cutaneous branch, ulnar nerve
- Ulnar nerve, palmar digital branches

(Top) *Axial graphic at the proximal forearm, below the level of the radial and ulnar tuberosities, is shown. Note that the muscles align into the anterior (flexor) and posterior (extensor) compartments.* (Bottom) *Vascular (red) and neural (yellow) structures of the forearm are shown.*

Forearm Radiographic Anatomy and MR Atlas

AXIAL T1 MR, RIGHT FOREARM

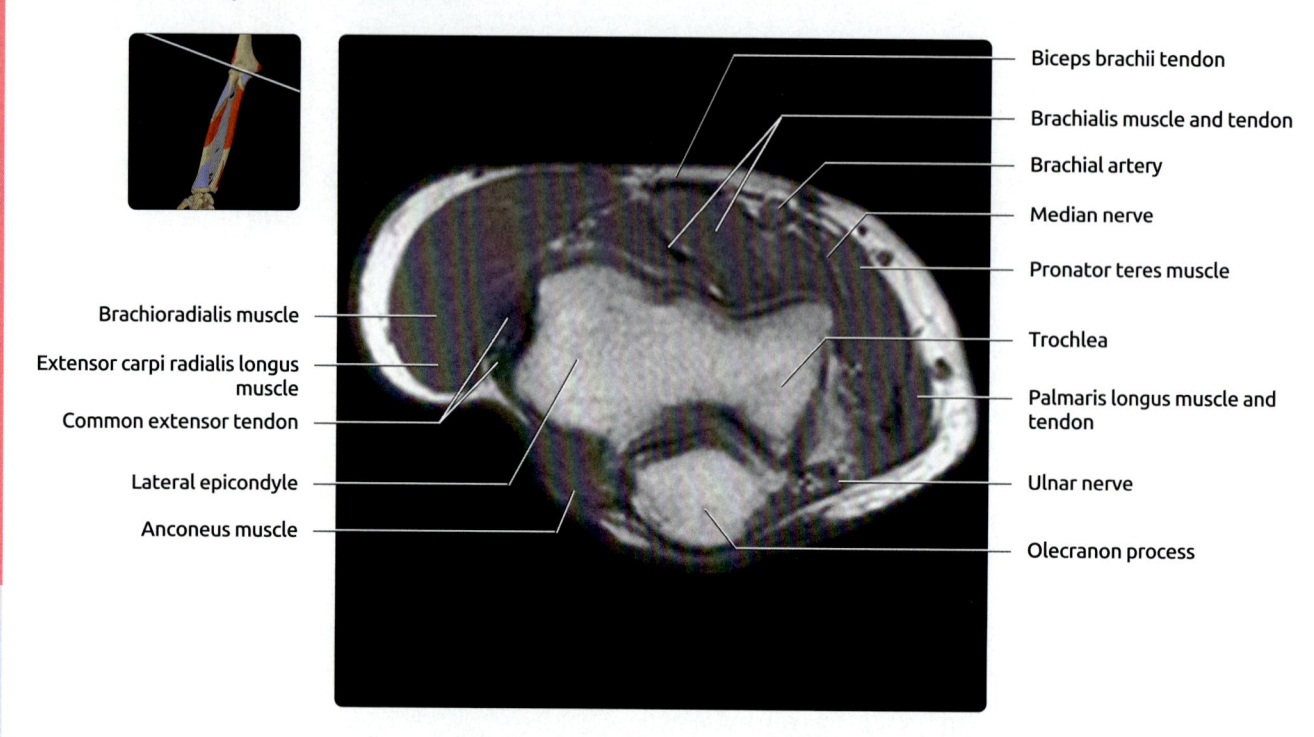

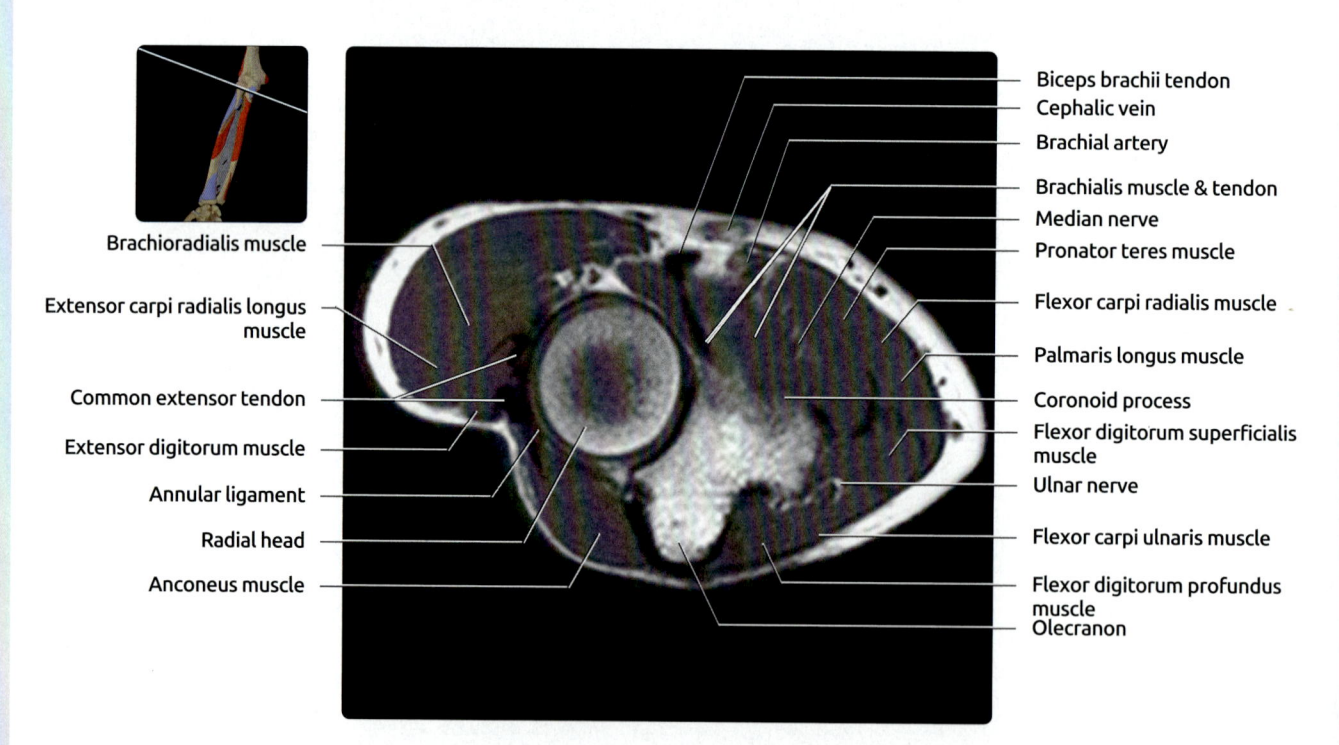

Top image labels (left side):
- Brachioradialis muscle
- Extensor carpi radialis longus muscle
- Common extensor tendon
- Lateral epicondyle
- Anconeus muscle

Top image labels (right side):
- Biceps brachii tendon
- Brachialis muscle and tendon
- Brachial artery
- Median nerve
- Pronator teres muscle
- Trochlea
- Palmaris longus muscle and tendon
- Ulnar nerve
- Olecranon process

Bottom image labels (left side):
- Brachioradialis muscle
- Extensor carpi radialis longus muscle
- Common extensor tendon
- Extensor digitorum muscle
- Annular ligament
- Radial head
- Anconeus muscle

Bottom image labels (right side):
- Biceps brachii tendon
- Cephalic vein
- Brachial artery
- Brachialis muscle & tendon
- Median nerve
- Pronator teres muscle
- Flexor carpi radialis muscle
- Palmaris longus muscle
- Coronoid process
- Flexor digitorum superficialis muscle
- Ulnar nerve
- Flexor carpi ulnaris muscle
- Flexor digitorum profundus muscle
- Olecranon

(Top) *Axial series through the forearm, proximal to distal, are shown. The proximal aspects of the flexor-pronator group and the extensor group are seen.* **(Bottom)** *At the level of the proximal radioulnar joint, there is a combination of muscles that act on the elbow, wrist, and hand.*

Forearm Radiographic Anatomy and MR Atlas

AXIAL T1 MR, LEFT FOREARM

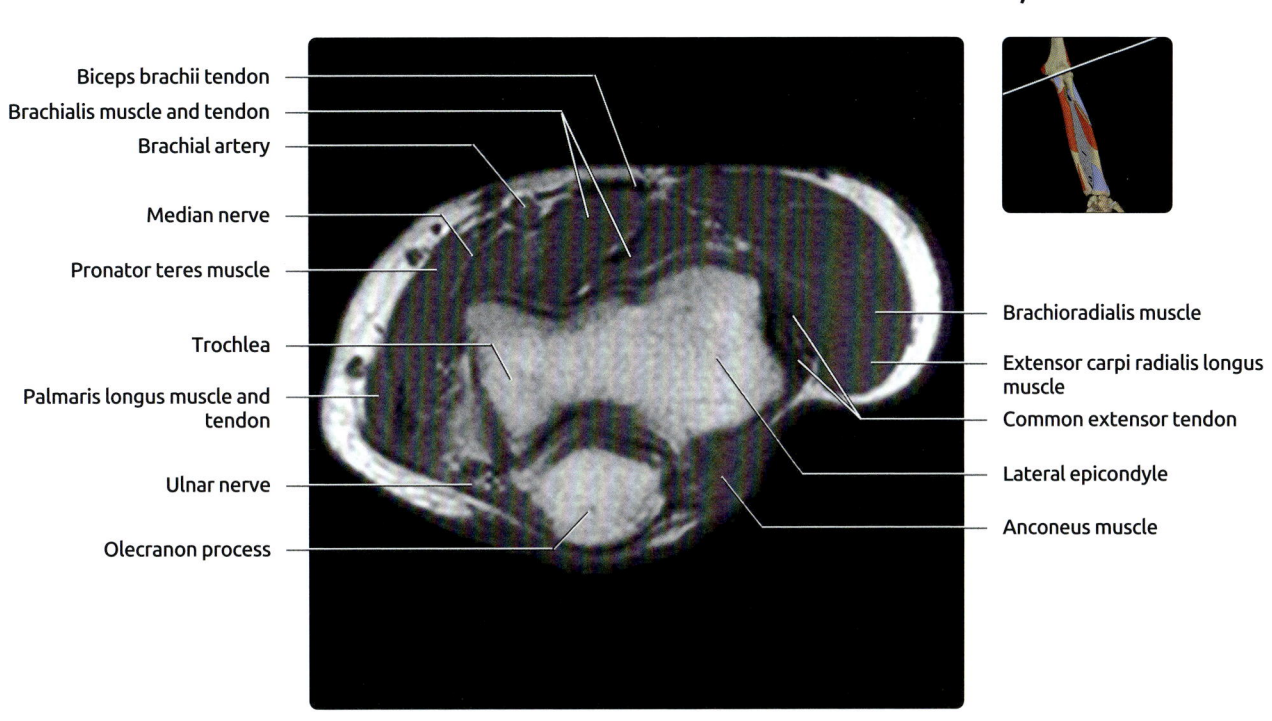

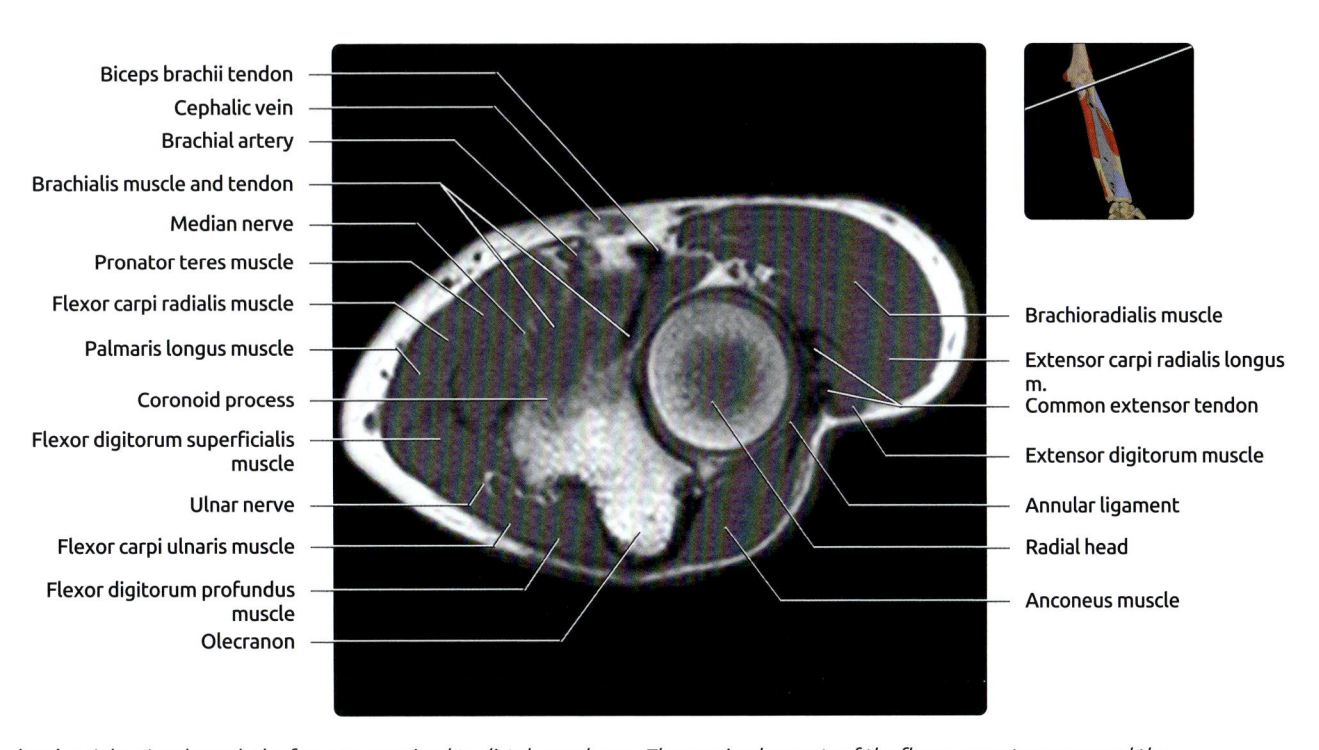

Labels (top image), left side:
- Biceps brachii tendon
- Brachialis muscle and tendon
- Brachial artery
- Median nerve
- Pronator teres muscle
- Trochlea
- Palmaris longus muscle and tendon
- Ulnar nerve
- Olecranon process

Labels (top image), right side:
- Brachioradialis muscle
- Extensor carpi radialis longus muscle
- Common extensor tendon
- Lateral epicondyle
- Anconeus muscle

Labels (bottom image), left side:
- Biceps brachii tendon
- Cephalic vein
- Brachial artery
- Brachialis muscle and tendon
- Median nerve
- Pronator teres muscle
- Flexor carpi radialis muscle
- Palmaris longus muscle
- Coronoid process
- Flexor digitorum superficialis muscle
- Ulnar nerve
- Flexor carpi ulnaris muscle
- Flexor digitorum profundus muscle
- Olecranon

Labels (bottom image), right side:
- Brachioradialis muscle
- Extensor carpi radialis longus m.
- Common extensor tendon
- Extensor digitorum muscle
- Annular ligament
- Radial head
- Anconeus muscle

(Top) *Axial series through the forearm, proximal to distal, are shown. The proximal aspects of the flexor-pronator group and the extensor group are seen.* **(Bottom)** *At the level of the proximal radioulnar joint, there is a combination of muscles that act on the elbow, wrist, and hand.*

Forearm Radiographic Anatomy and MR Atlas

AXIAL T1 MR, RIGHT FOREARM

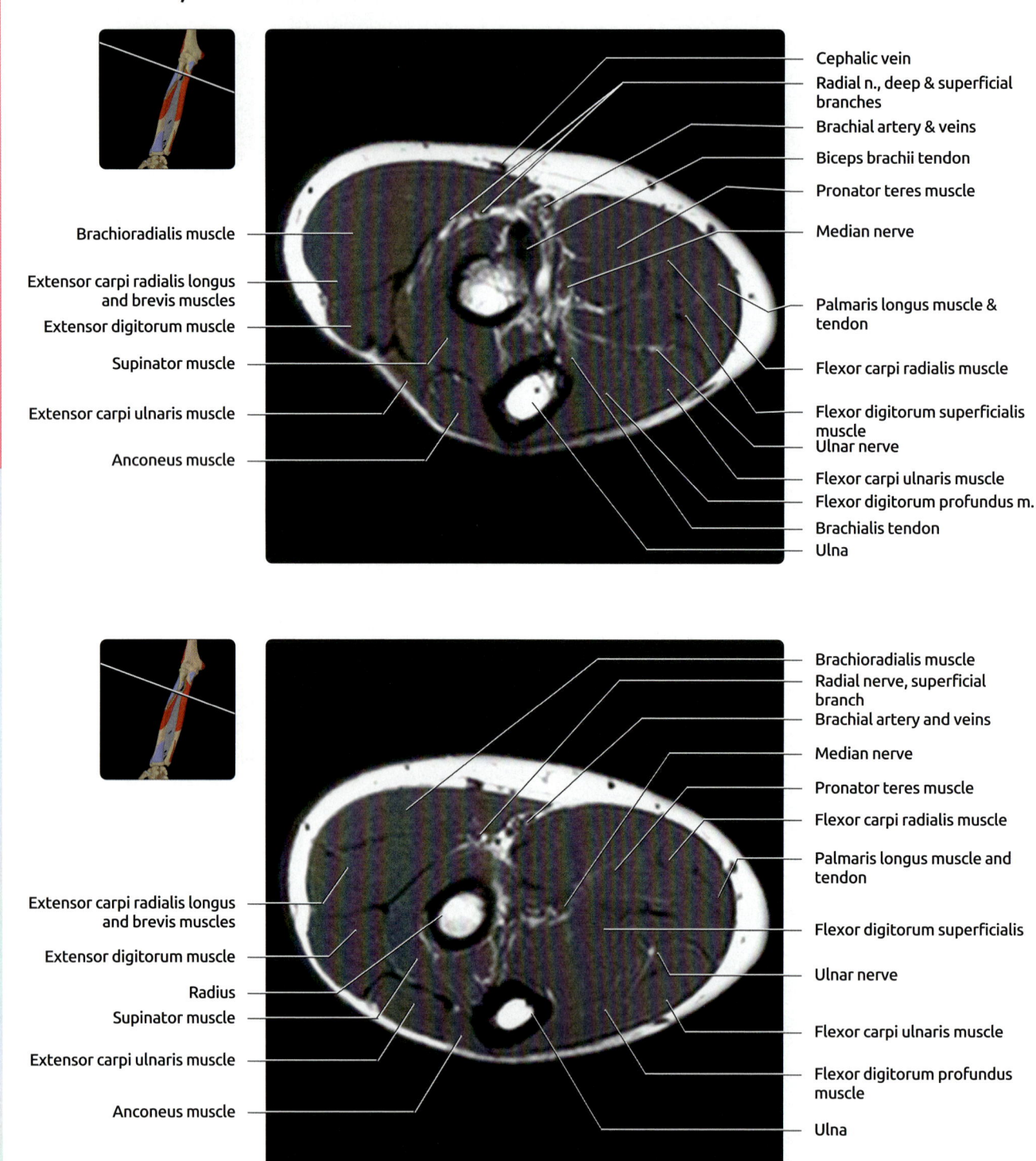

Top image labels (left):
- Brachioradialis muscle
- Extensor carpi radialis longus and brevis muscles
- Extensor digitorum muscle
- Supinator muscle
- Extensor carpi ulnaris muscle
- Anconeus muscle

Top image labels (right):
- Cephalic vein
- Radial n., deep & superficial branches
- Brachial artery & veins
- Biceps brachii tendon
- Pronator teres muscle
- Median nerve
- Palmaris longus muscle & tendon
- Flexor carpi radialis muscle
- Flexor digitorum superficialis muscle
- Ulnar nerve
- Flexor carpi ulnaris muscle
- Flexor digitorum profundus m.
- Brachialis tendon
- Ulna

Bottom image labels (left):
- Extensor carpi radialis longus and brevis muscles
- Extensor digitorum muscle
- Radius
- Supinator muscle
- Extensor carpi ulnaris muscle
- Anconeus muscle

Bottom image labels (right):
- Brachioradialis muscle
- Radial nerve, superficial branch
- Brachial artery and veins
- Median nerve
- Pronator teres muscle
- Flexor carpi radialis muscle
- Palmaris longus muscle and tendon
- Flexor digitorum superficialis
- Ulnar nerve
- Flexor carpi ulnaris muscle
- Flexor digitorum profundus muscle
- Ulna

(Top) The flexor muscles are grouped anteriorly and the extensors posteriorly. **(Bottom)** The deep branch of the radial nerve has entered the supinator muscle on its way toward the posterior compartment of the forearm and is not discernible.

Forearm Radiographic Anatomy and MR Atlas

AXIAL T1 MR, LEFT FOREARM

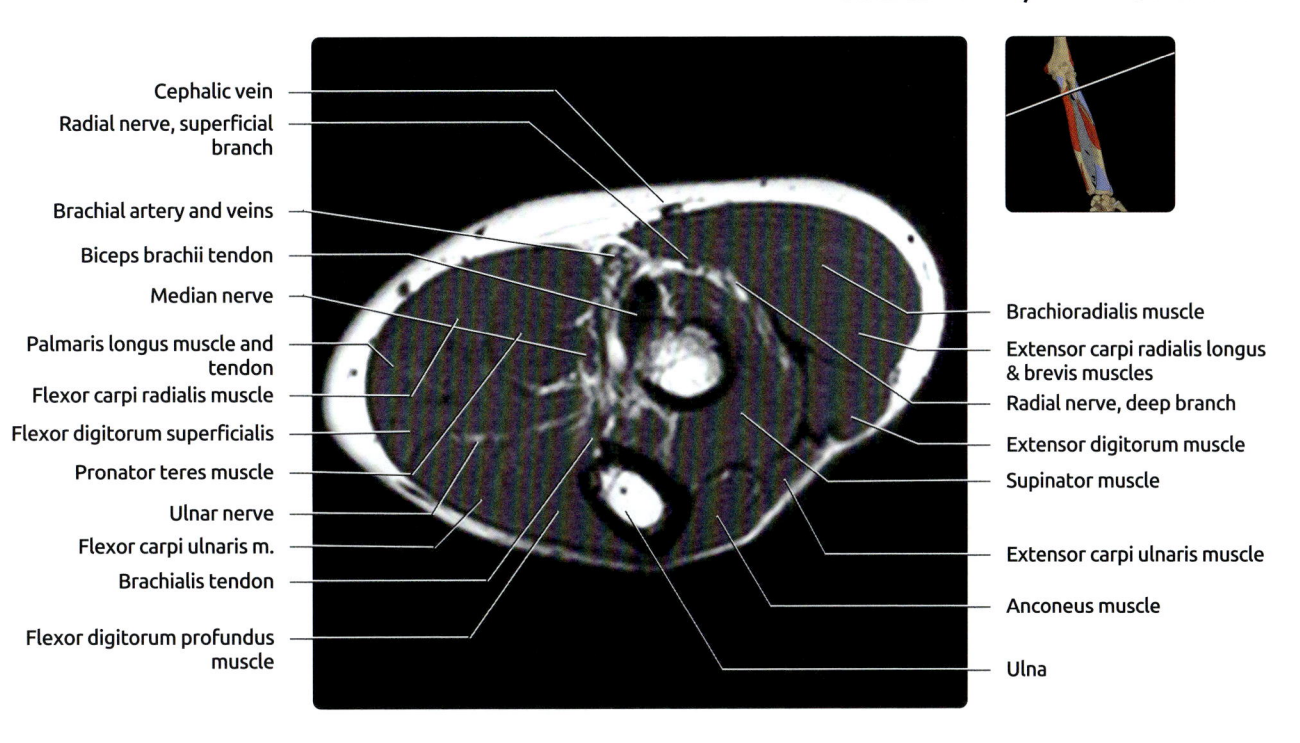

Top image labels:
- Cephalic vein
- Radial nerve, superficial branch
- Brachial artery and veins
- Biceps brachii tendon
- Median nerve
- Palmaris longus muscle and tendon
- Flexor carpi radialis muscle
- Flexor digitorum superficialis
- Pronator teres muscle
- Ulnar nerve
- Flexor carpi ulnaris m.
- Brachialis tendon
- Flexor digitorum profundus muscle
- Brachioradialis muscle
- Extensor carpi radialis longus & brevis muscles
- Radial nerve, deep branch
- Extensor digitorum muscle
- Supinator muscle
- Extensor carpi ulnaris muscle
- Anconeus muscle
- Ulna

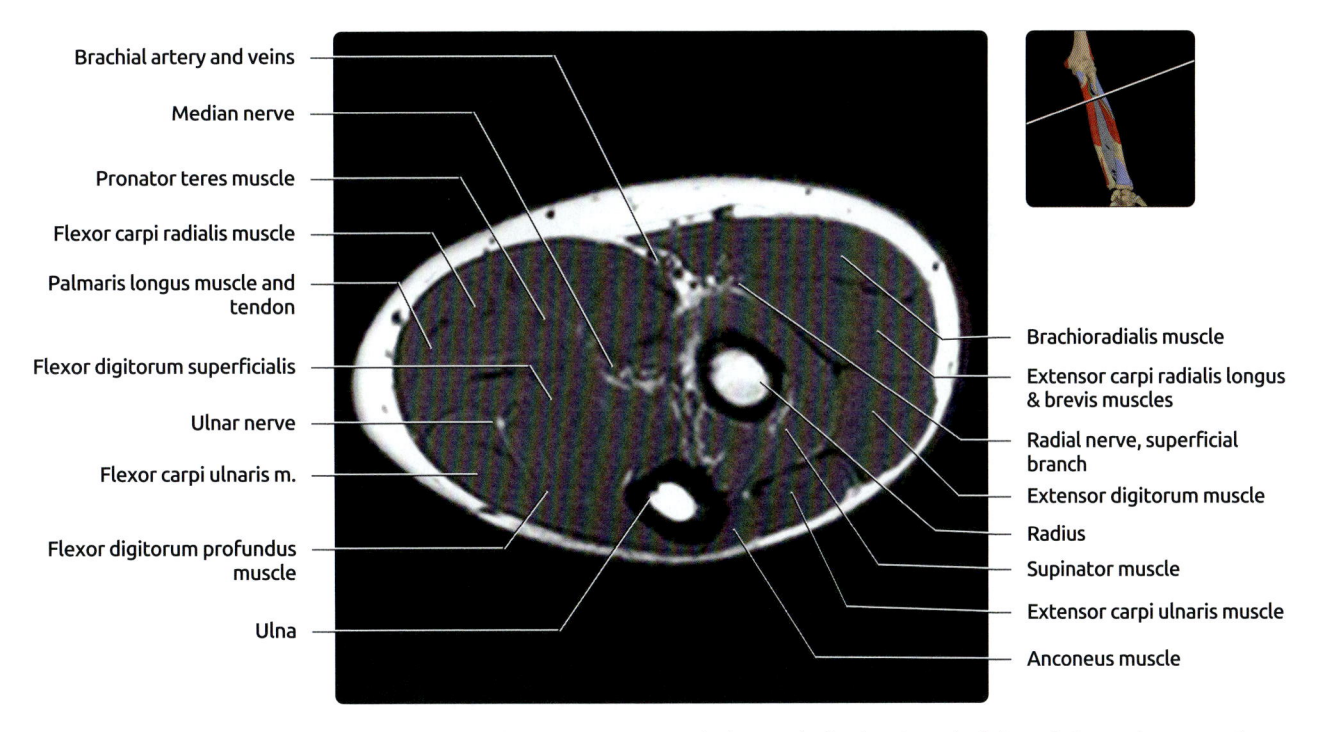

Bottom image labels:
- Brachial artery and veins
- Median nerve
- Pronator teres muscle
- Flexor carpi radialis muscle
- Palmaris longus muscle and tendon
- Flexor digitorum superficialis
- Ulnar nerve
- Flexor carpi ulnaris m.
- Flexor digitorum profundus muscle
- Ulna
- Brachioradialis muscle
- Extensor carpi radialis longus & brevis muscles
- Radial nerve, superficial branch
- Extensor digitorum muscle
- Radius
- Supinator muscle
- Extensor carpi ulnaris muscle
- Anconeus muscle

(Top) The flexor muscles are grouped anteriorly and the extensors posteriorly. (Bottom) The deep branch of the radial nerve has entered the supinator muscle on its way toward the posterior compartment of the forearm and is not discernible.

Forearm Radiographic Anatomy and MR Atlas

AXIAL T1 MR, RIGHT FOREARM

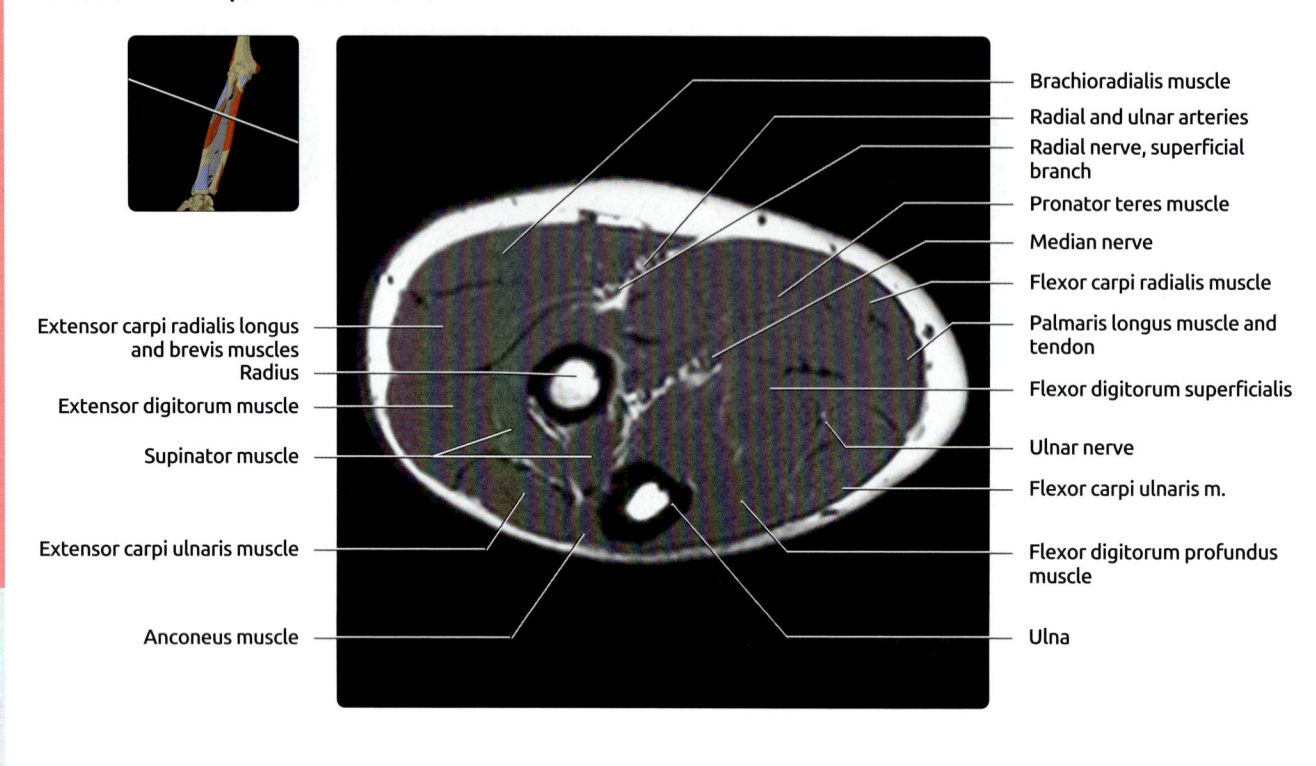

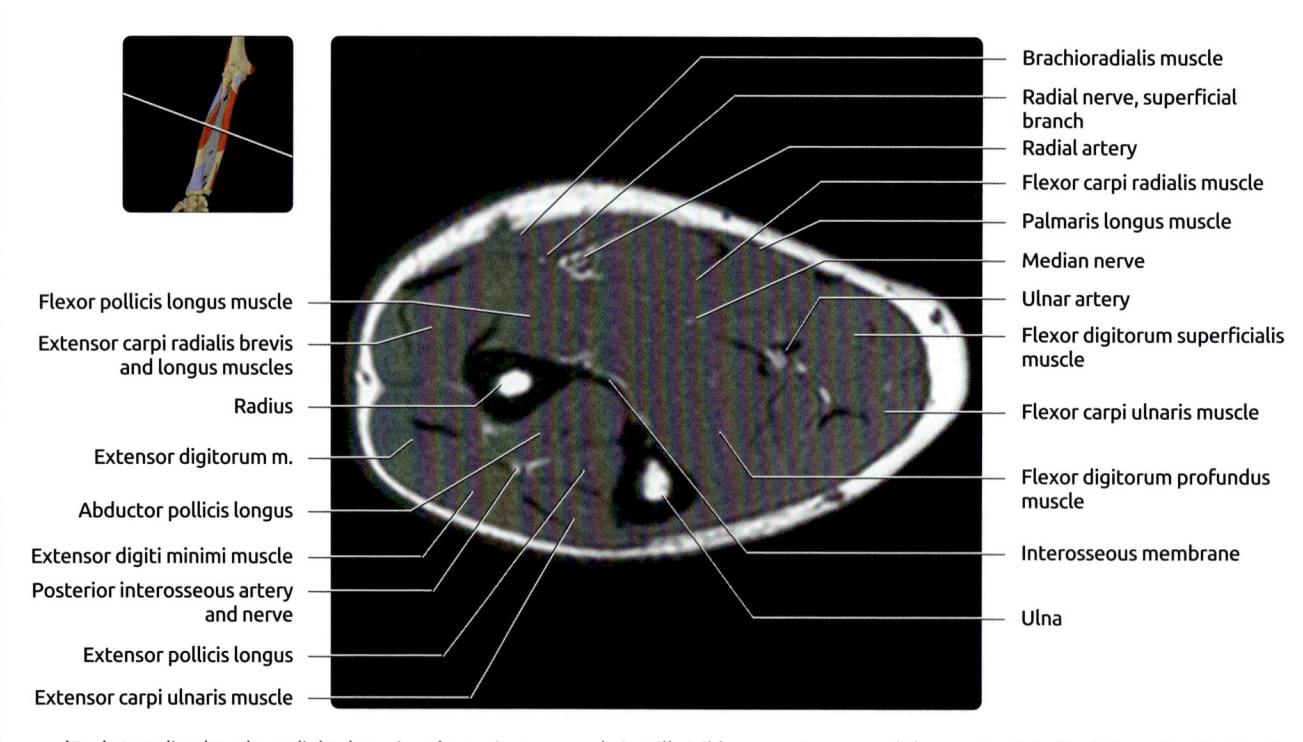

Labels (top image):
- Brachioradialis muscle
- Radial and ulnar arteries
- Radial nerve, superficial branch
- Pronator teres muscle
- Median nerve
- Flexor carpi radialis muscle
- Palmaris longus muscle and tendon
- Flexor digitorum superficialis
- Ulnar nerve
- Flexor carpi ulnaris m.
- Flexor digitorum profundus muscle
- Ulna
- Extensor carpi radialis longus and brevis muscles
- Radius
- Extensor digitorum muscle
- Supinator muscle
- Extensor carpi ulnaris muscle
- Anconeus muscle

Labels (bottom image):
- Brachioradialis muscle
- Radial nerve, superficial branch
- Radial artery
- Flexor carpi radialis muscle
- Palmaris longus muscle
- Median nerve
- Ulnar artery
- Flexor digitorum superficialis muscle
- Flexor carpi ulnaris muscle
- Flexor digitorum profundus muscle
- Interosseous membrane
- Ulna
- Flexor pollicis longus muscle
- Extensor carpi radialis brevis and longus muscles
- Radius
- Extensor digitorum m.
- Abductor pollicis longus
- Extensor digiti minimi muscle
- Posterior interosseous artery and nerve
- Extensor pollicis longus
- Extensor carpi ulnaris muscle

(Top) *Just distal to the radial tuberosity, the supinator muscle is still visible, wrapping around the proximal shaft of the radius.* **(Bottom)** *The interosseous membrane is now visible, helping to separate the anterior and posterior compartments.*

Forearm Radiographic Anatomy and MR Atlas

AXIAL T1 MR, LEFT FOREARM

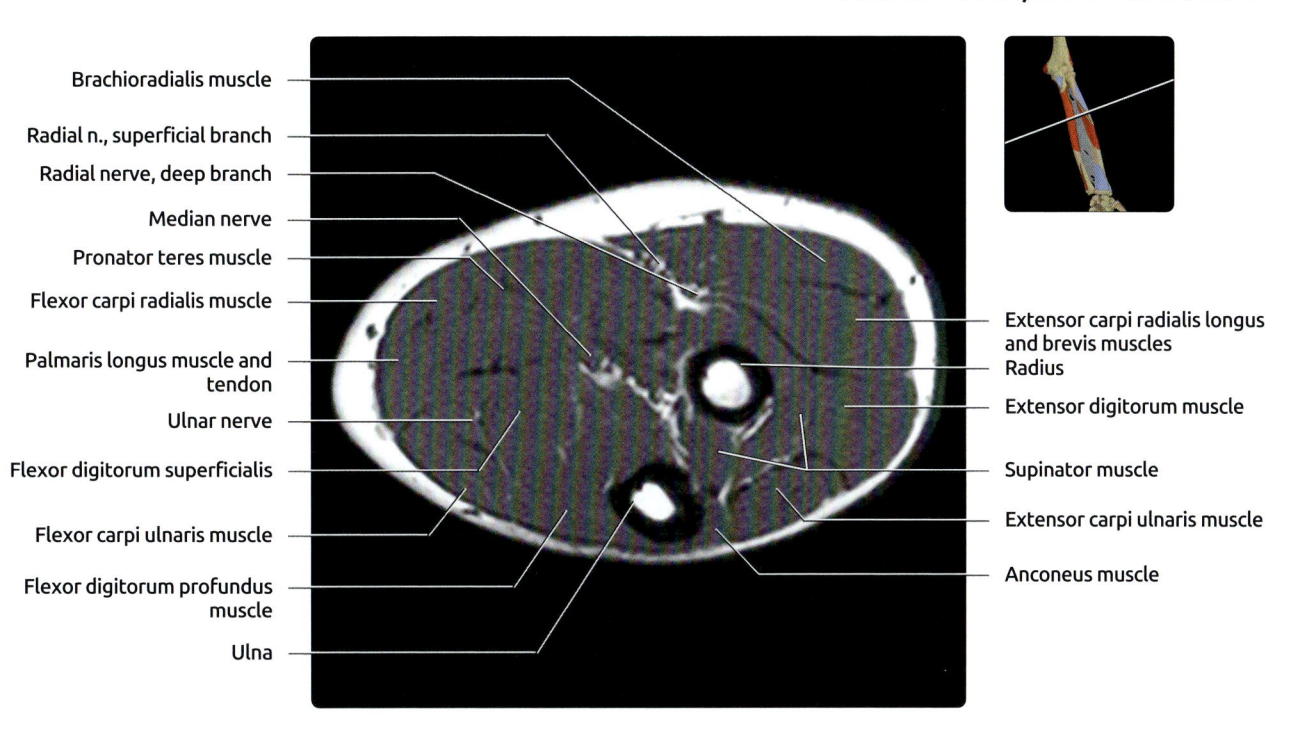

Top image labels:
- Brachioradialis muscle
- Radial n., superficial branch
- Radial nerve, deep branch
- Median nerve
- Pronator teres muscle
- Flexor carpi radialis muscle
- Palmaris longus muscle and tendon
- Ulnar nerve
- Flexor digitorum superficialis
- Flexor carpi ulnaris muscle
- Flexor digitorum profundus muscle
- Ulna
- Extensor carpi radialis longus and brevis muscles
- Radius
- Extensor digitorum muscle
- Supinator muscle
- Extensor carpi ulnaris muscle
- Anconeus muscle

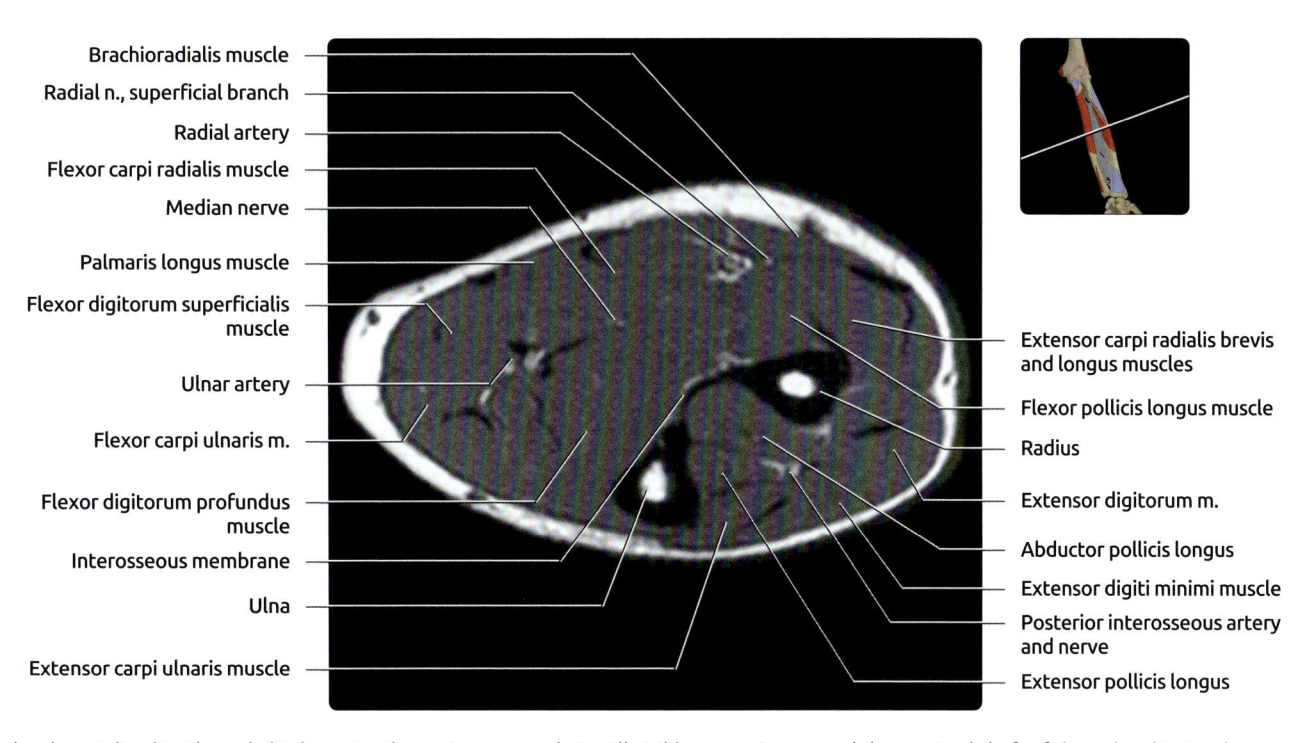

Bottom image labels:
- Brachioradialis muscle
- Radial n., superficial branch
- Radial artery
- Flexor carpi radialis muscle
- Median nerve
- Palmaris longus muscle
- Flexor digitorum superficialis muscle
- Ulnar artery
- Flexor carpi ulnaris m.
- Flexor digitorum profundus muscle
- Interosseous membrane
- Ulna
- Extensor carpi ulnaris muscle
- Extensor carpi radialis brevis and longus muscles
- Flexor pollicis longus muscle
- Radius
- Extensor digitorum m.
- Abductor pollicis longus
- Extensor digiti minimi muscle
- Posterior interosseous artery and nerve
- Extensor pollicis longus

(Top) Just distal to the radial tuberosity, the supinator muscle is still visible, wrapping around the proximal shaft of the radius. (Bottom) The interosseous membrane is now visible, helping to separate the anterior and posterior compartments.

Forearm Radiographic Anatomy and MR Atlas

AXIAL T1 MR, RIGHT FOREARM

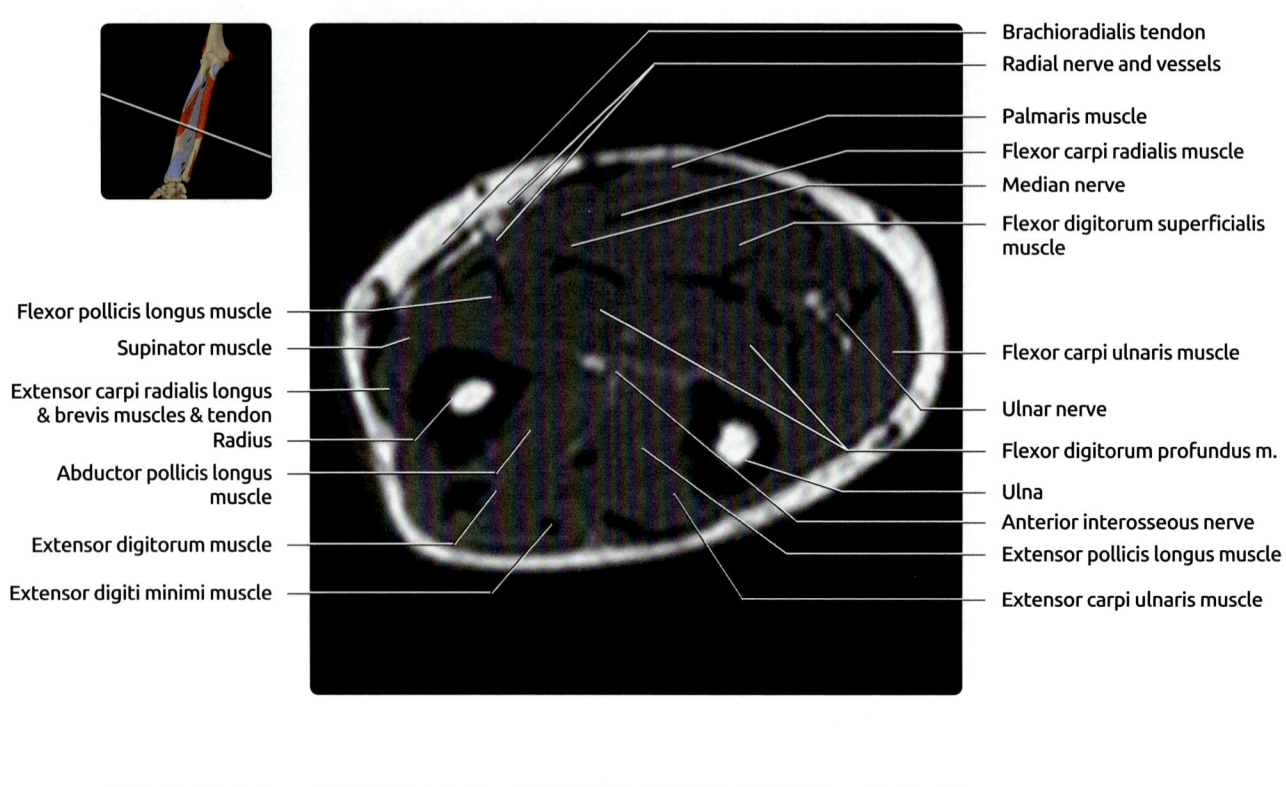

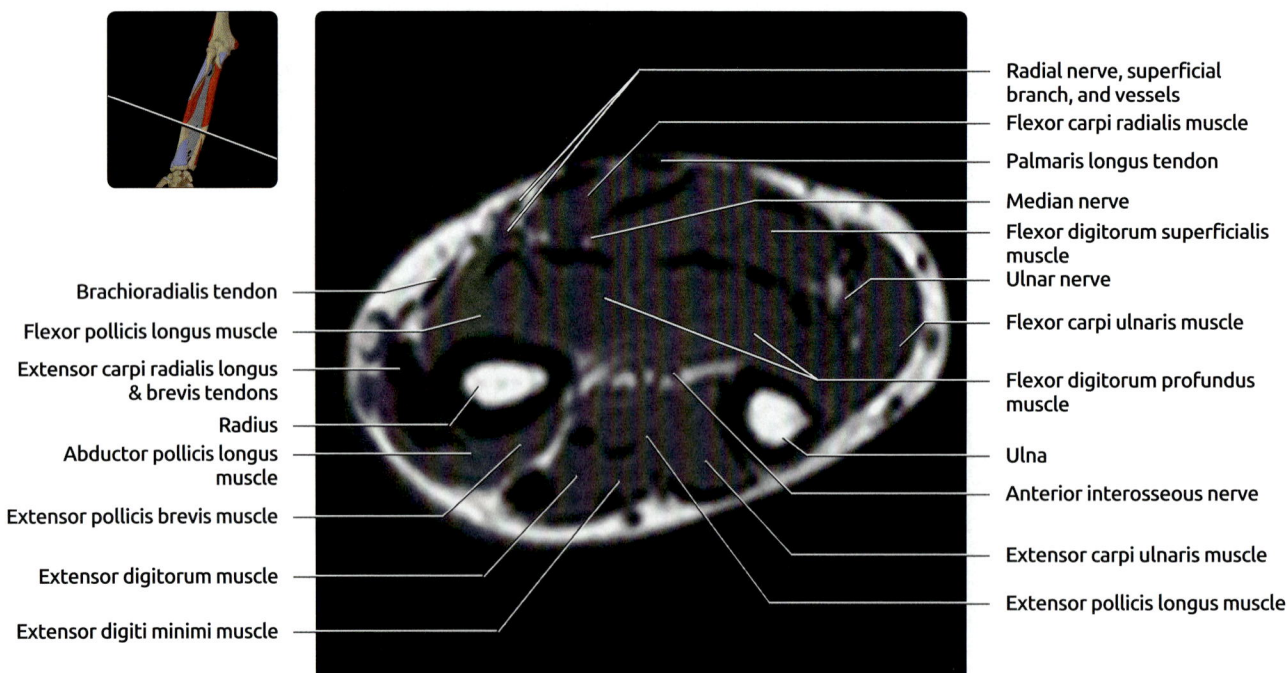

Top image labels (left side):
- Flexor pollicis longus muscle
- Supinator muscle
- Extensor carpi radialis longus & brevis muscles & tendon
- Radius
- Abductor pollicis longus muscle
- Extensor digitorum muscle
- Extensor digiti minimi muscle

Top image labels (right side):
- Brachioradialis tendon
- Radial nerve and vessels
- Palmaris muscle
- Flexor carpi radialis muscle
- Median nerve
- Flexor digitorum superficialis muscle
- Flexor carpi ulnaris muscle
- Ulnar nerve
- Flexor digitorum profundus m.
- Ulna
- Anterior interosseous nerve
- Extensor pollicis longus muscle
- Extensor carpi ulnaris muscle

Bottom image labels (left side):
- Brachioradialis tendon
- Flexor pollicis longus muscle
- Extensor carpi radialis longus & brevis tendons
- Radius
- Abductor pollicis longus muscle
- Extensor pollicis brevis muscle
- Extensor digitorum muscle
- Extensor digiti minimi muscle

Bottom image labels (right side):
- Radial nerve, superficial branch, and vessels
- Flexor carpi radialis muscle
- Palmaris longus tendon
- Median nerve
- Flexor digitorum superficialis muscle
- Ulnar nerve
- Flexor carpi ulnaris muscle
- Flexor digitorum profundus muscle
- Ulna
- Anterior interosseous nerve
- Extensor carpi ulnaris muscle
- Extensor pollicis longus muscle

(Top) The interosseous membrane is not as prominent in this image. The ulnar nerve and median nerve are located in the intermuscular septum between the deep flexors (flexor digitorum and flexor pollicis longus) and the more superficial flexors of the anterior compartment. **(Bottom)** The anterior interosseous nerve and accompanying vessels are well seen anterior to the interosseous membrane.

Forearm Radiographic Anatomy and MR Atlas

AXIAL T1 MR, LEFT FOREARM

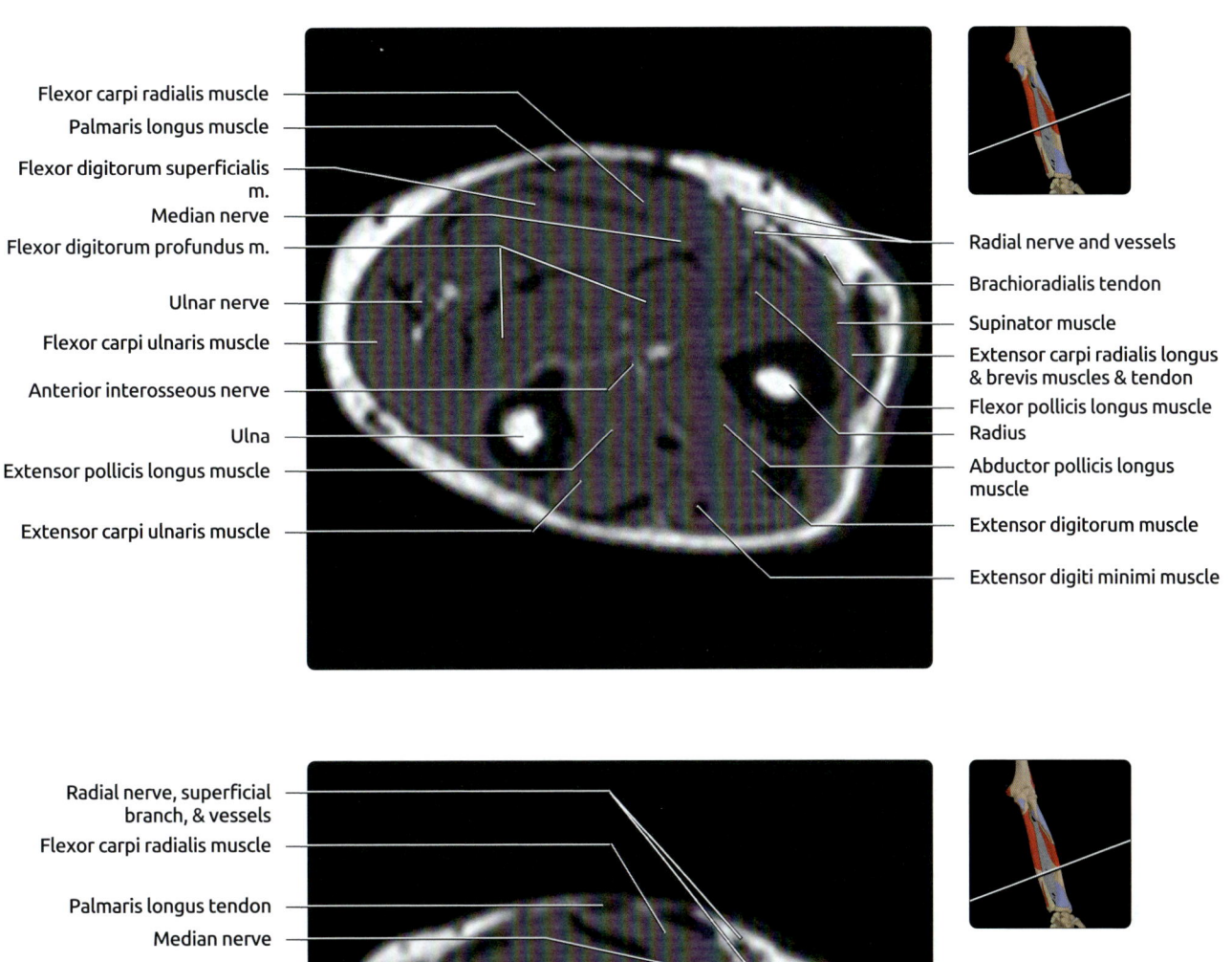

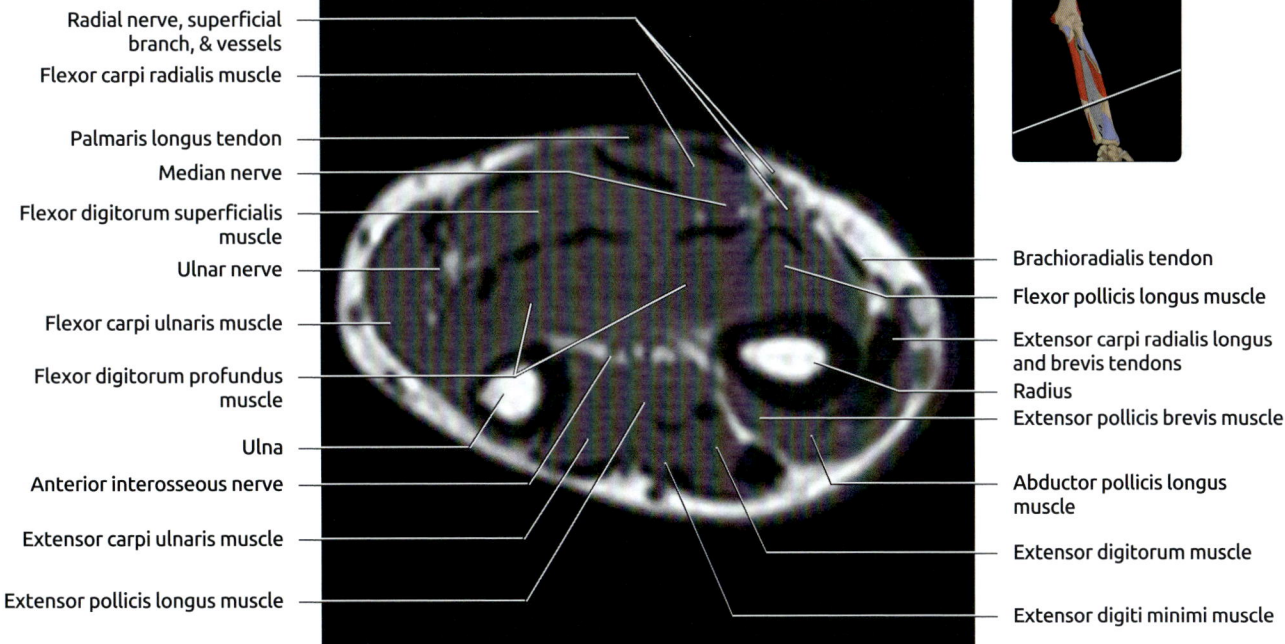

Top image labels:
- Flexor carpi radialis muscle
- Palmaris longus muscle
- Flexor digitorum superficialis m.
- Median nerve
- Flexor digitorum profundus m.
- Ulnar nerve
- Flexor carpi ulnaris muscle
- Anterior interosseous nerve
- Ulna
- Extensor pollicis longus muscle
- Extensor carpi ulnaris muscle
- Radial nerve and vessels
- Brachioradialis tendon
- Supinator muscle
- Extensor carpi radialis longus & brevis muscles & tendon
- Flexor pollicis longus muscle
- Radius
- Abductor pollicis longus muscle
- Extensor digitorum muscle
- Extensor digiti minimi muscle

Bottom image labels:
- Radial nerve, superficial branch, & vessels
- Flexor carpi radialis muscle
- Palmaris longus tendon
- Median nerve
- Flexor digitorum superficialis muscle
- Ulnar nerve
- Flexor carpi ulnaris muscle
- Flexor digitorum profundus muscle
- Ulna
- Anterior interosseous nerve
- Extensor carpi ulnaris muscle
- Extensor pollicis longus muscle
- Brachioradialis tendon
- Flexor pollicis longus muscle
- Extensor carpi radialis longus and brevis tendons
- Radius
- Extensor pollicis brevis muscle
- Abductor pollicis longus muscle
- Extensor digitorum muscle
- Extensor digiti minimi muscle

(**Top**) *The interosseous membrane is not as prominent in this image. The ulnar nerve and median nerve are located in the intermuscular septum between the deep flexors (flexor digitorum and flexor pollicis longus) and the more superficial flexors of the anterior compartment.* (**Bottom**) *The anterior interosseous nerve and accompanying vessels are well seen anterior to the interosseous membrane.*

Forearm Radiographic Anatomy and MR Atlas

AXIAL T1 MR, RIGHT FOREARM

Labels (top image):
- Flexor carpi radialis tendon
- Palmaris longus tendon
- Median nerve
- Flexor digitorum superficialis m.
- Flexor carpi ulnari muscle
- Ulnar nerve
- Flexor digitorum profundus muscle
- Pronator quadratus muscle
- Ulna
- Extensor digiti minimi muscle
- Extensor indicis muscle
- Extensor digitorum muscle
- Flexor pollicis longus muscle
- Radius
- Extensor pollicis brevis tendon
- Abductor pollicis longus tendon
- Extensor carpi radialis longus and brevis muscles and tendon
- Extensor pollicis longus tendon

Labels (bottom image):
- Flexor carpi radialis tendon
- Palmaris longus tendon
- Median nerve
- Flexor digitorum superficialis muscle
- Flexor carpi ulnari muscle
- Ulnar nerve
- Flexor digitorum profundus muscle
- Pronator quadratus muscle
- Ulna
- Extensor digiti minimi tendon
- Extensor indicis tendon
- Extensor digitorum muscle
- Flexor pollicis longus tendon
- Radius
- Extensor pollicis brevis tendon
- Abductor pollicis longus tendon
- Extensor carpi radialis brevis and longus tendons
- Extensor pollicis longus tendon

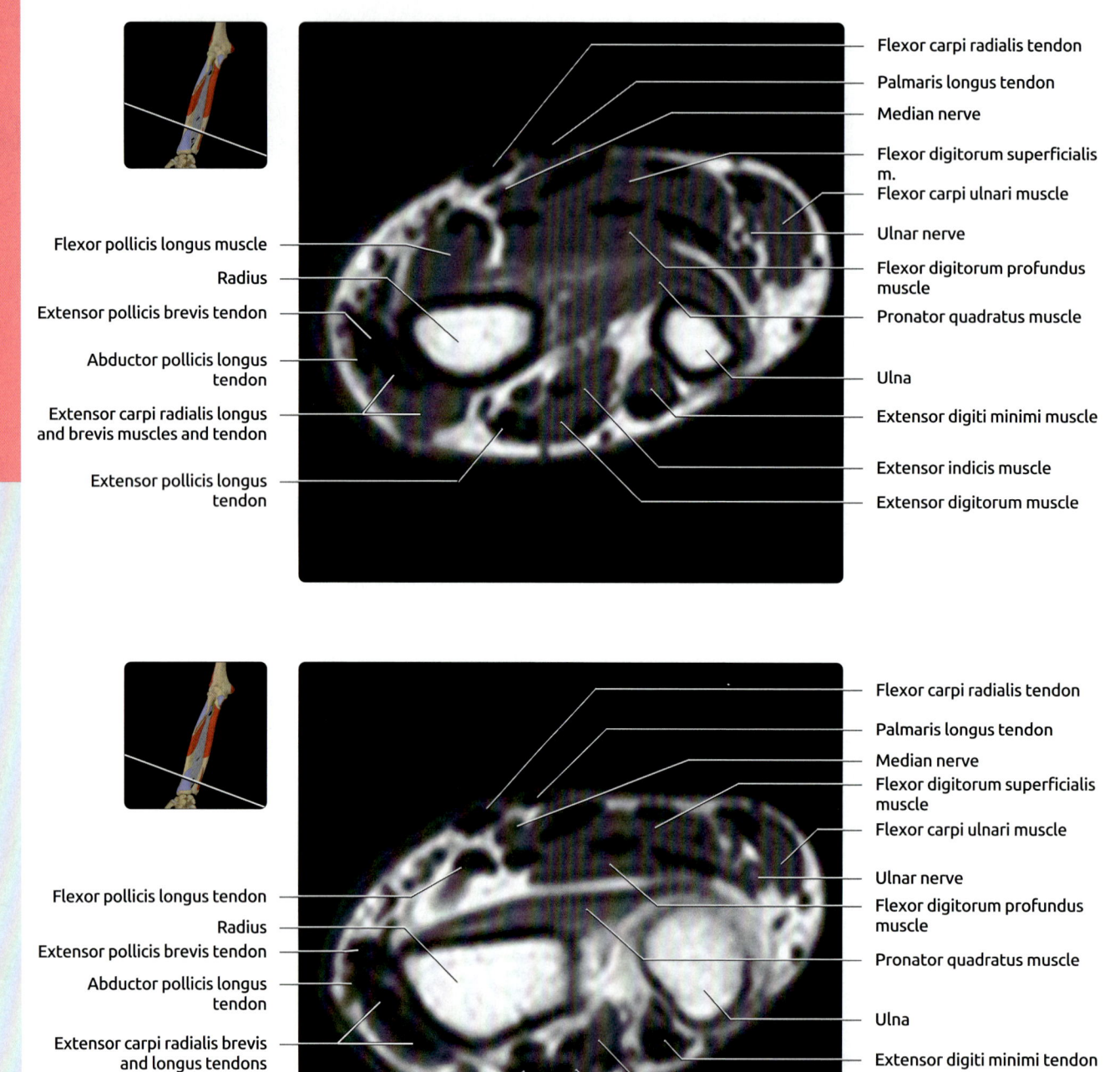

(Top) The tendons of the abductor pollicis longus and extensor pollicis brevis cross superficial and anterior to the tendons of the extensor carpi radialis brevis and longus. At this level of the distal forearm, the pronator quadratus is now visible. **(Bottom)** The extensor tendons are starting to align themselves into the 6 extensor compartments of the wrist.

Forearm Radiographic Anatomy and MR Atlas

AXIAL T1 MR, LEFT FOREARM

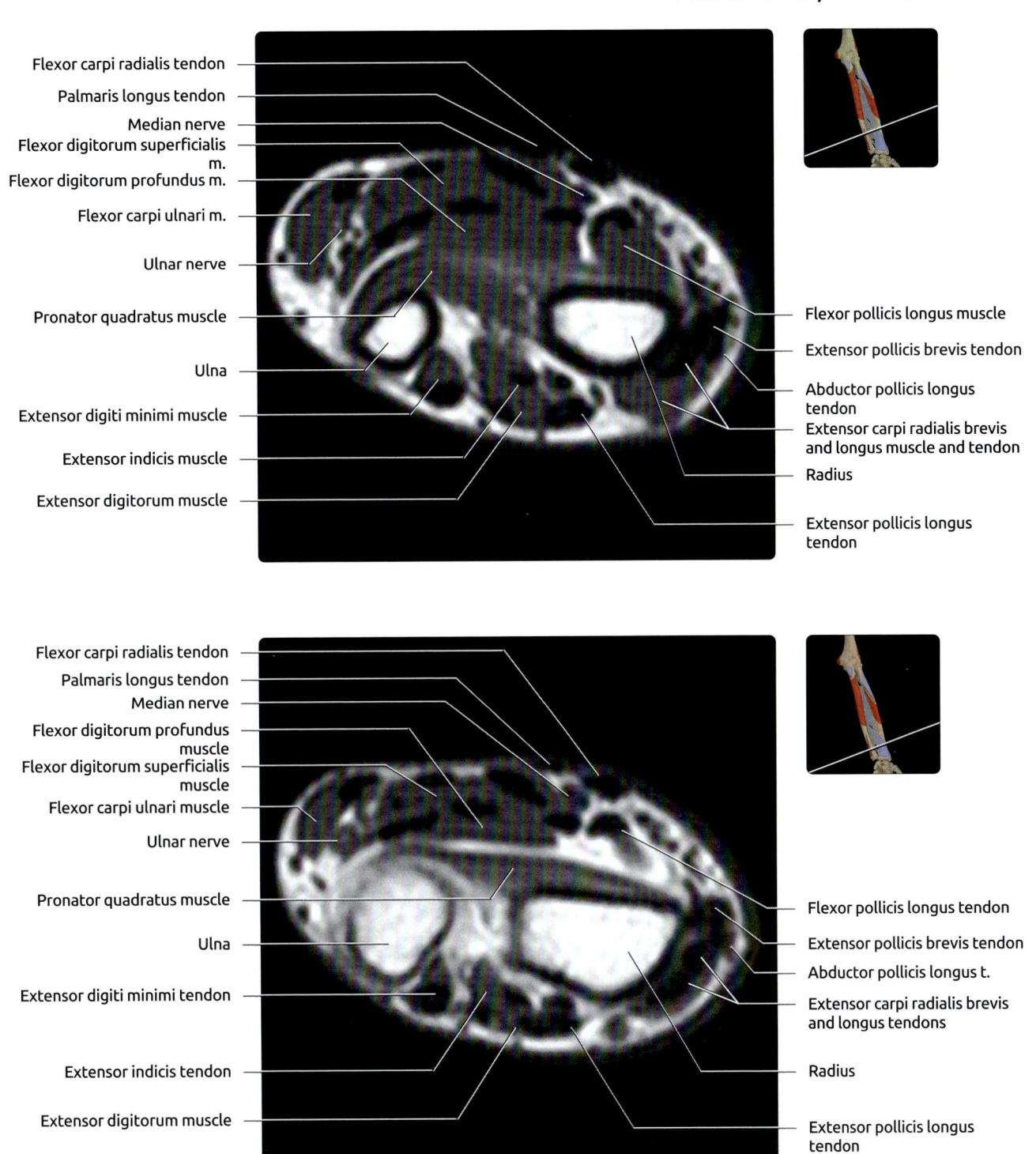

(Top) The tendons of the abductor pollicis longus and extensor pollicis brevis cross superficial and anterior to the tendons of the extensor carpi radialis brevis and longus. At this level of the distal forearm, the pronator quadratus is now visible. **(Bottom)** The extensor tendons are starting to align themselves into the 6 extensor compartments of the wrist.

Forearm Radiographic Anatomy and MR Atlas

AXIAL T1 MR, RIGHT FOREARM

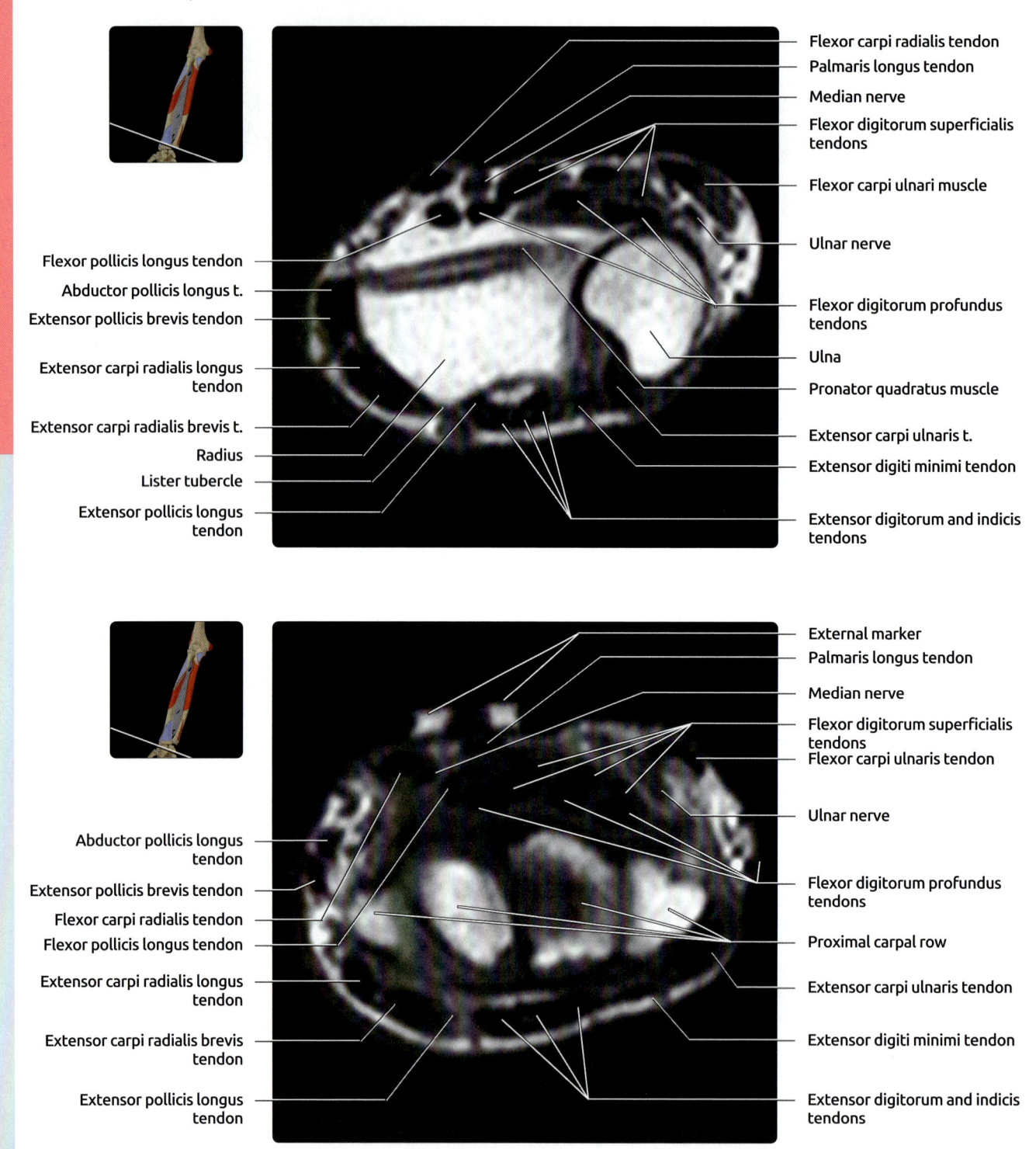

Labels (top image):
- Flexor carpi radialis tendon
- Palmaris longus tendon
- Median nerve
- Flexor digitorum superficialis tendons
- Flexor carpi ulnari muscle
- Ulnar nerve
- Flexor digitorum profundus tendons
- Ulna
- Pronator quadratus muscle
- Extensor carpi ulnaris t.
- Extensor digiti minimi tendon
- Extensor digitorum and indicis tendons
- Flexor pollicis longus tendon
- Abductor pollicis longus t.
- Extensor pollicis brevis tendon
- Extensor carpi radialis longus tendon
- Extensor carpi radialis brevis t.
- Radius
- Lister tubercle
- Extensor pollicis longus tendon

Labels (bottom image):
- External marker
- Palmaris longus tendon
- Median nerve
- Flexor digitorum superficialis tendons
- Flexor carpi ulnaris tendon
- Ulnar nerve
- Flexor digitorum profundus tendons
- Proximal carpal row
- Extensor carpi ulnaris tendon
- Extensor digiti minimi tendon
- Extensor digitorum and indicis tendons
- Abductor pollicis longus tendon
- Extensor pollicis brevis tendon
- Flexor carpi radialis tendon
- Flexor pollicis longus tendon
- Extensor carpi radialis longus tendon
- Extensor carpi radialis brevis tendon
- Extensor pollicis longus tendon

(Top) The wrist is supinated. The 6 extensor compartments are visualized. **(Bottom)** The tendons of the forearm muscles have now passed into the wrist.

Forearm Radiographic Anatomy and MR Atlas

AXIAL T1 MR, LEFT FOREARM

Top image labels:
- Flexor carpi radialis tendon
- Palmaris longus tendon
- Median nerve
- Flexor digitorum superficialis tendons
- Flexor carpi ulnari muscle
- Ulnar nerve
- Flexor digitorum profundus t.
- Ulna
- Extensor carpi ulnaris tendon
- Extensor digiti minimi tendon
- Extensor digitorum and indicis tendons
- Flexor pollicis longus t.
- Abductor pollicis longus tendon
- Pronator quadratus m.
- Extensor pollicis brevis tendon
- Extensor carpi radialis longus tendon
- Extensor carpi radialis brevis t.
- Radius
- Lister tubercle
- Extensor pollicis longus tendon

Bottom image labels:
- External marker
- Palmaris longus tendon
- Median nerve
- Flexor digitorum superficialis tendons
- Flexor carpi ulnaris tendon
- Ulnar nerve
- Flexor digitorum profundus tendons
- Proximal carpal row
- Extensor carpi ulnaris tendon
- Extensor digiti minimi tendon
- Extensor digitorum and indicis tendons
- Abductor pollicis longus t.
- Flexor carpi radialis t.
- Extensor pollicis brevis tendon
- Flexor pollicis longus tendon
- Extensor carpi radialis longus t.
- Extensor carpi radialis brevis tendon
- Extensor pollicis longus tendon

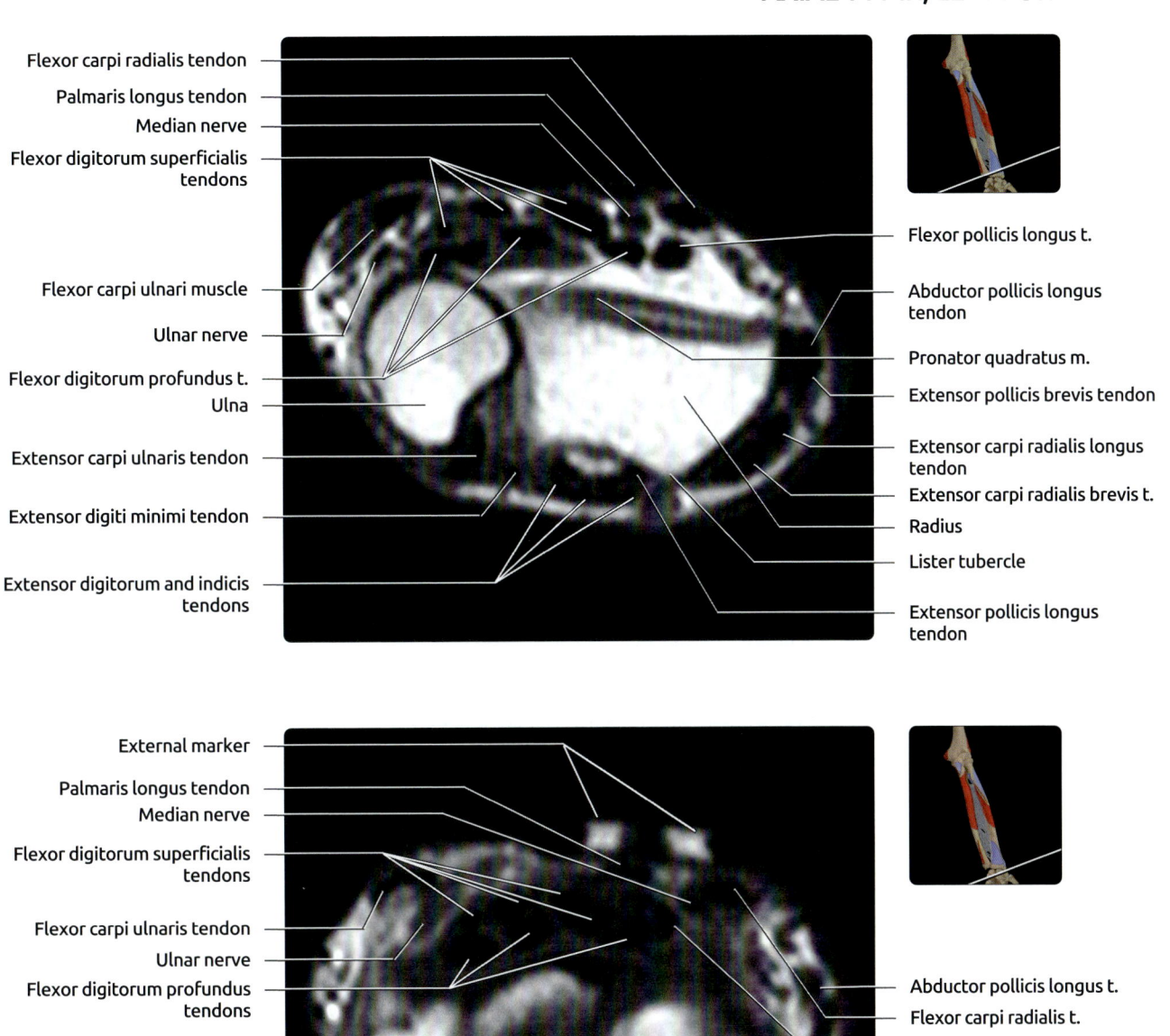

(**Top**) *The wrist is supinated. The 6 extensor compartments are visualized.* (**Bottom**) *The tendons of the forearm muscles have now passed into the wrist.*

Forearm Radiographic Anatomy and MR Atlas

CORONAL T1 MR, RIGHT FOREARM

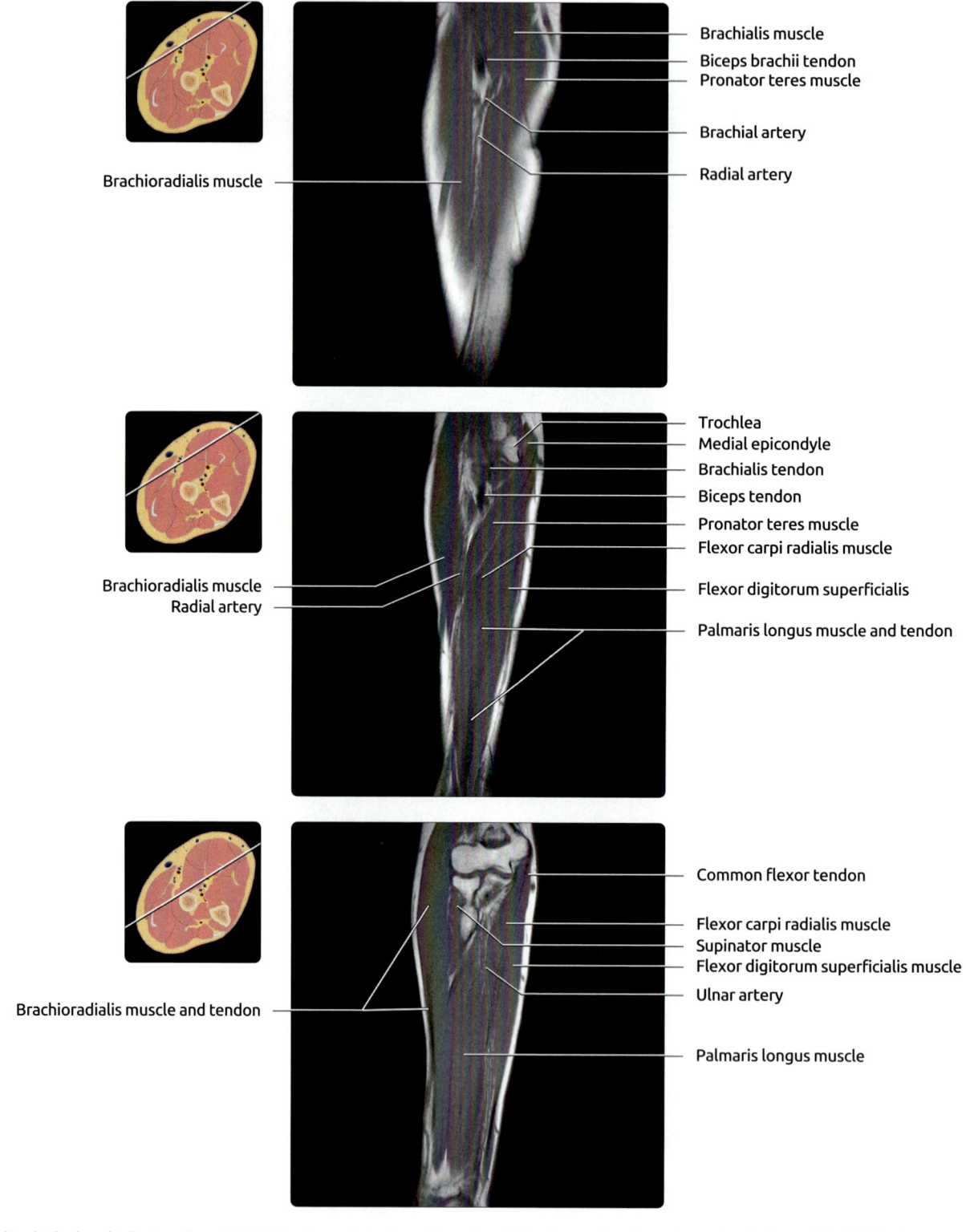

Brachialis muscle
Biceps brachii tendon
Pronator teres muscle
Brachial artery
Radial artery
Brachioradialis muscle

Trochlea
Medial epicondyle
Brachialis tendon
Biceps tendon
Pronator teres muscle
Flexor carpi radialis muscle
Flexor digitorum superficialis
Palmaris longus muscle and tendon
Brachioradialis muscle
Radial artery

Common flexor tendon
Flexor carpi radialis muscle
Supinator muscle
Flexor digitorum superficialis muscle
Ulnar artery
Palmaris longus muscle
Brachioradialis muscle and tendon

(**Top**) *The brachial artery has divided into the radial artery (shown) and the ulnar artery (not shown in this image).* (**Middle**) *The pronator teres sweeps from the medial epicondyle to the proximal radius. Note the brachialis tendon located medial to the biceps tendon.* (**Bottom**) *The brachioradialis muscle is the most lateral of all the forearm muscles.*

Forearm Radiographic Anatomy and MR Atlas

CORONAL T1 MR, LEFT FOREARM

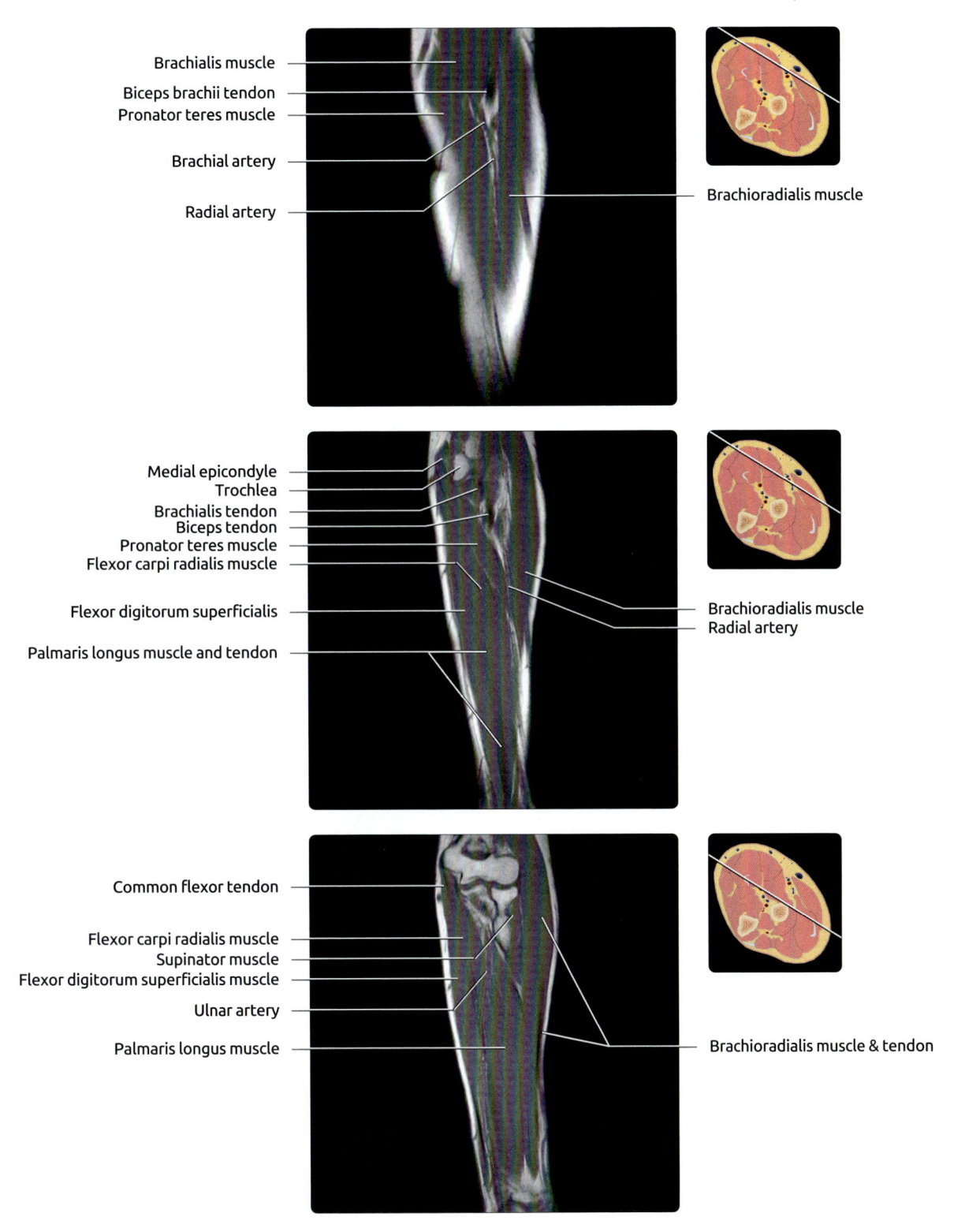

- Brachialis muscle
- Biceps brachii tendon
- Pronator teres muscle
- Brachial artery
- Radial artery
- Brachioradialis muscle

- Medial epicondyle
- Trochlea
- Brachialis tendon
- Biceps tendon
- Pronator teres muscle
- Flexor carpi radialis muscle
- Flexor digitorum superficialis
- Palmaris longus muscle and tendon
- Brachioradialis muscle
- Radial artery

- Common flexor tendon
- Flexor carpi radialis muscle
- Supinator muscle
- Flexor digitorum superficialis muscle
- Ulnar artery
- Palmaris longus muscle
- Brachioradialis muscle & tendon

(Top) The brachial artery has divided into the radial artery (shown) and the ulnar artery (not shown in this image). (Middle) The pronator teres sweeps from the medial epicondyle to the proximal radius. Note the brachialis tendon located medial to the biceps tendon. (Bottom) The brachioradialis muscle is the most lateral of all the forearm muscles.

Forearm Radiographic Anatomy and MR Atlas

CORONAL T1 MR, RIGHT FOREARM

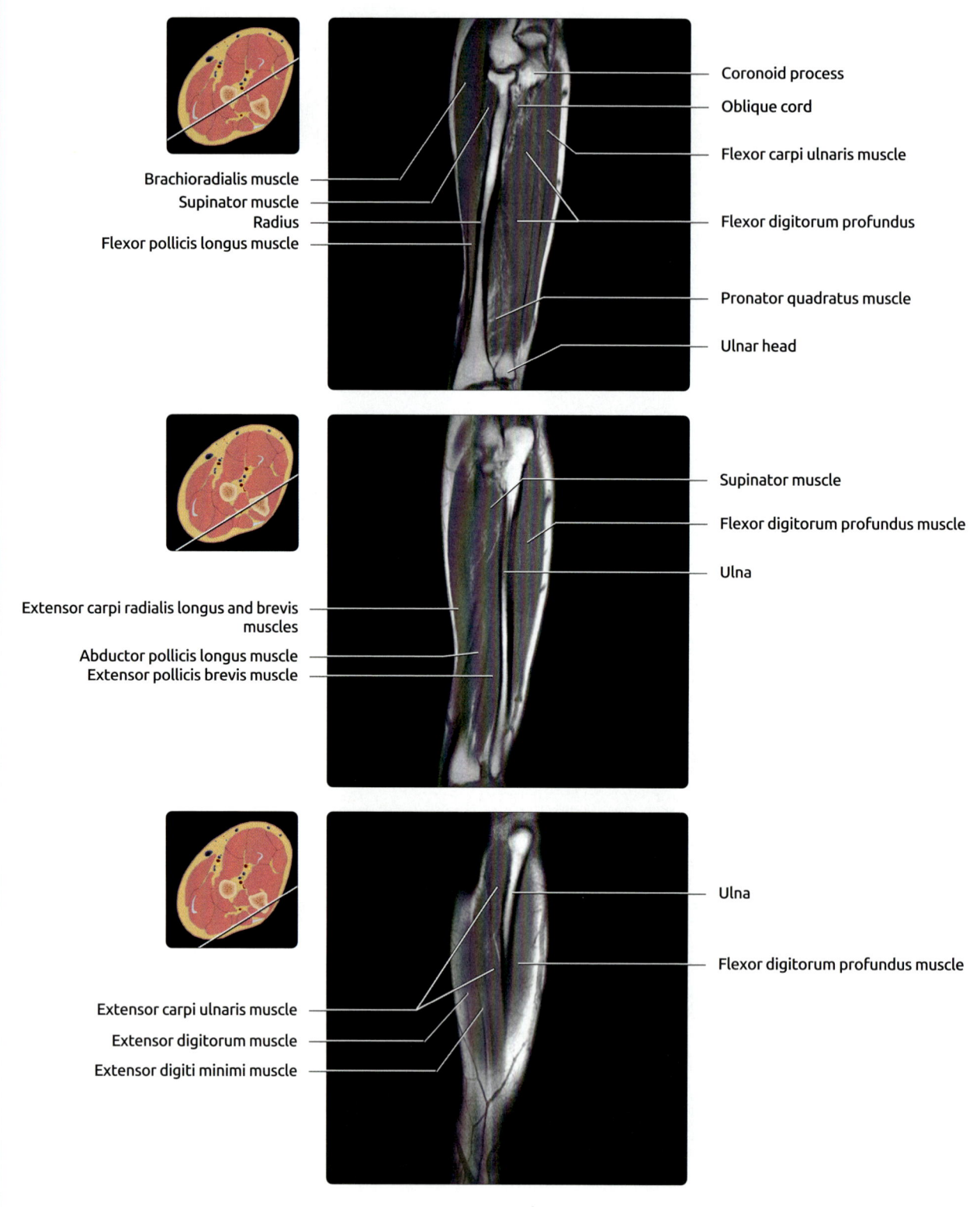

Labels (top image):
- Brachioradialis muscle
- Supinator muscle
- Radius
- Flexor pollicis longus muscle
- Coronoid process
- Oblique cord
- Flexor carpi ulnaris muscle
- Flexor digitorum profundus
- Pronator quadratus muscle
- Ulnar head

Labels (middle image):
- Extensor carpi radialis longus and brevis muscles
- Abductor pollicis longus muscle
- Extensor pollicis brevis muscle
- Supinator muscle
- Flexor digitorum profundus muscle
- Ulna

Labels (bottom image):
- Extensor carpi ulnaris muscle
- Extensor digitorum muscle
- Extensor digiti minimi muscle
- Ulna
- Flexor digitorum profundus muscle

(**Top**) *Just anterior to the ulna and interosseous membrane, the 3 deep muscles of the anterior compartment are seen: Flexor carpi ulnaris, flexor digitorum profundus, and pronator quadratus.* (**Middle**) *The flexor digitorum profundus muscle drapes over the medial aspect of the ulna and is separated from the extensor muscles of the posterior compartment by the posterior ridge of the ulna.* (**Bottom**) *The extensor carpi ulnaris muscle is the most medial muscle of the posterior compartment.*

Forearm Radiographic Anatomy and MR Atlas

CORONAL T1 MR, LEFT FOREARM

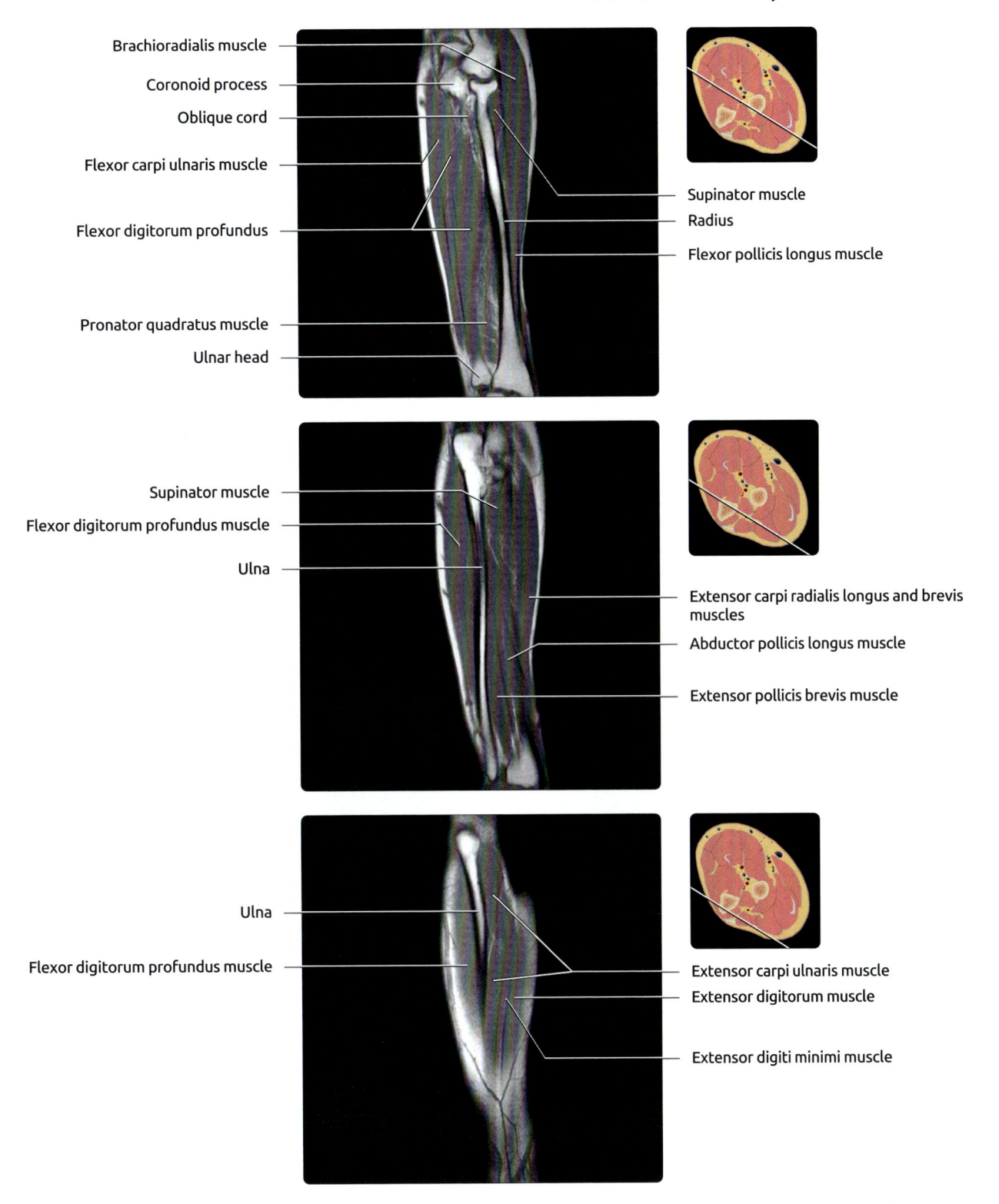

Labels (top image):
- Brachioradialis muscle
- Coronoid process
- Oblique cord
- Flexor carpi ulnaris muscle
- Flexor digitorum profundus
- Pronator quadratus muscle
- Ulnar head
- Supinator muscle
- Radius
- Flexor pollicis longus muscle

Labels (middle image):
- Supinator muscle
- Flexor digitorum profundus muscle
- Ulna
- Extensor carpi radialis longus and brevis muscles
- Abductor pollicis longus muscle
- Extensor pollicis brevis muscle

Labels (bottom image):
- Ulna
- Flexor digitorum profundus muscle
- Extensor carpi ulnaris muscle
- Extensor digitorum muscle
- Extensor digiti minimi muscle

(**Top**) *Just anterior to the ulna and interosseous membrane, the 3 deep muscles of the anterior compartment are seen: Flexor carpi ulnaris, flexor digitorum profundus, and pronator quadratus.* (**Middle**) *The flexor digitorum profundus muscle drapes over the medial aspect of the ulna and is separated from the extensor muscles of the posterior compartment by the posterior ridge of the ulna.* (**Bottom**) *The extensor carpi ulnaris muscle is the most medial muscle of the posterior compartment.*

Forearm Radiographic Anatomy and MR Atlas

SAGITTAL T1 MR, LEFT FOREARM

Brachioradialis muscle

Extensor carpi radialis brevis muscle

Brachioradialis muscle
Extensor carpi radialis longus muscle

Extensor carpi radialis brevis muscle

Radius

Brachioradialis muscle

Extensor carpi radialis longus muscle
Extensor carpi radialis brevis muscle

Radius

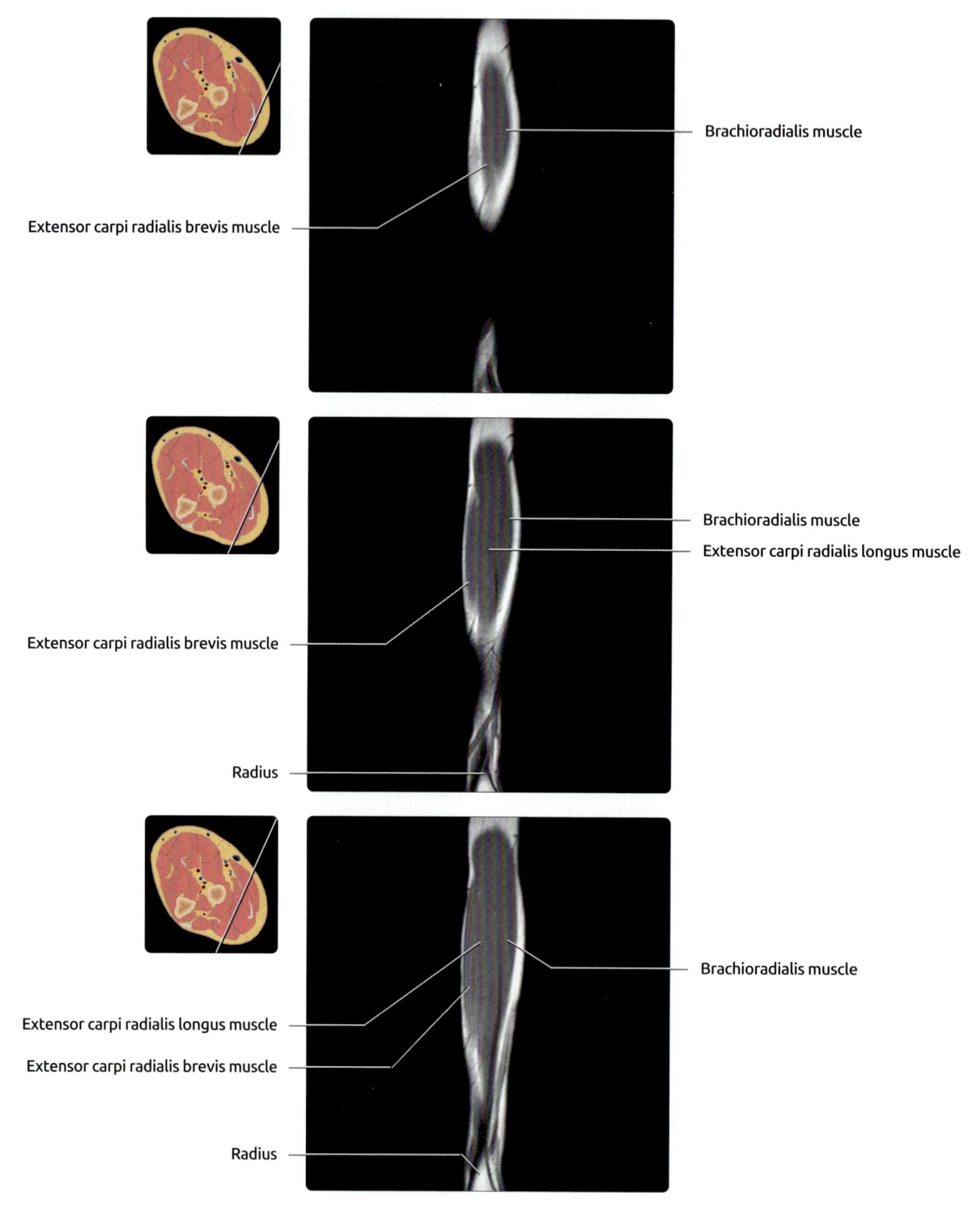

(Top) Sagittal series of the forearm, lateral to medial, are shown. At the extreme lateral aspect of the forearm, only the brachioradialis muscle anteriorly and the extensor carpi radialis brevis muscle posteriorly are visualized. (Middle) The extensor carpi radialis longus muscle is now visible, anterior to the brevis muscle. (Bottom) The brachioradialis tendon will insert on the distal aspect of the radius, while the tendons of the extensor carpi radialis longus and brevis will pass into the wrist via the 2nd extensor compartment.

Forearm Radiographic Anatomy and MR Atlas

SAGITTAL T1 MR, LEFT FOREARM

Top image labels:
- Extensor carpi radialis longus muscle
- Extensor carpi radialis brevis muscle
- Extensor digitorum
- Radius
- Brachioradialis muscle
- Pronator teres muscle
- Flexor pollicis longus muscle

Middle image labels:
- Capitellum
- Radial head
- Supinator muscle
- Brachioradialis muscle
- Radius
- Abductor pollicis longus muscle
- Extensor digitorum muscle
- Distal radius
- Pronator teres muscle
- Flexor pollicis longus muscle
- Flexor carpi radialis muscle
- Palmaris longus tendon

Bottom image labels:
- Brachialis muscle
- Biceps brachii tendon
- Capitellum
- Radial head
- Anconeus muscle
- Abductor pollicis longus muscle
- Extensor digitorum and digiti minimi muscles
- Interosseous membrane
- Cephalic vein
- Supinator muscle
- Flexor pollicis longus muscle
- Flexor carpi radialis muscle
- Palmaris longus tendon

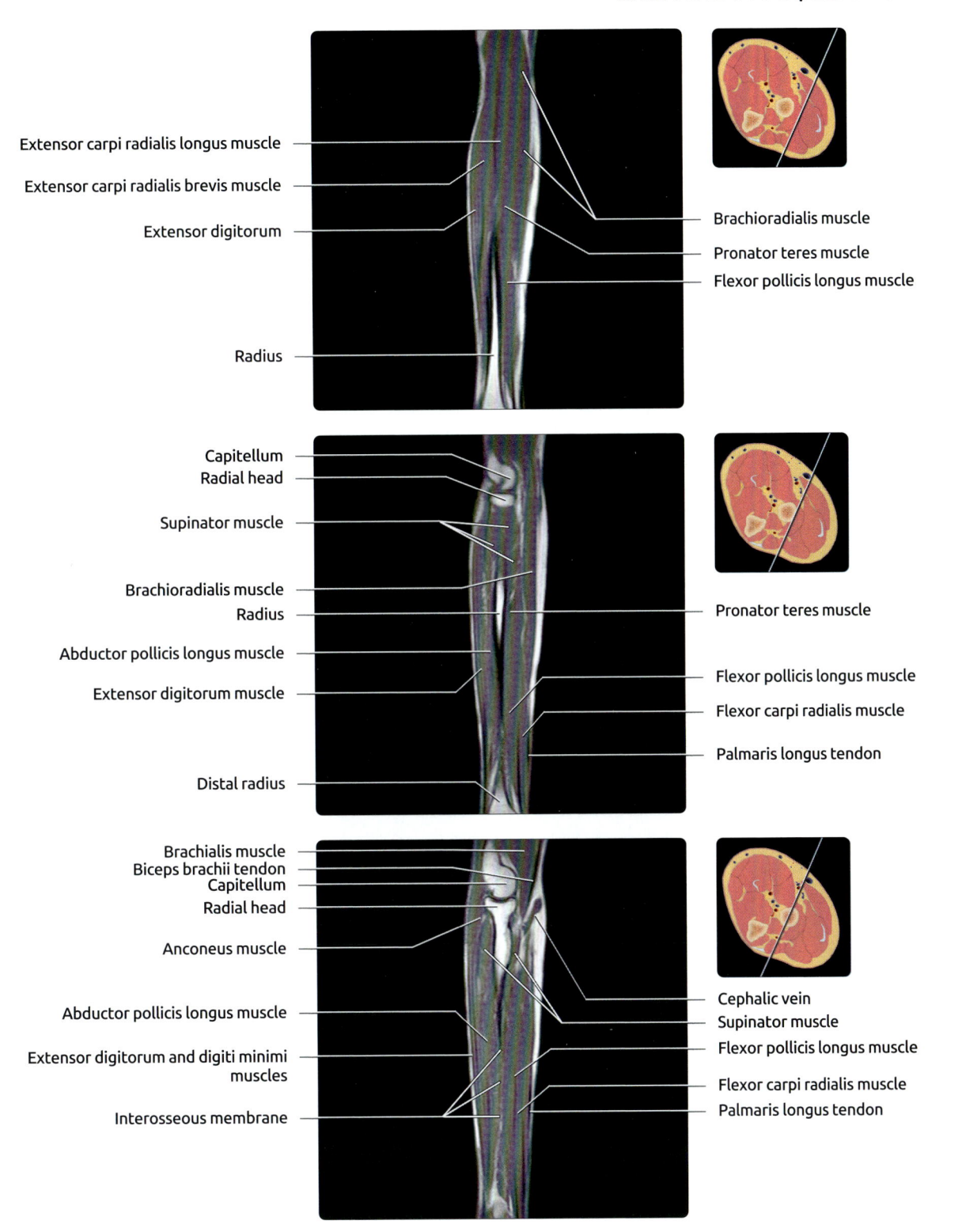

(**Top**) *The brachioradialis muscle is a flexor of the elbow, the pronator teres is a rotator of the radioulnar joints, and the other muscles seen in this image act on the wrist or fingers.* (**Middle**) *The palmaris longus muscle has a long tendon in the extreme anterior aspect of the forearm. This tendon is often harvested for surgical grafts.* (**Bottom**) *The thin cross section of the interosseous membrane is seen, dividing the forearm into anterior (flexor) and posterior (extensor) compartments.*

Forearm Radiographic Anatomy and MR Atlas

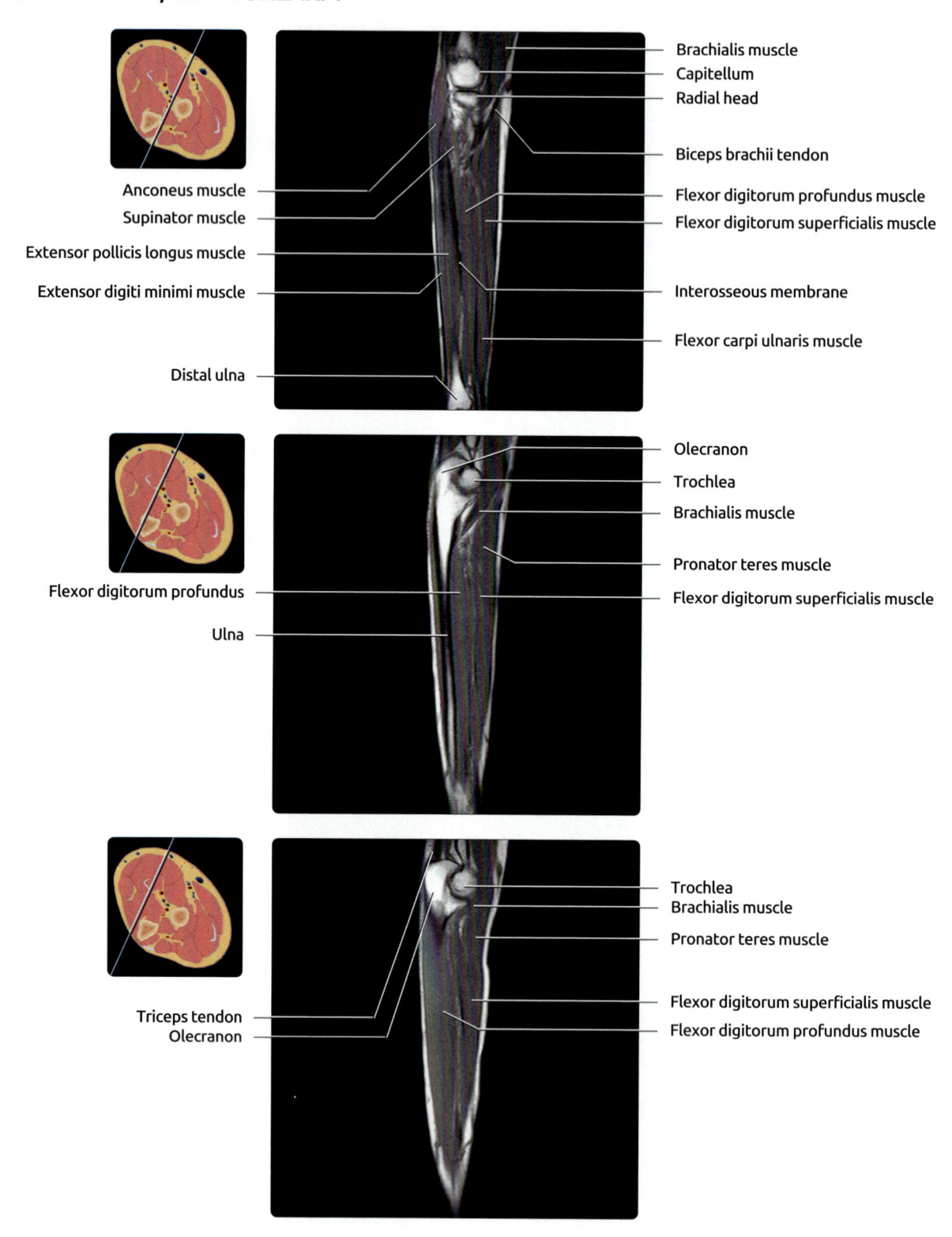

SAGITTAL T1 MR, LEFT FOREARM

Anconeus muscle
Supinator muscle
Extensor pollicis longus muscle
Extensor digiti minimi muscle

Distal ulna

Brachialis muscle
Capitellum
Radial head

Biceps brachii tendon
Flexor digitorum profundus muscle
Flexor digitorum superficialis muscle

Interosseous membrane

Flexor carpi ulnaris muscle

Flexor digitorum profundus
Ulna

Olecranon
Trochlea
Brachialis muscle

Pronator teres muscle
Flexor digitorum superficialis muscle

Triceps tendon
Olecranon

Trochlea
Brachialis muscle
Pronator teres muscle

Flexor digitorum superficialis muscle
Flexor digitorum profundus muscle

(Top) *The flexor digitorum profundus is the deepest and largest muscle of the anterior compartment.* (Middle) *The pronator teres muscle is seen in cross section as it courses obliquely across the proximal aspect of the forearm from its humeroulnar origins to its radial insertion.* (Bottom) *Medial to the posterior ridge of the ulna, all the muscles are flexors.*

Forearm Radiographic Anatomy and MR Atlas

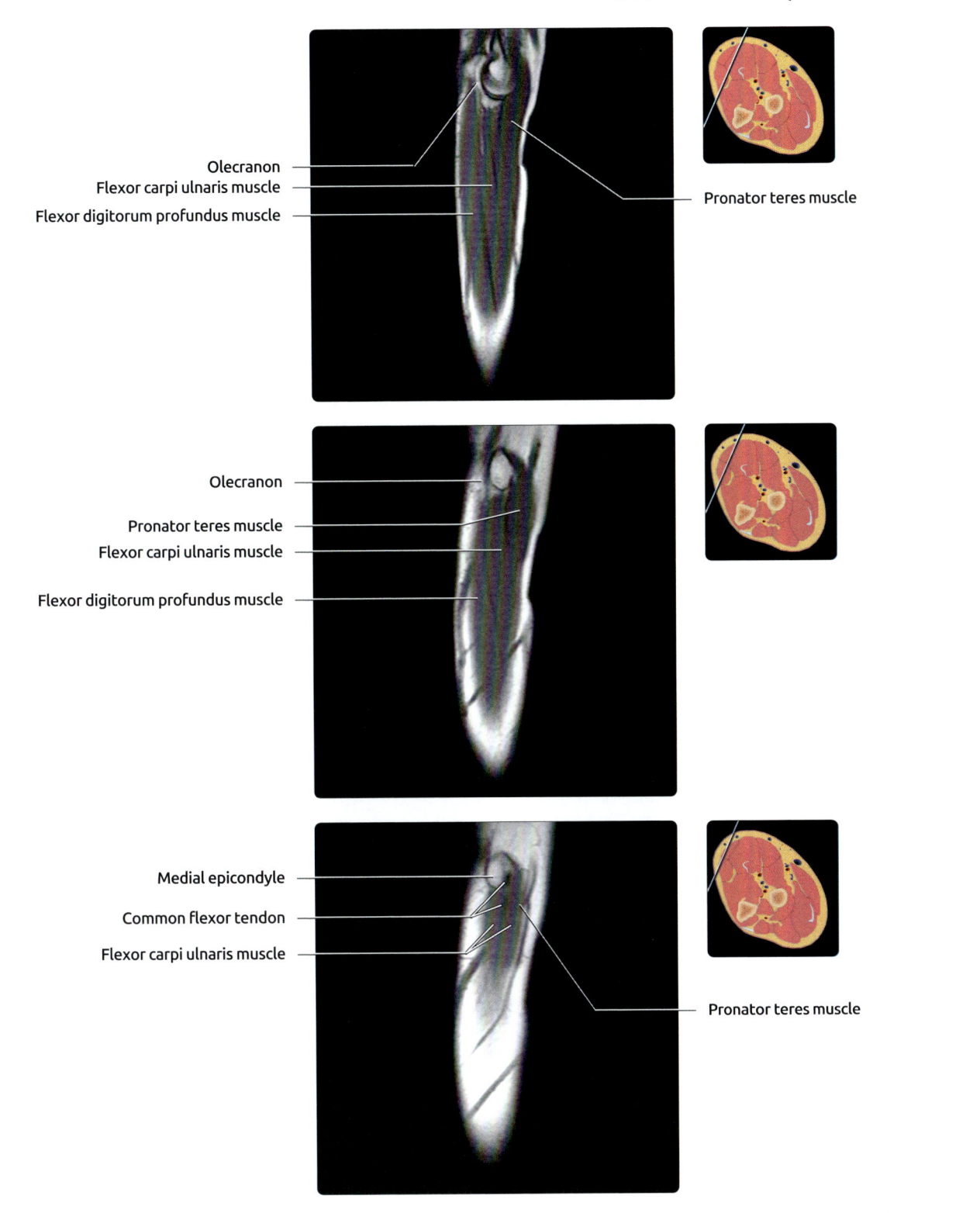

SAGITTAL T1 MR, LEFT FOREARM

Olecranon
Flexor carpi ulnaris muscle
Flexor digitorum profundus muscle
Pronator teres muscle

Olecranon
Pronator teres muscle
Flexor carpi ulnaris muscle
Flexor digitorum profundus muscle

Medial epicondyle
Common flexor tendon
Flexor carpi ulnaris muscle
Pronator teres muscle

(Top) The flexor digitorum profundus muscle drapes over the medial side of the ulna and is, therefore, both anterior and medial to the ulnar shaft. **(Middle)** The pronator teres muscle, seen here in cross section, originates on the medial side of the elbow at the medial epicondyle and proximal ulna and sweeps anterior and distal across the forearm to insert on the midshaft of the radius. **(Bottom)** The flexor carpi ulnaris muscle is the most medial of the forearm muscles.

SECTION 5
Wrist

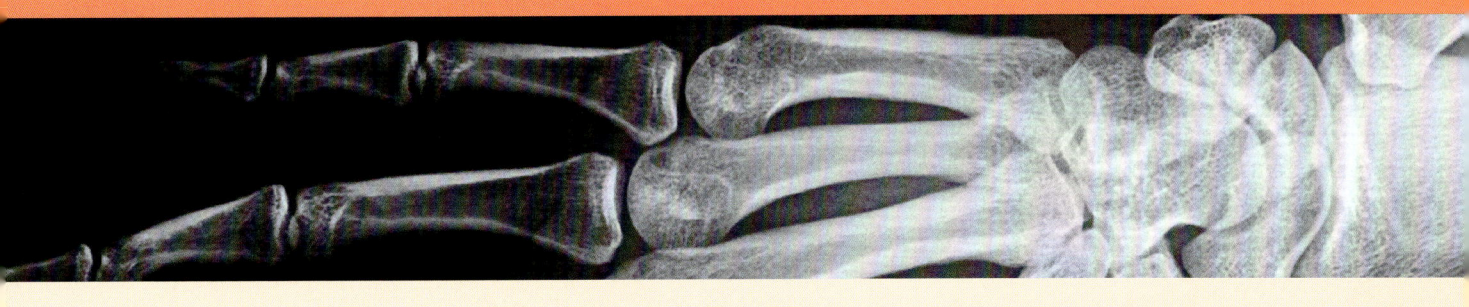

Wrist Overview	**326**
Wrist Radiographic and Arthrographic Anatomy	**334**
Wrist MR Atlas	**342**
Wrist Ligaments	**388**
Wrist Tendons	**398**
Wrist and Hand Normal Variants and Imaging Pitfalls	**418**
Wrist Measurements and Lines	**428**

Wrist Overview

TERMINOLOGY

Definitions
- Volar = palmar
- Ulnar = medial
- Radial = lateral

GROSS ANATOMY

Osseous Structures
- **Distal radius**: Articulates with scaphoid, lunate, and ulna
  - Radial styloid forms arc around radial side of scaphoid
  - Radial fossa is slight indentation for articulation with scaphoid
  - Lunate fossa is slight indentation for articulation with lunate
  - Radial and lunate fossae are separated by ridge
  - Lister tubercle is dorsal prominence proximal to joint
    - Extensor pollicis longus (EPL) wraps around tubercle as it courses radially toward thumb
  - Sigmoid notch is medial concavity in which ulna sits
    - Margin of distal radioulnar joint
- **Distal ulna**: Articulates with radius, triangular fibrocartilage
  - Head of ulna is the distal portion
    - Lateral margin articulates with radius in distal radioulnar joint
    - Distal margin articulates with triangular fibrocartilage
  - Ulnar styloid is small distal projection from ulnar head
  - Ulnar variance refers to length of distal ulna relative to distal radius
    - Ulnar minus is ulna > 2 mm shorter than radius
    - Ulnar plus is ulna longer than radius
- **Proximal carpal row**: Scaphoid, lunate, triquetrum, pisiform
  - **Scaphoid**: Articulates with radius, lunate, capitate, trapezium, trapezoid
    - Divided into proximal pole, waist, and distal pole
    - Tuberosity is a volar prominence from distal pole
    - Blood supply retrograde from scaphoid waist to proximal pole
  - **Lunate**: Articulates with scaphoid, radius, triangular fibrocartilage, triquetrum, capitate
    - Has lunar or crescent moon shape
  - **Triquetrum**: Articulates with articular disc triangular fibrocartilage, lunate, pisiform, hamate
  - **Pisiform**: Articulates with triquetrum
    - Sesamoid in flexor carpi ulnaris tendon
    - Flexor carpi ulnaris attaches to pisiform and continues distally as pisohamate and pisometacarpal ligaments
- **Distal carpal row**: Trapezium, trapezoid, capitate, hamate
  - **Trapezium** (greater multangular): Articulates with 1st, 2nd metacarpals, scaphoid, trapezoid
    - Has concave, saddle shape on its distal margin
      - Curvature of saddle has led to description as a saddle for a scoliotic horse
    - Link between carpals and thumb
  - **Trapezoid** (lesser multangular): Articulates with trapezium, scaphoid, capitate, 2nd metacarpal
  - **Capitate**: Articulates with scaphoid, lunate, hamate, trapezoid, 2nd, 3rd metacarpals
    - Divided into proximal portion, neck (or waist) and body (distal portion)
  - **Hamate**: Articulates with triquetrum, capitate, 4th, 5th metacarpals
    - Wedge shaped
    - Hook (hamulus) is prominent volar projection

Joints
- **4 separate joint cavities**: Distal radioulnar joint, carpometacarpal joint, intermetacarpal/midcarpal/carpometacarpal joint, 1st carpometacarpal joint
- **Distal (inferior) radioulnar joint**
  - Separate joint capsule separated from radiocarpal joint by triangular fibrocartilage
  - Pivot joint: Distal radius rotates around distal ulna
  - Radius moves dorsal to ulna in supination
- **Radiocarpal**: Ellipsoid joint created by proximal carpal row articulating with distal radius and ulna
  - Scaphoid articulates with scaphoid fossa of distal radius
  - Lunate articulates 50% with lunate fossa of distal radius, 50% with triangular fibrocartilage
  - Triquetrum articulates with triangular fibrocartilage
  - Motion: Flexion, extension, abduction, adduction, circumduction
- **Pisotriquetral**: Gliding joint created by pisiform and triquetrum
  - Usually joint recess from radiocarpal joint
  - Separate joint cavity in 10-25%
  - Minimal range of motion
- **Midcarpal**: Gliding joint created by articulation of proximal and distal carpal rows
  - Motion: Extension, abduction, minimal rotation
  - Communicates with intercarpal joints and carpometacarpal joints 2-5
- **Carpometacarpal**: 2nd-5th carpometacarpal joints communicate with midcarpal joint
  - 1st carpometacarpal (CMC) (thumb base)
    - Separate joint cavity
    - Saddle joint, highly mobile
    - Motion: Flexion, extension, abduction, adduction, circumduction, rotation, opposition
  - Carpometacarpal 2nd-5th: Gliding joints
    - Motion: Limited mobility of 2nd-3rd, increasing mobility of 4th-5th carpometacarpal joints
- **Intercarpal:** gliding articulations between individual carpal bones
  - Intercarpal, midcarpal, and carpometacarpal form a single joint cavity
- **Intermetacarpal** communicate with carpometacarpal, midcarpal
  - Small, vertically oriented facets between metacarpal bases
  - Minimal motion

Wrist Motion
- **Tendon contribution** to motion
  - Flexion: Flexor carpi ulnaris and radialis, palmaris longus, abductor pollicis longus
    - Flexor digitorum superficialis and profundus may assist when fingers are in full extension

Wrist Overview

- Extension: Extensor carpi radialis and brevis, ulnaris
  - Extensor digitorum and extensor pollicis longus may assist when fingers are in clenched fist
- Radial deviation (wrist abduction): Primarily by abductor polis longus and extensor pollicis brevis
  - Contributions by flexor carpi radialis, extensor carpi radialis longus and brevis, extensor pollicis longus
- Ulnar deviation (wrist adduction): Flexor carpi ulnaris, extensor carpi ulnaris
- Pronation: Pronator quadratus, pronator teres
- Supination: Supinator, biceps brachii
- Motions of wrist are complex, usually combinations of multiple simple motion vectors
  - Circumduction: Includes all 6 basic motions as wrist moves in circle
  - Dart thrower's motion: Wrist movement from position of combined extension and radial deviation to position of combined flexion and ulnar deviation

Nerves of Wrist Joints

- 3 major nerves serve wrist region
- **Median**
  - Origin: Brachial plexus lateral and medial cords
  - Course in wrist: Anterolateral margin of carpal tunnel
  - Supplies: Flexors (except flexor carpi ulnaris, ulnar 1/2 of flexor digitorum profundus)
- **Ulnar**
  - Origin: Brachial plexus medial cord
  - Course in wrist: Medial to ulnar artery, superficial to flexor retinaculum; bifurcates in Guyon canal
  - Supplies: Flexor carpi ulnaris, ulnar 1/2 of flexor digitorum profundus
- **Radial**
  - Origin: Brachial plexus posterior cord; multiple branches; terminates in superficial and deep branches
  - **Superficial** branch course in wrist: Passes under brachioradialis tendon into dorsal wrist and divides
    - **Lateral** branch: Supplies radial wrist and thumb skin
    - **Medial** branch: Supplies dorsal wrist skin; divides to dorsal digital nerves
  - **Deep** branch course in wrist: Enters supinator muscle ventrally; exits distally and posteriorly
    - Supplies extensor carpi radialis brevis, supinator
  - **Posterior interosseous** nerve is distal extension of deep branch
    - Supplies remaining extensors, abductor pollicis longus

Vessels of Wrist Joint

- Supplied by 3 major arteries
- **Common interosseous**: Branch of ulnar artery
  - Branches into **anterior** and **posterior** interosseous arteries
- **Ulnar**: Terminal branch of brachial artery
- **Radial**: Terminal branch of brachial artery
- Vessels create 3 major volar arches and 1 major dorsal arch

Ligaments

- **Extrinsic** (connect radius, ulna to carpals or carpals to metacarpals) or **intrinsic** (interconnect carpals)
- Summary by location
  - **Volar radiocarpal**: Radioscaphocapitate, long radiolunate, radioscapholunate, short radiolunate
  - **Ulnocarpal**: Ulnolunate, ulnotriquetral; lunocapitate
  - **Dorsal radiocarpal**: Dorsal radiocarpal, dorsal intercarpal, dorsal scaphotriquetral
  - **Volar midcarpal**: Scaphotrapeziotrapezoid, scaphocapitate, triquetrocapitate, triquetrohamate
  - **Proximal interosseous**: Scapholunate, lunotriquetral
  - **Distal interosseous**: Trapeziotrapezoid, trapeziocapitate, capitohamate
  - **Distal radioulnar**: Dorsal radioulnar, volar (palmar) radioulnar, articular disc (TFC)

Muscles and Tendons

- Muscles acting on wrist joint or tendons crossing wrist joints (listed by action on wrist)
- **Flexors, deep**
  - **Flexor digitorum profundus**: Origin ulna, insertion index, middle, ring, and little finger distal phalangeal bases
  - **Flexor pollicis longus**: Origin radius, interosseous membrane, and coronoid process ulna, insertion thumb distal phalangeal base
  - **Pronator quadratus**: Origin ulna and aponeurosis, insertion distal radius
- **Flexors, superficial**
  - **Flexor carpi radialis**: Origin medial epicondyle, insertion 2nd metacarpal base with slip to 3rd metacarpal
  - **Palmaris longus**: Origin medial epicondyle, insertion superficial flexor retinaculum and palmar aponeurosis
  - **Flexor carpi ulnaris**: Origin (humeral head) medial epicondyle and (ulnar head) medial olecranon/proximal ulna, insertion pisiform and flexor retinaculum
  - **Flexor digitorum superficialis**: Origin (humeroulnar head) medial epicondyle and coronoid process of ulna and (radial head) anterior radius, insertion index through little finger middle phalangeal bases
- **Extensors, deep**
  - **Abductor pollicis longus**: Origin ulna, insertion radial 1st metacarpal base with slips to trapezium and abductor pollicis brevis
  - **Extensor pollicis brevis**: Origin radius, insertion thumb proximal phalangeal base
  - **Extensor pollicis longus**: Origin mid ulna, insertion thumb distal phalangeal base
  - **Extensor indicis** (proprius): Origin mid ulna, insertion joins with ulnar side of extensor digitorum tendon inserting into 2nd digit extensor hood
- **Extensors, superficial**
  - **Brachioradialis**: Origin proximal humerus, insertion radial styloid base
  - **Extensor carpi radialis longus**: Origin lateral supracondylar ridge of humerus, insertion dorsal radial 2nd metacarpal base
  - **Extensor carpi radialis brevis**: Origin lateral humeral epicondyle, insertion dorsal radial 3rd metacarpal base
  - **Extensor digitorum** (communis): Origin lateral humeral epicondyle, insertion into middle and distal phalanges
  - **Extensor digiti minimi** (ex digiti quinti [V] proprius): Origin common extensor tendon of lateral humeral epicondyle, insertion extensor hood little finger
  - **Extensor carpi ulnaris**: Origin common extensor tendon of lateral humeral epicondyle, insertion 5th MC base
- **Thenar**

Wrist Overview

- ○ **Abductor pollicis brevis**: Origin flexor retinaculum, scaphoid tuberosity and trapezium ridge, insertion thumb proximal phalanx
- ○ **Opponens pollicis**: Origin trapezium and flexor retinaculum, insertion 1st metacarpal
- ○ **Flexor pollicis brevis**: Superficial origin flexor retinaculum and trapezium, deep origin trapezoid and capitate, insertion thumb proximal phalanx
- ○ **Adductor pollicis**: Origin capitate, 2nd and 3rd metacarpal bases, insertion ulnar thumb proximal phalanx
- **Hypothenar**
  - ○ **Palmaris brevis**: Origin flexor retinaculum and palmar aponeurosis, insertion skin of palm
  - ○ **Adductor digiti minimi**: Origin pisiform and flexor carpi ulnaris, insertion little finger proximal phalanx
  - ○ **Flexor digiti minimi brevis**: Origin hamate hook and flexor retinaculum, insertion ulnar little finger proximal phalanx
  - ○ **Opponens digiti minimi**: Origin hamate hook and flexor retinaculum, insertion 5th metacarpal

Retinacula

- **Flexor retinaculum**
  - ○ Superficial (volar carpal ligament or ligamentum carpi palmare): Attached to styloid processes of ulna and radius; merges with deep component distally
  - ○ Deep (transverse carpal ligament or ligamentum flexorum): Attached to pisiform and hook of hamate medially, scaphoid and trapezium laterally
- **Extensor retinaculum**
  - ○ Attaches to ulnar styloid process, triquetrum and pisiform medially, crosses obliquely to attach Lister tubercle and radial styloid process laterally
    - Sends septa to radius creating 6 compartments for extensor tendons
    - Compartment 1: Abductor pollicis longus, extensor pollicis brevis
    - Compartment 2: Extensor carpi radialis longus, extensor carpi radialis brevis
    - Compartment 3: Extensor pollicis longus
    - Compartment 4: Extensor digitorum, extensor indicis
    - Compartment 5: Extensor digiti minimi
    - Compartment 6: Extensor carpi ulnaris

Anatomic Spaces

- **Anatomic snuffbox**
  - ○ Contains cephalic vein, radial nerve, (superficial branch), radial artery
  - ○ Between radial styloid and base of thumb; margins are abductor pollicis longus and extensor pollicis longus
- **Carpal tunnel**
  - ○ Between pisiform and hook of hamate medial, scaphoid, and trapezium laterally
  - ○ Contains deep and superficial flexors, median nerve
- **Guyon canal**
  - ○ Contains ulnar artery and vein, ulnar nerve
  - ○ Between deep and superficial flexor retinaculum, pisiform, and flexor carpi ulnaris

Central Axis of Wrist

- Longitudinal axis formed by radius, lunate, capitate, and 3rd metacarpal

ANATOMY IMAGING ISSUES

Imaging Recommendations

- Radiography: For alignment, joint space width, mineralization, range of motion
- CT: Acquire thin section (0.5-1 mm) with 2D and 3D reformation; for alignment, cortical integrity
- MR: Dedicated coils, 8-10 cm field of view, thin sections essential for imaging small, complex wrist anatomy
  - ○ Structures best visualized (by plane)
    - Coronal: Osseous structures, alignment, intrinsic and extrinsic ligaments, triangular fibrocartilage complex (TFCC)
    - Axial: Tendons, neurovascular structures, distal radioulnar joint, pisotriquetral joint
    - Sagittal: Alignment, cross section ligaments, pisotriquetral joint
- Ultrasound: Dynamic evaluation of tendons, ligaments, neurovascular structures

Imaging Pitfalls

- Many tendon variations, including split or duplicated tendons
- Small amount of extensor tendon sheath fluid is common (particularly 2nd compartment); should not be mistaken for tenosynovitis
- TFCC attachments may mimic tears: Radial attachments to hyaline cartilage rather than cortex; ulnar attachment to ulna fossa often intermediate signal due to magic angle or volume averaging
  - ○ Articular disc may develop asymptomatic attritional tears
- Scapholunate and lunotriquetral ligaments may attach to articular cartilage rather than cortex
- Malpositioning: Ulnar or radial deviation may create apparent instability patterns
- Magic angle effect: Organized fibers (tendon or ligament) crossing at 55° to main magnetic field may have intermediate signal on short TE imaging (T1, PD, GRE)
  - ○ Examples: Extensor carpi ulnaris crossing dorsum of ulna; extensor pollicis longus crossing dorsal wrist obliquely

SELECTED REFERENCES

1. Moritomo H et al: 2007 IFSSH committee report of wrist biomechanics committee: biomechanics of the so-called dart-throwing motion of the wrist. J Hand Surg Am. 32(9):1447-53, 2007
2. Kobayashi M et al: Normal kinematics of carpal bones: a three-dimensional analysis of carpal bone motion relative to the radius. J Biomech. 30(8):787-93, 1997

Wrist Overview

3D RECONSTRUCTION CT

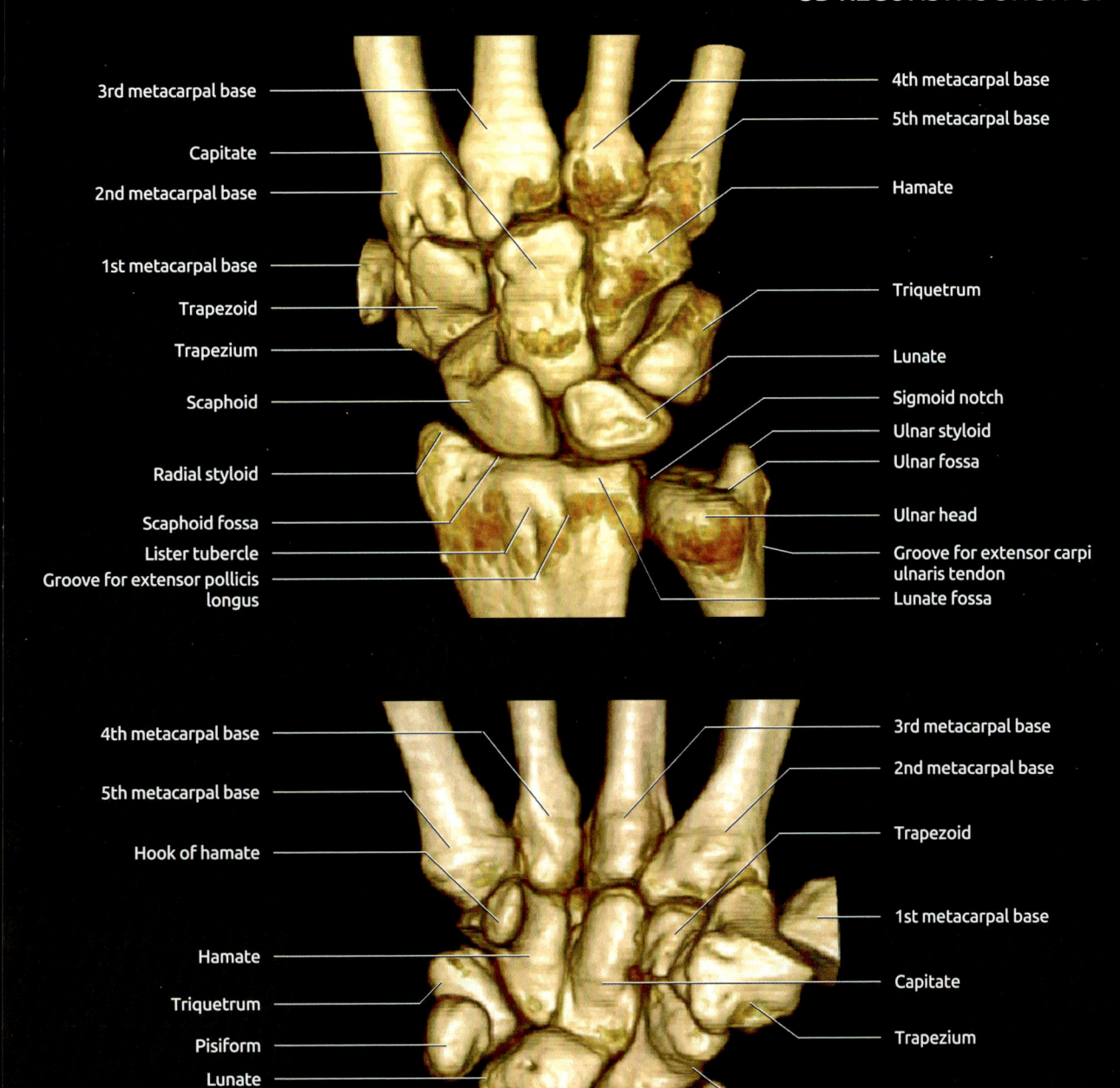

(Top) A 3D surface rendering of the dorsal wrist positioned in pronation is shown. (Bottom) Volar wrist, positioned in pronation, is shown.

Wrist Overview

GRAPHICS, WRIST LIGAMENTS

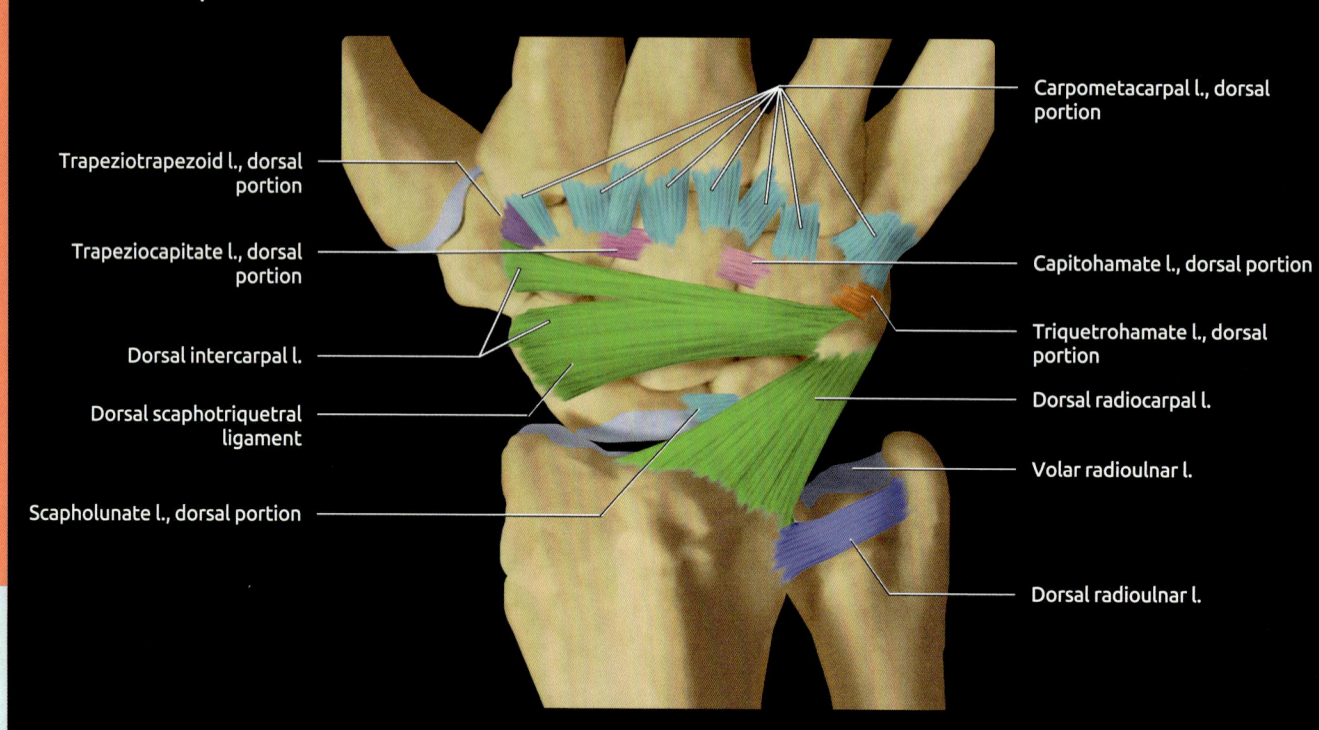

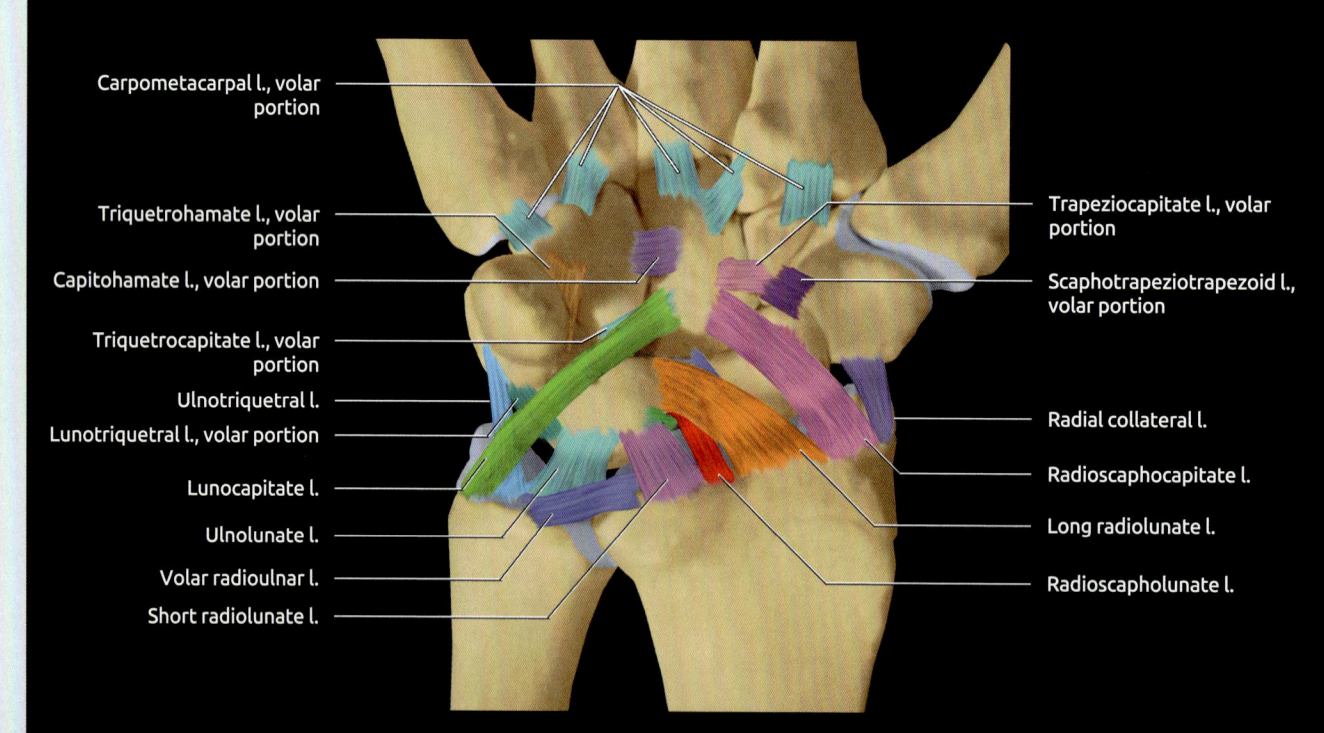

(Top) Intrinsic and extrinsic ligaments of dorsal wrist by location are shown. Dorsal radiocarpal: Dorsal radiocarpal, dorsal scaphotriquetral, dorsal intercarpal are seen. Proximal interosseous: Scapholunate, lunotriquetral are seen. Distal interosseous: Trapeziotrapezoid, trapeziocapitate, capitohamate are seen. Distal radioulnar volar and dorsal ligaments are seen. (Bottom) Extrinsic and intrinsic ligaments of the volar wrist by location are shown. Volar radiocarpal: Radioscaphocapitate, long radiolunate, radioscapholunate, short radiolunate are seen. Ulnocarpal: Ulnolunate, ulnotriquetral, lunocapitate are seen. Volar midcarpal: Scaphotrapeziotrapezoid, scaphocapitate, triquetrocapitate, triquetrohamate are seen. Proximal interosseous: Scapholunate, lunotriquetral are seen. Distal interosseous: Trapeziotrapezoid, trapeziocapitate, capitohamate are seen. Distal radioulnar volar and dorsal ligaments are seen.

Wrist Overview

GRAPHICS, WRIST TENDONS & RETINACULA

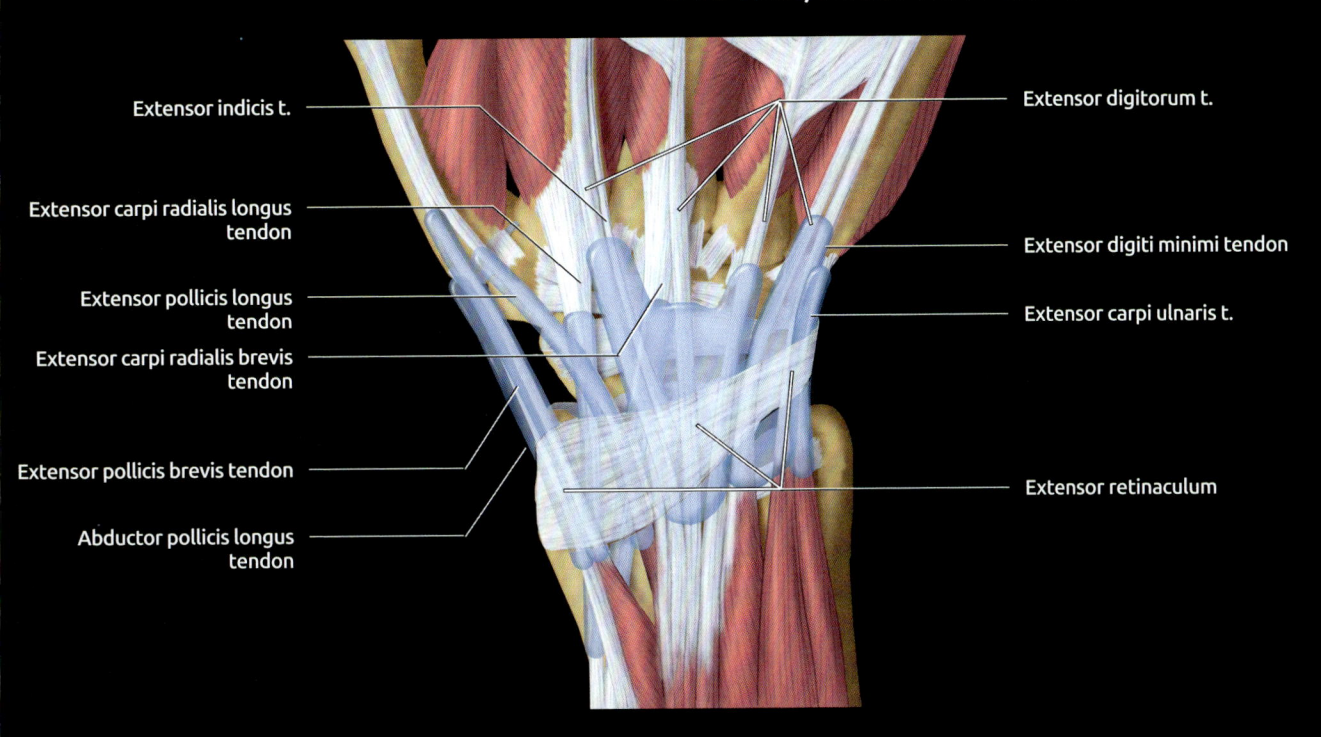

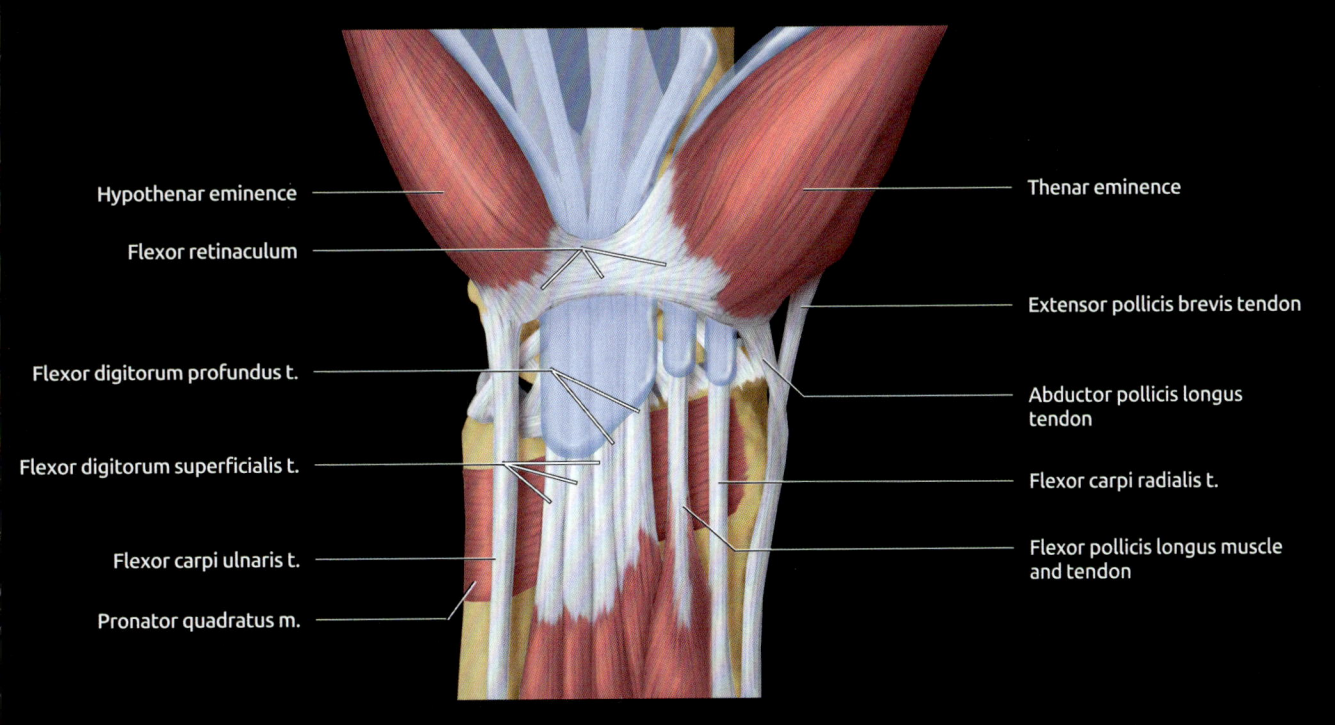

(Top) Tendons and retinaculum of the dorsal wrist are shown. The extensor retinaculum attaches to the triquetrum and pisiform medially, crossing obliquely to attach to Lister tubercle and the radial styloid laterally, creating a series of compartments, which separate the various tendons and their associated sheaths. Extensor tendons are enclosed in individual tenosynovial sheaths as they pass under the extensor retinaculum. (Bottom) Tendons and retinaculum of the volar wrist are shown. The flexor retinaculum spans the palmar arch, attaching to the radial and ulnar styloid processes. The thenar eminence musculature includes abductor pollicis brevis, opponens pollicis, flexor pollicis brevis, and adductor pollicis. The hypothenar musculature includes palmaris brevis, adductor digiti minimi, flexor digiti minimi brevis, and opponens digiti minimi.

Wrist Overview

GRAPHICS, WRIST ARTERIES & VEINS

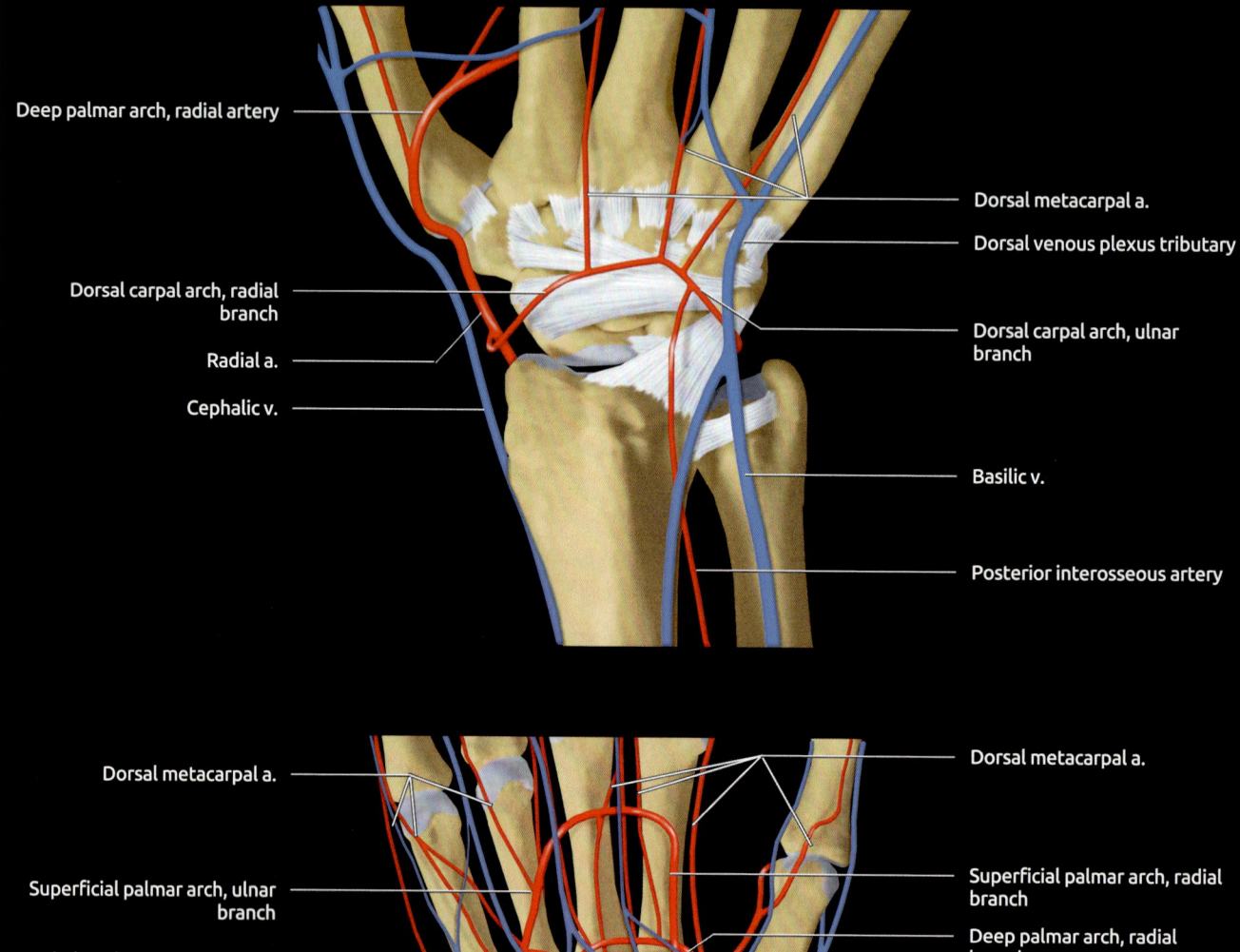

Labels (top image):
- Deep palmar arch, radial artery
- Dorsal carpal arch, radial branch
- Radial a.
- Cephalic v.
- Dorsal metacarpal a.
- Dorsal venous plexus tributary
- Dorsal carpal arch, ulnar branch
- Basilic v.
- Posterior interosseous artery

Labels (bottom image):
- Dorsal metacarpal a.
- Superficial palmar arch, ulnar branch
- 5th dorsal metacarpal artery
- Deep palmar arch, ulnar branch
- Palmar carpal arch, ulnar branch
- Basilic v.
- Anterior interosseous a.
- Ulnar a.
- Dorsal metacarpal a.
- Superficial palmar arch, radial branch
- Deep palmar arch, radial branch
- Cephalic v.
- Radial a., superficial palmar branch, radial artery
- Radial a.
- Palmar carpal arch, radial branch
- Median a.
- Radial a.

(**Top**) *Vasculature of the dorsal wrist is shown. The dorsal carpal arch supplies the distal radius, distal carpal row, and lateral proximal carpal row. The venous plexus drains into 2 main venous systems, the cephalic and basilic, with multiple anastomotic communications.*
(**Bottom**) *Vasculature of the volar wrist is shown. Three major arterial arches are contributed to by the radial, ulnar, and interosseous arteries: Palmar (volar) carpal and deep and superficial palmar arches. A dorsal venous plexus drains into the cephalic and basilic veins.*

Wrist Overview

GRAPHICS, WRIST NERVES

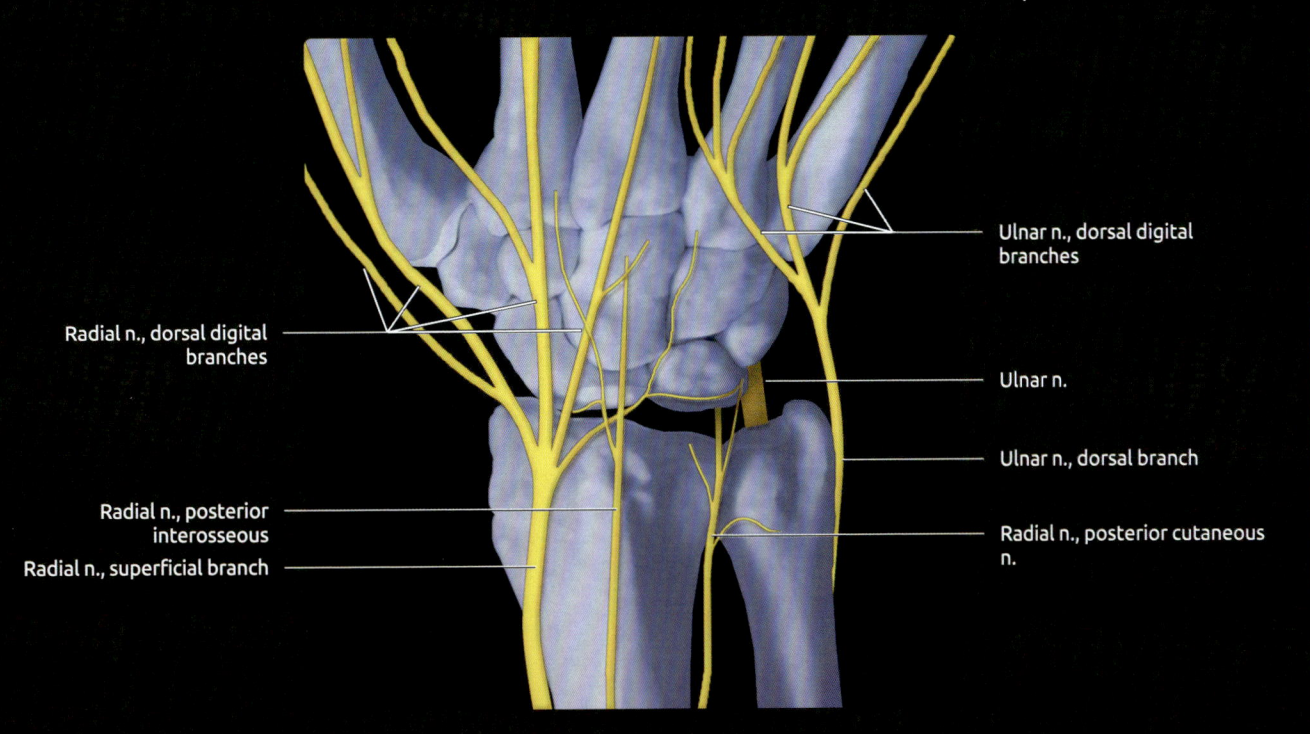

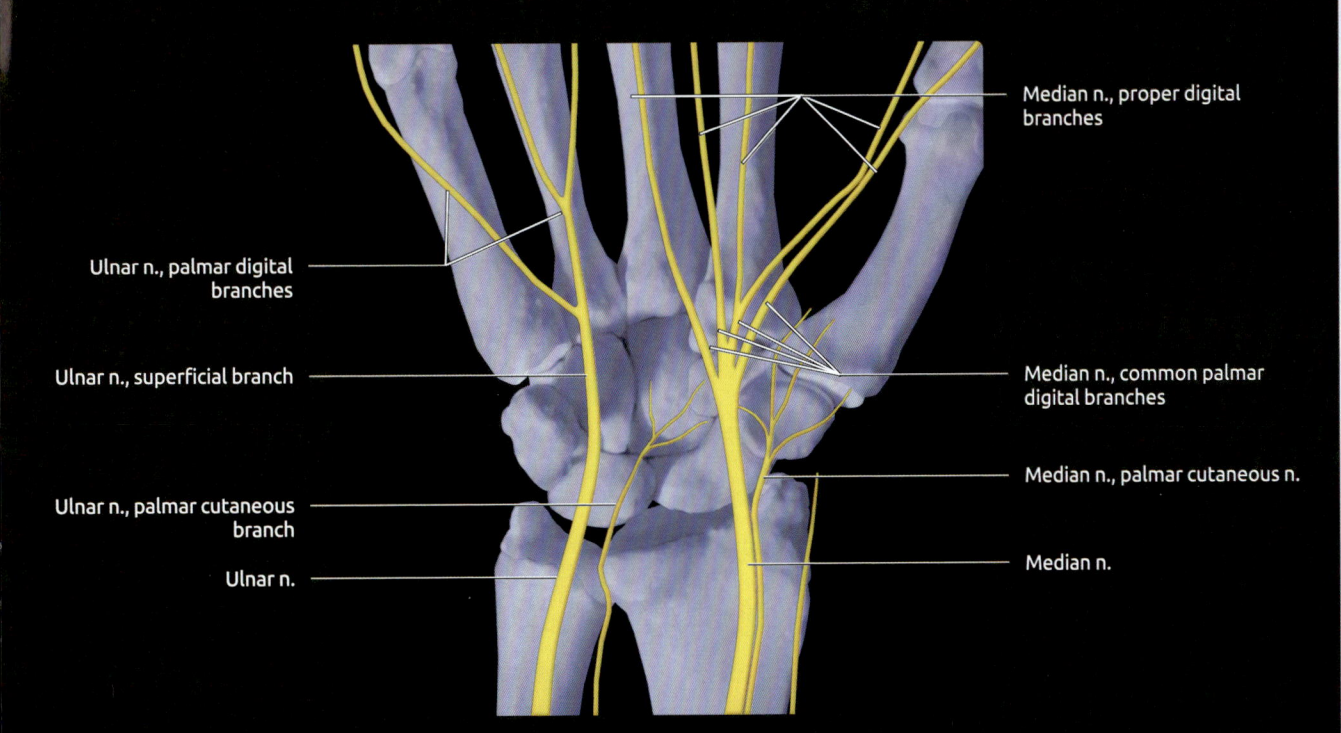

Labels (top image):
- Radial n., dorsal digital branches
- Radial n., posterior interosseous
- Radial n., superficial branch
- Ulnar n., dorsal digital branches
- Ulnar n.
- Ulnar n., dorsal branch
- Radial n., posterior cutaneous n.

Labels (bottom image):
- Ulnar n., palmar digital branches
- Ulnar n., superficial branch
- Ulnar n., palmar cutaneous branch
- Ulnar n.
- Median n., proper digital branches
- Median n., common palmar digital branches
- Median n., palmar cutaneous n.
- Median n.

(**Top**) Nerves of the dorsal wrist are shown. The radial nerve branches in the forearm with the superficial, posterior cutaneous, and posterior interosseous branches serving the wrist and hand. The ulnar nerve provides branches to dorsal and volar wrist. (**Bottom**) Nerves of the volar wrist are shown. The ulnar nerve provides motor and sensory branches to the ulnar aspect of the wrist. The median nerve passes through the carpal tunnel, with several branches serving the palmar and radial aspects of the wrist and hand.

Wrist Radiographic and Arthrographic Anatomy

IMAGING ANATOMY

Overview

- 4 separate joint compartments in wrist
  - **Distal radioulnar joint (DRUJ)**
    - Wide range of motion
    - Pronation/supination: Radius rotates around ulna
    - Ulna articulates with sigmoid notch of radius
    - In pronation, head of ulna moves up to 50% dorsal to radius
  - **Radiocarpal joint (RCJ)**
    - Proximal margin: Radius and triangular fibrocartilage complex (TFCC)
    - Distal margin: Proximal carpal row
    - Joint capsule attaches laterally to scaphoid, medially to triquetrum
    - Prestyloid recess: Volar to ulnar styloid
    - Pisotriquetral recess: Usually communicates with radiocarpal joint, but occasionally forms a separate compartment
    - In neutral position, lunate articulates 1/2 with radius, 1/2 with triangular fibrocartilage
  - **Midcarpal joint**
    - Synovial cavity extends between all of carpal bones except between pisiform and triquetrum
    - Scapholunate (SL) and lunatotriquetral (LT) ligaments and joint capsule separate from RCJ
    - Communicates normally with 2nd-5th carpometacarpal joints
  - **1st carpometacarpal joint**
- Distal radius articulates with scaphoid, lunate
  - Separate fossa for each bone
  - Ulnar 50% of lunate articulates with triangular fibrocartilage
- Ulna does not directly articulate with carpal bones
  - Triangular fibrocartilage is interposed

ANATOMY IMAGING ISSUES

Imaging Recommendations

- Wrist radiographs
  - 3 standard views: PA, PA oblique, lateral; also multiple specialty views
  - Posteroanterior (PA)
    - Elbow and wrist at same height as shoulder
      - This gives most accurate measurement of ulnar variance
    - Line drawn through distal radius should extend along axis of 3rd metacarpal
      - Radial or ulnar deviation will change relative alignment of carpal bones
  - PA oblique: 45° rotation
    - Often only view that will show chip fracture of dorsal triquetrum
  - Lateral view
    - On well-positioned lateral, pisiform should overlie distal pole of scaphoid
    - Lister tubercle a useful landmark on posterior radius
      - Occasionally, the only sign of nondisplaced radial fracture is irregularity of Lister tubercle
    - For evaluation of hardware in distal radius fractures an "elevated lateral" is useful
      - Clarifies position of screws relative to radial styloid
  - Radial deviation (PA)
    - Volar flexes scaphoid, creates foreshortened signet ring appearance
  - Ulnar deviation (PA)
    - Dorsiflexes scaphoid, creates elongated appearance
    - Shows scaphoid waist fractures well
    - Improves visualization of scapholunate dissociation
  - Semisupinated view
    - Anteroposterior (AP) view with 45° of supination
    - Shows hook of hamate & pisiform
  - Carpal tunnel view
    - Wrist dorsiflexed, volar forearm against image detector
    - Beam directed at midcarpal region
    - Shows hook of hamate
  - Clenched fist view (AP)
    - Action of clenching fist stresses scapholunate ligament
    - Scapholunate distance increases when ligament is torn
- Wrist arthrography
  - Radiocarpal injection
    - Wrist flexed, supported with rolled-up washcloth
    - Needle at proximal pole of scaphoid or lunate
    - Angled slightly proximally to avoid dorsal lip of radius
  - In past, triple compartment arthrography performed to look for "1-way valve" perforations
    - Injection of midcarpal joint at 4 corners region where lunate, triquetrum, capitate, and hamate meet
    - Injection of distal radioulnar joint
    - Followed several hours later (to allow contrast in other compartments to dissipate) by injection of radiocarpal joint
    - No longer felt to be necessary
  - Followed by CT or MR to improve visualization of ligaments
- MR arthrogram findings
  - Triangular fibrocartilage should have smooth distal margin
    - Volar recess by styloid process is normal finding
  - Contrast should not extend beyond contour of proximal carpal row margin
  - Radially, contrast extends to scaphoid waist
  - Ulnarly, contrast extends to proximal, ulnar margin of triquetrum

Imaging Pitfalls

- Small communications between compartments (i.e., ligament perforations) increase in incidence with age and may not be symptomatic
  - Central, membranous portion of triangular fibrocartilage
  - Central portion of scapholunate or lunatotriquetral ligament
- Small volar radiocarpal recesses are often seen and are a normal finding

Wrist Radiographic and Arthrographic Anatomy

PA RADIOGRAPH: NEUTRAL, RADIAL, AND ULNAR DEVIATION

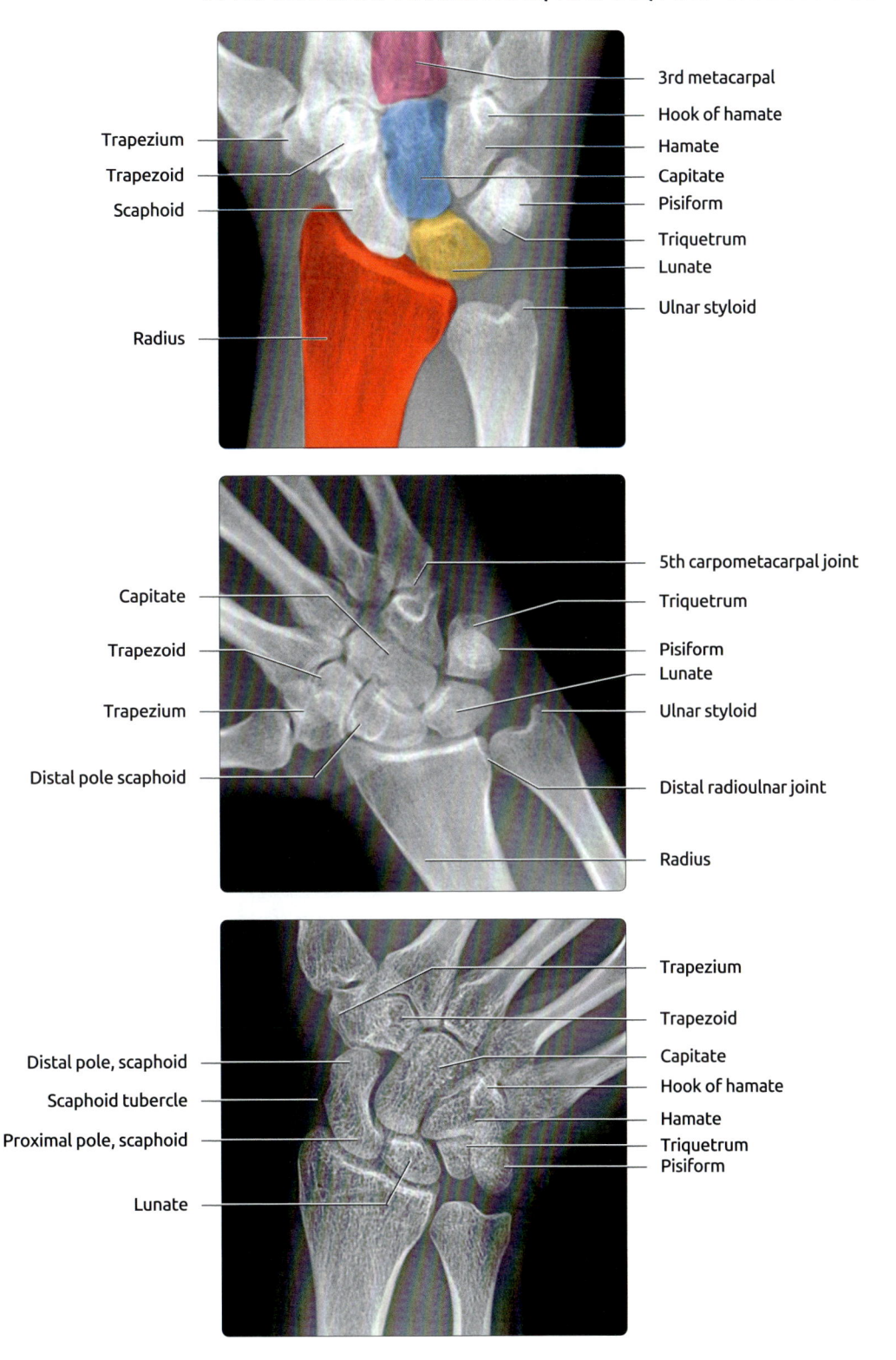

(Top) PA radiograph in a neutral position shows the lunate articulating 50% with the radius and 50% with triangular fibrocartilage. *(Middle)* PA radial deviation with positioned palm flat on cassette and wrist in maximum abduction without flexion or extension. The beam is perpendicular to the cassette and centered on capitate head. The scaphoid is volarflexed, resulting in apparent shortening of the bone and obscuring the scaphoid waist. *(Bottom)* Ulnar deviation view shows the elongated appearance of the scaphoid, reflecting dorsiflexion of the scaphoid. Also note the relative shift of the capitate and hamate compared to the proximal carpal row.

Wrist Radiographic and Arthrographic Anatomy

LATERAL RADIOGRAPH: NEUTRAL, EXTENSION, FLEXION

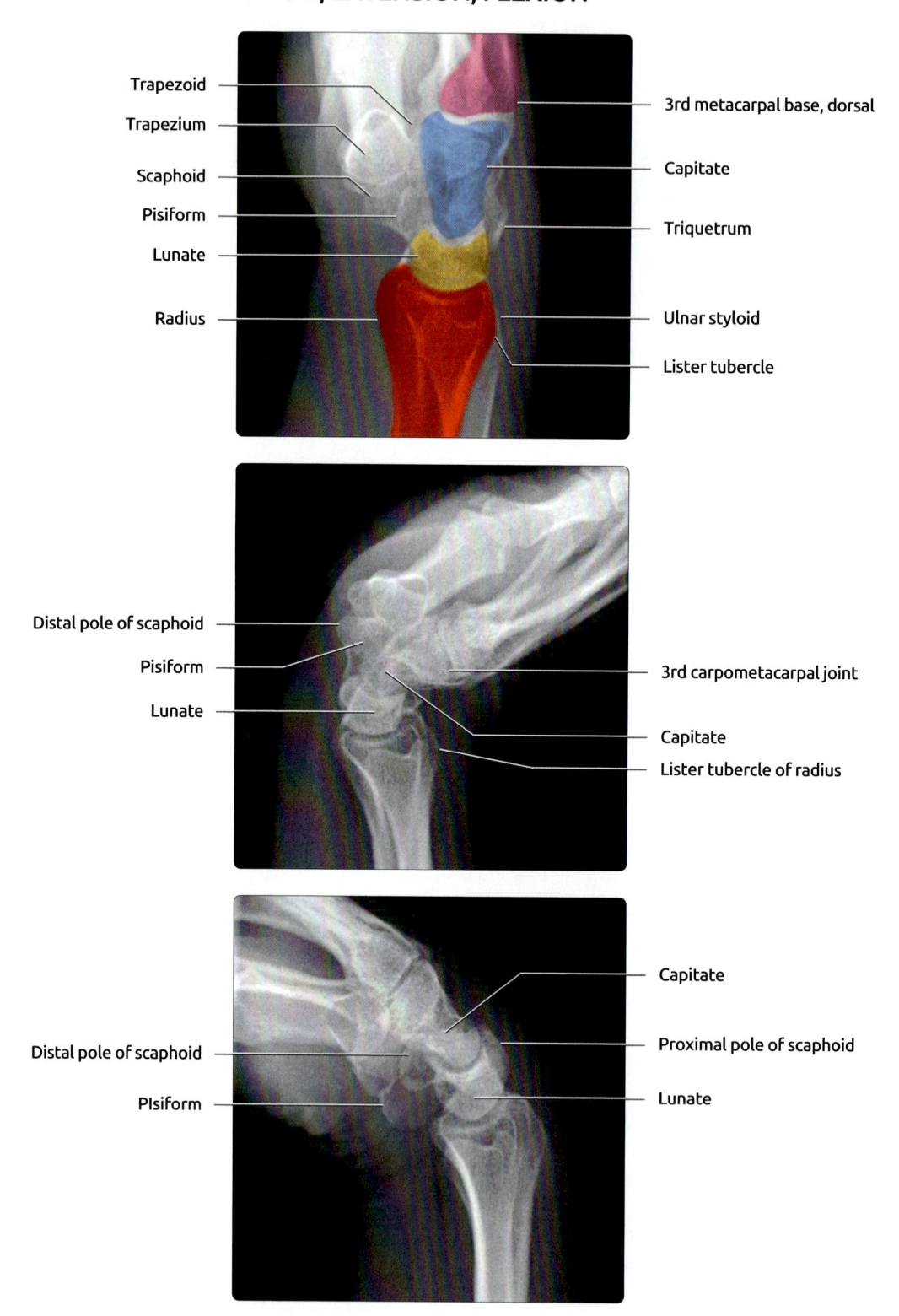

(Top) Lateral radiograph obtained in zero-rotation position is color-coded to facilitate key structure identification. Third metacarpal: Magenta; capitate: Blue; lunate: Yellow; radius: Red. (Middle) Lateral dorsiflexion is shown. The wrist placed in a neutral lateral position on the cassette and is maximally dorsiflexed. The center beam is perpendicular to the cassette and centered on the scaphoid waist. (Bottom) Lateral volarflexion is shown. The wrist is placed in the neutral lateral position on the on cassette and is maximally volarflexed. The center beam is perpendicular to the cassette and is centered on the scaphoid waist.

Wrist Radiographic and Arthrographic Anatomy

SPECIAL VIEWS OF WRIST

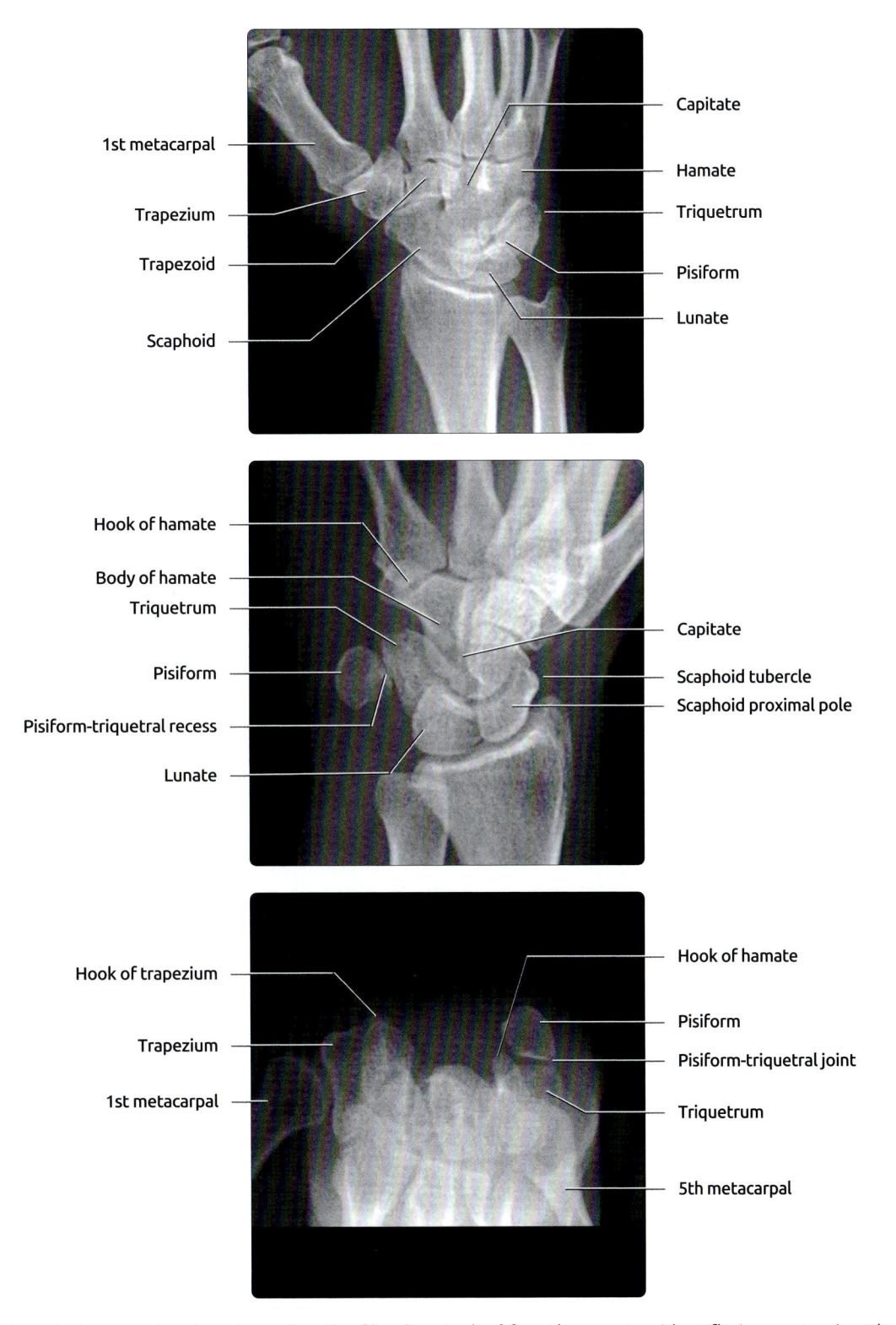

(Top) PA semipronated oblique view shows the radial side of hand is raised 45° from the cassette without flexion or extension. The beam is perpendicular to the cassette and centered on the capitate head. *(Middle)* Semisupinated oblique view shows the ulnar wrist is placed with 30-45° supination from the neutral lateral position. The center beam is perpendicular to the cassette and is centered on the capitate head. Supinated oblique view is ideal for evaluation of the hook of hamate, pisiform, or triquetral fractures. *(Bottom)* Carpal tunnel view is shown. The pisiform is a useful structure for orienting yourself on this view. Note that the trapezium has a hook, smaller than the hook of the hamate.

Wrist Radiographic and Arthrographic Anatomy

COMPARTMENTS OF WRIST

Labels (top diagram): 1st carpometacarpal compartment; Midcarpal compartment; Radiocarpal compartment; Common carpometacarpal compartment; Pisotriquetral recess; Distal radioulnar compartment.

Labels (middle arthrogram): Common carpometacarpal compartment; 1st carpometacarpal compartment; Scapholunate ligament; Lunatotriquetral ligament; Triangular fibrocartilage; Distal radioulnar joint.

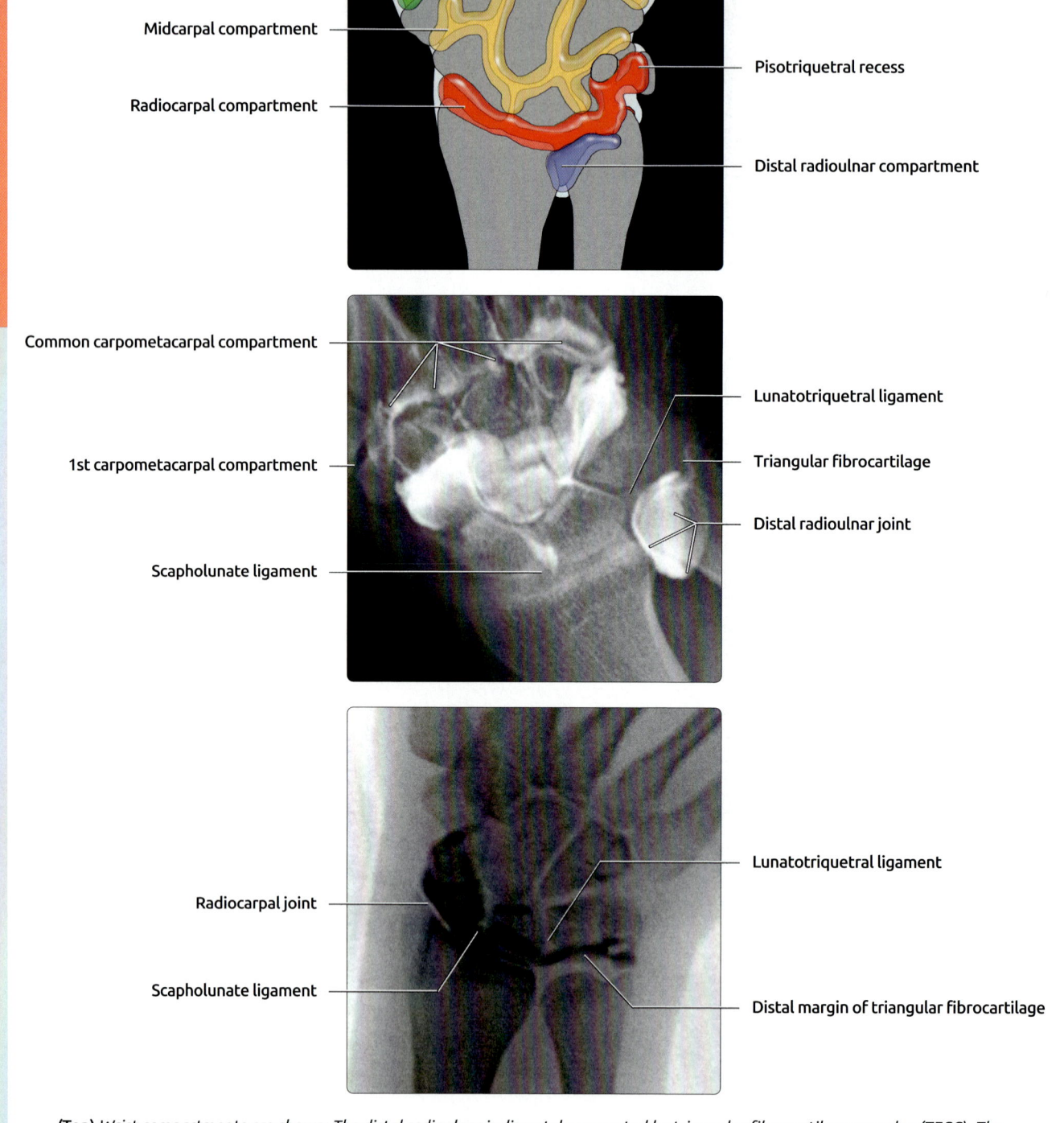

Labels (bottom arthrogram): Radiocarpal joint; Scapholunate ligament; Lunatotriquetral ligament; Distal margin of triangular fibrocartilage.

(Top) Wrist compartments are shown: The distal radioulnar is discretely separated by triangular fibrocartilage complex (TFCC). The radiocarpal is separated by proximal scapholunate and lunatotriquetral ligaments, as well as TFCC. The midcarpal, separated by the scapholunate and lunatotriquetral ligaments, typically communicates with carpometacarpal joint. The 1st carpometacarpal is separated from the common carpometacarpal by the trapeziometacarpal ligament. **(Middle)** Anteroposterior arthrogram was taken following injection of the midcarpal and distal radioulnar compartments. The midcarpal injection fills the midcarpal and common carpometacarpal compartments. A separate injection into the distal radioulnar joint has also been performed and shows contrast between radius and ulna, filling dorsal and volar recesses and outlining the smooth undersurface of triangular fibrocartilage. **(Bottom)** Anteroposterior arthrogram shows radiocarpal joint injection and the normal extent of the radiocarpal joint.

Wrist Radiographic and Arthrographic Anatomy

CORONAL MR ARTHROGRAM

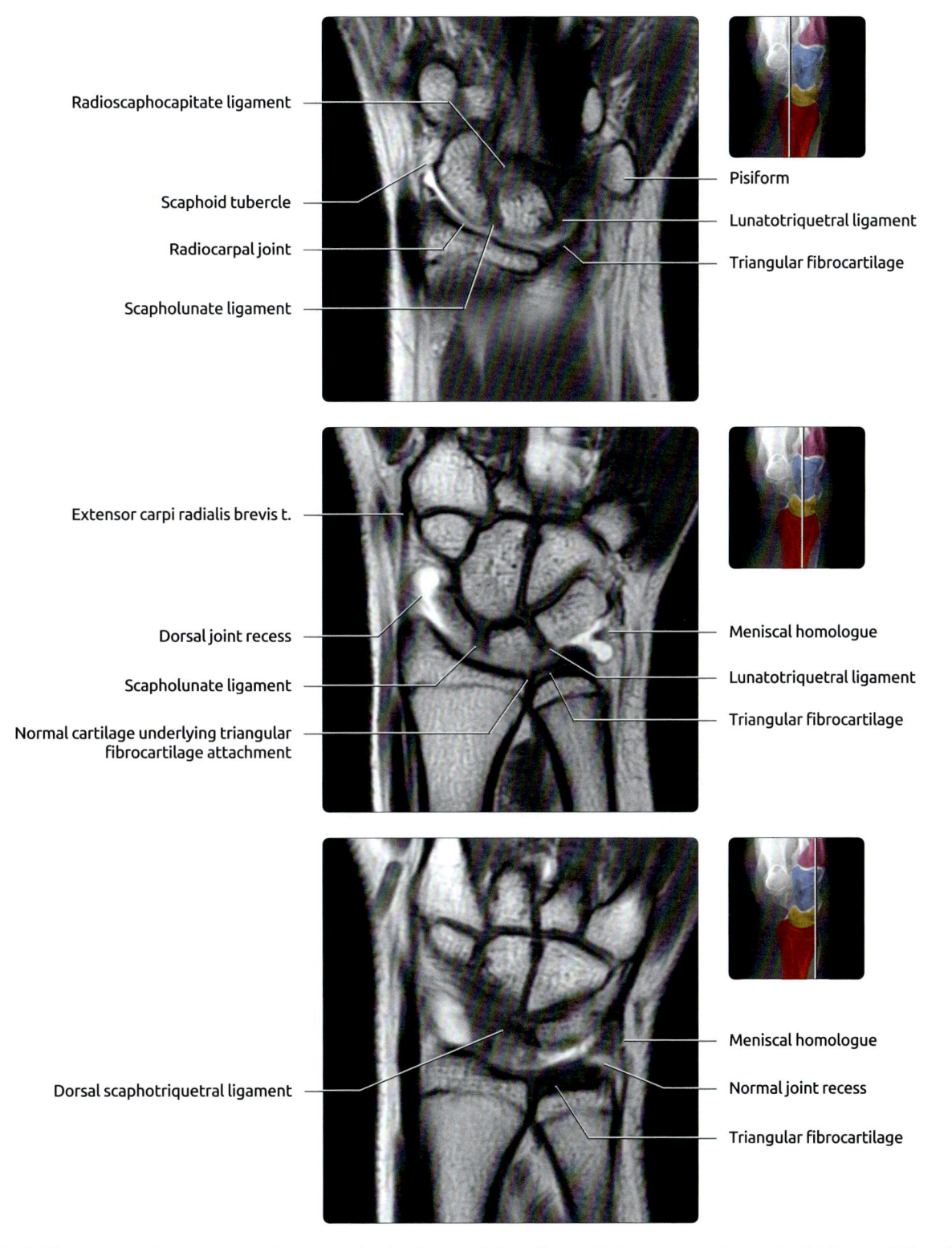

Labels (Top): Radioscaphocapitate ligament; Scaphoid tubercle; Radiocarpal joint; Scapholunate ligament; Pisiform; Lunatotriquetral ligament; Triangular fibrocartilage

Labels (Middle): Extensor carpi radialis brevis t.; Dorsal joint recess; Scapholunate ligament; Normal cartilage underlying triangular fibrocartilage attachment; Meniscal homologue; Lunatotriquetral ligament; Triangular fibrocartilage

Labels (Bottom): Dorsal scaphotriquetral ligament; Meniscal homologue; Normal joint recess; Triangular fibrocartilage

(**Top**) *MR arthrogram in a teenage patient shows the attachment of the radiocarpal joint capsule to the scaphoid tubercle. At the volar margin of the joint, the scapholunate and lunatotriquetral ligaments are thick, homogeneously low signal intensity structures.* (**Middle**) *Coronal T1 MR through the mid-dorsal wrist shows the normal appearance of the meniscal homologue, a variably present structure. The dorsal bands of the scapholunate and lunatotriquetral ligaments are seen as they wrap around the dorsal margins of the bones.* (**Bottom**) *Coronal T1 MR through the most dorsal aspect of the radiocarpal joint shows a portion of an extrinsic ligament: The dorsal scaphotriquetral ligament.*

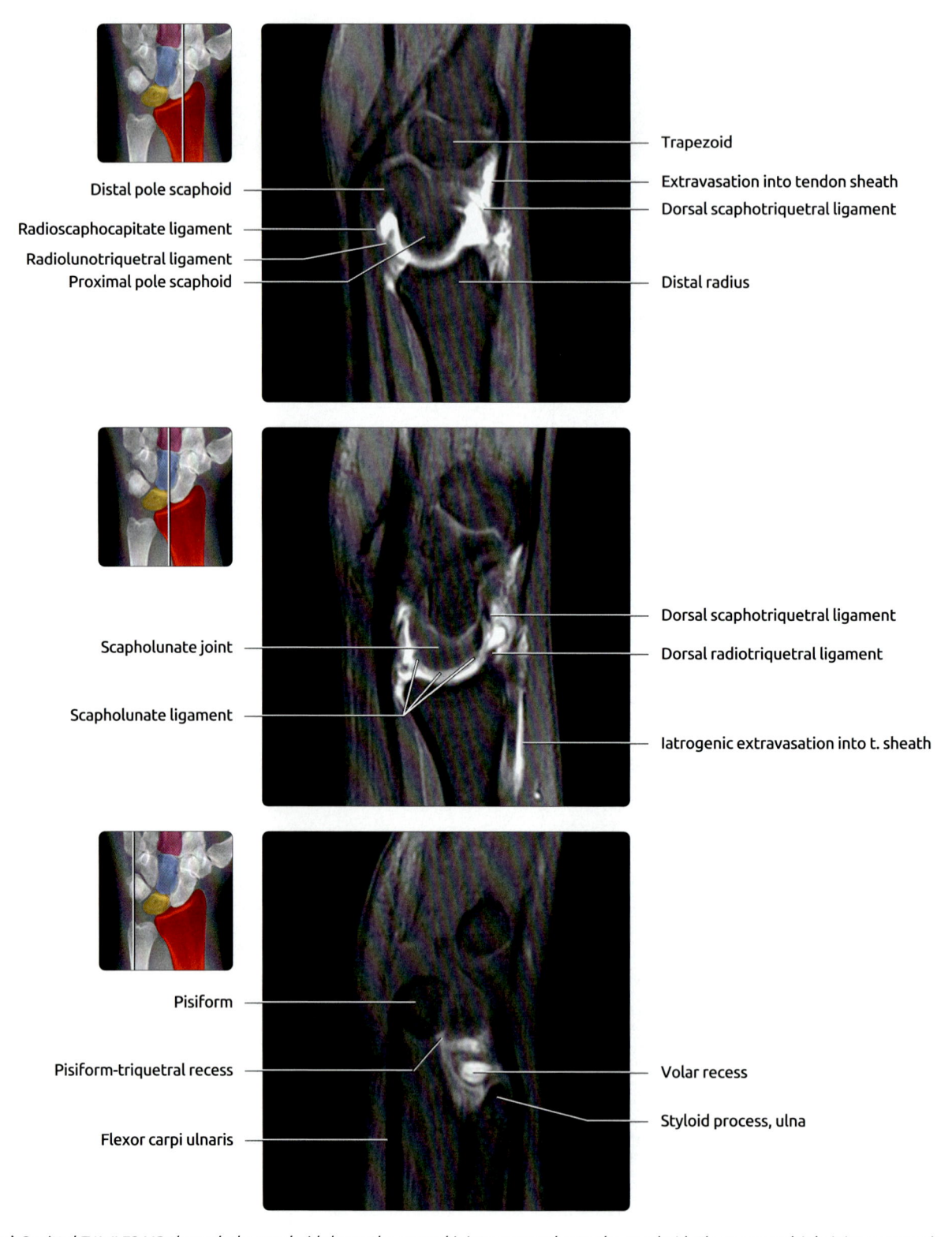

Wrist Radiographic and Arthrographic Anatomy

SAGITTAL T1 FS MR ARTHROGRAM

Distal pole scaphoid
Radioscaphocapitate ligament
Radiolunotriquetral ligament
Proximal pole scaphoid

Trapezoid
Extravasation into tendon sheath
Dorsal scaphotriquetral ligament
Distal radius

Scapholunate joint
Scapholunate ligament

Dorsal scaphotriquetral ligament
Dorsal radiotriquetral ligament
Iatrogenic extravasation into t. sheath

Pisiform
Pisiform-triquetral recess
Flexor carpi ulnaris

Volar recess
Styloid process, ulna

(**Top**) *Sagittal T1WI FS MR through the scaphoid shows the normal joint recess volar to the scaphoid. There are multiple joint recesses in the wrist, which can be distinguished from synovial cysts by their wide communication with the underlying joint.* (**Middle**) *Sagittal T1 FS MR arthrogram through the scapholunate joint shows the U-shaped scapholunate ligament.* (**Bottom**) *Sagittal T1 FS MR arthrogram through the ulnar margin of the wrist shows the normal volar recess adjacent to the styloid process of the ulna.*

Wrist Radiographic and Arthrographic Anatomy

AXIAL IMAGES

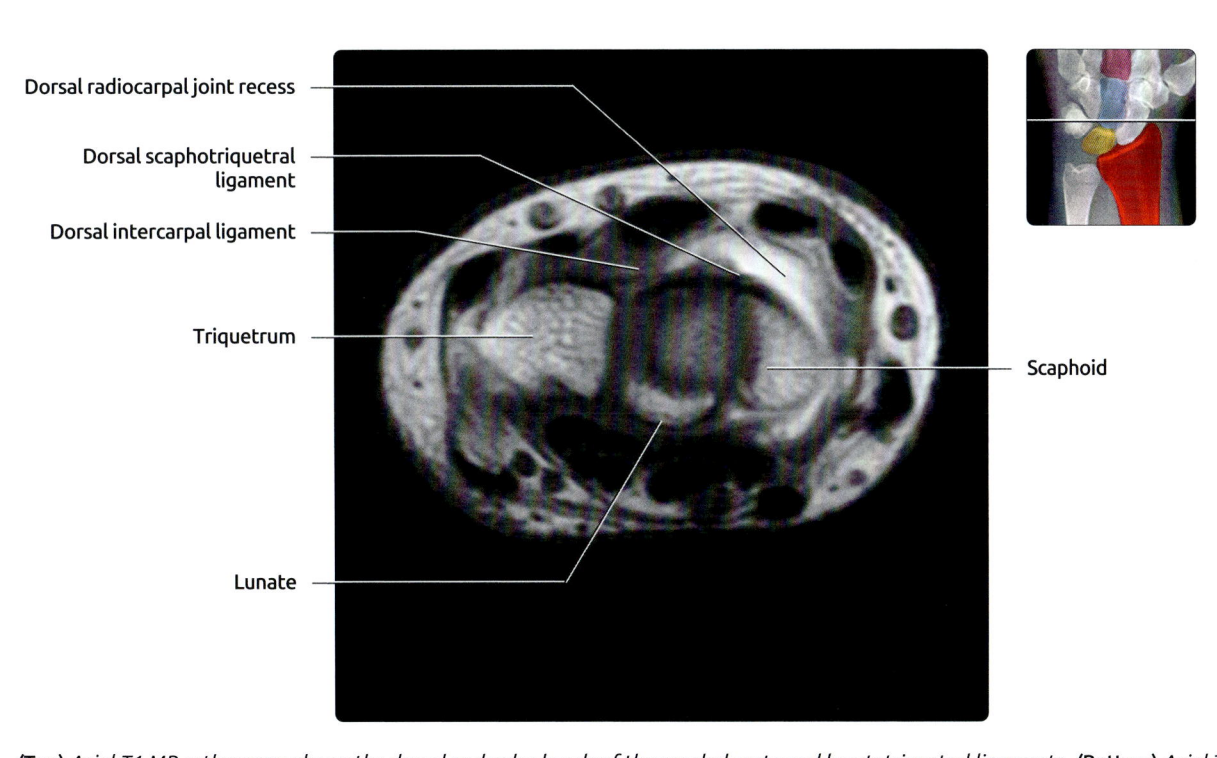

(Top) Axial T1 MR arthrogram shows the dorsal and volar bands of the scapholunate and lunatotriquetral ligaments. (Bottom) Axial T1 MR arthrogram slightly distal to the prior image shows the normal joint recesses.

Wrist MR Atlas

TERMINOLOGY

Definitions
- Volar = palmar; ulnar = medial; radial = lateral

IMAGING ANATOMY

Anatomy Relationships
- 6 dorsal compartments of wrist
  - Remember order of first 3 compartments by remembering "longus-brevis-longus-brevis-longus"
    - 1st tendon of 1st compartment is an abductor: Abductor pollicis longus (all other dorsal tendons are extensors)
    - Following the rule of alternating longus and brevis tendons, 2nd tendon of 1st compartment must be extensor pollicis brevis
    - 2nd compartment has the extensor carpi muscles: Longus & brevis
    - 3rd compartment has only 1 tendon: Extensor pollicis longus
- Compartment 4 has 4 tendons, all extensor digiti
- Compartments 5 and 6 have 1 tendon each, extensor digiti minimi and extensor carpi ulnaris

Retinacula
- **Flexor retinaculum**
  - Superficial (volar carpal ligament or ligamentum carpi palmare): Attached to styloid processes of ulna & radius; merges with deep component distally
  - Deep (transverse carpal ligament or ligamentum flexorum): Attached to pisiform & hook of hamate medially, scaphoid & trapezium laterally
- **Extensor retinaculum**
  - Attaches to ulnar styloid process, triquetrum & pisiform medially, crosses obliquely to attach Lister tubercle & radial styloid process laterally
    - Sends septa to radius creating compartments for extensor tendons
  - Compartment contents: (1) APL, EPB; (2) ECRL, ECRB; (3) EPL; (4) ED, EI; (5) EDM; (6) ECU

Anatomic Spaces
- **Anatomic snuffbox**: Concavity at radial side of wrist, from radial styloid to base of thumb
  - **Margins**: Outlined by extensor pollicis longus, abductor pollicis longus tendons
  - **Contents**: Cephalic vein, radial nerve, (superficial branch), radial artery
- **Carpal tunnel**
  - **Margins**: Carpals (dorsal margin), flexor retinaculum (volar margin); pisiform & hook of the hamate (medial margin), scaphoid & trapezium (lateral margin), radiocarpal joint (proximal margin) & metacarpal base (distal margin)
  - Contents: Flexor digitorum superficialis and profundus, flexor pollicis longus, median nerve
  - Median nerve lies at volar and radial side of tunnel
- **Guyon canal**
  - **Margins**: Superficial flexor retinaculum (volar carpal ligament or ligamentum carpi palmare) (ventral margin), pisiform & FCU (medial margin), deep flexor retinaculum (transverse carpal ligament or ligamentum flexorum) (lateral & dorsal margin)
  - **Contents**: Ulnar artery & vein, ulnar nerve

ANATOMY IMAGING ISSUES

Imaging Recommendations
- MR: Dedicated coils, 8-10 cm field of view, thin sections essential for imaging small, complex wrist anatomy
  - T1: Axial plane; for anatomy, marrow, spaces
  - PD FS or GRE (T2*): Coronal plane; for ligaments, articular cartilage
    - PD FS highest signal to noise
    - GRE has greater magic angle effect, susceptibility artifact
      - Often see increased signal intensity in normal ligaments
  - T2FS: Sagittal plane; for synovitis, marrow, masses
  - PD/T2FS: Axial plane; marrow, cartilage, ligaments, fluid collections
  - Structures best visualized (by plane)
    - Coronal: Osseous structures, alignment, intrinsic & extrinsic ligaments, triangular fibrocartilage
    - Axial: Tendons, neurovascular structures, distal radioulnar joint, pisotriquetral joint
    - Sagittal: Alignment, cross section ligaments, pisotriquetral joint

Imaging Pitfalls
- Many tendon variations, including split or duplicated tendons
- Small amount extensor tendon sheath fluid is common (particularly 2nd compartment); should not be mistaken for tenosynovitis
- Triangular fibrocartilage attachments may mimic tears: Radial attachments to hyaline cartilage rather than cortex; ulnar attachment to ulna fossa often intermediate signal due to magic angle or volume averaging
  - Articular disc may develop asymptomatic attritional tears
- Scapholunate & lunotriquetral ligaments may attach to articular cartilage rather than cortex
- Malpositioning: Ulnar or radial deviation may mimic appearance of instability patterns
- Magic angle effect: Organized fibers (t. or l.) crossing at 55° to main magnetic field may have intermediate signal on short TE imaging (T1, PD, GRE)
  - Examples: Extensor carpi ulnaris crossing dorsum of ulna; extensor pollicis longus crossing dorsal wrist obliquely

Wrist MR Atlas

3D CT ANATOMY

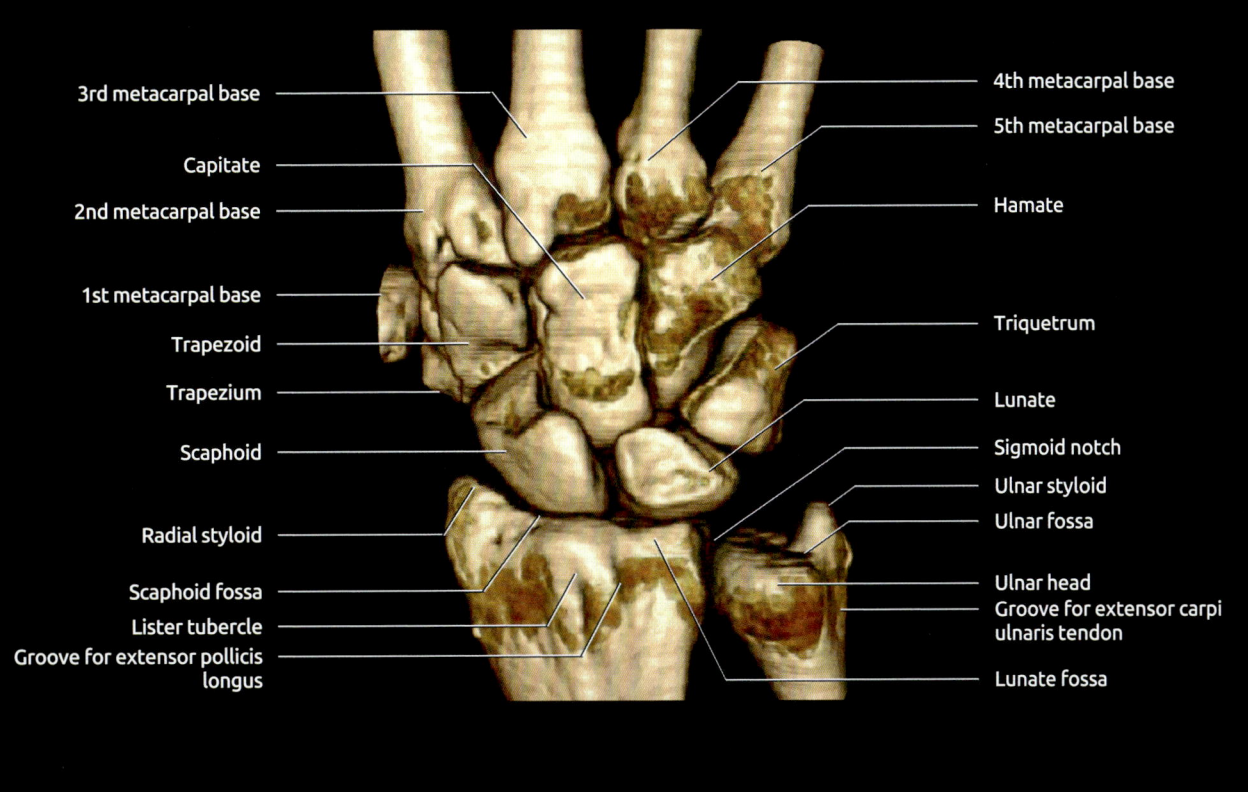

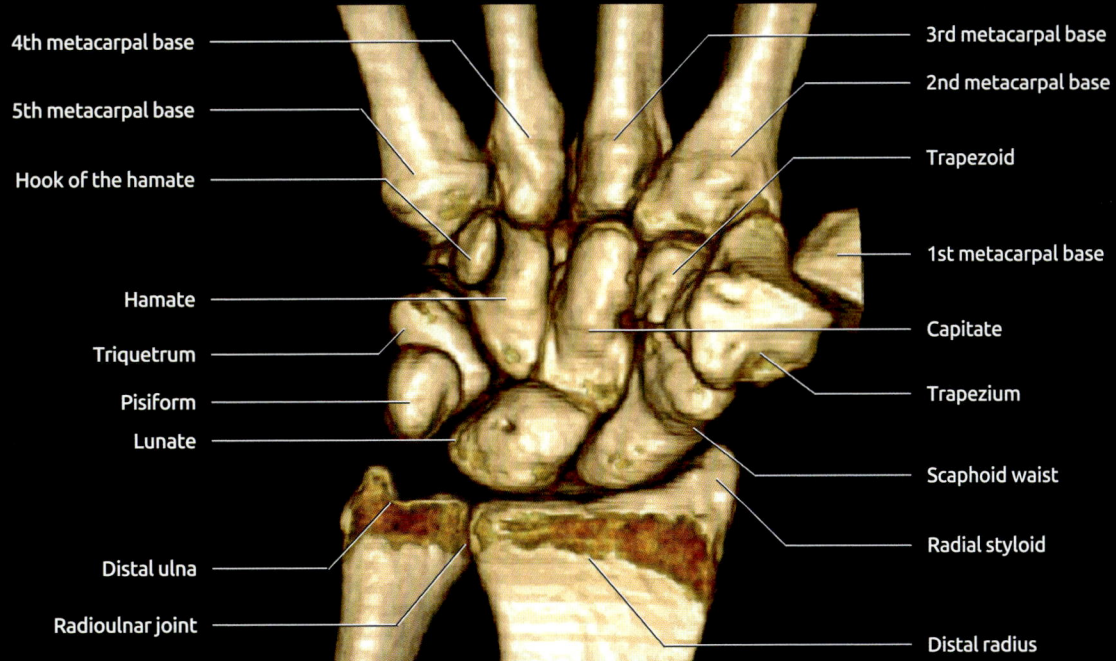

- 3rd metacarpal base
- Capitate
- 2nd metacarpal base
- 1st metacarpal base
- Trapezoid
- Trapezium
- Scaphoid
- Radial styloid
- Scaphoid fossa
- Lister tubercle
- Groove for extensor pollicis longus
- 4th metacarpal base
- 5th metacarpal base
- Hamate
- Triquetrum
- Lunate
- Sigmoid notch
- Ulnar styloid
- Ulnar fossa
- Ulnar head
- Groove for extensor carpi ulnaris tendon
- Lunate fossa

- 4th metacarpal base
- 5th metacarpal base
- Hook of the hamate
- Hamate
- Triquetrum
- Pisiform
- Lunate
- Distal ulna
- Radioulnar joint
- 3rd metacarpal base
- 2nd metacarpal base
- Trapezoid
- 1st metacarpal base
- Capitate
- Trapezium
- Scaphoid waist
- Radial styloid
- Distal radius

(**Top**) *3D surface rendering shows dorsal wrist, positioned in pronation.* (**Bottom**) *Volar wrist, positioned in pronation, is shown.*

Wrist MR Atlas

AXIAL T1 MR, RIGHT WRIST

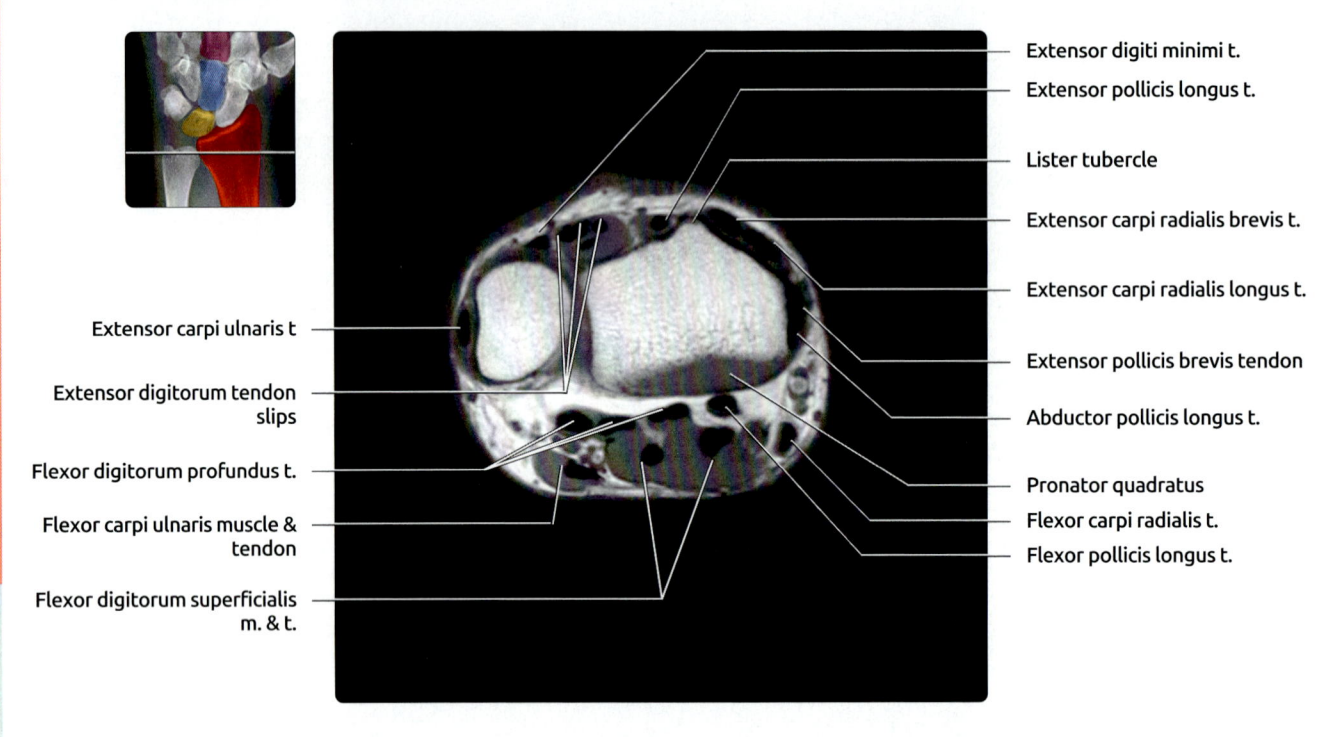

Extensor digiti minimi t.
Extensor pollicis longus t.
Lister tubercle
Extensor carpi radialis brevis t.
Extensor carpi radialis longus t.
Extensor pollicis brevis tendon
Abductor pollicis longus t.
Pronator quadratus
Flexor carpi radialis t.
Flexor pollicis longus t.

Extensor carpi ulnaris t
Extensor digitorum tendon slips
Flexor digitorum profundus t.
Flexor carpi ulnaris muscle & tendon
Flexor digitorum superficialis m. & t.

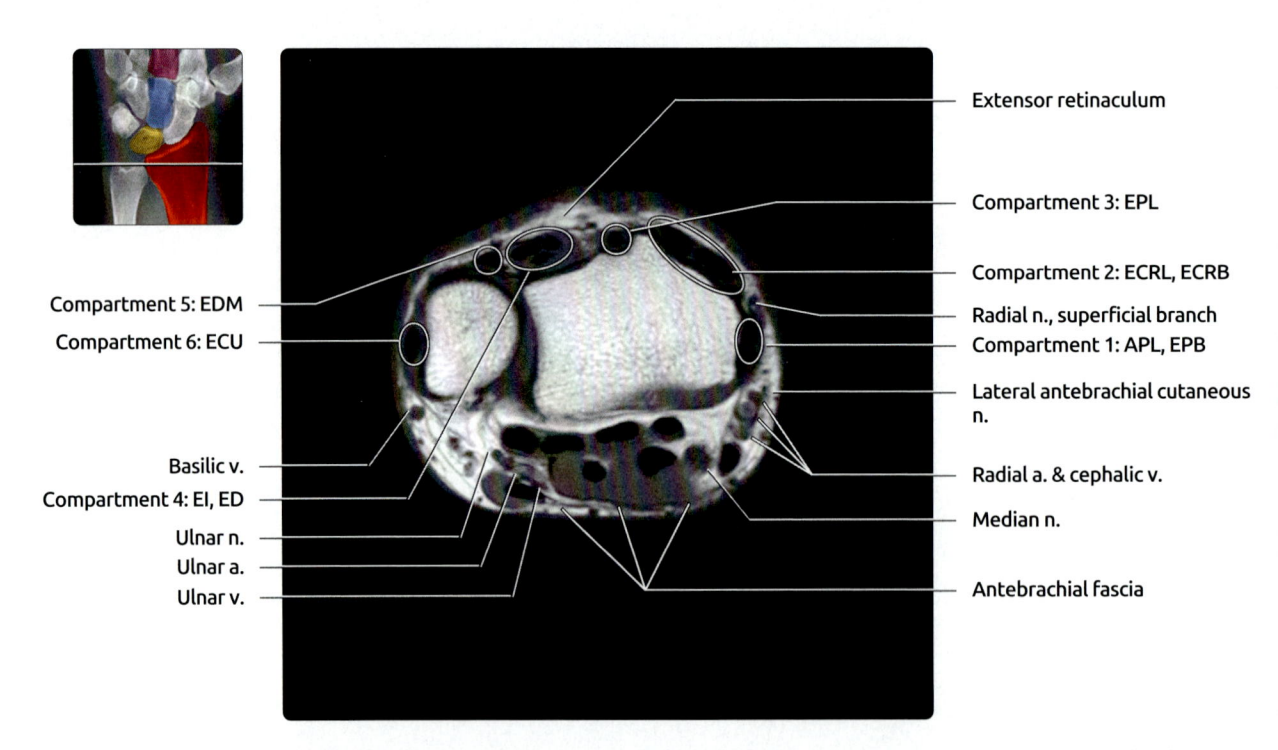

Extensor retinaculum
Compartment 3: EPL
Compartment 2: ECRL, ECRB
Radial n., superficial branch
Compartment 1: APL, EPB
Lateral antebrachial cutaneous n.
Radial a. & cephalic v.
Median n.
Antebrachial fascia

Compartment 5: EDM
Compartment 6: ECU
Basilic v.
Compartment 4: EI, ED
Ulnar n.
Ulnar a.
Ulnar v.

(Top) First of 2 sequential T1 axial images of right wrist, from proximal to distal, displays tendons & musculature at Lister tubercle. Lister tubercle is a useful landmark in understanding extensor compartment anatomy. **(Bottom)** Slightly distal, at level of ulnar head & distal radius, neurovascular structures & fascia are annotated. The extensor retinaculum creates 6 separate tunnels or compartments as it attaches to underlying bone. Each compartment contains 1 or more tendons as follows: (1) abductor pollicis longus, extensor pollicis brevis; (2) extensor carpi radialis longus & brevis; (3) extensor pollicis longus; (4) extensor indicis, extensor digitorum; (5) extensor digiti minimi; (6) extensor carpi ulnaris.

AXIAL T1 MR, LEFT WRIST

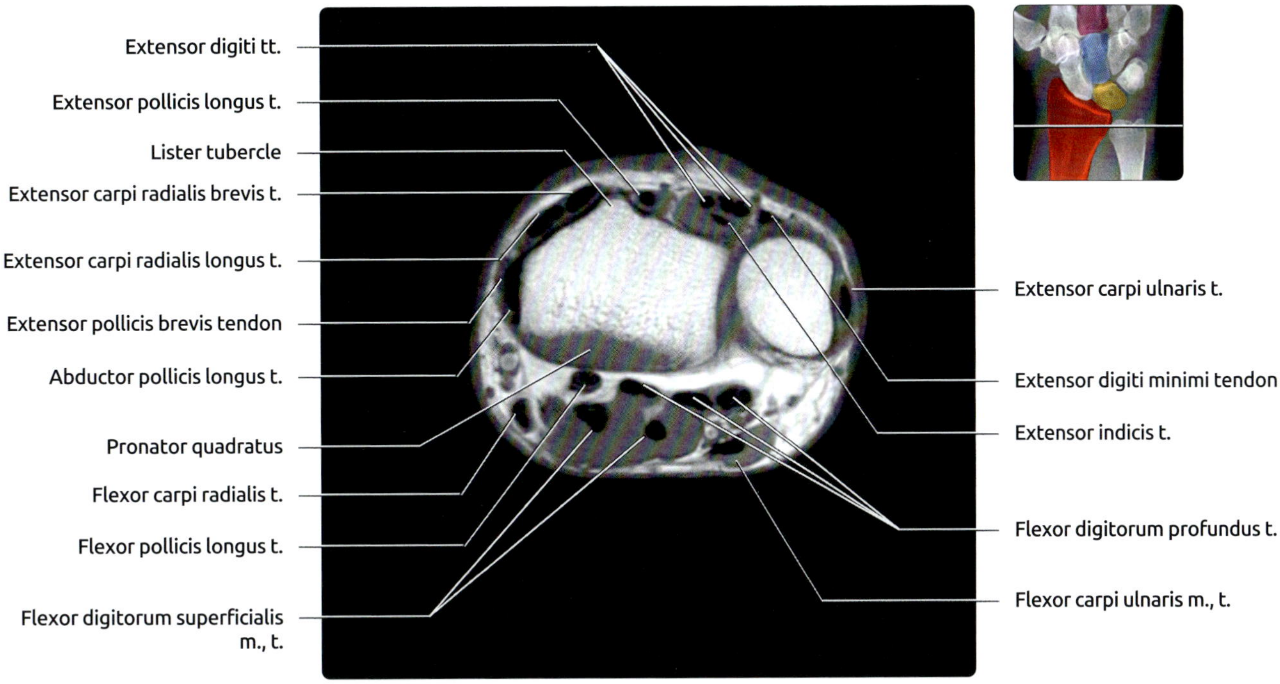
Extensor digiti tt.
Extensor pollicis longus t.
Lister tubercle
Extensor carpi radialis brevis t.
Extensor carpi radialis longus t.
Extensor pollicis brevis tendon
Abductor pollicis longus t.
Pronator quadratus
Flexor carpi radialis t.
Flexor pollicis longus t.
Flexor digitorum superficialis m., t.
Extensor carpi ulnaris t.
Extensor digiti minimi tendon
Extensor indicis t.
Flexor digitorum profundus t.
Flexor carpi ulnaris m., t.

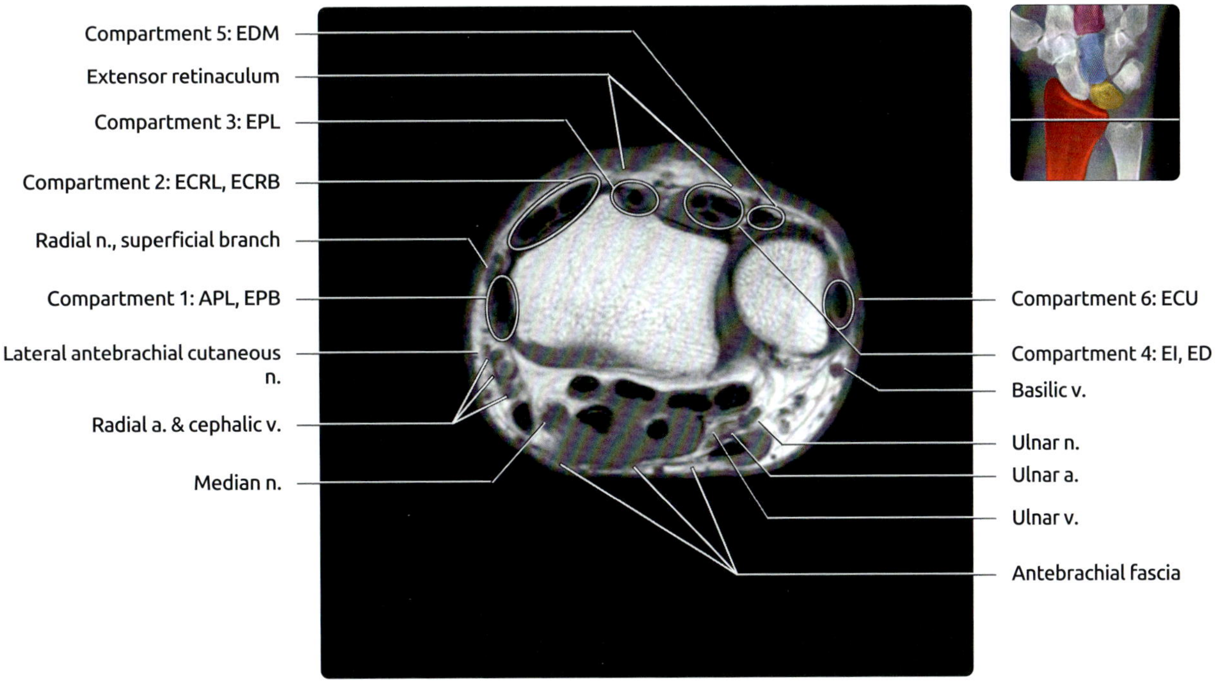
Compartment 5: EDM
Extensor retinaculum
Compartment 3: EPL
Compartment 2: ECRL, ECRB
Radial n., superficial branch
Compartment 1: APL, EPB
Lateral antebrachial cutaneous n.
Radial a. & cephalic v.
Median n.
Compartment 6: ECU
Compartment 4: EI, ED
Basilic v.
Ulnar n.
Ulnar a.
Ulnar v.
Antebrachial fascia

(Top) *First of 18 sequential T1 axial images of left wrist, from proximal to distal, displays tendons & musculature at Lister tubercle.* **(Bottom)** *Slightly distal, at level of ulnar head & distal radius, neurovascular structures, & fascia are annotated. The extensor retinaculum creates 6 separate tunnels or compartments as it attaches to underlying bone. Each compartment contains 1 or more tendons as follows: 1) abductor pollicis longus, extensor pollicis brevis; 2) extensor carpi radialis longus & brevis; 3) extensor pollicis longus; 4) extensor indicis, extensor digitorum; 5) extensor digiti minimi; 6) extensor carpi ulnaris.*

Wrist MR Atlas

AXIAL T1 MR, RIGHT WRIST

Top image labels (left side):
- Extensor digitorum tt., extensor indicis t.
- Extensor carpi ulnaris t.
- Ulnar styloid
- Sigmoid notch
- Volar radioulnar l.
- Flexor carpi ulnaris muscle & tendon
- Flexor digitorum profundus t.

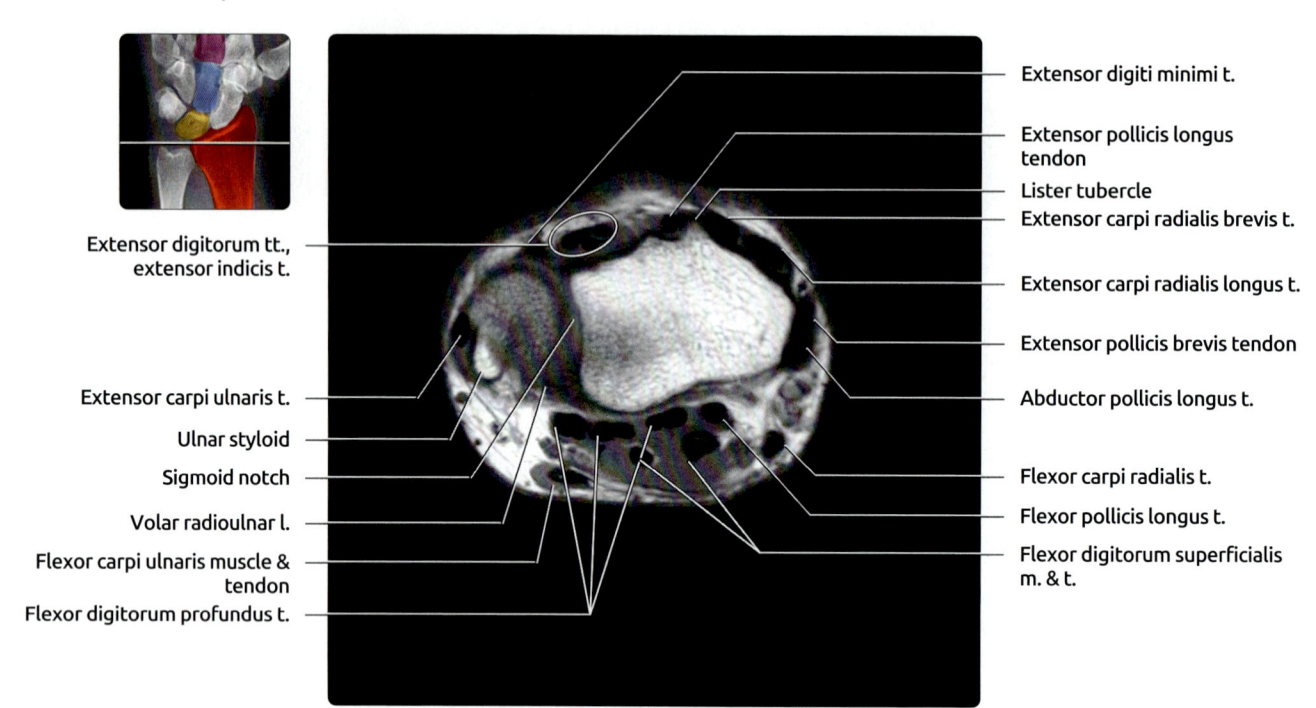

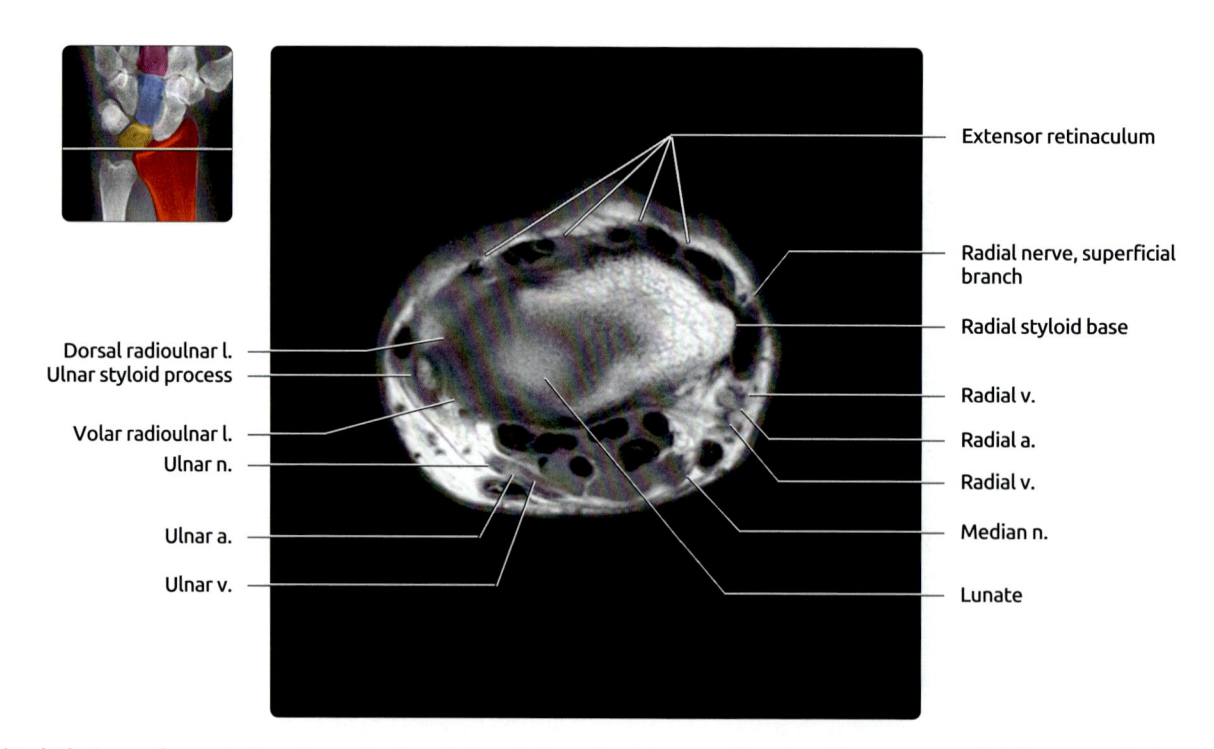

Top image labels (right side):
- Extensor digiti minimi t.
- Extensor pollicis longus tendon
- Lister tubercle
- Extensor carpi radialis brevis t.
- Extensor carpi radialis longus t.
- Extensor pollicis brevis tendon
- Abductor pollicis longus t.
- Flexor carpi radialis t.
- Flexor pollicis longus t.
- Flexor digitorum superficialis m. & t.

Bottom image labels (left side):
- Dorsal radioulnar l.
- Ulnar styloid process
- Volar radioulnar l.
- Ulnar n.
- Ulnar a.
- Ulnar v.

Bottom image labels (right side):
- Extensor retinaculum
- Radial nerve, superficial branch
- Radial styloid base
- Radial v.
- Radial a.
- Radial v.
- Median n.
- Lunate

(Top) The image demonstrates extensor tendons that are tethered by extensor retinaculum. The extensor pollicis longus tendon lies within a dorsal osseous groove ulnar to Lister tubercle. Flexor musculotendinous junctions are visualized proximal to carpal tunnel. Palmaris longus tendon is absent as it is in ~ 10% of the general population. **(Bottom)** Extensor retinaculum is identifiable at ulnar styloid tip & radial styloid base. Median & ulnar nerves are readily visualized as is superficial branch of radial nerve.

Wrist MR Atlas

AXIAL T1 MR, LEFT WRIST

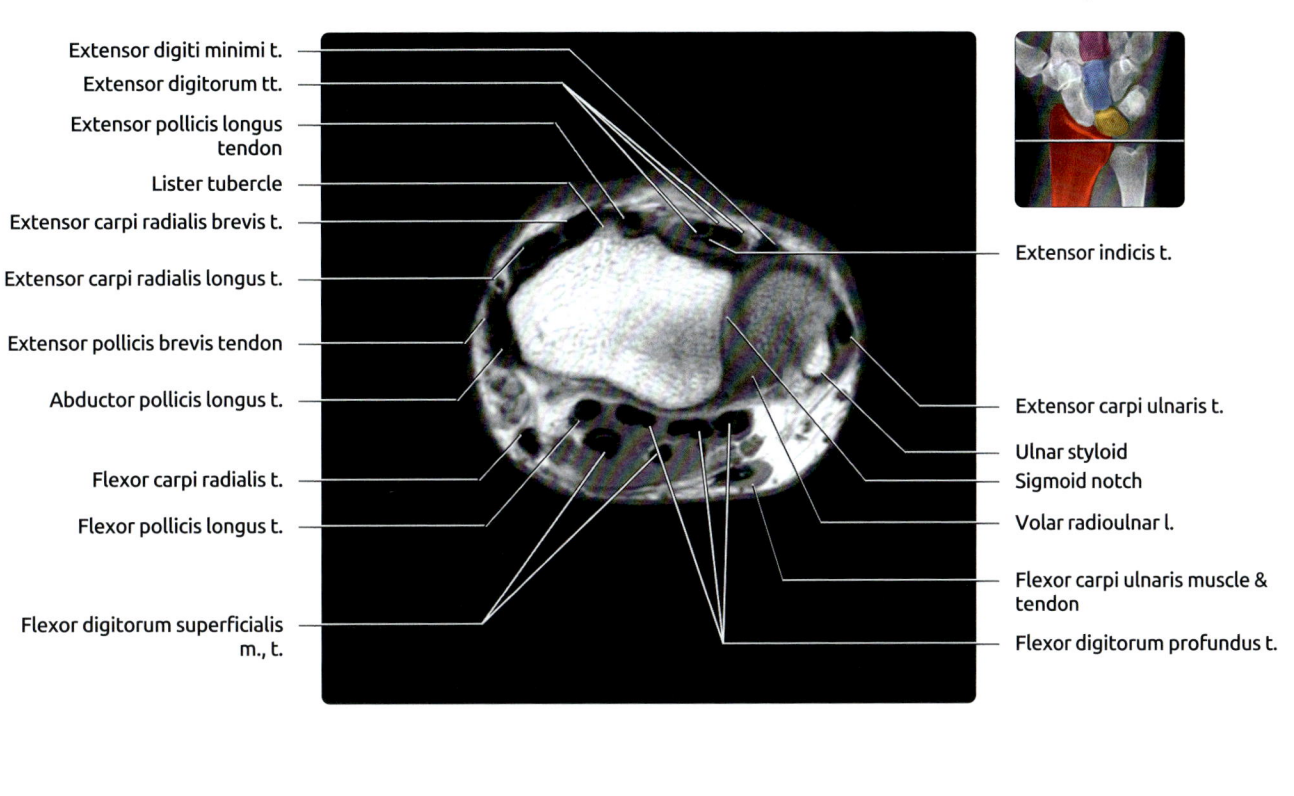

Labels (top image):
- Extensor digiti minimi t.
- Extensor digitorum tt.
- Extensor pollicis longus tendon
- Lister tubercle
- Extensor carpi radialis brevis t.
- Extensor carpi radialis longus t.
- Extensor pollicis brevis tendon
- Abductor pollicis longus t.
- Flexor carpi radialis t.
- Flexor pollicis longus t.
- Flexor digitorum superficialis m., t.
- Extensor indicis t.
- Extensor carpi ulnaris t.
- Ulnar styloid
- Sigmoid notch
- Volar radioulnar l.
- Flexor carpi ulnaris muscle & tendon
- Flexor digitorum profundus t.

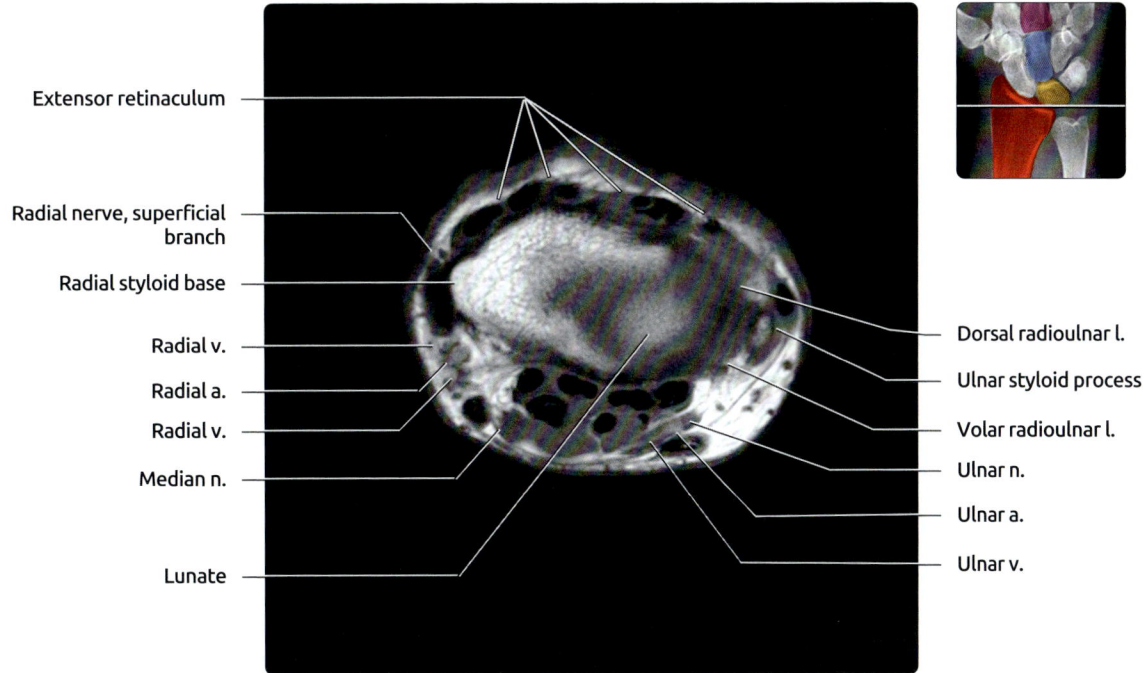

Labels (bottom image):
- Extensor retinaculum
- Radial nerve, superficial branch
- Radial styloid base
- Radial v.
- Radial a.
- Radial v.
- Median n.
- Lunate
- Dorsal radioulnar l.
- Ulnar styloid process
- Volar radioulnar l.
- Ulnar n.
- Ulnar a.
- Ulnar v.

(Top) *Extensor tendons are tethered by extensor retinaculum. Extensor pollicis longus tendon lies within a dorsal osseous groove ulnar to Lister tubercle. Flexor musculotendinous junctions are visualized proximal to carpal tunnel. Palmaris longus tendon is absent as it is in ~ 10% of the general population.* (Bottom) *Extensor retinaculum is identifiable at ulnar styloid tip & radial styloid base. Median & ulnar nerves are readily visualized as is superficial branch of radial nerve.*

Wrist MR Atlas

AXIAL T1 MR, RIGHT WRIST

Extensor digitorum t. slips
Extensor indicis t.
Extensor pollicis longus tendon
Extensor carpi radialis brevis t.
Extensor carpi radialis longus t.
Radial styloid process
Extensor pollicis brevis tendon
Abductor pollicis longus t.
Scaphoid
Flexor carpi radialis t.
Flexor pollicis longus t.
Flexor digitorum superficialis t.

Extensor digiti minimi tendon
Extensor carpi ulnaris t.
Dorsal radioulnar l.
Volar radioulnar l.
Lunate
Flexor carpi ulnaris t.
Flexor digitorum profundus t.

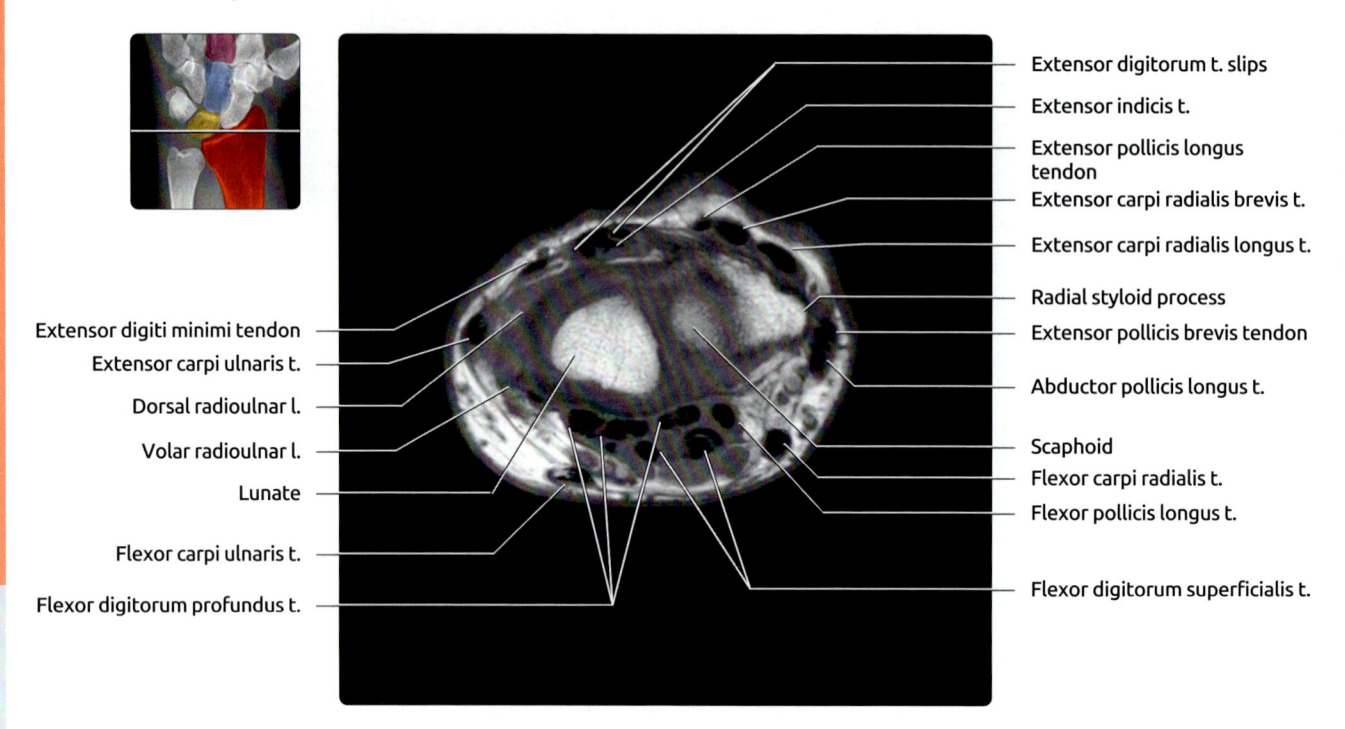

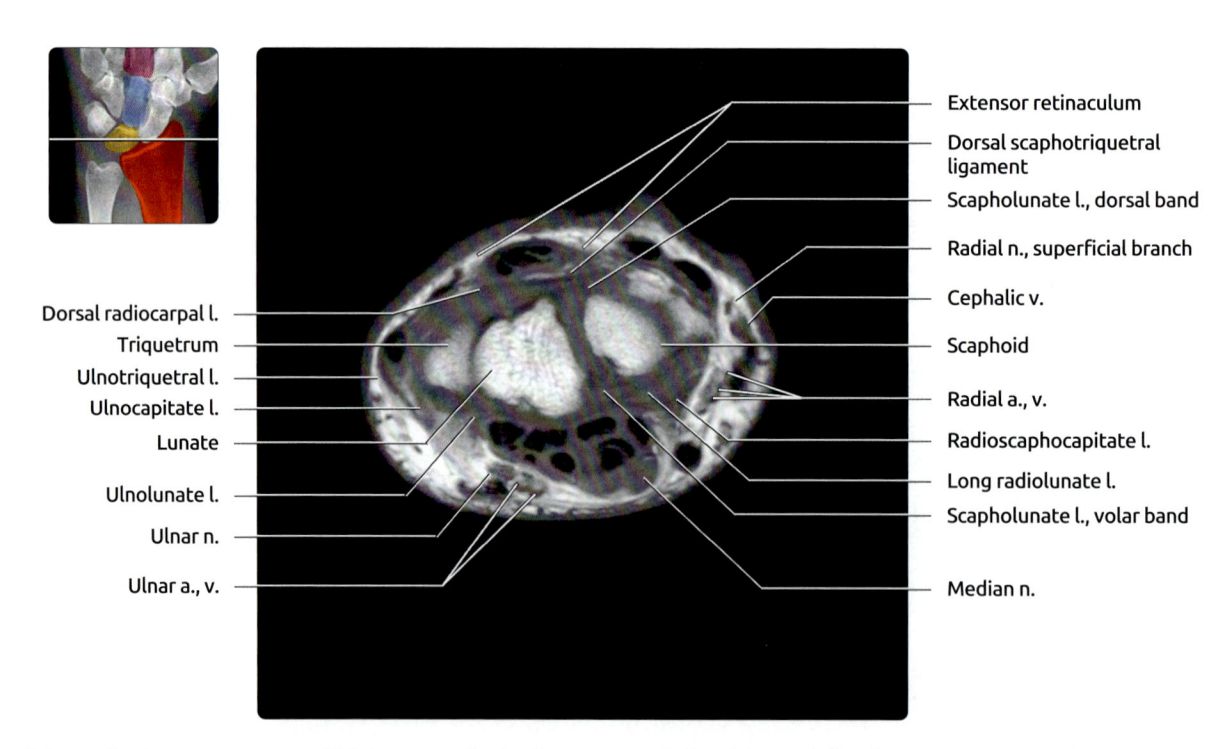

Extensor retinaculum
Dorsal scaphotriquetral ligament
Scapholunate l., dorsal band
Radial n., superficial branch
Cephalic v.
Scaphoid
Radial a., v.
Radioscaphocapitate l.
Long radiolunate l.
Scapholunate l., volar band
Median n.

Dorsal radiocarpal l.
Triquetrum
Ulnotriquetral l.
Ulnocapitate l.
Lunate
Ulnolunate l.
Ulnar n.
Ulnar a., v.

(Top) *At proximal lunate, extensor pollicis longus tendon begins to cross radially. Abductor pollicis longus & extensor pollicis brevis tendons are dividing into multiple slips. Extensor carpi ulnaris tendon has some intermediate intrasubstance signal intensity normally. This does not represent a tear. Dorsal & volar radioulnar ligaments, components of triangular fibrocartilage complex, are evident.*
(Bottom) *Volar & dorsal extrinsic ligaments & ulnocarpal ligaments are evident at level of mid lunate. Median nerve is rounded prior to entering carpal tunnel with signal intensity equal to muscle.*

Wrist MR Atlas

AXIAL T1 MR, LEFT WRIST

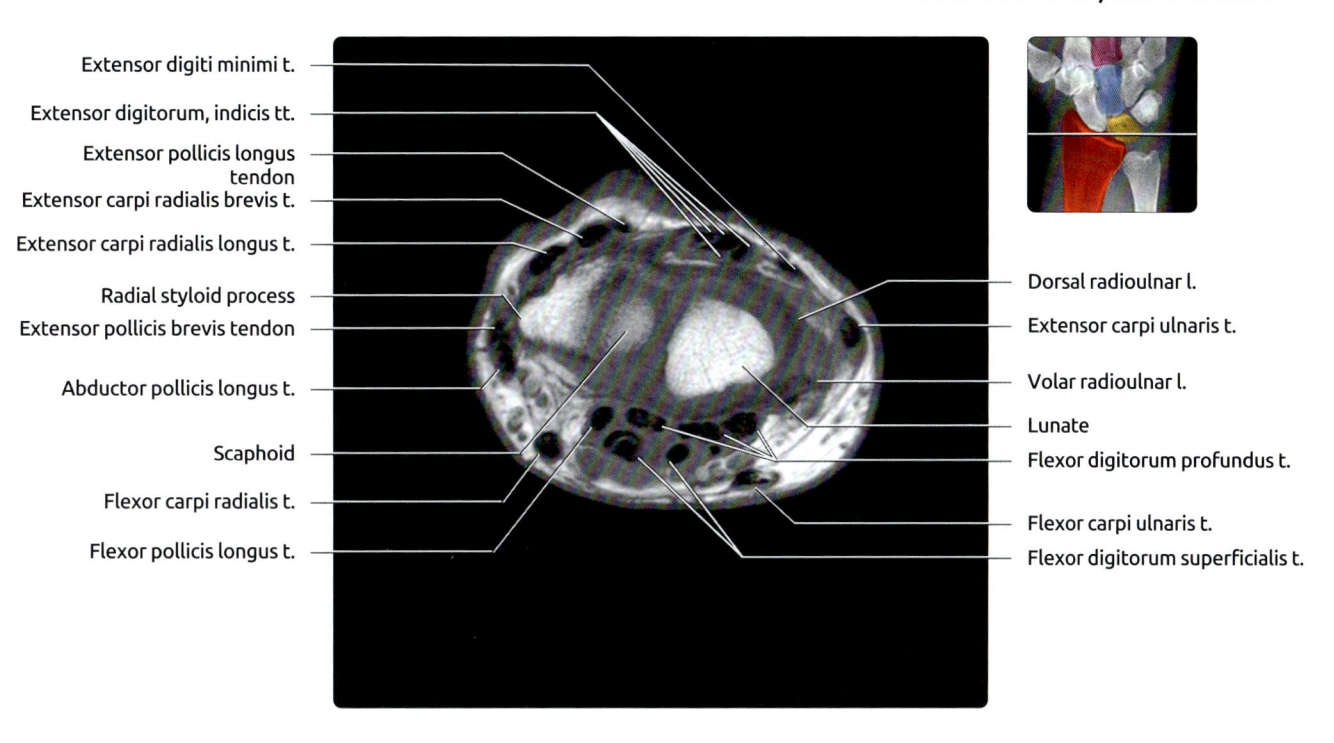

Top image labels (left):
- Extensor digiti minimi t.
- Extensor digitorum, indicis tt.
- Extensor pollicis longus tendon
- Extensor carpi radialis brevis t.
- Extensor carpi radialis longus t.
- Radial styloid process
- Extensor pollicis brevis tendon
- Abductor pollicis longus t.
- Scaphoid
- Flexor carpi radialis t.
- Flexor pollicis longus t.

Top image labels (right):
- Dorsal radioulnar l.
- Extensor carpi ulnaris t.
- Volar radioulnar l.
- Lunate
- Flexor digitorum profundus t.
- Flexor carpi ulnaris t.
- Flexor digitorum superficialis t.

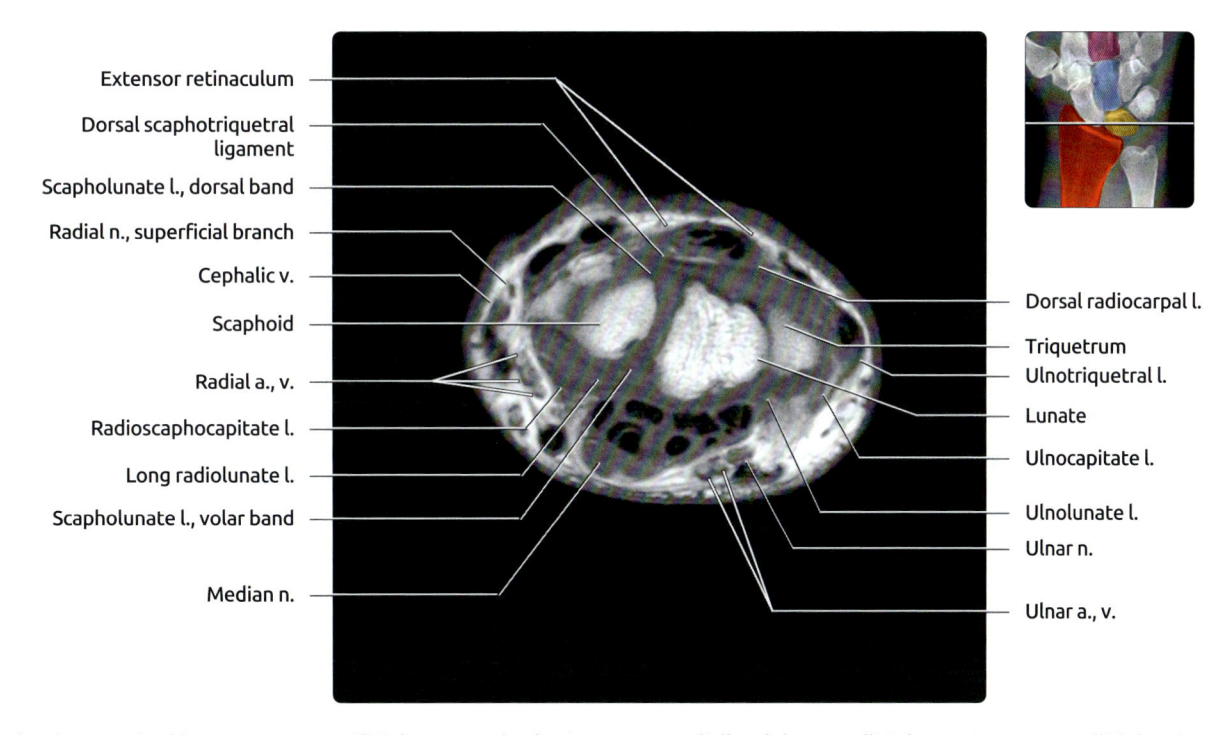

Bottom image labels (left):
- Extensor retinaculum
- Dorsal scaphotriquetral ligament
- Scapholunate l., dorsal band
- Radial n., superficial branch
- Cephalic v.
- Scaphoid
- Radial a., v.
- Radioscaphocapitate l.
- Long radiolunate l.
- Scapholunate l., volar band
- Median n.

Bottom image labels (right):
- Dorsal radiocarpal l.
- Triquetrum
- Ulnotriquetral l.
- Lunate
- Ulnocapitate l.
- Ulnolunate l.
- Ulnar n.
- Ulnar a., v.

(**Top**) *At proximal lunate, extensor pollicis longus tendon begins to cross radially. Abductor pollicis longus & extensor pollicis brevis tendons are dividing into multiple slips. Extensor carpi ulnaris tendon has some intermediate intrasubstance signal intensity normally. This does not represent a tear. Dorsal & volar radioulnar ligaments, components of triangular fibrocartilage complex, are evident.* (**Bottom**) *Volar & dorsal extrinsic ligaments & ulnocarpal ligaments are evident at level of mid lunate. Median nerve is rounded prior to entering carpal tunnel with signal intensity equal to muscle.*

AXIAL T1 MR, RIGHT WRIST

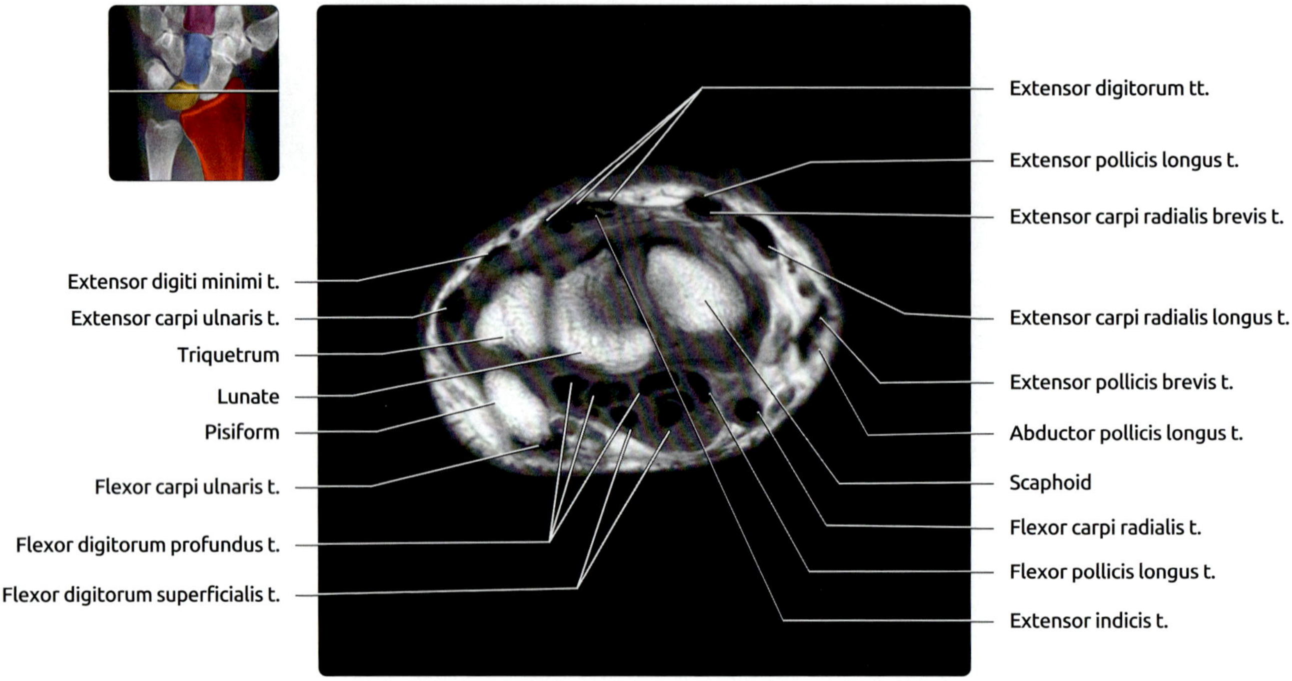
Extensor digitorum tt.
Extensor pollicis longus t.
Extensor carpi radialis brevis t.
Extensor digiti minimi t.
Extensor carpi ulnaris t.
Triquetrum
Lunate
Pisiform
Flexor carpi ulnaris t.
Flexor digitorum profundus t.
Flexor digitorum superficialis t.
Extensor carpi radialis longus t.
Extensor pollicis brevis t.
Abductor pollicis longus t.
Scaphoid
Flexor carpi radialis t.
Flexor pollicis longus t.
Extensor indicis t.

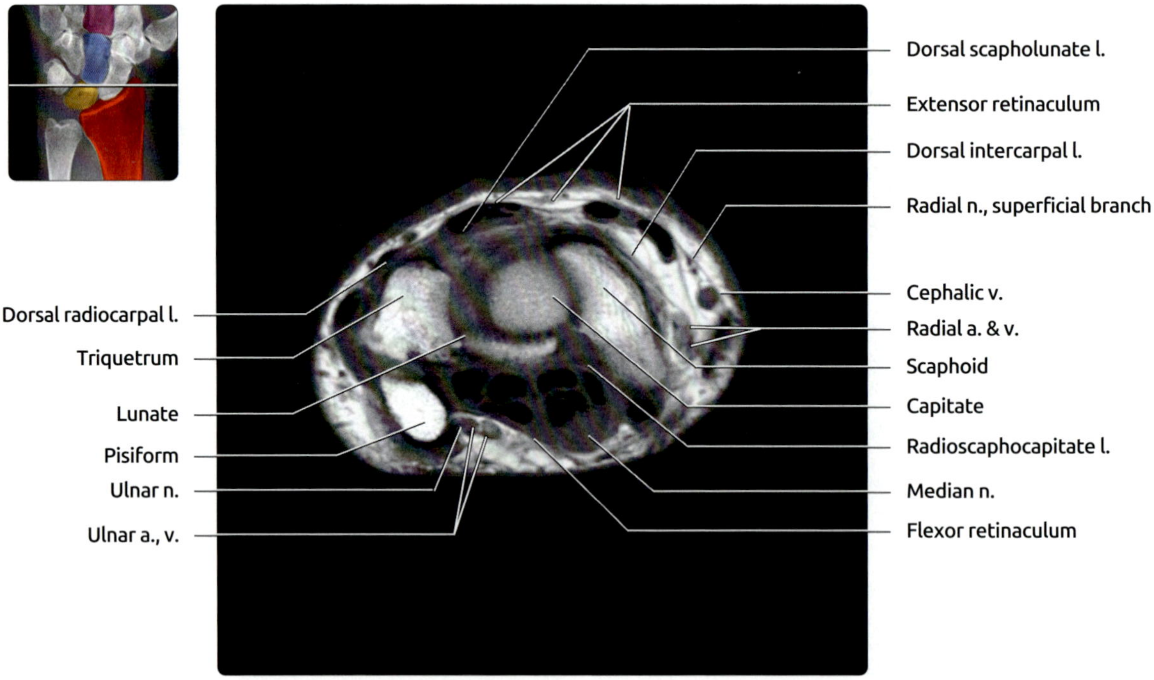
Dorsal scapholunate l.
Extensor retinaculum
Dorsal intercarpal l.
Radial n., superficial branch
Dorsal radiocarpal l.
Triquetrum
Lunate
Pisiform
Ulnar n.
Ulnar a., v.
Cephalic v.
Radial a. & v.
Scaphoid
Capitate
Radioscaphocapitate l.
Median n.
Flexor retinaculum

(Top) *Slightly more distal, at level of distal lunate & proximal pisiform, extensor pollicis longus tendon appears thin and ribbon-like as it crosses dorsal to extensor carpi radialis brevis tendon.* **(Bottom)** *Extensor retinaculum distal fibers are visualized at level of lunocapitate articulation. Extrinsic dorsal & volar ligaments are apparent as components of capsule. Median nerve remains rounded as it enters proximal carpal tunnel. Guyon canal is bordered by pisiform, deep, & superficial bands of flexor retinaculum, transverse carpal ligament proximally, & volar carpal ligament.*

Wrist MR Atlas

AXIAL T1 MR, LEFT WRIST

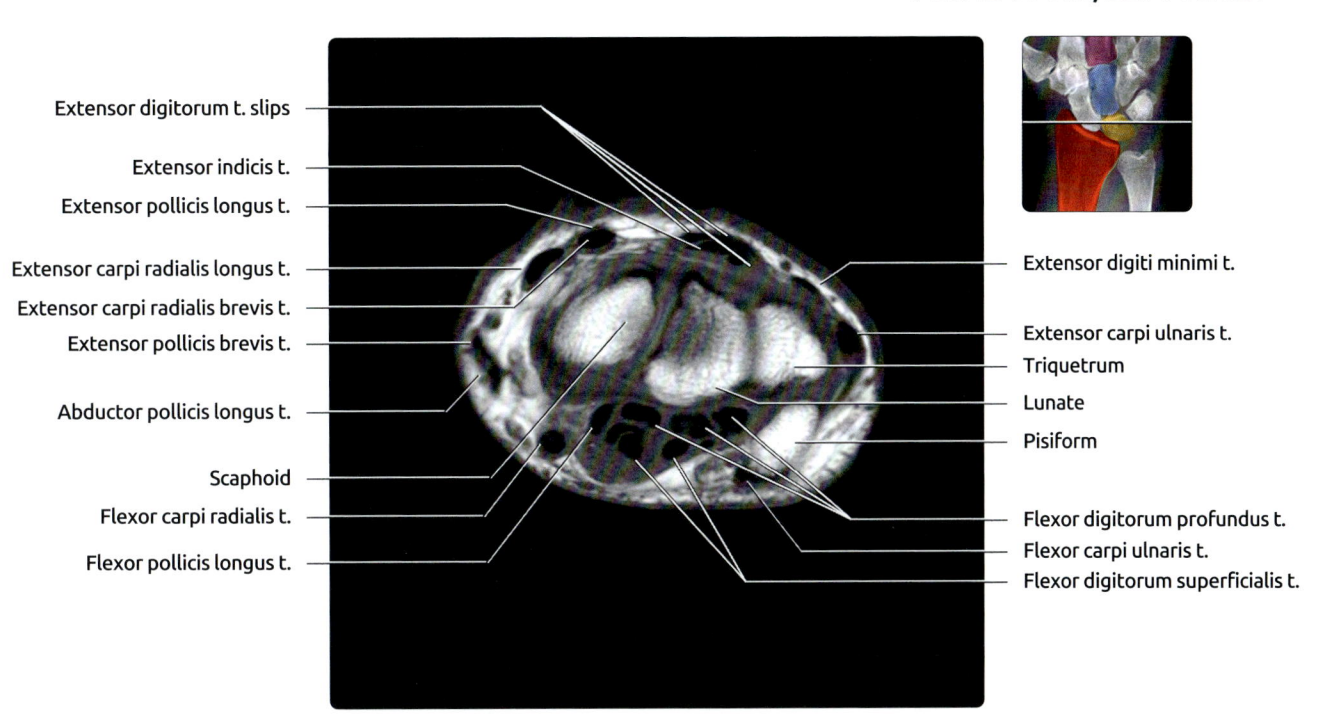

Labels (top image):
- Extensor digitorum t. slips
- Extensor indicis t.
- Extensor pollicis longus t.
- Extensor carpi radialis longus t.
- Extensor carpi radialis brevis t.
- Extensor pollicis brevis t.
- Abductor pollicis longus t.
- Scaphoid
- Flexor carpi radialis t.
- Flexor pollicis longus t.
- Extensor digiti minimi t.
- Extensor carpi ulnaris t.
- Triquetrum
- Lunate
- Pisiform
- Flexor digitorum profundus t.
- Flexor carpi ulnaris t.
- Flexor digitorum superficialis t.

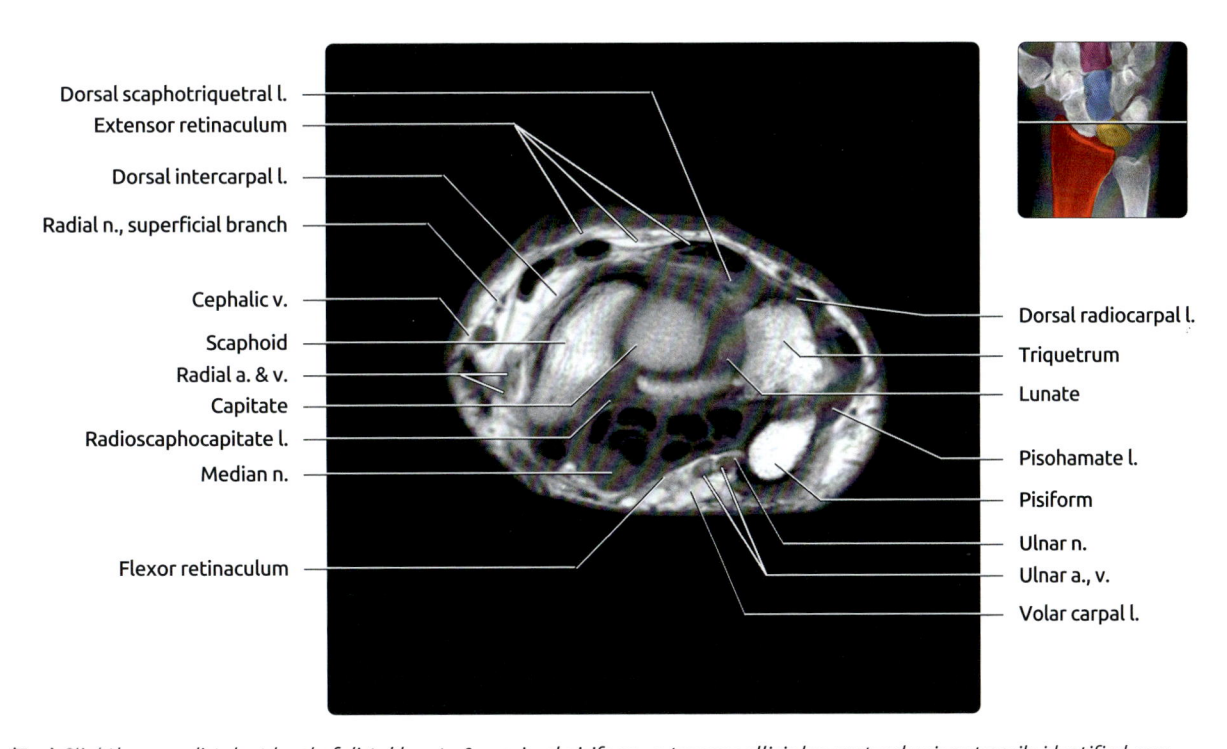

Labels (bottom image):
- Dorsal scaphotriquetral l.
- Extensor retinaculum
- Dorsal intercarpal l.
- Radial n., superficial branch
- Cephalic v.
- Scaphoid
- Radial a. & v.
- Capitate
- Radioscaphocapitate l.
- Median n.
- Flexor retinaculum
- Dorsal radiocarpal l.
- Triquetrum
- Lunate
- Pisohamate l.
- Pisiform
- Ulnar n.
- Ulnar a., v.
- Volar carpal l.

(Top) *Slightly more distal, at level of distal lunate & proximal pisiform, extensor pollicis longus tendon is not easily identified as a separate structure as it crosses dorsal to extensor carpi radialis brevis tendon.* (Bottom) *Extensor retinaculum distal fibers are visualized at level of lunocapitate articulation. Extrinsic dorsal & volar ligaments are apparent as components of capsule. Median nerve remains rounded as it enters proximal carpal tunnel. Guyon canal is bordered by pisiform, deep & superficial bands of flexor retinaculum, transverse carpal ligament proximally, & volar carpal ligament.*

Wrist MR Atlas

AXIAL T1 MR, RIGHT WRIST

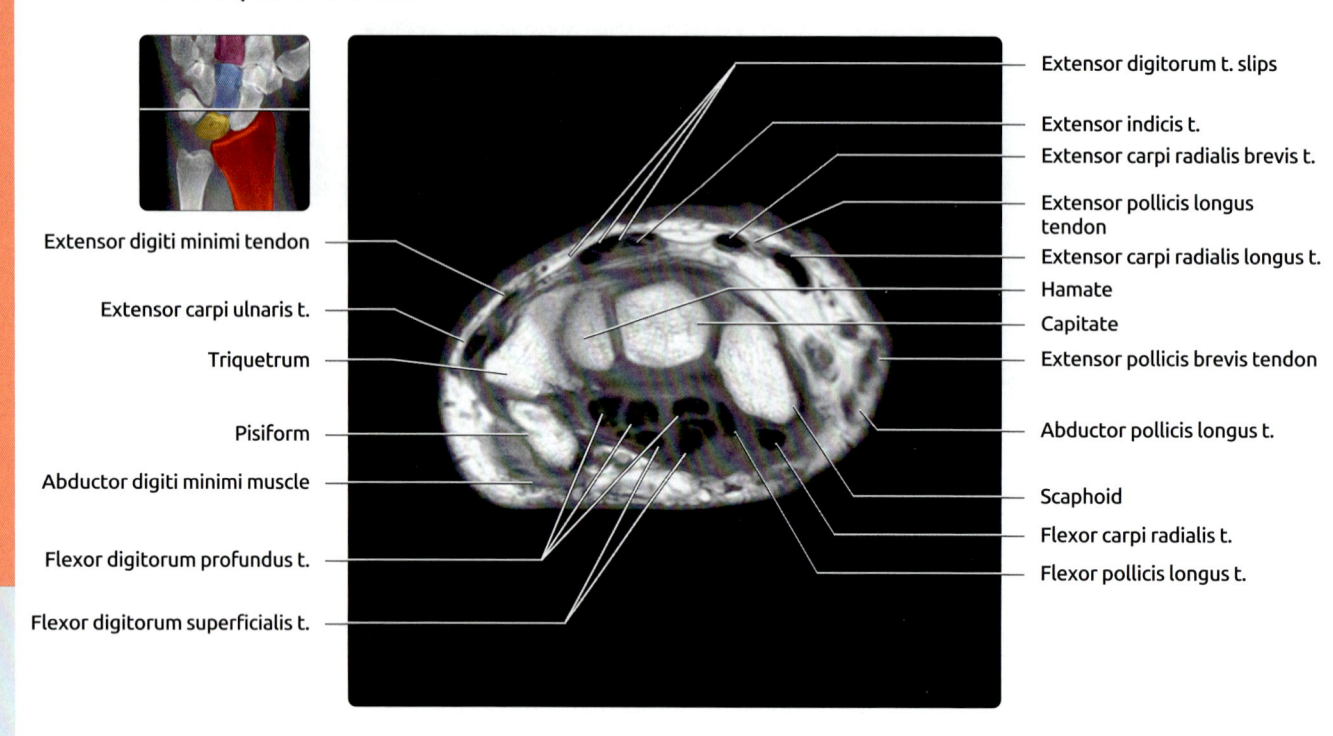

Labels (top image):
- Extensor digitorum t. slips
- Extensor indicis t.
- Extensor carpi radialis brevis t.
- Extensor pollicis longus tendon
- Extensor carpi radialis longus t.
- Hamate
- Capitate
- Extensor pollicis brevis tendon
- Abductor pollicis longus t.
- Scaphoid
- Flexor carpi radialis t.
- Flexor pollicis longus t.
- Extensor digiti minimi tendon
- Extensor carpi ulnaris t.
- Triquetrum
- Pisiform
- Abductor digiti minimi muscle
- Flexor digitorum profundus t.
- Flexor digitorum superficialis t.

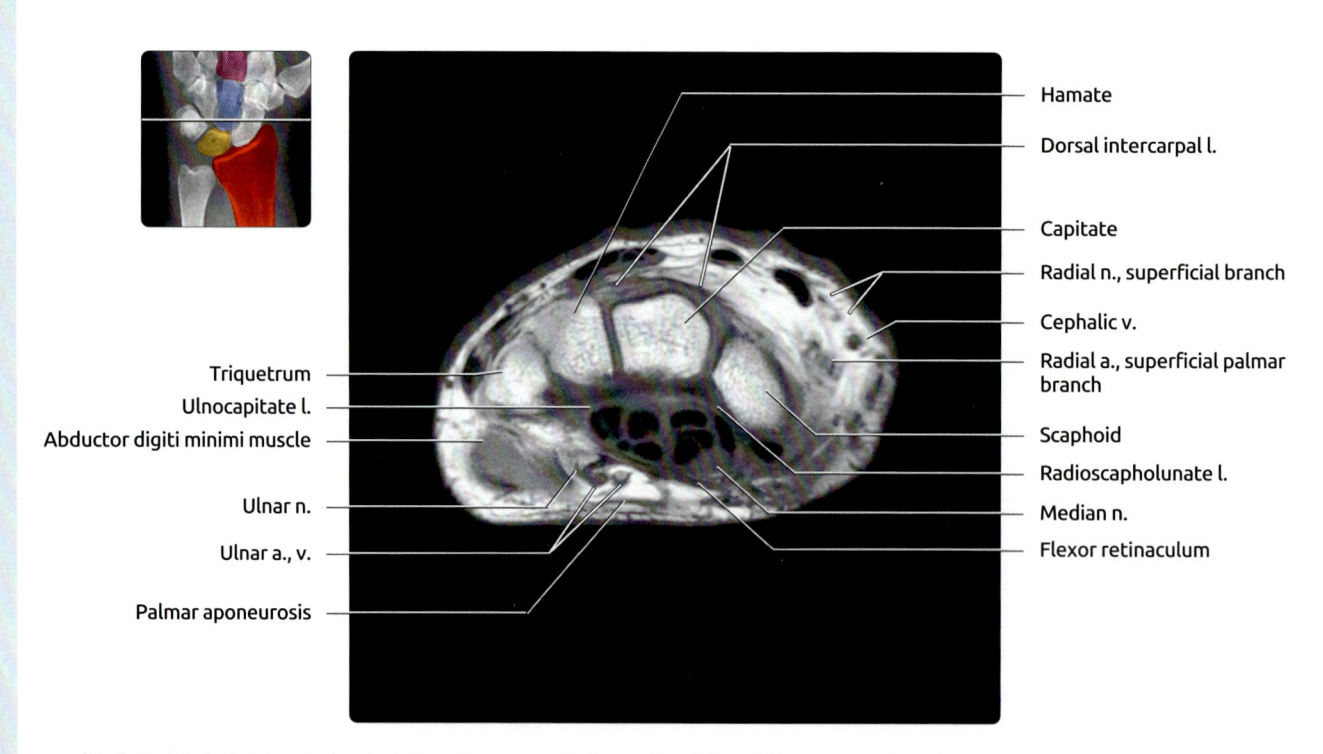

Labels (bottom image):
- Hamate
- Dorsal intercarpal l.
- Capitate
- Radial n., superficial branch
- Cephalic v.
- Radial a., superficial palmar branch
- Scaphoid
- Radioscapholunate l.
- Median n.
- Flexor retinaculum
- Triquetrum
- Ulnocapitate l.
- Abductor digiti minimi muscle
- Ulnar n.
- Ulnar a., v.
- Palmar aponeurosis

(Top) At distal pisotriquetral articulation, Guyon canal is located radial to pisiform & contains ulnar nerve, artery, & vein. Extensor pollicis longus tendon crosses dorsal to extensor carpi radialis brevis tendon & its obliquity makes it difficult to distinguish as a separate tendon. **(Bottom)** At the level of distal triquetrum & distal pole of scaphoid, ulnar nerve branches into deep & superficial branches. Note the beginning of thenar & hypothenar muscles, which originate from flexor retinaculum.

Wrist MR Atlas

AXIAL T1 MR, LEFT WRIST

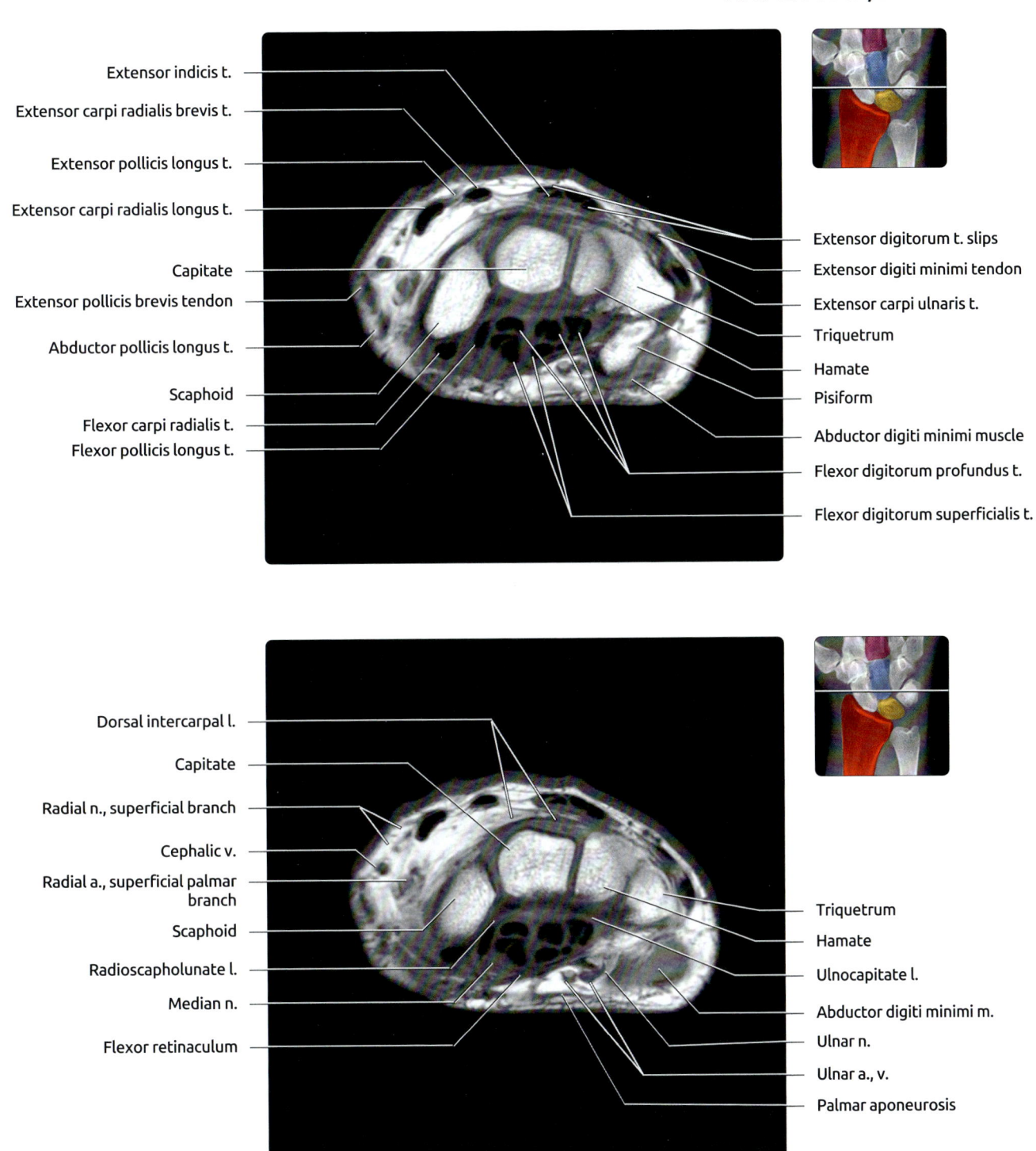

Extensor indicis t.
Extensor carpi radialis brevis t.
Extensor pollicis longus t.
Extensor carpi radialis longus t.
Capitate
Extensor pollicis brevis tendon
Abductor pollicis longus t.
Scaphoid
Flexor carpi radialis t.
Flexor pollicis longus t.

Extensor digitorum t. slips
Extensor digiti minimi tendon
Extensor carpi ulnaris t.
Triquetrum
Hamate
Pisiform
Abductor digiti minimi muscle
Flexor digitorum profundus t.
Flexor digitorum superficialis t.

Dorsal intercarpal l.
Capitate
Radial n., superficial branch
Cephalic v.
Radial a., superficial palmar branch
Scaphoid
Radioscapholunate l.
Median n.
Flexor retinaculum

Triquetrum
Hamate
Ulnocapitate l.
Abductor digiti minimi m.
Ulnar n.
Ulnar a., v.
Palmar aponeurosis

(Top) At distal pisotriquetral articulation, Guyon canal is located radial to pisiform & contains ulnar nerve, artery, & vein. Extensor pollicis longus tendon crosses dorsal to extensor carpi radialis brevis tendon & its obliquity makes it difficult to distinguish as a separate tendon. **(Bottom)** At the level of distal triquetrum & distal pole of scaphoid, ulnar nerve branches into deep & superficial branches. Note the beginning of thenar & hypothenar muscles, which originate from flexor retinaculum.

Wrist MR Atlas

AXIAL T1 MR, RIGHT WRIST

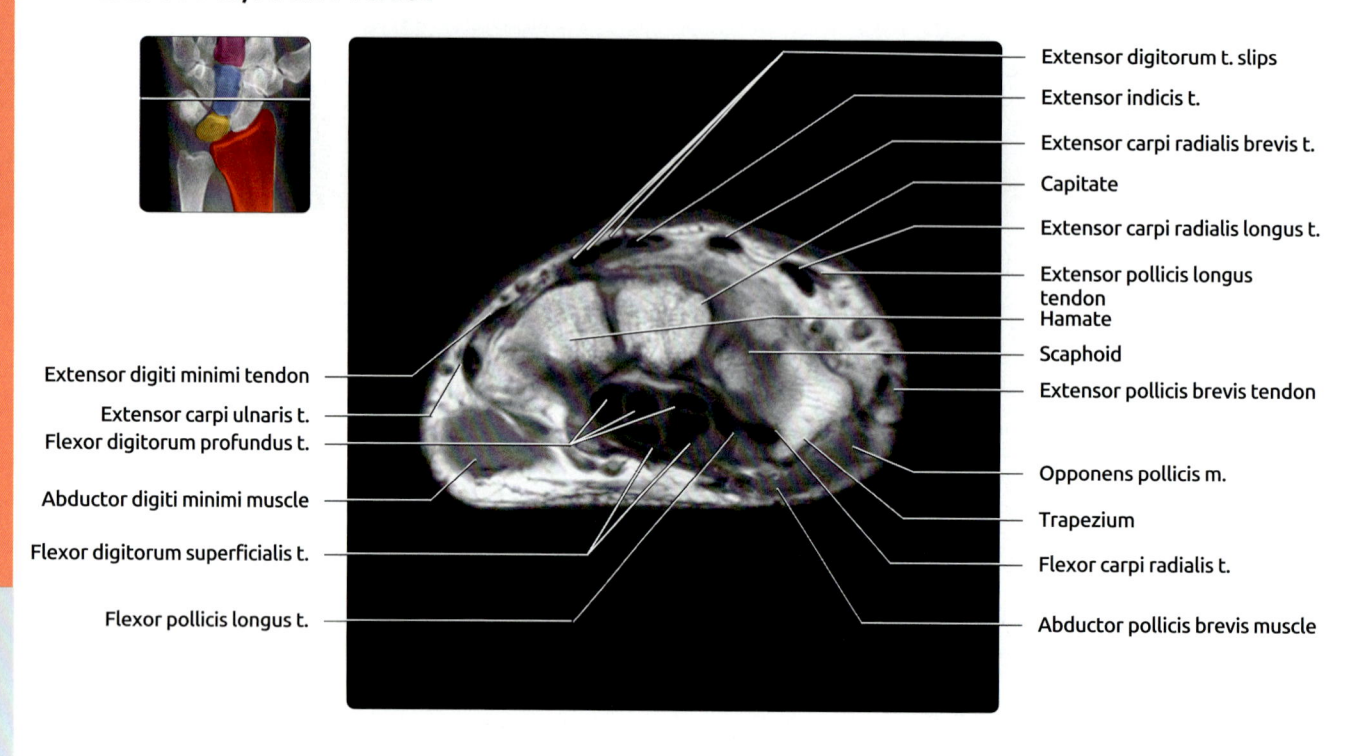

Labels (top image):
- Extensor digitorum t. slips
- Extensor indicis t.
- Extensor carpi radialis brevis t.
- Capitate
- Extensor carpi radialis longus t.
- Extensor pollicis longus tendon
- Hamate
- Scaphoid
- Extensor pollicis brevis tendon
- Opponens pollicis m.
- Trapezium
- Flexor carpi radialis t.
- Abductor pollicis brevis muscle
- Extensor digiti minimi tendon
- Extensor carpi ulnaris t.
- Flexor digitorum profundus t.
- Abductor digiti minimi muscle
- Flexor digitorum superficialis t.
- Flexor pollicis longus t.

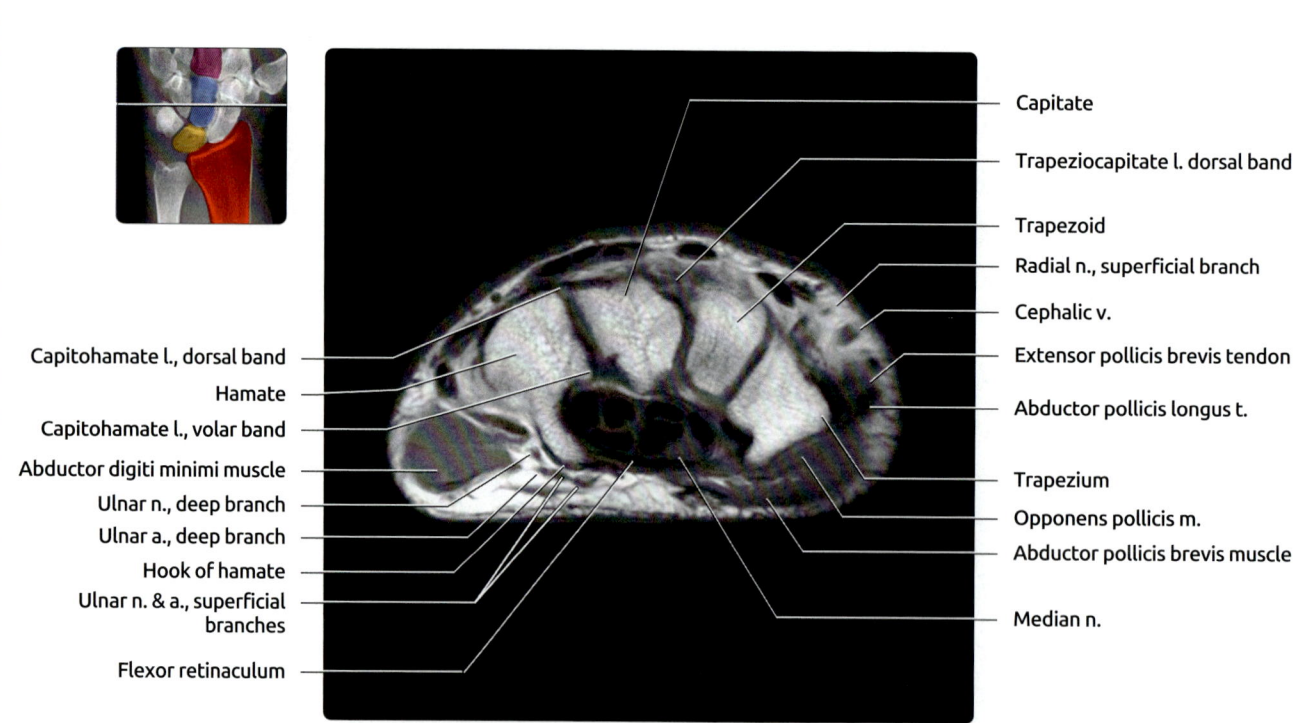

Labels (bottom image):
- Capitate
- Trapeziocapitate l. dorsal band
- Trapezoid
- Radial n., superficial branch
- Cephalic v.
- Extensor pollicis brevis tendon
- Abductor pollicis longus t.
- Trapezium
- Opponens pollicis m.
- Abductor pollicis brevis muscle
- Median n.
- Capitohamate l., dorsal band
- Hamate
- Capitohamate l., volar band
- Abductor digiti minimi muscle
- Ulnar n., deep branch
- Ulnar a., deep branch
- Hook of hamate
- Ulnar n. & a., superficial branches
- Flexor retinaculum

(**Top**) Hamate body (proximal to hook) & scaphotrapeziotrapezoid articulation correspond to midlevel carpal tunnel. EPL tendon intersects dorsally with ECRL tendon. The median nerve is slightly flattened. (**Bottom**) At hook of hamate & trapezium tubercle, ulnar nerve branches into deep & superficial branches with deep branch passing dorsal & ulnar to hamate hook. Portions of volar & dorsal interosseous ligaments are visualized.

Wrist MR Atlas

AXIAL T1 MR, LEFT WRIST

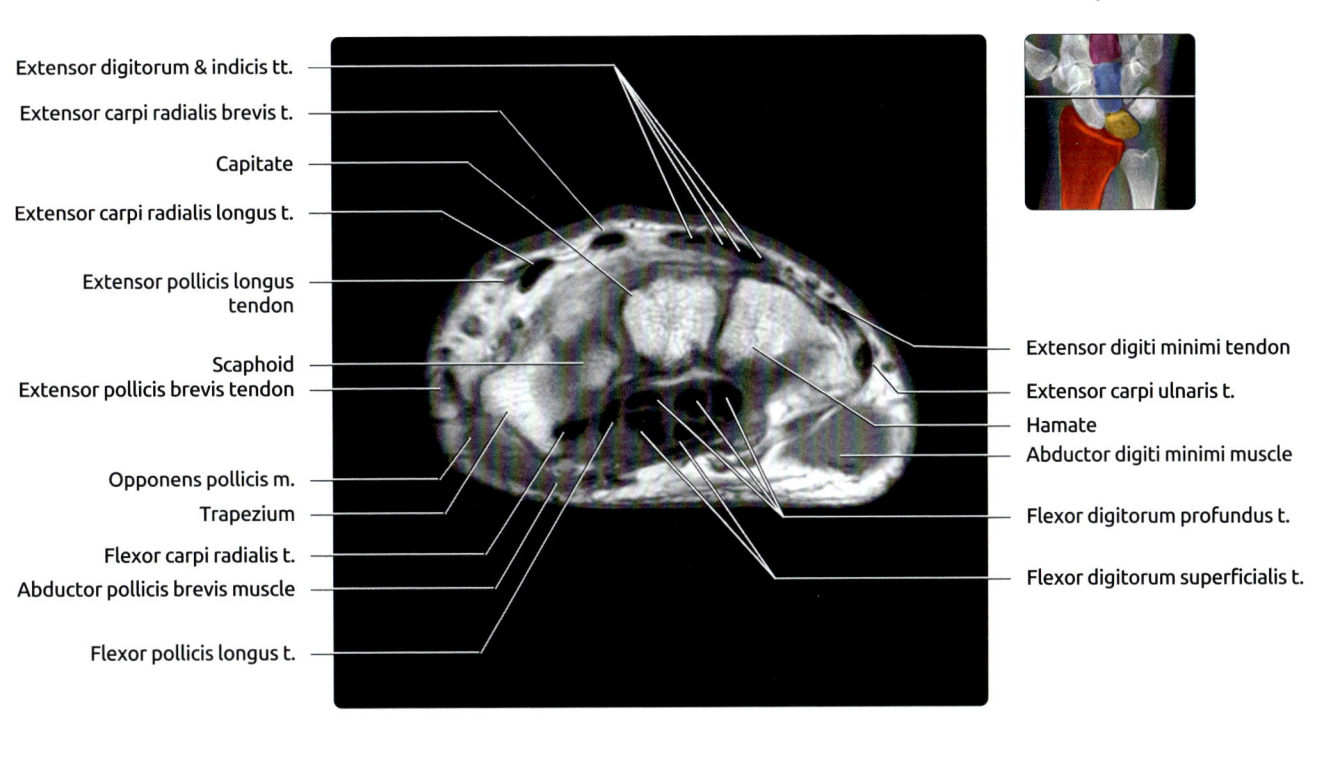

Labels (top image):
- Extensor digitorum & indicis tt.
- Extensor carpi radialis brevis t.
- Capitate
- Extensor carpi radialis longus t.
- Extensor pollicis longus tendon
- Scaphoid
- Extensor pollicis brevis tendon
- Opponens pollicis m.
- Trapezium
- Flexor carpi radialis t.
- Abductor pollicis brevis muscle
- Flexor pollicis longus t.
- Extensor digiti minimi tendon
- Extensor carpi ulnaris t.
- Hamate
- Abductor digiti minimi muscle
- Flexor digitorum profundus t.
- Flexor digitorum superficialis t.

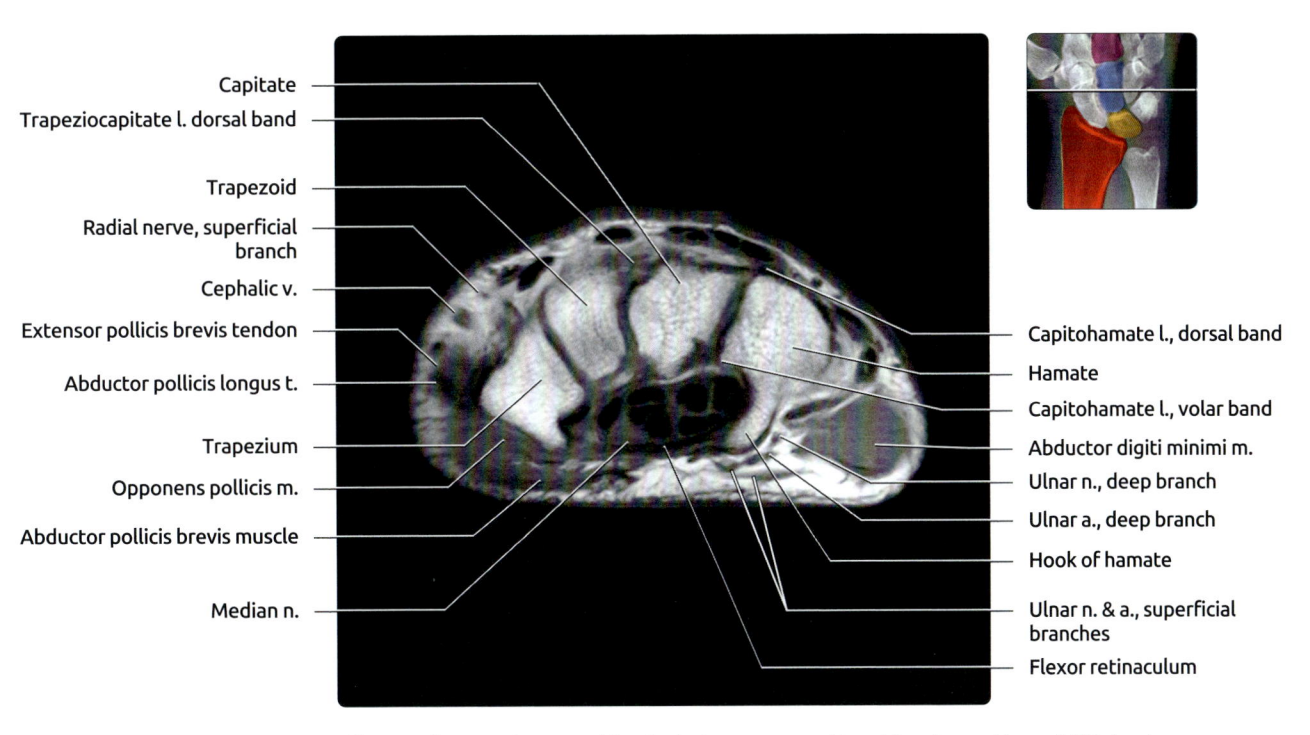

Labels (bottom image):
- Capitate
- Trapeziocapitate l. dorsal band
- Trapezoid
- Radial nerve, superficial branch
- Cephalic v.
- Extensor pollicis brevis tendon
- Abductor pollicis longus t.
- Trapezium
- Opponens pollicis m.
- Abductor pollicis brevis muscle
- Median n.
- Capitohamate l., dorsal band
- Hamate
- Capitohamate l., volar band
- Abductor digiti minimi m.
- Ulnar n., deep branch
- Ulnar a., deep branch
- Hook of hamate
- Ulnar n. & a., superficial branches
- Flexor retinaculum

(Top) Hamate body (proximal to hook) & scaphotrapeziotrapezoid articulation correspond to midlevel carpal tunnel. EPL tendon intersects dorsally with ECRL tendon. The median nerve is slightly flattened. (Bottom) At hook of hamate & trapezium tubercle, ulnar nerve branches into deep & superficial branches with deep branch passing dorsal & ulnar to hamate hook. Portions of volar & dorsal interosseous ligaments are visualized.

Wrist MR Atlas

AXIAL T1 MR, RIGHT WRIST

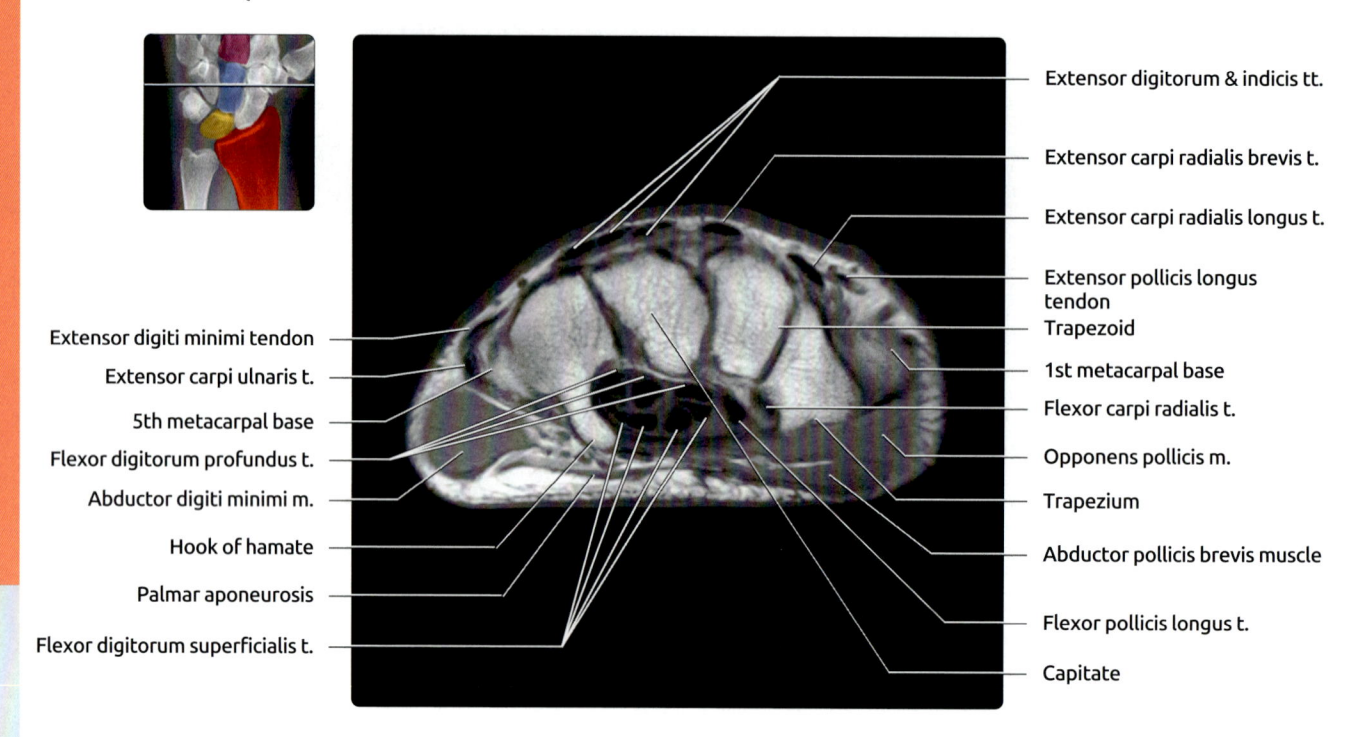

Labels (top image):
- Extensor digitorum & indicis tt.
- Extensor carpi radialis brevis t.
- Extensor carpi radialis longus t.
- Extensor pollicis longus tendon
- Trapezoid
- 1st metacarpal base
- Flexor carpi radialis t.
- Opponens pollicis m.
- Trapezium
- Abductor pollicis brevis muscle
- Flexor pollicis longus t.
- Capitate
- Extensor digiti minimi tendon
- Extensor carpi ulnaris t.
- 5th metacarpal base
- Flexor digitorum profundus t.
- Abductor digiti minimi m.
- Hook of hamate
- Palmar aponeurosis
- Flexor digitorum superficialis t.

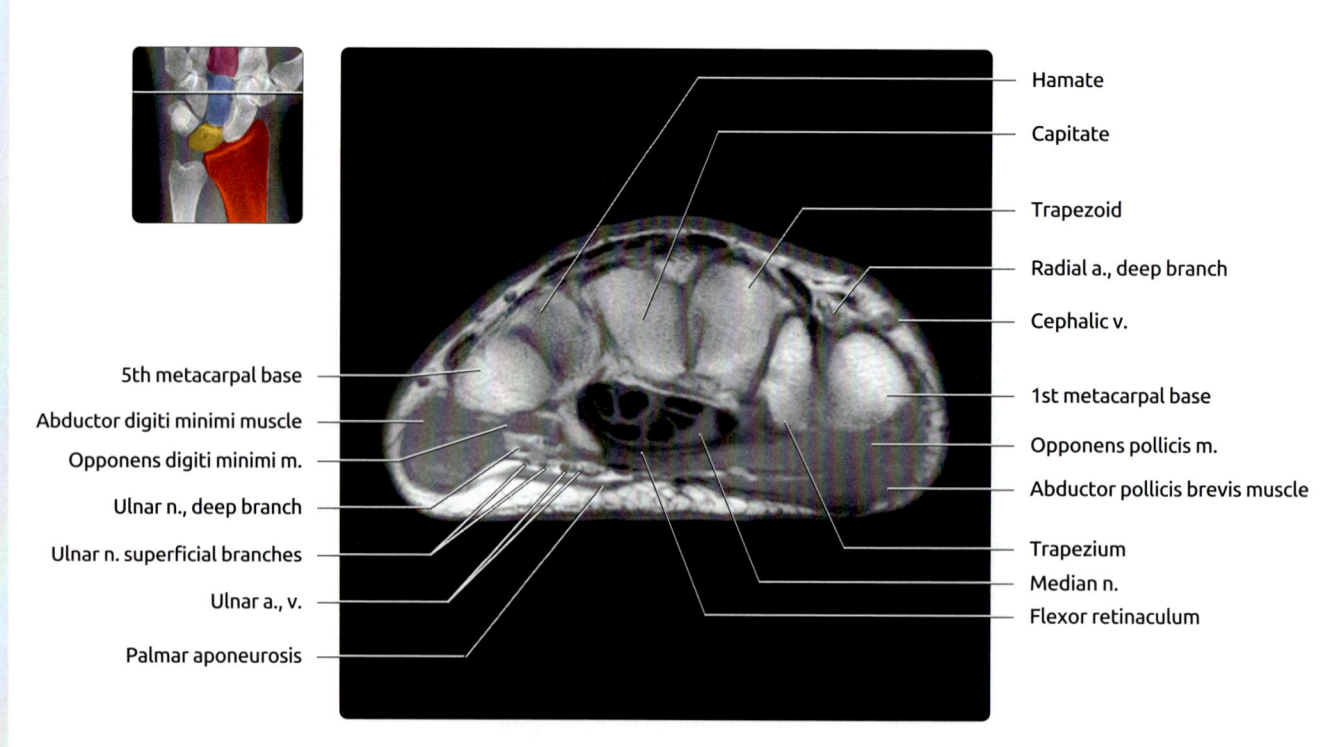

Labels (bottom image):
- Hamate
- Capitate
- Trapezoid
- Radial a., deep branch
- Cephalic v.
- 1st metacarpal base
- Opponens pollicis m.
- Abductor pollicis brevis muscle
- Trapezium
- Median n.
- Flexor retinaculum
- 5th metacarpal base
- Abductor digiti minimi muscle
- Opponens digiti minimi m.
- Ulnar n., deep branch
- Ulnar n. superficial branches
- Ulnar a., v.
- Palmar aponeurosis

(Top) At distal hook of hamate, flexor digitorum tendons pass through carpal tunnel with 2 most superficial tendons extending to long & ring fingers, 2 intermediate tendons to index & small fingers, & profundus tendons comprising deep layer. **(Bottom)** Distal carpal tunnel contents are passing through narrowest portion of carpal tunnel at level of carpometacarpal articulations. Ulnar nerve deep branches pass dorsal & distal to hook of hamate. Ulnar nerve superficial branches continue distally into palm. A portion of deep palmar arch (radial artery, deep branch) is visualized. However, major dorsal & volar vascular arches are typically not readily visualized.

Wrist MR Atlas

AXIAL T1 MR, LEFT WRIST

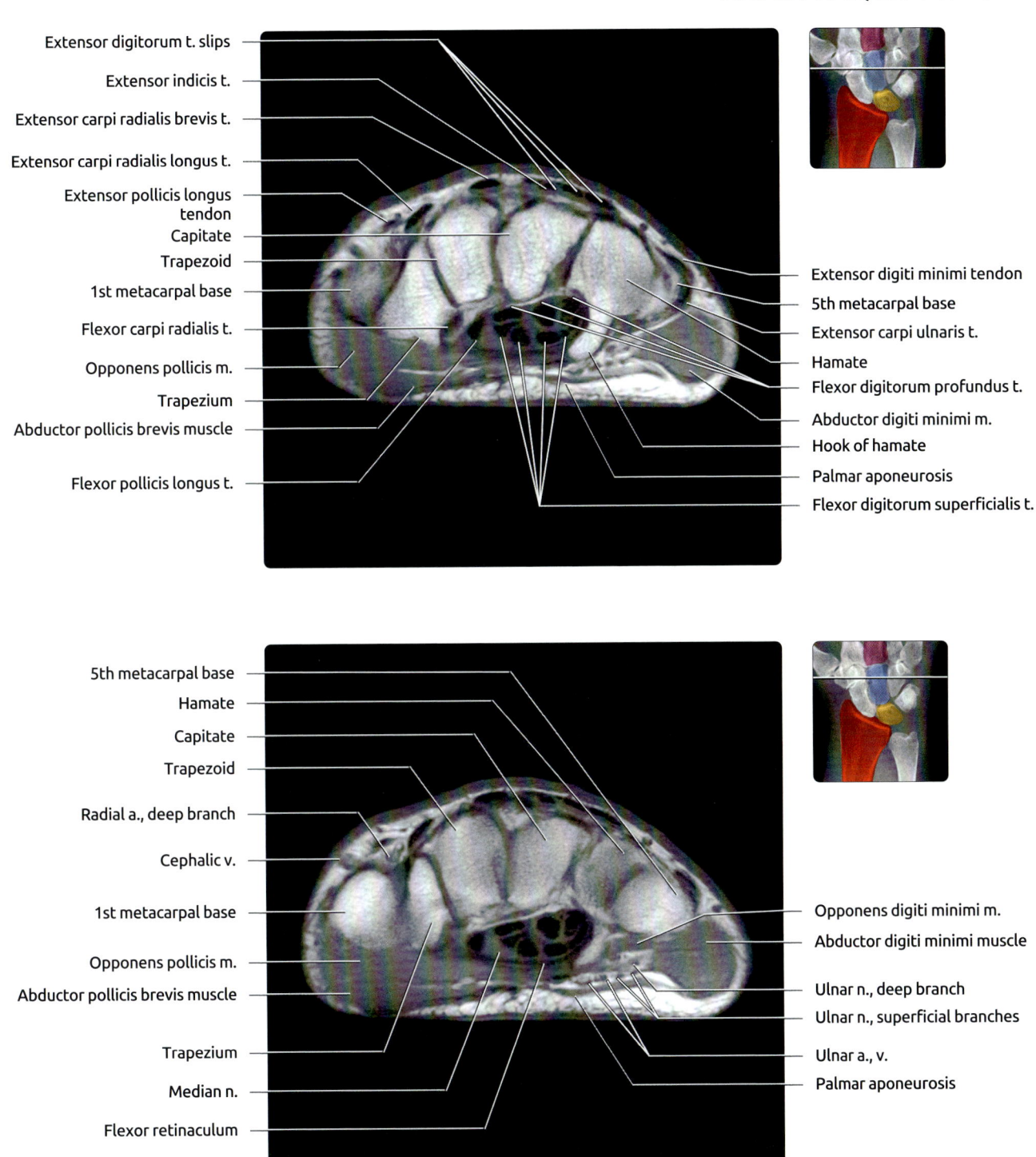

Labels (top image):
- Extensor digitorum t. slips
- Extensor indicis t.
- Extensor carpi radialis brevis t.
- Extensor carpi radialis longus t.
- Extensor pollicis longus tendon
- Capitate
- Trapezoid
- 1st metacarpal base
- Flexor carpi radialis t.
- Opponens pollicis m.
- Trapezium
- Abductor pollicis brevis muscle
- Flexor pollicis longus t.
- Extensor digiti minimi tendon
- 5th metacarpal base
- Extensor carpi ulnaris t.
- Hamate
- Flexor digitorum profundus t.
- Abductor digiti minimi m.
- Hook of hamate
- Palmar aponeurosis
- Flexor digitorum superficialis t.

Labels (bottom image):
- 5th metacarpal base
- Hamate
- Capitate
- Trapezoid
- Radial a., deep branch
- Cephalic v.
- 1st metacarpal base
- Opponens pollicis m.
- Abductor pollicis brevis muscle
- Trapezium
- Median n.
- Flexor retinaculum
- Opponens digiti minimi m.
- Abductor digiti minimi muscle
- Ulnar n., deep branch
- Ulnar n., superficial branches
- Ulnar a., v.
- Palmar aponeurosis

(Top) At distal hook of hamate, flexor digitorum tendons pass through carpal tunnel with 2 most superficial tendons extending to long & ring fingers, 2 intermediate tendons to index & small fingers, & profundus tendons comprising deep layer. **(Bottom)** Distal carpal tunnel contents are passing through narrowest portion of carpal tunnel at level of carpometacarpal articulations. Ulnar nerve deep branches pass dorsal & distal to hook of hamate. Ulnar nerve superficial branches continue distally into palm. A portion of deep palmar arch (radial artery, deep branch) is visualized. However, major dorsal & volar vascular arches are typically not readily visualized.

Wrist MR Atlas

AXIAL T1 MR, RIGHT WRIST

Extensor digitorum t. slips
3rd metacarpal base
Extensor carpi radialis brevis t.
2nd metacarpal base
Extensor carpi radialis longus t.
Extensor pollicis longus tendon
Flexor digitorum profundus tt.
Flexor pollicis longus t.
Adductor pollicis m.
Flexor pollicis brevis m.
1st metacarpal base
Abductor pollicis brevis muscle
Opponens pollicis m.
Flexor digitorum superficialis t.

Extensor digiti minimi tendon
5th metacarpal base
4th metacarpal base
Abductor digiti minimi m.
Flexor digit minimi brevis m.
Opponens digiti minimi m.
Ulnar n., superficial branch
Ulnar a.
Palmar aponeurosis

4th metacarpal base
3rd metacarpal base
2nd metacarpal base
Intermetacarpal l., volar bands
Deep palmar arch
1st metacarpal base
Median n.
Flexor retinaculum

5th metacarpal base
Ulnar n., superficial branch
Ulnar v.
Ulnar a.
Palmar aponeurosis

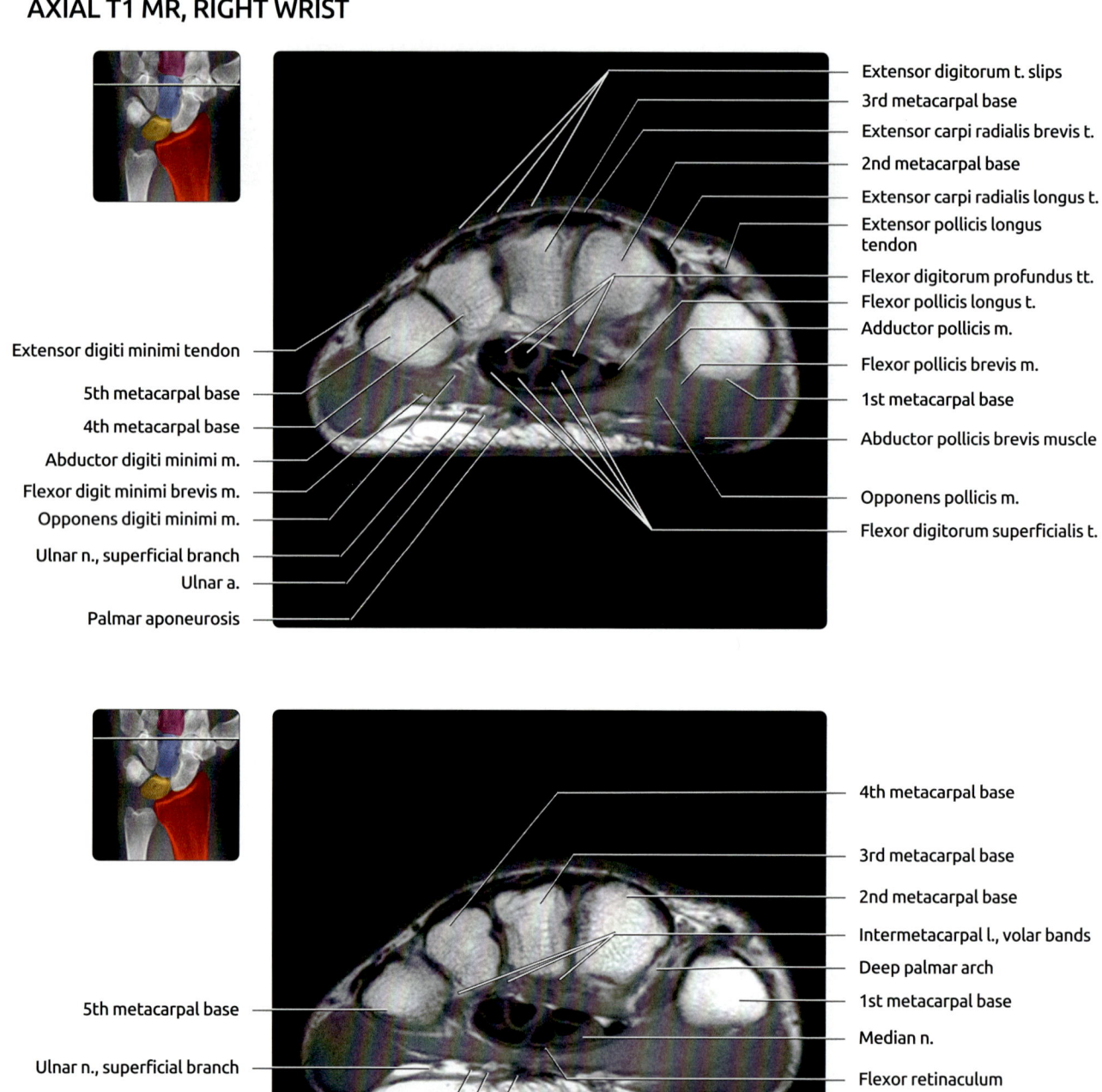

(**Top**) Thenar & hypothenar musculature is well developed at carpometacarpal articulation. Extensor pollicis longus tendon now becomes evident again as its course becomes more perpendicular to axial plane. Extensor digitorum tendons are becoming flattened near insertion sites. (**Bottom**) At distal flexor retinaculum & metacarpal bases, the carpal tunnel ends with median nerve branching into muscular branches & digital nerves. Ulnar nerve, superficial branch, remains evident. A small portion of radial contribution to deep palmar arch is seen between 1st & 2nd metacarpal bases.

Wrist MR Atlas

AXIAL T1 MR, LEFT WRIST

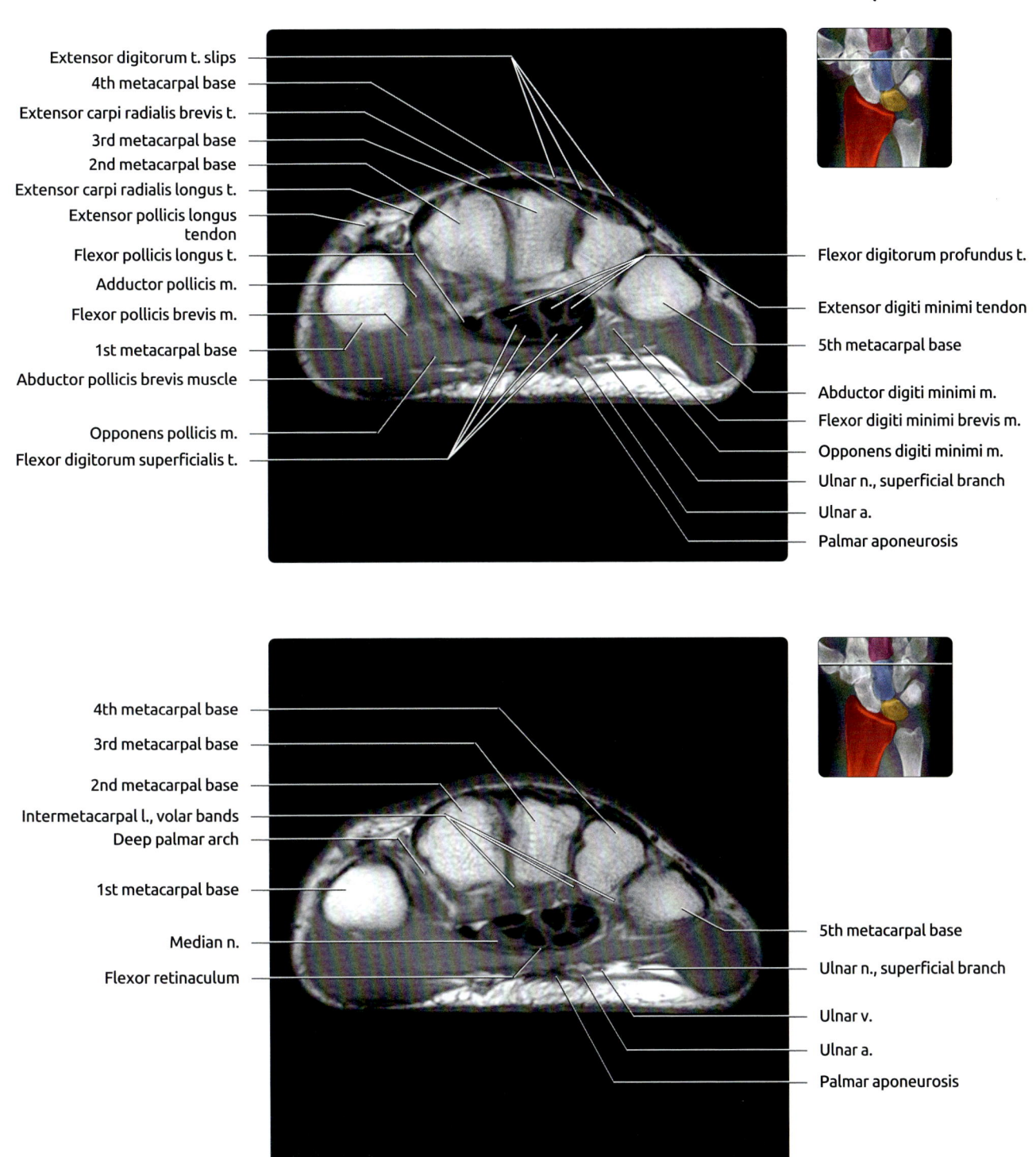

Top labels (left):
- Extensor digitorum t. slips
- 4th metacarpal base
- Extensor carpi radialis brevis t.
- 3rd metacarpal base
- 2nd metacarpal base
- Extensor carpi radialis longus t.
- Extensor pollicis longus tendon
- Flexor pollicis longus t.
- Adductor pollicis m.
- Flexor pollicis brevis m.
- 1st metacarpal base
- Abductor pollicis brevis muscle
- Opponens pollicis m.
- Flexor digitorum superficialis t.

Top labels (right):
- Flexor digitorum profundus t.
- Extensor digiti minimi tendon
- 5th metacarpal base
- Abductor digiti minimi m.
- Flexor digiti minimi brevis m.
- Opponens digiti minimi m.
- Ulnar n., superficial branch
- Ulnar a.
- Palmar aponeurosis

Bottom labels (left):
- 4th metacarpal base
- 3rd metacarpal base
- 2nd metacarpal base
- Intermetacarpal l., volar bands
- Deep palmar arch
- 1st metacarpal base
- Median n.
- Flexor retinaculum

Bottom labels (right):
- 5th metacarpal base
- Ulnar n., superficial branch
- Ulnar v.
- Ulnar a.
- Palmar aponeurosis

(Top) Thenar & hypothenar musculature is well developed at carpometacarpal articulation. Extensor pollicis longus tendon now becomes evident again as its course becomes more perpendicular to axial plane. Extensor digitorum tendons are becoming flattened near insertion sites. *(Bottom)* At distal flexor retinaculum & metacarpal bases, the carpal tunnel ends with median nerve branching into muscular branches & digital nerves. Ulnar nerve, superficial branch, remains evident. A small portion of radial contribution to deep palmar arch is seen between 1st & 2nd metacarpal bases.

Wrist MR Atlas

AXIAL T1 MR, RIGHT WRIST

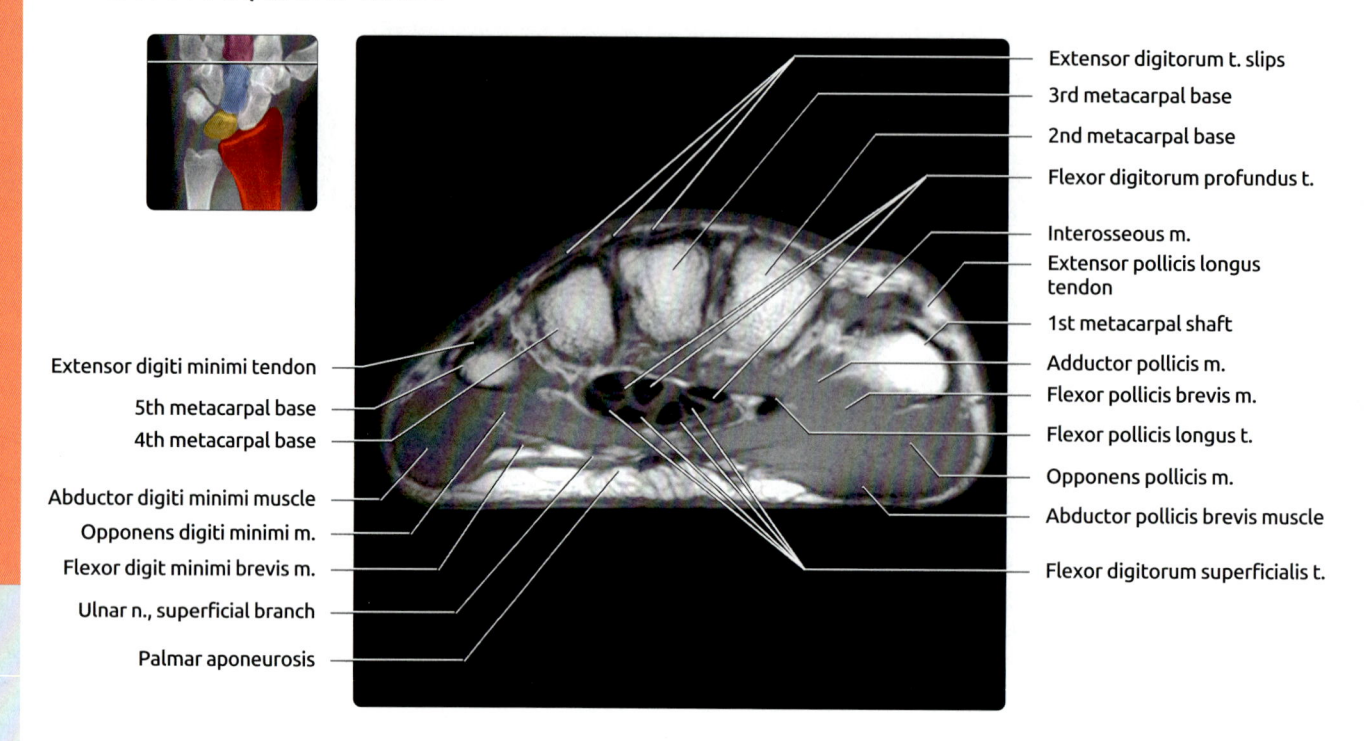

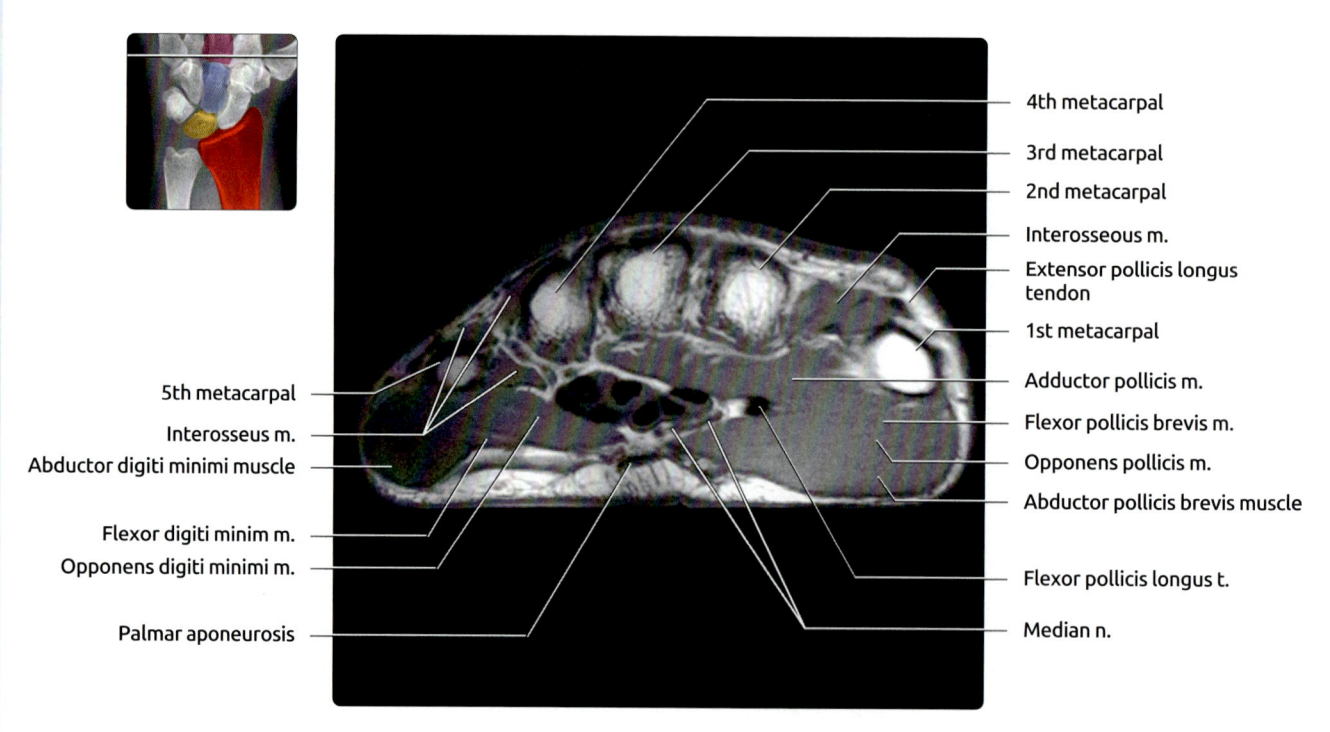

Labels (top image):
- Extensor digitorum t. slips
- 3rd metacarpal base
- 2nd metacarpal base
- Flexor digitorum profundus t.
- Interosseous m.
- Extensor pollicis longus tendon
- 1st metacarpal shaft
- Adductor pollicis m.
- Flexor pollicis brevis m.
- Flexor pollicis longus t.
- Opponens pollicis m.
- Abductor pollicis brevis muscle
- Flexor digitorum superficialis t.
- Extensor digiti minimi tendon
- 5th metacarpal base
- 4th metacarpal base
- Abductor digiti minimi muscle
- Opponens digiti minimi m.
- Flexor digit minimi brevis m.
- Ulnar n., superficial branch
- Palmar aponeurosis

Labels (bottom image):
- 4th metacarpal
- 3rd metacarpal
- 2nd metacarpal
- Interosseous m.
- Extensor pollicis longus tendon
- 1st metacarpal
- Adductor pollicis m.
- Flexor pollicis brevis m.
- Opponens pollicis m.
- Abductor pollicis brevis muscle
- Flexor pollicis longus t.
- Median n.
- 5th metacarpal
- Interosseus m.
- Abductor digiti minimi muscle
- Flexor digiti minim m.
- Opponens digiti minimi m.
- Palmar aponeurosis

(Top) Metacarpal bases mark transition from wrist into hand. Extensor digitorum tendons flatten & spread across dorsum of metacarpal bases. (Bottom) Interosseous musculature is evident at metacarpal bases. Thenar & hypothenar musculature is well developed. Distal branches of radial & ulnar nerves are not discernible, but median nerve branches are visible.

Wrist MR Atlas

AXIAL T1 MR, LEFT WRIST

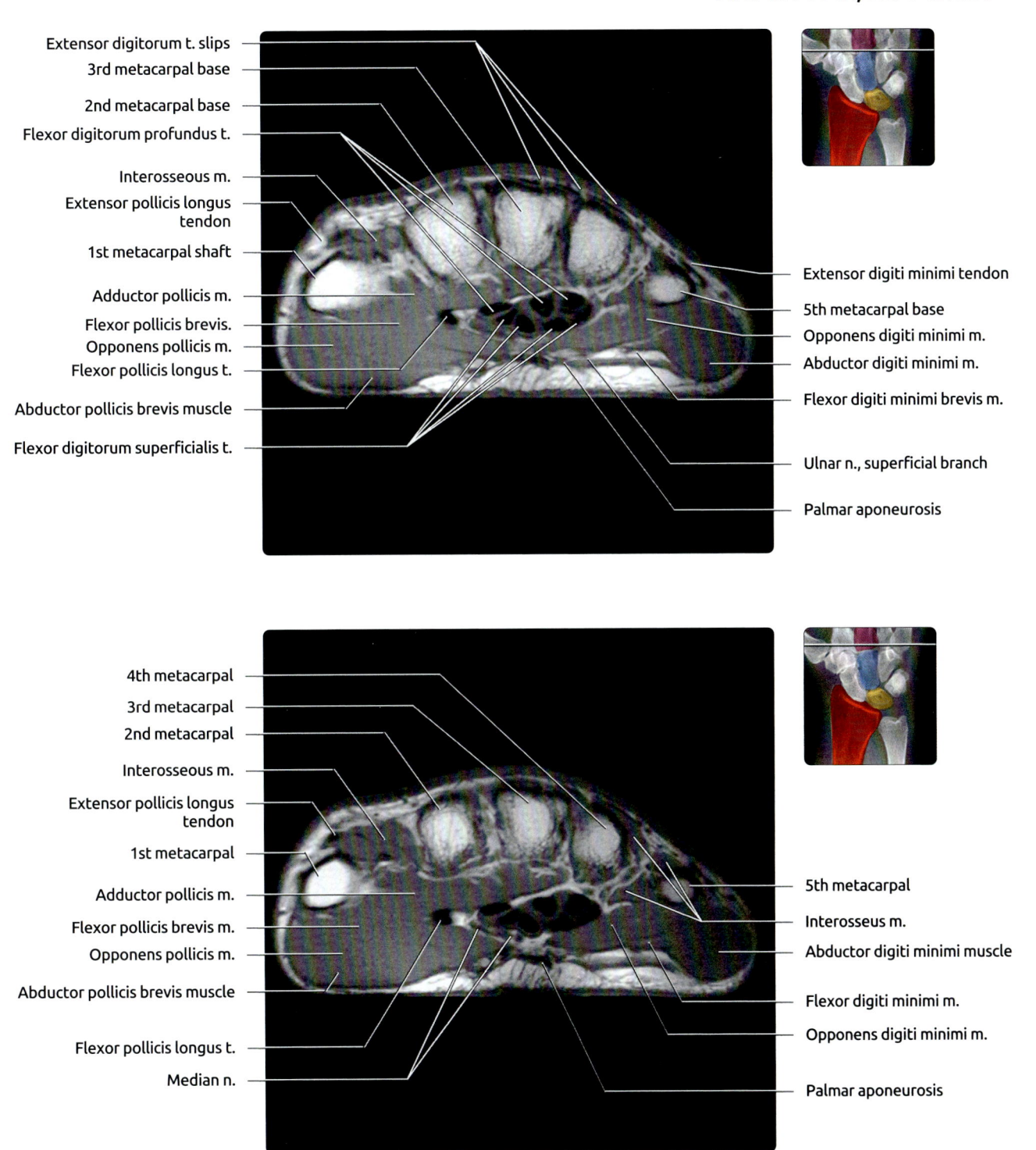

(Top) Metacarpal bases mark transition from wrist into hand. Extensor digitorum tendons flatten & spread across dorsum of metacarpal bases. (Bottom) Interosseous musculature is evident at metacarpal bases. Thenar & hypothenar musculature is well developed. Distal branches of radial & ulnar nerves are not discernible, but median nerve branches are visible.

CORONAL T1 MR, RIGHT WRIST

Dorsal vein

Dorsal vein

Dorsal vein

3rd metacarpal base

Extensor pollicis longus tendon

Ulnar styloid

Lister tubercle

Extensor digitorum t.

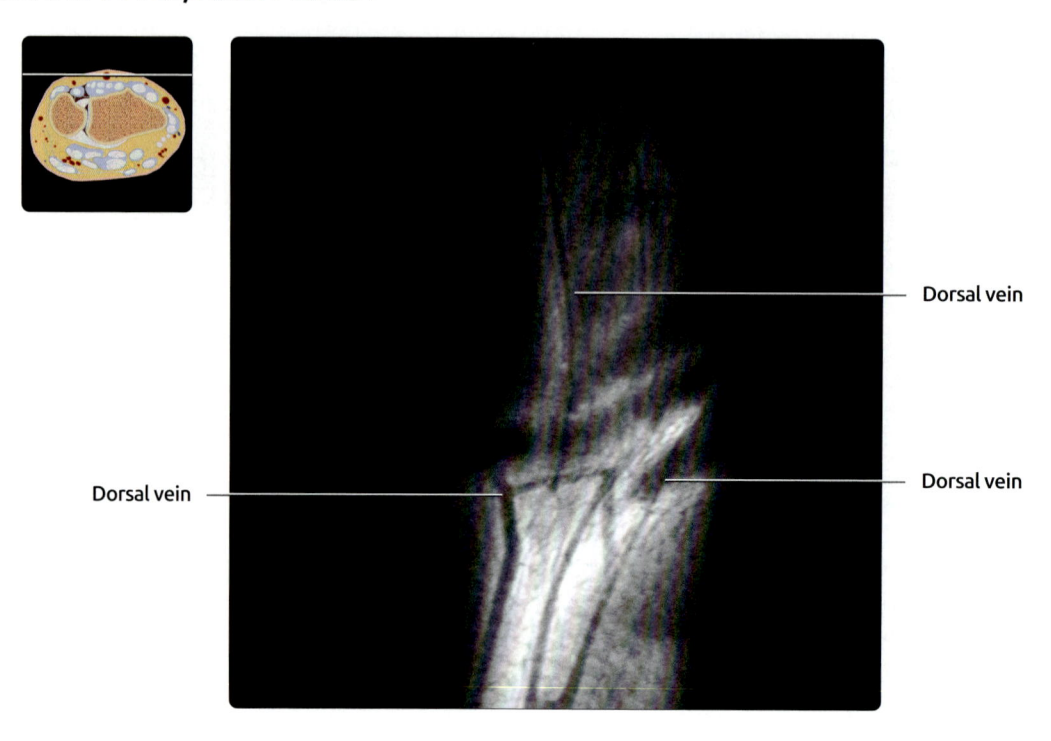

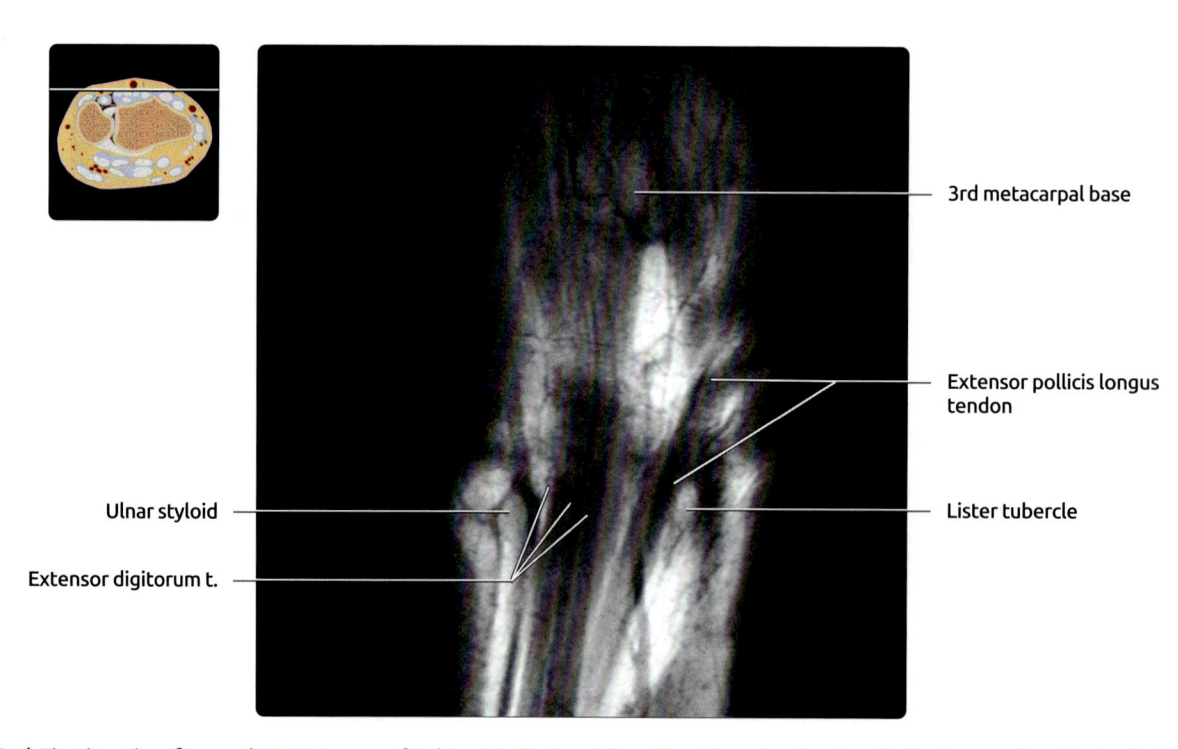

(Top) First in series of coronal T1 MR images of right wrist, displayed from dorsal to volar. A network of veins over dorsal wrist drains into cephalic vein radially & basilic vein ulnarly. (Bottom) Extensor digitorum tendons are most dorsal wrist structures. Dorsal portions of ulnar styloid, dorsal radius (Lister tubercle), & 3rd metacarpal base are seen.

Wrist MR Atlas

CORONAL T1 MR, LEFT WRIST

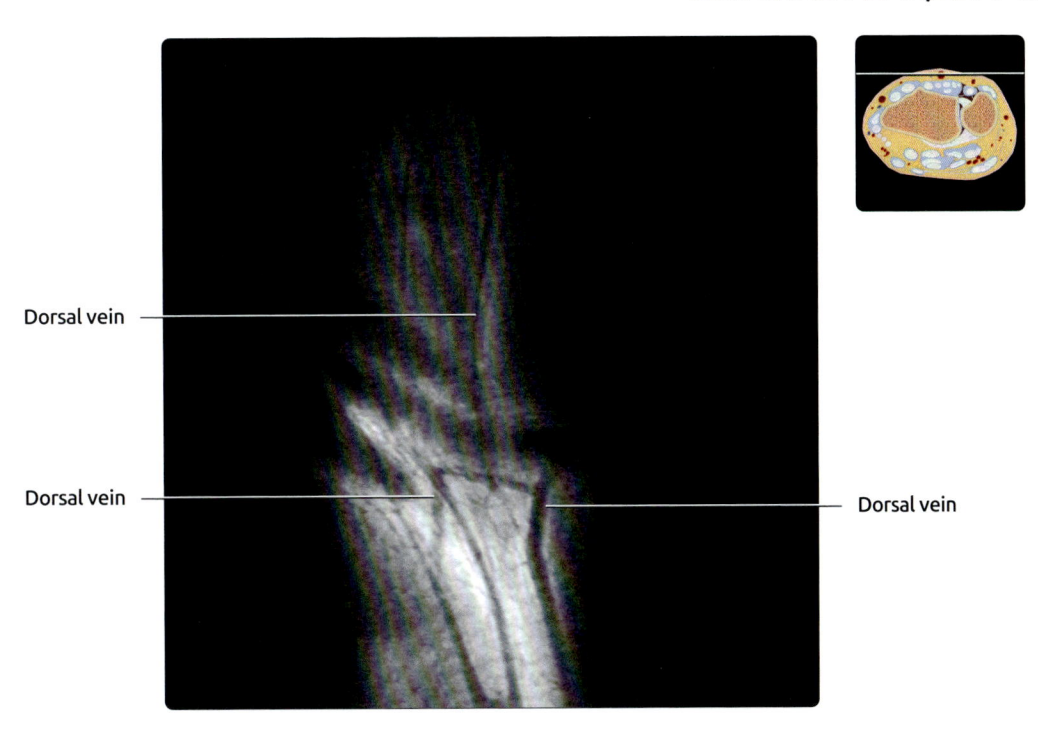

Dorsal vein

Dorsal vein

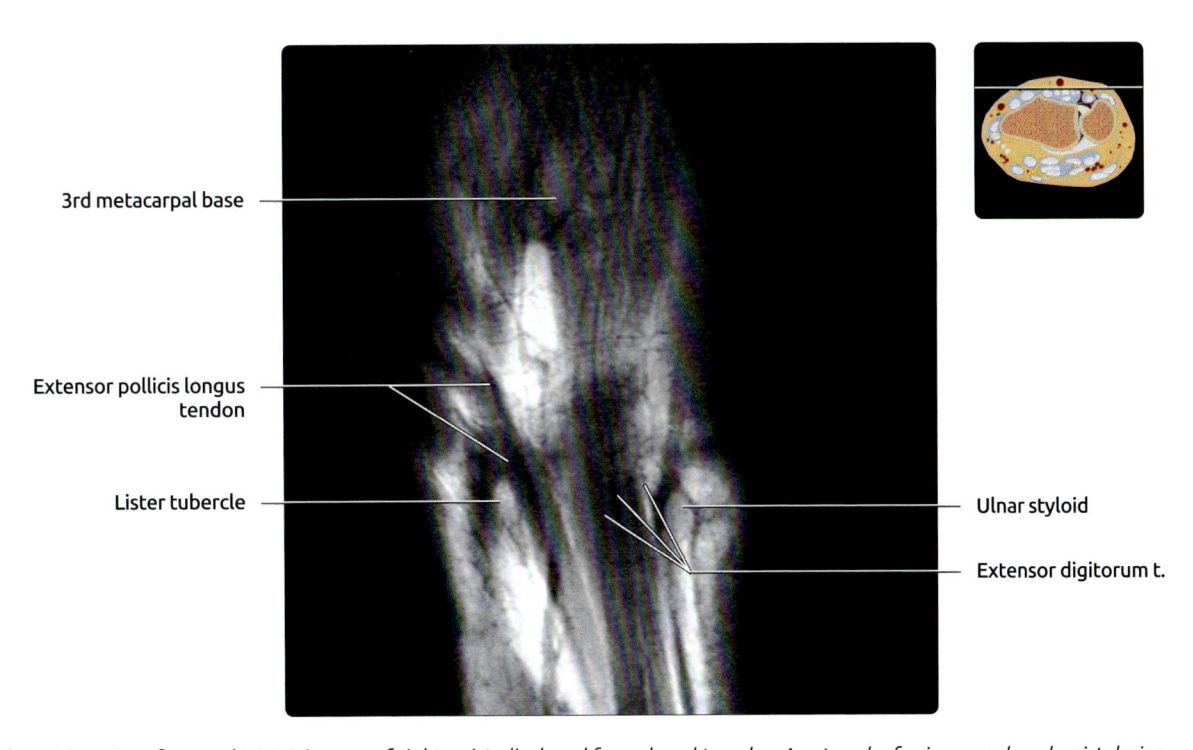

Dorsal vein

3rd metacarpal base

Extensor pollicis longus tendon

Lister tubercle

Ulnar styloid

Extensor digitorum t.

(Top) First in series of coronal T1 MR images of right wrist, displayed from dorsal to volar. A network of veins over dorsal wrist drains into cephalic vein radially & basilic vein ulnarly. (Bottom) Extensor digitorum tendons are most dorsal wrist structures. Dorsal portions of ulnar styloid, dorsal radius (Lister tubercle), & 3rd metacarpal base are seen.

Wrist MR Atlas

CORONAL T1 MR, RIGHT WRIST

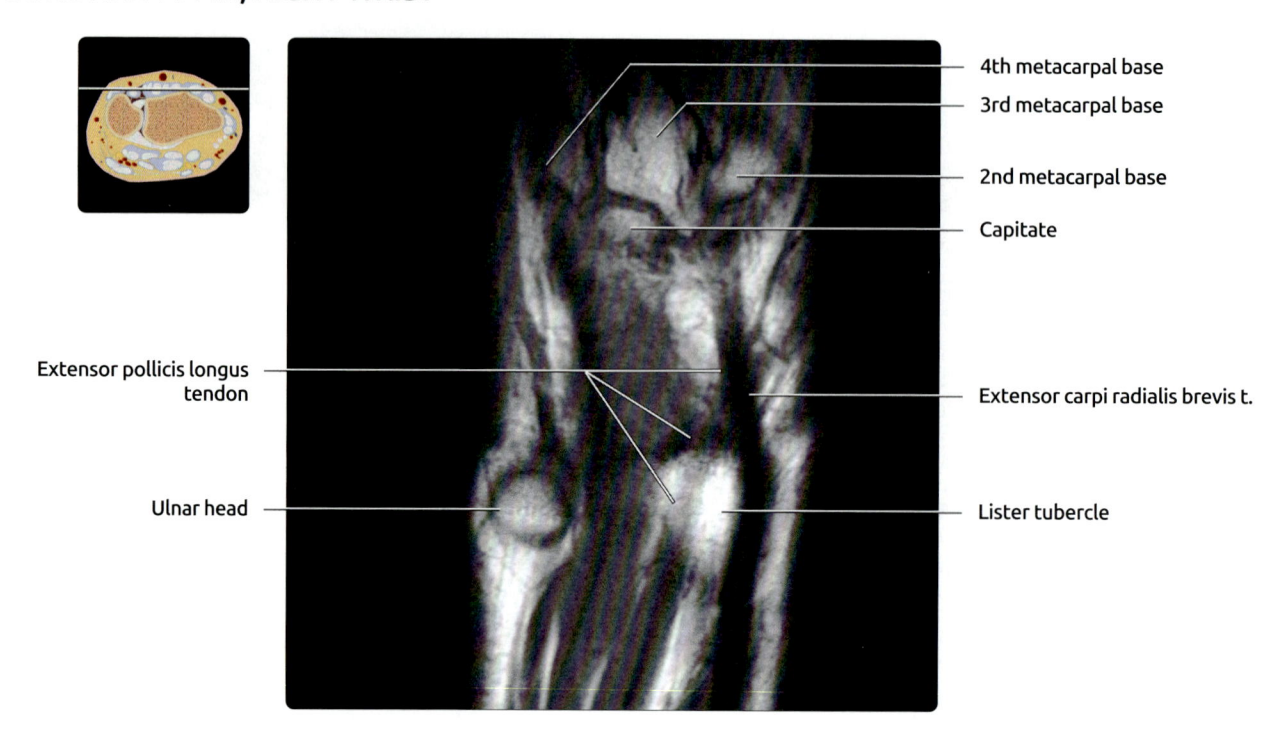

Labels (top image):
- 4th metacarpal base
- 3rd metacarpal base
- 2nd metacarpal base
- Capitate
- Extensor pollicis longus tendon
- Extensor carpi radialis brevis t.
- Ulnar head
- Lister tubercle

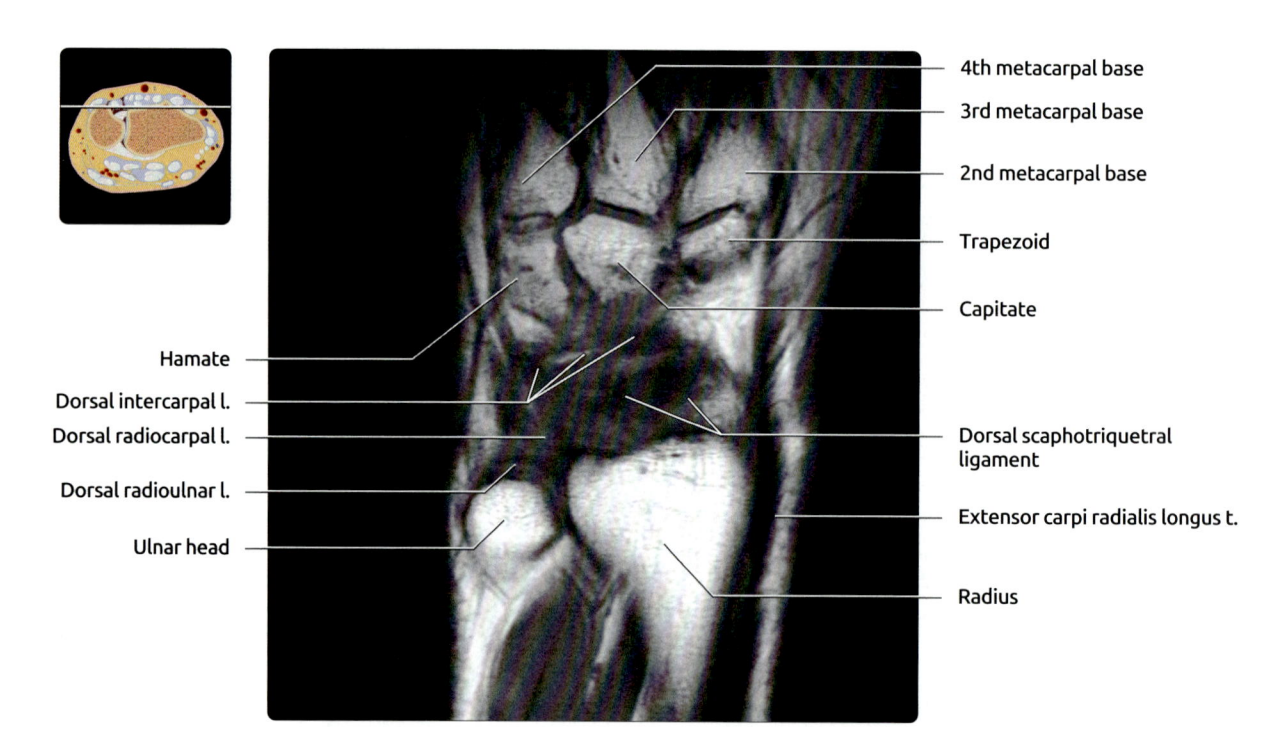

Labels (bottom image):
- 4th metacarpal base
- 3rd metacarpal base
- 2nd metacarpal base
- Trapezoid
- Capitate
- Hamate
- Dorsal intercarpal l.
- Dorsal radiocarpal l.
- Dorsal radioulnar l.
- Ulnar head
- Dorsal scaphotriquetral ligament
- Extensor carpi radialis longus t.
- Radius

(Top) Lister tubercle & ulnar head are dorsally positioned with extensor pollicis longus tendon passing ulnar to tubercle in a shallow groove & coursing radially over ECR tendon. ECR passes radial to tubercle. **(Bottom)** Dorsal extrinsic & intrinsic ligaments are visualized as thin low signal intensity bands coursing horizontally across wrist. Though many of these small, thin ligaments may be difficult to identify as discrete structures, dorsal intercarpal & dorsal radiocarpal ligaments are routinely seen.

Wrist MR Atlas

CORONAL T1 MR, LEFT WRIST

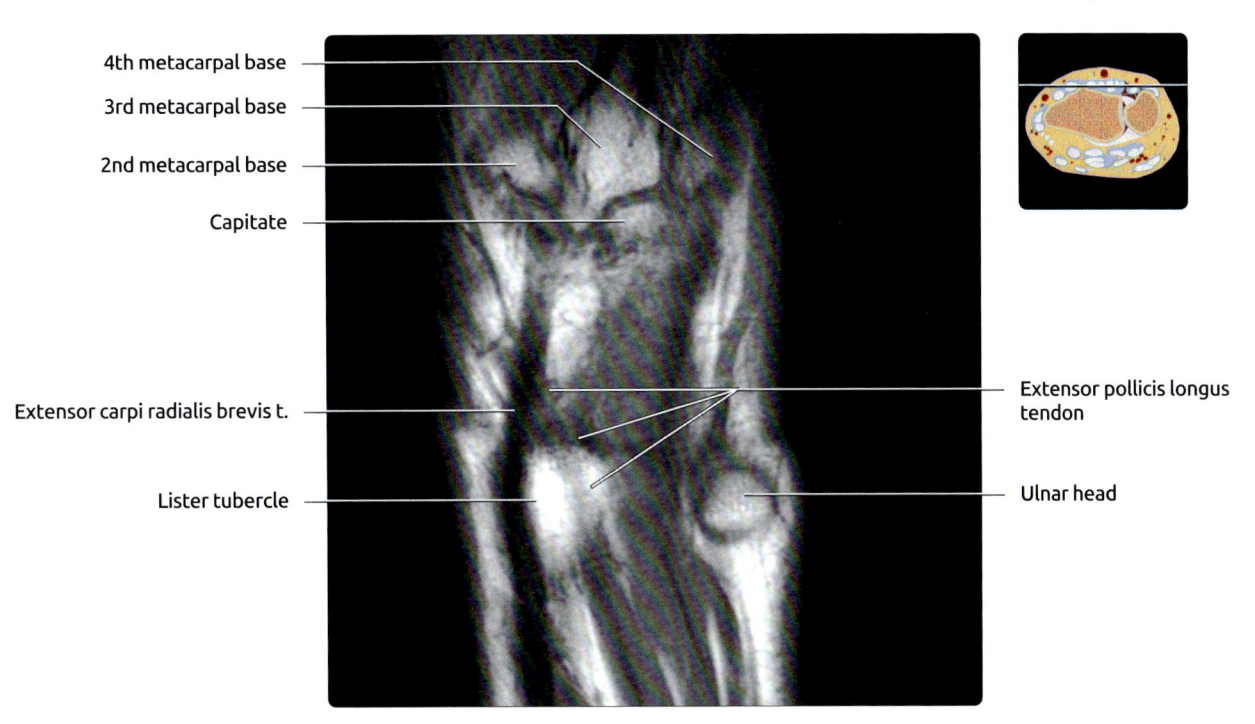

Labels (top image):
- 4th metacarpal base
- 3rd metacarpal base
- 2nd metacarpal base
- Capitate
- Extensor carpi radialis brevis t.
- Lister tubercle
- Extensor pollicis longus tendon
- Ulnar head

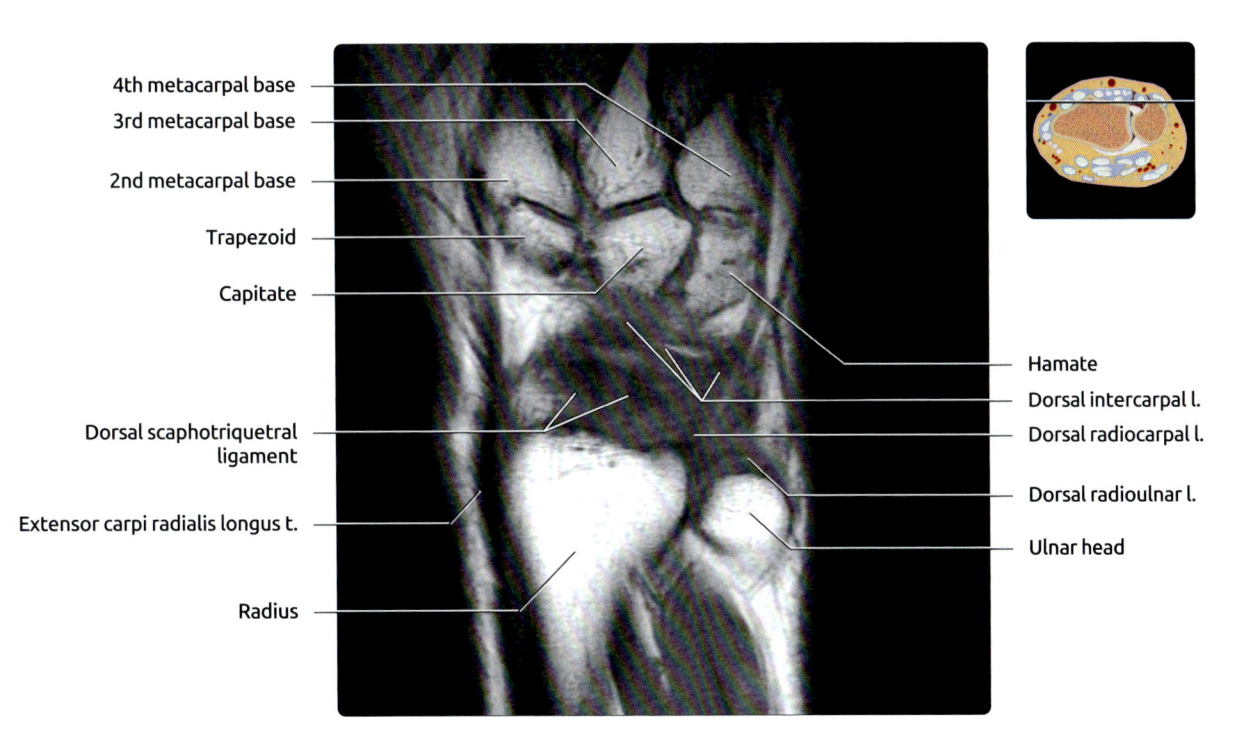

Labels (bottom image):
- 4th metacarpal base
- 3rd metacarpal base
- 2nd metacarpal base
- Trapezoid
- Capitate
- Dorsal scaphotriquetral ligament
- Extensor carpi radialis longus t.
- Radius
- Hamate
- Dorsal intercarpal l.
- Dorsal radiocarpal l.
- Dorsal radioulnar l.
- Ulnar head

(Top) *Lister tubercle & ulnar head are dorsally positioned with extensor pollicis longus tendon passing ulnar to tubercle in a shallow groove & coursing radially over extensor carpi radialis (ECR) tendon. ECR passes radial to tubercle.* (Bottom) *Dorsal extrinsic & intrinsic ligaments are visualized as thin low signal intensity bands coursing horizontally across wrist. Though many of these small, thin ligaments may be difficult to identify as discrete structures, dorsal intercarpal & dorsal radiocarpal ligaments are routinely seen.*

Wrist MR Atlas

CORONAL T1 MR, RIGHT WRIST

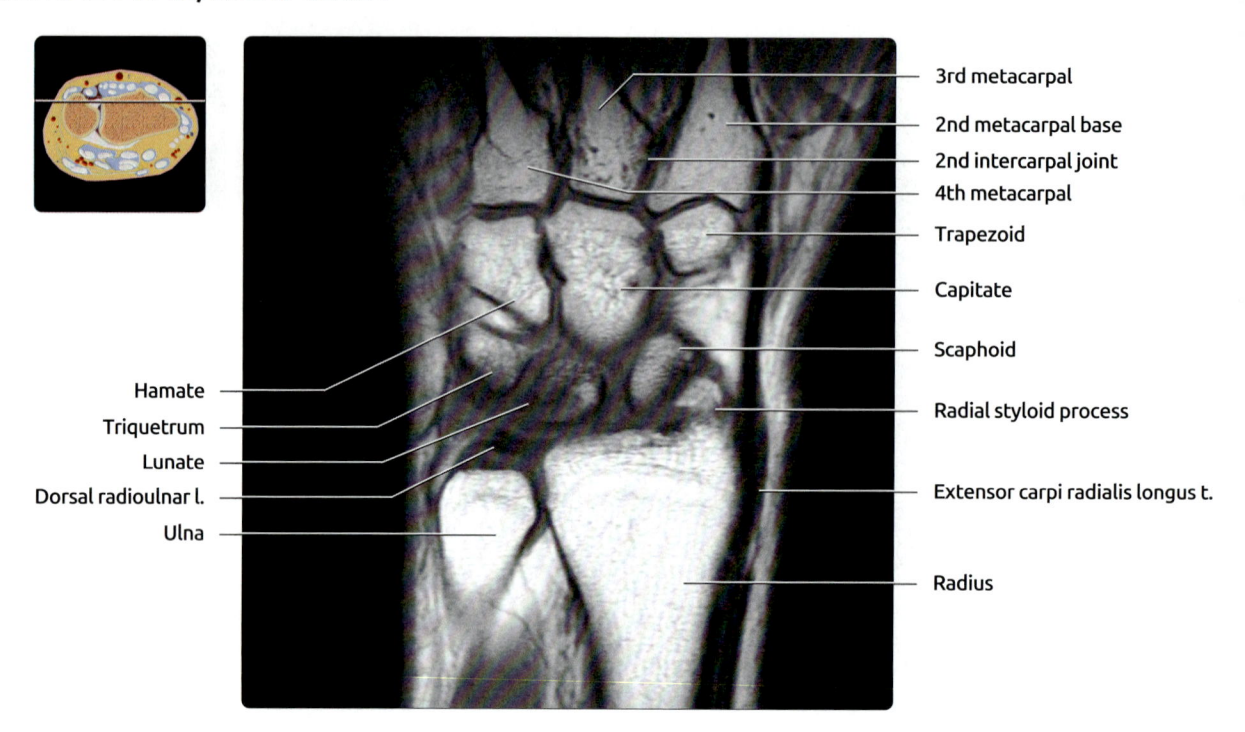

Labels (top image):
- 3rd metacarpal
- 2nd metacarpal base
- 2nd intercarpal joint
- 4th metacarpal
- Trapezoid
- Capitate
- Scaphoid
- Radial styloid process
- Extensor carpi radialis longus t.
- Radius
- Hamate
- Triquetrum
- Lunate
- Dorsal radioulnar l.
- Ulna

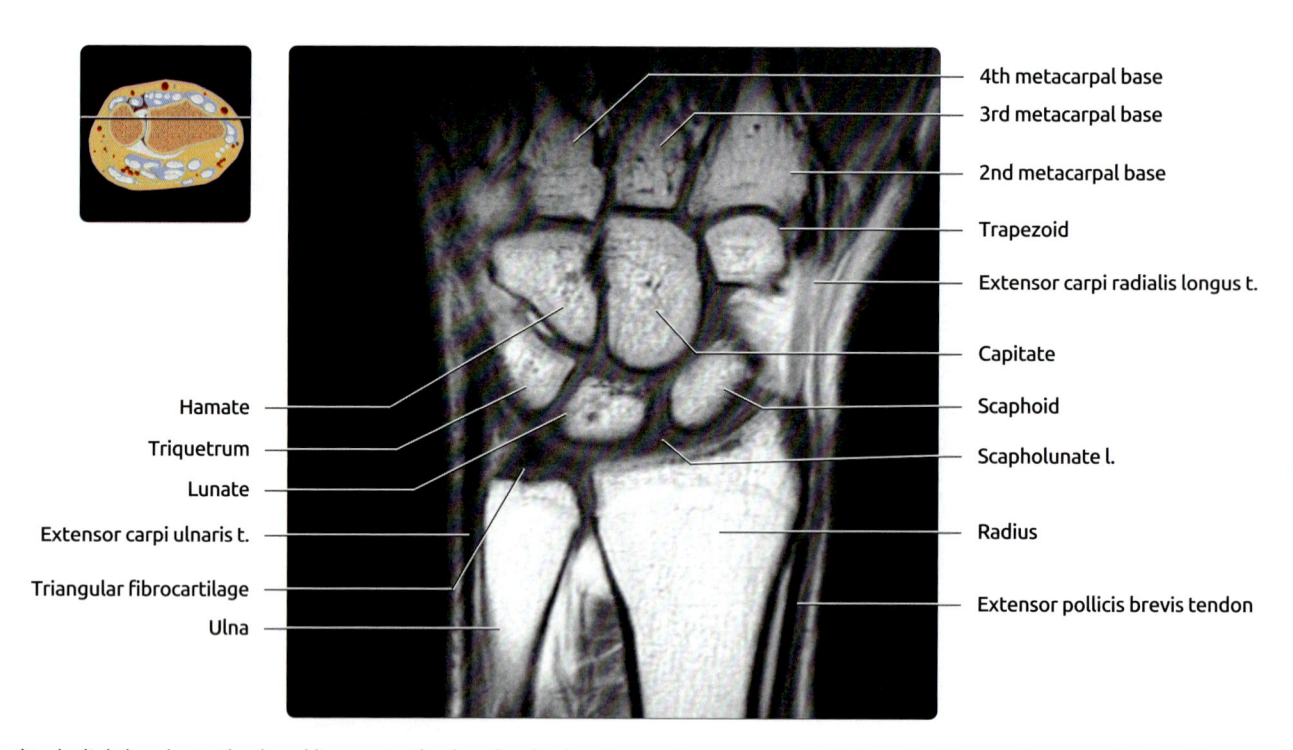

Labels (bottom image):
- 4th metacarpal base
- 3rd metacarpal base
- 2nd metacarpal base
- Trapezoid
- Extensor carpi radialis longus t.
- Capitate
- Scaphoid
- Scapholunate l.
- Radius
- Extensor pollicis brevis tendon
- Hamate
- Triquetrum
- Lunate
- Extensor carpi ulnaris t.
- Triangular fibrocartilage
- Ulna

(Top) Slightly volar to the dorsal ligaments, the dorsal radioulnar ligament, a component of triangular fibrocartilage complex is evident, as are dorsal proximal & distal row carpi. Extensor carpi radialis tendon courses distally to attach to 2nd metacarpal base. **(Bottom)** Ulnar head is seated in sigmoid notch of distal radius. Triangular fibrocartilage articular disc is readily visualized. Extensor carpi ulnaris (ECU) tendon passes dorsally in ECU ulnar groove. Small intrinsic carpal row ligaments, scapholunate & lunotriquetral, are present but poorly seen on T1 imaging.

Wrist MR Atlas

CORONAL T1 MR, LEFT WRIST

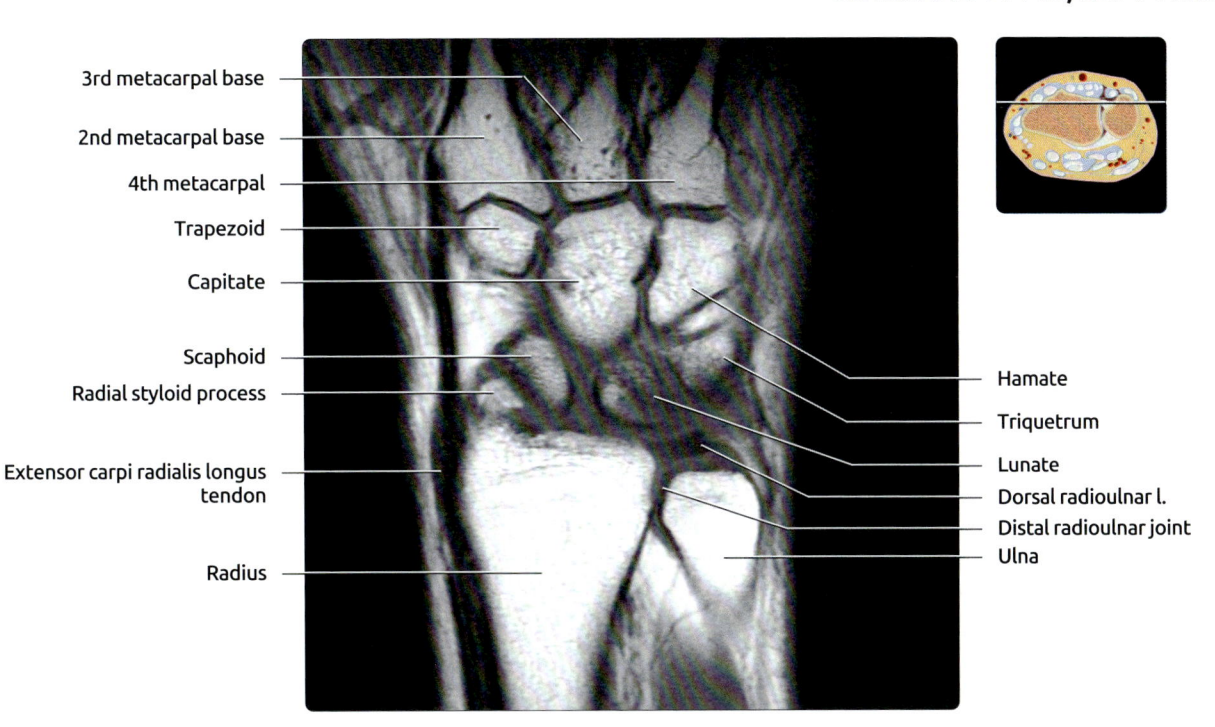

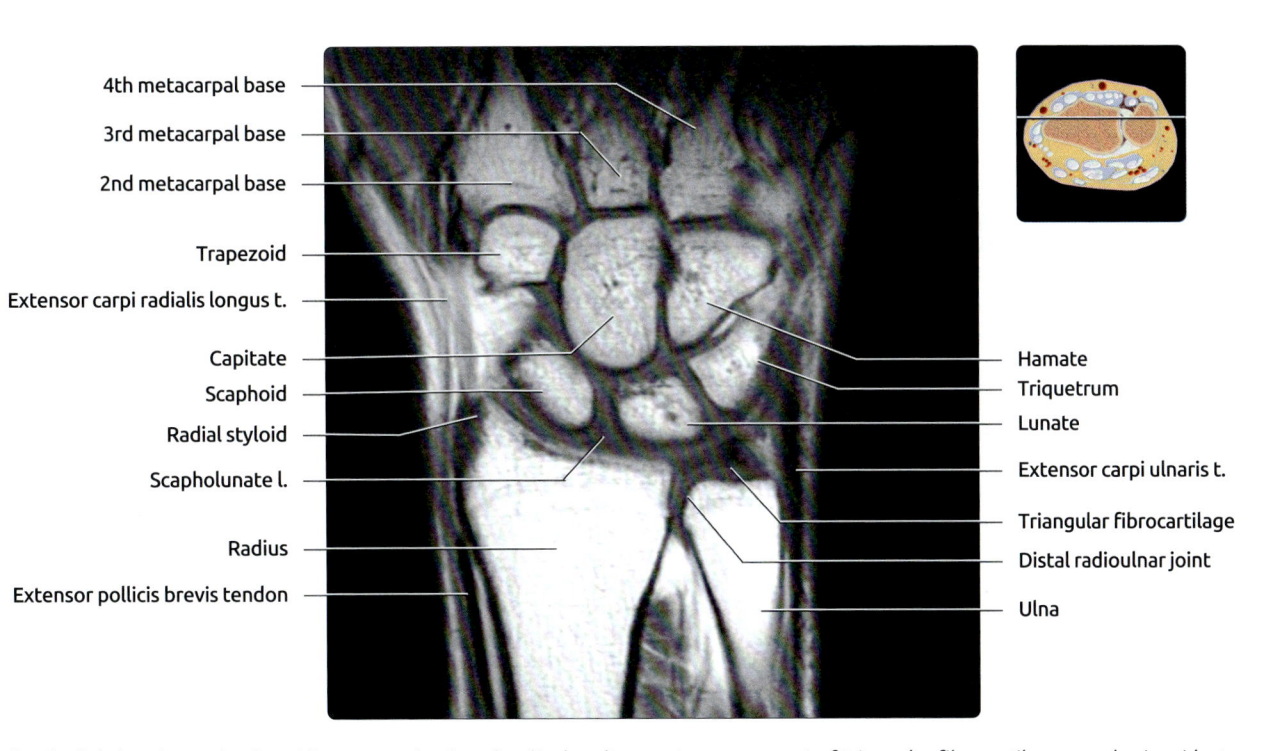

Labels (top image):
- 3rd metacarpal base
- 2nd metacarpal base
- 4th metacarpal
- Trapezoid
- Capitate
- Scaphoid
- Radial styloid process
- Extensor carpi radialis longus tendon
- Radius
- Hamate
- Triquetrum
- Lunate
- Dorsal radioulnar l.
- Distal radioulnar joint
- Ulna

Labels (bottom image):
- 4th metacarpal base
- 3rd metacarpal base
- 2nd metacarpal base
- Trapezoid
- Extensor carpi radialis longus t.
- Capitate
- Scaphoid
- Radial styloid
- Scapholunate l.
- Radius
- Extensor pollicis brevis tendon
- Hamate
- Triquetrum
- Lunate
- Extensor carpi ulnaris t.
- Triangular fibrocartilage
- Distal radioulnar joint
- Ulna

(Top) *Slightly volar to the dorsal ligaments, the dorsal radioulnar ligament, a component of triangular fibrocartilage complex is evident, as are dorsal proximal & distal row carpi. Extensor carpi radialis tendon courses distally to attach to 2nd metacarpal base.* **(Bottom)** *Ulnar head is seated in sigmoid notch of distal radius. Triangular fibrocartilage articular disc is readily visualized. ECU tendon passes dorsally in ECU ulnar groove. Small intrinsic carpal row ligaments, scapholunate & lunotriquetral, are present but poorly seen on T1 imaging.*

CORONAL T1 MR, RIGHT WRIST

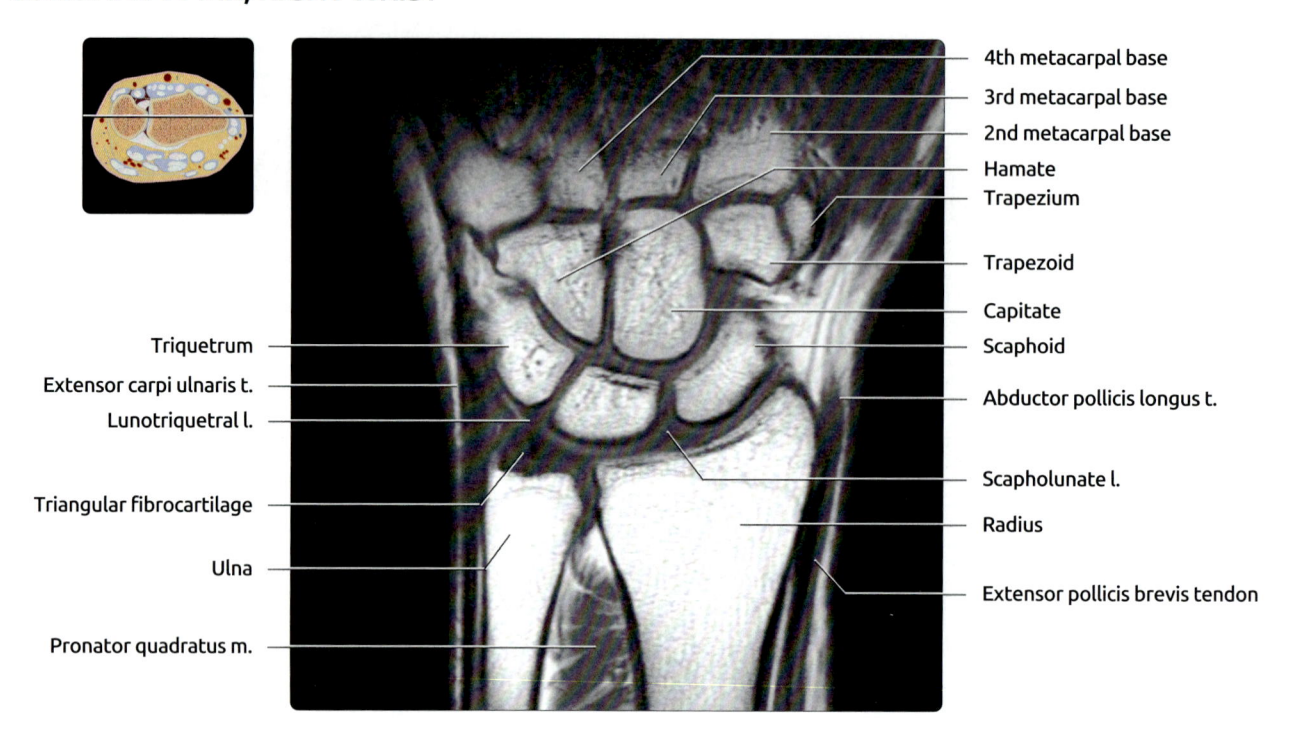

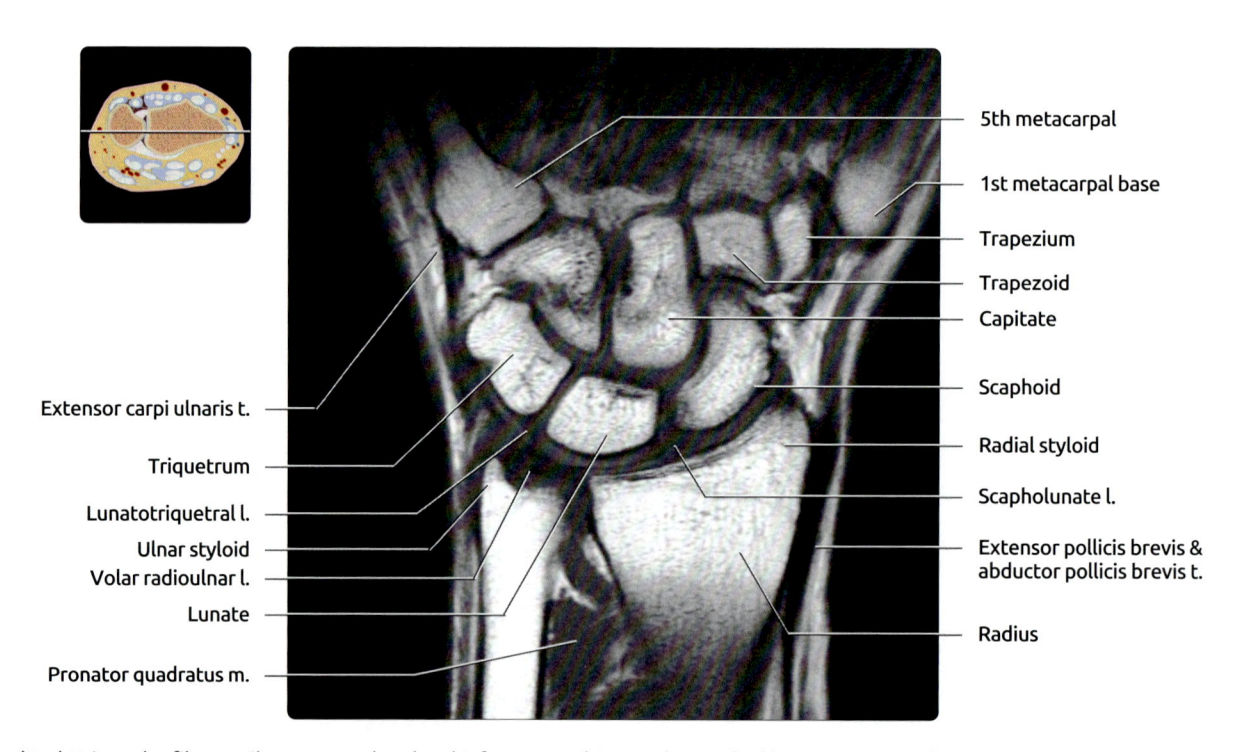

Labels (top image):
- 4th metacarpal base
- 3rd metacarpal base
- 2nd metacarpal base
- Hamate
- Trapezium
- Trapezoid
- Capitate
- Scaphoid
- Abductor pollicis longus t.
- Scapholunate l.
- Radius
- Extensor pollicis brevis tendon
- Triquetrum
- Extensor carpi ulnaris t.
- Lunotriquetral l.
- Triangular fibrocartilage
- Ulna
- Pronator quadratus m.

Labels (bottom image):
- 5th metacarpal
- 1st metacarpal base
- Trapezium
- Trapezoid
- Capitate
- Scaphoid
- Radial styloid
- Scapholunate l.
- Extensor pollicis brevis & abductor pollicis brevis t.
- Radius
- Extensor carpi ulnaris t.
- Triquetrum
- Lunatotriquetral l.
- Ulnar styloid
- Volar radioulnar l.
- Lunate
- Pronator quadratus m.

(Top) Triangular fibrocartilage covers ulnar head & fossa, attaching to ulnar styloid base. Extensor pollicis brevis tendon combines with (& is often indistinguishable from) abductor pollicis longus tendon in extensor compartment 1. Inflammation of this compartment is De Quervain tenosynovitis. **(Bottom)** Pronator quadratus muscle arises from ulna at this level. The volar triangular fibrocartilage complex component seen here is the volar radioulnar ligament. Small interosseous ligaments, such as scapholunate & lunotriquetral ligaments, are present but not well visualized.

Wrist MR Atlas

CORONAL T1 MR, LEFT WRIST

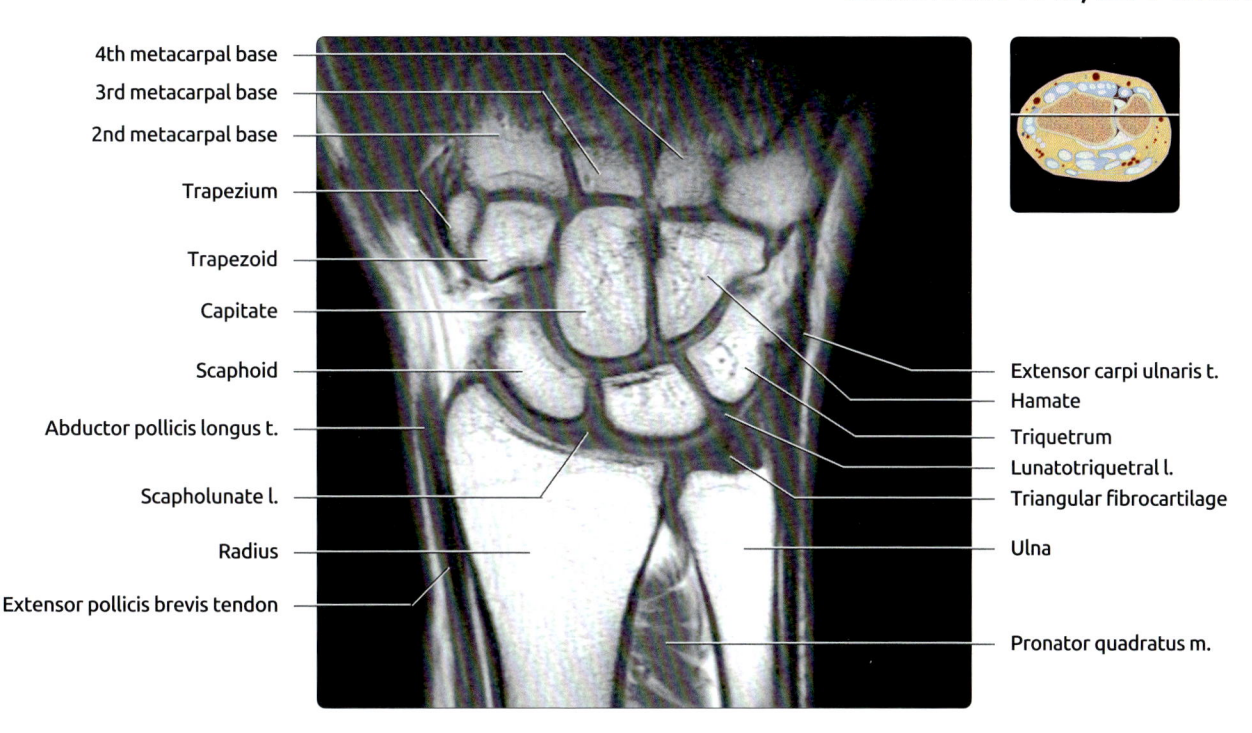

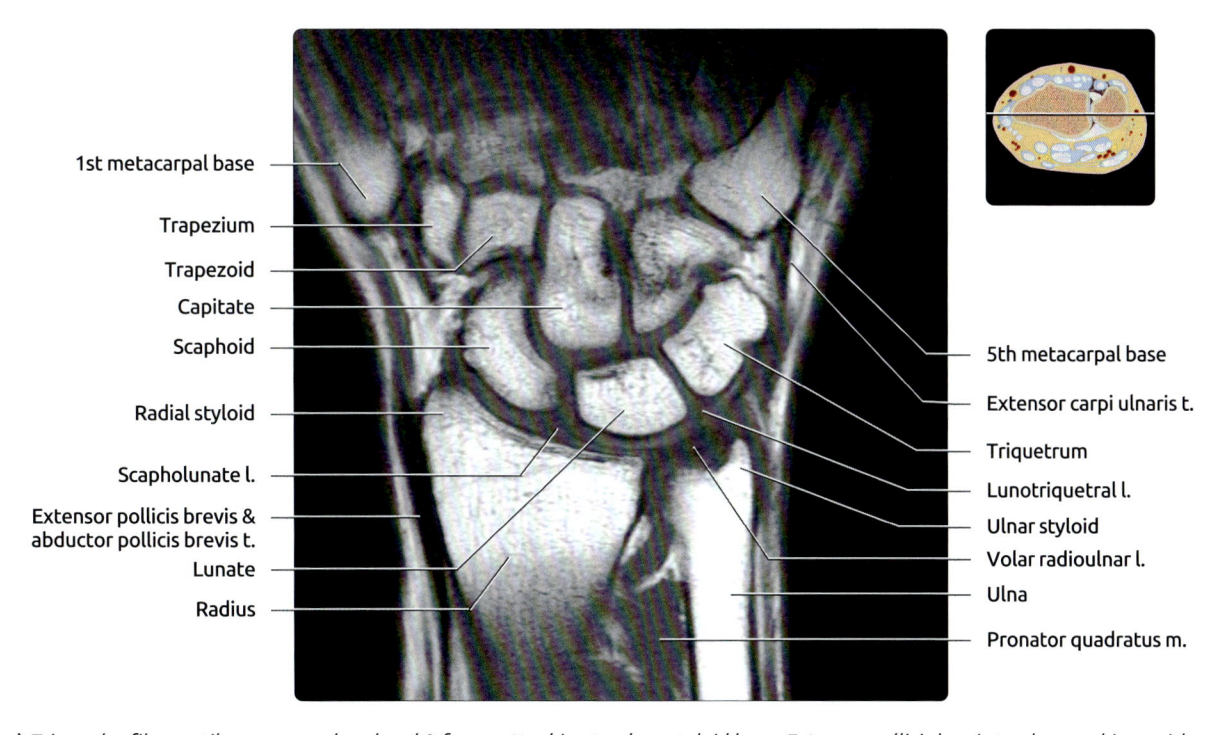

Labels (top image):
- 4th metacarpal base
- 3rd metacarpal base
- 2nd metacarpal base
- Trapezium
- Trapezoid
- Capitate
- Scaphoid
- Abductor pollicis longus t.
- Scapholunate l.
- Radius
- Extensor pollicis brevis tendon
- Extensor carpi ulnaris t.
- Hamate
- Triquetrum
- Lunatotriquetral l.
- Triangular fibrocartilage
- Ulna
- Pronator quadratus m.

Labels (bottom image):
- 1st metacarpal base
- Trapezium
- Trapezoid
- Capitate
- Scaphoid
- Radial styloid
- Scapholunate l.
- Extensor pollicis brevis & abductor pollicis brevis t.
- Lunate
- Radius
- 5th metacarpal base
- Extensor carpi ulnaris t.
- Triquetrum
- Lunotriquetral l.
- Ulnar styloid
- Volar radioulnar l.
- Ulna
- Pronator quadratus m.

(Top) *Triangular fibrocartilage covers ulnar head & fossa, attaching to ulnar styloid base. Extensor pollicis brevis tendon combines with (& is often indistinguishable from) abductor pollicis longus tendon in extensor compartment 1. Inflammation of this compartment is De Quervain tenosynovitis.* **(Bottom)** *Pronator quadratus muscle arises from ulna at this level. The volar triangular fibrocartilage complex component seen here is the volar radioulnar ligament. Small interosseous ligaments, such as scapholunate & lunotriquetral ligaments, are present but not well visualized.*

Wrist MR Atlas

CORONAL T1 MR, RIGHT WRIST

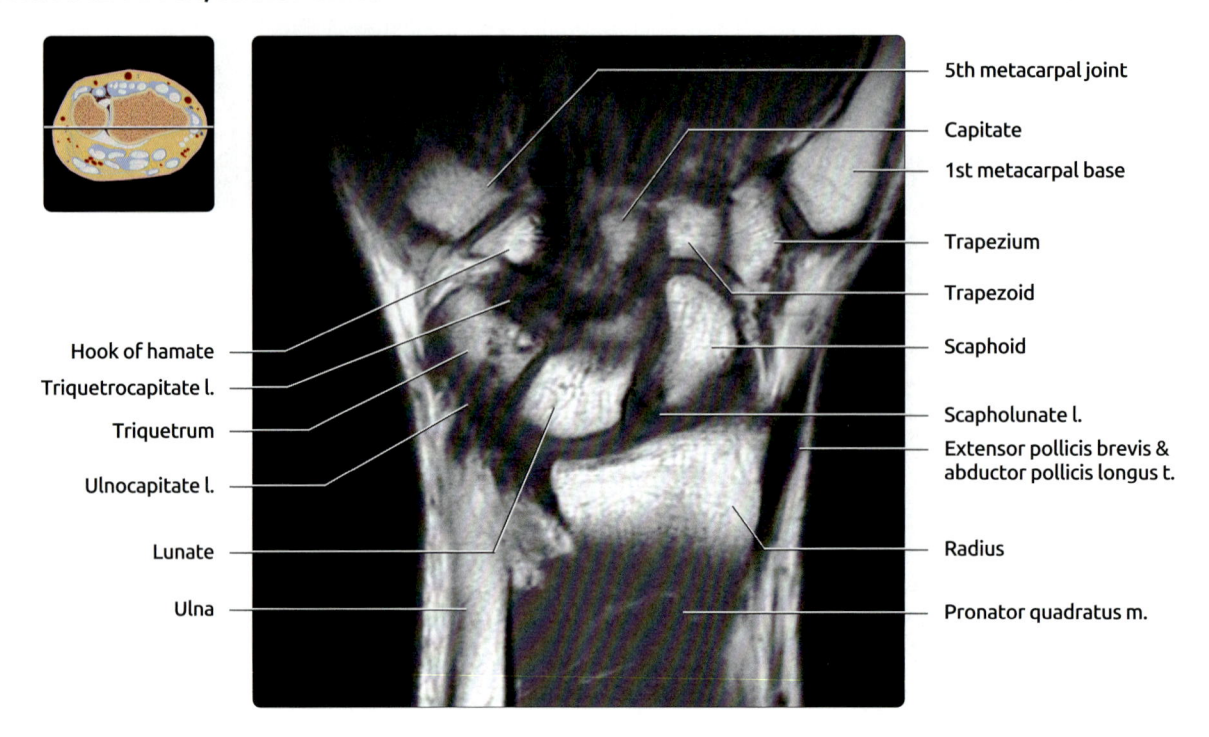

Labels (top image):
- 5th metacarpal joint
- Capitate
- 1st metacarpal base
- Trapezium
- Trapezoid
- Scaphoid
- Scapholunate l.
- Extensor pollicis brevis & abductor pollicis longus t.
- Radius
- Pronator quadratus m.
- Hook of hamate
- Triquetrocapitate l.
- Triquetrum
- Ulnocapitate l.
- Lunate
- Ulna

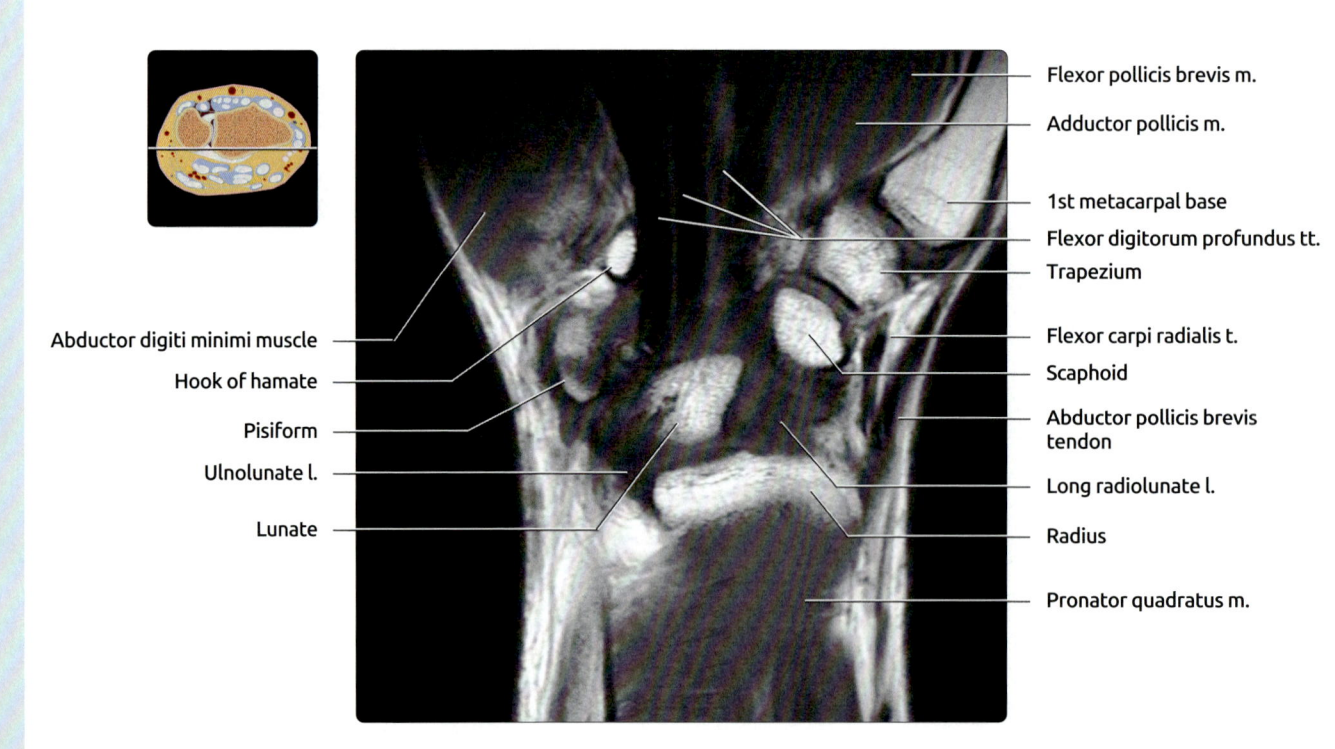

Labels (bottom image):
- Flexor pollicis brevis m.
- Adductor pollicis m.
- 1st metacarpal base
- Flexor digitorum profundus tt.
- Trapezium
- Flexor carpi radialis t.
- Scaphoid
- Abductor pollicis brevis tendon
- Long radiolunate l.
- Radius
- Pronator quadratus m.
- Abductor digiti minimi muscle
- Hook of hamate
- Pisiform
- Ulnolunate l.
- Lunate

(Top) At the level of dorsal pisotriquetral joint & base of scaphoid tubercle, portions of volar ligaments are noted, including ulnocapitate & triquetrocapitate ligaments. Extensor pollicis brevis & abductor pollicis longus tendons pass through snuffbox region of wrist. The hook of the hamate is evident. **(Bottom)** At level of volar side of pisotriquetral joint & scaphoid tubercle, pronator quadratus muscle belly is visualized. Flexor digitorum profundus tendons pass through dorsal carpal tunnel.

Wrist MR Atlas

CORONAL T1 MR, LEFT WRIST

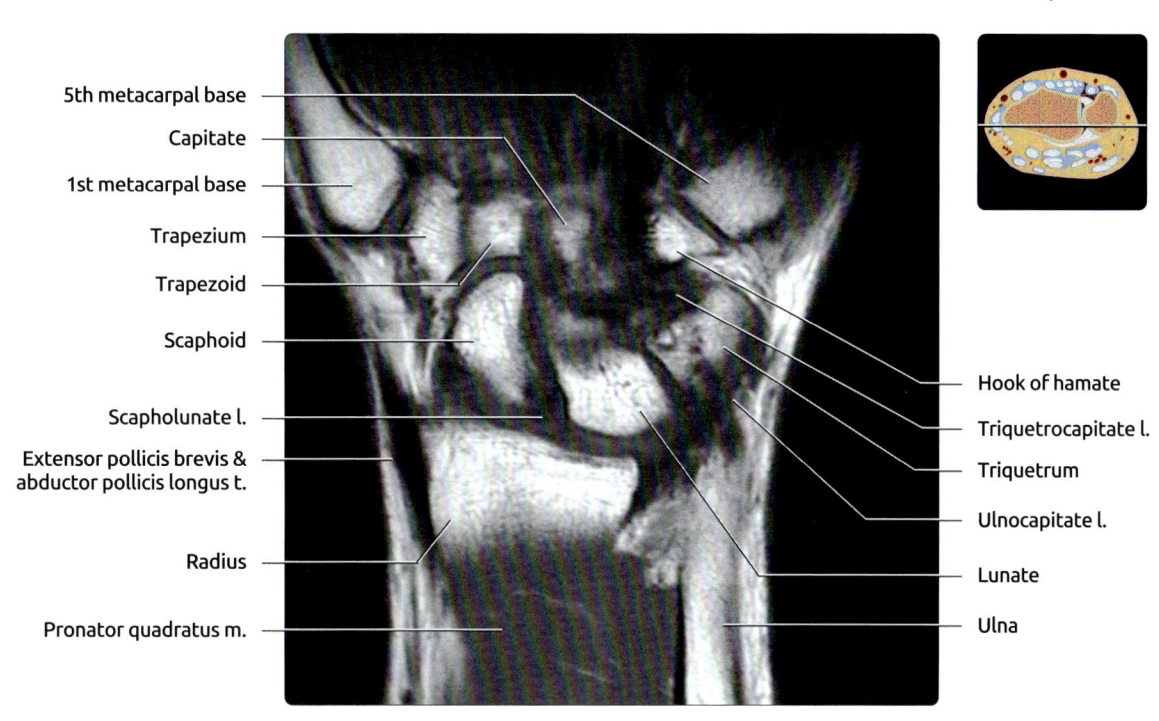

Top image labels (left):
- 5th metacarpal base
- Capitate
- 1st metacarpal base
- Trapezium
- Trapezoid
- Scaphoid
- Scapholunate l.
- Extensor pollicis brevis & abductor pollicis longus t.
- Radius
- Pronator quadratus m.

Top image labels (right):
- Hook of hamate
- Triquetrocapitate l.
- Triquetrum
- Ulnocapitate l.
- Lunate
- Ulna

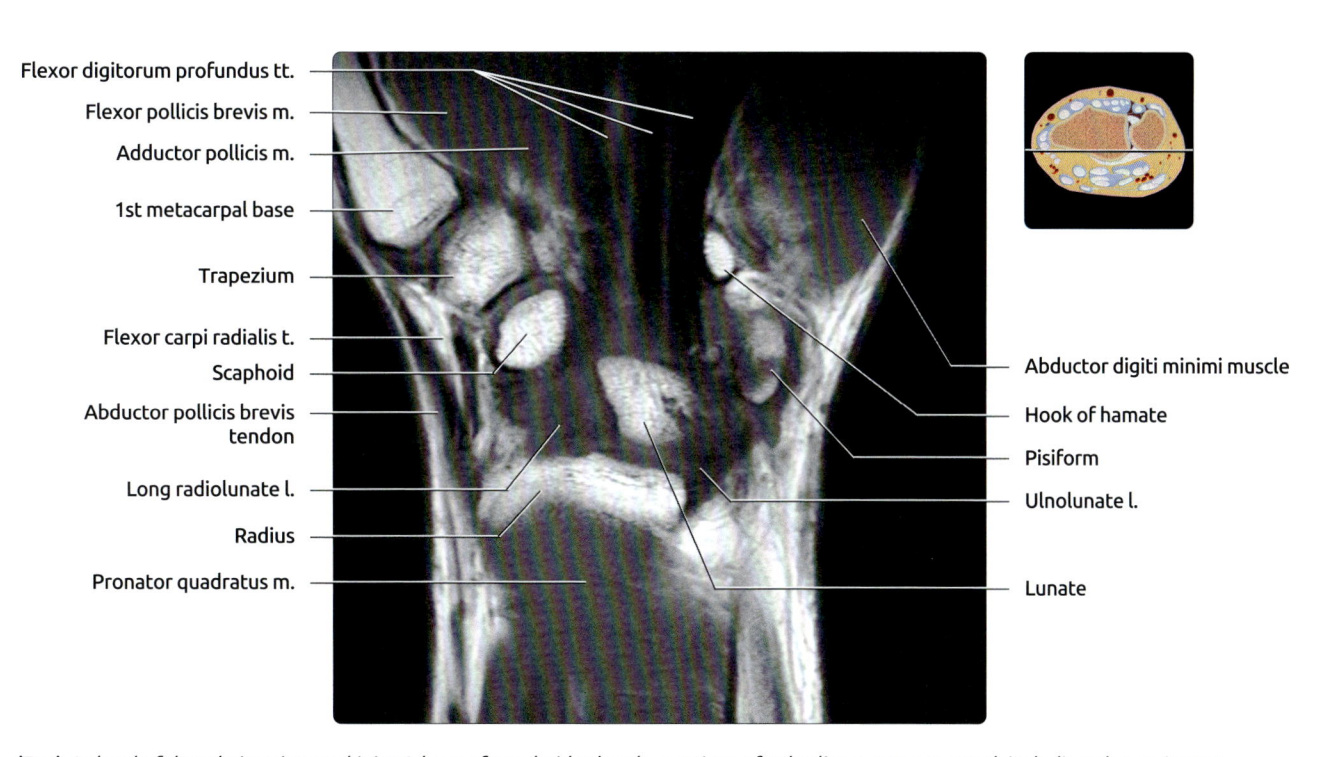

Bottom image labels (left):
- Flexor digitorum profundus tt.
- Flexor pollicis brevis m.
- Adductor pollicis m.
- 1st metacarpal base
- Trapezium
- Flexor carpi radialis t.
- Scaphoid
- Abductor pollicis brevis tendon
- Long radiolunate l.
- Radius
- Pronator quadratus m.

Bottom image labels (right):
- Abductor digiti minimi muscle
- Hook of hamate
- Pisiform
- Ulnolunate l.
- Lunate

(Top) *At level of dorsal pisotriquetral joint & base of scaphoid tubercle, portions of volar ligaments are noted, including ulnocapitate & triquetrocapitate ligaments. Extensor pollicis brevis & abductor pollicis longus tendons pass through snuffbox region of wrist. The hook of the hamate is evident.* **(Bottom)** *At level of volar side of pisotriquetral joint & scaphoid tubercle, pronator quadratus muscle belly is visualized. Flexor digitorum profundus tendons pass through dorsal carpal tunnel.*

CORONAL T1 MR, RIGHT WRIST

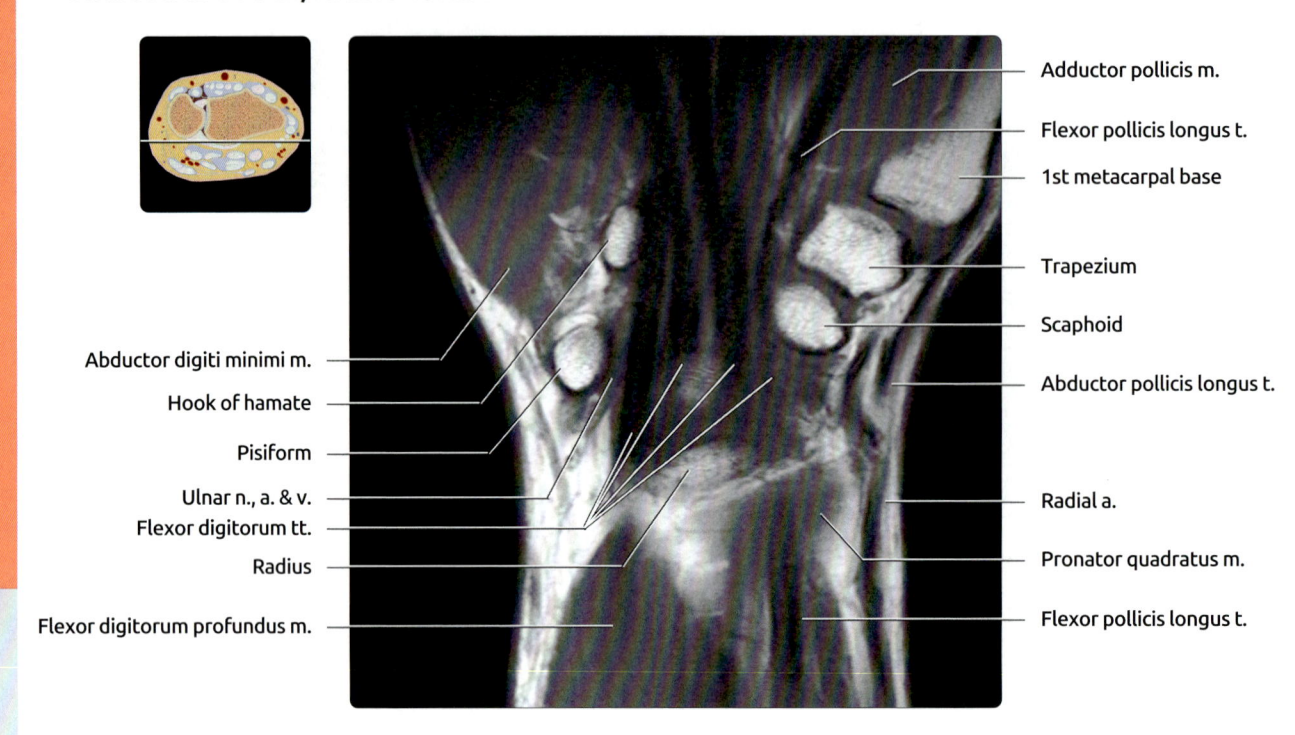

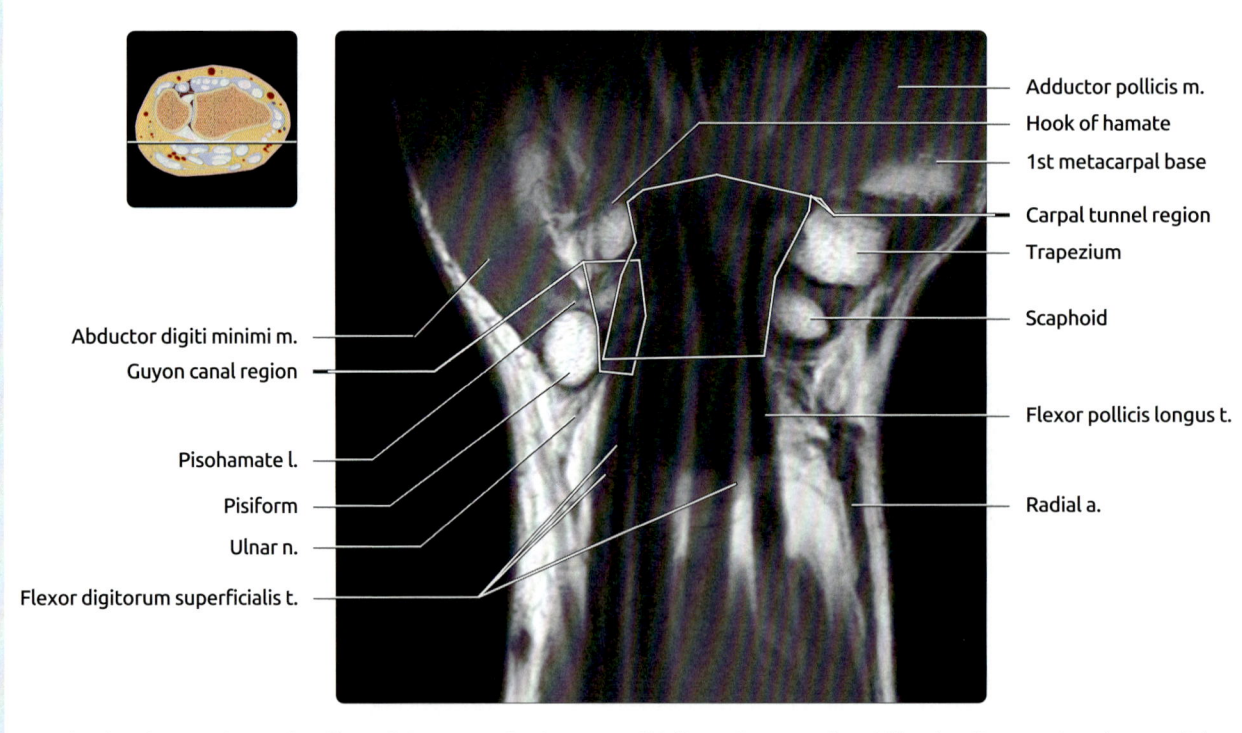

Labels (top image):
- Adductor pollicis m.
- Flexor pollicis longus t.
- 1st metacarpal base
- Trapezium
- Scaphoid
- Abductor pollicis longus t.
- Radial a.
- Pronator quadratus m.
- Flexor pollicis longus t.
- Abductor digiti minimi m.
- Hook of hamate
- Pisiform
- Ulnar n., a. & v.
- Flexor digitorum tt.
- Radius
- Flexor digitorum profundus m.

Labels (bottom image):
- Adductor pollicis m.
- Hook of hamate
- 1st metacarpal base
- Carpal tunnel region
- Trapezium
- Scaphoid
- Flexor pollicis longus t.
- Radial a.
- Abductor digiti minimi m.
- Guyon canal region
- Pisohamate l.
- Pisiform
- Ulnar n.
- Flexor digitorum superficialis t.

(Top) Volar to radius & ulna, flexor digitorum profundus & superficialis tendons pass dorsal (deep) to flexor retinaculum. Radial & ulnar arteries are visualized in proximal wrist but rapidly branch into smaller vessels, which may not be evident on routine MR imaging. (Bottom) Guyon canal region is defined by pisiform & deep & superficial components of medial flexor retinaculum. It contains ulnar nerve, artery, & veins as well as fat. Carpal tunnel region is dorsal (deep) to Guyon canal & contains flexor digitorum profundus & superficialis tendons, flexor pollicis longus tendon, & median nerve.

Wrist MR Atlas

CORONAL T1 MR, LEFT WRIST

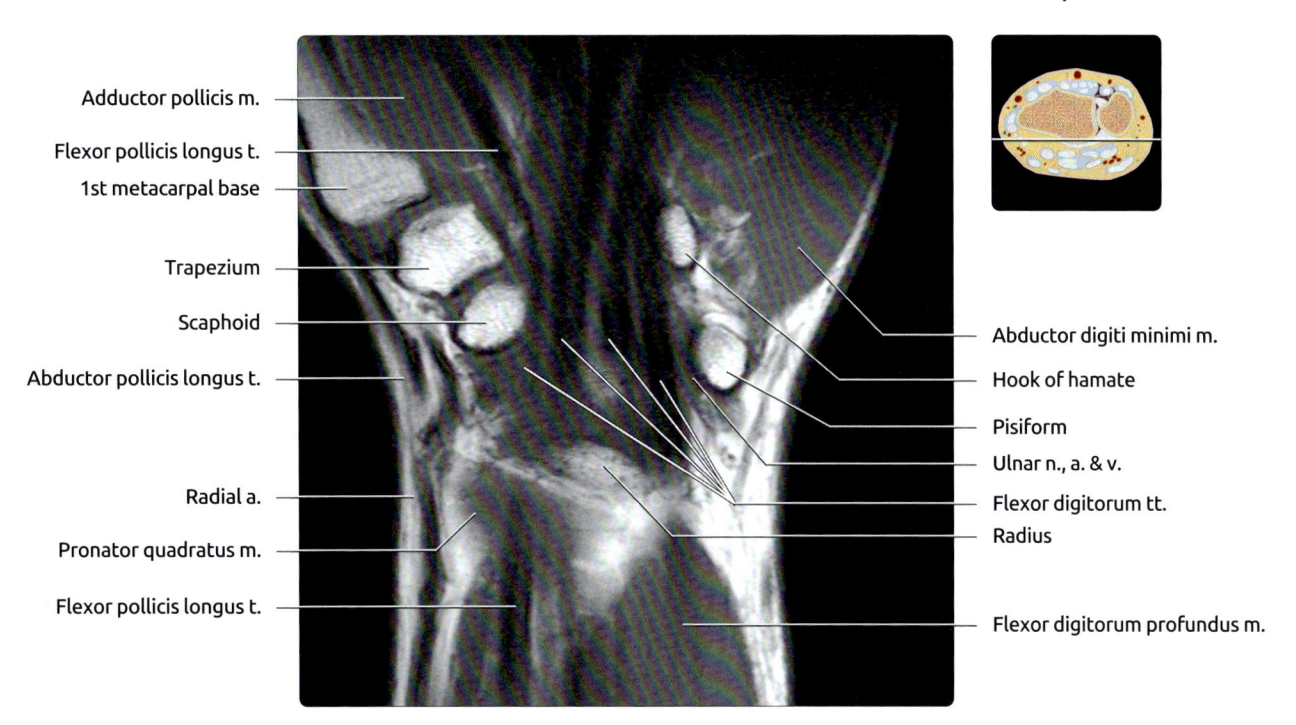

Labels (top image):
- Adductor pollicis m.
- Flexor pollicis longus t.
- 1st metacarpal base
- Trapezium
- Scaphoid
- Abductor pollicis longus t.
- Radial a.
- Pronator quadratus m.
- Flexor pollicis longus t.
- Abductor digiti minimi m.
- Hook of hamate
- Pisiform
- Ulnar n., a. & v.
- Flexor digitorum tt.
- Radius
- Flexor digitorum profundus m.

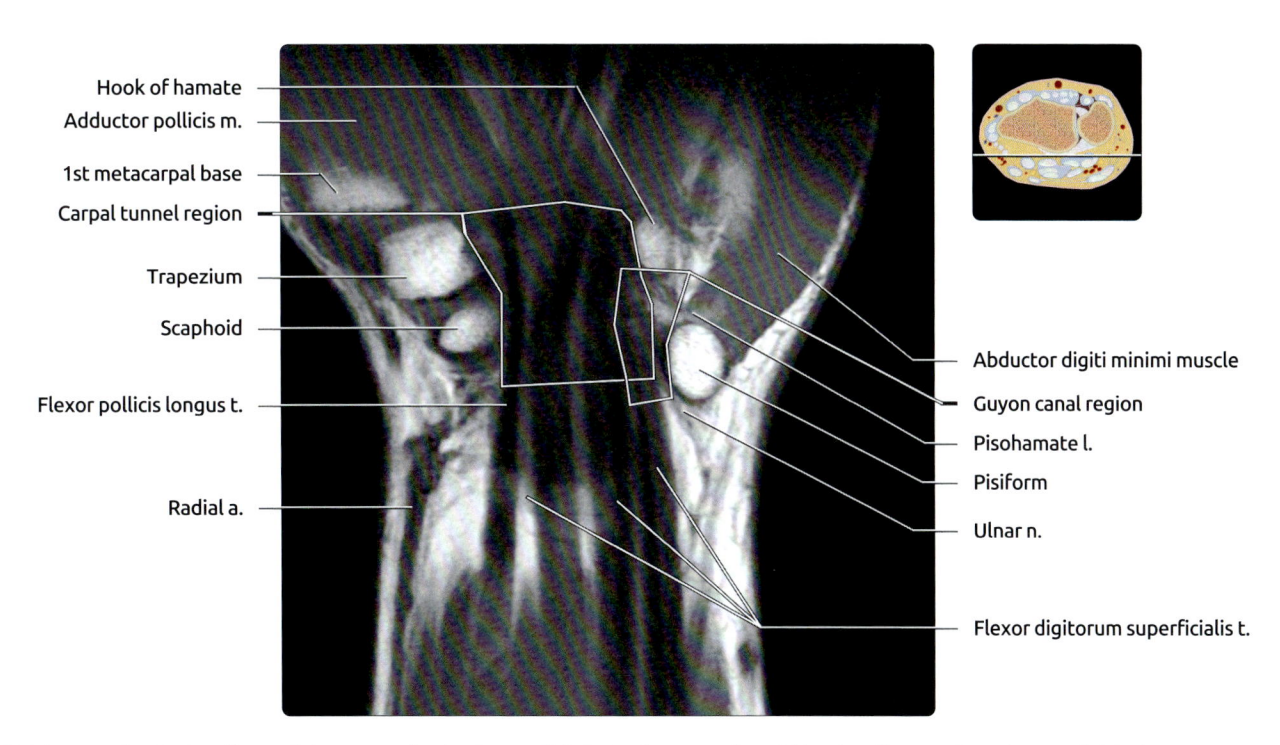

Labels (bottom image):
- Hook of hamate
- Adductor pollicis m.
- 1st metacarpal base
- Carpal tunnel region
- Trapezium
- Scaphoid
- Flexor pollicis longus t.
- Radial a.
- Abductor digiti minimi muscle
- Guyon canal region
- Pisohamate l.
- Pisiform
- Ulnar n.
- Flexor digitorum superficialis t.

(Top) *Volar to radius & ulna, flexor digitorum profundus & superficialis tendons pass dorsal (deep) to flexor retinaculum. Radial & ulnar arteries are visualized in proximal wrist but rapidly branch into smaller vessels, which may not be evident on routine MR imaging.*
(Bottom) *Guyon canal region is defined by pisiform & deep & superficial components of medial flexor retinaculum. It contains ulnar nerve, artery & veins as well as fat. Carpal tunnel region is dorsal (deep) to Guyon canal & contains flexor digitorum profundus & superficialis tendons, flexor pollicis longus tendon, & median nerve.*

Wrist MR Atlas

CORONAL T1 MR, RIGHT WRIST

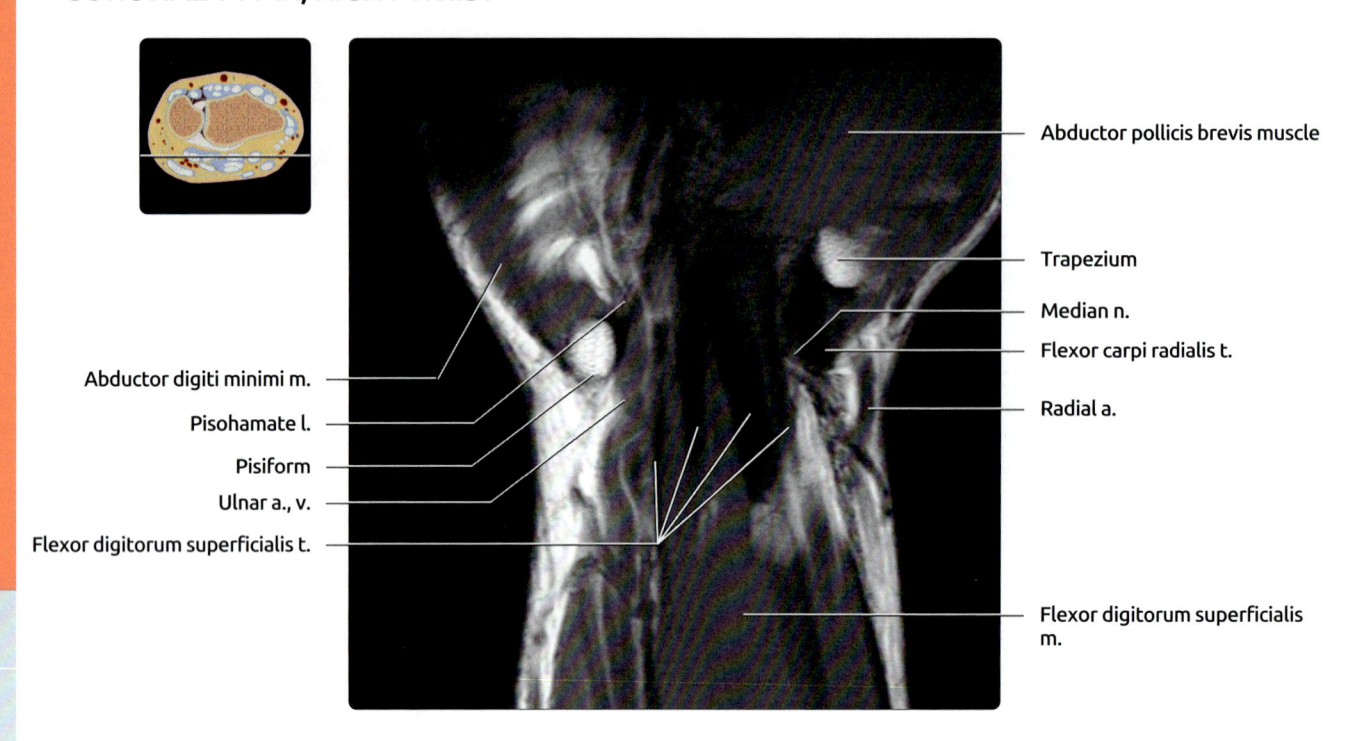

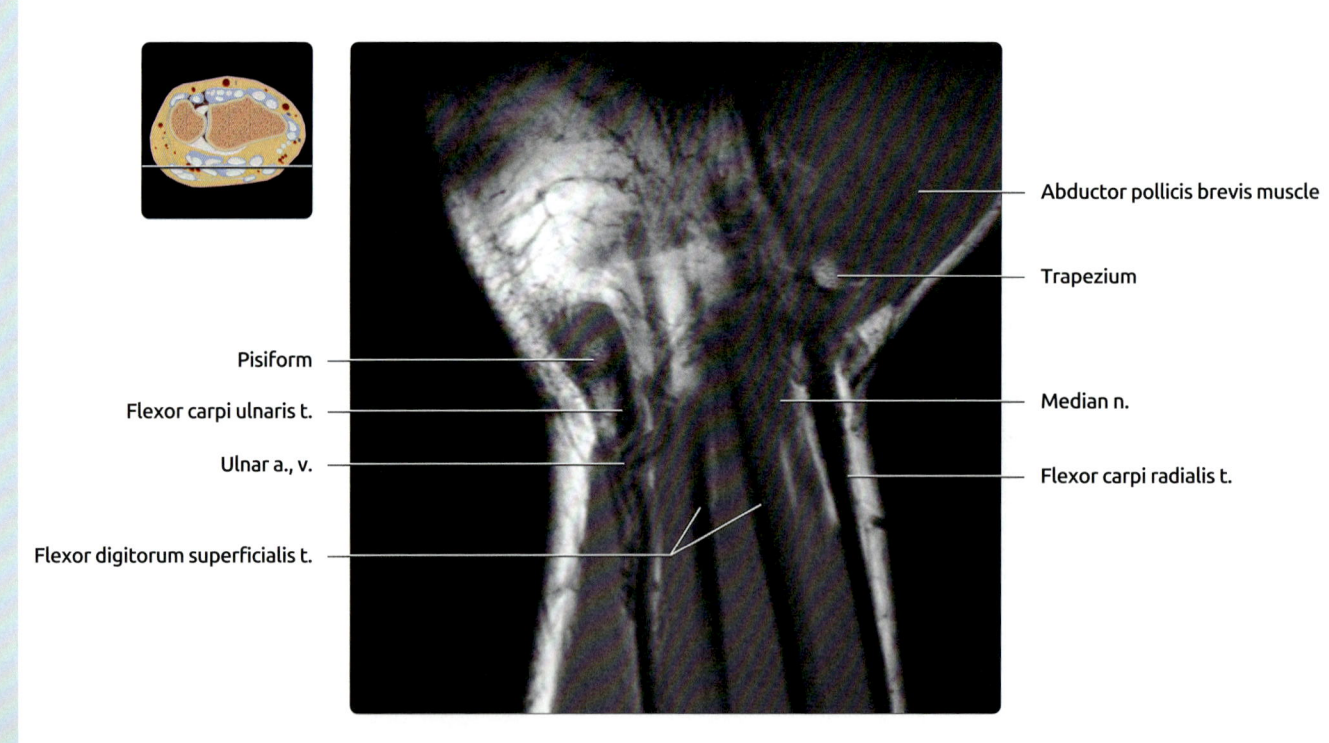

Abductor pollicis brevis muscle
Trapezium
Median n.
Flexor carpi radialis t.
Radial a.

Abductor digiti minimi m.
Pisohamate l.
Pisiform
Ulnar a., v.
Flexor digitorum superficialis t.

Flexor digitorum superficialis m.

Abductor pollicis brevis muscle
Trapezium

Pisiform
Flexor carpi ulnaris t.
Ulnar a., v.

Median n.
Flexor carpi radialis t.

Flexor digitorum superficialis t.

(Top) Small slips of flexor retinaculum pass horizontally from scaphoid toward hamate & pisiform. The flexor digitorum superficialis tendons are just dorsal to flexor retinaculum. Ulnar nerve is ulnar to ulnar artery & vein as it passes through Guyon canal. **(Bottom)** Median nerve is superficial & radial in carpal tunnel & is typically isointense to muscle, which may make it difficult to distinguish on T1 imaging.

Wrist MR Atlas

CORONAL T1 MR, LEFT WRIST

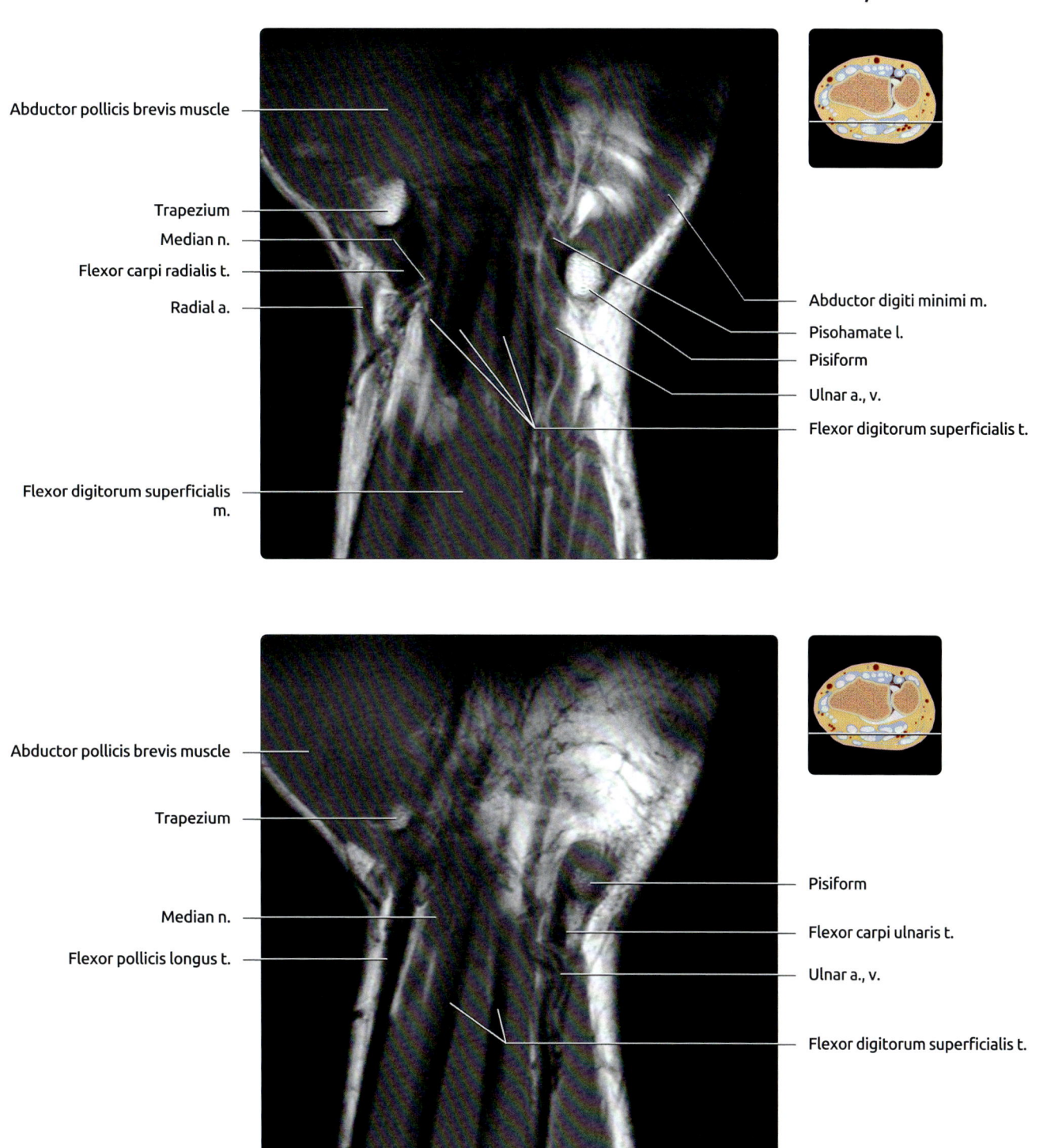

Abductor pollicis brevis muscle
Trapezium
Median n.
Flexor carpi radialis t.
Radial a.
Flexor digitorum superficialis m.

Abductor digiti minimi m.
Pisohamate l.
Pisiform
Ulnar a., v.
Flexor digitorum superficialis t.

Abductor pollicis brevis muscle
Trapezium
Median n.
Flexor pollicis longus t.

Pisiform
Flexor carpi ulnaris t.
Ulnar a., v.
Flexor digitorum superficialis t.

(Top) *Small slips of flexor retinaculum pass horizontally from scaphoid toward hamate & pisiform. The flexor digitorum superficialis tendons are just dorsal to flexor retinaculum. Ulnar nerve is ulnar to ulnar artery & vein as it passes through Guyon canal.* **(Bottom)** *Median nerve is superficial & radial in carpal tunnel & is typically isointense to muscle, which may make it difficult to distinguish on T1 imaging.*

CORONAL T1 MR, RIGHT WRIST

Abductor pollicis brevis muscle

Flexor carpi ulnaris t.

Flexor digitorum superficialis m.

Flexor carpi radialis t.

Superficial veins

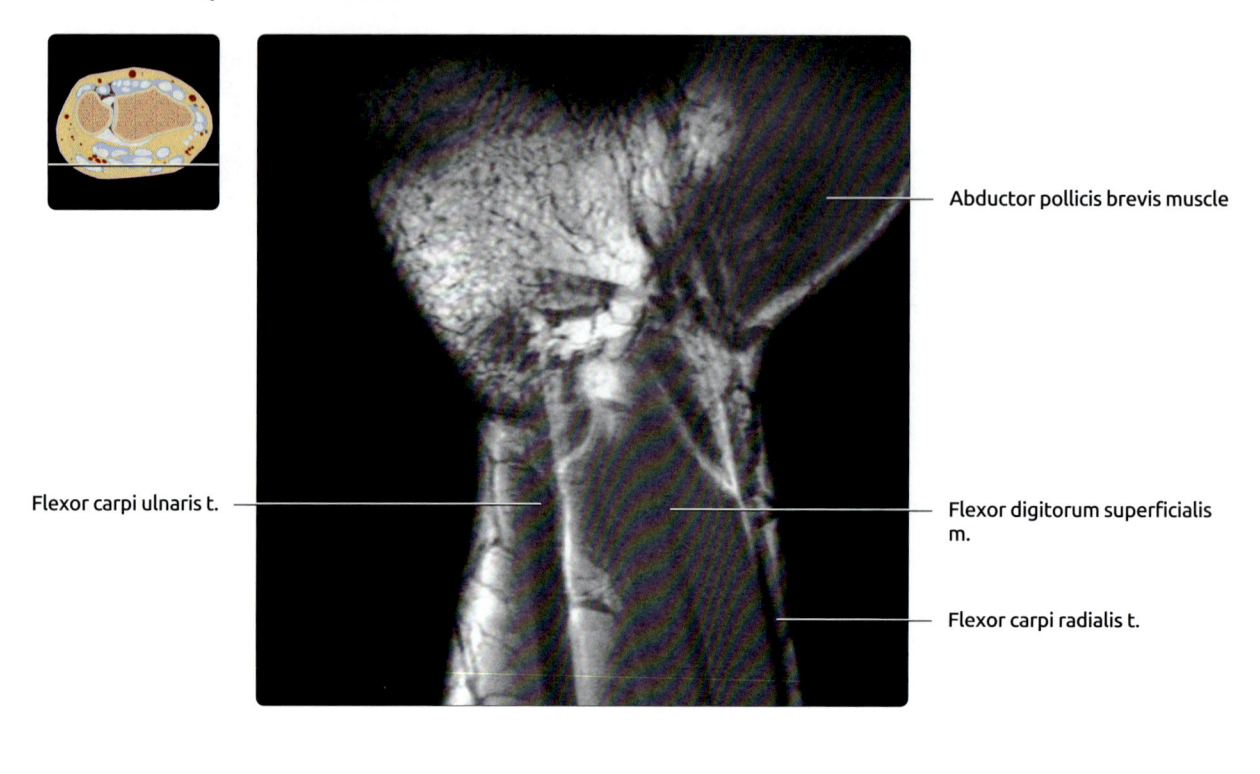

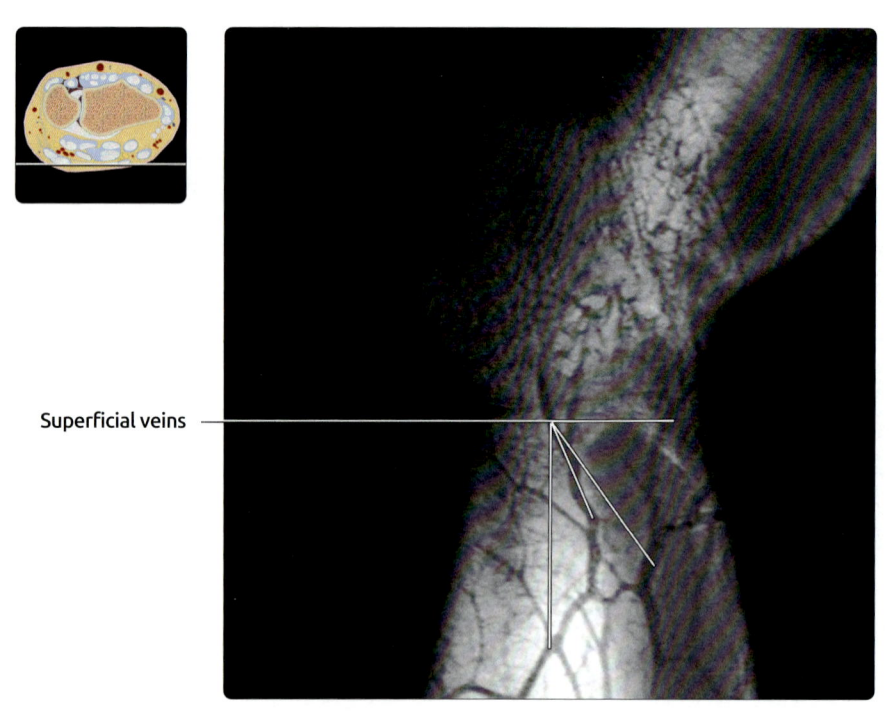

(Top) Volar musculature of distal forearm & thenar eminence is readily seen. *(Bottom)* A network of veins over the volar wrist drains into cephalic vein radially & basilic vein ulnarly.

Wrist MR Atlas

CORONAL T1 MR, LEFT WRIST

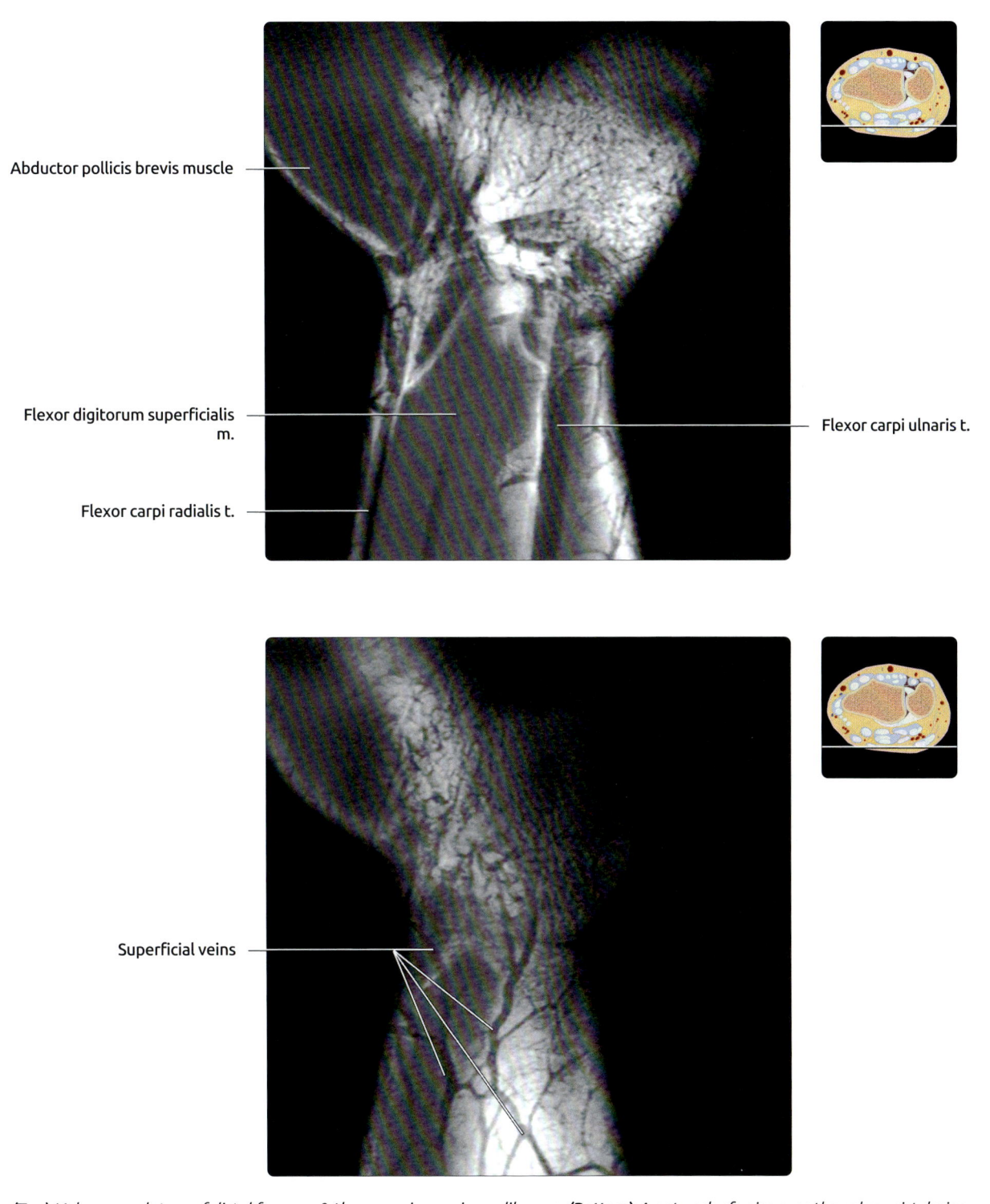

Abductor pollicis brevis muscle

Flexor digitorum superficialis m.

Flexor carpi radialis t.

Flexor carpi ulnaris t.

Superficial veins

(Top) *Volar musculature of distal forearm & thenar eminence is readily seen.* **(Bottom)** *A network of veins over the volar wrist drains into cephalic vein radially & basilic vein ulnarly.*

SAGITTAL T1 MR, WRIST

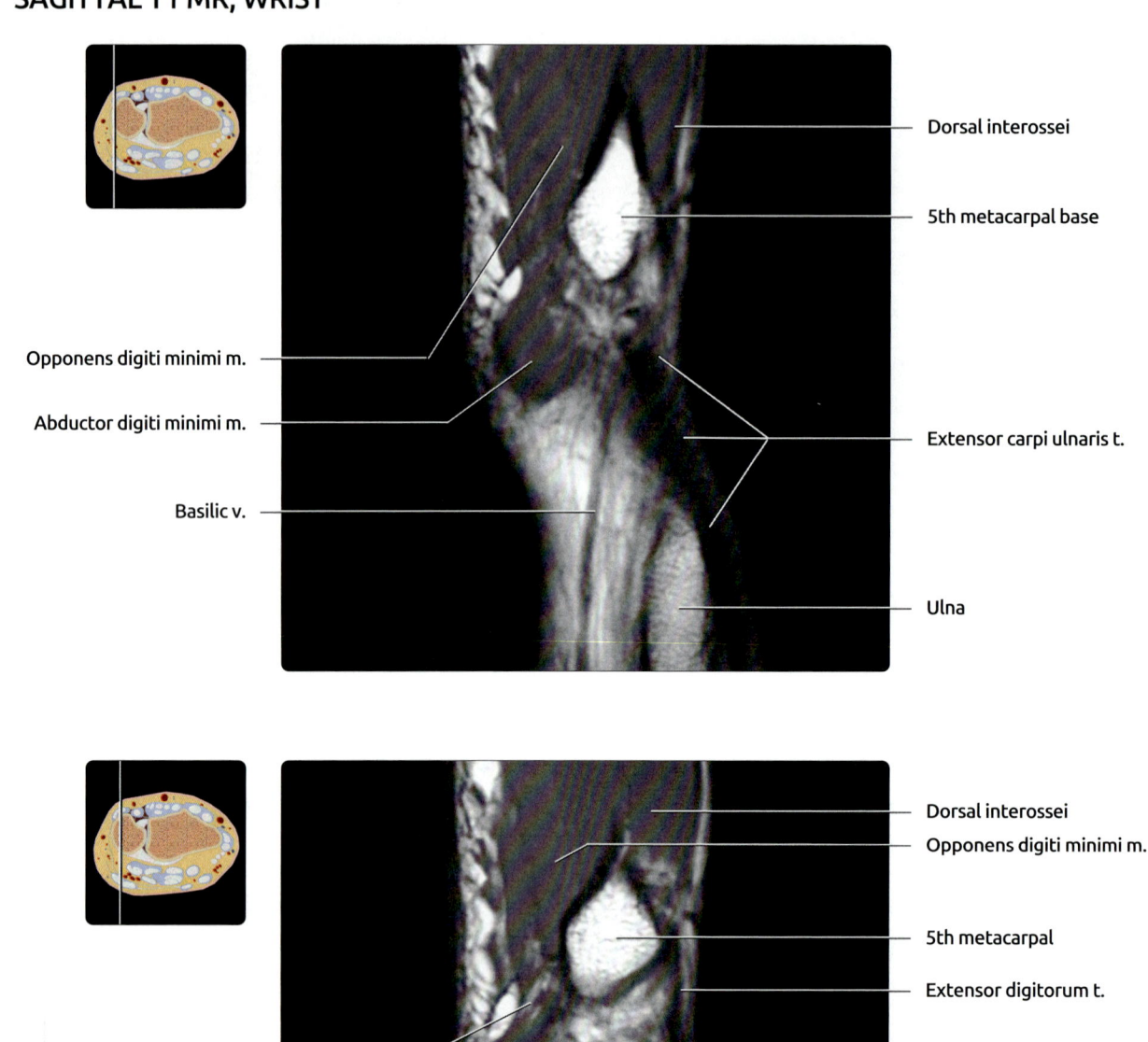

Labels (top image):
- Dorsal interossei
- 5th metacarpal base
- Opponens digiti minimi m.
- Abductor digiti minimi m.
- Extensor carpi ulnaris t.
- Basilic v.
- Ulna

Labels (bottom image):
- Dorsal interossei
- Opponens digiti minimi m.
- 5th metacarpal
- Extensor digitorum t.
- Abductor digiti minimi muscle
- Triquetrum
- Pisometacarpal l.
- Pisohamate ligament
- Extensor carpi ulnaris t.
- Pisiform
- Ulnar styloid process

(Top) First of 20 sequential T1 coronal images of the wrist, displayed from ulnar (medial) to radial (lateral). ECU tendon passes over distal ulna in ECU ulnar groove. The abductor digiti minimi is the most ulnar and ventral of the hypothenar muscles. (Bottom) Pisometacarpal ligament attaches the pisiform to the 5th metacarpal. It is adjacent to the pisohamate ligament (next image).

Wrist MR Atlas

SAGITTAL T1 MR, WRIST

Labels (top image, left): Dorsal interossei; Opponens digiti minimi m.; Flexor digiti minimi m.; Abductor digiti minimi muscle; Pisohamate ligament; Pisiform; Pisotriquetral joint; Flexor carpi ulnaris t.

Labels (top image, right): 5th metacarpal base; Hamate; Triquetrum; Extensor carpi ulnaris t.; Ulna

Labels (bottom image, left): Palmar interossei; Extensor digitorum t.; Opponens digiti minimi m.; 4th metacarpal base; Palmaris brevis; Pisohamate l.; Pisiform; Flexor carpi ulnaris t.; Ulnotriquetral l.; Flexor digitorum profundus m. & t.

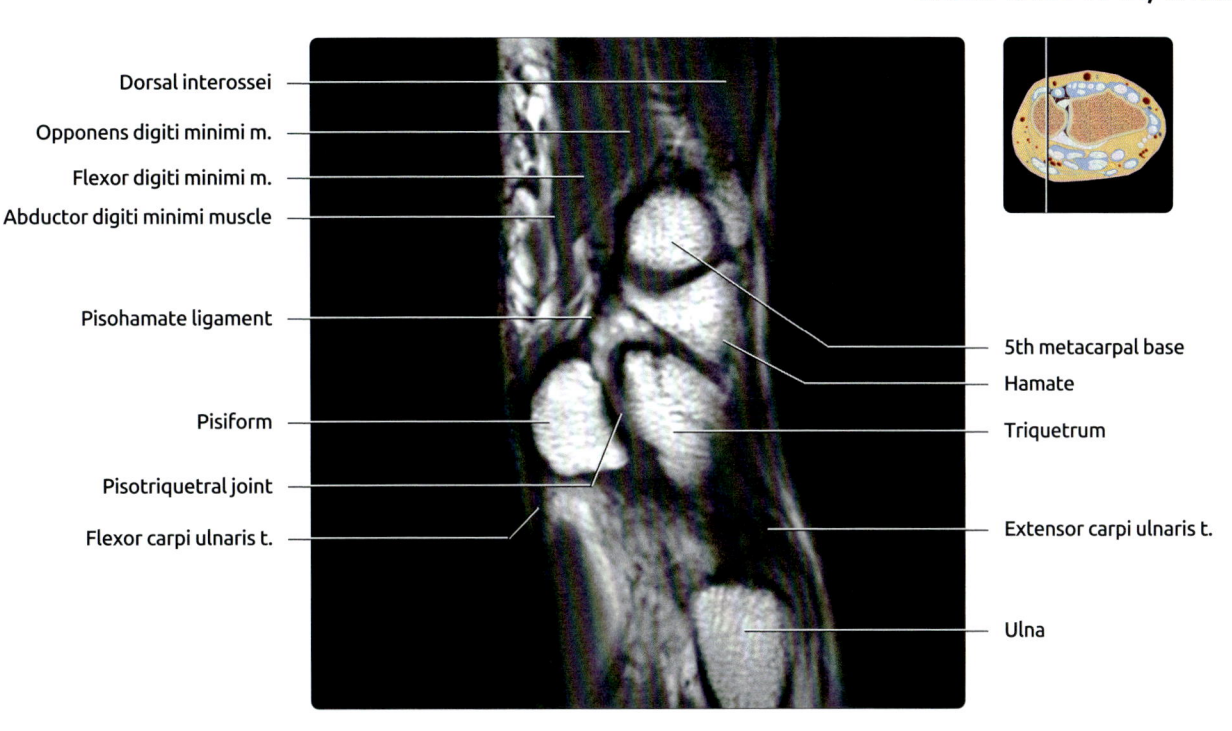

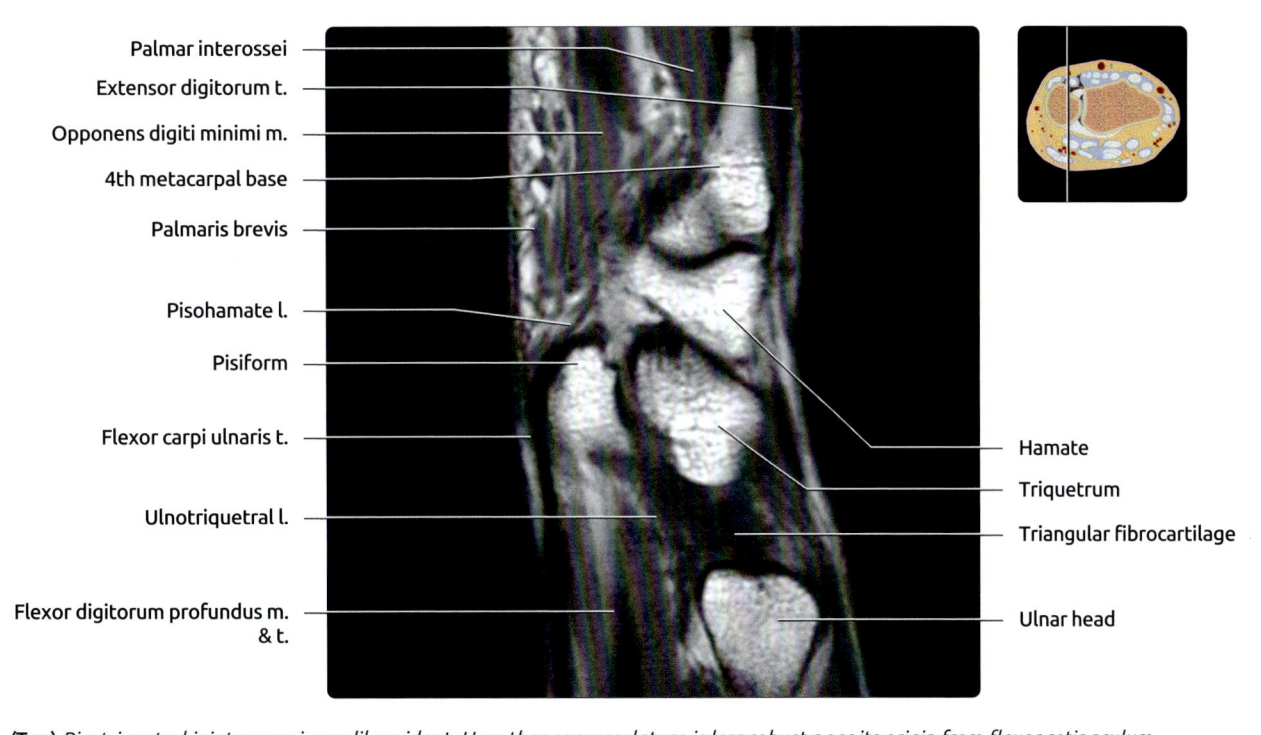

Labels (bottom image, right): Hamate; Triquetrum; Triangular fibrocartilage; Ulnar head

(Top) *Pisotriquetral joint recess is readily evident. Hypothenar musculature is less robust near its origin from flexor retinaculum.*
(Bottom) *Flexor carpi ulnaris tendon inserts on pisiform. Ulnotriquetral ligament arises from volar radioulnar ligament, inserting on volar triquetrum.*

Wrist MR Atlas

SAGITTAL T1 MR, WRIST

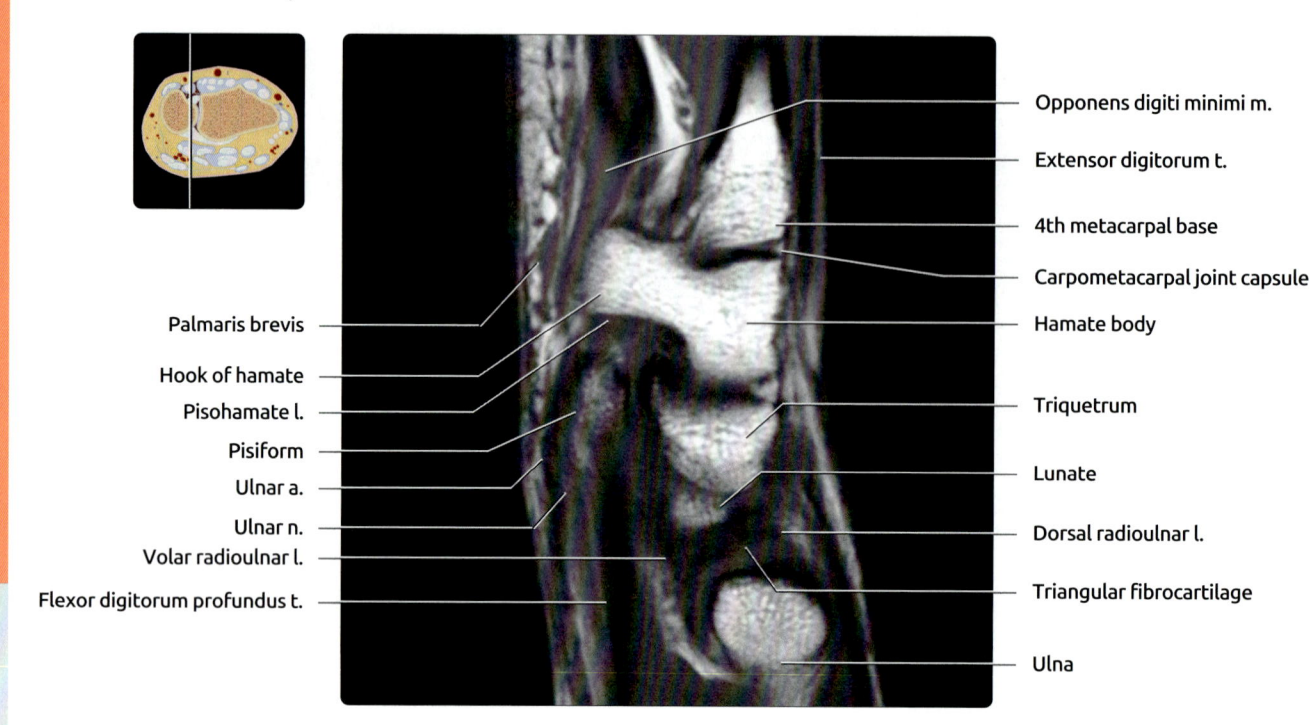

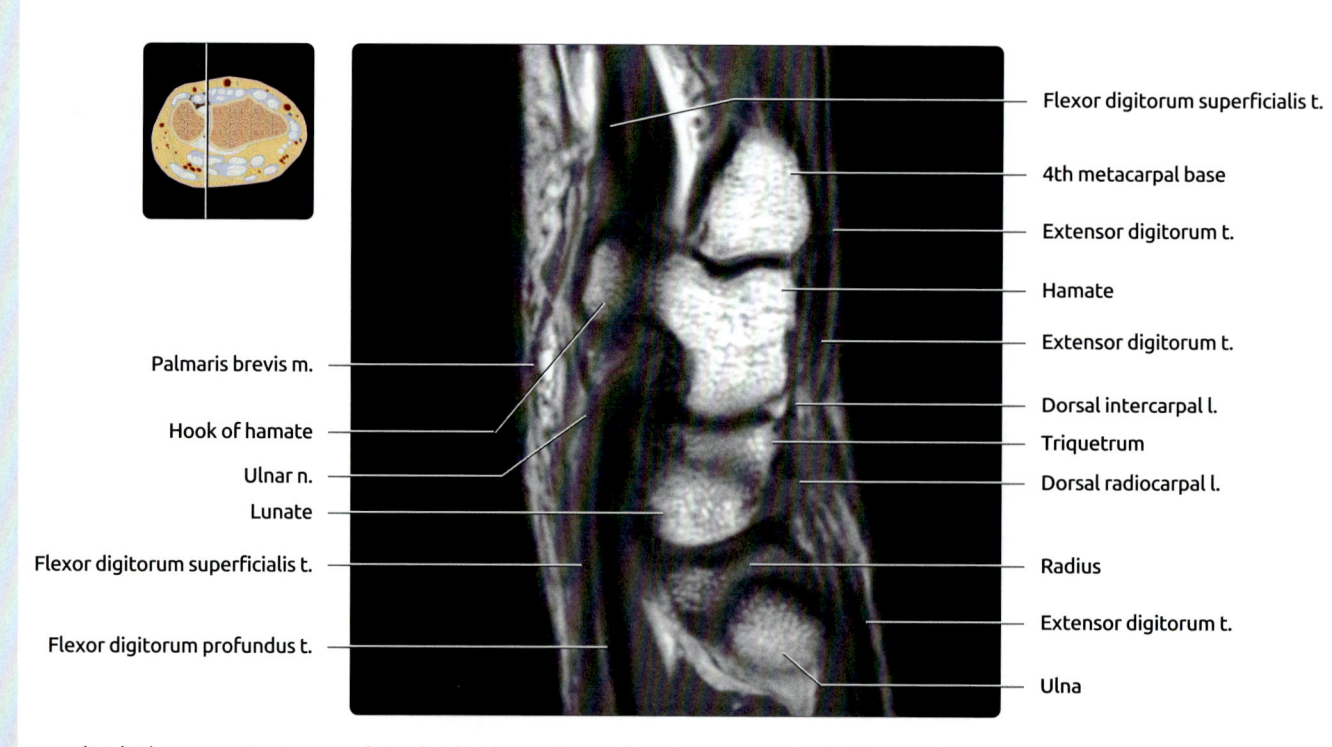

Labels (top image):
- Opponens digiti minimi m.
- Extensor digitorum t.
- 4th metacarpal base
- Carpometacarpal joint capsule
- Palmaris brevis
- Hamate body
- Hook of hamate
- Pisohamate l.
- Triquetrum
- Pisiform
- Ulnar a.
- Lunate
- Ulnar n.
- Dorsal radioulnar l.
- Volar radioulnar l.
- Triangular fibrocartilage
- Flexor digitorum profundus t.
- Ulna

Labels (bottom image):
- Flexor digitorum superficialis t.
- 4th metacarpal base
- Extensor digitorum t.
- Hamate
- Extensor digitorum t.
- Palmaris brevis m.
- Dorsal intercarpal l.
- Hook of hamate
- Triquetrum
- Ulnar n.
- Dorsal radiocarpal l.
- Lunate
- Flexor digitorum superficialis t.
- Radius
- Extensor digitorum t.
- Flexor digitorum profundus t.
- Ulna

(Top) Ulnar nerve & artery pass lateral & distal to pisiform within Guyon canal. Hook of hamate is prominent. Triangular fibrocartilage (TFC) is visualized as a low signal intensity disc interposed between ulnar head & triquetrum. Volar & dorsal radioulnar ligaments combine with TFC & adjacent structures to form triangular fibrocartilage complex. **(Bottom)** Intrinsic & extrinsic ligaments may be difficult to identify as individual structures, particularly in the absence of joint distension. Ligaments are labeled where visible or in the region of an expected ligament. Dorsal intercarpal ligament is a key dorsal wrist stabilizer but is visualized in only limited fashion.

Wrist MR Atlas

SAGITTAL T1 MR, WRIST

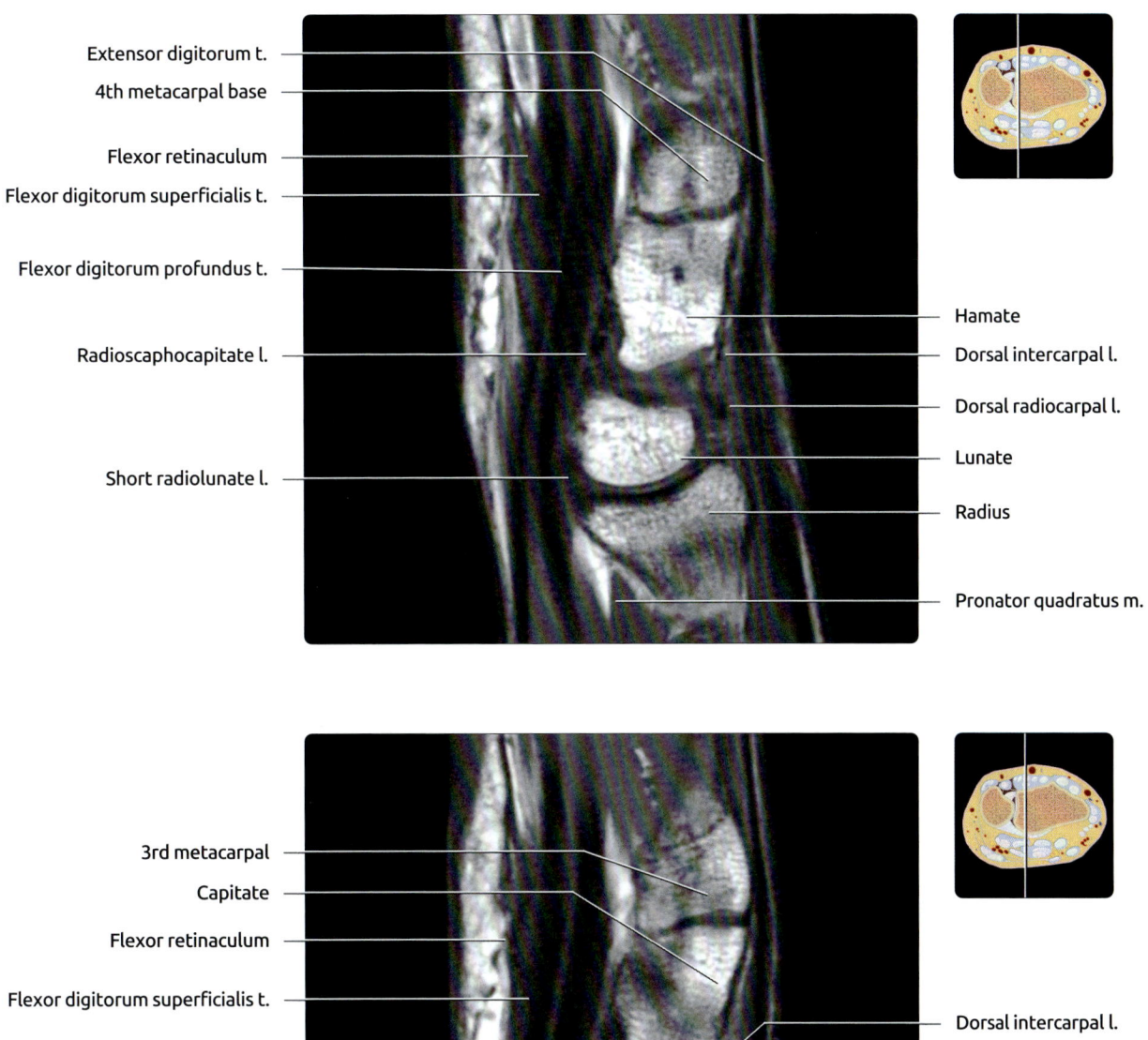

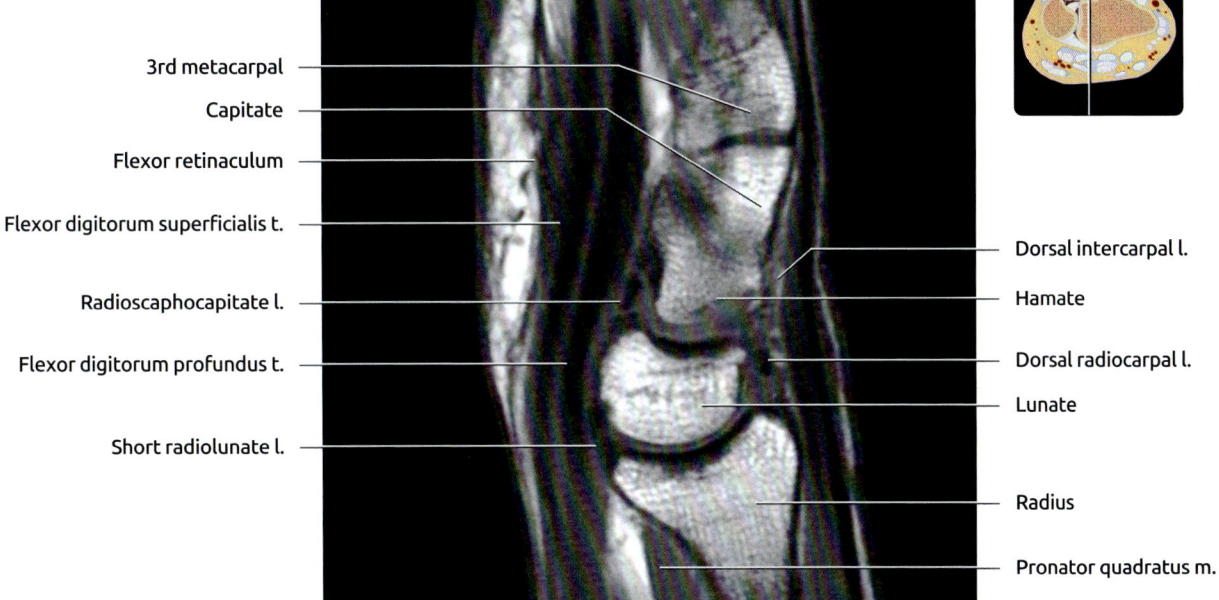

Top image labels:
- Extensor digitorum t.
- 4th metacarpal base
- Flexor retinaculum
- Flexor digitorum superficialis t.
- Flexor digitorum profundus t.
- Radioscaphocapitate l.
- Short radiolunate l.
- Hamate
- Dorsal intercarpal l.
- Dorsal radiocarpal l.
- Lunate
- Radius
- Pronator quadratus m.

Bottom image labels:
- 3rd metacarpal
- Capitate
- Flexor retinaculum
- Flexor digitorum superficialis t.
- Radioscaphocapitate l.
- Flexor digitorum profundus t.
- Short radiolunate l.
- Dorsal intercarpal l.
- Hamate
- Dorsal radiocarpal l.
- Lunate
- Radius
- Pronator quadratus m.

(**Top**) *Flexor digitorum superficialis & profundus tendons pass deep to the horizontally oriented flexor retinaculum. Extensor digitorum tendons course through 4th extensor compartment & are stabilized by extensor retinaculum.* (**Bottom**) *Portions of radioscapholunate & short radiolunate ligaments are visualized volarly. The dorsal radiocarpal ligament is seen dorsally & region of dorsal intercarpal ligament is marked. Dorsal lip of radius is more distal than volar lip, creating the characteristic volar tilt of the distal radius (12 degrees).*

Wrist MR Atlas

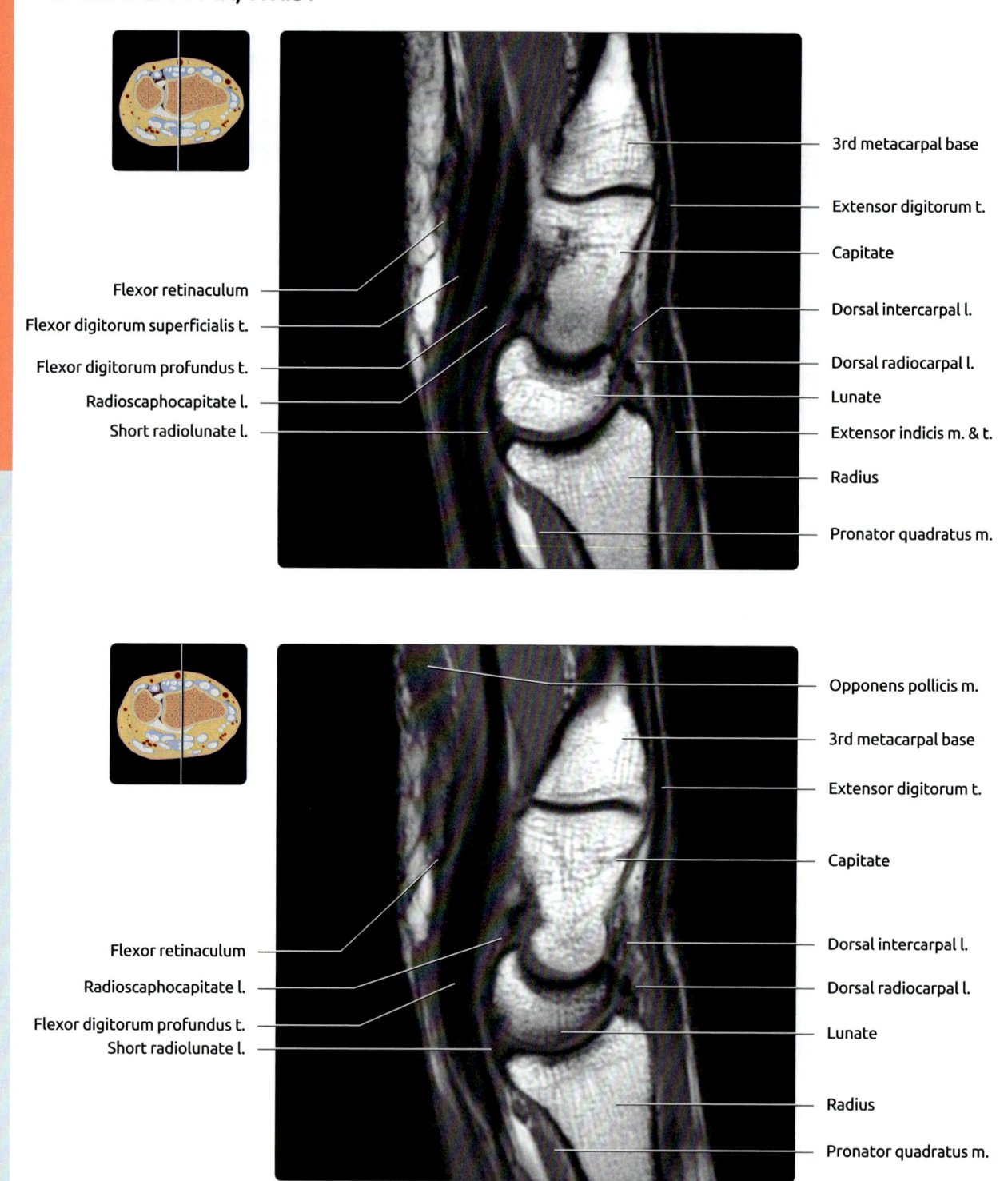

SAGITTAL T1 MR, WRIST

Top image labels:
- Flexor retinaculum
- Flexor digitorum superficialis t.
- Flexor digitorum profundus t.
- Radioscaphocapitate l.
- Short radiolunate l.
- 3rd metacarpal base
- Extensor digitorum t.
- Capitate
- Dorsal intercarpal l.
- Dorsal radiocarpal l.
- Lunate
- Extensor indicis m. & t.
- Radius
- Pronator quadratus m.

Bottom image labels:
- Flexor retinaculum
- Radioscaphocapitate l.
- Flexor digitorum profundus t.
- Short radiolunate l.
- Opponens pollicis m.
- 3rd metacarpal base
- Extensor digitorum t.
- Capitate
- Dorsal intercarpal l.
- Dorsal radiocarpal l.
- Lunate
- Radius
- Pronator quadratus m.

(Top) Third metacarpal base, capitate, lunate and lunate fossa of radius align, creating the central axis of wrist. **(Bottom)** Extensor indicis tendon is radial-most tendon in 4th extensor compartment. Opponens pollicis tendon originates from flexor retinaculum at this level.

Wrist MR Atlas

SAGITTAL T1 MR, WRIST

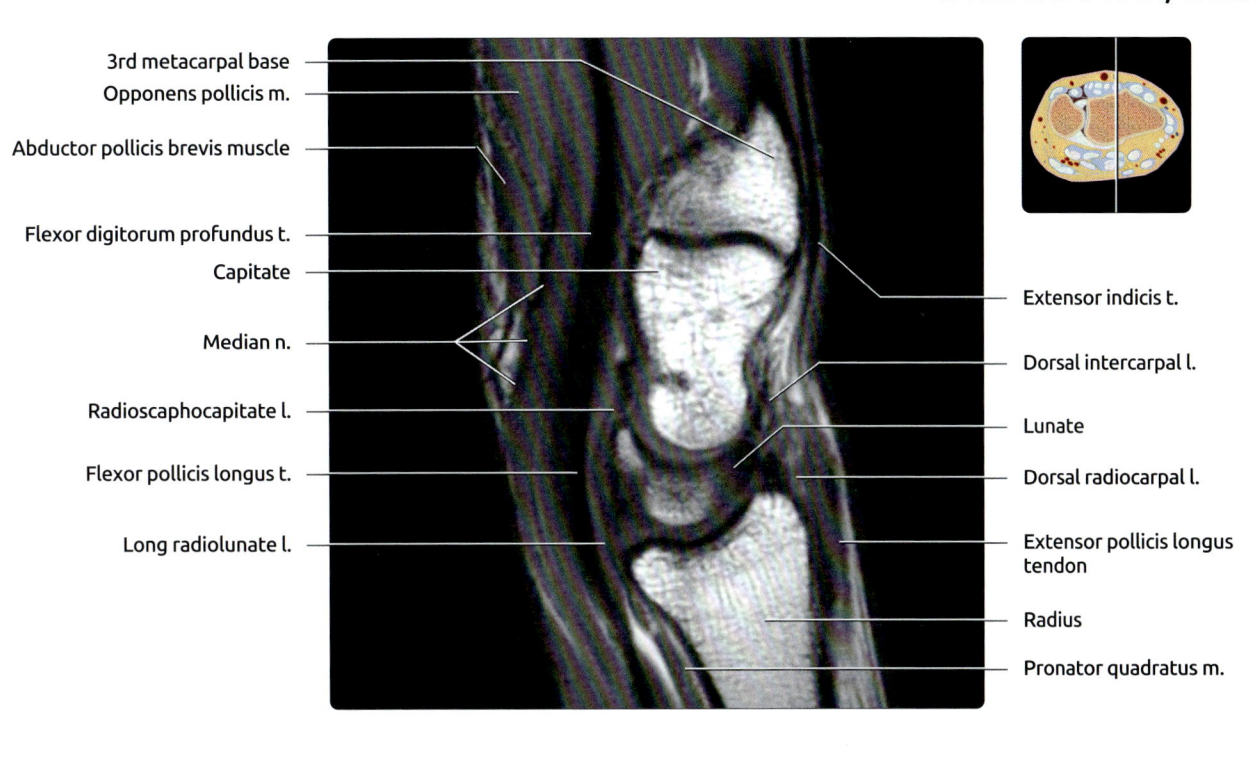

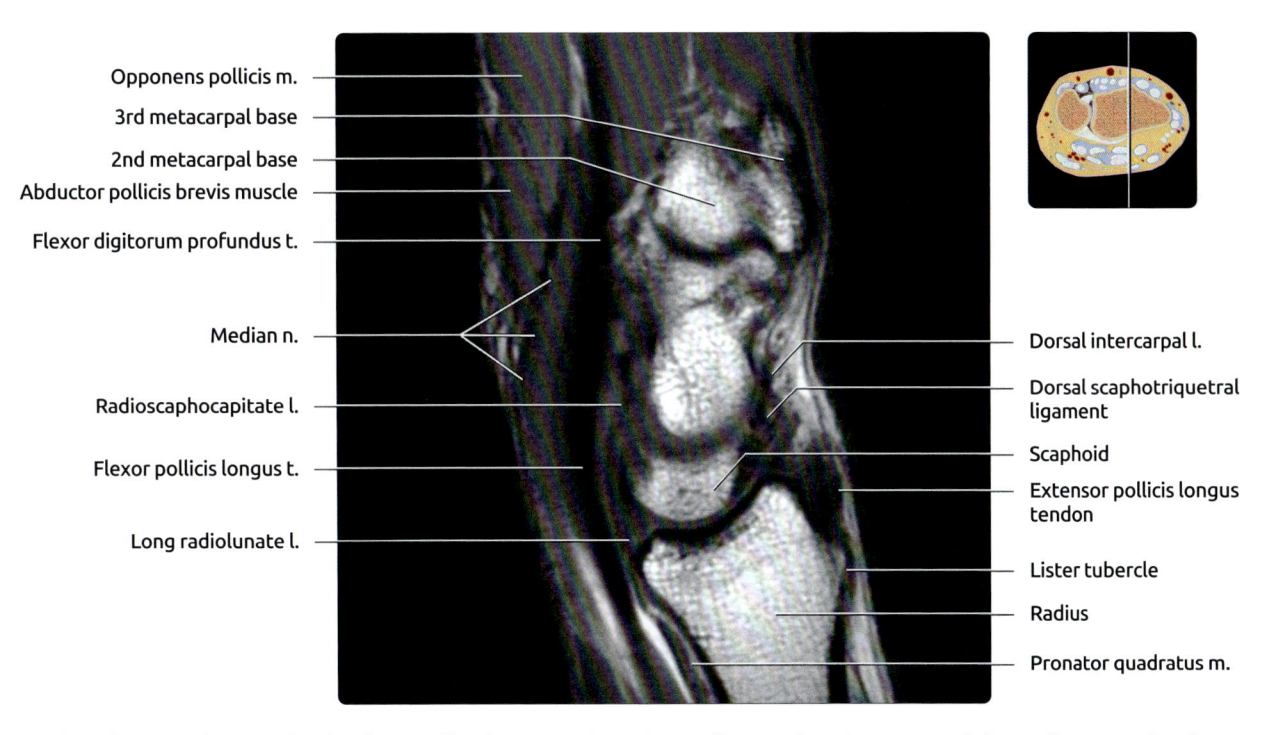

Top image labels (left):
- 3rd metacarpal base
- Opponens pollicis m.
- Abductor pollicis brevis muscle
- Flexor digitorum profundus t.
- Capitate
- Median n.
- Radioscaphocapitate l.
- Flexor pollicis longus t.
- Long radiolunate l.

Top image labels (right):
- Extensor indicis t.
- Dorsal intercarpal l.
- Lunate
- Dorsal radiocarpal l.
- Extensor pollicis longus tendon
- Radius
- Pronator quadratus m.

Bottom image labels (left):
- Opponens pollicis m.
- 3rd metacarpal base
- 2nd metacarpal base
- Abductor pollicis brevis muscle
- Flexor digitorum profundus t.
- Median n.
- Radioscaphocapitate l.
- Flexor pollicis longus t.
- Long radiolunate l.

Bottom image labels (right):
- Dorsal intercarpal l.
- Dorsal scaphotriquetral ligament
- Scaphoid
- Extensor pollicis longus tendon
- Lister tubercle
- Radius
- Pronator quadratus m.

(Top) *Median nerve lies superficial to flexor pollicis longus tendon & deep to flexor retinaculum. Long radiolunate ligament arises from radius just radial to radioscaphoid & short radiolunate ligaments.* **(Bottom)** *Extensor pollicis longus tendon lies ulnar to Lister tubercle crossing distally & radially over extensor carpi radialis brevis & longus tendons as it extends to thumb.*

Wrist MR Atlas

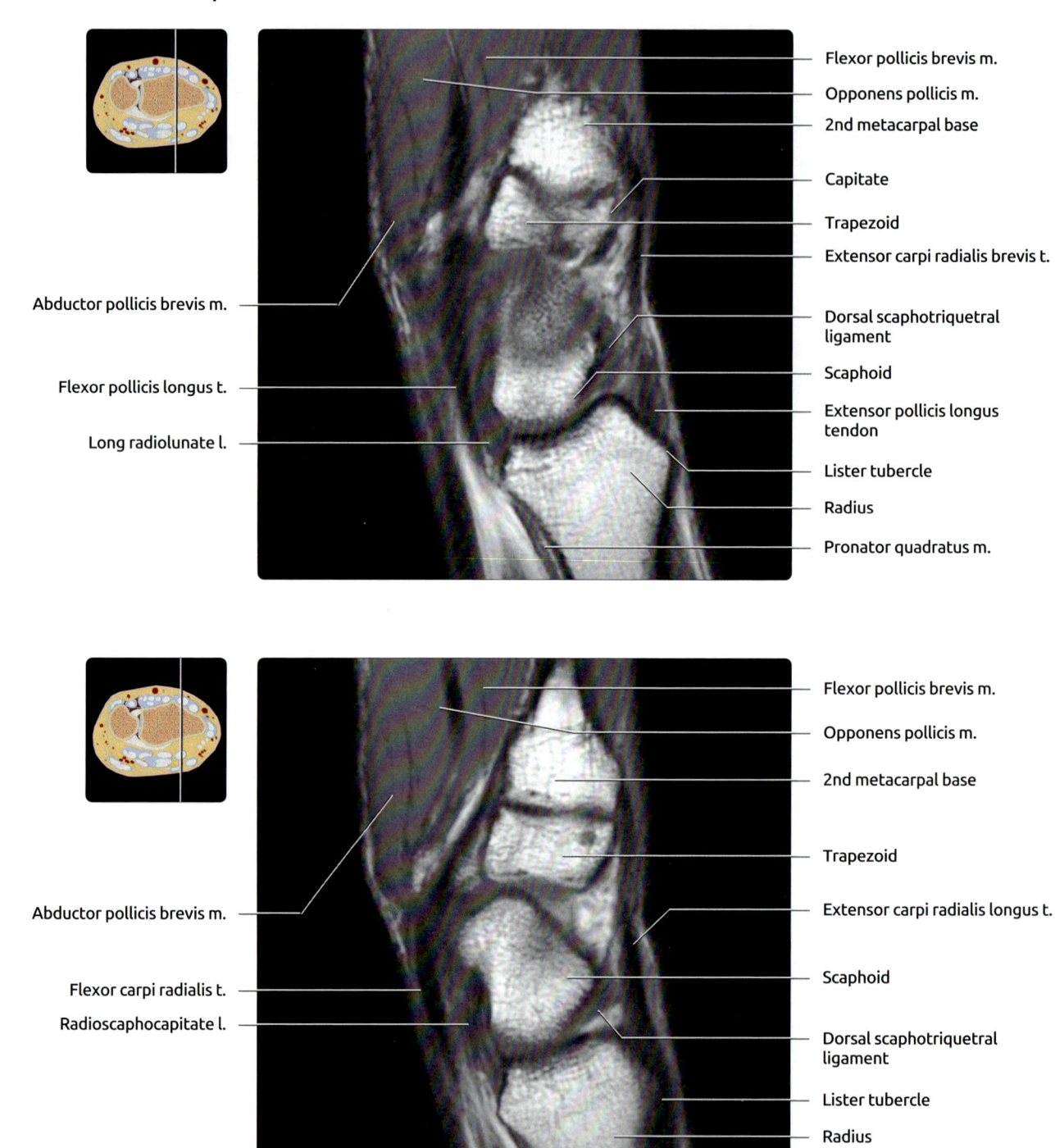

SAGITTAL T1 MR, WRIST

Labels (top image):
- Flexor pollicis brevis m.
- Opponens pollicis m.
- 2nd metacarpal base
- Capitate
- Trapezoid
- Extensor carpi radialis brevis t.
- Dorsal scaphotriquetral ligament
- Scaphoid
- Extensor pollicis longus tendon
- Lister tubercle
- Radius
- Pronator quadratus m.
- Abductor pollicis brevis m.
- Flexor pollicis longus t.
- Long radiolunate l.

Labels (bottom image):
- Flexor pollicis brevis m.
- Opponens pollicis m.
- 2nd metacarpal base
- Trapezoid
- Extensor carpi radialis longus t.
- Scaphoid
- Dorsal scaphotriquetral ligament
- Lister tubercle
- Radius
- Abductor pollicis brevis m.
- Flexor carpi radialis t.
- Radioscaphocapitate l.

(Top) This section demonstrates articular intersection of trapezoid, capitate, & scaphoid. Flexor pollicis longus tendon is deep to ulnar nerve & just ulnar to flexor carpi radialis tendon. Extensor carpi radialis brevis t. inserts on the base of the 3rd metacarpal. (Bottom) Flexor carpi radialis tendon passes superficial to scaphoid tubercle to insert on 2nd metacarpal base. Radioscaphocapitate ligament originates from volar radial lip.

Wrist MR Atlas

SAGITTAL T1 MR, WRIST

Top image labels:
- Opponens pollicis m.
- Flexor pollicis brevis m.
- Abductor pollicis brevis m.
- Flexor carpi radialis t.
- Trapezium
- Distal pole of scaphoid
- Radioscaphocapitate l.
- 2nd metacarpal base
- Trapezoid
- Extensor carpi radialis brevis t.

Bottom image labels:
- Flexor pollicis brevis m.
- 2nd metacarpal base
- Abductor pollicis brevis m.
- Trapezium
- Scaphoid distal pole
- Radioscaphocapitate l.
- Radial collateral l.
- Trapezoid
- Extensor carpi radialis longus t.
- Radial styloid

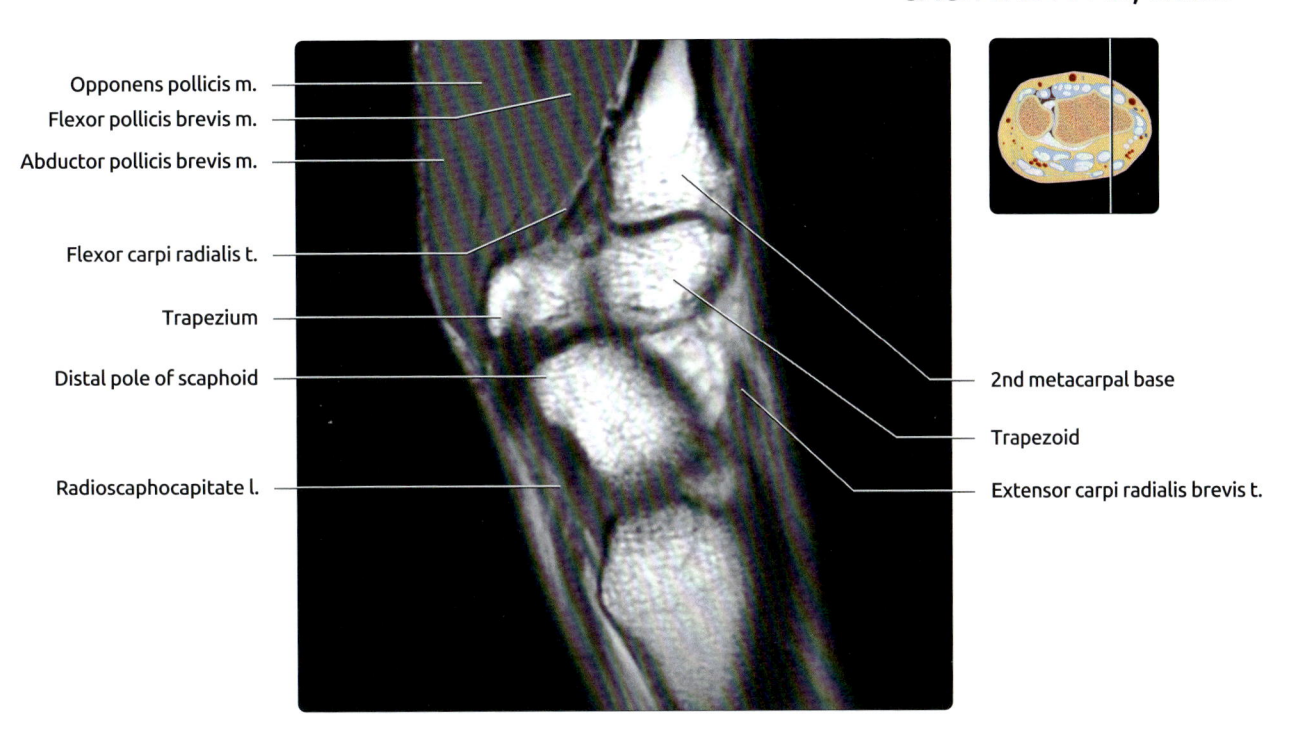

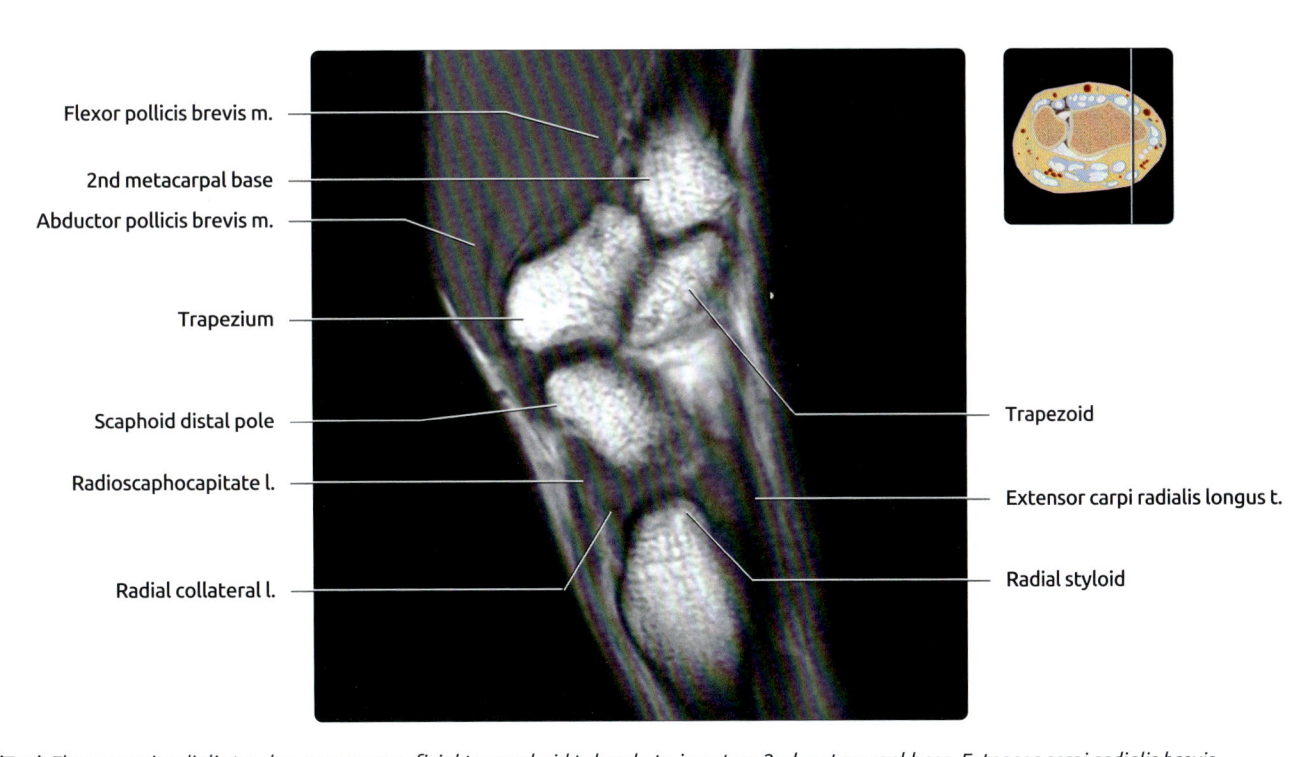

(**Top**) *Flexor carpi radialis tendon passes superficial to scaphoid tubercle to insert on 2nd metacarpal base. Extensor carpi radialis brevis tendon crosses dorsum of wrist to insert on dorsal 3rd metacarpal base.* (**Bottom**) *Radial-most component of radioscaphocapitate ligament is sometimes called radial collateral ligament. Extensor carpi radialis longus tendon crosses dorsum of wrist to insert on 2nd metacarpal base.*

SAGITTAL T1 MR, WRIST

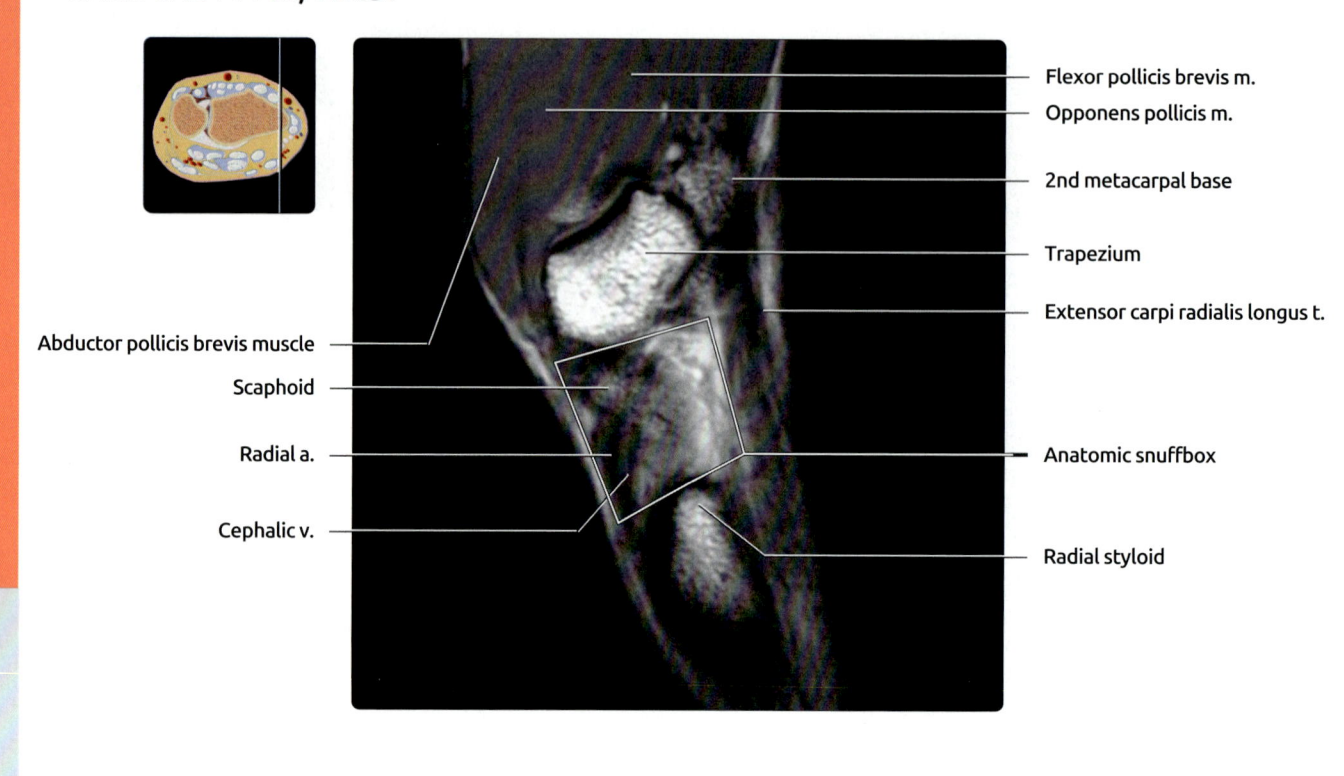

- Flexor pollicis brevis m.
- Opponens pollicis m.
- 2nd metacarpal base
- Trapezium
- Extensor carpi radialis longus t.
- Abductor pollicis brevis muscle
- Scaphoid
- Radial a.
- Anatomic snuffbox
- Cephalic v.
- Radial styloid

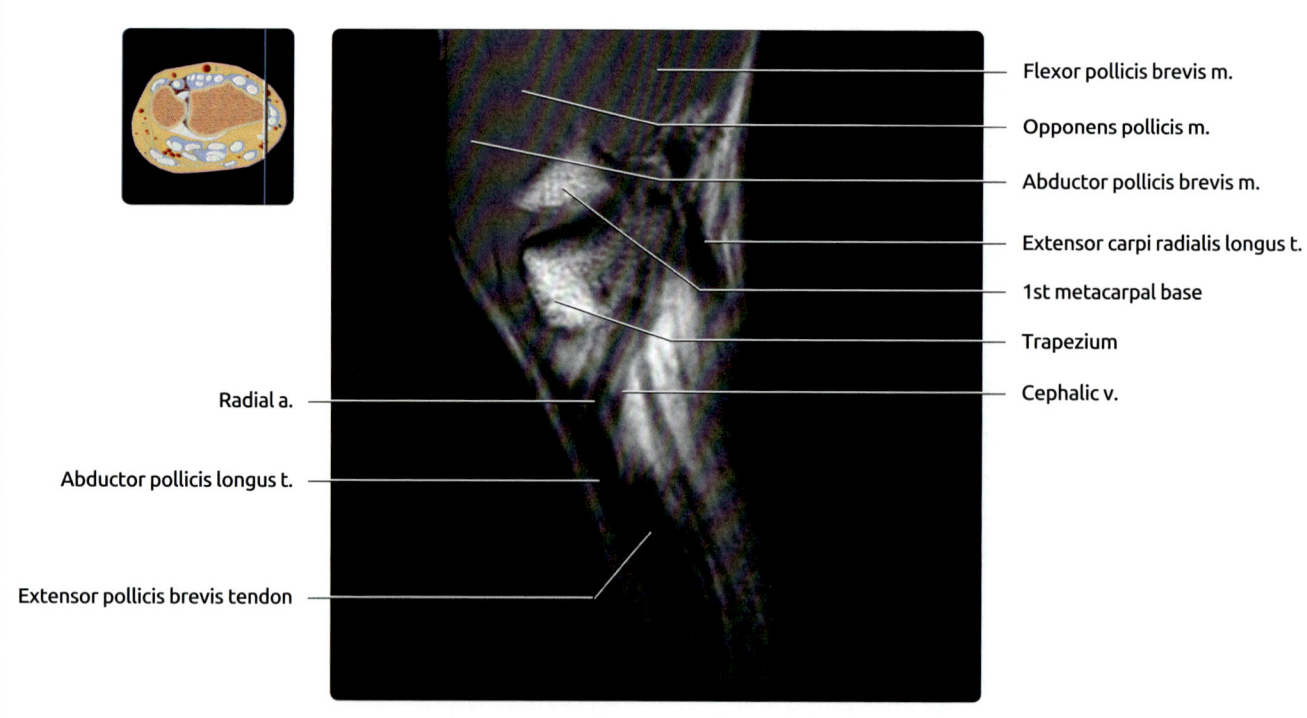

- Flexor pollicis brevis m.
- Opponens pollicis m.
- Abductor pollicis brevis m.
- Extensor carpi radialis longus t.
- 1st metacarpal base
- Trapezium
- Cephalic v.
- Radial a.
- Abductor pollicis longus t.
- Extensor pollicis brevis tendon

(**Top**) Radial artery, superficial radial nerve, & cephalic vein pass through anatomic snuff box, which is bounded by trapezium, scaphoid, & radial styloid. Abductor pollicis longus & extensor pollicis brevis tendons form volar margin of snuffbox & extensor pollicis longus tendon forms dorsal margin. (**Bottom**) Abductor pollicis longus & extensor pollicis brevis tendons form distal margin of snuffbox as they convergence just distal to 1st carpometacarpal joint.

SAGITTAL T1 MR, WRIST

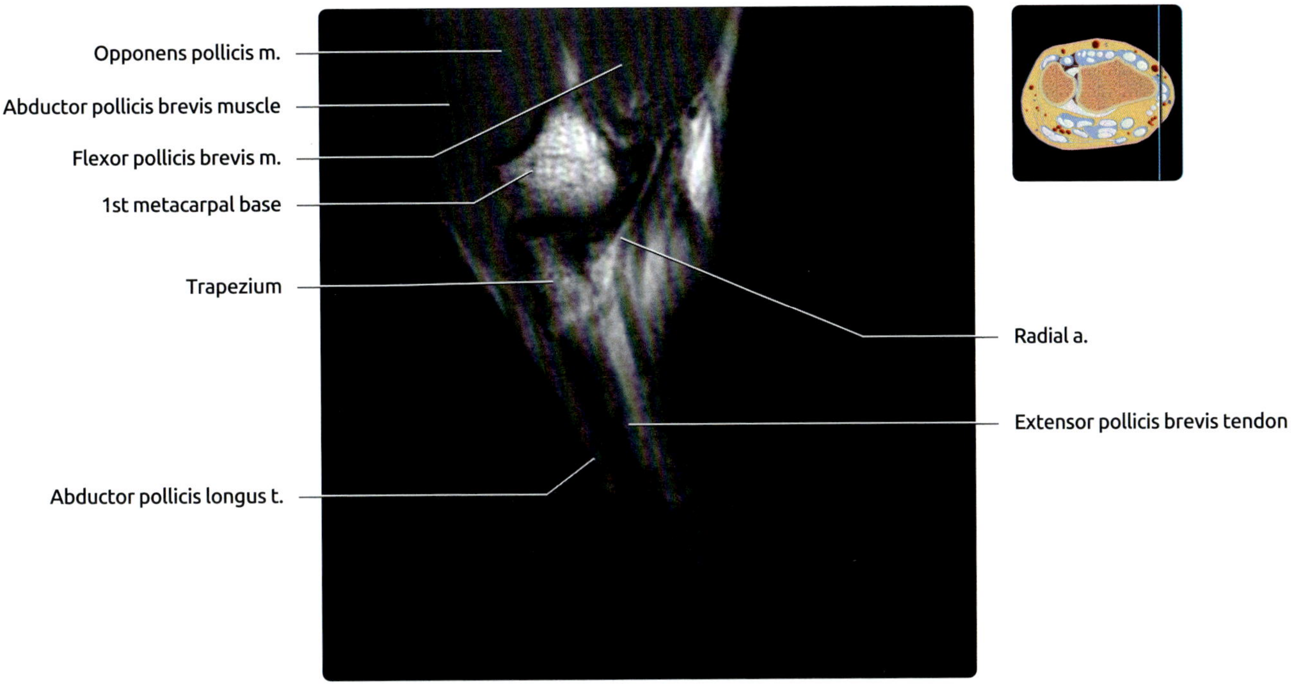
Opponens pollicis m.
Abductor pollicis brevis muscle
Flexor pollicis brevis m.
1st metacarpal base
Trapezium
Abductor pollicis longus t.
Radial a.
Extensor pollicis brevis tendon

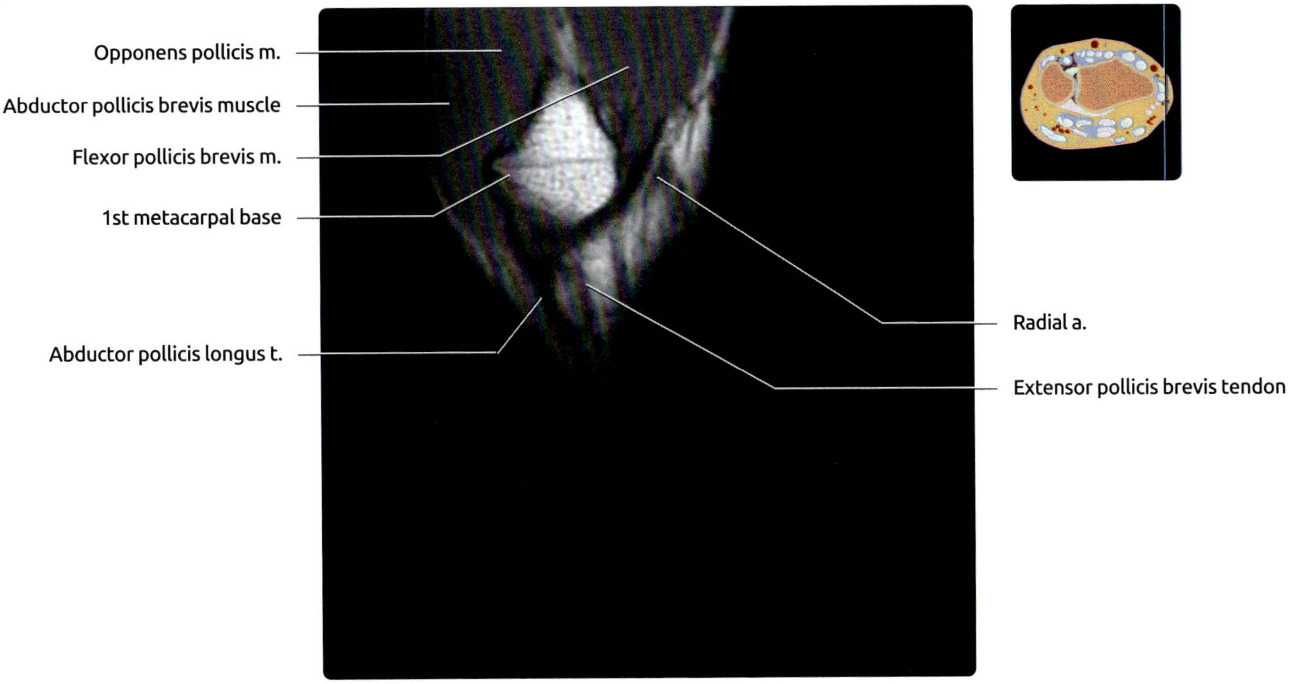
Opponens pollicis m.
Abductor pollicis brevis muscle
Flexor pollicis brevis m.
1st metacarpal base
Abductor pollicis longus t.
Radial a.
Extensor pollicis brevis tendon

(Top) *Radial artery branches & continues distally to form deep palmar arch.* **(Bottom)** *Abductor pollicis longus & extensor pollicis brevis tendon converge to insert on 1st metacarpal base.*

Wrist Ligaments

TERMINOLOGY

Abbreviations
- Carpometacarpal (CMC)
- Dorsal radiocarpal (DRC)
- Dorsal radioulnar (DRU)
- Extensor carpi radialis longus (ECRL)
- Extensor carpi ulnaris (ECU)
- Flexor carpi ulnaris (FCU)
- Long radiolunate ligament (LRL)
- Lunotriquetral (LT)
- Metacarpal (MC)
- Radioscaphocapitate ligament (RSC)
- Scapholunate (SL)
- Scaphotrapezium-trapezoid (STT)
- Short radiolunate ligament (SRL)
- Triangular fibrocartilage (TFC)
- Triangular fibrocartilage complex (TFCC)
- Triquetrocapitate (TC)
- Ulnocapitate (UC)
- Ulnolunate (UL)
- Ulnotriquetral (UT)
- Volar radioulnar (VRU)

Definitions
- Intrinsic ligaments: Connect carpals to carpals
- Extrinsic ligaments: Connect radius/ulna to carpals; carpals to metacarpals

IMAGING ANATOMY

Volar Radiocarpal Ligaments
- **Radioscaphocapitate** (RSC, sling, radiocapitate)
  - Origin: Distal radius, radial styloid
  - Course: Passes across scaphoid waist with minimal attachment
  - Insertion: Capitate body (10% of fibers); arcs around distal lunate, interdigitates with ulnocapitate & triquetrocapitate to form arcuate ligament
  - Action: Constrains radiocarpal pronation, ulnocarpal translocation; stabilizes distal scaphoid pole; creates sling for scaphoid
  - Radial collateral: Radial-most fibers of RSC; existence as separate ligament debated
- **Long radiolunate** (volar radiolunotriquetral, volar radiotriquetral ligament)
  - May appear as 2 separate ligaments: Radiolunate & LT
  - Origin: Radius ulnar to radioscaphocapital ligament
  - Course: Passes volar to scaphoid & SL ligament
  - Insertion: Volar lunate rim; continues to triquetrum
  - Action: Constrains ulnar translocation & distal translation of lunate; creates sling for lunate
- **Radioscapholunate** (ligament of Testut; intraarticular fat pad)
  - Origin: Volar radius ulnar to long radiolunate
  - Insertion: Proximal scaphoid, lunate, and SL ligament
  - Action: Mechanoreceptor of scapholunate relationship
  - Not true ligament: Contains fat, arterioles, venules, & small nerves
- **Short radiolunate**
  - Origin: Volar radius ulnar to long radiolunate ligament
  - Insertion: Volar lunate (radial 2/3)
  - Action: Stabilizes lunate; facilitates motion in flexion/extension
- **Arcuate ("V" ligament)**
  - Confluence of ligaments on volar surface of capitate
  - Includes radioscaphocapitate, ulnocapitate, and triquetrocapitate ligaments

Dorsal Radiocarpal Ligament
- **Dorsal radiocarpal** (dorsal radiotriquetral; dorsal radiolunotriquetral)
  - Origin: Broad attachment to dorsal radius from Lister tubercle to sigmoid notch
  - Insertion: Dorsal lunate & triquetrum
  - Action: Reinforces dorsal lunatotriquetral ligament; constrains ulnar translocation of carpals; creates dorsal sling for triquetrum

Volar Midcarpal Ligaments
- **Scaphotrapezium-trapezoid**
  - Origin: Scaphoid tubercle
  - Insertion: Volar trapezium; few fibers to trapezoid
  - Action: Maintains scaphoid in volar flexion; stabilizes scaphoid, trapezium, & trapezoid
- **Scaphocapitate**
  - Origin: Volar scaphoid distal pole
  - Insertion: Volar capitate body
  - Action: Stabilizer of scaphoid; balances volar flexion tendency of scaphotrapezium-trapezoid ligament
- **Triquetrocapitate**
  - Origin: Volar triquetrum
  - Insertion: Volar capitate body
  - Action: Midcarpal stabilization
- **Triquetrohamate**
  - Origin: Volar triquetrum
  - Insertion: Volar hamate body at hook base
  - Action: Midcarpal stabilization
- **Pisohamate**
  - Origin: Volar pisiform
  - Insertion: Hook of hamate
  - Action: Transmits pull of flexor carpi ulnaris on pisiform to carpals; considered a prolongation of FCU
- **Deltoid**
  - Confluence of scaphocapitate & TC ligaments
  - Parallels arcuate ligament

Dorsal Midcarpal Ligaments
- **Dorsal intercarpal**
  - Origin: Dorsal triquetrum, interdigitating with DRC ligament
  - Insertion: Scaphoid & dorsal trapezoid
  - Action: Envelops radial artery in anatomic snuffbox; constrains midcarpal rotation; acts as labrum to capitate head & proximal hamate
- **Dorsal scaphotriquetral**
  - Origin: Scaphoid, extending dorsal & distal to SL/LT ligaments
  - Insertion: Dorsal triquetrum
  - Action: Stabilizes SL/LT ligaments; labrum for capitate head & hamate proximal pole

Wrist Ligaments

Proximal Interosseous Ligaments

- **Scapholunate**
  - Origin/insertion: Ulnar scaphoid to radial lunate
    - Attaches to hyaline cartilage
  - Action
    - Dorsal portion resists volar-dorsal translation
    - Volar portion limits flexion/extension rotation
    - Proximal (central) portion accommodates compression & shear forces across radiocarpal joint
  - U-shaped ligament with dorsal, proximal, & volar components
    - Dorsal component thicker (5 mm) than volar (1-2 mm)
    - Proximal component is meniscus-like avascular fibrocartilage; triangular shape
    - Dorsal component most important functionally
  - Attritional tears occur with age, usually involve proximal component
- **Lunotriquetral**
  - **Origin/insertion**: Ulnar lunate to radial triquetrum
    - Attaches to hyaline cartilage
  - Action
    - Volar portion limits translation of lunate & triquetrum
    - Dorsal portion stabilizes joint
  - U-shaped ligament with dorsal, proximal, & volar components
    - Volar component thicker (2.3 mm) than dorsal (1 mm); functionally more important than proximal portion
    - Proximal component is meniscus-like avascular fibrocartilage; triangular shape
  - Attritional tears occur with age, usually involve proximal component

Distal Interosseous Ligaments

- **Trapeziotrapezoid**
  - Dorsal & volar components: Thickness 2 mm
  - Action: Stabilizes distal carpals; maintains carpal arch
  - Forms floor of extensor carpi radialis longus tendon sheath
- **Trapeziocapitate**
  - Dorsal, volar, and deep components: Thickness 1-2 mm
  - Deep portion connects dorsal trapezoid to volar capitate
  - Action: Stabilizes distal carpals; maintains carpal arch
- **Capitohamate**
  - Dorsal, volar, & deep components: Thickness 1-2 mm
  - Volar aspect contiguous with volar ligaments, contributing to ligamentous ring of carpal tunnel
  - Action: Stabilizes distal carpals; maintains carpal arch

Carpometacarpal Ligaments

- **Pisometacarpal**
  - Origin: Volar pisiform
  - Insertion: Volar 5th metacarpal
  - Action: Transmits pull of FCU on pisiform to metacarpals
  - Considered a prolongation of flexor carpi ulnaris tendon
- **Carpometacarpal ligaments of thumb**
  - Origin: Dorsal, lateral, & radial trapezium
  - Insertion: Dorsal, volar, & lateral thumb metacarpal base
  - Action: Stabilizes highly mobile thumb base
- **Dorsal carpometacarpal**
  - Origin: Adjacent carpals give 2-3 ligament slips each
  - Insertion: 2nd-5th dorsal metacarpal bases
  - Action: Stabilizes carpometacarpal joints sliding motion
- **Volar carpometacarpal**
  - Origin: Adjacent carpals give 1-2 ligament slips each
  - Insertion: 2nd-5th dorsal metacarpal bases
  - Action: Stabilizes carpometacarpal joints sliding motion

Distal Radioulnar Ligaments

- **Dorsal radioulnar**
  - Origin: Dorsal sigmoid notch, bone attachment
  - Insertion: Dorsal fibers form ECU sheath & attach to styloid process; volar fibers attach to ulnar fovea
  - Action: Stabilizes distal ulna, preventing volar subluxation during supination
- **Volar radioulnar**
  - Origin: Volar sigmoid notch, bone attachment
  - Action: Serves as base for ulnolunate & ulnotriquetral ligament origins; stabilizes distal ulna, preventing dorsal subluxation during pronation
  - Insertion: Ulnar fovea; joins with volar fibers of dorsal radioulnar ligament & creates "ring" (apparent on MR)

Ulnocarpal Structures

- **Ulnolunate**
  - Origin: Arises from volar radioulnar ligament; ulnar to short radiolunate ligament
    - Arises from ligament rather than bone, reducing effect of forearm rotation to carpals
  - Insertion: Lunate (ulnar 1/3) adjacent to short radiolunate ligament
  - Action: Stabilizes lunate through wrist range of motion
- **Ulnotriquetral**
  - **Lateral band**
    - Origin: Arises from volar radioulnar ligament, ulnar to ulnolunate ligament
    - Insertion: Triquetrum, medial to LT ligament
    - Action: Restricts & stabilizes triquetrum
  - **Medial band (ulnar collateral ligament)**
    - Actual existence of ulnar collateral ligament is debated
    - Origin: Arises from dorsal radioulnar ligament at its insertion on ulnar styloid
    - Action: Forms floor of ECU tendon sheath; constrains distal translation of triquetrum
    - Insertion: Lateral triquetrum
  - Arises from ligament rather than bone, reducing effects of forearm rotation on carpals
  - Lateral & medial bands separate just distal to prestyloid recess; lead to pisotriquetral joint (in 90%)
- **Ulnocapitate**
  - Origin: Ulnar fovea, bone attachment
  - Insertion: Fibers interdigitate with volar LT ligament; continue distally to capitate; blend with RSC to form arcuate ligament
  - Action: Reinforces ulnocarpal joint capsule & LT joint; anchors carpals to ulna; creates volar sling for triquetrum
- **Ulnocarpal meniscal homologue**
  - Capsular thickening, triangular shape; variably present

Wrist Ligaments

- Lies distal to ulnar triangular fibrocartilage & ulnar styloid tip; between dorsal radioulnar ligament & radial volar extensor carpi ulnaris tendon sheath; separated from triangular fibrocartilage by prestyloid recess opening
- **Triangular fibrocartilage (articular disc)**
  - Origin: Arises from radial sigmoid notch, attaching to hyaline cartilage
  - Insertion: 2 struts, extend to ulnar fovea & styloid tip
  - Variable thickness proportional to ulnar length (thicker with ulnar minus, thinner with ulnar plus); ulnar portion 2-3x thicker than radial
  - Ulnar portion is vascularized; radial & central portions are not
  - Attritional tears common aging phenomenon
- **Triangular fibrocartilage complex**
  - Complex includes articular disc, DRU, VRU, UL, UT, & extensor carpi ulnaris tendon sheath
  - Action: Transmits portion of axial load from ulnar carpals to distal ulna; stabilizer of distal radioulnar joint; stabilizer of ulnar carpals

Recesses

- May be seen arthrographically &/or arthroscopically
- **Interligamentous sulcus**
  - Arthroscopic landmark
  - Separates RSC from long radiolunate ligament
  - Allows motion between these ligaments on radial & ulnar deviation
- **Space of Poirier**
  - Area of weakness in volar capsule accessed via interligamentous sulcus
  - Located just proximal to deltoid ligament
  - Volar lunate dislocation can occur through this area
- **Radioscaphocapitate ligament region**
  - Space between volar scaphoid proximal pole & radioscaphocapitate deep surface
- **Prestyloid recess**
  - Located at apex of dorsal radioulnar & volar radioulnar ligaments just distal to ulnar fovea
  - Lined with synovium; variably communicates with ulnar styloid tip
- **Dorsal transverse recess**
  - Located between dorsal capitate head/neck, hamate & dorsal midcarpal joint capsule, dorsal distal scaphoid
- **Ulnar recess**
  - Located medial to triquetrohamate articulation
- **Radial recess**
  - Located lateral to STT & palmar recess anterior to capitate

ANATOMY IMAGING ISSUES

Imaging Recommendations

- **MR appearance**
  - Extrinsic ligaments: Low signal or striated bands on all sequences
  - Interosseous ligaments: Low signal bands; variably visualized, especially in midcarpal & distal rows; deep components tend to be thick, short ligaments
    - Scapholunate/lunotriquetral ligaments: Dorsal & volar contours band-like with proximal (central) portion triangular in shape
    - Normal signal varies from uniform low to striated intermediate signal; may be amorphous in proximal portion
    - Attach to cartilage rather than bone; should not be mistaken for a tear
    - Visualized on coronal & axial; important to scrutinize axial imaging as disruption of dorsal, volar components correlates with instability
  - TFCC: Low signal intensity articular disc attaches to cartilage along sigmoid notch
- **Arthrography**
  - Good evaluation for integrity of SL, LT, and TFC; limited for extrinsic ligaments
  - Injections spaced to allow contrast resorption 1st compartment before 2nd injected
    - Radiocarpal joint injected 1st (most likely to document with single injection); if no tear, wait 30-60 minutes & proceed sequentially with DRU & midcarpal injections
  - Digital subtraction allows dynamic evaluation of ligament status & sequential compartment injection without delay
  - Injectate: Iodinated contrast (180-300 mg I/mL); volumes: Midcarpal, 4-5 cc; radiocarpal, 2-3 cc; DRU, 1-2 cc; pisotriquetral, 1-2 cc
- **MR imaging**
  - GRE (T2*) imaging maximizes visualization of ligaments in absence of intraarticular fluid
    - Normal ligaments have more heterogeneous appearance on GRE T2* than on spin-echo T2
  - Coronal: SL, LT, triangular fibrocartilage, extrinsic ligaments
  - Axial: Triangular fibrocartilage, dorsal, and volar SL and lunato triquetral, extrinsic ligaments
  - Sagittal: Extrinsic ligaments
  - MR arthrography: Injectate: 1/200 normal saline (NS):Gd; volumes as noted above
- **CT imaging**
  - Ligaments not seen in absence of contrast
  - CT arthrography allows evaluation of ligament integrity; diagnostic efficacy equal to MR
  - Injectate: 1:1 NS:iodinated contrast; allows standard arthrography & CT arthrography
- **Ultrasound**
  - Described for evaluation of extrinsic ligament tears; performed with standoff pad; 15mHz transducer

Imaging Pitfalls

- Fenestrations of triangular fibrocartilage, scapholunate and lunatotriquetral ligaments common, often asymptomatic
- Ligament attachments to cartilage rather than bone mimics tears
  - Triangular fibrocartilage, scapholunate, lunatotriquetral
- Satisfaction of search: If intrinsic ligament tear seen, examine extrinsic ligaments carefully for accompanying abnormalities

SELECTED REFERENCES

1. Theumann NH et al: Extrinsic carpal ligaments: normal MR arthrographic appearance in cadavers. Radiology. 226(1):171-9, 2003

Wrist Ligaments

VOLAR EXTRINSIC LIGAMENTS

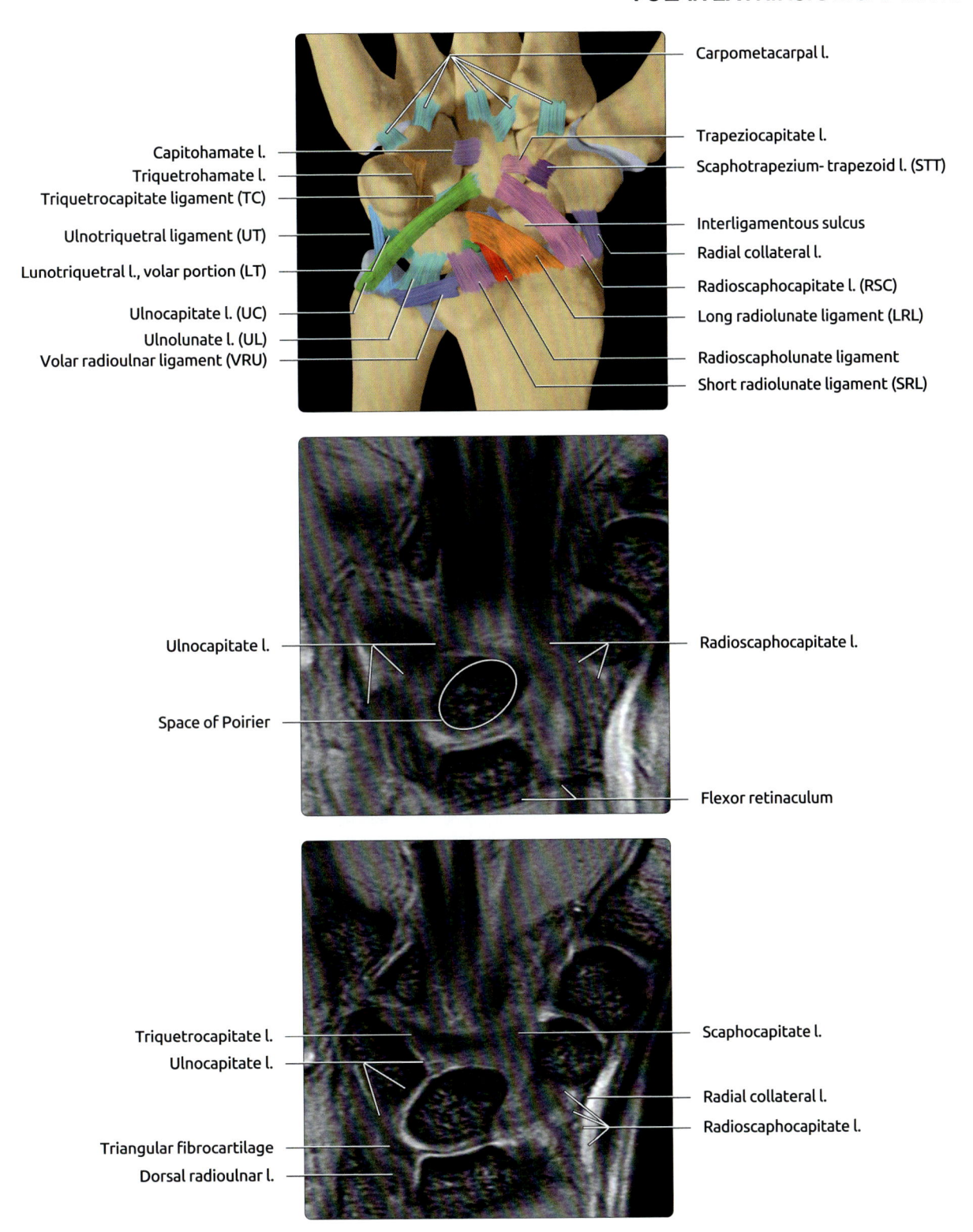

Labels (top illustration):
- Capitohamate l.
- Triquetrohamate l.
- Triquetrocapitate ligament (TC)
- Ulnotriquetral ligament (UT)
- Lunotriquetral l., volar portion (LT)
- Ulnocapitate l. (UC)
- Ulnolunate l. (UL)
- Volar radioulnar ligament (VRU)
- Carpometacarpal l.
- Trapeziocapitate l.
- Scaphotrapezium- trapezoid l. (STT)
- Interligamentous sulcus
- Radial collateral l.
- Radioscaphocapitate l. (RSC)
- Long radiolunate ligament (LRL)
- Radioscapholunate ligament
- Short radiolunate ligament (SRL)

Labels (middle image):
- Ulnocapitate l.
- Space of Poirier
- Radioscaphocapitate l.
- Flexor retinaculum

Labels (bottom image):
- Triquetrocapitate l.
- Ulnocapitate l.
- Triangular fibrocartilage
- Dorsal radioulnar l.
- Scaphocapitate l.
- Radial collateral l.
- Radioscaphocapitate l.

(Top) Volar intrinsic & extrinsic ligaments are shown. Extrinsic ligaments connect carpals to bones of the forearm (radius & ulna) & hand (metacarpals) & are often capsular. Intrinsic ligaments connect carpals to carpals. Note that the arcuate ligament (not labeled) is formed by interdigitating fibers of the radioscaphocapitate, ulnocapitate, & triquetrocapitate. Note that the deltoid ligament, running parallel to the arcuate ligament, lies deep to these structures and is not shown here. (Middle) Volar extrinsic ligaments are shown on GRE coronal MR. Radioscaphocapitate & ulnocapitate ligaments blend with triquetrocapitate ligaments to create arcuate (inverted "V") ligament. The lunate is immediately proximal to this confluence of ligaments which creates a vulnerable place in volar capsule, the space of Poirier. (Bottom) Image deep to prior image shows more of extrinsic ligaments. They are thin, wispy structures.

Wrist Ligaments

DORSAL EXTRINSIC LIGAMENTS

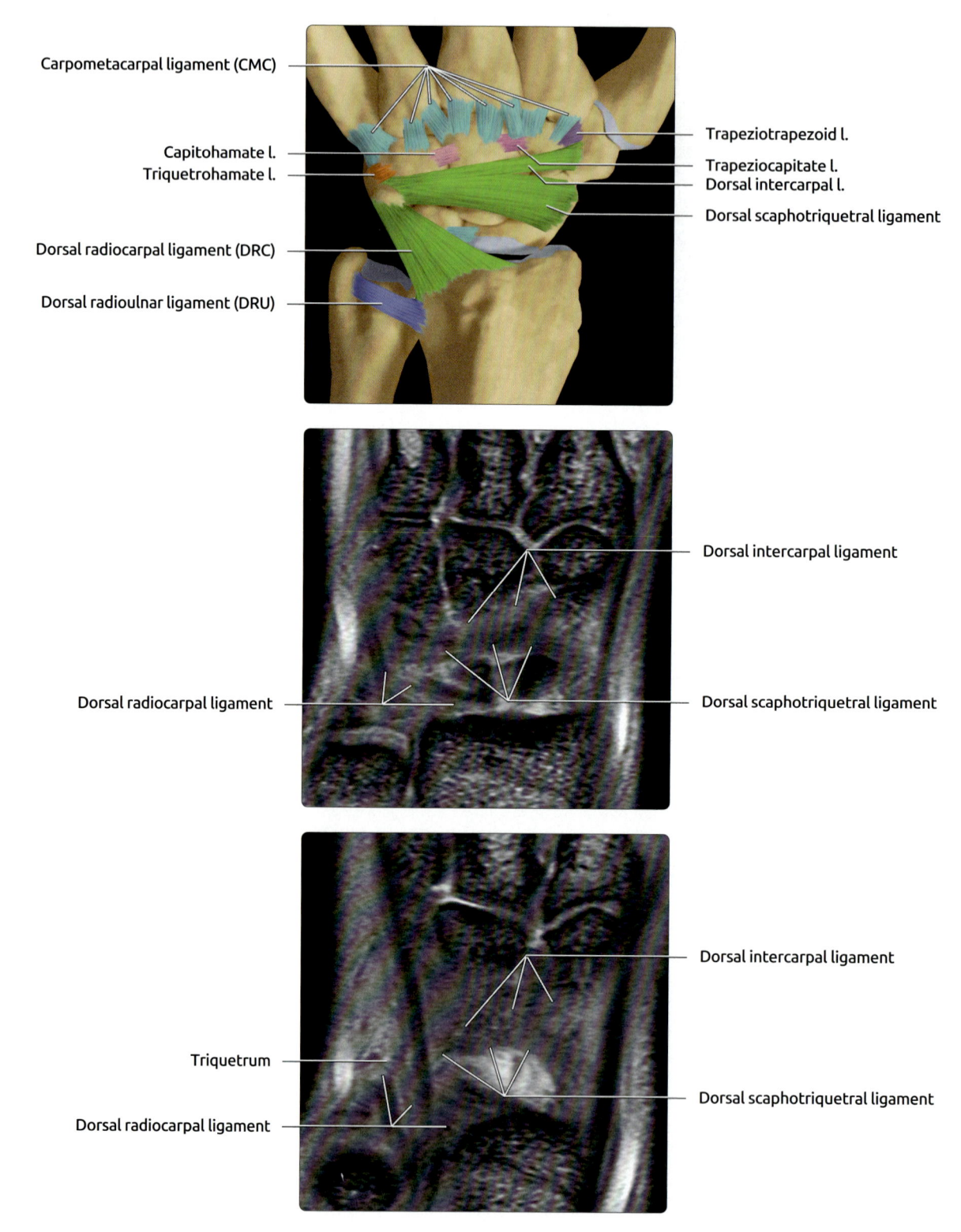

Labels (top illustration):
- Carpometacarpal ligament (CMC)
- Capitohamate l.
- Triquetrohamate l.
- Dorsal radiocarpal ligament (DRC)
- Dorsal radioulnar ligament (DRU)
- Trapeziotrapezoid l.
- Trapeziocapitate l.
- Dorsal intercarpal l.
- Dorsal scaphotriquetral ligament

Labels (middle image):
- Dorsal radiocarpal ligament
- Dorsal intercarpal ligament
- Dorsal scaphotriquetral ligament

Labels (bottom image):
- Triquetrum
- Dorsal radiocarpal ligament
- Dorsal intercarpal ligament
- Dorsal scaphotriquetral ligament

(Top) Extrinsic dorsal ligaments stabilize and restrict motion but are less critical to the stability of wrist structures than volar ligaments. (Middle) Dorsal stabilizing ligaments include dorsal radiocarpal, scaphotriquetral, & intercarpal ligaments. (Bottom) Coronal GRE MR arthrogram shows the triquetrum serves as an anchor point for the major dorsal midcarpal ligaments.

Wrist Ligaments

TRIANGULAR FIBROCARTILAGE COMPLEX

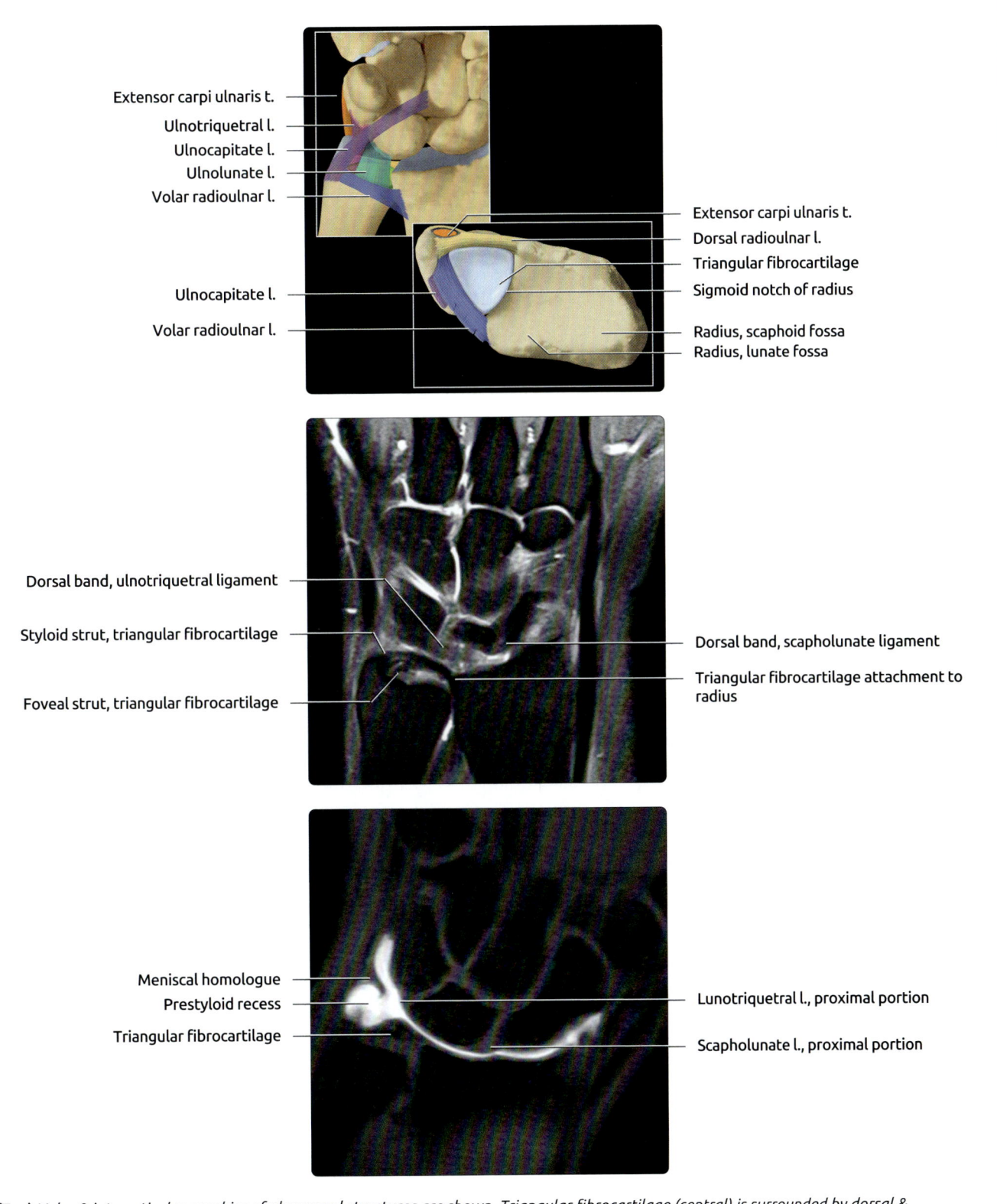

Labels (top graphic): Extensor carpi ulnaris t.; Ulnotriquetral l.; Ulnocapitate l.; Ulnolunate l.; Volar radioulnar l.; Ulnocapitate l.; Volar radioulnar l.; Extensor carpi ulnaris t.; Dorsal radioulnar l.; Triangular fibrocartilage; Sigmoid notch of radius; Radius, scaphoid fossa; Radius, lunate fossa

Labels (middle MR): Dorsal band, ulnotriquetral ligament; Styloid strut, triangular fibrocartilage; Foveal strut, triangular fibrocartilage; Dorsal band, scapholunate ligament; Triangular fibrocartilage attachment to radius

Labels (bottom MR): Meniscal homologue; Prestyloid recess; Triangular fibrocartilage; Lunotriquetral l., proximal portion; Scapholunate l., proximal portion

(**Top**) Volar & intraarticular graphics of ulnocarpal structures are shown. Triangular fibrocartilage (central) is surrounded by dorsal & volar radioulnar ligaments (periphery). Fibers of dorsal radioulnar ligament contribute to extensor carpi ulnaris sheath. Triangular fibrocartilage complex includes these structures as well as ulnolunate & ulnotriquetral ligaments. (**Middle**) This coronal T2WI MR shows the ulnar styloid and foveal struts of the triangular fibrocartilage. (**Bottom**) Coronal T1 fat-suppressed radiocarpal arthrogram accentuates meniscal homologue. Triangular fibrocartilage, scapholunate, & lunotriquetral ligaments are intact, and therefore no contrast extends into the midcarpal compartment.

Wrist Ligaments

INTRINSIC LIGAMENTS OF PROXIMAL CARPAL ROW

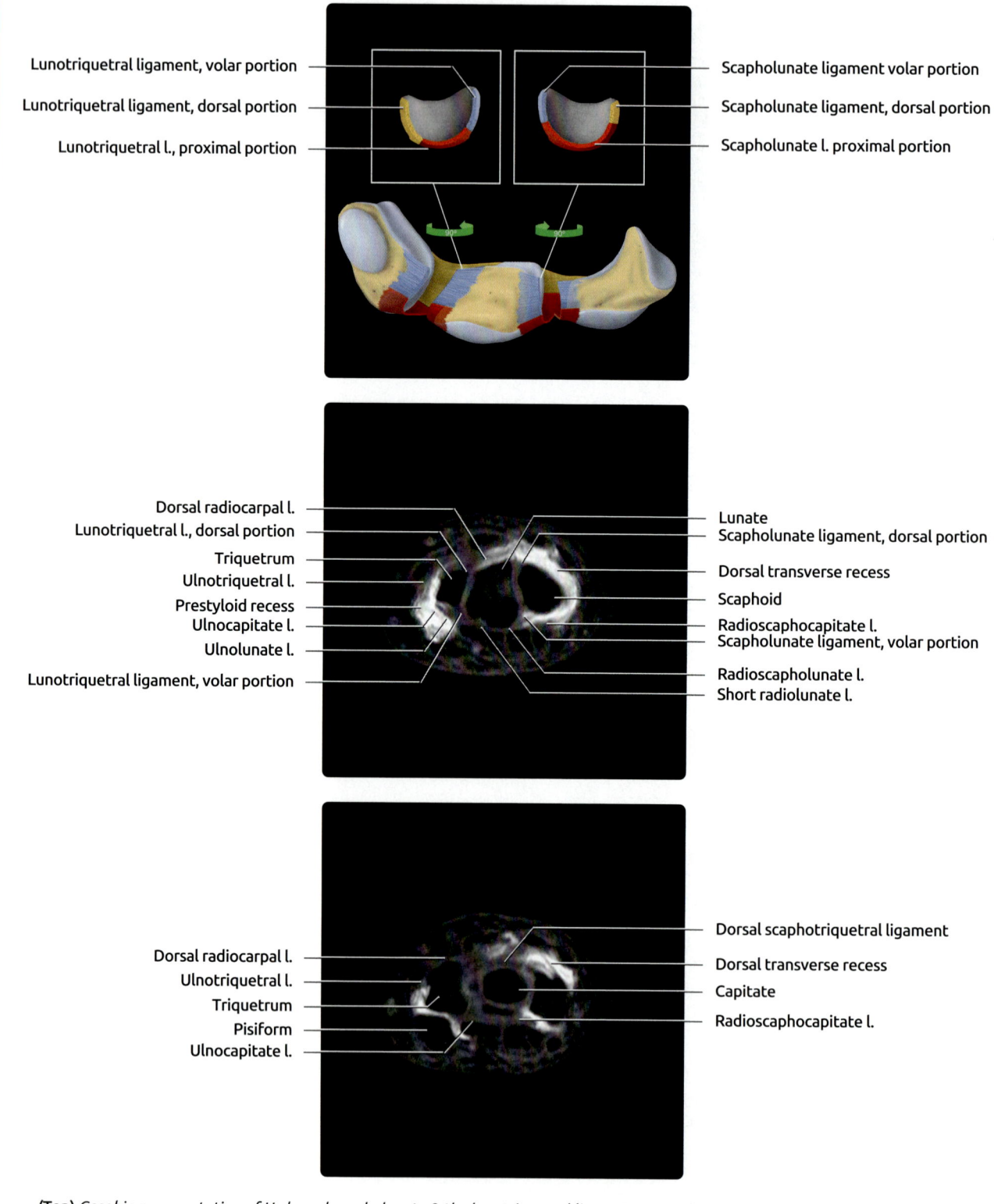

Lunotriquetral ligament, volar portion
Lunotriquetral ligament, dorsal portion
Lunotriquetral l., proximal portion

Scapholunate ligament volar portion
Scapholunate ligament, dorsal portion
Scapholunate l. proximal portion

Dorsal radiocarpal l.
Lunotriquetral l., dorsal portion
Triquetrum
Ulnotriquetral l.
Prestyloid recess
Ulnocapitate l.
Ulnolunate l.
Lunotriquetral ligament, volar portion

Lunate
Scapholunate ligament, dorsal portion
Dorsal transverse recess
Scaphoid
Radioscaphocapitate l.
Scapholunate ligament, volar portion
Radioscapholunate l.
Short radiolunate l.

Dorsal radiocarpal l.
Ulnotriquetral l.
Triquetrum
Pisiform
Ulnocapitate l.

Dorsal scaphotriquetral ligament
Dorsal transverse recess
Capitate
Radioscaphocapitate l.

(**Top**) *Graphic representation of U-shaped scapholunate & the lunotriquetral ligaments reveals volar portion, thicker in the lunotriquetral than scapholunate; proximal portion & dorsal portion, thicker in scapholunate than lunotriquetral ligament. Volar (blue) and part of proximal portions (red) are depicted as cut in this graphic.* (**Middle**) *Proximal row carpal ligaments are U-shaped with dorsal, volar, & proximal portions. Prestyloid & dorsal transverse recesses are evident.* (**Bottom**) *Ulnotriquetral ligament may be seen as two bands. Medial band forms the ECU tendon sheath floor & is sometimes referred to as ulnar collateral ligament.*

Wrist Ligaments

INTRINSIC LIGAMENTS ON CORONAL IMAGES

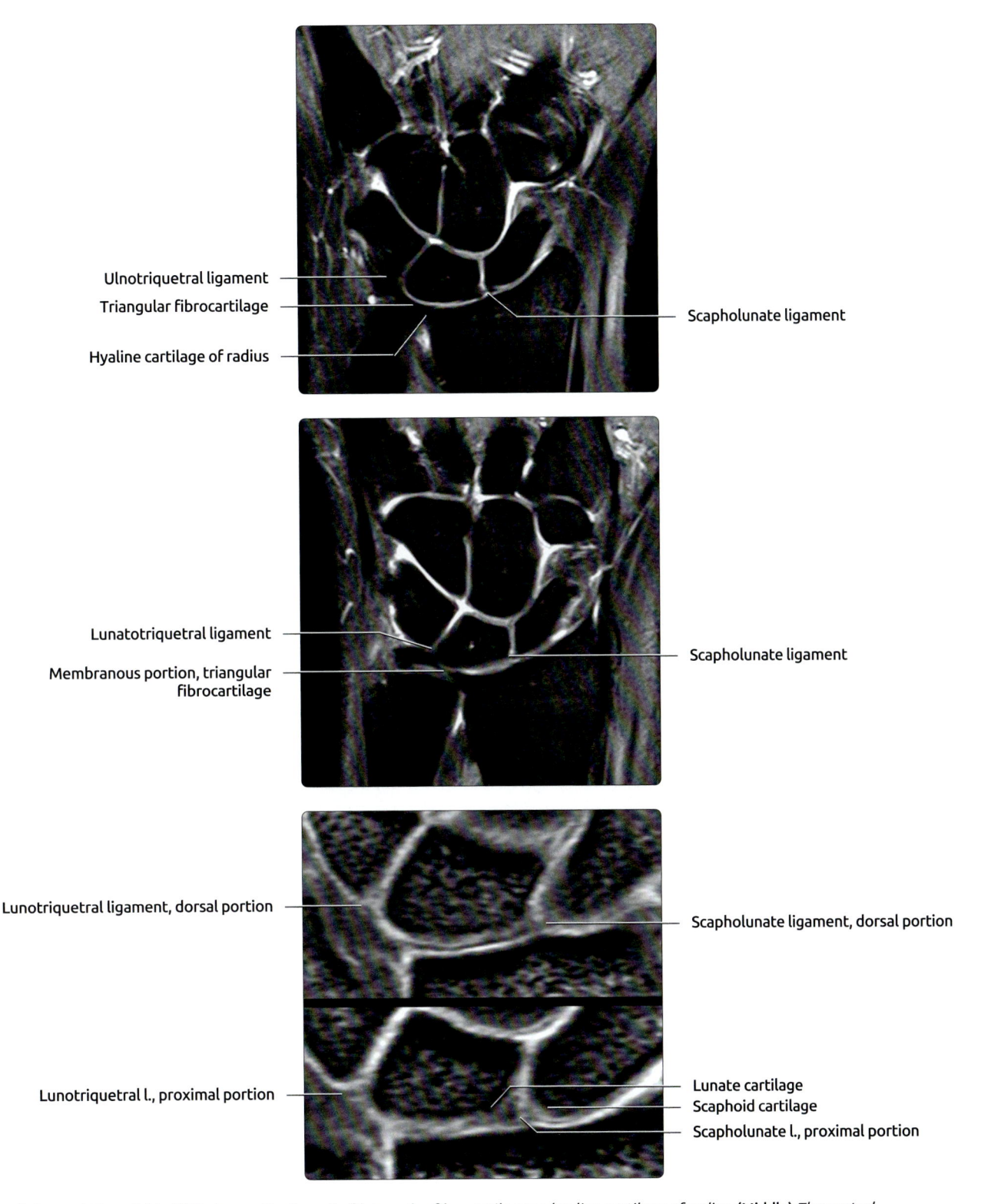

Ulnotriquetral ligament
Triangular fibrocartilage
Hyaline cartilage of radius
Scapholunate ligament

Lunatotriquetral ligament
Membranous portion, triangular fibrocartilage
Scapholunate ligament

Lunotriquetral ligament, dorsal portion
Scapholunate ligament, dorsal portion

Lunotriquetral l., proximal portion
Lunate cartilage
Scaphoid cartilage
Scapholunate l., proximal portion

(Top) Coronal T2-weighted MR shows attachment of triangular fibrocartilage to hyaline cartilage of radius. (Middle) The central, membranous portion of the triangular fibrocartilage is usually thin, as in this case, and there may be asymptomatic perforations of this portion of the ligament. (Bottom) Two coronal GRE images are shown, located dorsal and midsection, coned down to demonstrate the interosseous ligaments. Note that the thick dorsal portion of scapholunate ligament is readily seen on the upper image while the thinner dorsal portion of lunotriquetral ligament is less well visualized. Proximal portions of both scapholunate & lunotriquetral ligaments are triangular in shape (lower image).

Wrist Ligaments

LIGAMENTS IN AXIAL PLANE

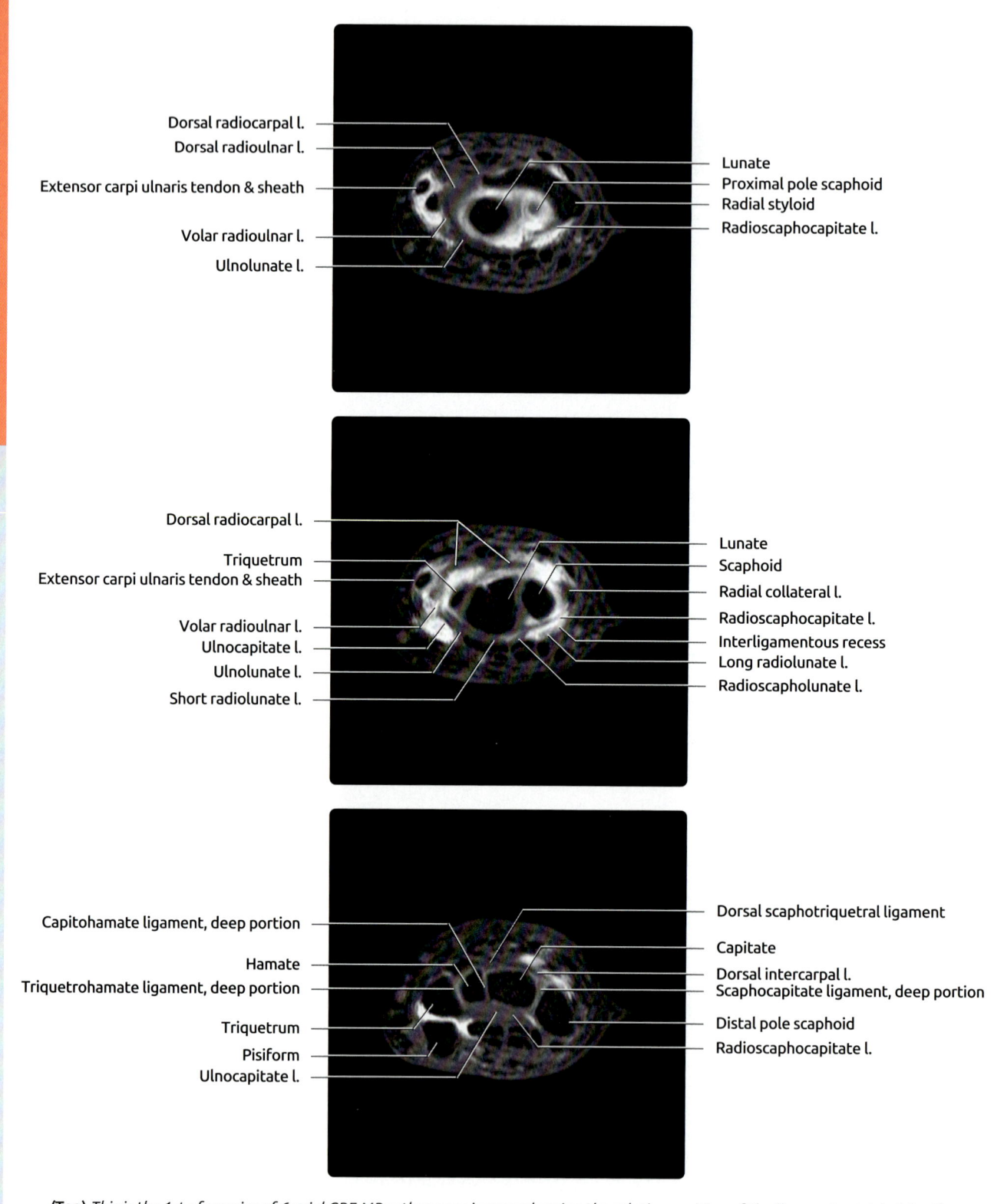

Dorsal radiocarpal l.
Dorsal radioulnar l.
Extensor carpi ulnaris tendon & sheath
Volar radioulnar l.
Ulnolunate l.

Lunate
Proximal pole scaphoid
Radial styloid
Radioscaphocapitate l.

Dorsal radiocarpal l.
Triquetrum
Extensor carpi ulnaris tendon & sheath
Volar radioulnar l.
Ulnocapitate l.
Ulnolunate l.
Short radiolunate l.

Lunate
Scaphoid
Radial collateral l.
Radioscaphocapitate l.
Interligamentous recess
Long radiolunate l.
Radioscapholunate l.

Capitohamate ligament, deep portion
Hamate
Triquetrohamate ligament, deep portion
Triquetrum
Pisiform
Ulnocapitate l.

Dorsal scaphotriquetral ligament
Capitate
Dorsal intercarpal l.
Scaphocapitate ligament, deep portion
Distal pole scaphoid
Radioscaphocapitate l.

(Top) This is the 1st of a series of 6 axial GRE MR arthrogram images showing the relative position of the ligaments. Joint distention accentuates volar & dorsal ligaments & associated recesses. The radiocarpal compartment may communicate with the ECU tendon sheath, as with this normal individual. (Middle) The dorsal radiocarpal ligament is the primary proximal dorsal stabilizer, spanning medial dorsal radial cortex & sweeping distally to the dorsal triquetrum. Volar stabilizers include radioscaphocapitate, long & short radiolunate, & ulnocarpal ligaments. (Bottom) Dorsal intercarpal ligament arises distal to scaphotriquetral ligament, spanning scaphoid & trapezoid (radially) to triquetrum (ulnarly).

Wrist Ligaments

LIGAMENTS IN AXIAL PLANE

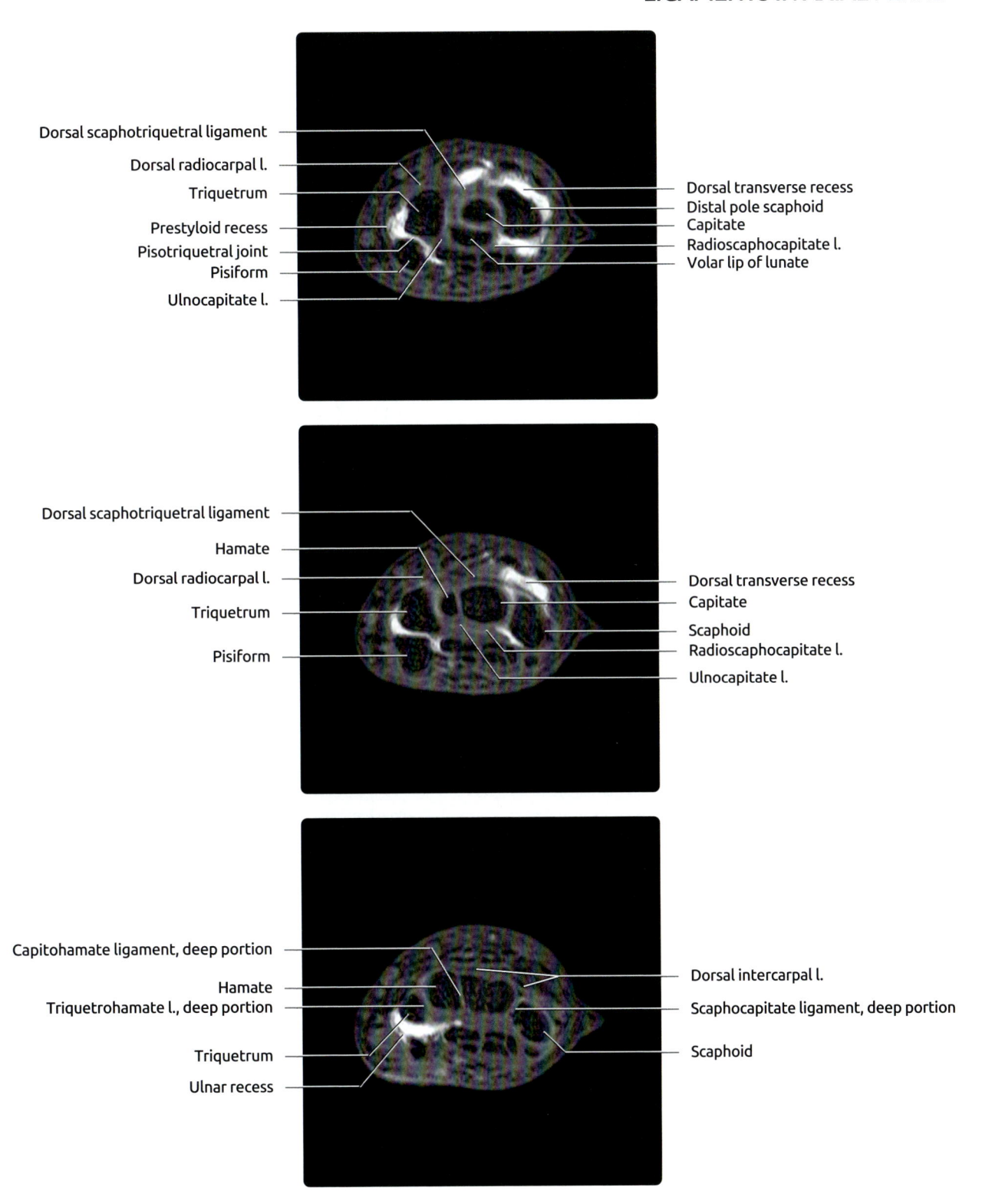

Top image labels:
- Dorsal scaphotriquetral ligament
- Dorsal radiocarpal l.
- Triquetrum
- Prestyloid recess
- Pisotriquetral joint
- Pisiform
- Ulnocapitate l.
- Dorsal transverse recess
- Distal pole scaphoid
- Capitate
- Radioscaphocapitate l.
- Volar lip of lunate

Middle image labels:
- Dorsal scaphotriquetral ligament
- Hamate
- Dorsal radiocarpal l.
- Triquetrum
- Pisiform
- Dorsal transverse recess
- Capitate
- Scaphoid
- Radioscaphocapitate l.
- Ulnocapitate l.

Bottom image labels:
- Capitohamate ligament, deep portion
- Hamate
- Triquetrohamate l., deep portion
- Triquetrum
- Ulnar recess
- Dorsal intercarpal l.
- Scaphocapitate ligament, deep portion
- Scaphoid

(Top) At the level of the junction of proximal and distal carpal rows, the dorsal & volar ligaments become less numerous. Radioscaphocapitate & ulnocapitate ligaments create arcuate or "V" ligament volarly. Dorsal scaphotriquetral ligament fibers span the dorsal proximal carpal row. (Middle) Volar extrinsic ligaments form the carpal tunnel floor. Small interosseous ligaments are present between all carpals, proximally, distally, medially, & laterally (except lunate-capitate relation, where there are no proximal-distal ligaments). (Bottom) Dorsal intercarpal ligament serves as dorsal distal stabilizing ligament, blending with the dorsal scaphotriquetral ligament at triquetrum. Ulnar recess is medial to triquetrohamate articulation.

Wrist Tendons

TERMINOLOGY

Definitions
- Palmar: Volar
- Ulnar: Medial
- Radial: Lateral
- Wrist abduction: Radial flexion
- Wrist adduction: Ulnar flexion

IMAGING ANATOMY

Flexors
- Deep flexor group
  - Flexor digitorum profundus
    - **Origin**: Proximal ulna
    - **Course**: Splits into 4 tendons proximal to pronator quadratus, passing through carpal tunnel
    - **Insertion**: Index, middle, ring, & little finger distal phalangeal bases
    - **Action**: Flexes distal phalanges; flexes other phalanges & hand with continued action
    - **Innervation**: Median, anterior interosseous, ulnar nerve
    - **Variants**: Duplicated slips
  - Flexor pollicis longus
    - **Origin**: Radius, interosseous membrane, coronoid process
    - **Course**: Passes deep to flexor retinaculum between flexor pollicis brevis & adductor pollicis
    - **Insertion**: Thumb distal phalangeal base
    - **Action**: Flexes thumb interphalangeal joint; flexes thumb metacarpal (MC) phalangeal joint with continued action
    - **Innervation**: Median nerve, anterior interosseous
    - **Variant**: Additional slip to index finger
  - Pronator quadratus
    - **Origin**: Medial distal volar ulna
    - **Course**: Passes medial to lateral
    - **Insertion**: Lateral distal dorsal radius
    - **Action**: Pronates hand
    - **Innervation**: Median nerve, anterior interosseous
    - **Variants**: May split into 2 or 3 layers; additional proximal or distal attachments
- Superficial
  - Flexor carpi radialis
    - **Origin**: Medial epicondyle/common flexor tendon
    - **Action**: Flexes hand at wrist; abducts wrist
    - **Innervation**: Median nerve
    - **Variants**: May attach to trapezium &/or 4th metacarpal
    - **Course**: Thin tendon passes through canal in lateral flexor retinaculum (FR) across volar trapezium groove
    - **Insertion**: 2nd metacarpal base; slip to 3rd metacarpal base
  - Palmaris longus
    - **Origin**: Medial epicondyle/common flexor tendon
    - **Course**: Thin tendon passes superficial to flexor retinaculum
    - **Insertion**: Volar distal flexor retinaculum & aponeurosis
    - **Action**: Flexes hand at wrist
    - **Innervation**: Median nerve
    - **Variants**: Absent in 10%; duplicated; complete or partial insertion on antebrachial fascia, flexor carpi ulnaris tendon, pisiform, or scaphoid; short tendon with low lying muscle belly may compress median n.
  - Flexor carpi ulnaris
    - **Origin**: Medial epicondyle/common flexor tendon (humeral head) & medial proximal ulna (ulnar head)
    - **Course**: Runs medial to ulnar neurovascular bundle
    - **Insertion**: Pisiform (continuing distally as pisohamate & pisometacarpal ligaments)
    - **Action**: Flexes hand; adducts wrist
    - **Innervation**: Ulnar nerve
  - Flexor digitorum superficialis
    - **Origin**: Medial epicondyle/common flexor tendon & ulnar coronoid process (humeroulnar head); volar proximal radius (radial head)
    - **Course**: Divides into superficial (tendons to middle & ring fingers) & deep (tendons to index & little fingers); passes deep to flexor retinaculum with superficial tendons volar to deep tendons
    - **Insertion**: Middle phalanges of index, middle, ring, & little fingers
    - **Action**: Flexes proximal interphalangeal and metacarpophalangeal joints of index, middle, ring, & little fingers
    - **Innervation**: Median nerve
    - **Variants**: Absent little finger slip; accessory slips to index & middle fingers; distal muscle belly along proximal phalanges may mimic mass

Extensors
- Superficial
  - Extensor carpi radialis longus
    - **Origin**: Lateral epicondyle/common extensor tendon
    - **Course**: Proximal to carpus, crosses beneath abductor pollicis longus & extensor pollicis brevis; passes deep to extensor retinaculum in compartment #2
    - **Insertion**: Dorsal radial 2nd metacarpal base
    - **Action**: Extends & abducts hand at wrist
    - **Innervation**: Radial nerve
    - **Variants**: Multiple tendons, insert on 2nd, 3rd, or 4th metacarpal
  - Extensor carpi radialis brevis
    - **Origin**: Lateral epicondyle/common extensor tendon
    - **Course**: Passes beneath abductor pollicis longus & extensor pollicis brevis; passes deep to extensor retinaculum in compartment #2
    - **Insertion**: Dorsal radial 3rd metacarpal base
    - **Action**: Extends & abducts hand at wrist
    - **Innervation**: Radial nerve
    - **Variants**: Multiple tendons, insert on 2nd, 3rd, or 4th MC
  - Extensor digitorum (communis)
    - **Origin**: Lateral epicondyle/common extensor tendon
    - **Action**: Extends index, middle, ring, little fingers; abducts index, ring, & little fingers away from middle finger; extends hand at wrist with continued action
    - **Innervation**: Deep radial nerve
    - **Variants**: Multiple slips; insertion on thumb

Wrist Tendons

- **Course**: Passes distally, dividing into 4 slips; passes deep to extensor retinaculum in compartment #4; extends into index, middle, ring, little fingers
- **Insertion**: Middle & distal phalanges of index, middle, ring, little fingers
- Extensor digiti minimi (extensor digiti quinti [V] proprius)
    - **Origin**: Lateral epicondyle/common extensor tendon
    - **Action**: Extends little finger; extends hand at wrist with continued action
    - **Course**: Passes medial to extensor digitorum & lateral to extensor carpi ulnaris; passes deep to extensor retinaculum in compartment #5
    - **Insertion**: Extensor hood of little finger proximal phalanx with slip to ring finger
    - **Innervation**: Deep radial nerve
    - **Variants**: Fused with extensor digitorum; absent ring finger slip
- Extensor carpi ulnaris
    - **Origin**: Common extensor tendon & dorsal ulna
    - **Course**: Passes into wrist deep to extensor retinaculum in compartment #6
    - **Insertion**: Dorsal ulnar 5th metacarpal base
    - **Action**: Extends & adducts hand
    - **Innervation**: Deep radial nerve
    - **Variants**: Insertion on 4th metacarpal

Deep

- **Abductor pollicis longus**
    - **Origin**: Dorsal lateral ulna, dorsal mid radius
    - **Action**: Abducts & extends thumb; abducts wrist; flexes wrist minimally
    - **Innervation**: Deep radial nerve, posterior interosseous branch
    - **Variants**: Multiple slips; insert on trapezium or flexor retinaculum
    - **Course**: Passes obliquely distal & lateral; crossing over extensor carpi radialis brevis & longus tt., passing into extensor compartment #1
        - Abductor pollicis longus & extensor pollicis brevis intersect extensor carpi radialis brevis & longus just proximal to extensor retinaculum; may impinge at musculotendinous intersection
    - **Insertion**: 1st metacarpal radial base with slips to trapezium & abductor pollicis brevis
- **Extensor pollicis brevis**
    - **Origin**: Dorsal mid radius
    - **Course**: Medial & contiguous with abductor pollicis longus; crossing over extensor carpi radialis longus & brevis to enter extensor compartment #1 with abductor pollicis longus
    - **Insertion**: Thumb proximal phalangeal base
    - **Action**: Extends thumb metacarpophalangeal joint; extends 1st metacarpal at carpometacarpal (CMC) joint with continued action; abducts wrist
    - **Innervation**: Deep radial nerve, posterior interosseous branch
    - **Variants**: May be absent; fused with extensor pollicis longus
- **Extensor pollicis longus**
    - **Origin**: Dorsal mid ulna
    - **Course**: Passes into wrist under extensor retinaculum in compartment #3; crosses lateral & superficial to extensor carpi radialis longus & brevis at 45°
    - **Insertion**: Thumb distal phalangeal base
    - **Action**: Extends thumb tip; extends thumb proximal phalanx & 1st MC by continued action
    - **Innervation**: Deep radial nerve, posterior interosseous branch
    - **Variant**: Fused with extensor pollicis brevis
- **Extensor indicis (proprius)**
    - **Origin**: Dorsal mid ulna & interosseous membrane
    - **Course**: Passes under extensor retinaculum in compartment #4, running deep & medial to extensor digitorum; joins tendon slip near ulnar index finger
    - **Insertion**: Extensor hood of index finger
    - **Action**: Extends & adducts index finger
    - **Innervation**: Deep radial nerve, posterior interosseous branch
    - **Variants**: Duplicated muscle; slip to middle finger

Muscles Originating at Wrist

- **Thenar**
    - Abductor pollicis brevis
        - **Origin**: Flexor retinaculum, scaphoid tuberosity, trapezium ridge
        - **Course**: Extends laterally
        - **Insertion**: Radial thumb proximal phalangeal base
        - **Action**: Abducts thumb at CMC & MC joints; draws thumb away from palm at right angle
        - **Innervation**: Median nerve
        - **Variants**: Absent or duplicated tendon slips
    - Opponens pollicis
        - **Origin**: FR, trapezium ridge
        - **Course**: Deep to abductor pollicis brevis
        - **Insertion**: Radial side of thumb metacarpal
        - **Action**: Abducts, flexes, & rotates 1st MC; draws thumbs across palm
        - **Innervation**: Median nerve
    - Flexor pollicis brevis
        - Consists of superficial (larger & lateral) & deep (smaller & medial) components
        - **Origin**: Superficial-distal flexor retinaculum & trapezium tubercle; deep trapezoid & capitate
        - **Course**: Located medial & distal to abductor pollicis brevis
        - **Insertion**: Common tendon inserts on radial thumb proximal phalangeal base
        - **Action**: Flexes thumb proximal phalanx; medially rotates thumb metacarpal
        - **Innervation**: Superficial median n.; deep ulnar n.
    - Adductor pollicis
        - **Origin**: Oblique head capitate, 2nd & 3rd MC bases, flexor carpi radialis (FCR) tendon sheath; transverse head 3rd metacarpal
        - **Action**: Abducts thumb proximal phalanx toward palm
        - **Innervation**: Ulnar nerve
        - **Course**: Oblique: Passes obliquely distally & converges to tendon (which contains sesamoid); transverse fibers converge laterally

Wrist Tendons

- Insertion: Oblique & transverse ulnar thumb proximal phalangeal base
- Hypothenar
  - Palmar brevis
    - Origin: Flexor retinaculum & palmar aponeurosis
    - Insertion: Skin of ulnar palm
    - Action: Draws skin of ulnarward palm toward middle
    - Innervation: Ulnar nerve, superficial branch
  - Abductor digiti minimi
    - Origin: Pisiform & flexor carpi ulnaris tendon
    - Insertion: Ulnar little finger proximal phalangeal base
    - Action: Abducts little finger away from ring finger; flexes proximal phalanx
    - Innervation: Ulnar nerve, deep branch
  - Flexor digiti minimi brevis
    - Origin: Hook of hamate & flexor retinaculum
    - Insertion: Ulnar little finger proximal phalangeal base
    - Action: Flexes little finger at metacarpophalangeal joint
    - Innervation: Ulnar nerve, deep branch
    - Variant: Anomalous origin may compress ulnar nerve
  - Opponens digiti minimi
    - Origin: Hook of hamate & flexor retinaculum
    - Insertion: Length of 5th metacarpal
    - Action: Abducts, flexes, & laterally rotates 5th metacarpal
    - Innervation: Ulnar nerve, deep branch

Anomalous Muscles

- May present as a soft tissue mass; may create neural compression
- **Accessory palmaris longus**: Superficial to flexor digitorum tendons, medial to flexor carpi radialis
- **Extensor digitorum manus brevis**
  - May be tender or present as mass
  - Origin: Distal radius or dorsal radiocarpal ligament
  - Insertion: 2nd metacarpal
- **Extensor carpi radialis intermedius**
  - Origin: Humerus or as accessory slip from extensor carpi radialis brevis or longus
  - Insertion: 2nd &/or 3rd metacarpal
- **Extensor carpi radialis accessory**
  - Origin: Humerus or extensor carpi radialis longus
  - Insertion: 1st metacarpal, abductor pollicis brevis, or 1st dorsal interosseous muscle
- **Accessory extensor pollicis longus**
  - Located in 3rd extensor compartment
  - May be tender, may mimic mass
- **Accessory abductor digiti minimi**: May compress ulnar or median n.
  - Origin: Flexor retinaculum or palmaris longus
  - Insertion: Adductor digiti minimi
- **Lumbrical muscle anomalous origin**
  - Usually arise from flexor digitorum tendons distal to carpal tunnel
  - If arising more proximally, within carpal tunnel, may cause carpal tunnel syndrome

Fascia & Retinacula

- Flexor retinaculum
  - Superficial (volar carpal ligament or ligamentum carpi palmare) portion
    - Thickened distal antebrachial fascia combined with transverse fibrous bundles
    - Attaches at ulnar styloid process & radial styloid process; blends distally with flexor retinaculum
    - Creates roof of Guyon canal; ulnar nerve, artery, & veins run deep to fascial layer but superficial to flexor retinaculum
  - Flexor retinaculum (transverse ligament or ligamentum flexorum)
    - Attaches at pisiform, hook of hamate, scaphoid tuberosity, trapezium palmar surface, & ridge; deep surface of palmar aponeurosis
    - Creates carpal tunnel & tunnel for FCR across trapezium
    - Hypothenar & thenar musculature arise from flexor retinaculum
    - Carpal tunnel release typically divides flexor retinaculum ulnarly near hook of hamate attachment
- **Extensor retinaculum (dorsal carpal ligament)**
  - Thickened distal antebrachial fascia combined with transverse fibrous bundles
  - Attaches to ulnar styloid process, medial margin of pisiform & triquetrum, lateral radius margin
  - Attaches to dorsal radial ridges, creating fibroosseous compartments (referred to by number)
    - #1: Abductor pollicis longus, extensor pollicis brevis; #2: Extensor carpi radialis longus & brevis; #3: Extensor pollicis longus; #4: Extensor digitorum, extensor indicis; #5: Extensor digiti minimi; #6: Extensor carpi ulnaris

Tendon Sheaths

- Wrist & hand synovial tendon sheaths are specialized bursae; tubular with visceral & parietal layers; intervening potential space contains minimal fluid & small blood vessels normally; fills with fluid when inflamed
- Flexor sheaths
  - **Common flexor tendon sheath** (ulnar bursa) encases flexor digitorum superficialis and profundus; arises 2.5 cm proximal to flexor retinaculum; index, middle, & ring sheaths terminate in palm, little finger sheath at distal phalanx
  - **Flexor pollicis longus tendon sheath** (radial bursa) encases flexor pollicis longus; arises 2.5 cm proximal to flexor retinaculum; terminates at thumb distal phalanx
- Extensor sheaths
  - 6 discrete tendon sheaths encase tendons of 6 extensor compartments; arise proximal to extensor retinaculum; terminate adjacent to dorsal MC base/shaft

ANATOMY IMAGING ISSUES

Imaging Issues

- Many variations of flexor & extensor muscles & tendons
- Multiple tendon slips can mimic longitudinal tendon tears
- Magic angle effect: Collagen bundle orientation so that images obtained 55° to main magnetic field may yield intermediate signal rather than expected low signal intensity (especially in short TE imaging: T1, PD, or GRE)
- Small amount of fluid in tendon sheaths is normal finding

Wrist Tendons

3D CT: VOLAR & DORSAL TENDONS

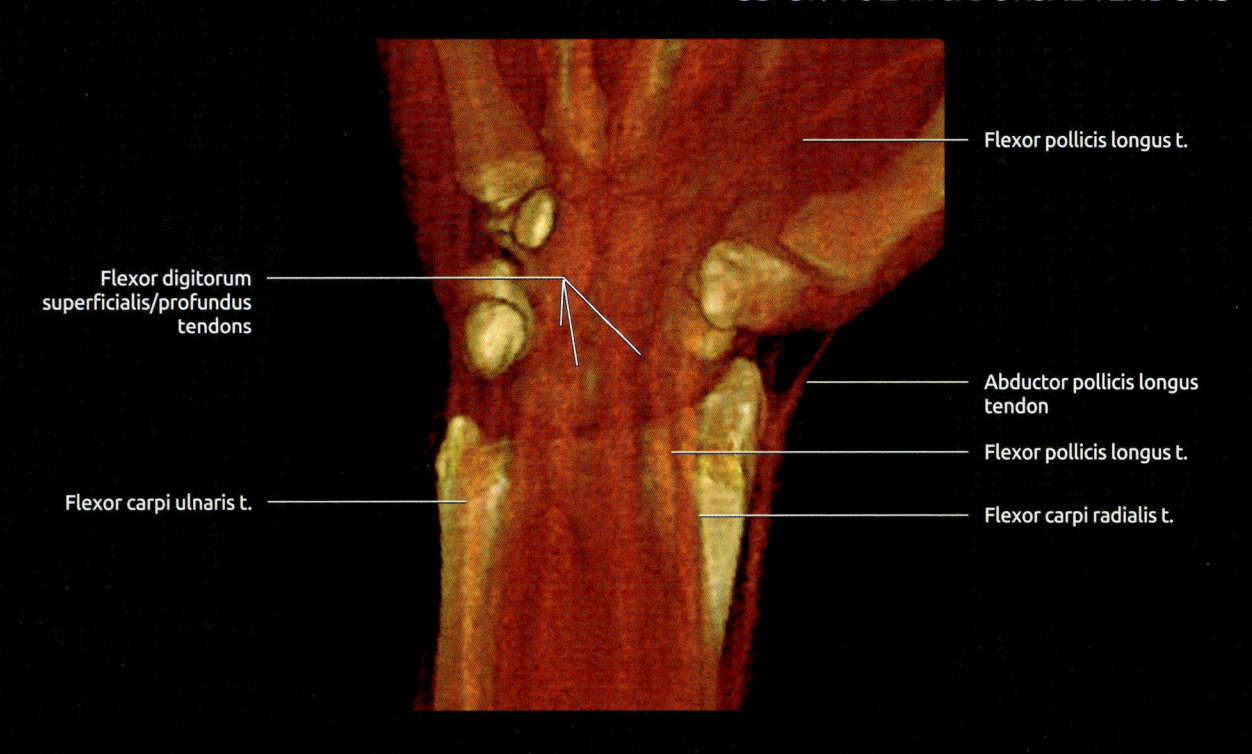

- Flexor pollicis longus t.
- Flexor digitorum superficialis/profundus tendons
- Abductor pollicis longus tendon
- Flexor pollicis longus t.
- Flexor carpi ulnaris t.
- Flexor carpi radialis t.

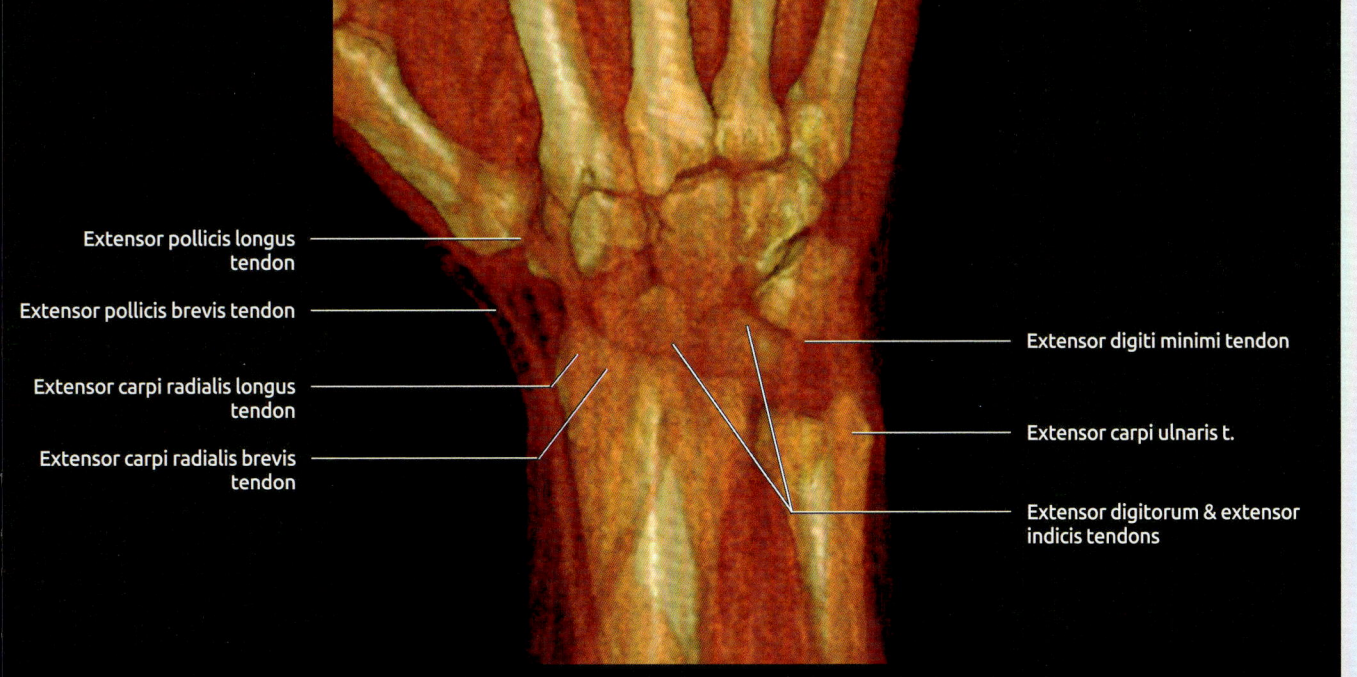

- Extensor pollicis longus tendon
- Extensor pollicis brevis tendon
- Extensor carpi radialis longus tendon
- Extensor carpi radialis brevis tendon
- Extensor digiti minimi tendon
- Extensor carpi ulnaris t.
- Extensor digitorum & extensor indicis tendons

(Top) *3D reconstruction with soft tissue overlay reveals volar tendons extending from forearm into wrist & hand.* **(Bottom)** *Dorsal tendons are similarly displayed.*

Wrist Tendons

GRAPHICS: VOLAR TENDONS

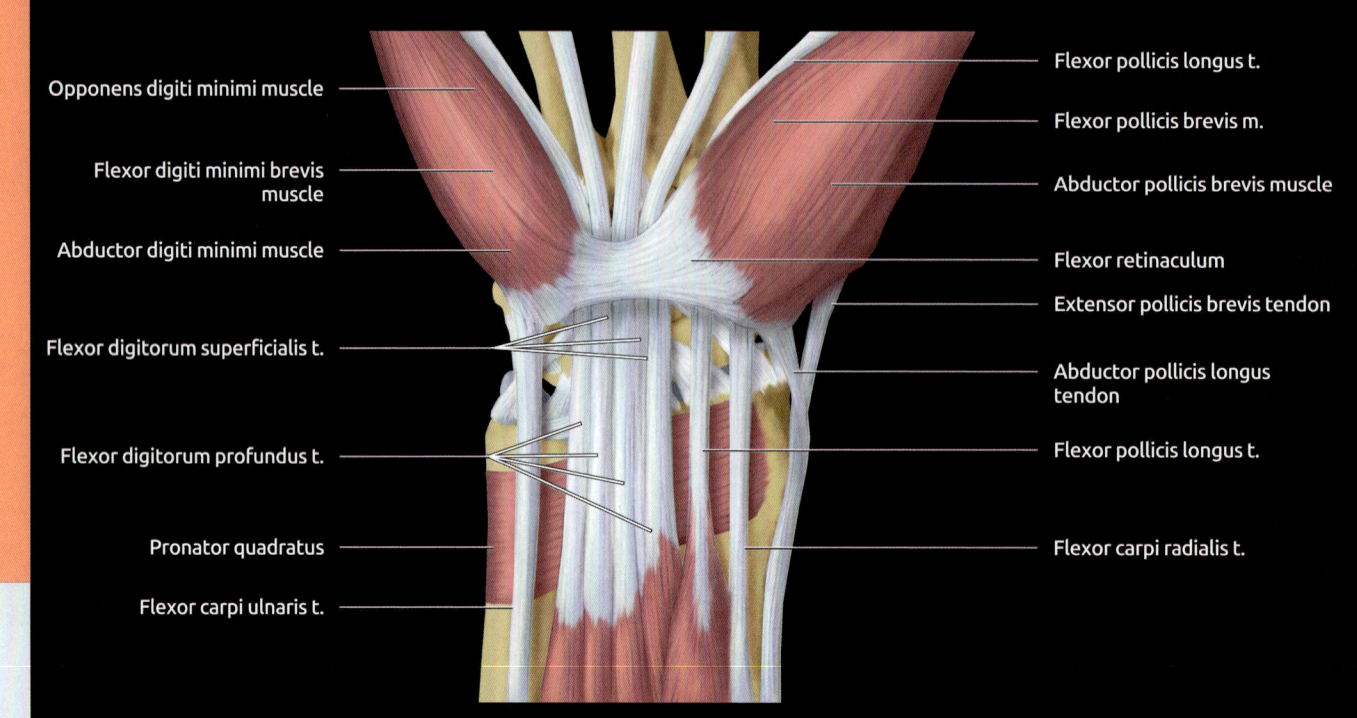

Labels (top image):
- Opponens digiti minimi muscle
- Flexor digiti minimi brevis muscle
- Abductor digiti minimi muscle
- Flexor digitorum superficialis t.
- Flexor digitorum profundus t.
- Pronator quadratus
- Flexor carpi ulnaris t.
- Flexor pollicis longus t.
- Flexor pollicis brevis m.
- Abductor pollicis brevis muscle
- Flexor retinaculum
- Extensor pollicis brevis tendon
- Abductor pollicis longus tendon
- Flexor pollicis longus t.
- Flexor carpi radialis t.

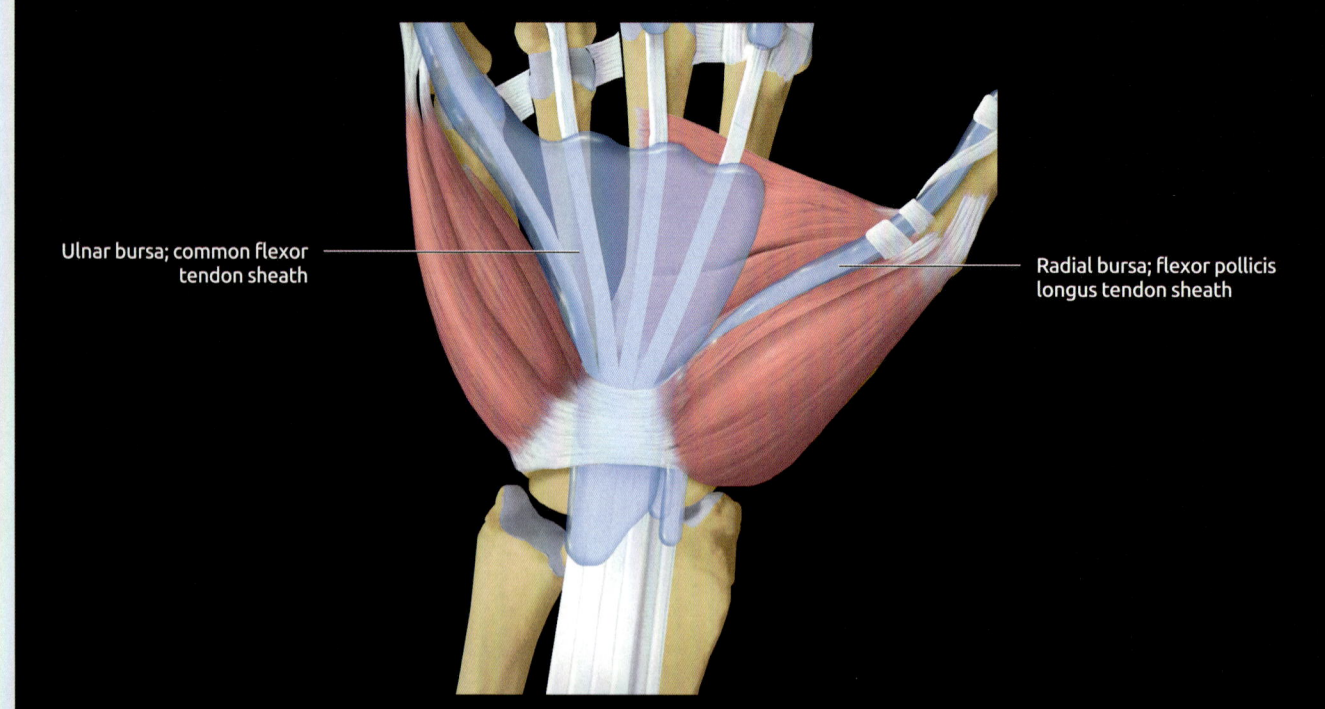

Labels (bottom image):
- Ulnar bursa; common flexor tendon sheath
- Radial bursa; flexor pollicis longus tendon sheath

(**Top**) *Volar muscles & tendons are displayed with their relation to flexor retinaculum. Note the muscles of thenar & hypothenar eminences arise from the retinaculum itself. Flexor digitorum & flexor pollicis longus tendons pass deep to the retinaculum while flexor carpi radialis is lateral but within fibers of lateral retinaculum.* (**Bottom**) *Volar bursae include ulnar & radial sheaths. Common flexor tendon sheath encases index, middle, ring, & little finger tendons, beginning proximal to flexor retinaculum & extending distally to midshaft metacarpals. Sheath also extends distally to the little finger distal phalanx. Flexor pollicis longus has a separate sheath.*

Wrist Tendons

GRAPHICS: DORSAL TENDONS

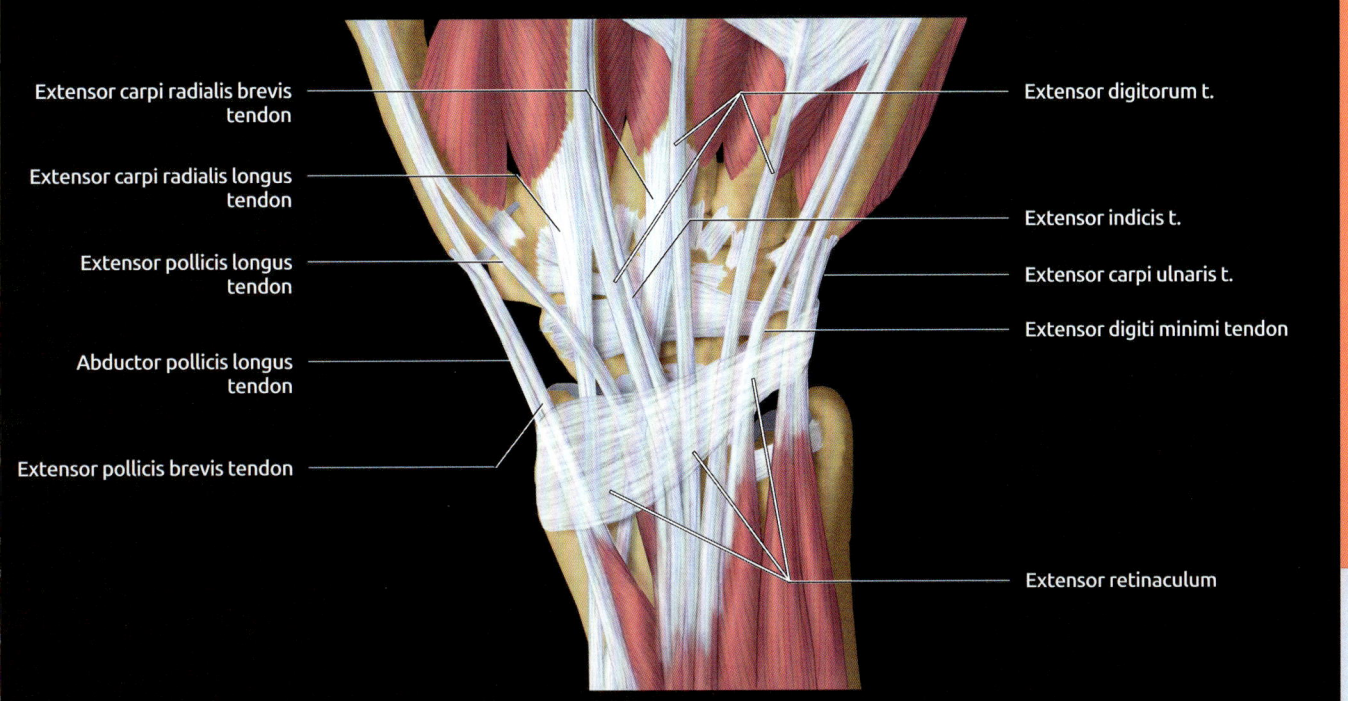

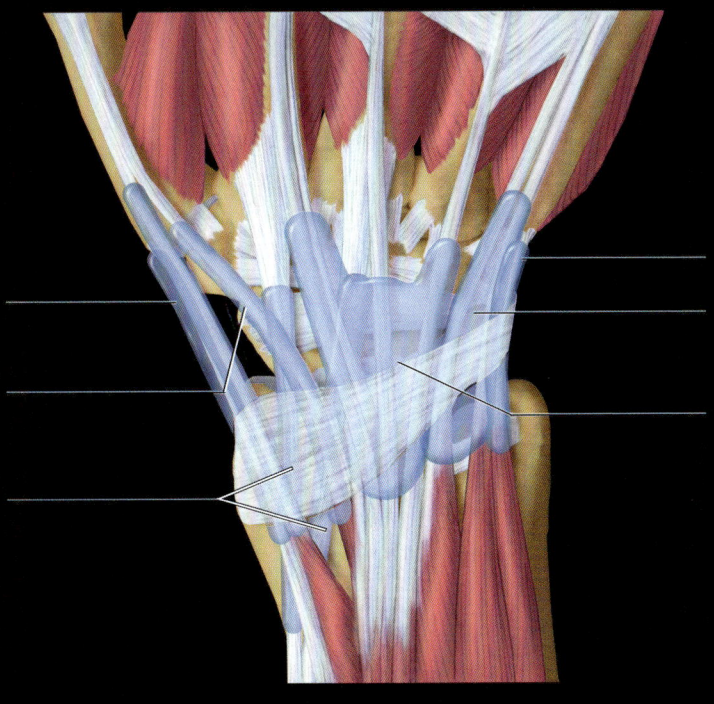

Extensor carpi radialis brevis tendon

Extensor carpi radialis longus tendon

Extensor pollicis longus tendon

Abductor pollicis longus tendon

Extensor pollicis brevis tendon

Extensor digitorum t.

Extensor indicis t.

Extensor carpi ulnaris t.

Extensor digiti minimi tendon

Extensor retinaculum

Compartment 1: Abductor pollicis longus & extensor pollicis brevis

Compartment 3: Extensor pollicis longus

Compartment 2: Extensor carpi radialis longus & brevis

Compartment 6: Extensor carpi ulnaris

Compartment 5: Extensor digiti minimi

Compartment 4: Extensor digitorum & extensor indicis

(Top) Dorsal extensor tendons pass deep to the extensor retinaculum, separated into 6 compartments by fibrous attachments of retinaculum to underlying bone. Compartment contents: #1: Abductor pollicis longus (APL), extensor pollicis brevis (EPB); #2: Extensor carpi radialis longus (ECRL), extensor carpi radialis brevis (ECRB); #3: Extensor pollicis longus (EPL); #4: Extensor digitorum (ED), extensor indicis (EI); #5: Extensor digiti minimi (EDM); #6: Extensor carpi ulnaris (ECU). **(Bottom)** Separate tendon sheaths enclose dorsal extensor tendons in compartments 1-6 individually.

Wrist Tendons

AXIAL GRAPHIC & MR: TENDONS AT DISTAL RADIUS

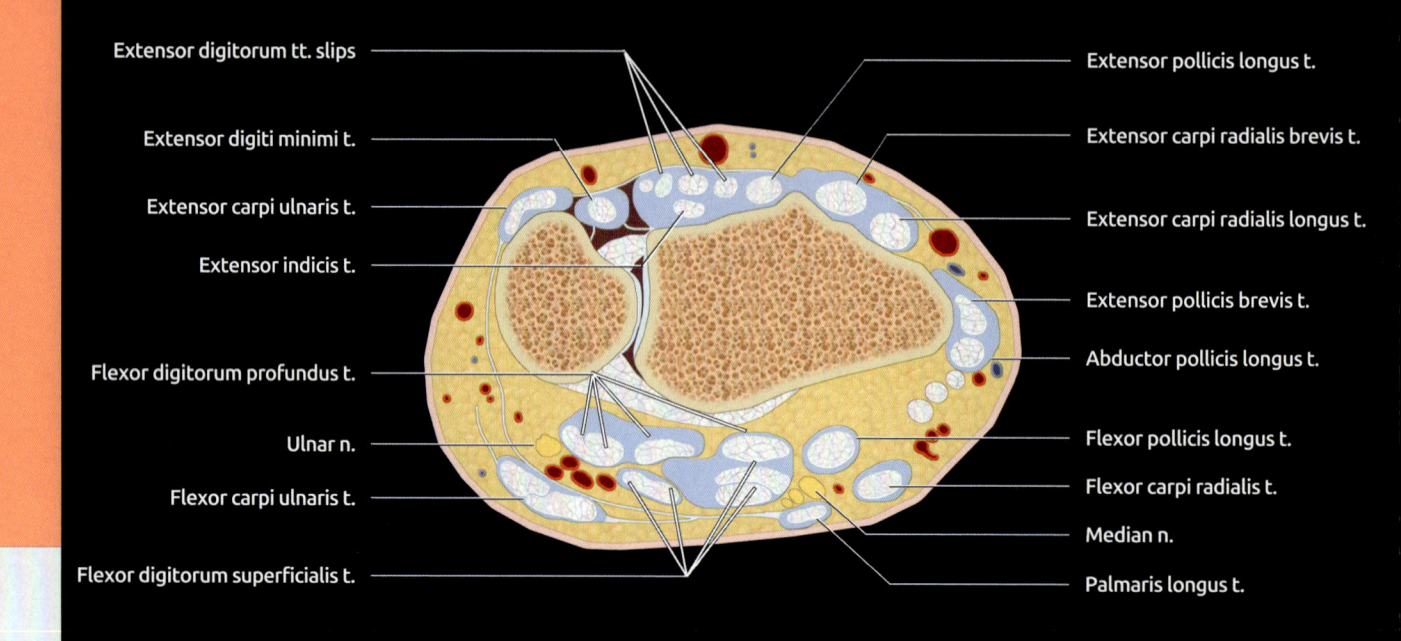

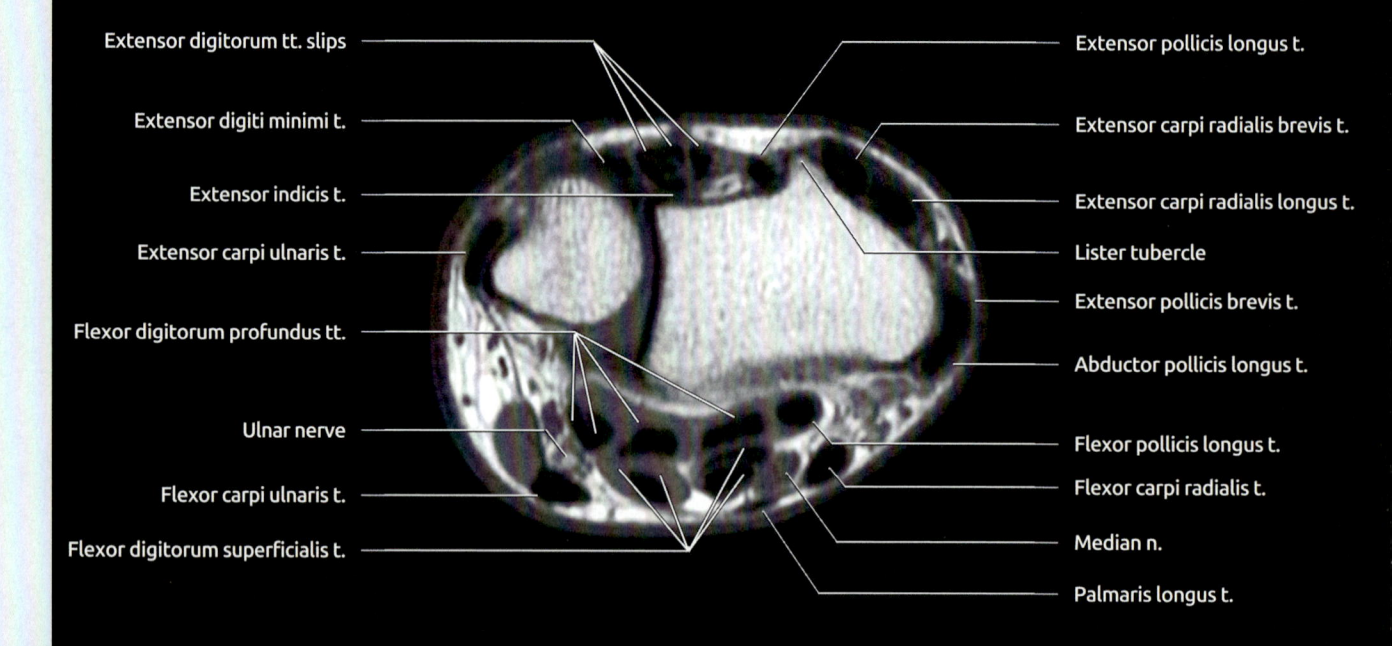

(Top) Graphic shows tendons in proximal wrist. Extensor tendons are deep to extensor retinaculum while flexor tendons are proximal to the flexor retinaculum at this level in the wrist. (Bottom) Corresponding axial MR demonstrates uniform low signal intensity of tendons.

Wrist Tendons

AXIAL GRAPHIC & MR: TENDONS AT MID WRIST

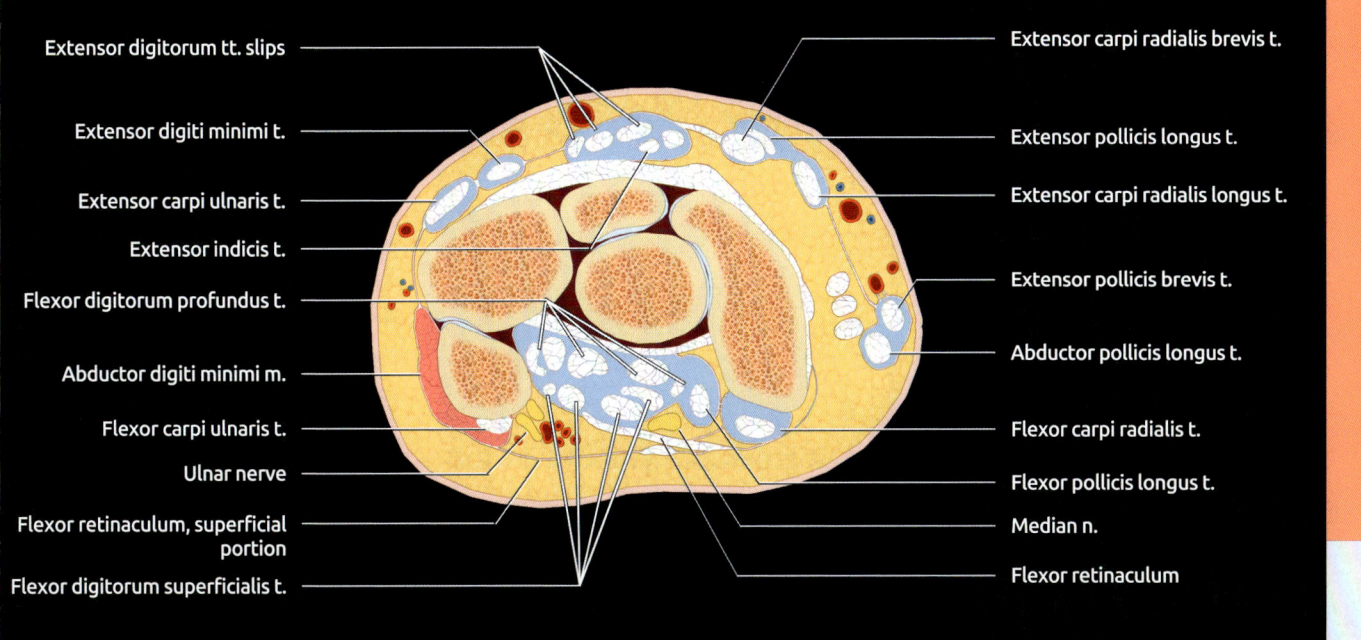

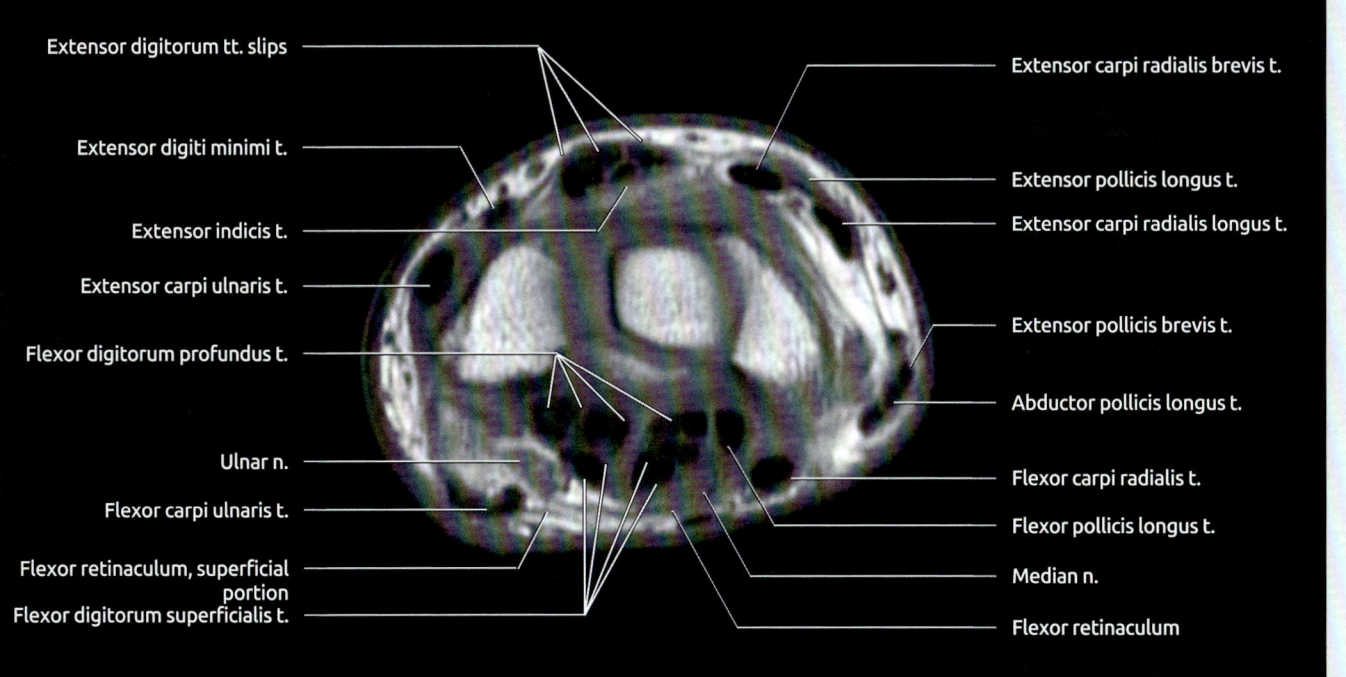

Labels (top graphic, left side):
- Extensor digitorum tt. slips
- Extensor digiti minimi t.
- Extensor carpi ulnaris t.
- Extensor indicis t.
- Flexor digitorum profundus t.
- Abductor digiti minimi m.
- Flexor carpi ulnaris t.
- Ulnar nerve
- Flexor retinaculum, superficial portion
- Flexor digitorum superficialis t.

Labels (top graphic, right side):
- Extensor carpi radialis brevis t.
- Extensor pollicis longus t.
- Extensor carpi radialis longus t.
- Extensor pollicis brevis t.
- Abductor pollicis longus t.
- Flexor carpi radialis t.
- Flexor pollicis longus t.
- Median n.
- Flexor retinaculum

Labels (bottom MR, left side):
- Extensor digitorum tt. slips
- Extensor digiti minimi t.
- Extensor indicis t.
- Extensor carpi ulnaris t.
- Flexor digitorum profundus t.
- Ulnar n.
- Flexor carpi ulnaris t.
- Flexor retinaculum, superficial portion
- Flexor digitorum superficialis t.

Labels (bottom MR, right side):
- Extensor carpi radialis brevis t.
- Extensor pollicis longus t.
- Extensor carpi radialis longus t.
- Extensor pollicis brevis t.
- Abductor pollicis longus t.
- Flexor carpi radialis t.
- Flexor pollicis longus t.
- Median n.
- Flexor retinaculum

(**Top**) *Graphic shows tendons in carpal tunnel. Flexor digitorum profundus tendons are ordered with little, ring, middle & index tendons side by side (ulnar to radial). Flexor digitorum superficialis tendons are organized with 2 deep tendons going to middle & ring fingers & 2 superficial tendons extending to little & index fingers. Extensor pollicis longus tendon is crossing superficial to extensor carpi radialis brevis tendon.* (**Bottom**) *Corresponding axial MR shows tendons in carpal tunnel. Note magic angle effect on EPL as it crosses over ECRB. The tendon is angled 55° to the main magnetic field, resulting in loss of normal low signal.*

Wrist Tendons

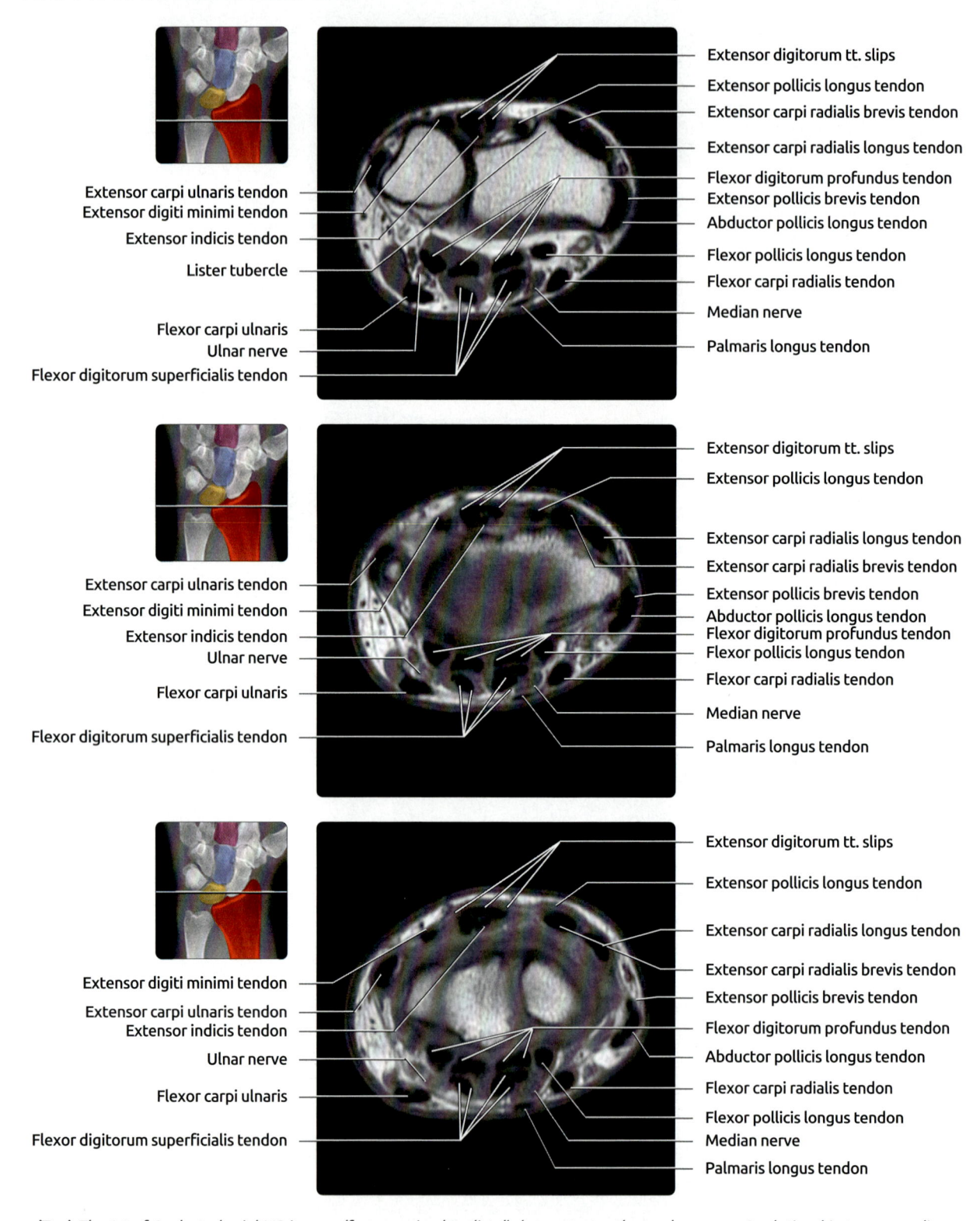

AXIAL T1 MR: WRIST TENDONS

(Top) The 1st of 6 selected axial MR images (from proximal to distal) demonstrates the tendon course & relationship to surrounding osseous structures. Lister tubercle is a useful bony landmark dividing the 2nd and 3rd compartments. (Middle) Extensor retinaculum secures the extensor tendons into 6 discrete compartments. (Bottom) The median nerve is rounded & lies superficial & lateral to the flexor digitorum tendons.

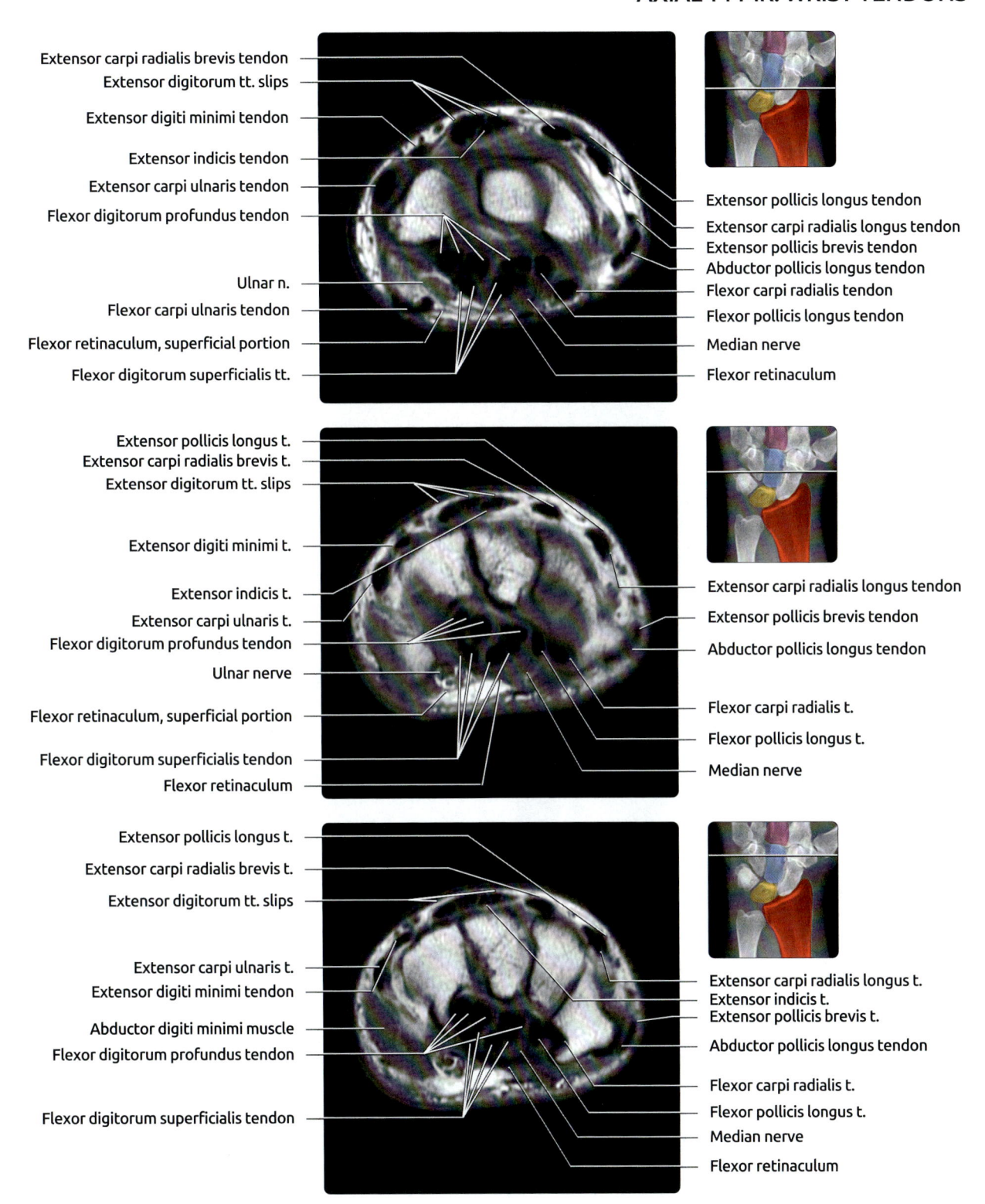

Wrist Tendons

AXIAL T1 MR: WRIST TENDONS

Extensor carpi radialis brevis tendon
Extensor digitorum tt. slips
Extensor digiti minimi tendon
Extensor indicis tendon
Extensor carpi ulnaris tendon
Flexor digitorum profundus tendon
Ulnar n.
Flexor carpi ulnaris tendon
Flexor retinaculum, superficial portion
Flexor digitorum superficialis tt.

Extensor pollicis longus tendon
Extensor carpi radialis longus tendon
Extensor pollicis brevis tendon
Abductor pollicis longus tendon
Flexor carpi radialis tendon
Flexor pollicis longus tendon
Median nerve
Flexor retinaculum

Extensor pollicis longus t.
Extensor carpi radialis brevis t.
Extensor digitorum tt. slips
Extensor digiti minimi t.
Extensor indicis t.
Extensor carpi ulnaris t.
Flexor digitorum profundus tendon
Ulnar nerve
Flexor retinaculum, superficial portion
Flexor digitorum superficialis tendon
Flexor retinaculum

Extensor carpi radialis longus tendon
Extensor pollicis brevis tendon
Abductor pollicis longus tendon
Flexor carpi radialis t.
Flexor pollicis longus t.
Median nerve

Extensor pollicis longus t.
Extensor carpi radialis brevis t.
Extensor digitorum tt. slips
Extensor carpi ulnaris t.
Extensor digiti minimi tendon
Abductor digiti minimi muscle
Flexor digitorum profundus tendon
Flexor digitorum superficialis tendon

Extensor carpi radialis longus t.
Extensor indicis t.
Extensor pollicis brevis t.
Abductor pollicis longus tendon
Flexor carpi radialis t.
Flexor pollicis longus t.
Median nerve
Flexor retinaculum

(Top) Note the magic angle effect on EPL as it crosses over the ECRB. **(Middle)** The carpal tunnel is spanned by the flexor retinaculum from the scaphoid tubercle to the hook of hamate. Its superficial fibers form the roof of Guyon canal. **(Bottom)** The flexor retinaculum attaches to the trapezial ridge radially & the hamate hook ulnarly.

Wrist Tendons

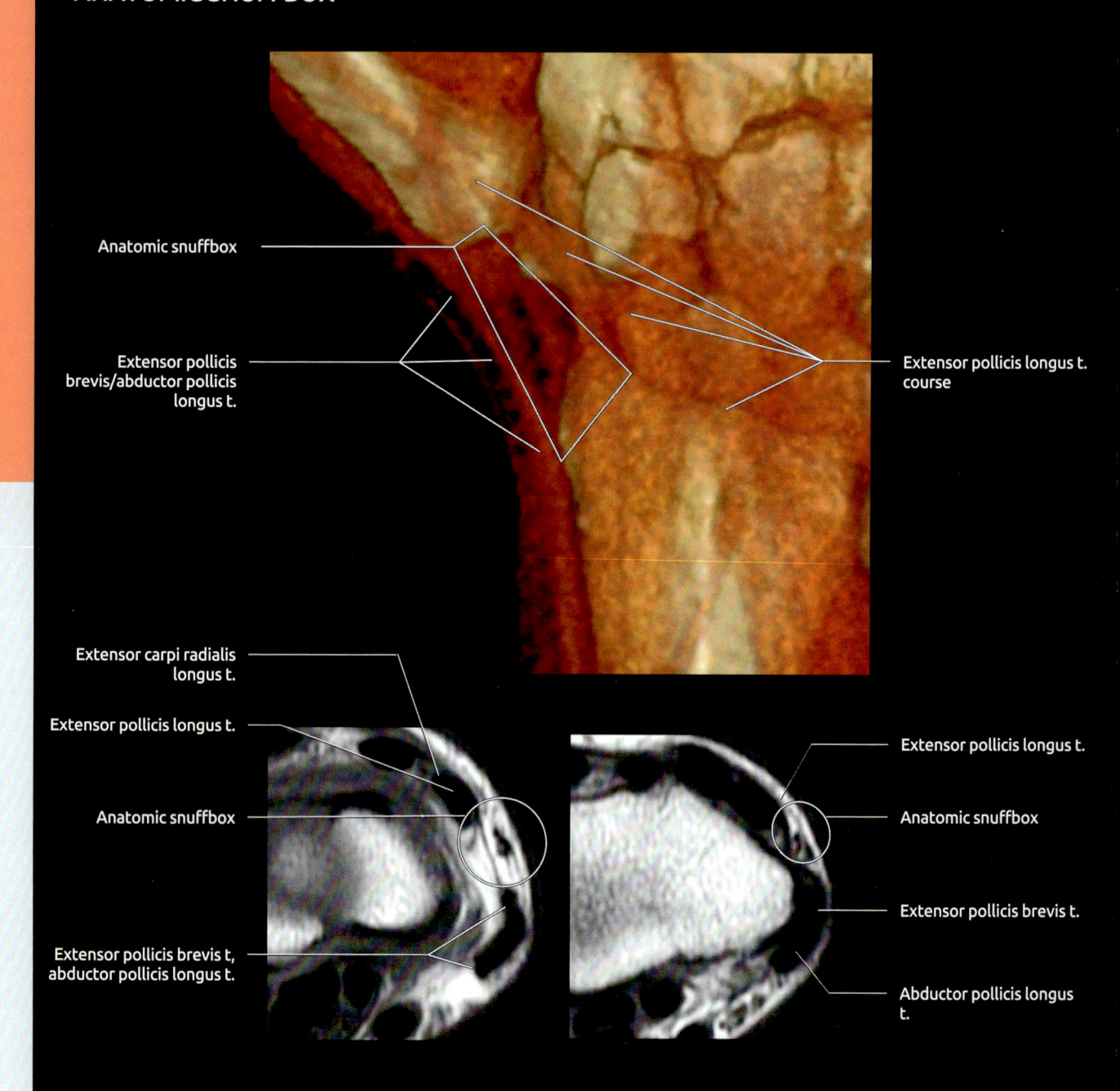

ANATOMIC SNUFFBOX

Anatomic snuffbox

Extensor pollicis brevis/abductor pollicis longus t.

Extensor pollicis longus t. course

Extensor carpi radialis longus t.

Extensor pollicis longus t.

Anatomic snuffbox

Extensor pollicis brevis t, abductor pollicis longus t.

Extensor pollicis longus t.

Anatomic snuffbox

Extensor pollicis brevis t.

Abductor pollicis longus t.

3D reconstruction CT with soft tissue overlay delineates margins of anatomic snuffbox with extensor pollicis longus (3rd compartment) crossing from medial to lateral over extensor carpi radialis brevis and longus tendons (2nd compartment), forming a dorsal margin, while abductor pollicis longus & extensor pollicis brevis tendons (1st compartment) form a volar margin. The radial nerve and superficial branch, as well as the arterial and venous branches, pass through snuffbox. MR images demonstrate snuffbox in axial plane.

Wrist Tendons

INTERSECTION ANATOMY

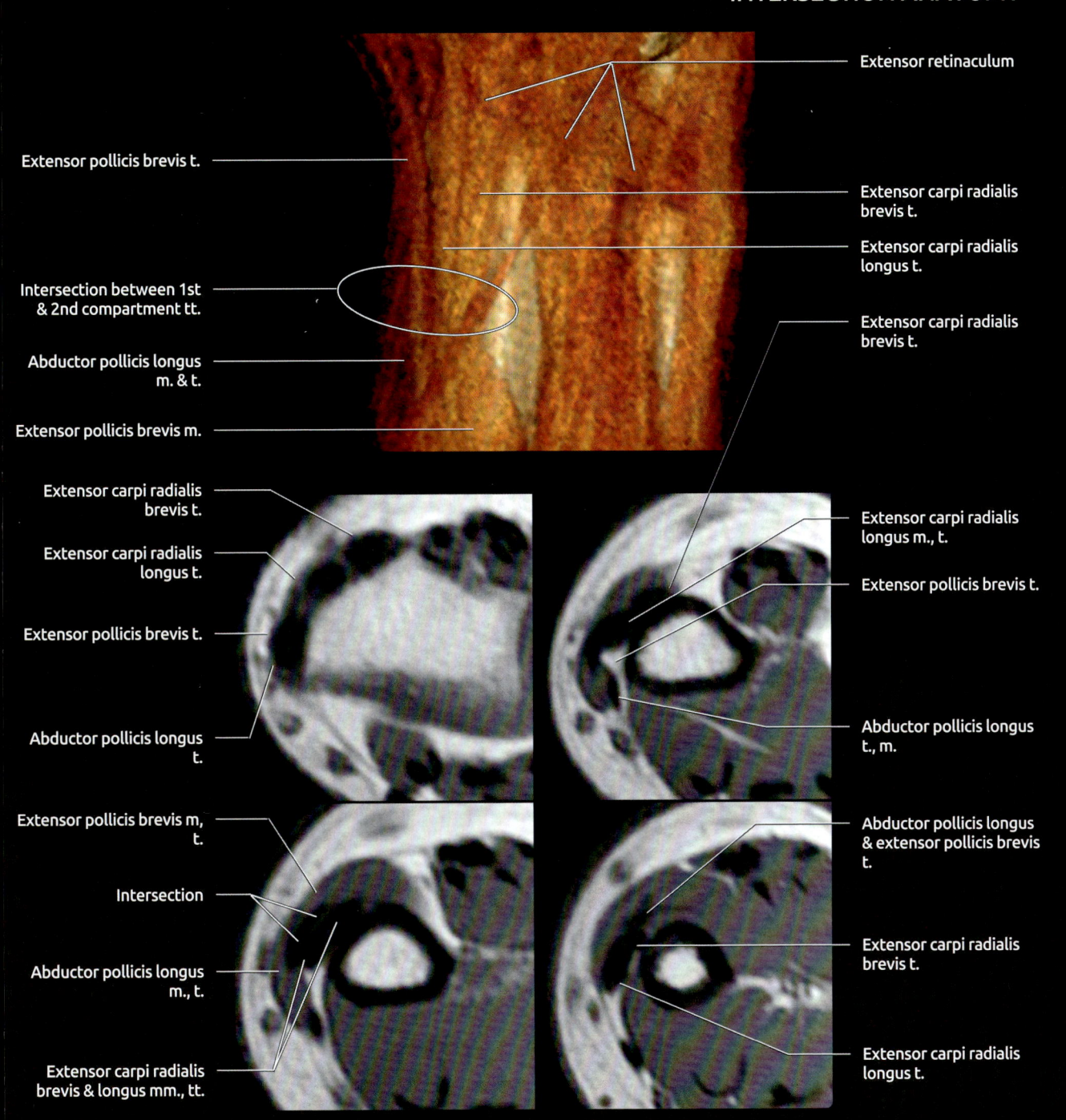

Extensor pollicis brevis t.

Extensor retinaculum

Extensor carpi radialis brevis t.

Extensor carpi radialis longus t.

Intersection between 1st & 2nd compartment tt.

Extensor carpi radialis brevis t.

Abductor pollicis longus m. & t.

Extensor pollicis brevis m.

Extensor carpi radialis brevis t.

Extensor carpi radialis longus m., t.

Extensor carpi radialis longus t.

Extensor pollicis brevis t.

Extensor pollicis brevis t.

Abductor pollicis longus t.

Abductor pollicis longus t., m.

Extensor pollicis brevis m, t.

Abductor pollicis longus & extensor pollicis brevis t.

Intersection

Abductor pollicis longus m., t.

Extensor carpi radialis brevis t.

Extensor carpi radialis brevis & longus mm., tt.

Extensor carpi radialis longus t.

3D reconstruction CT with soft tissue overlay demonstrates abductor pollicis longus & extensor pollicis brevis musculotendinous junctions sweeping distally & laterally, crossing over extensor carpi radialis longus & brevis tendons just proximal to extensor retinaculum. Axial MR demonstrates this complex relationship in cross section. Lower right MR is in the distal forearm and shows abductor pollicis longus & extensor pollicis brevis to be superficial & slightly dorsal to the extensor carpi radialis longus & brevis tendons. Lower left & upper right MRs show abductor pollicis longus & extensor pollicis brevis crossing over extensor carpi radialis longus & brevis to lie on the lateral aspect of the radius. Upper left MR is the most distal of this set, at the level of the Lister tubercle. The crossover is complete at this point & tendons are in their carpal positions.

SAGITTAL T1 MR: WRIST TENDONS

Radial styloid

Extensor pollicis longus tendon

Extensor carpi radialis longus tendon

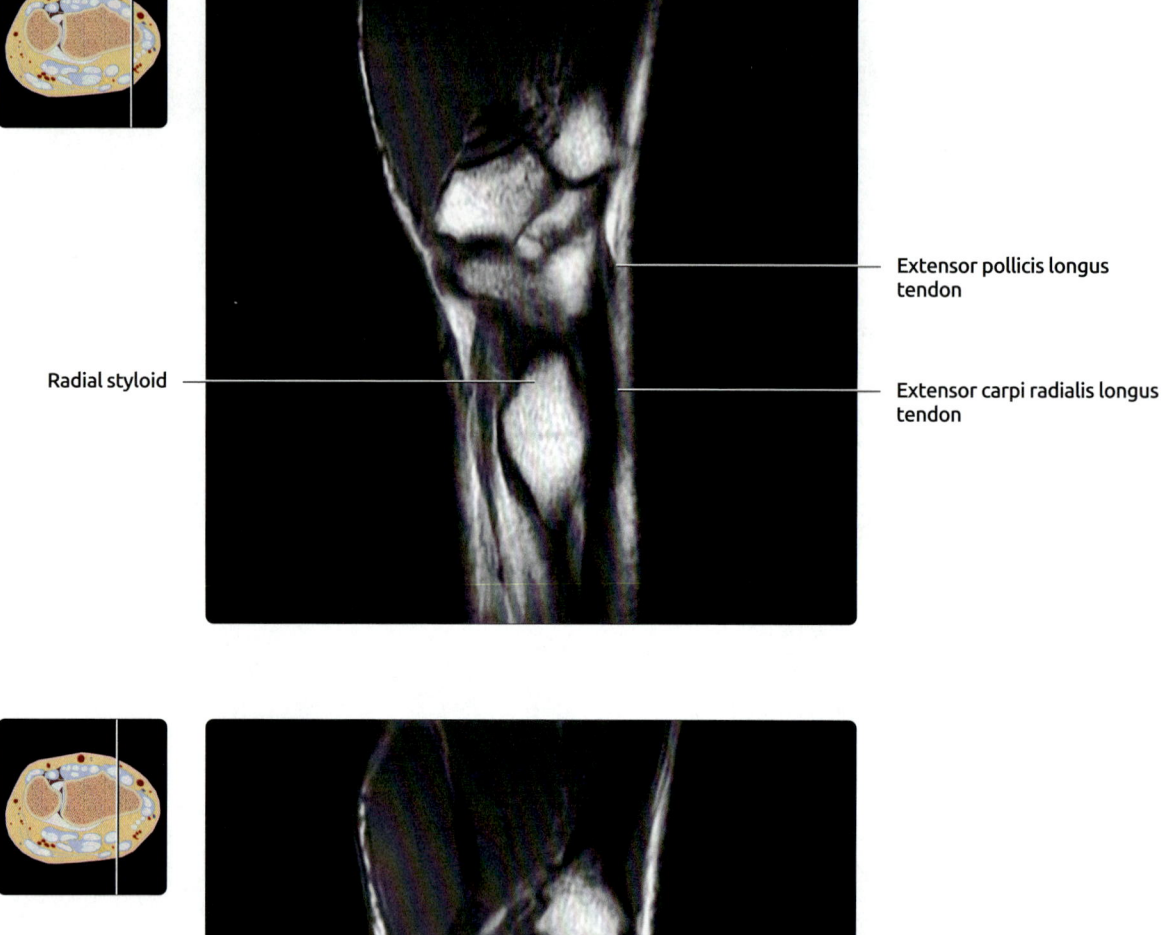

Flexor carpi radialis tendon

Extensor pollicis longus tendon

Extensor carpi radialis brevis tendon

(Top) The 1st of 8 sagittal images (from radial to ulnar) shows the relative position of wrist tendons. Extensor carpi radialis longus extends distal to the 2nd metacarpal base. Extensor pollicis longus is a thin tendon passing superficial & distal to the extensor carpi radialis longus & brevis tendons. (Bottom) Flexor carpi radialis is shown medial to scaphoid & along trapezium volar groove. Extensor carpi radialis brevis is medial to the extensor carpi radialis longus & extends to the 3rd metacarpal base.

Wrist Tendons

SAGITTAL T1 MR: WRIST TENDONS

Abductor pollicis brevis m.

Median n.

Flexor digitorum profundus t.

Flexor digitorum superficialis t.

Extensor digitorum t. slip

Abductor pollicis brevis m.

Flexor digitorum profundus t.

Flexor digitorum superficialis t.

Extensor digitorum t. slip

Extensor indicis t.

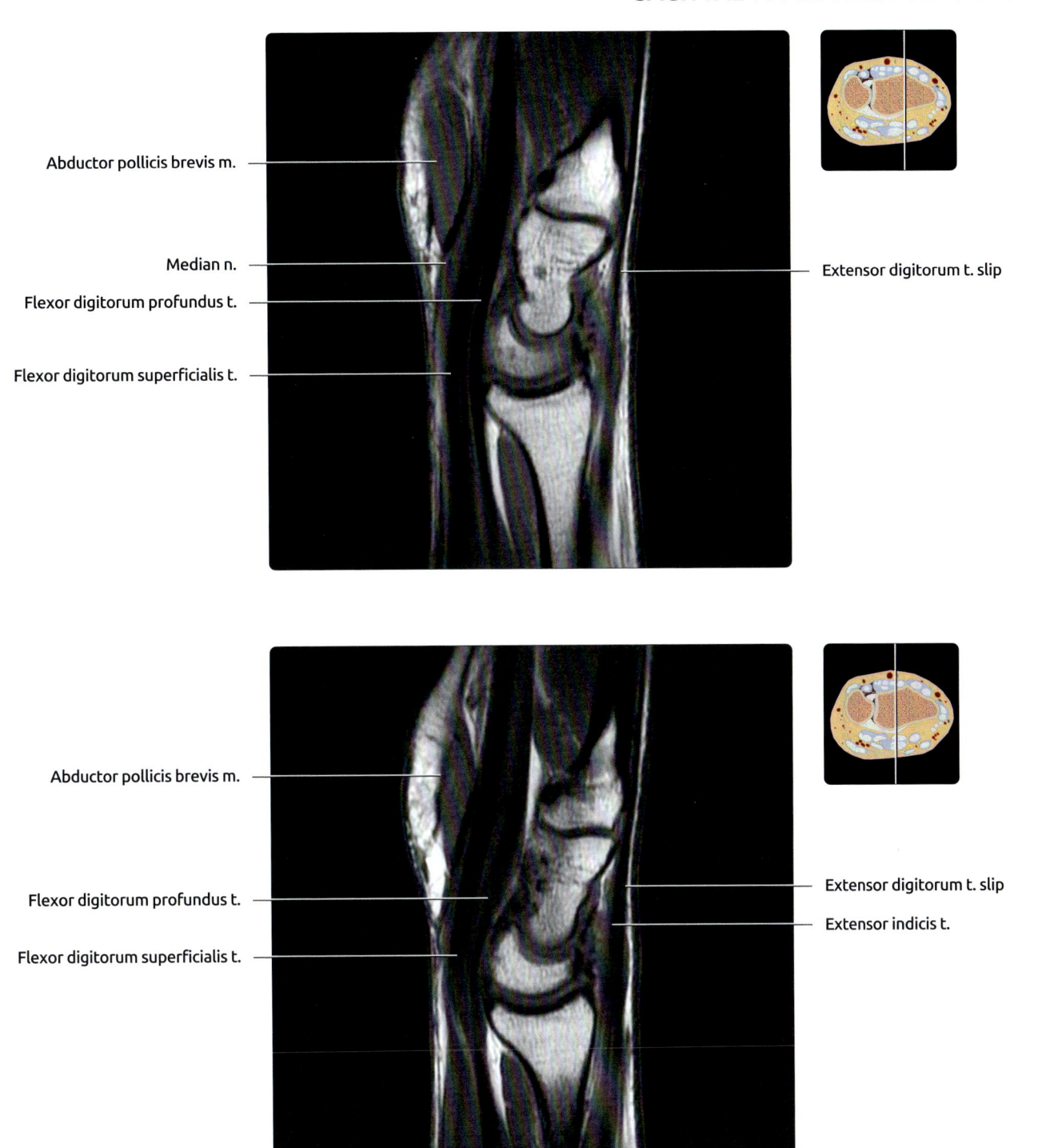

(Top) Flexor digitorum superficialis & profundus tendons are apparent in lateral carpal tunnel. Abductor pollicis brevis muscle arises from flexor retinaculum. (Bottom) Slightly medially, the extensor indicis tendon is deep to extensor digitorum tendon slips.

Wrist Tendons

SAGITTAL T1 MR: WRIST TENDONS

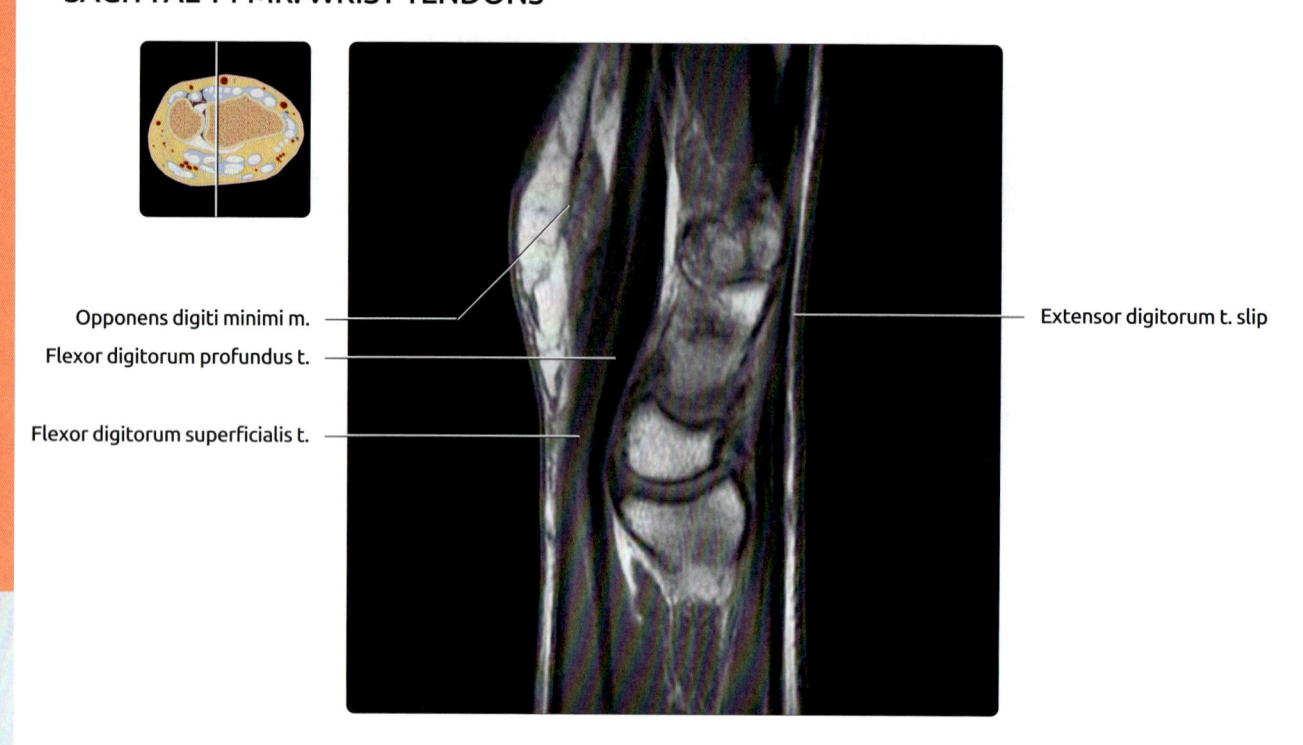

Opponens digiti minimi m.
Flexor digitorum profundus t.
Flexor digitorum superficialis t.
Extensor digitorum t. slip

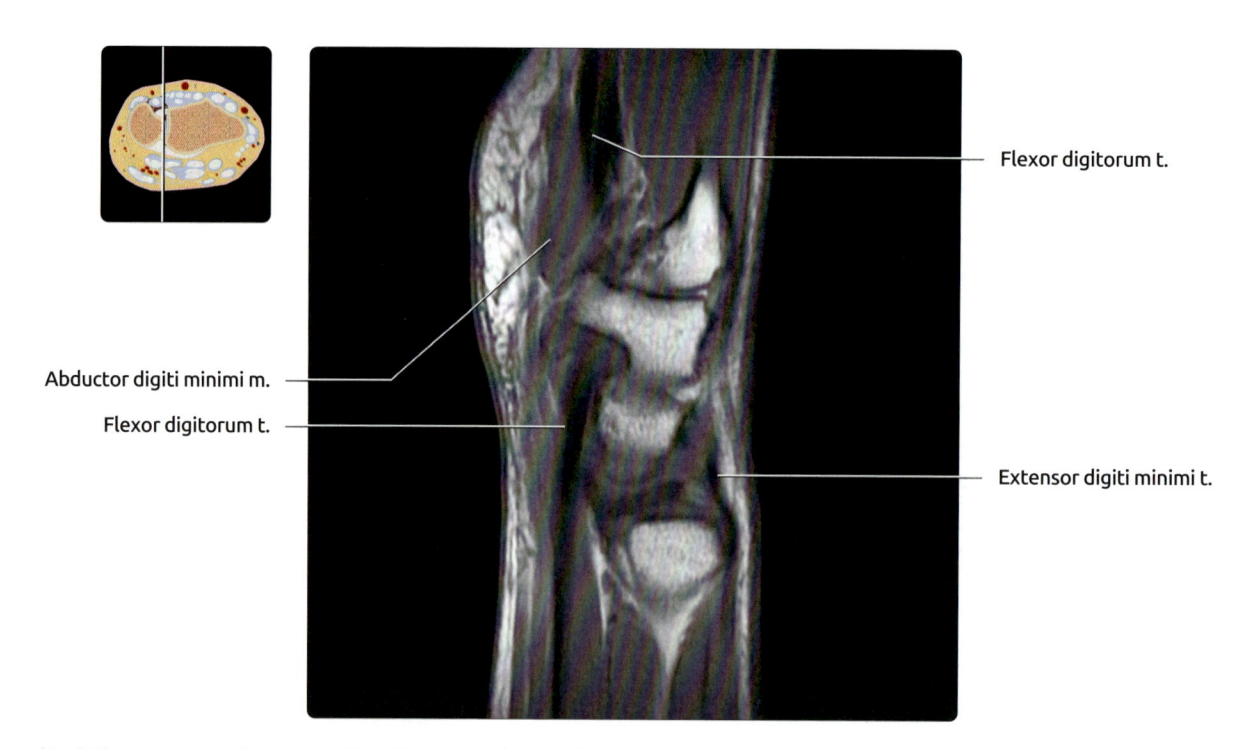

Abductor digiti minimi m.
Flexor digitorum t.
Flexor digitorum t.
Extensor digiti minimi t.

(Top) Flexor tendons of the ring & little finger pass deep to the flexor retinaculum in medial carpal tunnel. Hypothenar muscles take rise from the flexor retinaculum. (Bottom) Abductor digiti minimi arises from the flexor retinaculum. Extensor digiti minimi passes through the 5th extensor compartment.

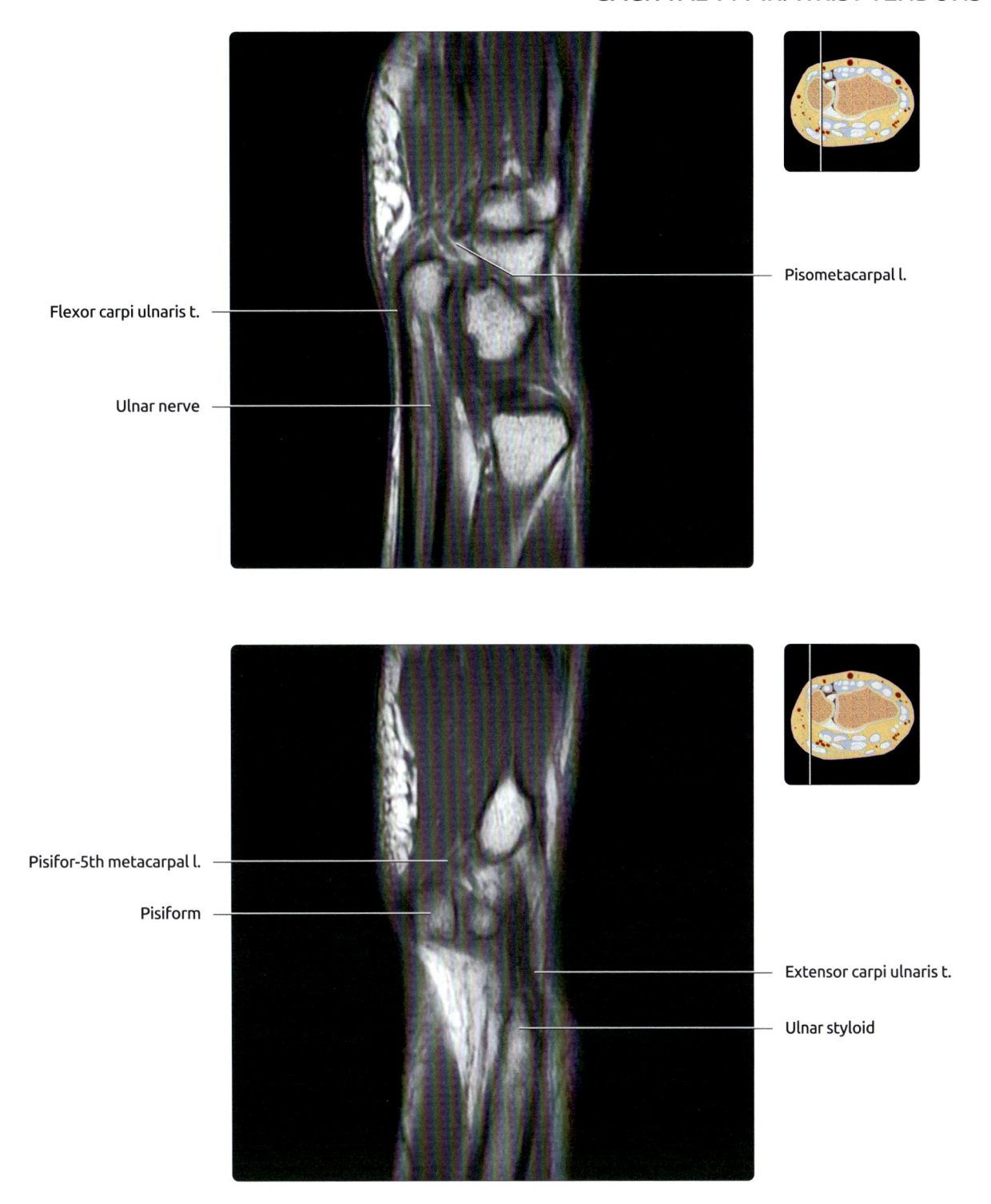

Wrist Tendons

SAGITTAL T1 MR: WRIST TENDONS

- Flexor carpi ulnaris t.
- Ulnar nerve
- Pisometacarpal l.

- Pisifor-5th metacarpal l.
- Pisiform
- Extensor carpi ulnaris t.
- Ulnar styloid

(Top) Flexor carpi ulnaris inserts on pisiform with fibers continuing distally as pisohamate & pisometacarpal ligaments. *(Bottom)* Extensor carpi ulnaris tendon passes over the dorsal groove of the distal ulna to insert on 5th metacarpal base.

Wrist Tendons

CORONAL GRE MR

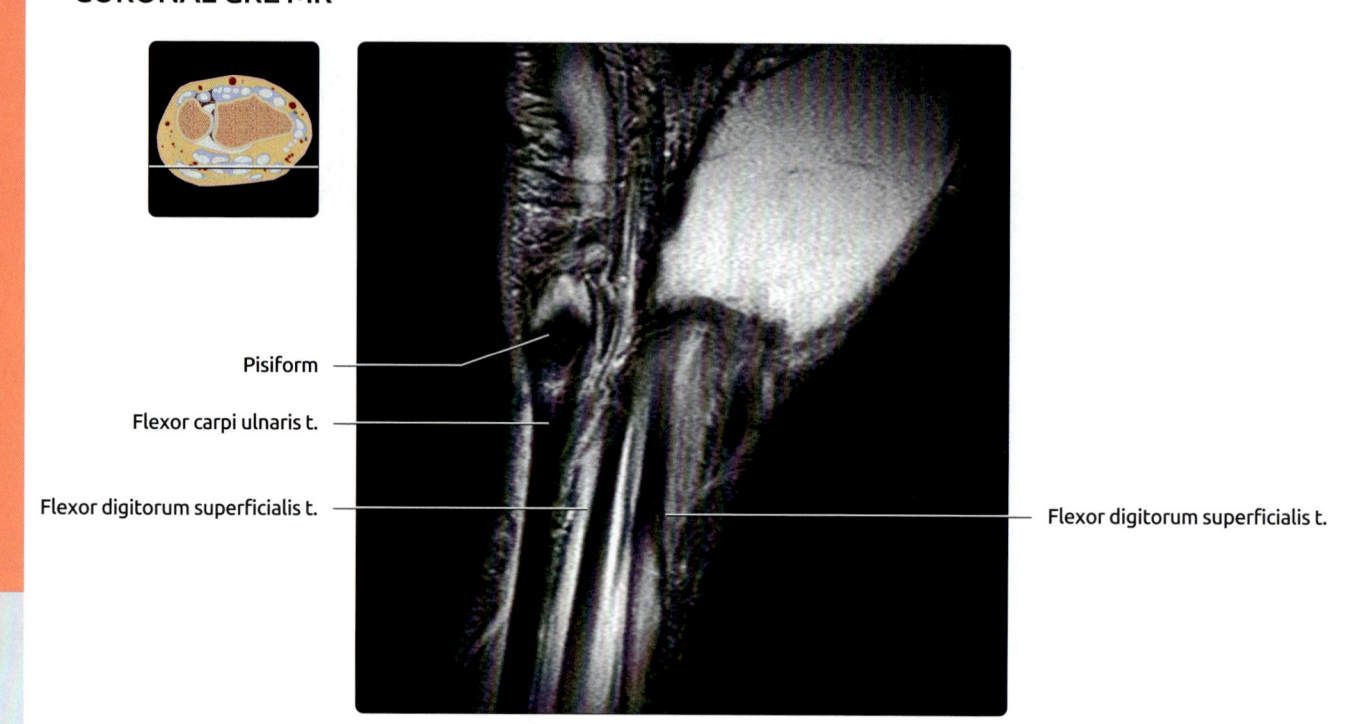

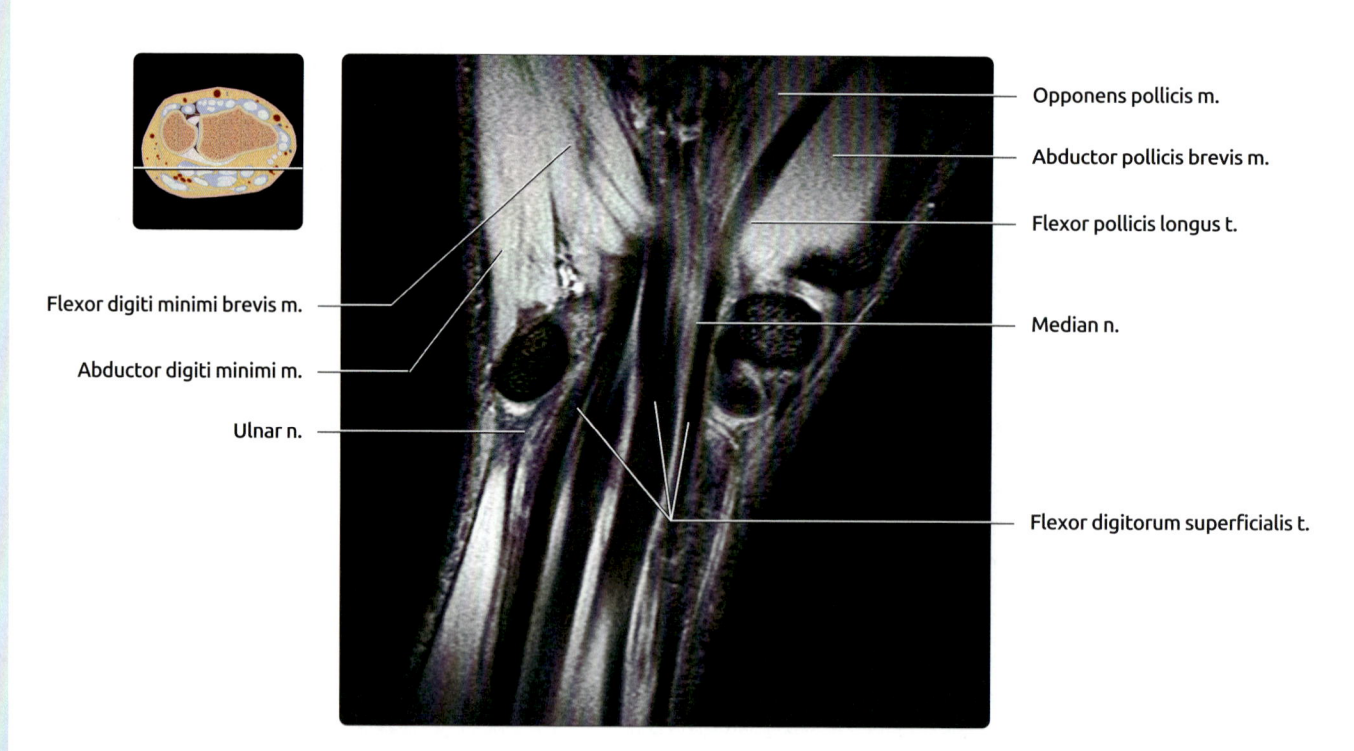

Pisiform

Flexor carpi ulnaris t.

Flexor digitorum superficialis t.

Flexor digitorum superficialis t.

Flexor digiti minimi brevis m.

Abductor digiti minimi m.

Ulnar n.

Opponens pollicis m.

Abductor pollicis brevis m.

Flexor pollicis longus t.

Median n.

Flexor digitorum superficialis t.

(Top) The 1st in a series of 8 selected coronal images (from volar to dorsal) is shown. Flexor carpi ulnaris inserts on pisiform while flexor digitorum superficialis tendons run deep to flexor retinaculum. *(Bottom)* Deep to the flexor retinaculum, the flexor digitorum profundus and superficialis tendons extend into hand. Hypothenar musculature arises from pisiform, hook of hamate, and flexor retinaculum. Thenar musculature arises from flexor retinaculum, scaphoid, trapezium, & trapezoid.

Wrist Tendons

CORONAL GRE MR

Flexor digiti minimi m.
Abductor digiti minimi tendon
Flexor digitorum profundus tendon
Pisohamate ligament
Ulnar nerve

Flexor pollicis longus tendon
Flexor digitorum superficialis tendon

Extensor carpi ulnaris tendon

Abductor pollicis longus tendon

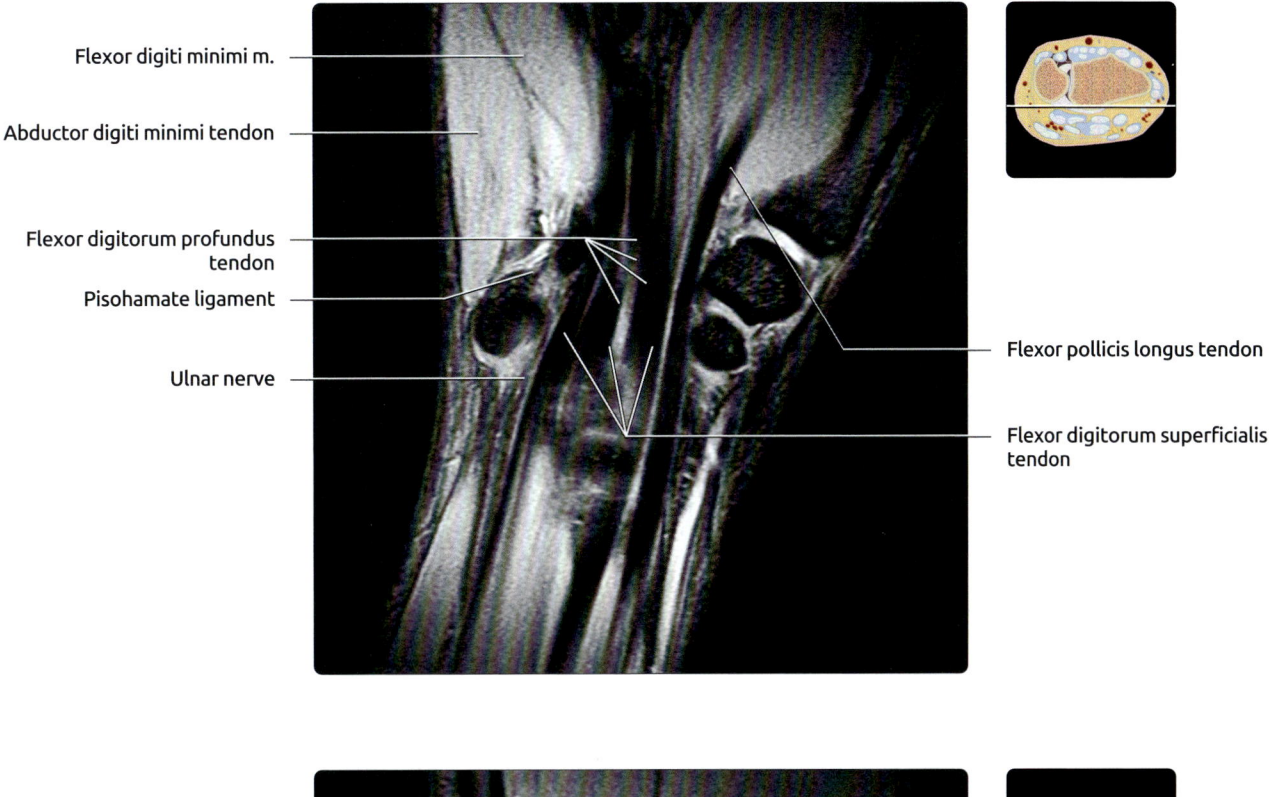

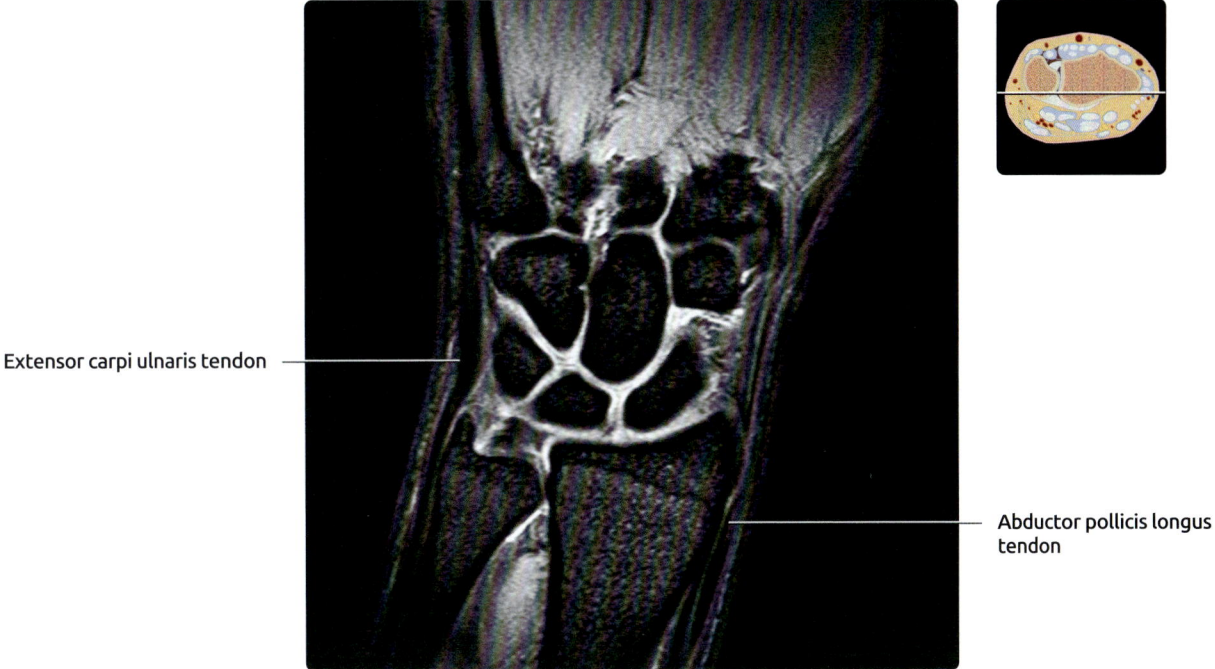

(Top) Carpal tunnel contains flexor digitorum tendons (profundus & superficialis) as well as flexor pollicis longus. *(Bottom)* Extensor carpi ulnaris passes over the FCU groove in the distal ulna, while abductor pollicis longus passes over the radial styloid.

Wrist Tendons

CORONAL GRE MR

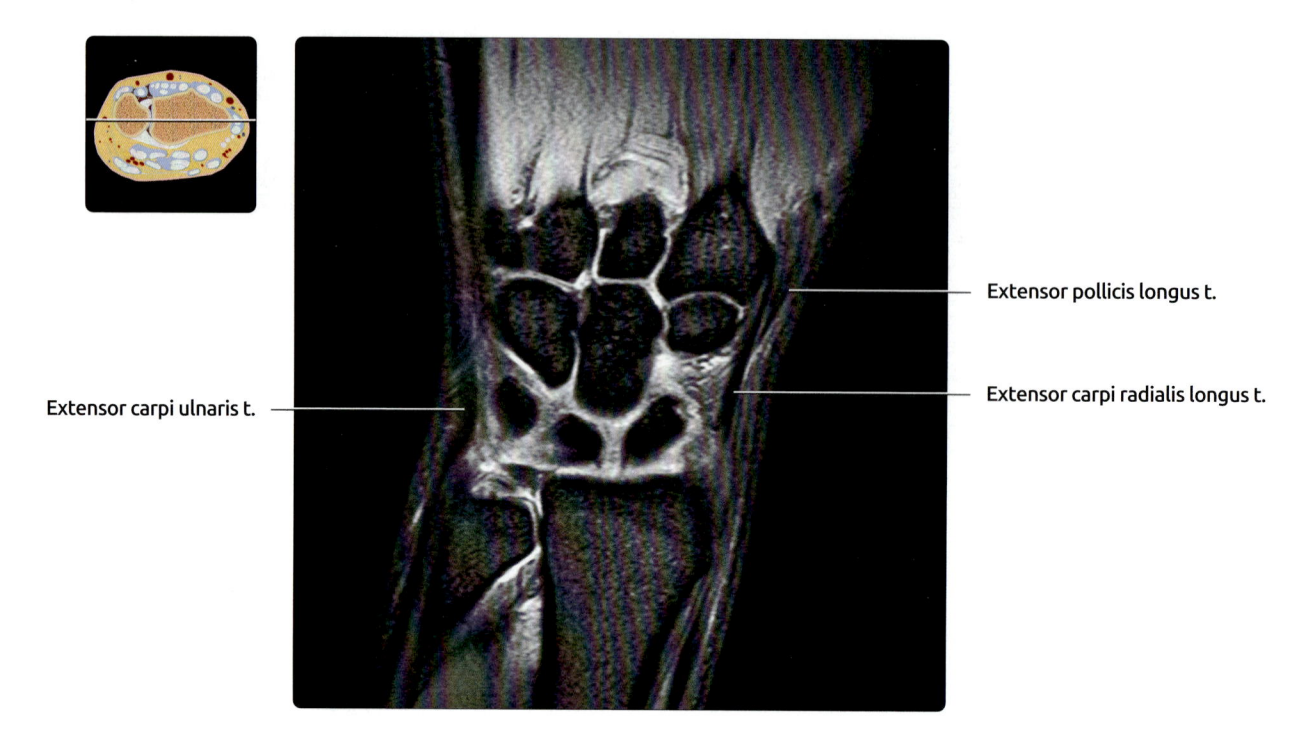

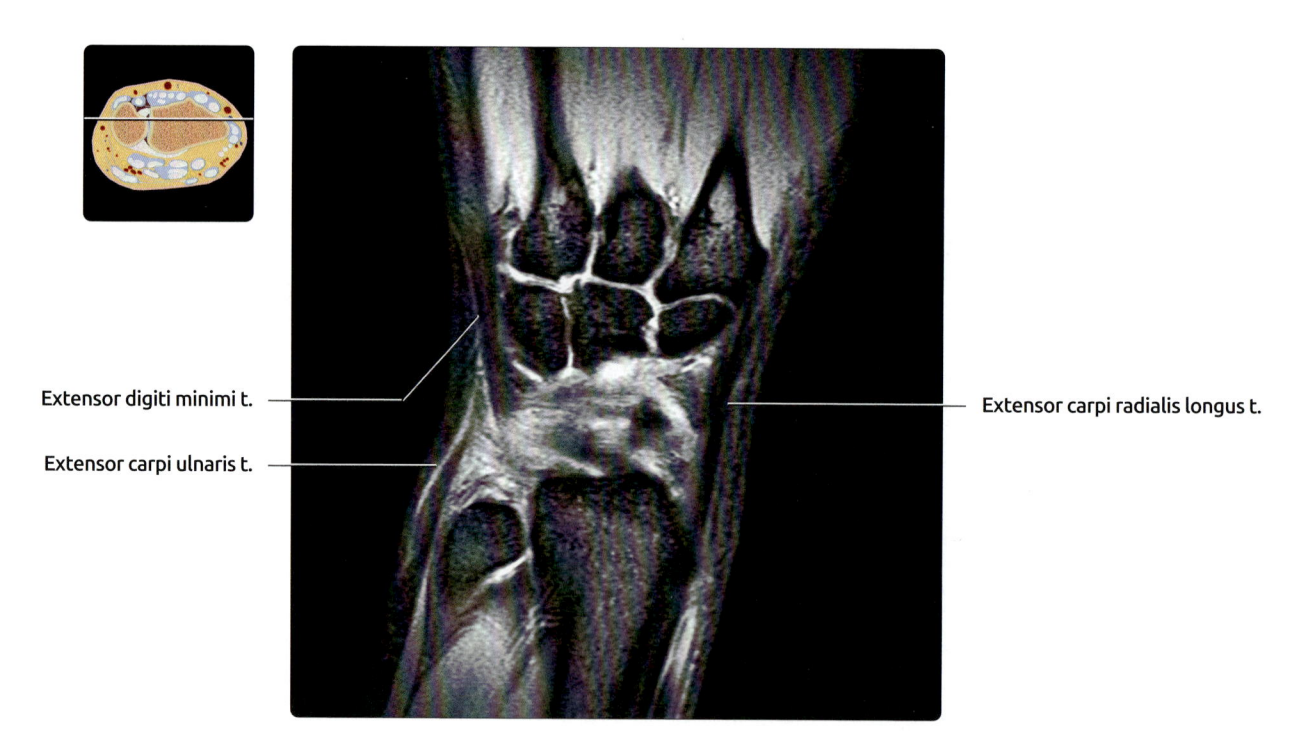

Extensor pollicis longus t.

Extensor carpi radialis longus t.

Extensor carpi ulnaris t.

Extensor digiti minimi t.

Extensor carpi ulnaris t.

Extensor carpi radialis longus t.

(Top) Dorsally, portions of extensor tendons become visible. *(Bottom)* Extensor digiti minimi sweeps distally & medially to insert on the little finger extensor hood. Extensor carpi radialis longus inserts on the 2nd metacarpal.

Wrist Tendons

CORONAL GRE MR

Extensor digitorum t. slip

Extensor digiti minimi t.

Extensor pollicis longus m., t.

Extensor carpi radialis brevis t.

Extensor carpi radialis longus t.

Lister tubercle

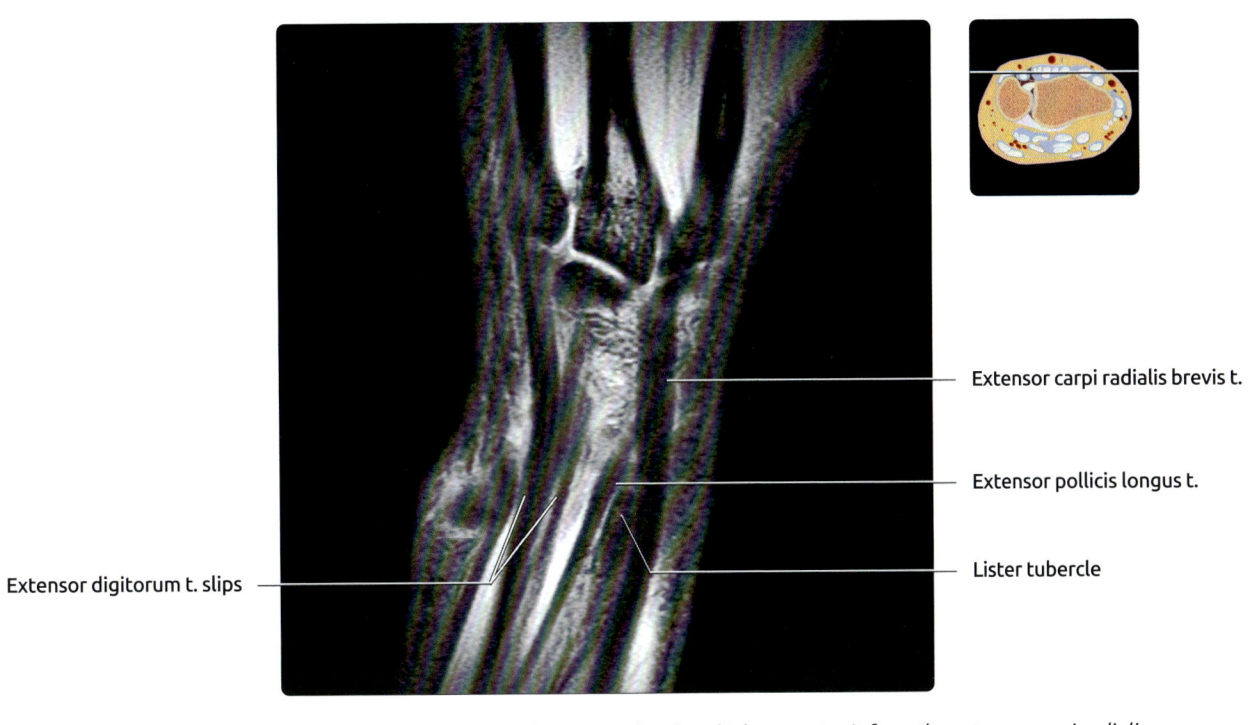

Extensor carpi radialis brevis t.

Extensor pollicis longus t.

Lister tubercle

Extensor digitorum t. slips

(Top) The extensor pollicis longus tendon is located medial to the Lister tubercle, which separates it from the extensor carpi radialis brevis at this level. Distal to the tubercle, the extensor pollicis longus crosses superficial to the extensor carpi radialis brevis, and courses laterally toward its insertion on the thumb. (Bottom) The extensor digitorum tendon slips pass through the 4th compartment. The extensor carpi radialis brevis inserts on the 2nd & 3rd metacarpals.

Wrist and Hand Normal Variants and Imaging Pitfalls

BONY VARIANTS

Type II Lunate
- Small facet at ulnar, distal margin of lunate articulates with tip of hamate
- Seen in 15% of population, usually asymptomatic
- Can present with impingement symptoms
  - Radiographs show sclerosis, cysts at site of abutment
  - MR shows chondromalacia, bone marrow edema

Carpal Coalitions (Uncommon)
- Between lunate & triquetrum
- Between pisiform, hook of hamate
- At radial side of wrist in cases of radial club hand

Accessory Centers of Ossification
- Much less common than in foot
- Many so-called accessory centers are probably old, nonunited fractures
- 2 most common accessory centers are os styloideum, trapezium secundarium, & os hamuli
- Trapezium secundarium
  - Accessory ossification center at ulnar aspect of 1st CMC joint
  - May be mistaken for an avulsion fracture, especially when small
- Os hamuli
  - Separate ossification for hook of hamate
- Os styloideum/carpal boss
  - Secondary center of ossification at base of 3rd metacarpal
  - Extensor carpi radialis brevis attaches here
  - Presents with bony prominence, occasionally pain due to muscle pull on synchondrosis
- Pseudoepiphysis
  - Normal ossification centers are at base of 1st metacarpal, neck of metacarpals 2-5
  - Accessory ossification centers (pseudoepiphysis) may occur at neck of 1st metacarpal, base of 2nd-5th metacarpals
    - May traverse entire bone or may be incomplete cleft in bone
    - Do not significantly contribute to bone growth
  - Occasionally mistaken for fracture

Pseudoerosions
- Small round or oval notches at margins of proximal phalangeal bases
- May be mistaken for erosions; however, they are smooth and well corticated

Sesamoids
- Up to 2 sesamoids can be present at each metacarpophalangeal joint and at 3rd distal interphalangeal joint
- 1 sesamoid can be present at each distal interphalangeal joint
- Sesamoids are usually embedded in volar plate

Bipartite Lunate
- Rare; lunate split in coronal plane into equal volar and dorsal parts

Duplication of Digits
- Fairly common isolated anomaly

TENDON AND MUSCLE VARIANTS

Accessory Abductor Digiti Minimi (24%)
- Muscle located palmar and lateral (radial) to pisiform is diagnostic

Proximal Origin of Lumbricals (22%)
- Lumbricals in carpal tunnel when fingers are extended is diagnostic
- Lumbricals may normally migrate proximally into carpal tunnel when fingers are flexed

Extensor Digitorum Manus Brevis (1-3%)
- Muscle belly associated with extensor digitorum tendons distal to carpometacarpal joint is diagnostic

Palmaris Longus Variants
- Normal muscle belly should be only in the proximal half of the forearm, and the tendon inserts on/in the palmar aponeurosis
- Variants may have a distal muscle belly, digastric muscle bellies, or muscle along almost entirety of the expected course of the tendon
- Muscle tissue in the midline superficial to the flexor retinaculum at the level of the carpus is diagnostic
- Not to be confused with the Palmaris brevis (normal structure) which is ulnar (not midline) and more distal (level of carpometacarpal joint)

Digastric Flexor Digitorum Superficialis of 2nd Digit
- A 2nd muscle belly is present in the mid-portion of the flexor digitorum superficialis tendon to the 2nd digit at mid-metacarpal level

NEUROVASCULAR VARIANTS

Persistent Median Artery
- Normally regresses in utero
- May persist, accompany median nerve through carpal tunnel

Median Nerve Variants
- Normally bifurcates after carpal tunnel, but may bifurcate in tunnel or proximal to tunnel
- Martin-Gruber anastomoses: Branches of the median nerve anastomoses with the ulnar nerve in forearm
- Riche-Cannieu anastomoses: Recurrent branch of the median nerve anastomoses with deep branch of the ulnar nerve.

Superficial Palmar Arterial Arch
- Superficial and deep arches normally are supplied from both radial & ulnar arteries
- Superficial arch may arise only from ulnar artery, which increases risk of ischemia

Wrist and Hand Normal Variants and Imaging Pitfalls

NORMAL VARIANT: TYPE II LUNATE

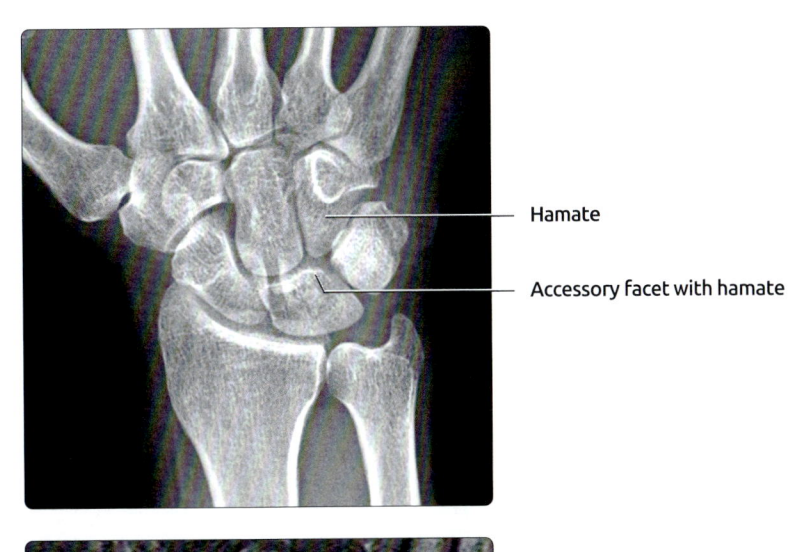

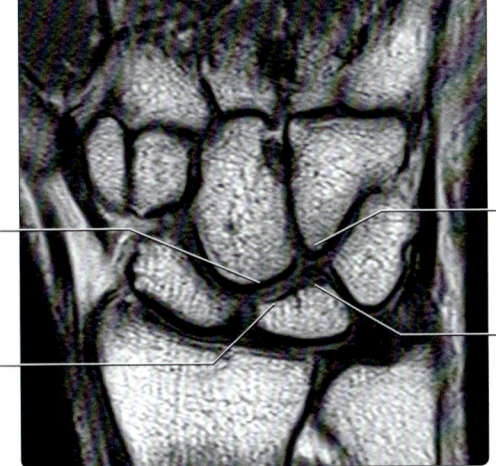

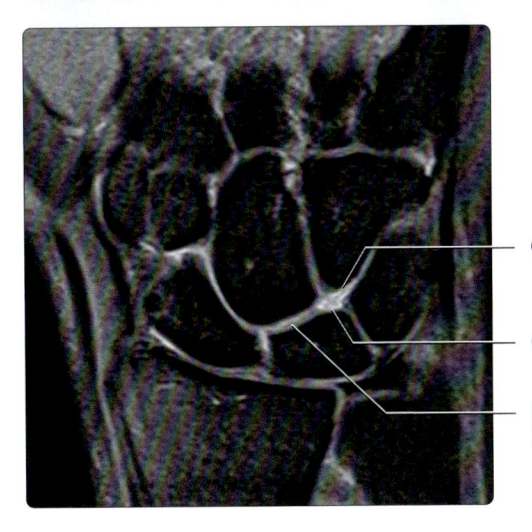

(Top) Type II lunate has an additional facet articulating with the hamate, and is seen in ~ 15% of the normal population. There can be resultant impingement of the hamate and lunate. Imaging signs of impingement on radiographs are cysts and sclerosis. MR shows bone marrow edema, cartilage loss, and subchondral cysts when impingement is present. *(Middle)* T1 MRI shows a Type II lunate. This morphology of the lunate has an "extra" facet that articulates with the hamate, often resulting in chondromalacia and arthritis. The remaining "normal" portion of the lunate mid-carpal articulation is concave, articulating with the capitate. *(Bottom)* T2FS MR of type II lunate shows chondromalacia at the extra lunate facet, and the adjacent hamate.

Wrist and Hand Normal Variants and Imaging Pitfalls

CARPAL COALITIONS

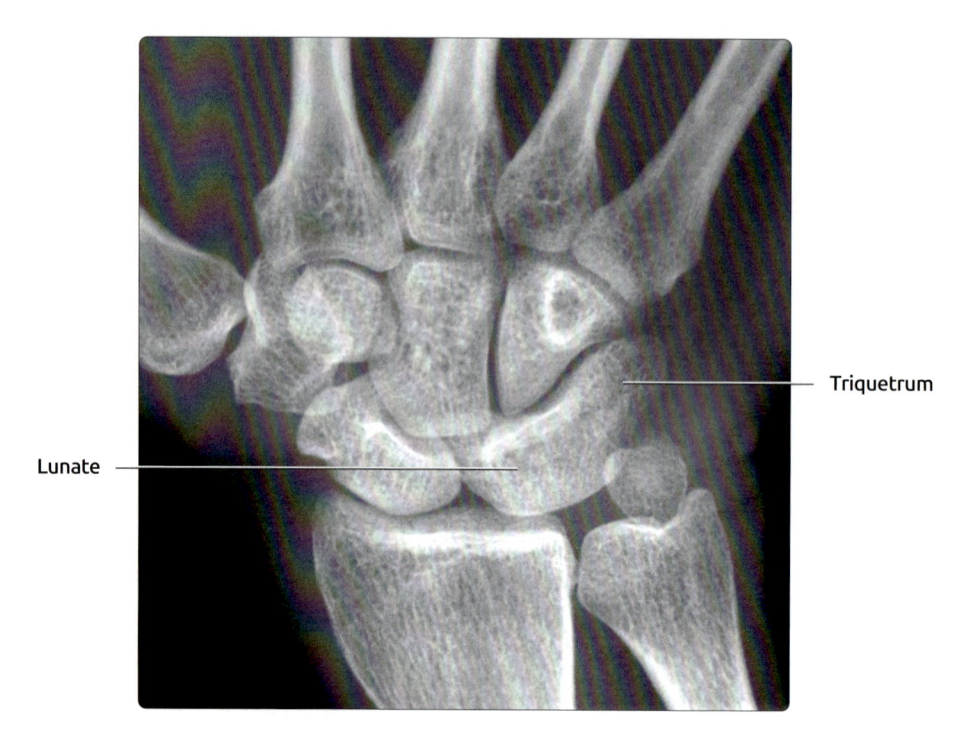

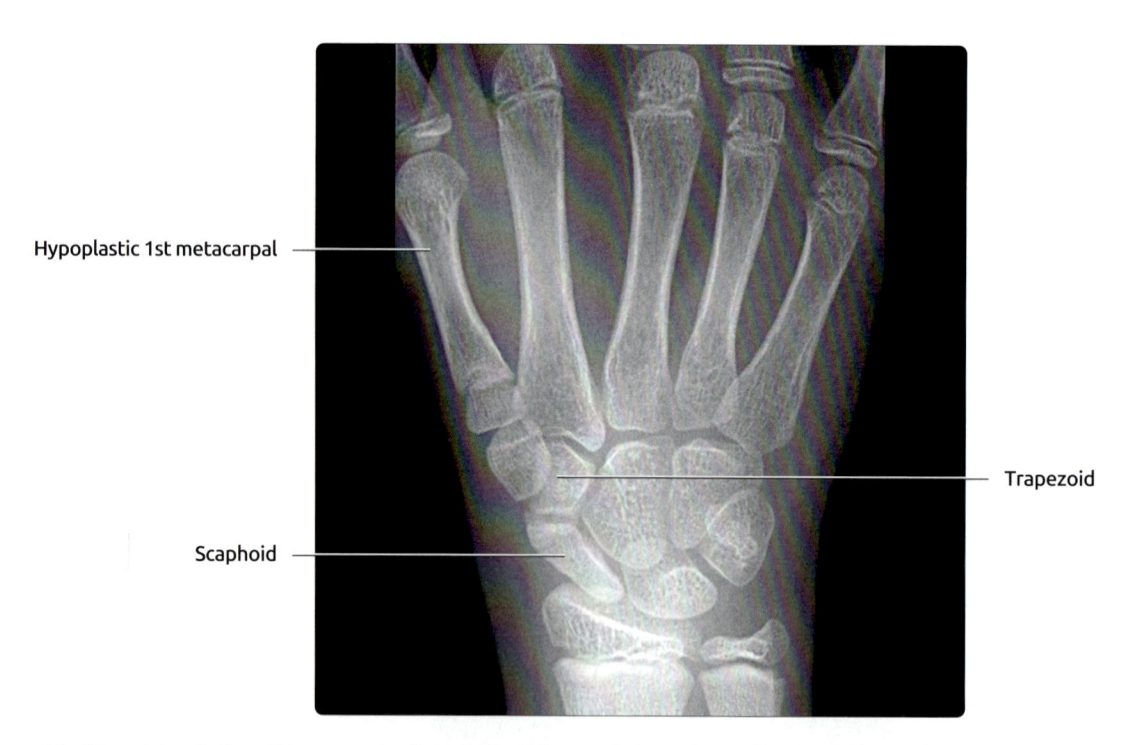

(Top) Lunotriquetral coalition occurs in about 0.1% of the population. It is usually asymptomatic, but possibly associated with increased risk of triangular fibrocartilage tear. *(Bottom)* Coalitions at the radial side of the wrist are usually associated with other anomalies. In this case, there is a coalition of the scaphoid and trapezoid, associated with hypoplasia of the thumb (part of the spectrum of radial club hand.)

Wrist and Hand Normal Variants and Imaging Pitfalls

HAMATE-PISIFORM COALITION

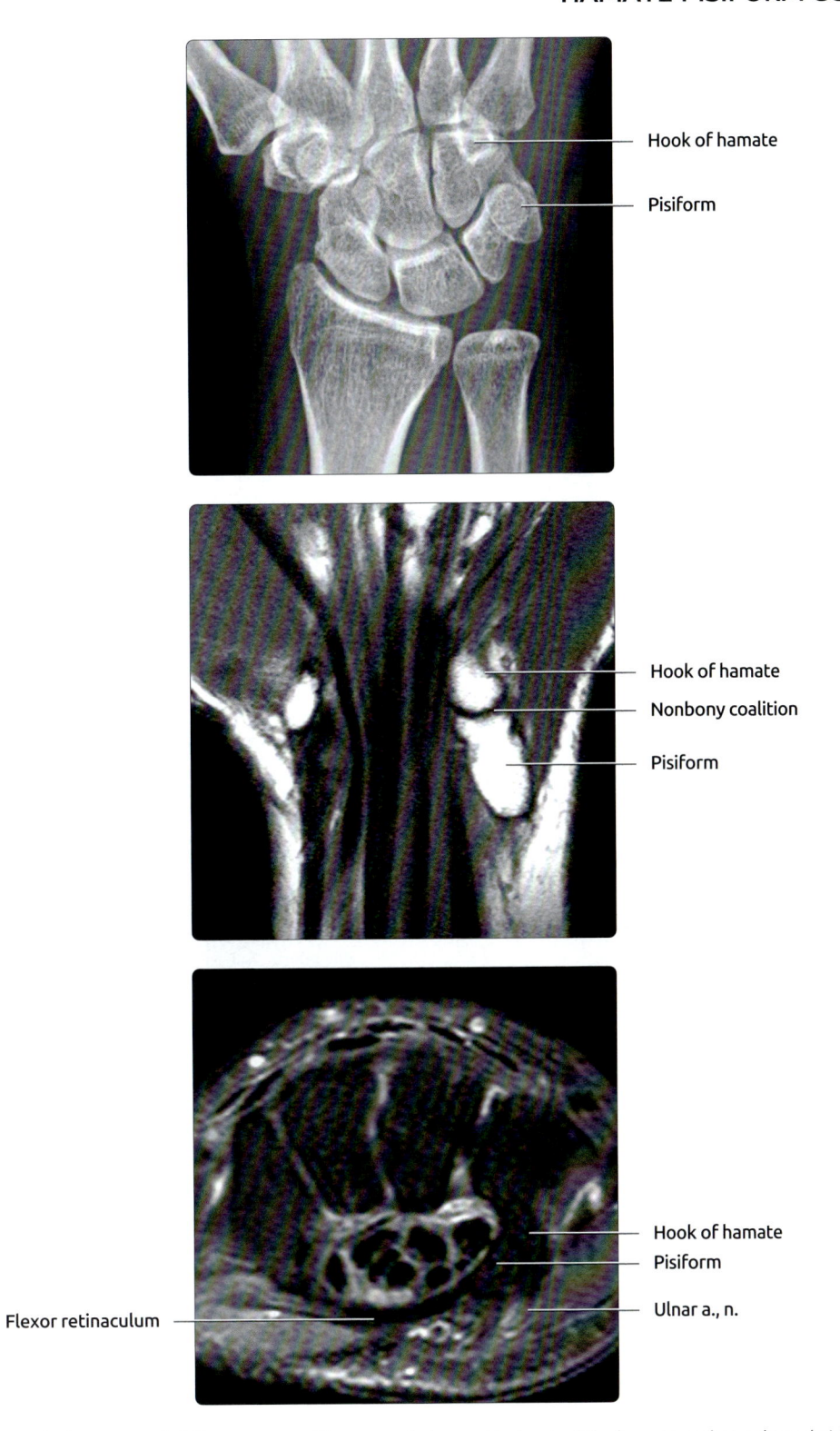

(Top) Coalitions between the hamate and pisiform are rare. They occur between the hook of the hamate and an enlarged pisiform. They may be osseous or fibrous. They are generally asymptomatic, but have been reported as a cause of both ulnar nerve impingement and carpal tunnel syndrome. (Middle) T1 MR shows the enlarged pisiform united to the hook of the hamate via a cartilaginous or fibrous coalition. (Bottom) Axial T2 FS MR shows elongated pisiform extending radially to partly cover the carpal tunnel.

Wrist and Hand Normal Variants and Imaging Pitfalls

CARPAL BOSS: OS STYLOIDEUM

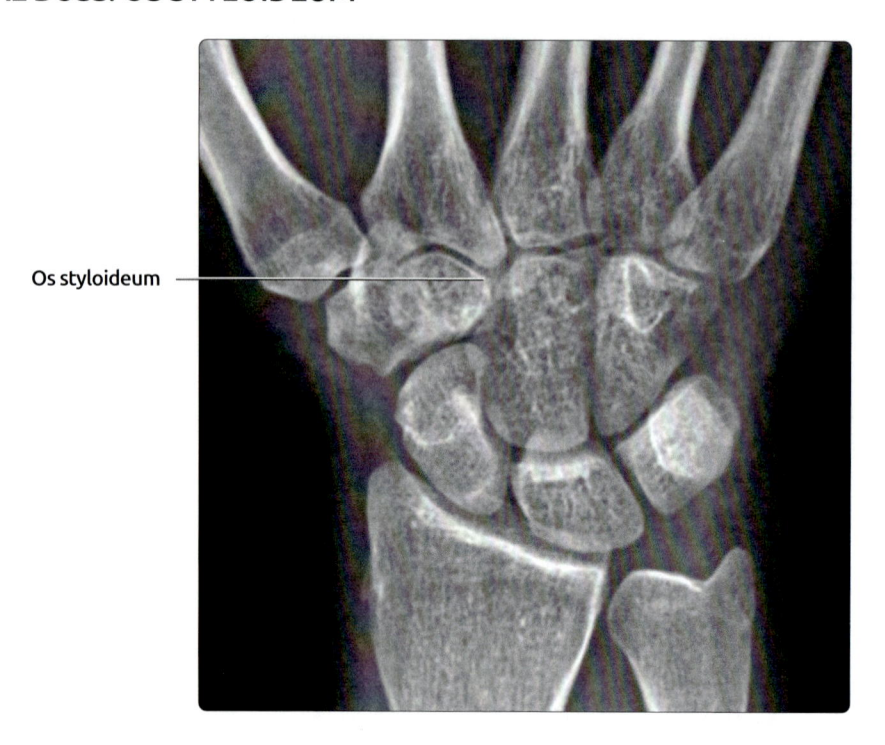

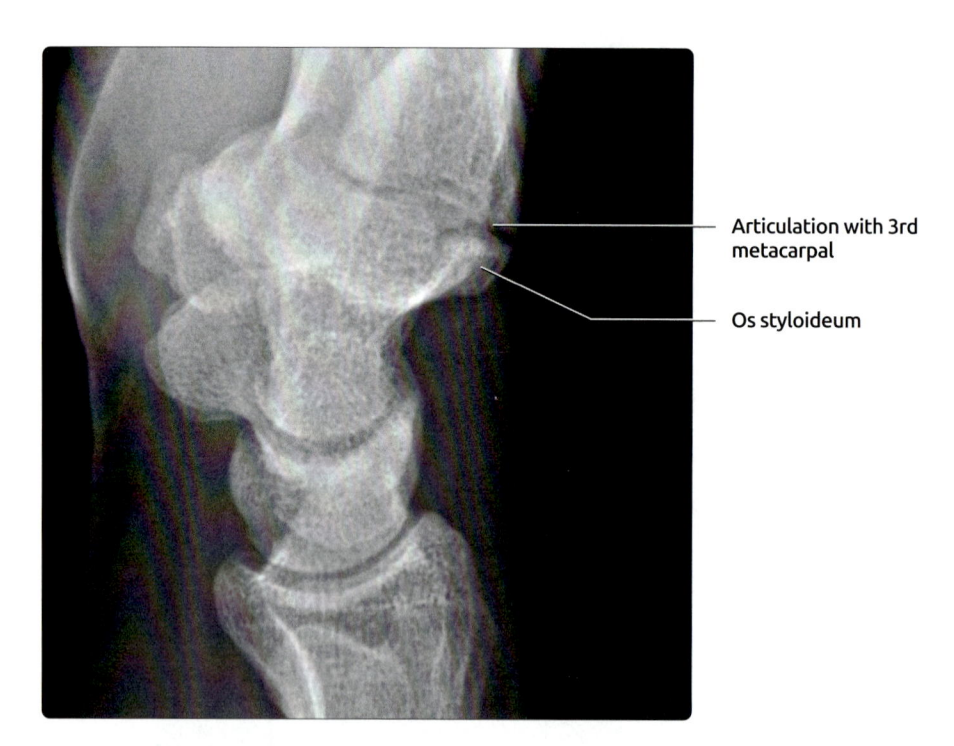

(Top) The enlarged styloid process at the base of the 3rd metacarpal has formed a secondary ossicle in this case, the os styloideum. Carpal boss refers to the resultant bony prominence palpable at the dorsum of the wrist. (Bottom) On the lateral view, the rounded bony prominence formed by the ossicle is more readily appreciable.

Wrist and Hand Normal Variants and Imaging Pitfalls

CARPAL BOSS, MR

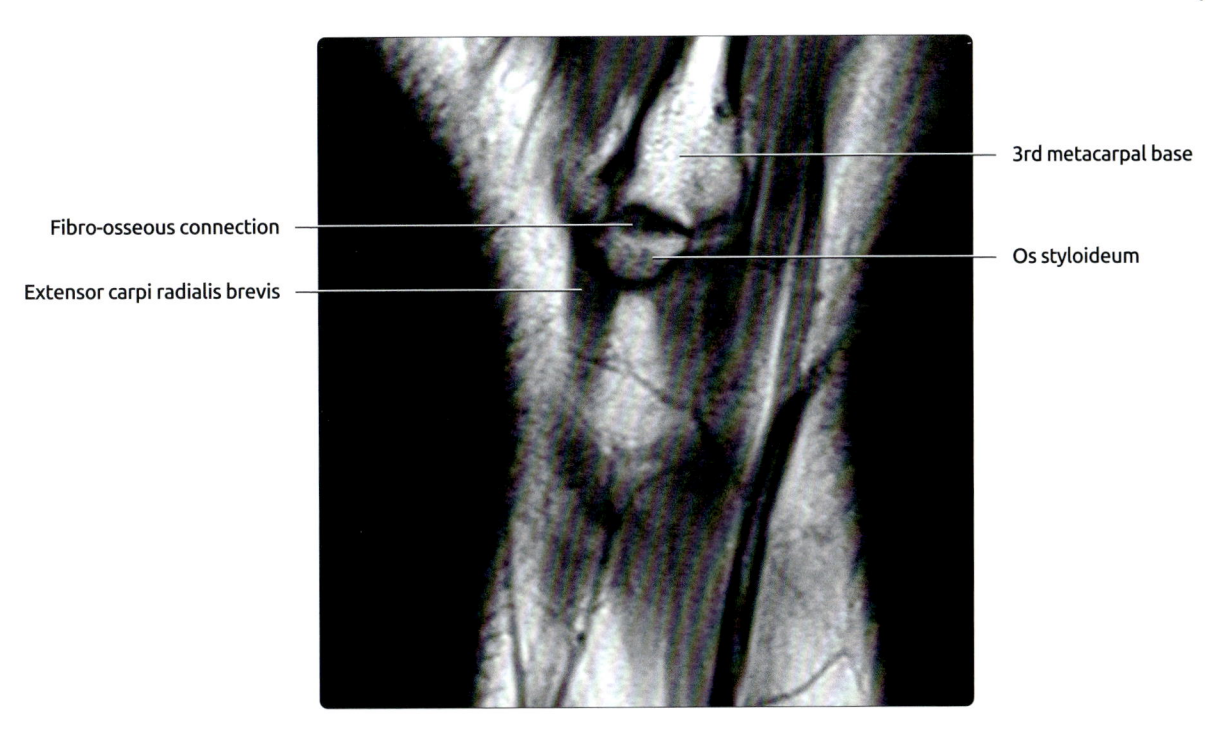

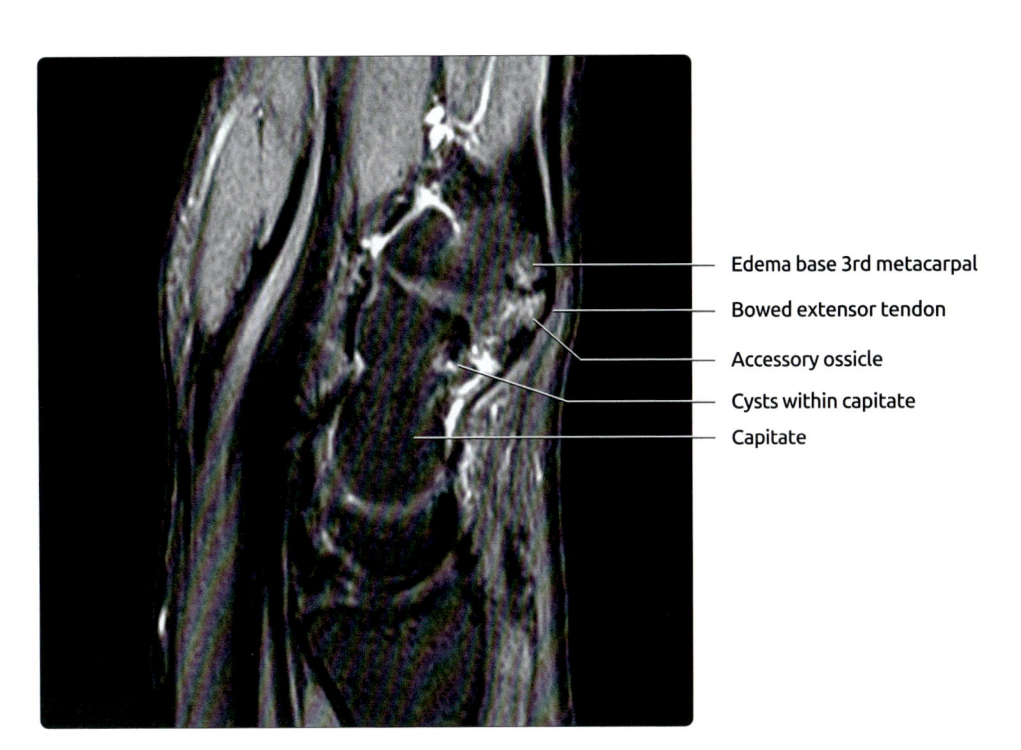

(Top) The extensor carpi radialis brevis tendon attaches primarily to the os styloideum. Rarely, an ossicle will present with pain related to increased stress on the extensor carpi radialis brevis. (Bottom) Sagittal T2 FS MR shows the accessory ossicle between the dorsal superior capitate and dorsal inferior 3rd metacarpal. There is edema within the ossicle and adjacent bones, as well as cyst formation in the adjacent capitate. The overlying extensor tendon is bowed.

OS HAMULI

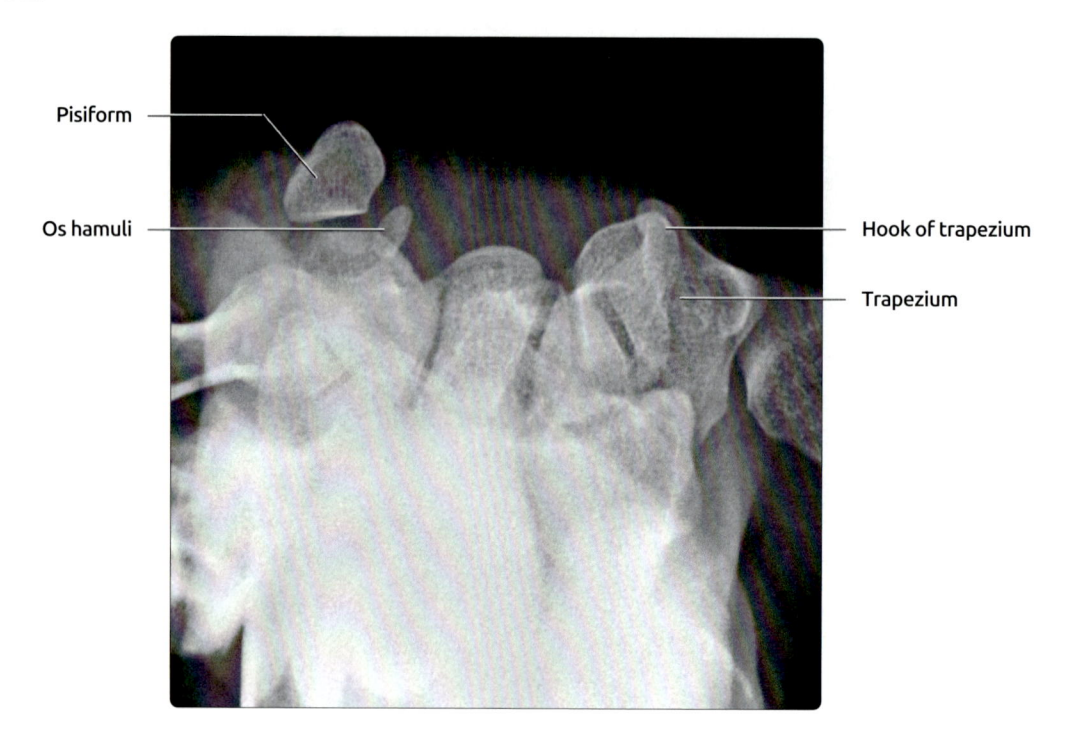

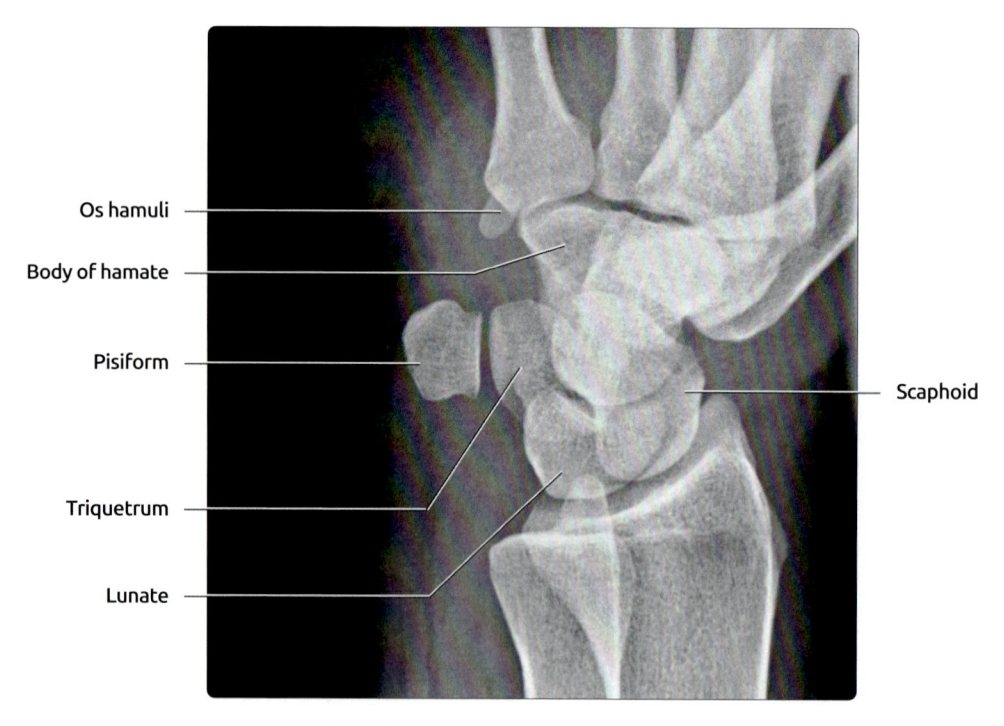

(Top) Carpal tunnel view shows an ovoid os hamuli. When evaluating a carpal tunnel view, it is useful to remember that the trapezium, as well as the hamate, has a volar hook (Bottom) Supinated view brings the hook of the hamate into profile and shows the os hamuli.

Wrist and Hand Normal Variants and Imaging Pitfalls

ANOMALOUS MUSCLES

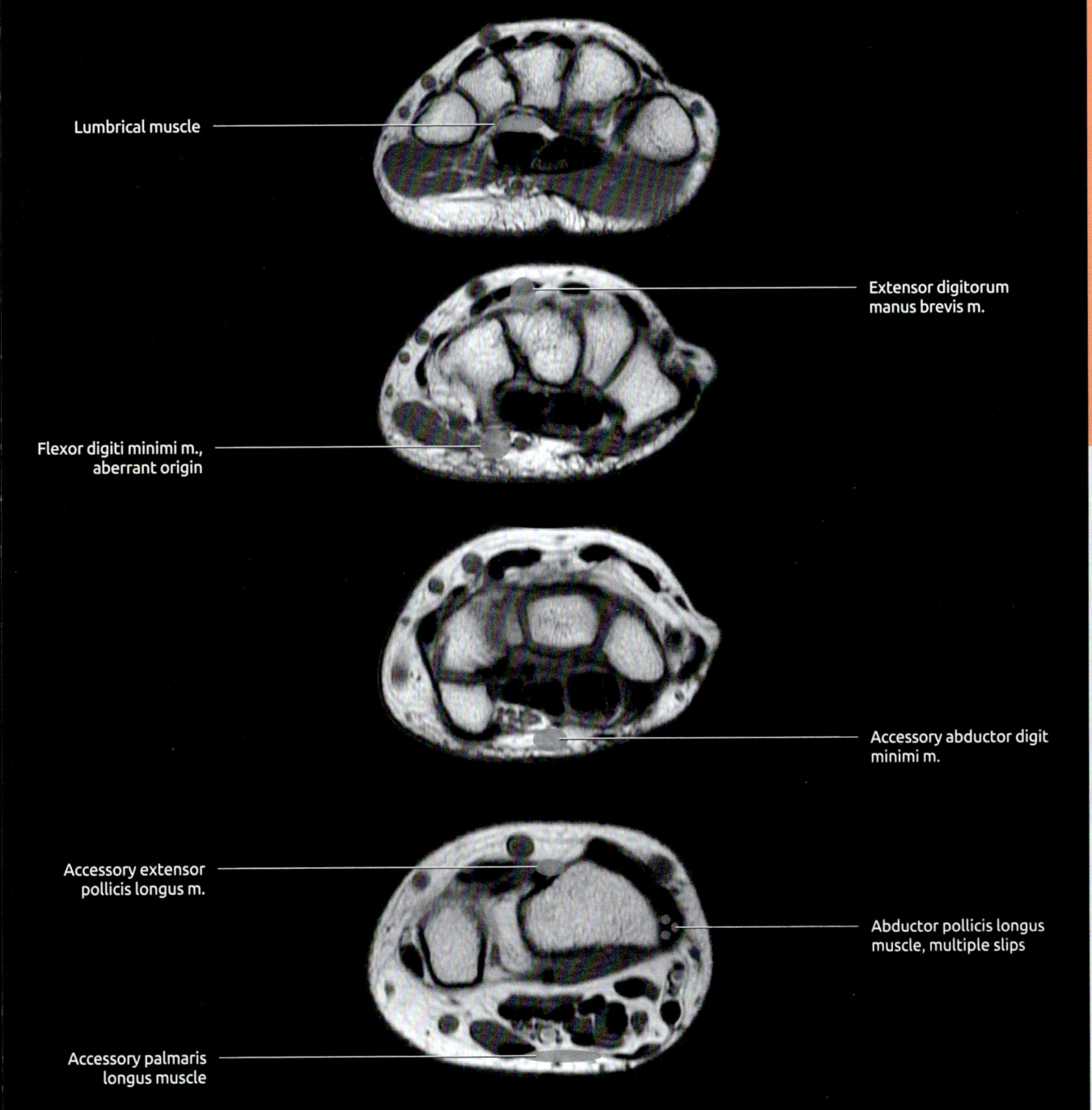

Lumbrical muscle

Extensor digitorum manus brevis m.

Flexor digiti minimi m., aberrant origin

Accessory abductor digit minimi m.

Accessory extensor pollicis longus m.

Abductor pollicis longus muscle, multiple slips

Accessory palmaris longus muscle

Anomalous muscle origins are shown. Lumbrical muscles may arise proximally within carpal tunnel, causing carpal tunnel syndrome. Extensor digitorum manus brevis may present as tender mass. Aberrant flexor digiti minimi origin may compress ulnar nerve. Accessory abductor digiti minimi may compress ulnar or median nerve. Accessory extensor pollicis longus may present as a tender mass. Abductor pollicis longus may have multiple slips & should not be mistaken for a tear. Palmaris longus has many variants; low-lying muscle bellies or multiple slips may compress median nerve.

Wrist and Hand Normal Variants and Imaging Pitfalls

PSEUDOEPIPHYSES (ACCESSORY EPIPHYSES)

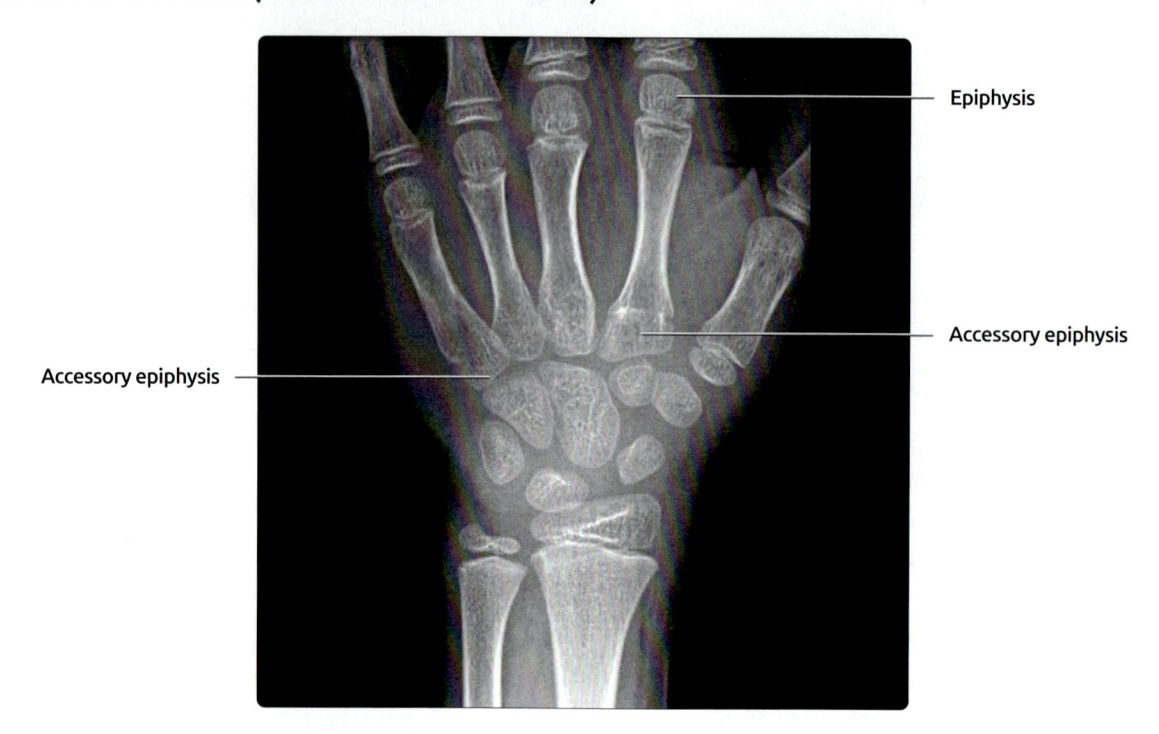

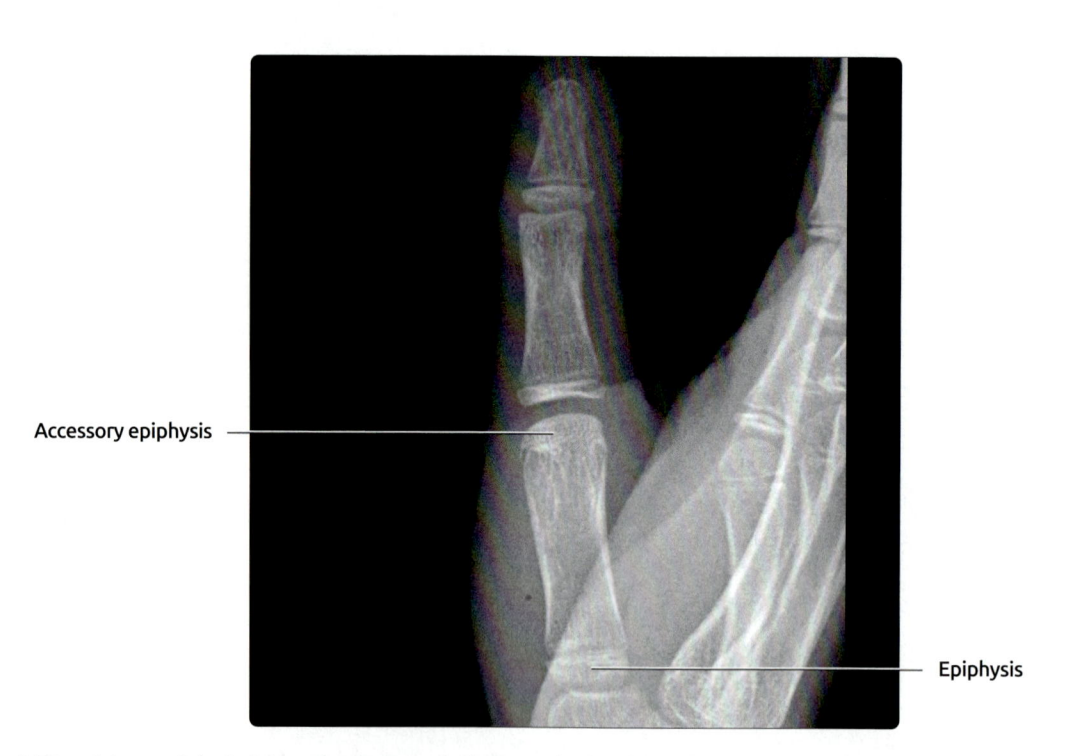

Epiphysis

Accessory epiphysis

Accessory epiphysis

Accessory epiphysis

Epiphysis

(Top) The epiphyses of the 2nd through 5th metacarpals are at the distal end of the metacarpal. Accessory epiphyses at the proximal end of the 2nd and 5th metacarpals are shown here. This is a common variant. **(Bottom)** The 1st metacarpal epiphysis is at the base of the metacarpal. This case shows an accessory epiphysis distally. The accessory epiphysis is always present in addition to the normal epiphysis, never instead of it.

Wrist and Hand Normal Variants and Imaging Pitfalls

MISCELLANEOUS BONY VARIANTS

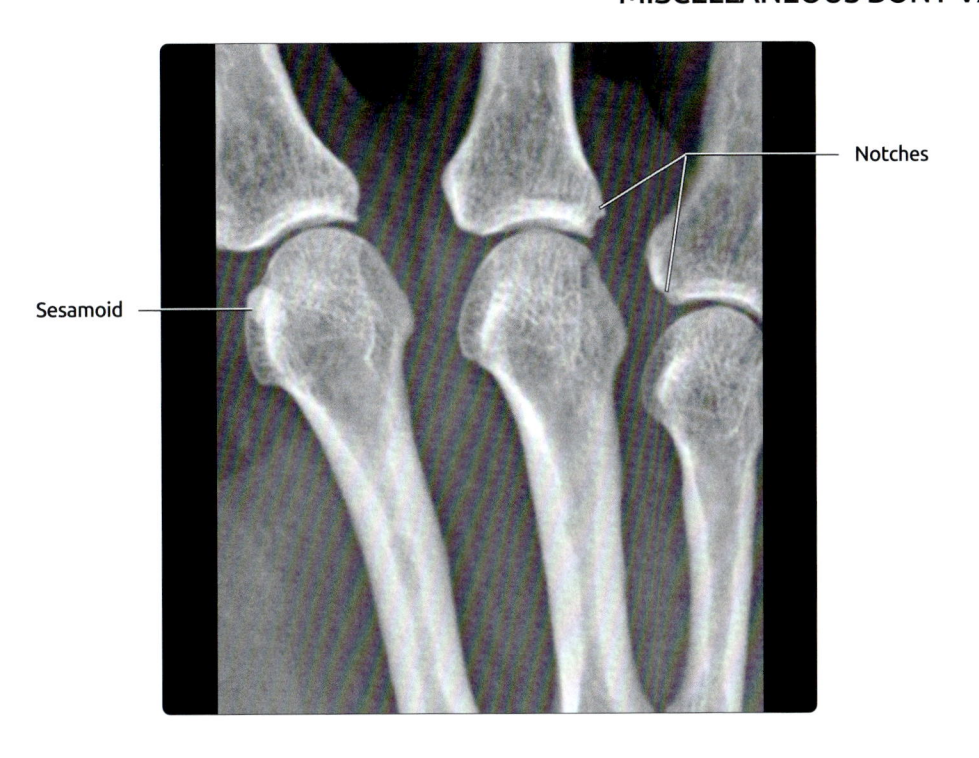

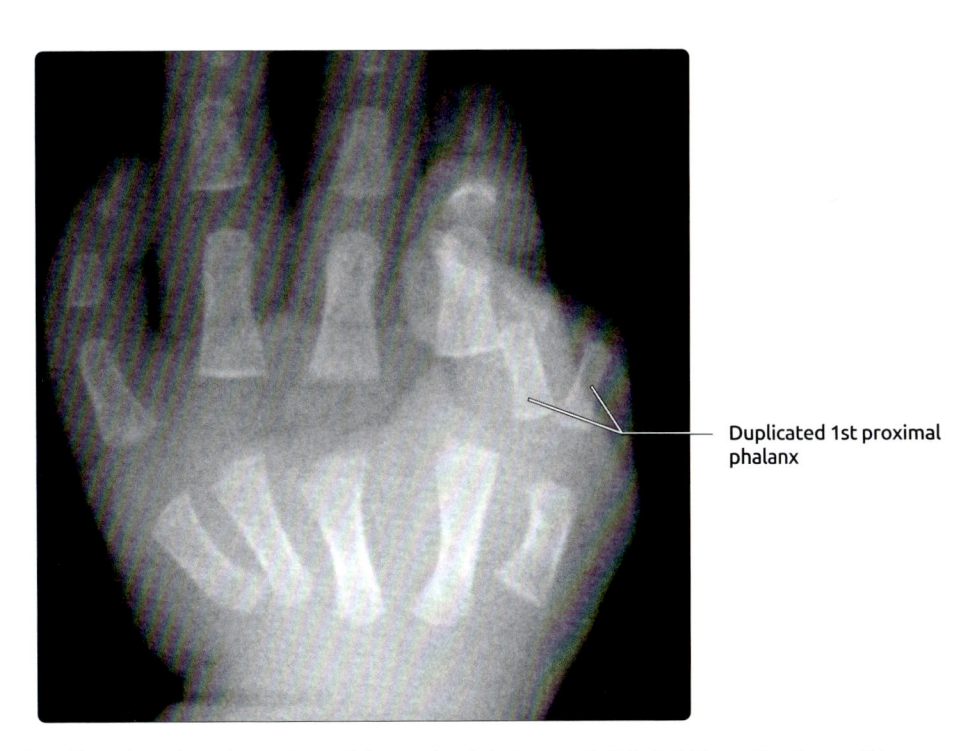

(Top) AP radiograph shows normal, well-corticated notches at base of the proximal phalanges of digits 3-4. The cortication and the absence of other signs suggesting inflammatory arthritis are the key to the diagnosis of pseudoerosion. Also note the sesamoid of the 2nd metacarpal, which is variably present. (Bottom) Supernumerary or partially duplicated digits are a common isolated anomaly.

Wrist Measurements and Lines

TERMINOLOGY

Definitions
- Ulnar variance: Ulna longer or shorter than radius
- Intercalated segment: Term for the proximal carpal row, indicating its position intercalated between radius and distal carpal row

ANATOMY IMAGING ISSUES

Imaging Approaches
- **Ulnar variance**: Careful positioning needed for accurate measurement
    - Elbow and wrist must be at same height as shoulder
    - Shoulder abducted 90°, elbow flexed 90°, forearm neutral
    - Hand flat against plate, beam centered on midcarpus
    - Ulnar positive variance defined as ulna ≥ 2 mm longer than radius
    - Ulnar negative variance defined as ulna ≥ 2 mm shorter than radius
    - Supination decreases ulnar variance
    - Pronation increases ulnar variance
    - Positive ulnar variance associated with triangular fibrocartilage tear, ulnar impaction syndrome
    - Negative ulnar variance associated with osteonecrosis of lunate
- **Relative position of radius and ulna on lateral radiograph**
    - On well-positioned radiograph, ulna should not be posterior to radius
    - Landmark for well-positioned lateral radiograph
        – Pisiform bone overlies distal pole of scaphoid
- **Radioulnar ratio (CT or MR)**
    - Ulna moves dorsally in pronation, should always remain < 30% dorsal to radius
    - Radioulnar ratio is used to evaluate radioulnar subluxation
    - Line drawn from center of ulnar head perpendicular to line across margins of sigmoid notch (CD)
    - Distance from this line to volar margin of sigmoid notch (AD) and total distance between margins of sigmoid notch (AB) expressed as a ratio
    - AD/AB = 0.6 ± 0.05 in pronation
    - AD/AB = 0.37 in supination
- **Ulnar head inclination: 11-27°**
    - Angle between sigmoid notch of radius and long axis of ulna
- **Ulnar styloid position**
    - Pronation: Styloid lies at medial margin of ulna
    - Supination: Styloid centered on head of ulna
- **Radial inclination (radial tilt): 21°-24°**
    - Radial styloid slopes distally compared to ulnar margin of radius
    - Angle between a line from tip of radial styloid to ulnar margin of radius, and a line perpendicular to radial shaft
- **Radial height: 10-13 mm**
    - Distance from line drawn perpendicular to radius at its ulnar margin and a parallel line drawn through the radial styloid
- **Radioulnar angle: 90°-111°**
    - Line from tip of radial styloid to ulnar margin of radial articular surface
    - Line along sigmoid notch
    - Angle between these is radioulnar angle
- **Radial volar (palmar) tilt**
    - Dorsal margin of radius is more distal than volar margin
    - Tilt is angle between a line drawn from dorsal to volar margin and a line perpendicular to radial shaft
    - Normal 11°-14°
- **Carpal translation**
    - In normal neutral position, lunate articulates 50% with radius, 50% with triangular fibrocartilage
    - With radial deviation, it moves ulnarly
    - With ulnar deviation, it moves radially
- **Central axis of wrist**
    - Radius, lunate, capitate and 3rd metacarpal form central axis of wrist
    - A line drawn through center of radial shaft should bisect lunate, capitate, and 3rd metacarpal
- **Gilula arcs/lines**
    - Method of assessing intercarpal relationships
    - 1st arc: Smooth arc around proximal margin of proximal carpal row
    - 2nd arc: Smooth arc around distal margin of proximal carpal row
    - 3rd arc: Smooth arc around proximal margins of capitate and hamate
    - Zigzag line: Carpometacarpal joints should be visible as a zigzag line, disrupted in carpometacarpal dislocation
- **Carpal angle**
    - Line drawn tangent to scaphoid and lunate
    - Line drawn tangent to lunate and triquetrum
    - Angle between these lines should be > 117°
- **Scapholunate angle**
    - Line drawn along axis of scaphoid, bisecting proximal and distal pole
    - Line bisecting proximal and distal surfaces of scaphoid
    - Angle between these lines is scapholunate angle and measures 30-60°
    - Angle is increased in dorsal intercalated segment instability (DISI)
    - Angle is increased in volar intercalated segment instability (VISI)
- **Lunotriquetral angle: 14-16°**
    - Secondary index for lunotriquetral ligament injury
- **Capitolunate angle: < 20°**
    - Wrist must be straight, without flexion or extension of hand
- **Scapholunate distance: < 4 mm**
    - Clenched fist view will help show widening in cases of scapholunate ligament injury
- **Carpal height ratio: 45-60% (mean: 54%)**
    - Carpal height is distance from distal margin of capitate to articular surface radius
    - Carpal height ratio is ratio of carpal height/length of 3rd metacarpal
    - Useful to quantify carpal collapse

Imaging Pitfalls
- Improper positioning will result in unreliable measurements

Wrist Measurements and Lines

DISTAL RADIOULNAR JOINT, SUPINATION VS. PRONATION

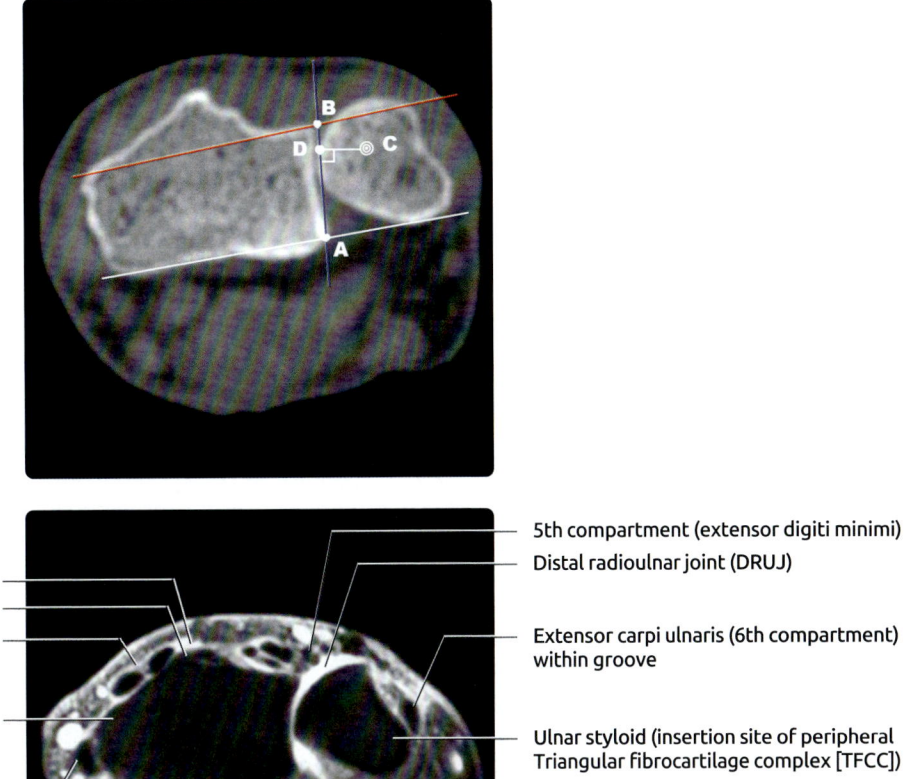

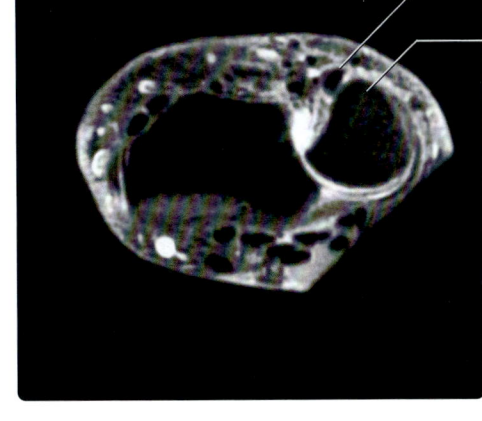

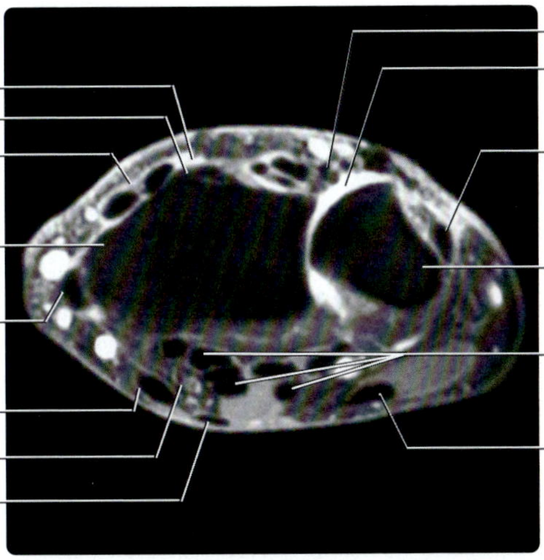

(Top) Radioulnar ratio (AD/AB), used to identify subluxation, is the ratio between ulnar head center (C) and length of sigmoid notch (AB). Line CD is perpendicular to AB. AD/AB = 0.6 ± 0.05 in pronation, 0.37 ± 0.09 in supination. Ulna moves dorsally in pronation but remains < 30% dorsal to radius. (From SI: Arthrography.) (Middle) Hand is shown in pronation. The radius rotates around the ulna on pronation/supination, resulting in different appearances on MR based on varying hand position. In order to align the ulnar styloid with the radius and position the triangular fibrocartilage complex (TFCC) optimally in the coronal plane, it is best to image the wrist with the hand in pronated position. Note that the extensor carpi ulnaris is positioned within a groove in the ulna. (From SI: Arthrography.) (Bottom) Hand is shown in supination. Note the excursion of the ulna relative to the radius. Also note the normal appearance of the extensor carpi ulnaris (ECU) at the margin of the ulnar groove. (From SI: Arthrography.)

Wrist Measurements and Lines

DISTAL RADIOULNAR JOINT, SUPINATION VS. PRONATION

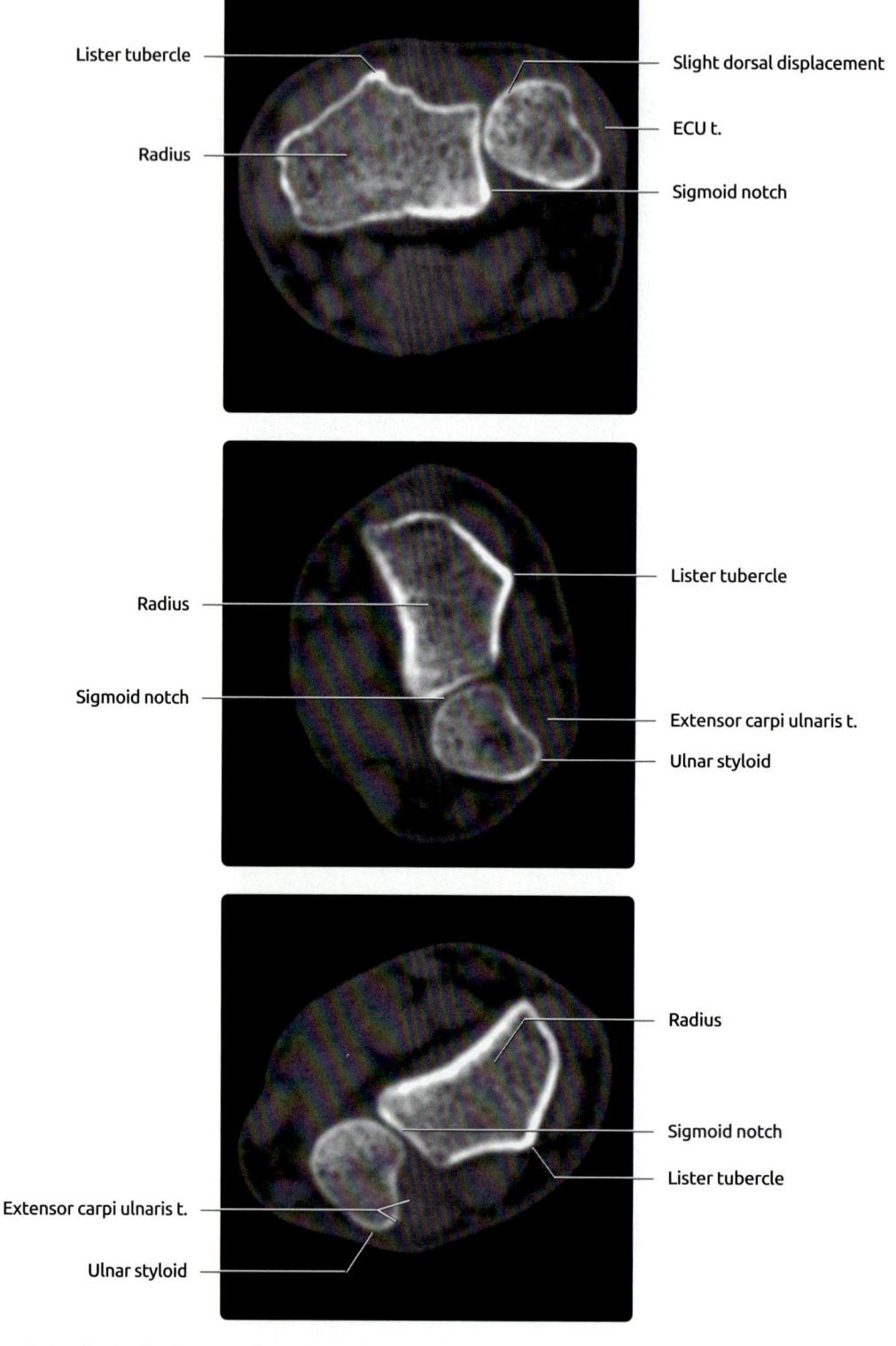

(Top) CT through the distal radioulnar joint shows the relationships of radius and ulna in full pronation. In this position there is slight dorsal position of ulna in sigmoid notch. ECU is seated within ulnar groove. Radius rotates around ulna. **(Middle)** CT of the distal radioulnar joint in neutral rotation shows that in this position the distal ulna is fully seated in radial sigmoid notch. The ECU is seated within ulnar groove. **(Bottom)** CT of the distal radioulnar joint in full supination shows that in this position the ulna is positioned slight volarly in the sigmoid notch. ECU is draped over medial rim of ulnar groove. Radius rotates around ulna.

Wrist Measurements and Lines

DISTAL RADIUS AND ULNA, LINES AND MEASUREMENTS

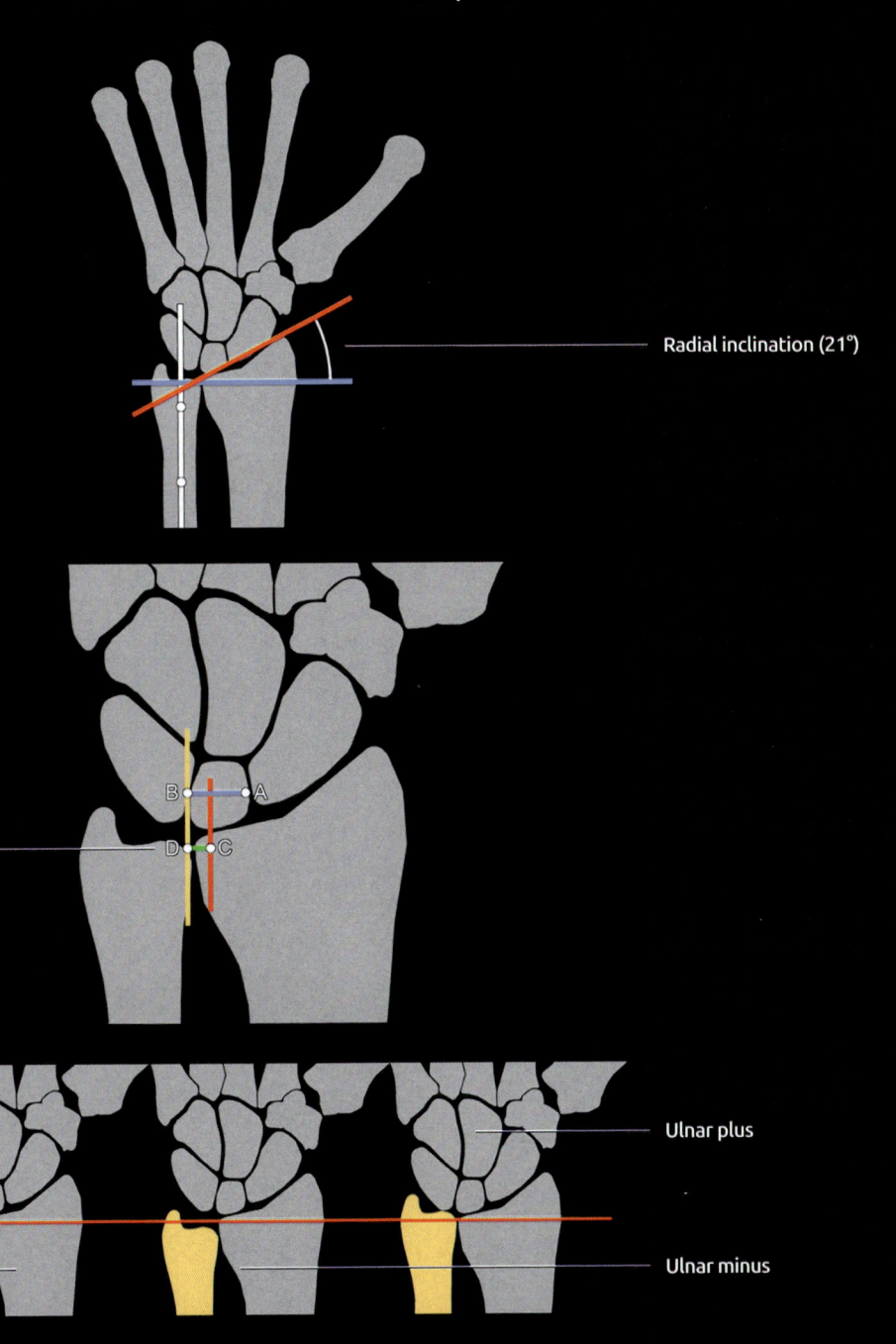

Radial inclination (21°)

Lunate overhang (CD/AB < 50%)

Ulnar plus

Ulnar neutral

Ulnar minus

First image: Radial tilt (inclination) measures normal distal radius angulation and may be disrupted in fractures. Normal tilt is 21°-25°. Second image: Ulnar carpal translation measures lunate overhang. AB is width of lunate and CD is overhang of medial lunate relative to sigmoid notch. Normal ratio is CD/AB < 50%, i.e., at least 50% of the lunate articular surface should articulate with the radius on a PA radiograph. Third image: Ulnar variance is measured as the length of distal ulna compared to distal radius. Ulnar neutral requires the ulna to be equal in length to the radius, or no more than 2 mm shorter. Ulnar minus occurs when the ulna is greater than 2 mm shorter than the radius. Ulnar plus variance occurs when the ulna is longer than the radius.

Wrist Measurements and Lines

CARPAL RELATIONSHIPS

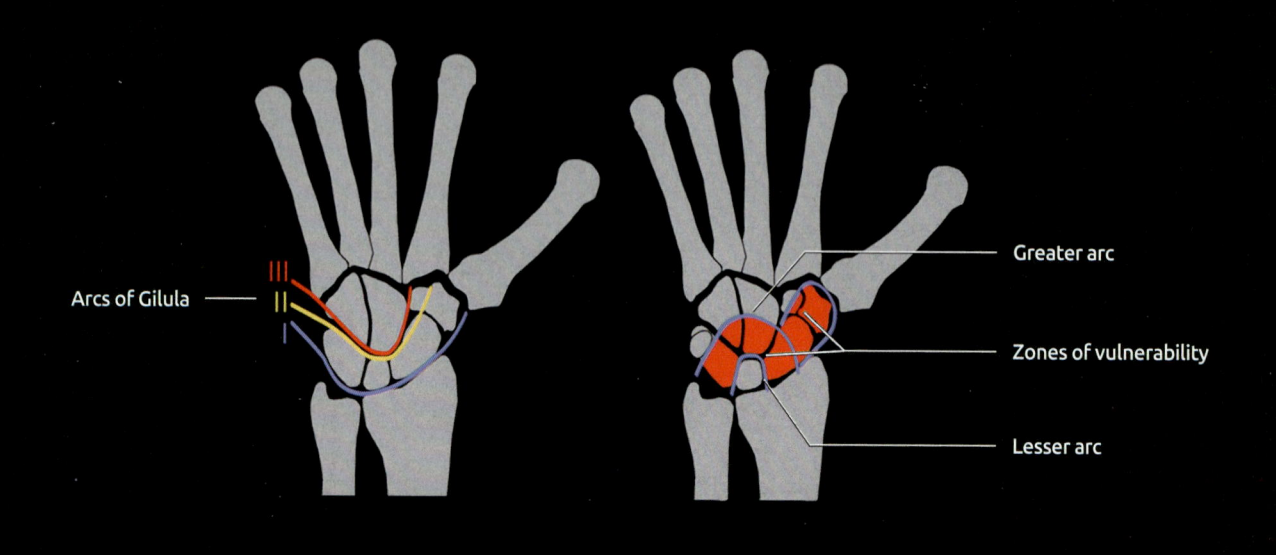

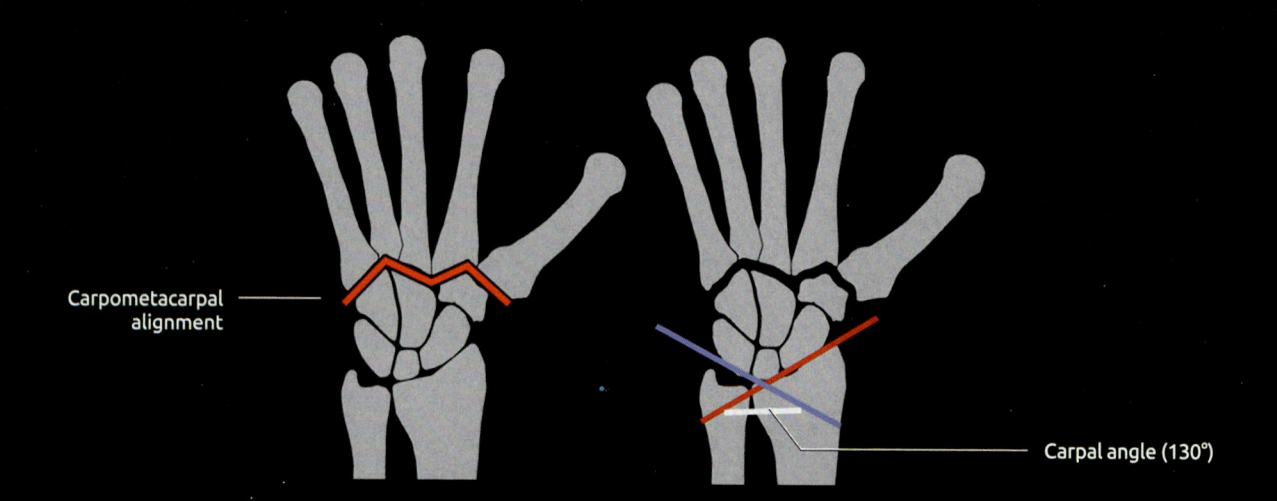

Images clockwise from upper left: Arcs of Gilula outline 3 smooth curves paralleling articular surfaces. Disruption of these smooth flowing arcs is an indication of trauma or carpal malalignment. Second image: Greater and lesser arcs describe joints around lunate (lesser arc) and mid scaphoid, capitate, hamate, and triquetrum. Vulnerable zone is the area encompassed by greater, lesser arcs, scaphoid, and trapezium; region where majority of fractures occur. Third image: Carpometacarpal alignment on PA wrist creates an "M." Disruption of contour suggests joint injury. Fourth image: Carpal angle evaluates developing carpal collapse related to arthritis or trauma.

Wrist Measurements and Lines

CARPAL LINES AND MEASUREMENTS

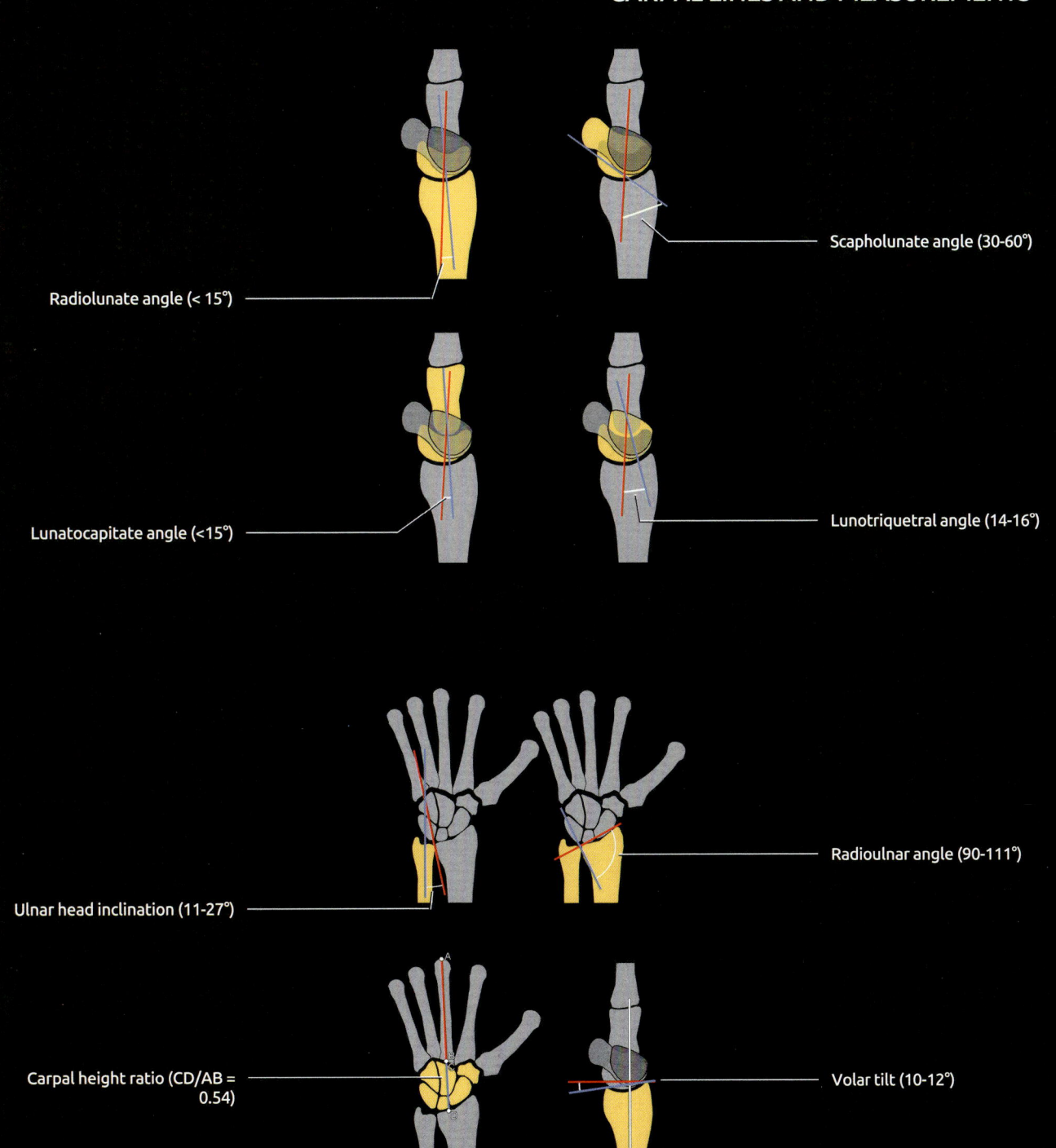

Radiolunate angle (< 15°)

Scapholunate angle (30-60°)

Lunatocapitate angle (<15°)

Lunotriquetral angle (14-16°)

Ulnar head inclination (11-27°)

Radioulnar angle (90-111°)

Carpal height ratio (CD/AB = 0.54)

Volar tilt (10-12°)

(Top) In the graphic, the lunate axis is colored red, and the axis against which it is being measured is blue. Disruption of these relationships are an indication of carpal instability. **(Bottom)** Ulnar head inclination assists in evaluating distal radioulnar joint injury. Radioulnar angle evaluates radiocarpal injury and carpal malalignment. Carpal height ratio measures CD/AB, is normally 0.54 and assists in evaluating of carpal collapse in arthropathies. Volar tilt measures normal radius volar angulation and may be disrupted in trauma.

SECTION 6
Hand

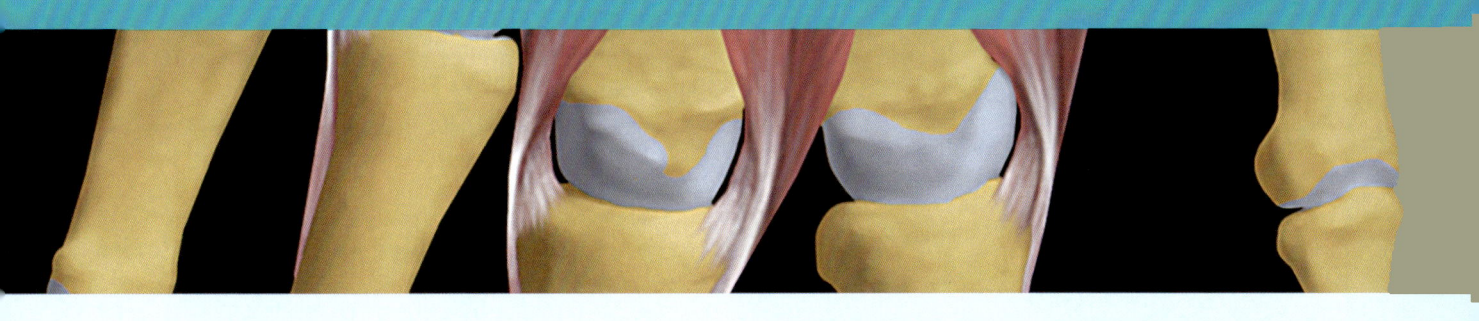

Hand Overview	**436**
Thumb Anatomy	**444**
Hand Radiographic Anatomy	**452**
Hand MR Atlas	**456**
Flexor and Extensor Mechanisms of Hand	**472**

Hand Overview

TERMINOLOGY

Definitions
- For this text, the hand will be defined as beginning at the carpometacarpal joint
- In anatomic position, the hand is in supination
- Radial: Toward radius and synonymous with lateral(ly)
- Ulnar: Toward ulna and synonymous with medial(ly)
- Mesial: Toward midline of structure
  - 3rd digit is midline of hand and therefore the most mesial structure
  - 2nd and 4th digits are more mesial than 1st and 5th digits
- Abduction is motion away from midline of structure
- Adduction is motion towards midline of structure

OSSEUS ANATOMY

Metacarpals
- Comprised of a base, diaphysis, neck and head (from proximal to distal)
- Normal ossification center (epiphysis) is distal (head) for digits 2-5 and proximal (base) for 1st digit
- Bases are trapezoidal in shape (broader dorsally) with concave articular surface
- 1st metacarpal articulates with trapezium
- 2nd-5th metacarpals articulate with trapezoid, capitate, and hamate (both 4th and 5th) respectively, as well as with one another
- Diaphysis is roughly triangular in cross section with apex volarly: Creating medial and lateral volar surfaces and dorsal surface
- Diaphysis is gently concave volarly (convex dorsally) throughout its proximal to distal course
- Head is relatively spherical with shallow groove volarly and short notches laterally and medially
- Volar groove of head transmits flexor tendons in extension and accommodates volar plate (especially in flexion)
- Lateral and medial notches are origin of collateral ligament complex

Phalanges
- 3 each (proximal, middle, and distal) for digits 2-5
- 2 (proximal and distal) for 1st digit
- Comprised of base, diaphysis, and head
- Ossification center (epiphysis) is proximal (base)
- Heads are bicondylar volarly with condyles separated by shallow groove
- Groove transmits flexor tendons in extension and accommodates volar plate (especially in flexion)
- Proximal articular surfaces of proximal phalanges are uniformly concave
- Proximal articular surfaces of middle and distal phalanges are biconcave with a median ridge running anteroposteriorly
- Median ridge tracks in groove between condyles: Helps prevent lateral translation

JOINTS OF HAND

1st Carpometacarpal Joint
- Saddle joint, highly mobile, critical for opposition and grasp
- Abducted and rotated volarly (pronated) compared to other carpometacarpal joints
- Allows thumb to abduct and adduct in a plane perpendicular to other digits
- Separate joint cavity

2nd-5th Carpometacarpal Joints & Intermetacarpal Joints
- Relatively flat configuration of articular surfaces
- Small recesses between metacarpals are the designated intermetacarpal joints
- Share common joint cavity with midcarpal joint
- 2nd-3rd carpometacarpal joints form stable base for hand motion
- 5th carpometacarpal joint has greatest mobility (assists in opposition)
- Motions: Flexion and extension, palmar cupping
- Ligaments: Longitudinal and transverse ligaments, dorsal, volar, and interosseous
- Intermetacarpal ligaments (dorsal, volar, and interosseous) link the bases of all metacarpals

Metacarpophalangeal Joints
- Rounded metacarpal head articulates with shallow concavity of proximal phalangeal base
- Motion: Flexion/extension & limited abduction/adduction
- Ligaments: Palmar and dorsal ligaments, collateral ligaments, & extensor hood + sagittal bands
- Palmar (volar) plate
  - Palmar thickening of joint capsule, helps prevent hyperextension
- Deep transverse palmar ligament
  - Between metacarpal heads
  - Interconnects 2nd-5th palmar plates
  - Flexor tendons pass volar to ligament, interossei pass dorsal
- Collateral ligaments
  - Stabilize abduction/adduction
- Sagittal bands: Connect extensor hood to collateral ligaments
  - Stabilize extensor tendon & joint
- Extensor hood: See "Flexor and Extensor Mechanism" chapter

Interphalangeal Joints
- Bicondylar phalangeal head has central concavity
- Middle and distal phalangeal bases have biconcave surface with central median ridge
- Motion: Flexion >> extension; proximal interphalangeal joint allows greater flexion than distal interphalangeal joint
- Ligaments: Volar (palmar) plate, extensor mechanism, collateral ligaments, joint capsule
- Palmar (volar) plate: Thickening of joint capsule
  - From neck of phalanx to base of phalanx distal to it
  - Prevents hyperextension
  - Palmar plate fracture common avulsion from attachment to base of phalanx

Hand Overview

MUSCLES OF HAND

See "Thumb Anatomy" and "Flexor and Extensor Mechanism" Chapters for Full Details of Muscle Function, Attachments, and Innervation

- Following summary is a guide to categorization of these complex muscles

Extrinsic Flexors
- Flexor digitorum superficialis, flexor digitorum profundus, flexor pollicis longus
- Pulley system maintains their position throughout flexion

Intrinsic Flexors
- Palmar interossei, lumbricals, flexor pollicis brevis, flexor digiti minimi
- Lumbricals flex metacarpophalangeal joint, extend interphalangeal joints

Thenar Muscles
- Opponens pollicis, abductor pollicis brevis, flexor pollicis brevis

Hypothenar Muscles
- Opponens digiti minimi, abductor digiti minimi, flexor digiti minimi

Extrinsic Extensors
- Extensor digitorum communis, extensor indicis, extensor pollicis longus, extensor digiti minimi
- Extensor hood maintains position throughout extension

Intrinsic Extensors
- Lumbricals, dorsal interossei, extensor pollicis brevis
- Lumbricals flex metacarpophalangeal joint, extend interphalangeal joints

Adductors
- Adductor pollicis, palmar interossei

Abductors
- Abductor pollicis, abductor digiti minimi, dorsal interossei

VESSELS OF HAND

Palmar Arches
- Both superficial palmar arch and deep palmar arch run from radial artery to ulnar artery
  - Ulnar artery primarily supplies the superficial palmar arch
  - Radial artery primarily supplies the deep palmar arch

Radial Artery: Proximal to Distal
- At radiocarpal joint level, gives off branch, which pierces abductor pollicis brevis before joining superficial palmar arch
- Travels superficially (superficial to extensor pollicis longus and extensor retinaculum) around radial aspect of wrist to travel dorsally in anatomic snuffbox
- Distal to snuffbox, gives off branch, which splits into princeps pollicis and radialis indicis arteries
- Dives deep in interspace between 1st and 2nd metacarpals
- Travels between heads of 1st dorsal interosseus and adductor pollicis muscles before forming deep palmar arch
- Deep palmar arch runs between flexor tendons and metacarpals

Ulnar Artery: Proximal to Distal
- Runs superficial to flexor retinaculum
- Passes radial to pisiform
- Gives off deep branch to deep palmar arch just proximal to hook of hamate
  - Runs between abductor digiti minimi and flexor digiti minimi
- Forms superficial palmar arch
  - Runs between palmar aponeurosis and flexor tendons
- Arterial supply to lateral aspect 5th digit usually entirely from ulnar artery

Common Palmar Digital Arteries
- Between metacarpal necks and heads in 2nd, 3rd, and 4th interspaces
- Variably supplied by superficial and deep palmar arches

Proper Digital Arteries
- Arise at metacarpophalangeal joint level
- Run in subcutaneous fat along lateral aspects of digits

NERVES OF HAND

Median Nerve
- Travels in carpal tunnel
- After exiting carpal tunnel, gives off recurrent branch (motor supply to thenars)
- Motor in hand
  - To thenar muscles (opponens pollicis, abductor pollicis brevis, flexor pollicis brevis)
  - To 1st & 2nd lumbrical muscles
- Sensory
  - Palmar surface: Radial 1/2 of palm, digits 1-3 and radial 1/2 4th digit
  - Dorsal surface: From just distal to proximal interphalangeal joint to fingertip, digits 1-3, and radial 1/2 of 4th digit

Ulnar Nerve
- Motor in hand
  - Hypothenars (opponens digiti minimi, abductor digiti minimi, flexor digiti minimi)
  - All interossei, 3rd & 4th lumbricals, and adductor pollicis
- Sensory
  - From radiocarpal joint to fingertips of 5th and ulnar 1/2 of 4th digits: Both volarly and dorsally

Radial Nerve
- **Not usually seen on routine imaging**
- No motor innervation in hand
- Sensory
  - Dorsal surface from radiocarpal joint to just distal to PIP joints for digits 1-3 and radial 1/2 of 4th digit

Hand Overview

ORIGINS AND INSERTIONS, VOLAR HAND

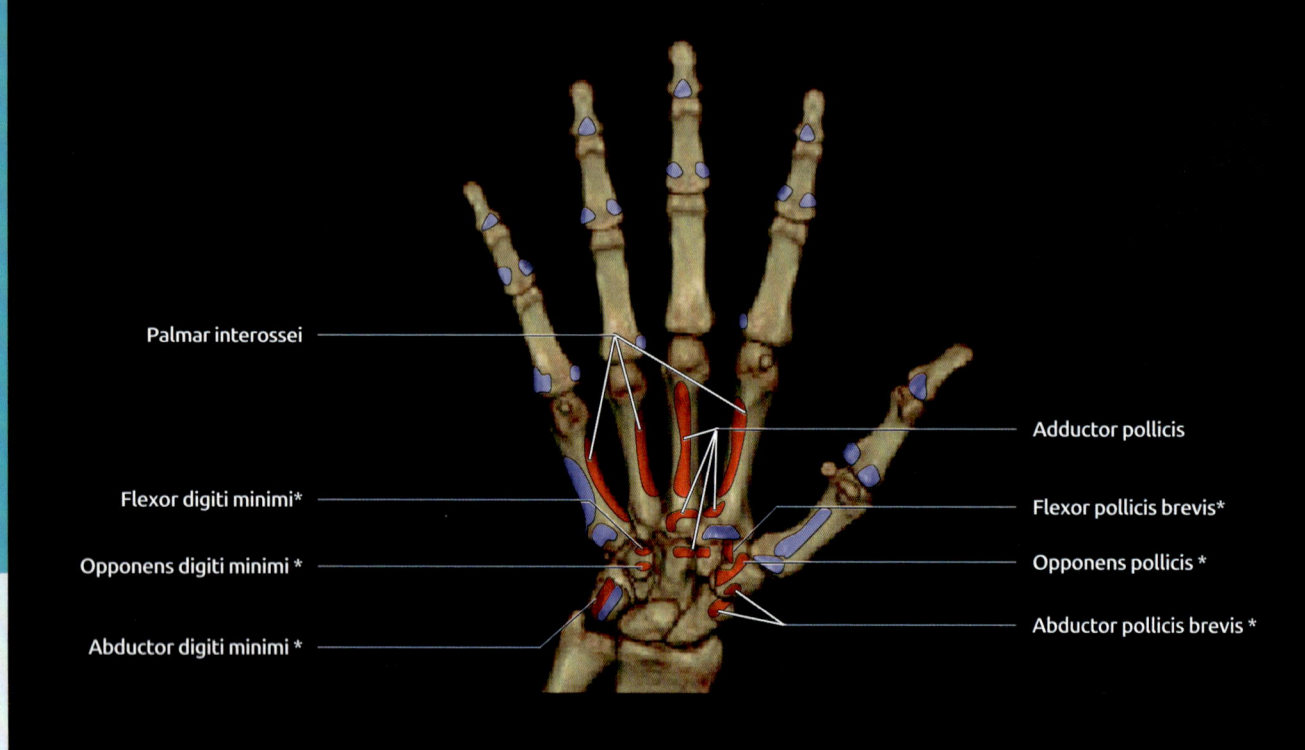

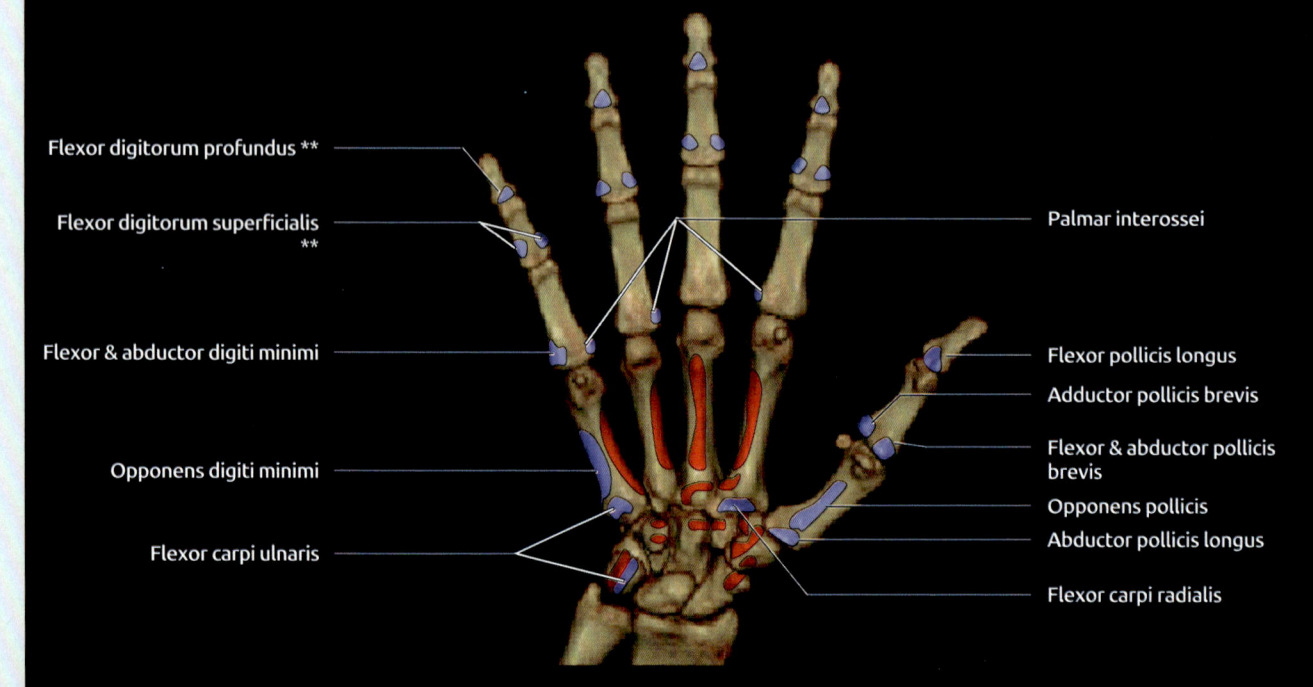

Labels (top image):
- Palmar interossei
- Flexor digiti minimi*
- Opponens digiti minimi *
- Abductor digiti minimi *
- Adductor pollicis
- Flexor pollicis brevis*
- Opponens pollicis *
- Abductor pollicis brevis *

Labels (bottom image):
- Flexor digitorum profundus **
- Flexor digitorum superficialis **
- Flexor & abductor digiti minimi
- Opponens digiti minimi
- Flexor carpi ulnaris
- Palmar interossei
- Flexor pollicis longus
- Adductor pollicis brevis
- Flexor & abductor pollicis brevis
- Opponens pollicis
- Abductor pollicis longus
- Flexor carpi radialis

(Top) *Volar surface origins of the intrinsic muscles are shown in red.* * *Indicates that in addition to bony origin as illustrated, muscle also arises from the flexor retinaculum.* (Bottom) *Volar surface tendon insertions are shown in blue.* ** *Indicates pattern is repeated on digits 2-5 despite lack of labels on image.*

Hand Overview

ORIGINS AND INSERTIONS, DORSAL HAND

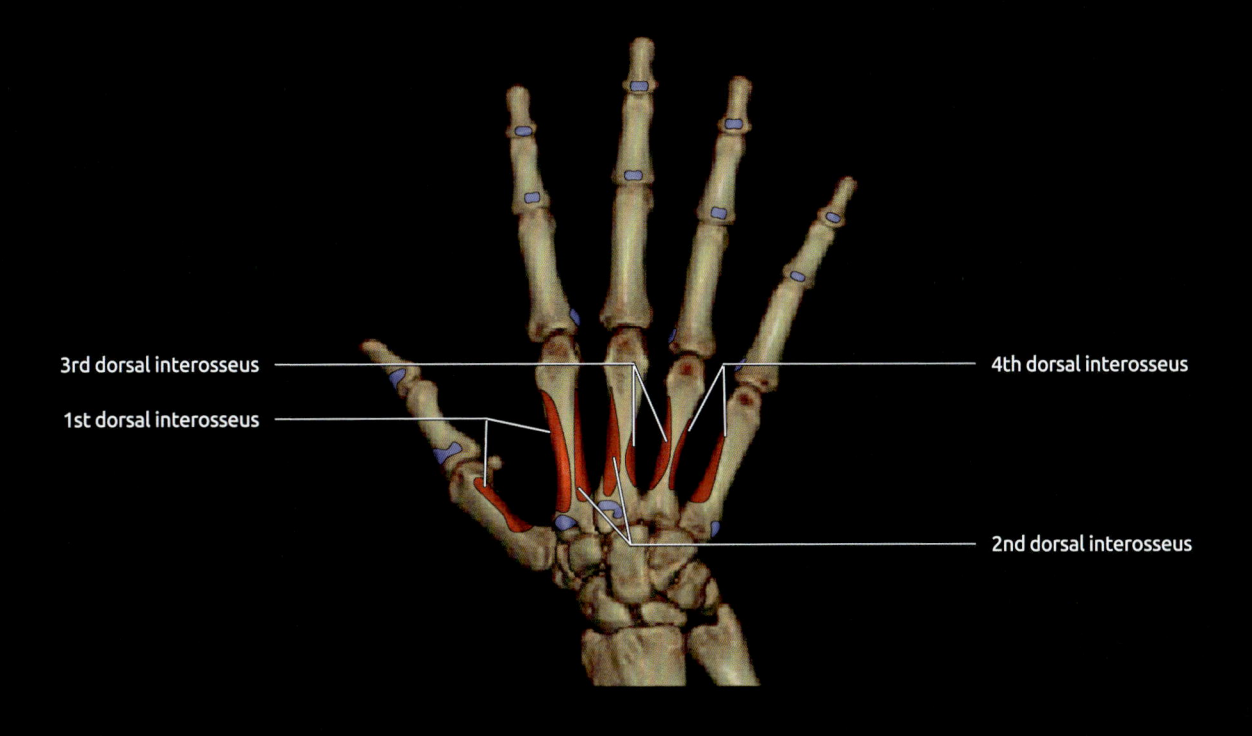

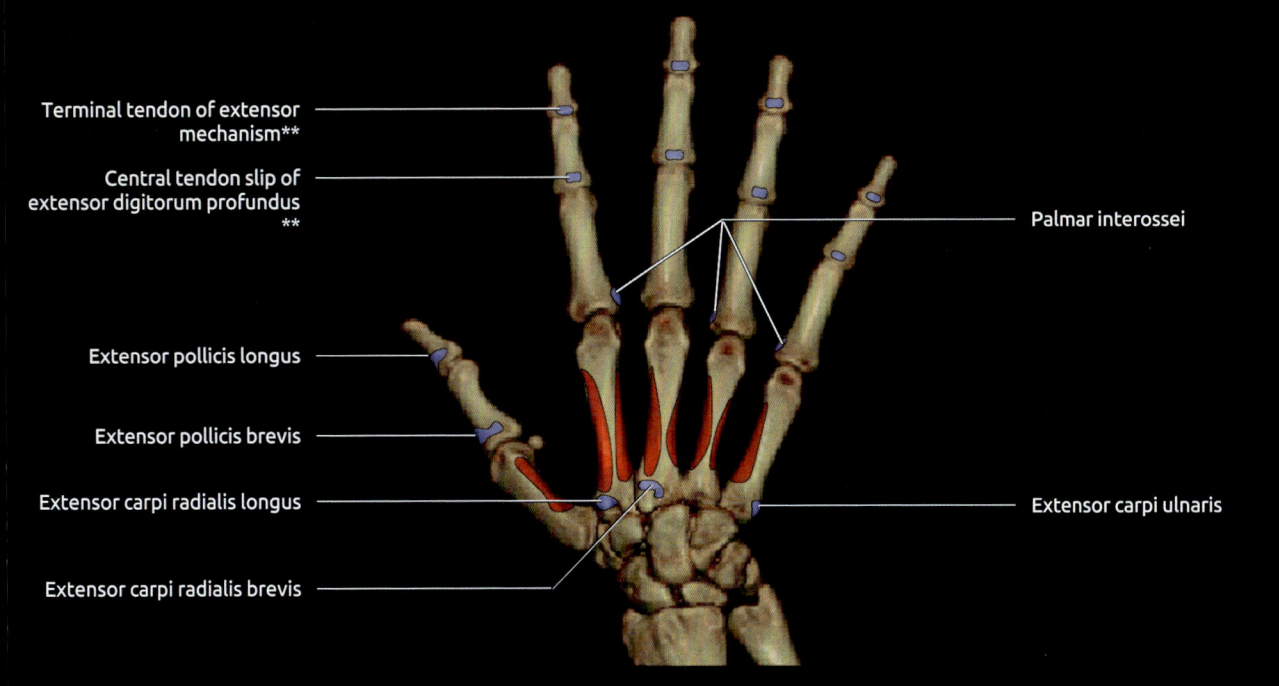

- 3rd dorsal interosseus
- 1st dorsal interosseus
- 4th dorsal interosseus
- 2nd dorsal interosseus

- Terminal tendon of extensor mechanism**
- Central tendon slip of extensor digitorum profundus**
- Extensor pollicis longus
- Extensor pollicis brevis
- Extensor carpi radialis longus
- Extensor carpi radialis brevis
- Palmar interossei
- Extensor carpi ulnaris

*(Top) Dorsal surface origins of the intrinsic muscles of the hand are shown in red. (Bottom) Dorsal surface tendon insertions are shown in blue. ** Indicates pattern is repeated on digits 2-5 despite lack of labels on image.*

Hand Overview

PALMAR INTRINSIC MUSCLES

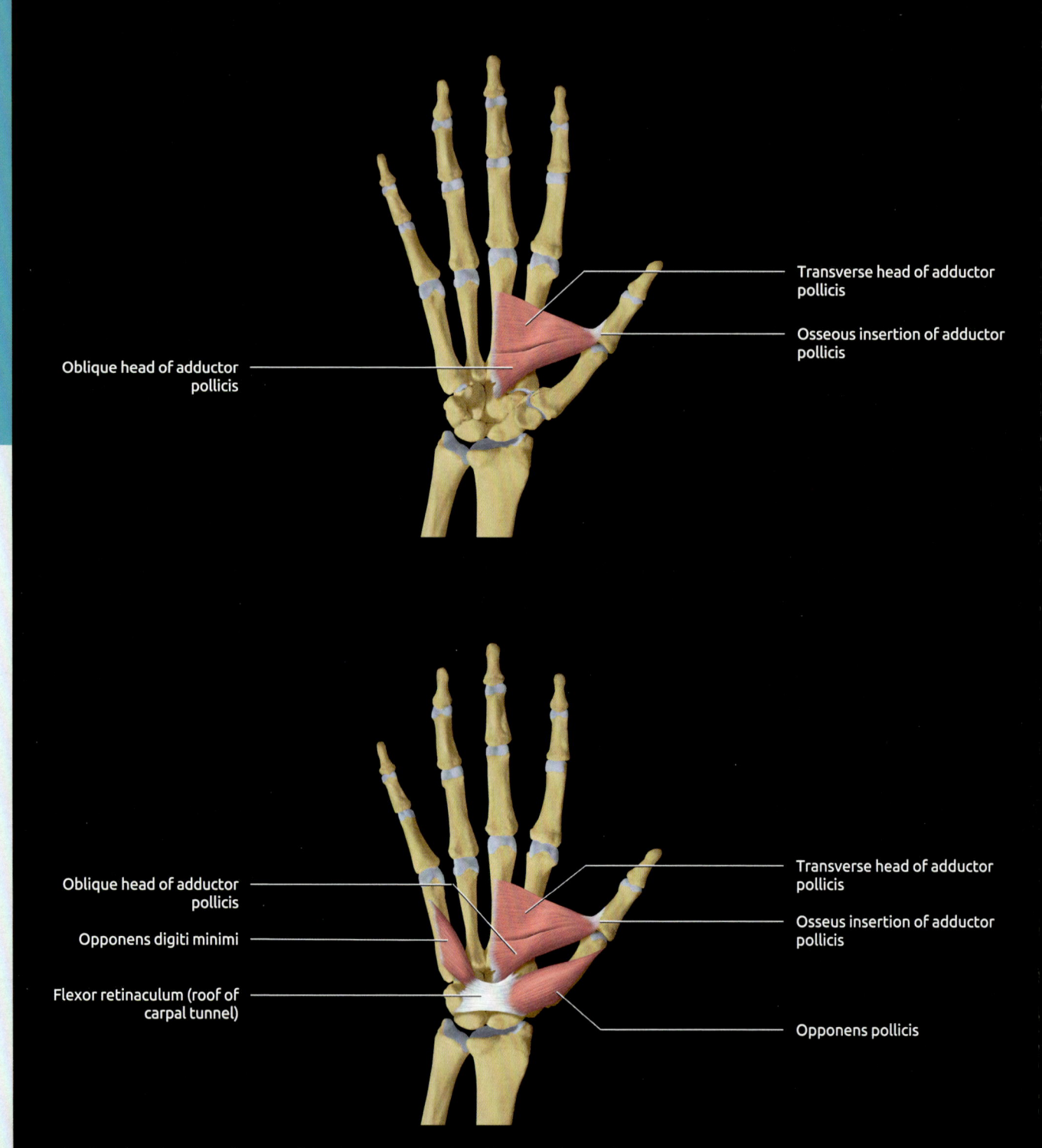

Oblique head of adductor pollicis

Transverse head of adductor pollicis

Osseous insertion of adductor pollicis

Oblique head of adductor pollicis

Opponens digiti minimi

Flexor retinaculum (roof of carpal tunnel)

Transverse head of adductor pollicis

Osseus insertion of adductor pollicis

Opponens pollicis

(Top) Although technically not 1 of the thenar muscles, the adductor pollicis is often grouped with them due to proximity. The osseus insertion is as shown on the graphic. The adductor pollicis also inserts on the volar plate and the extensor hood of the thumb. The contribution of the adductor pollicis to the extensor hood of the 1st digit cannot be seen here, as it is dorsal and lateral to the MCP joint in this projection. The radial artery passes between the 2 heads of the adductor pollicis from dorsal to volar before forming the deep palmar arch. (Bottom) The 2 opponens (pollicis and digiti minimi) muscles have been added. Note that in addition to their osseous origins, these muscles also arise from the flexor retinaculum (which is the roof of the carpal tunnel).

Hand Overview

PALMAR INTRINSIC MUSCLES

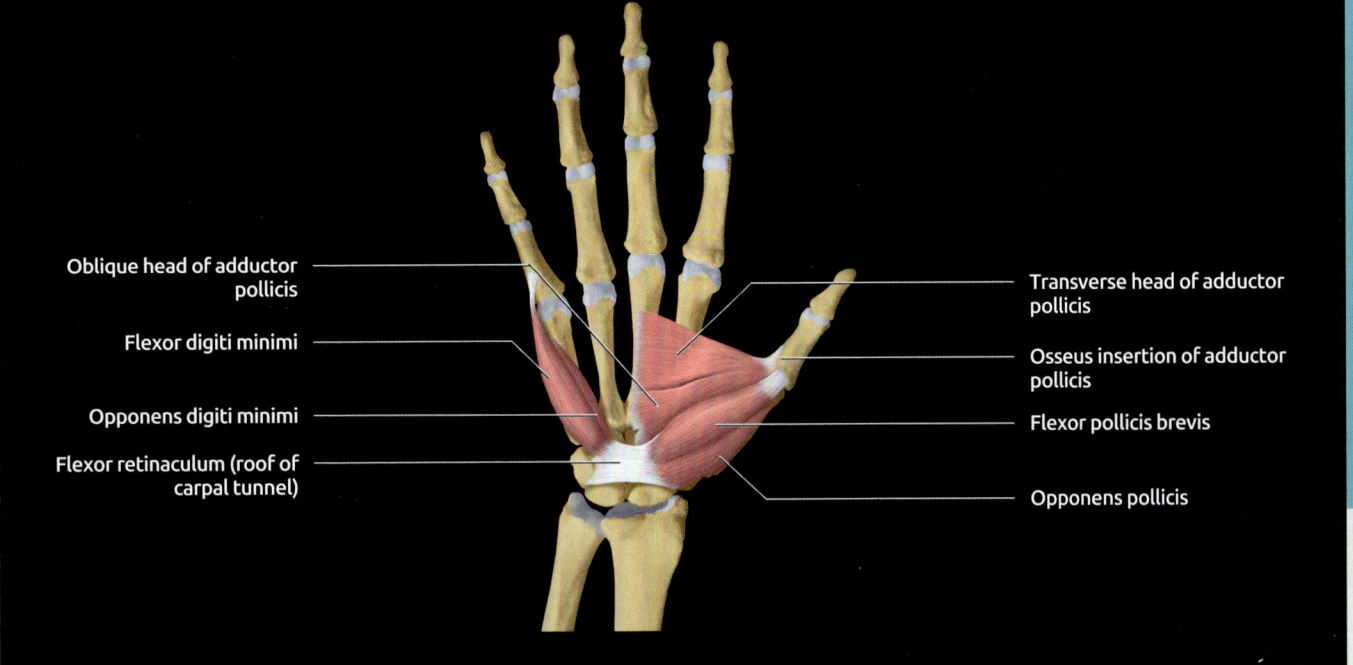

Oblique head of adductor pollicis

Flexor digiti minimi

Opponens digiti minimi

Flexor retinaculum (roof of carpal tunnel)

Transverse head of adductor pollicis

Osseus insertion of adductor pollicis

Flexor pollicis brevis

Opponens pollicis

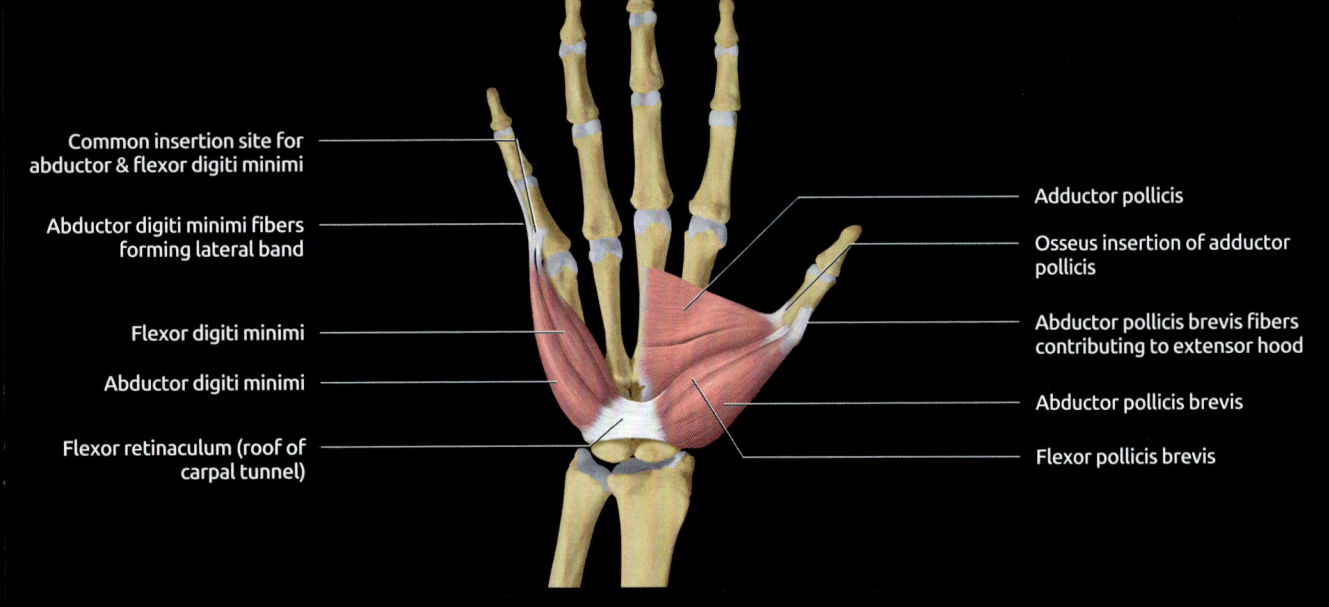

Common insertion site for abductor & flexor digiti minimi

Abductor digiti minimi fibers forming lateral band

Flexor digiti minimi

Abductor digiti minimi

Flexor retinaculum (roof of carpal tunnel)

Adductor pollicis

Osseus insertion of adductor pollicis

Abductor pollicis brevis fibers contributing to extensor hood

Abductor pollicis brevis

Flexor pollicis brevis

(Top) *In this graphic, the 2 flexor (pollicis brevis and digiti minimi) muscles have been added. As before, they originate from the flexor retinaculum as well as from their osseous origins.* (Bottom) *In this graphic, the abductor (pollicis brevis and digiti minimi) muscles have been added. Note that the abductor digiti minimi shares a combined osseous insertion at the base of the 5th proximal phalanx with the flexor digiti minimi. In addition, it gives off fibers to form the ulnar lateral band for the 5th digit. Similarly, the abductor pollicis brevis shares an osseous insertion with the flexor pollicis brevis as well as contributing fibers to the extensor hood of the 1st digit.*

Hand Overview

LUMBRICALS AND INTEROSSEI

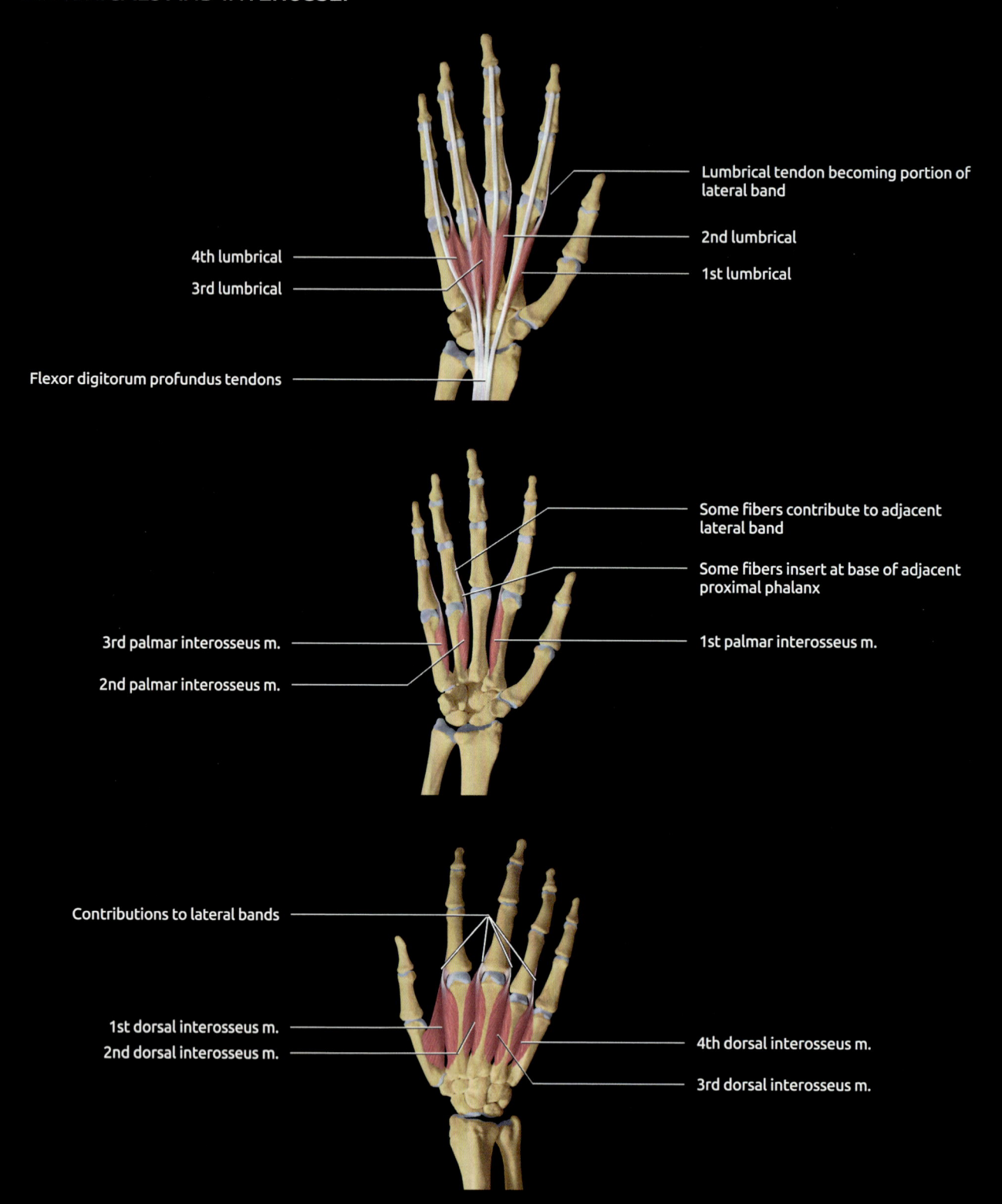

- Lumbrical tendon becoming portion of lateral band
- 2nd lumbrical
- 4th lumbrical
- 1st lumbrical
- 3rd lumbrical
- Flexor digitorum profundus tendons

- Some fibers contribute to adjacent lateral band
- Some fibers insert at base of adjacent proximal phalanx
- 3rd palmar interosseus m.
- 1st palmar interosseus m.
- 2nd palmar interosseus m.

- Contributions to lateral bands
- 1st dorsal interosseus m.
- 2nd dorsal interosseus m.
- 4th dorsal interosseus m.
- 3rd dorsal interosseus m.

(**Top**) *The lumbricals originate from the flexor digitorum profundus tendons as shown. Note how the 1st and 2nd lumbricals arise only from the tendons to the 2nd and 3rd digits, respectively (unipennate), whereas the 3rd and 4th lumbrical arise from the tendons to both the 3rd & 4th and the 4th & 5th digits, respectively (bipennate).* (**Middle**) *The palmar interossei insert at both the bases of the adjacent proximal phalanges as well as the adjacent lateral bands. The 2nd and 3rd palmar interossei contribute to the radial lateral bands of the 4th and 5th digits, respectively, whereas the 1st palmar interosseus contributes to the ulnar lateral band of the 2nd digit.* (**Bottom**) *The tendons of the dorsal interossei (along with the tendons of the palmar interossei and tendons of the lumbricals) help form the lateral bands. Note how each interosseus muscle only contributes fibers to the mesial-most adjacent lateral band. The dorsal interossei do not contribute any lateral band fibers to the 1st or 5th digits.*

Hand Overview

ARTERIES AND NERVES

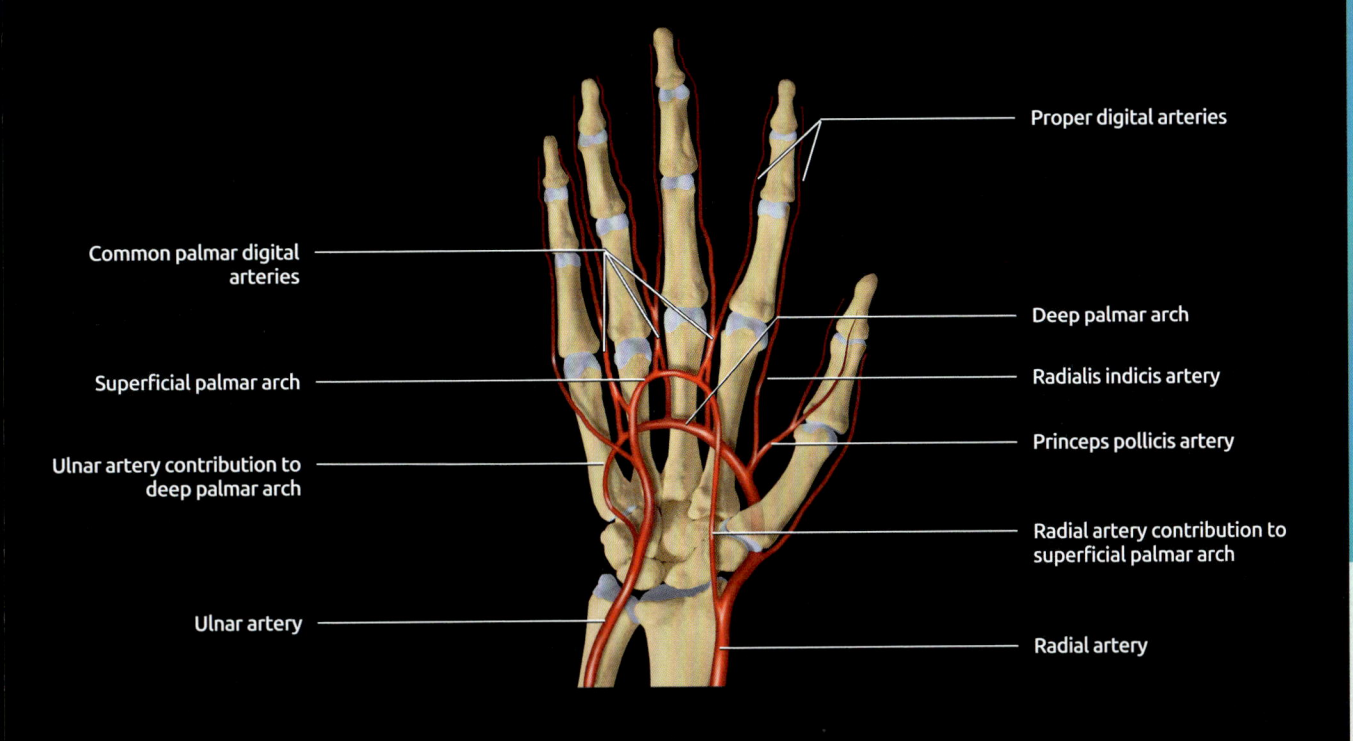

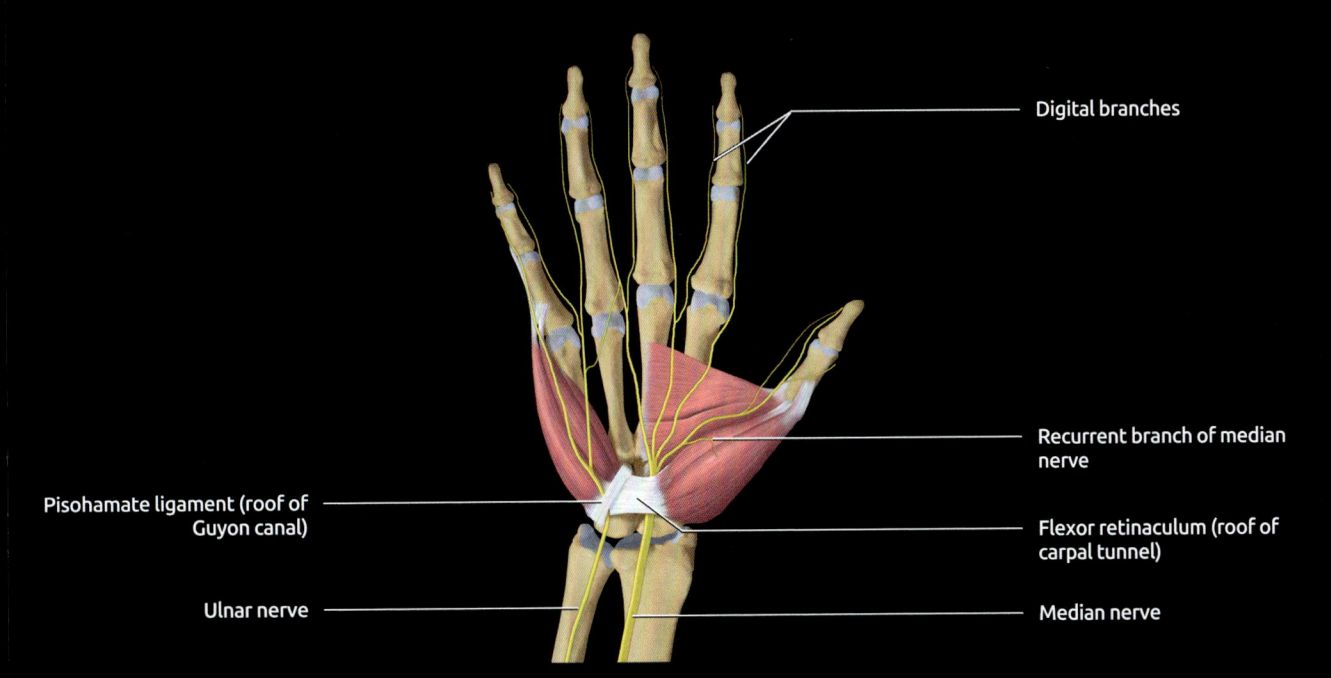

- Proper digital arteries
- Common palmar digital arteries
- Deep palmar arch
- Superficial palmar arch
- Radialis indicis artery
- Princeps pollicis artery
- Ulnar artery contribution to deep palmar arch
- Radial artery contribution to superficial palmar arch
- Ulnar artery
- Radial artery

- Digital branches
- Recurrent branch of median nerve
- Pisohamate ligament (roof of Guyon canal)
- Flexor retinaculum (roof of carpal tunnel)
- Ulnar nerve
- Median nerve

(**Top**) *After giving off its contribution to the superficial palmar arch, the radial artery travels around the radial aspect of the wrist to the dorsum of the hand where it travels in the anatomic snuffbox. It then dives into the 1st interspace between the heads of the 1st dorsal interosseus as well as between the transverse and oblique heads of the adductor pollicis before forming the deep palmar arch.* (**Bottom**) *The median nerve travels deep to the flexor retinaculum (within the carpal tunnel). The ulnar nerve travels superficial to the flexor retinaculum and deep to the pisohamate ligament (within the Guyon canal). Both are prone to compression syndromes within these fibroosseous tunnels. Motor supply of the median nerve is to the thenars (via the recurrent branch) and the 1st & 2nd lumbricals. Ulnar nerve motor supply is to all the intrinsic muscles of the hand not supplied by the median nerve. Muscle atrophy should prompt an evaluation of the supplying nerve.*

Thumb Anatomy

TERMINOLOGY

Definitions
- Abduction: Movement away from 2nd digit
- Adduction: Movement toward 2nd digit
- Opposition: Thumb comes in contact with other fingers; combination of flexion and abduction
- Reposition: Return from opposition to anatomic position

GROSS ANATOMY

Features Distinguishing Thumb From Other Digits
- Thumb is biphalangeal, other digits are triphalangeal
- Thumb has much greater range of motion
  - Opposition a critically important motion seen in man and some primates

1st Carpometacarpal Joint
- Saddle joint: Concave trapezium articulating with convex 1st metacarpal base
- Stabilized by multiple ligaments
- Anterior oblique ligament: Thickening of joint capsule
  - Origin: Palmar tubercle of trapezium
  - Insertion: Ulnar margin of volar base of 1st metacarpal
- Ulnar collateral ligament: Ulnar to anterior oblique ligament
  - Origin: Flexor retinaculum
  - Insertion: Ulnopalmar tubercle of 1st metacarpal
- 1st intermetacarpal ligament
  - Origin and insertion: 1st and 2nd metacarpal bases
- Posterior oblique ligament (minor importance)
  - Connects posterior margin of trapezium to ulnopalmar tubercle of 1st metacarpal
- Dorsoradial ligament
  - Connects dorsal and radial margins of trapezium and 1st metacarpal

1st Metacarpophalangeal Joint: Hinge Joint
- Ulnar and radial collateral ligaments stabilize thumb in abduction and adduction respectively
  - Accessory collateral ligaments are separate structures volar to primary collateral ligaments, link to sesamoids
- Extensor hood: Aids in interphalangeal joint extension
  - Formed by fibers from adductor pollicis and abductor pollicis

1st Interphalangeal Joint
- Pure hinge joint

Intrinsic Thenar Muscles
- Opponens pollicis
  - Origin: Flexor retinaculum and trapezium tubercle
  - Insertion: Proximal 2/3 of volar diaphysis of 1st metacarpal
  - Actions: Opposition, adduction
  - Innervation: Recurrent branch of median nerve
- Abductor pollicis brevis
  - Origin: Flexor retinaculum and tubercle of scaphoid
  - Insertion: Radial sesamoid of 1st metacarpophalangeal joint and lateral base of proximal phalanx of 1st digit
  - Action: Abducts thumb, aids in extension of the joints of 1st digit via its contributions to the extensor hood
  - Innervation: Recurrent branch of median nerve
- Flexor pollicis brevis
  - Superficial head origin: Flexor retinaculum
  - Deep head origin: Trapezium, trapezoid, capitate
  - Insertion: Radial sesamoid of 1st metacarpophalangeal joint, base 1st metacarpal
  - Action: Flexion, abduction, adduction
  - Innervation: Superficial head by recurrent branch of median nerve, deep head by ulnar nerve

Other Intrinsic Muscles
- Adductor pollicis
  - Transverse head origin: 3rd metacarpal
  - Oblique head: Capitate, 2nd-3rd metacarpal, volar ligaments of wrist
  - Insertion: Ulnar sesamoid of 1st metacarpophalangeal joint and medial base of proximal phalanx of 1st digit
    - Joins with flexor pollicis brevis to form **adductor aponeurosis**
  - Action: Adduction; innervation: Deep branch, ulnar nerve
- Dorsal interosseous
  - Origin: Base of 1st and 2nd metacarpals (bipennate)
  - Insertion: Radial side of 2nd proximal phalanx
  - Action: Thumb adduction, 2nd digit abduction; innervation: Median nerve

Extrinsic Muscles
- Flexor pollicis longus
  - Origin: Volar radius and interosseous membrane
  - Insertion: Base of distal phalanx of 1st digit
  - Action: Flexes 1st digit interphalangeal and metacarpophalangeal joints
  - Innervation: Anterior interosseous branch, median nerve
  - Tendon sheath (radial bursa) from slightly proximal to carpal tunnel to tendon insertion on distal phalanx of the thumb
- Extensor pollicis longus
  - Origin: Dorsal ulna and interosseous membrane
  - Insertion: Dorsal side of base of 1st metacarpal
  - Innervation: Radial nerve (posterior interosseous branch)
  - Action: Extends metacarpophalangeal and interphalangeal joints
- Extensor pollicis brevis
  - Origin: Distal to extensor pollicis longus on ulna, interosseous membrane, radius
  - Insertion: Base of 1st proximal phalanx
  - Innervation: Radial nerve (posterior interosseous branch)
- Abductor pollicis longus
  - Origin: Dorsal ulna and radius and interosseous membrane
  - Insertion: Radial side of 1st metacarpal base and trapezium, sometimes into thenar muscles
  - Innervation: Radial nerve (posterior interosseous branch)

Flexor Pulleys
- Fibrous bands, which stabilize flexor mechanism
- A1 pulley: At metacarpophalangeal joint
- Oblique pulley: From ulnar aspect of proximal phalanx to radial aspect of distal phalanx
- A2 pulley: At interphalangeal joint: Most important pulley
- Av pulley: Variable in position, at proximal 1/2 of proximal phalanx

Thumb Anatomy

GRAPHICS, INTRINSIC THUMB MUSCLES

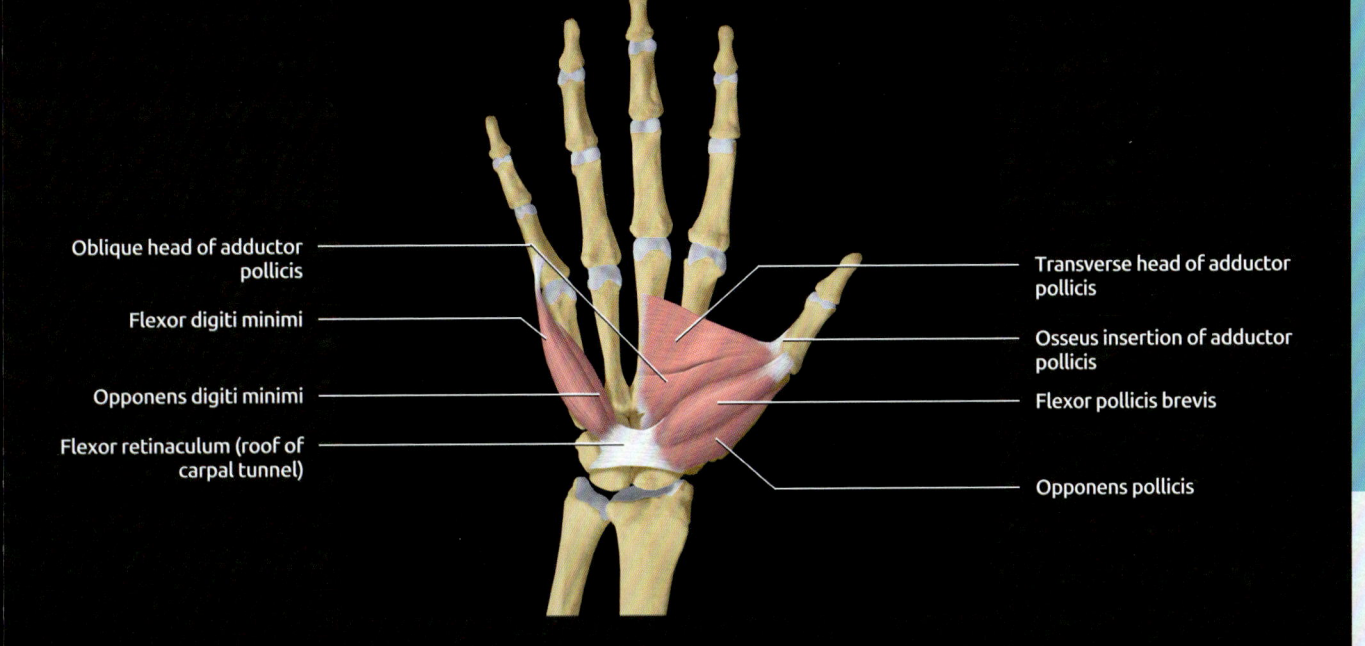

Labels (top image):
- Oblique head of adductor pollicis
- Flexor digiti minimi
- Opponens digiti minimi
- Flexor retinaculum (roof of carpal tunnel)
- Transverse head of adductor pollicis
- Osseus insertion of adductor pollicis
- Flexor pollicis brevis
- Opponens pollicis

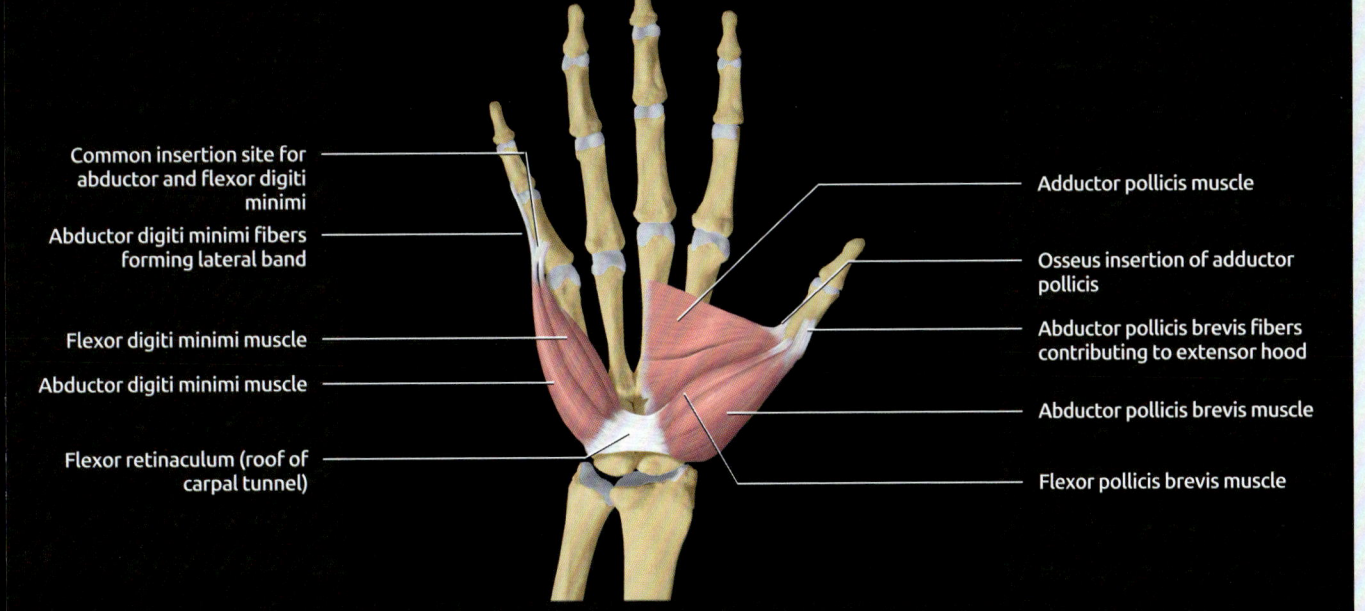

Labels (bottom image):
- Common insertion site for abductor and flexor digiti minimi
- Abductor digiti minimi fibers forming lateral band
- Flexor digiti minimi muscle
- Abductor digiti minimi muscle
- Flexor retinaculum (roof of carpal tunnel)
- Adductor pollicis muscle
- Osseus insertion of adductor pollicis
- Abductor pollicis brevis fibers contributing to extensor hood
- Abductor pollicis brevis muscle
- Flexor pollicis brevis muscle

(**Top**) *Graphic of the hand shows the 2 heads of the adductor pollicis muscle, extending from the 3rd metacarpal to the 1st proximal phalanx. The flexor pollicis brevis and opponens pollicis originate from the flexor retinaculum and trapezium; the former inserts on the base of the 1st proximal phalanx and the latter on the 1st metacarpal.* (**Bottom**) *The abductor pollicis brevis is superficial to the flexor pollicis brevis. They share an osseus insertion on the base of the 1st proximal phalanx. The abductor pollicis brevis also contributes fibers to the extensor hood of the 1st digit.*

Thumb Anatomy

RADIOGRAPHS OF THE THUMB

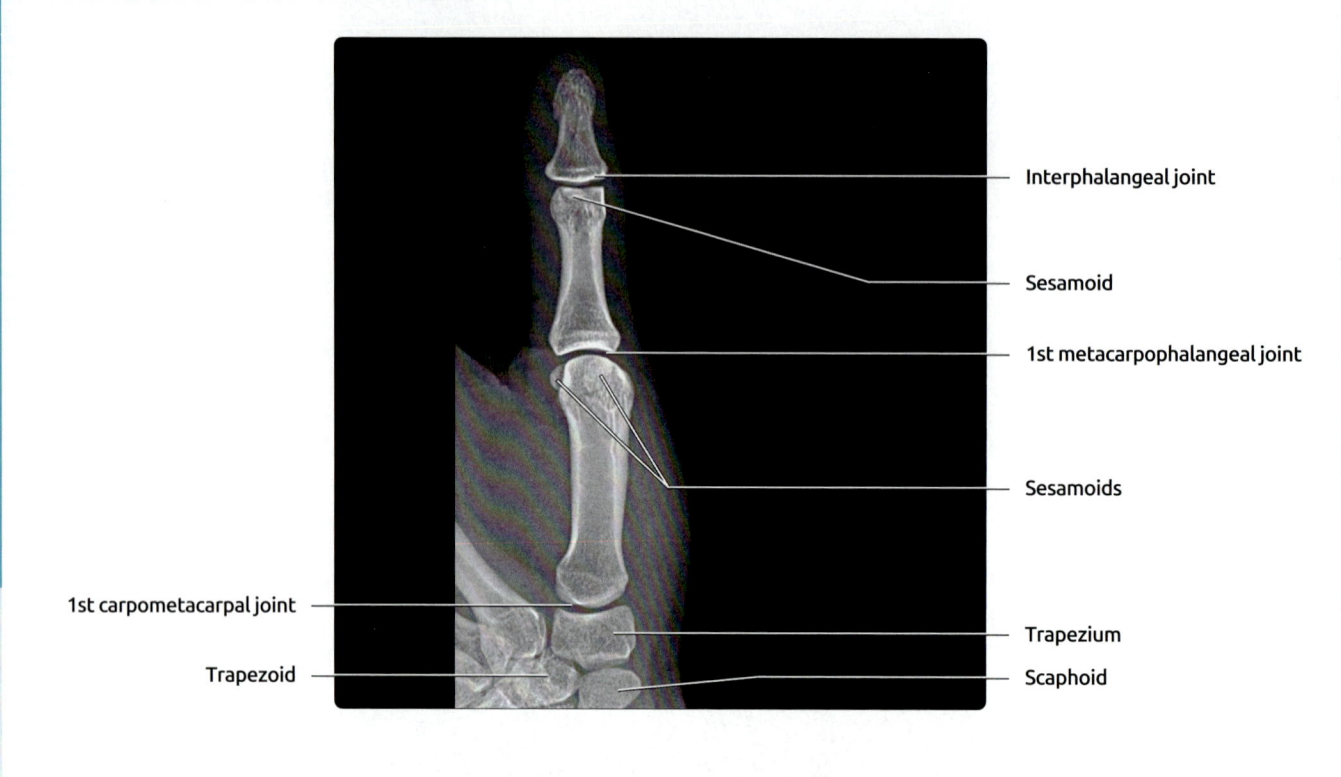

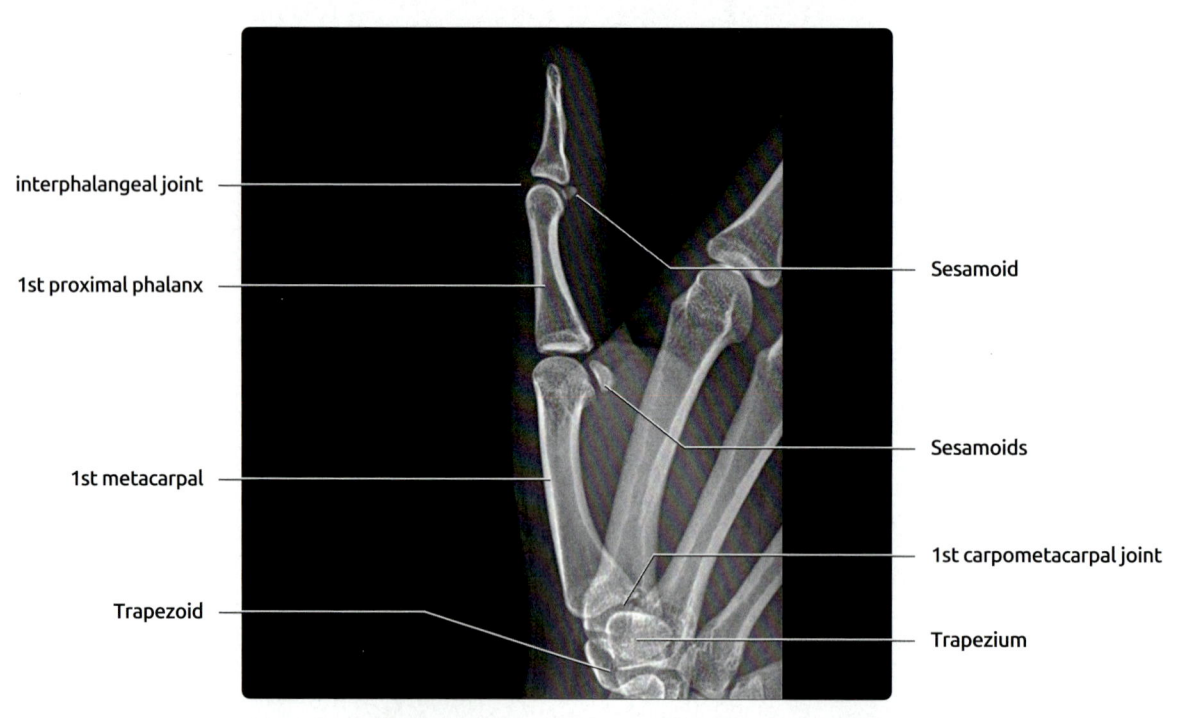

(Top) AP radiograph of the thumb shows the 2 sesamoids at the 1st metacarpophalangeal joint and the single sesamoid at the interphalangeal joint. The relationship of the trapezium to the trapezoid and scaphoid is well seen. *(Bottom)* Lateral view of the thumb shows slight volar subluxation of the 1st metacarpophalangeal joint and slight flexion of the interphalangeal joint. The base of the thumb is subluxated slightly lateral to the trapezius. All of these findings are normal in a resting thumb.

Thumb Anatomy

SAGITTAL MR OF THUMB

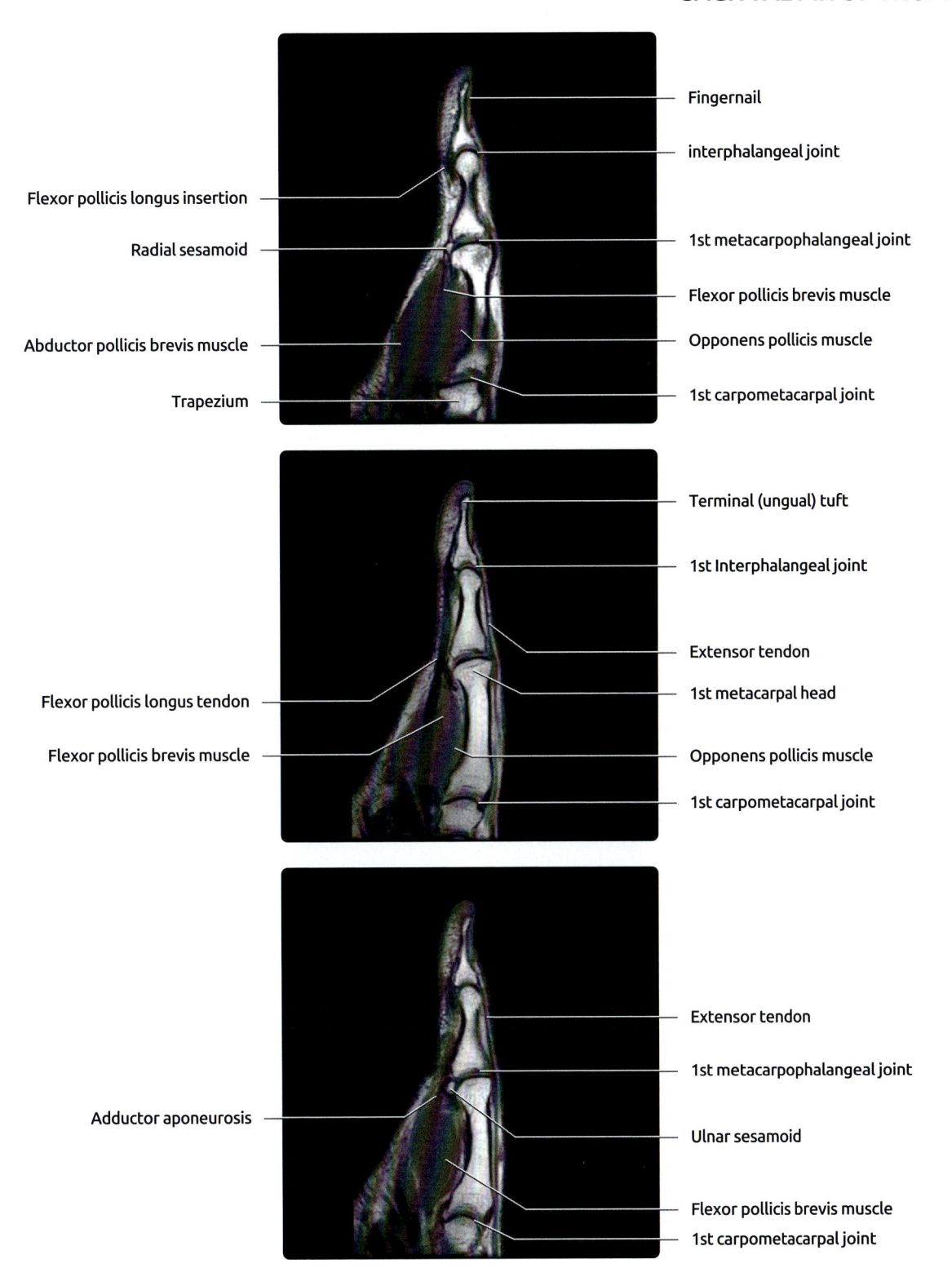

- Flexor pollicis longus insertion
- Radial sesamoid
- Abductor pollicis brevis muscle
- Trapezium
- Fingernail
- Interphalangeal joint
- 1st metacarpophalangeal joint
- Flexor pollicis brevis muscle
- Opponens pollicis muscle
- 1st carpometacarpal joint

- Flexor pollicis longus tendon
- Flexor pollicis brevis muscle
- Terminal (ungual) tuft
- 1st Interphalangeal joint
- Extensor tendon
- 1st metacarpal head
- Opponens pollicis muscle
- 1st carpometacarpal joint

- Adductor aponeurosis
- Extensor tendon
- 1st metacarpophalangeal joint
- Ulnar sesamoid
- Flexor pollicis brevis muscle
- 1st carpometacarpal joint

(Top) This is the 1st of 3 sagittal T1 MR images of the thumb showing the radial sesamoid. The sesamoid lies within the volar plate of the metacarpophalangeal joint. The flexor pollicis brevis inserts on this sesamoid. Opponens pollicis muscle inserts on radial side of 1st metacarpal. **(Middle)** This image is through the central portion of the 1st metacarpophalangeal joint. Note that the 1st metacarpal head is more flat and broad than the heads of the 2nd-5th metacarpals. **(Bottom)** This image is through the ulnar sesamoid of the thumb. The adductor aponeurosis is seen at its volar margin.

Thumb Anatomy

AXIAL ANATOMY OF THUMB

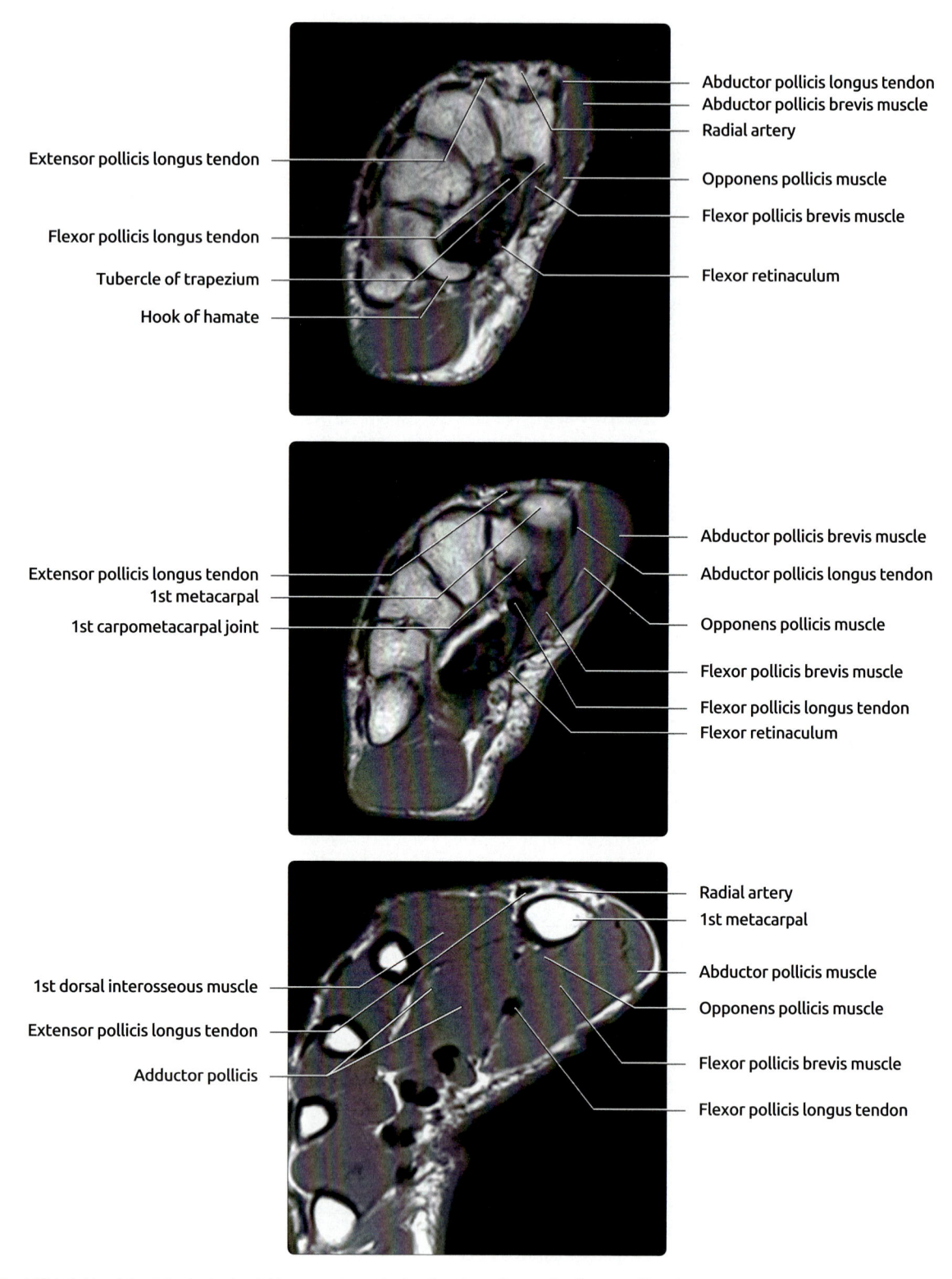

Extensor pollicis longus tendon

Flexor pollicis longus tendon

Tubercle of trapezium

Hook of hamate

Abductor pollicis longus tendon
Abductor pollicis brevis muscle
Radial artery
Opponens pollicis muscle
Flexor pollicis brevis muscle
Flexor retinaculum

Extensor pollicis longus tendon
1st metacarpal
1st carpometacarpal joint

Abductor pollicis brevis muscle
Abductor pollicis longus tendon
Opponens pollicis muscle
Flexor pollicis brevis muscle
Flexor pollicis longus tendon
Flexor retinaculum

1st dorsal interosseous muscle
Extensor pollicis longus tendon
Adductor pollicis

Radial artery
1st metacarpal
Abductor pollicis muscle
Opponens pollicis muscle
Flexor pollicis brevis muscle
Flexor pollicis longus tendon

(Top) *This is the 1st of 6 selected axial images through the thumb. It shows the flexor pollicis longus tendon passing adjacent to the tubercle of the trapezium. The flexor pollicis brevis lies deep to the opponens pollicis muscle, both arising from the trapezium and he flexor retinaculum.* **(Middle)** *This image is through the 1st carpometacarpal joint. The abductor pollicis longus tendon is seen at its insertion. The abductor pollicis brevis is the farthest lateral of the thenar muscles.* **(Bottom)** *This image is through the proximal 1st metacarpal shaft and shows the broad adductor pollicis. The transverse head of the muscle arises from the 3rd metacarpal, while the oblique head arises from the capitate and 2nd-3rd metacarpals.*

Thumb Anatomy

AXIAL MR OF THUMB

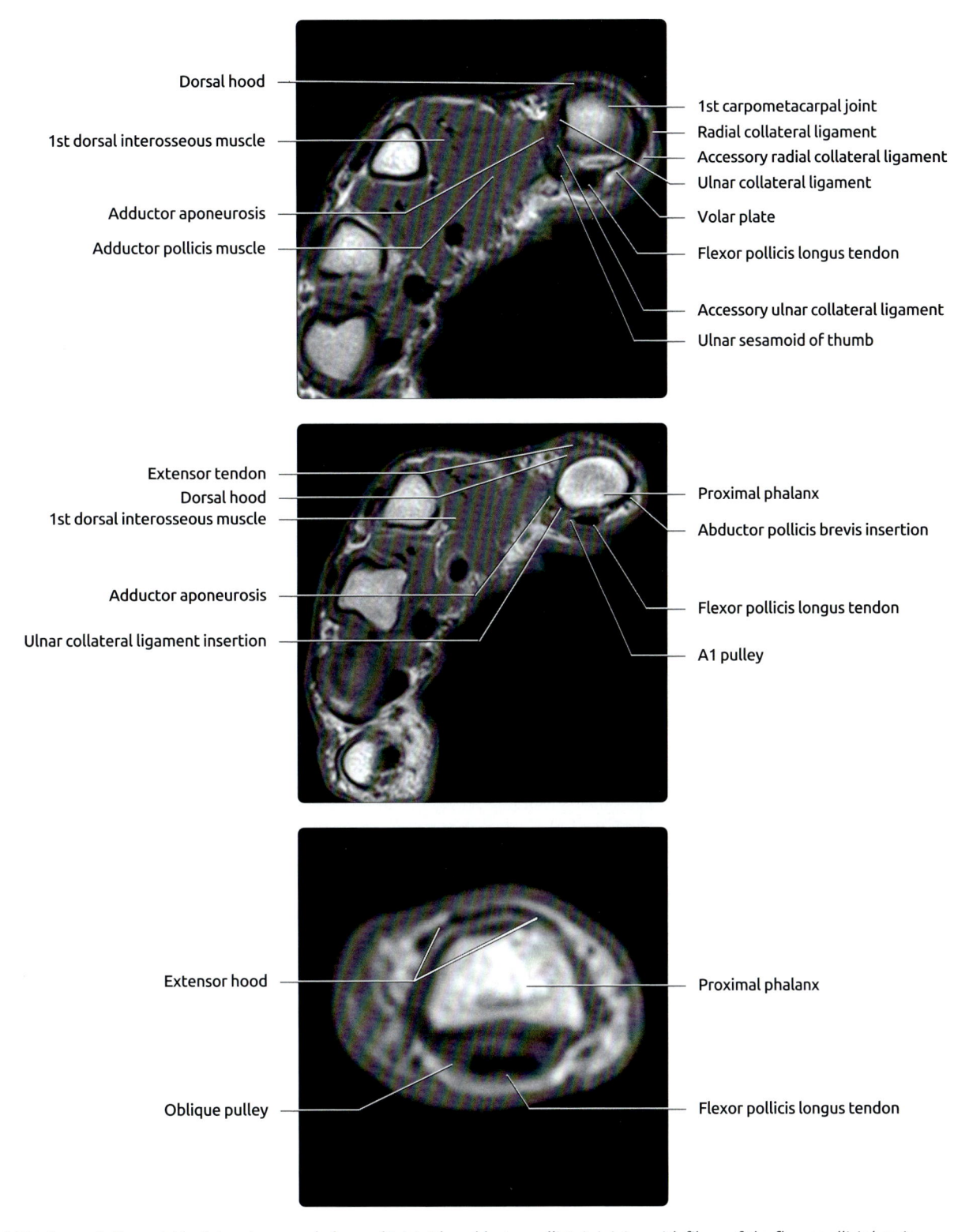

Labels (top image):
- Dorsal hood
- 1st dorsal interosseous muscle
- Adductor aponeurosis
- Adductor pollicis muscle
- 1st carpometacarpal joint
- Radial collateral ligament
- Accessory radial collateral ligament
- Ulnar collateral ligament
- Volar plate
- Flexor pollicis longus tendon
- Accessory ulnar collateral ligament
- Ulnar sesamoid of thumb

Labels (middle image):
- Extensor tendon
- Dorsal hood
- 1st dorsal interosseous muscle
- Adductor aponeurosis
- Ulnar collateral ligament insertion
- Proximal phalanx
- Abductor pollicis brevis insertion
- Flexor pollicis longus tendon
- A1 pulley

Labels (bottom image):
- Extensor hood
- Oblique pulley
- Proximal phalanx
- Flexor pollicis longus tendon

(Top) This image is through the 1st metacarpophalangeal joint. The adductor pollicis is joining with fibers of the flexor pollicis brevis. They contain the ulnar sesamoid of the 1st metacarpophalangeal joint and form the adductor aponeurosis, which inserts on the base of the proximal phalanx. (Middle) At the base of the proximal phalanx, the insertion of the abductor pollicis brevis tendon is seen. The extensor tendon has widened to form the dorsal hood. (Bottom) This image through the proximal phalangeal shaft shows the flexor and extensor pollicis longus tendons as they course to their insertions on the base of the 1st distal phalanx.

Thumb Anatomy

CORONAL MR OF THUMB

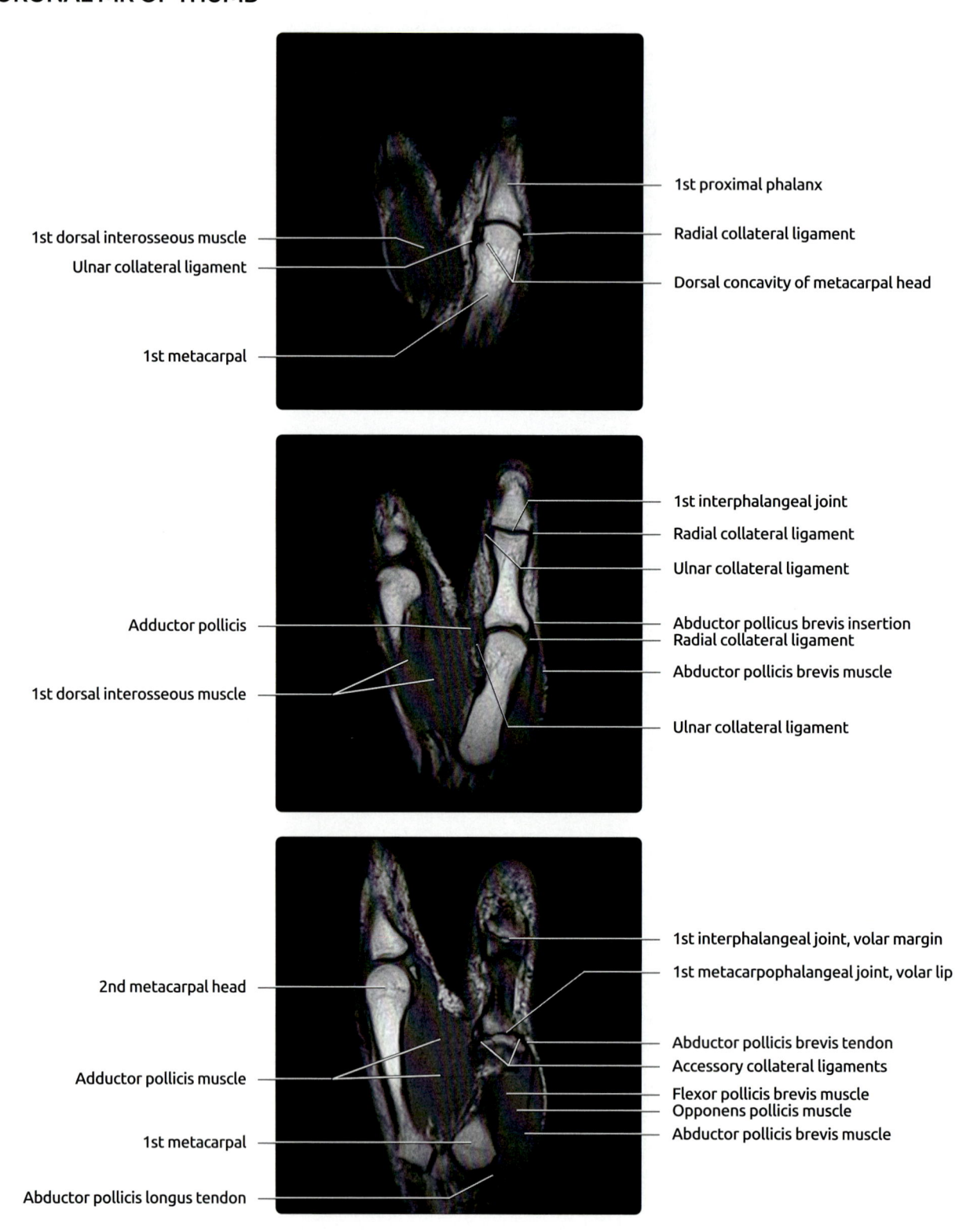

- 1st proximal phalanx
- 1st dorsal interosseous muscle
- Ulnar collateral ligament
- Radial collateral ligament
- Dorsal concavity of metacarpal head
- 1st metacarpal

- 1st interphalangeal joint
- Radial collateral ligament
- Ulnar collateral ligament
- Adductor pollicis
- Abductor pollicus brevis insertion
- Radial collateral ligament
- 1st dorsal interosseous muscle
- Abductor pollicis brevis muscle
- Ulnar collateral ligament

- 1st interphalangeal joint, volar margin
- 1st metacarpophalangeal joint, volar lip
- 2nd metacarpal head
- Adductor pollicis muscle
- Abductor pollicis brevis tendon
- Accessory collateral ligaments
- Flexor pollicis brevis muscle
- Opponens pollicis muscle
- 1st metacarpal
- Abductor pollicis brevis muscle
- Abductor pollicis longus tendon

(**Top**) This is the 1st in a series of 6 coronal images through the thumb from dorsal to volar. The dorsal contour of the 1st metacarpal head shows concave margins at both the radial and ulnar sides. (**Middle**) This image is through the midportion of the 1st metacarpophalangeal joint. The 1st dorsal interosseous muscle arises from the 1st and 2nd metacarpals and inserts on the base of the proximal phalanx as well as the extensor expansion of the 2nd digit. (**Bottom**) This image is through the volar lip of the 1st metacarpophalangeal joint. The accessory radial collateral ligaments of the metacarpophalangeal joints are volar to the primary collateral ligaments.

Thumb Anatomy

CORONAL MR OF THUMB

Labels (Top): Adductor aponeurosis; Adductor pollicis muscle; Opponens pollicis; Articulation between trapezium and 2nd metacarpal; Flexor pollicis longus tendon; Ulnar sesamoid; Radial sesamoid; Flexor pollicis brevis muscle; Abductor pollicis brevis muscle

Labels (Middle): Adductor aponeurosis; Adductor pollicis muscle; ulnar sesamoid; Flexor pollicis longus tendon; Flexor hallucis brevis muscle; Opponens pollicis muscle

Labels (Bottom): 2nd proximal phalanx; Adductor pollicus muscle; Anterior oblique ligament; Trapezoid; Flexor pollicis longus tendon; Flexor pollicis brevis; Opponens pollicis muscle; Abductor pollicis brevis muscle; 1st carpometacarpal joint; Trapezium

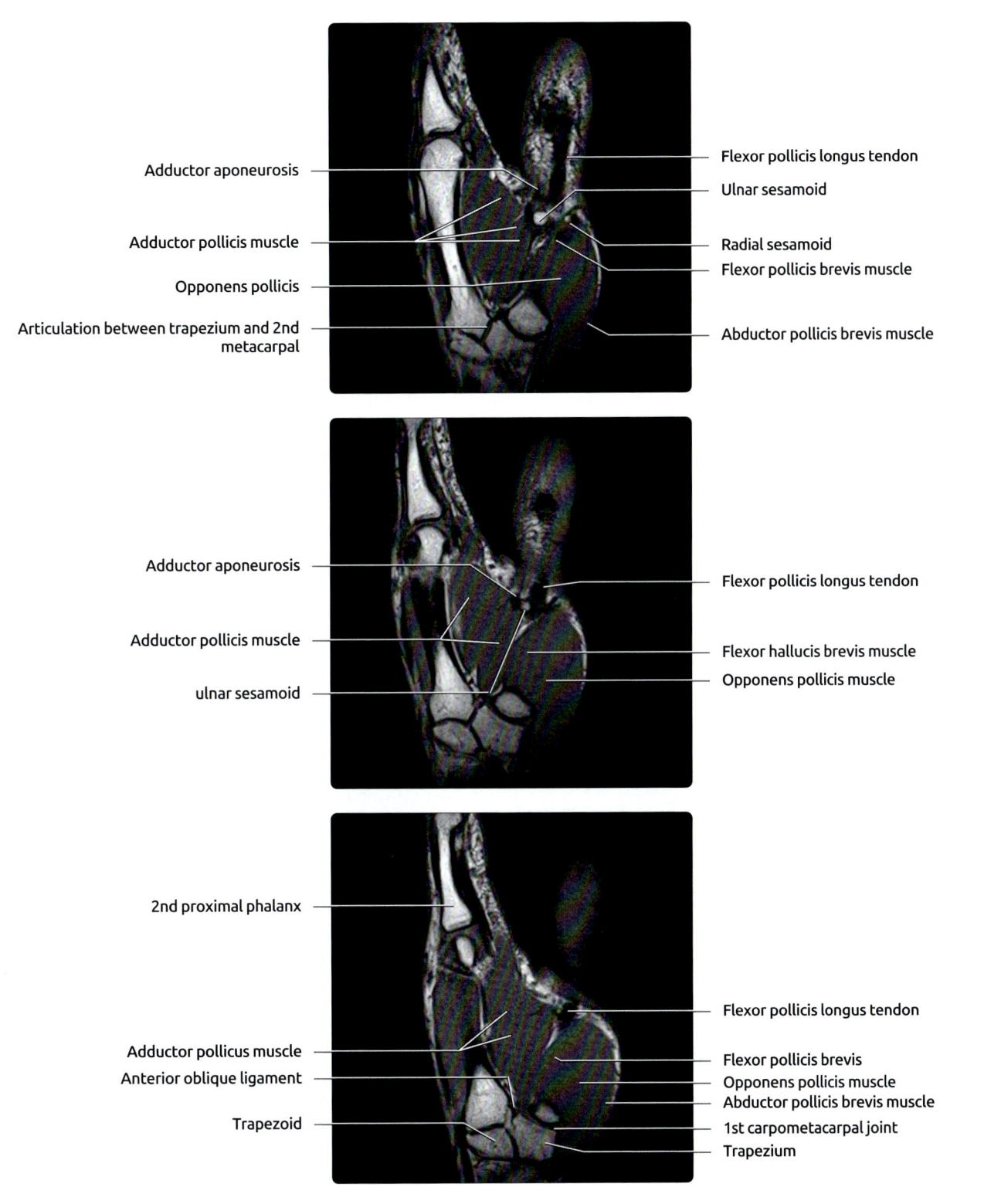

(**Top**) *Volar to the metacarpal head, the radial and ulnar sesamoid of the 1st metacarpophalangeal joints are seen. The opponens pollicis sits at the radial margin of the flexor pollicis brevis.* (**Middle**) *The transverse and oblique heads of the adductor pollicis are seen together with the proximal portion of the adductor aponeurosis.* (**Bottom**) *This image through the volar portion of the thumb shows the flexor pollicis longus tendon between the adductor pollicis and the flexor pollicis brevis. The anterior oblique ligament extends from the tubercle of the trapezium to the ulnar and volar margin of the 2nd metacarpal base and is an important stabilizer of the joint.*

Hand Radiographic Anatomy

TERMINOLOGY

Definitions
- In anatomic position, hand is in supination
  - Thumb points away from body, palm faces forward
- Radial: Toward radius and synonymous with lateral(ly)
- Ulnar: Toward ulna and synonymous with medial(ly)

IMAGING ANATOMY

Orientation of Thumb
- Thumb is abducted and rotated relative to other digits
- Posteroanterior view of hand is near lateral view of thumb

Metacarpals
- Comprised of a base, diaphysis, neck, and head
- Ossification center (epiphysis) is at base of 1st digit
- Ossification center is at head of digits 2-5
- Combined width of diaphyseal cortexes should be equal to width of metacarpal shaft medullary cavity
  - Cortical thinning seen in chronic osteopenia
- 1st metacarpal articulates with trapezium
- 2nd-5th metacarpals articulate with trapezoid, capitate, and hamate (both 4th and 5th) respectively, as well as with one another
- Diaphysis is roughly triangular in cross section with volar apex
  - 3 surfaces: Dorsal, medial volar, & lateral volar
- Diaphysis is gently concave volarly (convex dorsally) throughout its proximal to distal course

Metacarpal Heads
- 2 separate cortical contours should be seen on PA view
- Dorsal cortex is concave, smaller than volar cortex
- Volar cortex convex, comes to sharp point at joint margin
- Erosions due to inflammatory/infections arthritis seen 1st at peripheral margin of volar cortex

Phalanges
- Digits 2-5 are triphalangeal
- 1st digit is biphalangeal
- Comprised of base, diaphysis, and head
- Ossification center (epiphysis) is at phalangeal base
- Heads are bicondylar with condyles separated by shallow groove
- Proximal articular surfaces of proximal phalanges form single concavity
- Proximal articular surfaces of middle and distal phalanges are biconcave with a median ridge running anteroposteriorly
- Nutrient grooves medially and laterally extend from midshaft toward head
  - Distinguished from fracture by their smooth contour, parallel margins

Appearance of Terminal Tufts
- May vary in size; cortical margins should always be distinct

Evaluating Joint Width
- Interphalangeal joints are normally narrow; this may be exaggerated by obliquity of x-ray beam
- Best to evaluate on lateral radiographs rather than posteroanterior view

ANATOMY IMAGING ISSUES

Imaging Pitfalls
- Thumb alignment
  - Slight radial subluxation at 1st carpometacarpal joint is normal
  - Slight volar subluxation at 1st metacarpophalangeal joint is normal
- Normal trabecular anatomy
  - Trabeculae are fairly sparse in normal phalanges
  - Look for normal interlacing of primary (vertical) and secondary (horizontal) trabeculae
    - Loss of secondary trabeculae a sign of osteopenia
  - Trabeculae on end sometimes mistaken for enchondroma calcifications
- Ulnar variance cannot be accurately assessed on hand series
  - Need series centered on wrist, shoulder abducted 90°, elbow and wrist at same level as shoulder

Evaluating Alignment
- Patient positioning may mimic malalignment, be cautious in diagnosis

Nutrient Grooves
- Smooth, parallel margins help distinguish from fracture

RADIOGRAPHIC VIEWS

Hand Series
- Proper positioning is key
- Standard hand series usually consists of PA, PA oblique, and lateral view

PA Oblique View
- 30-45° rotation, thumb up, 5th finger against imaging plate
- Allows visualization of "bare area" of metacarpal heads
  - Margin of joint, intrasynovial but not covered by cartilage
  - Early site where rheumatoid arthritis can be seen

Lateral View
- 5th finger against imaging plate
- Fingers fanned: Thumb and 2nd finger touch, other fingers arranged fanning back
- Important not to dorsiflex the wrist in order to optimize visualization of anatomic relationships
- Best for visualization of interphalangeal joint space
  - Slight flexion of digit on AP or oblique may cause spurious appearance of joint narrowing
- Joint subluxations/dislocations may be best seen on this view

AP Oblique View
- Palm up, hand rotated 30-45°
- 5th finger against imaging plate
- Especially useful as additional view of metacarpophalangeal joints
  - Evaluation of rheumatoid arthritis
- Often useful for serendipitous evaluation of carpus
  - Obliquity of the beam may show abnormalities not visible on wrist radiographs

Hand Radiographic Anatomy

PA & LATERAL RADIOGRAPHS OF HAND

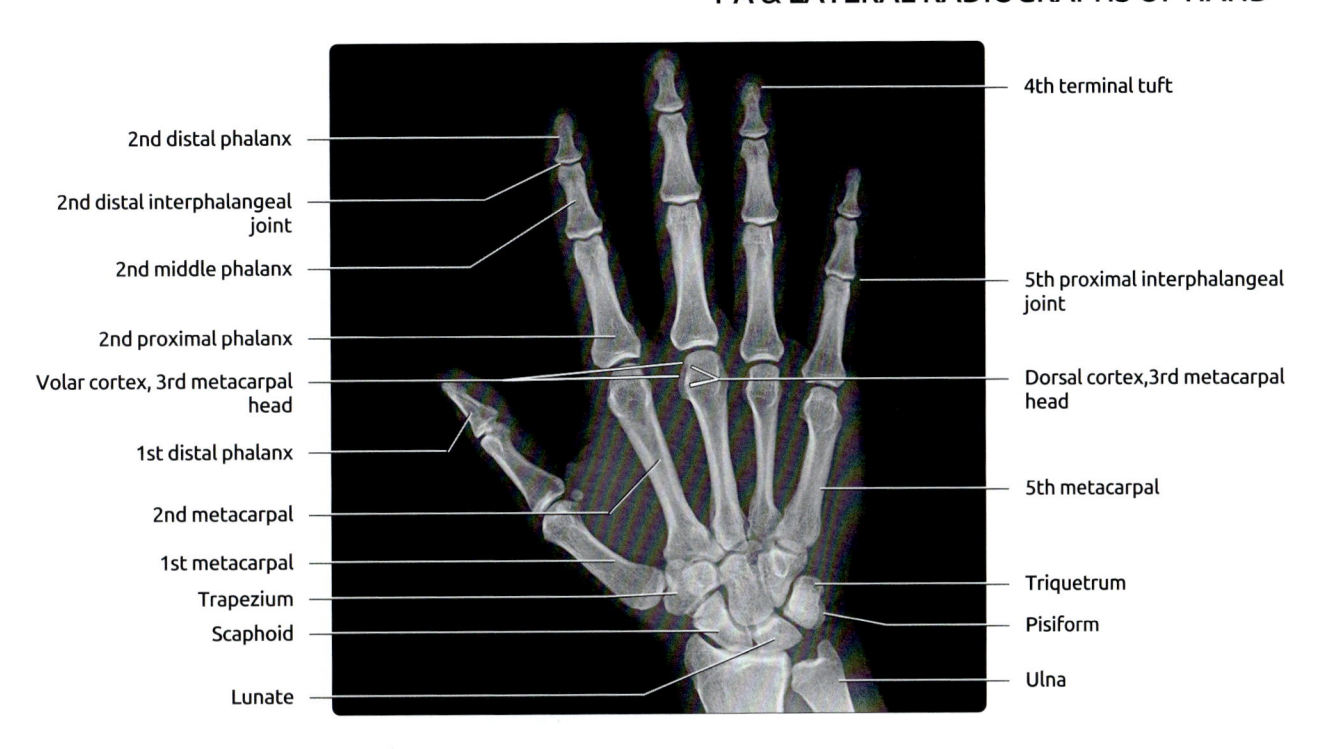

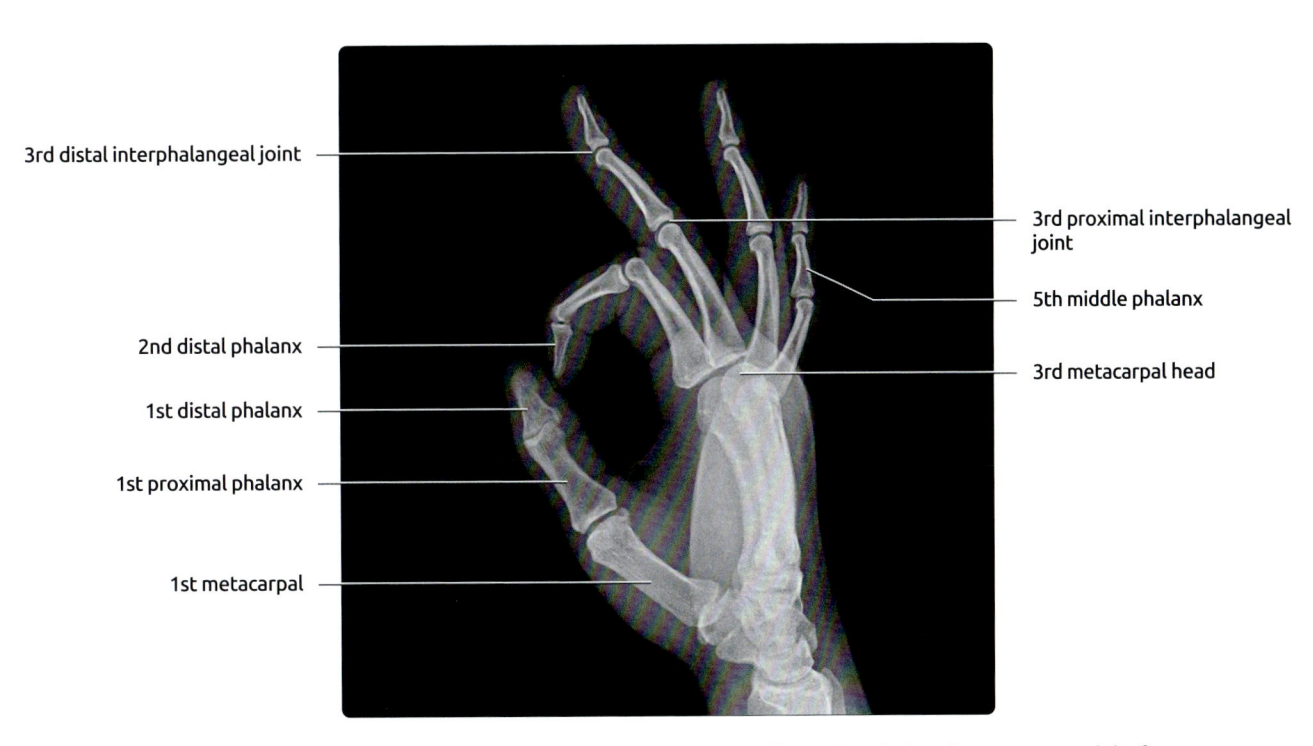

(Top) Posteroanterior view of the hand is performed with the hand as flat as possible against the imaging cassette, and the fingers straight. The divergent position of the thumb is well appreciated. Note 2 separate contours of the 2nd-5th metacarpal heads: The concave dorsal contour, and the convex volar contour. **(Bottom)** Lateral view of the hand is obtained with the fingers fanned. The index finger is brought to the thumb, creating an "O," while the 3rd-5th fingers are progressively fanned posteriorly. The 3rd metacarpal is the longest of the metacarpals.

Hand Radiographic Anatomy

ADDITIONAL VIEWS OF HAND

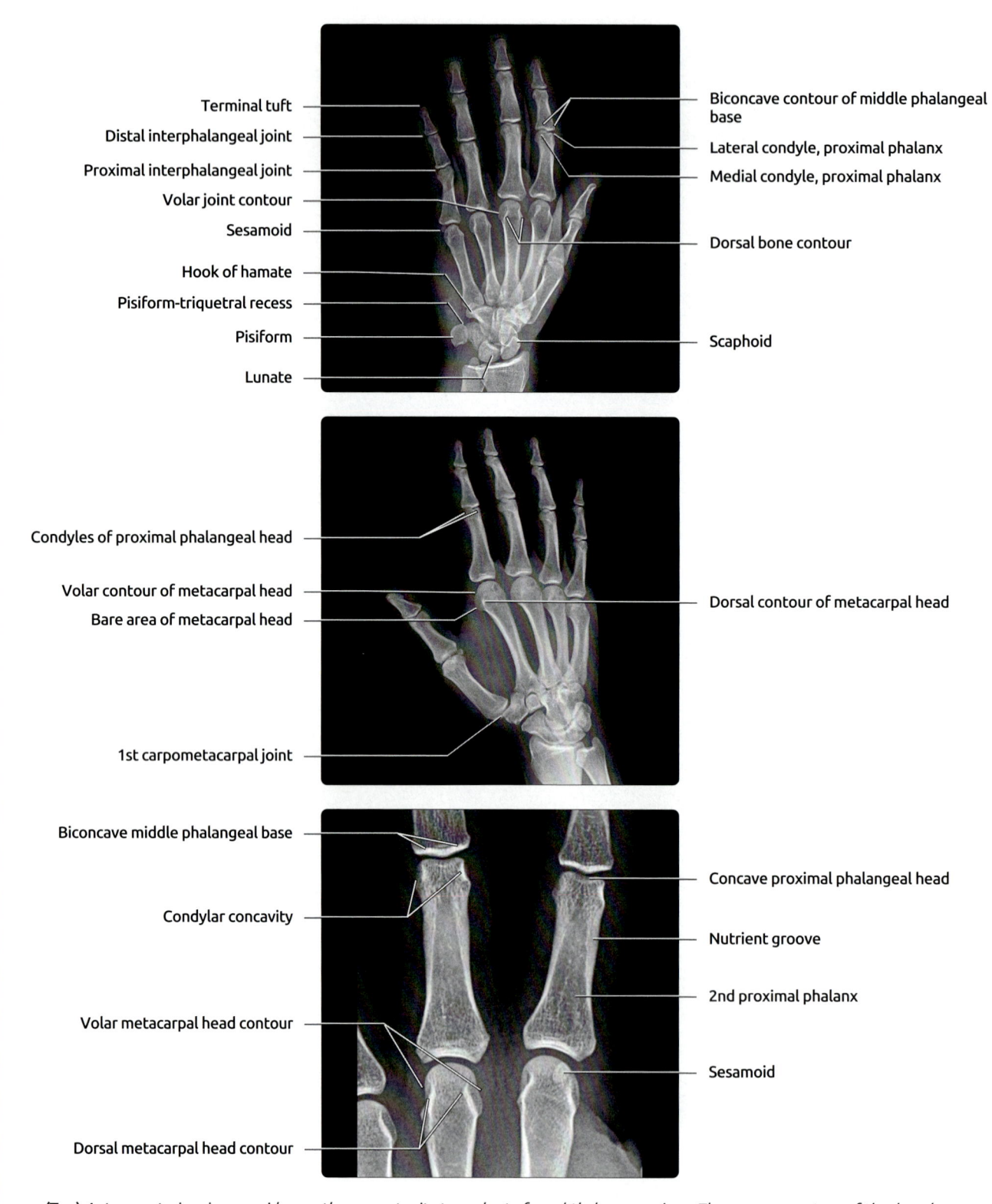

Labels (top image):
- Terminal tuft
- Distal interphalangeal joint
- Proximal interphalangeal joint
- Volar joint contour
- Sesamoid
- Hook of hamate
- Pisiform-triquetral recess
- Pisiform
- Lunate
- Biconcave contour of middle phalangeal base
- Lateral condyle, proximal phalanx
- Medial condyle, proximal phalanx
- Dorsal bone contour
- Scaphoid

Labels (middle image):
- Condyles of proximal phalangeal head
- Volar contour of metacarpal head
- Bare area of metacarpal head
- 1st carpometacarpal joint
- Dorsal contour of metacarpal head

Labels (bottom image):
- Biconcave middle phalangeal base
- Condylar concavity
- Volar metacarpal head contour
- Dorsal metacarpal head contour
- Concave proximal phalangeal head
- Nutrient groove
- 2nd proximal phalanx
- Sesamoid

(**Top**) *Anteroposterior view provides another opportunity to evaluate for subtle bone erosions. The concave contour of the dorsal margin of the metacarpal heads is well seen on this view. Although radiographs centered on the wrist are usually preferred for evaluation of wrist abnormalities, they may show up by serendipity on hand views and the wrist should be included in the search pattern of hand radiographs.* (**Middle**) *The oblique view of the hand is useful in evaluation of arthritis. It shows the volar cortex of the metacarpal heads in profile. The margin of the metacarpal head lies within the synovial cavity but is not covered by cartilage (bare area) and is often the 1st site where erosive arthritis can be detected. Slight subluxation of 1st carpometacarpal joint is seen, and is within normal range.* (**Bottom**) *Coned view of the 2nd-3rd digits shows the concave dorsal metacarpal head contour superimposed on the rounded, volar contour.*

Hand Radiographic Anatomy

RADIOGRAPHS OF THUMB

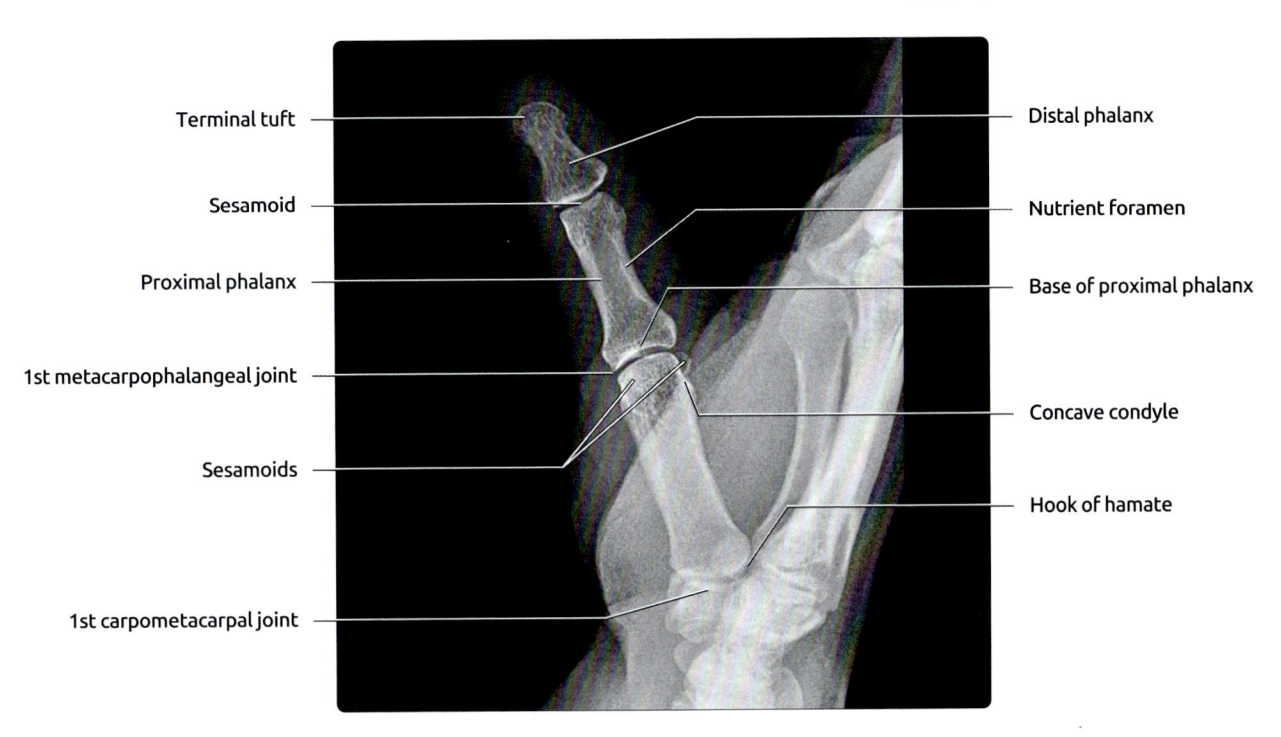

Top image labels:
- Terminal tuft
- Sesamoid
- Proximal phalanx
- 1st metacarpophalangeal joint
- Sesamoids
- 1st carpometacarpal joint
- Distal phalanx
- Nutrient foramen
- Base of proximal phalanx
- Concave condyle
- Hook of hamate

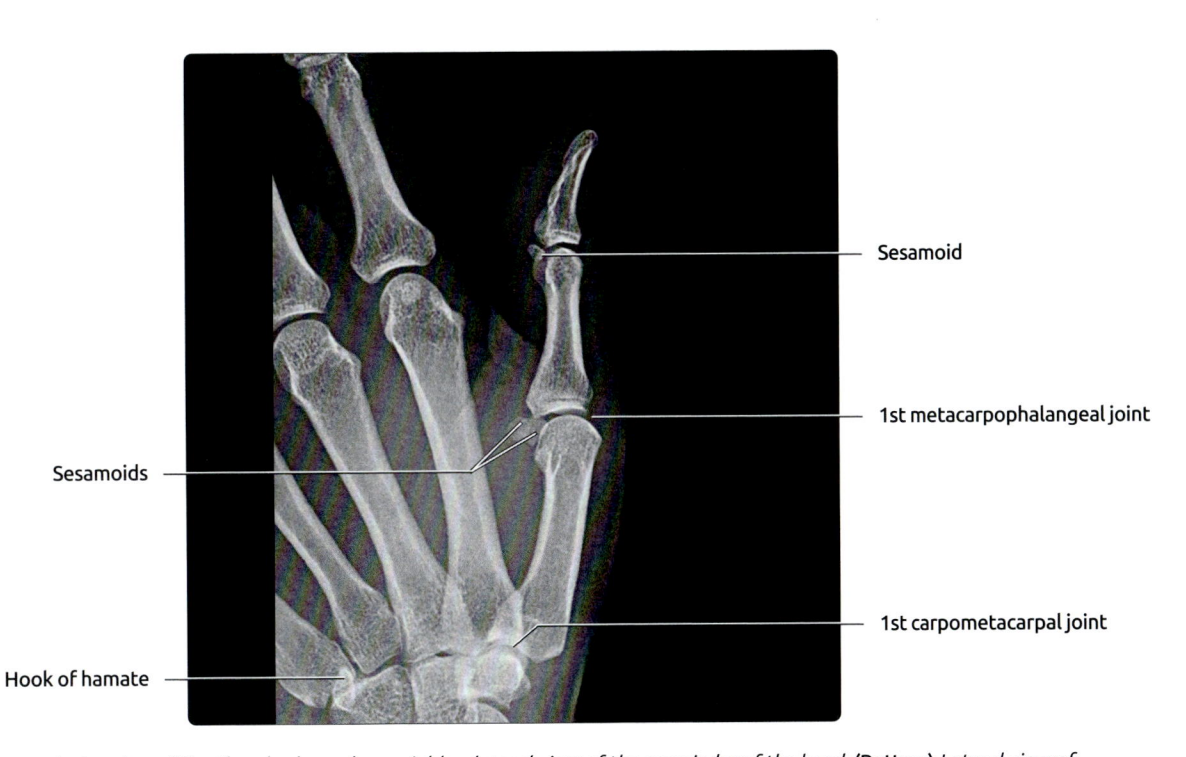

Bottom image labels:
- Sesamoids
- Hook of hamate
- Sesamoid
- 1st metacarpophalangeal joint
- 1st carpometacarpal joint

(**Top**) The posteroanterior view of the thumb, shown here, yields a lateral view of the remainder of the hand. (**Bottom**) Lateral view of the thumb shows slight volar position of the 1st proximal phalanx relative to metacarpal. This is a common, normal finding.

Hand MR Atlas

TERMINOLOGY

Definitions
- For this text, hand will be defined as beginning at carpometacarpal joint
- In anatomic position, hand is in supination
- Radial: Toward radius and synonymous with lateral(ly)
- Ulnar: Toward ulna and synonymous with medial(ly)
- Mesial: Toward midline of structure
  - In the hand, for example, 3rd digit is more mesial than 2nd and 4th digits, which are more mesial than 1st and 5th digits
- Opposition: Motion bringing thumb toward other digits; critical motion for grasping objects

SUMMARY OF MUSCLES OF HAND

2nd-5th Digits
- More detailed information is found in "Flexor and Extensor Mechanisms of Hand" chapter
- Flexor digitorum superficialis: Inserts base of middle phalanx, flexes metacarpophangeal joint, and proximal interphalangeal joint
- Flexor digitorum profundus: Inserts distal phalanx, flexes primarily distal interphalangeal joint but also proximal interphalangeal and metacarpophalangeal joints
- Lumbricals: Insert on extensor expansion, flex metacarpophalangeal joints, and extend interphalangeal joints
- Palmar interossei: Insert on extensor expansion and base of proximal phalanx
  - Present on index, ring, and little fingers and adduct these digits toward long finger
  - Flex metacarpophalangeal joints and extend interphalangeal joints
- Dorsal interossei: Insert on extensor expansion and base of proximal phalanx
  - Abduct fingers away from the long finger
  - Flex metacarpophalangeal joints and extend interphalangeal joints at digit index, long and ring fingers
- Abductor digiti minimi: Inserts ulnar side of base of middle phalanx; abducts little finger
- Extensor digitorum communis, extensor indicis, extensor digiti minimi
  - Extensive attachments along extensor expansion, middle phalanx, and distal phalanx
- Opponens digiti minimi: Inserts 5th metacarpal, brings 5th finger toward thumb (opposition)

1st Digit
- More detailed information is found in "Thumb" chapter
- Extensor pollicis longus: Inserts distal phalanx, extends metacarpophalangeal and interphalangeal joints
- Extensor pollicis brevis: Inserts proximal phalanx, extends metacarpophalangeal joint
- Adductor pollicis: Inserts base proximal phalanx, adducts thumb
- Abductor pollicis brevis: Inserts lateral margin base proximal phalanx; abducts, opposes, and extends thumb
- Abductor pollicis longus: Multiple insertions, on lateral margin base of metacarpal, also joint capsule and abductor pollicis brevis; abducts thumb
- Opponens pollicis: Inserts lateral side of metacarpal, opposes thumb

MR TIPS

Best Planes for Imaging
- Flexor tendons: Axial and sagittal
- Extensor tendons: Axial and sagittal
- Tendon sheaths: Axial > sagittal
- Musculature: Axial > coronal and sagittal
- Pulleys: Axial > sagittal
- Collateral ligaments: Coronal and axial
- Volar plate: Sagittal > axial

Coils
- Circumferential coils are generally preferred
  - Dedicated combined hand and wrist coils available
  - Knee coils can be used if nothing else available: Place hand on pads to center in coil

Patient Positioning
- Hand as close as possible to center of magnet (superoinferior as well as mediolateral)
- Prone or semiprone, arm over head
- Care to patient comfort minimizes motion

IMAGING PITFALLS

Inhomogeneous Fat Saturation
- Can be mistaken for abnormal signal
- More likely to be seen when
  - Coil not in center of magnet
  - At ends of field of view
  - Coil not circumferential

Magic Angle Phenomenon
- Seen with short TE sequences
- Occurs when structures composed of parallel fibers (almost exclusively tendons) are oriented at 55° to main magnetic vector
- **Lack of increased signal in same location on long TE (usually T2 or STIR) sequences confirms magic angle**

Fluid in Tendon Sheaths
- A small amount of fluid is normal
- Circumferential fluid around a tendon is usually abnormal

Heterogeneous Appearance of Collateral Ligament Complex
- Commonly seen in normal digits
- Compare to other collateral ligaments and evaluate continuity

Hand MR Atlas

ARTERIAL ANATOMY

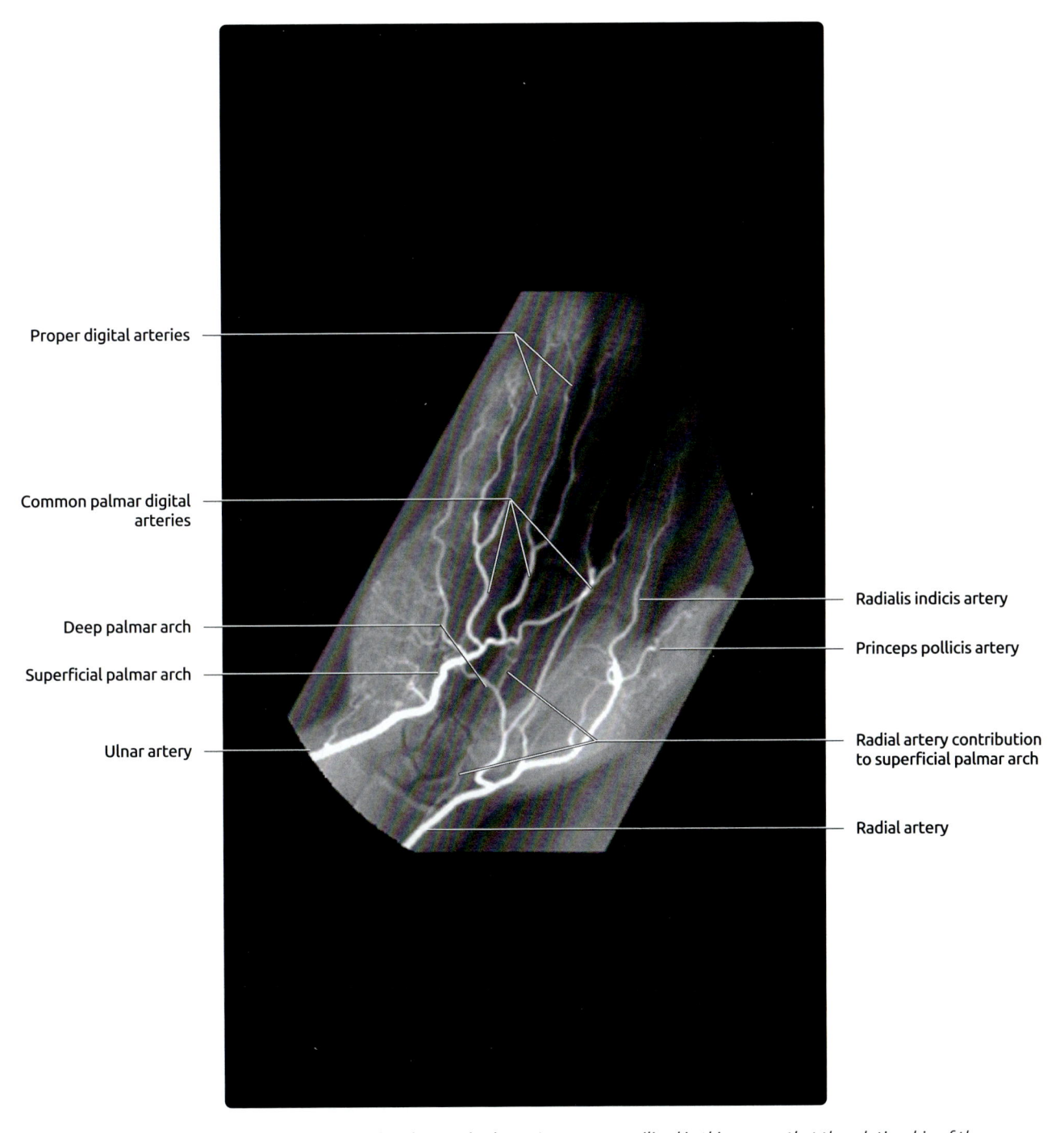

- Proper digital arteries
- Common palmar digital arteries
- Deep palmar arch
- Superficial palmar arch
- Ulnar artery
- Radialis indicis artery
- Princeps pollicis artery
- Radial artery contribution to superficial palmar arch
- Radial artery

Conventional angiogram shows the arteries of the hand. Digital subtraction was not utilized in this case so that the relationship of the arteries to the underlying bony architecture could be demonstrated.

Hand MR Atlas

AXIAL T1 MR, LEFT HAND

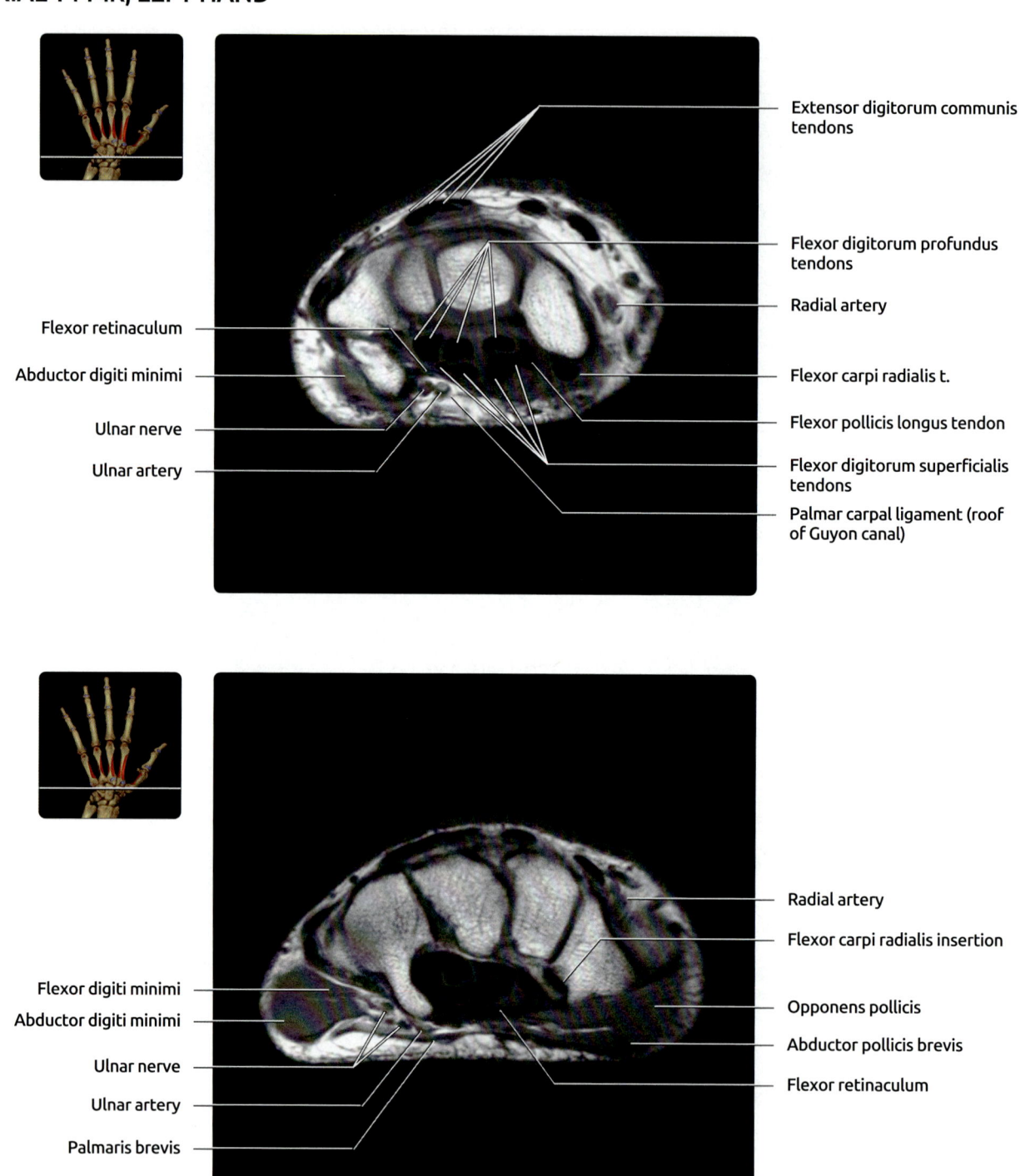

Labels (top image):
- Extensor digitorum communis tendons
- Flexor digitorum profundus tendons
- Radial artery
- Flexor carpi radialis t.
- Flexor pollicis longus tendon
- Flexor digitorum superficialis tendons
- Palmar carpal ligament (roof of Guyon canal)
- Flexor retinaculum
- Abductor digiti minimi
- Ulnar nerve
- Ulnar artery

Labels (bottom image):
- Radial artery
- Flexor carpi radialis insertion
- Opponens pollicis
- Abductor pollicis brevis
- Flexor retinaculum
- Flexor digiti minimi
- Abductor digiti minimi
- Ulnar nerve
- Ulnar artery
- Palmaris brevis

(Top) *This is the 1st in series of selected axial T1 MR images of the left hand. Note the ulnar artery and nerve in Guyon canal. Also note the ghosting (pulsation) artifact from the radial artery at the radial aspect of the dorsal wrist. This artifact can occasionally help locate the normal vascular structures.* **(Bottom)** *This axial MR image of the left hand is at the level of hook of hamate. Note the thenar muscles originating from the flexor retinaculum. At the level of the hook of the hamate, the ulnar artery generally passes anterior or anteromedial to the hook, whereas the ulnar nerve and its branches generally pass lateral to the hook.*

Hand MR Atlas

AXIAL T1 MR, RIGHT HAND

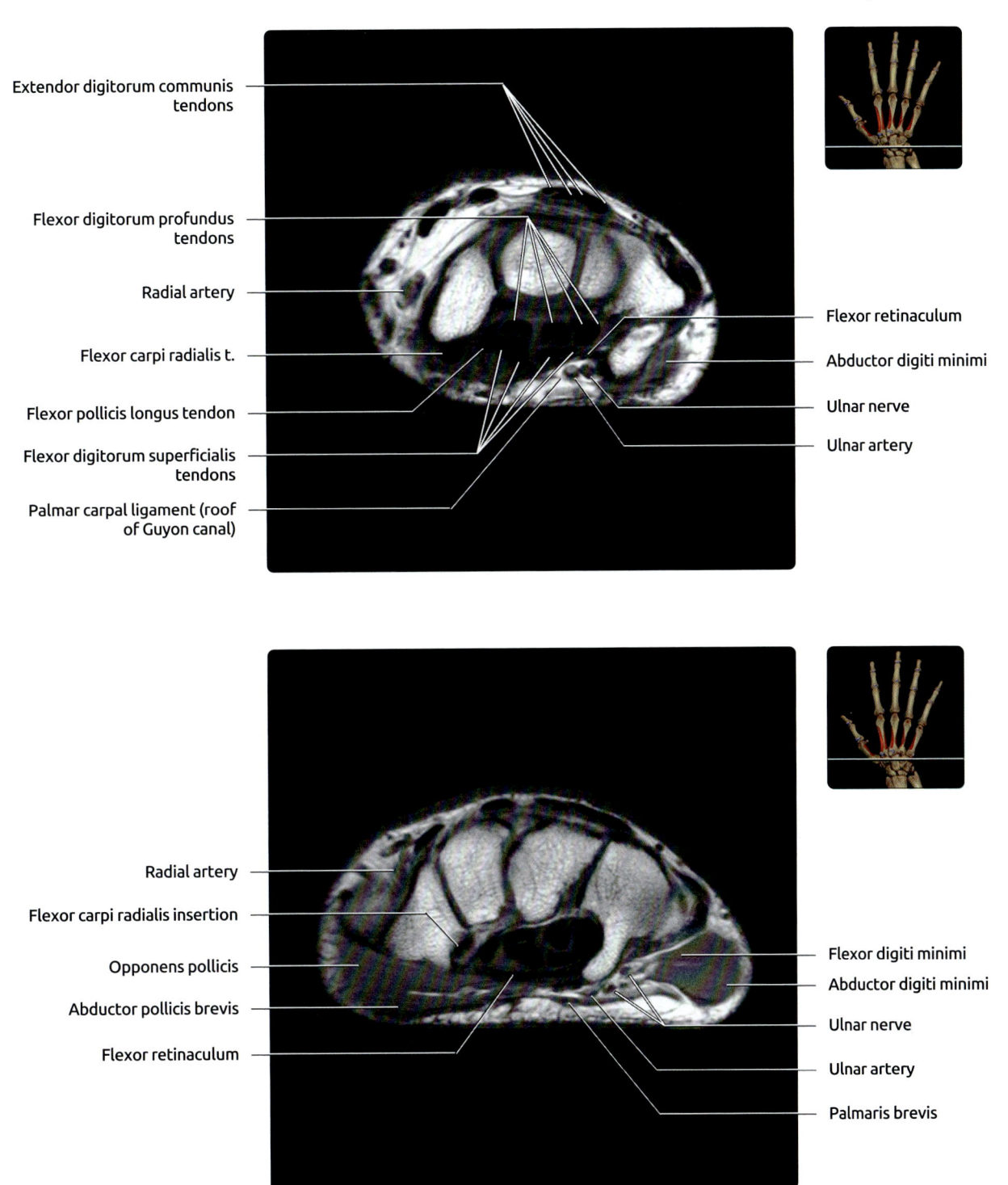

Labels (Top image):
- Extendor digitorum communis tendons
- Flexor digitorum profundus tendons
- Radial artery
- Flexor carpi radialis t.
- Flexor pollicis longus tendon
- Flexor digitorum superficialis tendons
- Palmar carpal ligament (roof of Guyon canal)
- Flexor retinaculum
- Abductor digiti minimi
- Ulnar nerve
- Ulnar artery

Labels (Bottom image):
- Radial artery
- Flexor carpi radialis insertion
- Opponens pollicis
- Abductor pollicis brevis
- Flexor retinaculum
- Flexor digiti minimi
- Abductor digiti minimi
- Ulnar nerve
- Ulnar artery
- Palmaris brevis

(Top) This is the 1st in series of selected axial T1 MR images of the right hand. Note the ulnar artery and nerve in Guyon canal. Also note the ghosting (pulsation) artifact from the radial artery at the radial aspect of the dorsal wrist. This artifact can occasionally help locate the normal vascular structures. **(Bottom)** This axial MR image is at the level of hook of hamate. Note the thenar muscles originating from the flexor retinaculum. At the level of the hook of the hamate, the ulnar artery generally passes anterior or anteromedial to the hook, whereas the ulnar nerve and its branches generally pass lateral to the hook.

Hand MR Atlas

AXIAL T1 MR, LEFT HAND

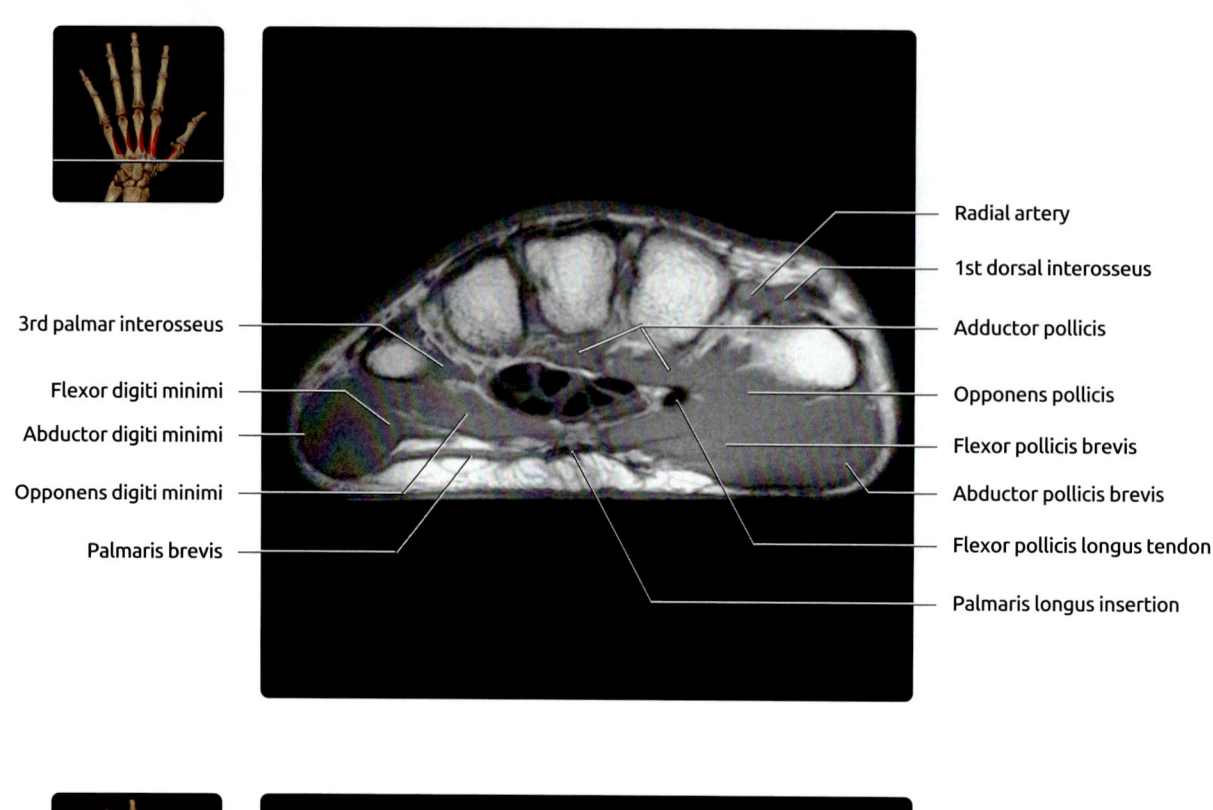

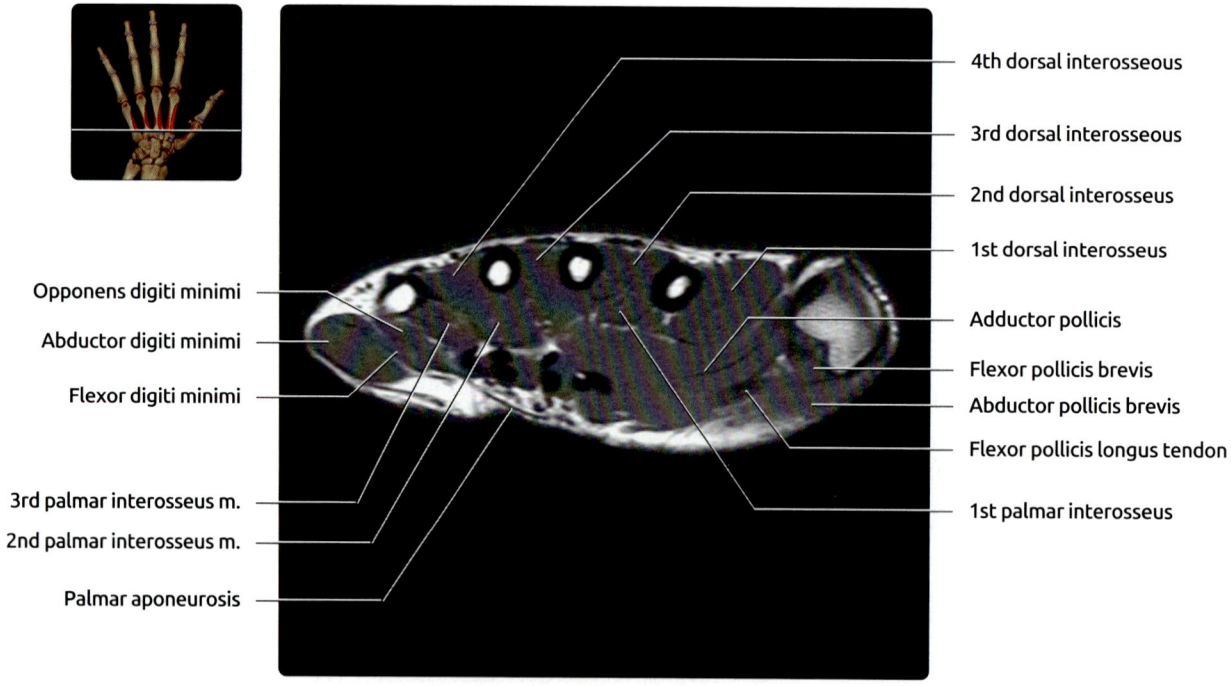

Labels (top image):
- 3rd palmar interosseus
- Flexor digiti minimi
- Abductor digiti minimi
- Opponens digiti minimi
- Palmaris brevis
- Radial artery
- 1st dorsal interosseus
- Adductor pollicis
- Opponens pollicis
- Flexor pollicis brevis
- Abductor pollicis brevis
- Flexor pollicis longus tendon
- Palmaris longus insertion

Labels (bottom image):
- Opponens digiti minimi
- Abductor digiti minimi
- Flexor digiti minimi
- 3rd palmar interosseus m.
- 2nd palmar interosseus m.
- Palmar aponeurosis
- 4th dorsal interosseous
- 3rd dorsal interosseous
- 2nd dorsal interosseus
- 1st dorsal interosseus
- Adductor pollicis
- Flexor pollicis brevis
- Abductor pollicis brevis
- Flexor pollicis longus tendon
- 1st palmar interosseus

(Top) *This axial T1 MR image of the left hand is through the level of the metacarpal bases. The palmaris longus inserts onto the palmar aponeurosis (a fascial layer superficial to the flexor retinaculum) and can be identified as a midline thickening of the palmar aponeurosis. It is a relatively insignificant muscle, and as such, its long tendon is often sacrificed for tendon repairs at other sites.*
(Bottom) *This axial T1 MR image of the left hand is through the mid metacarpals. At this level, we are beyond the carpal tunnel. The lumbricals are beginning to come into view adjacent to the flexor tendons.*

Hand MR Atlas

AXIAL T1 MR, RIGHT HAND

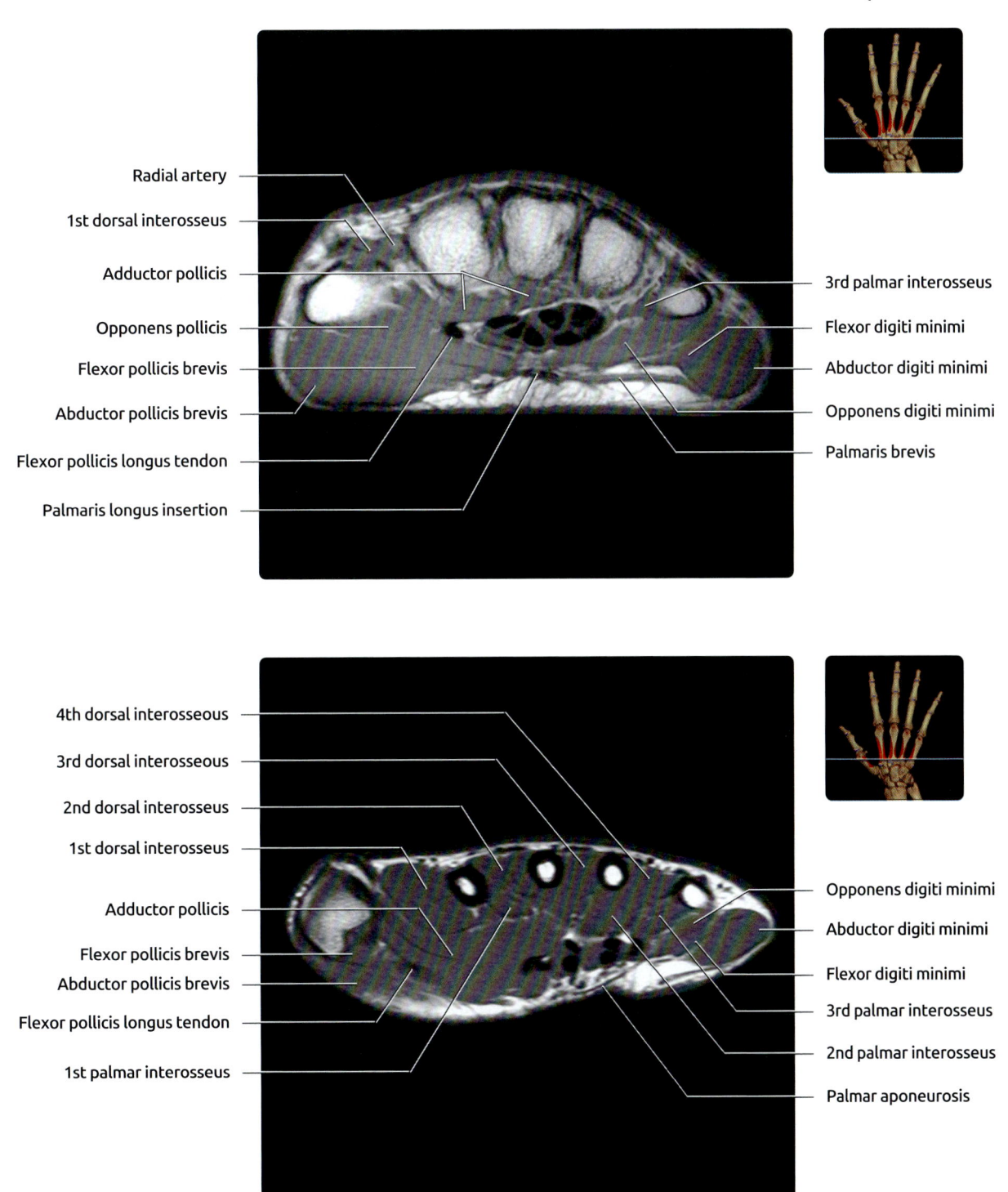

(Top) This axial T1 MR image of the right hand is through the level of the metacarpal bases. The palmaris longus inserts onto the palmar aponeurosis (a fascial layer superficial to the flexor retinaculum) and can be identified as a midline thickening of the palmar aponeurosis. It is a relatively insignificant muscle, and as such, its long tendon is often sacrificed for tendon repairs at other sites. **(Bottom)** This axial T1 MR image of the right hand is through the mid metacarpals. At this level, we are beyond the carpal tunnel. The lumbricals are beginning to come into view adjacent to the flexor tendons.

Hand MR Atlas

AXIAL T1 MR, LEFT HAND

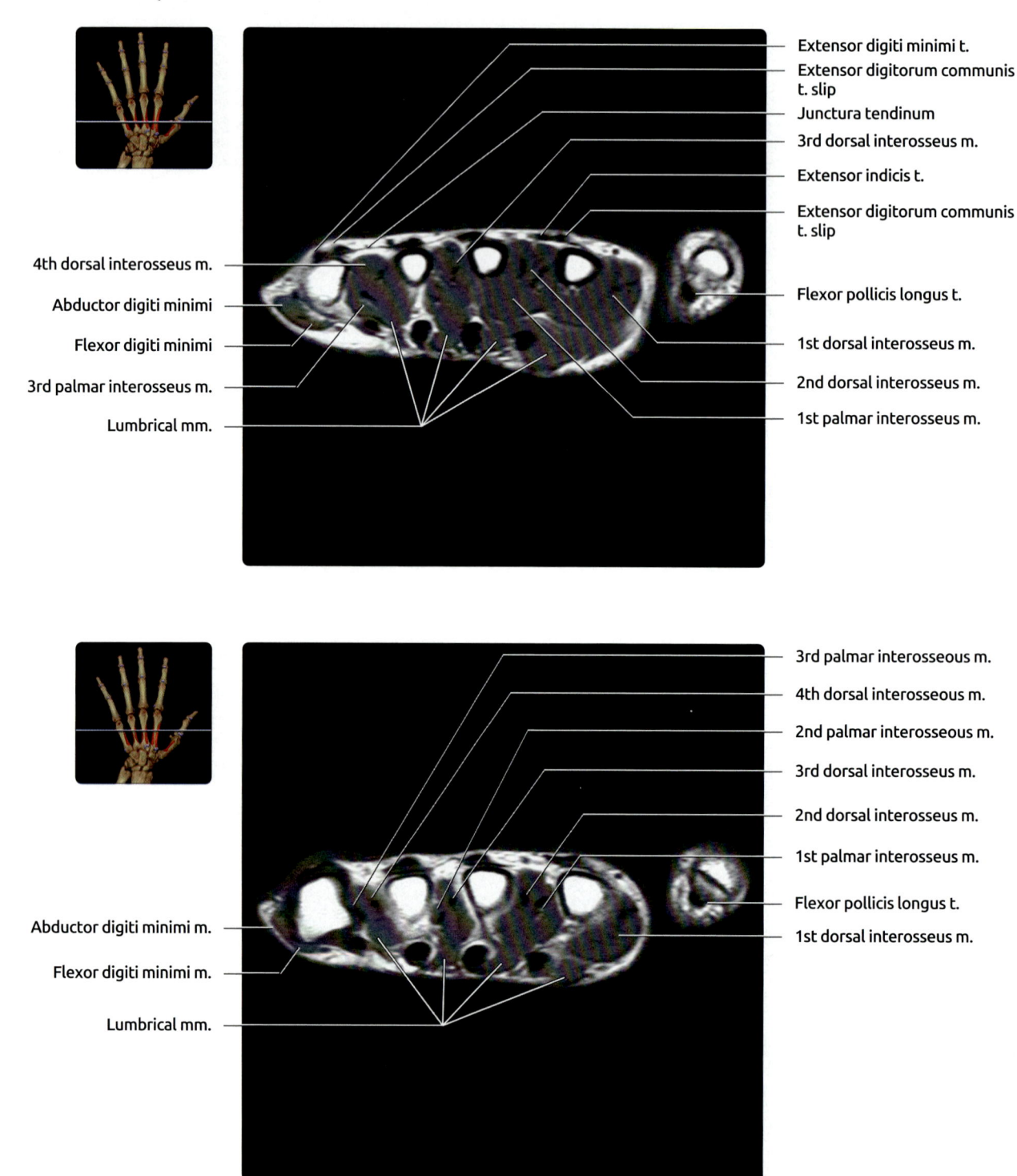

Labels (top image):
- Extensor digiti minimi t.
- Extensor digitorum communis t. slip
- Junctura tendinum
- 3rd dorsal interosseus m.
- Extensor indicis t.
- Extensor digitorum communis t. slip
- Flexor pollicis longus t.
- 1st dorsal interosseus m.
- 2nd dorsal interosseus m.
- 1st palmar interosseus m.
- 4th dorsal interosseus m.
- Abductor digiti minimi
- Flexor digiti minimi
- 3rd palmar interosseus m.
- Lumbrical mm.

Labels (bottom image):
- 3rd palmar interosseous m.
- 4th dorsal interosseous m.
- 2nd palmar interosseous m.
- 3rd dorsal interosseus m.
- 2nd dorsal interosseus m.
- 1st palmar interosseus m.
- Flexor pollicis longus t.
- 1st dorsal interosseus m.
- Abductor digiti minimi m.
- Flexor digiti minimi m.
- Lumbrical mm.

(Top) *Axial T1 MR image of the left hand shows the distal metacarpal diaphyses. The juncturae tendinum are fibrous bands, which interconnect the extensor tendons of digits 2-5 just proximal to the MCP joints. These fibrous bands help prevent lateral translation of the extensor tendons over the metacarpals. Because of these interconnections, digital extension can be relatively preserved in the face of a complete transection of a single extensor digitorum communis tendon proximal to the juncturae, and such an injury may not be evident clinically.* (Bottom) *Axial T1 MR image of the left hand shows the 5th metacarpal head and the 2nd-4th metacarpal distal shafts.*

Hand MR Atlas

AXIAL T1 MR, RIGHT HAND

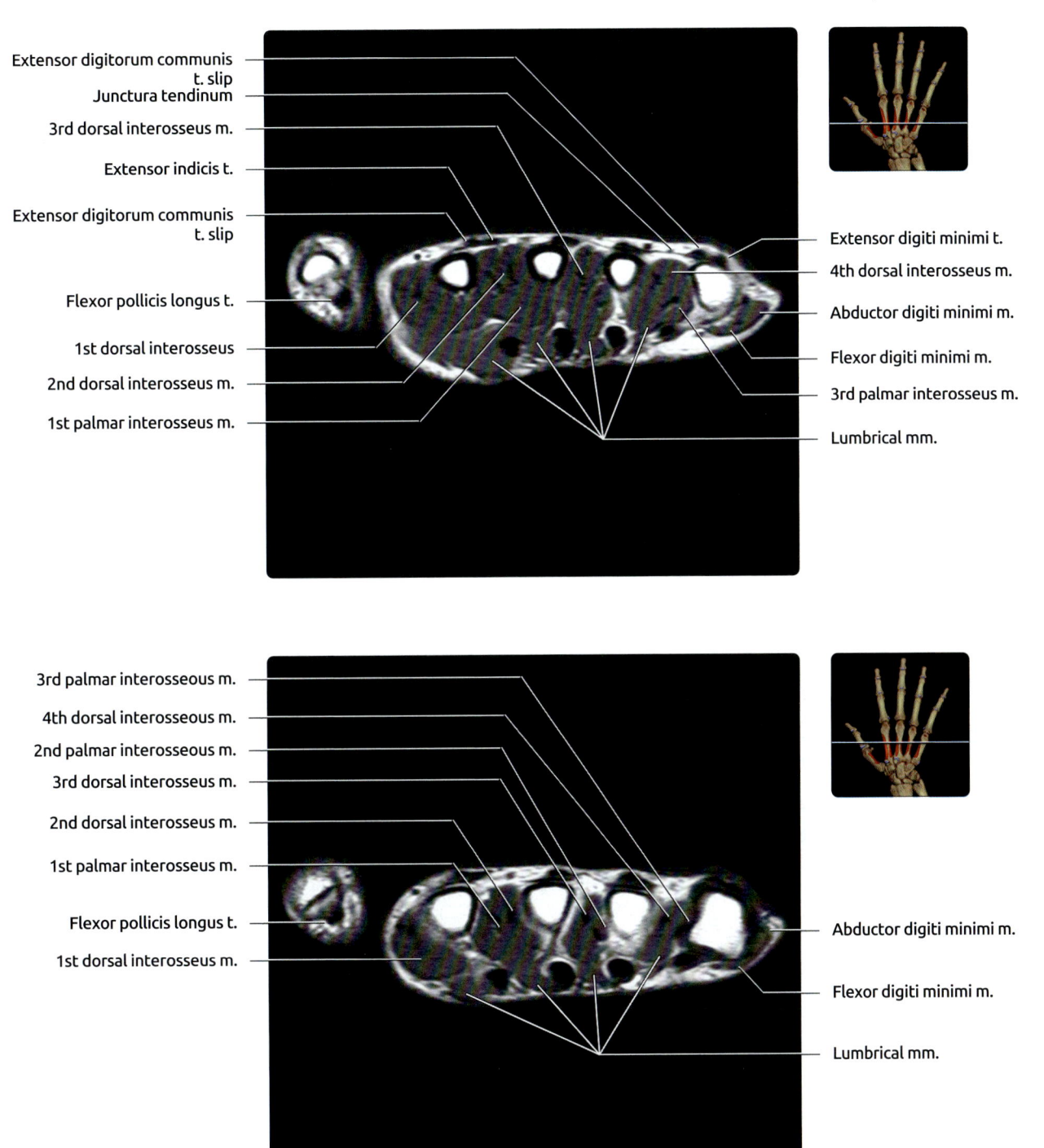

Extensor digitorum communis t. slip
Junctura tendinum
3rd dorsal interosseus m.
Extensor indicis t.
Extensor digitorum communis t. slip
Flexor pollicis longus t.
1st dorsal interosseus
2nd dorsal interosseus m.
1st palmar interosseus m.

Extensor digiti minimi t.
4th dorsal interosseus m.
Abductor digiti minimi m.
Flexor digiti minimi m.
3rd palmar interosseus m.
Lumbrical mm.

3rd palmar interosseous m.
4th dorsal interosseous m.
2nd palmar interosseous m.
3rd dorsal interosseus m.
2nd dorsal interosseus m.
1st palmar interosseus m.
Flexor pollicis longus t.
1st dorsal interosseus m.

Abductor digiti minimi m.
Flexor digiti minimi m.
Lumbrical mm.

(Top) Axial T1 MR image of the right hand shows the distal metacarpal diaphyses. The juncturae tendinum are fibrous bands, which interconnect the extensor tendons of digits 2-5 just proximal to the MCP joints. These fibrous bands help prevent lateral translation of the extensor tendons over the metacarpals. Because of these interconnections, digital extension can be relatively preserved in the face of a complete transection of a single extensor digitorum communis tendon proximal to the juncturae, and such an injury may not be evident clinically. **(Bottom)** Axial T1 MR image of the right hand shows the 5th metacarpal head and the 2nd-4th metacarpal distal shafts.

Hand MR Atlas

AXIAL T1 MR, LEFT HAND

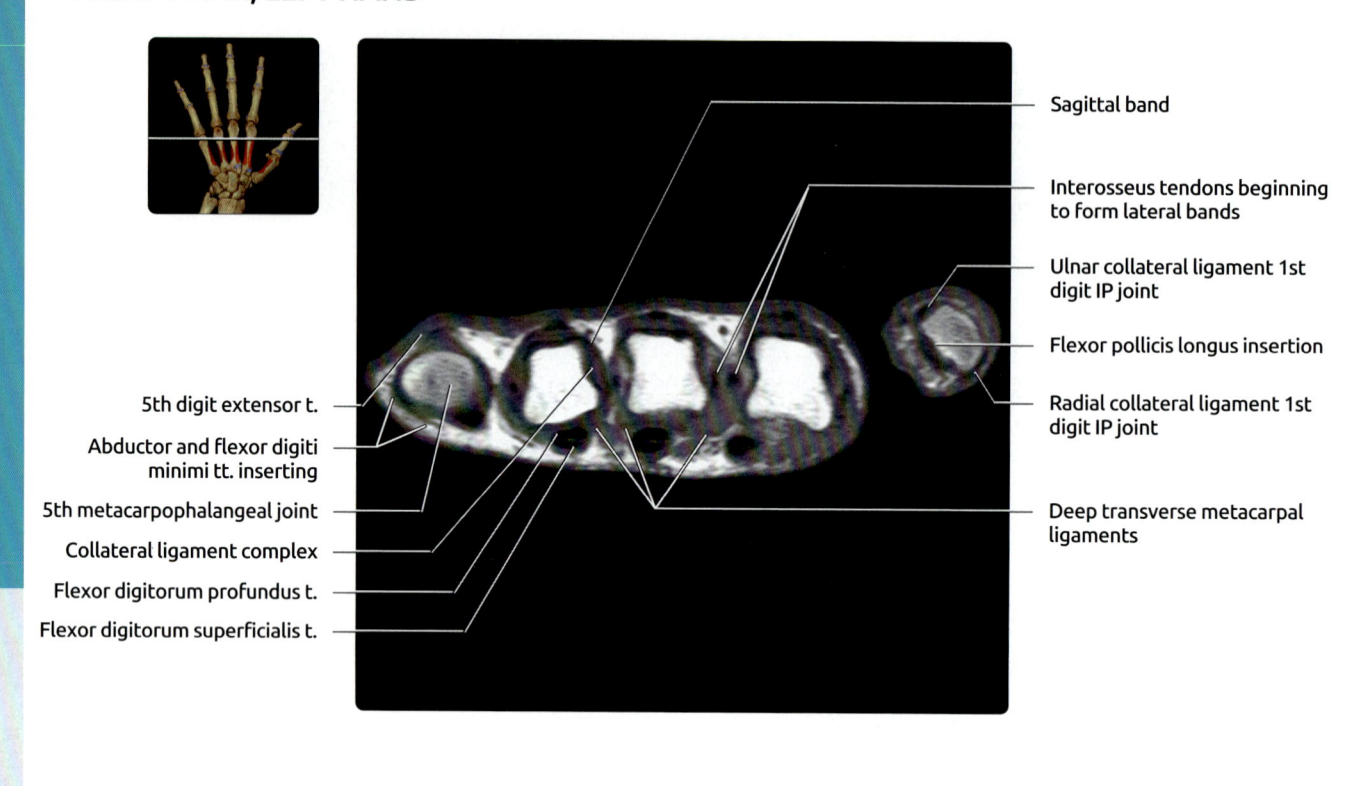

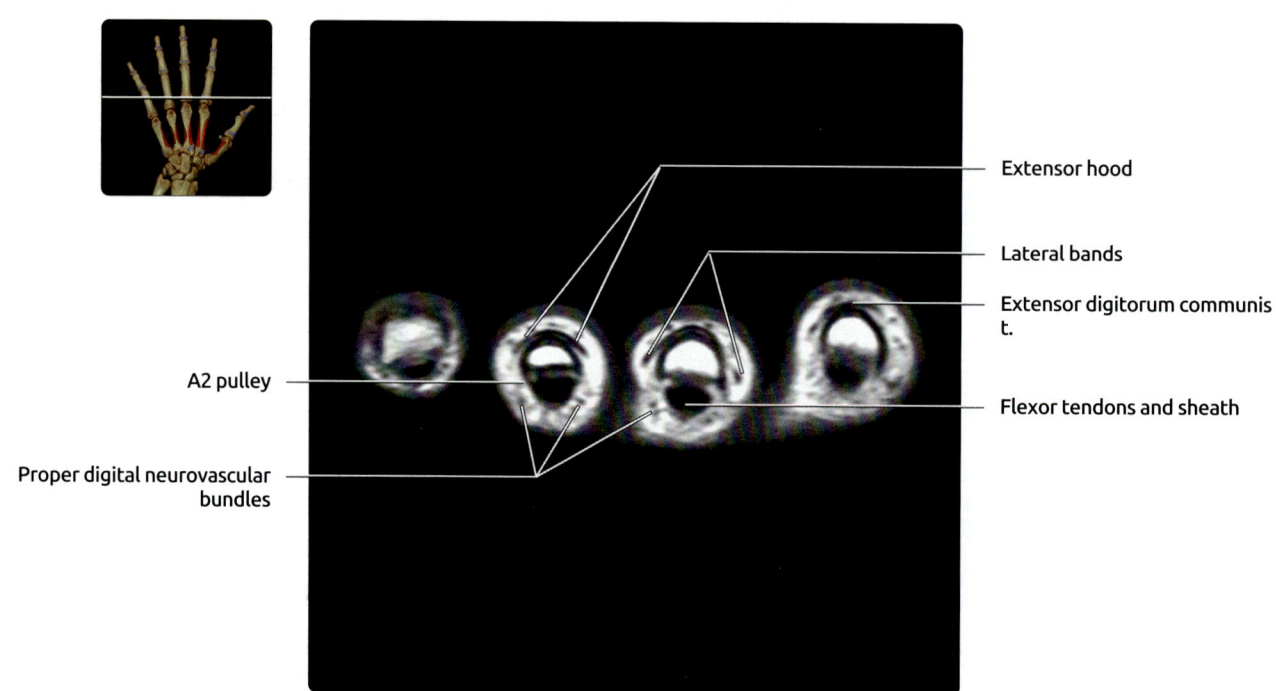

(Top) Axial T1 MR image of the left hand slightly shows the 2nd-4th metacarpal heads. The lateral notches of the metacarpal (MC) heads are the sites of origin of the collateral ligaments, which are the intermediate signal structures deep to the sagittal and lateral bands. The deep transverse metacarpal ligaments connect the volar plates of digits 2-5. **(Bottom)** Axial T1 MR image of the left hand shows the proximal phalanges. The lateral bands can be defined as the lateral thickenings of the extensor hood, and the extensor digitorum communis (EDC) tendon can be defined as the central thickening of the extensor hood. We know we are still in the lateral bands instead of the conjoined tendons as we are still proximal to the PIP joints.

Hand MR Atlas

AXIAL T1 MR, RIGHT HAND

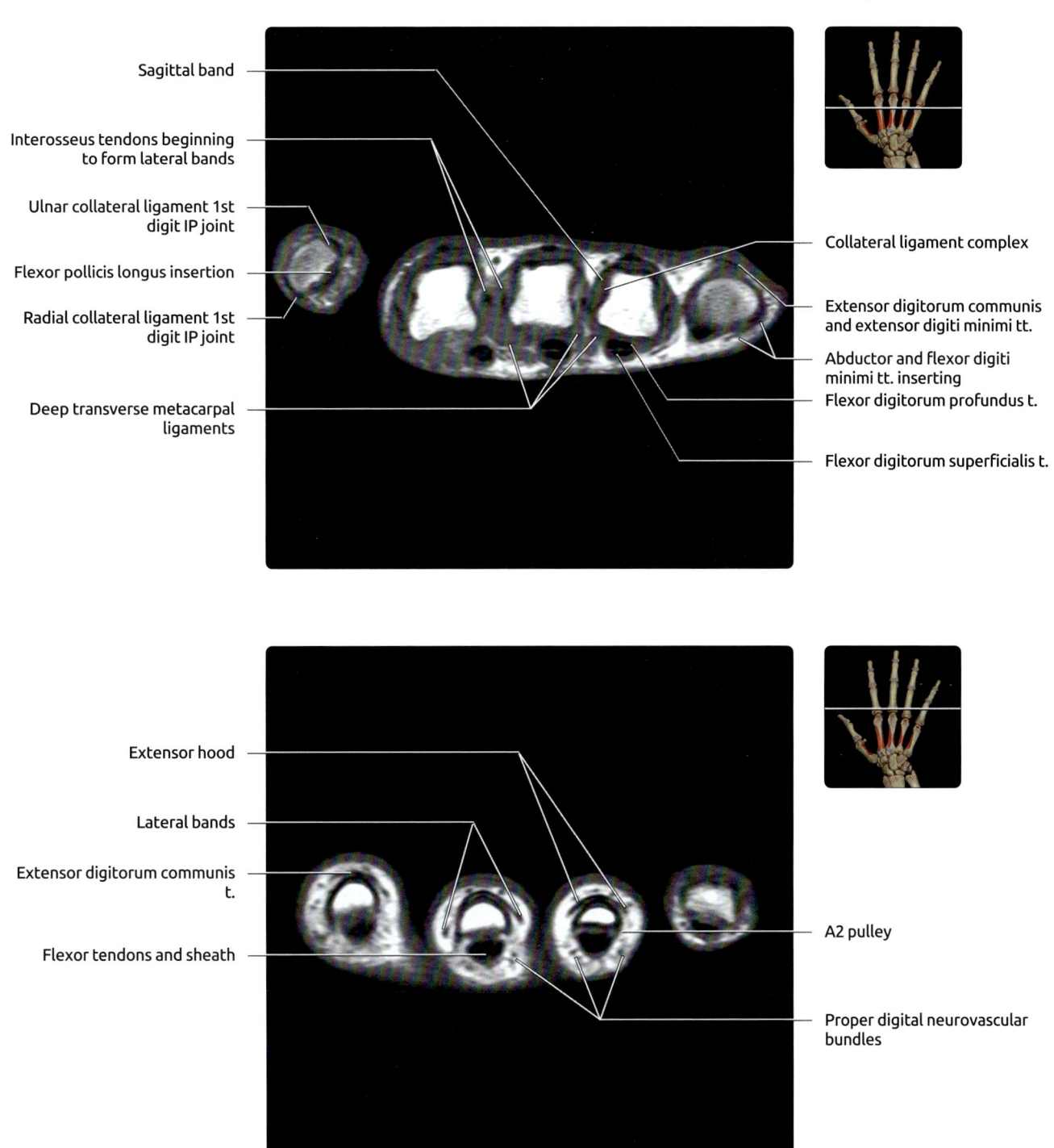

Labels (Top image):
- Sagittal band
- Interosseus tendons beginning to form lateral bands
- Ulnar collateral ligament 1st digit IP joint
- Flexor pollicis longus insertion
- Radial collateral ligament 1st digit IP joint
- Deep transverse metacarpal ligaments
- Collateral ligament complex
- Extensor digitorum communis and extensor digiti minimi tt.
- Abductor and flexor digiti minimi tt. inserting
- Flexor digitorum profundus t.
- Flexor digitorum superficialis t.

Labels (Bottom image):
- Extensor hood
- Lateral bands
- Extensor digitorum communis t.
- Flexor tendons and sheath
- A2 pulley
- Proper digital neurovascular bundles

(Top) Axial T1 MR image shows the right hand slightly more distally through the metacarpal heads. The lateral notches of the MC heads are the sites of origin of the collateral ligaments, which are the intermediate signal structures deep to the sagittal and lateral bands. The deep transverse metacarpal ligaments connect the volar plates of digits 2-5. **(Bottom)** Axial T1 MR image of the right hand shows the proximal phalanges. The lateral bands can be defined as the lateral thickenings of the extensor hood, and the extensor digitorum tendon can be defined as the central thickening of the extensor hood. We know we are still in the lateral bands instead of the conjoined tendons as we are still proximal to the proximal interphalangeal joints.

Hand MR Atlas

CORONAL T1 MR, LEFT HAND

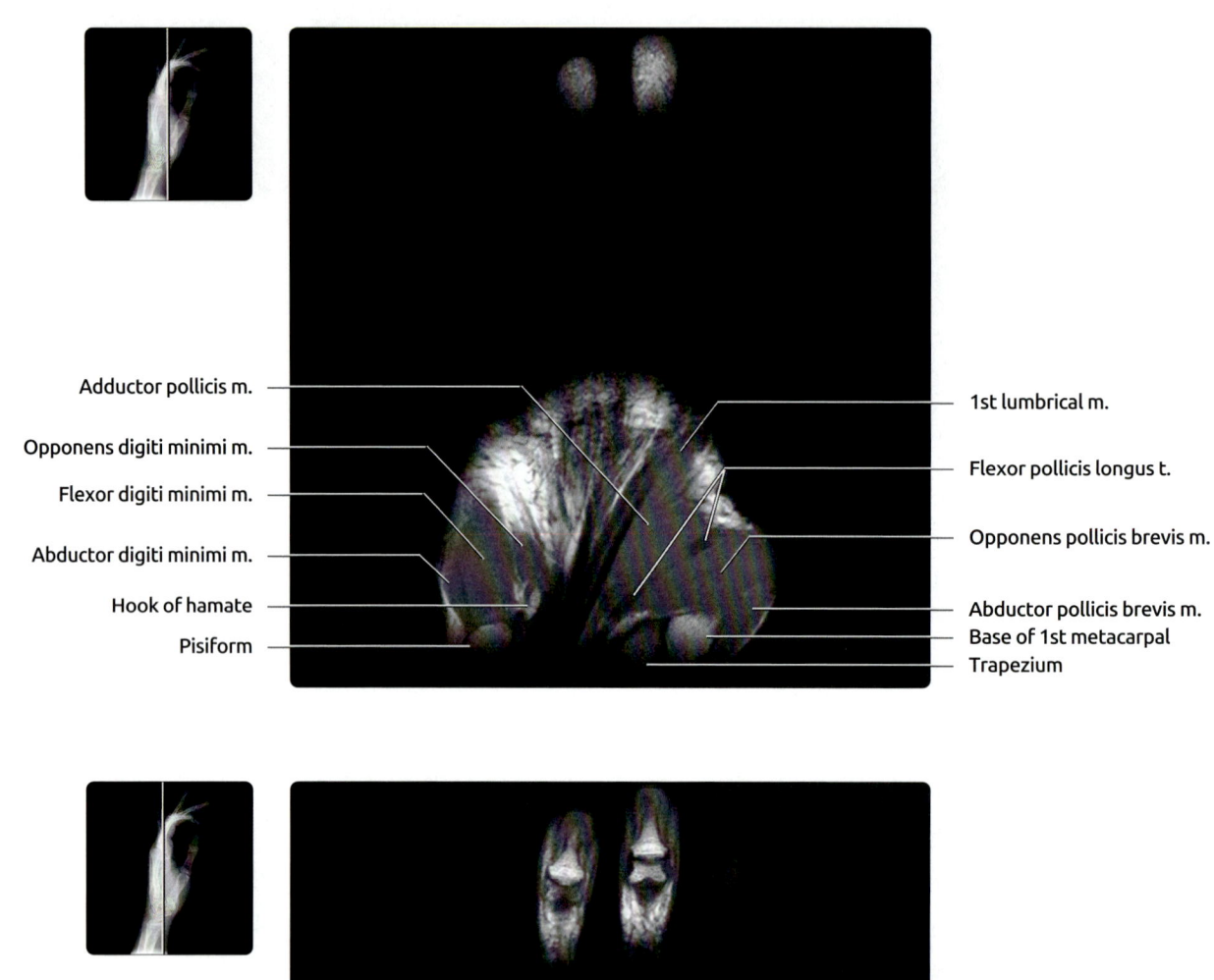

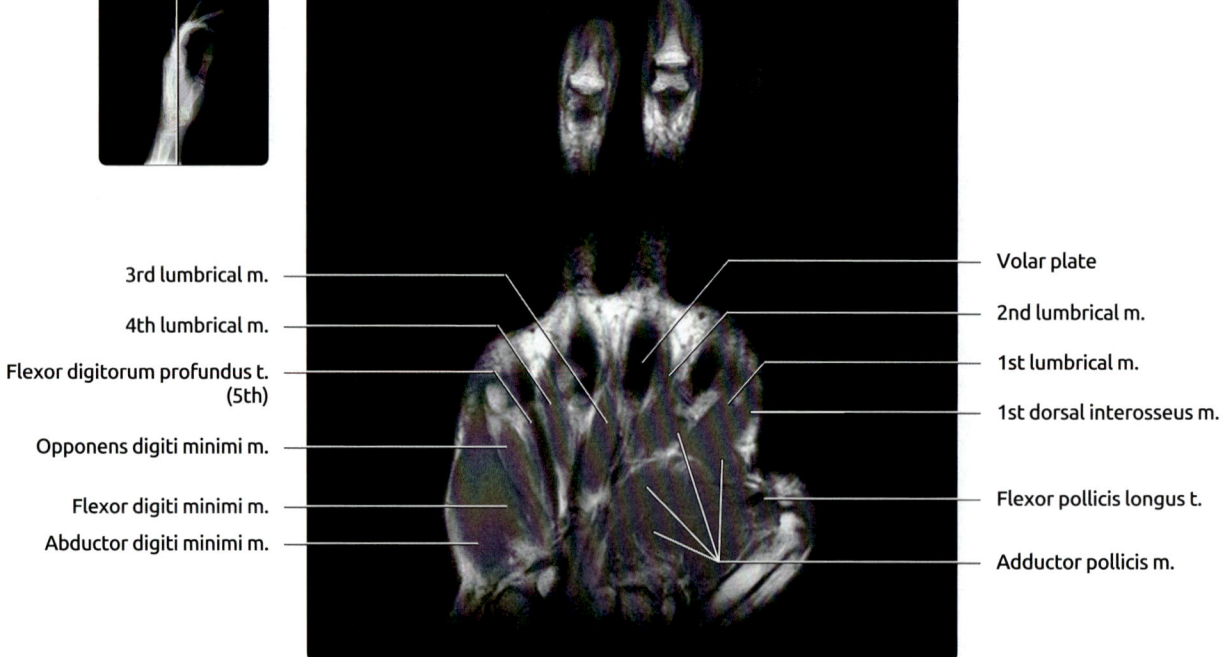

Labels (top image):
- Adductor pollicis m.
- Opponens digiti minimi m.
- Flexor digiti minimi m.
- Abductor digiti minimi m.
- Hook of hamate
- Pisiform
- 1st lumbrical m.
- Flexor pollicis longus t.
- Opponens pollicis brevis m.
- Abductor pollicis brevis m.
- Base of 1st metacarpal
- Trapezium

Labels (bottom image):
- 3rd lumbrical m.
- 4th lumbrical m.
- Flexor digitorum profundus t. (5th)
- Opponens digiti minimi m.
- Flexor digiti minimi m.
- Abductor digiti minimi m.
- Volar plate
- 2nd lumbrical m.
- 1st lumbrical m.
- 1st dorsal interosseus m.
- Flexor pollicis longus t.
- Adductor pollicis m.

(Top) *1st in series of coronal T1 MR images of the left hand shows the superficial volar structures.* **(Bottom)** *Coronal T1 MR image of the left hand shows the deeper palmar structures. At this level, we happen to catch a portion of the metacarpophalangeal volar plates of digits 2-5 (only labeled on the 3rd digit in this image). It can be determined that these are volar plates by their location and thickness. Note how much thicker they are compared to the flexor tendons.*

Hand MR Atlas

CORONAL T1 MR, RIGHT HAND

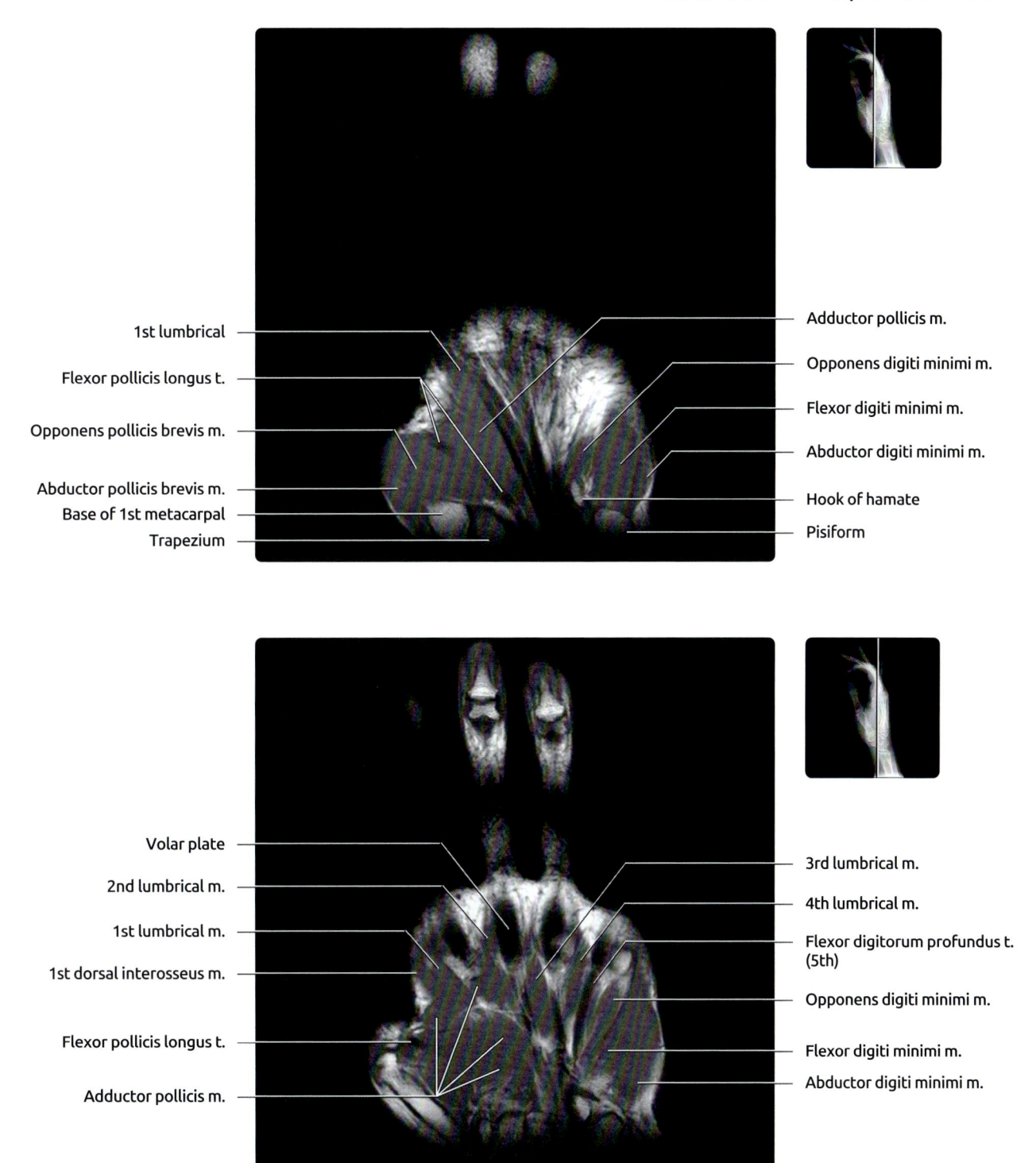

Labels (top image):
- 1st lumbrical
- Flexor pollicis longus t.
- Opponens pollicis brevis m.
- Abductor pollicis brevis m.
- Base of 1st metacarpal
- Trapezium
- Adductor pollicis m.
- Opponens digiti minimi m.
- Flexor digiti minimi m.
- Abductor digiti minimi m.
- Hook of hamate
- Pisiform

Labels (bottom image):
- Volar plate
- 2nd lumbrical m.
- 1st lumbrical m.
- 1st dorsal interosseus m.
- Flexor pollicis longus t.
- Adductor pollicis m.
- 3rd lumbrical m.
- 4th lumbrical m.
- Flexor digitorum profundus t. (5th)
- Opponens digiti minimi m.
- Flexor digiti minimi m.
- Abductor digiti minimi m.

(Top) 1st in series of coronal T1 MR images of the right hand shows the superficial volar structures. **(Bottom)** Coronal T1 MR image of the right hand shows the deeper palmar structures. At this level, we happen to catch a portion of the MCP volar plates of digits 2-5 (only labeled on the 3rd digit in this image). It can be determined that these are volar plates by their location and thickness. Note how much thicker they are compared to the flexor tendons.

467

CORONAL T1 MR, LEFT HAND

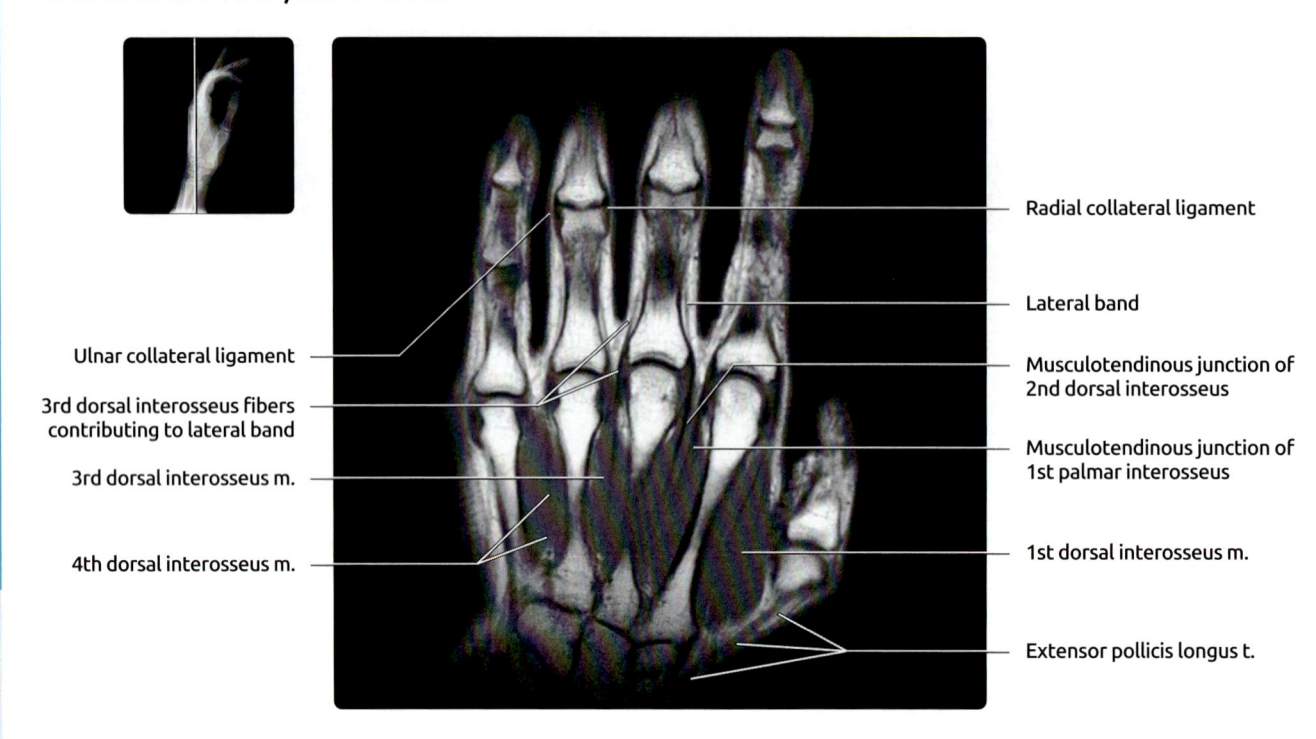

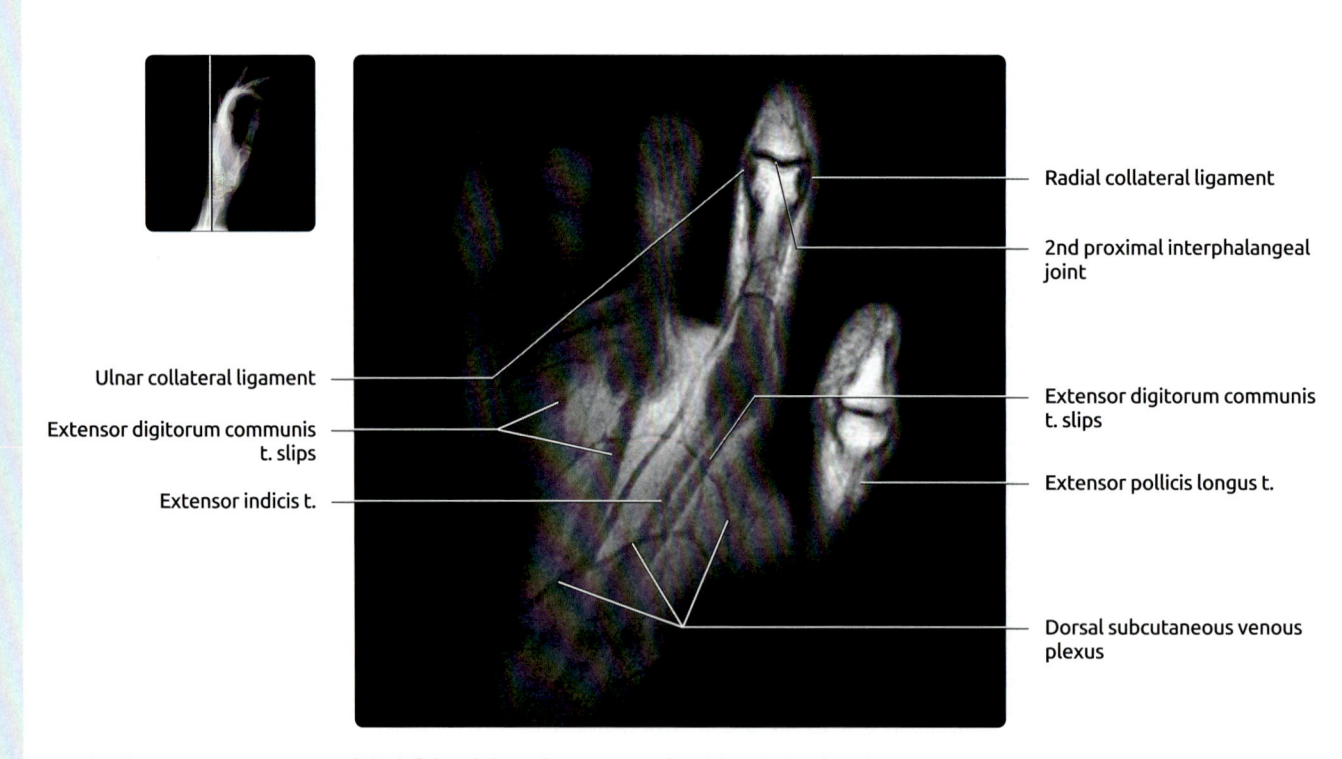

Labels (top image):
- Ulnar collateral ligament
- 3rd dorsal interosseus fibers contributing to lateral band
- 3rd dorsal interosseus m.
- 4th dorsal interosseus m.
- Radial collateral ligament
- Lateral band
- Musculotendinous junction of 2nd dorsal interosseus
- Musculotendinous junction of 1st palmar interosseus
- 1st dorsal interosseus m.
- Extensor pollicis longus t.

Labels (bottom image):
- Ulnar collateral ligament
- Extensor digitorum communis t. slips
- Extensor indicis t.
- Radial collateral ligament
- 2nd proximal interphalangeal joint
- Extensor digitorum communis t. slips
- Extensor pollicis longus t.
- Dorsal subcutaneous venous plexus

(Top) Coronal T1 MR image of the left hand show the metacarpals. Although the dorsal interossei are predominately imaged in this plane, some of the 1st palmar interosseus is visible in the 2nd interspace. You can tell that this is palmar interosseus since it is contributing fibers from its musculotendinous junction to the ulnar lateral band of the 2nd digit instead of the radial lateral band of the 3rd digit (as the 2nd dorsal interosseus does). **(Bottom)** Coronal T1 MR image of the left hand (dorsal) demonstrates a few of the extensor digitorum communis tendons as well as the extensor indicis tendon. Note that the collateral ligaments of the PIP joints (and DIP joints as well, although not seen here) do not arise from the lateral notches of the heads of the phalanges as they do in their counterparts (the lateral notches of the metacarpal heads) at the MCP joints.

Hand MR Atlas

CORONAL T1 MR, RIGHT HAND

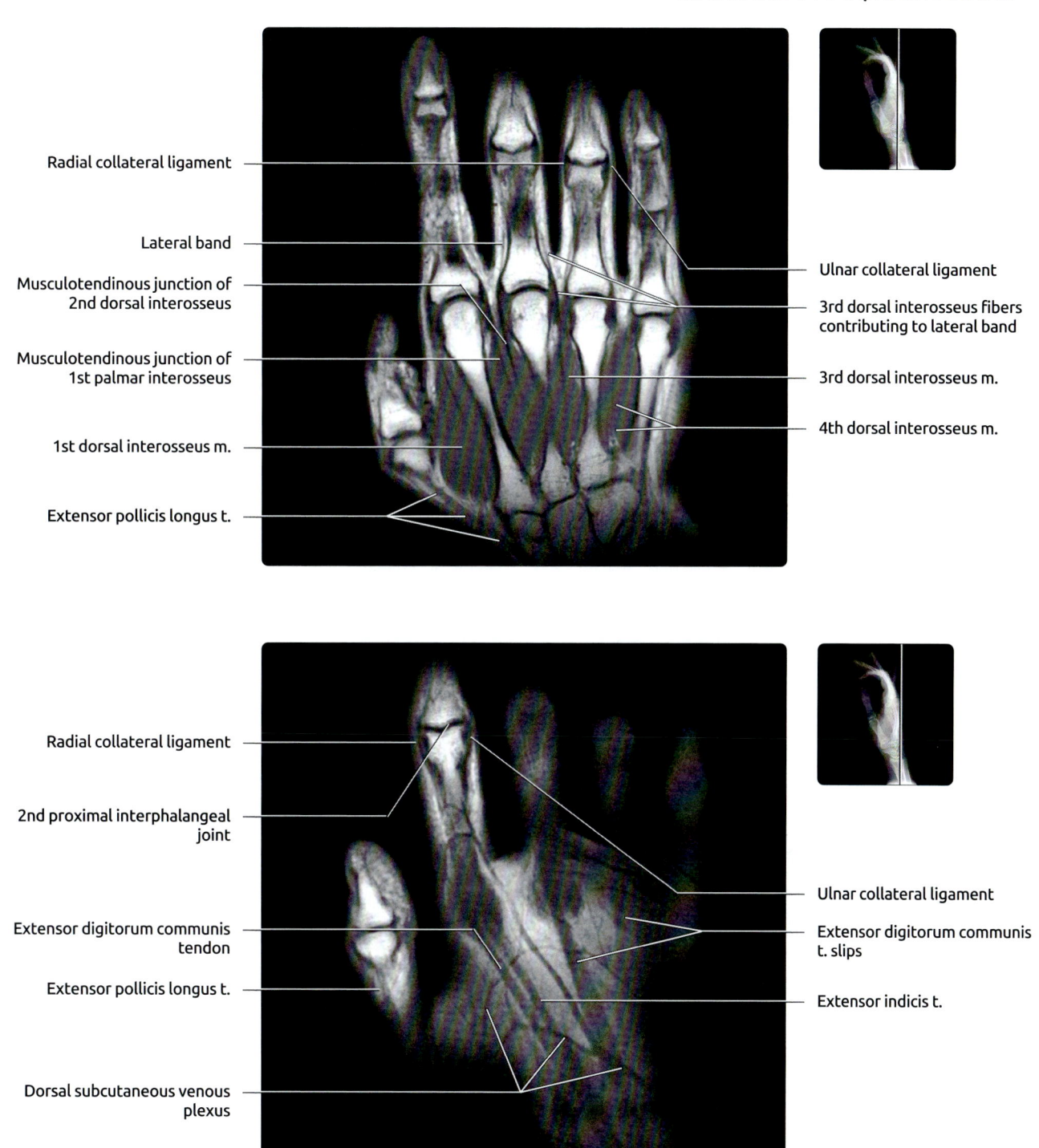

(Top) Coronal T1 MR image of the right hand shows the metacarpals. Although the dorsal interossei are predominately imaged in this plane, some of the 1st palmar interosseus is visible in the 2nd interspace. You can tell that this is palmar interosseus since it is contributing fibers from its musculotendinous junction to the ulnar lateral band of the 2nd digit instead of the radial lateral band of the 3rd digit (as the 2nd dorsal interosseus does). **(Bottom)** Coronal T1 MR image of the right hand (dorsal) demonstrates a few of the extensor digitorum communis tendons as well as the extensor indicis tendon. Note that the collateral ligaments of the PIP joints (and DIP joints as well, although not seen here) do not arise from the lateral notches of the heads of the phalanges as they do in their counterparts (the lateral notches of the metacarpal heads) at the MCP joints.

Hand MR Atlas

SAGITTAL T1 MR, RIGHT HAND

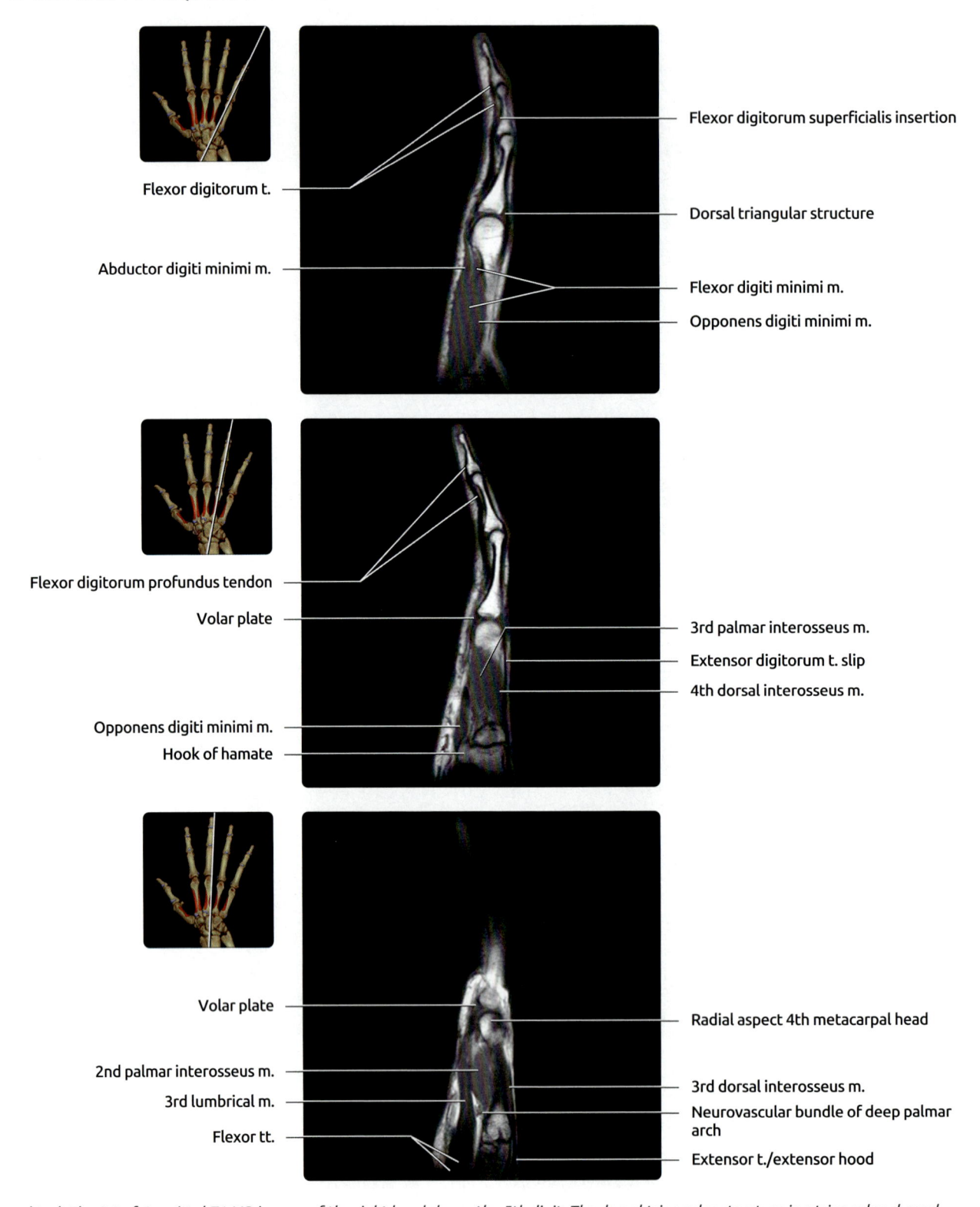

Flexor digitorum t.

Abductor digiti minimi m.

Flexor digitorum superficialis insertion

Dorsal triangular structure

Flexor digiti minimi m.

Opponens digiti minimi m.

Flexor digitorum profundus tendon

Volar plate

Opponens digiti minimi m.

Hook of hamate

3rd palmar interosseus m.

Extensor digitorum t. slip

4th dorsal interosseus m.

Volar plate

2nd palmar interosseus m.

3rd lumbrical m.

Flexor tt.

Radial aspect 4th metacarpal head

3rd dorsal interosseus m.

Neurovascular bundle of deep palmar arch

Extensor t./extensor hood

(Top) The 1st of 6 sagittal T1 MR images of the right hand shows the 5th digit. The dorsal triangular structure is a triangular-shaped vascularized fibrous structure of unknown significance, which can be identified on MR and ultrasound imaging. *(Middle)* Sagittal T1 MR image of the right hand shows the 4th digit. *(Bottom)* Sagittal T1 MR image of the right hand shows the 3rd interspace between the 3rd and 4th digits.

Hand MR Atlas

SAGITTAL T1 MR, RIGHT HAND

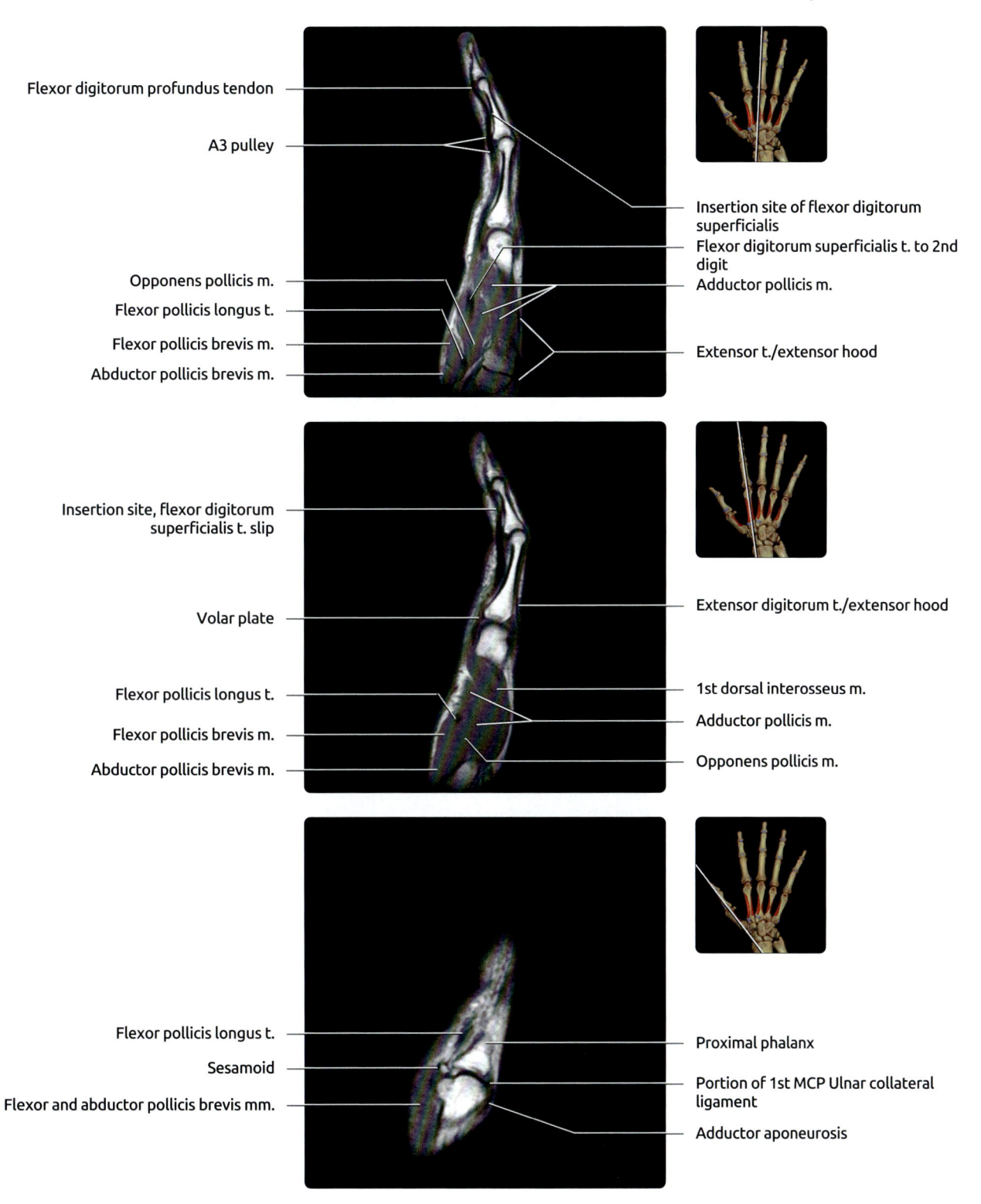

Labels (Top image):
- Flexor digitorum profundus tendon
- A3 pulley
- Opponens pollicis m.
- Flexor pollicis longus t.
- Flexor pollicis brevis m.
- Abductor pollicis brevis m.
- Insertion site of flexor digitorum superficialis
- Flexor digitorum superficialis t. to 2nd digit
- Adductor pollicis m.
- Extensor t./extensor hood

Labels (Middle image):
- Insertion site, flexor digitorum superficialis t. slip
- Volar plate
- Flexor pollicis longus t.
- Flexor pollicis brevis m.
- Abductor pollicis brevis m.
- Extensor digitorum t./extensor hood
- 1st dorsal interosseus m.
- Adductor pollicis m.
- Opponens pollicis m.

Labels (Bottom image):
- Flexor pollicis longus t.
- Sesamoid
- Flexor and abductor pollicis brevis mm.
- Proximal phalanx
- Portion of 1st MCP Ulnar collateral ligament
- Adductor aponeurosis

(Top) Sagittal T1 MR image of the right hand shows the 3rd digit. Although not routinely seen, the A3 pulley can be identified in this image as a slight, focal thickening of the flexor tendons just superficial to the PIP joint. (Middle) Sagittal T1 MR image of the right hand shows the 2nd digit. Note the slight prominence of low signal on the volar surface of the middle phalanx. This is the insertion site of the flexor digitorum superficialis. (Bottom) Sagittal T1 MR image of the right hand was obtained obliquely through the thumb metacarpal phalangeal joint. As this is a true sagittal image with respect to the hand, it is an oblique plane midway between sagittal and coronal with respect to the true axis of the thumb (1st digit). As such, the ulnar aspect of the MCP joint of the thumb is image right.

Flexor and Extensor Mechanisms of Hand

TERMINOLOGY

Definitions
- This chapter discusses digits 2-5; thumb musculature is discussed in the "Thumb Anatomy" chapter

EXTRINSIC FLEXOR MUSCULATURE: DIGITS 2-5

Flexor Digitorum Superficialis (FDS)
- Origin: Common flexor tendon (medial humeral epicondyle) of elbow and mid-radius
- Insertion: Volar plates of the proximal interphalangeal joints as well as the bases of the middle phalanges of digits 2 through 5
- Innervation: Median nerve
- Superficialis tendons split at level of the bases of proximal phalanges, forming 2 distinct tendon slips
  - Slips pass circumferentially around the lateral aspects of flexor digitorum profundus tendon before inserting deep to the FDP tendon
  - This forms a "tunnel" through which the flexor digitorum profundus tendon passes
  - Just proximal to their insertion level, some fibers from each slip of FDS tendon decussate to the contralateral insertion site of the same digit
- Flexes both the metacarpophalangeal joints (aided by lumbricals and interossei) and proximal interphalangeal joints of digits 2 through 5

Flexor Digitorum Profundus (FDP)
- Origin: Proximal and mid-radius, as well as the interosseus membrane
- Insertion: Volar plates of the distal interphalangeal joints as well as the bases of the distal phalanges of digits 2 through 5
- Innervation: Ulnar and median nerves
- Flexes the distal interphalangeal joints, and to lesser extent, the metacarpophalangeal (aided by lumbricals and interossei) and proximal interphalangeal joints of digits 2 through 5

Vinculum Breve and Longum
- Focal fibrovascular bands, which course between the flexor tendons and volar surfaces of the phalanges
- Each of the flexor digitorum superficialis and flexor digitorum profundus tendons has 1 vinculum breve (distally) and 1 vinculum longum (proximally)
- Although not usually seen on routine imaging, these are important structures as they provide nutrients (via small vascular channels) to the flexor tendons

FLEXOR PULLEYS: DIGITS 2-5

Critical Stabilizers of Flexor Mechanism
- Focal thickening of fibrous tissue of the common digital tendon sheaths
- Focally anchor tendon sheaths to volar surface of their respective digits at mechanically strategic points
- 2 types: Annular and cruciform

Annular Pulleys
- Denoted with **A for annular** and a number
  - Numbered 1 through 5 from proximal to distal
- **Odd** numbered pulleys are at the joints, attach to volar plates
  - A1 pulley is located at level of metacarpophalangeal joint
  - A3 pulley is located at level of proximal interphalangeal joint
  - A5 pulley is located at level of distal interphalangeal joint
- **Even** numbered pulleys are at the metaphyses, attach to periosteum
  - A2 pulley is located at level of mid-diaphysis of proximal phalanx
  - A4 pulley is located at level of mid-diaphysis of middle phalanx
- A2 and A4 pulleys are the **most important clinically** (for normal finger flexion)

Cruciform Pulleys
- Not identified on routine imaging
  - Denoted with **C for cruciform** and a number
    - Numbered 1 through 3 from proximal to distal

FLEXOR TENDON SHEATHS: DIGITS 2-5

Common Flexor Tendon Sheath
- Extends to just beyond the level of the carpal tunnel over digits 2 through 4
- Encompasses the 5th digit flexor tendons over their entire course (to level of distal interphalangeal joint)
- Begins just proximal to the carpal tunnel
- Contains the flexor digitorum superficialis and profundus tendons
- Tendon sheaths are lined by synovium

Digital Flexor Tendon Sheaths (Digits 2-4)
- Encompass the flexor tendons from the level of the metacarpal necks to the bases of the distal phalanges
- Common digital sheaths may connect to the ulnar bursa (common flexor sheath) proximally in up to 10% of population
  - This possible connection is important as **it may provide a route for spread of infection** from digits 2 through 4 to common flexor sheath (and vice versa)

EXTENSOR MECHANISM: DIGITS 2-5

Extensor Digitorum Communis (EDC)
- Origin: Common extensor tendon (lateral humeral epicondyle)
  - Distinct extensor digitorum communis tendon to 5th digit is present in only approximately 50% of population
  - When distinct 5th digit EDC tendon is absent, fiber contributions from 4th digit EDC tendon and junctura tendinum form a "makeshift" 5th digit EDC tendon
- Insertion: Inserts as central slip on dorsal bases of middle phalanges and proximal interphalangeal joint capsules
  - Just proximal to proximal interphalangeal joints, extensor digitorum communis tendons trifurcate into a central slip and 2 lateral slips
  - Lateral slips each fuse with their adjacent lateral band to form conjoined tendons

Flexor and Extensor Mechanisms of Hand

- o Disruption of central slip (via laceration or avulsion) can allow proximal interphalangeal joint to flex and herniate between EDC tendon lateral slips and lateral bands during extension resulting in a boutonnière deformity
- Innervation: Posterior interosseus nerve (branch of radial nerve)

Extensor Indicis (EI)
- Origin: Posterior, distal ulna, and interosseus membrane
- Insertion: Extensor indicis tendon blends with 2nd digit extensor digitorum communis tendon and extensor hood
- Innervation: Posterior interosseus nerve (branch of radial nerve)

Extensor Digiti Minimi (EDM)
- Origin: Common extensor tendon (lateral humeral epicondyle)
  - o In most cases, exists as 2 distinct tendons over wrist and 5th metacarpal
- Insertion
  - o 2 tendons of extensor digiti minimi fuse with one another and with 5th digit extensor digitorum communis tendon (if it exists) or, in its absence, with its "makeshift" counterpart
  - o This combined extensor tendon inserts on dorsal base of proximal phalanx of 5th digit and also blends with joint capsule of 5th proximal interphalangeal joint
- Innervation: Posterior interosseus branch of radial nerve

Lateral Bands/Conjoined Tendons
- Lateral bands are formed by lumbrical and interosseus muscle tendons
  - o Exception: Abductor digiti minimi forms ulnar lateral band of 5th digit
- Lateral bands fuse with lateral slips of extensor digitorum communis tendons at proximal interphalangeal joints to form conjoined tendons
- Conjoined tendons fuse at distal phalangeal joints to form terminal tendons
- Terminal tendons insert on dorsal bases of distal phalanges
- Triangular ligament connects conjoined tendons just proximal to distal interphalangeal joint
- Sudden forced flexion of an extended distal interphalangeal joint may cause terminal tendon to avulse its osseous insertion (a.k.a. mallet finger or baseball finger)

Extensor Hood
- Begins just proximal to metacarpophalangeal joints and terminates just proximal to proximal interphalangeal joints
- Dorsal hood of fibers oriented nearly perpendicular to long axis of extensor tendons
- Fibers of extensor hood interdigitate with extensor digitorum communis (and extensor indicis and digiti minimi) tendons to help prevent lateral translation
- Sagittal bands
  - o Located at metacarpophalangeal joints
  - o Extend form extensor hood to volar plate
  - o Prevent lateral translation of extensor digitorum communis tendons at metacarpophalangeal joint level

INTRINSIC FLEXORS AND EXTENSORS: DIGITS 2-5

Lumbricals
- Numbered 1-4 from radial to ulnar
- Origin: Flexor digitorum profundus tendons just distal to carpal tunnel
- Insertion: Radial lateral bands of digits 2-5
- Innervation
  - o 1st and 2nd lumbricals: Median nerve
  - o 3rd and 4th lumbricals: Ulnar nerve
- Extend interphalangeal joints and flexes metacarpophalangeal joints of digits 2-5

Dorsal Interossei
- Numbered 1-4 from radial to ulnar
- Origin: Dorsolateral metacarpal diaphyses, bipennate
- Insertion: Mesial-most (in hand) adjacent lateral bands of digits 2-4
- Innervation: Ulnar nerve
- Flexes 2nd-4th metacarpophalangeal joints, extends 2nd-4th interphalangeal joints and abducts digits 2-4

Palmar Interosseous Muscles
- Denoted 1 through 3 from radial to ulnar
- Origin: Mesial palmar diaphyses of the 2nd, 4th, and 5th metacarpals
- Insertion: Mesial lateral bands and mesial aspect of the bases of proximal phalanges of the same digit from which they originate
- Innervation: Ulnar nerve
- Actions: Adduct digits and assists lumbricals with flexion of the metacarpophalangeal joints and extension of the interphalangeal joints of digits 2, 4, and 5

Hypothenar Muscles: Opponens Digiti Minimi, Abductor Digiti Minimi, and Flexor Digiti Minimi
- Origin: Flexor digiti minimi and opponens digiti minimi originate from the flexor retinaculum and the hook of the hamate
- Origin: Abductor digiti minimi originates from the pisiform
- Insertion: Flexor digiti minimi and abductor digiti minimi share a combined insertion on the ulnar base of the proximal phalanx of the 5th digit
  - o Abductor digiti minimi also contributes fibers to the ulnar lateral band and extensor hood of the 5th digit
- Insertion: Opponens digiti minimi inserts on the proximal and mid diaphysis of the 5th metacarpal
- Innervation: All by ulnar nerve
- Actions
  - o Abductor digiti minimi aids flexion of the metacarpophalangeal joint and extension of the interphalangeal joint of the 5th digit via its contributions to the 5th digit ulnar lateral band and extensor hood
  - o Actions of the hypothenars are otherwise, as their name implies

Flexor and Extensor Mechanisms of Hand

FLEXOR MECHANISM OF HAND

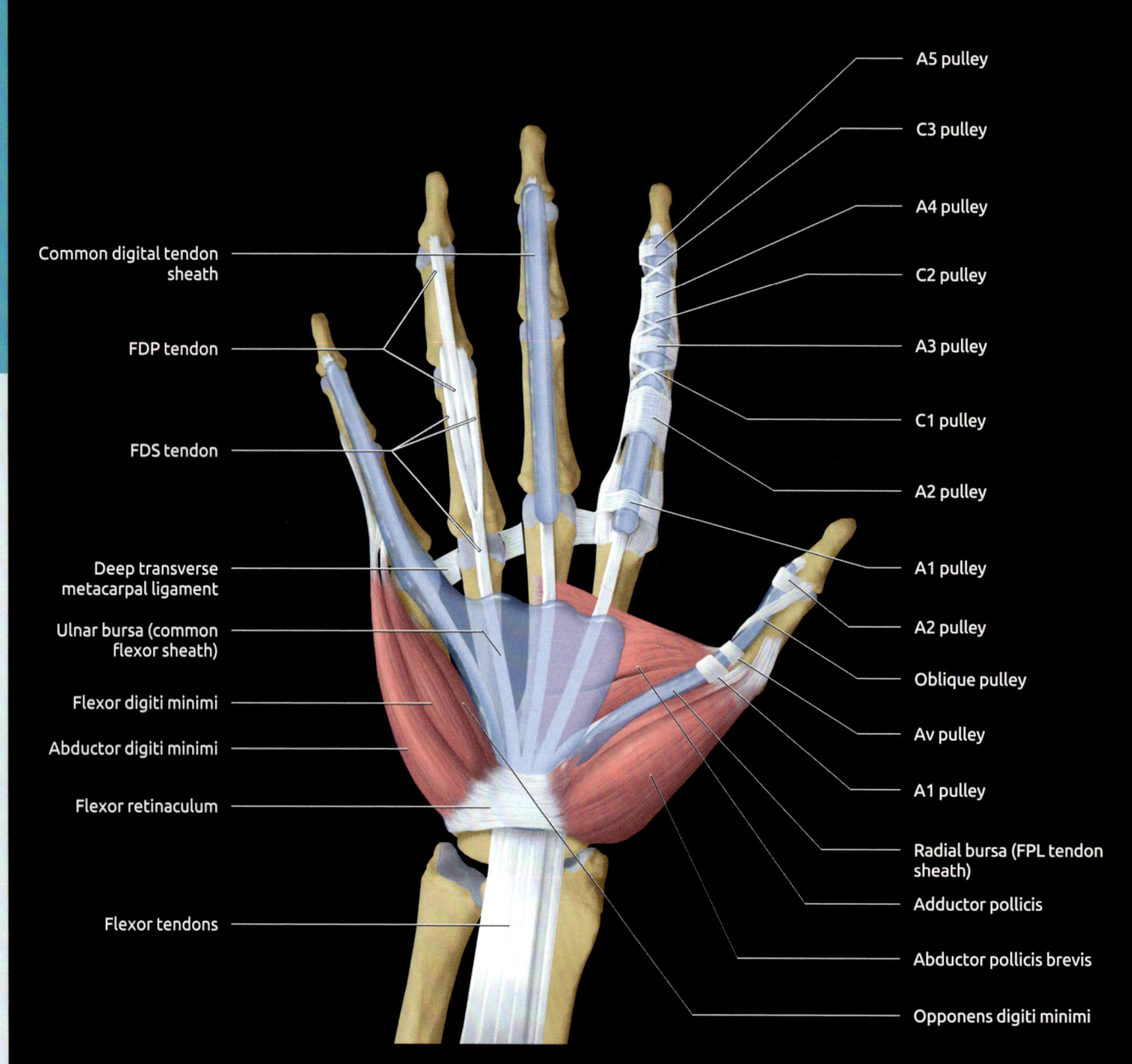

Labels (left side):
- Common digital tendon sheath
- FDP tendon
- FDS tendon
- Deep transverse metacarpal ligament
- Ulnar bursa (common flexor sheath)
- Flexor digiti minimi
- Abductor digiti minimi
- Flexor retinaculum
- Flexor tendons

Labels (right side):
- A5 pulley
- C3 pulley
- A4 pulley
- C2 pulley
- A3 pulley
- C1 pulley
- A2 pulley
- A1 pulley
- A2 pulley
- Oblique pulley
- Av pulley
- A1 pulley
- Radial bursa (FPL tendon sheath)
- Adductor pollicis
- Abductor pollicis brevis
- Opponens digiti minimi

Pulley system for the 3rd-5th digits is identical to that demonstrated for the 2nd digit. Common digital sheath of the 4th digit is removed to show the relationship of the flexor digitorum superficialis (FDS) and flexor digitorum profundus (FDP) tendons. The deep transverse metacarpal ligaments connect the volar plates (not shown) of digits 2-5. Although there is overlap of the radial and ulnar bursae in this image, these structures normally do not communicate. It is, however, important to know that the radial and ulnar bursae may communicate as a normal variation in a small percentage of the population. Similarly, any 1 or more of the common digital sheaths may communicate with the ulnar bursa in up to 10% of the normal population. These normal variant bursal communications are important, as they can provide routes for more extensive spread of infection.

Flexor and Extensor Mechanisms of Hand

FLEXOR MECHANISM OF DIGITS 2-5

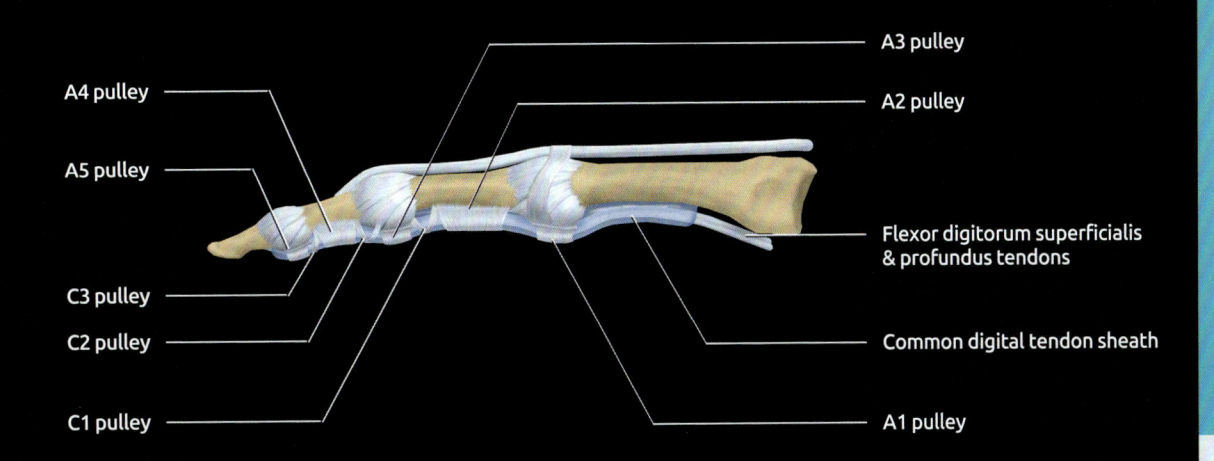

- A3 pulley
- A4 pulley
- A2 pulley
- A5 pulley
- Flexor digitorum superficialis & profundus tendons
- C3 pulley
- C2 pulley
- Common digital tendon sheath
- C1 pulley
- A1 pulley

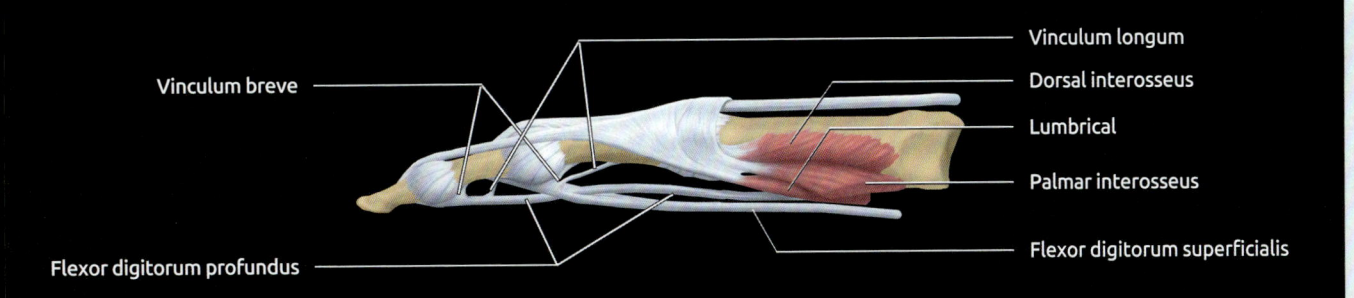

- Vinculum longum
- Vinculum breve
- Dorsal interosseus
- Lumbrical
- Palmar interosseus
- Flexor digitorum superficialis
- Flexor digitorum profundus

(Top) Graphic of the lateral finger shows the flexor pulley system and common digital sheath. (Bottom) Graphic of the lateral finger shows the relationship of the 2 separate flexor tendons. Note how the FDP tendon passes through the "split" of the FDS tendon. Each FDS and FDP tendon has a vinculum longum and a vinculum breve. Although not normally seen on routine imaging, these structures are important as they provide vascular supply and a portion of the nutrients to the flexor tendons. Synovial fluid produced by the tendon sheaths also provides nutrients for the tendons.

Flexor and Extensor Mechanisms of Hand

EXTENSOR MECHANISM OF HAND

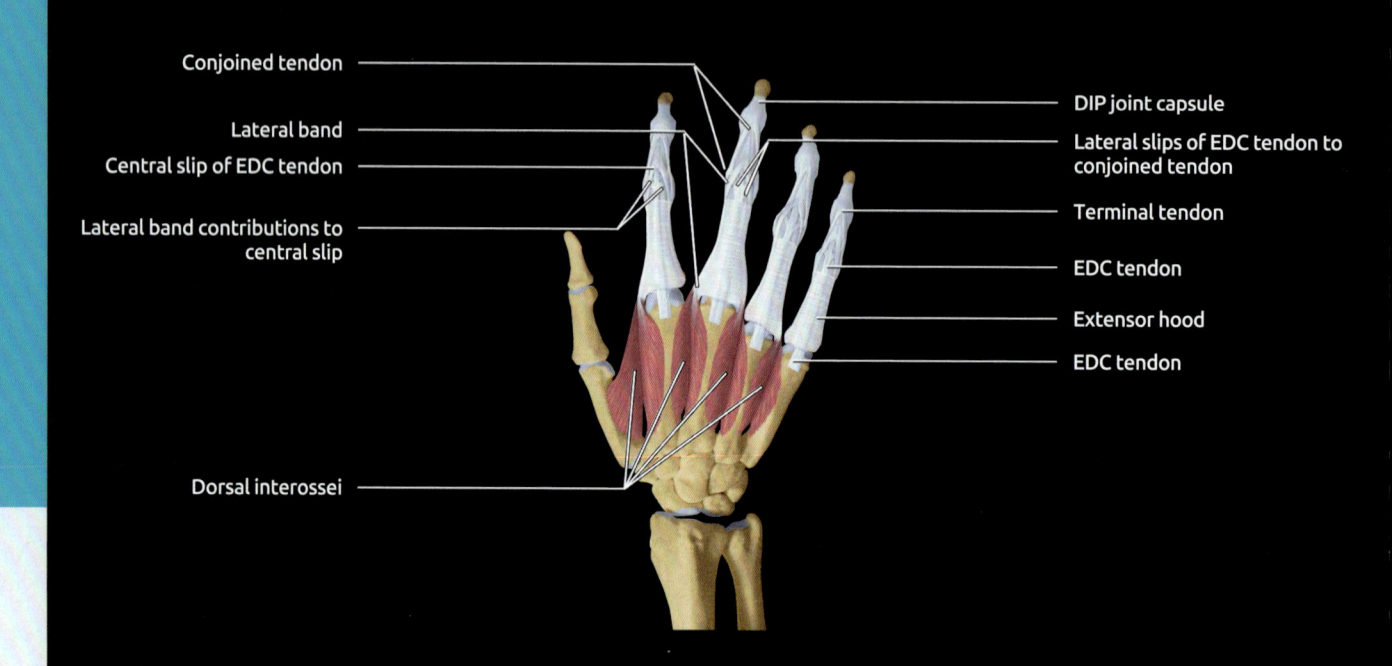

Conjoined tendon
Lateral band
Central slip of EDC tendon
Lateral band contributions to central slip
Dorsal interossei

DIP joint capsule
Lateral slips of EDC tendon to conjoined tendon
Terminal tendon
EDC tendon
Extensor hood
EDC tendon

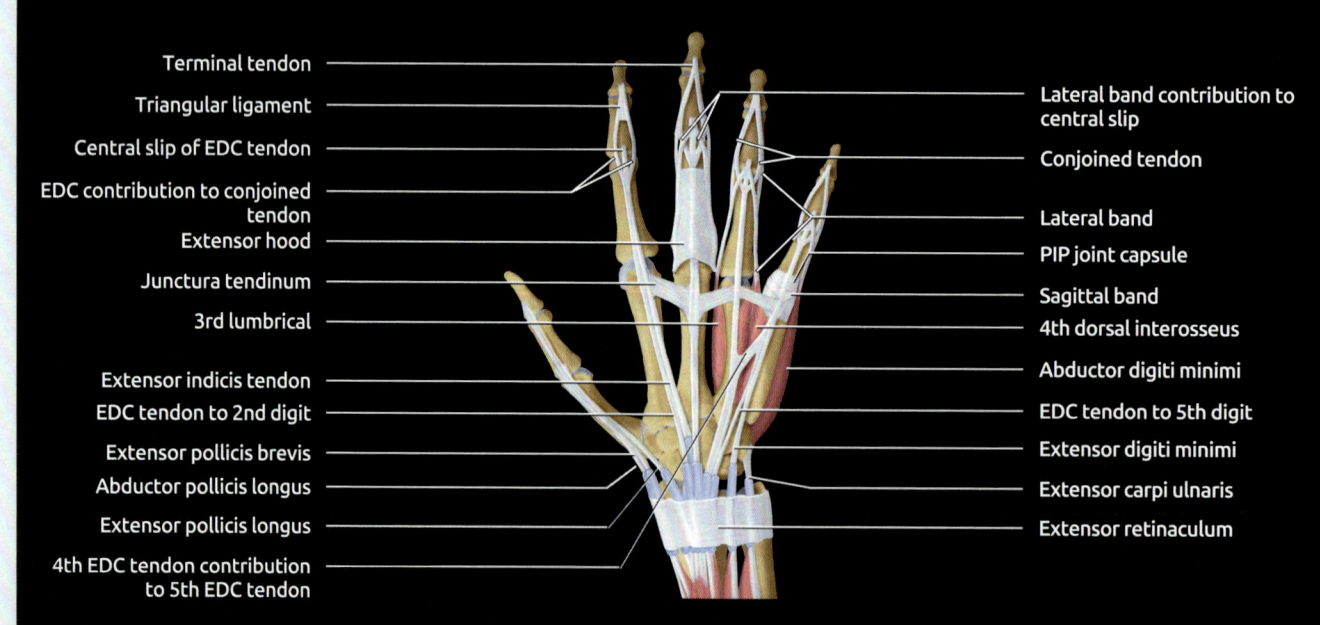

Terminal tendon
Triangular ligament
Central slip of EDC tendon
EDC contribution to conjoined tendon
Extensor hood
Junctura tendinum
3rd lumbrical
Extensor indicis tendon
EDC tendon to 2nd digit
Extensor pollicis brevis
Abductor pollicis longus
Extensor pollicis longus
4th EDC tendon contribution to 5th EDC tendon

Lateral band contribution to central slip
Conjoined tendon
Lateral band
PIP joint capsule
Sagittal band
4th dorsal interosseus
Abductor digiti minimi
EDC tendon to 5th digit
Extensor digiti minimi
Extensor carpi ulnaris
Extensor retinaculum

(Top) This dorsal surface graphic of the extensor mechanism of digits 2-5 demonstrates the complex relationship of the various fiber bands. As in imaging, distinction of individual fiber bands is often difficult and must be inferred by knowledge of where the structure "should" be with respect to more easily identifiable structures (such as bones and joints). *(Bottom)* Extensor mechanism composite shows different components of extensor mechanism on different digits. With the exception of the extensor indicis, extensor digiti minimi, abductor digiti minimi, and 4th EDC tendon contribution to the 5th EDC tendon, any structure on any of the 2nd-5th digits can be extrapolated to any and all of the other 2nd-5th digits. Note that the 2nd extensor retinaculum compartment and its contents (the extensor carpi radialis longus and brevis tendons) are not included in this graphic.

Flexor and Extensor Mechanisms of Hand

EXTENSOR MECHANISM OF DIGITS

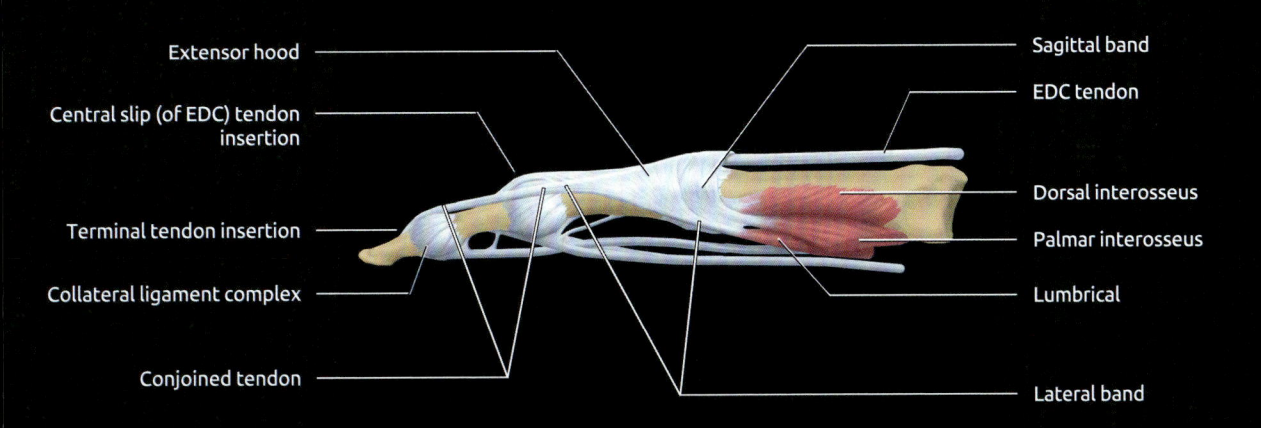

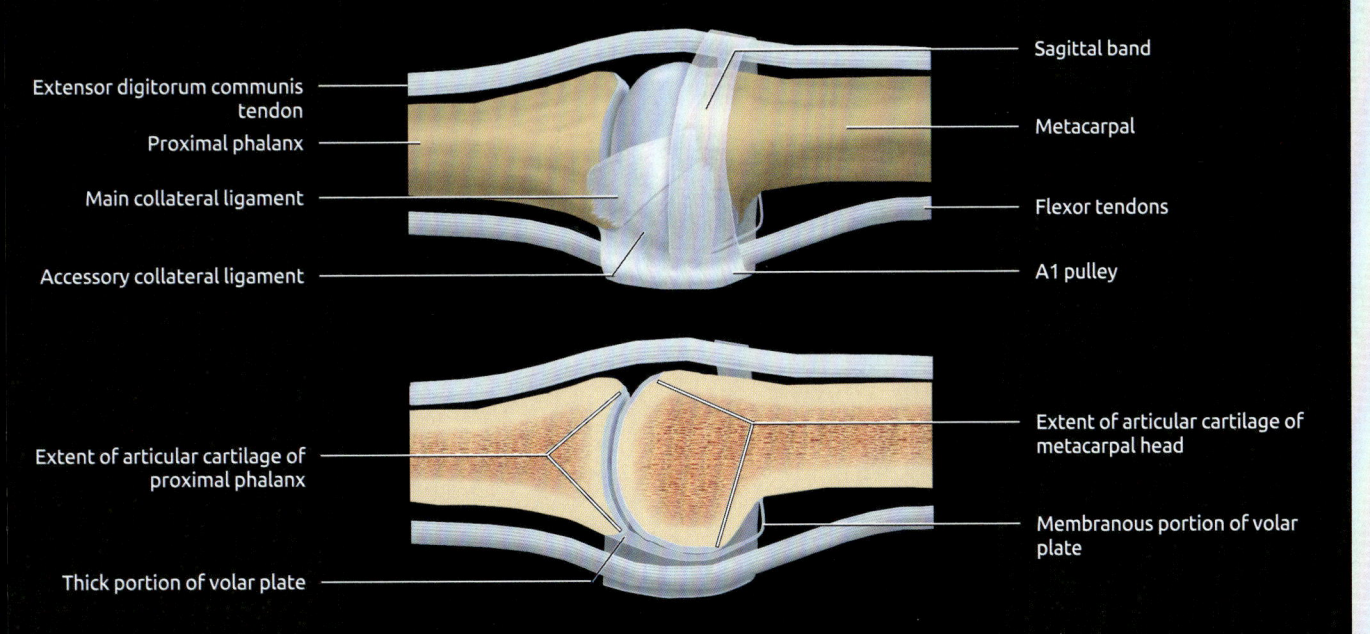

(Top) Lateral view of the extensor components of the finger is shown. The lateral band becomes the conjoined tendon after it receives the lateral slips of the EDC tendon (roughly at the level of the mid to distal PIP joint). The proximal-most fibers of the extensor hood known as the sagittal band run at a slightly different obliquity than those of the remainder of the extensor hood. (Bottom) Surface and cut-section graphics of the MCP joint are shown. The collateral ligament complex is composed of 2 separate fiber bands. The main collateral ligament inserts on the base of the adjacent phalanx. The accessory collateral ligament inserts on the volar plate. The volar plate is thick distally; thin and redundant proximally. With the exception of the sagittal band (present only at the MCP joints), the anatomy in this graphic is duplicated in all MCP and IP joints in the hand.

Flexor and Extensor Mechanisms of Hand

TENDON INJURY ZONES

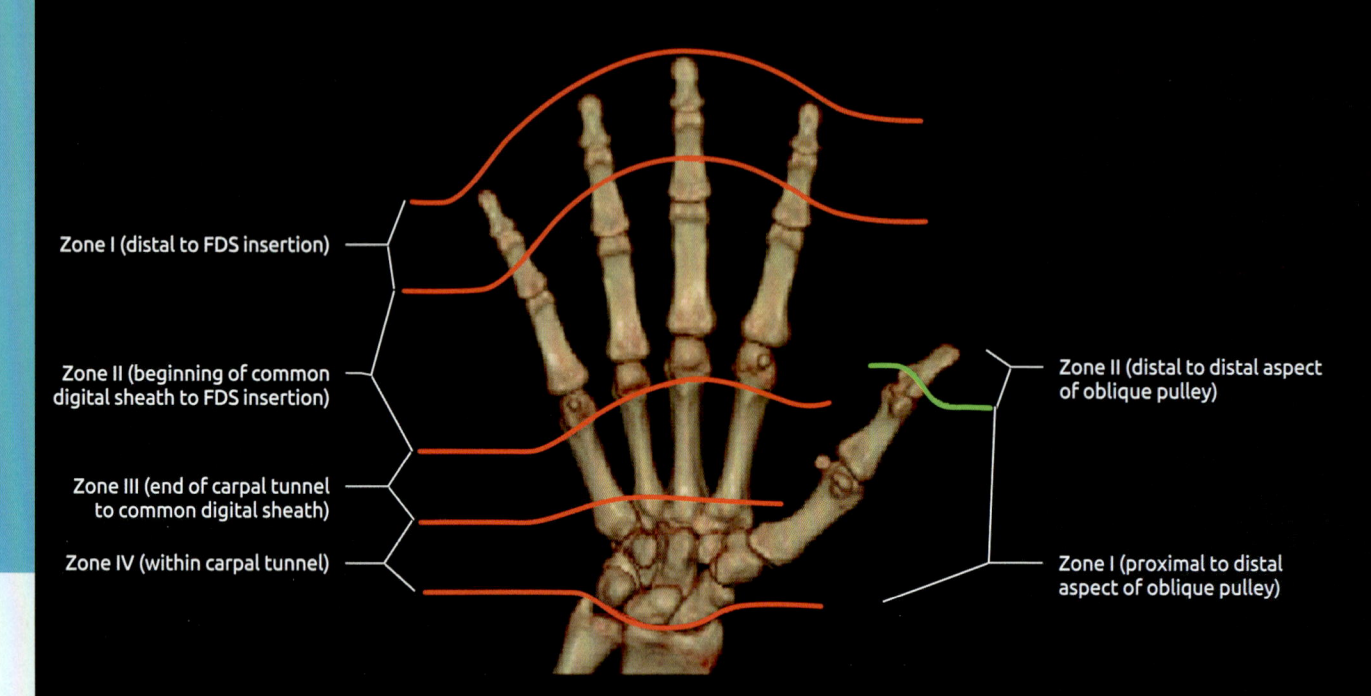

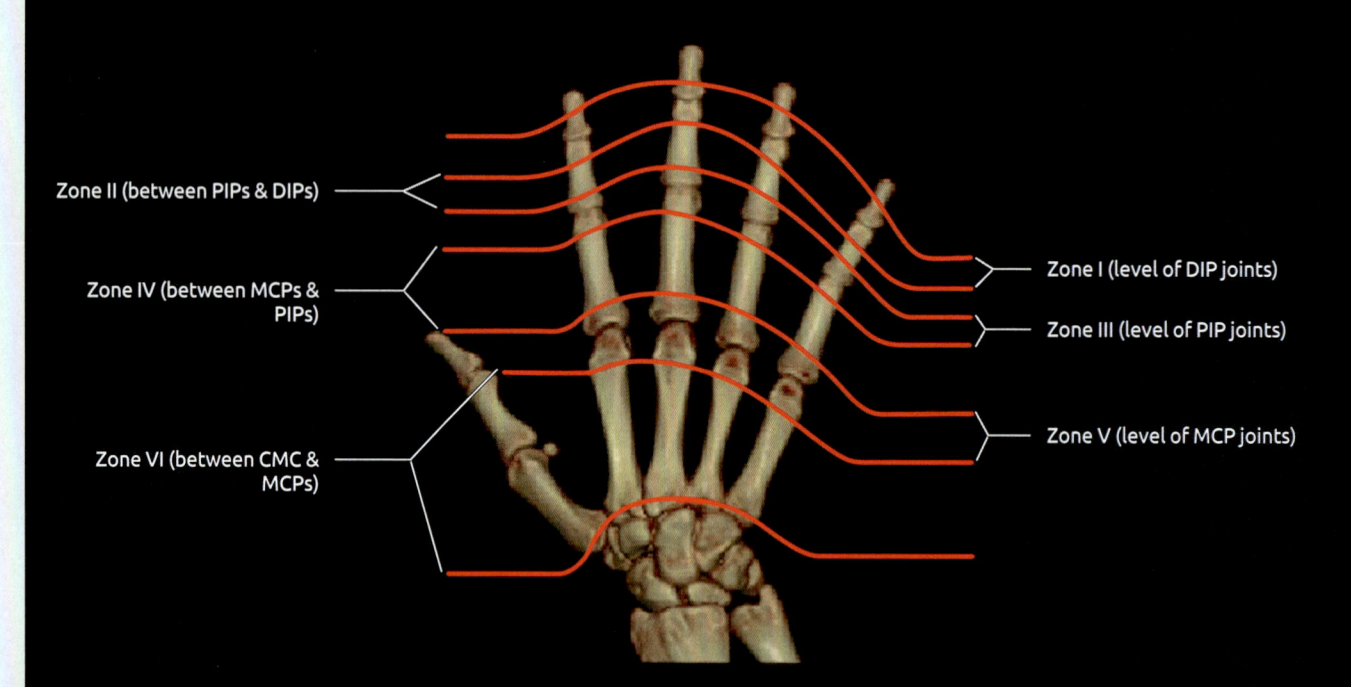

Zone I (distal to FDS insertion)

Zone II (beginning of common digital sheath to FDS insertion)

Zone III (end of carpal tunnel to common digital sheath)

Zone IV (within carpal tunnel)

Zone II (distal to distal aspect of oblique pulley)

Zone I (proximal to distal aspect of oblique pulley)

Zone II (between PIPs & DIPs)

Zone IV (between MCPs & PIPs)

Zone VI (between CMC & MCPs)

Zone I (level of DIP joints)

Zone III (level of PIP joints)

Zone V (level of MCP joints)

(Top) A modification of Verdan original tendon injury zones is now utilized for flexor tendon injuries. Establishing the zone of injury can be useful for the hand surgeon. Additional useful information includes: Complete vs. incomplete disruption (when incomplete, the transverse width of the tendon disruption should be estimated), when complete disruption is encountered, the level to which the tendon ends are retracted, and the distance between the tendon ends should be given. Injury zones for the thumb are not widely accepted. The most referenced zoning system for the thumb is illustrated. **(Bottom)** Verdan extensor injury zones are shown. When extensor mechanism injury is encountered, information for the flexor injury zones should be given. No established zone classification for the thumb exists.

Flexor and Extensor Mechanisms of Hand

AXIAL T1 MR OF LEFT HAND

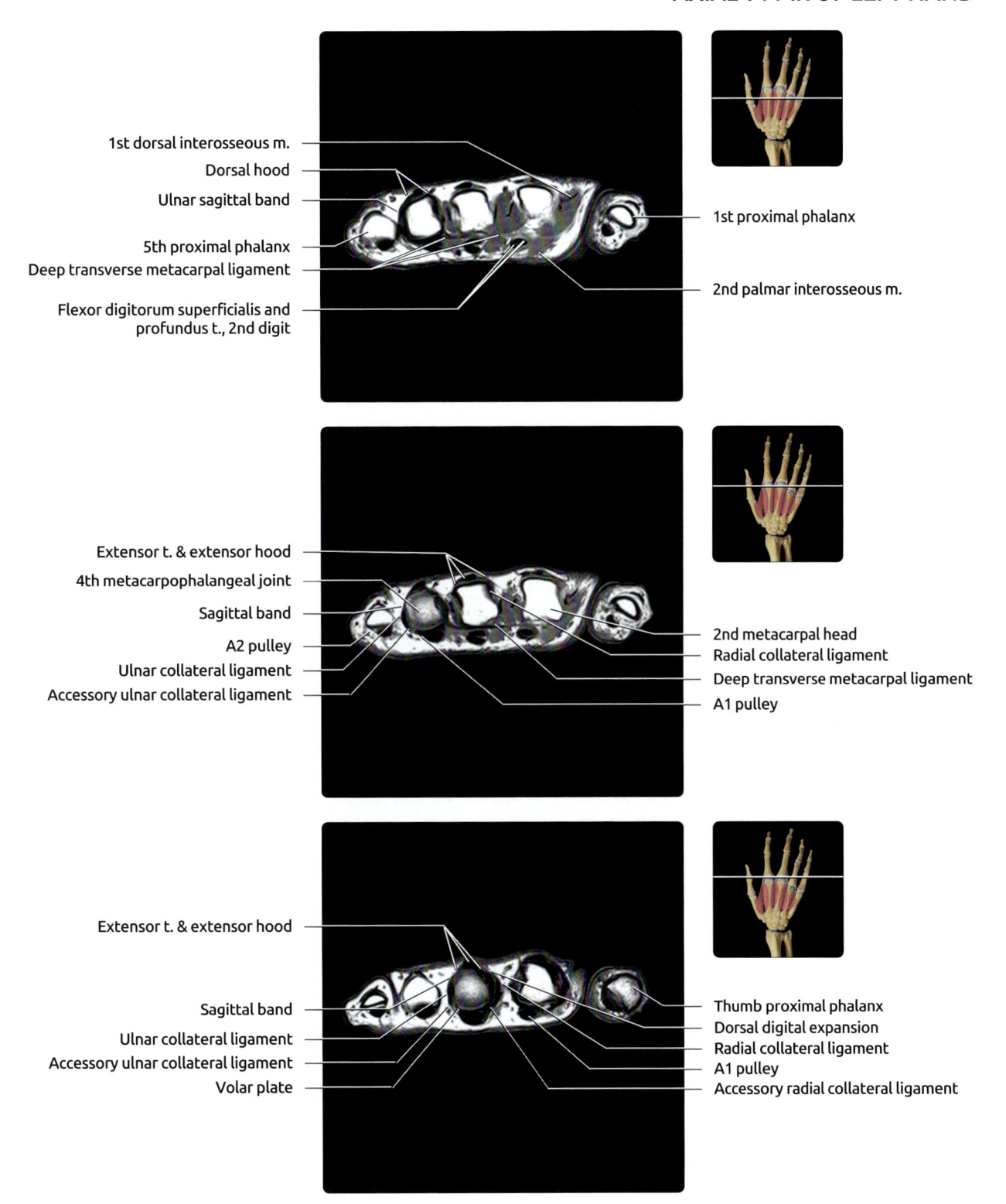

Labels (Top image):
- 1st dorsal interosseous m.
- Dorsal hood
- Ulnar sagittal band
- 5th proximal phalanx
- Deep transverse metacarpal ligament
- Flexor digitorum superficialis and profundus t., 2nd digit
- 1st proximal phalanx
- 2nd palmar interosseous m.

Labels (Middle image):
- Extensor t. & extensor hood
- 4th metacarpophalangeal joint
- Sagittal band
- A2 pulley
- Ulnar collateral ligament
- Accessory ulnar collateral ligament
- 2nd metacarpal head
- Radial collateral ligament
- Deep transverse metacarpal ligament
- A1 pulley

Labels (Bottom image):
- Extensor t. & extensor hood
- Sagittal band
- Ulnar collateral ligament
- Accessory ulnar collateral ligament
- Volar plate
- Thumb proximal phalanx
- Dorsal digital expansion
- Radial collateral ligament
- A1 pulley
- Accessory radial collateral ligament

(Top) This is the 1st of 6 selected axial images through the digits. Because of the varying length of the digits, different portions of the flexor and extensor mechanisms will be seen on a single image. This image is at the base of the 5th proximal phalanx, but at the 3rd and 4th metacarpal heads. The deep transverse metacarpal ligaments interconnect the volar plates of digits 2-4. Palmar interossei are volar to this ligament, while dorsal interossei lie dorsal to it. (Middle) At the level of the 4th metacarpophalangeal joint, the A1 pulley is seen surrounding the flexor tendons. The A2 pulley of the 5th digit, which is at the level of the middle of the proximal phalanx, is also seen. (Bottom) Slightly more distally, the 3rd metacarpophalangeal joint is in plane. The relationships of the extensor hood, sagittal bands, collateral ligaments, accessory collateral ligaments, and volar plate are well seen as they form a ring around the joint. Dorsal digital expansion of 2nd dorsal interosseous muscle is nearing its insertion on the radial side of the base of the 3rd proximal phalanx.

Flexor and Extensor Mechanisms of Hand

AXIAL T1 MR OF LEFT HAND

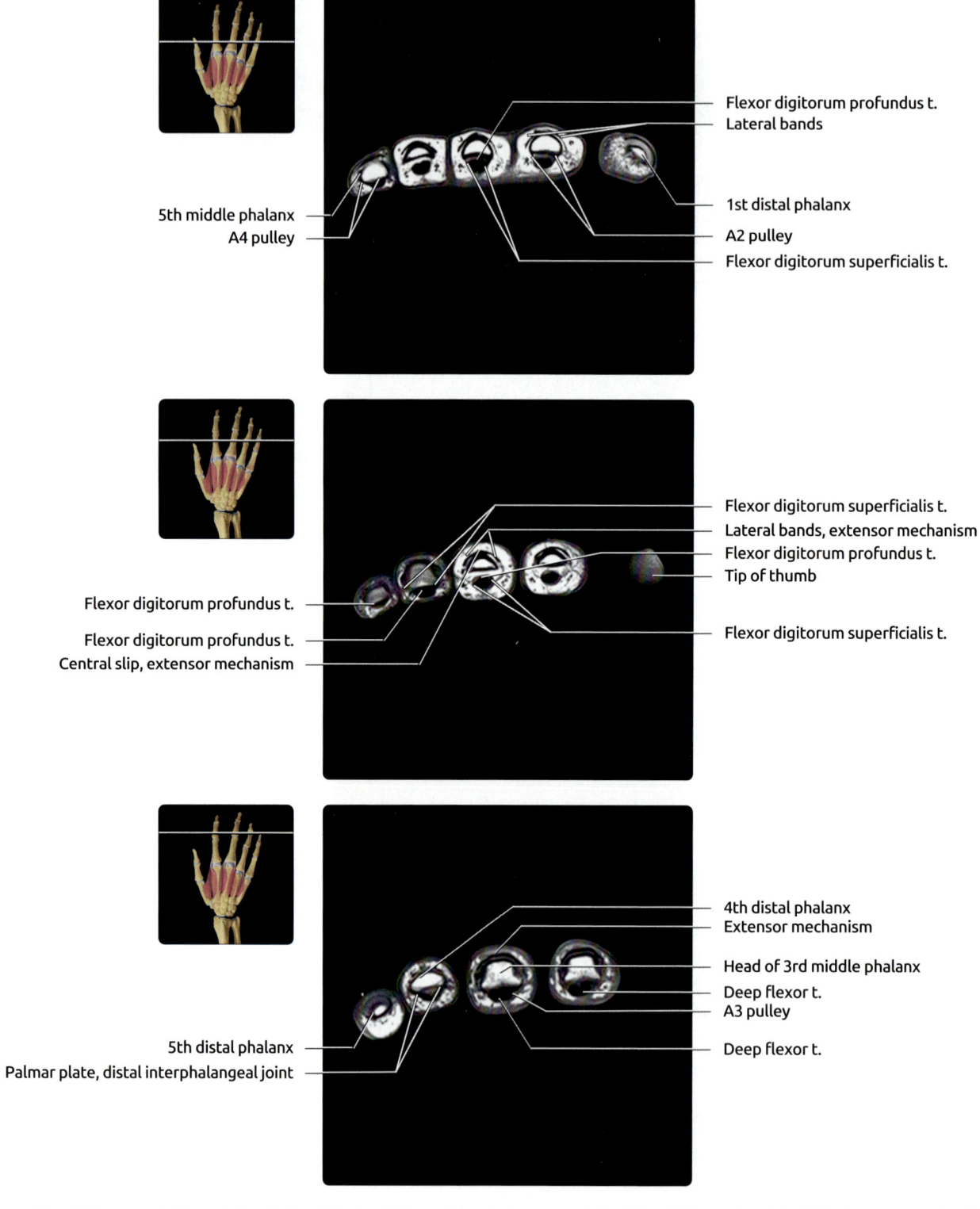

Labels (Top image):
- Flexor digitorum profundus t.
- Lateral bands
- 5th middle phalanx
- A4 pulley
- 1st distal phalanx
- A2 pulley
- Flexor digitorum superficialis t.

Labels (Middle image):
- Flexor digitorum superficialis t.
- Lateral bands, extensor mechanism
- Flexor digitorum profundus t.
- Tip of thumb
- Flexor digitorum profundus t.
- Flexor digitorum profundus t.
- Central slip, extensor mechanism
- Flexor digitorum superficialis t.

Labels (Bottom image):
- 4th distal phalanx
- Extensor mechanism
- Head of 3rd middle phalanx
- Deep flexor t.
- A3 pulley
- 5th distal phalanx
- Palmar plate, distal interphalangeal joint
- Deep flexor t.

(Top) This image is through the shafts of the 2nd-4th proximal phalanges, and the 5th middle phalanx. It is difficult on T1 weighted images to distinguish the deep and superficial flexor tendons; at this point in the 3rd digit the superficial tendons have split and moved lateral to the deep tendon. Lateral bands arise from sides of the extensor tendon in the distal portion of the proximal phalanx, and are supplemented by attachments of the interossei (radially and ulnarly) and by the lumbricals on the radial side of the digit. (Middle) This image is at the level of the 4th proximal interphalangeal joint. In this digit, the flexor digitorum's superficialis tendons have moved laterally toward their attachment on the base of the middle phalanx. The 3rd digit is seen at the proximal phalanx, at a point where the flexor digitorum superficialis has split and flanks the profundus tendon. (Bottom) This image is at the level of the 5th distal phalanx, the base of the 4th distal phalanx, and the middle phalanges of the 3rd-4th digits.

Flexor and Extensor Mechanisms of Hand

AXIAL PD FS MR, RIGHT HAND

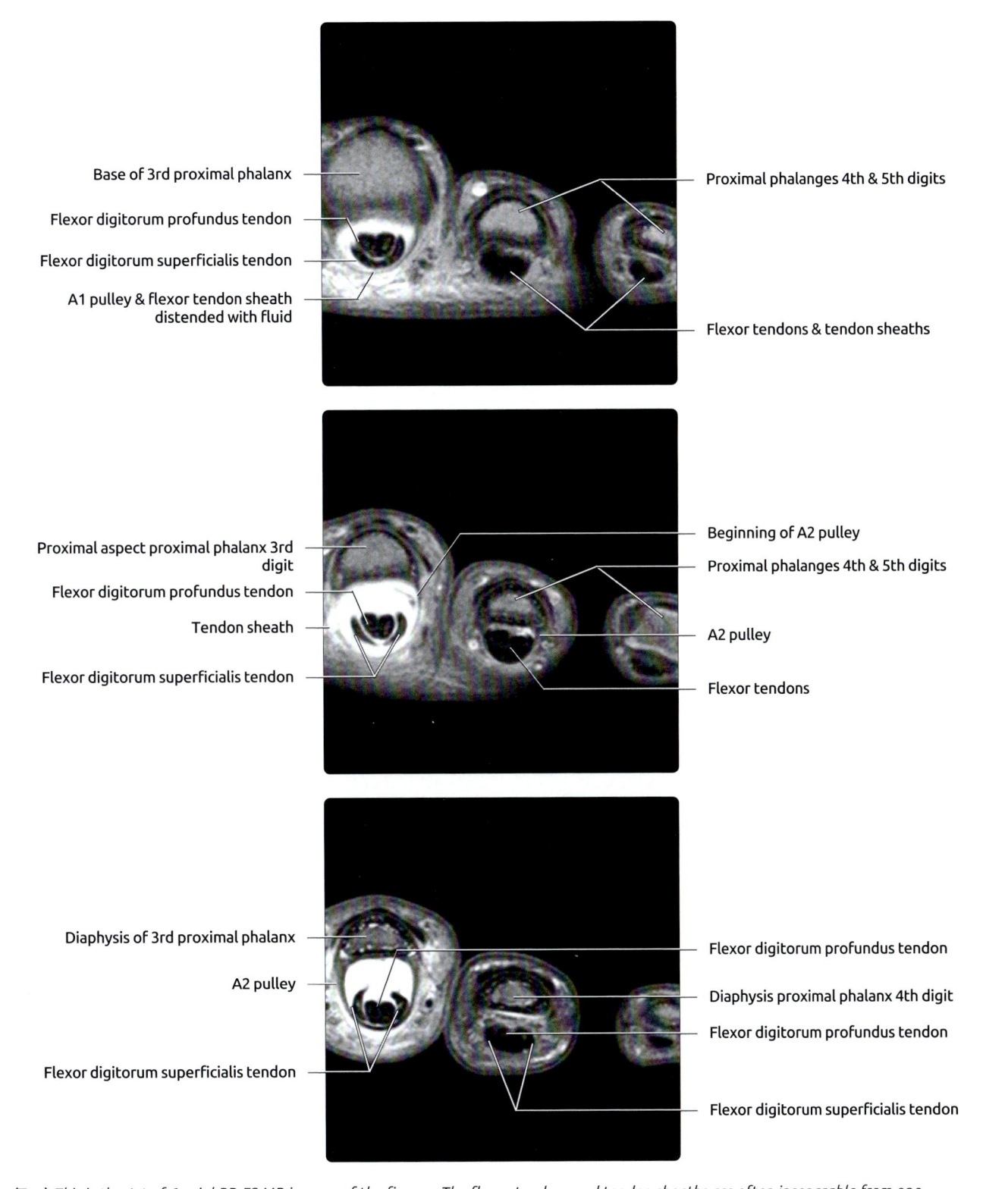

- Base of 3rd proximal phalanx
- Flexor digitorum profundus tendon
- Flexor digitorum superficialis tendon
- A1 pulley & flexor tendon sheath distended with fluid
- Proximal phalanges 4th & 5th digits
- Flexor tendons & tendon sheaths

- Proximal aspect proximal phalanx 3rd digit
- Flexor digitorum profundus tendon
- Tendon sheath
- Flexor digitorum superficialis tendon
- Beginning of A2 pulley
- Proximal phalanges 4th & 5th digits
- A2 pulley
- Flexor tendons

- Diaphysis of 3rd proximal phalanx
- A2 pulley
- Flexor digitorum superficialis tendon
- Flexor digitorum profundus tendon
- Diaphysis proximal phalanx 4th digit
- Flexor digitorum profundus tendon
- Flexor digitorum superficialis tendon

(**Top**) *This is the 1st of 6 axial PD FS MR images of the fingers. The flexor tendons and tendon sheaths are often inseparable from one another on routine imaging unless outlined by increased fluid (as in the 3rd digit in this example).* (**Middle**) *The FDS tendon splits at the proximal aspect of the proximal phalanx, as demonstrated in the 3rd digit. The same relationship exists in the 4th digit in this image, but delineation of the tendons as separate structures is difficult without the pathologic tendon sheath fluid present in the 3rd digit.* (**Bottom**) *After the FDS tendon splits, it travels laterally around the FDP tendon from superficial to deep. In the 4th digit here, even without pathologic fluid for contrast, the flexor tendons can be seen as separate structures. The A2 pulley can be identified by its location and thickness (compare to thickness of tendon sheath on the next image).*

Flexor and Extensor Mechanisms of Hand

AXIAL PD FS MR, RIGHT HAND

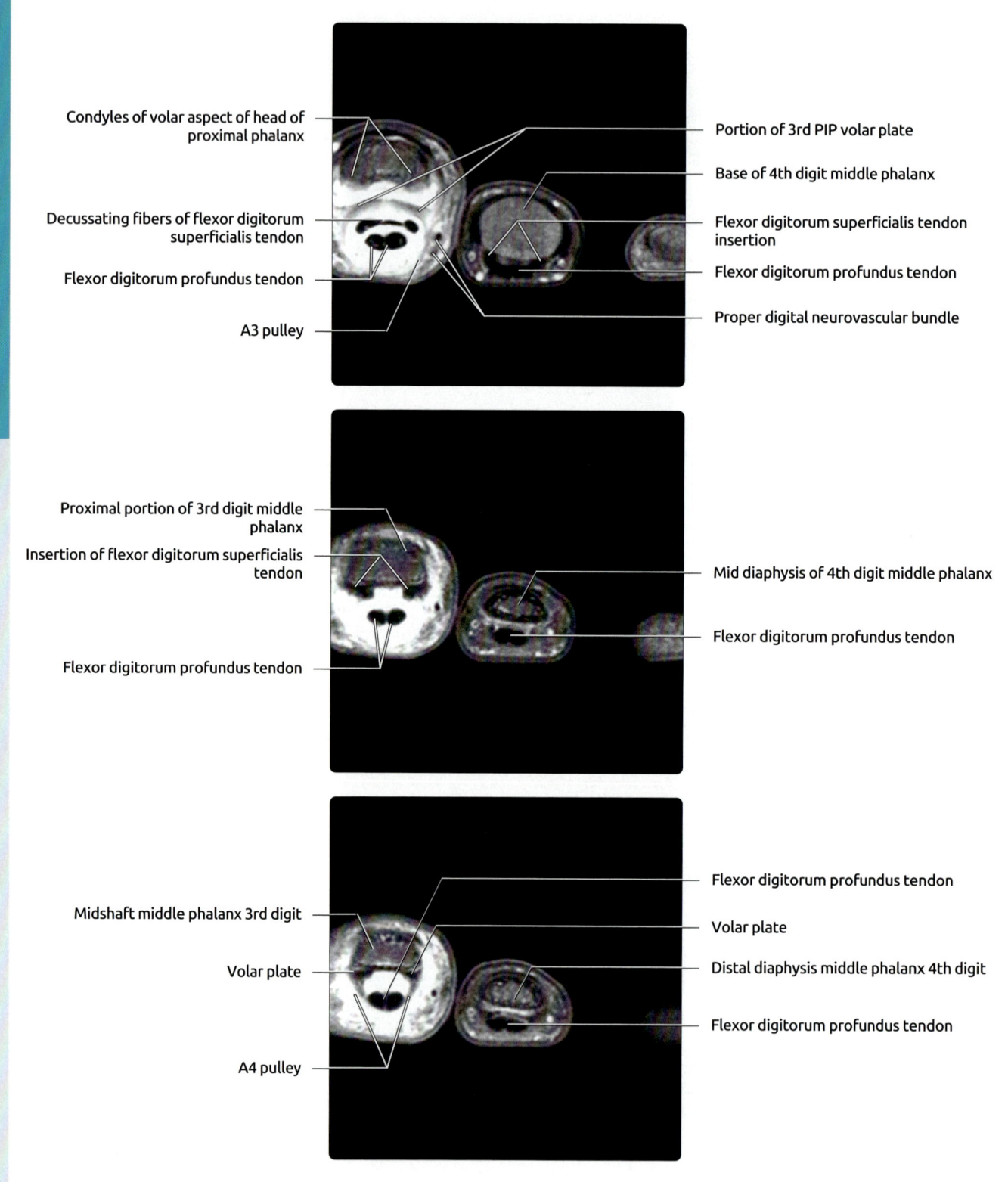

Labels (top image):
- Condyles of volar aspect of head of proximal phalanx
- Decussating fibers of flexor digitorum superficialis tendon
- Flexor digitorum profundus tendon
- A3 pulley
- Portion of 3rd PIP volar plate
- Base of 4th digit middle phalanx
- Flexor digitorum superficialis tendon insertion
- Flexor digitorum profundus tendon
- Proper digital neurovascular bundle

Labels (middle image):
- Proximal portion of 3rd digit middle phalanx
- Insertion of flexor digitorum superficialis tendon
- Flexor digitorum profundus tendon
- Mid diaphysis of 4th digit middle phalanx
- Flexor digitorum profundus tendon

Labels (bottom image):
- Midshaft middle phalanx 3rd digit
- Volar plate
- A4 pulley
- Flexor digitorum profundus tendon
- Volar plate
- Distal diaphysis middle phalanx 4th digit
- Flexor digitorum profundus tendon

(Top) In the 4th digit, the slips of the FDS tendon are beginning to insert on the volar aspect of the proximal portion of the middle phalanx. In the 3rd digit, the decussation of fibers from 1 slip of the FDS tendon to the other can be seen. Note the volar bicondylar shape of the head of the 3rd proximal phalanx vs. the oval shape of the base of 4th middle phalanx. (Middle) In the 3rd digit, the FDS tendons insert on the volar aspect of the proximal portion of the middle phalanx. In the 4th digit, we are already beyond the insertion of the FDS tendon, and accordingly, only 1 tendon (the FDP tendon) is seen. (Bottom) Understanding the normal location of the pulleys allows identification of the A4 pulley at the midshaft of the middle phalanx 3rd digit. Additionally, note that the pulley is thicker than the normal tendon sheath: Compare to previous image where the normal tendon sheath is barely (if at all) discernible.

Flexor and Extensor Mechanisms of Hand

SAGITTAL PD FS MR, RIGHT HAND

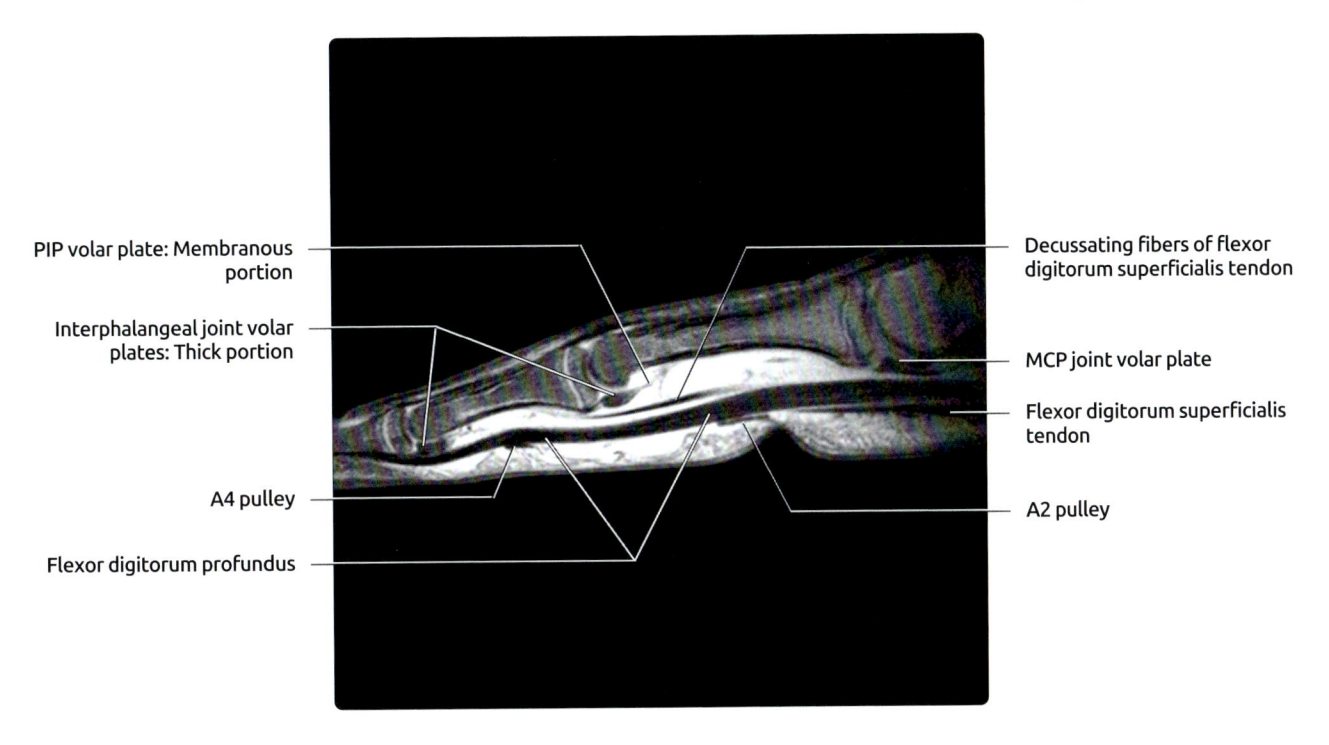

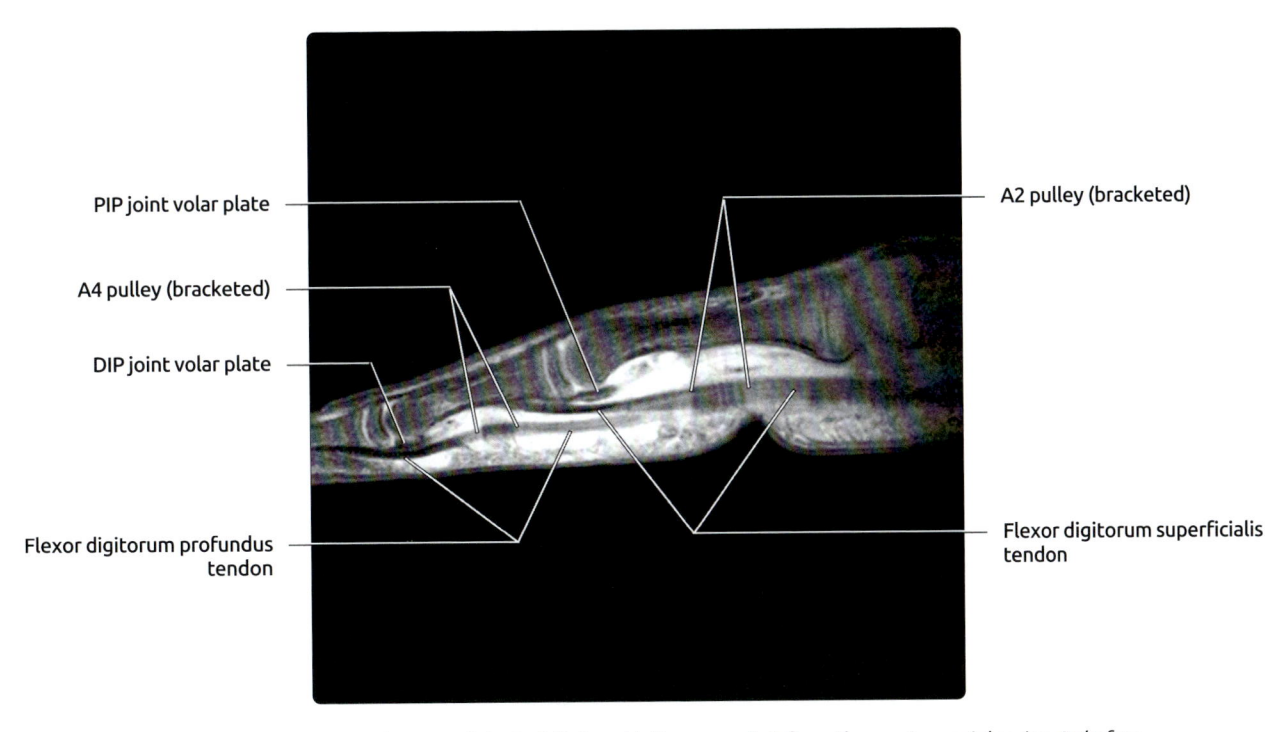

Labels (top image):
- PIP volar plate: Membranous portion
- Interphalangeal joint volar plates: Thick portion
- A4 pulley
- Flexor digitorum profundus
- Decussating fibers of flexor digitorum superficialis tendon
- MCP joint volar plate
- Flexor digitorum superficialis tendon
- A2 pulley

Labels (bottom image):
- PIP joint volar plate
- A4 pulley (bracketed)
- DIP joint volar plate
- Flexor digitorum profundus tendon
- A2 pulley (bracketed)
- Flexor digitorum superficialis tendon

(Top) This is the 1st of 2 sagittal PD FS MR images of the 3rd digit and is the same digit from the previous axial series. As before, pathologic fluid is present within and about the common digital tendon sheath, providing excellent contrast for delineation of normal structures. In this image, the FDS tendon appears discontinuous; however, remember that the FDS tendon splits and it slips pass lateral to the FDP tendon from just distal to the MCP joint until its decussation. Note the thin membranous portion of the volar plate of the PIP joint (not normally seen). In this plane, only the volar-most portions of the A2 and A4 pulleys can be seen. **(Bottom)** This image is slightly more lateral than the previous image. In this plane, we see that the FDS tendon is intact. We are also just lateral enough to catch some of the lateral portions of the A2 and A4 pulleys.

SECTION 7
Pelvis and Hip

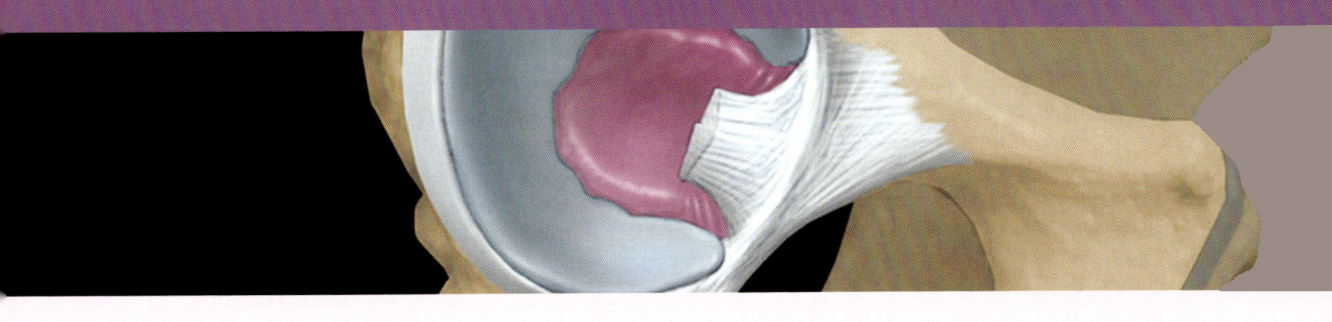

Pelvis Overview	**486**
Pelvis MR Atlas	**494**
Anterior Pelvis	**528**
Hip Overview	**554**
Hip MR Anatomy	**558**
Pelvis and Hip Radiographic and Arthrographic Anatomy	**574**
Pelvis and Hip Normal Variants and Imaging Pitfalls	**590**
Pelvis and Hip Measurements and Lines	**598**

Pelvis Overview

GROSS ANATOMY

Basic Concepts of Pelvic Anatomy

- Pelvic ring composed of sacrum, coccyx, hip bone
  - Articulations: Lumbosacral, sacrococcygeal, sacroiliac, symphysis pubis
- Transmits body weight to lower extremities and absorbs forces from lower extremity
- Anatomic boundaries between pelvis and lower limb
  - External surfaces of pelvic bones/sacrum/coccyx, iliac crest, inguinal ligament, symphysis pubis, ischiopubic rami, ischial tuberosity, sacrotuberous ligament
- Anteriorly tilted
  - Pelvic inlet 50° from horizontal
  - Anterior superior iliac spine (ASIS) and anterosuperior pubis along same vertical axis
- Acetabulum faces inferomedially
  - Acetabular notch opens inferiorly
- Hip bone: Ischium, ilium, pubis
  - Articulation: Ball and socket hip joint
- **Greater (false) and lesser (true) pelvis**
  - Greater pelvis: Part of abdominal cavity
  - Lesser pelvis: Between pelvic inlet and pelvic outlet
  - **Pelvic inlet**: Pelvic brim, sacral promontory, sacral ala, **linea terminalis** (arcuate line of ilium, pecten pubis, pubic crest)
  - **Pelvic outlet**: Pubic arch, ischial tuberosities, sacrotuberous ligament, tip of coccyx
- **Obturator foramen**: Covered by obturator membrane
  - Boundaries: Pubis, ischium, superior pubic, and ischiopubic rami
  - Reduces weight of pelvis
  - **Obturator canal**: Obturator vessels and nerve through membrane

Bones

- **Sacrum**
  - Triangular, concave anterior, convex posterior
  - Contains 5-6 fused vertebra
    - Transitional lumbosacral vertebra common
    - 1st coccygeal segment often fused with sacrum
  - 4 ridges and 4 anterior (ventral) neural foramina
    - Ridges remnants intervertebral discs
  - **Sacral ala** (wings): Lateral aspect
  - Lamina fused posteriorly; cover spinal canal to level of S4
  - **Lumbosacral angle**: 130-160°
  - **Median sacral crest**: Fusion of spinous processes S1-S3, ± S4
  - **Sacral hiatus**: Dorsal defect in posterior coverage of spinal canal below S3 or S4 level
    - Utilized as access point for caudal epidural injections
  - **Intermediate sacral crest**: Fusion articular processes
  - **Lateral sacral crest**: Tips fused transverse processes
  - **Sacral cornua**: Inferior articular facets S5
    - Articulate with coccyx (may be fibrous or fused)
  - Lateral surface: Sacroiliac joint (SI)
  - **Sacral promontory**: Anterior superior corner of S1
- **Coccyx**
  - Triangular shape, 3-5 rudimentary vertebra
  - Coccygeal cornua articulates with sacrum
- **Innominate bone**
  - Forms from 3 primary centers
    - Ischium, ilium, pubis
    - Joined by triradiate cartilage; matures by 15-16 years old
- **Ilium**
  - **Iliac wing** is large, flat, superior portion
    - Concave internal **iliac fossa**
    - Convex external **auricular surface** (gluteal fossa)
  - **Iliac crest** is superior margin of iliac wing, extends from anterior ASIS to posterior superior iliac spine (PSIS)
    - **Tubercle** of iliac crest at anterosuperior margin
    - L4-L5 disc is usually at level of iliac crest
  - **Iliac crest accessory ossification center**
    - 1st appears at lateral margin of crest
    - Develops medially as skeletal maturation progresses
    - Usually completed by age 14 in girls, age 16 in boys
  - **Anterior superior iliac spine (ASIS)**
    - Anterior margin of iliac crest
    - Site of origin of sartorius muscle
  - **Anterior inferior iliac spine (AIIS)**
    - Has a rounded contour
    - Site of origin of straight head rectus femoris muscle, iliofemoral ligament
  - **Anterior inferior iliac spine ossification center**
    - Ossification begins by age 13-15
    - Fusion complete by age 20-25
  - **Posterior superior iliac spine (PSIS)**
    - Posterior margin of iliac crest
    - Site of attachment of dorsal SIs, multifidus muscle
  - **Posterior inferior iliac spine (PIIS)**
    - Posterior margin of greater sciatic notch
  - **Iliac portion of acetabulum**
    - Posterior-superior portion of acetabulum is part of ilium
    - ~ 2/5 of acetabulum
- **Ischium**
  - **Ischial spine**: Posterior margin of ischium
    - Greater sciatic notch is posterior to ischial spine
    - Lesser sciatic notch is anterior to ischial spine
  - **Ischial portion of acetabulum**
    - Forms posterior, inferior 2/5 of acetabulum
  - **Ischial tuberosity**
    - Rounded, inferior portion of ischium
    - In seated position, ischial tuberosities bear all body weight
  - **Ischial tuberosity ossification center**
    - Ossification begins by age 14-16
    - Fuses by age 20-25
  - **Ischial ramus**
    - Joins inferior pubic ramus forming ischiopubic ramus
- **Pubis**
  - Body and 2 rami
  - Rami meet midline at symphysis pubis
  - **Pubic body**
    - Lateral portion of pubis, forming superomedial 1/5 of acetabulum
  - **Iliopubic (iliopectineal) eminence** at junction with ilium
  - **Superior pubic ramus**

Pelvis Overview

- Extends into pubic portion of acetabulum
- Lateral portion often designated as "root" of ramus
  - **Inferior ramus** continuous with ischial ramus
  - **Pubic crest** along anterior superior border of symphysis and pubic bodies
  - **Pubic tubercle**: Lateral aspect of pubic crest
    - Attachment inguinal ligament
  - **Pecten**: Lateral ridge along superior ramus from pubic tubercle to arcuate line
  - **Secondary ossification center**
    - Medial margin of pubic bones
    - Arises at puberty, ossifies in early adulthood

Muscle Groups

- Hip adductors
  - Pectineus, adductors brevis, longus and magnus, obturator externus, quadratus femoris
- Hip flexors
  - Iliopsoas, rectus femoris, sartorius
- Hip abductors
  - Gluteus medius, gluteus minimus, tensor fascia lata, sartorius, tensor fascia lata
- Hip external rotators
  - Piriformis, gemelli, quadratus femoris, obturator internus, obturator externus
- Hip internal rotators
  - Piriformis (when hip flexed)
- Hip extensors
  - Gluteus maximus, long head biceps femoris, semimembranosus, semitendinosus

Vessels

- **Iliac artery**
  - Originates at inferior terminus of aorta
  - Level of L4
  - Bifurcates into internal and external iliac arteries at pelvic brim
- **Internal iliac artery**: Supplies pelvic wall, pelvic organs, buttock, medial compartment of thigh
  - 3-4 cm long, divides into anterior and posterior divisions
  - Posterior division: Iliolumbar, lateral sacral, superior gluteal artery
  - Anterior division: Inferior gluteal, internal pudendal, inferior vesical (or uterine), middle rectal, vaginal, umbilical artery
- **Superior gluteal artery**: Continuation of posterior division internal iliac artery
  - Passes between lumbosacral trunk and S1 nerve
  - Exits pelvis superior to piriformis muscle
  - Divides and supplies musculature
    - Superficial: Gluteus maximus muscle
    - Deep: Gluteus medius and minimus muscle, tensor fascia lata
  - **Superior gluteal vein**: Travels with artery, drains into internal iliac vein
- **Inferior gluteal artery**: Larger terminal branch anterior division internal iliac artery
  - Passes between S1 and S2 or S2 and S3
  - Exits pelvis through sciatic notch inferior to piriformis muscle
  - Posteromedial to sciatic nerve
  - Supplies pelvic diaphragm, piriformis, quadratus femoris, upper hamstring and gluteus maximus muscle, sciatic nerve
  - **Inferior gluteal vein** travels with artery, drains into internal iliac vein
- **Obturator artery**: Branch anterior division internal iliac artery
  - Travels lateral pelvic wall; lateral to ureter, ductus deferens, peritoneum
  - Leaves pelvis via obturator canal, enters medial thigh
  - Acetabular branch via acetabular notch to ligamentum fovea capitis
  - 20% incidence aberrant artery from inferior epigastric artery
  - **Obturator vein** with artery, drains into internal iliac vein
- **External iliac artery**
  - Branches: Inferior epigastric artery, deep circumflex iliac artery
  - Becomes femoral artery after passing beneath inguinal ligament

Nerves

- Preaxial: Anterior to bone
- Postaxial: Posterior to bone
- **Lumbar plexus**: Ventral rami L1, L2, L3, portion of L4
  - Forms along anterior transverse processes within psoas major muscle
  - Branches: Iliohypogastric: L1 ± T12; ilioinguinal: L1; genitofemoral: L1, L2 (pre-axial); lateral femoral cutaneous: L2, L3 (postaxial); obturator: L2, L3, L4 (preaxial); accessory obturator: L3, L4 (preaxial); femoral: L2, L3, L4 (postaxial)
    - Obturator and femoral nerves
- **Sacral plexus**: **Lumbosacral trunk** (descending L4, anterior ramus L5), S1, S2, S3
  - Forms anterior surface piriformis and coccygeus muscles
  - Branches
    - Sciatic nerve divides into tibial nerve: L4, L5, S1, S2, S3 (preaxial); common peroneal nerve: L4, L5, S1, S2 (postaxial)
    - Muscular branches: Piriformis: S1, S2; levator ani and coccygeus: S3, S4; quadratus femoris and inferior gemellus: L4, L5, S1; obturator internus and superior gemellus: L5, S1, S2
    - Superior gluteal nerve: L4, L5, S1; inferior gluteal nerve: L5, S1, S2; posterior femoral cutaneous nerve: S1, S2, S3; perforating cutaneous nerve: S2, S3; pudendal nerve: S3, S4; pelvic splanchnic nerve: S2, S3, S4; perineal branch S4
- **Coccygeal plexus**: S4, S5, coccygeal nerves
  - Supplies coccygeus and levator ani muscles
  - Branch: Anococcygeal nerve

Pelvis Overview

PELVIC BONES AND LIGAMENTS

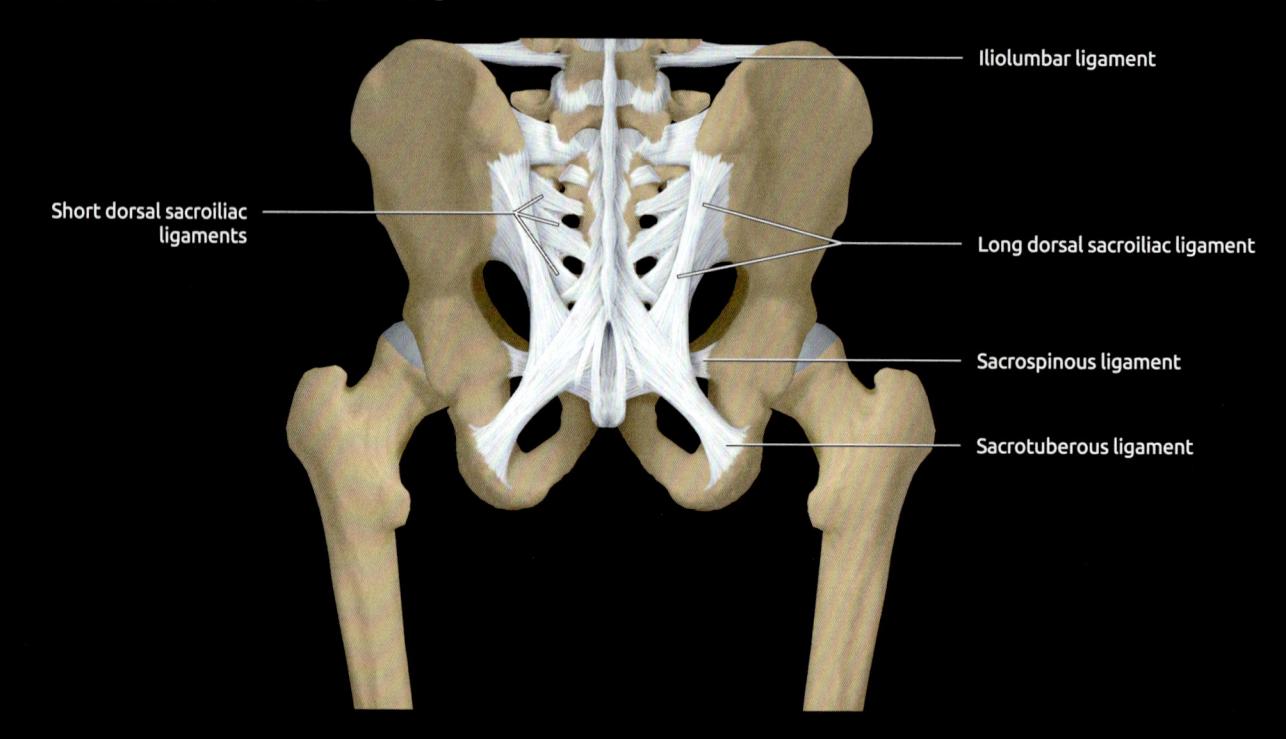

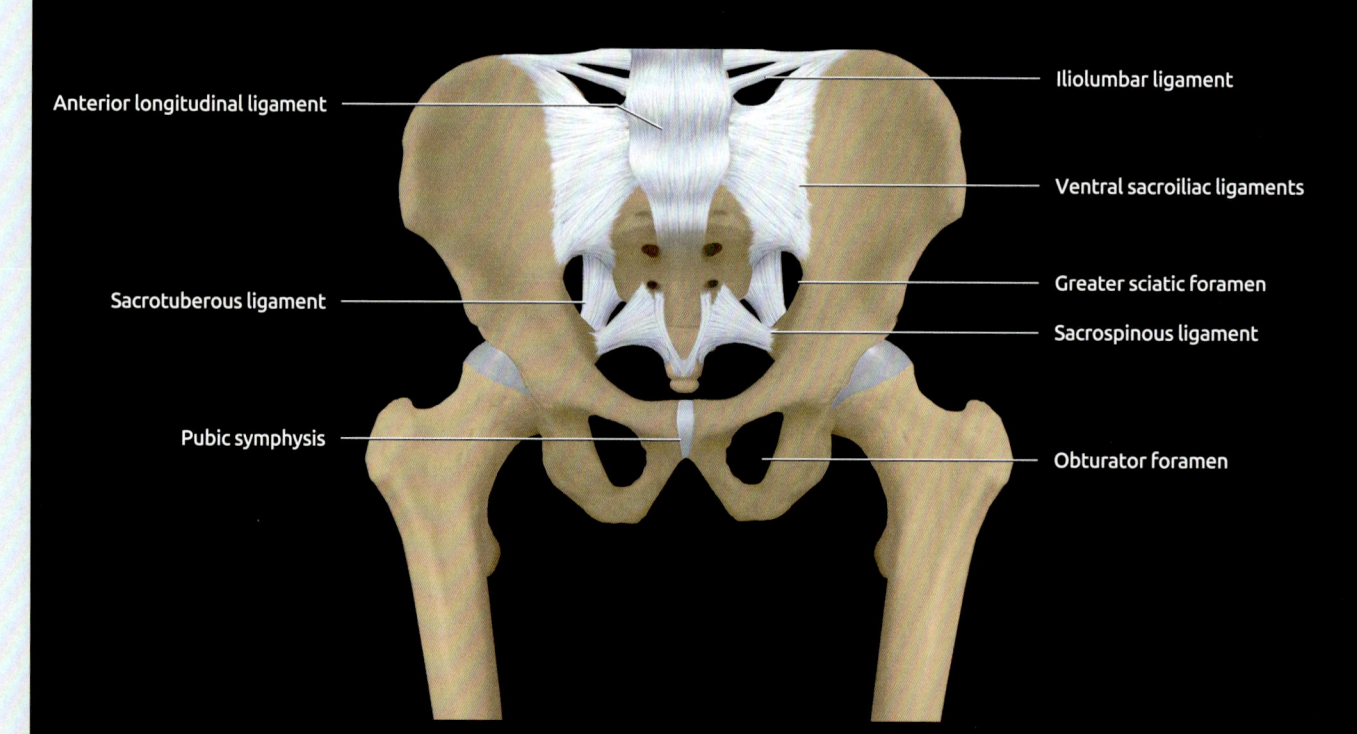

- Iliolumbar ligament
- Short dorsal sacroiliac ligaments
- Long dorsal sacroiliac ligament
- Sacrospinous ligament
- Sacrotuberous ligament

- Anterior longitudinal ligament
- Iliolumbar ligament
- Ventral sacroiliac ligaments
- Sacrotuberous ligament
- Greater sciatic foramen
- Sacrospinous ligament
- Pubic symphysis
- Obturator foramen

(**Top**) *Posterior view of the sacroiliac ligaments demonstrates the horizontal short dorsal sacroiliac ligaments and the vertically oriented long dorsal sacroiliac ligaments. The horizontally oriented iliolumbar ligaments are part of the posterior sacroiliac ligament complex. The posterior sacroiliac ligament complex is crucial in pelvic stability.* (**Bottom**) *Graphic shows anterior view of the ligaments of the sacroiliac joint and pelvis. The ventral ligaments of the sacroiliac joint are weak and composed primarily of joint capsule.*

Pelvis Overview

EXTERNAL SURFACE OF INNOMINATE BONE

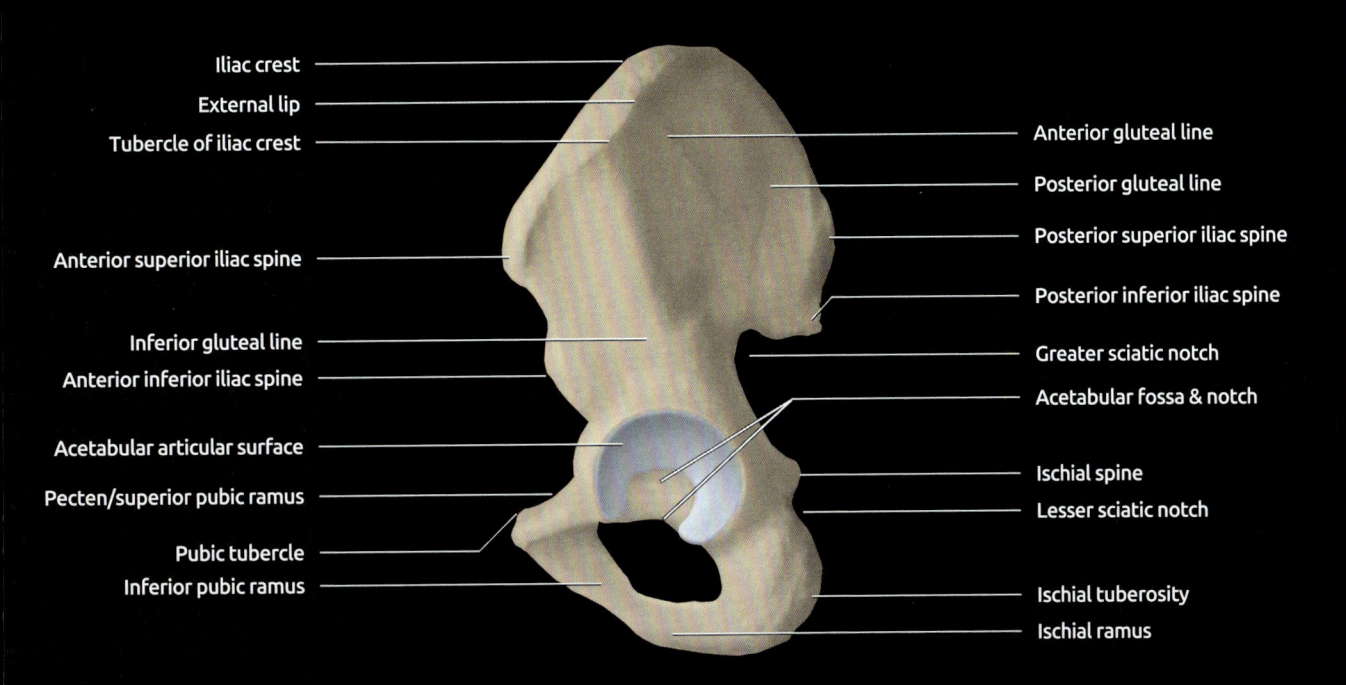

Labels (top figure):
- Iliac crest
- External lip
- Tubercle of iliac crest
- Anterior superior iliac spine
- Inferior gluteal line
- Anterior inferior iliac spine
- Acetabular articular surface
- Pecten/superior pubic ramus
- Pubic tubercle
- Inferior pubic ramus
- Anterior gluteal line
- Posterior gluteal line
- Posterior superior iliac spine
- Posterior inferior iliac spine
- Greater sciatic notch
- Acetabular fossa & notch
- Ischial spine
- Lesser sciatic notch
- Ischial tuberosity
- Ischial ramus

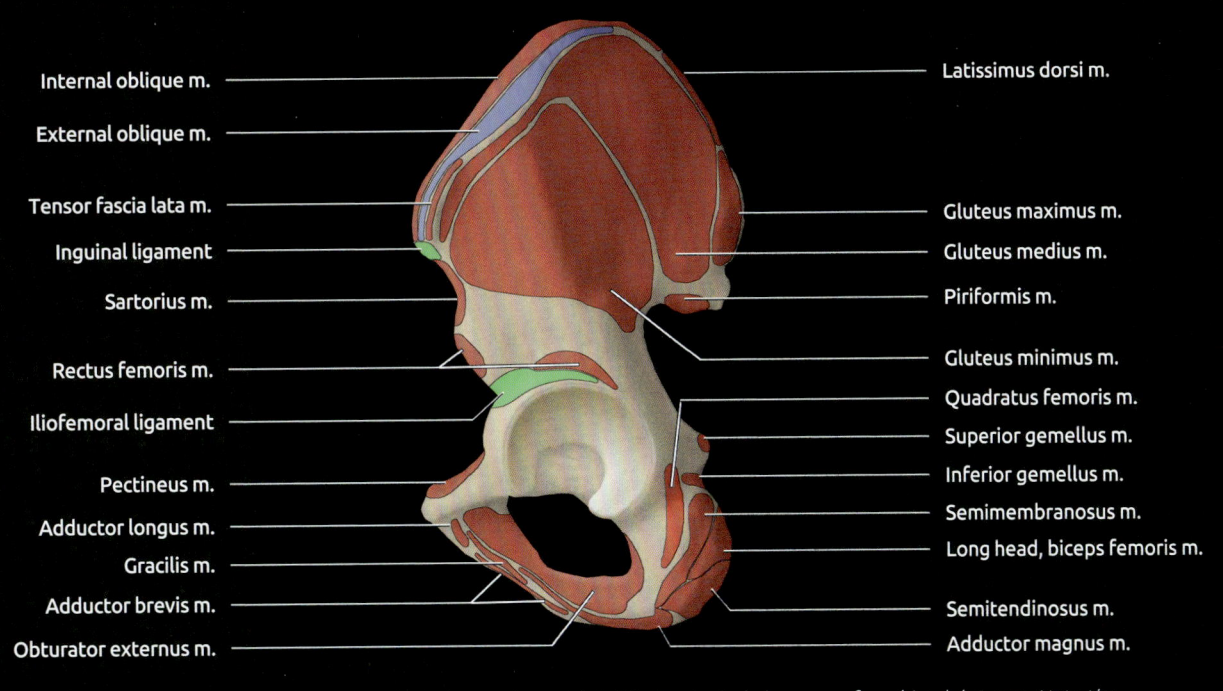

Labels (bottom figure):
- Internal oblique m.
- External oblique m.
- Tensor fascia lata m.
- Inguinal ligament
- Sartorius m.
- Rectus femoris m.
- Iliofemoral ligament
- Pectineus m.
- Adductor longus m.
- Gracilis m.
- Adductor brevis m.
- Obturator externus m.
- Latissimus dorsi m.
- Gluteus maximus m.
- Gluteus medius m.
- Piriformis m.
- Gluteus minimus m.
- Quadratus femoris m.
- Superior gemellus m.
- Inferior gemellus m.
- Semimembranosus m.
- Long head, biceps femoris m.
- Semitendinosus m.
- Adductor magnus m.

(**Top**) *Graphic shows external surface of the innominate bone. The pelvis is tilted anteriorly because of our bipedal stance. Note the orientation with anterior superior iliac spine and symphysis pubis along the same vertical axis, acetabular notch inferior.* (**Bottom**) *Graphic shows muscle and ligament attachments to the external surface of the innominate bone. Note the relatively small origin of the tendon of the adductor longus muscle. The adductor brevis muscle is just deep to the longus muscle. The origin of the gracilis muscle is lateral to the adductor brevis muscle. The adductor magnus muscle has 2 heads. The small head (adductor minimus or pubofemoral portion) arises from the ischiopubic ramus, and the larger head (ischiocondylar portion) arises from the ischial tuberosity.*

Pelvis Overview

INTERNAL SURFACE OF INNOMINATE BONE

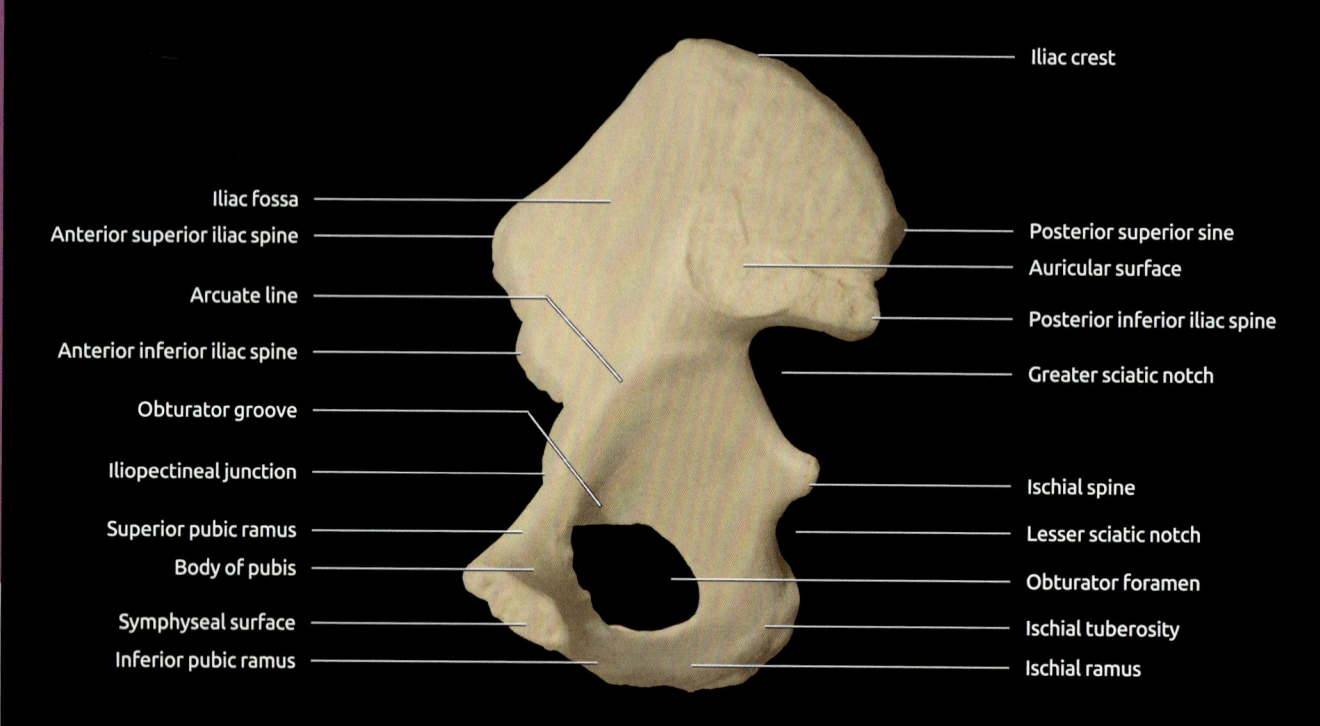

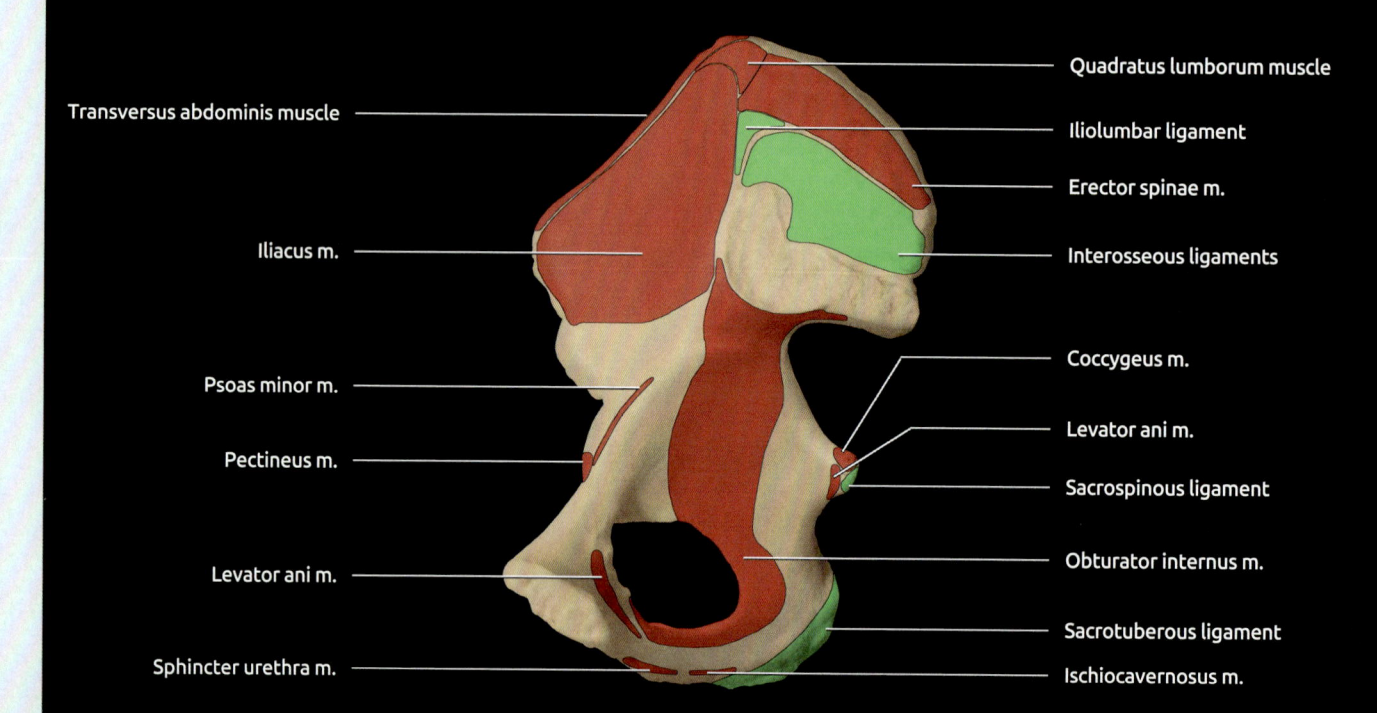

Labels (top graphic):
- Iliac crest
- Iliac fossa
- Anterior superior iliac spine
- Arcuate line
- Anterior inferior iliac spine
- Obturator groove
- Iliopectineal junction
- Superior pubic ramus
- Body of pubis
- Symphyseal surface
- Inferior pubic ramus
- Posterior superior sine
- Auricular surface
- Posterior inferior iliac spine
- Greater sciatic notch
- Ischial spine
- Lesser sciatic notch
- Obturator foramen
- Ischial tuberosity
- Ischial ramus

Labels (bottom graphic):
- Transversus abdominis muscle
- Iliacus m.
- Psoas minor m.
- Pectineus m.
- Levator ani m.
- Sphincter urethra m.
- Quadratus lumborum muscle
- Iliolumbar ligament
- Erector spinae m.
- Interosseous ligaments
- Coccygeus m.
- Levator ani m.
- Sacrospinous ligament
- Obturator internus m.
- Sacrotuberous ligament
- Ischiocavernosus m.

(**Top**) *Graphic shows internal surface of the pelvis. Note the relationships of the greater and lesser sciatic notch, separated by the ischial spine.* (**Bottom**) *Graphic shows muscle and ligament attachments to the internal surface of the pelvis. The muscles of the lower extremity include the iliacus, psoas, pectineus, and obturator internus muscles.*

Pelvis Overview

INTERNAL SURFACE OF PELVIC WALL

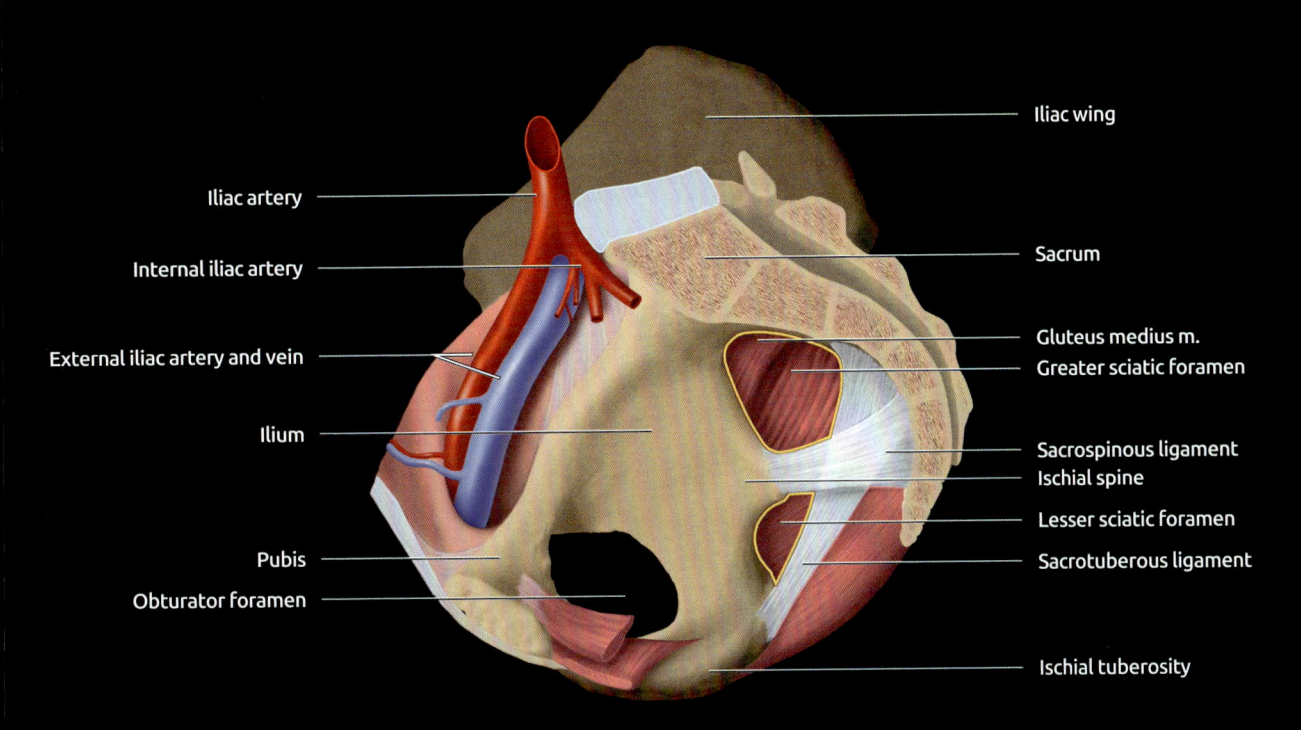

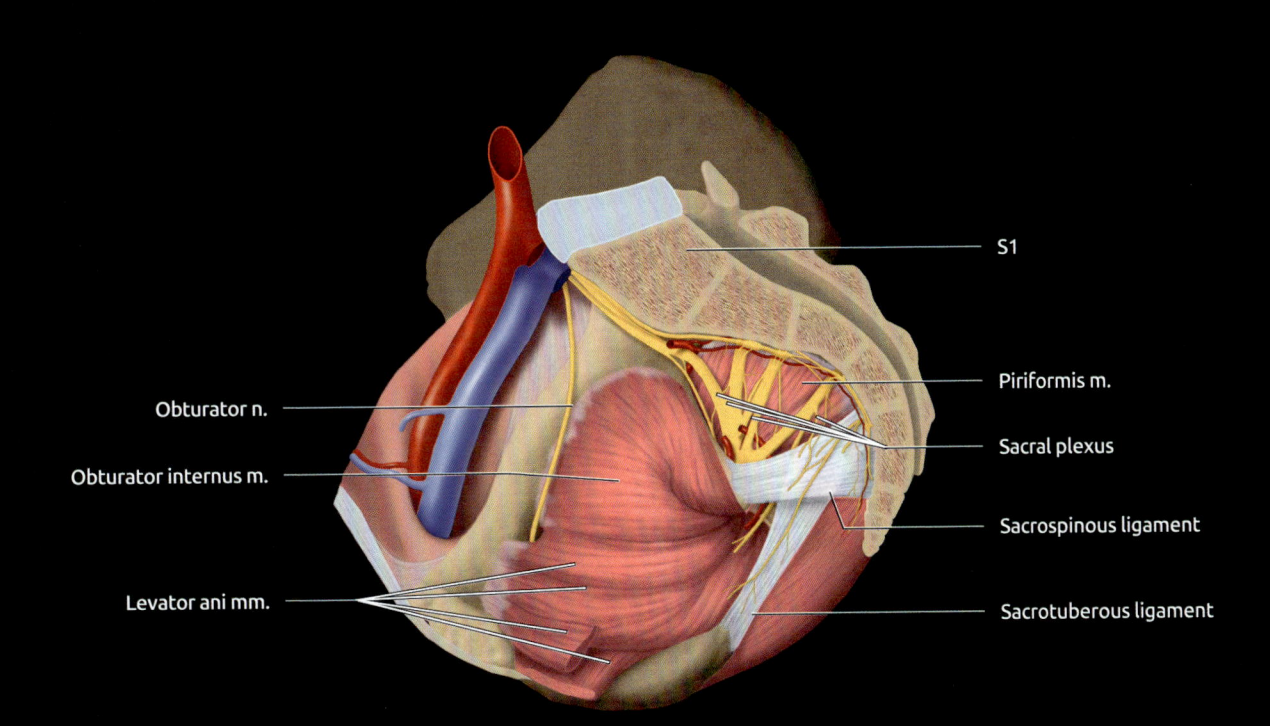

(Top) This view of the pelvis from the internal surface demonstrates the framework of the sciatic foramen. Each sciatic foramen is outlined in yellow. The greater sciatic notch is converted into a foramen by the vertically oriented sacrotuberous ligament. The intersection of the sacrotuberous and sacrospinous ligaments converts the lesser sciatic notch into a foramen. (Bottom) The obturator internus, piriformis muscles, and sacral plexus now overlay the framework. The obturator nerve is not part of the sacral plexus but arises from the 2nd-4th lumbar ventral rami. The levator ani muscles arise from the ischium, fascia of the obturator internus muscle, and pubic bone.

Pelvis Overview

SACRUM

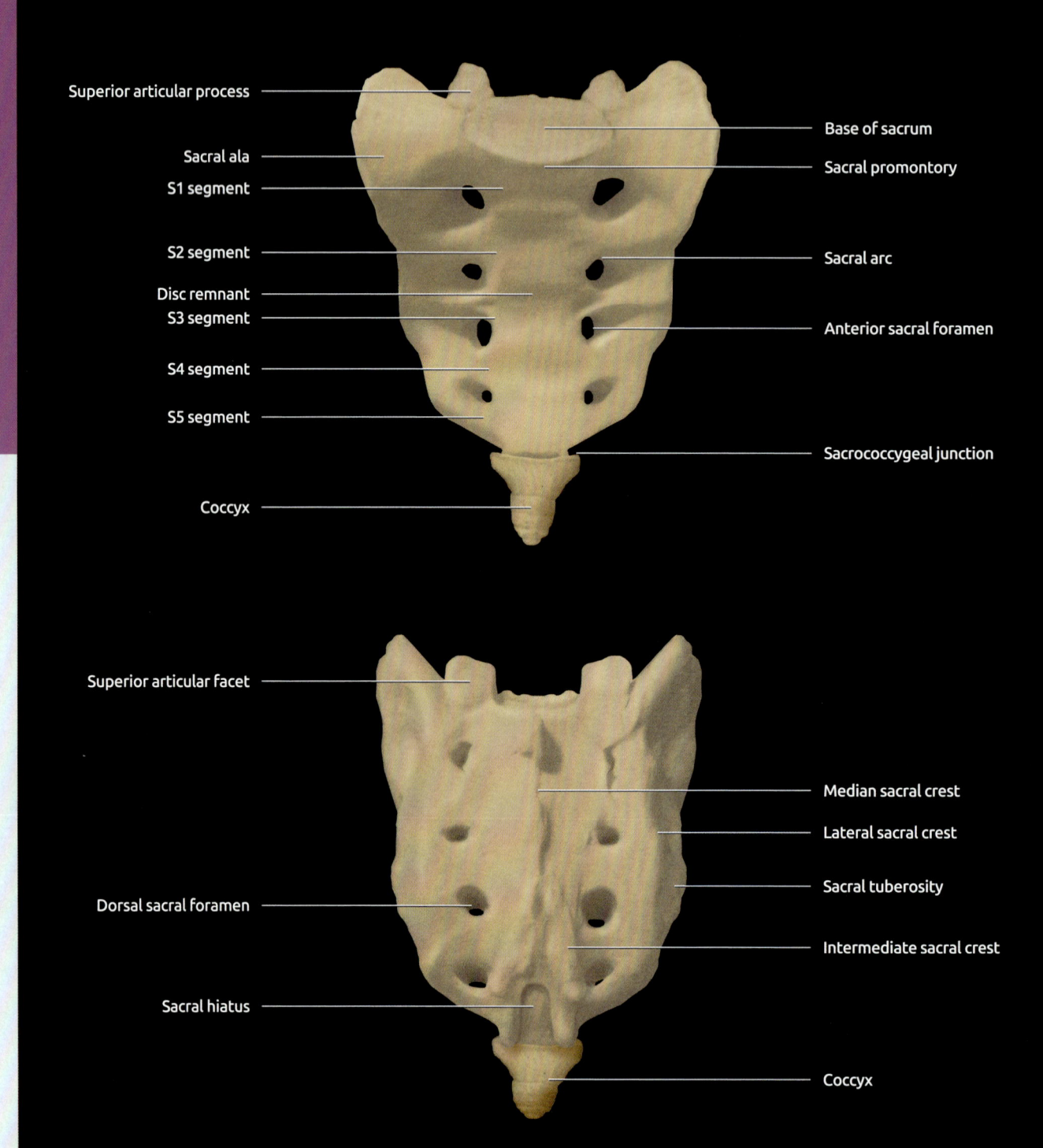

Labels (anterior view, top):
- Superior articular process
- Sacral ala
- S1 segment
- S2 segment
- Disc remnant
- S3 segment
- S4 segment
- S5 segment
- Coccyx
- Base of sacrum
- Sacral promontory
- Sacral arc
- Anterior sacral foramen
- Sacrococcygeal junction

Labels (posterior view, bottom):
- Superior articular facet
- Dorsal sacral foramen
- Sacral hiatus
- Median sacral crest
- Lateral sacral crest
- Sacral tuberosity
- Intermediate sacral crest
- Coccyx

(**Top**) *Graphic shows the anterior view of the sacrum. The sacral promontory is the upper aspect of the S1 segment. The sacral ala are the lateral "wings" of the sacrum. Note the residual structures of the vertebral bodies, including the disc remnants and neural foramina between each segment.* (**Bottom**) *Graphic shows the posterior view of the sacrum. The vestigial divisions of the vertebral bodies are not as readily appreciated as anteriorly. The medial sacral crest of the fused spinous processes, the intermediate sacral crest of the fused articular processes, and the lateral sacral crest of the fused transverse processes are all visible. The long and short dorsal sacroiliac ligaments attach to the lateral sacral crests. The incomplete fusion of the laminae in the lower sacrum creates the sacral hiatus. The hiatus is used as an access portal to the epidural space.*

Pelvis Overview

POSTERIOR PELVIS AND SACRAL PLEXUS

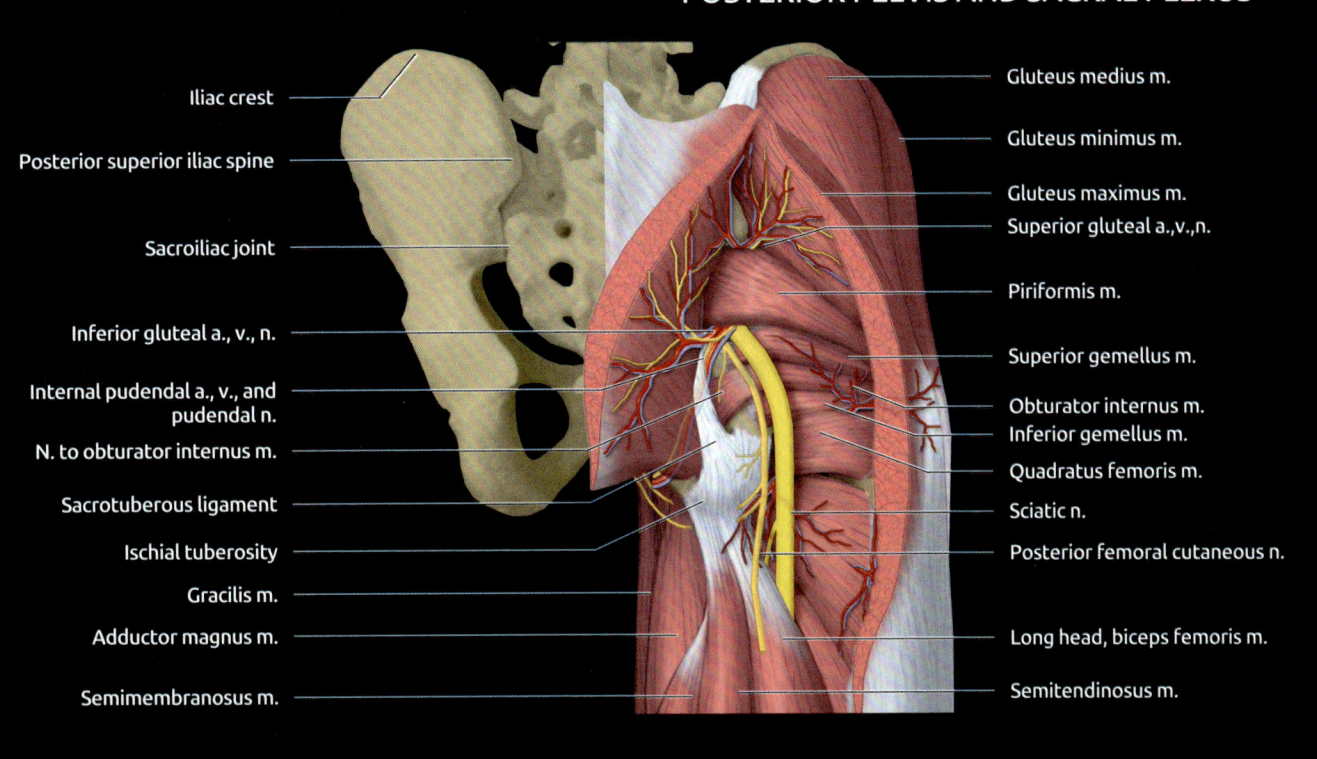

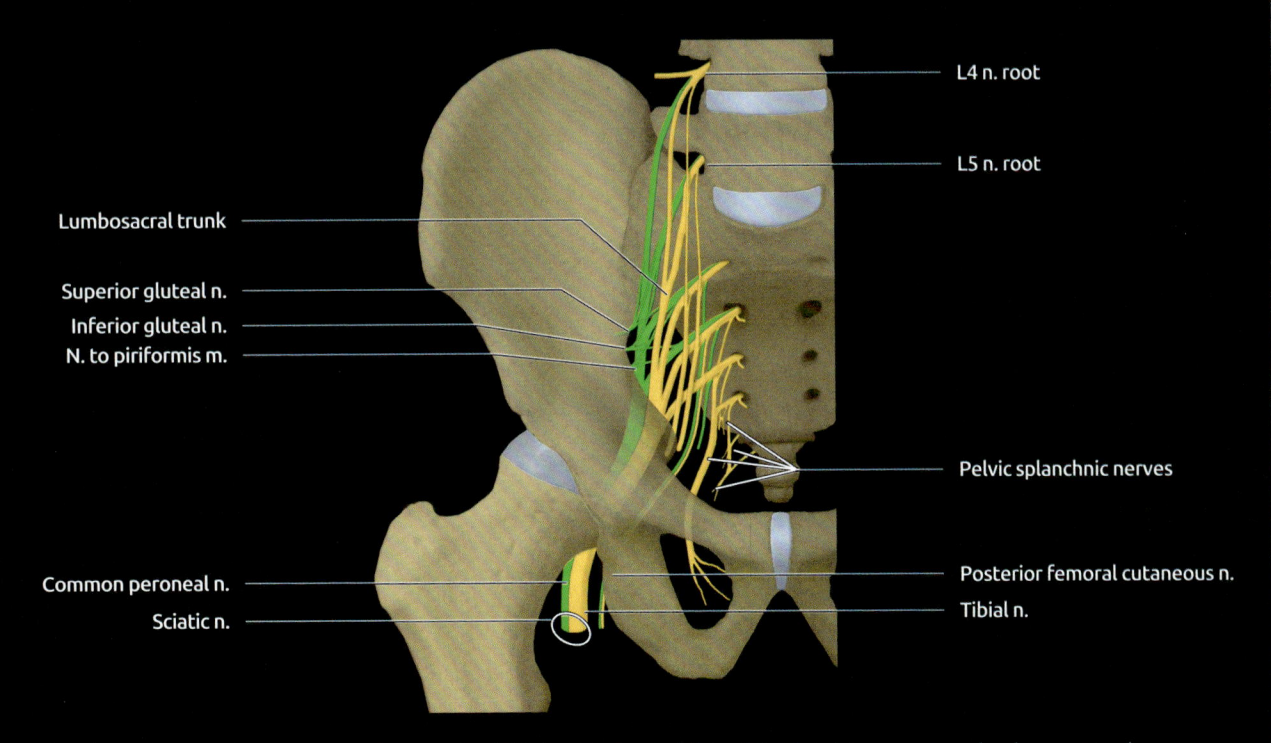

Labels (top image):
- Iliac crest
- Posterior superior iliac spine
- Sacroiliac joint
- Inferior gluteal a., v., n.
- Internal pudendal a., v., and pudendal n.
- N. to obturator internus m.
- Sacrotuberous ligament
- Ischial tuberosity
- Gracilis m.
- Adductor magnus m.
- Semimembranosus m.
- Gluteus medius m.
- Gluteus minimus m.
- Gluteus maximus m.
- Superior gluteal a., v., n.
- Piriformis m.
- Superior gemellus m.
- Obturator internus m.
- Inferior gemellus m.
- Quadratus femoris m.
- Sciatic n.
- Posterior femoral cutaneous n.
- Long head, biceps femoris m.
- Semitendinosus m.

Labels (bottom image):
- Lumbosacral trunk
- Superior gluteal n.
- Inferior gluteal n.
- N. to piriformis m.
- Common peroneal n.
- Sciatic n.
- L4 n. root
- L5 n. root
- Pelvic splanchnic nerves
- Posterior femoral cutaneous n.
- Tibial n.

(Top) Graphic shows the posterior structures of the proximal thigh at the level of the pelvis. The gluteus maximus has been cut to show the external rotators of the hip. The sciatic nerve emerges from the pelvis through the greater sciatic foramen and lies posterior to the external rotators. The pudendal nerve also exits the pelvis through the greater sciatic foramen but reenters it through the lesser sciatic foramen into the pudendal canal on the lateral wall of the ischioanal fossa. *(Bottom)* The sacral plexus lies anterior to the piriformis muscle. The anterior (yellow) and posterior (green) divisions of the respective nerves are denoted. The common peroneal nerve is a postaxial nerve and the tibial nerve is a preaxial nerve. The peroneal and tibial nerves travel together as the sciatic nerve but are clearly distinguishable on axial MR.

Pelvis MR Atlas

ANATOMY IMAGING ISSUES

Imaging Recommendations

- MR of pelvis should
  - Cover iliac crests to lesser trochanter
  - Include all musculature, not usually necessary to do skin-to-skin on all 3 planes
- Useful to evaluate entire pelvis even when hip MR is requested
  - Many centers perform screening coronal T1, STIR of entire pelvis
    - Hip pain is difficult to localize and full field-of-view pelvis images often show unsuspected pathology
  - Use torso coil or body coil
- Axial, sagittal images often performed on painful side only
  - Use surface coil
    - Ideal to have scanner where use torso coil for whole pelvis
    - Turn off torso coil and switch to hip coil for affected side
  - Allows higher resolution of area of greatest concern
  - Sagittal, axial, coronal, oblique axial planes

Imaging Pitfalls

- Nerves are often difficult to see
  - Use T1 or PD to locate nerve
  - Correlate with fluid-sensitive sequences
  - T1 or PD help distinguish fluid in vessels from nerve
  - Fat fascicles are especially prominent in sciatic nerve
    - Tibial and peroneal nerves are distinct from origin to bifurcation in popliteal fossa
- Muscles can be difficult to separate on any one plane
  - Cross checking between planes is useful
  - Utilize information regarding relative positions of muscles to accurately distinguish

Anatomic Spaces in Pelvis

- Horizontal division into true and false pelvis
- **False pelvis**: Iliac crest to pelvic brim
  - Part of abdominal cavity
- **True pelvis**: Pelvic brim to ischial tuberosity
- **Greater sciatic notch**
  - Concavity along inferior border of ilium between posteroinferior margin of ilium and ischial spine
  - Sacrospinous ligament along inferior border of notch converts notch to greater sciatic foramen
  - Much of foramen is occupied by piriformis muscle
  - Superior to piriformis muscle: Superior gluteal vessels and nerve
  - Inferior to piriformis muscle: Inferior gluteal vessels, internal pudendal vessels, sciatic nerve, posterior femoral cutaneous nerve, nerve to obturator internus, nerve to quadratus femoris muscle
- **Lesser sciatic notch**
  - Small notch anterior to ischial spine
  - Sacrospinous and sacrotuberous ligaments convert notch to lesser sciatic foramen
  - Contains obturator internus, nerve to obturator internus, internal pudendal vessels and nerve
- **Obturator ring/foramen**
  - Bony ring formed from pubic body, superior and inferior pubic rami, and ischium
  - Majority of foramen is covered by obturator membrane
  - Superior portion of foramen not covered by obturator membrane
    - Designated obturator canal
    - Obturator artery, vein, and nerve pass out of pelvis through obturator canal
  - Obturator internus muscle arises from internal margin of obturator ring and obturator membrane
  - Obturator externus muscle arises from external margin of obturator ring and obturator membrane
- **Inguinal canal**
  - Anterior: Lower border internal oblique muscle: External oblique aponeurosis and internal oblique muscle
  - Posterior wall: Transversalis fascia and conjoined tendon
  - Roof: Lower border internal oblique muscle
  - Floor
    - Lateral portion: Iliopubic tract
    - Midportion: Inguinal ligament
    - Medial: Lacunar ligament
  - Entrance: Deep inguinal ring
    - Located midinguinal ligament
    - Opening of transversalis fascia
  - Exit: Superficial inguinal ring
    - Division of external oblique aponeurosis lateral to pubic tubercle
    - Lateral crus: Inserts pubic tubercle
    - Medial crus: Inserts pubic crest
    - Intercrural fibers: Superficial to canal; run medial crus to lateral crus
  - Contains: Ilioinguinal nerve, spermatic cord (males) or round ligament (females), associated vessels
- **Subinguinal space**
  - Deep to inguinal ligament
  - Contains femoral vessels and nerve, iliopsoas muscle
  - Dividing point between femoral (caudal to ligament) and external iliac vessels (cephalad to ligament)

CLINICAL IMPLICATIONS

Clinical Importance

- Pelvis is bridge from torso to lower extremity
- Problems in lumbar spine often misdiagnosed as pelvic and vice versa
- Be careful to include lumbar spine and abdominal wall in search pattern when reviewing pelvic MR
- SI joint abnormalities may present as back or hip pain
  - Arthritis involves synovial portion
    - Primarily inferior portion of joint
    - Small synovial extension to anterosuperior joint
  - Sacroiliac joints completely unstable when trauma disrupts
    - Often also see disruption of iliolumbar ligament
- Sciatica may be due to piriformis syndrome rather than intervertebral disc abnormality
  - Sciatic nerve takes abnormal course through piriformis muscle
  - Piriformis muscle may have duplicated muscle belly
  - Signal intensity of piriformis muscle is almost always normal in this syndrome

Pelvis MR Atlas

AXIAL T1 MR, UPPER PELVIS

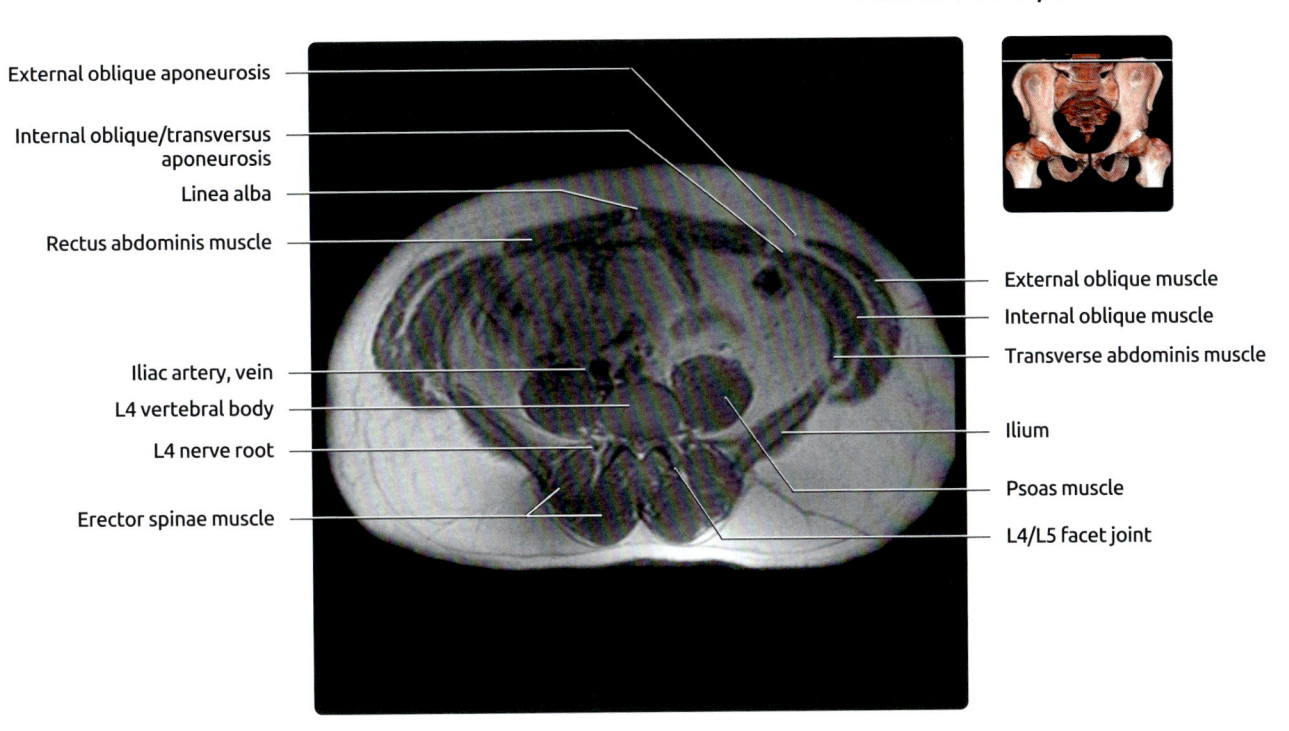

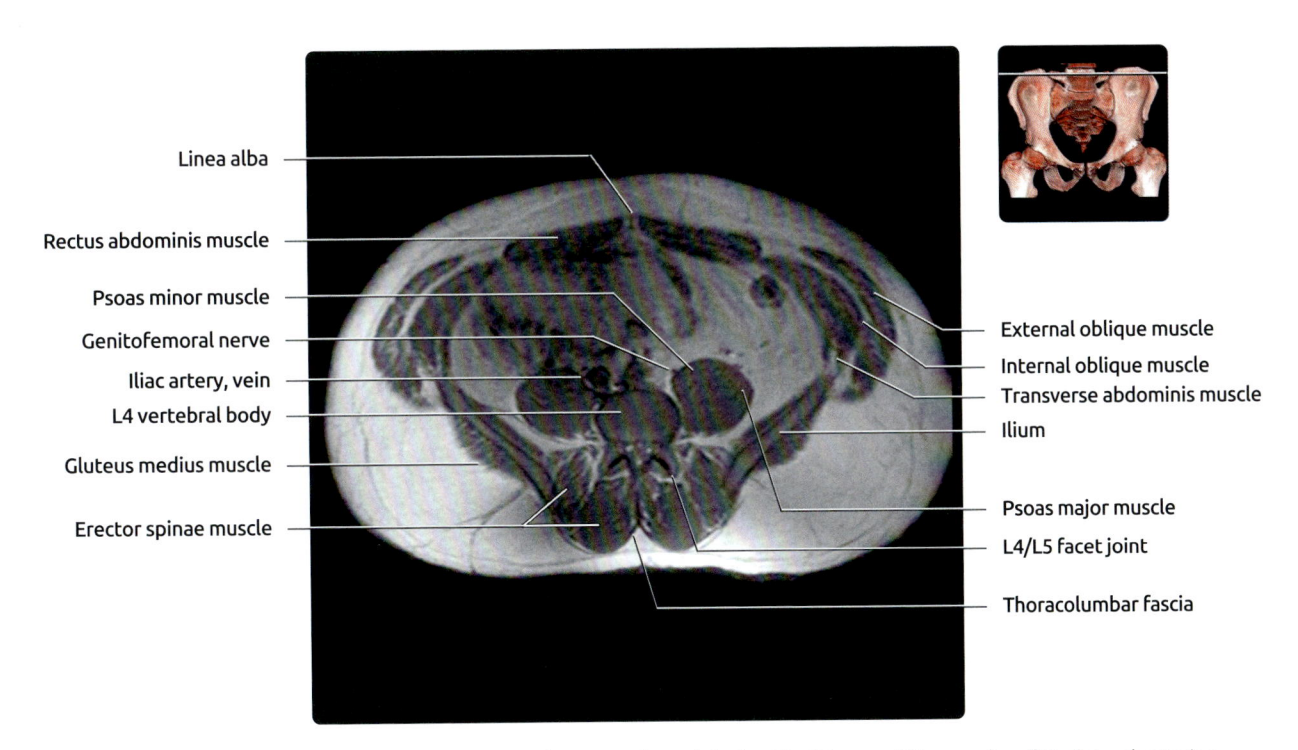

Top image labels:
- External oblique aponeurosis
- Internal oblique/transversus aponeurosis
- Linea alba
- Rectus abdominis muscle
- Iliac artery, vein
- L4 vertebral body
- L4 nerve root
- Erector spinae muscle
- External oblique muscle
- Internal oblique muscle
- Transverse abdominis muscle
- Ilium
- Psoas muscle
- L4/L5 facet joint

Bottom image labels:
- Linea alba
- Rectus abdominis muscle
- Psoas minor muscle
- Genitofemoral nerve
- Iliac artery, vein
- L4 vertebral body
- Gluteus medius muscle
- Erector spinae muscle
- External oblique muscle
- Internal oblique muscle
- Transverse abdominis muscle
- Ilium
- Psoas major muscle
- L4/L5 facet joint
- Thoracolumbar fascia

(Top) First in a series of 34 axial images of the pelvis, shown from superior to inferior. The 3 layers of the muscles of the lateral anterior abdominal wall are clearly visible. The psoas muscle courses inferiorly from its multifaceted spinal origin. The superior most aspect of the iliac crest corresponds to the L4/L5 intervertebral disc space. **(Bottom)** The aorta has just bifurcated. The paired rectus abdominis muscles in the center of the abdomen are joined by the dense fibrous band known as the linea alba.

Pelvis MR Atlas

AXIAL T1 MR, UPPER PELVIS

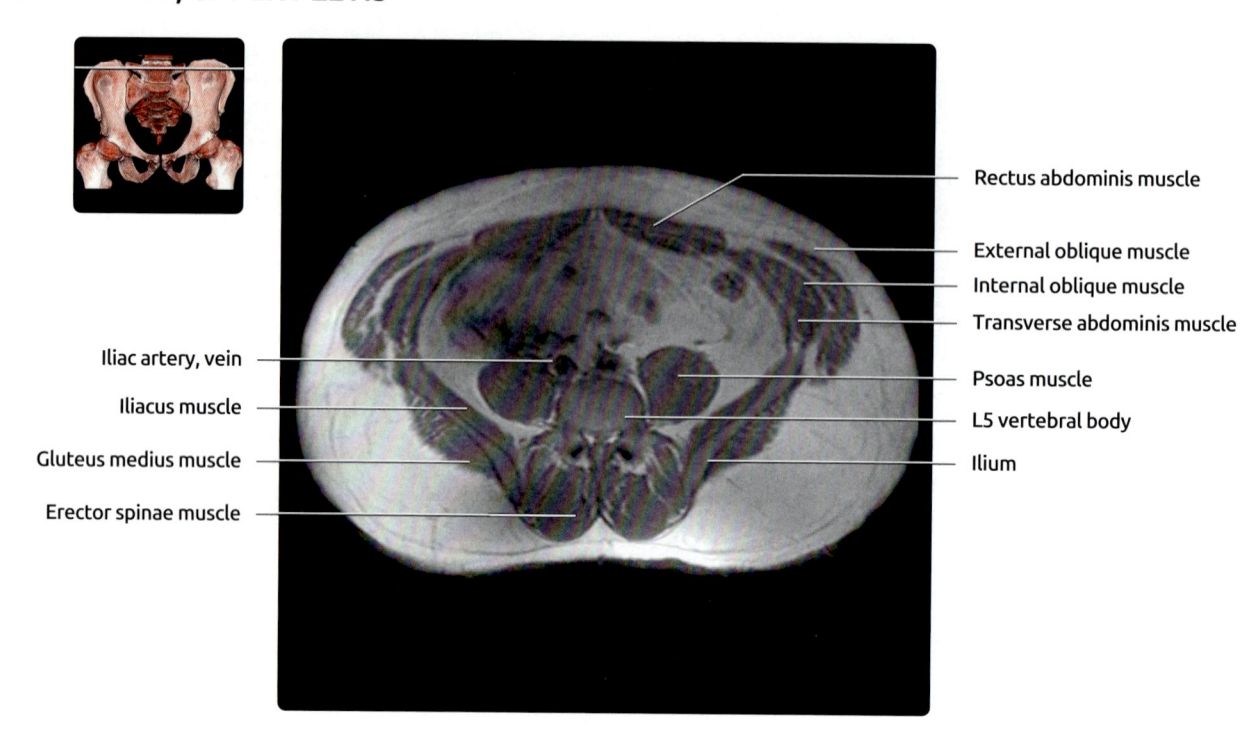

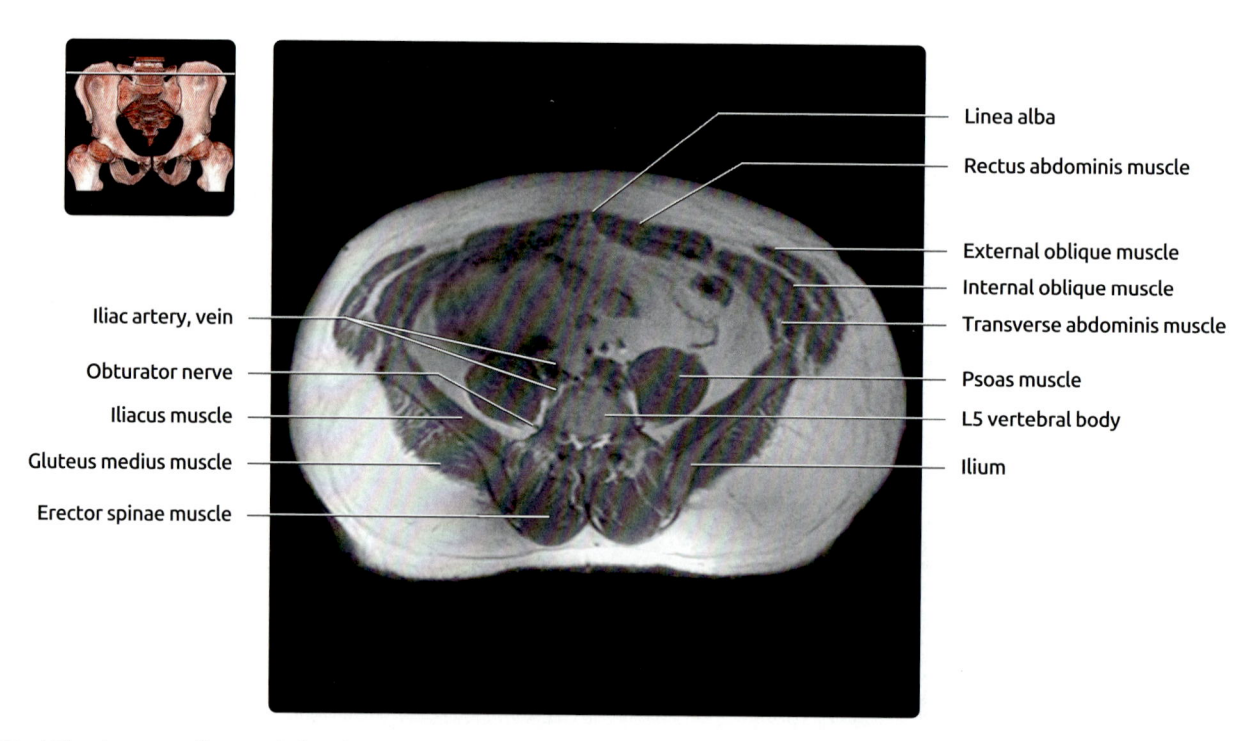

Labels (top image):
- Rectus abdominis muscle
- External oblique muscle
- Internal oblique muscle
- Transverse abdominis muscle
- Psoas muscle
- L5 vertebral body
- Ilium
- Iliac artery, vein
- Iliacus muscle
- Gluteus medius muscle
- Erector spinae muscle

Labels (bottom image):
- Linea alba
- Rectus abdominis muscle
- External oblique muscle
- Internal oblique muscle
- Transverse abdominis muscle
- Psoas muscle
- L5 vertebral body
- Ilium
- Iliac artery, vein
- Obturator nerve
- Iliacus muscle
- Gluteus medius muscle
- Erector spinae muscle

(Top) The gluteus medius muscle has the most superior origin of the gluteus muscles. The erector spinae muscles are a paired longitudinal muscle complex along the posterior aspect of the spine. **(Bottom)** The iliacus muscle has a broad origin from the deep surface of the ilium. The iliac artery and vein lie on the medial border of the psoas muscle with the artery anterior to the vein. Obturator nerve is medial to the psoas muscle at the pelvic brim.

Pelvis MR Atlas

AXIAL T1 MR, UPPER PELVIS

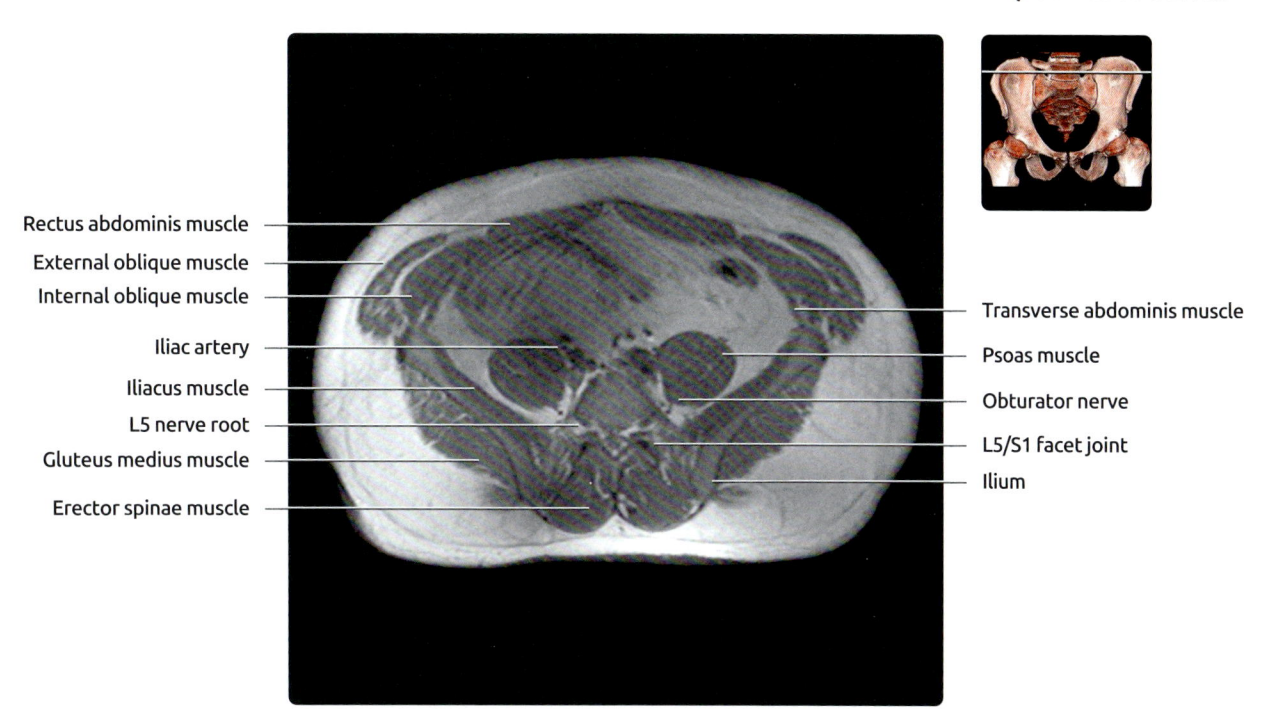

Top image labels (left):
- Rectus abdominis muscle
- External oblique muscle
- Internal oblique muscle
- Iliac artery
- Iliacus muscle
- L5 nerve root
- Gluteus medius muscle
- Erector spinae muscle

Top image labels (right):
- Transverse abdominis muscle
- Psoas muscle
- Obturator nerve
- L5/S1 facet joint
- Ilium

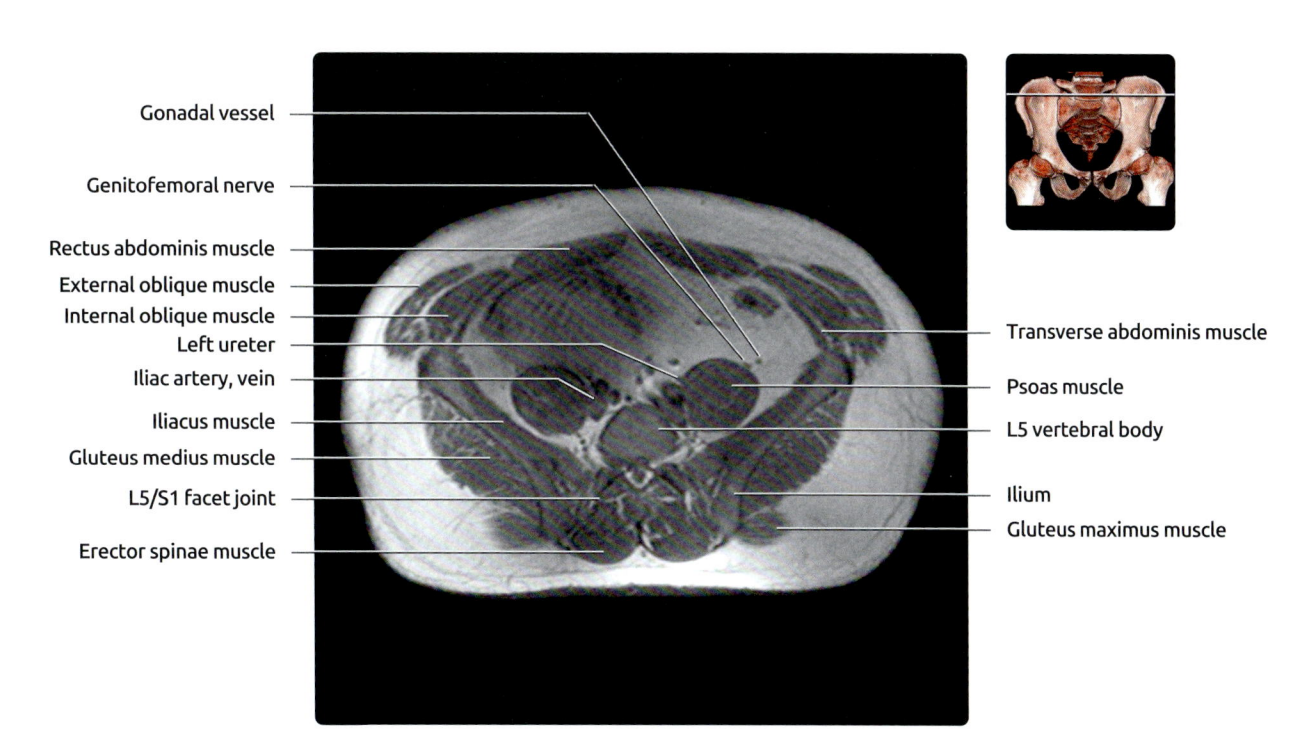

Bottom image labels (left):
- Gonadal vessel
- Genitofemoral nerve
- Rectus abdominis muscle
- External oblique muscle
- Internal oblique muscle
- Left ureter
- Iliac artery, vein
- Iliacus muscle
- Gluteus medius muscle
- L5/S1 facet joint
- Erector spinae muscle

Bottom image labels (right):
- Transverse abdominis muscle
- Psoas muscle
- L5 vertebral body
- Ilium
- Gluteus maximus muscle

(**Top**) *The L5 nerve root exits the neural foramina. The iliac vessels course along the medial aspect of the psoas muscle. Note that the iliacus and psoas remain separate through the majority of their pelvic course.* (**Bottom**) *The gluteus maximus muscle originates from the external surface of the ilium posterior to the gluteus medius muscle.*

AXIAL T1 MR, UPPER PELVIS

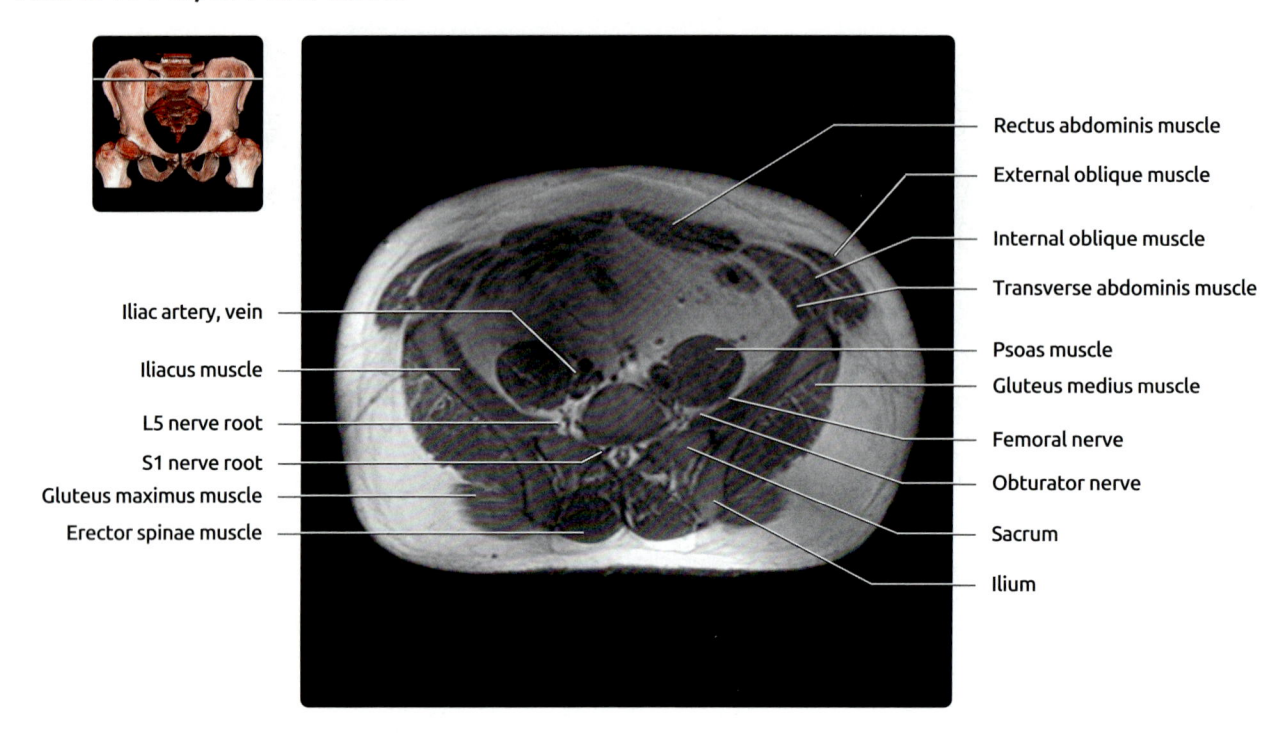

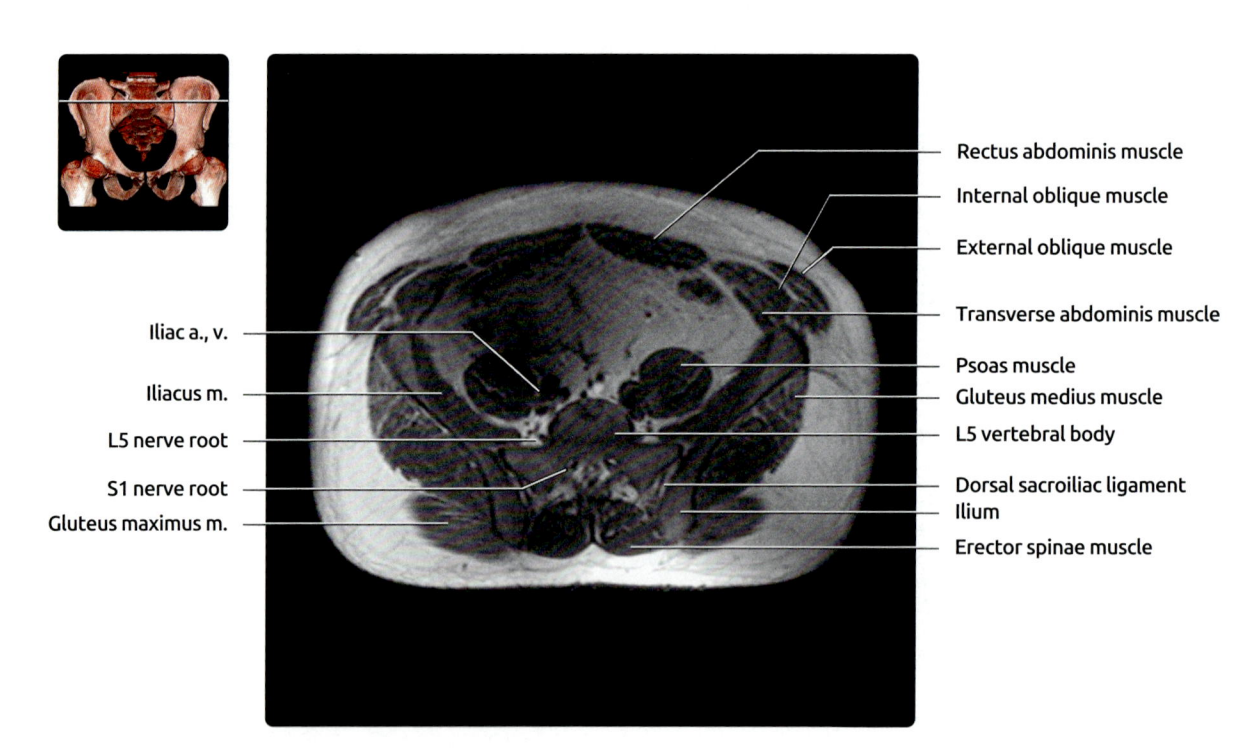

Labels (top image):
- Iliac artery, vein
- Iliacus muscle
- L5 nerve root
- S1 nerve root
- Gluteus maximus muscle
- Erector spinae muscle
- Rectus abdominis muscle
- External oblique muscle
- Internal oblique muscle
- Transverse abdominis muscle
- Psoas muscle
- Gluteus medius muscle
- Femoral nerve
- Obturator nerve
- Sacrum
- Ilium

Labels (bottom image):
- Iliac a., v.
- Iliacus m.
- L5 nerve root
- S1 nerve root
- Gluteus maximus m.
- Rectus abdominis muscle
- Internal oblique muscle
- External oblique muscle
- Transverse abdominis muscle
- Psoas muscle
- Gluteus medius muscle
- L5 vertebral body
- Dorsal sacroiliac ligament
- Ilium
- Erector spinae muscle

(Top) The femoral nerve runs in the iliopsoas notch. The obturator nerve is posterior to the psoas muscle. The transverse abdominis and internal oblique muscles share a conjoined tendon/aponeurosis. The external oblique muscle is a more distinct muscle. **(Bottom)** Note the course of the L5 nerve root along the anterior aspect of the sacrum. The sacroiliac articulation is ligamentous at this level.

Pelvis MR Atlas

AXIAL T1 MR, UPPER PELVIS

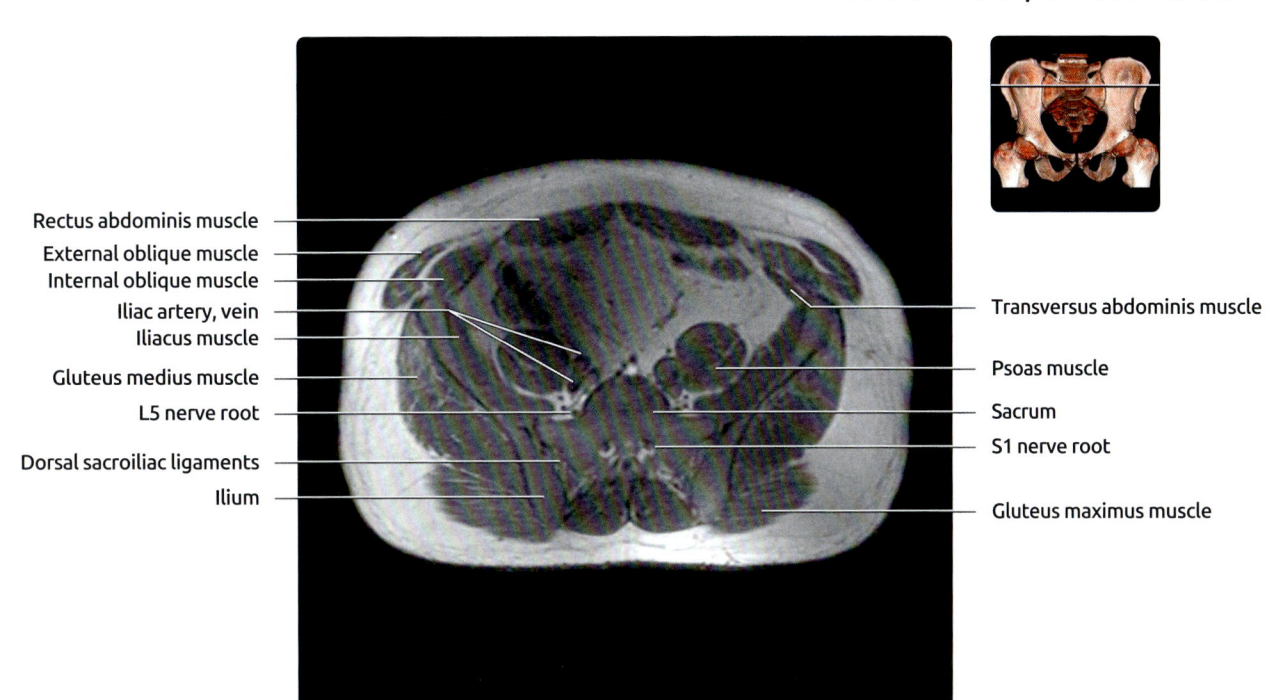

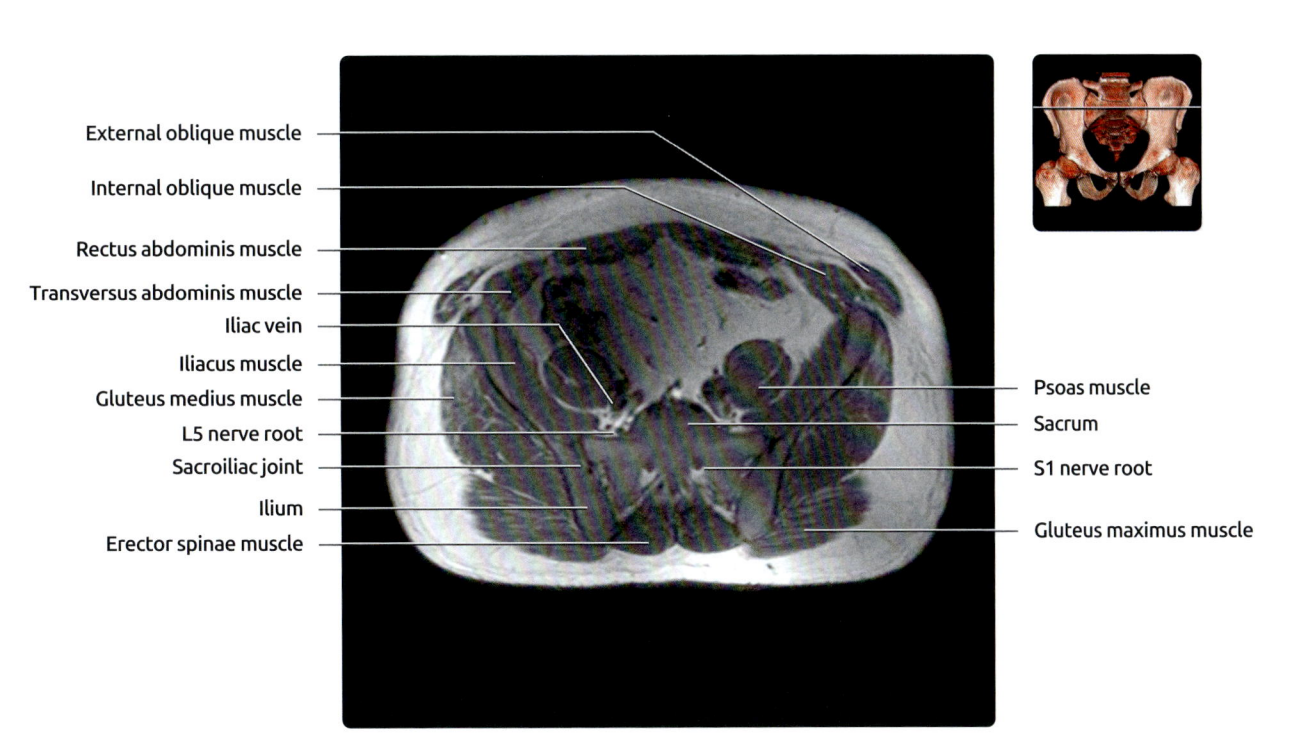

Labels (top image):
- Rectus abdominis muscle
- External oblique muscle
- Internal oblique muscle
- Iliac artery, vein
- Iliacus muscle
- Gluteus medius muscle
- L5 nerve root
- Dorsal sacroiliac ligaments
- Ilium
- Transversus abdominis muscle
- Psoas muscle
- Sacrum
- S1 nerve root
- Gluteus maximus muscle

Labels (bottom image):
- External oblique muscle
- Internal oblique muscle
- Rectus abdominis muscle
- Transversus abdominis muscle
- Iliac vein
- Iliacus muscle
- Gluteus medius muscle
- L5 nerve root
- Sacroiliac joint
- Ilium
- Erector spinae muscle
- Psoas muscle
- Sacrum
- S1 nerve root
- Gluteus maximus muscle

(Top) *The gluteus maximus has an inferior and lateral course. At its superior aspect only a small portion of the muscle is visible.*
(Bottom) *The erector spinae muscle complex diminishes in size as they near their inferior extent.*

Pelvis MR Atlas

AXIAL T1 MR, UPPER PELVIS

Labels (top image):
- Rectus abdominis muscle
- Inferior epigastric vein
- External oblique aponeurosis
- External oblique muscle
- Internal oblique muscle
- Genitofemoral nerve
- Femoral nerve
- Synovial portion sacroiliac joint
- Dorsal sacroiliac ligament
- Gluteus maximus muscle
- Iliacus muscle
- Gluteus minimus muscle
- Iliac vessels
- Gluteus medius muscle
- Sacroiliac joint
- S2 nerve root

Labels (bottom image):
- Rectus abdominis muscle
- External oblique aponeurosis
- Internal oblique muscle
- Transversus abdominis muscle
- External oblique muscle
- Genitofemoral nerve
- Left ureter
- Femoral nerve
- Psoas muscle
- Sacrum
- S1 nerve root
- Ilium
- Gluteus maximus muscle
- Anterior superior iliac spine
- Iliacus muscle
- Gluteus minimus muscle
- Gluteus medius muscle
- Sacroiliac joint
- Erector spinae muscle

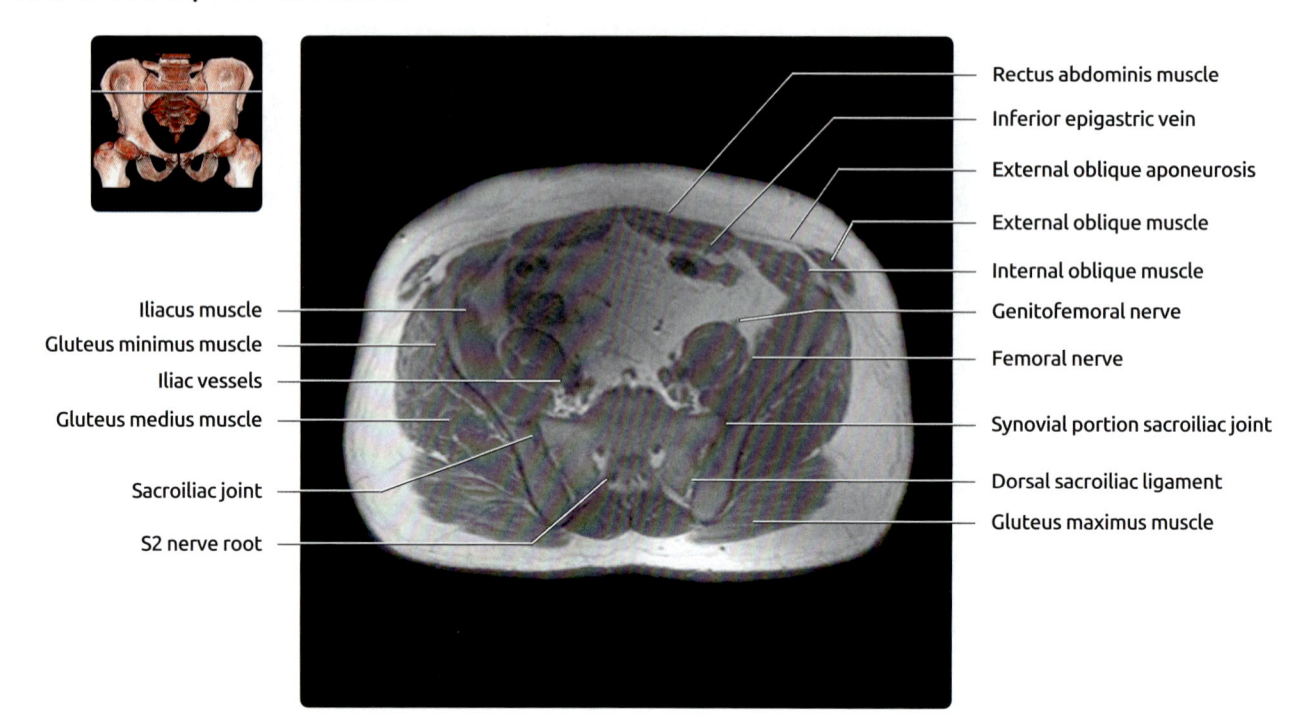

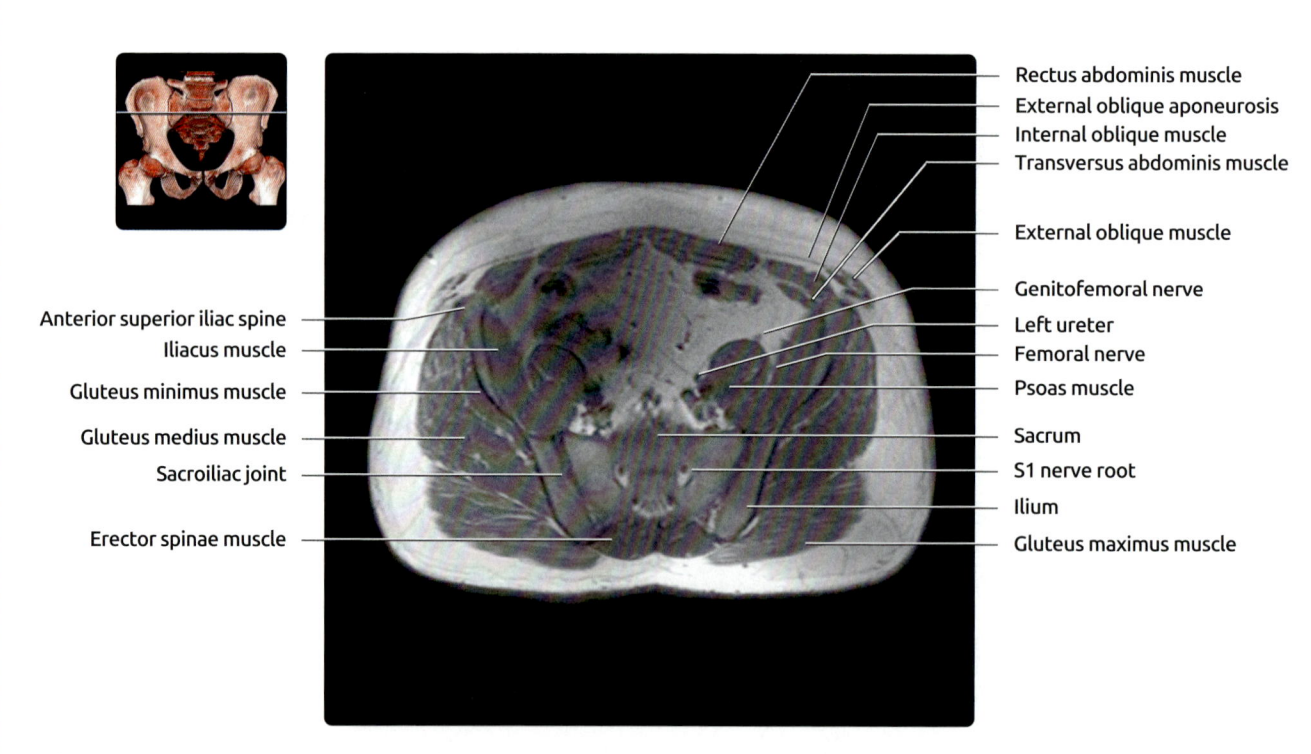

(Top) The S2 nerve root is now apparent. There is a small anterior synovial sacroiliac joint at this level, but the majority of the articulation is composed of strong dorsal ligaments. **(Bottom)** Gluteus minimus muscle has the most anterior origin of the gluteal muscles. The anterior superior iliac spine is seen as a bulbous enlargement from the anterior aspect of the ilium. It serves as the site of origin of sartorius muscle and inguinal ligament. The ligament is the inferior edge of the external oblique aponeurosis.

AXIAL T1 MR, MID PELVIS

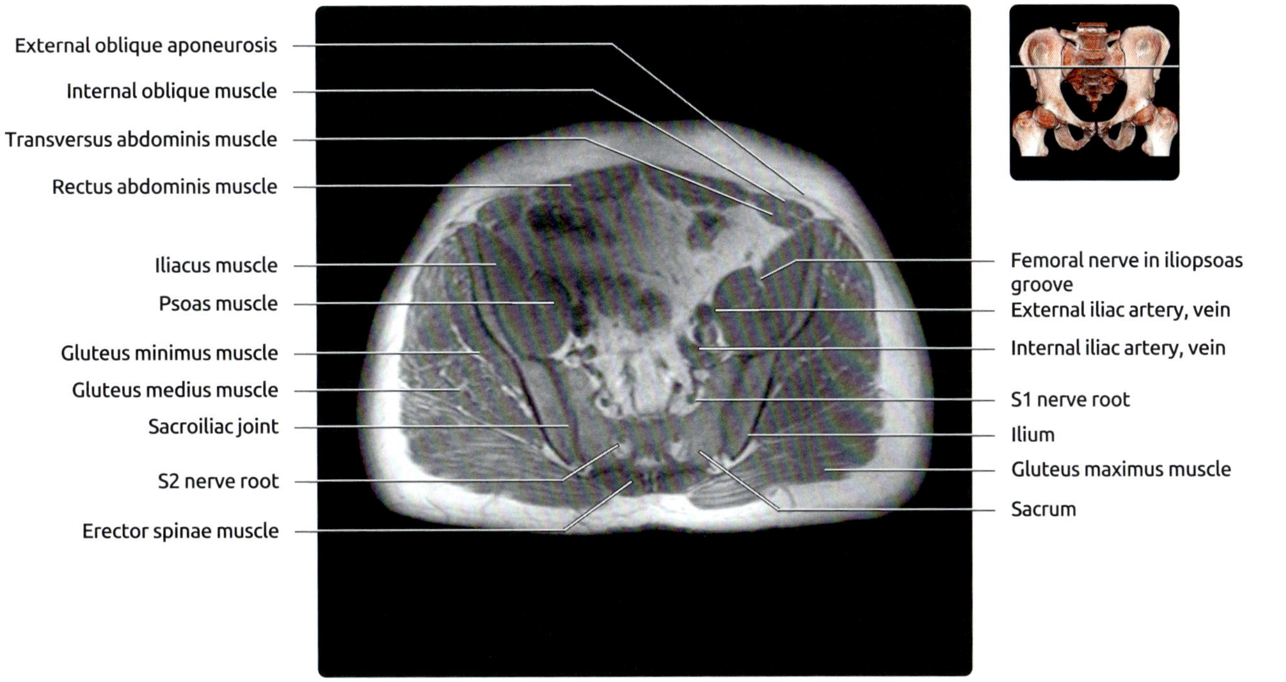
External oblique aponeurosis
Internal oblique muscle
Transversus abdominis muscle
Rectus abdominis muscle
Iliacus muscle
Psoas muscle
Gluteus minimus muscle
Gluteus medius muscle
Sacroiliac joint
S2 nerve root
Erector spinae muscle
Femoral nerve in iliopsoas groove
External iliac artery, vein
Internal iliac artery, vein
S1 nerve root
Ilium
Gluteus maximus muscle
Sacrum

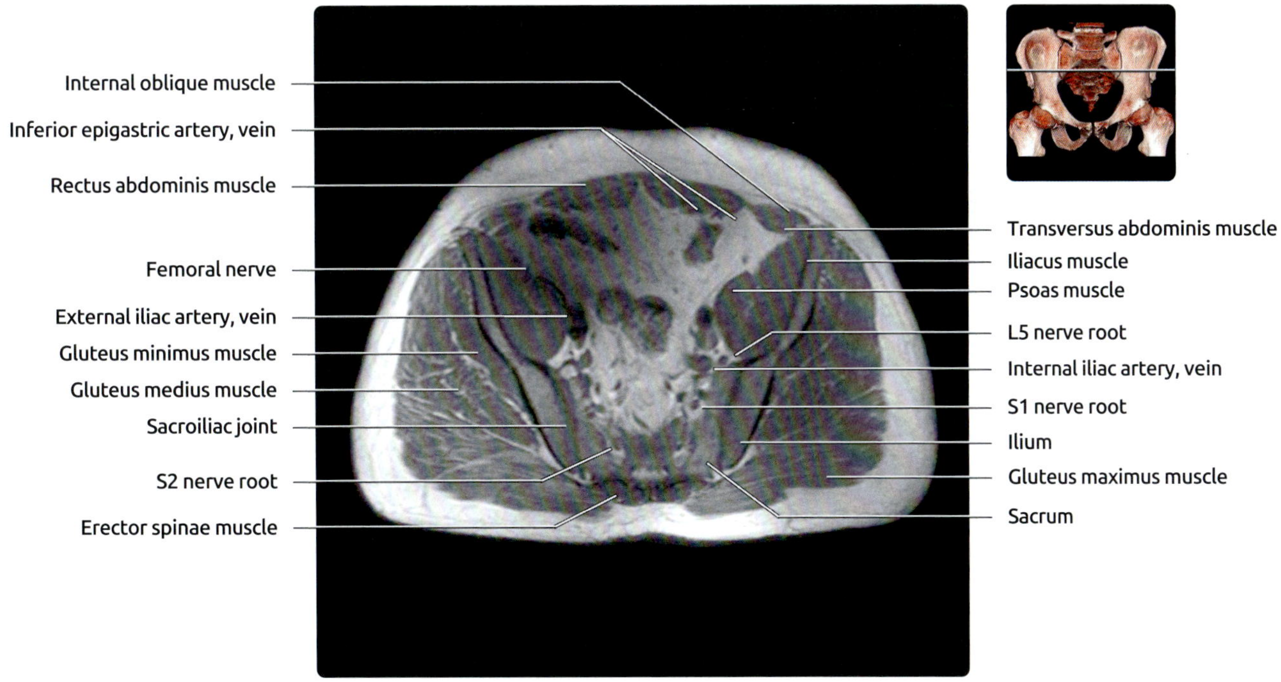
Internal oblique muscle
Inferior epigastric artery, vein
Rectus abdominis muscle
Femoral nerve
External iliac artery, vein
Gluteus minimus muscle
Gluteus medius muscle
Sacroiliac joint
S2 nerve root
Erector spinae muscle
Transversus abdominis muscle
Iliacus muscle
Psoas muscle
L5 nerve root
Internal iliac artery, vein
S1 nerve root
Ilium
Gluteus maximus muscle
Sacrum

(Top) *The S1 nerve roots have exited their foramina and are coursing inferolaterally, while S2 nerve roots still lie within their foramina.* **(Bottom)** *The iliacus and psoas muscles are becoming more tightly apposed, but retain a shallow anterior notch between them that contains the femoral nerve.*

Pelvis MR Atlas

AXIAL T1 MR, MID PELVIS

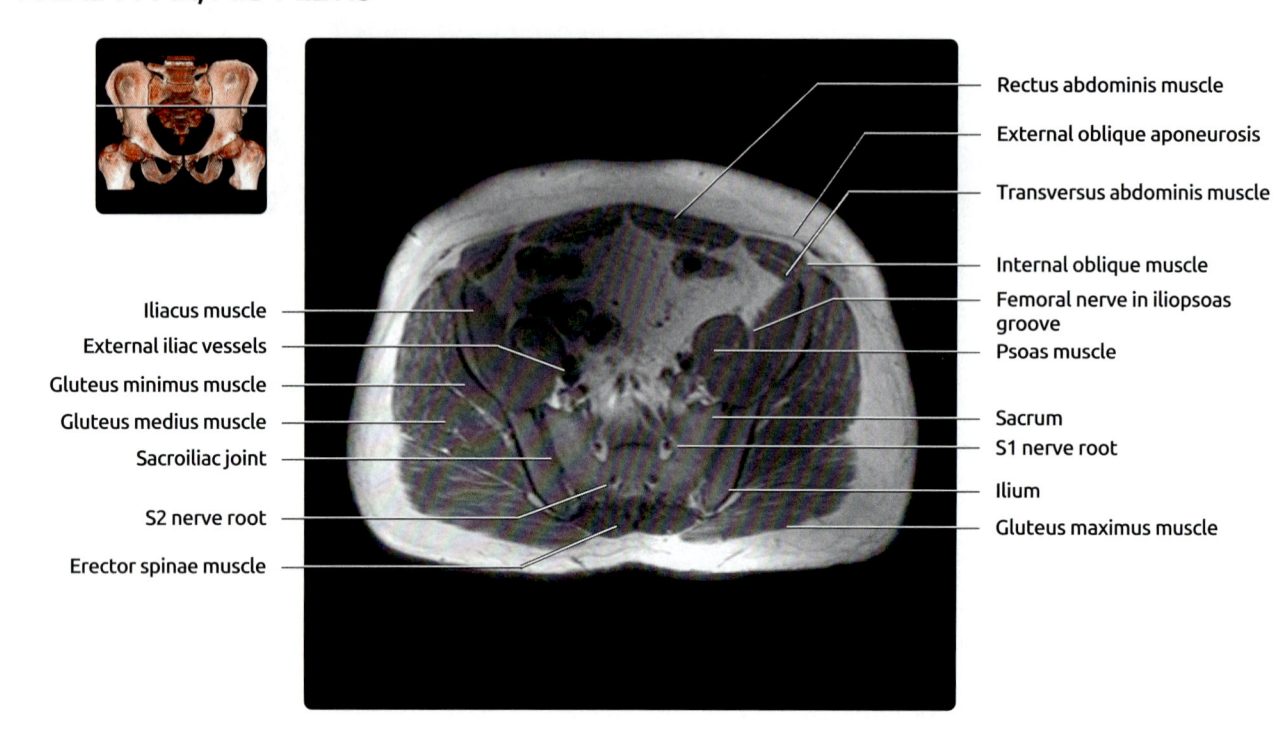

Top image labels:
- Rectus abdominis muscle
- External oblique aponeurosis
- Transversus abdominis muscle
- Internal oblique muscle
- Femoral nerve in iliopsoas groove
- Psoas muscle
- Sacrum
- S1 nerve root
- Ilium
- Gluteus maximus muscle
- Iliacus muscle
- External iliac vessels
- Gluteus minimus muscle
- Gluteus medius muscle
- Sacroiliac joint
- S2 nerve root
- Erector spinae muscle

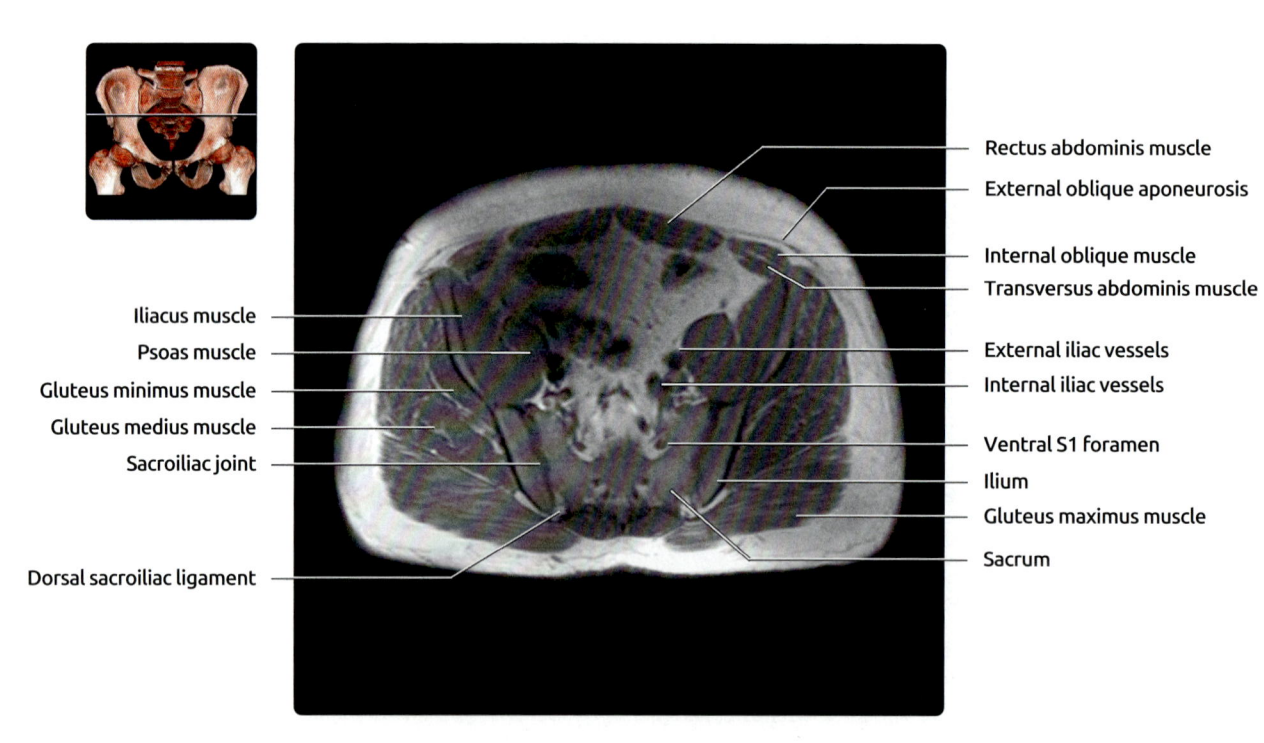

Bottom image labels:
- Rectus abdominis muscle
- External oblique aponeurosis
- Internal oblique muscle
- Transversus abdominis muscle
- External iliac vessels
- Internal iliac vessels
- Ventral S1 foramen
- Ilium
- Gluteus maximus muscle
- Sacrum
- Iliacus muscle
- Psoas muscle
- Gluteus minimus muscle
- Gluteus medius muscle
- Sacroiliac joint
- Dorsal sacroiliac ligament

(Top) The iliacus and psoas are now apposed but retain a well-defined iliopsoas groove between them, in which the femoral nerve courses. **(Bottom)** The iliac vessels have bifurcated. The internal iliac vessels will course posteriorly as they traverse the pelvis. The sacroiliac joint is primarily synovial at this more inferior level. Dorsal sacroiliac ligaments are visible posterior to the synovial joint and are important stabilizers of the pelvis.

Pelvis MR Atlas

AXIAL T1 MR, MID PELVIS

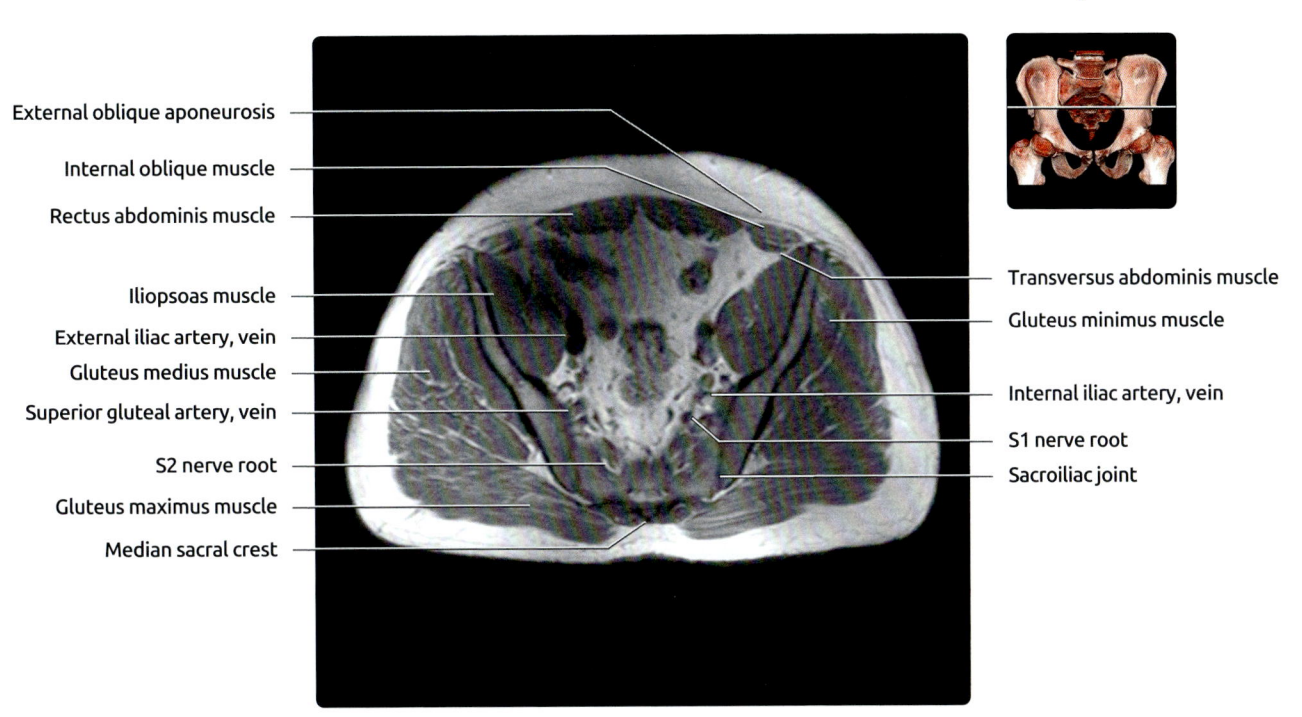

Top image labels (left side):
- External oblique aponeurosis
- Internal oblique muscle
- Rectus abdominis muscle
- Iliopsoas muscle
- External iliac artery, vein
- Gluteus medius muscle
- Superior gluteal artery, vein
- S2 nerve root
- Gluteus maximus muscle
- Median sacral crest

Top image labels (right side):
- Transversus abdominis muscle
- Gluteus minimus muscle
- Internal iliac artery, vein
- S1 nerve root
- Sacroiliac joint

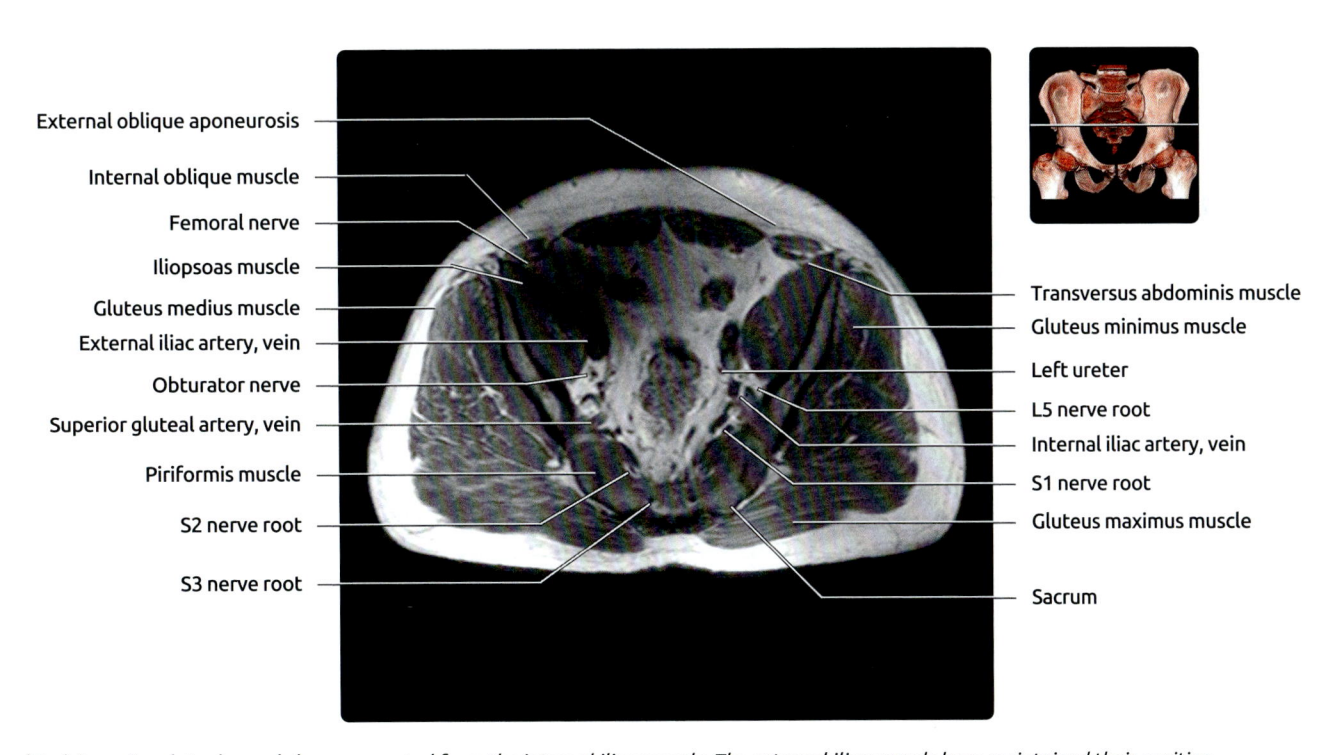

Bottom image labels (left side):
- External oblique aponeurosis
- Internal oblique muscle
- Femoral nerve
- Iliopsoas muscle
- Gluteus medius muscle
- External iliac artery, vein
- Obturator nerve
- Superior gluteal artery, vein
- Piriformis muscle
- S2 nerve root
- S3 nerve root

Bottom image labels (right side):
- Transversus abdominis muscle
- Gluteus minimus muscle
- Left ureter
- L5 nerve root
- Internal iliac artery, vein
- S1 nerve root
- Gluteus maximus muscle
- Sacrum

(Top) Superior gluteal vessels have separated from the internal iliac vessels. The external iliac vessels have maintained their position along the medial aspect of the psoas muscle. The iliacus and psoas remain distinct to their insertions but are often called the iliopsoas muscle from this point inferiorly. **(Bottom)** The obturator nerve is visible along the medial border of the psoas muscle posterior to the external iliac vessels.

AXIAL T1 MR, MID PELVIS

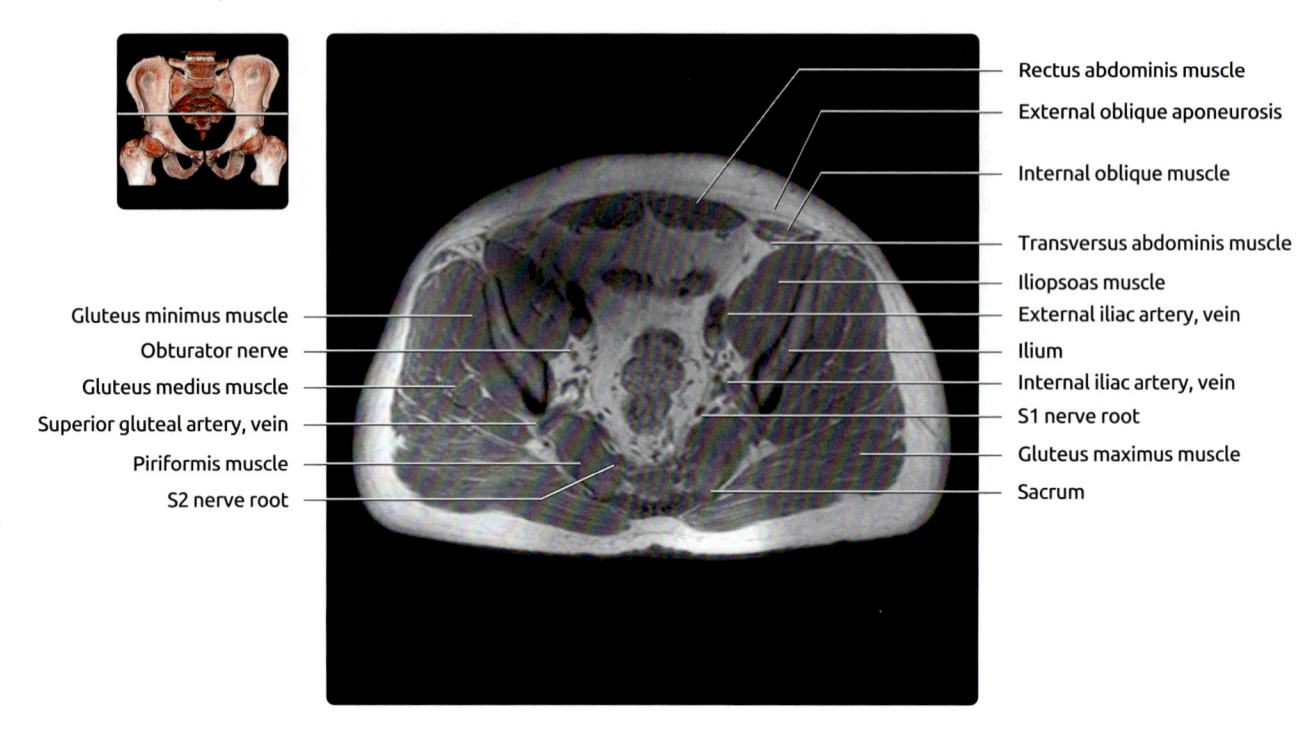

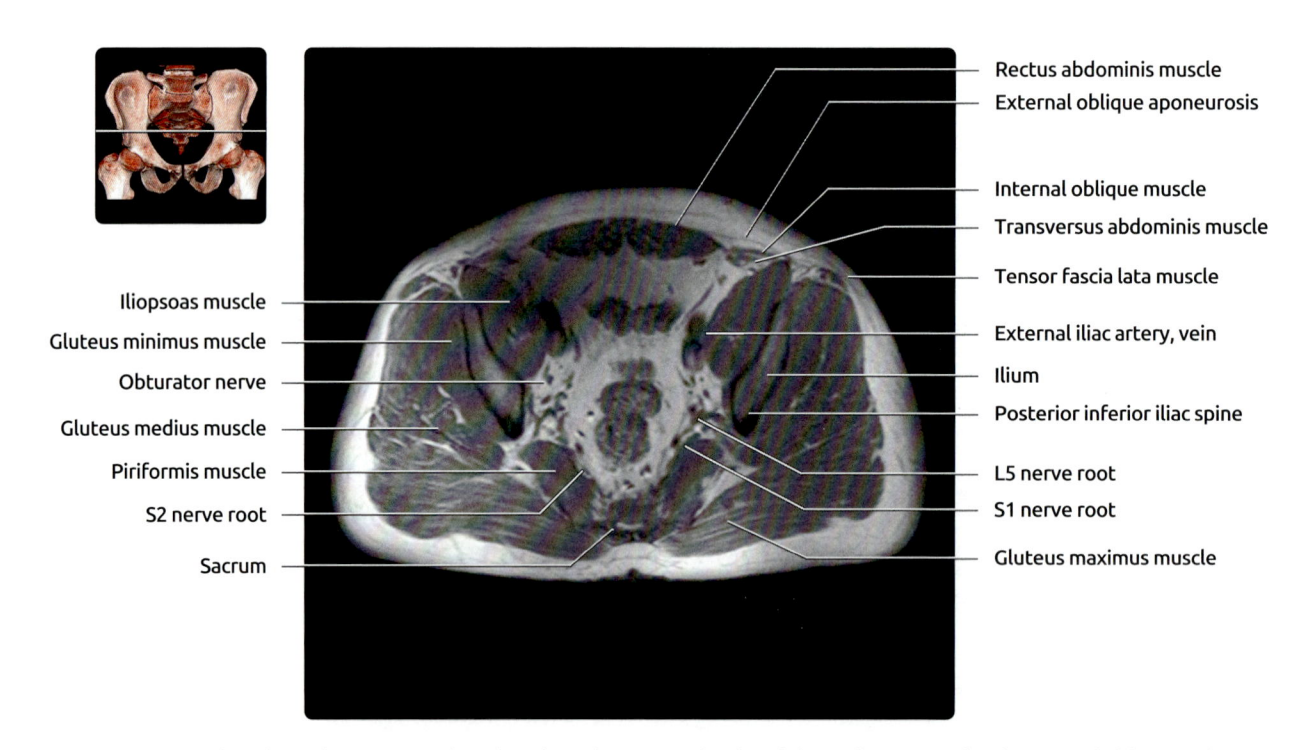

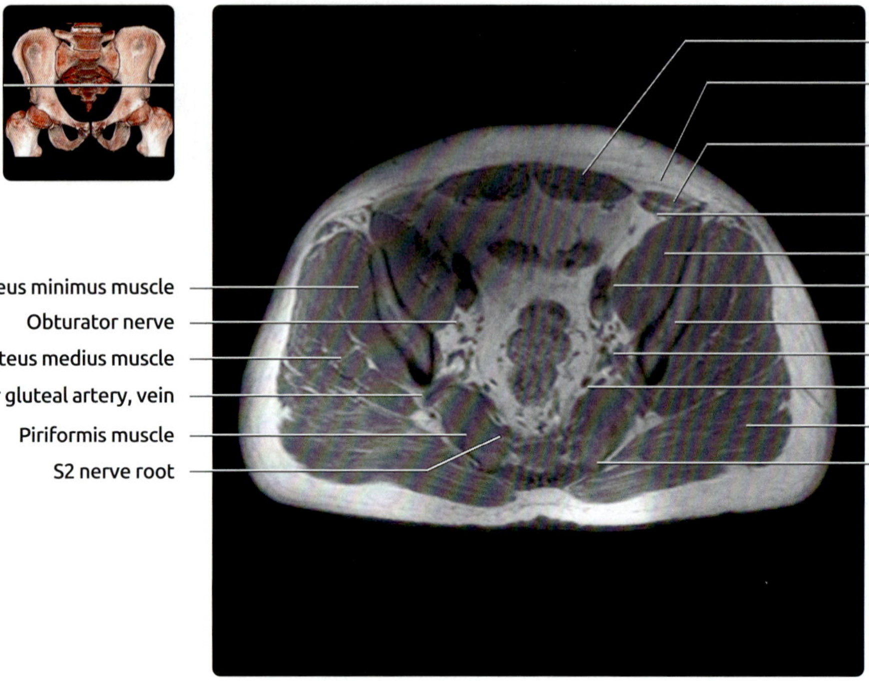
Rectus abdominis muscle
External oblique aponeurosis
Internal oblique muscle
Transversus abdominis muscle
Iliopsoas muscle
External iliac artery, vein
Ilium
Internal iliac artery, vein
S1 nerve root
Gluteus maximus muscle
Sacrum
Gluteus minimus muscle
Obturator nerve
Gluteus medius muscle
Superior gluteal artery, vein
Piriformis muscle
S2 nerve root

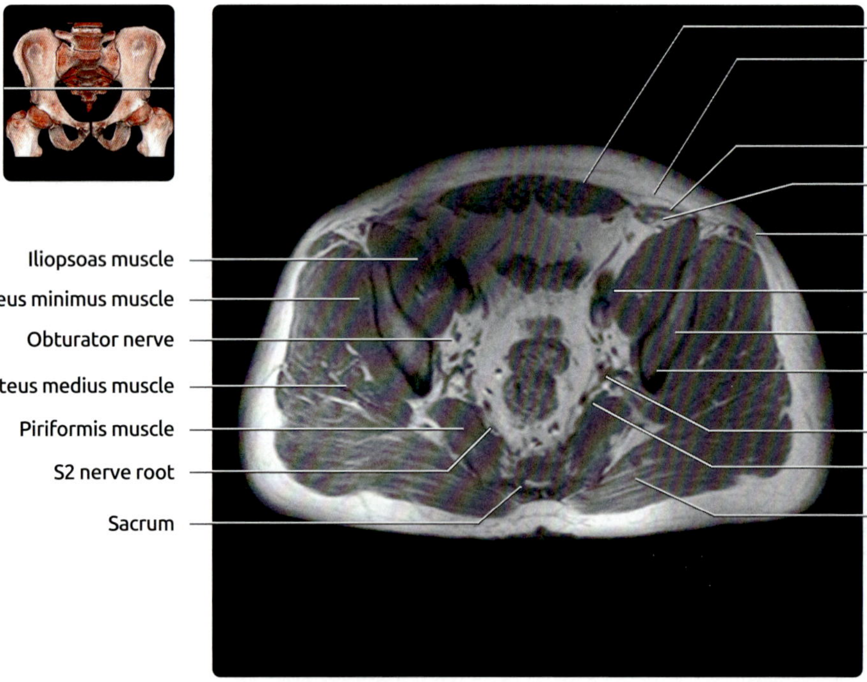
Rectus abdominis muscle
External oblique aponeurosis
Internal oblique muscle
Transversus abdominis muscle
Tensor fascia lata muscle
External iliac artery, vein
Ilium
Posterior inferior iliac spine
L5 nerve root
S1 nerve root
Gluteus maximus muscle
Iliopsoas muscle
Gluteus minimus muscle
Obturator nerve
Gluteus medius muscle
Piriformis muscle
S2 nerve root
Sacrum

(Top) *The superior gluteal vessels are exiting the pelvis along the superior border of the piriformis muscle. The internal oblique and transverse abdominis muscles are now more medially located than in more superior images. This position is consistent with their medial and inferior course.* **(Bottom)** *Muscle fibers of the tensor fascia lata are now visible. The posterior inferior iliac spine marks the superior anterior margin of the greater sciatic notch.*

AXIAL T1 MR, MID PELVIS

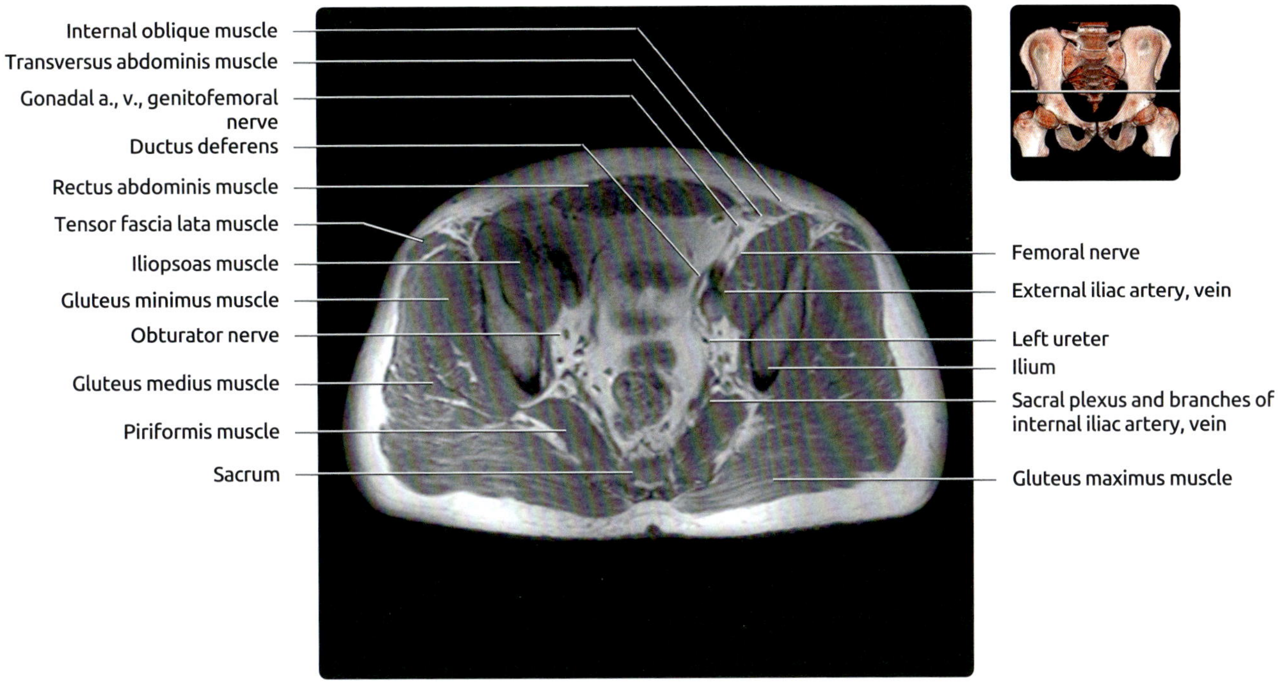
Internal oblique muscle
Transversus abdominis muscle
Gonadal a., v., genitofemoral nerve
Ductus deferens
Rectus abdominis muscle
Tensor fascia lata muscle
Iliopsoas muscle
Gluteus minimus muscle
Obturator nerve
Gluteus medius muscle
Piriformis muscle
Sacrum
Femoral nerve
External iliac artery, vein
Left ureter
Ilium
Sacral plexus and branches of internal iliac artery, vein
Gluteus maximus muscle

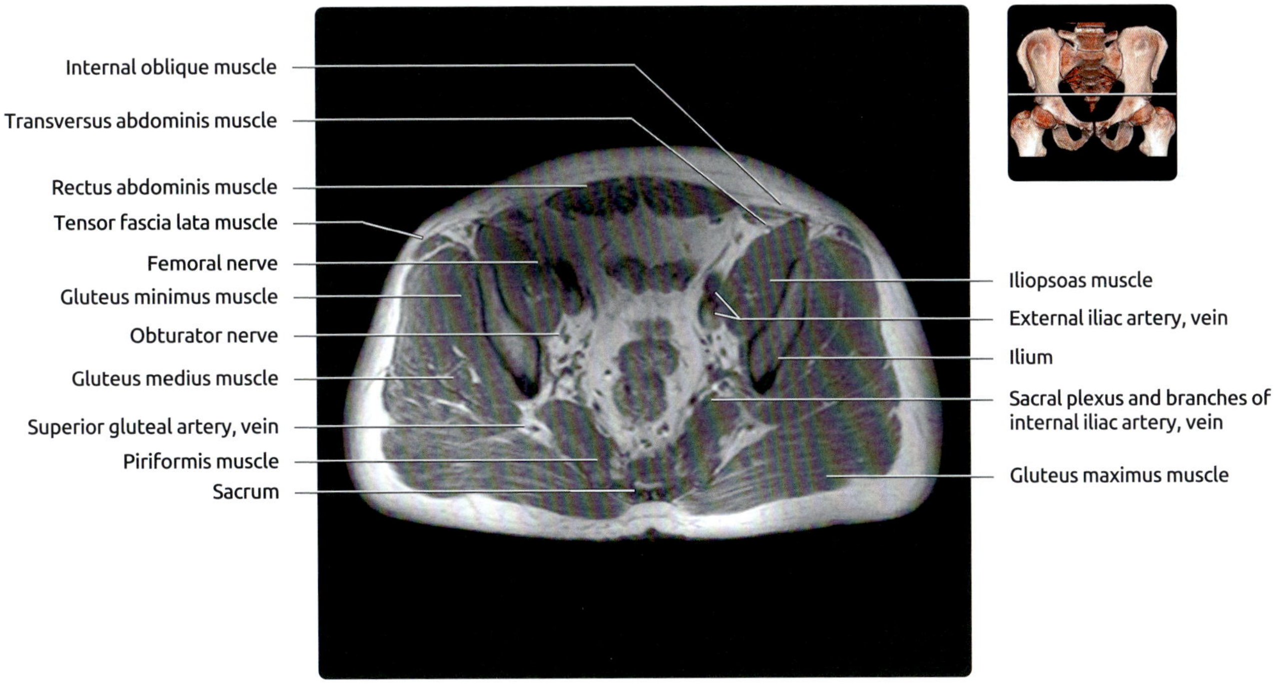
Internal oblique muscle
Transversus abdominis muscle
Rectus abdominis muscle
Tensor fascia lata muscle
Femoral nerve
Gluteus minimus muscle
Obturator nerve
Gluteus medius muscle
Superior gluteal artery, vein
Piriformis muscle
Sacrum
Iliopsoas muscle
External iliac artery, vein
Ilium
Sacral plexus and branches of internal iliac artery, vein
Gluteus maximus muscle

(Top) *A complex relationship exists between the branches of the internal iliac vessels and the nerve roots of the sacral plexus along the deep surface of the piriformis muscle.* **(Bottom)** *Once they exit the pelvis the superior gluteal vessels travel in the fat plane deep to the gluteus maximus muscle.*

Pelvis MR Atlas

AXIAL T1 MR, MID PELVIS

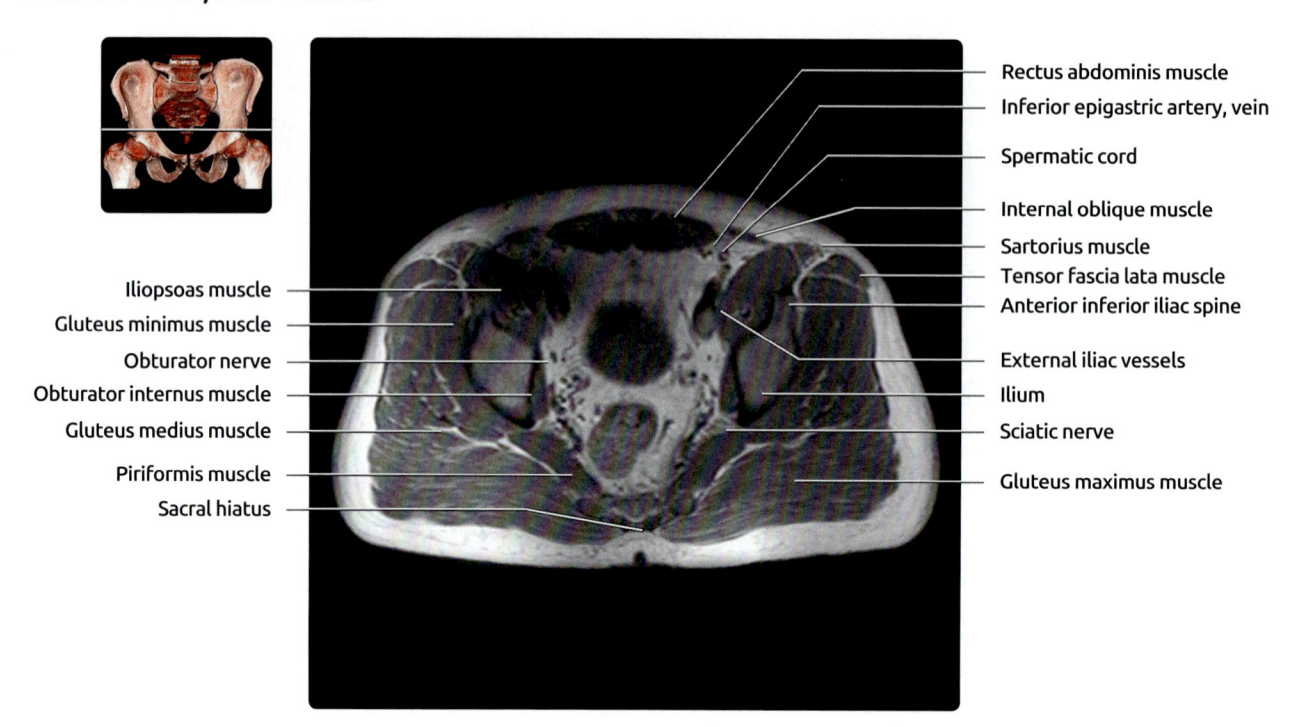

Top image labels (left):
- Iliopsoas muscle
- Gluteus minimus muscle
- Obturator nerve
- Obturator internus muscle
- Gluteus medius muscle
- Piriformis muscle
- Sacral hiatus

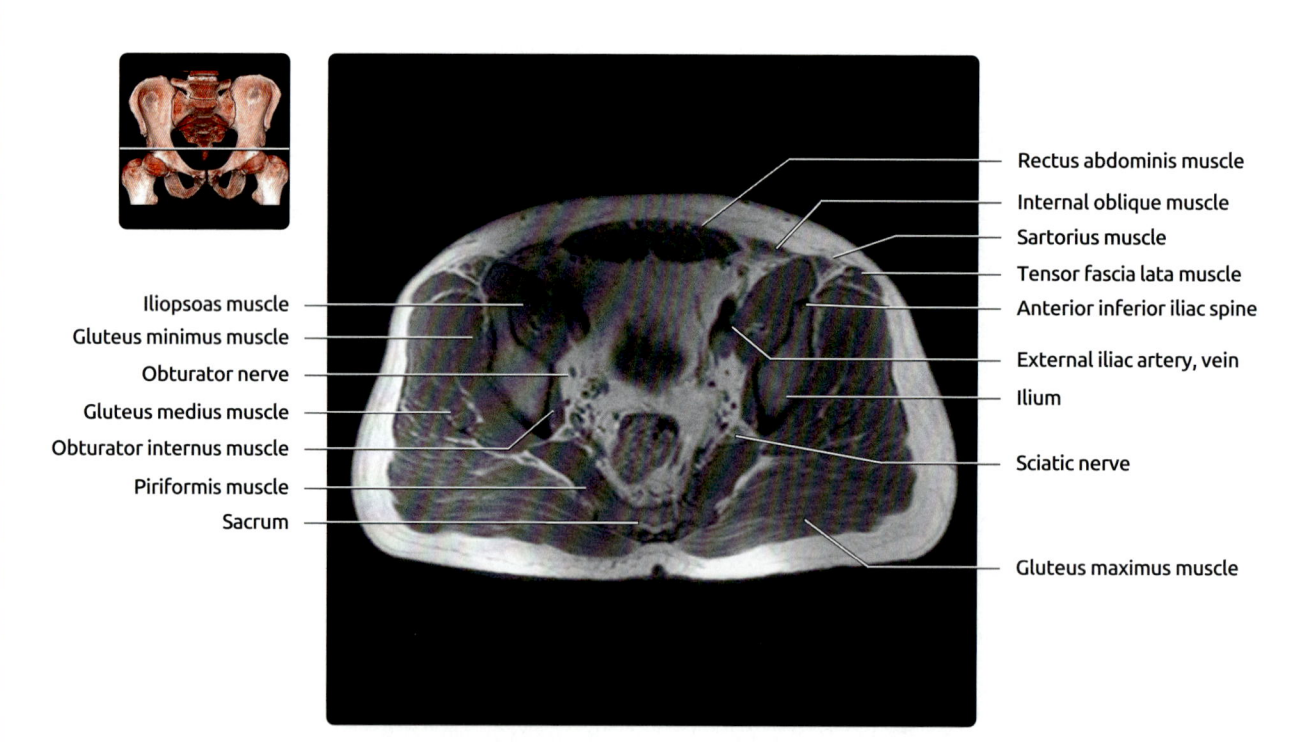

Top image labels (right):
- Rectus abdominis muscle
- Inferior epigastric artery, vein
- Spermatic cord
- Internal oblique muscle
- Sartorius muscle
- Tensor fascia lata muscle
- Anterior inferior iliac spine
- External iliac vessels
- Ilium
- Sciatic nerve
- Gluteus maximus muscle

Bottom image labels (left):
- Iliopsoas muscle
- Gluteus minimus muscle
- Obturator nerve
- Gluteus medius muscle
- Obturator internus muscle
- Piriformis muscle
- Sacrum

Bottom image labels (right):
- Rectus abdominis muscle
- Internal oblique muscle
- Sartorius muscle
- Tensor fascia lata muscle
- Anterior inferior iliac spine
- External iliac artery, vein
- Ilium
- Sciatic nerve
- Gluteus maximus muscle

(Top) The piriformis muscle originates from the sacrum and courses laterally through the greater sciatic notch, with the sciatic nerve along its anterior margin. The sartorius muscle is now apparent, inferior to its origin from the anterior superior iliac spine. **(Bottom)** The anterior inferior iliac spine is present just superior to the acetabulum. It is the origin of the straight head of the rectus femoris muscle. The iliofemoral ligament arises from its inferior margin.

Pelvis MR Atlas

AXIAL T1 MR, LOWER PELVIS

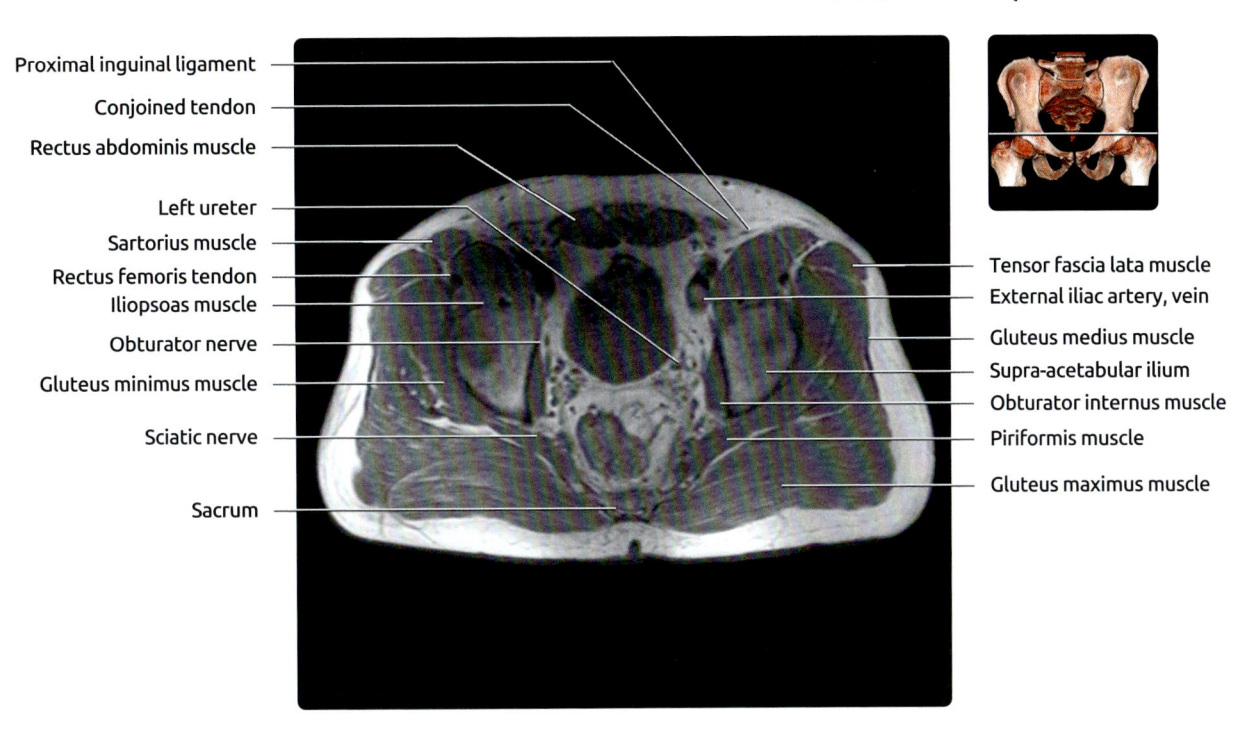

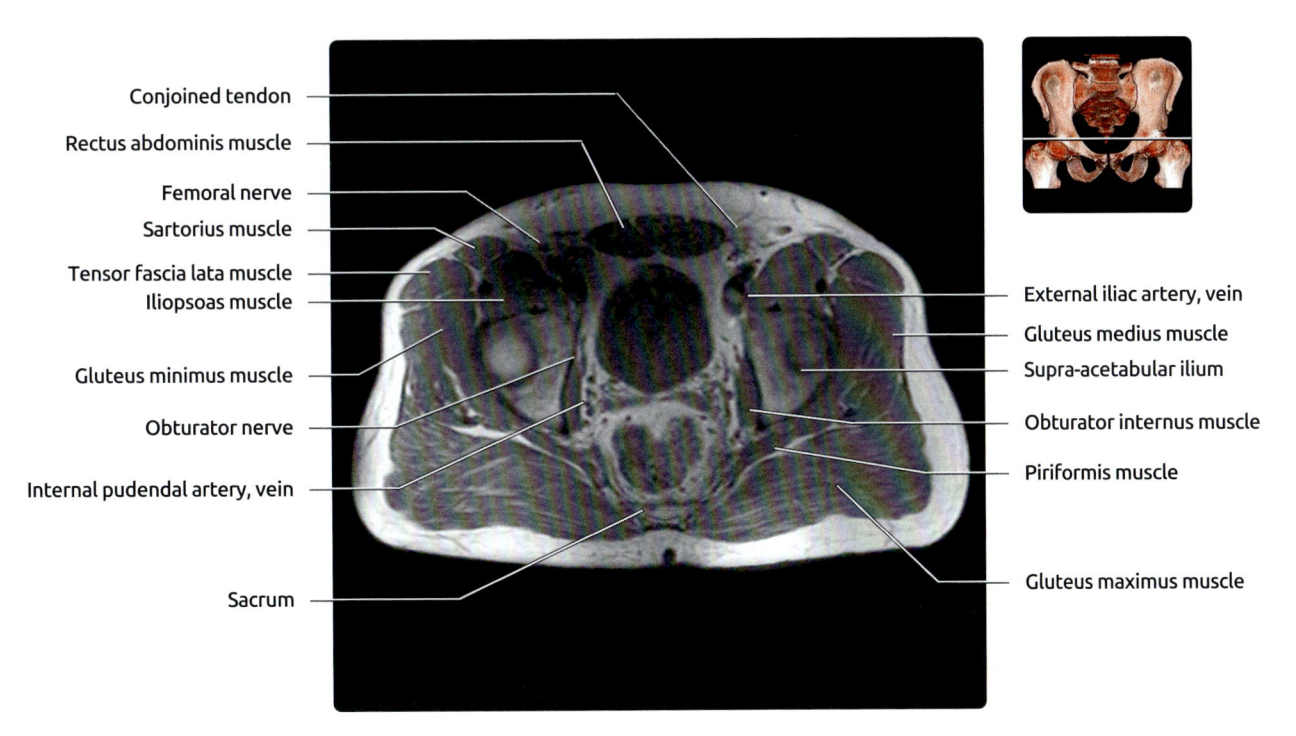

Labels (top image):
- Proximal inguinal ligament
- Conjoined tendon
- Rectus abdominis muscle
- Left ureter
- Sartorius muscle
- Rectus femoris tendon
- Iliopsoas muscle
- Obturator nerve
- Gluteus minimus muscle
- Sciatic nerve
- Sacrum
- Tensor fascia lata muscle
- External iliac artery, vein
- Gluteus medius muscle
- Supra-acetabular ilium
- Obturator internus muscle
- Piriformis muscle
- Gluteus maximus muscle

Labels (bottom image):
- Conjoined tendon
- Rectus abdominis muscle
- Femoral nerve
- Sartorius muscle
- Tensor fascia lata muscle
- Iliopsoas muscle
- Gluteus minimus muscle
- Obturator nerve
- Internal pudendal artery, vein
- Sacrum
- External iliac artery, vein
- Gluteus medius muscle
- Supra-acetabular ilium
- Obturator internus muscle
- Piriformis muscle
- Gluteus maximus muscle

(**Top**) The sartorius muscle is anterior to the psoas muscle. The rectus femoris straight head tendon is a narrow structure lateral to the iliopsoas muscle. (**Bottom**) The inferior medial-most portions of the transverse abdominis and internal oblique muscles form the conjoined tendon. Below this level, the tendons are not distinct from the rectus abdominis muscle. The internal pudendal vessels are located posterior to the obturator nerve.

Pelvis MR Atlas

AXIAL T1 MR, LOWER PELVIS

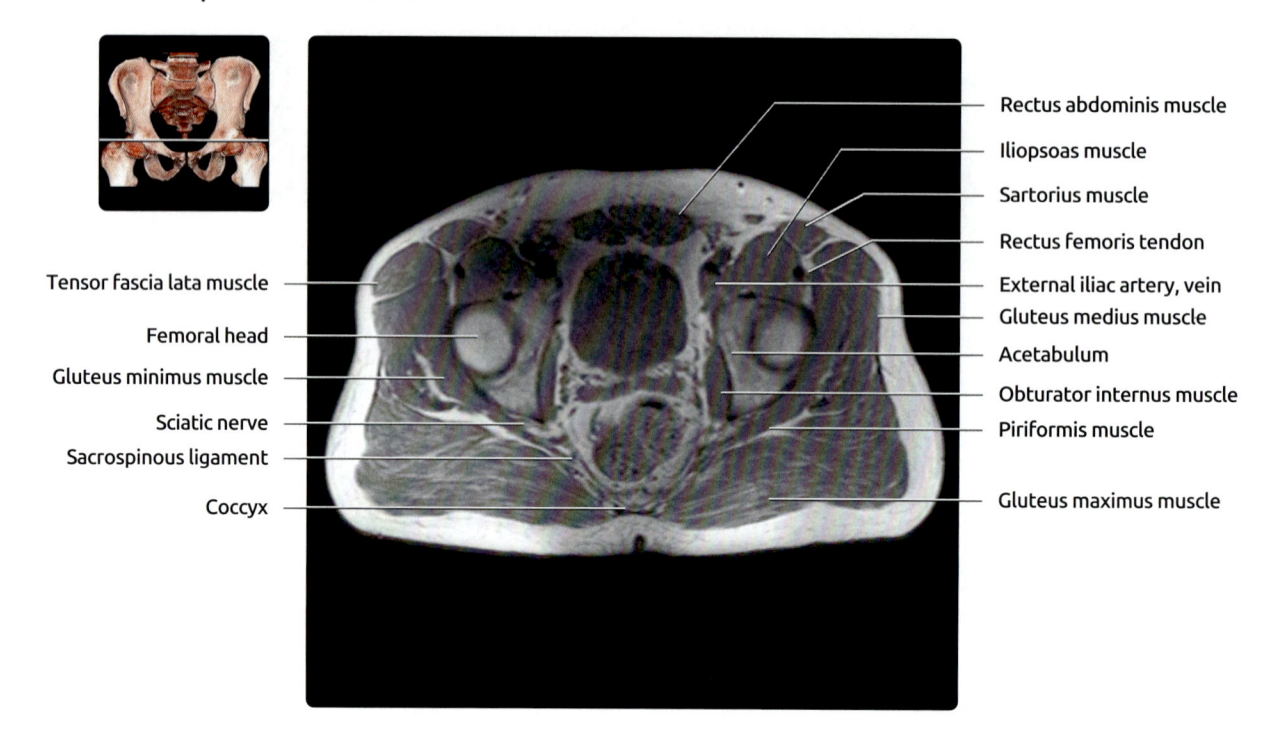

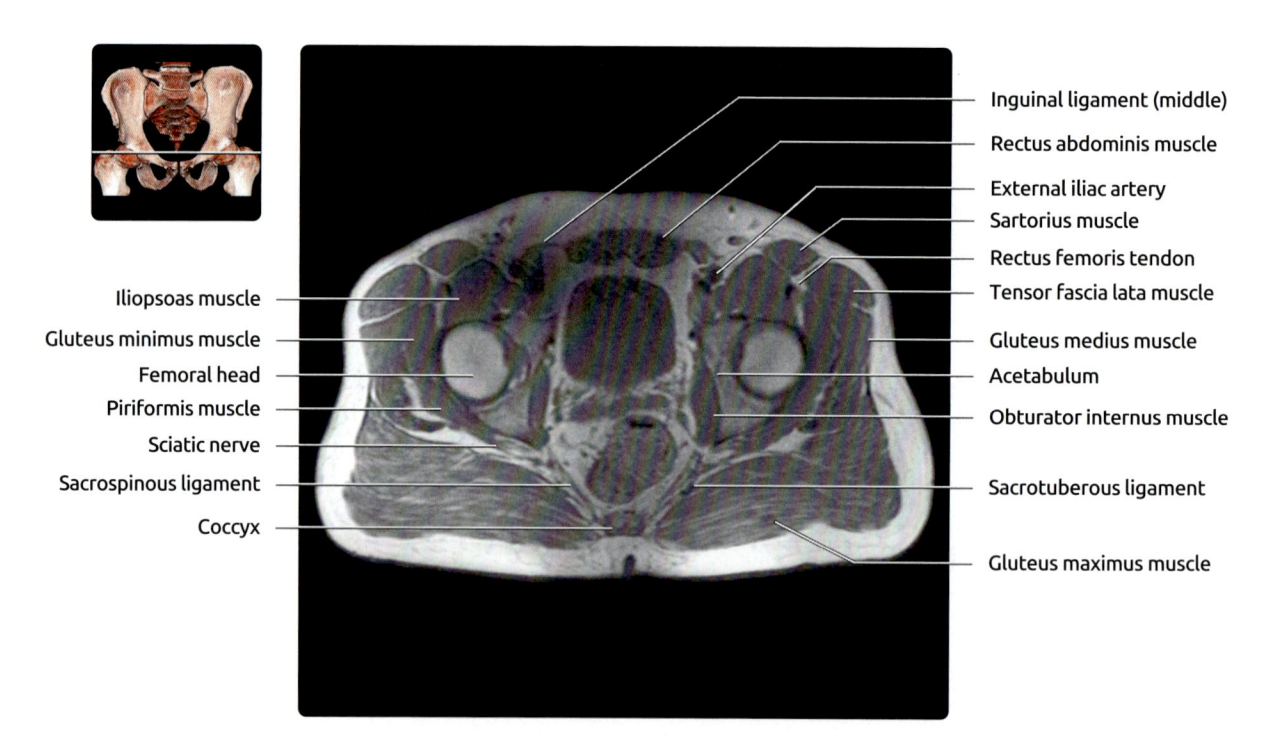

Labels (top image):
- Rectus abdominis muscle
- Iliopsoas muscle
- Sartorius muscle
- Rectus femoris tendon
- External iliac artery, vein
- Gluteus medius muscle
- Acetabulum
- Obturator internus muscle
- Piriformis muscle
- Gluteus maximus muscle
- Tensor fascia lata muscle
- Femoral head
- Gluteus minimus muscle
- Sciatic nerve
- Sacrospinous ligament
- Coccyx

Labels (bottom image):
- Inguinal ligament (middle)
- Rectus abdominis muscle
- External iliac artery
- Sartorius muscle
- Rectus femoris tendon
- Tensor fascia lata muscle
- Gluteus medius muscle
- Acetabulum
- Obturator internus muscle
- Sacrotuberous ligament
- Gluteus maximus muscle
- Iliopsoas muscle
- Gluteus minimus muscle
- Femoral head
- Piriformis muscle
- Sciatic nerve
- Sacrospinous ligament
- Coccyx

(Top) The sacrospinous ligament is visible; it lies anterior to the sacrotuberous ligament. The iliopsoas muscle is intimately related to the anterior aspect of the hip joint, and immediately lateral to the femoral artery and vein. **(Bottom)** The sciatic nerve has exited the greater sciatic notch and lies posterior to the acetabulum.

Pelvis MR Atlas

AXIAL T1 MR, LOWER PELVIS

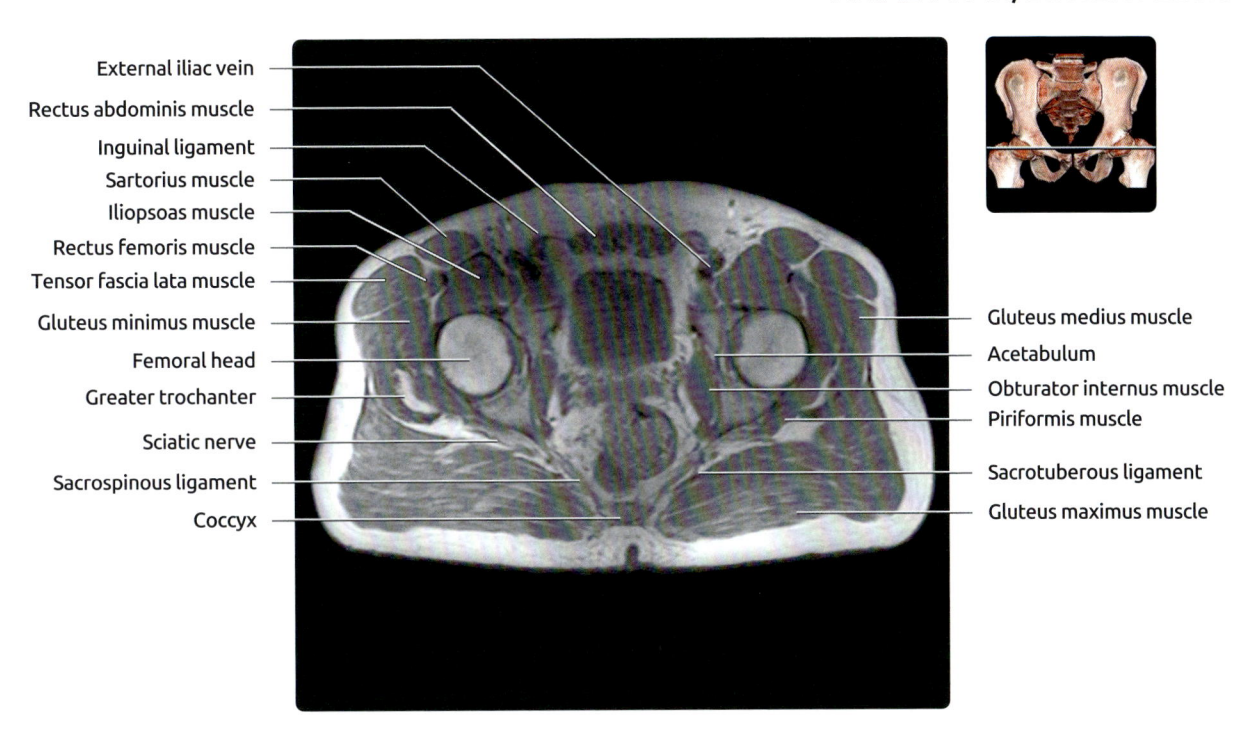

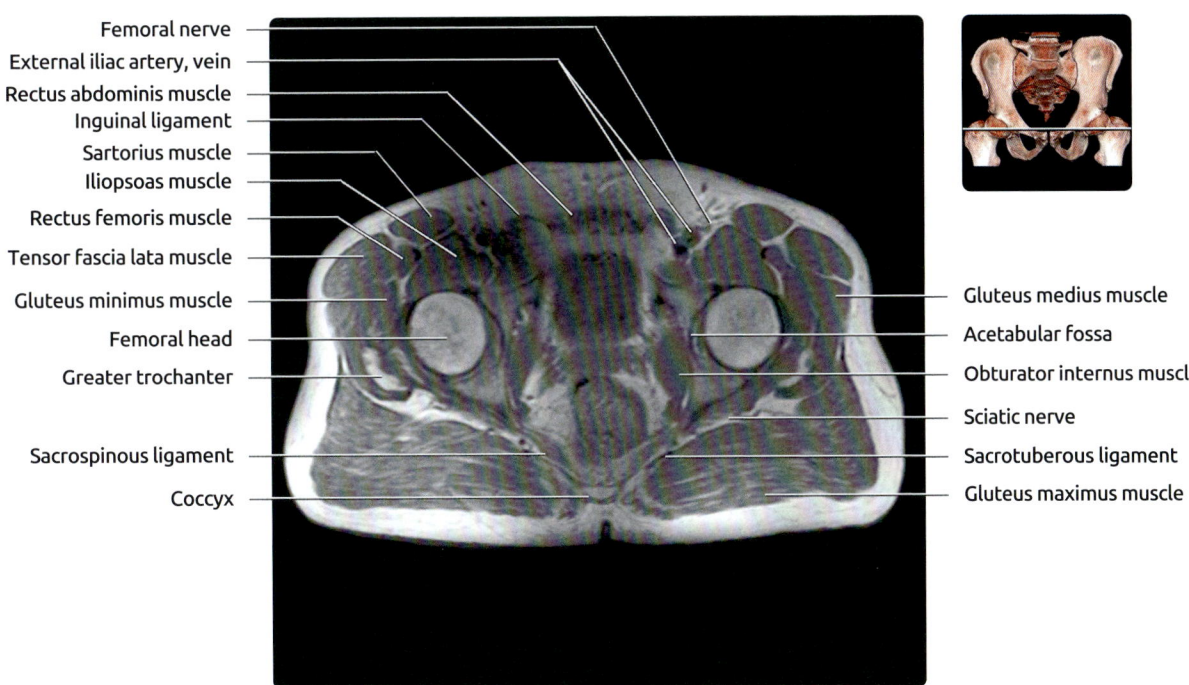

Top image labels (left): External iliac vein, Rectus abdominis muscle, Inguinal ligament, Sartorius muscle, Iliopsoas muscle, Rectus femoris muscle, Tensor fascia lata muscle, Gluteus minimus muscle, Femoral head, Greater trochanter, Sciatic nerve, Sacrospinous ligament, Coccyx

Top image labels (right): Gluteus medius muscle, Acetabulum, Obturator internus muscle, Piriformis muscle, Sacrotuberous ligament, Gluteus maximus muscle

Bottom image labels (left): Femoral nerve, External iliac artery, vein, Rectus abdominis muscle, Inguinal ligament, Sartorius muscle, Iliopsoas muscle, Rectus femoris muscle, Tensor fascia lata muscle, Gluteus minimus muscle, Femoral head, Greater trochanter, Sacrospinous ligament, Coccyx

Bottom image labels (right): Gluteus medius muscle, Acetabular fossa, Obturator internus muscle, Sciatic nerve, Sacrotuberous ligament, Gluteus maximus muscle

(Top) The inguinal ligament is present just lateral to the rectus abdominis muscle. Like the muscles, this structure also has an oblique, inferior medial course so that we only see segments and its most inferior extent will be medially located. **(Bottom)** Segments of the sacrotuberous ligament are present along the deep surface of the gluteus maximus muscle. The vertical orientation of this ligament means that only segments will be visible on axial image.

Pelvis MR Atlas

AXIAL T1 MR, LOWER PELVIS

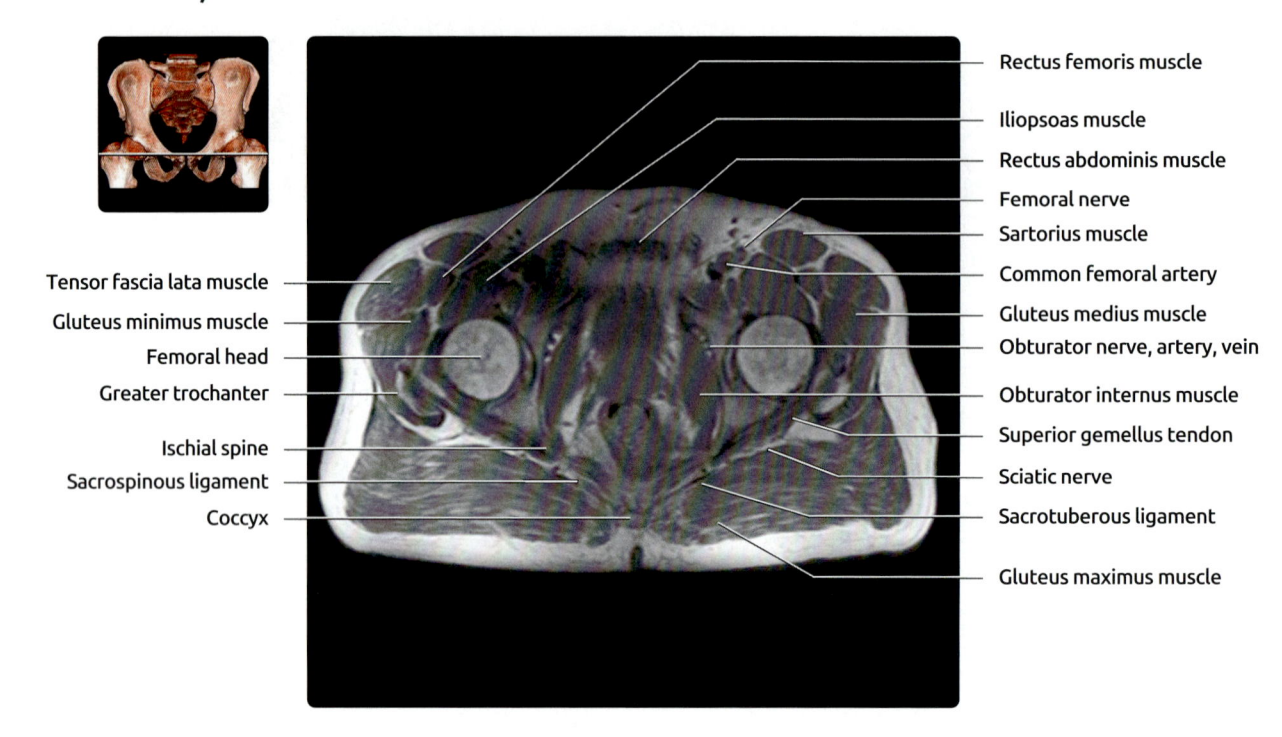

Labels (top image):
- Rectus femoris muscle
- Iliopsoas muscle
- Rectus abdominis muscle
- Femoral nerve
- Sartorius muscle
- Common femoral artery
- Gluteus medius muscle
- Obturator nerve, artery, vein
- Obturator internus muscle
- Superior gemellus tendon
- Sciatic nerve
- Sacrotuberous ligament
- Gluteus maximus muscle
- Tensor fascia lata muscle
- Gluteus minimus muscle
- Femoral head
- Greater trochanter
- Ischial spine
- Sacrospinous ligament
- Coccyx

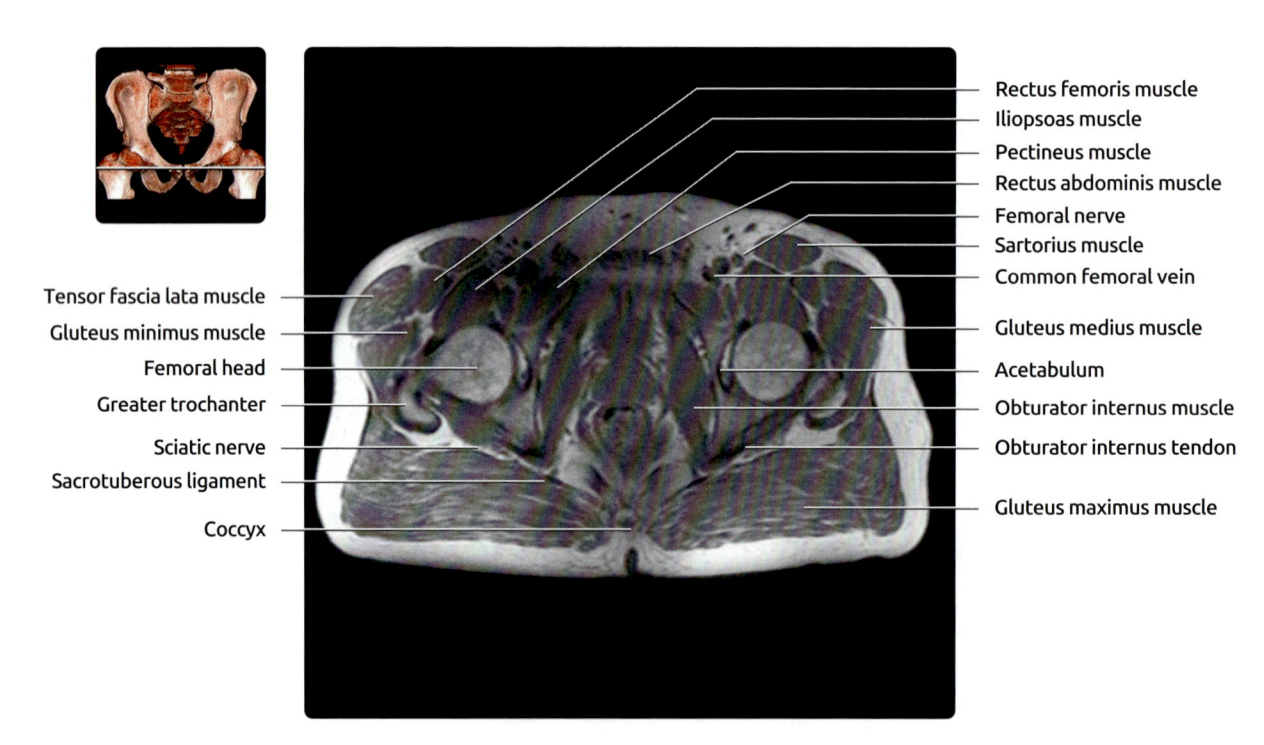

Labels (bottom image):
- Rectus femoris muscle
- Iliopsoas muscle
- Pectineus muscle
- Rectus abdominis muscle
- Femoral nerve
- Sartorius muscle
- Common femoral vein
- Gluteus medius muscle
- Acetabulum
- Obturator internus muscle
- Obturator internus tendon
- Gluteus maximus muscle
- Tensor fascia lata muscle
- Gluteus minimus muscle
- Femoral head
- Greater trochanter
- Sciatic nerve
- Sacrotuberous ligament
- Coccyx

(Top) At this point the external iliac vessels have crossed beneath the inguinal ligament and have become the common femoral vessels. The vein lies medial to the artery and the femoral n. lies lateral to the artery **(Bottom)** Note the dramatic change in course of the obturator internus muscle as it exits the pelvis, wrapping around the posterior margin of the acetabulum. The sciatic nerve is closely applied to the posterior aspect of the obturator internus tendon and is difficult to identify as a separate structure. The rectus abdominis muscles are nearing their origin from the pubic crest.

Pelvis MR Atlas

AXIAL T1 MR, LOWER PELVIS

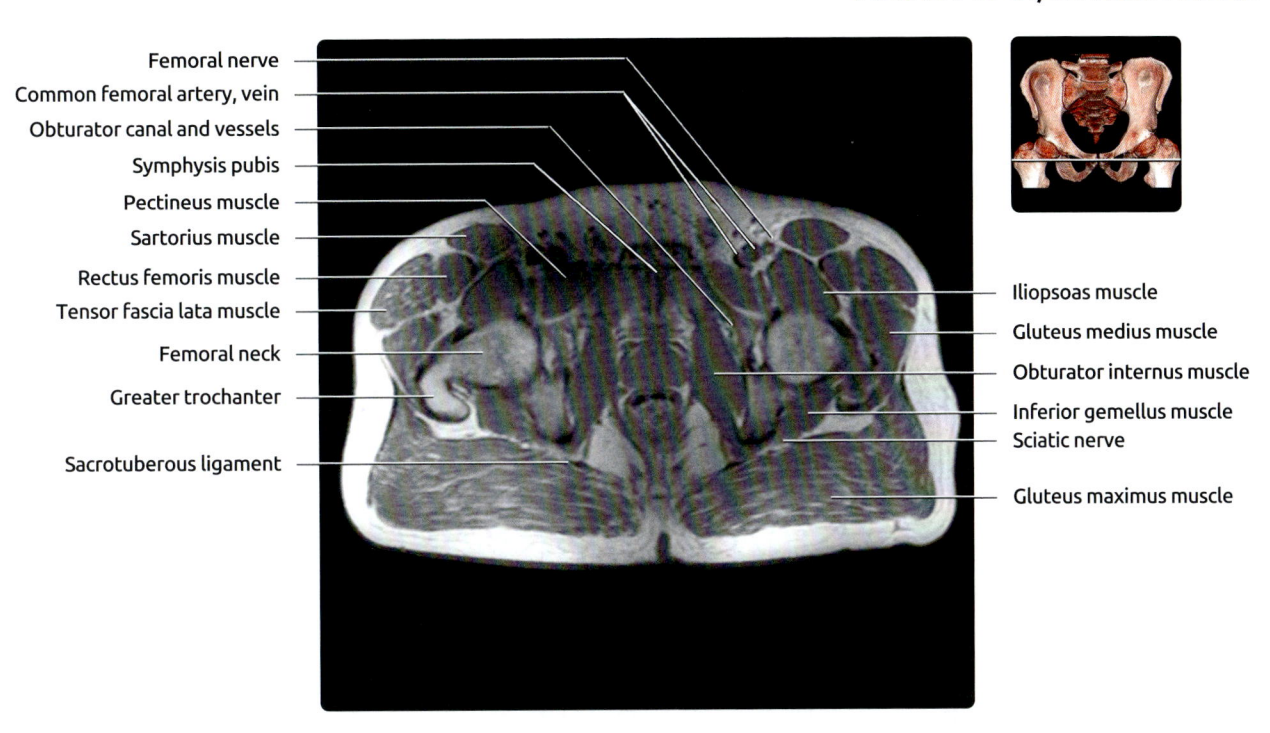

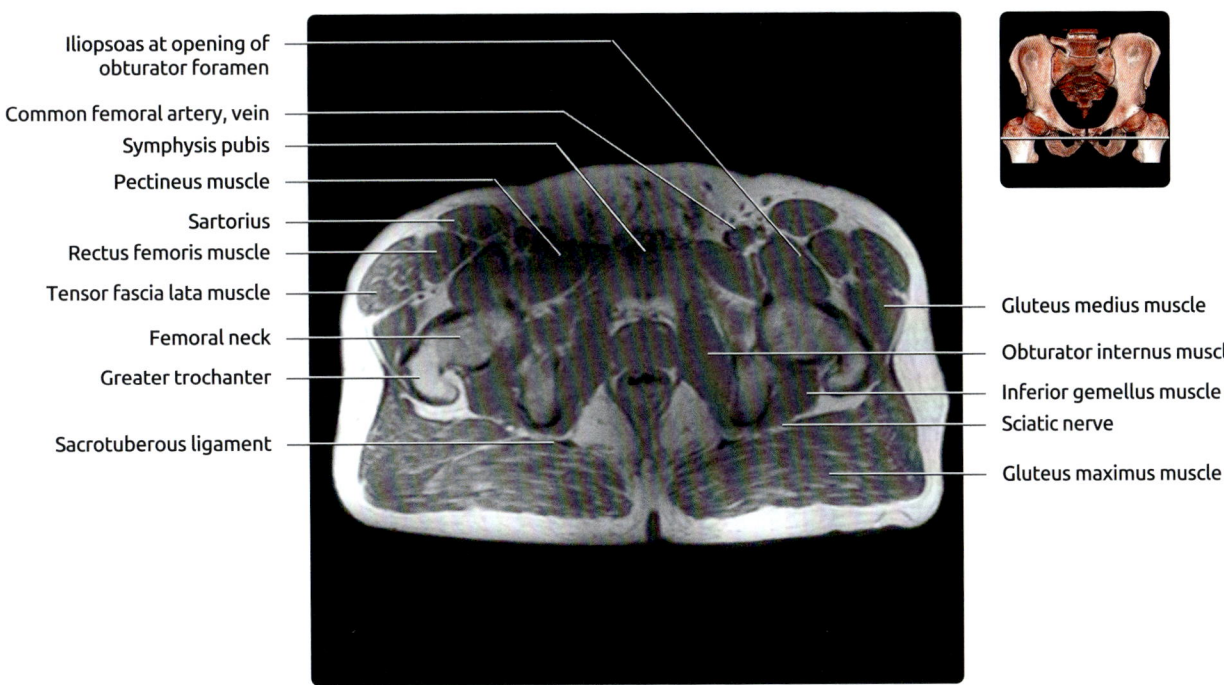

(Top) *Note the extension of tendon slips from the rectus abdominis along the anterior aspect of the symphysis pubis, joining the adductor aponeurosis which is continuous with the adductor longus origin. The adductor muscles of the thigh are now visible. The pectineus muscle is the most superior of these muscles.* (Bottom) *At the opening of the obturator foramen the obturator internus covers the entire deep surface. The sciatic nerve is now lateral to the acetabulum, along the deep surface of the gluteus maximus.*

Pelvis MR Atlas

CORONAL T1 MR, POSTERIOR PELVIS

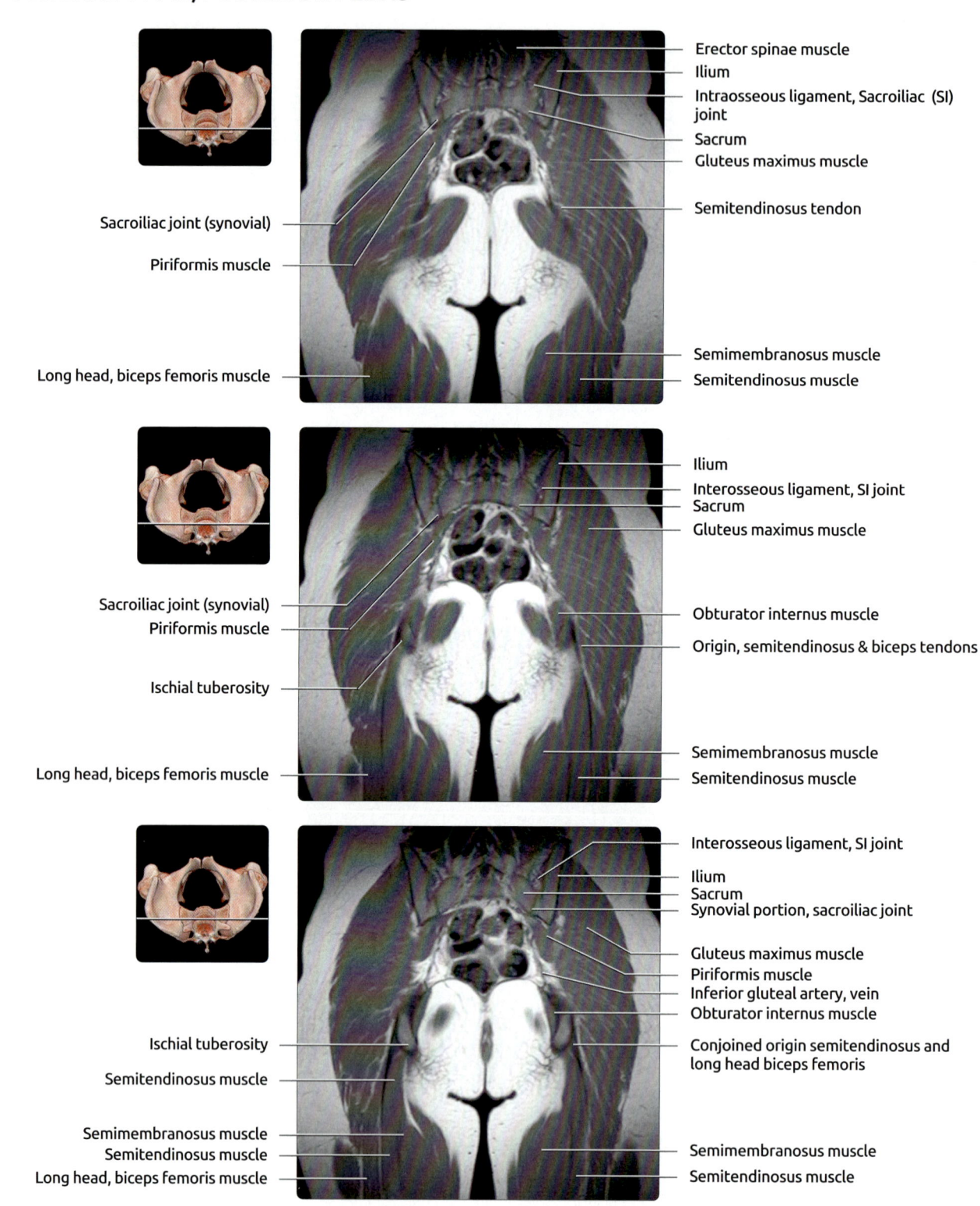

Top image labels:
- Erector spinae muscle
- Ilium
- Intraosseous ligament, Sacroiliac (SI) joint
- Sacrum
- Gluteus maximus muscle
- Semitendinosus tendon
- Sacroiliac joint (synovial)
- Piriformis muscle
- Semimembranosus muscle
- Semitendinosus muscle
- Long head, biceps femoris muscle

Middle image labels:
- Ilium
- Interosseous ligament, SI joint
- Sacrum
- Gluteus maximus muscle
- Sacroiliac joint (synovial)
- Piriformis muscle
- Obturator internus muscle
- Origin, semitendinosus & biceps tendons
- Ischial tuberosity
- Semimembranosus muscle
- Semitendinosus muscle
- Long head, biceps femoris muscle

Bottom image labels:
- Interosseous ligament, SI joint
- Ilium
- Sacrum
- Synovial portion, sacroiliac joint
- Gluteus maximus muscle
- Piriformis muscle
- Inferior gluteal artery, vein
- Obturator internus muscle
- Conjoined origin semitendinosus and long head biceps femoris
- Ischial tuberosity
- Semitendinosus muscle
- Semimembranosus muscle
- Semitendinosus muscle
- Long head, biceps femoris muscle
- Semimembranosus muscle
- Semitendinosus muscle

(**Top**) *First of 24 coronal images of the pelvis from posterior to anterior. The broad expanse of the gluteus maximus muscle is easy to appreciate on this image.* (**Middle**) *The piriformis muscle is seen arising from anterior surface of sacrum. The sciatic nerve lies on its anterior margin.* (**Bottom**) *The inferior gluteal vessels follow the same course as the sciatic nerve. The vessels are located medial to the nerve.*

Pelvis MR Atlas

CORONAL T1 MR, POSTERIOR PELVIS

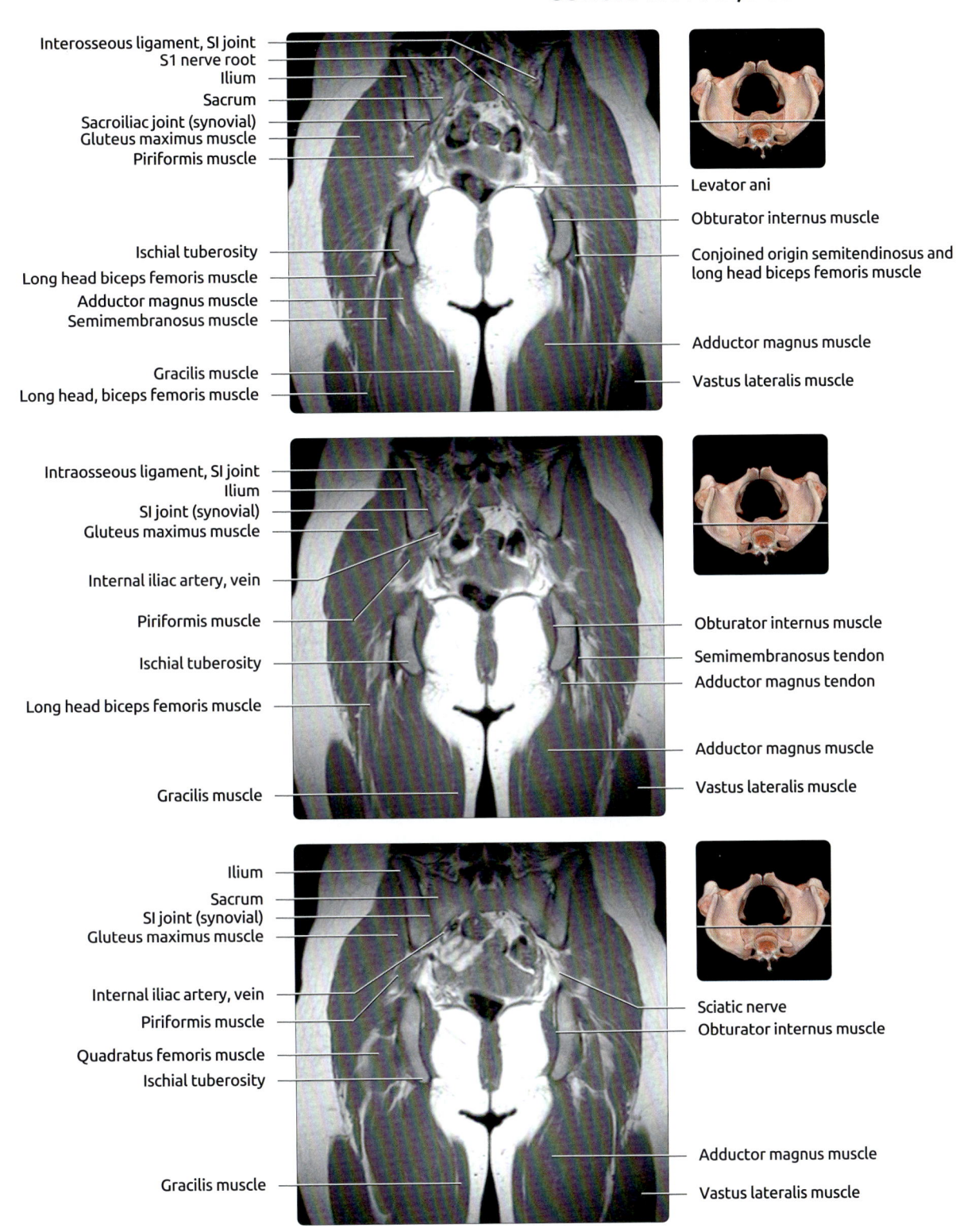

(Top) The semitendinosus and long head of biceps tendon have a conjoined origin from the posterior portion of the ischial tuberosity. The semimembranosus tendon originates slightly more anteriorly and laterally (Middle) The sacroiliac joint is primarily ligamentous in its superior portion, with only a small synovial extension anteriorly. More inferiorly, the majority of the joint is synovial, although there are still strong dorsal interosseous ligaments. (Bottom) The adductor magnus muscle dominates the posterior thigh. The gracilis muscle is the most medial muscle of the thigh. The vastus lateralis muscle occupies a large section of the lateral thigh.

CORONAL T1 MR, POSTERIOR PELVIS

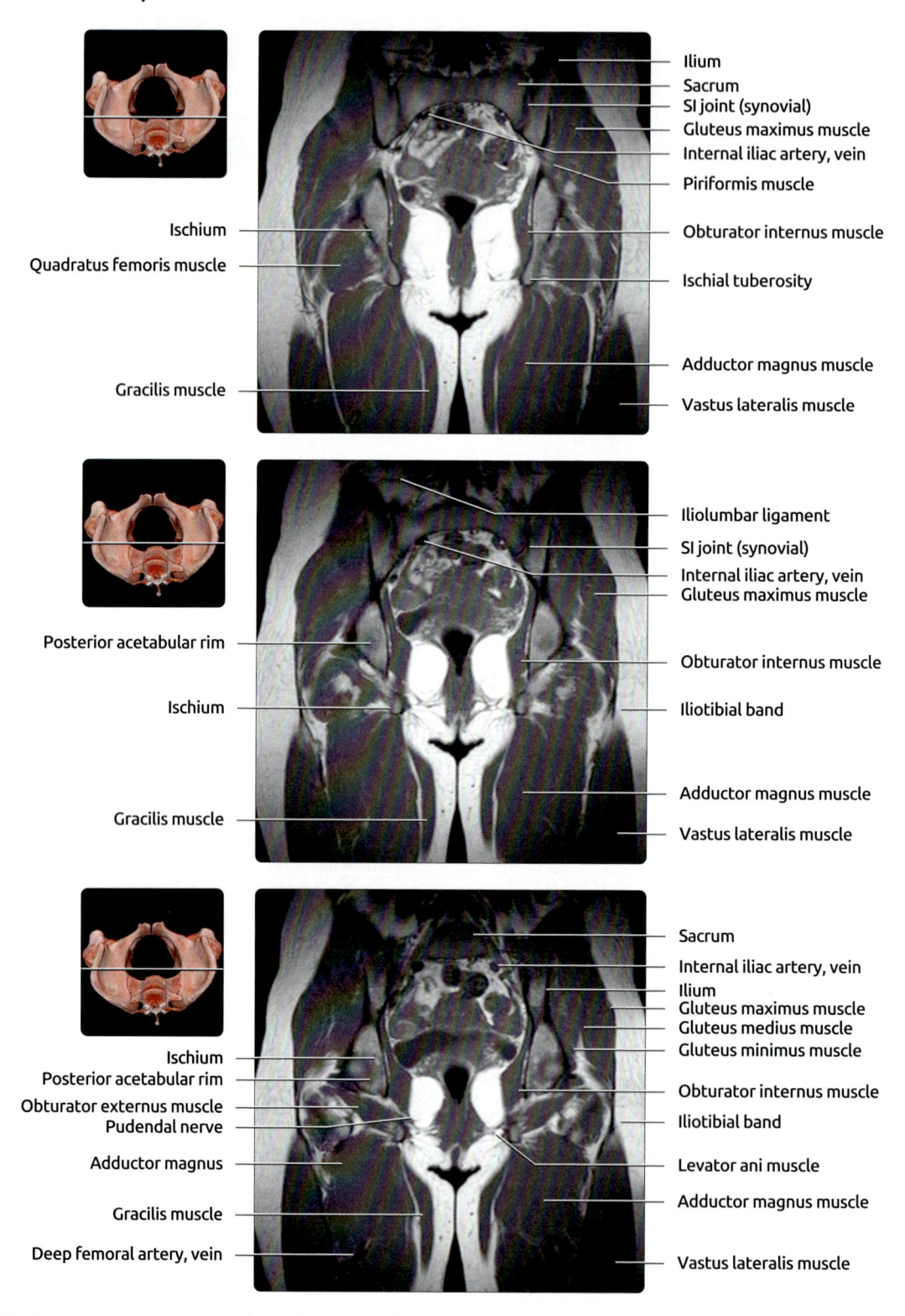

Labels (Top image):
- Ilium
- Sacrum
- SI joint (synovial)
- Gluteus maximus muscle
- Internal iliac artery, vein
- Piriformis muscle
- Obturator internus muscle
- Ischial tuberosity
- Adductor magnus muscle
- Vastus lateralis muscle
- Ischium
- Quadratus femoris muscle
- Gracilis muscle

Labels (Middle image):
- Iliolumbar ligament
- SI joint (synovial)
- Internal iliac artery, vein
- Gluteus maximus muscle
- Obturator internus muscle
- Iliotibial band
- Adductor magnus muscle
- Vastus lateralis muscle
- Posterior acetabular rim
- Ischium
- Gracilis muscle

Labels (Bottom image):
- Sacrum
- Internal iliac artery, vein
- Ilium
- Gluteus maximus muscle
- Gluteus medius muscle
- Gluteus minimus muscle
- Obturator internus muscle
- Iliotibial band
- Levator ani muscle
- Adductor magnus muscle
- Vastus lateralis muscle
- Ischium
- Posterior acetabular rim
- Obturator externus muscle
- Pudendal nerve
- Adductor magnus
- Gracilis muscle
- Deep femoral artery, vein

(**Top**) The broad, nearly horizontal quadratus femoris muscle is seen coursing from the ischial tuberosity to the posterior aspect of the femur. (**Middle**) The synovial portion of the sacroiliac joint is now seen and has a curved contour. The iliolumbar ligament extends from the transverse process of L5 to the ilium. Avulsion of the transverse process by this ligament is a useful sign of posterior pelvic instability. (**Bottom**) Nearly the entire extent of the obturator externus muscle is visible from its origin at the obturator foramen to its insertion onto the piriformis fossa. It is separated from the obturator internus by the obturator membrane.

Pelvis MR Atlas

CORONAL T1 MR, MID PELVIS

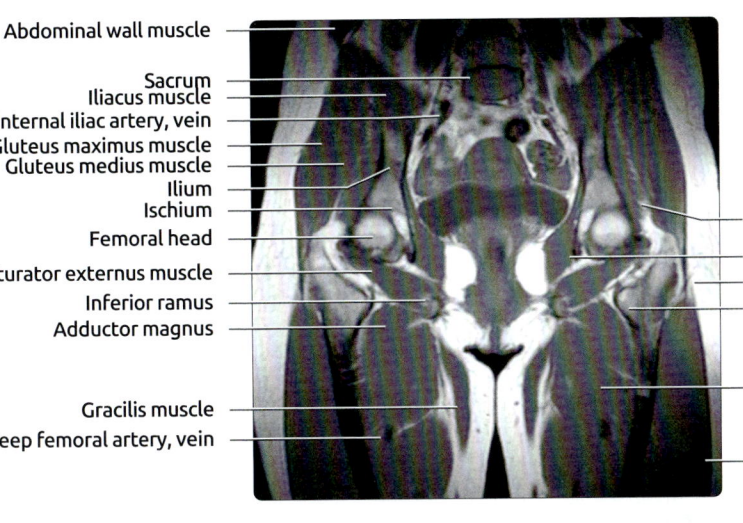

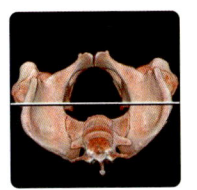

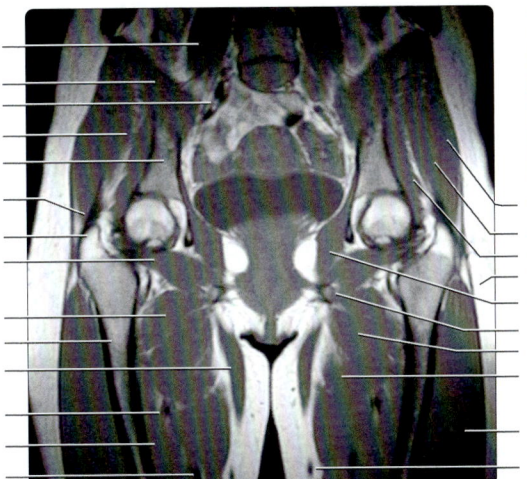

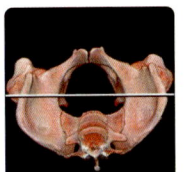

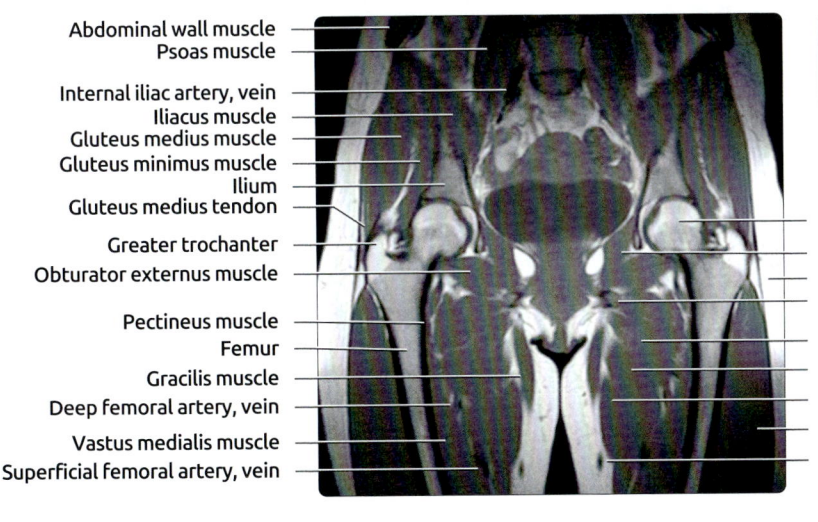

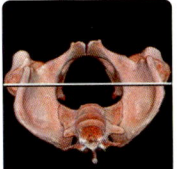

Image labels (Top):
- Abdominal wall muscle
- Sacrum
- Iliacus muscle
- Internal iliac artery, vein
- Gluteus maximus muscle
- Gluteus medius muscle
- Ilium
- Ischium
- Femoral head
- Obturator externus muscle
- Inferior ramus
- Adductor magnus
- Gracilis muscle
- Deep femoral artery, vein
- Gluteus minimus muscle
- Obturator internus muscle
- Iliotibial band
- Lesser trochanter
- Adductor magnus muscle
- Vastus lateralis muscle

Image labels (Middle):
- Psoas muscle
- Iliacus muscle
- Internal iliac artery, vein
- Superior gluteal artery, vein
- Ilium
- Gluteus medius tendon
- Greater trochanter
- Obturator externus muscle
- Adductor magnus muscle
- Femur
- Gracilis muscle
- Deep femoral artery, vein
- Vastus medialis muscle
- Superficial femoral artery, vein
- Gluteus maximus muscle
- Gluteus medius muscle
- Gluteus minimus muscle
- Iliotibial band
- Obturator internus muscle
- Inferior ramus
- Adductor brevis muscle
- Adductor magnus muscle
- Vastus lateralis muscle
- Greater saphenous vein

Image labels (Bottom):
- Abdominal wall muscle
- Psoas muscle
- Internal iliac artery, vein
- Iliacus muscle
- Gluteus medius muscle
- Gluteus minimus muscle
- Ilium
- Gluteus medius tendon
- Greater trochanter
- Obturator externus muscle
- Pectineus muscle
- Femur
- Gracilis muscle
- Deep femoral artery, vein
- Vastus medialis muscle
- Superficial femoral artery, vein
- Femoral head
- Obturator internus muscle
- Iliotibial band
- Inferior ramus
- Adductor brevis muscle
- Adductor longus muscle
- Adductor magnus muscle
- Vastus lateralis muscle
- Greater saphenous vein

(Top) *The images are now entering the adductor musculature. The adductor magnus has 2 heads. The short, superior head shown here is sometimes called the adductor minimus. It extends from the ischiopubic ramus to the posterior femur.* **(Middle)** *The adductor musculature is now coming into view. The pectineus muscle has the most superior insertion of the adductor muscles onto the posterior femur. Segments of the deep femoral vessels are visible.* **(Bottom)** *Note the general relationship of the major vessels of the thigh. The greater saphenous vein is medial within the subcutaneous fat. The superficial femoral vessels are medial to the deep femoral vessels.*

Pelvis MR Atlas

CORONAL T1 MR, MID PELVIS

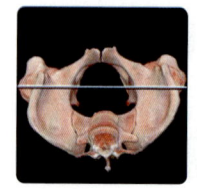

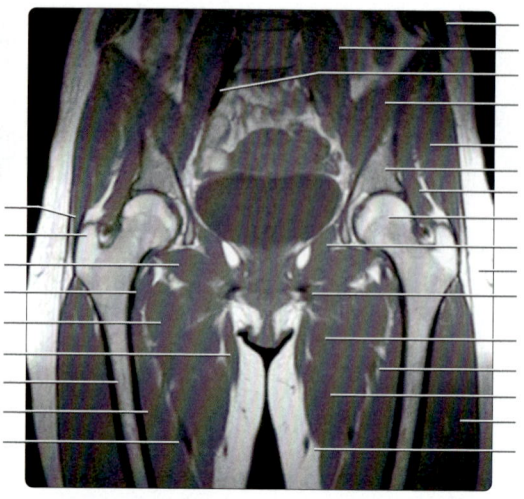

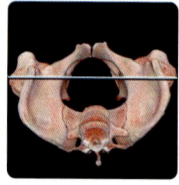

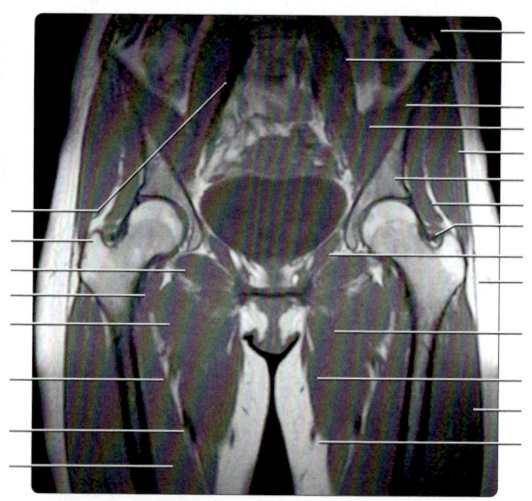

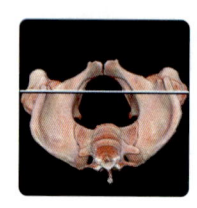

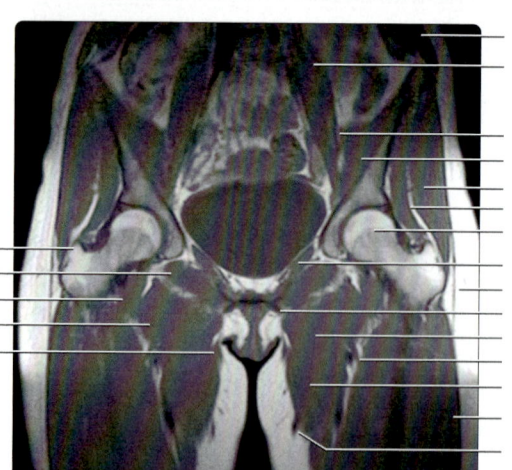

Top image labels (left): Gluteus medius tendon; Greater trochanter; Obturator externus muscle; Iliopsoas muscle; Pectineus muscle; Gracilis muscle; Femur; Vastus medialis muscle; Superficial femoral artery, vein

Top image labels (right): Abdominal wall muscle; Psoas muscle; Internal iliac artery, vein; Iliacus muscle; Gluteus medius muscle; Ilium; Gluteus minimus muscle; Femoral head; Obturator internus muscle; Iliotibial band; Inferior ramus; Adductor brevis muscle; Deep femoral artery, vein; Adductor longus muscle.; Vastus lateralis muscle; Greater saphenous vein

Middle image labels (left): Internal iliac artery, vein; Greater trochanter; Obturator externus muscle; Iliopsoas muscle; Pectineus muscle; Deep femoral artery, vein; Superficial femoral artery, vein; Vastus medialis muscle

Middle image labels (right): Abdominal wall muscle; Psoas muscle; Iliacus muscle; Femoral nerve; Gluteus medius muscle; Ilium; Gluteus minimus muscle; Posterior circumflex artery; Obturator internus muscle; Iliotibial band; Adductor brevis muscle; Adductor longus muscle; Vastus lateralis muscle; Greater saphenous vein

Bottom image labels (left): Greater trochanter; Obturator externus muscle; Iliopsoas muscle; Pectineus muscle; Gracilis muscle

Bottom image labels (right): Abdominal wall muscle; Psoas muscle; Femoral nerve; Iliacus muscle; Gluteus medius muscle; Gluteus minimus muscle; Femoral head; Obturator internus muscle; Iliotibial band; Inferior ramus; Adductor brevis muscle; Deep femoral artery, vein; Adductor longus muscle; Vastus lateralis muscle; Greater saphenous vein

(**Top**) *The gluteus medius tendon inserts onto the lateral facet of the greater trochanter. The gluteus maximus courses more distally to insert on the iliotibial band, the fascia of the vastus lateralis and the posterior femur.* (**Middle**) *The femoral nerve lies between iliacus and psoas muscles, in the iliopsoas groove. The gluteus medius is seen inserting on the lateral margin of the greater trochanter. The gluteus minimus inserts more anteriorly on the anterior margin of the greater trochanter.* (**Bottom**) *The obturator internus and externus muscles are separated by the fat plane of the obturator foramen.*

Pelvis MR Atlas

CORONAL T1 MR, ANTERIOR PELVIS

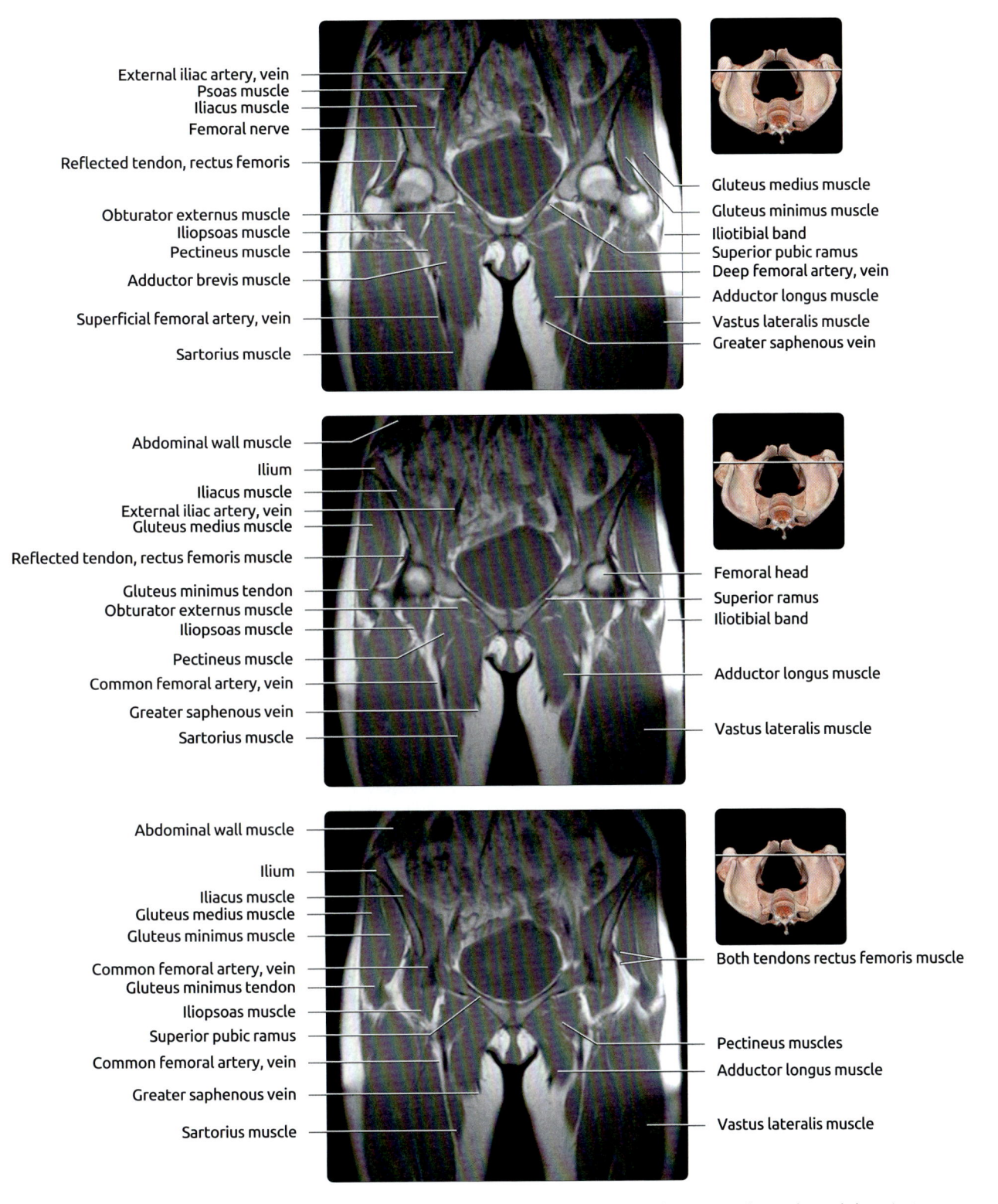

Top image labels (left): External iliac artery, vein; Psoas muscle; Iliacus muscle; Femoral nerve; Reflected tendon, rectus femoris; Obturator externus muscle; Iliopsoas muscle; Pectineus muscle; Adductor brevis muscle; Superficial femoral artery, vein; Sartorius muscle

Top image labels (right): Gluteus medius muscle; Gluteus minimus muscle; Iliotibial band; Superior pubic ramus; Deep femoral artery, vein; Adductor longus muscle; Vastus lateralis muscle; Greater saphenous vein

Middle image labels (left): Abdominal wall muscle; Ilium; Iliacus muscle; External iliac artery, vein; Gluteus medius muscle; Reflected tendon, rectus femoris muscle; Gluteus minimus tendon; Obturator externus muscle; Iliopsoas muscle; Pectineus muscle; Common femoral artery, vein; Greater saphenous vein; Sartorius muscle

Middle image labels (right): Femoral head; Superior ramus; Iliotibial band; Adductor longus muscle; Vastus lateralis muscle

Bottom image labels (left): Abdominal wall muscle; Ilium; Iliacus muscle; Gluteus medius muscle; Gluteus minimus muscle; Common femoral artery, vein; Gluteus minimus tendon; Iliopsoas muscle; Superior pubic ramus; Common femoral artery, vein; Greater saphenous vein; Sartorius muscle

Bottom image labels (right): Both tendons rectus femoris muscle; Pectineus muscles; Adductor longus muscle; Vastus lateralis muscle

(**Top**) *The gluteus minimus tendon inserts onto the anterior facet of the greater trochanter. The common femoral vessels have just bifurcated into deep femoral and superficial femoral vessels.* (**Middle**) *The common femoral vessels course along the anterior surface of the adductor longus muscle, which forms the floor of the femoral triangle.* (**Bottom**) *The crossing point of the sartorius muscle and the adductor longus muscle forms the apex of the femoral triangle. From this point inferior, the vessels traverse the adductor canal. The course of the vessels through the canal is depicted on more posterior images. The tensor fascia lata muscle is located along the anterior border of the iliotibial band.*

Pelvis MR Atlas

CORONAL T1 MR, ANTERIOR PELVIS

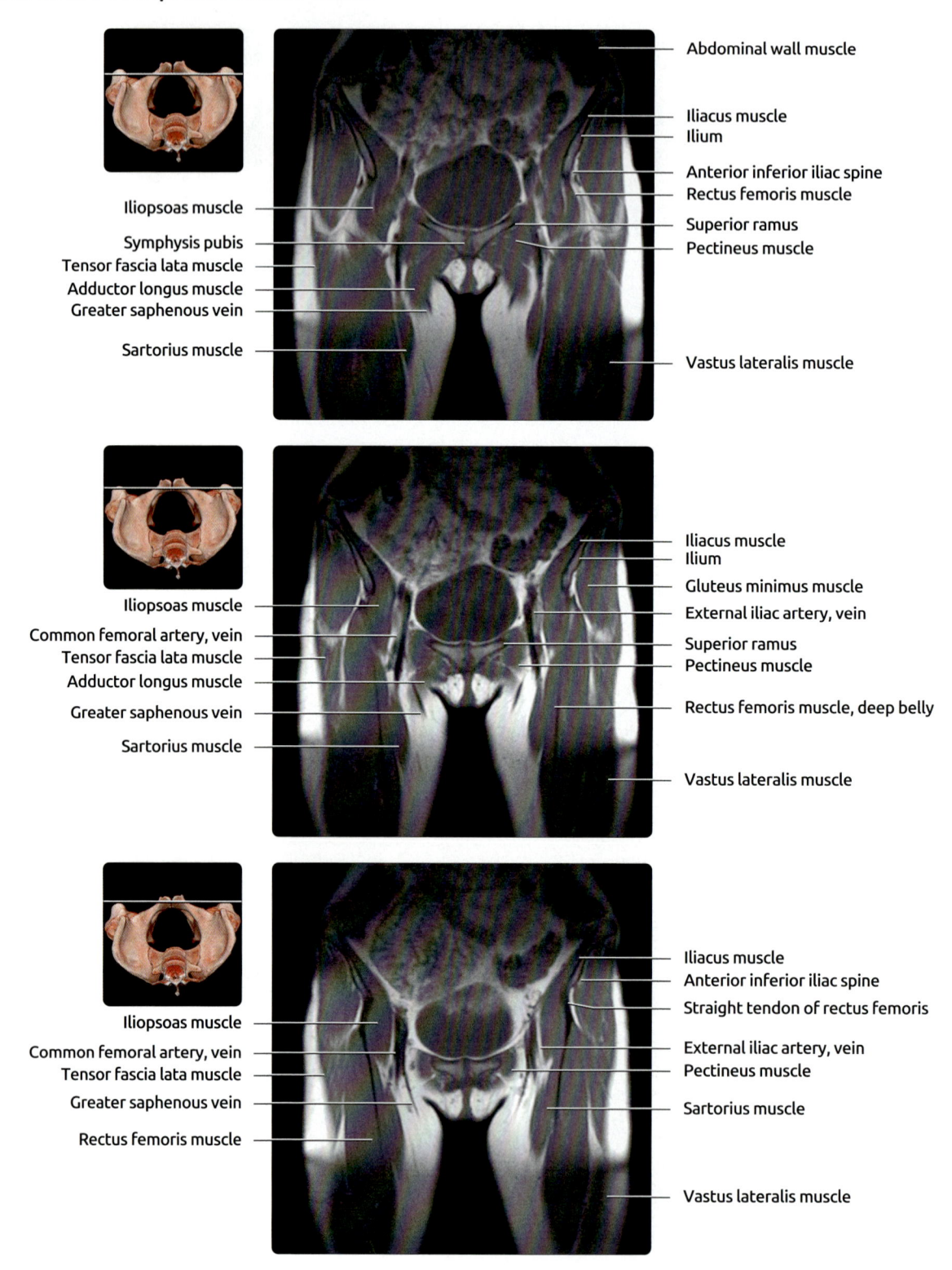

Top image labels (left): Iliopsoas muscle; Symphysis pubis; Tensor fascia lata muscle; Adductor longus muscle; Greater saphenous vein; Sartorius muscle
Top image labels (right): Abdominal wall muscle; Iliacus muscle; Ilium; Anterior inferior iliac spine; Rectus femoris muscle; Superior ramus; Pectineus muscle; Vastus lateralis muscle

Middle image labels (left): Iliopsoas muscle; Common femoral artery, vein; Tensor fascia lata muscle; Adductor longus muscle; Greater saphenous vein; Sartorius muscle
Middle image labels (right): Iliacus muscle; Ilium; Gluteus minimus muscle; External iliac artery, vein; Superior ramus; Pectineus muscle; Rectus femoris muscle, deep belly; Vastus lateralis muscle

Bottom image labels (left): Iliopsoas muscle; Common femoral artery, vein; Tensor fascia lata muscle; Greater saphenous vein; Rectus femoris muscle
Bottom image labels (right): Iliacus muscle; Anterior inferior iliac spine; Straight tendon of rectus femoris; External iliac artery, vein; Pectineus muscle; Sartorius muscle; Vastus lateralis muscle

(Top) The symphysis pubis is the articulation of the anterior aspect of the pelvis. The straight head of the rectus femoris muscle originates from the anterior inferior iliac spine, while the reflected head originates immediately superior to the acetabulum. **(Middle)** The external iliac vessels are medial to the iliopsoas muscle as those structures enter the thigh. The vessels become the common femoral vessels as they pass beneath the inguinal ligament. The femoral nerve is the most lateral structure entering the femoral triangle. It is not identifiable on this examination. **(Bottom)** The junction of the greater saphenous vein and common femoral vein is nicely seen on this image. External iliac vessels change name to common femoral as they pass beneath the inguinal ligament.

Pelvis MR Atlas

CORONAL T1 MR, ANTERIOR PELVIS

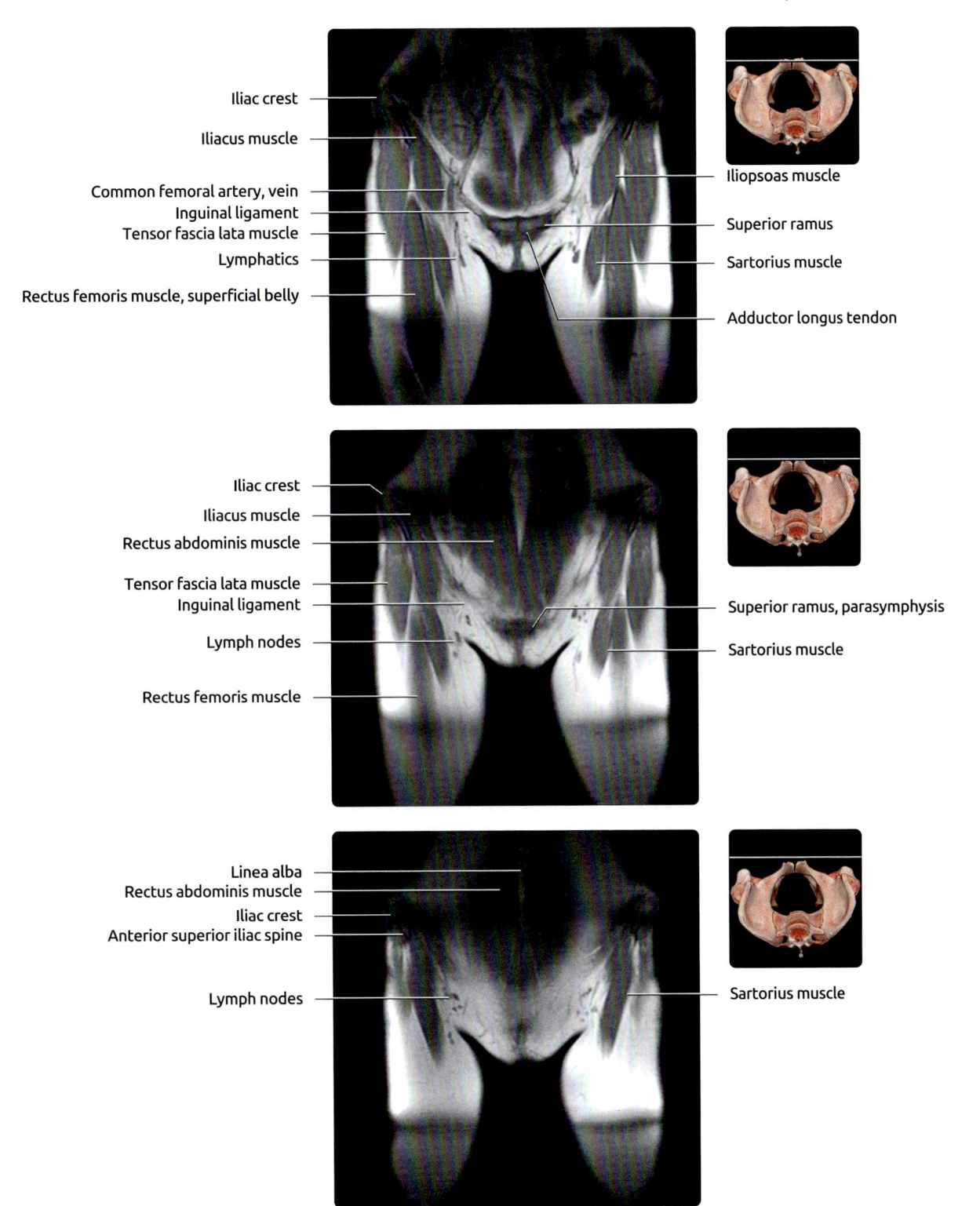

Labels (top image):
- Iliac crest
- Iliacus muscle
- Common femoral artery, vein
- Inguinal ligament
- Tensor fascia lata muscle
- Lymphatics
- Rectus femoris muscle, superficial belly
- Iliopsoas muscle
- Superior ramus
- Sartorius muscle
- Adductor longus tendon

Labels (middle image):
- Iliac crest
- Iliacus muscle
- Rectus abdominis muscle
- Tensor fascia lata muscle
- Inguinal ligament
- Lymph nodes
- Rectus femoris muscle
- Superior ramus, parasymphysis
- Sartorius muscle

Labels (bottom image):
- Linea alba
- Rectus abdominis muscle
- Iliac crest
- Anterior superior iliac spine
- Lymph nodes
- Sartorius muscle

(Top) A short segment of the inguinal ligament is visible near its attachment to the pubic tubercle. The lymphatics are the most lateral structures at the entrance to the femoral triangle. (Middle) The sartorius and rectus femoris muscles are the most anterior of the thigh muscles. The sartorius has a diagonal orientation from its origin on the anterior superior iliac spine to its insertion as part of the pes anserinus on the medial tibia. A rich supply of lymphatics is present in the anterior thigh. (Bottom) The paired midline rectus abdominis muscles are visible. The muscles originate (not insert) from the superior pubic ramus and pubic crest.

Pelvis MR Atlas

SAGITTAL T1 MR, MID PELVIS

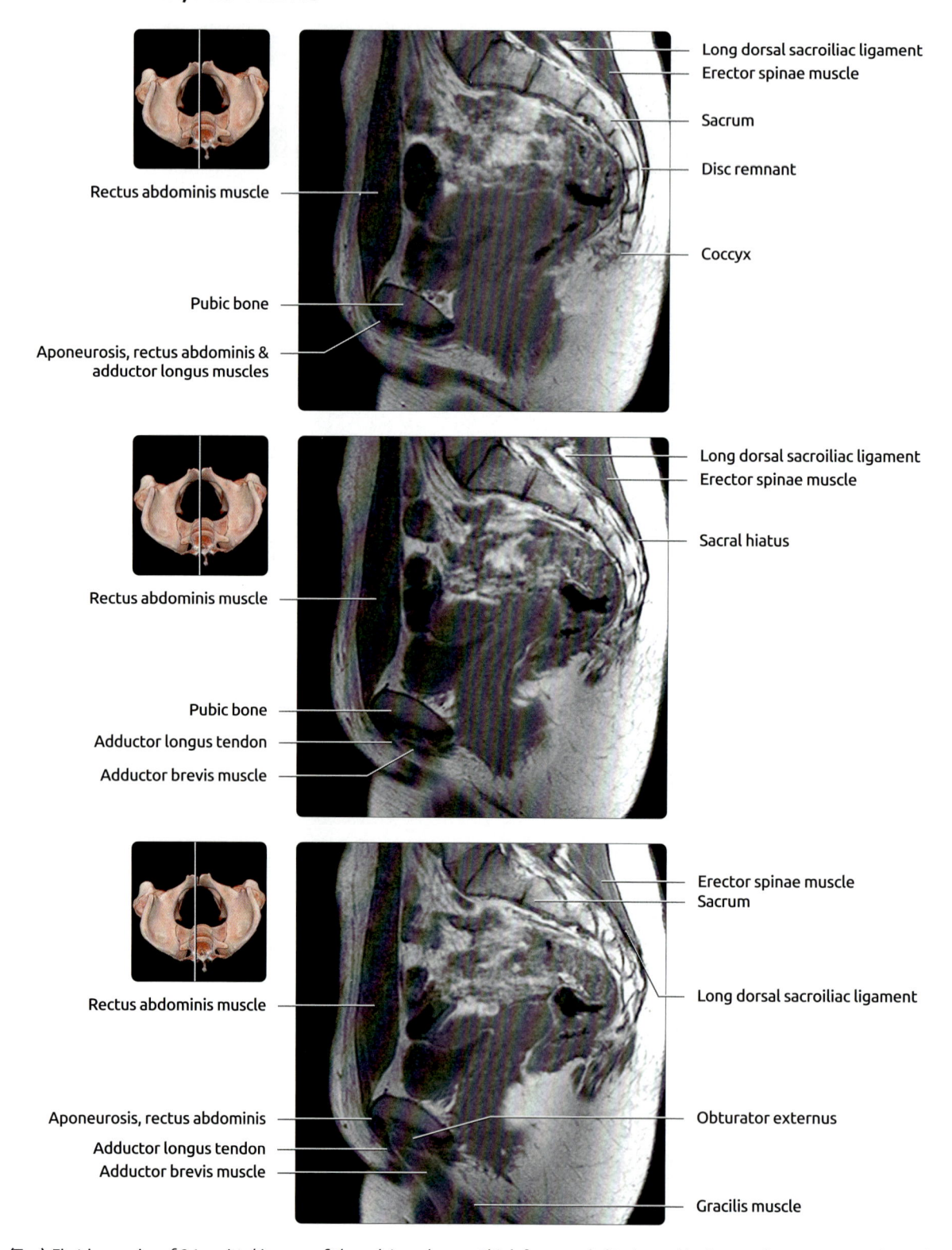

Labels (Top image):
- Rectus abdominis muscle
- Pubic bone
- Aponeurosis, rectus abdominis & adductor longus muscles
- Long dorsal sacroiliac ligament
- Erector spinae muscle
- Sacrum
- Disc remnant
- Coccyx

Labels (Middle image):
- Rectus abdominis muscle
- Pubic bone
- Adductor longus tendon
- Adductor brevis muscle
- Long dorsal sacroiliac ligament
- Erector spinae muscle
- Sacral hiatus

Labels (Bottom image):
- Rectus abdominis muscle
- Aponeurosis, rectus abdominis
- Adductor longus tendon
- Adductor brevis muscle
- Erector spinae muscle
- Sacrum
- Long dorsal sacroiliac ligament
- Obturator externus
- Gracilis muscle

(**Top**) *First in a series of 24 sagittal images of the pelvis and upper thigh from medial to lateral is shown. There are 6 sacral vertebrae in this patient, reflecting incorporation of the 1st coccygeal segment, a common variant.* (**Middle**) *The dorsal bony plate of the sacrum is absent at S4 (sometimes S5) and below, forming the sacral hiatus, which allows caudal needle access to the epidural space.* (**Bottom**) *The rectus abdominis muscle forms an aponeurosis which inserts along the anterior margin of the pubic bone and is continuous with the origin of the adductor longus tendon. Muscular forces concentrated in this region during athletic activity can cause detachment of the aponeurosis in the syndrome known as athletic pubalgia.*

Pelvis MR Atlas

SAGITTAL T1 MR, MIDPELVIS

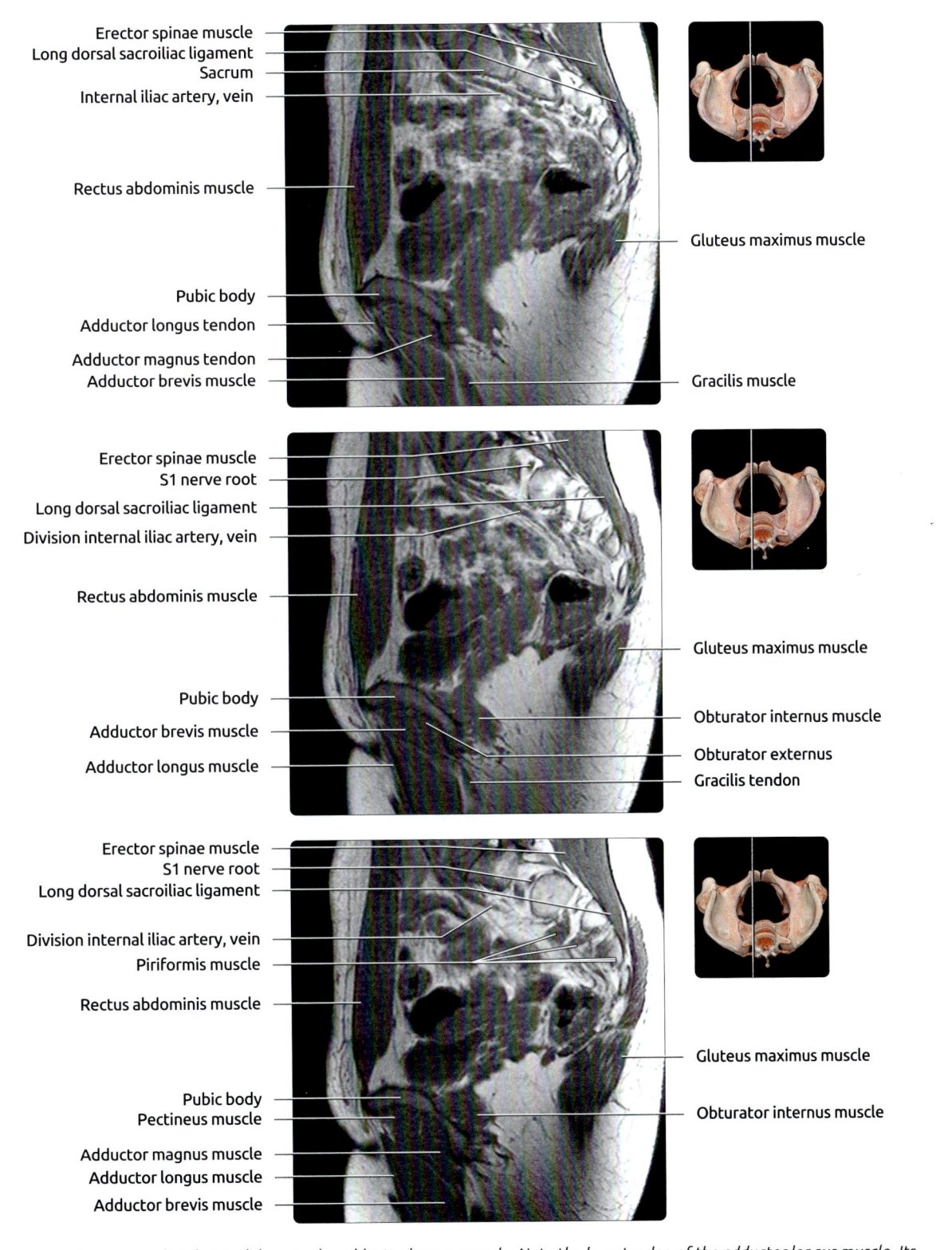

(Top) Adductor brevis muscle is located deep to the adductor longus muscle. Note the long tendon of the adductor longus muscle. Its origin is a small footprint on the anterior aspect of the pubic body. **(Middle)** The gracilis muscle is the most medial of the adductor muscles. It has a thin tendinous origin from the medial aspect of the inferior pubic ramus. **(Bottom)** The obturator internus muscles lines almost the entire deep surface of the pelvis. The adductor magnus has the most inferior origin of the adductor muscles, originating from the inferior portion of the pubic body and the ischium.

Pelvis MR Atlas

SAGITTAL T1 MR, MID PELVIS

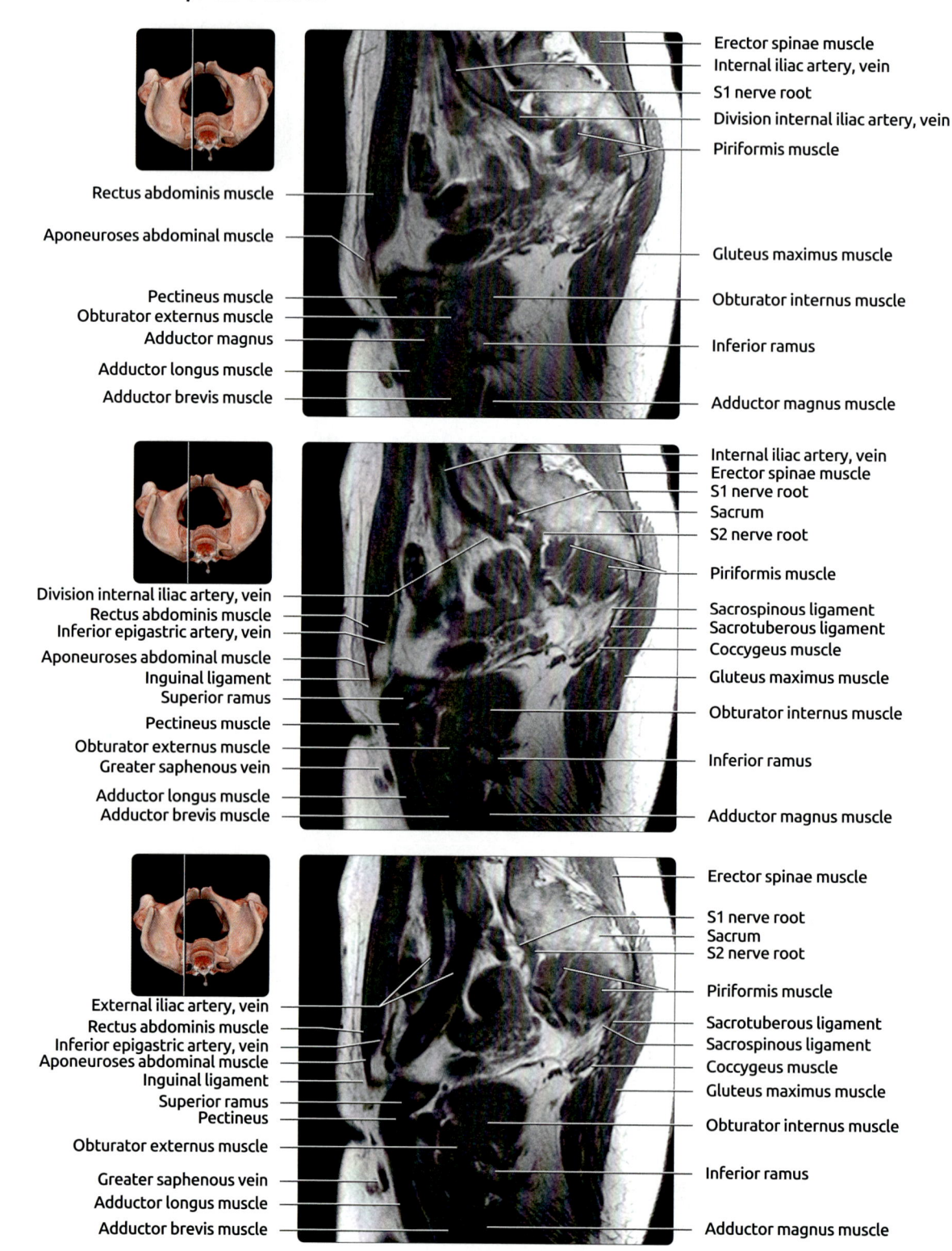

Erector spinae muscle
Internal iliac artery, vein
S1 nerve root
Division internal iliac artery, vein
Piriformis muscle

Rectus abdominis muscle
Aponeuroses abdominal muscle

Gluteus maximus muscle

Pectineus muscle
Obturator externus muscle
Adductor magnus
Adductor longus muscle
Adductor brevis muscle

Obturator internus muscle

Inferior ramus

Adductor magnus muscle

Internal iliac artery, vein
Erector spinae muscle
S1 nerve root
Sacrum
S2 nerve root
Piriformis muscle

Division internal iliac artery, vein
Rectus abdominis muscle
Inferior epigastric artery, vein
Aponeuroses abdominal muscle
Inguinal ligament
Superior ramus
Pectineus muscle
Obturator externus muscle
Greater saphenous vein
Adductor longus muscle
Adductor brevis muscle

Sacrospinous ligament
Sacrotuberous ligament
Coccygeus muscle
Gluteus maximus muscle
Obturator internus muscle

Inferior ramus

Adductor magnus muscle

Erector spinae muscle
S1 nerve root
Sacrum
S2 nerve root

External iliac artery, vein
Rectus abdominis muscle
Inferior epigastric artery, vein
Aponeuroses abdominal muscle
Inguinal ligament
Superior ramus
Pectineus
Obturator externus muscle
Greater saphenous vein
Adductor longus muscle
Adductor brevis muscle

Piriformis muscle
Sacrotuberous ligament
Sacrospinous ligament
Coccygeus muscle
Gluteus maximus muscle
Obturator internus muscle

Inferior ramus

Adductor magnus muscle

(Top) The adductor magnus muscle occupies the position assumed by the gracilis muscle on more medial images. The aponeuroses of the external and internal oblique and transversus abdominis muscles are present just lateral to the rectus abdominis muscle. **(Middle)** The transverse abdominis and internal oblique tendons are present just lateral to the rectus abdominis muscle. The somewhat horizontal fibers of the sacrospinous ligament are deep to the more vertical fibers of the sacrotuberous ligament. **(Bottom)** This image bisects the long axis of the external iliac vessels. The inguinal ligament is the inferior edge of the aponeurosis of the external oblique muscle. The cross section of the pubic rami is presented.

Pelvis MR Atlas

SAGITTAL T1 MR, MID PELVIS

Labels (Top image):
- Erector spinae muscle
- Interosseous ligament of SI joint
- Sacrum
- Rectus abdominis muscle
- External iliac artery, vein
- Piriformis muscle
- Transverse abdominis muscle
- Internal oblique muscle
- Aponeuroses abdominal muscle
- Inguinal ligament
- Superior ramus
- Pectineus muscle
- Pectineus muscle
- Adductor longus muscle
- Adductor brevis muscle
- Sacrotuberous ligament
- Sacrospinous ligament
- Coccygeus muscle
- Gluteus maximus muscle
- Obturator internus muscle
- Obturator externus muscle
- Inferior ramus
- Adductor magnus muscle

Labels (Middle image):
- Interosseous ligament SI joint
- Ilium
- Sacrum
- Rectus abdominis muscle
- Iliopsoas muscle
- Transverse abdominis muscle
- Piriformis muscle
- Internal oblique muscle
- External iliac artery, vein
- Aponeuroses abdominal muscle
- Inguinal ligament
- Superior ramus
- Pectineus muscle
- Greater saphenous vein
- Adductor longus muscle
- Adductor brevis muscle
- Sacrotuberous ligament
- Sacrospinous ligament
- Coccygeus muscle
- Gluteus maximus muscle
- Obturator internus muscle
- Inferior ramus
- Adductor magnus muscle

Labels (Bottom image):
- Interosseous ligaments SI joint
- Ilium
- Sacrum
- Transverse abdominis muscle
- Internal oblique muscle
- Iliopsoas muscle
- Piriformis muscle
- External iliac artery, vein
- Aponeuroses abdominal muscle
- Inguinal ligament
- Iliopectineal junction
- Common femoral artery, vein
- Pectineus muscle
- Sartorius muscle
- Adductor brevis muscle
- Sciatic nerve
- Sacrospinous ligament
- Sacrotuberous ligament
- Gluteus maximus muscle
- Obturator internus muscle
- Obturator externus muscle
- Inferior ramus
- Adductor magnus muscle

(**Top**) *The transition between the rectus abdominis muscle and the more lateral muscles is indistinct on sagittal images. The rectus abdominis muscle is wider superiorly than it is inferiorly, thus it extends onto more lateral images. The interosseous ligaments of the sacroiliac joint are seen in cross section.* (**Middle**) *The adductor magnus muscle has 2 separate origins both of which are visible on this image. The ischiocondylar portion originates from the ischial tuberosity while the adductor portion originates from the inferior pubic ramus. This is the most lateral image on which the greater saphenous vein is present. It drains into the common femoral vein through the saphenous hiatus.* (**Bottom**) *The external iliac vessels have crossed under the inguinal ligament to become the common femoral vessels. The sacroiliac joint is obliquely oriented and thus short segments will be seen on multiple images. The cross section of the iliopectineal junction is larger than the superior pubic ramus indicating transition from superior pubic ramus to acetabulum.*

Pelvis MR Atlas

SAGITTAL T1 MR, LATERAL PELVIS

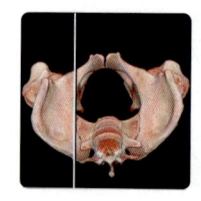

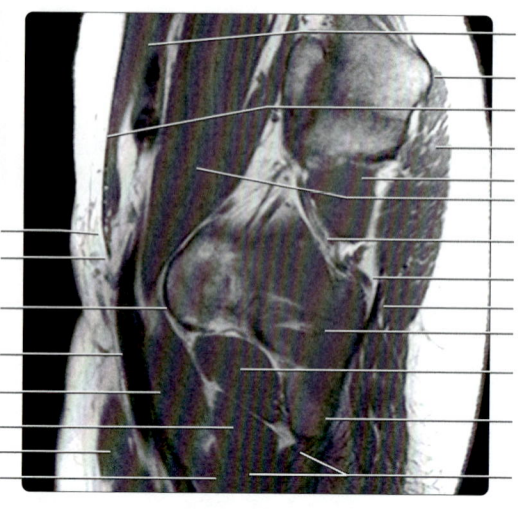

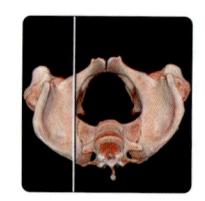

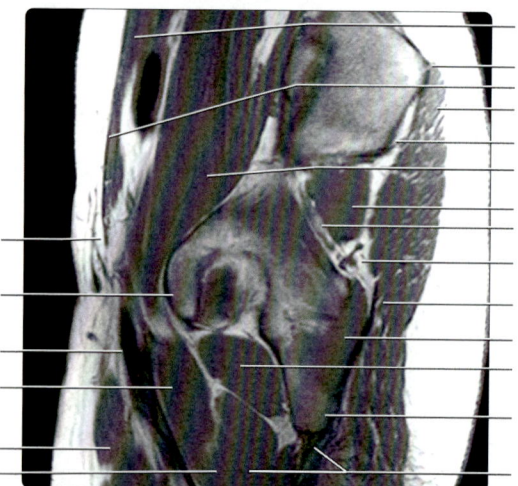

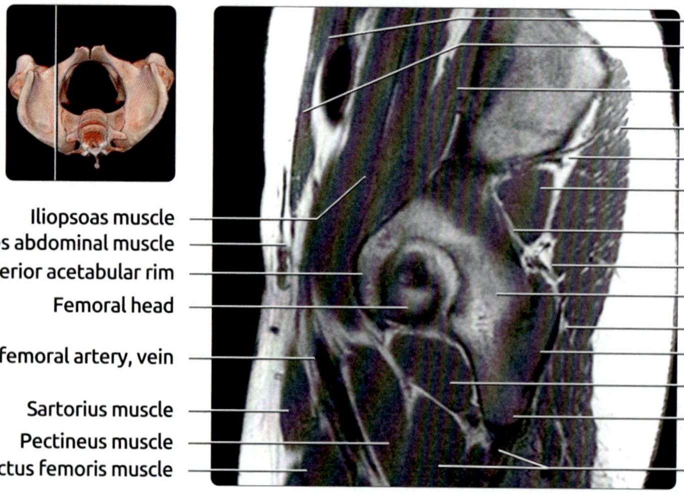

Top image labels (left): Aponeuroses abdominal muscle; Inguinal ligament; Iliopectineal junction; Common femoral artery, vein; Pectineus muscle; Adductor magnus muscle; Sartorius muscle; Adductor brevis muscle

Top image labels (right): Transverse abdominis muscle; Posterior superior iliac spine; Internal oblique muscle; Gluteus maximus muscle; Piriformis muscle; Iliopsoas muscle; Sciatic nerve; Inferior gluteal artery, vein; Sacrotuberous ligament; Obturator internus muscle; Obturator externus muscle; Ischial tuberosity; Adductor magnus muscle

Middle image labels (left): Aponeuroses abdominal muscle; Anterior acetabular rim; Common femoral artery, vein; Pectineus muscle; Sartorius muscle; Adductor brevis muscle

Middle image labels (right): Transverse abdominis muscle; Posterior superior iliac spine; Internal oblique muscle; Gluteus maximus muscle; Posterior inferior iliac spine; Iliopsoas muscle; Piriformis muscle; Sciatic nerve; Inferior gluteal artery, vein; Sacrotuberous ligament; Obturator internus muscle; Obturator externus muscle; Ischial tuberosity; Adductor magnus muscle

Bottom image labels (left): Iliopsoas muscle; Aponeuroses abdominal muscle; Anterior acetabular rim; Femoral head; Common femoral artery, vein; Sartorius muscle; Pectineus muscle; Rectus femoris muscle

Bottom image labels (right): Transverse abdominis muscle; Internal oblique muscle; Iliacus muscle; Gluteus maximus muscle; Superior gluteal artery, vein; Piriformis muscle; Sciatic nerve; Inferior gluteal artery, vein; Ischium; Sacrotuberous ligament; Obturator internus muscle; Obturator externus muscle; Ischial tuberosity; Adductor magnus muscle

(Top) *A long segment of the inferior aspect of the sacrotuberous ligament as it attaches to the ischial tuberosity is nicely demonstrated. A long segment of the sciatic nerve on the deep surface of the piriformis muscle is also visible. The inferior gluteal vessels are located just medial to the sciatic nerve.* **(Middle)** *The posterior superior and inferior iliac spines are apparent. The inferior iliac spine marks the superior aspect of the greater sciatic notch.* **(Bottom)** *The superior gluteal vessels exit the pelvis through the greater sciatic notch above the superior border of the piriformis muscle. The sciatic nerve and inferior gluteal vessels exit inferiorly. The sciatic nerve lies along the anterior border of the piriformis muscle.*

Pelvis MR Atlas

SAGITTAL T1 MR, LATERAL PELVIS

Top image labels (left): Transverse abdominis muscle; Gluteus maximus muscle; Superior gluteal artery, vein; Internal oblique muscle; Psoas muscle; Iliacus muscle; Aponeuroses abdominal muscle; Anterior acetabular rim; Femoral head; Common femoral artery, vein; Pectineus muscle; Sartorius muscle; Rectus femoris muscle

Top image labels (right): Piriformis muscle; Inferior gluteal artery, vein; Ischium; Sacrotuberous ligament; Obturator internus muscle; Obturator externus muscle; Ischial tuberosity; Adductor magnus muscle

Middle image labels (left): Gluteus medius muscle; Ilium; Internal oblique muscle; Gluteus maximus muscle; Transverse abdominis muscle; Psoas muscle; Iliacus muscle; Aponeuroses abdominal muscle; Anterior rim; Femoral head; Iliopsoas muscle; Sartorius muscle; Lateral circumflex femoral artery, vein; Pectineus muscle; Rectus femoris muscle

Middle image labels (right): Superior gluteal artery, vein; Piriformis muscle; Inferior gluteal artery, vein; Ischium; Sacrotuberous ligament; Obturator internus muscle; Obturator externus muscle; Ischial tuberosity; Medial circumflex femoral artery, vein; Adductor magnus muscle

Bottom image labels (left): Gluteus medius muscle; External oblique muscle; Internal oblique muscle; Iliacus muscle; Transverse abdominis muscle; Iliopsoas muscle; Aponeuroses abdominal muscle; Anterior rim; Femoral head; Iliopsoas muscle; Sartorius muscle; Lateral circumflex femoral artery, vein; Pectineus muscle; Rectus femoris muscle

Bottom image labels (right): Gluteus maximus muscle; Superior gluteal artery, vein; Piriformis muscle; Sciatic nerve; Ischium; Obturator internus muscle; Obturator externus muscle; Ischial tuberosity; Medial circumflex femoral artery, vein; Adductor magnus muscle

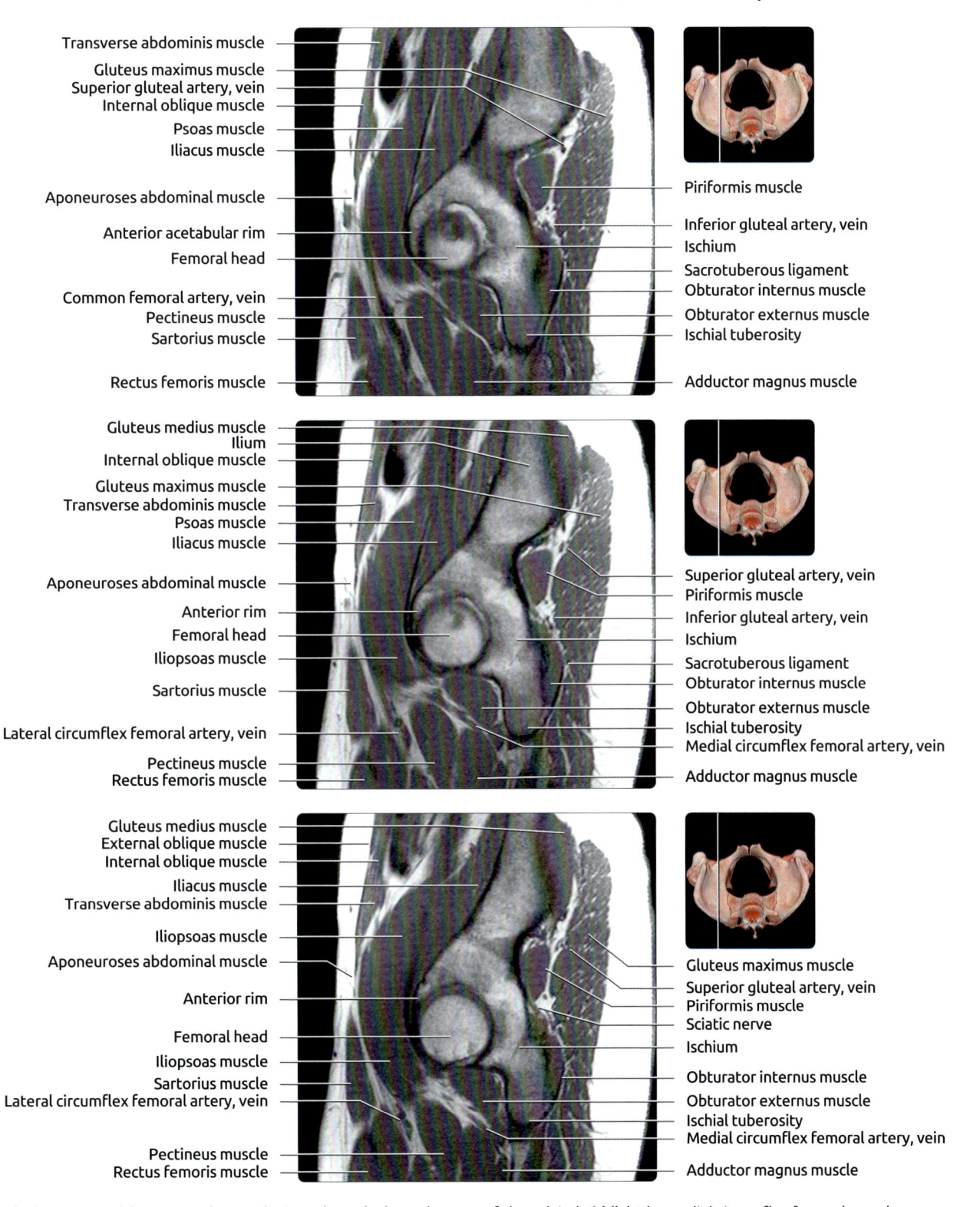

(Top) The psoas and iliacus muscles are distinct along the lateral aspect of the pelvis. (Middle) The medial circumflex femoral vessels are found between the pectineus and iliopsoas muscles while the lateral circumflex femoral vessels are located deep to the sartorius and rectus femoris muscles. (Bottom) The rectus femoris muscle is now visible along the anterior aspect of the thigh. Note the inverted "Y" appearance of the ilium and acetabulum. The stem is the ilium and the anterior limb is the anterior acetabulum and the posterior limb is the posterior column extending from the ilium through the ischium.

SAGITTAL T1 MR, LATERAL PELVIS

Top image labels (left): Internal oblique muscle; Transverse abdominis muscle; Femoral head; Iliopsoas muscle; Sartorius muscle; Lateral circumflex femoral artery, vein; Pectineus muscle; Rectus femoris muscle

Top image labels (right): External oblique muscle; Gluteus medius muscle; Ilium; Gluteus maximus muscle; Iliopsoas muscle; Acetabular roof; Piriformis muscle; Sciatic nerve; External rotators; Obturator internus muscle; Obturator externus muscle; Quadratus femoris muscle; Semimembranosus tendon; Adductor magnus muscle

Middle image labels (left): Iliopsoas muscle; Acetabular roof; Femoral head; Iliopsoas muscle; Sartorius muscle; Lateral circumflex femoral artery, vein; Rectus femoris muscle; Pectineus muscle

Middle image labels (right): External oblique muscle; Gluteus medius muscle; Ilium; Transverse abdominis muscle; Internal oblique muscle; Gluteus maximus muscle; Posterior rim; External rotators; Obturator externus muscle; Semimembranosus tendon; Conjoined origin semitendinous and long head biceps femoris muscle

Bottom image labels (left): Iliopsoas muscle; Acetabular roof; Sartorius muscle; Femoral head; Iliopsoas muscle; Lateral circumflex femoral artery, vein; Lesser trochanter; Rectus femoris muscle

Bottom image labels (right): External oblique muscle; Transverse abdominis muscle; Internal oblique muscle; Gluteus maximus muscle; Gluteus medius muscle; Ilium; Gluteus minimus muscle; Posterior rim; External rotators; Obturator externus muscle; Semimembranosus tendon; Quadratus femoris muscle

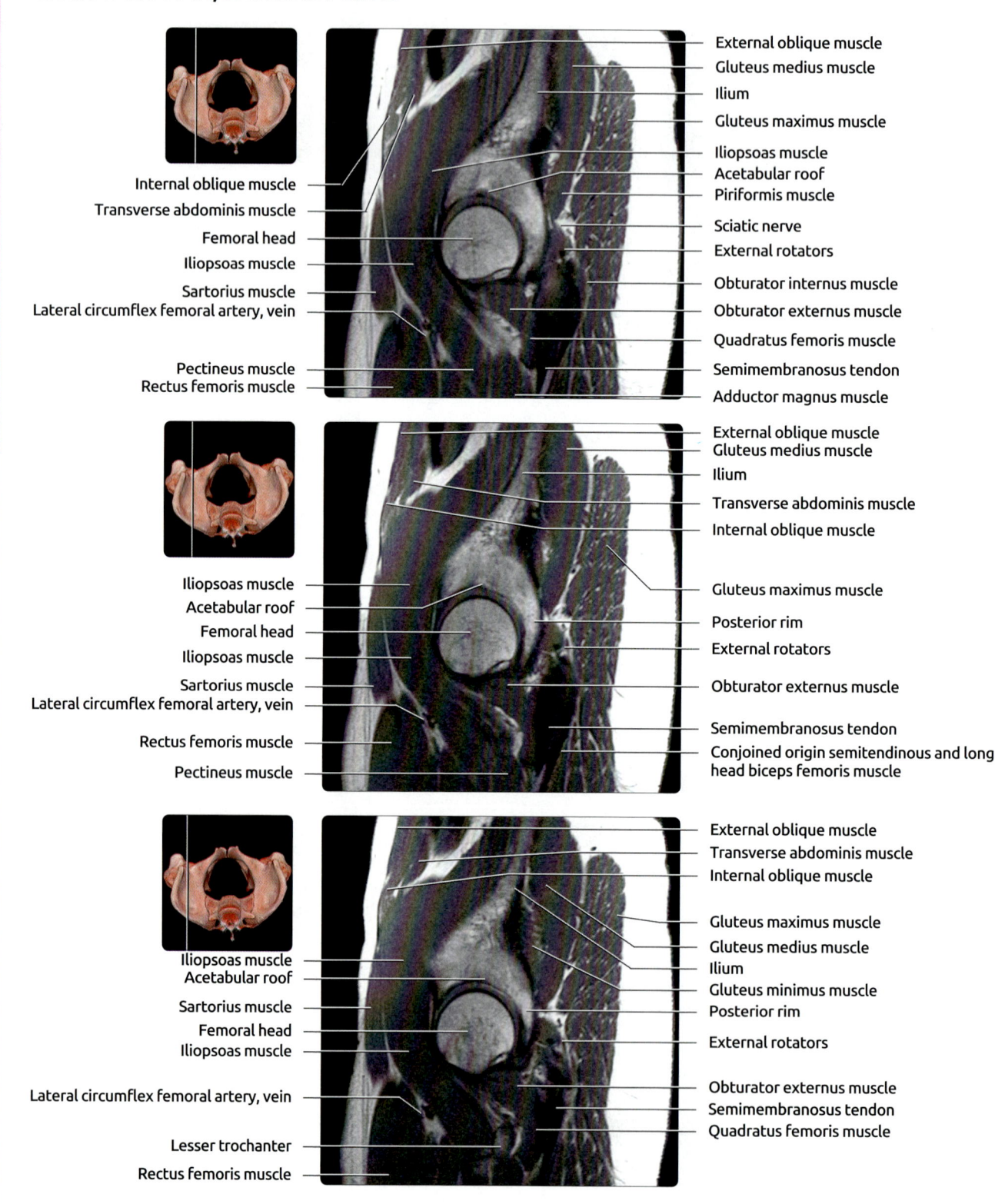

(Top) The external rotators of the hip are present along the posterior surface of the acetabulum. Note also the origin of the semimembranosus from the lateral portion of the ischial tuberosity. **(Middle)** The sciatic nerve is not identifiable as a separate structure due to its close approximation to the external rotators of the hip. The conjoined origin of the semitendinosus and long head of the biceps femoris muscles takes origin from the ischial tuberosity posterior to the semimembranosus muscle origin. The quadratus femoris muscle also originates from the ischial tuberosity. The quadratus femoris muscle is deep to the hamstring tendons. **(Bottom)** The relationship of the gluteal muscles is well seen on sagittal images, and the wide span of the gluteus maximus can be appreciated.

Pelvis MR Atlas

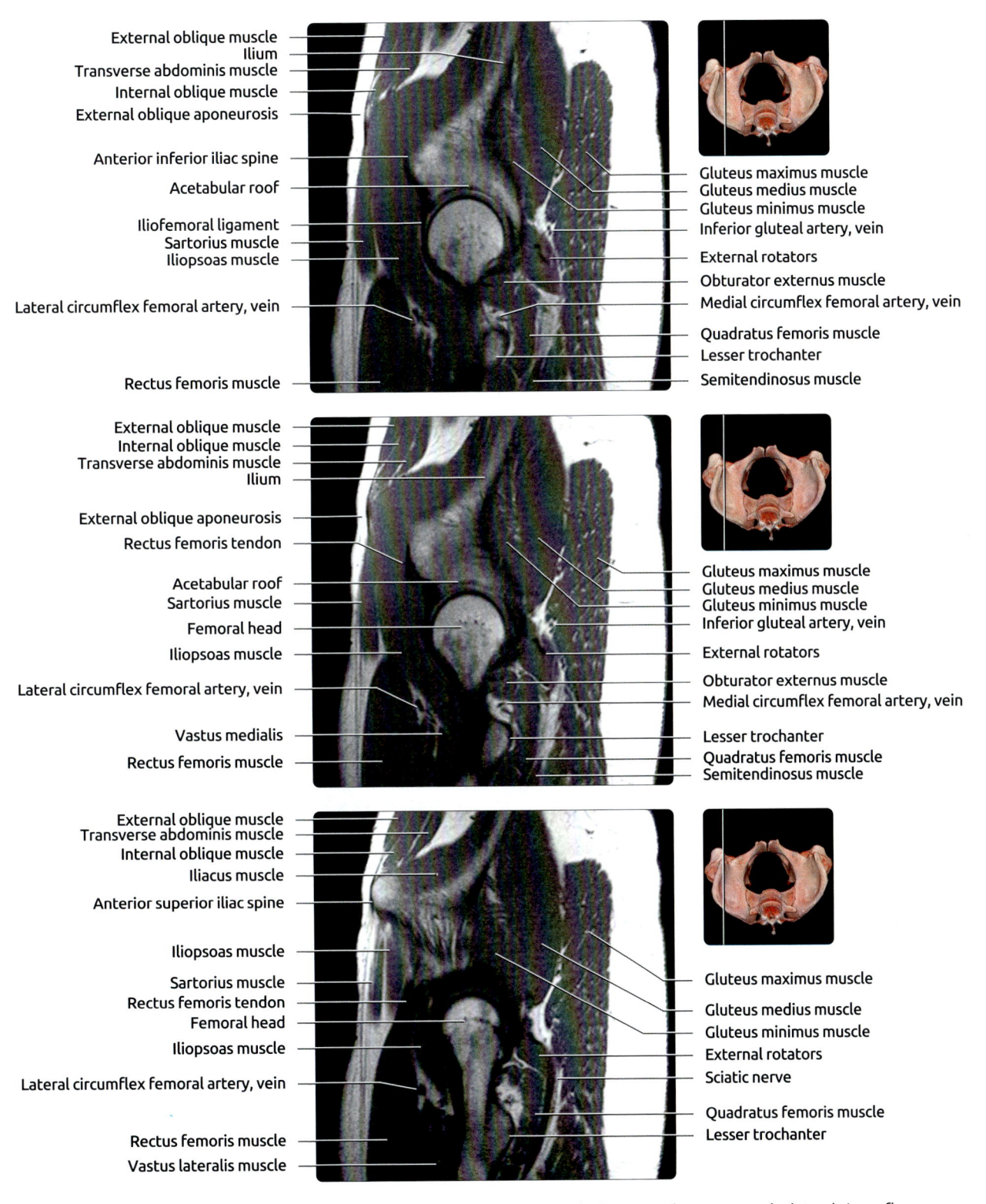

SAGITTAL T1 MR, LATERAL PELVIS

(Top) The Iliopsoas muscle is anterior to the femoral head and neck and inserts on the lesser trochanter. Note the lateral circumflex femoral vessels anterior to the femoral neck, and medial circumflex posterior to the neck. **(Middle)** The rectus femoris muscle originates from the anterior inferior iliac spine. The inferior gluteal vessels are still apparent along the deep surface of the gluteus maximus muscle. Although a discrete nerve is still not discernible, the wisps of tissue adjacent to the inferior gluteal vessels are the sciatic nerve. The inguinal ligament is the most inferior edge of the external oblique aponeurosis. **(Bottom)** The sciatic nerve is seen closely applied to the posterior surface of the quadratus femoris tendon.

Anterior Pelvis

IMAGING ANATOMY

Osseous Anatomy

- **Pubic bone consists of body plus superior and inferior rami**
- Bodies of pubic bones articulate at symphysis pubis
- **Superior and inferior rami** extend from pubis
  - Superior pubic ramus extends to acetabulum
  - Inferior pubic ramus merges with ischium
- **Pecten**: Ridge posterior aspect superior pubic body
  - Origin of pectineus muscle (m.)
  - Insertion of conjoined tendon of abdominal wall
- **Pubic crest**: Superior surface anterior aspect pubic body
  - Insertion of transversus abdominis and external oblique muscles
  - Origin of rectus abdominis m.
- **Pubic tubercle**: Small protuberance lateral border pubic crest
  - Attachment of inguinal ligament
- **Pubic arch**: Undersurface of ischiopubic (inferior) rami
- **Pubic angle**: Between ischiopubic (inferior) rami
  - Major differential feature between male and female pelvis
  - Wider (near 90°) in women

Symphysis Pubis

- Synovial joint between pubic bodies
- Hyaline cartilage along articular surfaces
- Fibrocartilaginous intraarticular disc
  - 10% of adults have cleft in disc
- Normal joint width 2- 7 mm
- Minimal motion occurs at joint
  - < 2 mm superoinferior motion
  - < 3° rotation
- **Superior pubic ligament**: Bridges joint, attaches to pubic tubercles
- **Inferior pubic ligament (arcuate pubic ligament)**
  - Fibrous arch along inferior margin of joint
  - Blends with articular disc
  - Merges inferiorly with aponeuroses of gracilis, adductor longus muscle
- Anterior pubic ligament
  - Deep layer: Merges with articular disk
  - Superficial layer: Merges with aponeurosis of external oblique and rectus abdominis muscles
- Posterior pubic ligament: Thin, few transverse fibers

Anterior Abdominal Wall Musculature

- All attach to pubic bones
- Muscle function (F): Trunk flexion, side to side bending, rotation; compress abdominal cavity, elevate diaphragm
- Nerve supply (N): Intercostal 7-11, subcostal, iliohypogastric, ilioinguinal
  - **Iliohypogastric nerve (n.)**: Traverses internal oblique m. anterior to anterior superior iliac spine (ASIS), traverses external oblique m. above superficial inguinal ring
  - **Ilioinguinal n.**: Traverses internal oblique m. adjacent to deep inguinal ring, courses through inguinal canal
- **Rectus abdominis**: Paired, vertically oriented paramedian strap muscles
  - Joined centrally by linea alba
  - Aponeurotic junction of rectus femoris, transverse abdominis, internal and external oblique muscles
  - Muscle origin (O): Superior pubic ramus, pubic crest
  - Muscle Insertion (I): Xiphoid process, costal cartilages 5-7
  - Surrounded by rectus sheath
    - Anterior sheath: Aponeuroses internal oblique, external oblique, transversus abdominis muscles
    - Posterior sheath: Peritoneum
  - Strain of rectus important in causing syndrome of athletic pubalgia
    - Aponeurosis of rectus continuous with anterior pubic fascia, which are continuous with origin of adductor longus
    - Imbalance between these muscles leads to detachment of anterior pubic fascia, strain/tear of adductor longus m.
- **External oblique**: Most superficial
  - O: Ribs 5-12
  - I: Pubic crest, anterior iliac crest, linea alba
  - Inguinal ligament: Lower border of aponeurosis
- **Internal oblique**: Between external oblique, transversus abdominis
  - O: Lateral inguinal ligament, iliac crest, thoracolumbar fascia
  - I: Pecten (conjoined tendon), pubic crest, inferior aspect ribs 10-12, linea alba
    - Insertion lateral to rectus abdominis m.
    - Insertion posterior and medial to superficial inguinal ring
  - Forms roof of inguinal canal
  - Origin anterior to deep inguinal ring
- **Transversus abdominis**: Deepest
  - O: Iliac crest, posterior aspect of lateral inguinal ligament, thoracolumbar fascia
  - I: Pubic crest, pecten (conjoined tendon), linea alba
  - Remains posterior to inguinal canal
  - **Transversalis fascia** along deep surface
- **Conjoined tendon (inguinal falx)**: Conjoined insertion internal oblique and transversus abdominis muscle onto pecten
  - Inconsistently present

Inguinal Ligament

- Thickening at inferior border of external oblique aponeurosis
- Separates lower extremity from pelvis
  - External iliac vessels become femoral vessels once pass beyond ligament
- **Reflected inguinal ligament (l.)**: Fibers of inguinal l. travel beyond pubic tubercle to interdigitate with contralateral external oblique aponeurosis
- **Lacunar ligament**: Deep fibers of inguinal l., arched and posteriorly directed to insert lateral to pubic tubercle
  - Medial wall subinguinal space
- **Pectineal ligament**: Lateral most fibers lacunar l., insert along pecten
- Attachments: ASIS and pubic tubercle
- Fascia lata attaches to inferior border
- **Iliopubic tract**
  - Thickening inferior border transversalis fascia
  - Deep and parallel to inguinal ligament

Anterior Pelvis

Subinguinal Space: Deep to Inguinal L.
- Passageway for femoral vessels and nerve, iliopsoas m. into femoral triangle

Inguinal Canal
- Anterior wall: External oblique aponeurosis and internal oblique m.
- Posterior wall: Transversalis fascia and conjoined tendon
- Roof: Lower border internal oblique m.
- Floor: Iliopubic tract lateral, inguinal ligament midportion, lacunar ligament medial
- Entrance: **Deep inguinal ring**
  - Located midinguinal ligament
  - Opening of evaginated transversalis fascia through which spermatic cord/round ligament pass
- Exit: Superficial inguinal ring
  - **Superficial inguinal ring**: Division of external oblique aponeurosis lateral to pubic tubercle
    - **Lateral crus**: Inserts pubic tubercle
    - **Medial crus**: Inserts pubic crest
    - **Intercrural fibers**: Superficial to canal; run medial crus to lateral crus
- Oblique orientation medial and inferior
  - Obliquity protects against hernia formation
  - Obliquity accounts for changing boundaries from lateral to medial
- Contents: Ilioinguinal nerve; male: Spermatic cord, female: Round ligament; associated vessels
  - Covered by evaginated transversalis fascia

Thigh Adductor Muscles
- **Pectineus m.**: Also flexes hip
  - Most superficial and cranial of hip adductors
  - O: Pubic tubercle, pecten pubis, and iliopectineal eminence
  - I: Posterior femur lateral to lesser trochanter, immediately inferior to iliopsoas t.
  - N: Femoral and accessory obturator nerves
- **Adductor longus m.**: Also flexes, internally rotates hip
  - O: Anterior pubis, below pubic crest, posterior to pectineus
  - I: Middle 1/3 linea aspera of femur
  - N: Obturator n.
- **Adductor brevis m.**
  - O: Anterior pubis and inferior pubic ramus, posterior to adductor longus
  - I: Proximal portion of linea aspera of femur
  - N: Obturator n.
- **Adductor magnus m.**: Divided into 2 portions
  - **Adductor minimus**: Small, superior and horizontal portion
    - Also called pubofemoral or adductor portion of adductor magnus
    - O: Inferior pubic ramus
    - I: Superior portion linea aspera of femur, medial to gluteus maximus
    - N: Obturator n. (posterior branch)
  - **Ischiocondylar (hamstring) portion**
    - O: Ischial tuberosity
    - I: Extended insertion from linea aspera in midfemur to adductor tubercle above medial femoral condyle
    - N: Tibial n.
- **Gracilis m.**: Also minor function in hip flexion, medial rotation
  - O: Anterior symphysis pubis and inferior pubic ramus
    - Origin medial to adductor brevis m., deep to adductor longus m.
  - I: Medial tibia as part of pes anserinus
  - N: Obturator n.

ANATOMY IMAGING ISSUES

Imaging Recommendations
- Oblique imaging helpful to separate muscles and explicate findings in athletic pubalgia

Imaging Pitfalls
- Adductor muscles can be difficult to separate on coronal images due to their varying obliquities

Sports Hernia
- Term superseded by more accurate concept of athletic pubalgia

Inguinal Hernias
- Exit superficial inguinal ring medial and superior to pubic tubercle
- **Direct inguinal hernia** from weak posterior inguinal wall
  - Medial to inferior epigastric artery (a.)
  - Lateral to spermatic cord
  - Not in deep inguinal ring
  - No preformed sac
  - Transversalis fascia covers
- **Indirect inguinal hernia** through patent processus vaginalis into deep inguinal ring
  - **Processus vaginalis**: Peritoneal diverticulum that follows descending testes, usually closes off
  - Lateral to inferior epigastric a.
  - Within spermatic cord
  - More common overall
  - More common in men
  - May enter scrotum/labia
- **Osteitis pubis**
  - Irregular, eroded bone contour of pubic symphysis
  - Consider: Athletic pubalgia, mulitparity, infection

Anterior Pelvis

SYMPHYSIS PUBIS

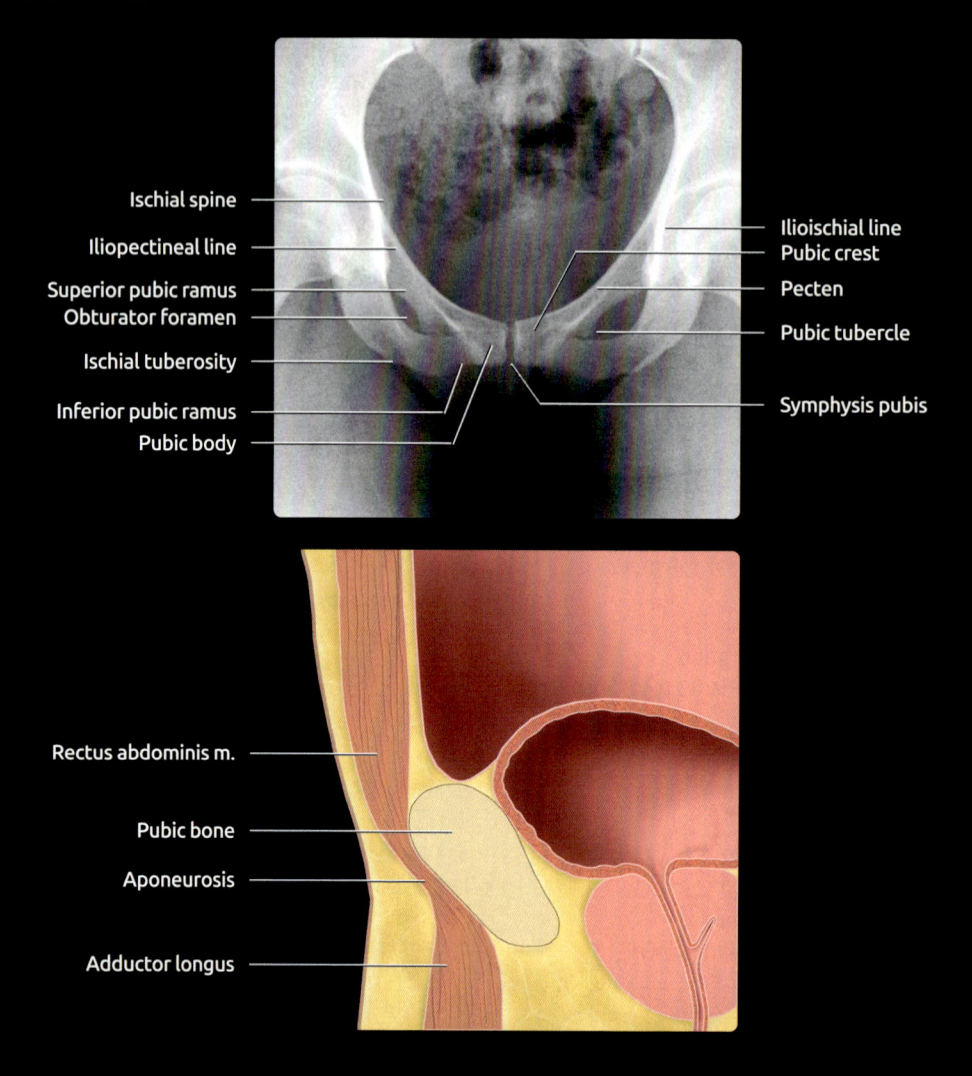

Ischial spine
Iliopectineal line
Superior pubic ramus
Obturator foramen
Ischial tuberosity
Inferior pubic ramus
Pubic body

Ilioischial line
Pubic crest
Pecten
Pubic tubercle
Symphysis pubis

Rectus abdominis m.
Pubic bone
Aponeurosis
Adductor longus

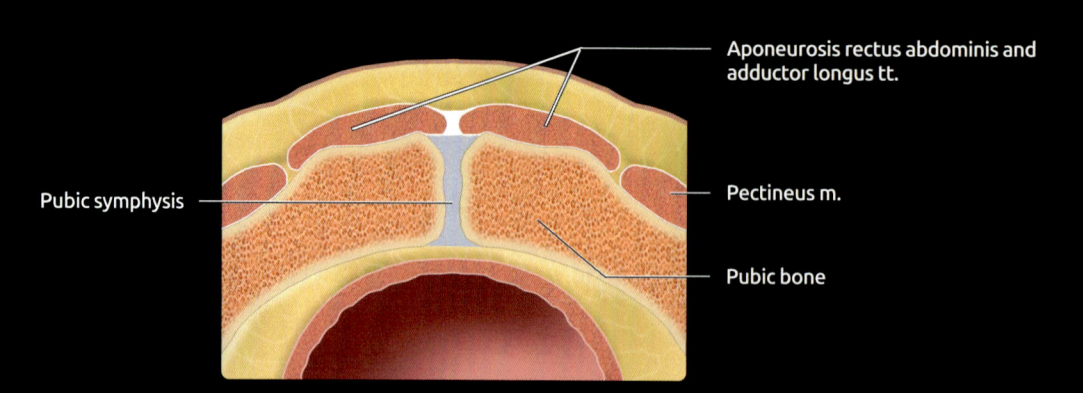

Aponeurosis rectus abdominis and adductor longus tt.
Pubic symphysis
Pectineus m.
Pubic bone

(**Top**) *AP radiograph coned down to the anterior pelvis is shown. The symphysis pubis and the different regions of the pubic body and the pubic rami are evident.* (**Middle**) *Sagittal graphic shows the relationship between the rectus abdominis and the adductor longus tendons via the aponeurosis, a fascial sheet at the anterior margin of the pubic bone. The aponeurosis is thinner than shown in this illustration. It is readily visible how asymmetric stress between the 2 muscles can result in detachment of the aponeurosis in the syndrome known as athletic pubalgia.* (**Bottom**) *Axial graphic shows the aponeurosis shared by the rectus abdominis and adductor longus tendons. Pectineus lies immediately lateral to the aponeurosis, originating from the anterior as well as the superior margin of the pubic bone.*

Anterior Pelvis

AXIAL T1 MR, SYMPHYSIS PUBIS AND ADDUCTORS

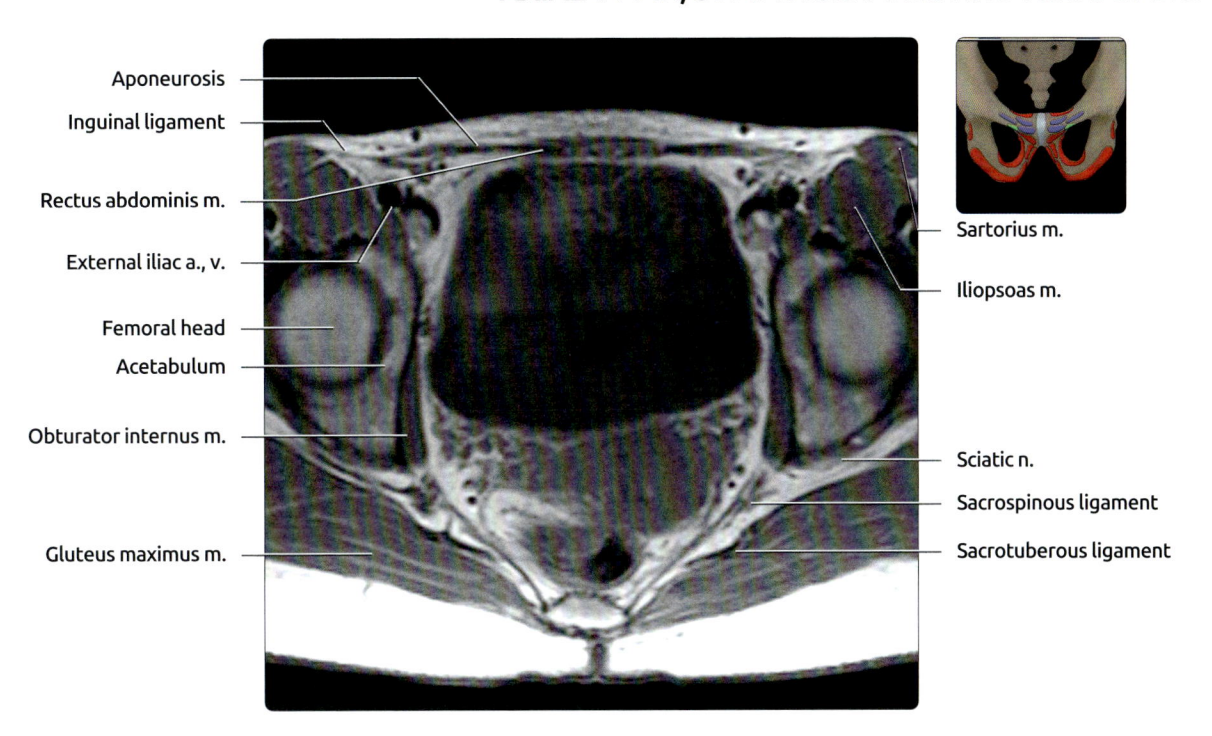

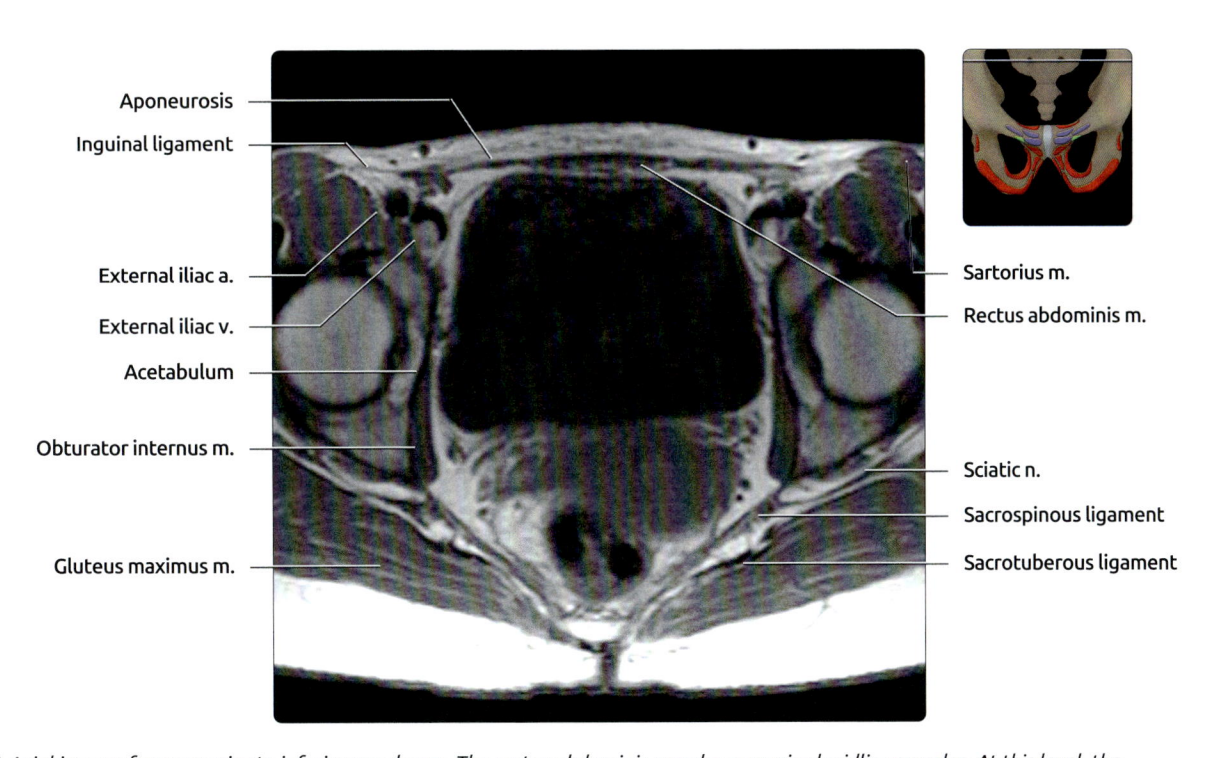

Top image labels:
- Aponeurosis
- Inguinal ligament
- Rectus abdominis m.
- External iliac a., v.
- Femoral head
- Acetabulum
- Obturator internus m.
- Gluteus maximus m.
- Sartorius m.
- Iliopsoas m.
- Sciatic n.
- Sacrospinous ligament
- Sacrotuberous ligament

Bottom image labels:
- Aponeurosis
- Inguinal ligament
- External iliac a.
- External iliac v.
- Acetabulum
- Obturator internus m.
- Gluteus maximus m.
- Sartorius m.
- Rectus abdominis m.
- Sciatic n.
- Sacrospinous ligament
- Sacrotuberous ligament

(Top) *Axial images from superior to inferior are shown. The rectus abdominis muscles are paired midline muscles. At this level, the external and internal abdominal oblique and transversus muscle bellies are no longer visible. The aponeuroses of these muscles have joined together.* **(Bottom)** *The inguinal ligament is the inferior border of the external oblique aponeurosis. Its orientation is from superolateral to inferomedial. On axial images, it is seen along the lateral edge of the fused aponeuroses.*

Anterior Pelvis

AXIAL T1 MR, SYMPHYSIS PUBIS AND ADDUCTORS

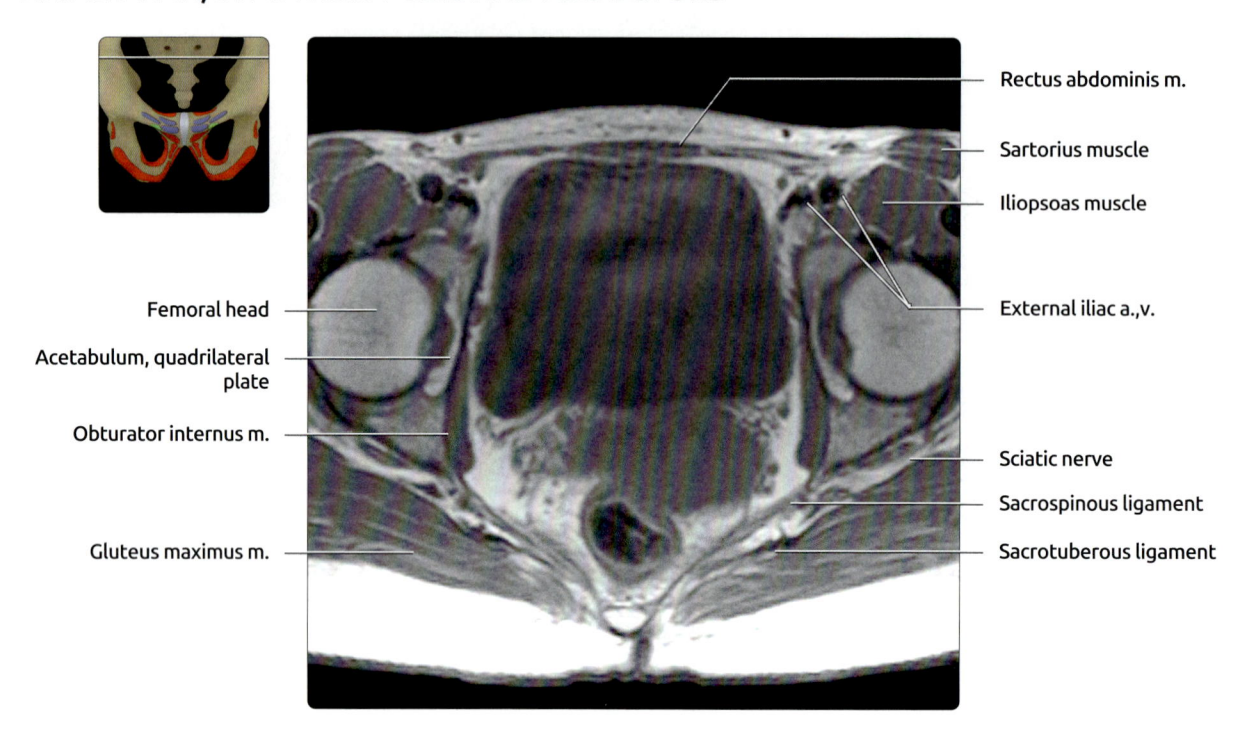

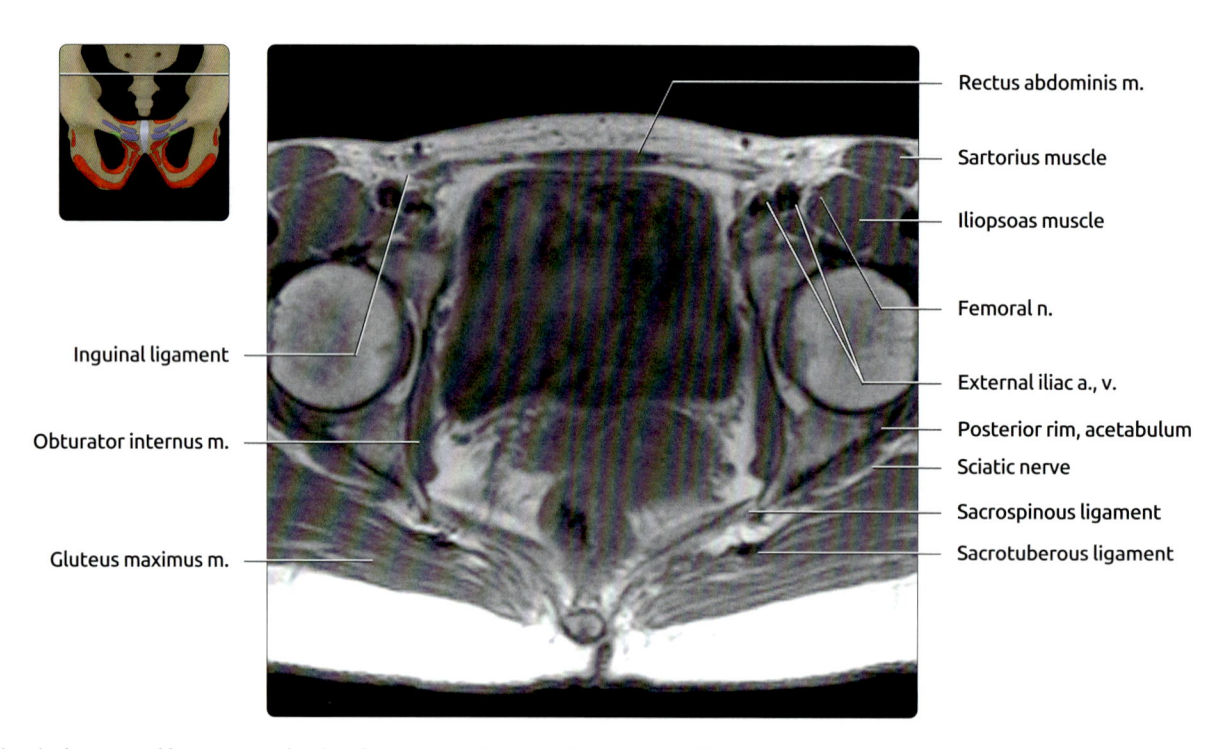

(Top) The inguinal ligament is a landmark separating the pelvis from thigh. In the axial plane, the structures lateral to the ligament are within the thigh. The structures medial and deep are within the pelvis. *(Bottom)* The external iliac vessels are deep to the inguinal ligament.

Anterior Pelvis

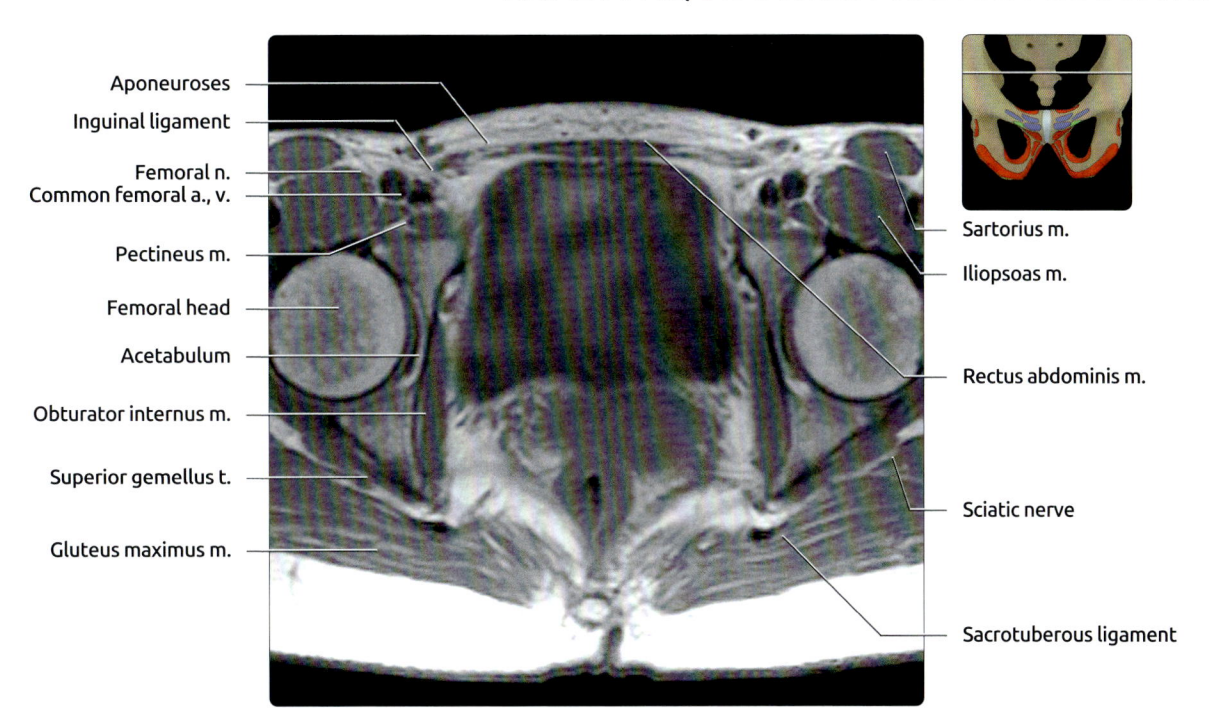

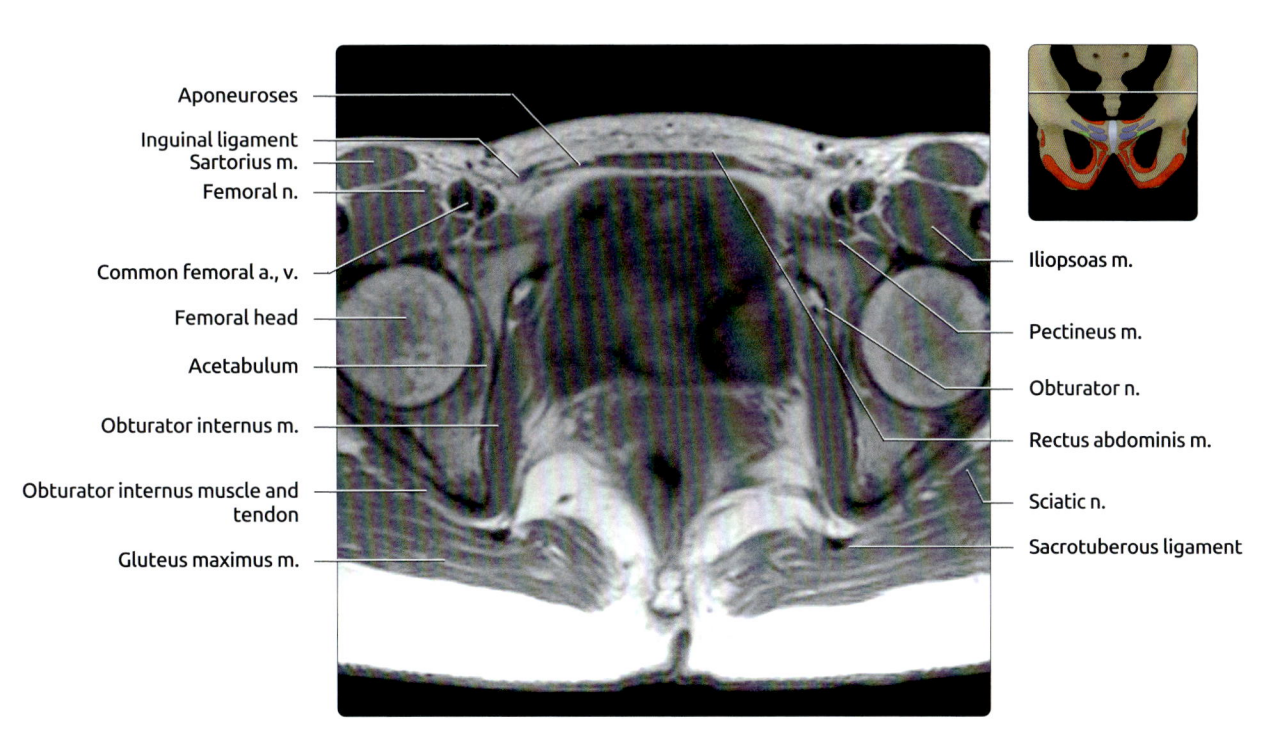

AXIAL T1 MR, SYMPHYSIS PUBIS AND ADDUCTORS

Labels (top image):
- Aponeuroses
- Inguinal ligament
- Femoral n.
- Common femoral a., v.
- Pectineus m.
- Femoral head
- Acetabulum
- Obturator internus m.
- Superior gemellus t.
- Gluteus maximus m.
- Sartorius m.
- Iliopsoas m.
- Rectus abdominis m.
- Sciatic nerve
- Sacrotuberous ligament

Labels (bottom image):
- Aponeuroses
- Inguinal ligament
- Sartorius m.
- Femoral n.
- Common femoral a., v.
- Femoral head
- Acetabulum
- Obturator internus m.
- Obturator internus muscle and tendon
- Gluteus maximus m.
- Iliopsoas m.
- Pectineus m.
- Obturator n.
- Rectus abdominis m.
- Sciatic n.
- Sacrotuberous ligament

(**Top**) *As the vessels pass by the inguinal ligament, they become the common femoral vessels of the thigh.* (**Bottom**) *The femoral vessels are now located within the femoral triangle. The femoral nerve is on the medial surface of iliopsoas and approaches the artery.*

Anterior Pelvis

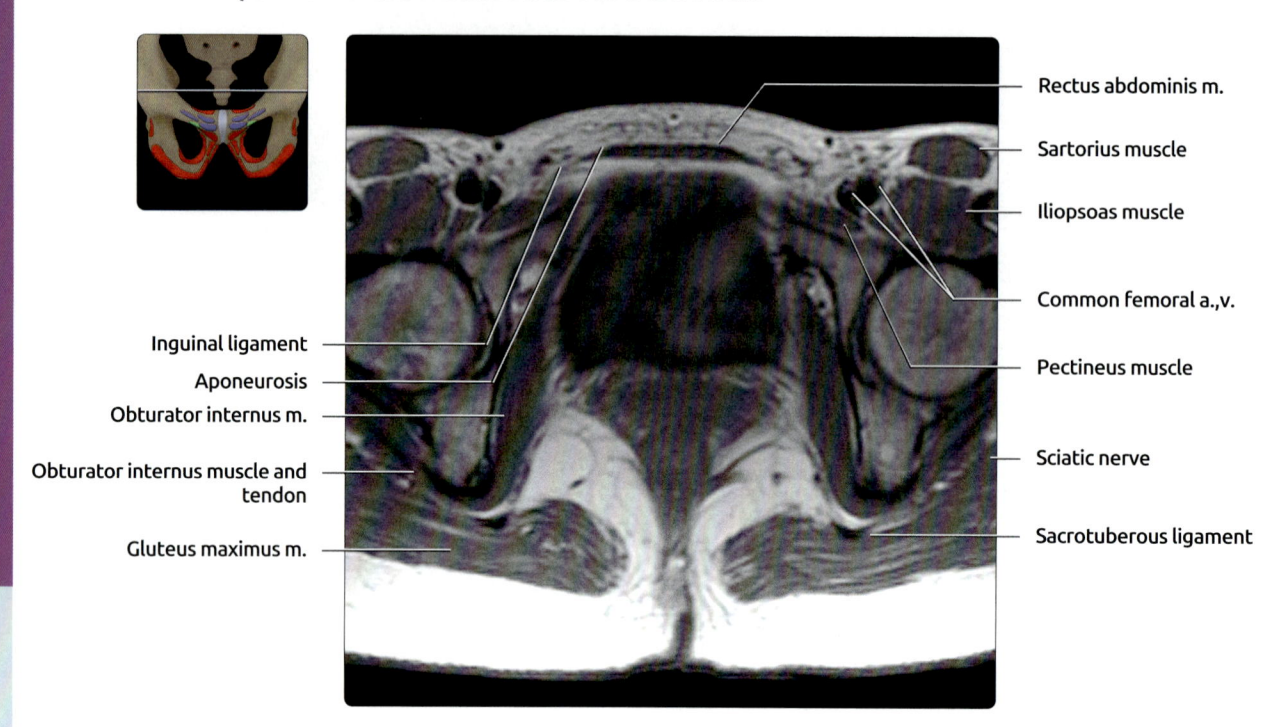

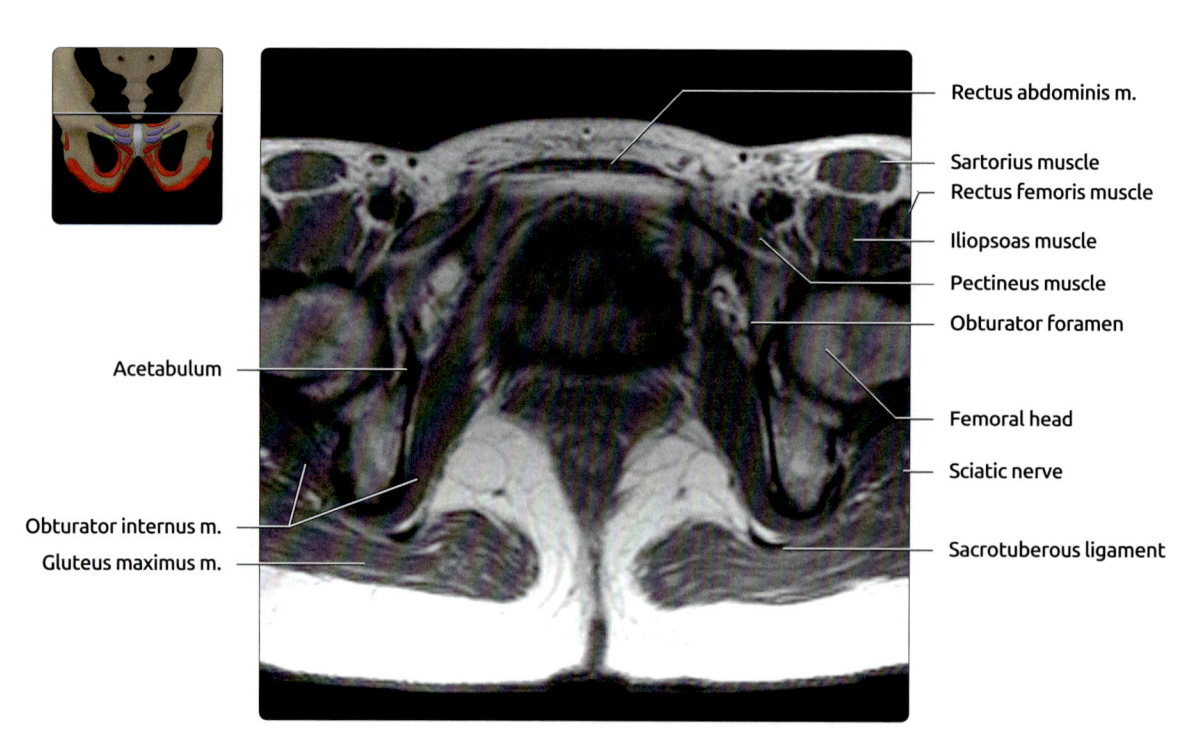

AXIAL T1 MR, SYMPHYSIS PUBIS AND ADDUCTORS

(Top) The pectineus origin from the pecten of the superior pubic ramus is the most superior of the adductor muscle origins. The muscle wraps around the superior and anterior surface of the superior pubic ramus. *(Bottom)* The obturator foramen is visible along the anterior aspect of the pelvis. Its contents are the obturator vessels and nerve.

Anterior Pelvis

AXIAL T1 MR, SYMPHYSIS PUBIS AND ADDUCTORS

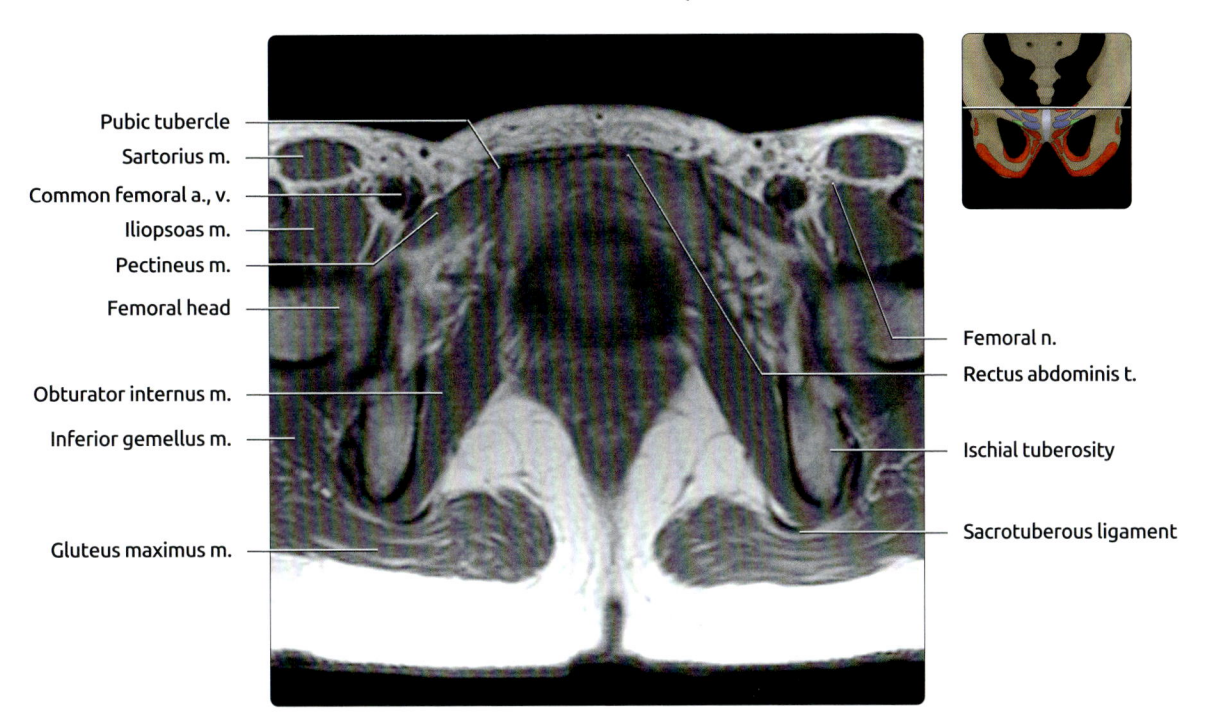

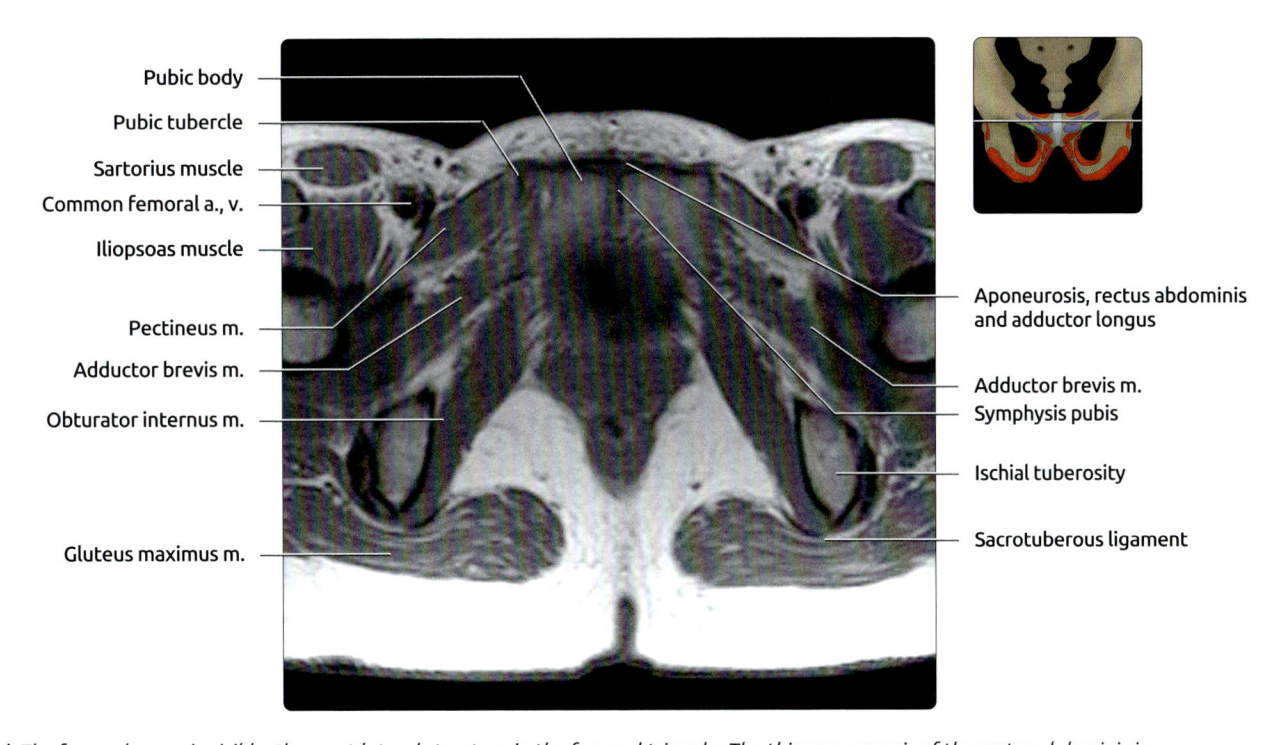

Labels (top image):
- Pubic tubercle
- Sartorius m.
- Common femoral a., v.
- Iliopsoas m.
- Pectineus m.
- Femoral head
- Obturator internus m.
- Inferior gemellus m.
- Gluteus maximus m.
- Femoral n.
- Rectus abdominis t.
- Ischial tuberosity
- Sacrotuberous ligament

Labels (bottom image):
- Pubic body
- Pubic tubercle
- Sartorius muscle
- Common femoral a., v.
- Iliopsoas muscle
- Pectineus m.
- Adductor brevis m.
- Obturator internus m.
- Gluteus maximus m.
- Aponeurosis, rectus abdominis and adductor longus
- Adductor brevis m.
- Symphysis pubis
- Ischial tuberosity
- Sacrotuberous ligament

(**Top**) The femoral nerve is visible, the most lateral structure in the femoral triangle. The thin aponeurosis of the rectus abdominis is seen along the anterior margin of the pubic bone. (**Bottom**) The protrusion of the pubic tubercle from the anterior surface of pubic body is apparent. This tubercle is the site of the medial attachment of the inguinal ligament.

Anterior Pelvis

AXIAL T1 MR, SYMPHYSIS PUBIS AND ADDUCTORS

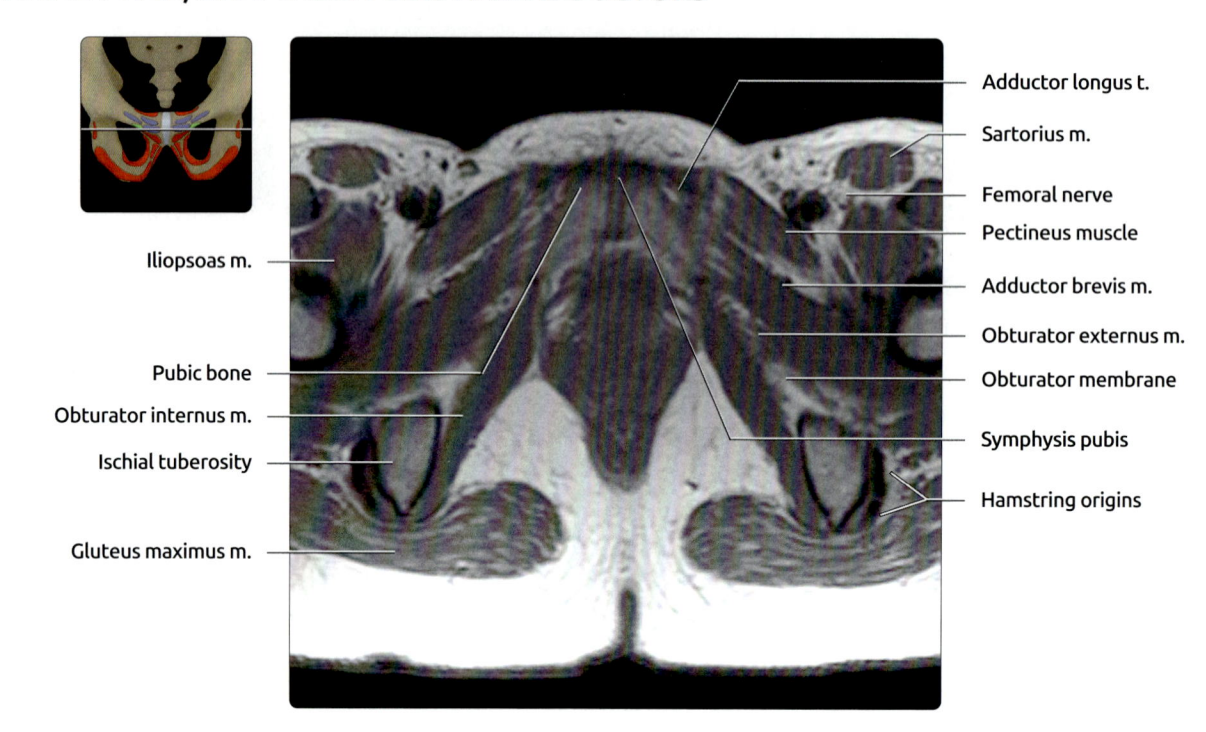

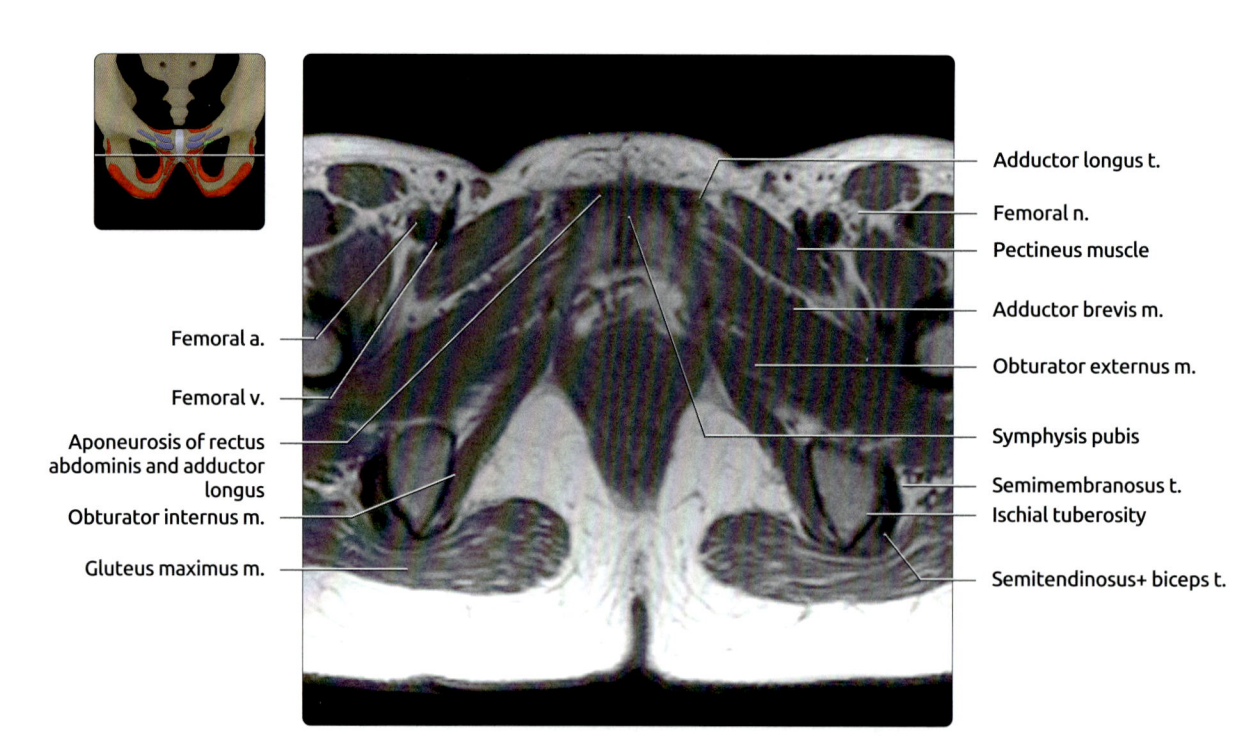

(Top) The origin of the obturator externus muscle includes the obturator membrane. Its origin from the pubic margin of the foramen is readily appreciated. *(Bottom)* The adductor longus muscle originates via a long tendon from a small region of the anterior pubic body inferior to the pubic crest. The conjoined aponeurosis of the rectus abdominis and adductor longus forms a low signal intensity band along the anterior margin of the pubic bones.

Anterior Pelvis

AXIAL T1 MR, SYMPHYSIS PUBIS AND ADDUCTORS

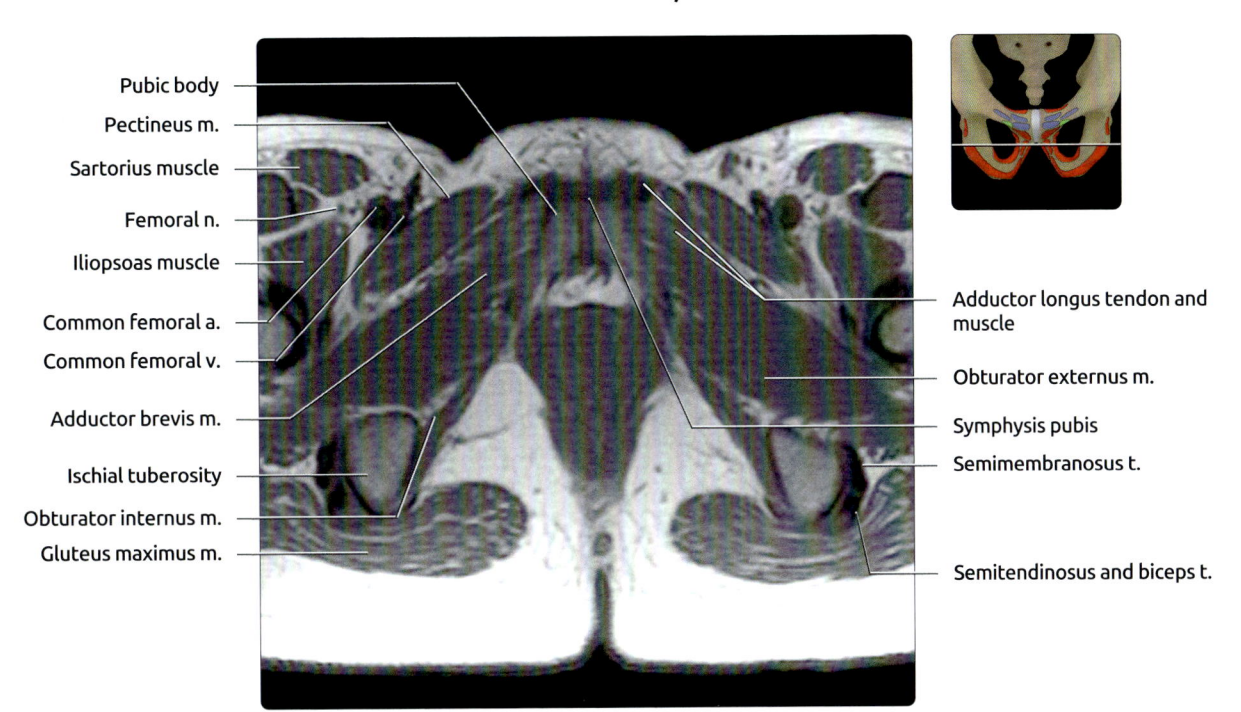

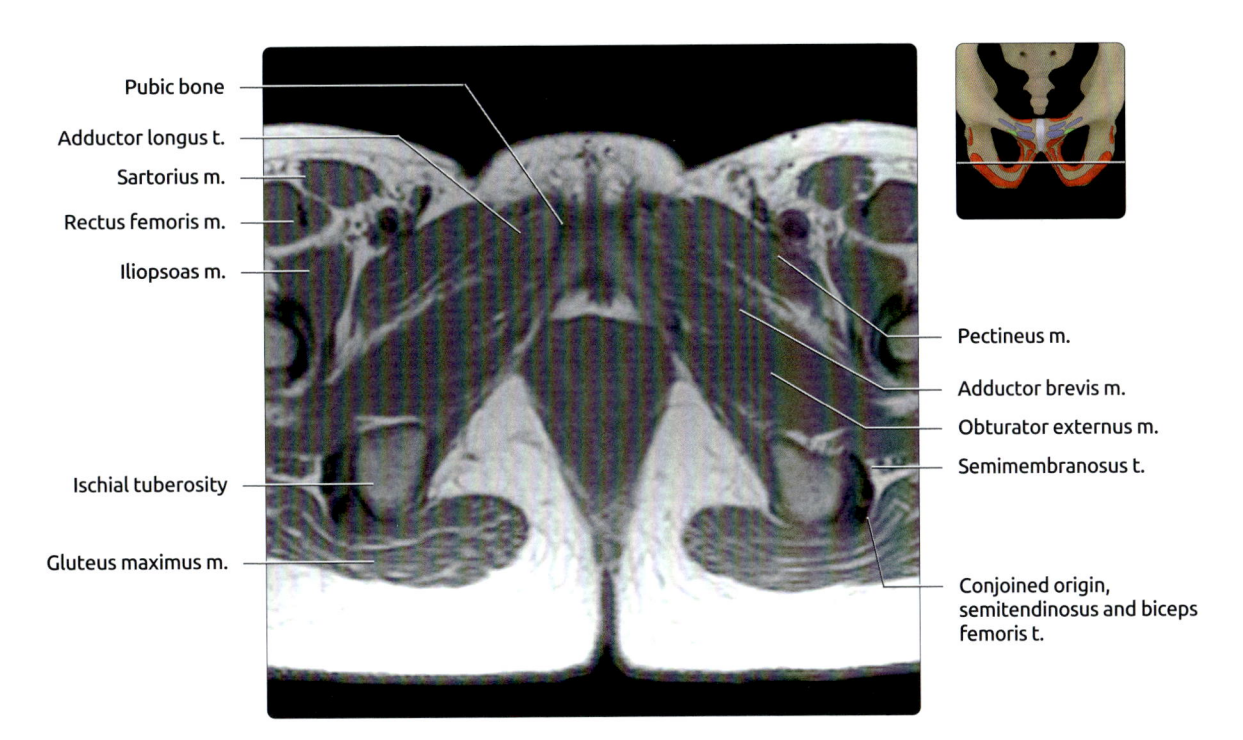

Top image labels:
- Pubic body
- Pectineus m.
- Sartorius muscle
- Femoral n.
- Iliopsoas muscle
- Common femoral a.
- Common femoral v.
- Adductor brevis m.
- Ischial tuberosity
- Obturator internus m.
- Gluteus maximus m.
- Adductor longus tendon and muscle
- Obturator externus m.
- Symphysis pubis
- Semimembranosus t.
- Semitendinosus and biceps t.

Bottom image labels:
- Pubic bone
- Adductor longus t.
- Sartorius m.
- Rectus femoris m.
- Iliopsoas m.
- Ischial tuberosity
- Gluteus maximus m.
- Pectineus m.
- Adductor brevis m.
- Obturator externus m.
- Semimembranosus t.
- Conjoined origin, semitendinosus and biceps femoris t.

(Top) The origin of the adductor brevis muscle is from the anterior surface of the inferior pubic ramus just distal to the symphysis pubis. The adductor brevis muscle is located deep and lateral to the adductor longus muscle. (Bottom) The adductor brevis muscle is located anterior to the obturator externus muscle and on axial images may be difficult to separate from that muscle.

Anterior Pelvis

AXIAL T1 MR, SYMPHYSIS PUBIS AND ADDUCTORS

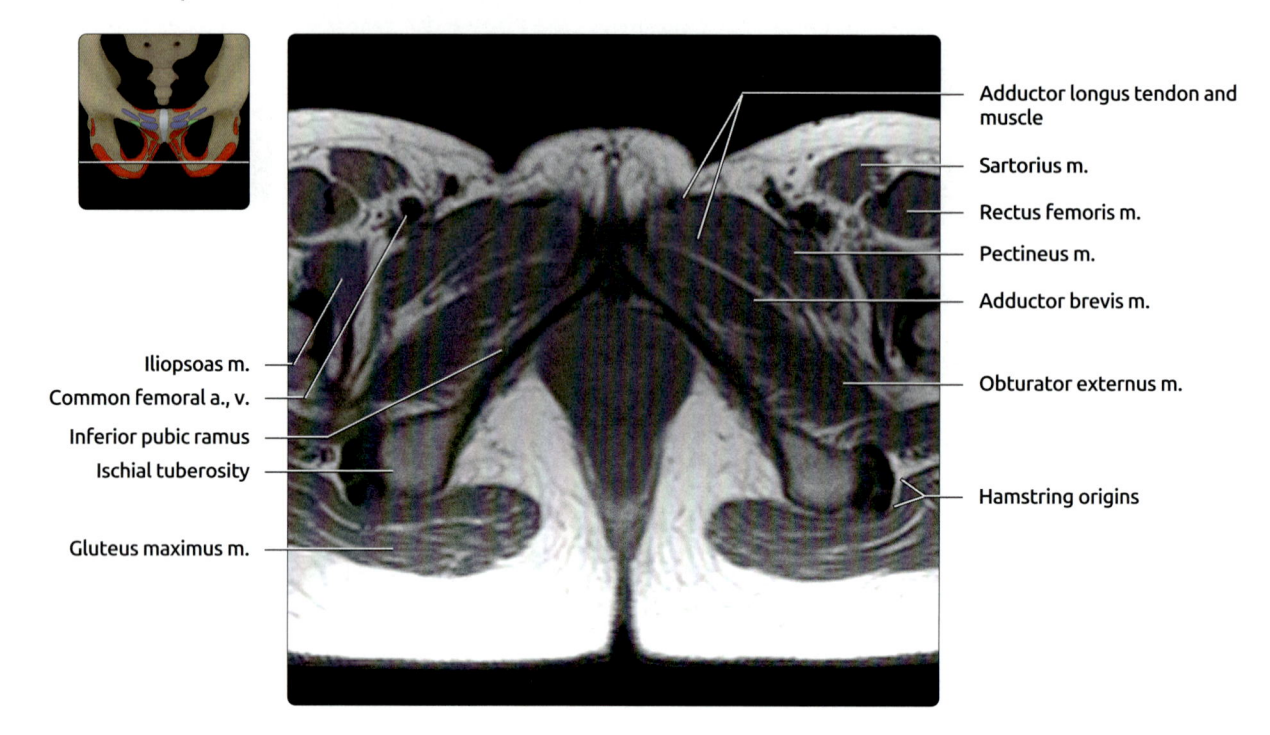

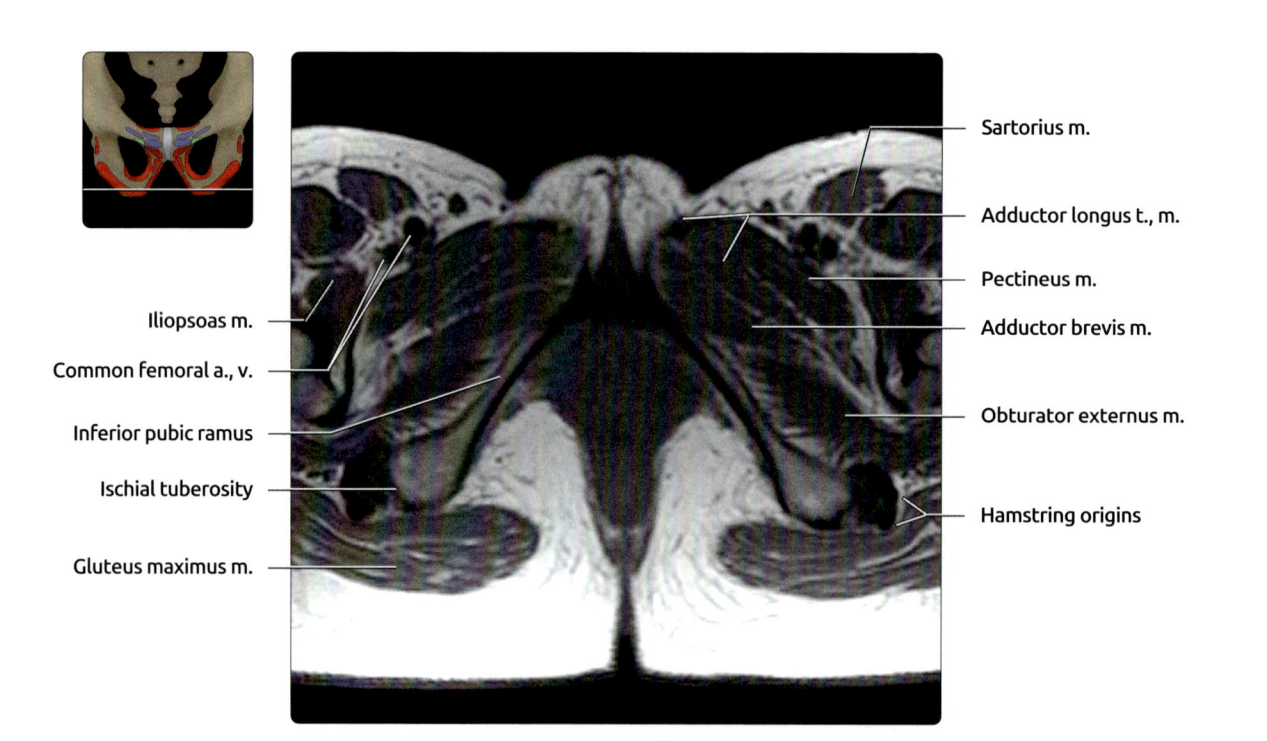

(Top) From anterior to posterior in the upper thigh, the adductor muscles are pectineus, adductor longus, and adductor brevis, respectively. *(Bottom)* In the coronal plane, the pectineus and adductor longus muscles lie in the same plane. Pectineus will insert on the posterior femur, just distal to the iliopsoas insertion.

Anterior Pelvis

CORONAL T1 MR, PUBIS AND ADDUCTORS

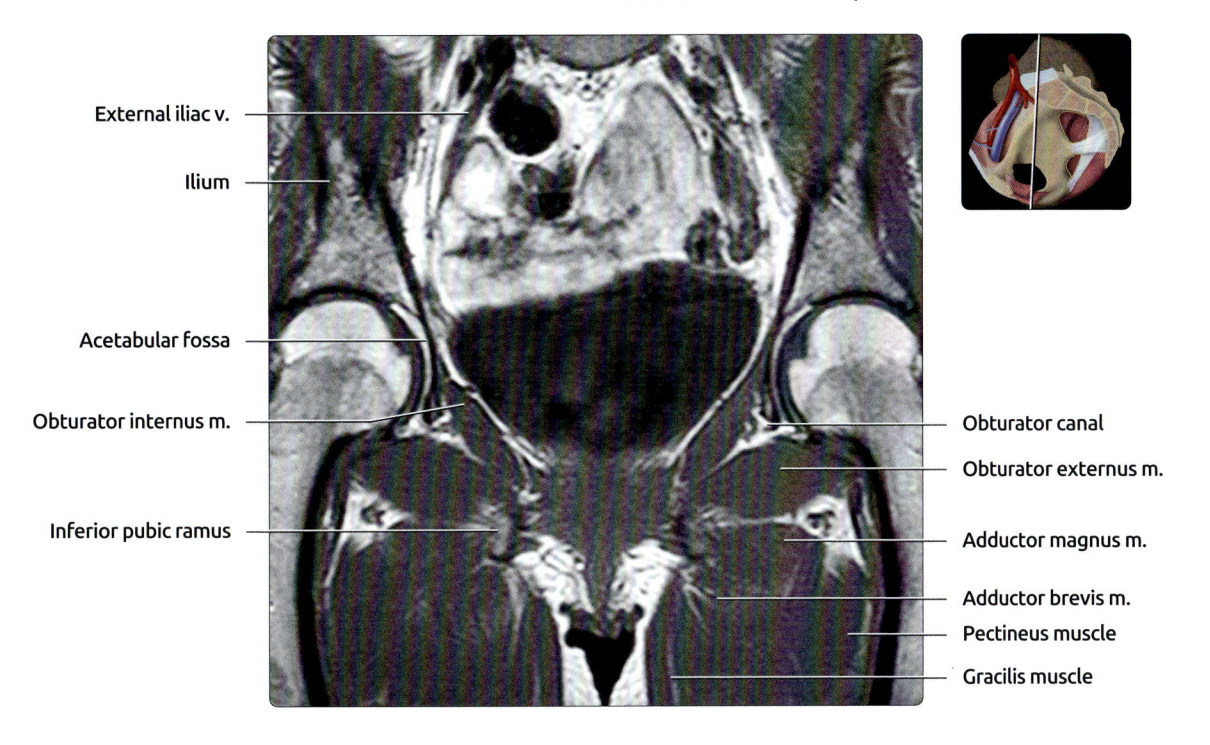

Labels (top image):
- External iliac v.
- Ilium
- Acetabular fossa
- Obturator internus m.
- Inferior pubic ramus
- Obturator canal
- Obturator externus m.
- Adductor magnus m.
- Adductor brevis m.
- Pectineus muscle
- Gracilis muscle

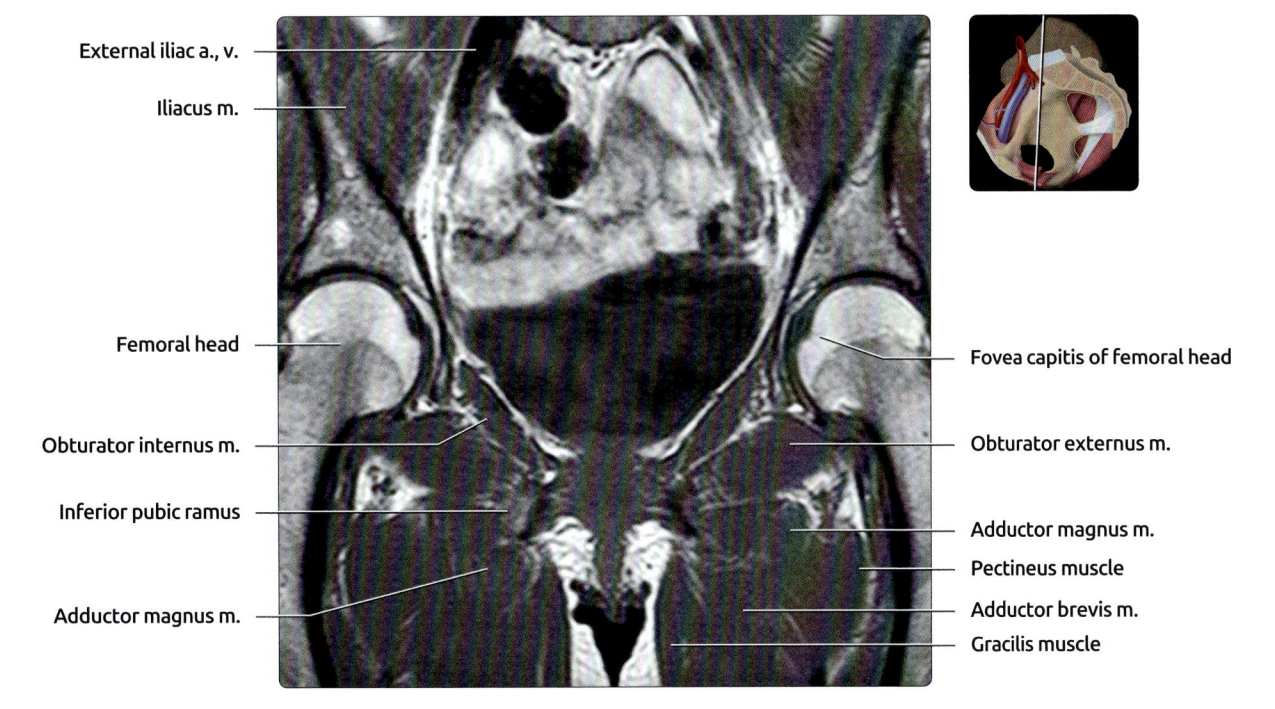

Labels (bottom image):
- External iliac a., v.
- Iliacus m.
- Femoral head
- Obturator internus m.
- Inferior pubic ramus
- Adductor magnus m.
- Fovea capitis of femoral head
- Obturator externus m.
- Adductor magnus m.
- Pectineus muscle
- Adductor brevis m.
- Gracilis muscle

(Top) Coronal images of the anterior pelvis from posterior to anterior are shown. The obturator externus and internus muscles are seen along the inner and outer margins of the foramen. The adductor magnus is the most posterior of the adductor muscles. Its uppermost fibers are horizontally oriented and insert on the proximal femur, medial to the insertion of the gluteus maximus. (Bottom) In the anterior to posterior direction, the adductor brevis muscle is located between the adductor magnus and adductor longus muscle. Therefore these 3 muscles may not be seen in the same coronal image. The adductor brevis fibers travel lateral and inferior.

Anterior Pelvis

CORONAL T1 MR, PUBIS AND ADDUCTORS

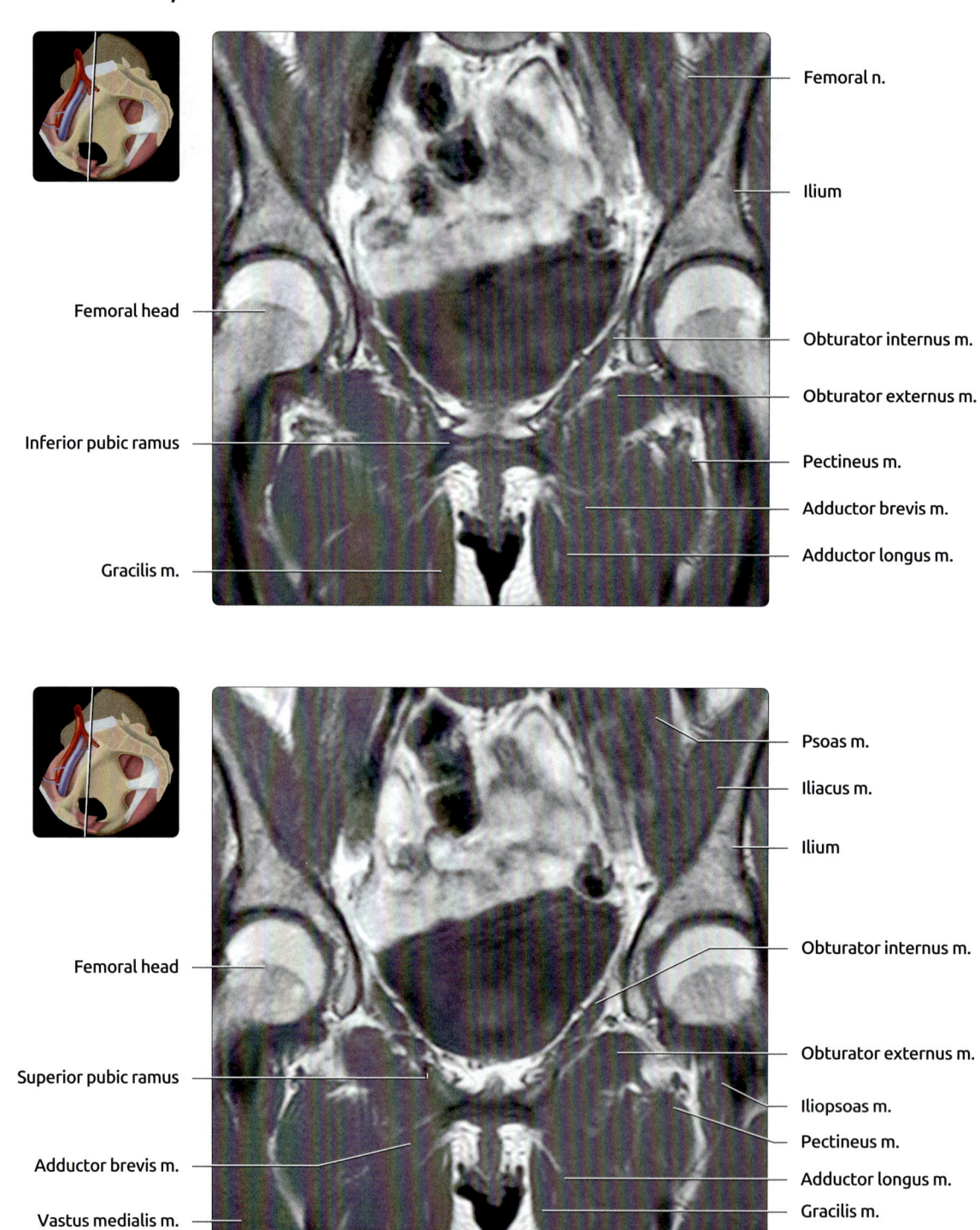

(Top) The femoral nerve lies in the iliopsoas groove between the muscle bellies and does not joint the vessels until it exits the pelvis. It courses lateral to the femoral artery in the femoral triangle. *(Bottom)* The pectineus muscle is located lateral to the adductor longus and brevis muscles. The pectineus muscle has the most medial insertion of these muscles onto the posterior aspect of the femur, inferior to the iliopsoas tendon.

Anterior Pelvis

CORONAL T1 MR, PUBIS AND ADDUCTORS

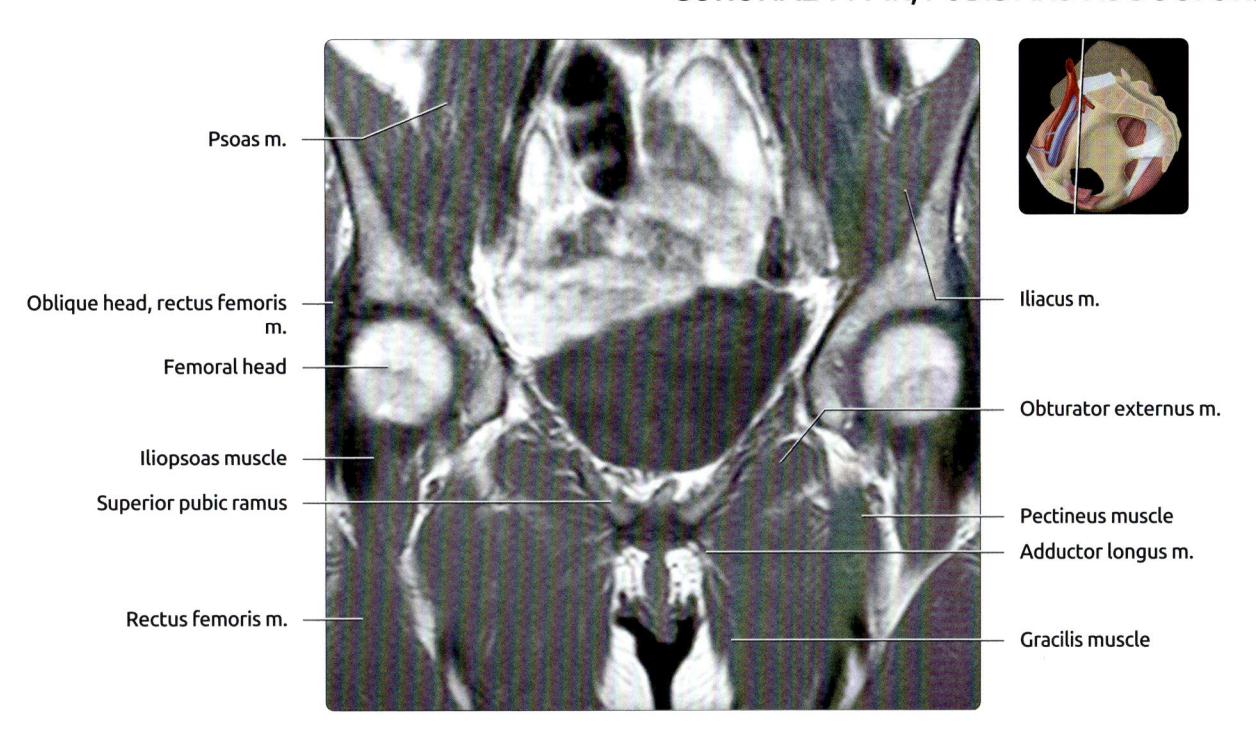

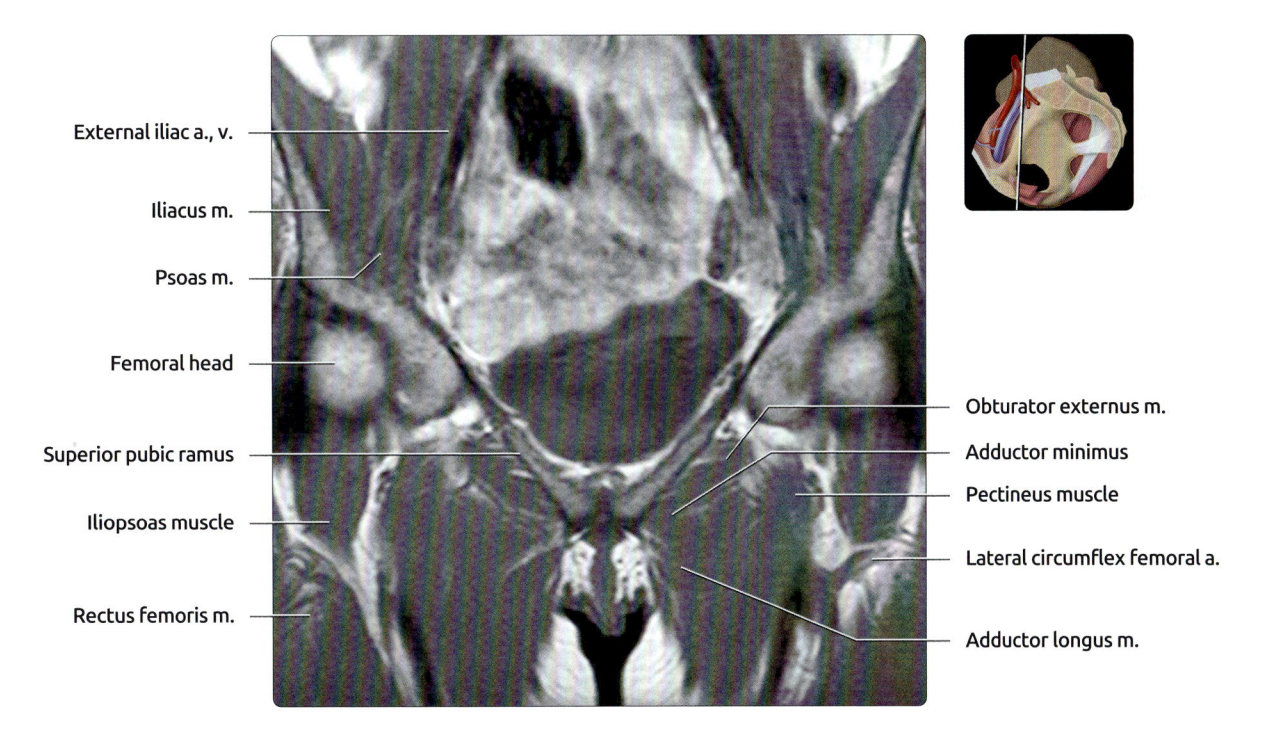

(Top) Recognition of the superior pubic ramus is 1 landmark that will help identify the adductor longus muscle and differentiate it from the adductor brevis muscle. (Bottom) The adductor longus muscle forms the medial border of the femoral triangle. Thus, the vessels may be used as landmarks for differentiation of the adductor longus and brevis muscles in the coronal plane. Adductor minimus is a variant term for the short, horizontal head of the adductor magnus.

Anterior Pelvis

CORONAL T1 MR, PUBIS AND ADDUCTORS

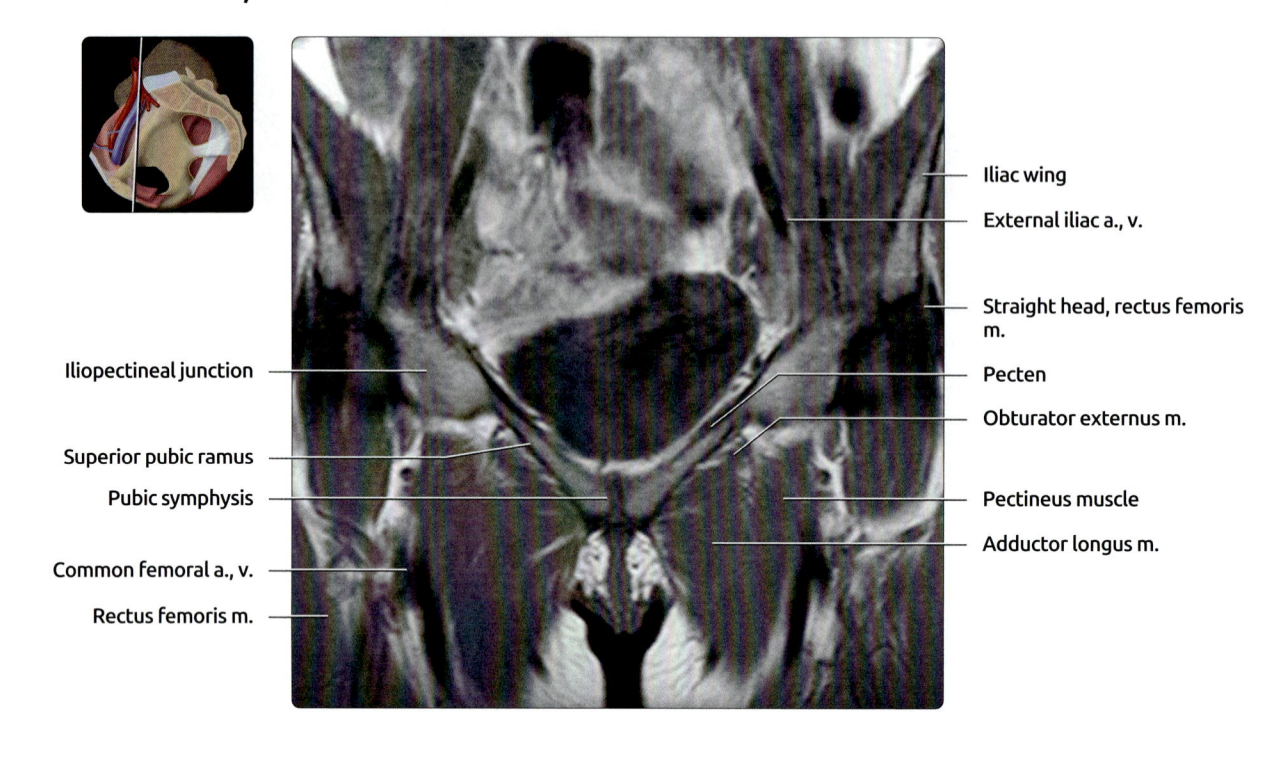

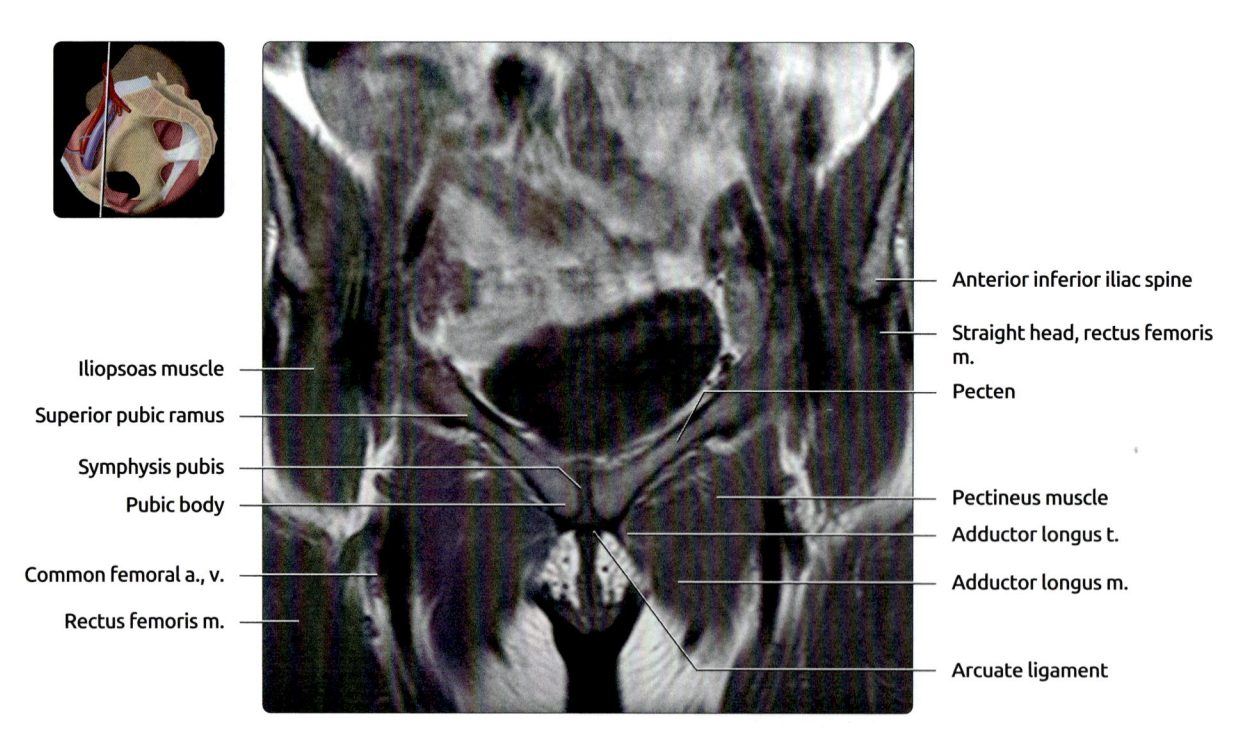

Labels (top image):
- Iliac wing
- External iliac a., v.
- Straight head, rectus femoris m.
- Pecten
- Obturator externus m.
- Pectineus muscle
- Adductor longus m.
- Iliopectineal junction
- Superior pubic ramus
- Pubic symphysis
- Common femoral a., v.
- Rectus femoris m.

Labels (bottom image):
- Anterior inferior iliac spine
- Straight head, rectus femoris m.
- Pecten
- Pectineus muscle
- Adductor longus t.
- Adductor longus m.
- Arcuate ligament
- Iliopsoas muscle
- Superior pubic ramus
- Symphysis pubis
- Pubic body
- Common femoral a., v.
- Rectus femoris m.

(Top) The arcuate ligament is a relatively thick structure that helps to reinforce the inferior aspect of the symphysis pubis. The ridge along the superior pubic ramus is known as the pecten. **(Bottom)** The adductor longus tendon is seen originating from the aponeurosis along the anterior margin of the pubic bone. The straight head of rectus femoris is seen originating from the anterior inferior iliac spine.

Anterior Pelvis

CORONAL T1 MR, PUBIS AND ADDUCTORS

Labels (top image):
- Iliacus m.
- External iliac a., v.
- Symphysis pubis
- Pubic crest
- Pubic body
- Common femoral a., v.
- Rectus femoris m.
- Greater saphenous v.
- Anterior inferior iliac spine
- Rectus femoris t.
- Superior pubic ramus
- Pectineus m.
- Adductor longus m.
- Arcuate ligament

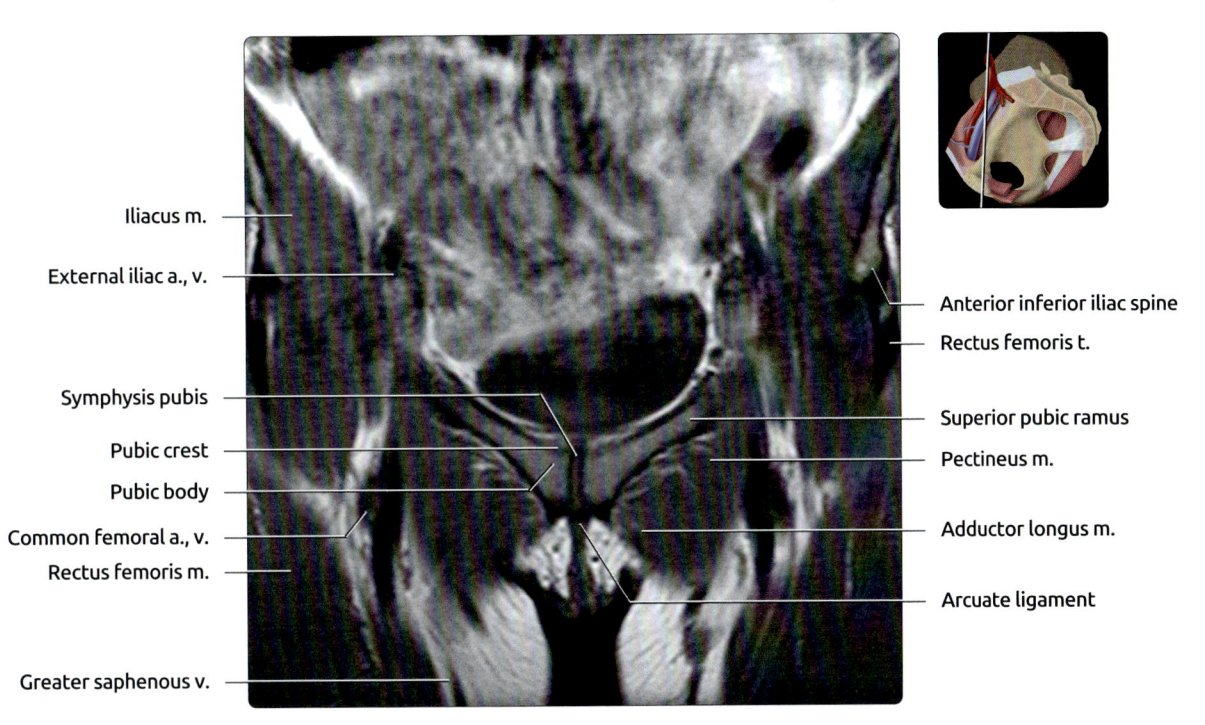

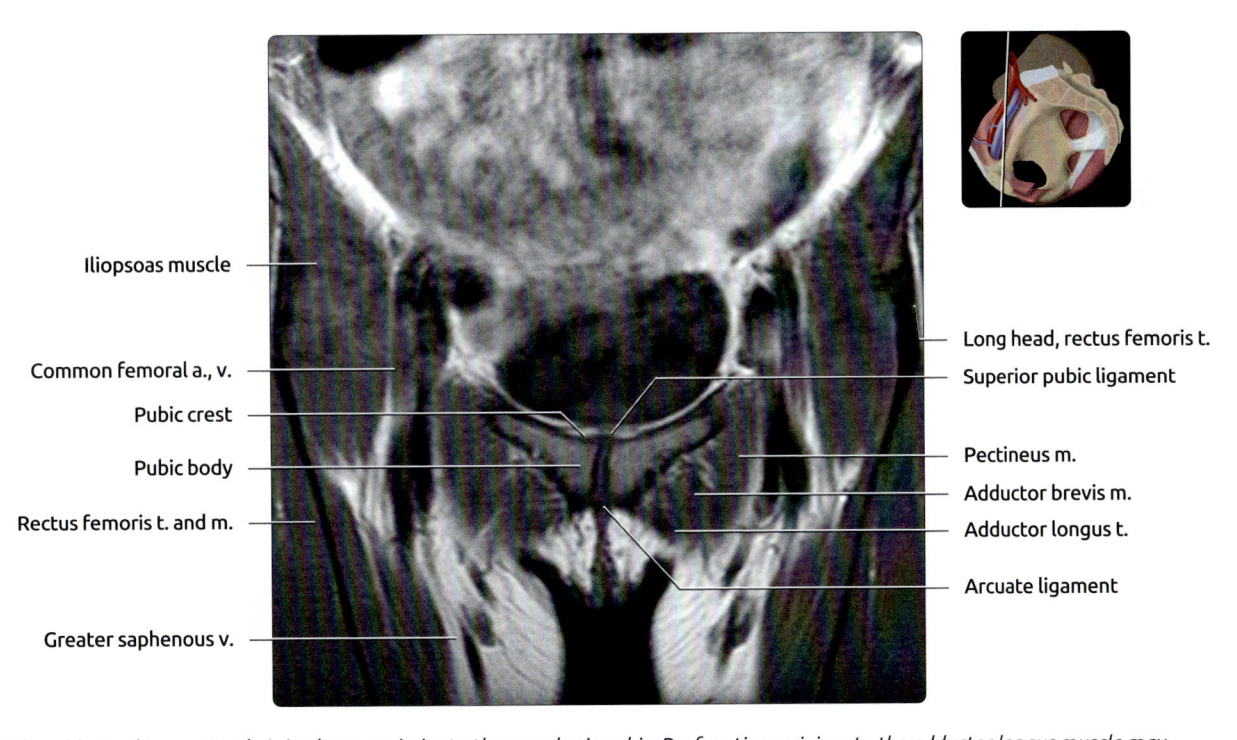

Labels (bottom image):
- Iliopsoas muscle
- Common femoral a., v.
- Pubic crest
- Pubic body
- Rectus femoris t. and m.
- Greater saphenous v.
- Long head, rectus femoris t.
- Superior pubic ligament
- Pectineus m.
- Adductor brevis m.
- Adductor longus t.
- Arcuate ligament

(Top) The adductor longus muscle is in close proximity to the symphysis pubis. Dysfunction or injury to the adductor longus muscle may contribute to instability of the symphysis. (Bottom) The relatively small superior pubic ligament is visible on this image. The long head of rectus femoris muscle arises from anterior inferior iliac spine. The reflected head arises from the anterolateral margin of the acetabulum, superior to the joint capsule.

Anterior Pelvis

CORONAL T1 MR, PUBIS AND ADDUCTORS

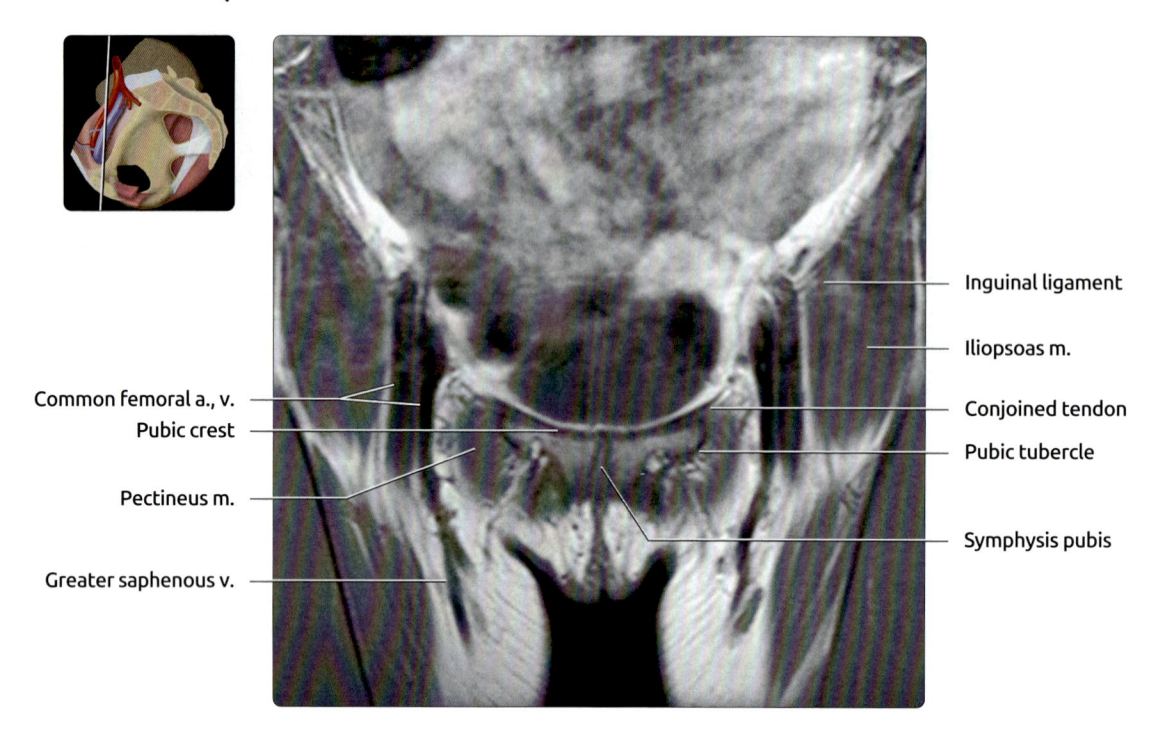

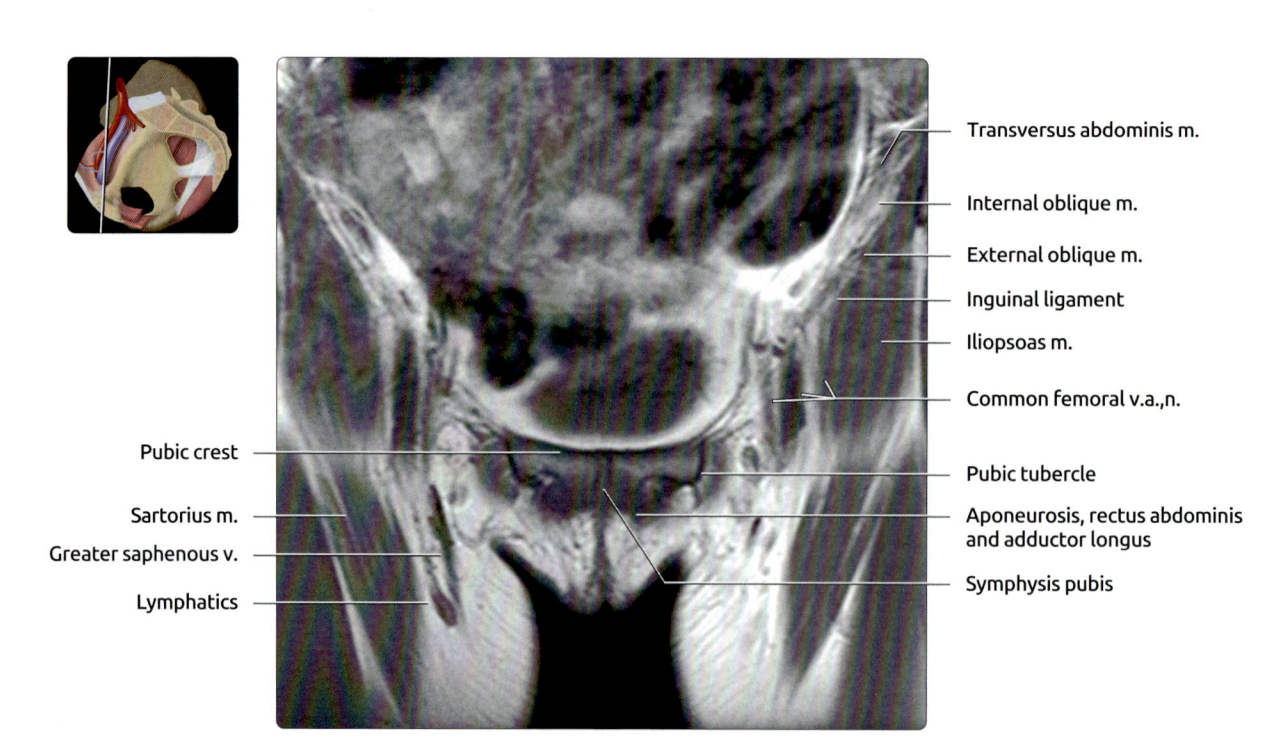

Labels (Top image):
- Common femoral a., v.
- Pubic crest
- Pectineus m.
- Greater saphenous v.
- Inguinal ligament
- Iliopsoas m.
- Conjoined tendon
- Pubic tubercle
- Symphysis pubis

Labels (Bottom image):
- Pubic crest
- Sartorius m.
- Greater saphenous v.
- Lymphatics
- Transversus abdominis m.
- Internal oblique m.
- External oblique m.
- Inguinal ligament
- Iliopsoas m.
- Common femoral v.a.,n.
- Pubic tubercle
- Aponeurosis, rectus abdominis and adductor longus
- Symphysis pubis

(Top) The pubic tubercles are easy to visualize on this image. The pubic crest is the superior portion of the pubic body medial to the tubercle. The conjoined tendon of the obturator internus and transversus abdominis muscles inserts onto the pubic crest. (Bottom) The inguinal ligament orientation from superolateral to inferomedial is easy to appreciate on this image. Note the vessels as they cross beneath the ligament to enter the femoral triangle.

Anterior Pelvis

CORONAL T1 MR, PUBIS AND ADDUCTORS

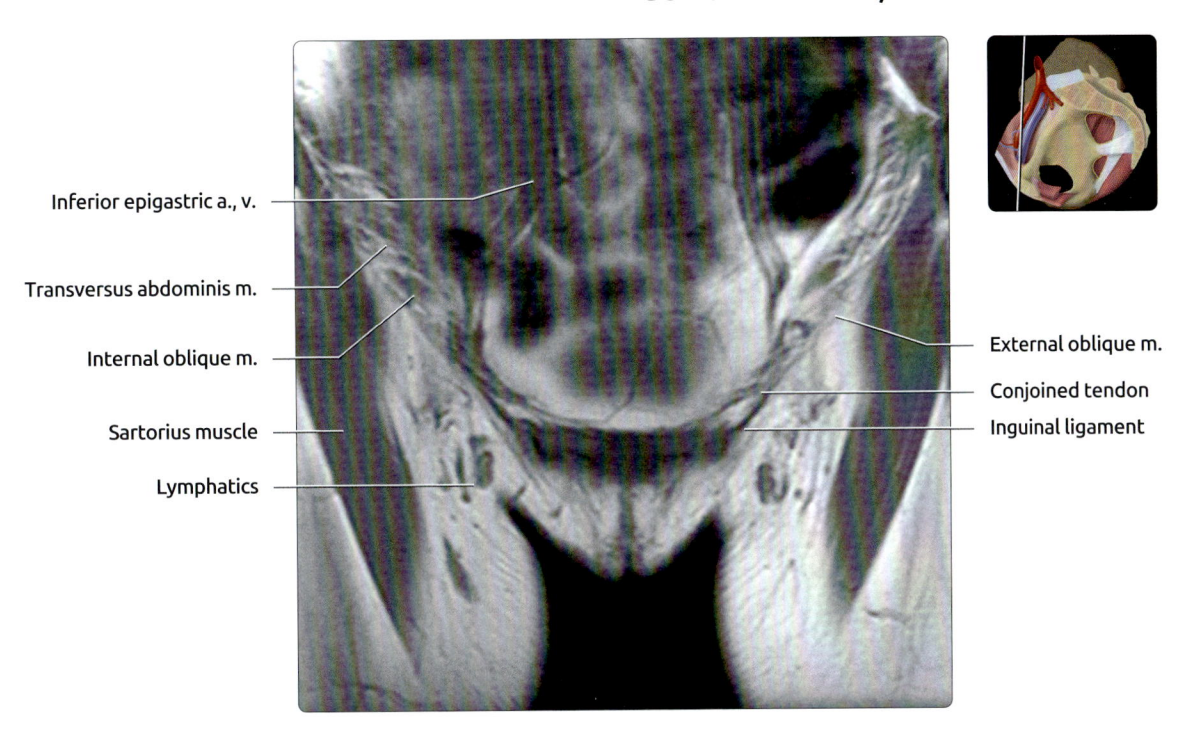

Labels (top image):
- Inferior epigastric a., v.
- Transversus abdominis m.
- Internal oblique m.
- Sartorius muscle
- Lymphatics
- External oblique m.
- Conjoined tendon
- Inguinal ligament

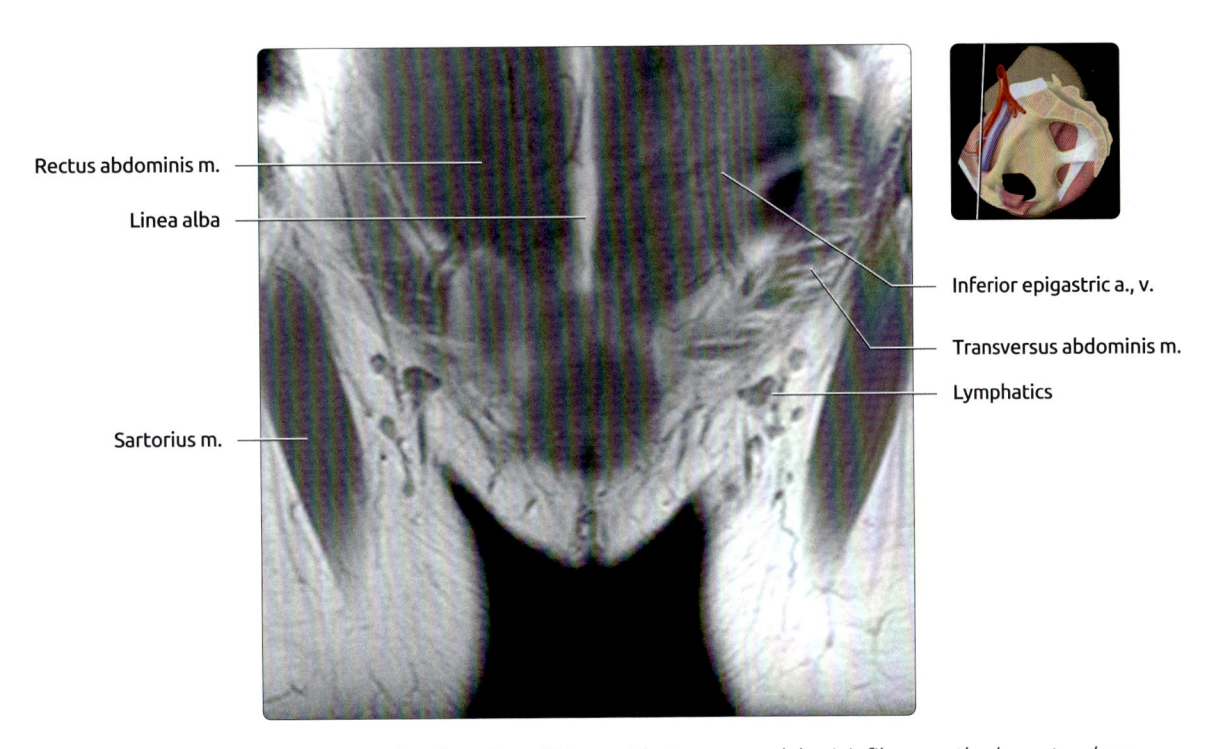

Labels (bottom image):
- Rectus abdominis m.
- Linea alba
- Sartorius m.
- Inferior epigastric a., v.
- Transversus abdominis m.
- Lymphatics

(Top) The lateral aspect of the anterior abdominal wall consists of 3 layers. The transverse abdominis fibers are the deepest and are horizontally oriented. The middle layer, internal oblique muscle, is comprised of muscle fibers that are oriented from the iliac crest upward and medially. The external oblique fibers are oriented from superolateral to inferomedial. (Bottom) The rectus abdominis muscles are the most medial of the abdominal wall musculature. They are separated in the midline by the linea alba. The inferior epigastric vessels are located along the lateral aspect of these muscle bellies.

Anterior Pelvis

SAGITTAL T1 MR, PUBIS AND ADDUCTORS

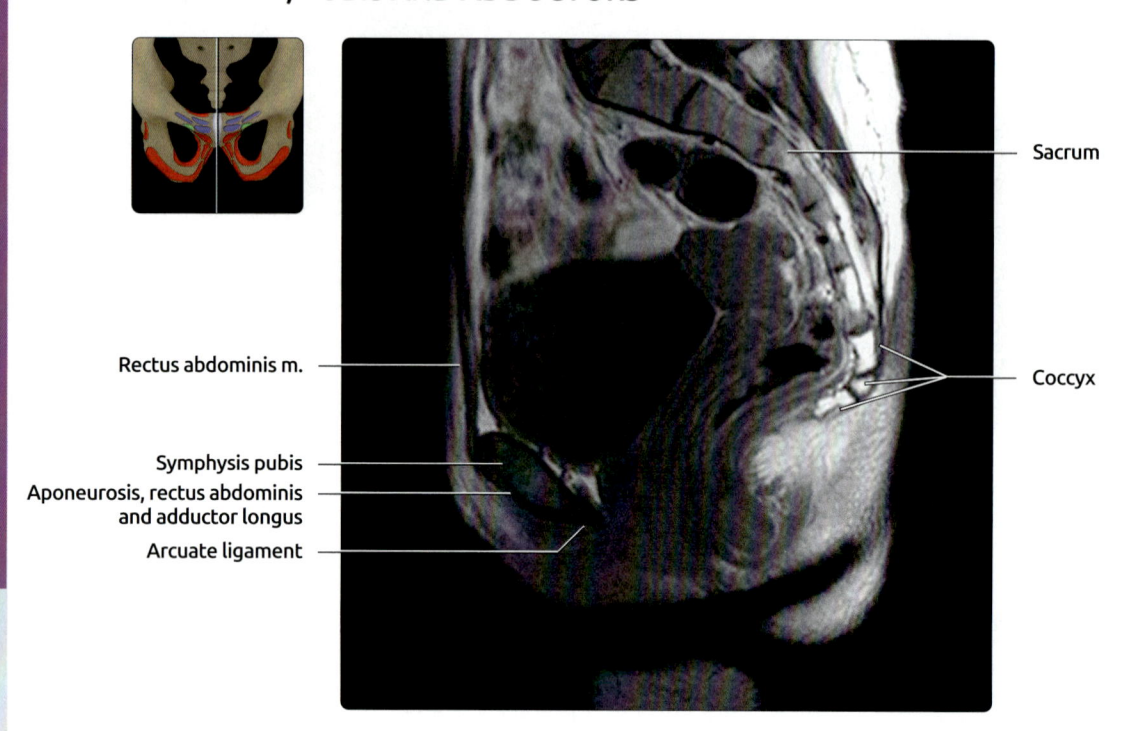

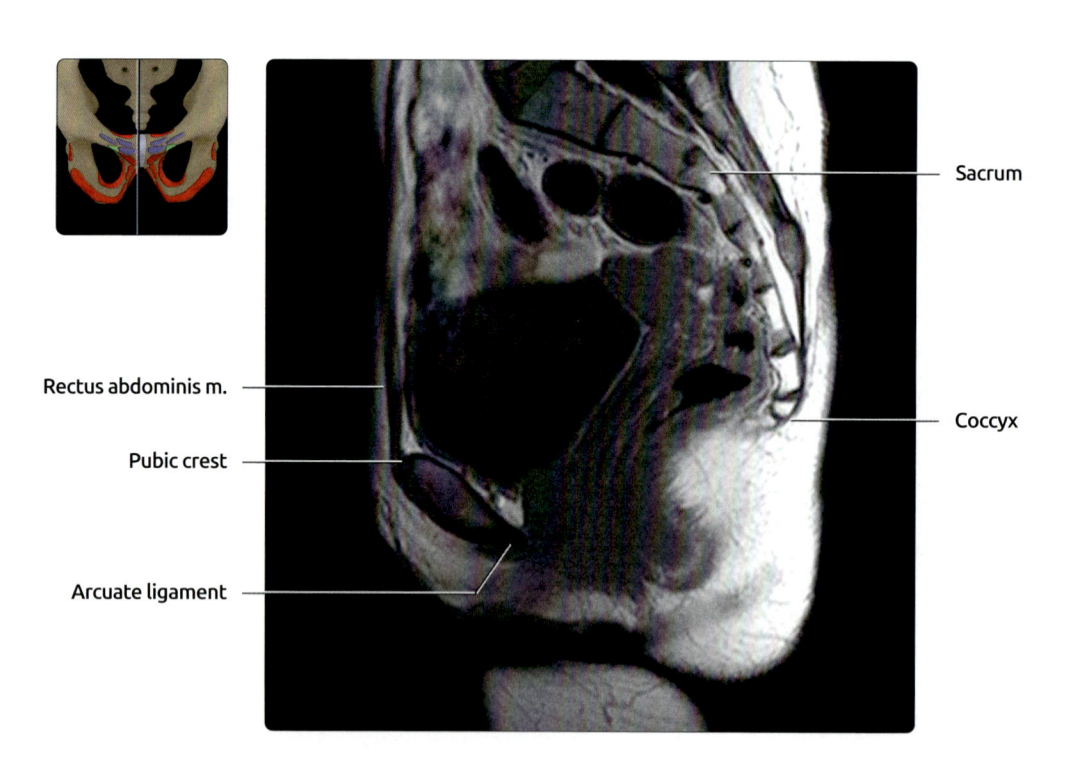

Rectus abdominis m.
Symphysis pubis
Aponeurosis, rectus abdominis and adductor longus
Arcuate ligament
Sacrum
Coccyx

Rectus abdominis m.
Pubic crest
Arcuate ligament
Sacrum
Coccyx

(Top) Sagittal images of the anterior pelvis from midline to lateral are shown. The symphysis pubis is present as partial volumed pubic bodies. There are 5 sacral segments in this patient and 3 separate coccygeal segments; segmentation in this region is variable. (Bottom) The thick arcuate ligament along the inferior aspect of the symphysis pubis is nicely seen. The rectus abdominis muscles arise from the pubic crest. Fibers from the rectus abdominis muscle merge with the aponeurosis of the adductor longus muscle along the anterior margin of the pubis.

Anterior Pelvis

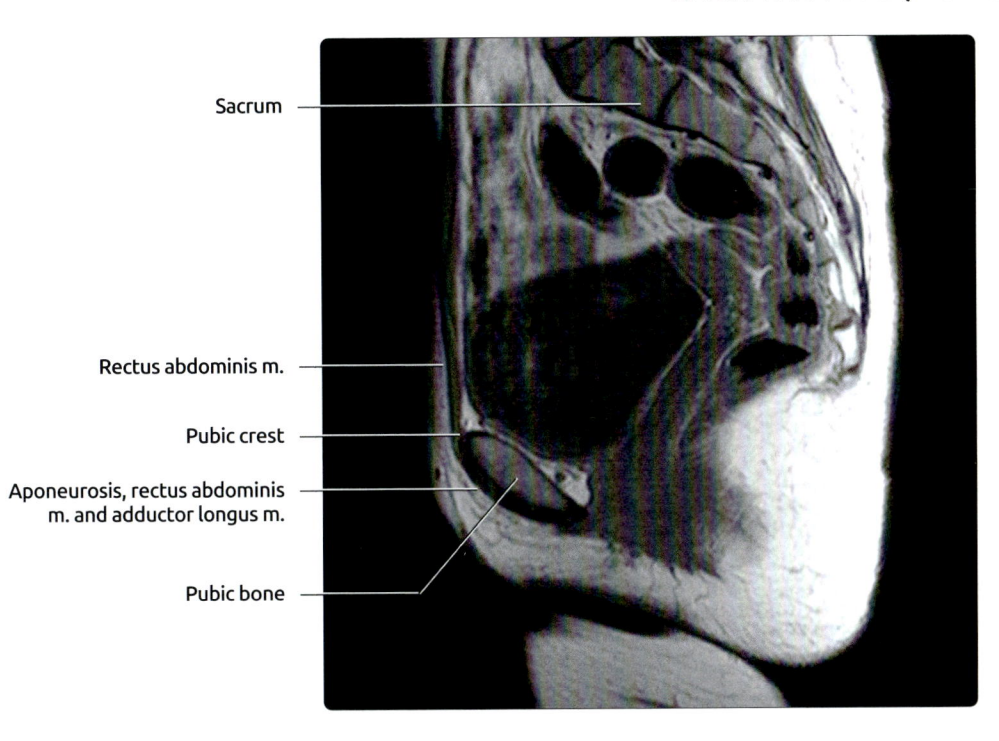

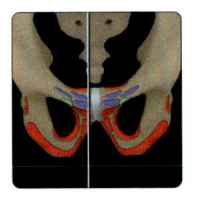

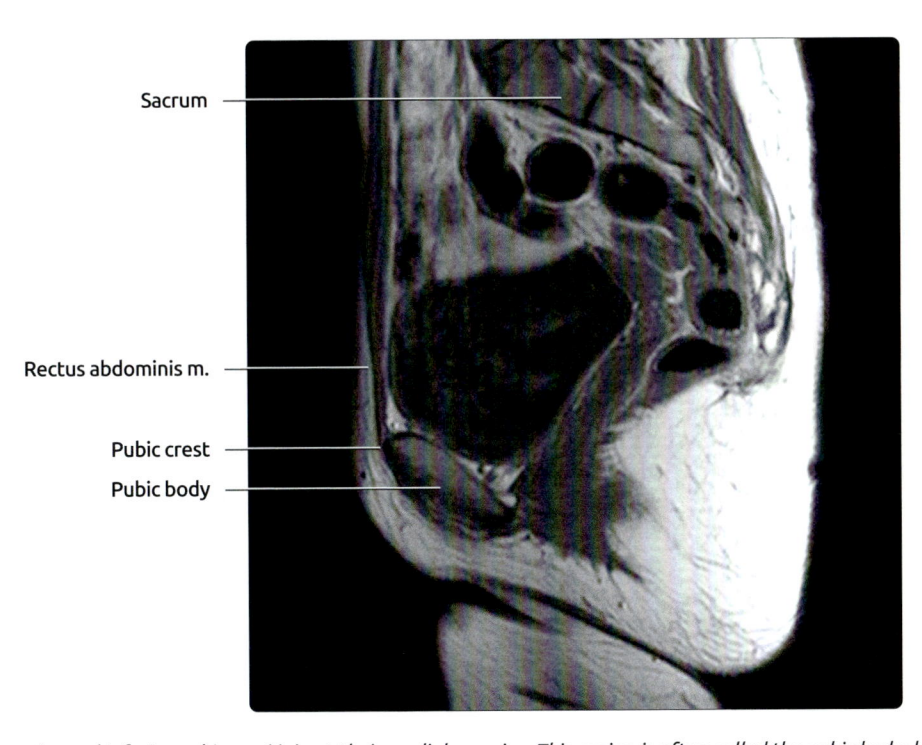

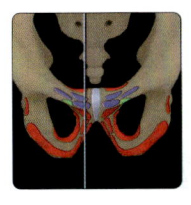

SAGITTAL T1 MR, PUBIS AND ADDUCTORS

(Top) Superior and inferior pubic rami join at their medial margins. This region is often called the pubic body; however, anatomists reserve that term for the extension of the pubic bone into the acetabulum. (Bottom) Note how the rectus abdominis muscle thins from superior to inferior. It originates on the pubic bone and inserts on the ribs.

SAGITTAL T1 MR, PUBIS AND ADDUCTORS

Rectus abdominis m.

Aponeurosis

Adductor longus t.

Adductor longus m.

Sacrum

Rectus abdominis m.

Pubic tubercle

Adductor longus t.

Adductor brevis m.

Adductor longus m.

Sacrum

Obturator externus m.

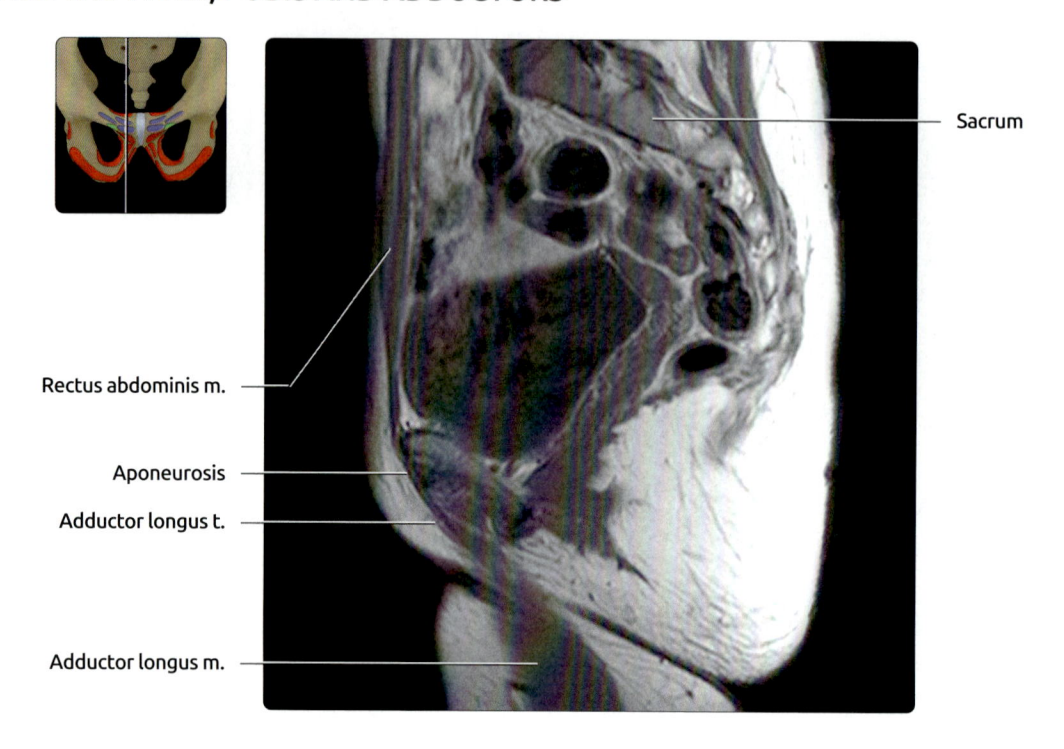

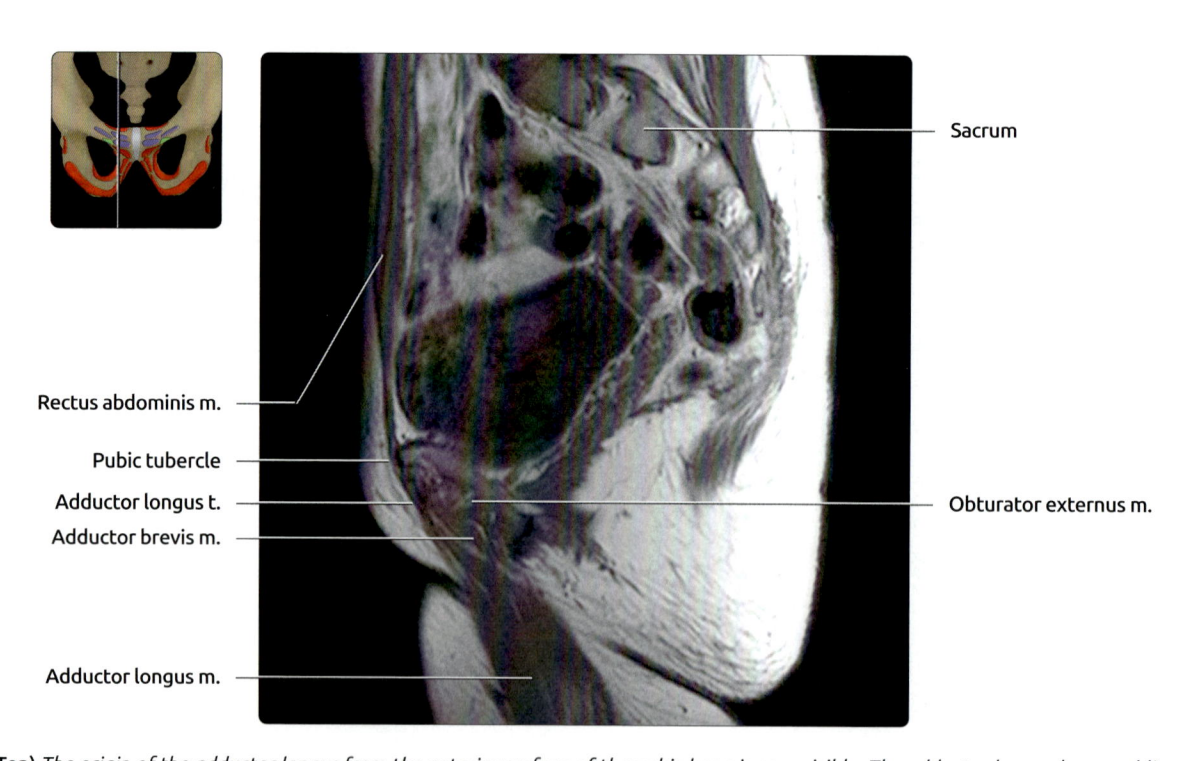

(Top) The origin of the adductor longus from the anterior surface of the pubic bone is now visible. The adductor longus has an oblique course and inserts on the mid femur at the medial aspect of the linea aspera. (Bottom) The anterior protrusion of the pubic tubercle is apparent. The adductor brevis muscle lies deep to the adductor longus muscle. The obturator externus muscle is deep to the adductor brevis muscle.

Anterior Pelvis

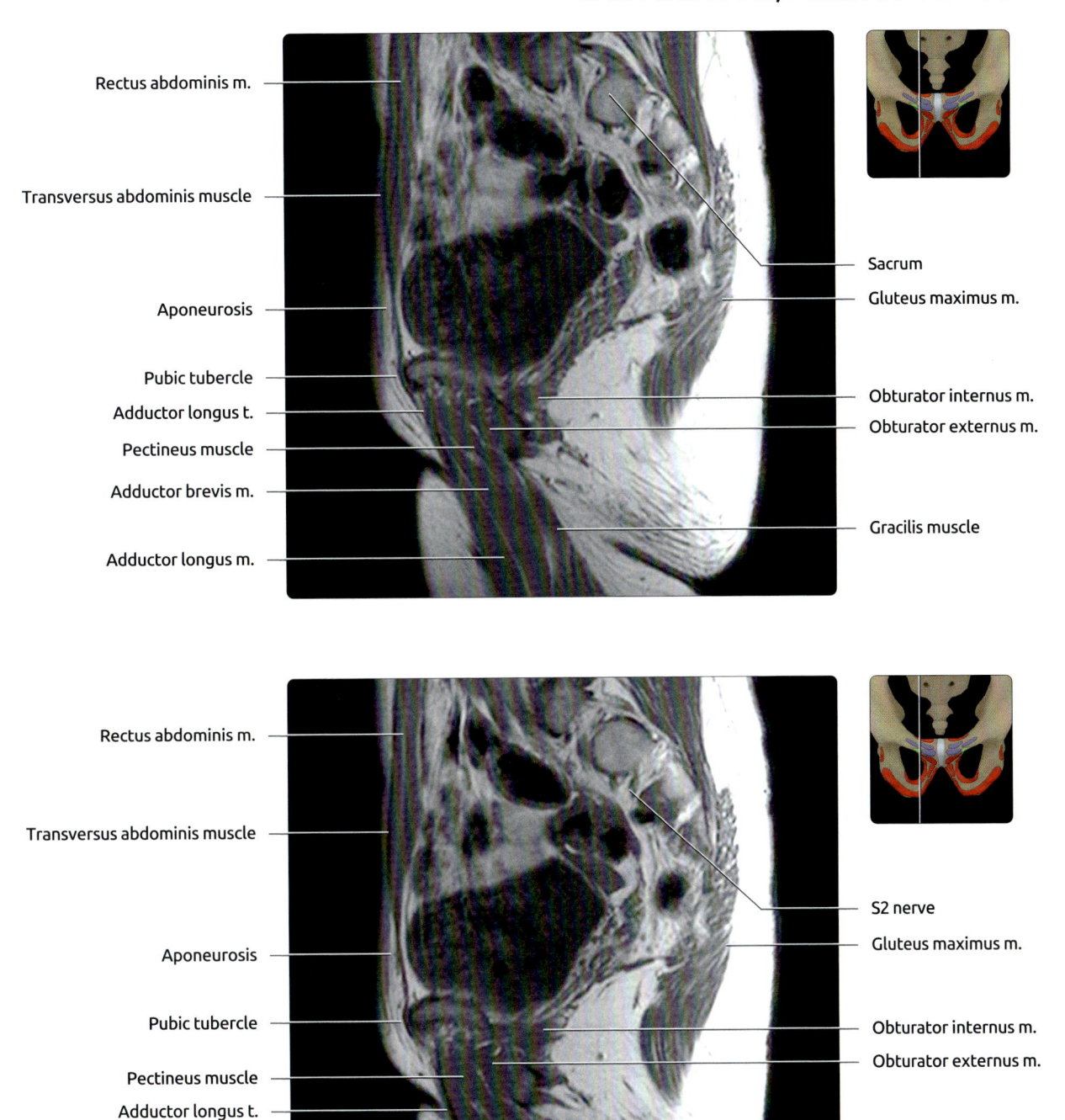

SAGITTAL T1 MR, PUBIS AND ADDUCTORS

(Top) The transition from the rectus abdominis muscle to the lateral abdominal muscles is not a distinct transition on sagittal MR. The gracilis muscle takes origin from the inferior pubic ramus and that origin is nicely seen on this image. (Bottom) The thin fused aponeuroses of the lateral abdominal muscles is located along the inferior and lateral aspect of the abdominal wall. The inguinal ligament is formed by the lower border of the external oblique aponeurosis. The attachment of that structure to the pubic tubercle is visualized here.

Anterior Pelvis

SAGITTAL T1 MR, PUBIS AND ADDUCTORS

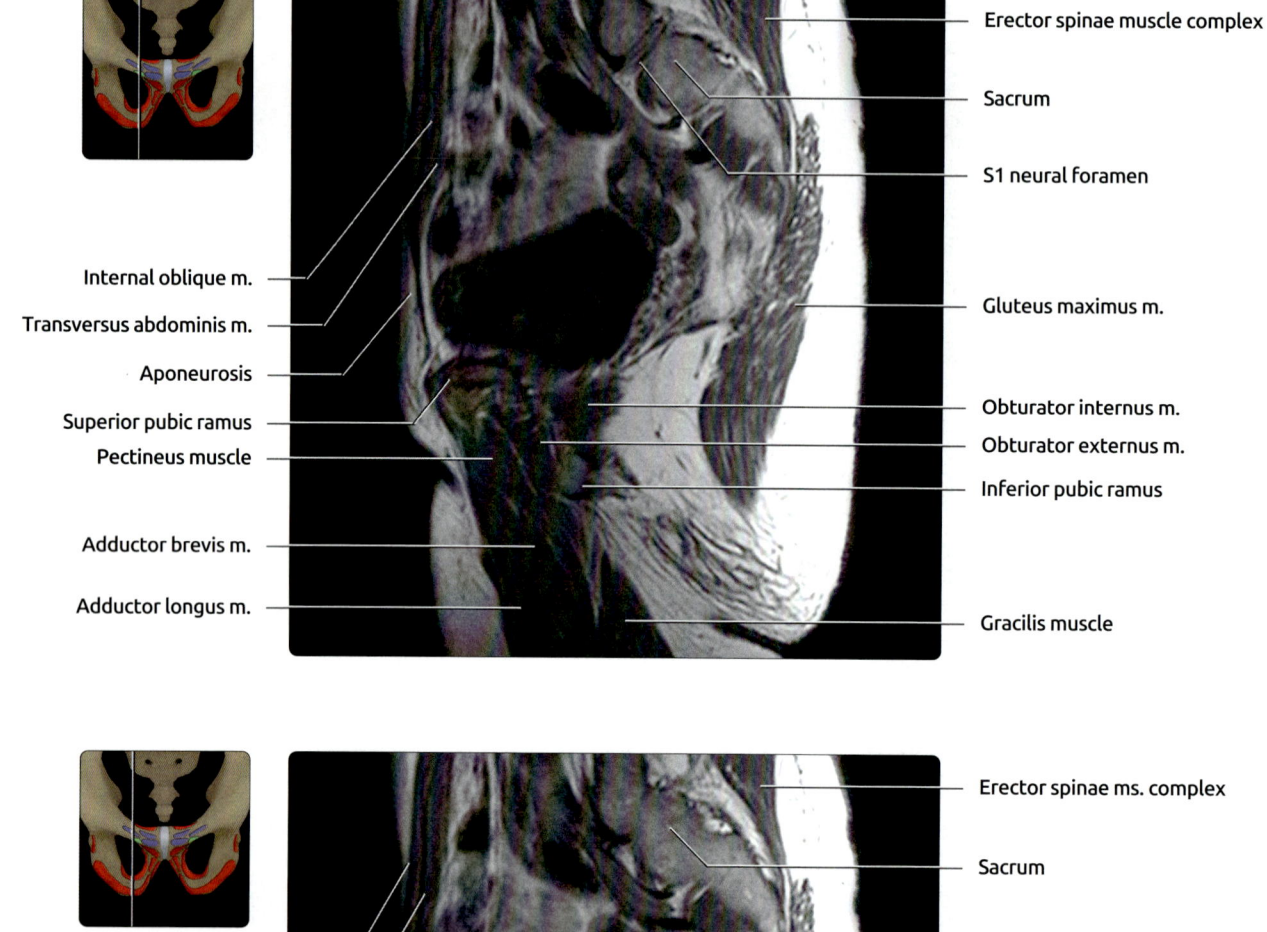

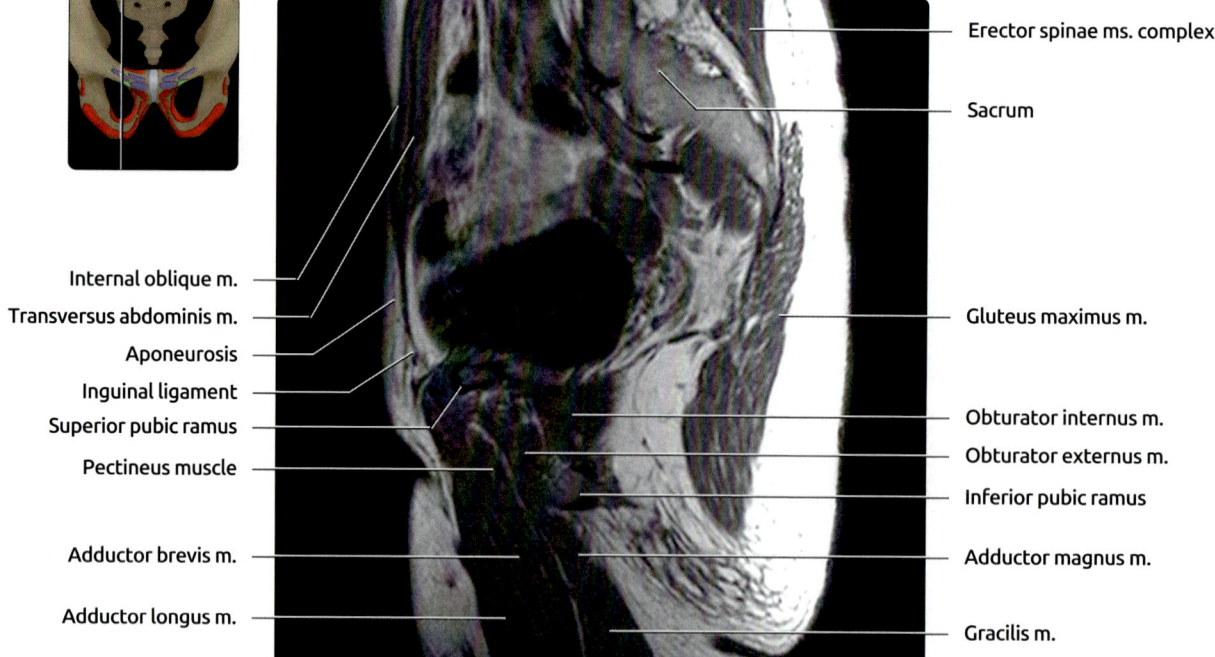

Labels (top image):
- Internal oblique m.
- Transversus abdominis m.
- Aponeurosis
- Superior pubic ramus
- Pectineus muscle
- Adductor brevis m.
- Adductor longus m.
- Erector spinae muscle complex
- Sacrum
- S1 neural foramen
- Gluteus maximus m.
- Obturator internus m.
- Obturator externus m.
- Inferior pubic ramus
- Gracilis muscle

Labels (bottom image):
- Internal oblique m.
- Transversus abdominis m.
- Aponeurosis
- Inguinal ligament
- Superior pubic ramus
- Pectineus muscle
- Adductor brevis m.
- Adductor longus m.
- Erector spinae ms. complex
- Sacrum
- Gluteus maximus m.
- Obturator internus m.
- Obturator externus m.
- Inferior pubic ramus
- Adductor magnus m.
- Gracilis m.

(Top) The superior pubic ramus is slightly anterior to the inferior pubic ramus. This relationship should be remembered when reviewing outlet views of the pelvis. (Bottom) The inguinal ligament is visible along the inferior aspect of the abdominal wall aponeurosis.

Anterior Pelvis

SAGITTAL T1 MR, PUBIS AND ADDUCTORS

Labels (top image, left): Internal oblique m.; Transversus abdominis muscle; Aponeurosis; Inguinal ligament; Superior pubic ramus; Pectineus muscle; Adductor brevis m.; Adductor longus m.

Labels (top image, right): Piriformis m.; Gluteus maximus m.; Obturator internus m.; Obturator externus m.; Inferior pubic ramus; Adductor magnus m.

Labels (bottom image, left): Internal oblique m.; Transversus abdominis muscle; Aponeurosis; Inguinal ligament; Superior pubic ramus; Pectineus m.; Adductor brevis m.; Adductor longus m.

Labels (bottom image, right): Piriformis m.; Gluteus maximus m.; Obturator internus m.; Obturator externus m.; Inferior pubic ramus; Adductor magnus m.

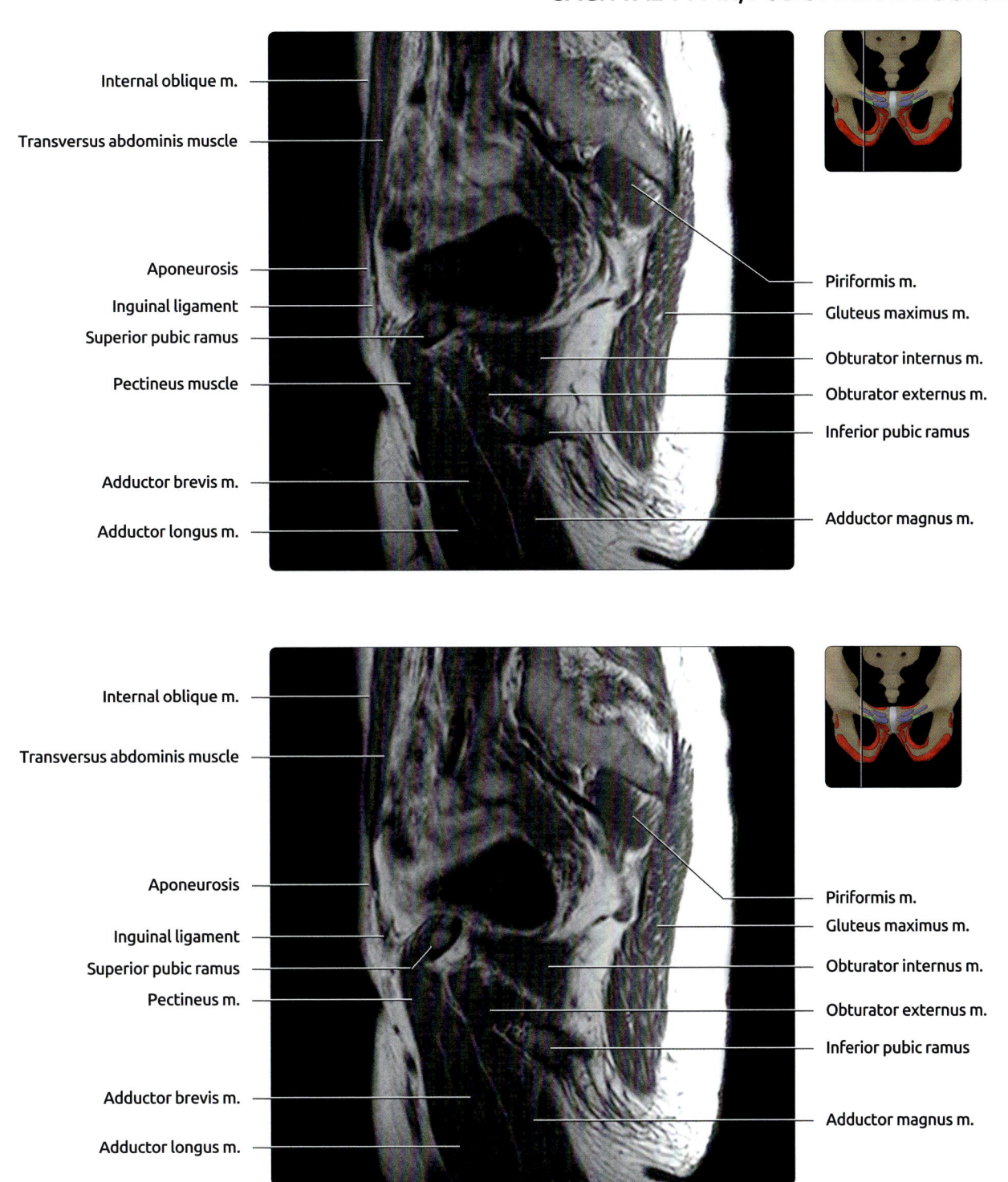

(Top) *Note the transition from gracilis muscle to the adductor magnus muscle as the images move from medial to lateral. The origin of the pectineus muscle from the pecten of the superior pubis ramus and its wrapping over the top of the ramus is well visualized on this image.* **(Bottom)** *Pectineus is seen originating from the superior and anterior margins of the superior pubic ramus.*

Anterior Pelvis

OBLIQUE AXIAL T1 MR, PUBIS AND ADDUCTORS

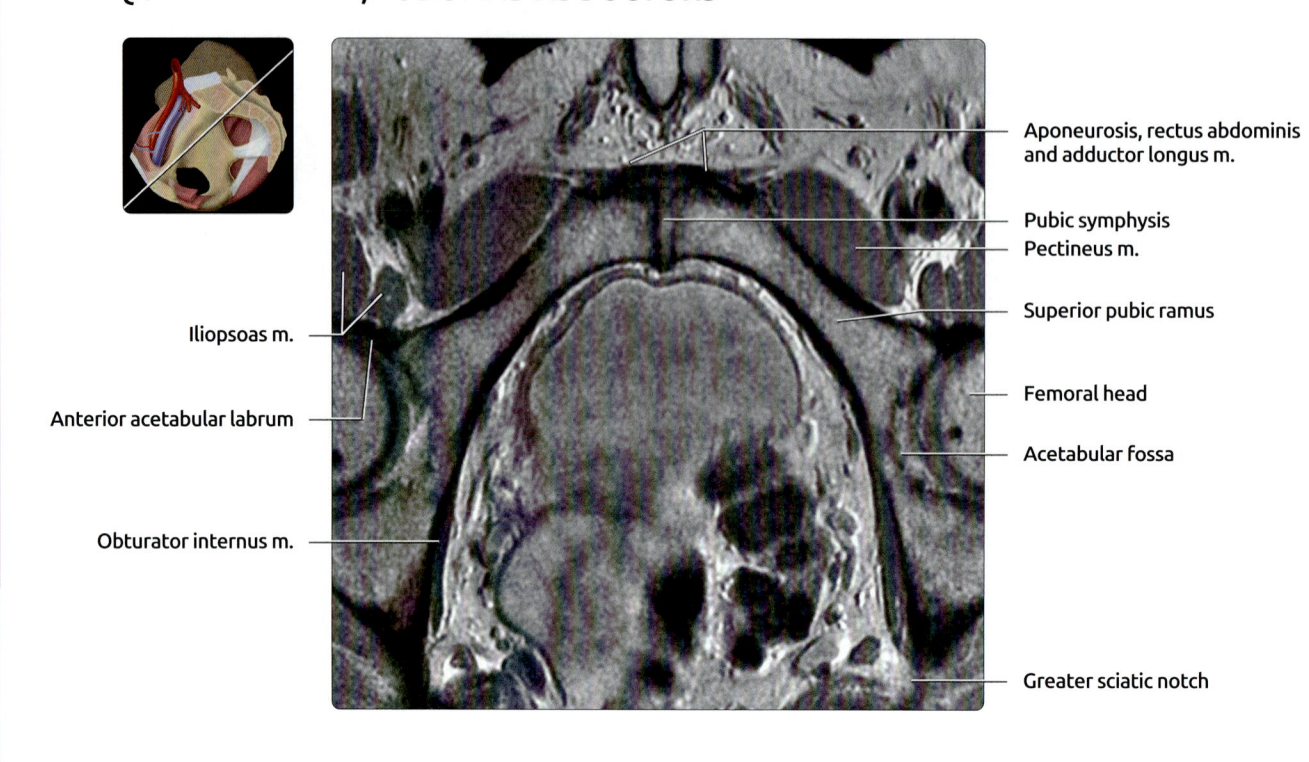

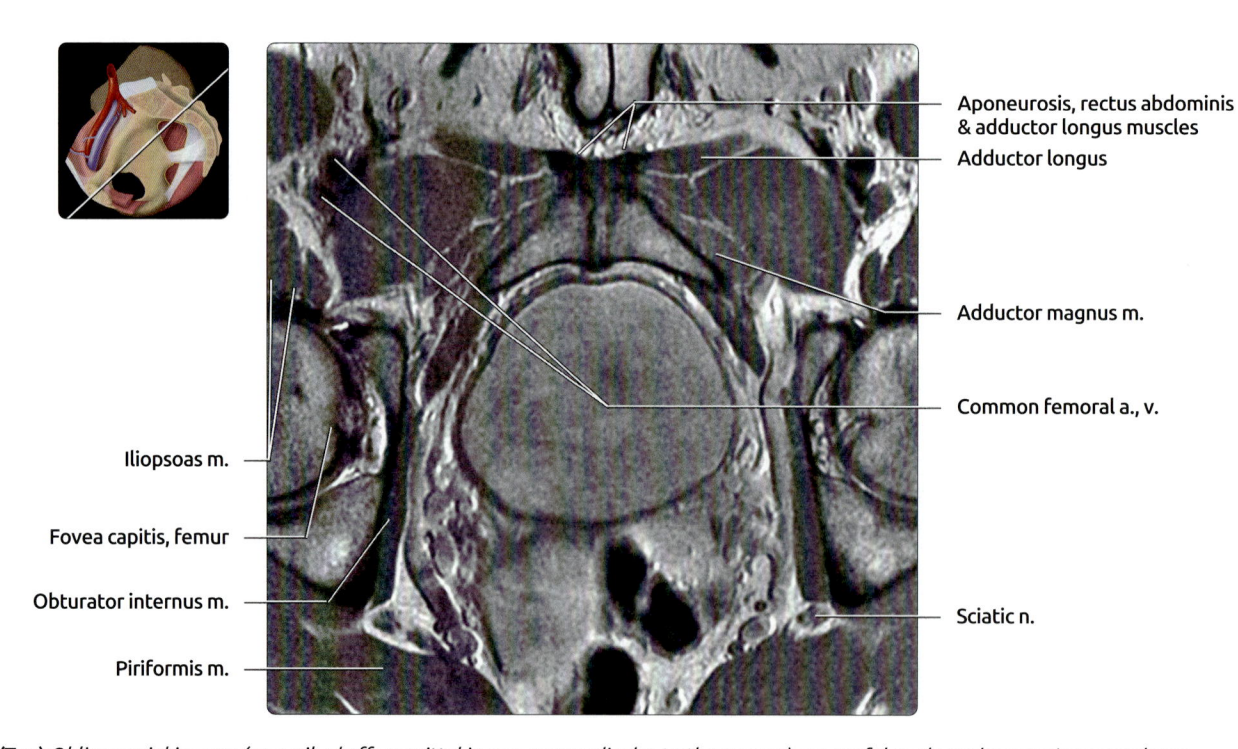

Labels (top image): Iliopsoas m.; Anterior acetabular labrum; Obturator internus m.; Aponeurosis, rectus abdominis and adductor longus m.; Pubic symphysis; Pectineus m.; Superior pubic ramus; Femoral head; Acetabular fossa; Greater sciatic notch

Labels (bottom image): Iliopsoas m.; Fovea capitis, femur; Obturator internus m.; Piriformis m.; Aponeurosis, rectus abdominis & adductor longus muscles; Adductor longus; Adductor magnus m.; Common femoral a., v.; Sciatic n.

(Top) Oblique axial images (prescribed off a sagittal image, perpendicular to the sacrum) are useful to show the anterior musculature. The rectus femoris and adductor longus muscles form a shared aponeurosis along the anterior margin of the pubic bone. Detachment of the aponeurosis is an important feature of athletic pubalgia. **(Bottom)** The pectineus muscle is moving posterolaterally, and the adductor longus muscle is now the most anterior adductor. The pectineus is medial to the common femoral vessels, and the iliopsoas is lateral to them, a useful landmark.

Anterior Pelvis

OBLIQUE AXIAL T1 MR, PUBIS AND ADDUCTORS

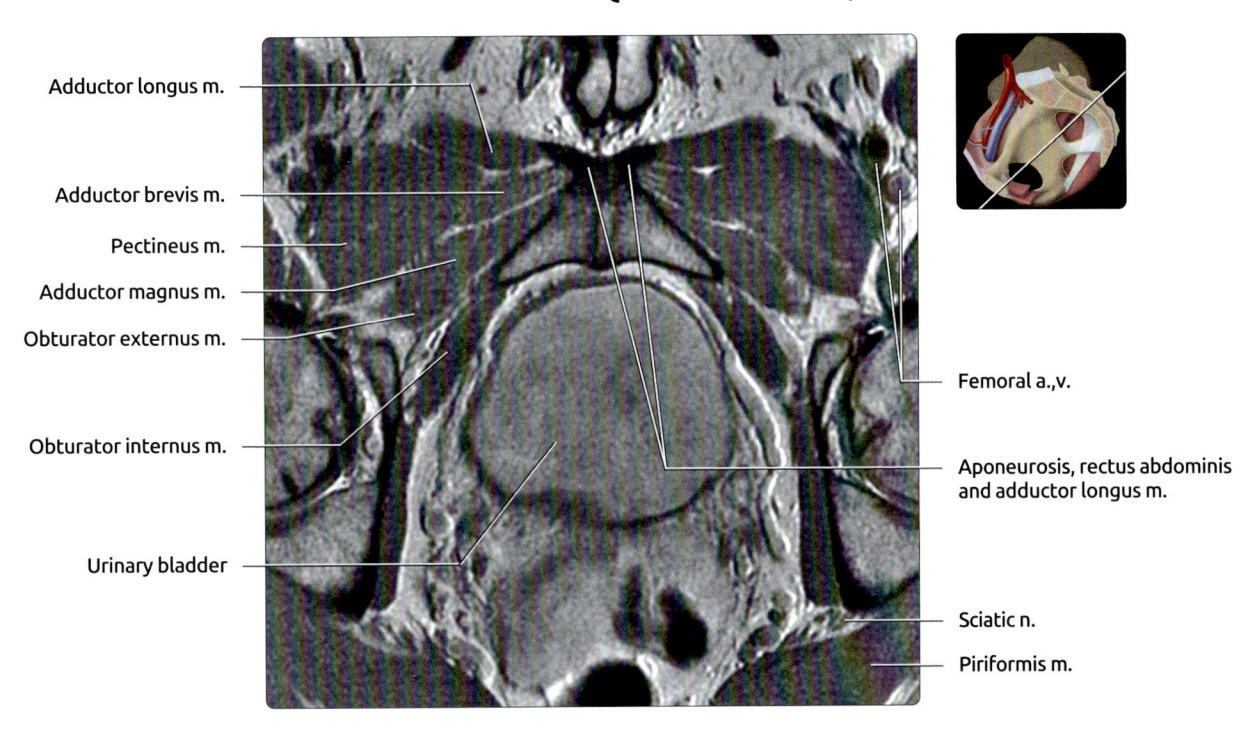

Labels (top image): Adductor longus m.; Adductor brevis m.; Pectineus m.; Adductor magnus m.; Obturator externus m.; Obturator internus m.; Urinary bladder; Femoral a., v.; Aponeurosis, rectus abdominis and adductor longus m.; Sciatic n.; Piriformis m.

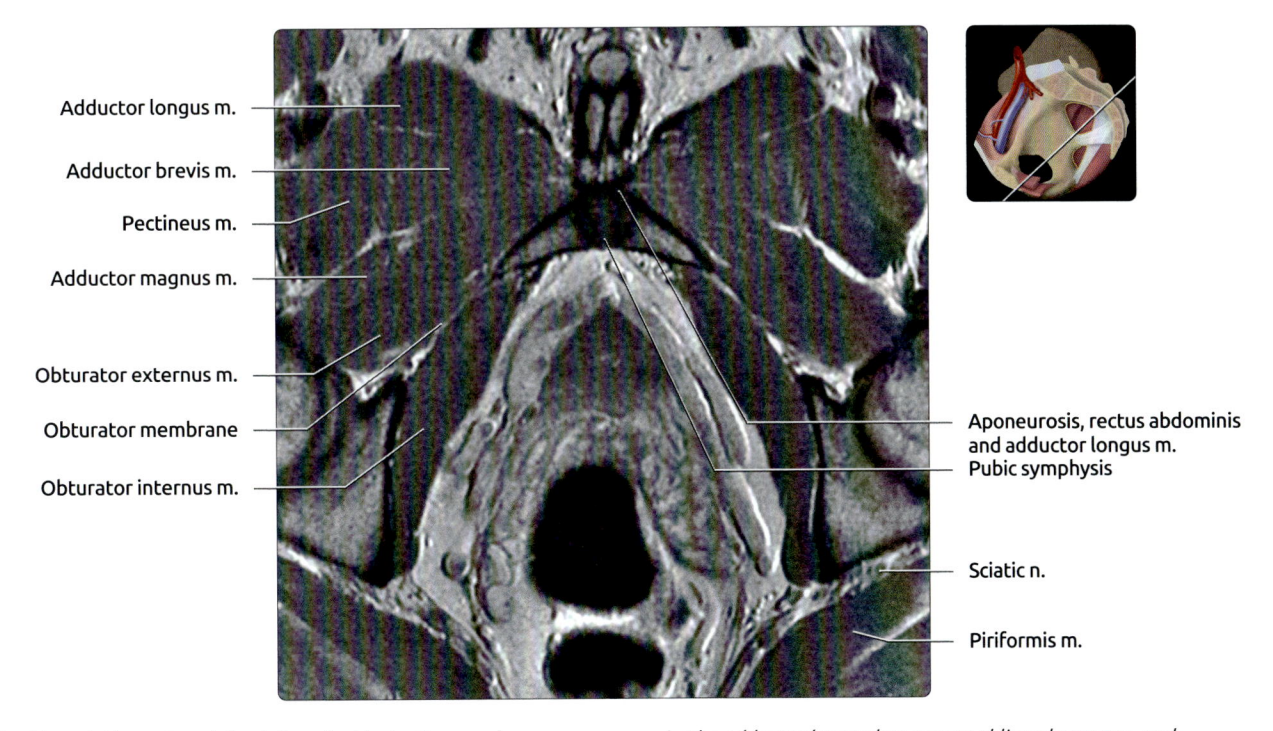

Labels (bottom image): Adductor longus m.; Adductor brevis m.; Pectineus m.; Adductor magnus m.; Obturator externus m.; Obturator membrane; Obturator internus m.; Aponeurosis, rectus abdominis and adductor longus m.; Pubic symphysis; Sciatic n.; Piriformis m.

(Top) Although the rectus abdominis and adductor longus share an aponeurosis, the adductor longus has a more oblique lever arm, and the different axes of the muscles can result in shear stress on the aponeurosis. (Bottom) Obturator externus is now visible, arising from the obturator membrane as well as the inferior pubic ramus. It is separated from the obturator internus by the obturator membrane.

Hip Overview

TERMINOLOGY

Abbreviations
- Muscle origin (O)
- Muscle insertion (I)
- Muscle innervation (N)
- Muscle function (F)

Definitions
- **Rotator cuff of hip**: Term for 3 gluteal muscles
  - May develop tendinopathy, degenerative tears similar to rotator cuff of shoulder
- **Triceps coxae:** Term that includes obturator internus and gemelli, which function as 1 unit

GROSS ANATOMY

Overview
- **Motion**
  - Most stable articulation in body
  - Greatest range of motion after glenohumeral joint
  - Flexion with knee flexed limited by abdomen
  - Flexion with knee extended limited by hamstrings
  - Extension limited to 30° past vertical
  - Abduction without limitation
  - Adduction limited by opposite extremity
  - External rotation > internal
  - Internal rotation weakest motion
  - Maximum stability in extension
- Muscle/ligament balance
  - Anterior ligaments stronger than internal rotators
  - External rotators stronger than posterior ligaments

Vascular Supply
- Branches of medial and lateral circumflex femoral, deep division superior gluteal, inferior gluteal arteries (a.), a. of ligamentum teres (branch of obturator a.)

Innervation
- Branches from multiple nerves (n): n. to rectus femoris, n. to quadratus femoris, anterior division obturator n., accessory obturator n., superior gluteal n.

Osseous Structures
- **Acetabulum**
  - Formed by pubis, ilium, ischium (innominate bone)
  - Oriented anterior, inferior, lateral
  - Posterior (Ilioischial) column transmits weight from torso to lower extremity
  - Anterior (iliopectineal or iliopubic) column connects to anterior pelvis
  - Covers > 50% femoral head
  - Articular surface is called lunate surface
    - Covered by horseshoe shaped articular cartilage
  - Central region (acetabular fossa) is not articular
  - **Acetabular fossa**: Central, medial region of hip joint
    - Depressed centrally relative to lunate surface
    - Covered by synovium: Extraarticular except for joint recess at superior margin of fossa
    - **Pulvinar**: Fibrofatty tissue filling most of acetabular fossa
    - Ligamentum teres attaches partly to fossa, primarily to transverse ligament
  - **Acetabular notch**: Osseous opening inferior margin
  - **Anterior and posterior rims**: Osseous margins of acetabulum
  - **Medial wall**: Quadrilateral plate ilium
    - Radiographic acetabular line
  - **Teardrop**: Radiographic conglomerate shadow
    - Lateral: Wall acetabular fossa
    - Medial: Anterior, inferior quadrilateral plate
- **Femoral Head**
  - 2/3 of sphere
    - Centered on column-like femoral neck
    - Normally have circumferential cutback from femoral head to femoral neck
  - Covered by articular cartilage except at fovea capitis
    - Cartilage thickest superiorly
    - Cartilage thins at head/neck junction
  - **Fovea capitis**: Bowl-shaped depression on superomedial femoral head
    - Attachment site of ligamentum teres

Acetabular Labrum
- Fibrocartilage
- Morphology
  - Triangular: 66-94%
    - Decreasing incidence with increasing age
  - Thickest posterior and superior
  - Widest anterior and superior
  - Variants: Rounded, blunted, absent
  - Absent labra: Constellation absent anterior labrum and small remnant superiorly
    - 10-14% asymptomatic individuals
  - Overlies articular cartilage
- Attaches to acetabular rim
  - Covers 270° of acetabulum, not present inferiorly
    - Transverse ligament traverses inferior margin of joint
  - Forms horse-shoe cushion around anterior, superior, and posterior acetabulum
- Inferiorly attaches to transverse ligament of acetabulum
  - **Labroligamentous sulci**: Junction ligament and labrum
- **Labrocartilaginous cleft**
  - Between articular cartilage and labrum
  - Anterosuperior, posteroinferior
  - Likely normal variant
- Vascular supply: Branches obturator, superior and inferior gluteal arteries
  - Mainly capsular surface
  - Articular surface avascular
    - Limited ability to repair
- Function
  - Separates superficial and deep portions of joint
  - Helps hold synovial fluid in deep portion of joint
    - This synovial fluid protects and nourishes cartilage
  - Prevents lateral translation femoral head

Synovial Joint Capsule
- Attachments
  - Acetabulum
    - Anterior: Base of labrum

Hip Overview

- Superior: Several mm above labrum
- Posterior: Base of labrum or several mm medial to it
- Inferior: Transverse ligament
  o Femur
    - Anterior: Intertrochanteric line
    - Posterior: Proximal to intertrochanteric crest
- Iliopectineal fold: Synovial fold along medial margin of femoral neck
- Synovial folds also enclose medial circumflex artery
  o Inferior to zona orbicularis

Ligaments of Hip Joint

- Ligaments are important stabilizers of hip
- Iliofemoral, pubofemoral, ischiofemoral, and zona orbicularis form outer layer of capsule, external to synovium
- **Iliofemoral (Bigelow ligament)**
  o Strongest ligament in body
  o Prevents anterior translation, hyperextension
  o Originates from inferior surface of anterior inferior iliac spine
  o Shaped like inverted V with broad attachment to femur
    - Lateral, medial limbs attach to intertrochanteric line
- **Pubofemoral**
  o Prevents hyperabduction
  o Anterior, inferior, longitudinal spiral
  o Medial attachment obturator crest pubis
  o Laterally merges with joint capsule
- **Ischiofemoral**: Posterior, longitudinal spiral
  o Weakest
- **Zona orbicularis**: Deep, circular
  o Around central portion of femoral neck
  o Causes central narrowing of hip joint
- **Ligamentum teres**
  o Attachments: Fovea capitis and transverse ligament and pulvinar
  o Lined by synovium: Intracapsular, extraarticular
  o Contains artery of ligamentum teres
    - Negligible supply to femoral head in adults
  o Narrow superior, wider inferior
  o May help stabilize hip
  o Tension in flexion, adduction, external rotation
  o May be pain generator
- **Transverse ligament**
  o Spans acetabular notch at inferior margin of acetabulum
    - Completes socket of acetabulum
  o Blends with labra at margins of notch
    - Labroligamentous sulci at junction

Muscles of Hip

- **Gluteal muscles: Maximus, medius, and minimus**
  o Often called rotator cuff of hip
  o **Maximus**
    - O: Posterior gluteal line of ilium, posterior sacrum and coccyx, sacrotuberous ligament
    - I: Iliotibial band, gluteal tuberosity of femur
    - N: Inferior gluteal n.
    - F: Extension, abduction, external rotation of hip
  o **Medius**
    - O: Posterior ilium
    - I: Superoposterior, lateral facets of greater trochanter
    - N: Superior gluteal n.
    - F: Abduction, internal rotation of hip
  o **Minimus**
    - O: Posterior ilium
    - I: Anterior facet of greater trochanter
    - N: Superior gluteal n.
    - F: Abduction, internal rotation of hip
- **Deep posterior muscles of hip**
  o **Piriformis**
    - O: Anterior sacrum, sacrotuberous ligament
    - I: Greater trochanter
    - N: S1, S2
    - F: External rotation, weak abduction of hip
  o **Gemellus superior**
    - O: Ischial spine
    - I: Piriformis fossa
    - N: N. to obturator internus muscle (m.)
    - F: External rotation, weak abduction of hip
  o **Gemellus inferior**
    - O: Ischial tuberosity
    - I: Piriformis fossa
    - N: N. to quadratus femoris m.
    - F: External rotation, weak abduction of hip
  o **Obturator internus**
    - O: Internal surface obturator foramen and membrane
    - I: Piriformis fossa
    - N: L5, S1, S2 (NOT obturator n.)
    - F: External rotation, weak abduction of hip
  o **Obturator externus**
    - O: External surface obturator foramen and membrane
    - I: Piriformis fossa
    - N: Obturator n.
    - F: External rotation of hip
  o **Quadratus femoris**
    - O: Lateral ischial tuberosity
    - I: Quadrate line, intertrochanteric crest of femur
    - N: L4, L5, S1
    - F: External rotation of hip

Bursae

- **Iliopsoas bursa**: Between muscle and hip joint capsule
  o Communicates with hip joint: 10-14%
- **Obturator externus bursa**: Outpouching between zona orbicularis and ischiofemoral ligaments
- **Greater trochanteric bursa**: Between lateral margin of trochanter and gluteus maximus muscle

SELECTED REFERENCES

1. Tan V et al: Contribution of acetabular labrum to articulating surface area and femoral head coverage in adult hip joints: an anatomic study in cadavera. Am J Orthop. 30(11):809-12, 2001
2. Abe I et al: Acetabular labrum: abnormal findings at MR imaging in asymptomatic hips. Radiology. 216(2):576-81, 2000
3. Cotten A et al: Acetabular labrum: MRI in asymptomatic volunteers. J Comput Assist Tomogr. 22(1):1-7, 1998

Hip Overview

LIGAMENTS OF THE HIP

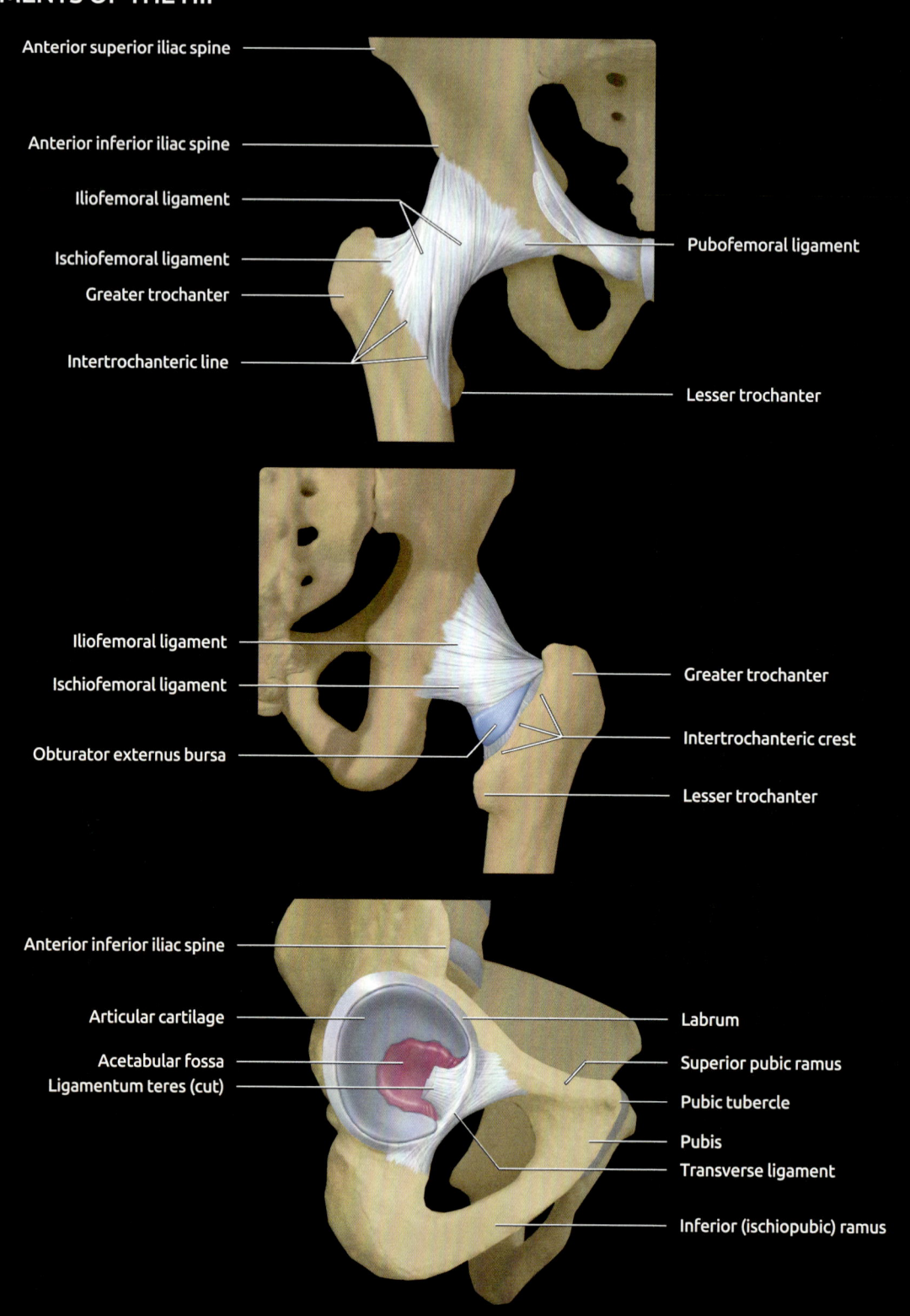

Anterior superior iliac spine

Anterior inferior iliac spine

Iliofemoral ligament

Ischiofemoral ligament

Greater trochanter

Intertrochanteric line

Pubofemoral ligament

Lesser trochanter

Iliofemoral ligament

Ischiofemoral ligament

Obturator externus bursa

Greater trochanter

Intertrochanteric crest

Lesser trochanter

Anterior inferior iliac spine

Articular cartilage

Acetabular fossa

Ligamentum teres (cut)

Labrum

Superior pubic ramus

Pubic tubercle

Pubis

Transverse ligament

Inferior (ischiopubic) ramus

(Top) Anterior view of the hip shows the longitudinal spirals of the iliofemoral and pubofemoral ligaments. Their attachments to the anterior inferior iliac spine and pubic aspect of the obturator foramen respectively are visible. The ischiofemoral ligament is primarily located along the posterior aspect of the joint, but wraps over the superior aspect of the femoral neck to attach to the anterior femoral neck. (Middle) Posterior view shows the longitudinal spiral of the ischiofemoral ligament. The obturator externus bursa protrudes from the joint along the inferior margin of the ischiofemoral ligament. (Bottom) External view of the acetabulum demonstrates the horseshoe-shaped articular cartilage surrounding the acetabular fossa. The acetabular fossa is filled with fatty tissue called the pulvinar. The labrum resides on the acetabular rim and blends at its inferior margins with the transverse ligament. The ligamentum teres attaches to the transverse ligament.

Hip Overview

MUSCLE ATTACHMENTS, INNOMINATE BONE

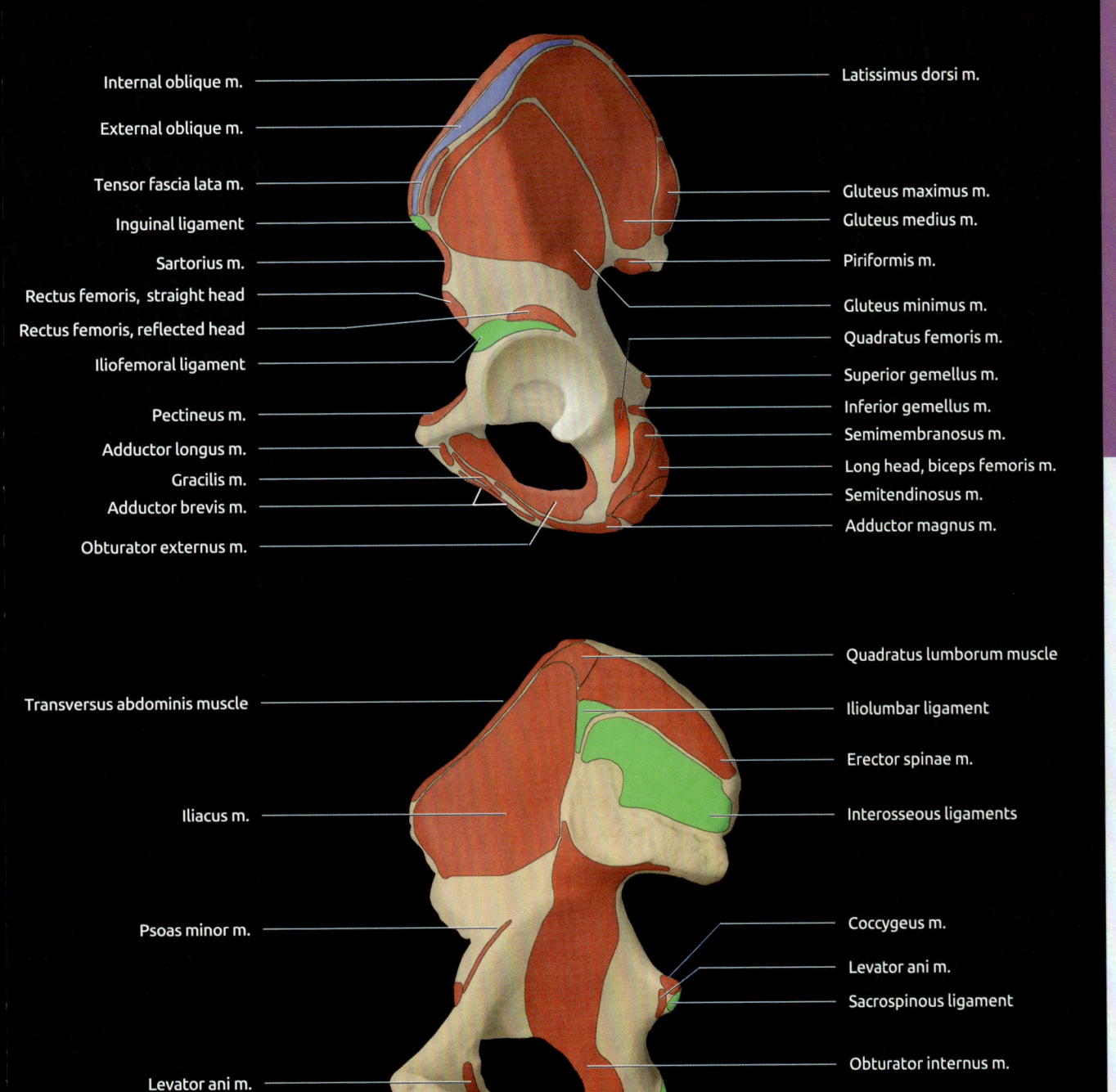

Labels (top figure, external surface):
- Internal oblique m.
- External oblique m.
- Tensor fascia lata m.
- Inguinal ligament
- Sartorius m.
- Rectus femoris, straight head
- Rectus femoris, reflected head
- Iliofemoral ligament
- Pectineus m.
- Adductor longus m.
- Gracilis m.
- Adductor brevis m.
- Obturator externus m.
- Latissimus dorsi m.
- Gluteus maximus m.
- Gluteus medius m.
- Piriformis m.
- Gluteus minimus m.
- Quadratus femoris m.
- Superior gemellus m.
- Inferior gemellus m.
- Semimembranosus m.
- Long head, biceps femoris m.
- Semitendinosus m.
- Adductor magnus m.

Labels (bottom figure, internal surface):
- Transversus abdominis muscle
- Iliacus m.
- Psoas minor m.
- Levator ani m.
- Sphincter urethra m.
- Quadratus lumborum muscle
- Iliolumbar ligament
- Erector spinae m.
- Interosseous ligaments
- Coccygeus m.
- Levator ani m.
- Sacrospinous ligament
- Obturator internus m.
- Sacrotuberous ligament
- Ischiocavernosus m.

(Top) Muscle and ligament attachments to the external surface of the innominate bone are seen. Note the relatively small origin of the tendon of the adductor longus muscle. The adductor brevis muscle is just deep to the longus muscle. The origin of the gracilis muscle is lateral to the adductor brevis muscle. The adductor magnus muscle has a broad origin with 2 heads. The fibers arising from the pubic body are sometimes called the adductor minimus and have a horizontal course. The fibers originating on the ischial tuberosity have a vertical orientation to the mid and distal femur. (Bottom) Muscle and ligament attachments to the internal surface of the pelvis are seen.

Hip MR Anatomy

ANATOMY IMAGING ISSUES

Imaging Recommendations
- Surface coil on affected hip
  - Field of view (FOV): 14-20 cm
  - Slice thickness: 3-5 mm
  - Axial plane
    - Include from above acetabular roof to lesser trochanter
  - Oblique axial plane
    - Oriented along axis of femoral neck
    - Include entire acetabulum and femoral neck
    - Originally designed to evaluate α angle for femoroacetabular impingement
    - Also useful for evaluation of labral tears
  - Sagittal plane
    - Include from midline of pelvis to lateral margin of musculature
    - Often best plane for visualizing labral tear, detachment
  - Coronal plane
    - Include all muscles
- Full FOV coronal T1 STIR of pelvis should be included with imaging of hip
  - Hip pain often due to abnormality at site beyond hip joint
  - FOV: 32-44 cm
  - Slice thickness: 4-6 mm
- Body coil slices through femoral condyle also useful
  - Allows determination of femoral anteversion

Imaging Pitfalls
- Labrum may be congenitally absent
- Sulci deep to labrum may mimic tear
  - May occur in any location
  - Smoothly marginated, parallel margins; contrast to jagged, irregular contour of tear
- Sulcus between labrum and capsule may mimic tear
- Labral degeneration almost universal, should not be diagnosed as tear
- Most labral tears occur in anterosuperior quadrant
  - Partial volume artifact in coronal plane may mimic or obscure tear
  - Tears are better seen on sagittal or oblique axial plane

CLINICAL IMPLICATIONS

Clinical Importance
- Multiple impingement syndromes can occur around hip due to variant anatomy
- Femoroacetabular impingement (FAI)
  - Pincer type: Acetabular overcoverage, may be global or focal
    - Evaluate global overcoverage on coronal and sagittal images
    - Evaluate superior rim retroversion on axial images at top of femoral head
  - Cam type: Femoral head/neck junction prominence
    - May be seen best on oblique axial images along femoral neck
    - **Or** may be seen best on sagittal images
  - Consequences of FAI
    - Labral tear
    - Juxtalabral cartilage loss
    - Fibrocystic changes anterior femoral head
    - Premature osteoarthritis
- Ischiofemoral impingement
  - Impingement of quadratus femoris between ischium and lesser trochanter
  - More common in women
  - Measurement of space less important than abnormal signal in muscle on fluid-sensitive images
  - Often related to prior trauma, bony overgrowth of ischium, or total hip arthroplasty position
- Psoas impingement
  - Impingement of psoas muscle with flexion, internal rotation
  - Muscle usually normal in morphology and signal intensity on MR
  - Suspect when labral tear at midanterior position is seen

Bursae of Hip
- **Iliopsoas bursa**
  - Deep to muscle
  - Centered at anterior wall of acetabulum
  - Rarely enlarged at MR
  - Injections may relieve psoas impingement
- **Greater trochanteric bursa**
  - Between gluteus medius and gluteus maximus
  - Clinical diagnosis of bursitis often incorrect
  - Pain in this region is often due to tendinopathy or tear of gluteal muscles
- **Obturator externus bursa**
  - Synovial outpouching from posterior hip joint
  - Between ischiofemoral ligament and zona orbicularis
  - Deep to obturator externus muscle
- **Subgluteus medius bursa**
  - Deep to gluteus medius tendon at its insertion
- **Subgluteus minimus bursa**
  - Deep to gluteus minimus tendon at its insertion

SELECTED REFERENCES

1. Kassarjian A et al: Obturator externus bursa: prevalence of communication with the hip joint and associated intra-articular findings in 200 consecutive hip MR arthrograms. Eur Radiol. 19(11):2779-82, 2009
2. Woodley SJ et al: Morphology of the bursae associated with the greater trochanter of the femur. J Bone Joint Surg Am. 90(2):284-94, 2008
3. Pfirrmann CW et al: Greater trochanter of the hip: attachment of the abductor mechanism and a complex of three bursae—MR imaging and MR bursography in cadavers and MR imaging in asymptomatic volunteers. Radiology. 221(2):469-77, 2001

Hip MR Anatomy

GRAPHICS OF HIP JOINT

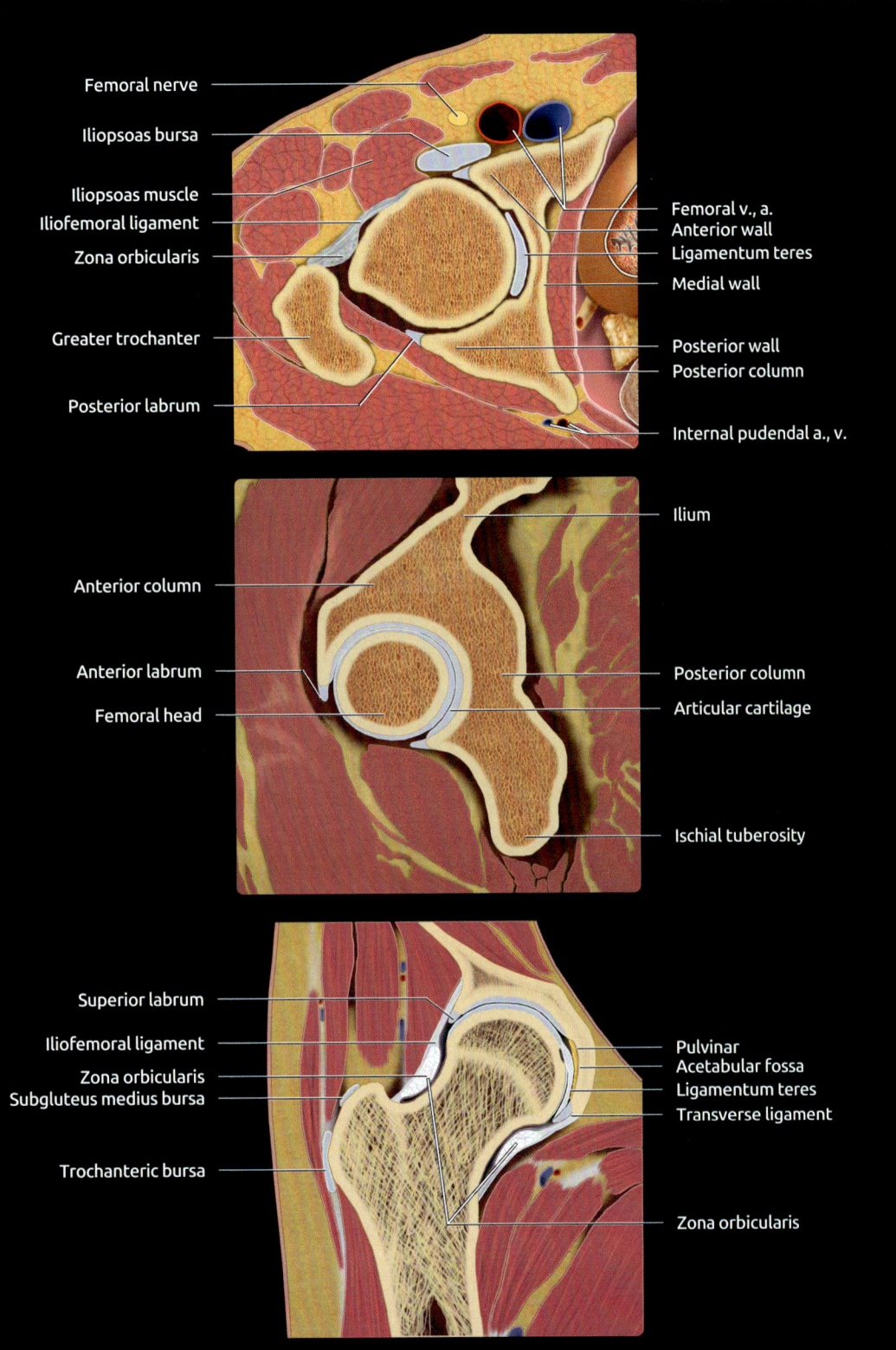

(Top) Axial representation of the hip joint is shown. The iliopsoas bursa is closely approximated to the joint anteriorly. The ligamentum teres is seen in profile as a flattened structure. The 2 layers of the external capsule are visible: The more superficial longitudinal fibers and deep circular fibers. (Middle) Sagittal representation of the hip joint nicely demonstrates the inverted Y of the acetabulum. The ilium is the stem, and the limbs are the anterior and posterior acetabular columns. (Bottom) Coronal graphic demonstrates many of the important structures of the hip joint. The longitudinally oriented fibers of the ligaments of the external joint capsule and the deeper circularly oriented fibers of the zona orbicularis are visible. Note the long axis of the ligamentum teres and its insertion onto the transverse ligament. The pulvinar fills the acetabular fossa.

Hip MR Anatomy

AXIAL T1 MR

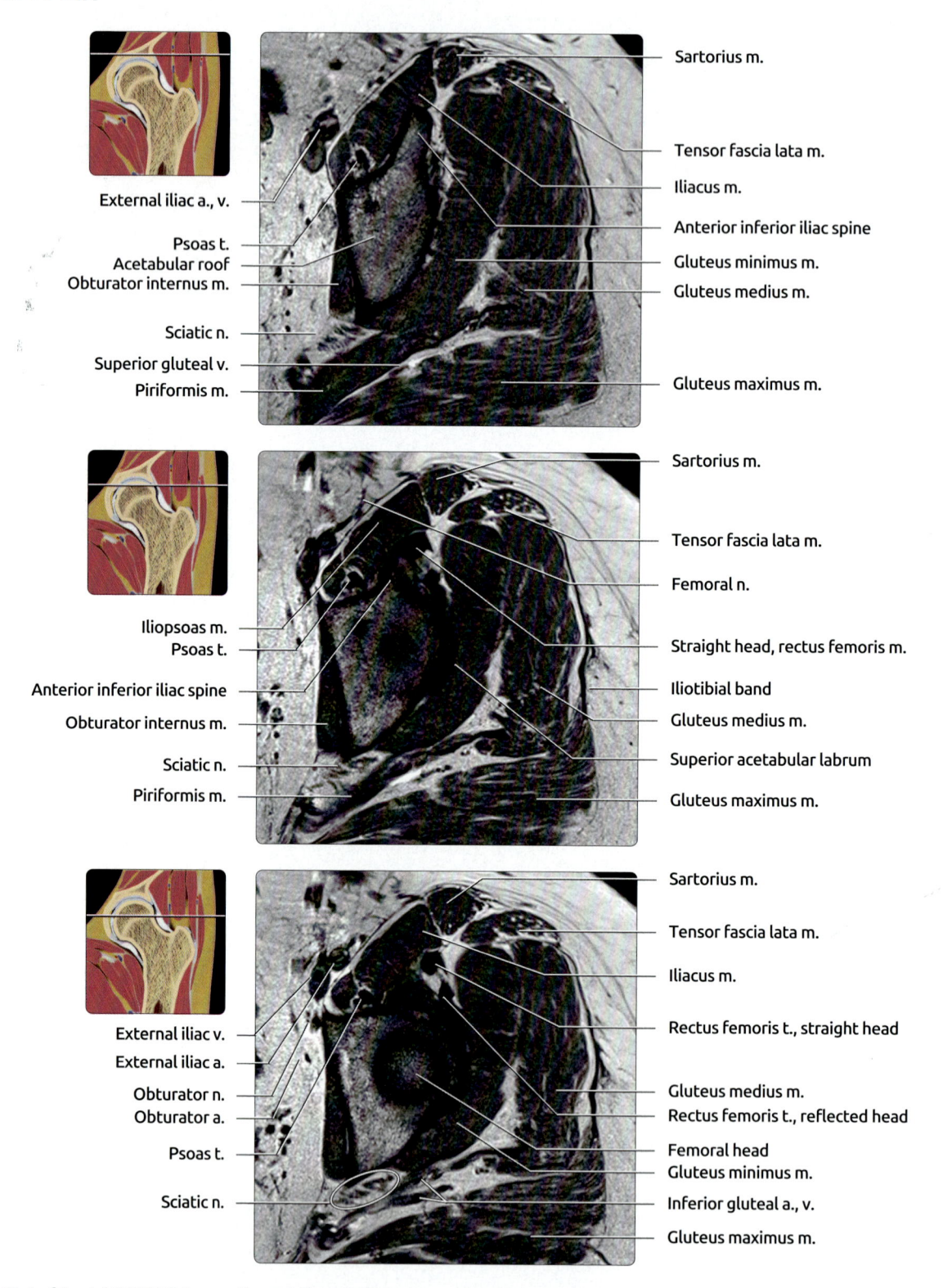

Top image labels:
- Sartorius m.
- Tensor fascia lata m.
- Iliacus m.
- Anterior inferior iliac spine
- Gluteus minimus m.
- Gluteus medius m.
- Gluteus maximus m.
- External iliac a., v.
- Psoas t.
- Acetabular roof
- Obturator internus m.
- Sciatic n.
- Superior gluteal v.
- Piriformis m.

Middle image labels:
- Sartorius m.
- Tensor fascia lata m.
- Femoral n.
- Straight head, rectus femoris m.
- Iliotibial band
- Gluteus medius m.
- Superior acetabular labrum
- Gluteus maximus m.
- Iliopsoas m.
- Psoas t.
- Anterior inferior iliac spine
- Obturator internus m.
- Sciatic n.
- Piriformis m.

Bottom image labels:
- Sartorius m.
- Tensor fascia lata m.
- Iliacus m.
- Rectus femoris t., straight head
- Gluteus medius m.
- Rectus femoris t., reflected head
- Femoral head
- Gluteus minimus m.
- Inferior gluteal a., v.
- Gluteus maximus m.
- External iliac v.
- External iliac a.
- Obturator n.
- Obturator a.
- Psoas t.
- Sciatic n.

(Top) First of 9 axial T1WI MR images through the left hip is shown. The obturator nerve overlies the obturator internus muscle. The sciatic nerve is exiting the pelvis through the greater sciatic notch. (Middle) The psoas tendon is visible as a distinct low signal intensity structure at the posterior margin of the iliopsoas muscle. The straight head of the rectus femoris is seen at its origin from the anterior inferior iliac spine. (Bottom) Both heads of the rectus femoris tendon are visible. The iliopsoas lies medial to the rectus femoris, and the sartorius extends diagonally across it.

Hip MR Anatomy

AXIAL T1 MR

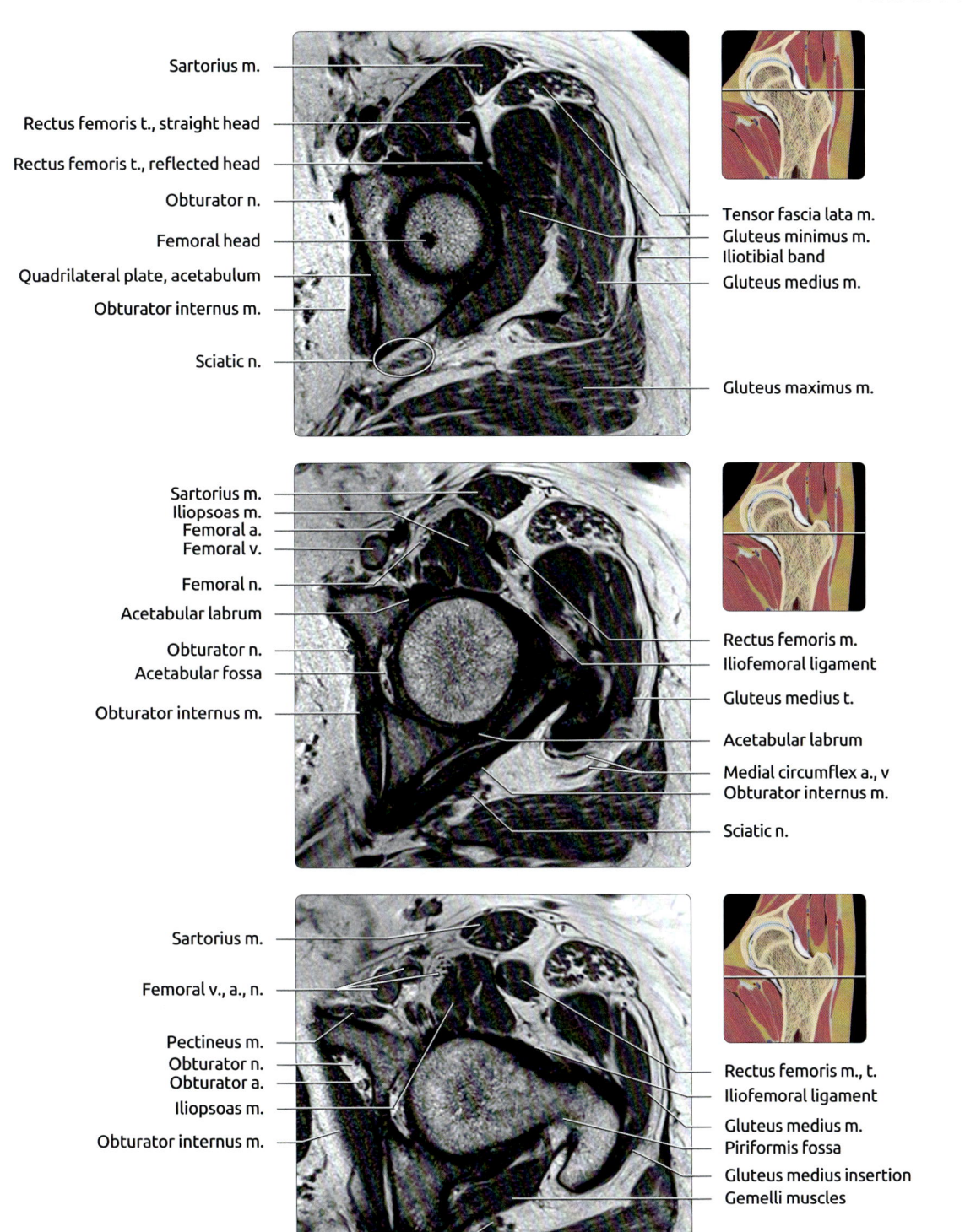

Top image labels:
- Sartorius m.
- Rectus femoris t., straight head
- Rectus femoris t., reflected head
- Obturator n.
- Femoral head
- Quadrilateral plate, acetabulum
- Obturator internus m.
- Sciatic n.
- Tensor fascia lata m.
- Gluteus minimus m.
- Iliotibial band
- Gluteus medius m.
- Gluteus maximus m.

Middle image labels:
- Sartorius m.
- Iliopsoas m.
- Femoral a.
- Femoral v.
- Femoral n.
- Acetabular labrum
- Obturator n.
- Acetabular fossa
- Obturator internus m.
- Rectus femoris m.
- Iliofemoral ligament
- Gluteus medius t.
- Acetabular labrum
- Medial circumflex a., v
- Obturator internus m.
- Sciatic n.

Bottom image labels:
- Sartorius m.
- Femoral v., a., n.
- Pectineus m.
- Obturator n.
- Obturator a.
- Iliopsoas m.
- Obturator internus m.
- Sciatic n.
- Rectus femoris m., t.
- Iliofemoral ligament
- Gluteus medius m.
- Piriformis fossa
- Gluteus medius insertion
- Gemelli muscles

(Top) The sciatic nerve has an oblique course as it exits the pelvis, and it appears ovoid on axial cross-sectional images. Straight and reflected heads of rectus femoris are seen joining on this image. (Middle) Medial circumflex vessels are wrapping around the posterior margin of the greater trochanter and supply the proximal femur. The obturator internus muscle is seen extending from the medial surface of the acetabulum, wrapping at an acute angle around the ischium and coursing in an anterolateral direction toward its insertion on the piriformis fossa. (Bottom) Gluteus minimus and medius tendons are reaching their insertions on the greater trochanter.

Hip MR Anatomy

AXIAL T1 MR

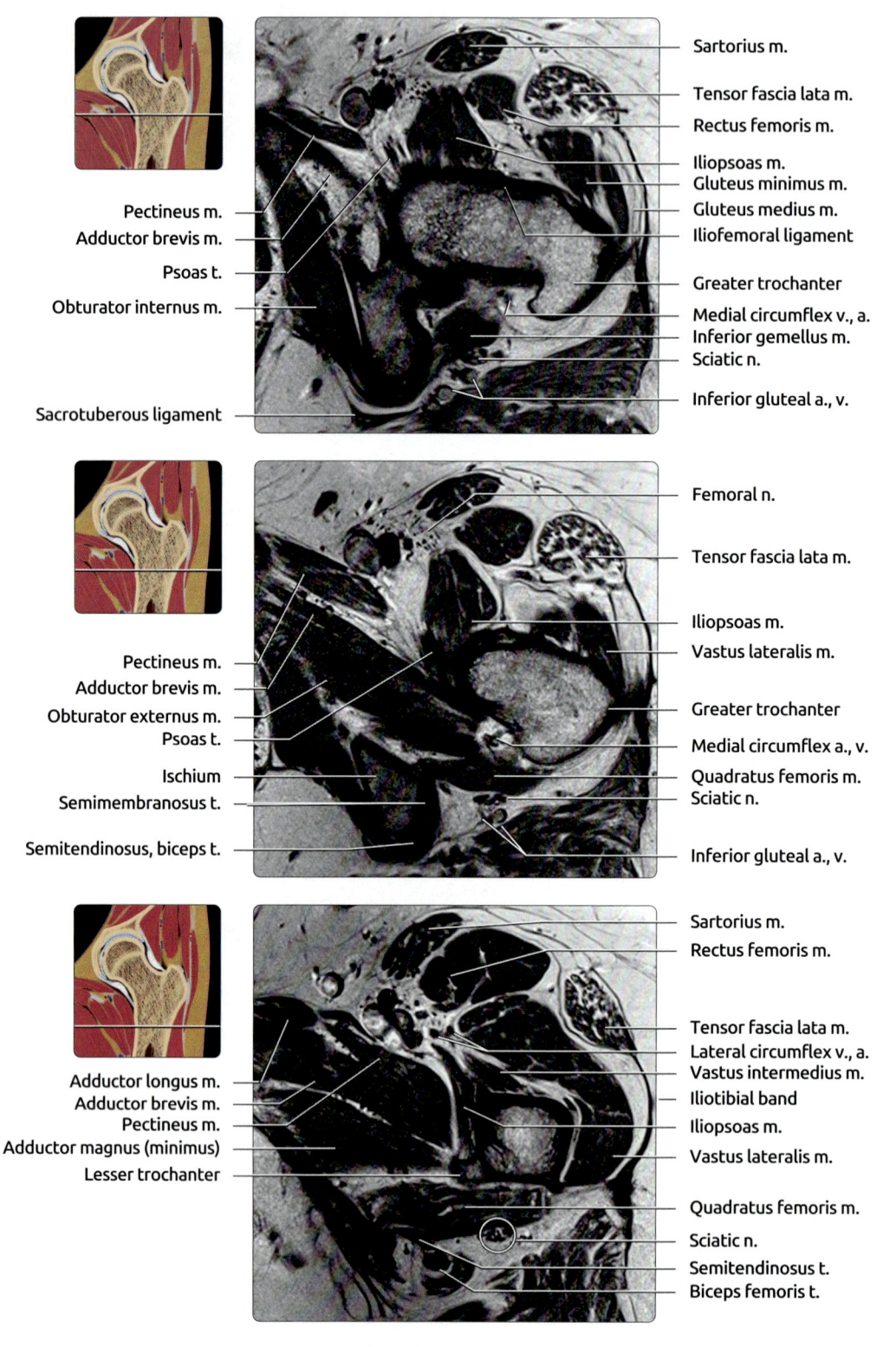

Labels (top image): Pectineus m.; Adductor brevis m.; Psoas t.; Obturator internus m.; Sacrotuberous ligament; Sartorius m.; Tensor fascia lata m.; Rectus femoris m.; Iliopsoas m.; Gluteus minimus m.; Gluteus medius m.; Iliofemoral ligament; Greater trochanter; Medial circumflex v., a.; Inferior gemellus m.; Sciatic n.; Inferior gluteal a., v.

Labels (middle image): Pectineus m.; Adductor brevis m.; Obturator externus m.; Psoas t.; Ischium; Semimembranosus t.; Semitendinosus, biceps t.; Femoral n.; Tensor fascia lata m.; Iliopsoas m.; Vastus lateralis m.; Greater trochanter; Medial circumflex a., v.; Quadratus femoris m.; Sciatic n.; Inferior gluteal a., v.

Labels (bottom image): Adductor longus m.; Adductor brevis m.; Pectineus m.; Adductor magnus (minimus); Lesser trochanter; Sartorius m.; Rectus femoris m.; Tensor fascia lata m.; Lateral circumflex v., a.; Vastus intermedius m.; Iliotibial band; Iliopsoas m.; Vastus lateralis m.; Quadratus femoris m.; Sciatic n.; Semitendinosus t.; Biceps femoris t.

(Top) The psoas tendon is a distinct structure at the posteromedial margin of the iliopsoas muscle. **(Middle)** Semimembranosus tendon originates anterior to conjoint tendon of semitendinosus and biceps femoris. **(Bottom)** The adductor magnus is perhaps best considered as 2 muscles. The upper portion shown here is nearly horizontal in orientation and is sometimes called the adductor minimus, and adducts the hip. The more vertically oriented portion is seen here originating from the ischial tuberosity. It has multiple insertions on the femoral shaft, and a small vertically oriented portion inserting on the adductor tubercle of the medial femoral condyle.

Hip MR Anatomy

OBLIQUE ANGLED AXIAL T1 MR

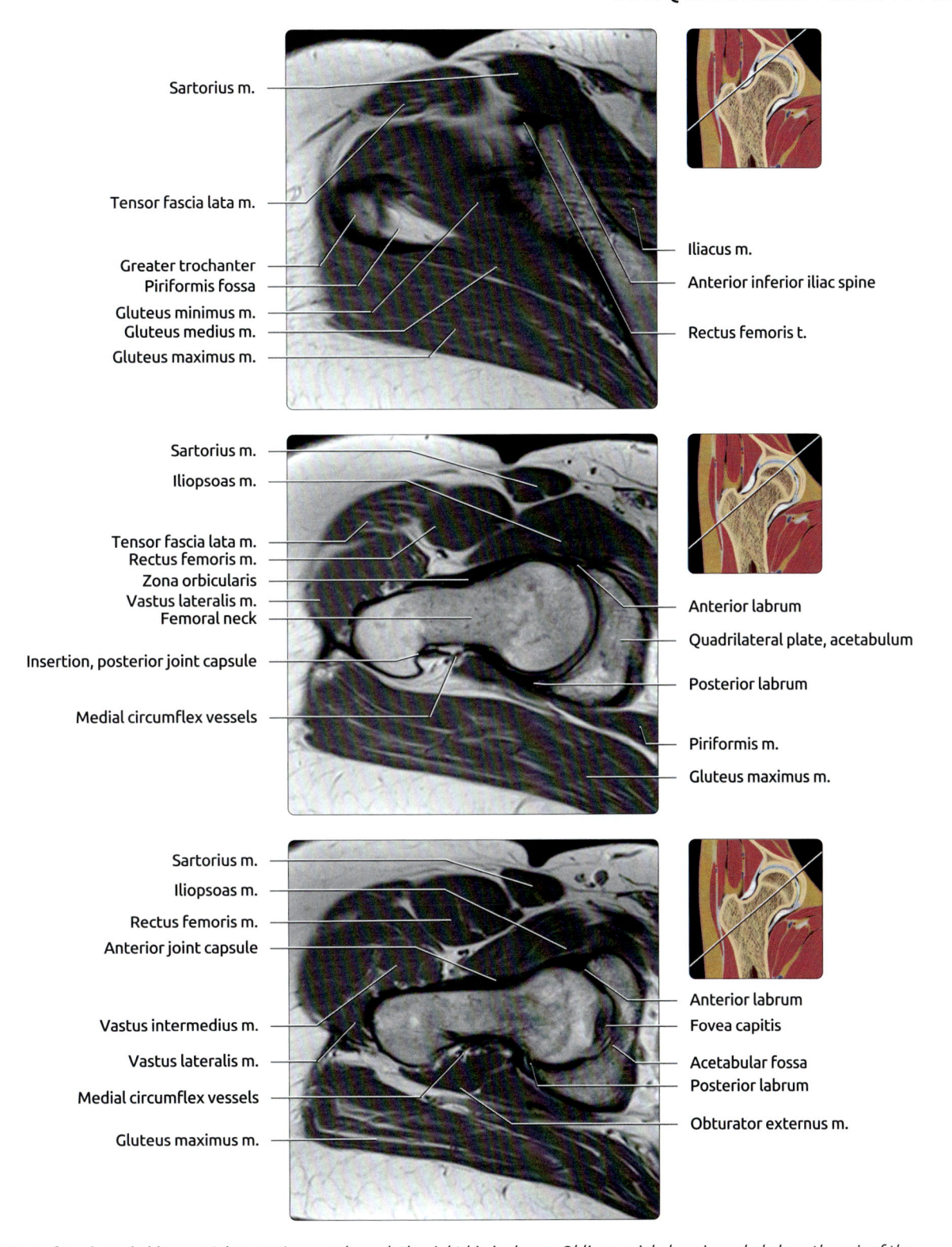

Labels (Top image):
- Sartorius m.
- Tensor fascia lata m.
- Greater trochanter
- Piriformis fossa
- Gluteus minimus m.
- Gluteus medius m.
- Gluteus maximus m.
- Iliacus m.
- Anterior inferior iliac spine
- Rectus femoris t.

Labels (Middle image):
- Sartorius m.
- Iliopsoas m.
- Tensor fascia lata m.
- Rectus femoris m.
- Zona orbicularis
- Vastus lateralis m.
- Femoral neck
- Insertion, posterior joint capsule
- Medial circumflex vessels
- Anterior labrum
- Quadrilateral plate, acetabulum
- Posterior labrum
- Piriformis m.
- Gluteus maximus m.

Labels (Bottom image):
- Sartorius m.
- Iliopsoas m.
- Rectus femoris m.
- Anterior joint capsule
- Vastus intermedius m.
- Vastus lateralis m.
- Medial circumflex vessels
- Gluteus maximus m.
- Anterior labrum
- Fovea capitis
- Acetabular fossa
- Posterior labrum
- Obturator externus m.

(**Top**) *First of 3 selected oblique axial T1 MR images through the right hip is shown. Oblique axial plane is angled along the axis of the femoral neck and is useful in evaluating for femoroacetabular impingement. The oblique plane is often useful for evaluation of musculature as well.* (**Middle**) *The zona orbicularis is a thickening and relative constriction of the joint capsule. The capsule inserts at the base of the femoral neck on the intertrochanteric line. The joint capsule is reinforced by iliofemoral, pubofemoral, and ischiofemoral ligaments.* (**Bottom**) *This image shows through the inferior margin of the fovea capitis. Anterior and posterior labra are seen as low signal intensity triangles deepening the acetabular fossa.*

Hip MR Anatomy

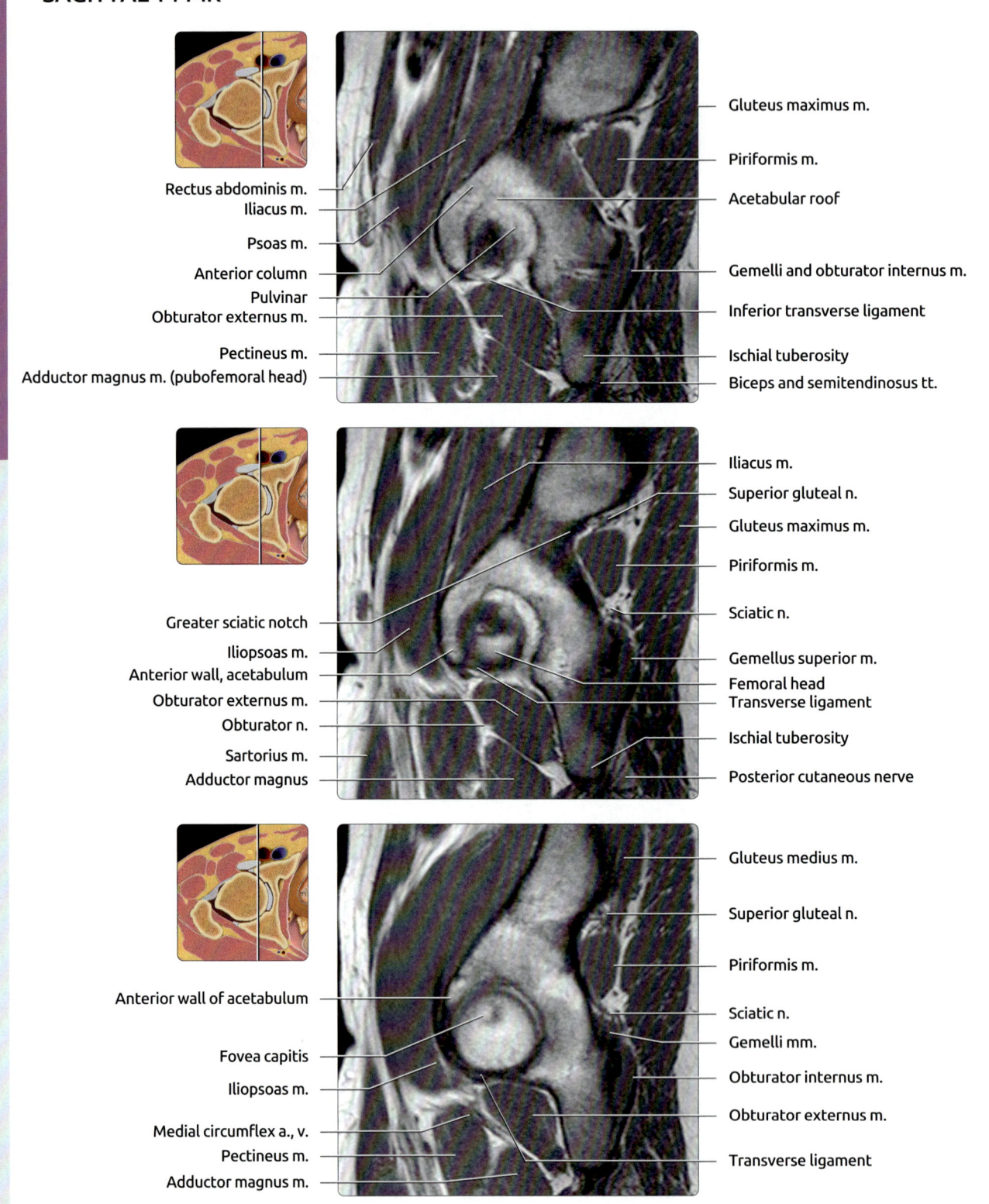

SAGITTAL T1 MR

Labels (top image, medial):
- Rectus abdominis m.
- Iliacus m.
- Psoas m.
- Anterior column
- Pulvinar
- Obturator externus m.
- Pectineus m.
- Adductor magnus m. (pubofemoral head)
- Gluteus maximus m.
- Piriformis m.
- Acetabular roof
- Gemelli and obturator internus m.
- Inferior transverse ligament
- Ischial tuberosity
- Biceps and semitendinosus tt.

Labels (middle image):
- Greater sciatic notch
- Iliopsoas m.
- Anterior wall, acetabulum
- Obturator externus m.
- Obturator n.
- Sartorius m.
- Adductor magnus
- Iliacus m.
- Superior gluteal n.
- Gluteus maximus m.
- Piriformis m.
- Sciatic n.
- Gemellus superior m.
- Femoral head
- Transverse ligament
- Ischial tuberosity
- Posterior cutaneous nerve

Labels (bottom image, lateral):
- Anterior wall of acetabulum
- Fovea capitis
- Iliopsoas m.
- Medial circumflex a., v.
- Pectineus m.
- Adductor magnus m.
- Gluteus medius m.
- Superior gluteal n.
- Piriformis m.
- Sciatic n.
- Gemelli mm.
- Obturator internus m.
- Obturator externus m.
- Transverse ligament

(**Top**) Sagittal T1 MR shows the appearance of the hip from medial to lateral. The fatty pulvinar at the medial aspect of the hip joint is seen. The acetabulum forms a horseshoe shape that opens inferiorly. A small portion of the inferior transverse ligament is visible as it traverses the inferior, open side of the acetabulum. (**Middle**) Superior gluteal nerve is exiting the sciatic notch superior to the piriformis muscle. Sciatic nerve lies between piriformis muscle and superior gemellus muscle. Posterior cutaneous nerve lies immediately posterior to ischial tuberosity. (**Bottom**) The sciatic nerve is located along the inferior border of the piriformis muscle as it enters the lower extremity. The muscle belly of the obturator internus tapers as it courses along the posterior aspect of the hip joint.

Hip MR Anatomy

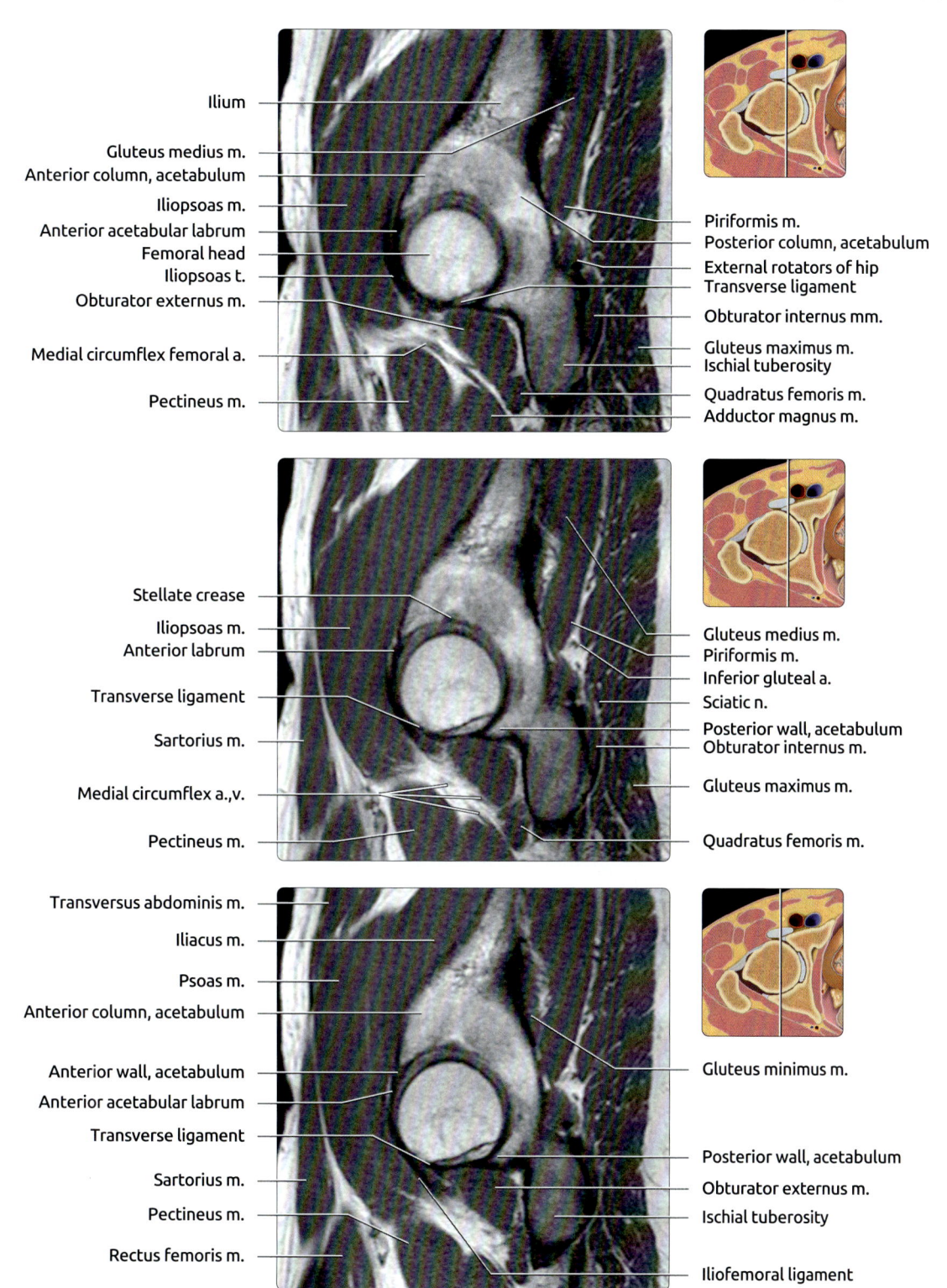

SAGITTAL T1 MR

Labels (Top image):
- Ilium
- Gluteus medius m.
- Anterior column, acetabulum
- Iliopsoas m.
- Anterior acetabular labrum
- Femoral head
- Iliopsoas t.
- Obturator externus m.
- Medial circumflex femoral a.
- Pectineus m.
- Piriformis m.
- Posterior column, acetabulum
- External rotators of hip
- Transverse ligament
- Obturator internus mm.
- Gluteus maximus m.
- Ischial tuberosity
- Quadratus femoris m.
- Adductor magnus m.

Labels (Middle image):
- Stellate crease
- Iliopsoas m.
- Anterior labrum
- Transverse ligament
- Sartorius m.
- Medial circumflex a., v.
- Pectineus m.
- Gluteus medius m.
- Piriformis m.
- Inferior gluteal a.
- Sciatic n.
- Posterior wall, acetabulum
- Obturator internus m.
- Gluteus maximus m.
- Quadratus femoris m.

Labels (Bottom image):
- Transversus abdominis m.
- Iliacus m.
- Psoas m.
- Anterior column, acetabulum
- Anterior wall, acetabulum
- Anterior acetabular labrum
- Transverse ligament
- Sartorius m.
- Pectineus m.
- Rectus femoris m.
- Gluteus minimus m.
- Posterior wall, acetabulum
- Obturator externus m.
- Ischial tuberosity
- Iliofemoral ligament

(Top) The inverted Y shape of the anterior and posterior columns of the acetabulum is seen forming a cup around the femoral head. The posterior column terminates inferiorly in the ischial tuberosity. **(Middle)** The sciatic nerve now lies between the obturator internus muscle and gluteus maximus muscle. The gluteus medius muscle is seen deep to the gluteus maximus and superior to the piriformis muscle. Stellate crease, a small indentation in the superior acetabulum, is visible. **(Bottom)** The acetabulum is anteverted, i.e., the anterior wall does not extend as far inferiorly as does the posterior wall. This allows the hip greater flexion than extension.

Hip MR Anatomy

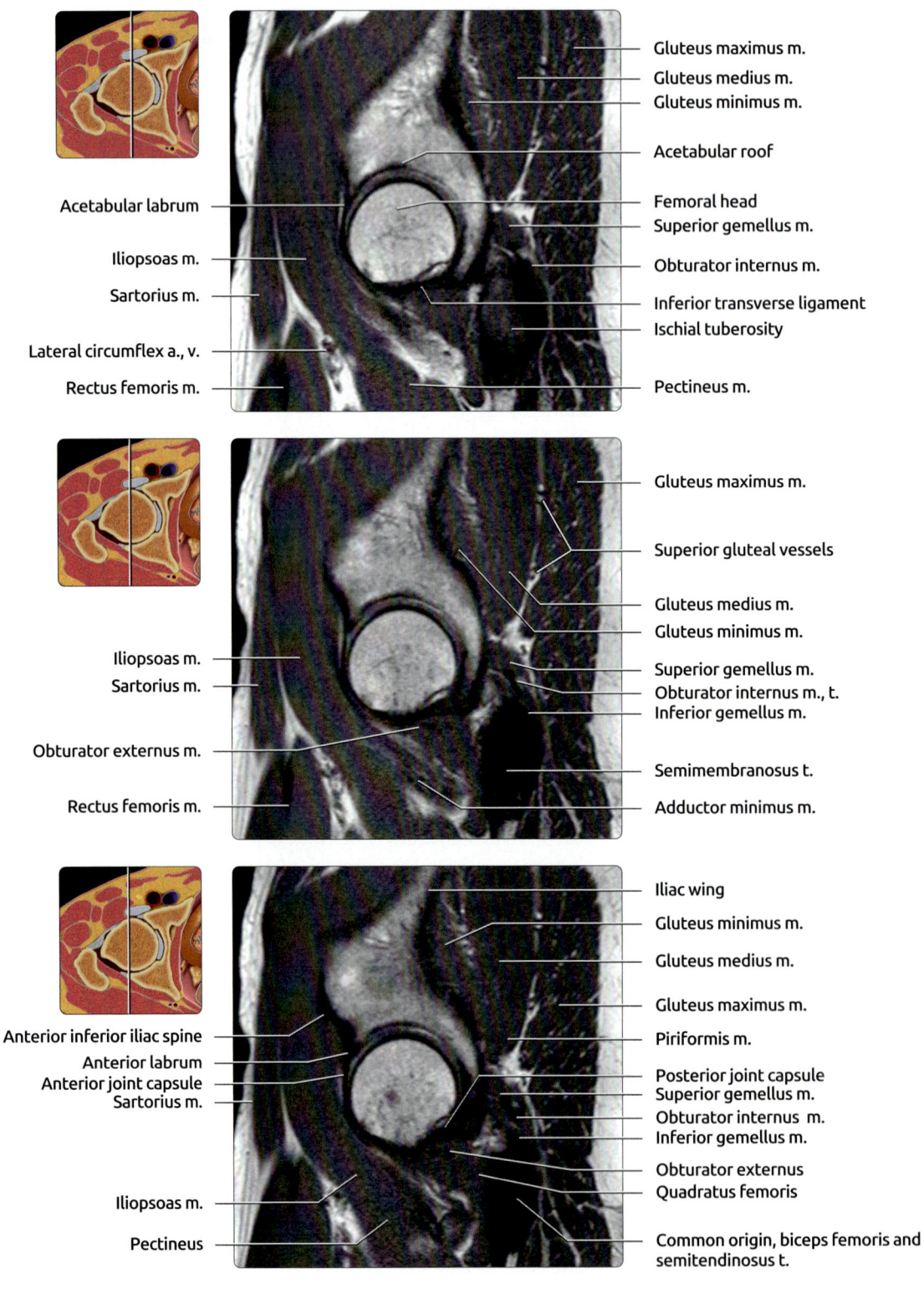

SAGITTAL T1 MR

Top image labels:
- Acetabular labrum
- Iliopsoas m.
- Sartorius m.
- Lateral circumflex a., v.
- Rectus femoris m.
- Gluteus maximus m.
- Gluteus medius m.
- Gluteus minimus m.
- Acetabular roof
- Femoral head
- Superior gemellus m.
- Obturator internus m.
- Inferior transverse ligament
- Ischial tuberosity
- Pectineus m.

Middle image labels:
- Iliopsoas m.
- Sartorius m.
- Obturator externus m.
- Rectus femoris m.
- Gluteus maximus m.
- Superior gluteal vessels
- Gluteus medius m.
- Gluteus minimus m.
- Superior gemellus m.
- Obturator internus m., t.
- Inferior gemellus m.
- Semimembranosus t.
- Adductor minimus m.

Bottom image labels:
- Anterior inferior iliac spine
- Anterior labrum
- Anterior joint capsule
- Sartorius m.
- Iliopsoas m.
- Pectineus
- Iliac wing
- Gluteus minimus m.
- Gluteus medius m.
- Gluteus maximus m.
- Piriformis m.
- Posterior joint capsule
- Superior gemellus m.
- Obturator internus m.
- Inferior gemellus m.
- Obturator externus
- Quadratus femoris
- Common origin, biceps femoris and semitendinosus t.

(Top) The acetabular labrum is well seen on sagittal images. In this case, it is small but normal in contour and signal intensity. **(Middle)** The gluteus minimus muscle origin is the deepest and most lateral of the gluteal muscles. The superior gluteal vessels are branching as they travel in the fat plane deep to the gluteus maximus muscle. Lateral to the ischium, the obturator externus muscle courses posteriorly to join the other external rotators of the hip. **(Bottom)** It is helpful to focus on key relationships of the complex muscles around the hip. The obturator externus is superior to the quadratus femoris. The iliopsoas is superior to the quadratus femoris at this level, and lateral to it on more medial sections. The gemelli muscles flank the obturator internus.

Hip MR Anatomy

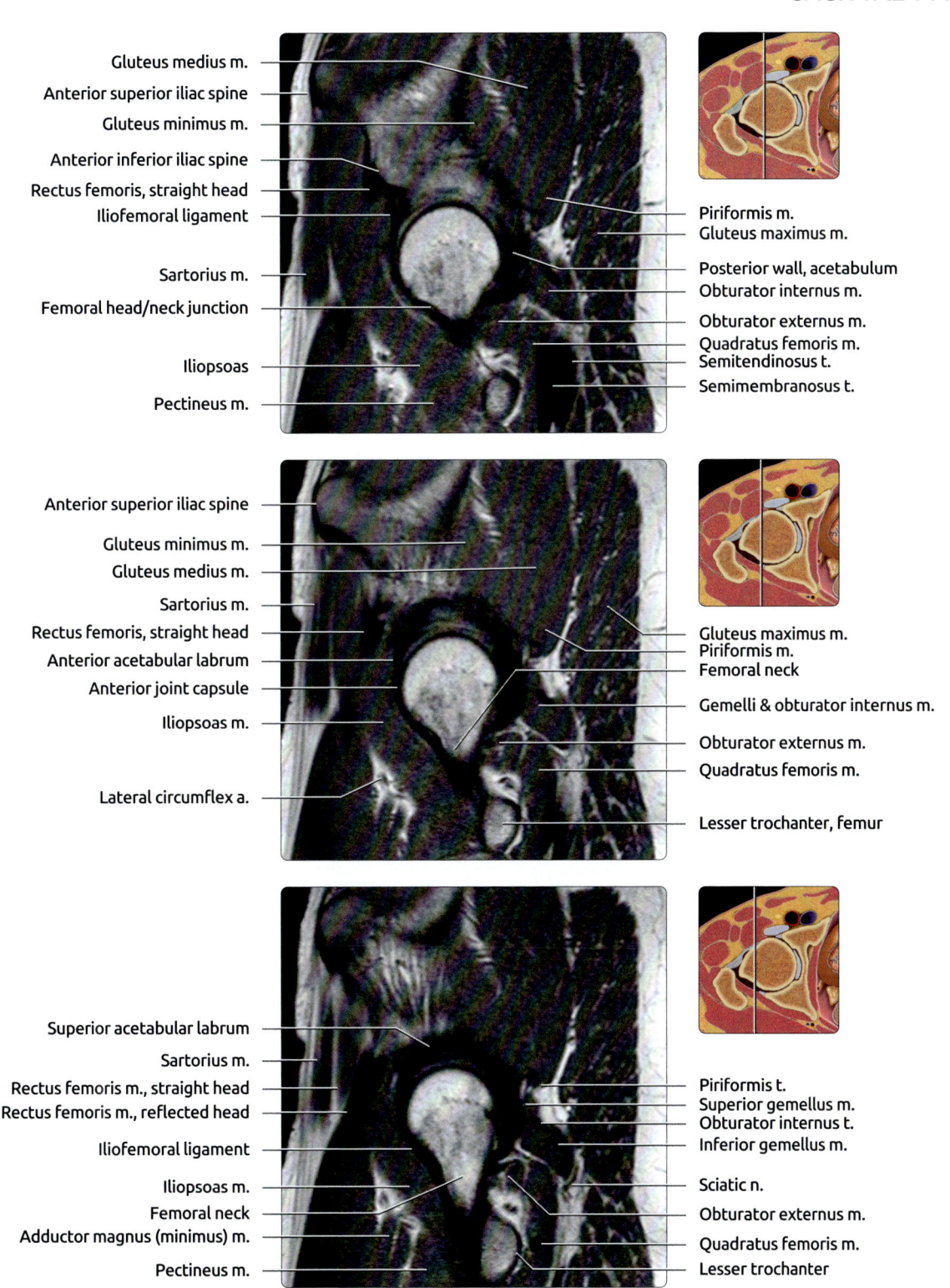

SAGITTAL T1 MR

Top image labels (left):
- Gluteus medius m.
- Anterior superior iliac spine
- Gluteus minimus m.
- Anterior inferior iliac spine
- Rectus femoris, straight head
- Iliofemoral ligament
- Sartorius m.
- Femoral head/neck junction
- Iliopsoas
- Pectineus m.

Top image labels (right):
- Piriformis m.
- Gluteus maximus m.
- Posterior wall, acetabulum
- Obturator internus m.
- Obturator externus m.
- Quadratus femoris m.
- Semitendinosus t.
- Semimembranosus t.

Middle image labels (left):
- Anterior superior iliac spine
- Gluteus minimus m.
- Gluteus medius m.
- Sartorius m.
- Rectus femoris, straight head
- Anterior acetabular labrum
- Anterior joint capsule
- Iliopsoas m.
- Lateral circumflex a.

Middle image labels (right):
- Gluteus maximus m.
- Piriformis m.
- Femoral neck
- Gemelli & obturator internus m.
- Obturator externus m.
- Quadratus femoris m.
- Lesser trochanter, femur

Bottom image labels (left):
- Superior acetabular labrum
- Sartorius m.
- Rectus femoris m., straight head
- Rectus femoris m., reflected head
- Iliofemoral ligament
- Iliopsoas m.
- Femoral neck
- Adductor magnus (minimus) m.
- Pectineus m.

Bottom image labels (right):
- Piriformis t.
- Superior gemellus m.
- Obturator internus t.
- Inferior gemellus m.
- Sciatic n.
- Obturator externus m.
- Quadratus femoris m.
- Lesser trochanter

(**Top**) Straight head of rectus femoris originates from anterior inferior iliac spine (AIIS). Iliofemoral ligament originates immediately inferior to it, from the undersurface of the AIIS. (**Middle**) Most tears of the acetabular labrum occur in the anterosuperior quadrant. They are often best visualized on sagittal images. (**Bottom**) The sciatic nerve is now visible as it travels below the border of the inferior gemellus muscle. Once it assumes its position along the posterior hip, the obturator externus muscle rapidly decreases in size.

Hip MR Anatomy

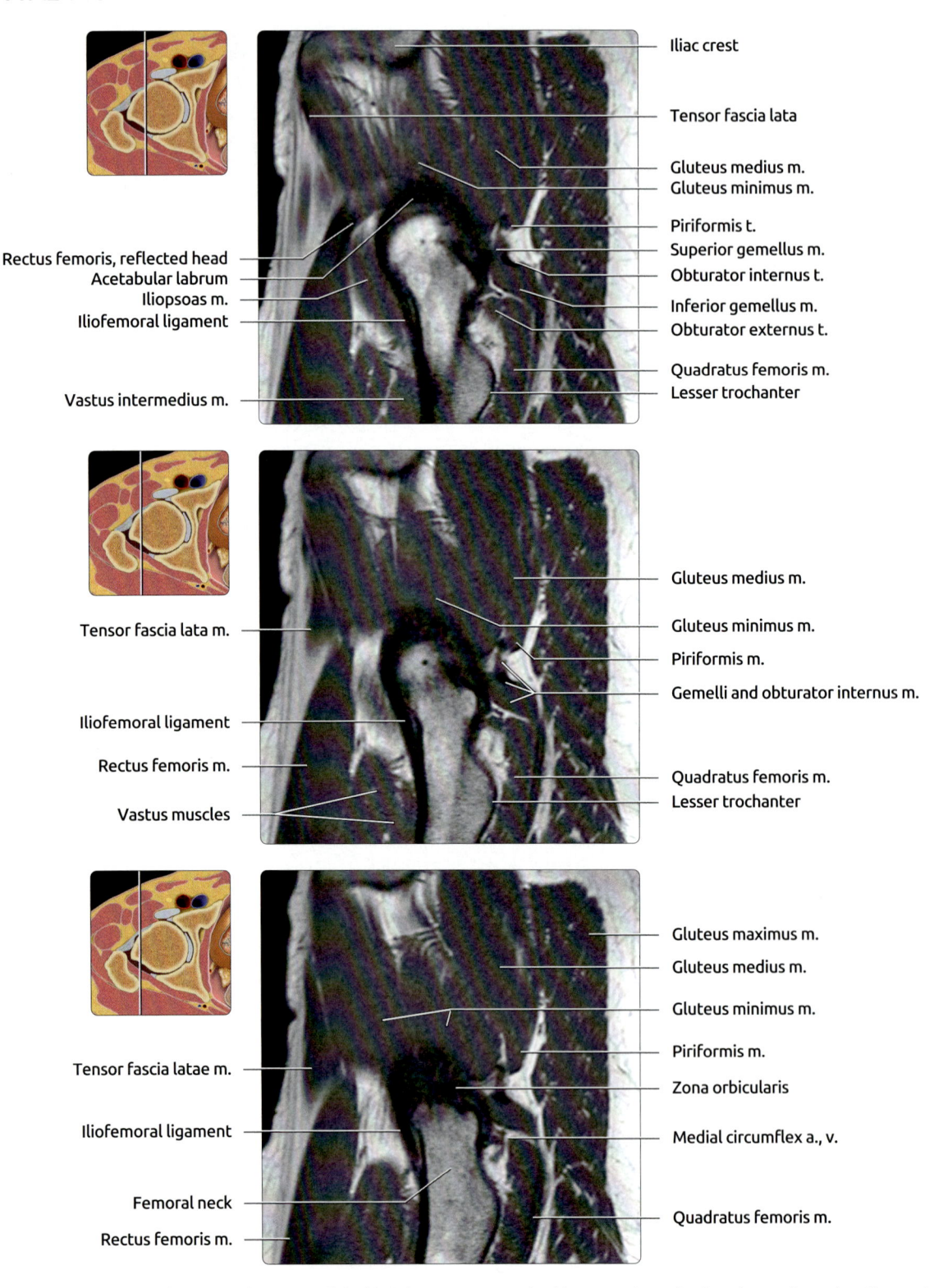

SAGITTAL T1 MR

Image 1 labels:
- Iliac crest
- Tensor fascia lata
- Gluteus medius m.
- Gluteus minimus m.
- Piriformis t.
- Superior gemellus m.
- Obturator internus t.
- Inferior gemellus m.
- Obturator externus t.
- Quadratus femoris m.
- Lesser trochanter
- Rectus femoris, reflected head
- Acetabular labrum
- Iliopsoas m.
- Iliofemoral ligament
- Vastus intermedius m.

Image 2 labels:
- Gluteus medius m.
- Gluteus minimus m.
- Piriformis m.
- Gemelli and obturator internus m.
- Quadratus femoris m.
- Lesser trochanter
- Tensor fascia lata m.
- Iliofemoral ligament
- Rectus femoris m.
- Vastus muscles

Image 3 labels:
- Gluteus maximus m.
- Gluteus medius m.
- Gluteus minimus m.
- Piriformis m.
- Zona orbicularis
- Medial circumflex a., v.
- Quadratus femoris m.
- Tensor fascia latae m.
- Iliofemoral ligament
- Femoral neck
- Rectus femoris m.

(**Top**) *The relationships of the external rotators of the hip is best seen on sagittal images. Along the deep layer of muscles, the most superior tendon is the piriformis, followed by superior gemellus, obturator internus, inferior gemellus, then obturator externus. These muscles all insert onto the piriformis fossa. The quadratus femoris muscle is deep to the gluteus maximus muscle and inserts medial to that muscle on the posterior aspect of the femur. The gluteus minimus and medius muscles both insert onto the greater trochanter.* (**Middle**) *The iliofemoral ligament is up to 10 mm thick. Because of its thickness, joint injections may be only partly intraarticular and partly into the substance of the ligament, especially if joint recesses are not distended. A slight cephalad or lateral angulation of the needle allows the bevel of the needle to lie completely within the joint.* (**Bottom**) *Branches of the medial circumflex femoral artery wrap around posterior femoral neck.*

Hip MR Anatomy

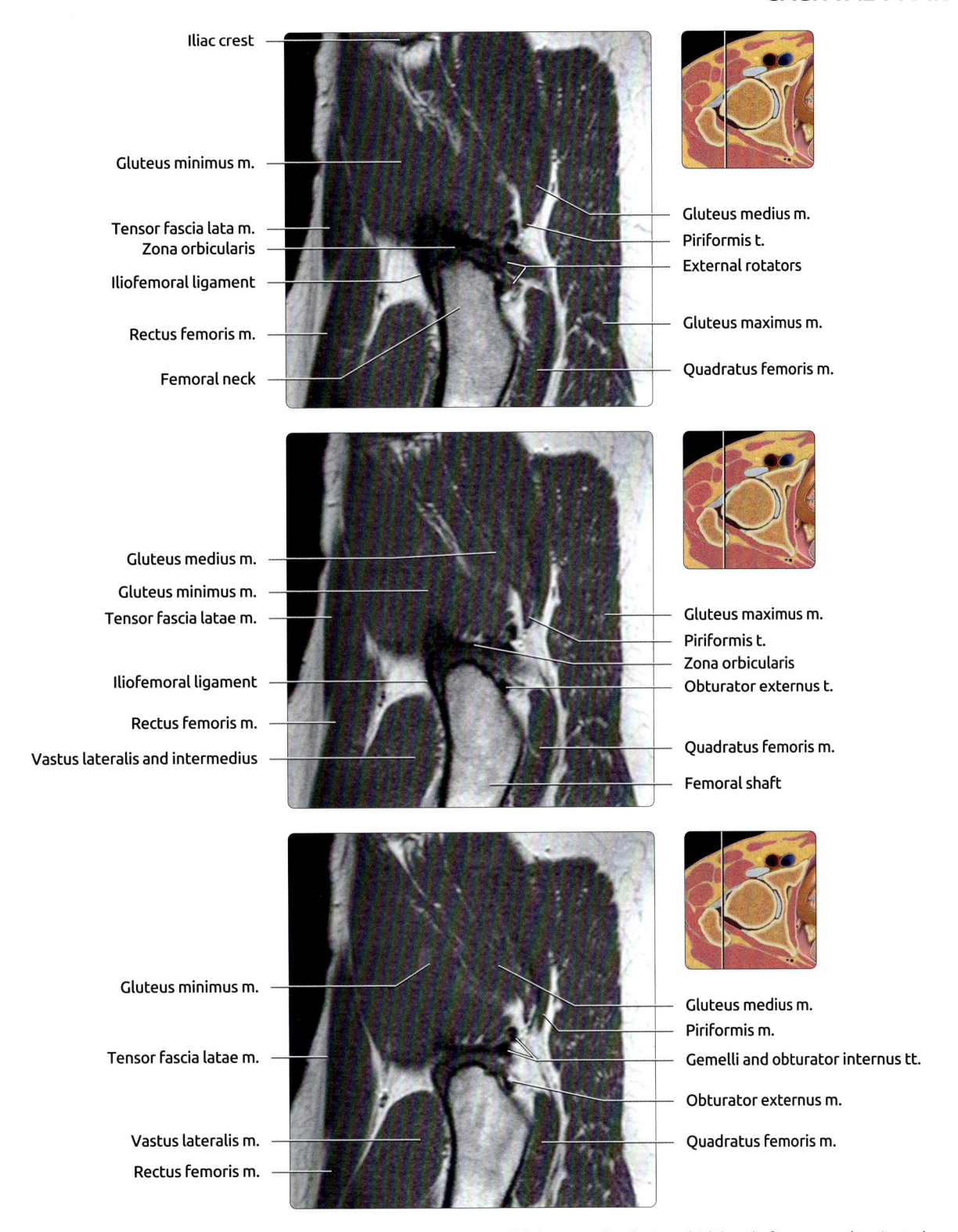

SAGITTAL T1 MR

(Top) The tensor fascia latae is the most anterolateral muscle of the hip. **(Middle)** Zona orbicularis, a thick band of transversely oriented fibers reinforcing the hip joint capsule, is seen here at the lateral margin of hip joint. **(Bottom)** The piriformis muscle is at the inferior margin of the gluteus medius muscle and it may be difficult to distinguish on sagittal images. On axial images, which are more aligned with the piriformis muscle, the muscle is more readily distinguished.

Hip MR Anatomy

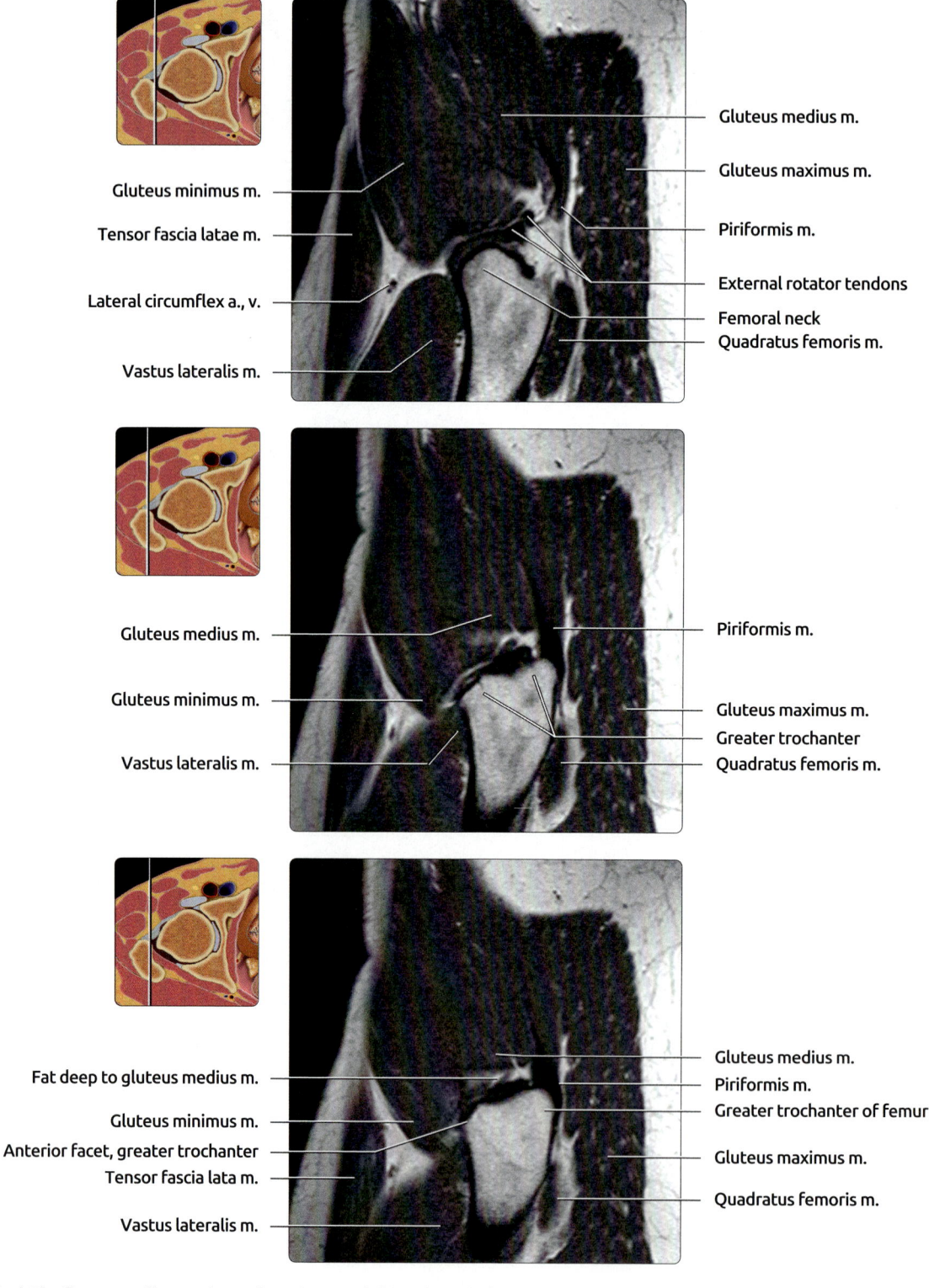

SAGITTAL T1 MR

(Top image labels):
- Gluteus minimus m.
- Tensor fascia latae m.
- Lateral circumflex a., v.
- Vastus lateralis m.
- Gluteus medius m.
- Gluteus maximus m.
- Piriformis m.
- External rotator tendons
- Femoral neck
- Quadratus femoris m.

(Middle image labels):
- Gluteus medius m.
- Gluteus minimus m.
- Vastus lateralis m.
- Piriformis m.
- Gluteus maximus m.
- Greater trochanter
- Quadratus femoris m.

(Bottom image labels):
- Fat deep to gluteus medius m.
- Gluteus minimus m.
- Anterior facet, greater trochanter
- Tensor fascia lata m.
- Vastus lateralis m.
- Gluteus medius m.
- Piriformis m.
- Greater trochanter of femur
- Gluteus maximus m.
- Quadratus femoris m.

(Top) The flat, strap-like quadratus femoris extends from the ischium to the posterior femur. It is the most inferiorly positioned of the external rotators of the hip. (Middle) The piriformis tendon and the obturator internus and gemelli muscles insert in close proximity on the greater trochanter at its posterior margin. The gluteus medius tendon inserts onto the lateral facet of the greater trochanter. The gluteus medius tendon has 2 components, one that is coronally oriented and the other more sagittally oriented. The coronally oriented component is visible here. (Bottom) The gluteus minimus is seen at the anterior margin of the femur, approaching its insertion on the anterior facet of the greater trochanter.

Hip MR Anatomy

SAGITTAL T1 MR

Labels (Top): Gluteus medius m.; Gluteus minimus m.; Tensor fascia latae m.; Vastus lateralis m.; Greater trochanter; Gluteus maximus m.

Labels (Middle): Gluteus minimus m.; Rectus femoris m.; Vastus lateralis m.; Gluteus medius m.; Gluteus maximus m.

Labels (Bottom): Gluteus medius m.; Gluteus minimus m.; Vastus lateralis m.; Gluteus maximus m.

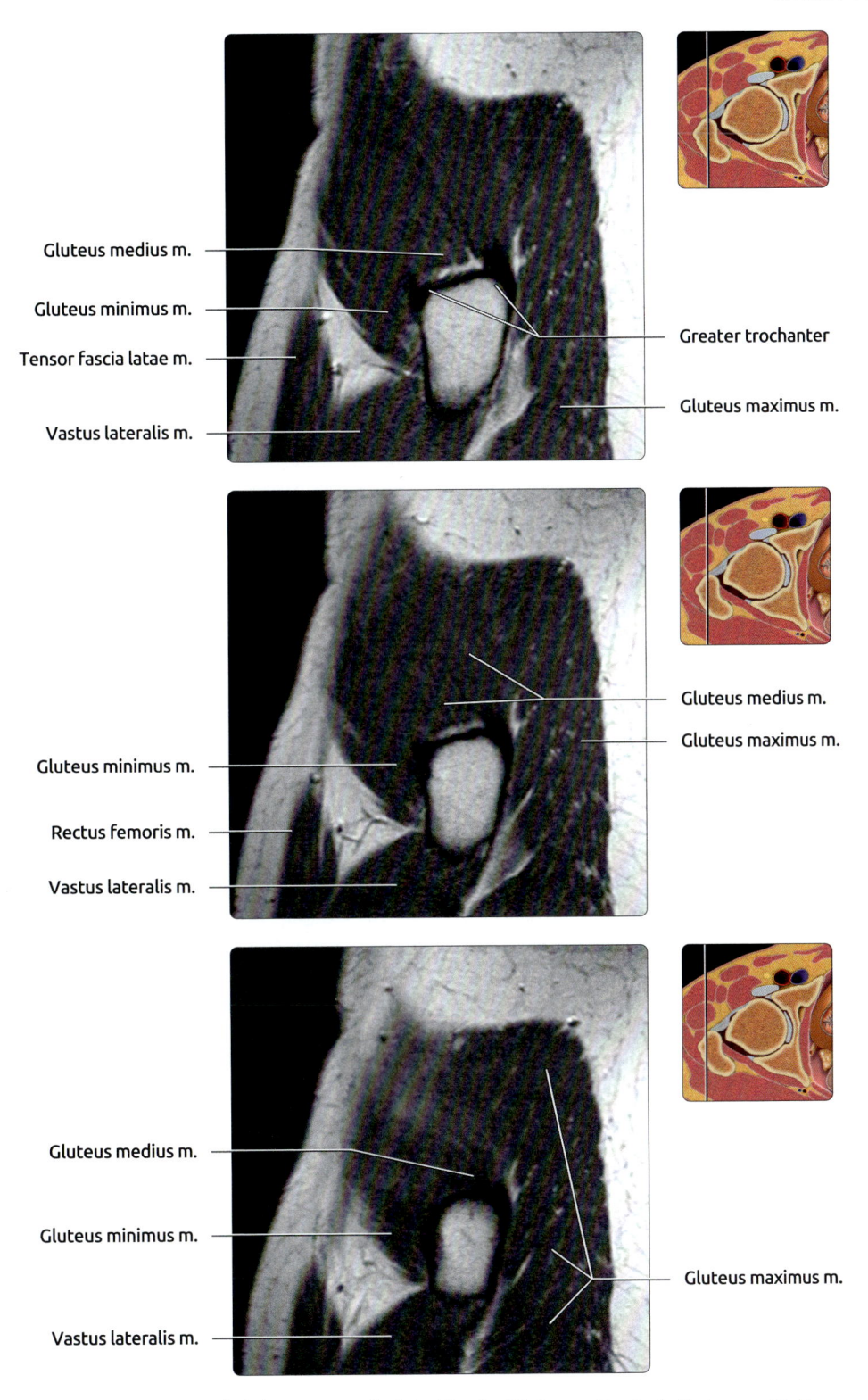

(**Top**) The gluteal muscles are sometimes called the rotator cuff of the hip. On this image, the similarity to a sagittal image of the rotator cuff of the shoulder is readily apparent. (**Middle**) The vastus lateralis wraps around the anterior and lateral portions of the femur. (**Bottom**) Gluteus minimus attaches to the anterior facet of the greater trochanter. Gluteus medius attaches to its superior facet and lateral margin. Gluteus maximus does not insert on the greater trochanter, sweeping beyond it, separated from the gluteus medius by the trochanteric bursa.

Hip MR Anatomy

CORONAL T1 MR

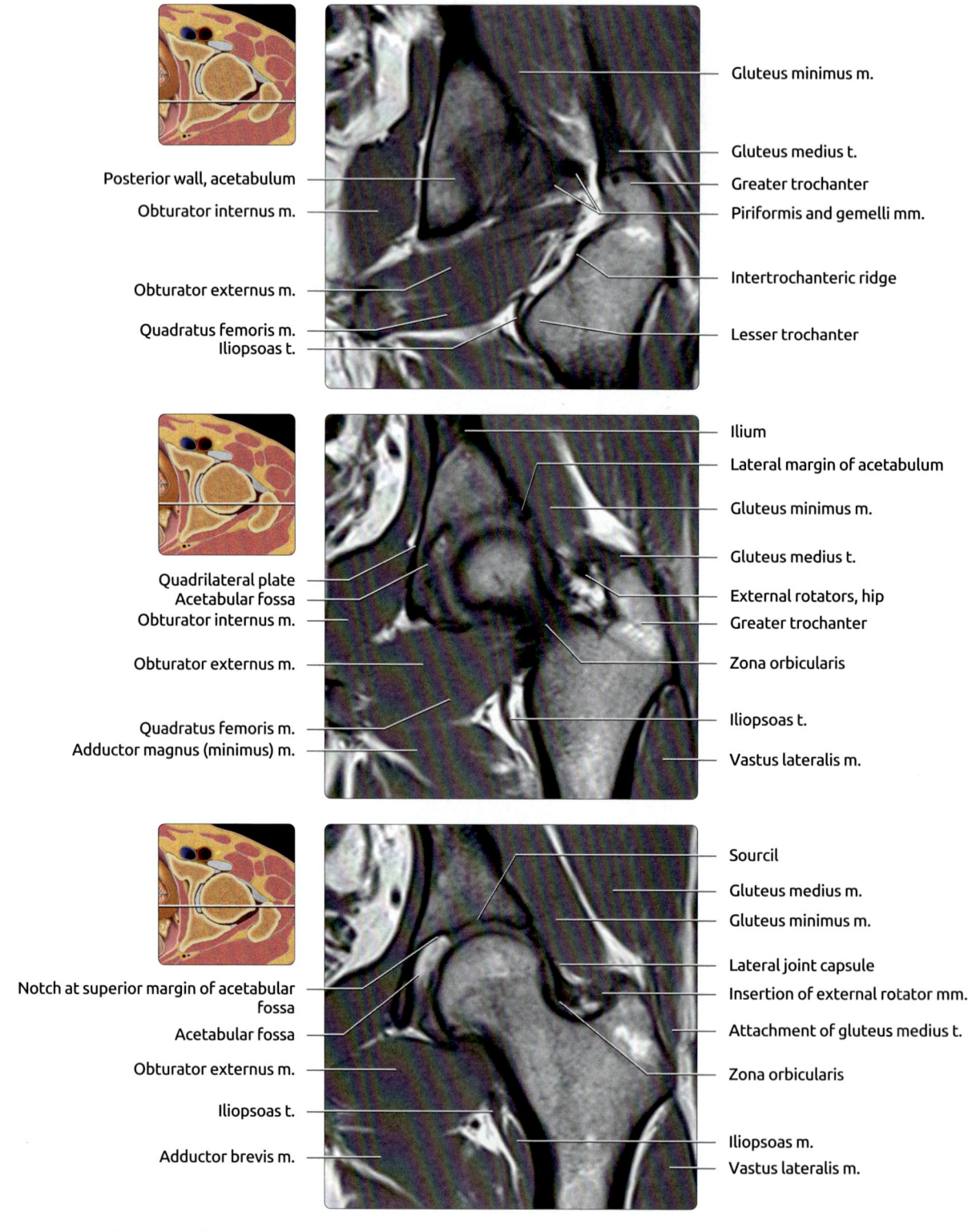

Labels (Top image):
- Posterior wall, acetabulum
- Obturator internus m.
- Obturator externus m.
- Quadratus femoris m.
- Iliopsoas t.
- Gluteus minimus m.
- Gluteus medius t.
- Greater trochanter
- Piriformis and gemelli mm.
- Intertrochanteric ridge
- Lesser trochanter

Labels (Middle image):
- Quadrilateral plate
- Acetabular fossa
- Obturator internus m.
- Obturator externus m.
- Quadratus femoris m.
- Adductor magnus (minimus) m.
- Ilium
- Lateral margin of acetabulum
- Gluteus minimus m.
- Gluteus medius t.
- External rotators, hip
- Greater trochanter
- Zona orbicularis
- Iliopsoas t.
- Vastus lateralis m.

Labels (Bottom image):
- Notch at superior margin of acetabular fossa
- Acetabular fossa
- Obturator externus m.
- Iliopsoas t.
- Adductor brevis m.
- Sourcil
- Gluteus medius m.
- Gluteus minimus m.
- Lateral joint capsule
- Insertion of external rotator mm.
- Attachment of gluteus medius t.
- Zona orbicularis
- Iliopsoas m.
- Vastus lateralis m.

(Top) The iliopsoas tendon is seen at its insertion on the lesser trochanter. The external rotators of the hip include the obturator internus and externus, the superior and inferior gemelli, the piriformis, and the quadratus femoris. **(Middle)** This image shows the relative positions of the obturator externus and internus muscles on either side of the obturator ring. **(Bottom)** Acetabular fossa is filled with fatty tissue called the pulvinar. The normal notch at the superior margin of the acetabular fossa is sometimes mistaken for cortical step-off due to fracture.

Hip MR Anatomy

CORONAL T1 MR

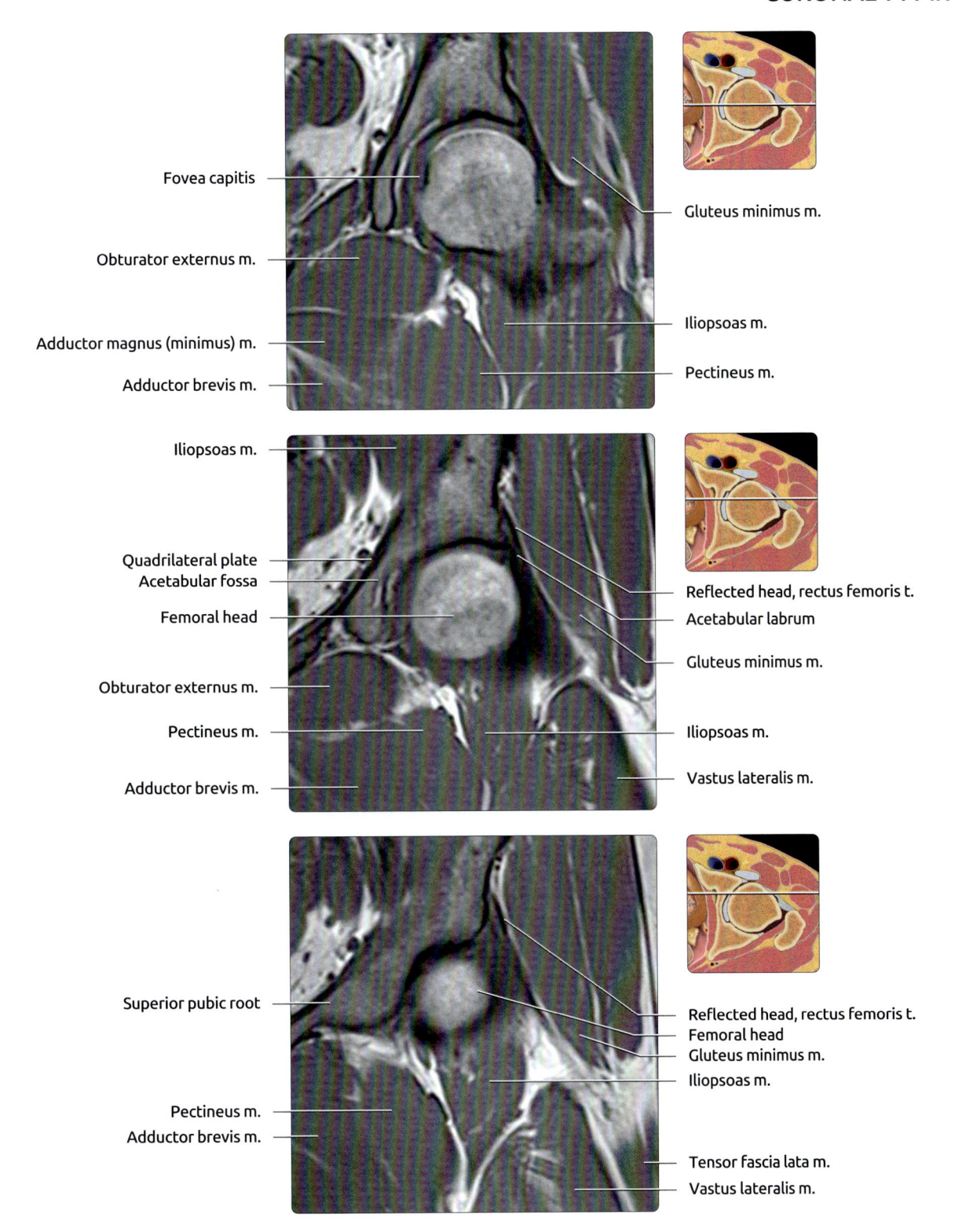

Labels (top image):
- Fovea capitis
- Obturator externus m.
- Adductor magnus (minimus) m.
- Adductor brevis m.
- Gluteus minimus m.
- Iliopsoas m.
- Pectineus m.

Labels (middle image):
- Iliopsoas m.
- Quadrilateral plate
- Acetabular fossa
- Femoral head
- Obturator externus m.
- Pectineus m.
- Adductor brevis m.
- Reflected head, rectus femoris t.
- Acetabular labrum
- Gluteus minimus m.
- Iliopsoas m.
- Vastus lateralis m.

Labels (bottom image):
- Superior pubic root
- Pectineus m.
- Adductor brevis m.
- Reflected head, rectus femoris t.
- Femoral head
- Gluteus minimus m.
- Iliopsoas m.
- Tensor fascia lata m.
- Vastus lateralis m.

(Top) The fovea capitis is a normal indentation on the medial femoral head, and the attachment site of the ligamentum teres. **(Middle)** The quadrilateral plate is the medial bony margin of the acetabulum. It has a central concavity along its lateral margin, called the acetabular fossa. **(Bottom)** The most lateral portion of the superior pubic ramus, adjacent to the acetabulum, is called the superior pubic root.

Pelvis and Hip Radiographic and Arthrographic Anatomy

IMAGING ANATOMY

Overview

- **AP pelvis**
  - Should be centered on pubic symphysis
  - Patient supine or upright, anteroposterior beam
  - Include iliac crest to below lesser trochanters
  - May be obtained standing or supine
  - Pelvic tilt should be neutral
  - Hips internally rotated 10°
- **Inlet view**
  - Patient supine, anteroposterior beam
  - Beam directed 25° caudally
  - Optimal visualization of contour of pelvic inlet
  - Allows visualization of anteroposterior fracture displacement
- **Outlet view**
  - Patient supine, anteroposterior beam
  - Beam directed 25° cephalad
  - Elongates pelvic outlet
  - Allows visualization of superoinferior fracture displacement
- **Judet view**
  - Patient upright or supine, anteroposterior beam
  - Pelvis rotated 45° posterior oblique
  - Obturator oblique: Shows obturator foramen of affected side en face
    - Allows visualization of ipsilateral anterior column, posterior wall of acetabulum
  - Iliac oblique: Shows iliac wing of affected side en face
    - Allows visualization of ipsilateral posterior column, anterior wall of acetabulum
- **Frog leg lateral view**
  - Patient supine, anteroposterior beam
  - Pelvis flat, hips abducted, knees flexed, soles of feet together
- **Dunn view**
  - Patient supine, anteroposterior beam
  - Hip abducted 90° or 45° (modified Dunn view)
  - Similar to frog but feet flat on table
- **False profile view**
  - Patient standing, anteroposterior beam
  - Rotated 45-65° posterior oblique
  - Centered on hip
- **Löwenstein lateral view**
  - Patient supine, anteroposterior beam
  - Pelvis rotated 45° posterior oblique
  - Knee flexed, lateral side of knee touches table
- **Cross-table lateral view**
  - Also known as true lateral, groin lateral, or Johnson lateral
  - Patient supine
  - Unaffected hip flexed
  - Beam directed cross-table through affected hip
  - 20° cephalad beam angulation from anterior to posterior
- **Ferguson view of sacrum**
  - Patient prone
  - Beam directed 15° caudal from posterior to anterior
- **AP view of sacrum**
  - Sacroiliac joints appear duplicated
  - Due to oblique orientation of joint
- **Lateral view of sacrum**
  - Patient in lateral decubitus or upright position
  - Centered at mid sacrum
- **Oblique sacroiliac joint view**
  - Patient supine, rotated 30° oblique

Arthrographic Approach to Hip

- Patient supine, hip slightly internally rotated
  - Internal rotation elongates femoral neck
- Best approach is at junction of lateral head and neck
  - Away from vessels, femoral nerve
  - In large patients, may need to tape pannus of abdomen above area of injection
- Alternate approach is oblique, along axis of femoral neck
  - Helps to avoid large abdominal pannus
- Contrast should flow away from needle and to medial side of joint
  - If contrast "puddles" at needle tip, needle is not intraarticular
  - Should outline zona orbicularis
- Be aware that potential spaces outside hip may also allow easy flow of contrast
  - But will not extend medially along zona orbicularis

Arthrographic Landmarks

- Contrasts outlines femoral head, neck
- Does not extend inferior to intertrochanteric line
- Does not fill acetabular fossa
- Recesses medially and laterally at femoral head/neck junction
- Recess superolaterally between labrum and capsule
- Joint constricted in mid neck at zona orbicularis

Arthrographic Approach to Sacroiliac Joints

- Patient prone
- Angle beam to show joint in profile
- Enter in lower 1/3 of joint

Arthrographic Approach to Pubic Symphysis

- Patient supine
- Enter joint slightly off midline to avoid fibrocartilage

ANATOMY IMAGING ISSUES

Imaging Recommendations

- Multiple lateral views of hip available
  - Use cross-table lateral to evaluate hip trauma
  - Each lateral shows slightly different view of acetabulum, femoral head/neck morphology
- Sacroiliac joints better seen on Ferguson PA view than AP view of pelvis
- Judet views used for acetabular trauma
- Inlet/outlet views used for pelvic ring disruption

Imaging Pitfalls

- Assessment of acetabular version is very dependent on pelvic position
  - Inlet view increases apparent retroversion
  - Outlet view increases apparent anteversion

Pelvis and Hip Radiographic and Arthrographic Anatomy

AP PELVIS AND HIP

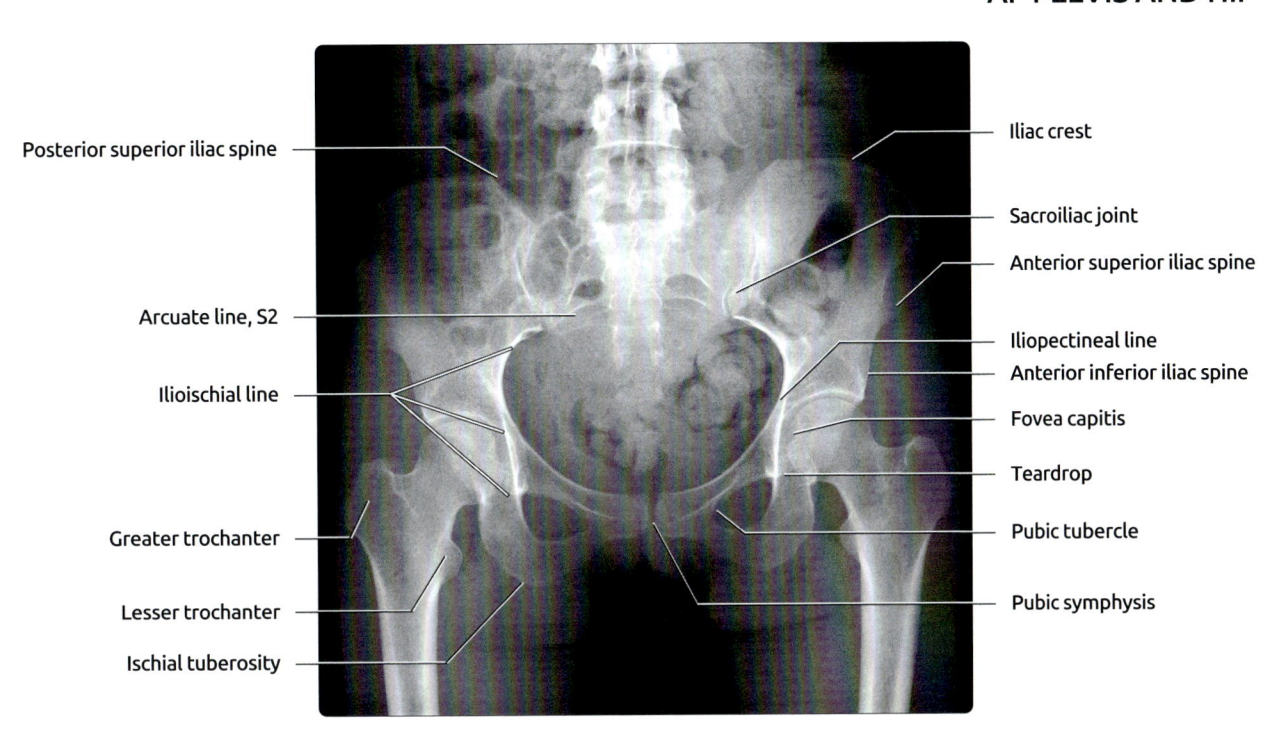

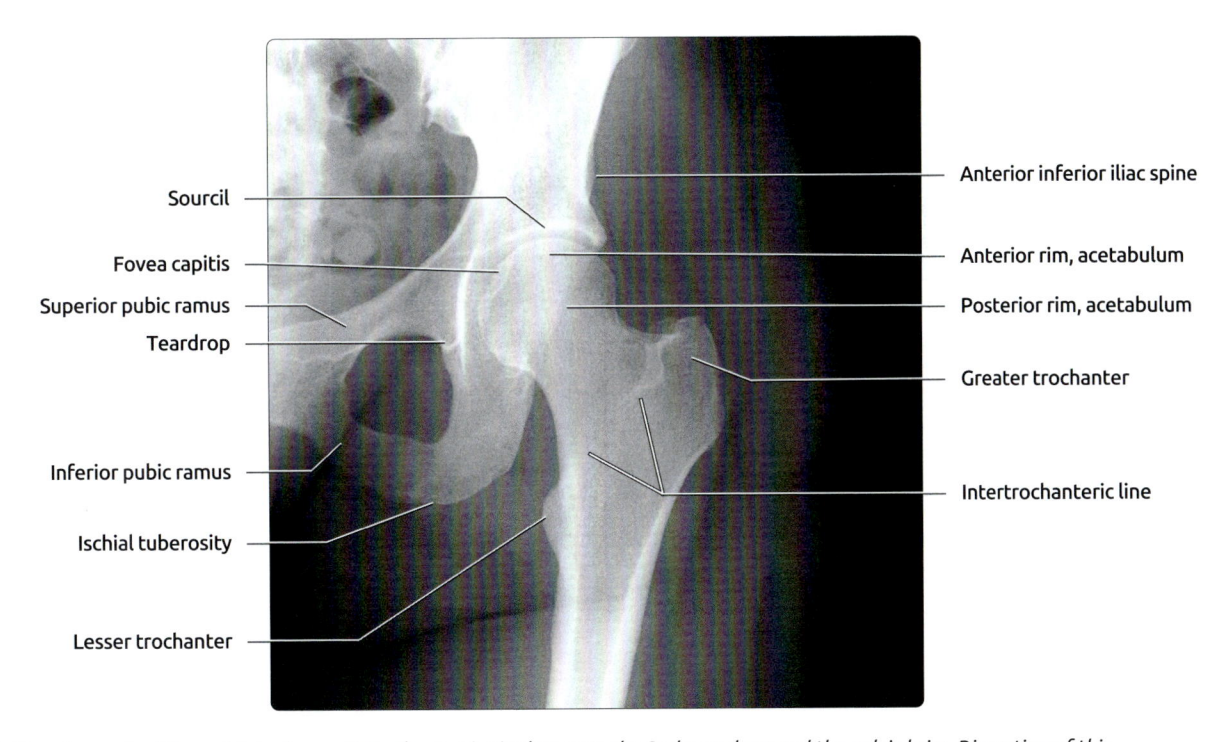

(Top) AP radiograph of the pelvis is shown. Note the continuity between the 2nd sacral arc and the pelvic brim. Disruption of this continuity is a sign of malalignment. The iliac crest extends from posterior to anterior superior iliac spines. (Bottom) AP radiograph of the hip shows the supraacetabular ilium is above the acetabular roof. The thin medial acetabular wall overlaps the ilioischial line. The teardrop is present at the inferior aspect of the medial wall. The sourcil is the condensation of cortical bone at the acetabular roof.

Pelvis and Hip Radiographic and Arthrographic Anatomy

INLET AND OUTLET PELVIS VIEWS

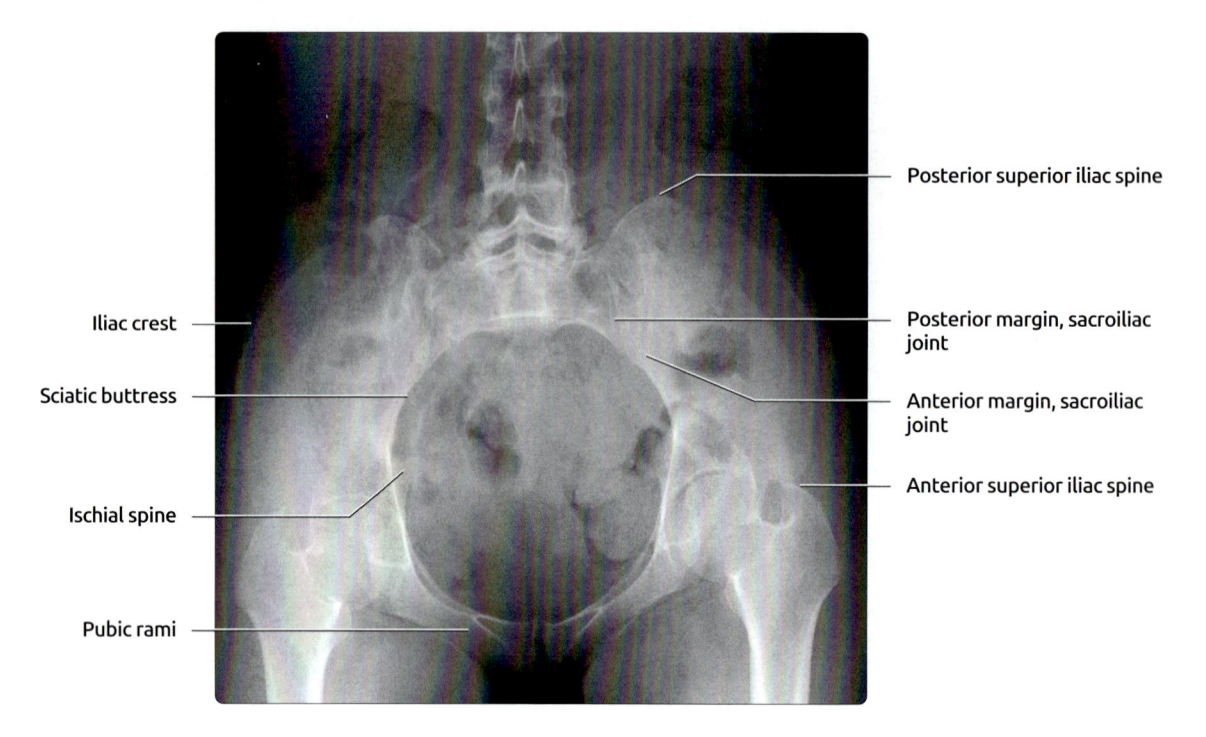

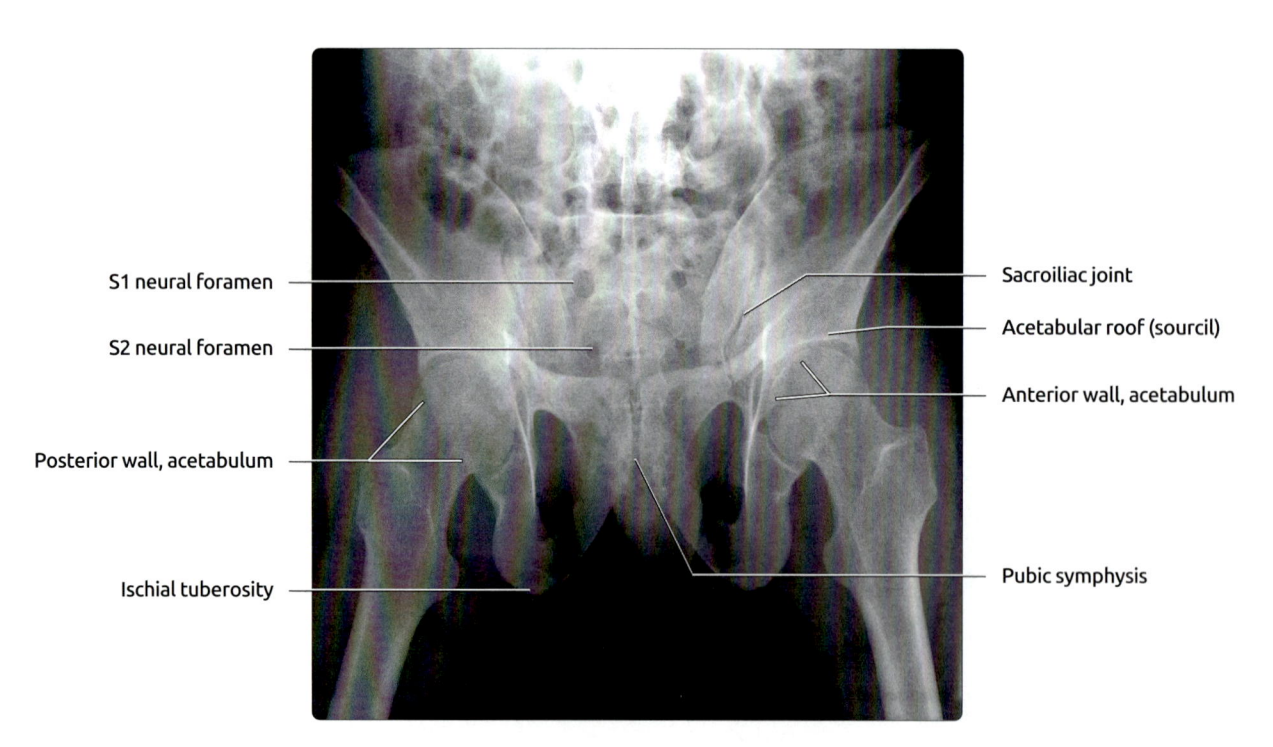

Labels (top image): Iliac crest; Sciatic buttress; Ischial spine; Pubic rami; Posterior superior iliac spine; Posterior margin, sacroiliac joint; Anterior margin, sacroiliac joint; Anterior superior iliac spine.

Labels (bottom image): S1 neural foramen; S2 neural foramen; Posterior wall, acetabulum; Ischial tuberosity; Sacroiliac joint; Acetabular roof (sourcil); Anterior wall, acetabulum; Pubic symphysis.

(**Top**) *Inlet view of the pelvis is used to assess anterior to posterior alignment within the pelvis. The pubic rami are nearly superimposed. The inferior ramus is slightly posterior to the superior ramus. The anterior and posterior iliac spines are well seen and the iliac crest between the 2 spines is laid out. The anterior margin of the sacroiliac joint projects lateral to the posterior margin due to obliquity of the joint.* (**Bottom**) *Outlet view of the pelvis is used to assess superior and inferior alignment of the pelvis. Obturator rings have an "owl's eye" appearance. Outlet view is usually the best view for evaluation of the sacral neural foramina.*

Pelvis and Hip Radiographic and Arthrographic Anatomy

JUDET VIEWS

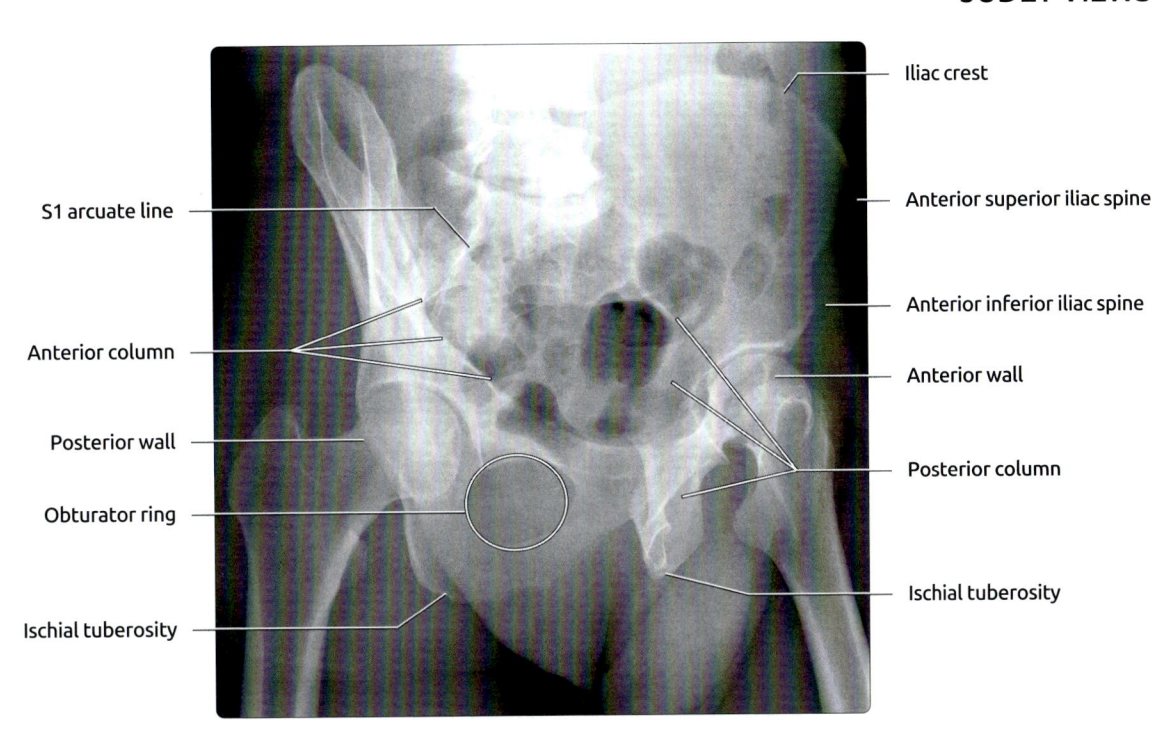

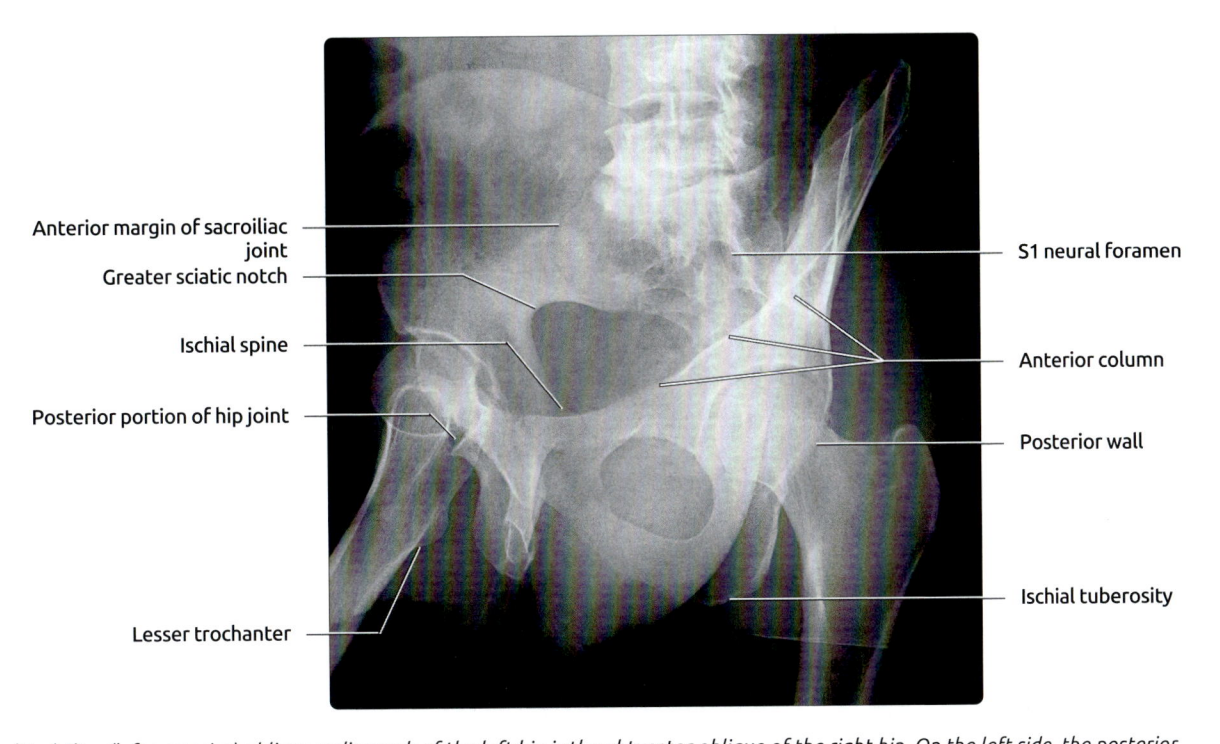

(Top) *Iliac (left posterior) oblique radiograph of the left hip is the obturator oblique of the right hip. On the left side, the posterior (ilioischial) column and the anterior acetacular rim are well seen.* **(Bottom)** *Obturator (left anterior) oblique of the left hip (iliac oblique right hip) is shown. On this view, the anterior or iliopectineal column of the acetabulum is seen in profile. The posterior acetabular rim is well visualized.*

Pelvis and Hip Radiographic and Arthrographic Anatomy

LATERAL VIEWS OF HIP

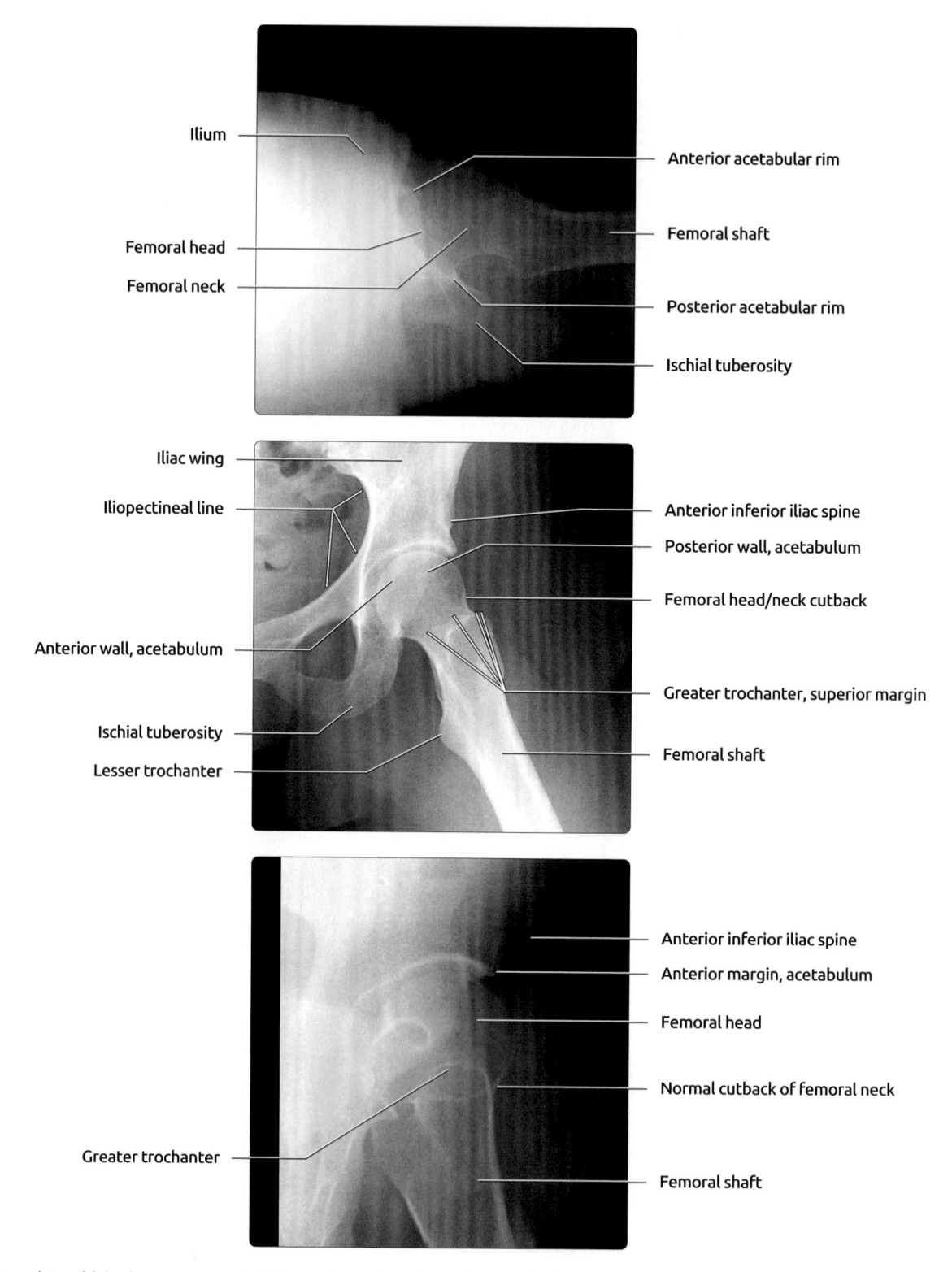

(Top) True lateral (also known as cross-table lateral or Johnson lateral) view of the hip is most commonly used for suspected fracture or evaluation of acetabular version after total hip replacement. The prominence of the ischial tuberosity identifies the posterior aspect of the hip. (Middle) Frog leg lateral radiograph of the hip shows the cutback of the anterolateral femoral head/neck junction. The greater trochanter and femoral neck overlap are seen. The femoral neck and shaft are oriented in a straight line. (Bottom) False profile view of the left hip was obtained with the patient standing and rotated approximately 65 degrees posterior oblique. This view shows coverage of anterior femoral head, morphology of acetabular roof, and morphology of anterior femoral head/neck junction. Lesser trochanter is en face and not distinctly seen. The femoral neck is anteverted relative to the femoral shaft

Pelvis and Hip Radiographic and Arthrographic Anatomy

SACROILIAC JOINT VIEWS

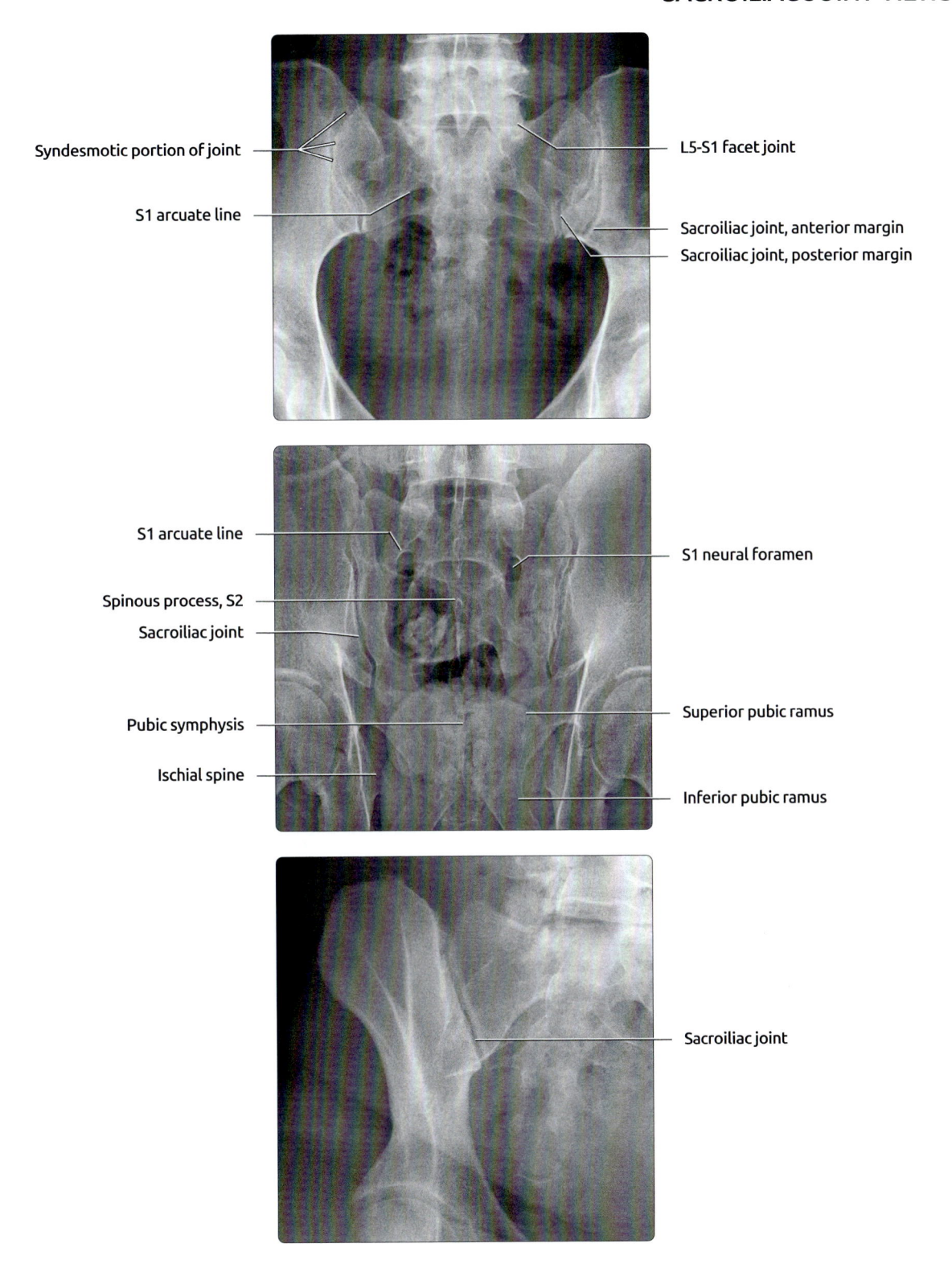

- Syndesmotic portion of joint
- S1 arcuate line
- L5-S1 facet joint
- Sacroiliac joint, anterior margin
- Sacroiliac joint, posterior margin

- S1 arcuate line
- Spinous process, S2
- Sacroiliac joint
- Pubic symphysis
- Ischial spine
- S1 neural foramen
- Superior pubic ramus
- Inferior pubic ramus

- Sacroiliac joint

(**Top**) AP radiograph of the sacroiliac joints is shown. Two joint margins are visible in the inferior 2/3 of each joint, reflecting the oblique orientation of the joint from posteromedial to anterolateral. The superior 1/3 of the joint is primarily syndesmotic and is oriented in a nearly coronal plane. (**Middle**) Ferguson view, PA sacral radiograph: The anterior and posterior joint margins are now seen as a single line, due to the orientation of the x-ray beam. The neural foramina are easily appreciated. The arcuate lines are the superior margins of each neural foramina. (**Bottom**) In the left posterior oblique (right anterior oblique), the right sacroiliac joint is profiled and the articular surfaces delineated. Cartilage is thinner on the iliac side of the joint; therefore, the earliest findings of sacroiliitis will be visible radiographically on the iliac side.

Pelvis and Hip Radiographic and Arthrographic Anatomy

HIP ARTHROGRAPHIC TECHNIQUE

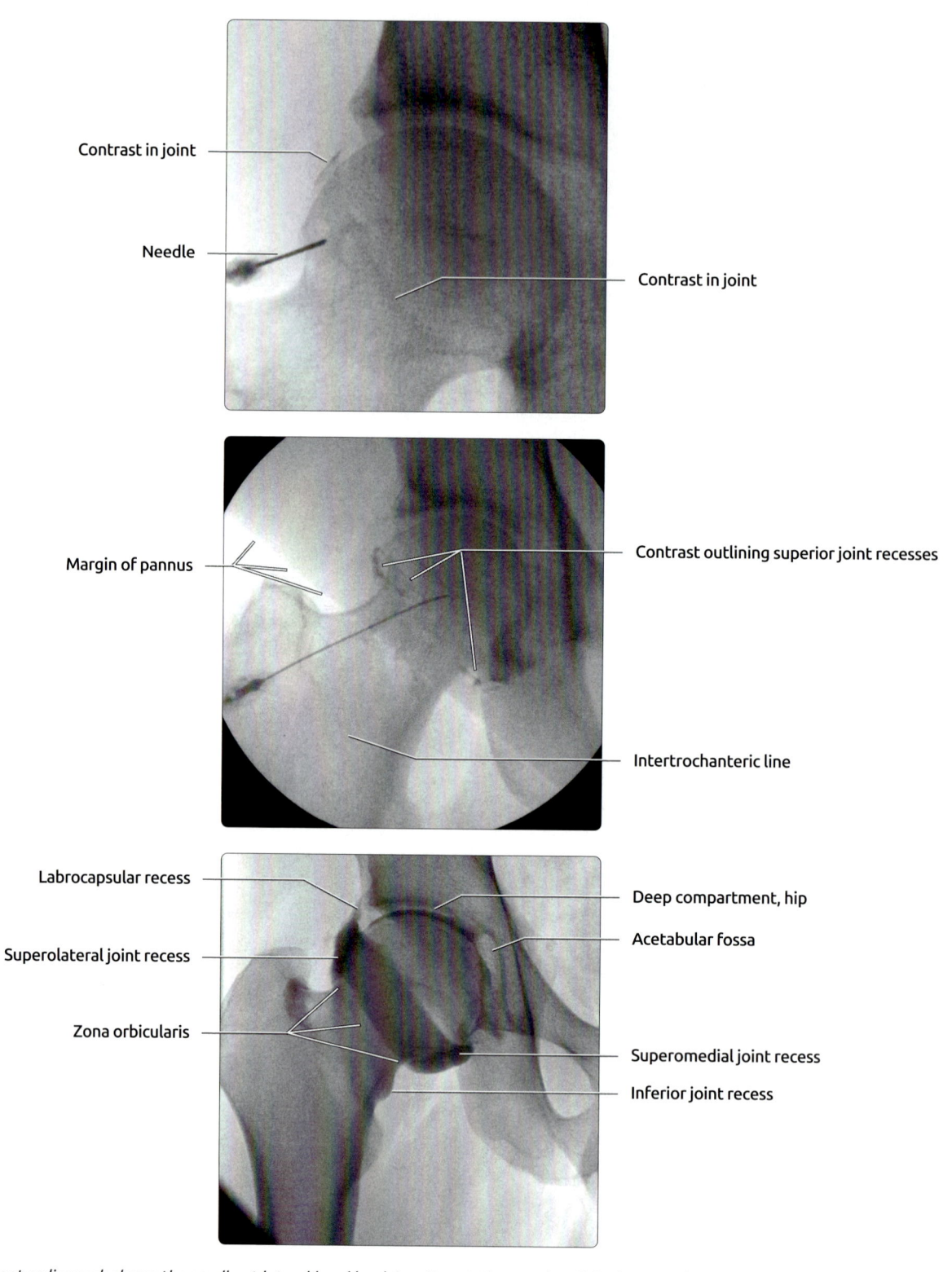

Contrast in joint
Needle
Contrast in joint

Margin of pannus
Contrast outlining superior joint recesses
Intertrochanteric line

Labrocapsular recess
Deep compartment, hip
Superolateral joint recess
Acetabular fossa
Zona orbicularis
Superomedial joint recess
Inferior joint recess

(Top) AP spot radiograph shows the needle at lateral head/neck junction. Arthrography of the hip is performed from anterior approach. This injection is early in the injection procedure; a small amount of contrast is present and proves its intraarticular location by flowing freely away from the needle. (Middle) AP fluoroscopic spot radiograph shows alternate approach to enter hip in larger patient. Taping the belly superiorly improves access to the joint, but in this case a large pannus could not be removed from the field. An oblique approach was used to avoid much of the pannus, with the needle entering at the artertrochanteric line, angling superomedially along the femoral neck axis. (Bottom) AP radiograph shows ideal filling of the hip joint. Passage of contrast into the deep compartment of the hip is facilitated by pulling on the leg, with the patient holding position on the proximal portion of the fluoroscopy table. The zona orbicularis is seen as a region of tight joint capsule. Contrast does not fill the majority of the acetabular fossa, which is extrasynovial.

Pelvis and Hip Radiographic and Arthrographic Anatomy

CORONAL MR ARTHROGRAM

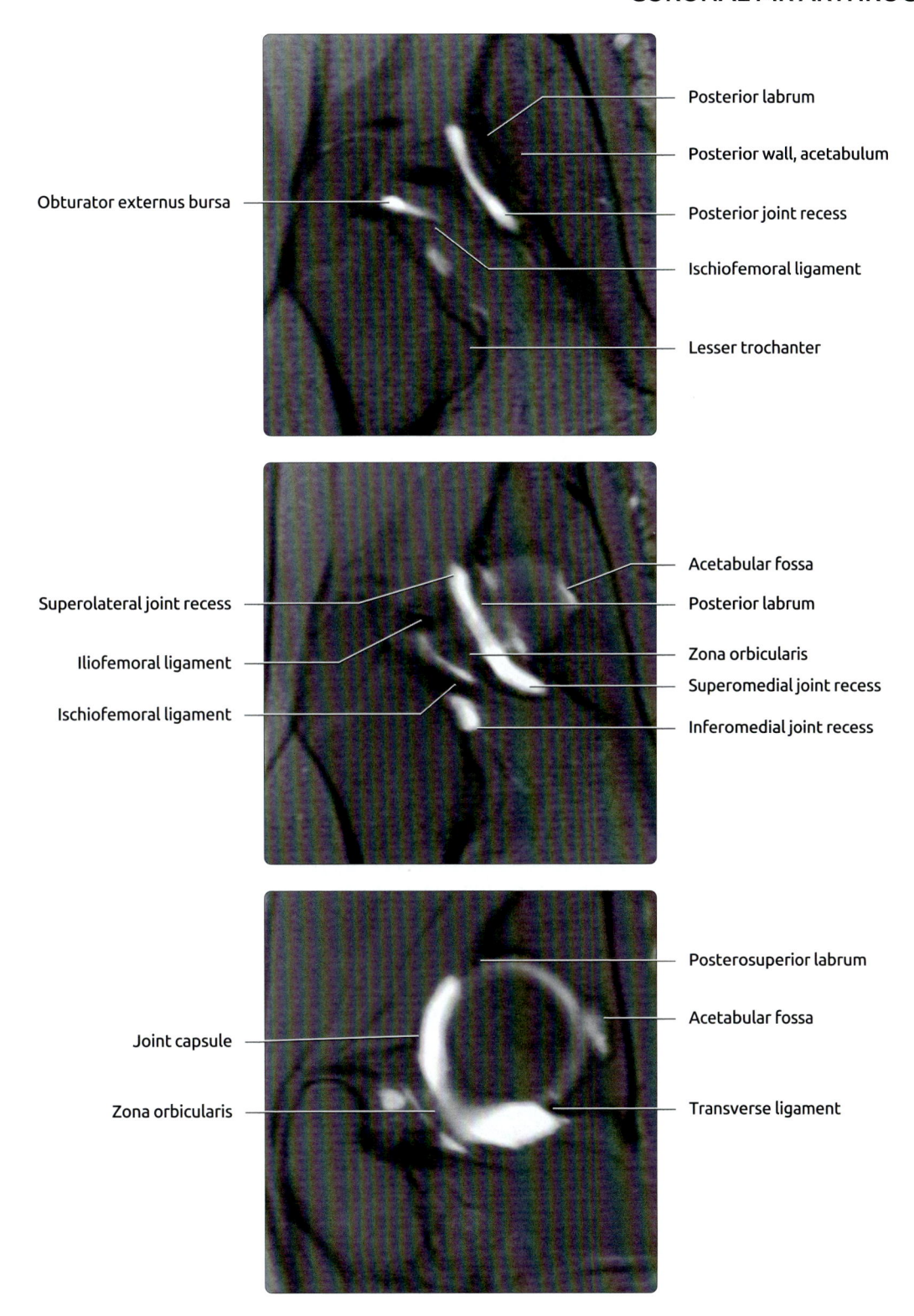

- Obturator externus bursa
- Posterior labrum
- Posterior wall, acetabulum
- Posterior joint recess
- Ischiofemoral ligament
- Lesser trochanter

- Superolateral joint recess
- Iliofemoral ligament
- Ischiofemoral ligament
- Acetabular fossa
- Posterior labrum
- Zona orbicularis
- Superomedial joint recess
- Inferomedial joint recess

- Joint capsule
- Zona orbicularis
- Posterosuperior labrum
- Acetabular fossa
- Transverse ligament

(Top) This is the 1st of a series of selected coronal T1WI FS MR arthrogram images showing a normal joint from posterior to anterior (different patients). This image shows the posterior joint recesses and posterior labrum. Obturator externus bursa is a joint recess located posteriorly, inferior to zona orbicularis. (Middle) The zona orbicularis is a waist-like constriction of the joint capsule at the mid femoral neck. Joint recesses are seen superior and inferior to the zona orbicularis. (Bottom) Acetabular fossa is a wide depression in the medial wall of the acetabulum. It is partially filled with a fatty pad called the pulvinar. It is normal for some fluid to extend partially around the pulvinar, but the majority of this region is extrasynovial.

CORONAL MR ARTHROGRAM

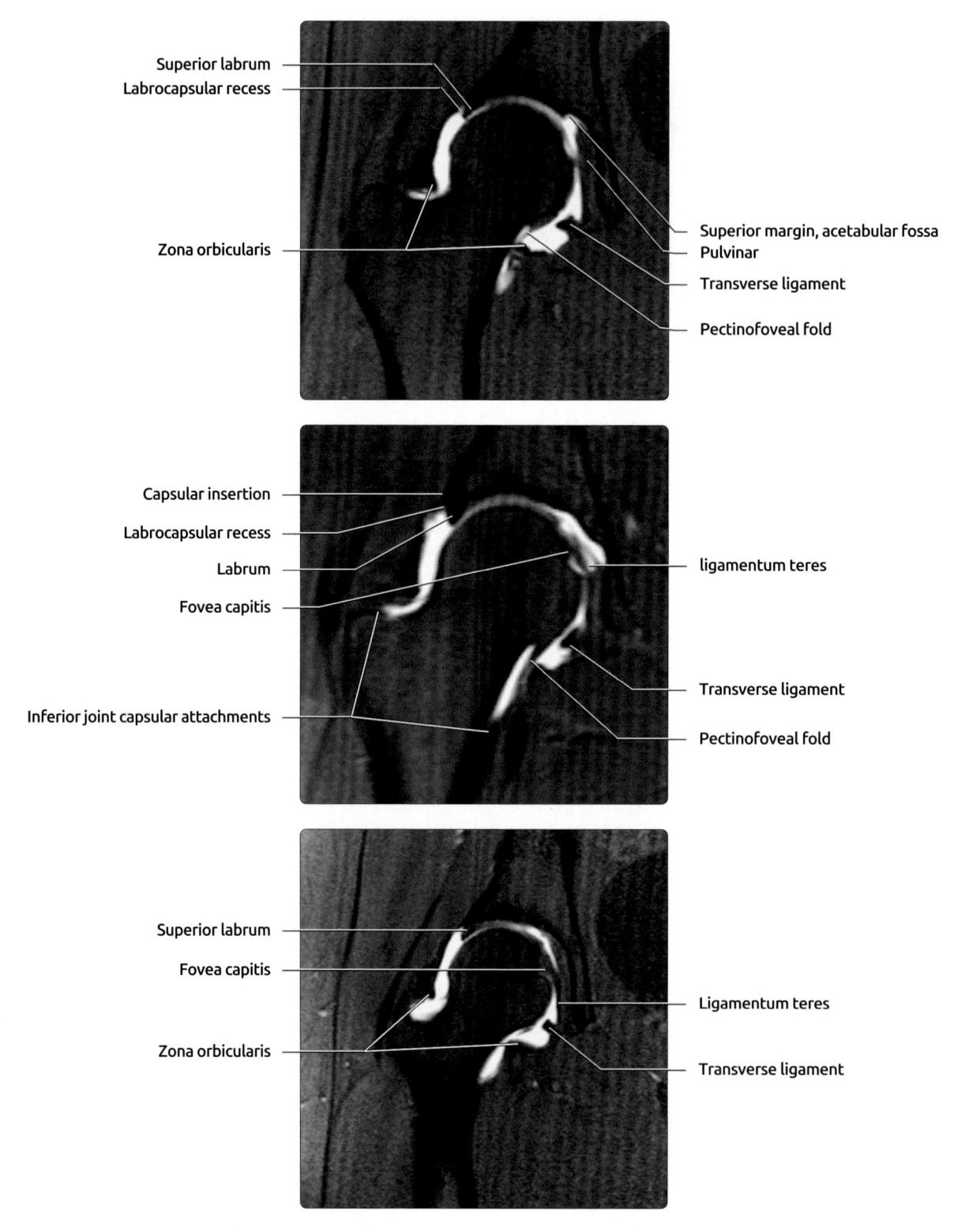

(Top) The articular surface of the acetabular roof terminates in a notch at the margin of the acetabular fossa, and this should not be mistaken for a cartilage defect. The acetabular fossa is not articular; the pulvinar filling the majority of the fossa is extrasynovial. (Middle) Origin of the ligament teres in the fovea capitis of the femur is now visible. A thin, normal fold of synovium parallels the femoral neck, inserting on the capsule or femur, and is known as pectinofoveal fold. (Bottom) The ligamentum teres is vertically oriented along medial joint margin abutting the pulvinar. It is narrow superiorly but widens into a fan shape inferiorly before its wide insertion on the transverse ligament.

Pelvis and Hip Radiographic and Arthrographic Anatomy

CORONAL MR ARTHROGRAM

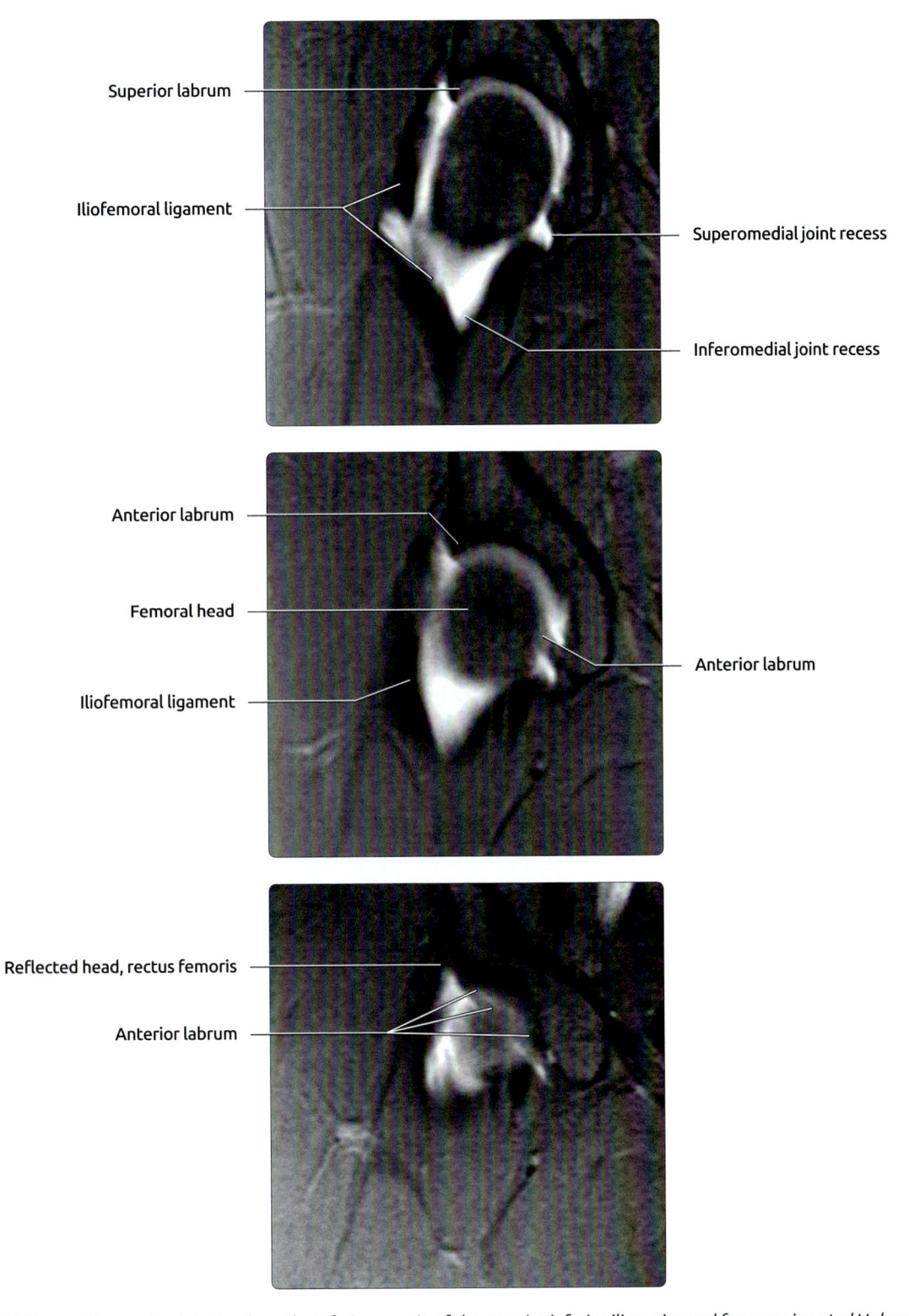

- Superior labrum
- Iliofemoral ligament
- Superomedial joint recess
- Inferomedial joint recess

- Anterior labrum
- Femoral head
- Iliofemoral ligament
- Anterior labrum

- Reflected head, rectus femoris
- Anterior labrum

(**Top**) *The iliofemoral ligament originates from the inferior margin of the anterior inferior iliac spine and forms an inverted V shape, with 1 band inserting laterally and 1 band inserting medially on the intertrochanteric line.* (**Middle**) *Due to anteversion of the acetabulum and normal curvature from superior to anterior, the anterosuperior labrum is obliquely seen. Careful correlation between coronal, sagittal, and axial images is needed for accurate evaluation. Most tears occur in this quadrant.* (**Bottom**) *The anterior labrum appears separated from the acetabulum on this image, but that is due to anterior curvature of the acetabulum.*

Pelvis and Hip Radiographic and Arthrographic Anatomy

AXIAL MR ARTHROGRAM

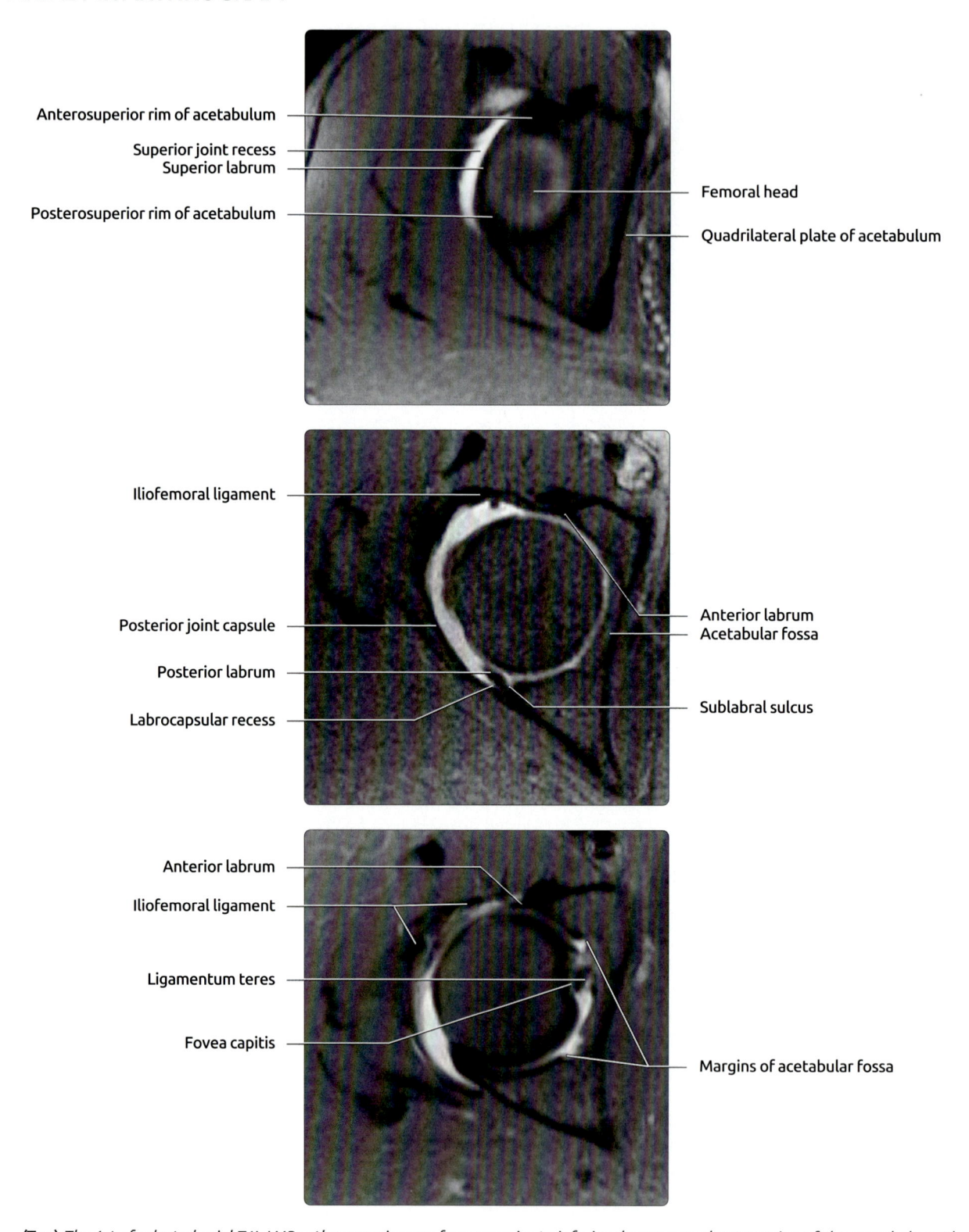

Anterosuperior rim of acetabulum
Superior joint recess
Superior labrum
Posterosuperior rim of acetabulum
Femoral head
Quadrilateral plate of acetabulum

Iliofemoral ligament
Posterior joint capsule
Posterior labrum
Labrocapsular recess
Anterior labrum
Acetabular fossa
Sublabral sulcus

Anterior labrum
Iliofemoral ligament
Ligamentum teres
Fovea capitis
Margins of acetabular fossa

(Top) The 1st of selected axial T1W MR arthrogram images from superior to inferior shows normal anteversion of the acetabulum. The labrum forms a smoothly curving arc, separating the superficial from the deep compartments; it helps to maintain fluid within the deep compartment. **(Middle)** Above the fovea capitis, the femoral head has a rounded medial contour. A sublabral sulcus is seen posteriorly; these may be present in any quadrant and are distinguished from tears by their smooth contour. **(Bottom)** The acetabular fossa occupies most of the medial wall of the acetabulum; it is only partly filled by fat (pulvinar). It is easy to see how it becomes a prime location for sequestration of loose bodies.

Pelvis and Hip Radiographic and Arthrographic Anatomy

OBLIQUE AXIAL MR ARTHROGRAM

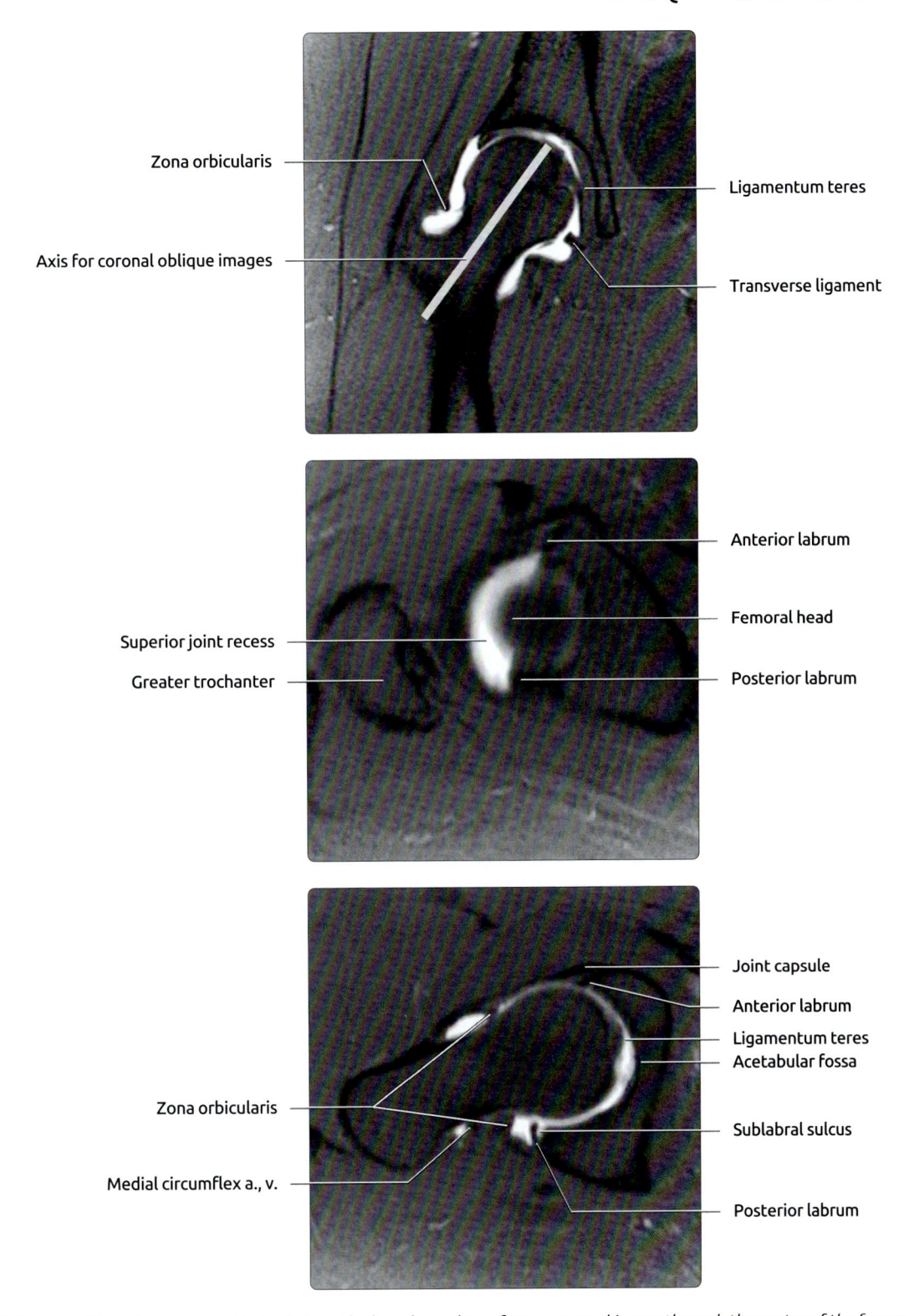

(Top) Coronal oblique images are obtained along the line shown here, from a coronal image through the center of the femoral head. (Middle) The coronal oblique plane is a useful secondary plane for evaluating abnormalities of the labrum. These most commonly occur in the anterosuperior portion of the labrum, where tears can be difficult to visualize due to curvature of the acetabulum. (Bottom) This image is along the central axis of the femur. Note the prominent sublabral sulcus, a normal variant.

Pelvis and Hip Radiographic and Arthrographic Anatomy

SAGITTAL MR ARTHROGRAM

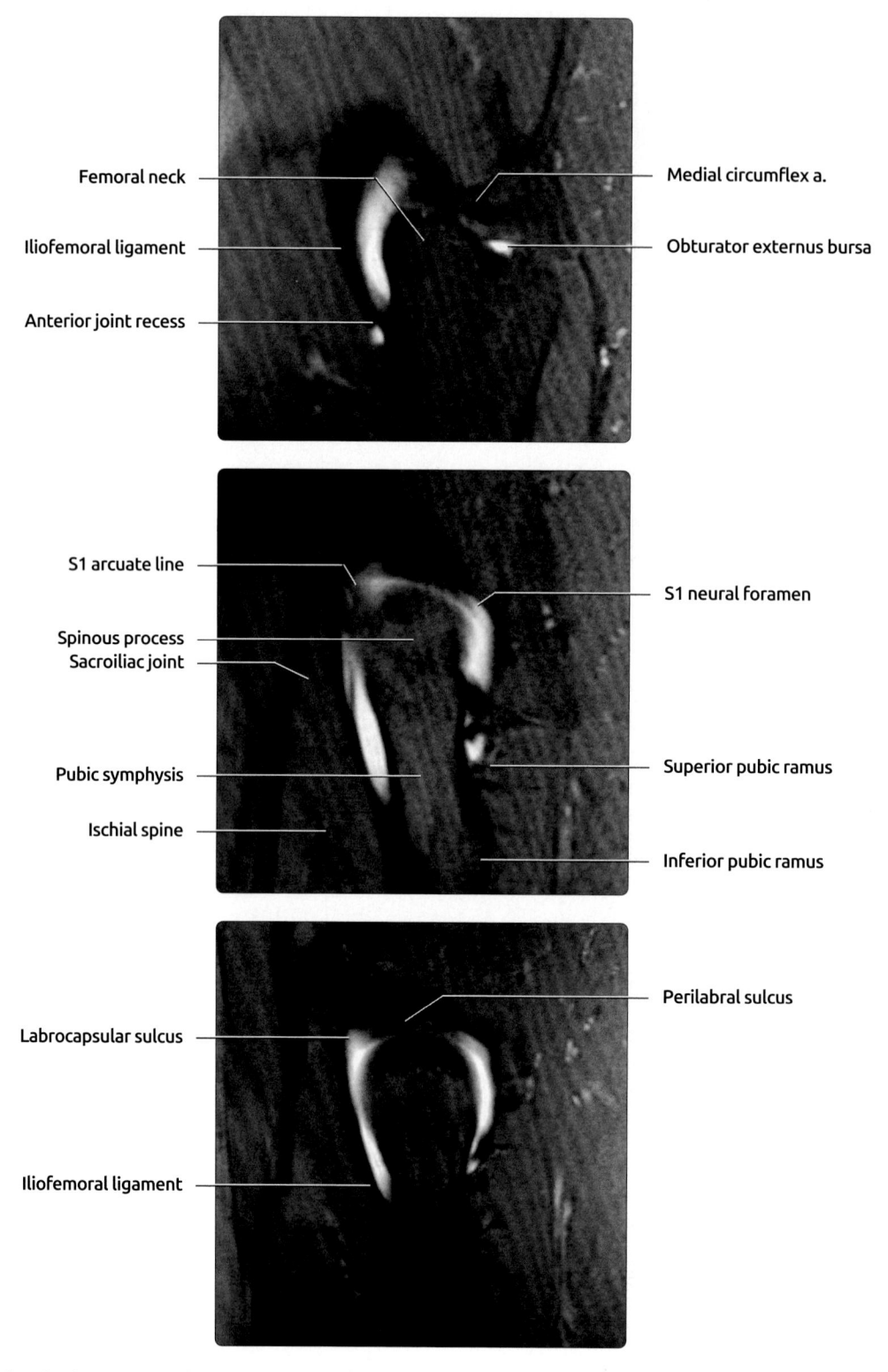

(Top) Selected sagittal PD FS MR arthrogram images are shown from lateral to medial (in different patients). (Middle) Ferguson view, PA sacral radiograph: The anterior and posterior joint margins are now seen as a single line, due to the orientation of the x-ray beam. The neural foramina are easily appreciated. The arcuate lines are the superior margins of each neural foramina. (Bottom) On sagittal images, the perilabral sulcus (recess) may be mistaken for a labral tear; correlate with coronal images. Note the thickness of the iliofemoral ligament; because of its thickness, injections may be partly intraarticular but partly into the substance of the ligament.

Pelvis and Hip Radiographic and Arthrographic Anatomy

SAGITTAL MR ARTHROGRAM

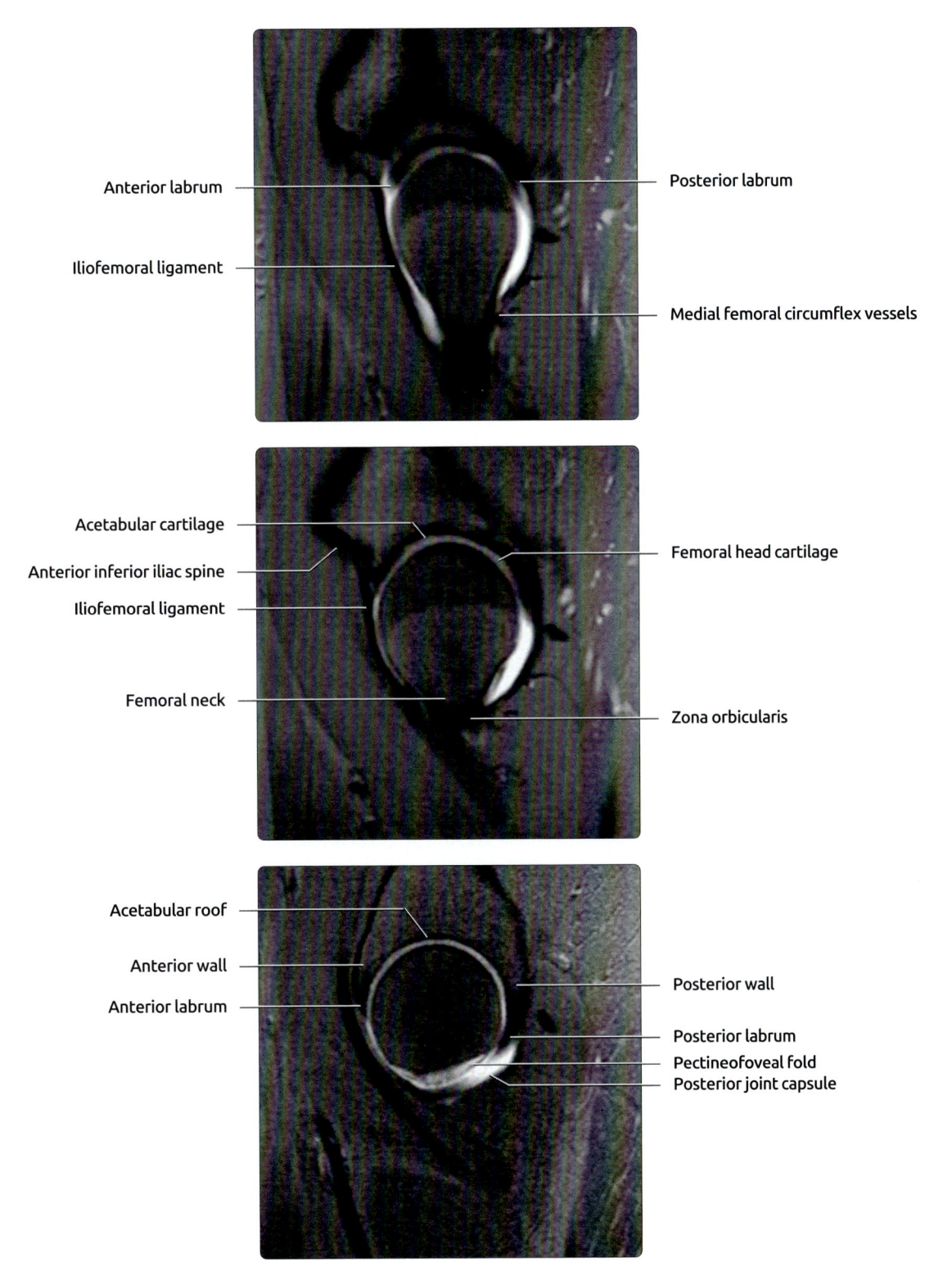

(Top) The glenoid labrum merges smoothly with adjacent hyaline cartilage. The labral contour may be triangular or rounded, or anterior labrum may be absent in what is probably a normal variant. The bony roof of acetabulum is also known as the sourcil. *(Middle)* Hyaline cartilage of the femoral head and acetabulum may not be visually distinguishable despite adequate joint distention. However, focal defects are usually visible. *(Bottom)* A thin pectinofoveal fold hugs the contour of the medial femoral neck, above the zona orbicularis.

Pelvis and Hip Radiographic and Arthrographic Anatomy

SAGITTAL MR ARTHROGRAM

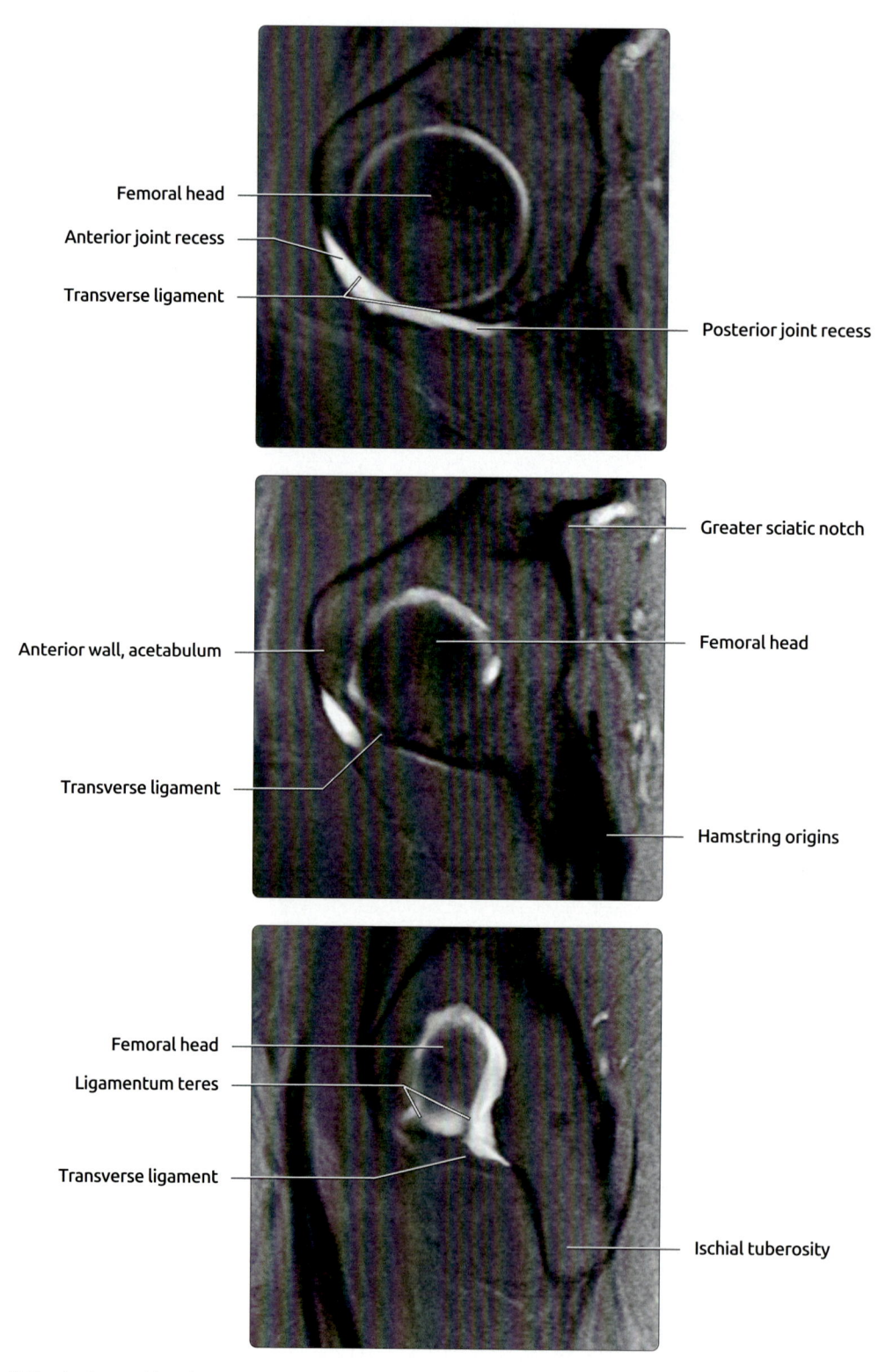

Femoral head
Anterior joint recess
Transverse ligament
Posterior joint recess

Greater sciatic notch
Anterior wall, acetabulum
Femoral head
Transverse ligament
Hamstring origins

Femoral head
Ligamentum teres
Transverse ligament
Ischial tuberosity

(Top) *Medially, the femoral head is surrounded by the acetabulum and transverse ligament.* **(Middle)** *The femoral head is partly out of view, as the acetabular fossa is entered.* **(Bottom)** *The fan shape of the ligamentum teres insertion on the transverse ligament is well seen. The ligamentum teres normally appears lax on MR arthrography. The acetabular fossa has an undulating contour, roughly horseshoe-shaped.*

Pelvis and Hip Radiographic and Arthrographic Anatomy

SACROILIAC AND PUBIC SYMPHYSIS ARTHROGRAPHY

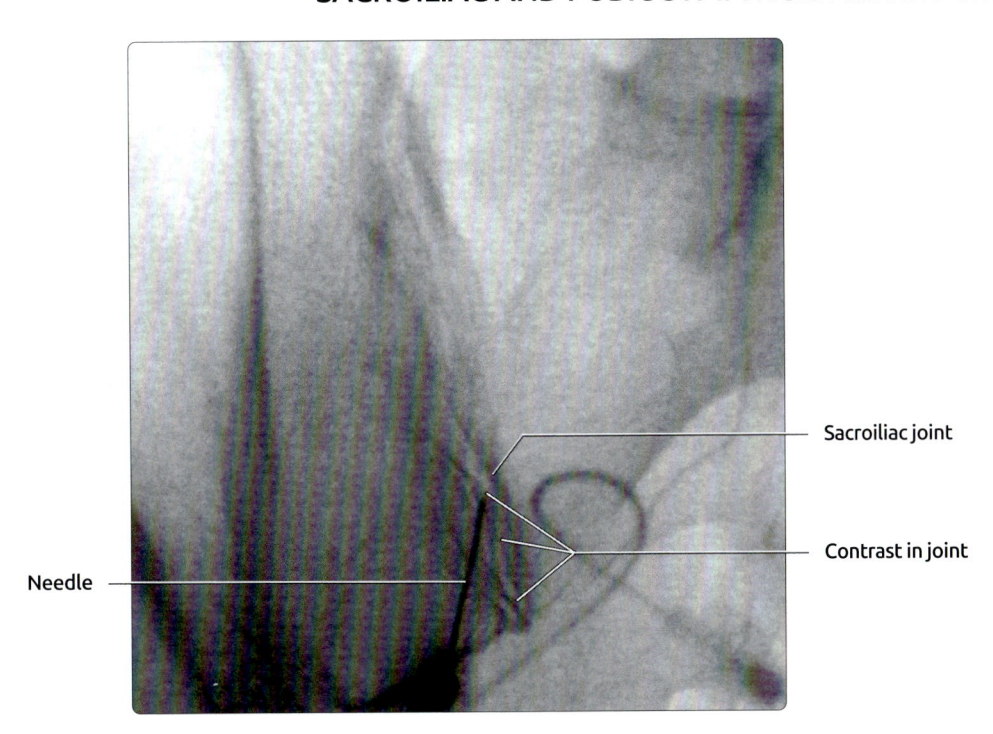

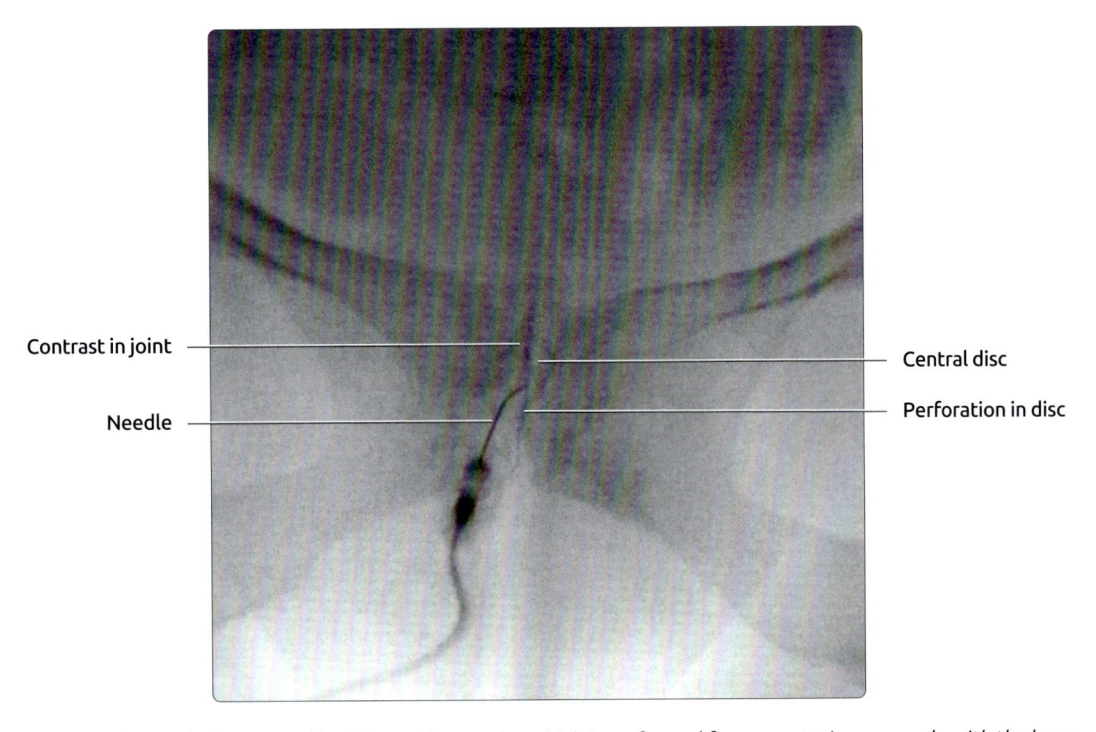

(Top) PA oblique spot radiograph shows sacroiliac joint arthrography, which is performed from a posterior approach, with the beam angled to show the joint in profile. The needle enters in the inferior 1/3 of the joint, where the majority of the synovial portion of the joint is found. (Bottom) AP spot radiograph shows arthrography of the pubic symphysis, which is performed from an anterior approach. Contrast outlines the cartilage and the central disc. A perforation in the disc is a common incidental finding and allows passage of contrast to the other side of the disc.

Pelvis and Hip Normal Variants and Imaging Pitfalls

IMAGING ANATOMY

Bony Variants

- **Transitional lumbosacral vertebra**
  - Most individuals have 12 thoracic, 5 lumbar, and 5 sacral vertebrae
  - May have transitional lumbosacral vertebra, with 4, 5, or 6 lumbar vertebrae
  - Transitional vertebra has features of both lumbar and sacral vertebrae
    - Transverse process may be enlarged and form articulation with sacrum (assimilation joint) **or**
    - Enlarged transverse process may fuse with sacrum
    - Variant may be unilateral or bilateral
    - May be pain generator (Bertolotti syndrome)
    - Present in 4.6% of 1 study of patients with low back pain, 11.4% of patients < 30 years old
- **Accessory sacroiliac joint**
  - Common variant
  - Usually extends from S2 neural foramen nearly horizontally to lateral margin of sacrum
- **Osteitis condensans ilii**
  - Sclerosis seen on iliac side of joint only
  - Related to multiparity
  - Asymptomatic
- **Paraglenoid fossa (or sulcus)**
  - Corticated concavity adjacent to sacroiliac joint, usually seen in women
  - Should not be mistaken for erosion
  - May be related to prominent superior gluteal artery
- **Superior acetabular notch**
  - Also called supraacetabular fossa, pseudocartilage defect
  - Notch found at superior, central acetabulum
  - May be filled with cartilage
  - Found in 10% of hips
  - May have plica extending from notch to pulvinar
- **Stellate crease/lesion**
  - Linear defect extending deep to superior acetabular notch
  - Term also used for rudimentary defect in location of superior acetabular notch
- **Os acetabuli**
  - Unfused secondary ossification center
  - May be mimicked by fatigue fracture in patients with developmental dysplasia or femoroacetabular impingement
  - May be mimicked by ossification of acetabular labrum
- **Cam morphology** of femur
  - Decreased offset of femoral head and neck
  - Can predispose to femoroacetabular impingement
  - Also common in asymptomatic population

Muscle and Nerve Variants

- Piriformis may be duplicated (2 muscle bellies)
- Associated with abnormal course of sciatic nerve (n.)
- Tibial or peroneal n. may pass between muscle bellies
- May lead to sciatica/piriformis syndrome

Acetabular Labral Variants

- Absent labrum reported in 3% of population
- Labrum normally triangular but may be rounded
- Sublabral sulci may occur in any location
  - Most common in superior labrum
  - Distinguished from labral tear by smooth, parallel margins

ANATOMY IMAGING ISSUES

Imaging Pitfalls

- **Accessory centers of ossification**
  - Iliac crest, ischial tuberosity, anterior inferior iliac spine, anterior superior iliac spine, pubic bone
  - Ossify in adolescence, fuse in early adulthood
  - Avulsion injuries may occur in adolescents
- **Acetabular fossa**
  - Extrasynovial depression in medial wall of acetabulum
  - Contains fat, which is designated "pulvinar"
  - Superior recess not filled by pulvinar normally fills during arthrography
- **Labrocapsular recess**
  - Normal recess between labrum and capsule
  - Up to several mm in depth
  - Often distended during arthrography
- **Sublabral recess**
  - Smooth indentation between labrum and hyaline cartilage
  - Described in all locations of labrum
  - Smooth contour helps distinguish from jagged tear
- **Labral degeneration**
  - Extremely common aging phenomenon, should not be mistaken for tear
  - Labrum may be small, blunt, irregular, &/or contain heterogeneous signal
  - Reserve term labral tear for linear signal abnormalities
- **Cam-type morphology** of femoral head may be present in asymptomatic individuals
- **Iliopectineal fold** can be mistaken for abnormality
  - Normal synovial fold along inferior femoral neck
- **Ligamentum teres**
  - May appear lax, appearance varies with hip rotation
- **Femoral head cartilage**
  - Thin at head-neck junction
  - May be difficult to detect cartilage loss
  - Look for fibrocystic change as secondary finding of cartilage damage

SELECTED REFERENCES

1. Hack K et al: Prevalence of cam-type femoroacetabular impingement morphology in asymptomatic volunteers. J Bone Joint Surg Am. 92(14):2436-44, 2010
2. Martinez AE et al: Os acetabuli in femoro-acetabular impingement: stress fracture or unfused secondary ossification centre of the acetabular rim? Hip Int. 16(4):281-6, 2006
3. Quinlan JF et al: Bertolotti's syndrome. A cause of back pain in young people. J Bone Joint Surg Br. 88(9):1183-6, 2006
4. Saddik D et al: Prevalence and location of acetabular sublabral sulci at hip arthroscopy with retrospective MRI review. AJR Am J Roentgenol. 187(5):W507-11, 2006

Pelvis and Hip Normal Variants and Imaging Pitfalls

BONY VARIANTS

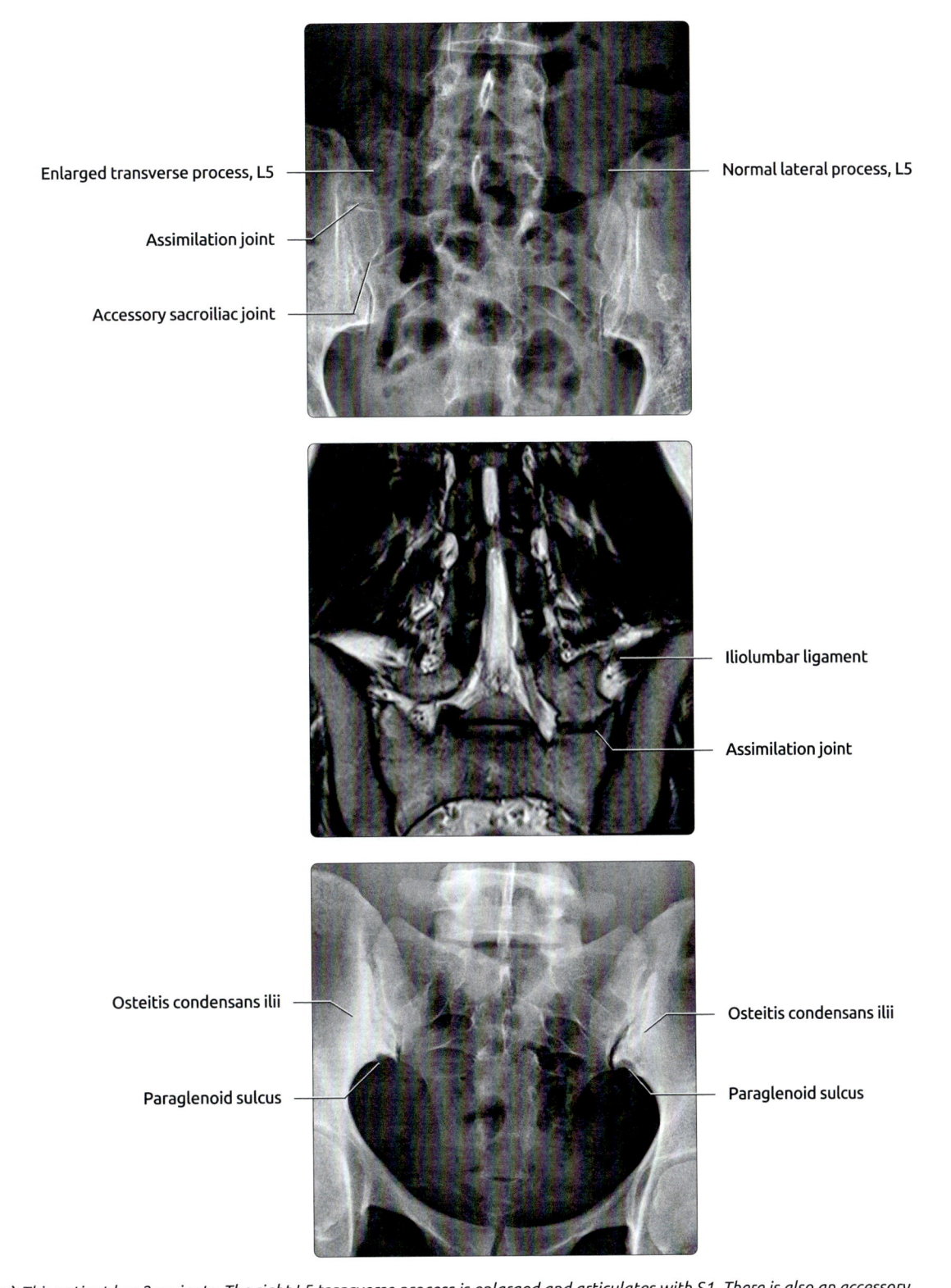

Enlarged transverse process, L5

Assimilation joint

Accessory sacroiliac joint

Normal lateral process, L5

Iliolumbar ligament

Assimilation joint

Osteitis condensans ilii

Paraglenoid sulcus

Osteitis condensans ilii

Paraglenoid sulcus

(Top) This patient has 2 variants. The right L5 transverse process is enlarged and articulates with S1. There is also an accessory sacroiliac joint. This joint usually extends from the lateral margin of the S2 neural foramen to a point just inferior to the posterior superior iliac spine, but, in this case, it is at the S1 level. **(Middle)** Coronal T2W MR shows an accessory sacroiliac joint with an irregular contour. Osteoarthritis of the assimilation joint is a common finding. Iliolumbar ligament is seen. This ligament usually is from the transverse process of L5 to the ilium and is a secondary indicator of spinal level. **(Bottom)** AP radiograph of the pelvis shows osteitis condensans ilii, sclerosis of the iliac side of the sacroiliac joint due to multiparity. Articular cortex is normal. This patient also has paraglenoid sulcus, another normal variant.

Pelvis and Hip Normal Variants and Imaging Pitfalls

BONY VARIANTS

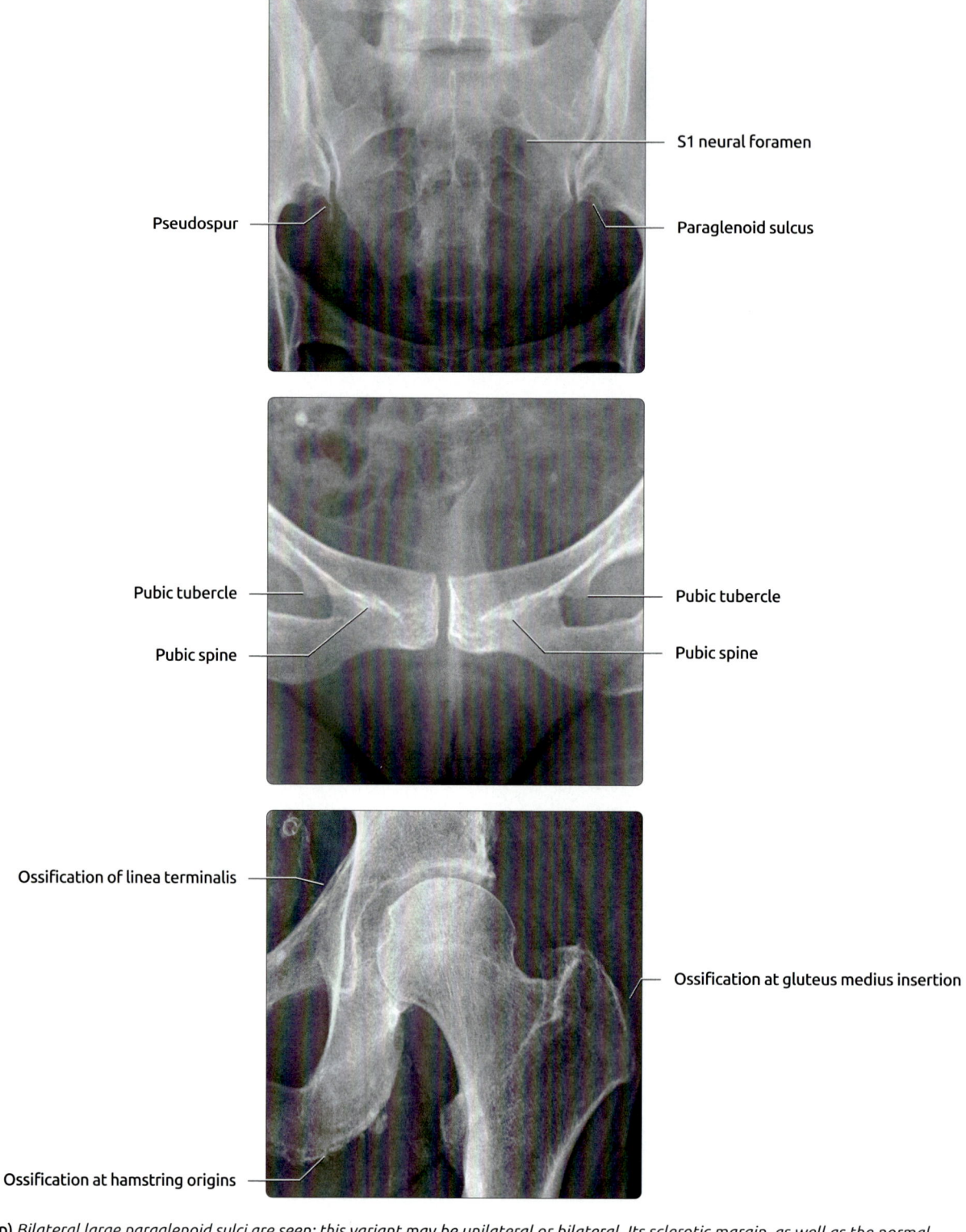

(Top) Bilateral large paraglenoid sulci are seen; this variant may be unilateral or bilateral. Its sclerotic margin, as well as the normal appearance of the adjacent sacroiliac joint, distinguish this normal variant from an erosion. The normal bone adjacent to the sulcus may form a pseudospur, which is sometimes mistaken for osteoarthritis. **(Middle)** AP radiograph shows bilateral prominence of the pubic tubercle, the site of attachment of the inguinal ligament. The pubic spine is the ridge that extends medially from the tubercle. **(Bottom)** Ossification of the fascia of the linea terminalis is common in older patients and is a manifestation of diffuse idiopathic skeletal hyperostosis (DISH). It is sometimes mistaken for a periosteal reaction due to stress fractures. Other manifestations of DISH, such as the hamstring origin ossification and gluteus medius insertional ossification seen in this case, are usually also present.

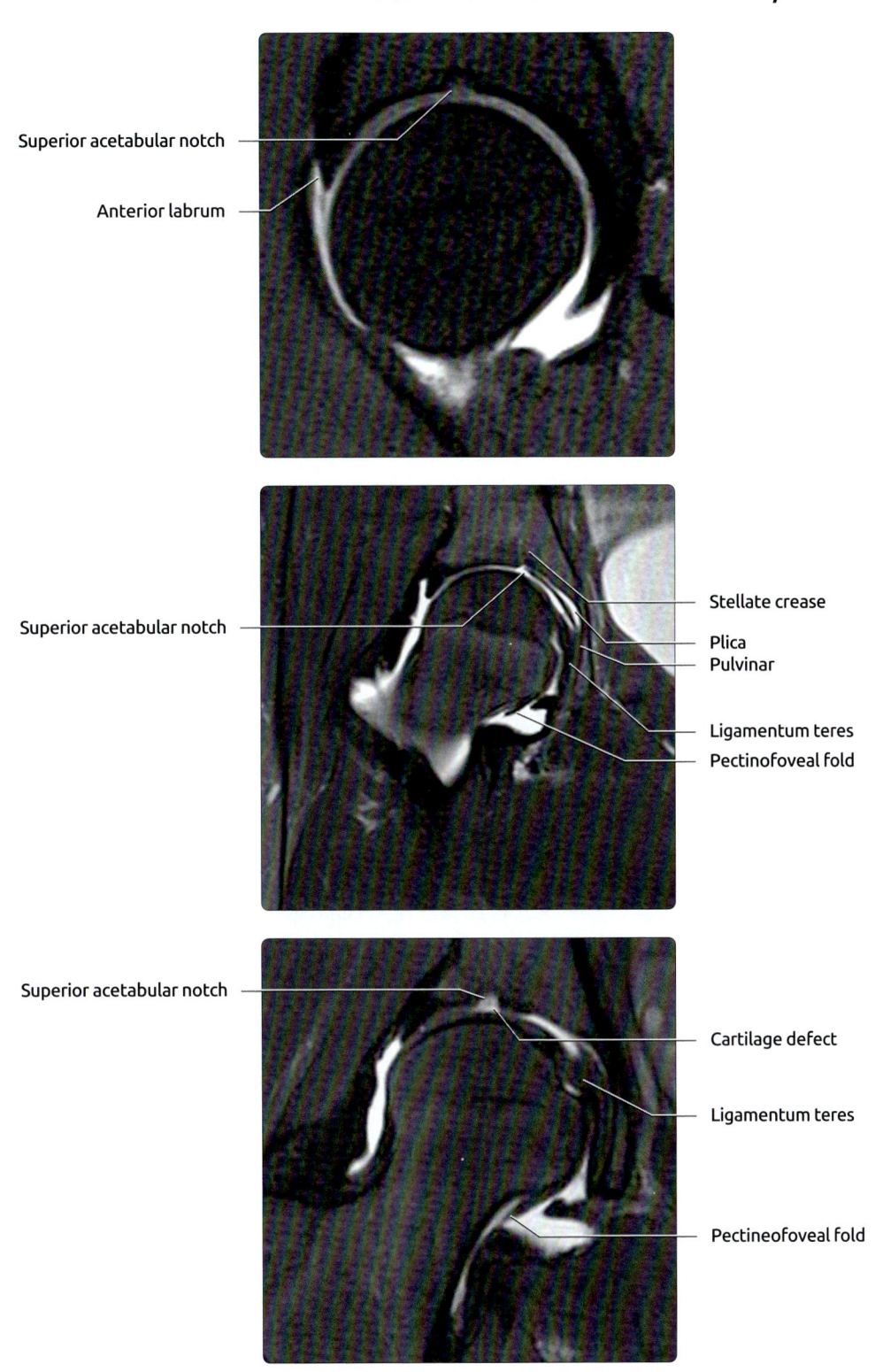

Pelvis and Hip Normal Variants and Imaging Pitfalls

SUPERIOR ACETABULAR NOTCH/STELLATE CREASE

Labels (Top): Superior acetabular notch; Anterior labrum

Labels (Middle): Superior acetabular notch; Stellate crease; Plica; Pulvinar; Ligamentum teres; Pectinofoveal fold

Labels (Bottom): Superior acetabular notch; Cartilage defect; Ligamentum teres; Pectineofoveal fold

(Top) Sagittal T1WI FS MR arthrogram shows a superior acetabular notch that is filled with cartilage. The notch can be quite variable in size and may be a bare area or filled with cartilage. (Middle) Coronal T2FS MR arthrogram shows a superior acetabular notch that does not contain cartilage and so fills with contrast. The stellate crease extends superior to the notch. A plica is sometimes seen, as in this case, going from the notch to the pulvinar. Pectineofoveal fold is a normal finding. (Bottom) Coronal T1WI FS MR arthrogram shows a superior acetabular notch/stellate lesion with a focal overlying cartilage defect. (Courtesy P. Tirman, MD.)

Pelvis and Hip Normal Variants and Imaging Pitfalls

OS ACETABULI

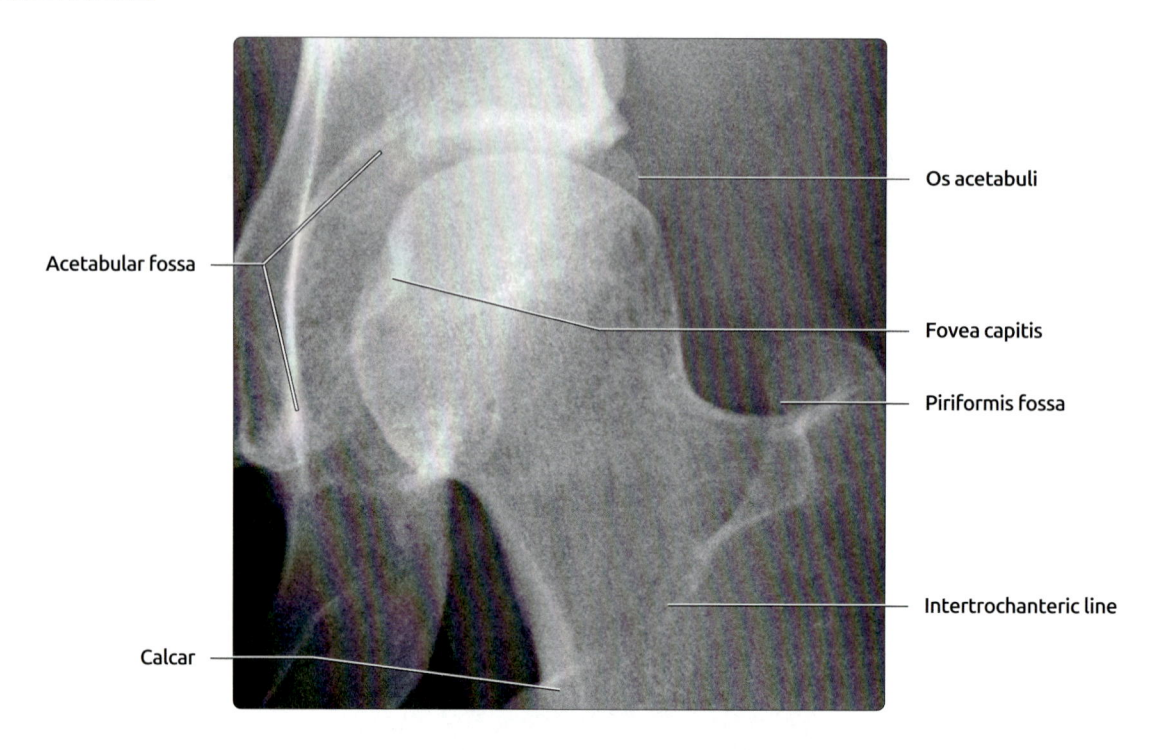

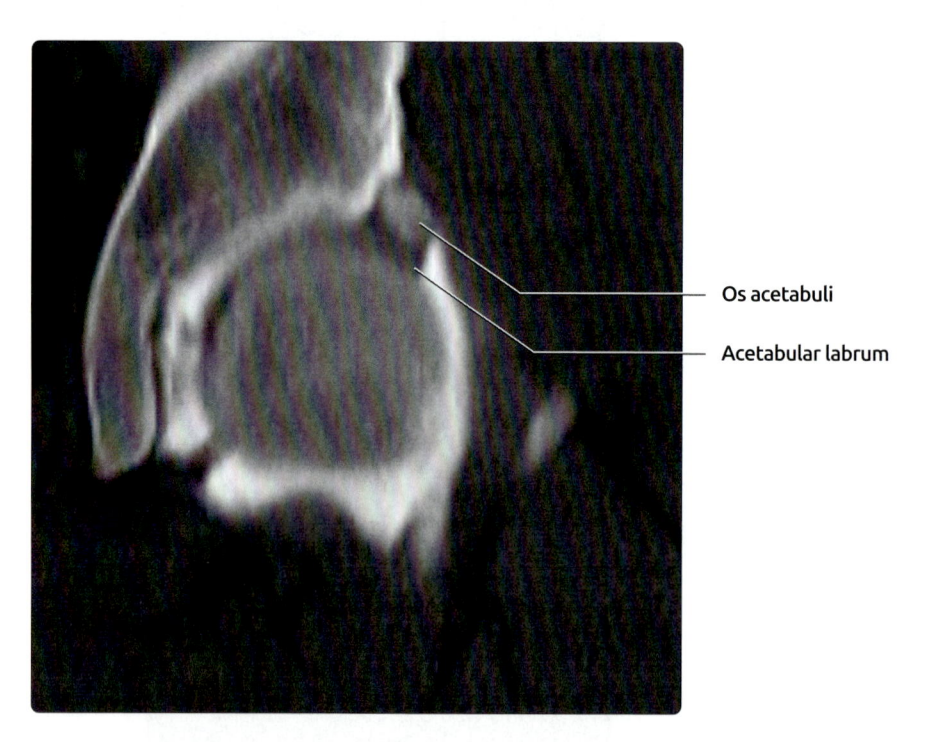

(Top) The os acetabuli is always located at the anterolateral margin of the acetabular roof. There is no definitive criteria to distinguish them from nonunited fractures; although, a rounded contour is a helpful finding. Ossification may also occur in the acetabular labrum. (Bottom) Rounded contour of the os acetabuli is well seen on this coronal CT arthrogram and helps to distinguish the ossicle from a nonunited rim fracture.

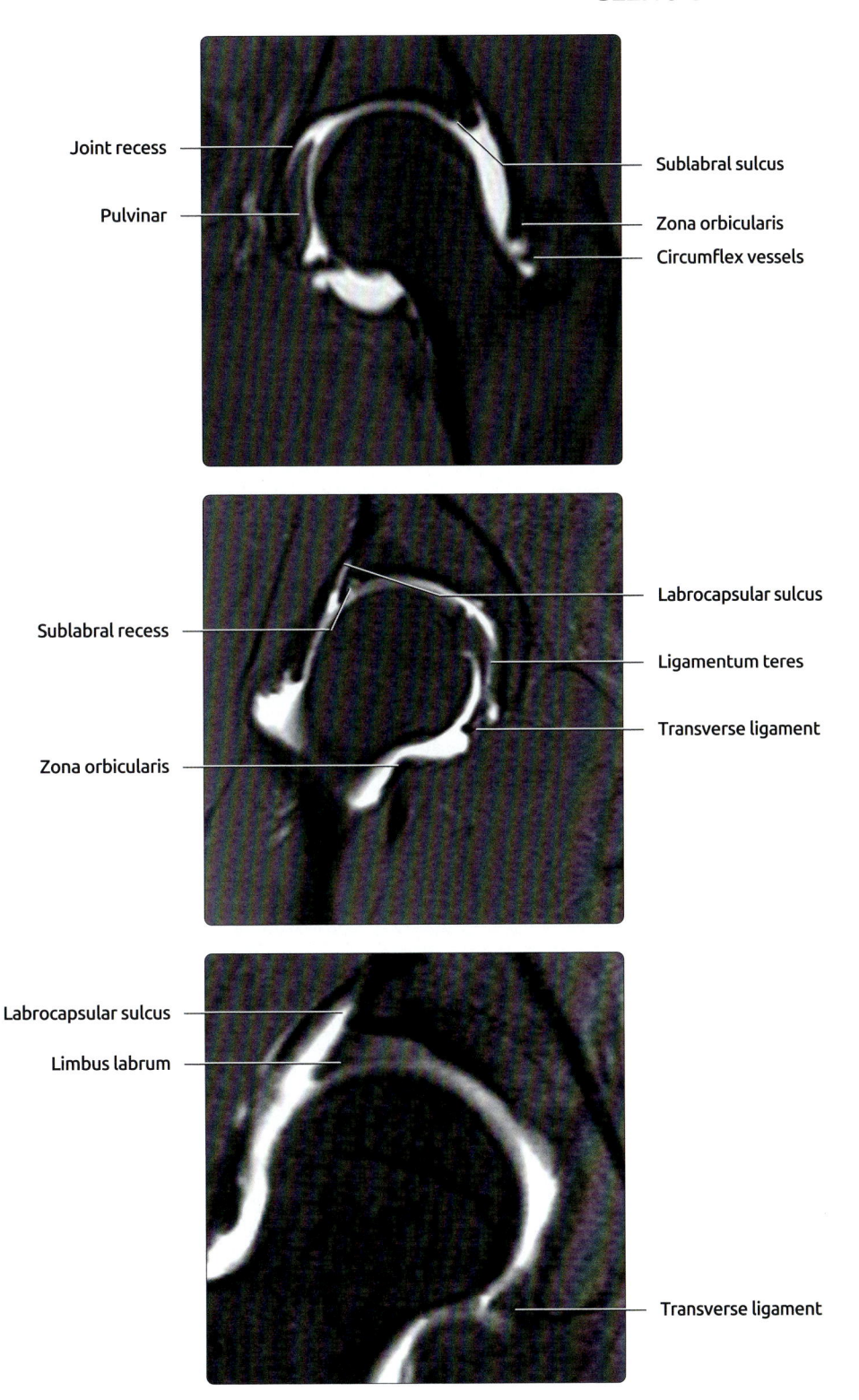

Pelvis and Hip Normal Variants and Imaging Pitfalls

GLENOID LABRUM VARIANTS

Joint recess — Sublabral sulcus
Pulvinar — Zona orbicularis
— Circumflex vessels

Sublabral recess — Labrocapsular sulcus
— Ligamentum teres
Zona orbicularis — Transverse ligament

Labrocapsular sulcus
Limbus labrum
— Transverse ligament

(Top) A sublabral sulcus is a common variant and can occur in any quadrant. Note that the fatty pulvinar fills the majority of the acetabular fossa, but there is a small joint recess superiorly, which normally fills with contrast during arthrography. (Middle) This sublabral recess is wider than many, but the fact that the margins are smooth and parallel allows distinction from labral tear. (Bottom) In this patient with mild developmental hip dysplasia, the labrum is enlarged (limbus labrum) and has an increased weight-bearing load. Labrocapsular sulcus is a normal finding, distended during arthrography.

Pelvis and Hip Normal Variants and Imaging Pitfalls

DUPLICATED PIRIFORMIS

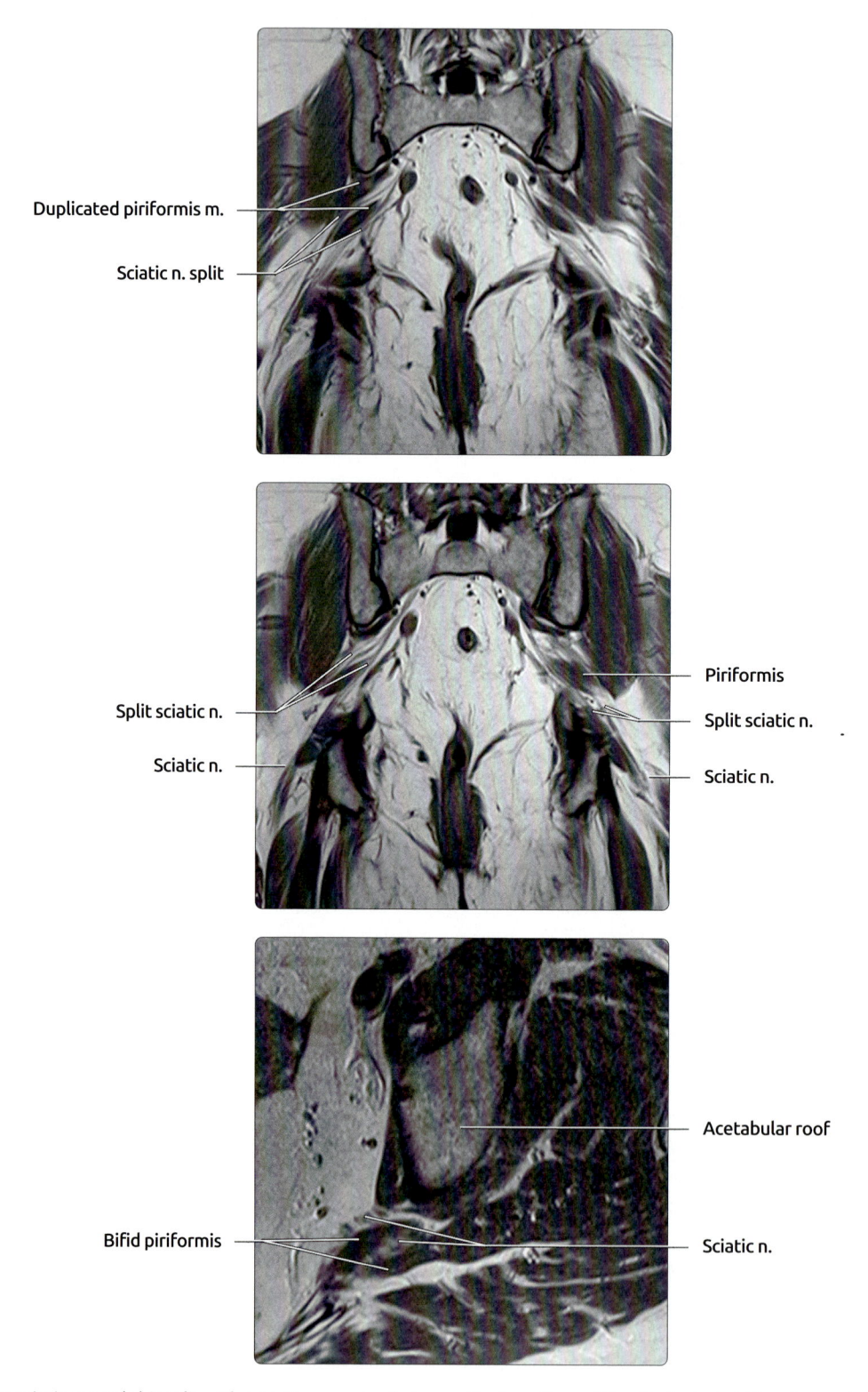

(Top) The sciatic nerve (n.) is split with a portion coursing between the 2 portions of the duplicated piriformis muscle (m.). The appearance is bilaterally symmetric in this patient but may be unilateral. (Middle) The split sciatic n. rejoins distal to the piriformis m. The 2 components of the sciatic n., the peroneal and tibial, are clearly distinguishable throughout the course of the sciatic n. in all persons and are not a result of the more proximal split in this patient. (Bottom) Two slips of the piriformis m. are seen. The sciatic n. is split with a portion between the piriformis slips and a 2nd portion anterior to the piriformis m. This configuration can cause sciatic n. impingement.

Pelvis and Hip Normal Variants and Imaging Pitfalls

PEDIATRIC VARIANTS

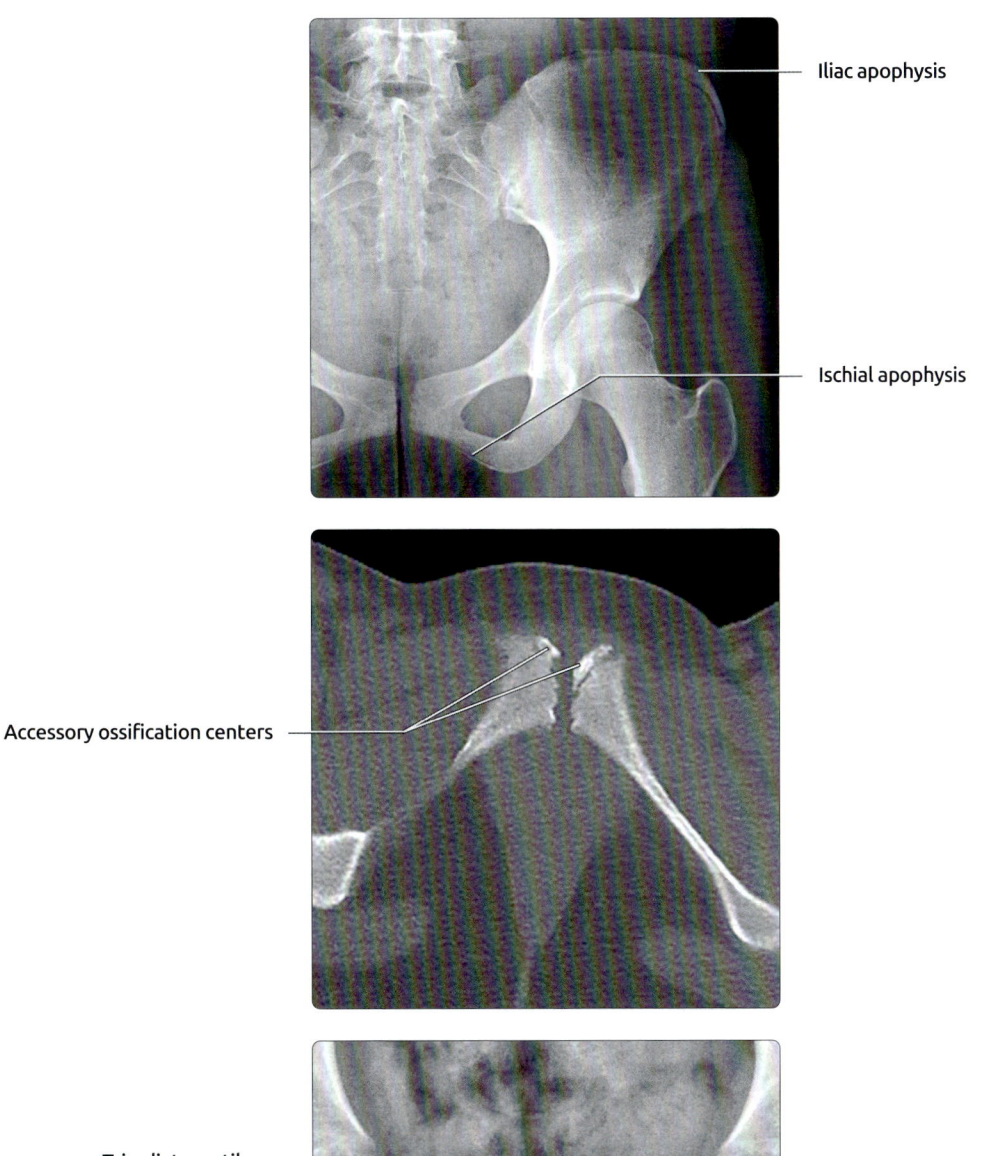

Iliac apophysis

Ischial apophysis

Accessory ossification centers

Triradiate cartilage

Ischiopubic synchondrosis

Pubic symphysis

(Top) Ossification centers in a 17-year-old female. The iliac apophysis at this age covers the entire iliac wing. Note that it is bipartite, a common variant. Ischial apophysis is thin and inconspicuous, the probable reason that avulsions of this apophysis are commonly missed. **(Middle)** Axial CT shows accessory centers of ossification for the pubis. Centers are frequently asymmetric, as in this case. The undulating contour of the bone at the symphysis posterior to the ossification center is normal in young adults. **(Bottom)** Asymmetric ossification of the ischiopubic synchondrosis in a 7-year-old girl. This normal variant is sometimes mistaken for fracture or tumor. Also note the mild bony irregularity of pubis at symphysis, normal before skeletal maturity.

Pelvis and Hip Measurements and Lines

TERMINOLOGY

Synonyms
- Center-edge angle = angle of Wiberg = lateral center-edge angle
- Anterior center-edge angle = vertical center anterior margin angle (VCA)

Definitions
- Acetabular depth: Coverage of femoral head by acetabulum
  - Measured by center-edge angle of Wiberg
    - Use both lateral and anterior center-edge angle
- Coxa profunda: Descriptor for deep acetabulum
  - Medial wall of acetabulum medial to ilioischial line
  - Center-edge angle > 40°
- Protrusio acetabulae: Descriptor for deep acetabulum
  - Medial cortex of femoral head medial to ilioischial line
- Acetabular version: Relationship of anterior and posterior rims of acetabulum
  - Anteversion: Anterior rim is medial to posterior rim
  - Retroversion: Anterior rim is lateral to posterior rim
- Femoral version: Rotation of femoral neck relative to femoral condyles
  - Anteversion: Femoral neck axis is anterior to axis of femoral condyle
  - Retroversion: Femoral neck axis is posterior to axis of femoral condyle
- Sourcil: Weight-bearing portion of acetabular roof
  - Demarcated by sclerotic subchondral bone plate
- Hilgenreiner line: Horizontal line joining superior margins of triradiate cartilage

IMAGING ANATOMY

Overview
- All measurements are dependent on careful patient positioning
- AP pelvis must be appropriately centered
- Inlet or outlet position will result in inappropriate measurements

Acetabular Roof Morphology
- 2 methods of assessing morphology of sourcil: Acetabular index and acetabular angle
  - Increase in either measurement is sign of developmental dysplasia
- **Acetabular index**
  - Measures contour of acetabular roof
  - Measured on AP radiograph pelvis
  - Measurement in pediatric population
    - Draw Hilgenreiner line bisecting top of triradiate cartilages of both hips
    - Draw line center medial margin of sourcil to lateral margin of sourcil
    - Acetabular angle is angle between these 2 lines
    - Measures up to 30° in neonates
    - Angle decreases with age
  - Measurement in adult population
    - Draw line from medial margin of sourcil to lateral margin of sourcil
    - Draw horizontal line from medial margin of sourcil
    - Angle between these lines is acetabular index
    - Normal acetabular index 3-13°
- **Acetabular angle**
  - Measures contour of acetabular roof
  - Measured on AP radiograph pelvis
    - Draw horizontal line along inferomedial margin of acetabulum
    - Draw line from inferomedial margin of acetabulum to lateral margin of sourcil
    - Angle between these lines is acetabular angle
    - Normal acetabular angle: 33-38°

Acetabular Depth
- **Measurements based on ilioischial line**
  - Measured on AP radiograph of pelvis or hip
  - Position of femoral head or acetabulum relative to ilioischial line
  - Protrusio acetabuli
    - Femoral head medial to ilioischial line
  - Coxa profunda
    - Medial wall of acetabulum medial to ilioischial line
    - Does not indicate overcoverage of femoral head
- **Center-edge angle**
  - Angle between center of femoral head and lateral or anterior margin of acetabulum
    - AP radiograph: Lateral center-edge angle (angle of Wiberg)
    - False profile radiograph: Anterior center-edge angle
  - Method of measurement
    - Locate center of femoral head
    - Draw vertical line from center
    - Draw line from center to lateral (or anterior) margin of acetabulum
    - Angle between these lines is center-edge angle
  - Normal lateral center-edge angle: 20-35°
    - Developmental dysplasia: Angle < 20° (some authors < 25°)
    - Femoral head overcoverage: Angle > 35° (some authors > 40°)
  - Normal anterior center-edge angle: > 20° (some authors > 25°)

Acetabular Version
- AP radiograph
  - Normal anterior and posterior rims form an inverted "V," with anterior rim medial to posterior rim
  - Retroversion present when anterior rim is lateral to posterior rim
  - Appearance of version susceptible to differences in patient positioning
    - Inlet view will overestimate retroversion
    - Outlet view will underestimate retroversion
  - Retroversion isolated to superior rim associated with femoroacetabular impingement
  - Radiographs provide only a qualitative evaluation of superior rim version
- CT or MR
  - Superior rim version
    - This is the location where pincer-type femoroacetabular impingement occurs

Pelvis and Hip Measurements and Lines

- Measure at most superior slice where femoral head is visible
- Angle between line bisecting posterior and anterior rims and horizontal line
- Normal is 15° anteversion
○ Global version
- Measure at equator
- Angle between line bisecting posterior and anterior rims and horizontal line
- Rarely retroverted unless prior surgery

Femoral Head Coverage
- **Perkin line (pediatric population)**
  ○ Measured on AP pelvis
  ○ Vertical line lateral acetabular roof perpendicular to Hilgenreiner line
  ○ Femoral head should lie in inferomedial quadrant formed by intersection of Hilgenreiner and Perkin lines
- **Shenton line (pediatric population)**
  ○ Arc measured on AP pelvis
  ○ Normal: Smooth arc from medial cortex femoral neck along superior and medial wall of obturator foramen
  ○ Developmental dysplasia: Line is interrupted
- **Extrusion index**
  ○ Percent of femoral head uncovered by acetabulum compared to total diameter of femoral head
  ○ Normal: 18-28%
  ○ Developmental dysplasia: Increased extrusion index

Femoral Head Morphology
- α (alpha) angle
  ○ Measure of femoral head-neck offset
    - Decreased offset, or bony prominence, between femoral head and neck may cause femoroacetabular impingement
  ○ Performed on oblique axial MR or CT
  ○ Slice along center of femoral neck axis
  ○ Create best fit circle of femoral head
  ○ Draw line bisecting femoral neck axis
  ○ Identify junction of femoral neck and circle outlining femoral head
  ○ α° is angle between femoral neck axis at center of femoral head and point where femoral neck intersects circle outlining femoral head
- 50° or less is normal
  ○ Larger angles associated with femoroacetabular impingement

Femur
- **Femoral angle of inclination (neck-shaft angle)**
  ○ Measured on AP radiograph of hip, femur, or pelvis
  ○ Angle between axis of femoral neck and axis of femoral shaft
  ○ Normal at birth: 140-150°
  ○ Normal in adulthood: 120-135°
  ○ Decreased angle = coxa vara
  ○ Increased angle = coxa valga
- **Measurement of femoral version**
  ○ Rotation of femoral neck relative to femoral condyles
  ○ Measured on axial CT or MR images through femoral neck and condyles
  - Angle between axis of femoral neck and posterior margins of femoral condyles
  ○ Normal: Femoral neck anteverted relative to femoral condyles
    - Normal at birth: 30-40° anteversion
    - Normal in adulthood: 8-15° (men < women) anteverted

Mechanical Axis of Lower Extremity
- Axis of weight transmission through lower extremity
  ○ Abnormal leads to osteoarthritis
  ○ Abnormal may result from arthritis
- Evaluated on standing radiograph including hip to ankle
  ○ Line drawn from center of femoral head to center of tibial plafond
  ○ Normal: Line passes through intercondylar notch
  ○ Varus: Line passes medial to notch
    - Mild medial deviation can be considered physiologic varus
  ○ Valgus: Line passes lateral to notch

ANATOMY IMAGING ISSUES

Acetabular Overcoverage
- Leads to pincer-type impingement
- 2 types
  ○ Global overcoverage: Increased center-edge angle
  ○ Superior rim retroversion

Acetabular Undercoverage
- Diagnostic of developmental dysplasia

Decreased Femoral Head-Neck Offset
- α° is less commonly used today
- Focal "bump" at head-neck junction or qualitative assessment of decreased femoral head-neck offset are more commonly used

SELECTED REFERENCES
1. Tannast M et al: What are the radiographic reference values for acetabular under- and overcoverage? Clin Orthop Relat Res. ePub, 2014
2. Nepple JJ et al: Coxa profunda is not a useful radiographic parameter for diagnosing pincer-type femoroacetabular impingement. J Bone Joint Surg Am. 95(5):417-23, 2013
3. Anderson LA et al: Coxa profunda: is the deep acetabulum overcovered? Clin Orthop Relat Res. 470(12):3375-82, 2012
4. Werner CM et al: Normal values of Wiberg's lateral center-edge angle and Lequesne's acetabular index--a coxometric update. Skeletal Radiol. 41(10):1273-8, 2012
5. Delaunay S et al: Radiographic measurements of dysplastic adult hips. Skeletal Radiol. 26(2):75-81, 1997
6. Notzli HP et al: The contour of the femoral head-neck junction as a predictor for the risk of anterior impingement. J Bone Joint Surg. 84:556-560, 2002
7. Reynolds D et al: Retroversion of the acetabulum. J Bone Joint Surg. 81-B:281-288, 1999

Pelvis and Hip Measurements and Lines

PROTRUSIO; FEMORAL INCLINATION: MECHANICAL AXIS

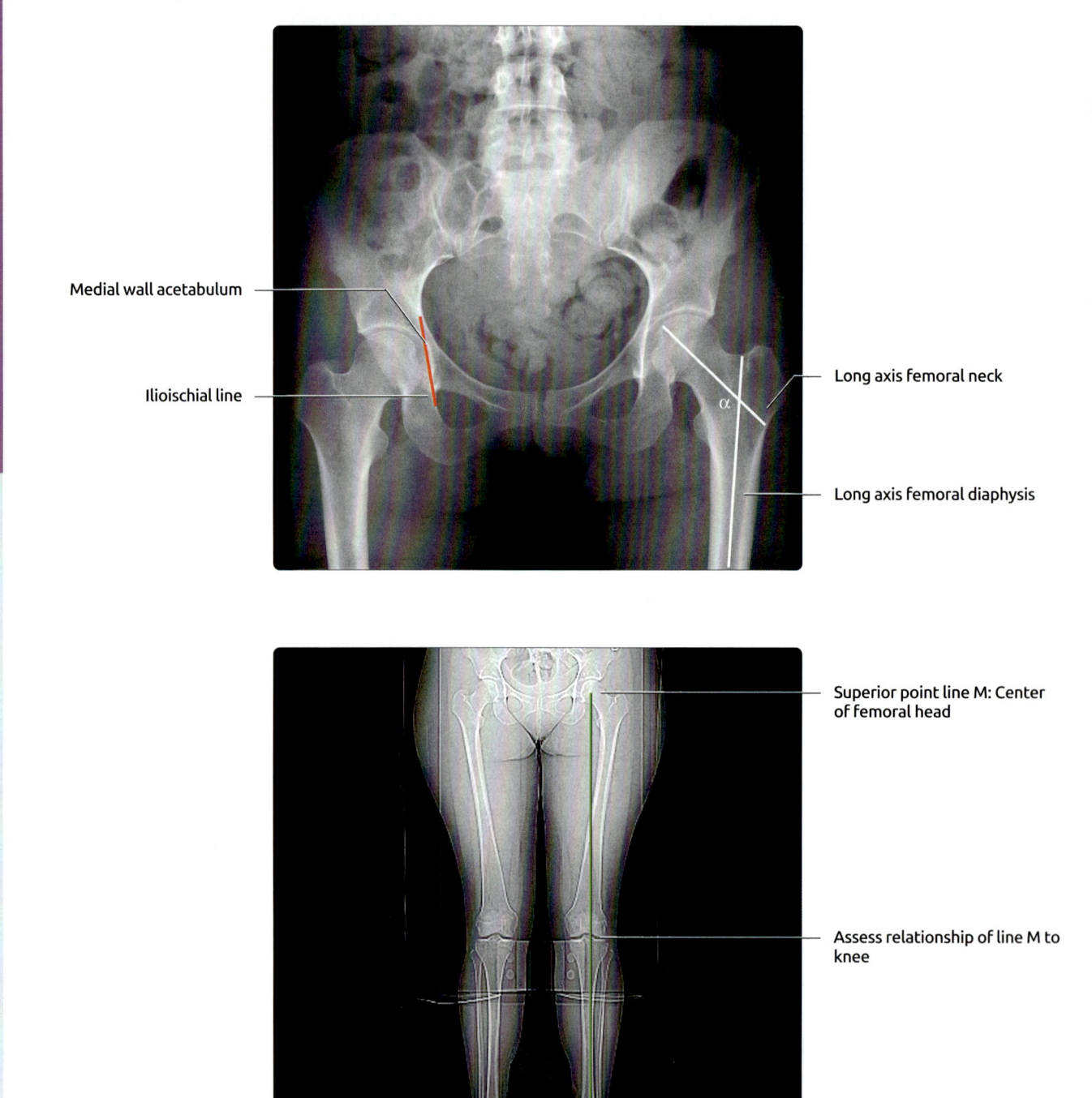

- Medial wall acetabulum
- Ilioischial line
- Long axis femoral neck
- Long axis femoral diaphysis
- Superior point line M: Center of femoral head
- Assess relationship of line M to knee
- Inferior point line M: Center of tibial plafond

(Top) Determination of neck-shaft angle, also known as femoral angle of inclination of the left hip, is demonstrated. The angle of inclination (angle alpha) is measured between the long axis of the femoral diaphysis and the long axis of the femoral neck. Coxa profunda is present when the medial wall of the acetabulum is medial to the ilioischial line. **(Bottom)** Determination of the mechanical axis (line M) is shown. With a normal mechanical axis the main force of weight is through the center of the knee.

Pelvis and Hip Measurements and Lines

ACETABULAR ANGLE, LATERAL MIGRATION, ALPHA ANGLE

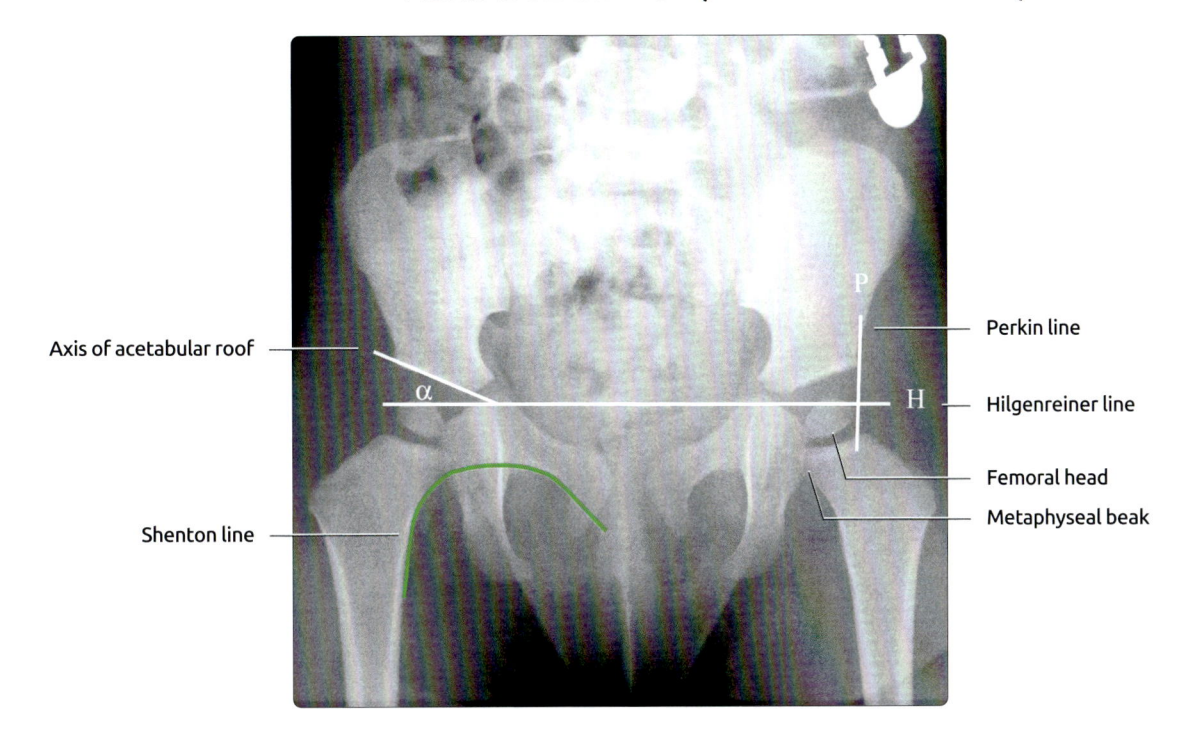

Axis of acetabular roof

Shenton line

Perkin line

Hilgenreiner line

Femoral head

Metaphyseal beak

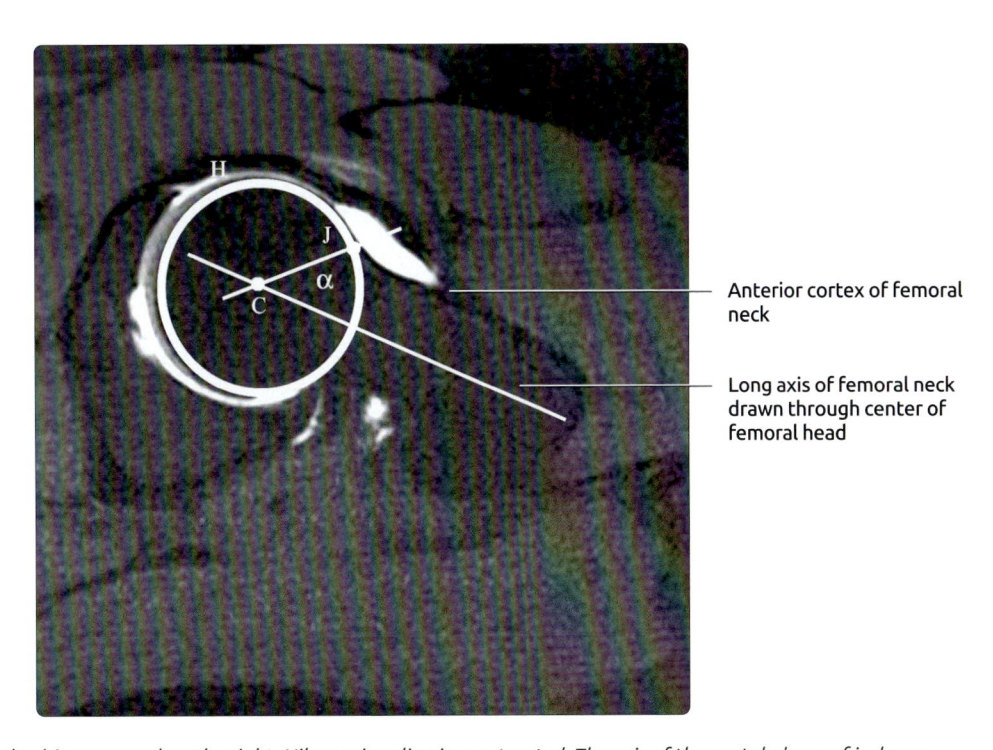

Anterior cortex of femoral neck

Long axis of femoral neck drawn through center of femoral head

(Top) The acetabular angle (angle a) is measured on the right. Hilgenreiner line is constructed. The axis of the acetabular roof is drawn (see left hip for anatomic reference). The angle formed by these 2 lines is measured. Lateral migration of the femoral head is determined on the left. Hilgenreiner and Perkin lines are constructed. In this normal hip the head and metaphyseal beak are in the inferior medial quadrant formed by these lines. A normal Shenton line is shown on the right, with continuous curvature extending from the obturator foramen to femoral metaphysis. **(Bottom)** The a angle is a measure of head-neck offset. Increased a angle is associated with femoroacetabular impingement. The a angle is constructed on oblique axial image. Critical points include: Circle H (best fit to circumference of femoral head), point C (center of femoral head), point J (point where circle H crosses the anterior femoral neck cortex), line CJ (from center of femoral head to point J). The a angle is the angle between the long axis of femoral neck and the line C-J.

Pelvis and Hip Measurements and Lines

AP & FALSE PROFILE, CENTER-EDGE ANGLE

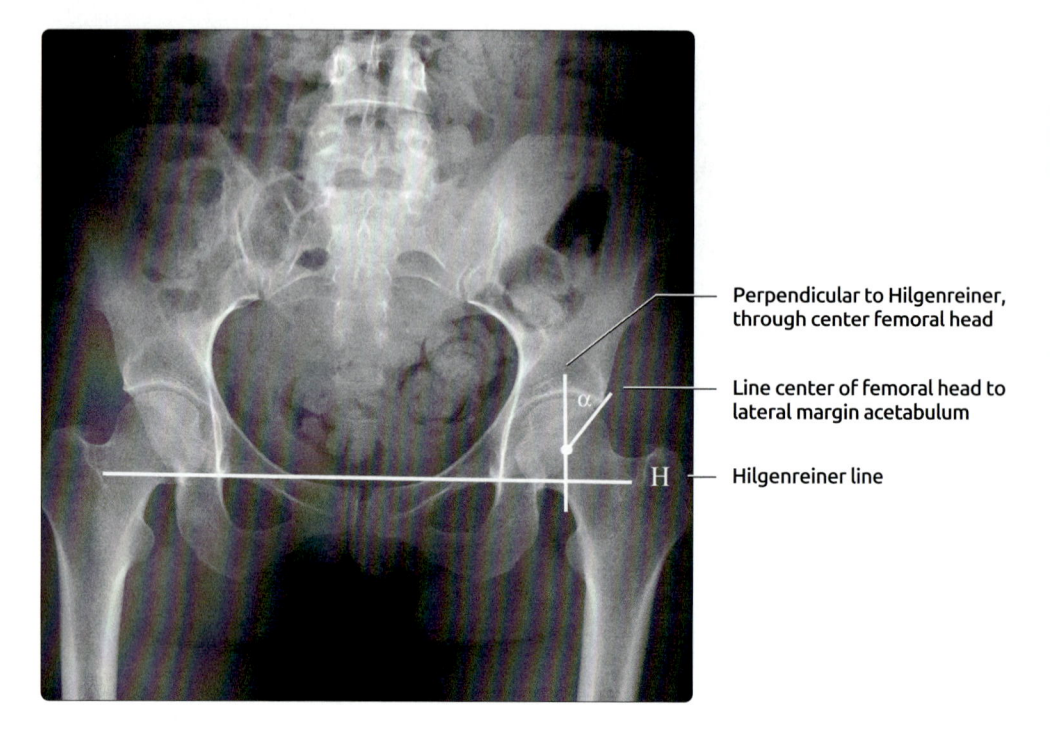

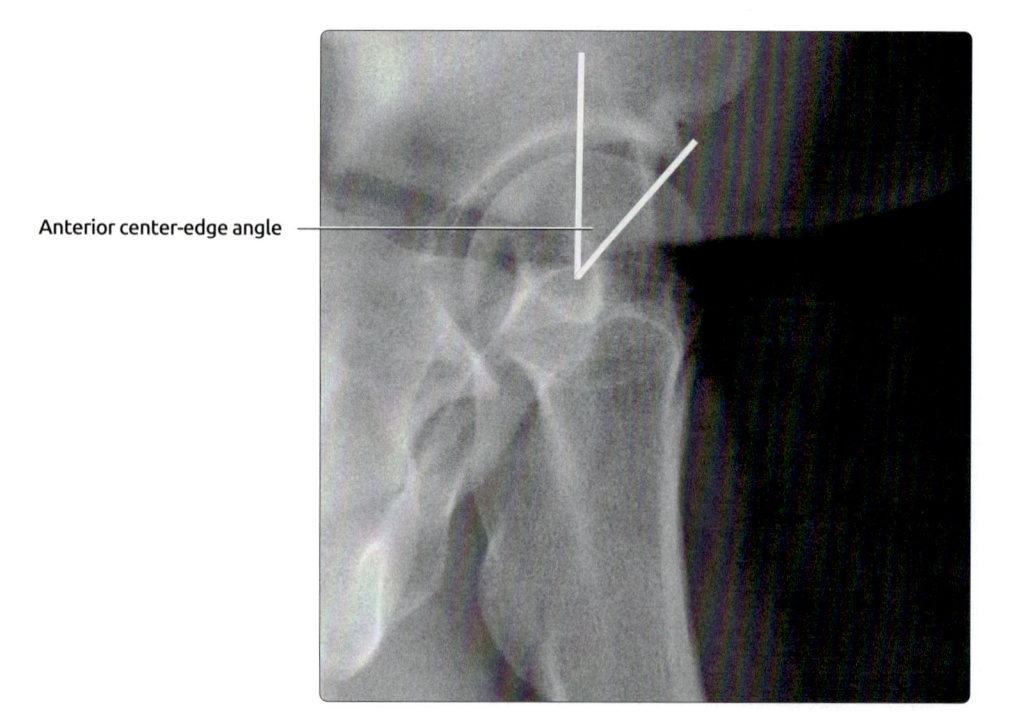

- Perpendicular to Hilgenreiner, through center femoral head
- Line center of femoral head to lateral margin acetabulum
- Hilgenreiner line

- Anterior center-edge angle

(Top) The center-edge angle (angle α) of the acetabulum is constructed on AP radiograph. This angle measures lateral acetabular coverage of the femoral head. **(Bottom)** The anterior center-edge angle is measured on the false profile view. Patient is standing, and rotated 65° posterior oblique. The angle is drawn between a vertical line through the center of the femoral head, and a line is drawn from the center of the femoral head to the anterior acetabular margin.

Pelvis and Hip Measurements and Lines

RADIOGRAPHIC MEASUREMENT OF ACETABULAR VERSION

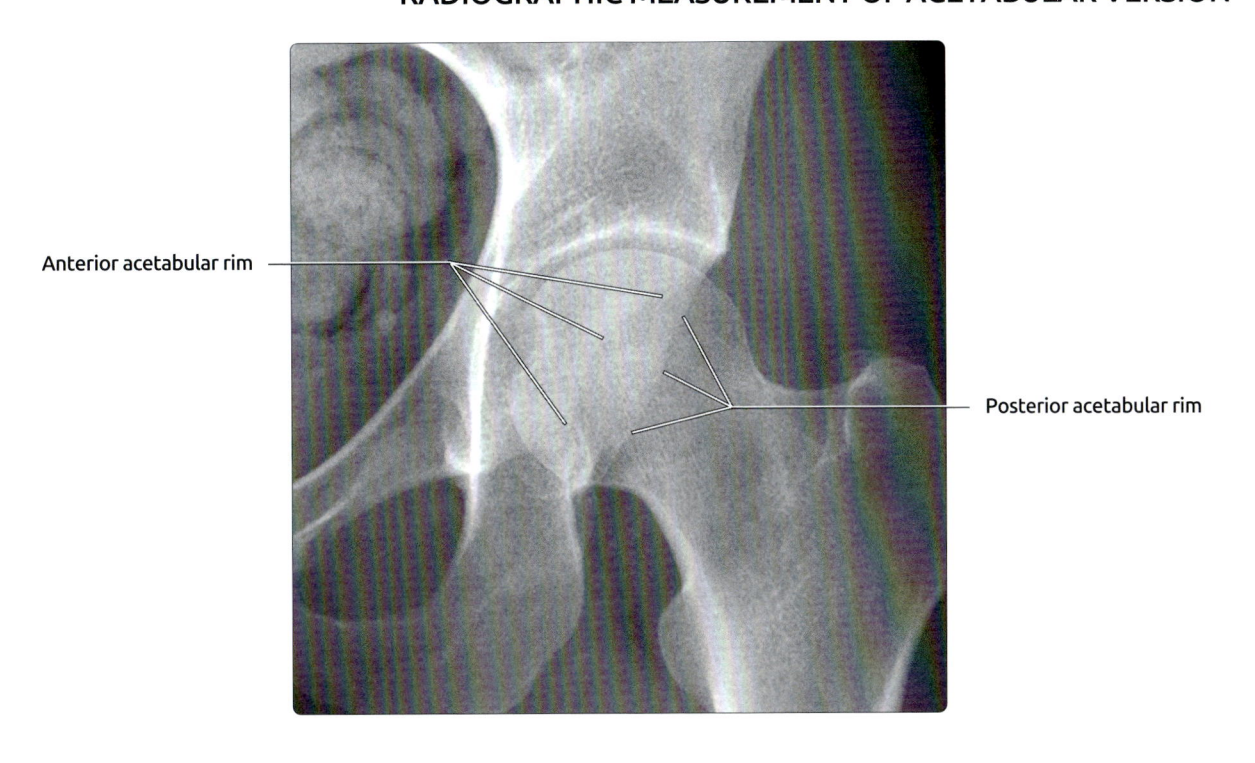

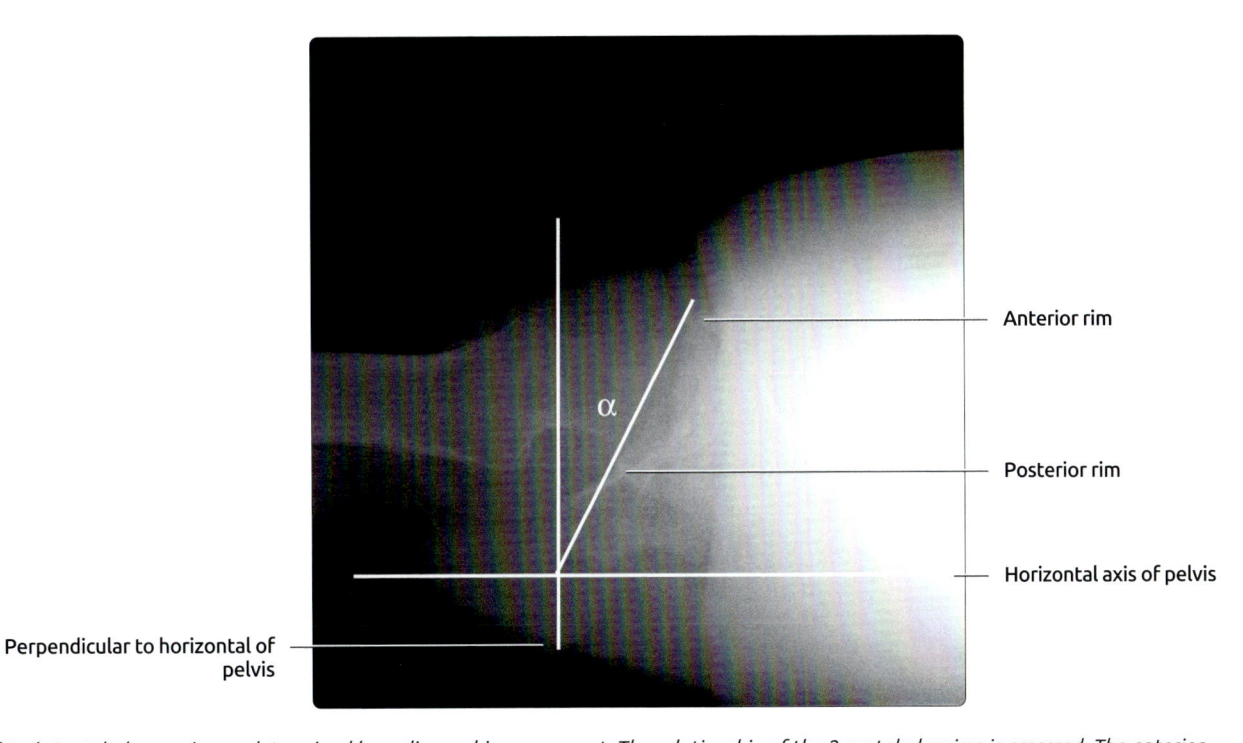

(Top) Acetabular version as determined by radiographic assessment. The relationship of the 2 acetabular rims is assessed. The anterior rim should be medial to the posterior rim. The posterior rim should be lateral to the center of the femoral head. Retroversion is usually limited to the most superior portion of the acetabulum, and results in crossover sign where the anterior rim projects lateral to the posterior rim of the acetabulum. (Bottom) Acetabular version (angle a) measured on an axiolateral view of the hip. The horizontal axis of the pelvis is assumed to be parallel to the edge of the film. A perpendicular line to this axis is drawn. A line is then drawn through the 2 rims of the acetabulum. This measurement is useful for hip arthroplasty evaluation. For impingement, the most superior portion of the rim, not evaluated here, is the area of concern.

SECTION 8
Thigh

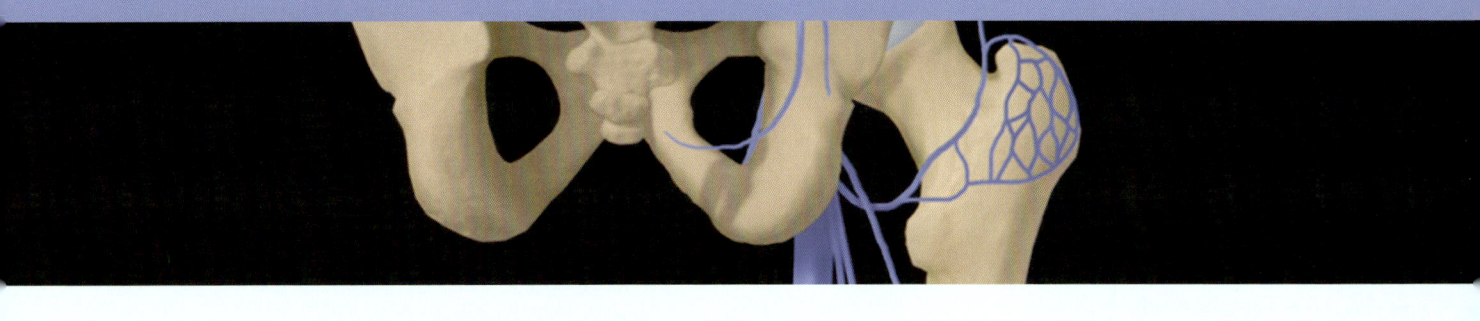

Thigh Radiographic Anatomy and MR Atlas — 606

Thigh Radiographic Anatomy and MR Atlas

TERMINOLOGY

Abbreviations
- Anterior superior iliac spine (ASIS)
- Function (F)
- Muscle insertion (I)
- Nerve supply (N)
- Muscle origin (O)
- Structure supplied by nerve or vessel (S)
- Sacroiliac joint (SI)

IMAGING ANATOMY

Bony Anatomy of Femur
- Femoral head
  - 2/3 of sphere sitting on cylindrical femoral neck
  - Fovea capitis: Medial concavity for attachment of ligamentum teres
- Femoral neck
  - Connects head to intertrochanteric region
- Trochanters
  - Greater: Superior/posterior projection from femoral neck/shaft junction
  - Lesser: Posterior/medial projection from femoral neck/shaft junction
  - Joined by intertrochanteric crest
- Shaft
  - Bowed anteriorly, inclined medially
  - Linea aspera on posterior surface; multiple muscle attachments
- Condyles
  - Medial and lateral condyles separated by intercondylar notch
  - Epicondyles superior margin of condyles

Compartment Anatomy
- Thigh divided into 3-4 soft tissue compartments
  - **Anterior compartment**: Iliotibial tract, tensor fascia lata m., quadriceps muscles (sartorius m.)
  - **Medial compartment**: Gracilis muscle, adductor muscles
  - **Posterior compartment**: Hamstring muscles, short head of biceps femoris muscle, sciatic nerve
  - **Sartorius** is often considered separate compartment
- Muscles at junction pelvis/thigh: Each considered separate compartment
  - Pectineus, iliopsoas, obturator externus, lateral femoral muscles
- Extensions from fascia lata divide compartments
  - Medial intermuscular septum: Anterior/medial
  - Lateral intermuscular septum: Anterior/lateral
  - Thin fascia separates medial, posterior compartments
- Clinical note: Compartment anatomy critical to tumor staging and biopsy planning
  - Cross compartment extension of tumor, contamination by biopsy may require change from limb salvage to amputation

Medial Thigh Muscles
- F: Hip adduction; assist hip flexion, internal rotation
  - Except obturator externus muscle (external rotation of hip)
- **Adductor longus**
  - O: Pubic body inferior to crest
  - I: Medial lip linea aspera
  - N: Posterior division of obturator nerve
- **Adductor brevis** lies posterior to adductor longus
  - O: Inferior pubic ramus
  - I: Inferior 2/3 of pectineal line, superior 1/2 of medial lip of linea aspera
  - N: Posterior division of obturator nerve
- **Adductor magnus**: Massive, posteromedial muscle can be divided into 3 parts
  - N: Posterior division obturator nerve, except ischiocondylar portion innervated by tibial nerve
  - Adductor minimus
    - O: Pubic ramus
    - I: Gluteal tuberosity of femur, medial to gluteus maximus
  - Adductor and ischiocondylar portion of adductor magnus
    - O: Ischiopubic ramus, ischial tuberosity
    - I: Wide insertion on medial lip linea aspera, medial supracondylar line
      - 5 aponeurotic openings in insertion sites
      - 4 openings transmit perforating branches and terminus of profunda femoris a.
      - Lowest opening is adductor hiatus, through which superficial femoral vessels pass into popliteal fossa
    - Ischiocondylar portion is most medial (hamstring) portion, inserts on medial supracondylar line
- **Gracilis**
  - O: Inferior pubic ramus, symphysis pubis
  - I: Medial proximal tibia (pes anserine)
  - F: Also assists knee flexion
- **Obturator externus**
  - O: External margins of obturator foramen and membrane
  - I: Piriformis fossa
  - F: Hip external rotation only
- **Pectineus**
  - O: Superior pubic ramus, pecten
  - I: Pectineal line femur
  - Femoral nerve ± accessory obturator nerve

Anterior Thigh Muscles
- Common innervation: Femoral nerve
- Common function: Knee extension (except sartorius)
- **Sartorius** (tailor's) muscle
  - O: ASIS, notch below
  - I: Proximal medial tibia (pes anserine)
  - F: Hip flexion, abduction, external rotation; knee flexion
  - Crosses hip and knee joints
  - Longest muscle in body
  - Separate fascial covering
- **Quadriceps femoris**: Rectus femoris, vastus lateralis, vastus medialis, vastus intermedius muscles
  - Common tendon of insertion onto superior, lateral, medial patella
- **Rectus femoris**
  - O: Straight head: Anterior inferior iliac spine

Thigh Radiographic Anatomy and MR Atlas

- o O: Reflected head: Lateral ilium, in groove above acetabulum
- o I: Superior patella, tibial tuberosity
- o F: Also hip flexion
- o Crosses hip and knee joints
- **Vastus lateralis**
  - o O: Superior intertrochanteric line femur, anterior and inferior greater trochanter, gluteal tuberosity, lateral lip linea aspera, lateral intermuscular septum
  - o I: Lateral patellar retinaculum, superolateral patella, rectus femoris tendon
  - o Largest quadriceps muscle
- **Vastus medialis**
  - o O: Entire medial lip linea aspera, inferior intertrochanteric line, medial intermuscular septum
  - o I: Tendon rectus femoris muscle, superomedial patella (quadriceps tendon), medial condyle tibia (medial patellar retinaculum)
- **Vastus intermedius**
  - o O: Anterior and lateral femoral shaft, inferior lateral lip linea aspera, lateral intermuscular septum
  - o I: Blends along deep aspect rectus femoris, vastus medialis, vastus lateralis muscles
- **Articularis genu**
  - o O: Anterior lower femur
  - o I: Synovial membrane knee
  - o N. to vastus intermedius

Iliotibial Tract/Band: Lateral Thickening Fascia Lata

- O: Tubercle iliac crest
- I: Lateral condyle tibia
- Insertion site of tensor fascia lata muscle and portion of gluteus maximus muscle

Posterior Thigh Muscles

- Common nerve: Sciatic nerve
  - o Tibial division: Long head of biceps femoris, semitendinosus, semimembranosus, ischiocondylar portion adductor magnus muscles
  - o Common peroneal division: Short head of biceps femoris muscle
- Common functions: Hip extension, knee flexion
- **Hamstrings**: Long head of biceps femoris, semimembranous, semitendinosus, ischiocondylar portion adductor magnus muscles
  - o Does not include short head of biceps femoris m.
- **Biceps femoris**
  - o Long head: O: Ischial tuberosity (inferior, medial)
    - Common tendon with semitendinosus muscle
  - o Short head: O: Lateral lip linea aspera femur, lateral supracondylar line, lateral intermuscular septum
    - Post-axial muscle
    - Not part of hamstring muscles
  - o I: Fibular head, lateral condyle tibia
  - o F: Also external rotation flexed knee
- **Semimembranosus**
  - o O: Ischial tuberosity (superior, lateral)
  - o I: Posterior medial condyle tibia, popliteal fascia
    - Some fibers extend to form oblique popliteal l. (see "Knee Medial Supporting Structures" chapter)
  - o F: Also internal rotation flexed knee

- o Membranous in upper thigh
- **Semitendinosus**
  - o O: Ischial tuberosity (inferior, medial)
    - Common tendon long head of biceps femoris m.
  - o I: Medial proximal tibia (pes anserine)
  - o F: Also internal rotation flexed knee
  - o Entirely tendinous in distal thigh

Hip Flexors

- Sartorius: Anterior femoral muscle
- Pectineus: Medial femoral muscle
- **Iliopsoas**: I: Lesser trochanter
  - o Iliacus
    - O: Iliac crest, iliac fossa, sacral ala, SI joint capsule
    - N: Femoral nerve
  - o Psoas major
    - O: Lateral vertebral body and intervertebral discs T12-L5, all lumbar transverse processes
    - N: L1, L2, L3
  - o Psoas minor
    - O: Lateral vertebral body T12, L1 and T12-L1 intervertebral disc
    - N: L1, L2

Femoral Triangle

- Anterior wall: Inguinal ligament
- Posterior wall: Adductor longus and pectineus muscles (medial), iliopsoas muscle (lateral)
- Medial border: Adductor longus muscle
- Lateral border: Sartorius muscle
- Apex: Crossing adductor longus and sartorius muscles
- Contents: Femoral nerve and branches, femoral vessels, lymph node (Cloquet node), femoral sheath
  - o Structures lateral to medial at entrance: NAVeL: Nerve, artery, vein, lymphatics
- Femoral artery/vein relationships
  - o Entrance: Artery lateral
  - o Apex: Artery anterior
- Femoral nerve branches within triangle
  - o Saphenous nerve, and nerve to vastus medialis only branches to exit triangle
- **Femoral sheath**: Transversalis fascia covers vessels proximally
  - o 3 compartments: Lateral (artery), middle (vein), medial (femoral canal)
- **Femoral canal**: Medial compartment femoral sheath
  - o Anterior border: Inguinal ligament
  - o Posterior border: Pubic bone
  - o Medial border: Lacunar ligament
  - o Lateral border: Femoral vein
  - o Entrance: **Femoral ring**
    - Anterior border: Medial inguinal ligament
    - Posterior border: Superior pubic ramus
    - Medial border: Lacunar ligament
    - Lateral border: Septum between femoral canal and femoral vein
    - Open to peritoneal cavity
  - o Contents: Lymphatic vessels and nodes (**Cloquet node**), fat, connective tissue

Thigh Radiographic Anatomy and MR Atlas

Adductor (Subsartorial or Hunter) Canal
- Vessel passageway from thigh to popliteal fossa
- Anteromedial border: Sartorius muscle
- Anterolateral border: Vastus medialis muscle
- Posterior border: Adductor longus and magnus muscles
- Entrance: Apex femoral triangle, exit adductor hiatus
  - **Adductor hiatus**: Gap in adductor magnus muscle between adductor portion and ischiocondylar portion distal thigh
- Contents: Femoral artery and vein, saphenous nerve
  - Nerve initially anterior to artery, then medial
  - Artery anterior to vein
  - Descending geniculate artery arises in canal

Femoral Vessels
- Enter thigh deep to inguinal ligament, midpoint between ASIS and symphysis pubis
- Upper thigh: Vessels within femoral triangle
  - Enter: Artery lateral to vein
  - Exit: Artery anterior
- Mid thigh: Vessels within adductor canal
  - Entrance: Artery anterior
  - Exit: Artery anterior
- Distal thigh: Exit adductor canal via adductor hiatus, enter popliteal fossa
- **Common femoral artery branches**
  - **Superficial epigastric, superficial circumflex iliac, superficial external pudendal** arise anteriorly
  - **Deep external pudendal** arises medially
    - May branch from medial circumflex femoral
  - Divides into superficial and deep branches
  - **Superficial femoral artery**
    - Branch: **Descending genicular**
  - **Deep femoral (profunda femoris)**
    - Arises laterally in femoral triangle
    - Dives between pectineus and adductor longus muscles
    - Medial to femur, deep to adductor longus muscle
    - Branches in femoral triangle: **Medial circumflex femoral** (main supply to femoral head and neck), lateral circumflex femoral, muscular branches
    - Branches in adductor canal: 3 perforating branches, descending genicular
    - Terminal branch: 4th perforating artery
- **Femoral vein**: Travels with artery
  - Tributaries: Deep femoral, descending genicular, lateral circumflex femoral, medial circumflex femoral, deep external pudendal, greater saphenous veins
  - **Greater saphenous vein**
    - Longest vein in body
    - Toes to saphenous opening (fascia lata)
    - Tributaries: Accessory saphenous, superficial epigastric, superficial circumflex femoral, superficial external pudendal veins

Femoral Nerve
- L2, L3, L4, L5; post axial
- Largest branch lumbar plexus
- Exits plexus lower psoas muscle
- Travels in groove between psoas and iliacus muscles
- Exits pelvis beneath inguinal ligament, lateral to femoral vessels, enters femoral triangle
- Multiple branches in femoral triangle
  - Muscular branches: To pectineus, sartorius, rectus femoris, vastus lateralis, vastus medialis, vastus intermedius muscles
  - Cutaneous nerves: Anterior femoral cutaneous, saphenous
    - Saphenous nerve exits triangle, enters adductor canal
  - Articular branches hip and knee

Obturator Nerve
- L2, L3, L4; pre axial
- Branch lumbar plexus
- Relationships
  - Posterior to iliac vessels
  - Medial to psoas muscle
  - Lateral to internal iliac vessels
- Via obturator foramen to thigh
- S: Adductor muscles, hip and knee joints, skin medial distal thigh
- Accessory obturator nerve: L3, L4
  - Present in 9%

Sciatic Nerve
- L4, L5, S1, S2, S3, largest branch of sacral plexus
- 2 nerves in 1 sheath
  - Tibial nerve (medial) and common peroneal nerve (lateral)
  - Separate in lower thigh
- Exits pelvis inferior to piriformis muscle
- Crosses over superior gemellus, obturator internus, inferior gemellus, quadratus femoris, adductor magnus muscles
- Deep to long head of biceps femoris muscle
- Branches arising in thigh: Articular to hip, nerves to hamstring muscles
- **Tibial nerve**: Larger division of sciatic nerve
  - S: Posterior femoral muscles except short head of biceps femoris muscle
- **Common peroneal nerve**
  - Oblique lateral course with biceps femoris muscle
  - S: Short head of biceps femoris muscle

Fascia of Thigh
- **Fascia lata**: Encase entire thigh
  - Superior attachment: Inguinal ligament
- **Iliotibial tract**: Lateral thickening of fascia lata
  - Superior attachment: Tubercle of iliac crest
  - Inferior attachment: Lateral tubercle of tibial condyle (Gerdy tubercle)
  - Insertion site of portions of gluteus maximus and tensor fascia lata muscles
- **Lateral intermuscular septum**: Separates vastus lateralis and biceps femoris muscles
- **Medial intermuscular septum**: Separates adductor and vastus medialis muscles

Thigh Radiographic Anatomy and MR Atlas

ANTERIOR THIGH

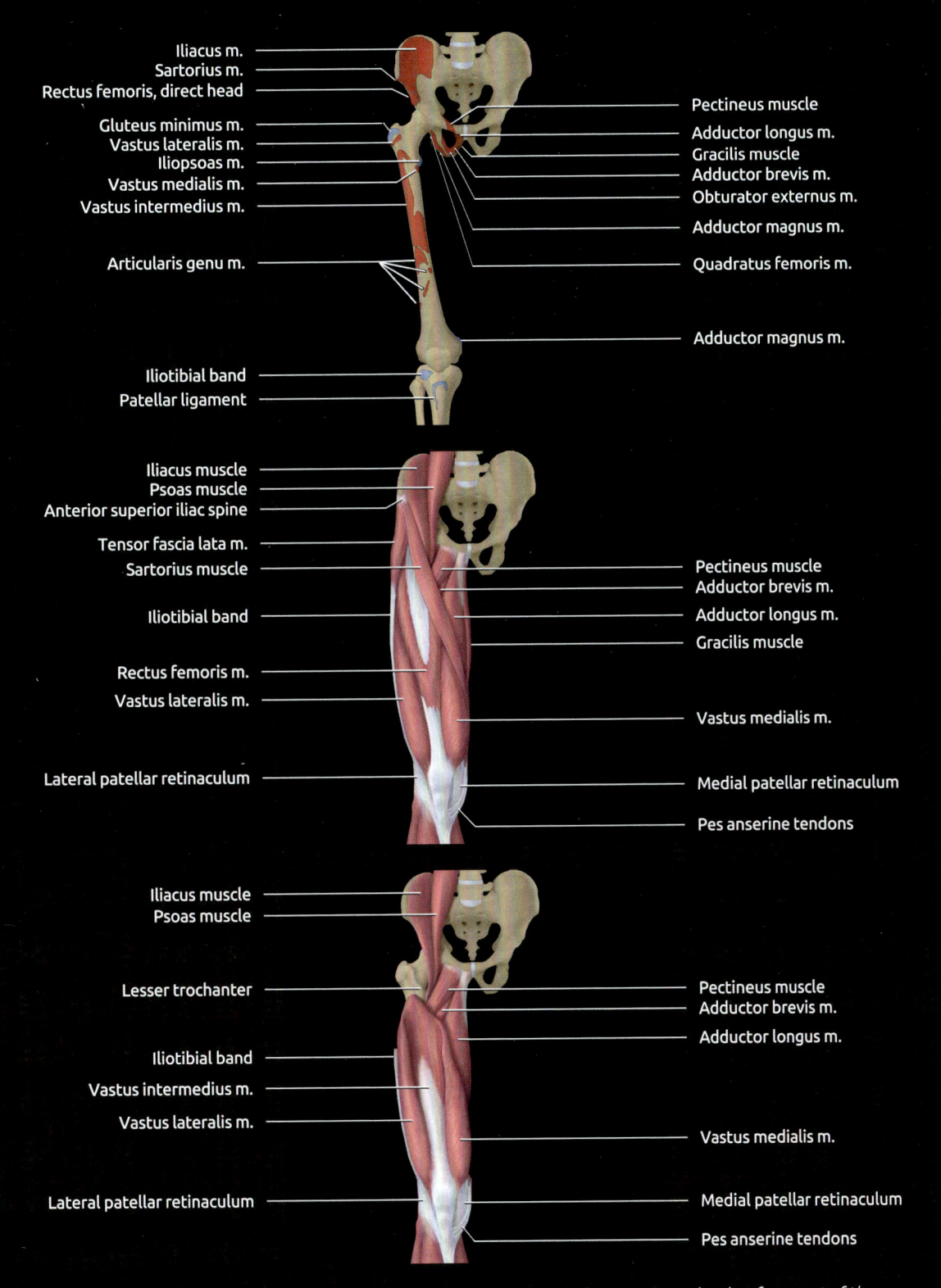

(Top) Muscle and ligament attachments of the anterior pelvis and femur are shown. The 3 vasti muscles that form part of the quadriceps group are the primary muscles arising from the anterior femur. Adductor magnus inserts on the adductor tubercle just above the medial femoral condyle. (Middle) Superficial muscles of the anterior thigh are shown. The oblique course of the sartorius muscle is easily appreciated. The adductor brevis muscle is deep to the adductor longus and pectineus muscles. The most medial muscle is the gracilis. The vastus lateralis and medialis muscles continue to their insertions on the lateral and medial patellar margins, respectively. (Bottom) Deep muscles of the anterior thigh are shown. The vastus intermedius muscle is deep to the rectus femoris muscle. With the removal of the sartorius muscle, a little more of the adductor brevis muscle is visible. The sartorius, gracilis, and semitendinosus tendons combine to form the pes anserinus, inserting on the tibia just distal and anterior to the medial collateral ligament.

Thigh Radiographic Anatomy and MR Atlas

POSTERIOR THIGH

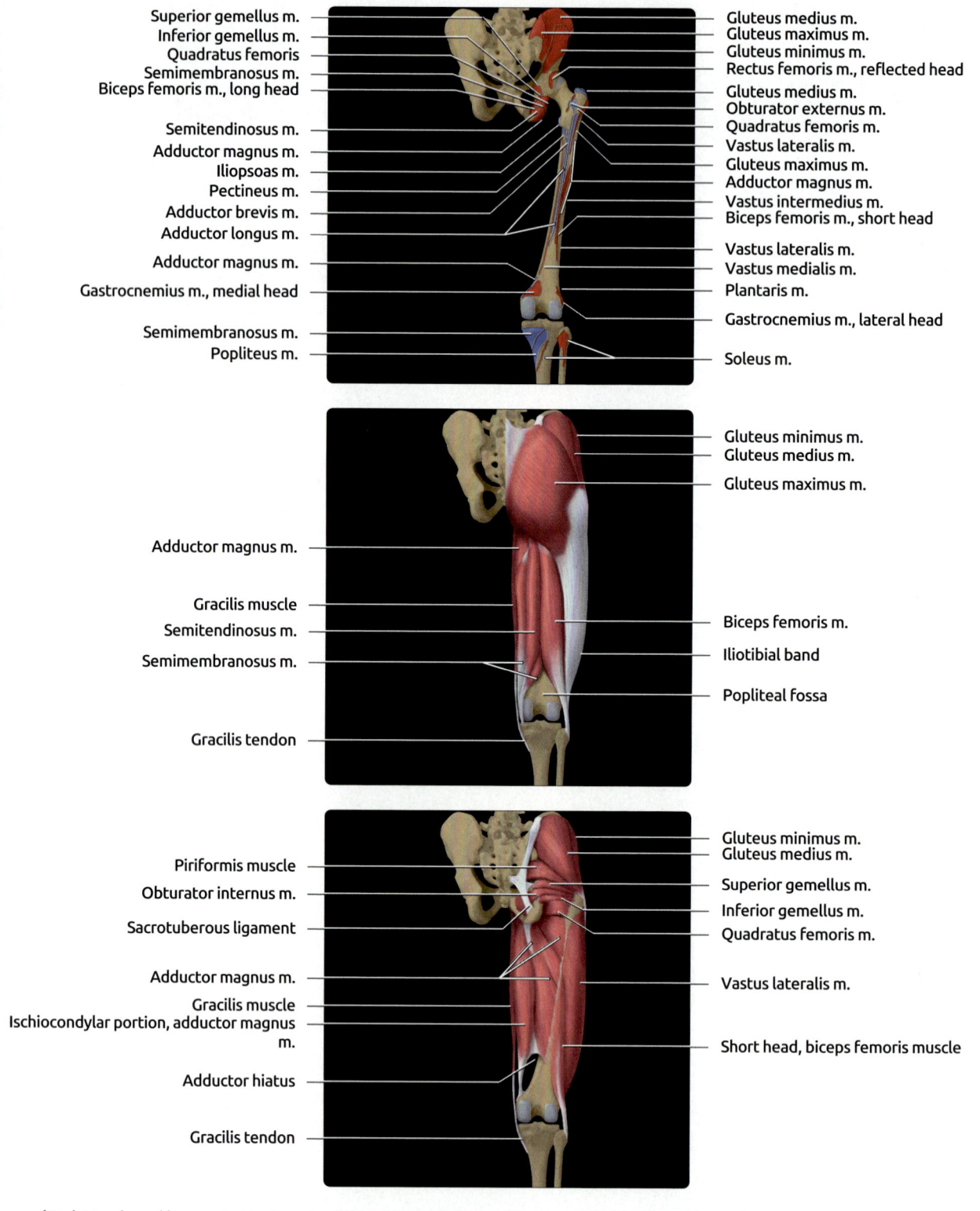

(Top) Muscle and ligament attachments of the posterior pelvis and femur are shown. The adductor brevis muscle insertion is superior to the adductor longus muscle. The transverse head of the adductor magnus (a.k.a. adductor minimus) inserts just medial to the gluteus maximus muscle. The ischiocondylar head has a long insertion on the posterior femur. (Middle) Superficial muscles of the posterior thigh are shown. The gluteus muscles from anterior to posterior and deep to superficial are gluteus minimus, medius, and maximus. The semitendinosus muscle is superficial to the semimembranosus muscle. The semimembranous muscle originates lateral to the conjoined origin of biceps and semitendinosus. (Bottom) Deep muscles of the posterior thigh are shown. With the removal of the hamstring muscles, the expansive adductor magnus muscle is visible. The separation of its 2 heads in the distal thigh forms the adductor hiatus. The femoral vessels pass through the hiatus into the popliteal fossa.

Thigh Radiographic Anatomy and MR Atlas

COMPARTMENTS OF THIGH

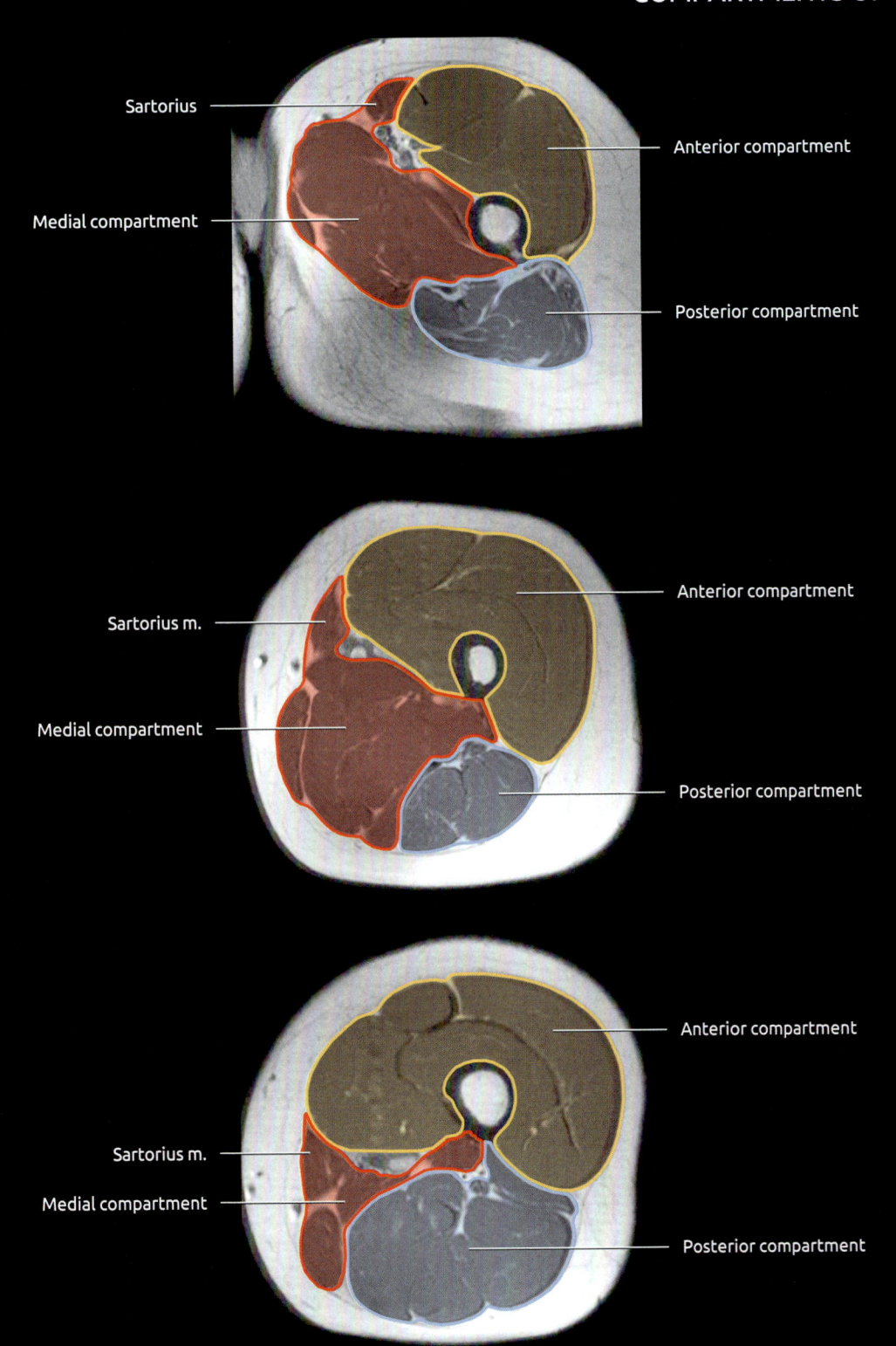

(Top) There are 3 soft tissue compartments of the thigh: Anterior, containing the quadriceps, medial, containing the adductors, and posterior, containing the hamstrings. The sartorius can be considered part of the anterior or medial compartments, but it has a separate fascial sheath and is often considered a separate compartment. (Middle) Fascial compartments at the level of the mid thigh are shown. The medial compartment has enlarged, whereas the posterior compartment has decreased in size. (Bottom) Compartments of the distal thigh are shown. Compartments of the thigh are an important anatomic consideration for tumor biopsy and resection, since care must be taken not to traverse more than 1 compartment to avoid wide contamination of the tumor.

Thigh Radiographic Anatomy and MR Atlas

ARTERIAL ANATOMY OF THIGH

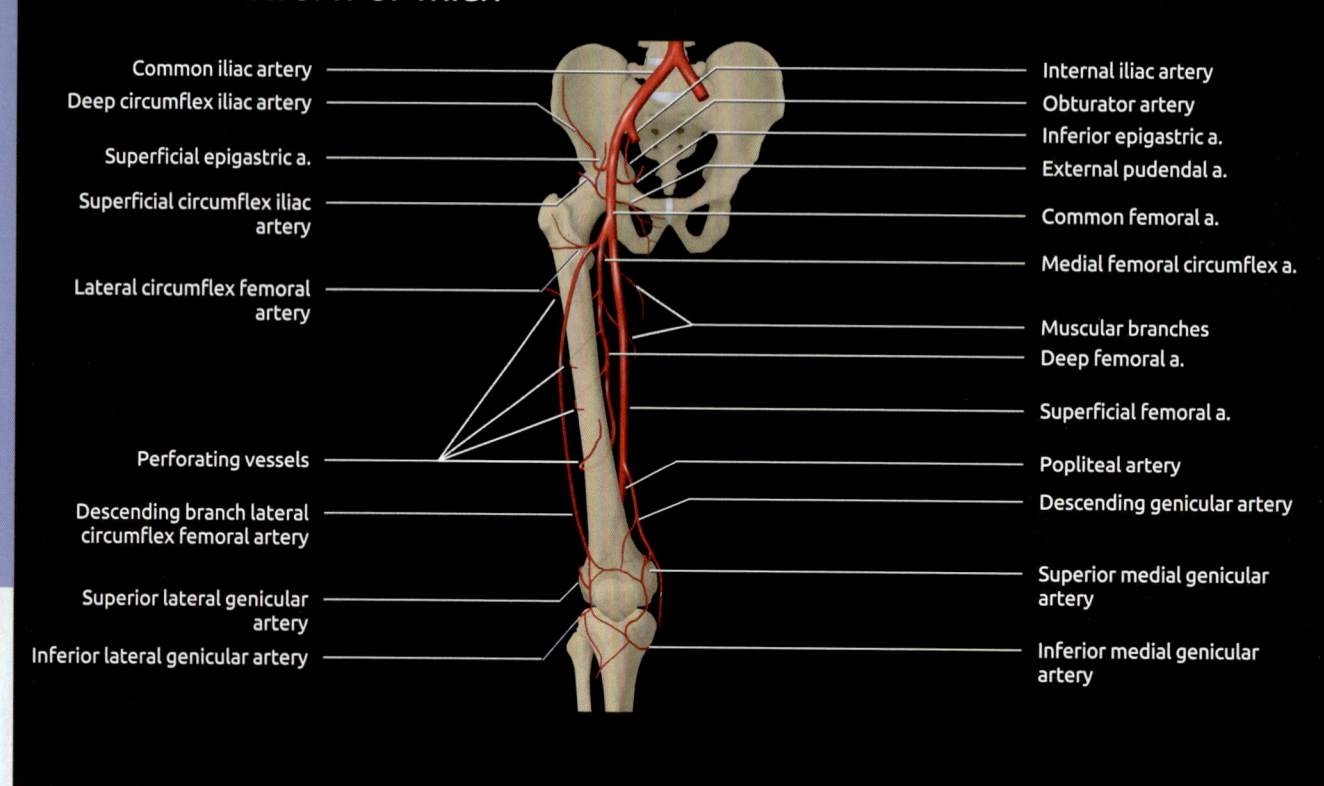

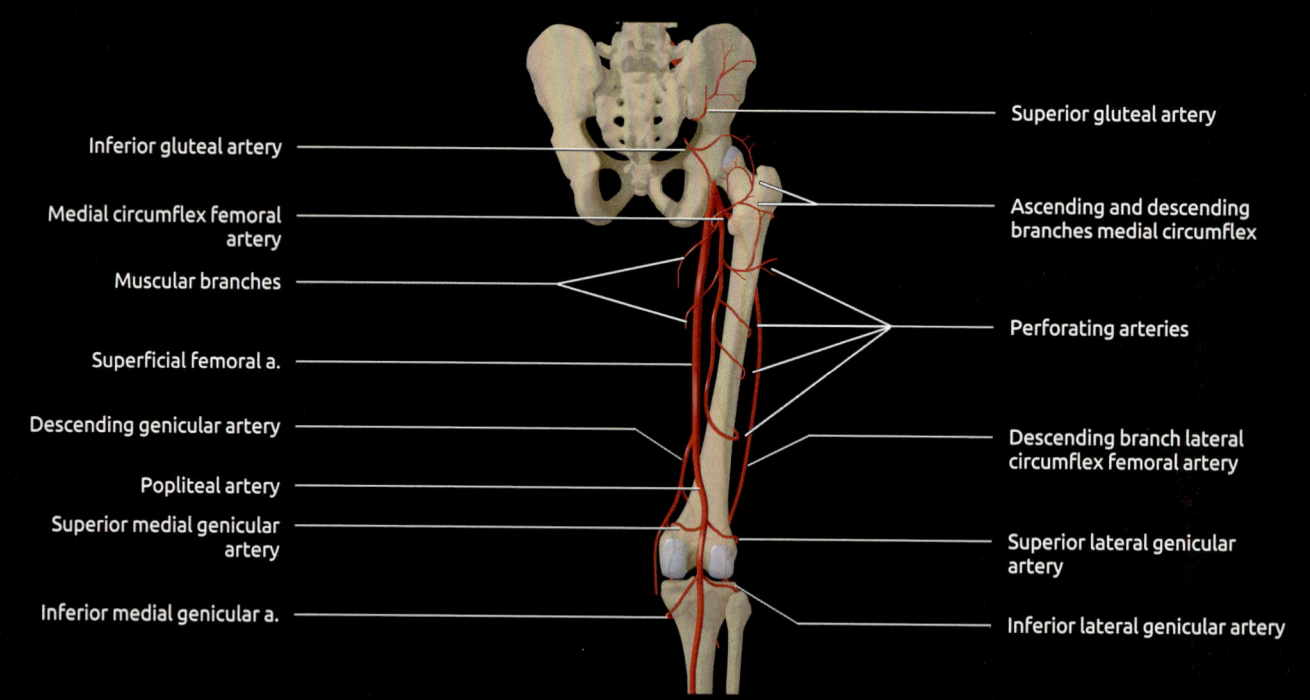

Labels (top, anterior view), left side: Common iliac artery; Deep circumflex iliac artery; Superficial epigastric a.; Superficial circumflex iliac artery; Lateral circumflex femoral artery; Perforating vessels; Descending branch lateral circumflex femoral artery; Superior lateral genicular artery; Inferior lateral genicular artery.

Labels (top, anterior view), right side: Internal iliac artery; Obturator artery; Inferior epigastric a.; External pudendal a.; Common femoral a.; Medial femoral circumflex a.; Muscular branches; Deep femoral a.; Superficial femoral a.; Popliteal artery; Descending genicular artery; Superior medial genicular artery; Inferior medial genicular artery.

Labels (bottom, posterior view), left side: Inferior gluteal artery; Medial circumflex femoral artery; Muscular branches; Superficial femoral a.; Descending genicular artery; Popliteal artery; Superior medial genicular artery; Inferior medial genicular a.

Labels (bottom, posterior view), right side: Superior gluteal artery; Ascending and descending branches medial circumflex; Perforating arteries; Descending branch lateral circumflex femoral artery; Superior lateral genicular artery; Inferior lateral genicular artery.

(Top) *Anterior view of the arteries of the thigh is shown. Deep femoral artery (a.k.a. profunda femoris artery) gives rise to the circumflex femoral arteries. It supplies the musculature of the thigh. Lateral femoral circumflex artery travels posterior to the rectus femoris muscle and wraps around the anterior portion of the femoral neck.* **(Bottom)** *Posterior view of the femoral and popliteal arteries and the superior and inferior gluteal arteries of the greater sciatic notch is shown. Medial circumflex femoral artery wraps around posterior femoral neck.*

Thigh Radiographic Anatomy and MR Atlas

VENOUS ANATOMY OF THIGH

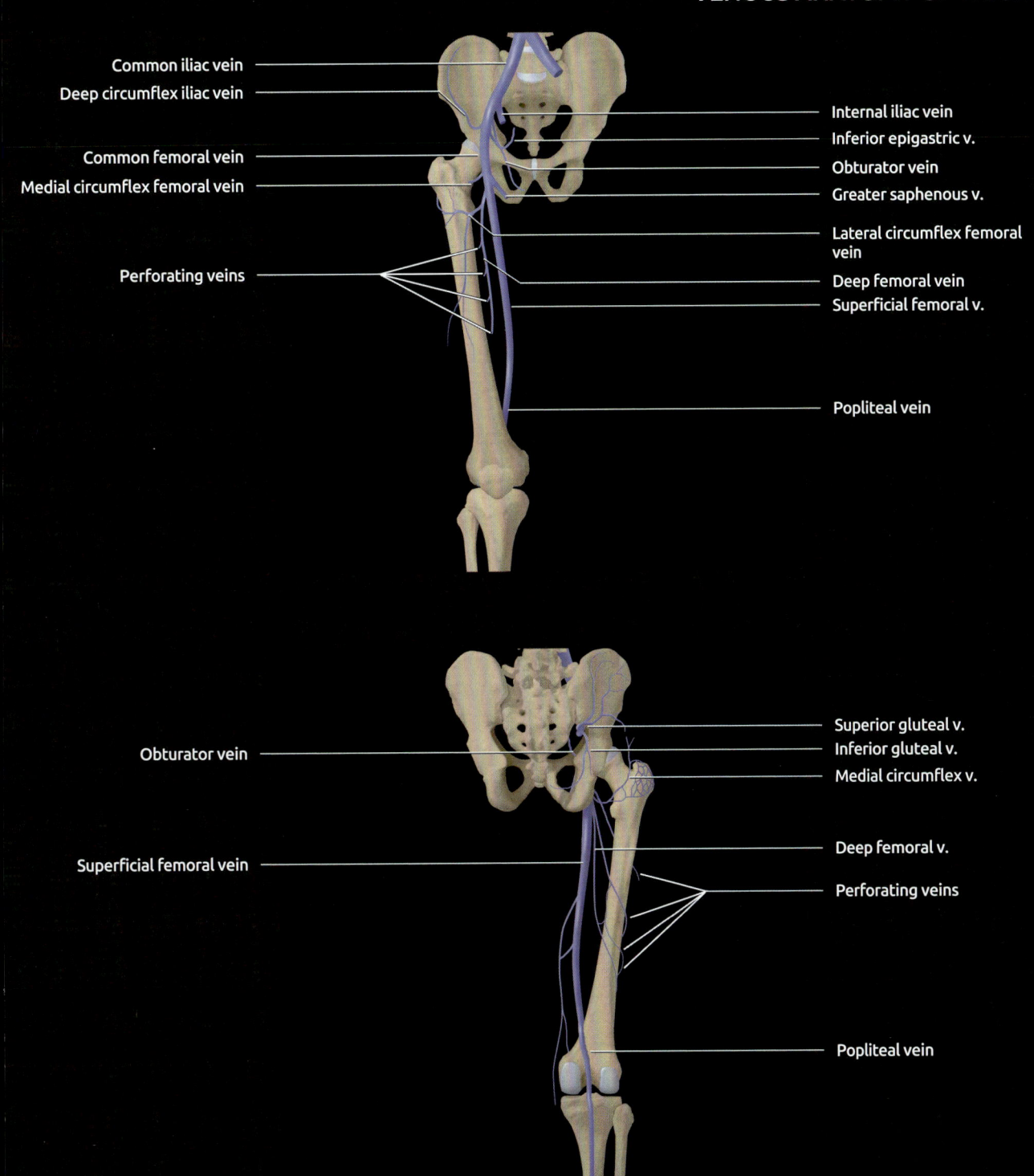

Common iliac vein
Deep circumflex iliac vein

Common femoral vein
Medial circumflex femoral vein

Perforating veins

Internal iliac vein
Inferior epigastric v.
Obturator vein
Greater saphenous v.
Lateral circumflex femoral vein
Deep femoral vein
Superficial femoral v.

Popliteal vein

Obturator vein

Superficial femoral vein

Superior gluteal v.
Inferior gluteal v.
Medial circumflex v.

Deep femoral v.
Perforating veins

Popliteal vein

(Top) *Anterior view of the deep veins of the thigh is shown. The deep veins typically follow the arterial tree. The main venous drainage is the superficial femoral vein, which is (confusingly) part of the deep venous system. Note the entrance of the greater saphenous vein into the femoral vein; it has no associated artery.* **(Bottom)** *Posterior view of the veins of the thigh and buttocks is shown. Superficial femoral vein becomes the popliteal vein in the popliteal fossa.*

Thigh Radiographic Anatomy and MR Atlas

SCIATIC NERVE AND DERMATOMES

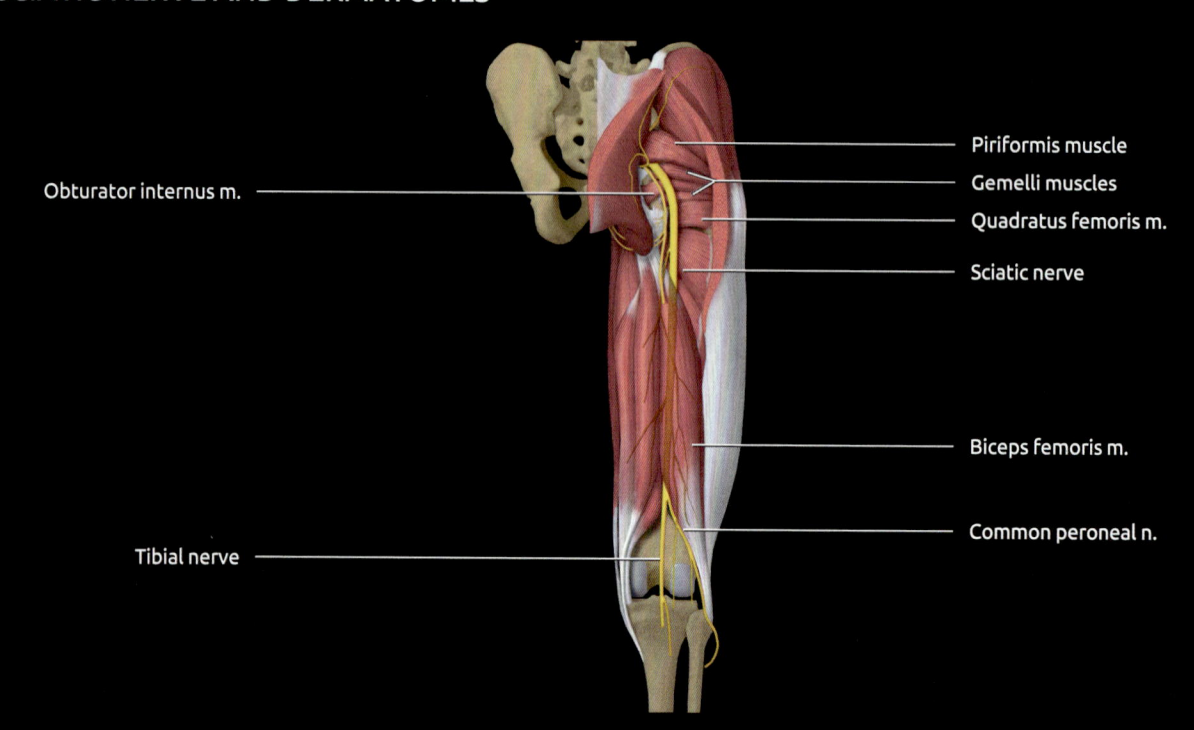

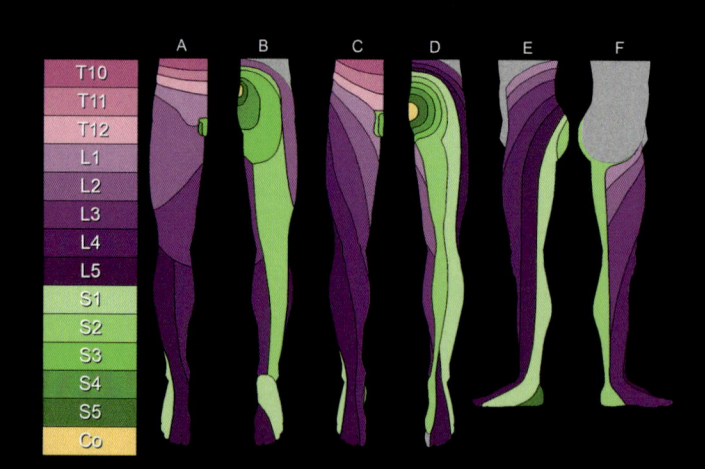

(Top) *The sciatic nerve enters the lower extremity by passing under the inferior border of the piriformis muscle. The sciatic nerve passes posterior to the external rotator tendons and then courses deep to the biceps femoris muscle. The tibial and peroneal divisions of the sciatic nerve are visible throughout its course. They diverge in the distal thigh. The tibial nerve bisects the popliteal fossa. The common peroneal nerve follows the biceps femoris muscle around the fibular head.* (Bottom) *Dermatomes of the anterior (A, C), posterior (B, D), lateral (E), and medial (F) thigh are shown. Two different patterns are recognized for the anterior and posterior thigh, as represented by the 2 diagrams.*

Thigh Radiographic Anatomy and MR Atlas

MEDIAL THIGH MUSCLES, FEMORAL TRIANGLE

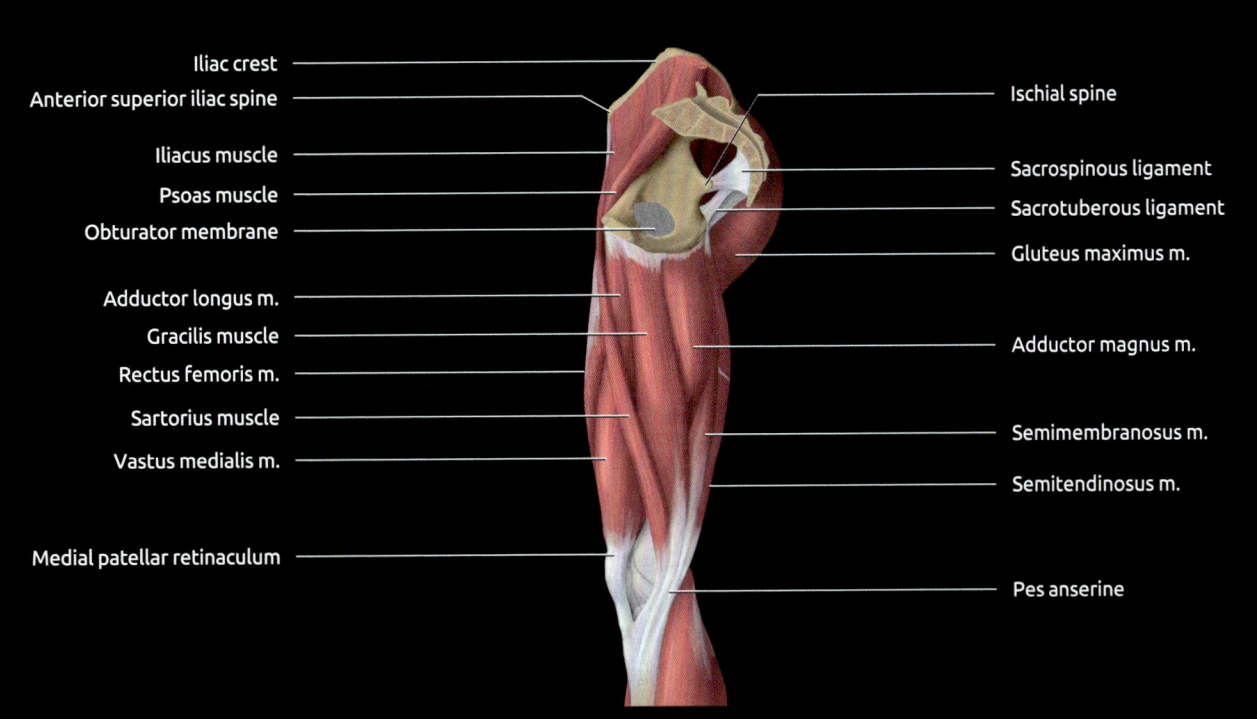

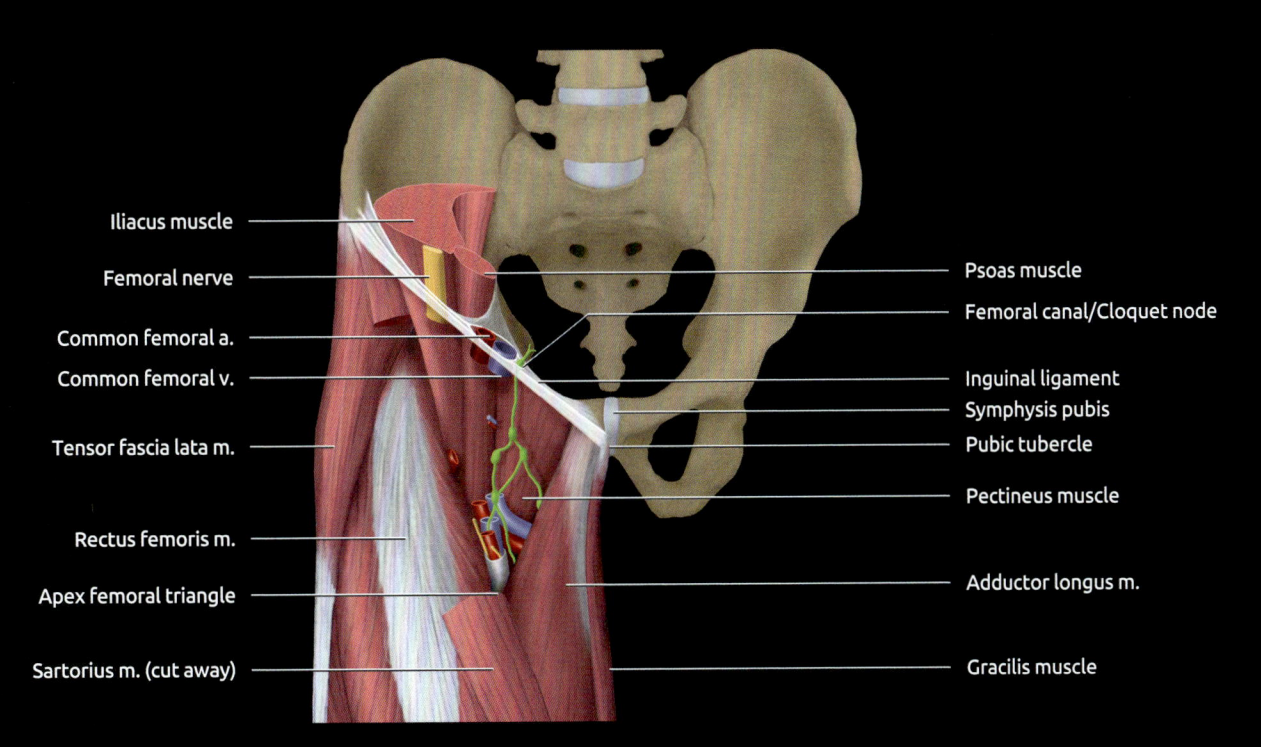

(Top) Medial muscles of the thigh are shown. The gracilis muscle has a thin profile when viewed from the front, however, when viewed from the side, it is quite broad. The semimembranosus muscle runs along the deep surface of the semitendinous muscle and inserts onto the tibia posterior to the pes anserine tendons. Its insertion is hidden on this image. The iliopsoas muscle courses over the pelvic brim on its course to the lesser trochanter. (Bottom) The contents of the femoral triangle from lateral to medial (NAVeL) are femoral nerve, femoral artery, femoral vein, and lymphatics. The nerve lies superficial to the iliopsoas muscle. The lateral border of the triangle is the sartorius muscle. The anterior wall is the inguinal ligament. The fascia lata encases the structures of the thigh. The femoral sheath is the fascial covering over the proximal vessels. At the cutaway proximal boundary, note the septa dividing the sheath into compartments. The femoral canal is the medial compartment.

Thigh Radiographic Anatomy and MR Atlas

PROXIMAL FEMUR RADIOGRAPHS

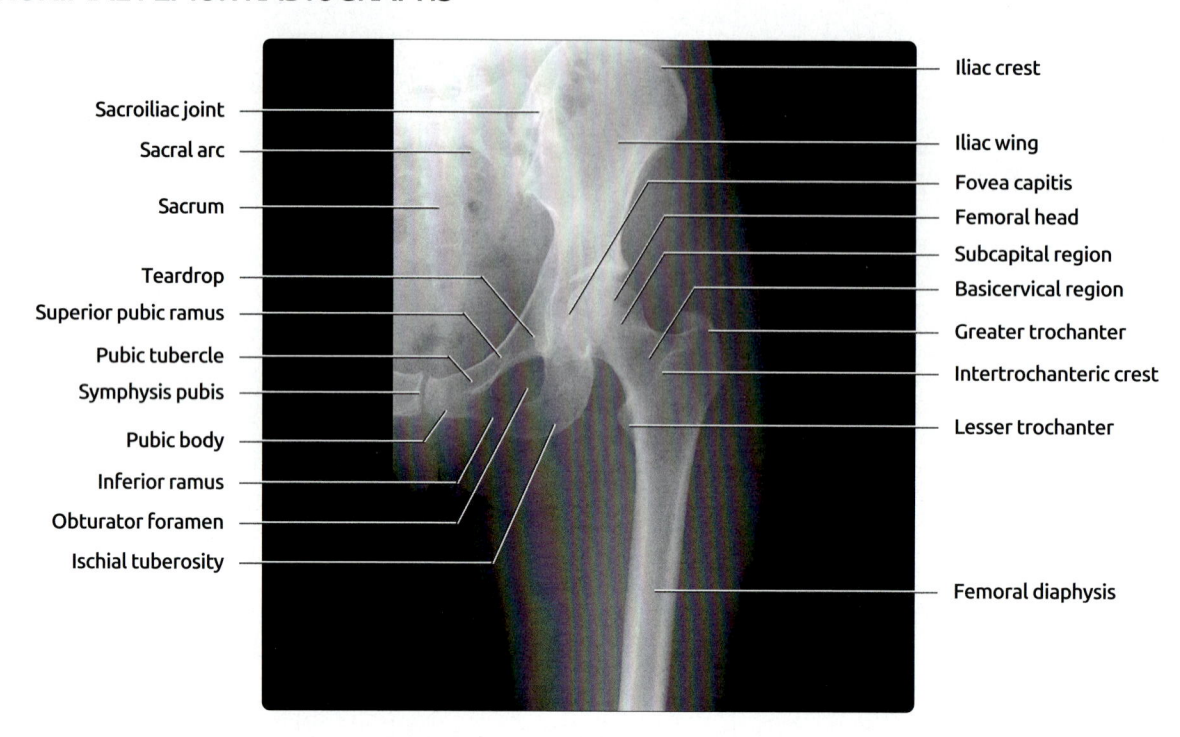

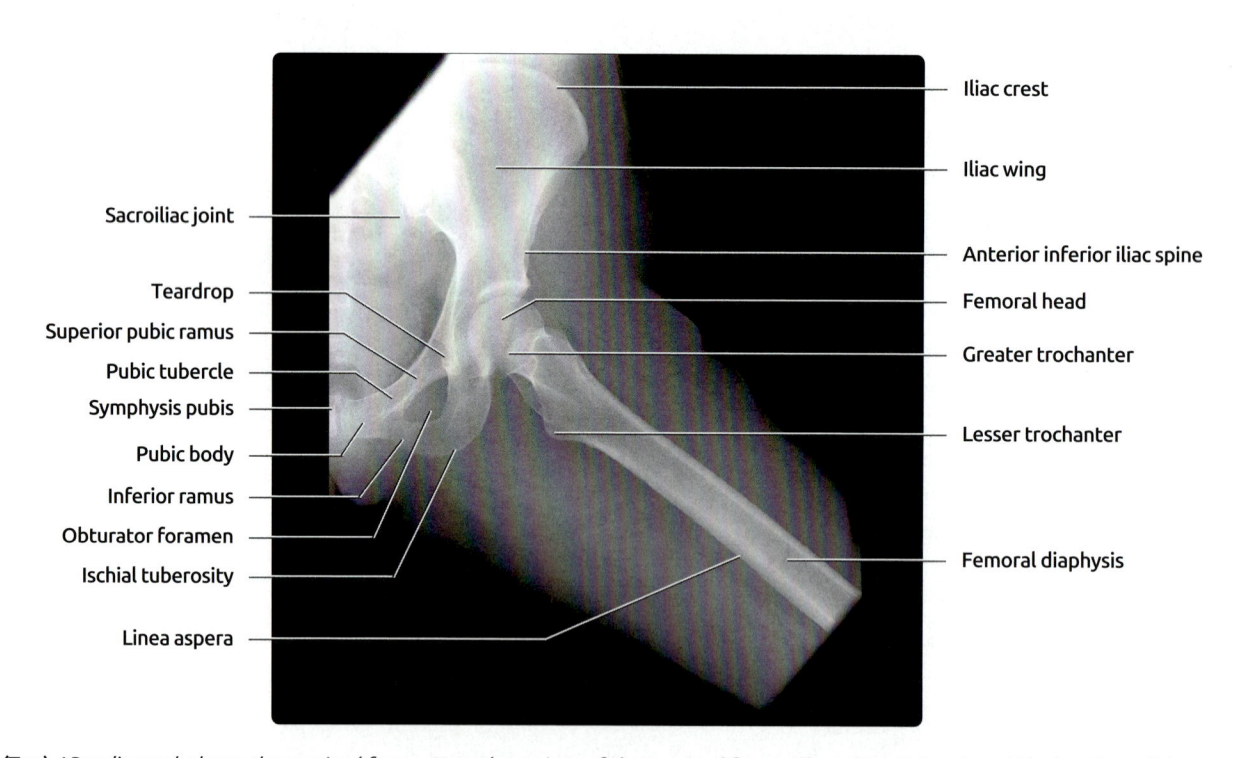

(Top) AP radiograph shows the proximal femur. Note the regions of the proximal femur: The subcapital region at the junction of the femoral head and neck, the basicervical region at the base of the femoral neck. For descriptive purposes, fractures between the basicervical and subcapital regions are referred to as transcervical (not labeled). In a well-positioned AP femur the lesser trochanter points medial and posterior. The intertrochanteric crest, a posterior prominence connecting the 2 trochanters, is visible. The fovea capitis appears as a central depression on the femoral head. (Bottom) Lateral view of the proximal femur is shown. With external rotation, the lesser trochanter is now seen in profile, its inferior cortex blending with the cortex of the adjacent femoral neck. The femoral head, neck, and greater trochanter are all overlapping.

Thigh Radiographic Anatomy and MR Atlas

DISTAL FEMUR RADIOGRAPHS

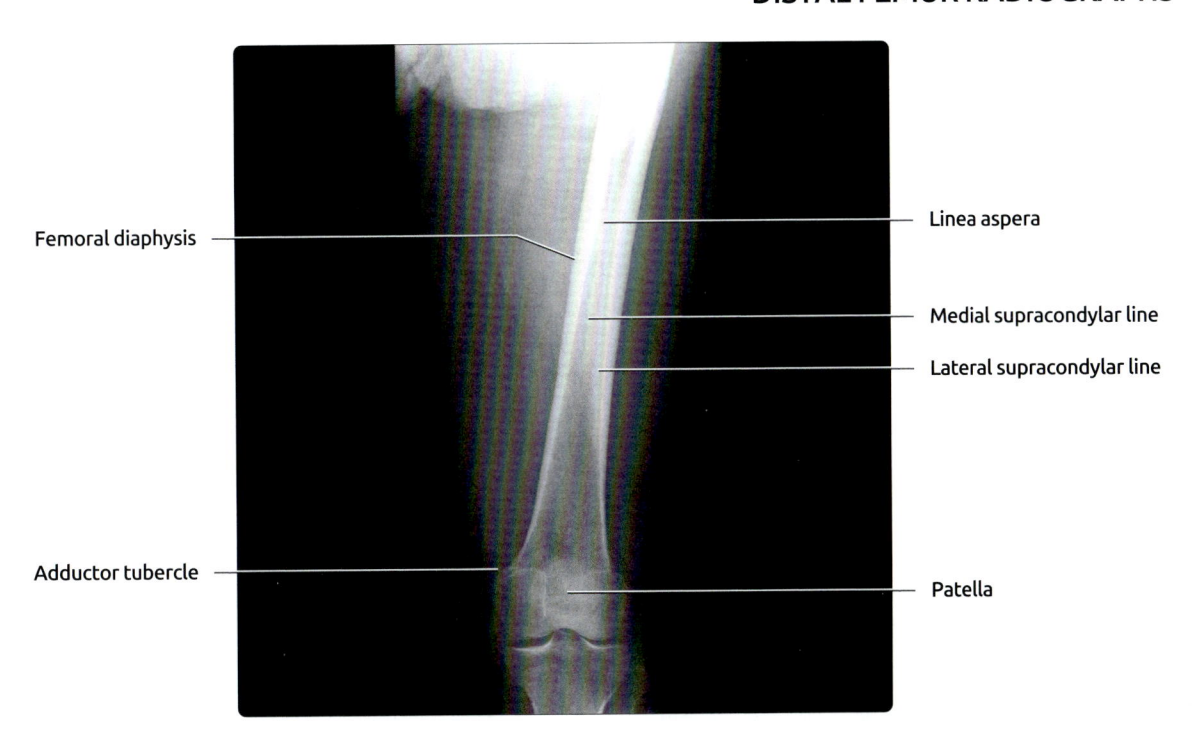

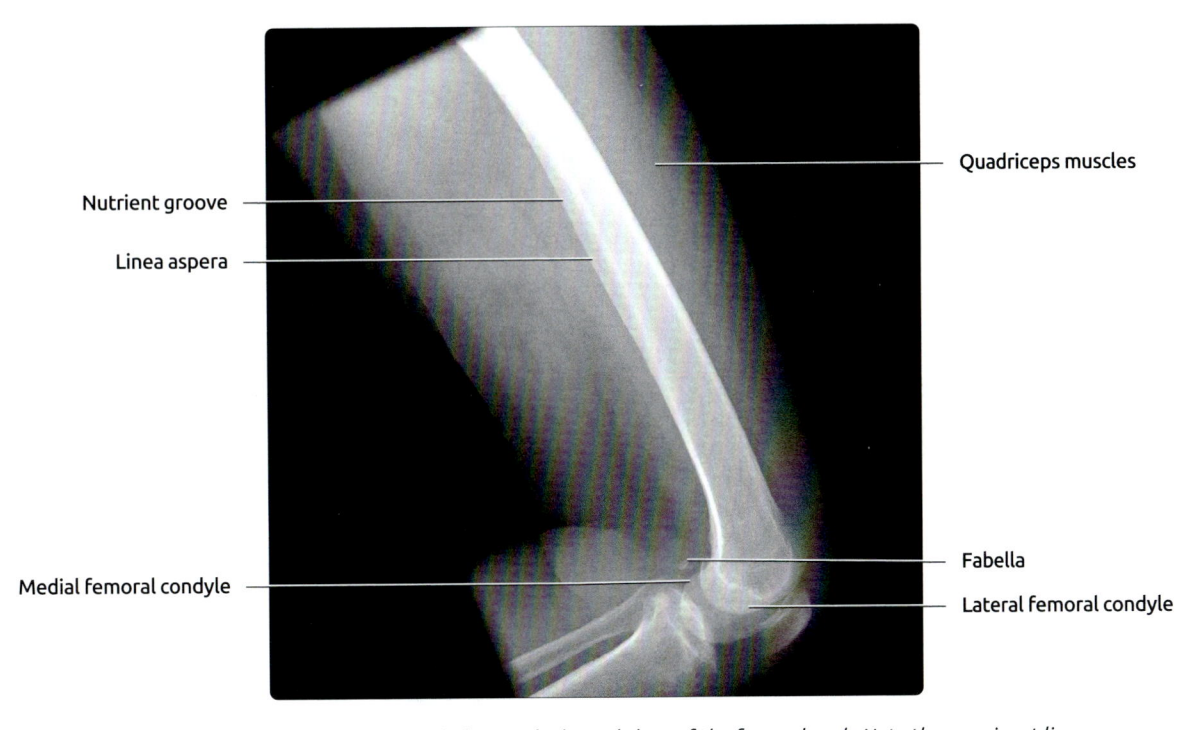

(Top) The femoral shaft has a slight medial slant that balances the lateral slant of the femoral neck. Note the prominent linea aspera, which divides inferiorly into medial and lateral supracondylar lines. Hyperostosis of the linea aspera is common in older patients. **(Bottom)** Lateral radiograph of the distal femur shows a posterior flange, known as the linea aspera. The linea aspera is a site of multiple muscle attachments. Nutrient groove enters the posterior femur at the midshaft and courses superiorly and anteriorly in the femoral shaft. Fabella is a variably present sesamoid in the lateral head of the gastrocnemius.

Thigh Radiographic Anatomy and MR Atlas

AXIAL T1 MR, UPPER RIGHT THIGH

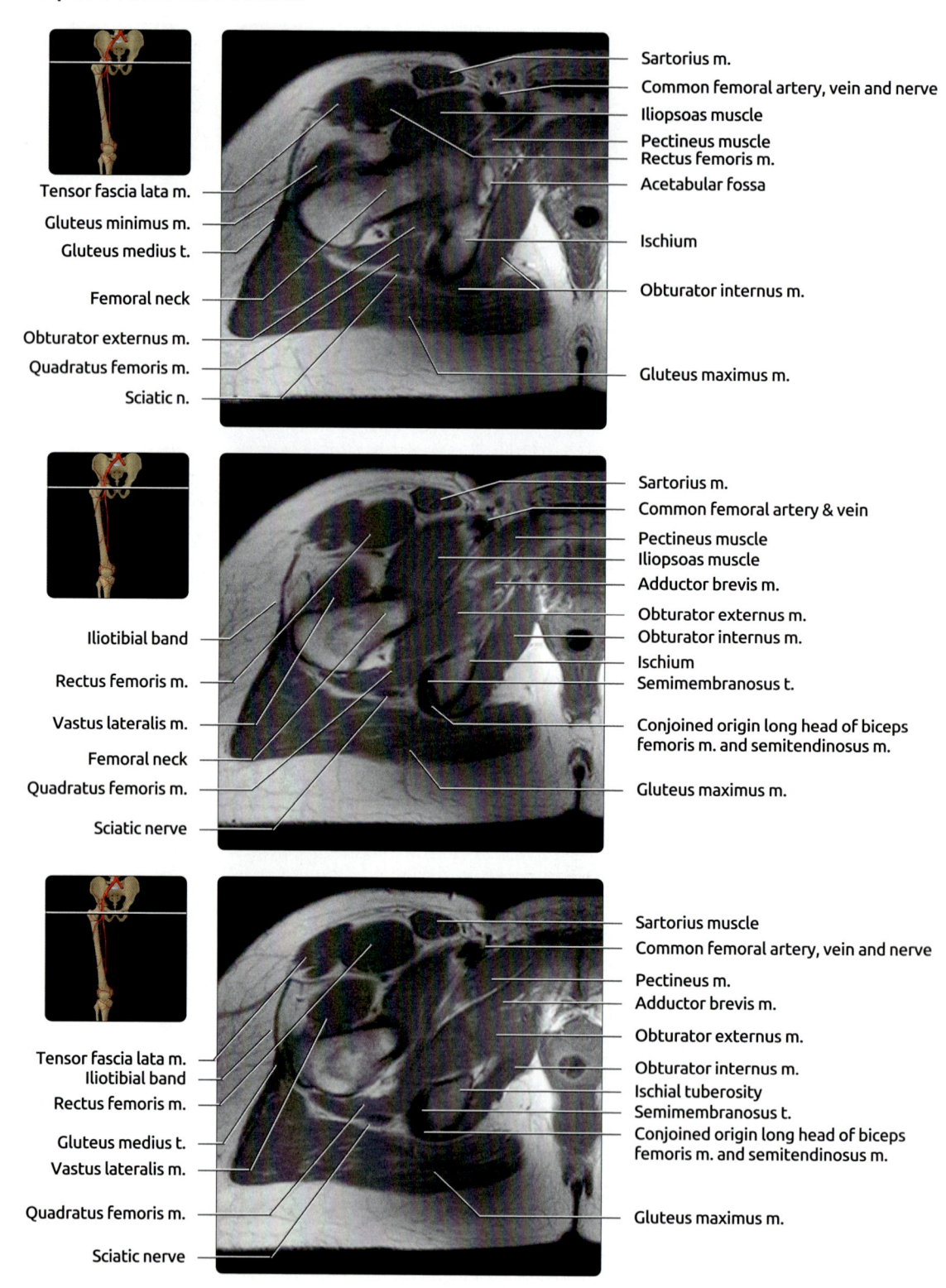

Labels (top image):
- Sartorius m.
- Common femoral artery, vein and nerve
- Iliopsoas muscle
- Pectineus muscle
- Rectus femoris m.
- Acetabular fossa
- Ischium
- Obturator internus m.
- Gluteus maximus m.
- Tensor fascia lata m.
- Gluteus minimus m.
- Gluteus medius t.
- Femoral neck
- Obturator externus m.
- Quadratus femoris m.
- Sciatic n.

Labels (middle image):
- Sartorius m.
- Common femoral artery & vein
- Pectineus muscle
- Iliopsoas muscle
- Adductor brevis m.
- Obturator externus m.
- Obturator internus m.
- Ischium
- Semimembranosus t.
- Conjoined origin long head of biceps femoris m. and semitendinosus m.
- Gluteus maximus m.
- Iliotibial band
- Rectus femoris m.
- Vastus lateralis m.
- Femoral neck
- Quadratus femoris m.
- Sciatic nerve

Labels (bottom image):
- Sartorius muscle
- Common femoral artery, vein and nerve
- Pectineus m.
- Adductor brevis m.
- Obturator externus m.
- Obturator internus m.
- Ischial tuberosity
- Semimembranosus t.
- Conjoined origin long head of biceps femoris m. and semitendinosus m.
- Gluteus maximus m.
- Tensor fascia lata m.
- Iliotibial band
- Rectus femoris m.
- Gluteus medius t.
- Vastus lateralis m.
- Quadratus femoris m.
- Sciatic nerve

(Top) Sciatic nerve lies between quadratus femoris muscle and gluteus maximus muscle. The tensor fascia lata and sartorius muscles are on a divergent course heading laterally and medially, respectively. **(Middle)** The obturator internus and externus muscles are seen on the inner and outer surfaces of the obturator foramen. The obturator membrane separates the muscles. The iliopsoas muscle is tapering toward its insertion onto the lesser trochanter. The gluteus maximus muscle continues its wide coverage of the inferior aspect of the buttocks. **(Bottom)** The semimembranosus muscle originates from the external surface of the ischial tuberosity, anterior to the conjoined origin of the semitendinous and long head of the biceps femoris muscles. The adductor brevis muscles lie deep to the pectineus muscle.

Thigh Radiographic Anatomy and MR Atlas

AXIAL T1 MR, UPPER LEFT THIGH

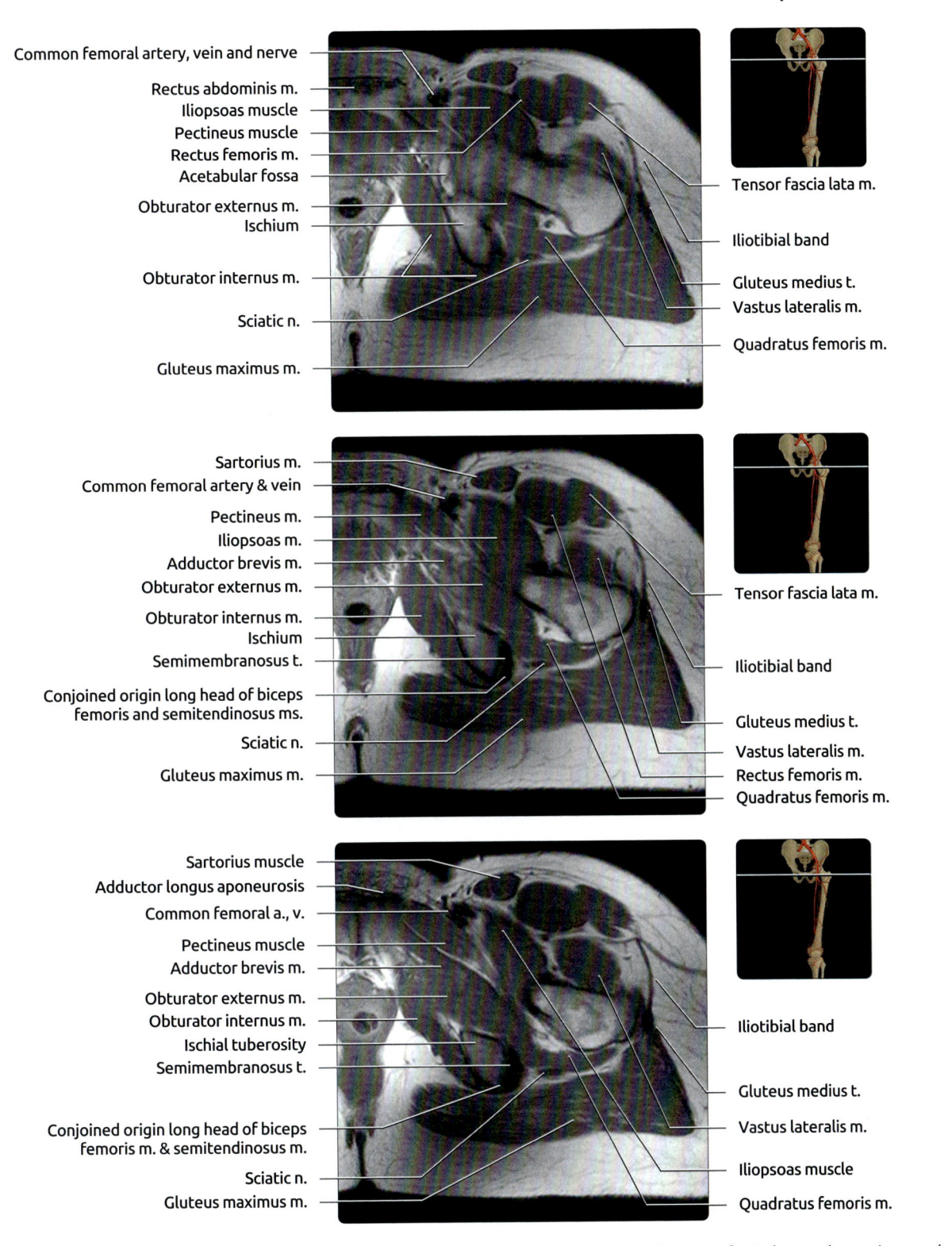

Top image labels (left): Common femoral artery, vein and nerve; Rectus abdominis m.; Iliopsoas muscle; Pectineus muscle; Rectus femoris m.; Acetabular fossa; Obturator externus m.; Ischium; Obturator internus m.; Sciatic n.; Gluteus maximus m.

Top image labels (right): Tensor fascia lata m.; Iliotibial band; Gluteus medius t.; Vastus lateralis m.; Quadratus femoris m.

Middle image labels (left): Sartorius m.; Common femoral artery & vein; Pectineus m.; Iliopsoas m.; Adductor brevis m.; Obturator externus m.; Obturator internus m.; Ischium; Semimembranosus t.; Conjoined origin long head of biceps femoris and semitendinosus ms.; Sciatic n.; Gluteus maximus m.

Middle image labels (right): Tensor fascia lata m.; Iliotibial band; Gluteus medius t.; Vastus lateralis m.; Rectus femoris m.; Quadratus femoris m.

Bottom image labels (left): Sartorius muscle; Adductor longus aponeurosis; Common femoral a., v.; Pectineus muscle; Adductor brevis m.; Obturator externus m.; Obturator internus m.; Ischial tuberosity; Semimembranosus t.; Conjoined origin long head of biceps femoris m. & semitendinosus m.; Sciatic n.; Gluteus maximus m.

Bottom image labels (right): Iliotibial band; Gluteus medius t.; Vastus lateralis m.; Iliopsoas muscle; Quadratus femoris m.

(**Top**) *Sciatic nerve lies between quadratus femoris muscle and gluteus maximus muscle. The tensor fascia lata and sartorius muscles are on a divergent course heading laterally and medially, respectively.* (**Middle**) *The obturator internus and externus muscles are seen on the inner and outer surfaces of the obturator foramen. The obturator membrane separates the muscles. The iliopsoas muscle tapers toward its insertion onto the lesser trochanter. The gluteus maximus muscle continues its wide coverage of the inferior aspect of the buttocks.* (**Bottom**) *The semimembranosus muscle originates from the external surface of the ischial tuberosity, anterior to the conjoined origin of the semitendinous and long head of the biceps femoris muscles. The adductor brevis muscles lies deep to the pectineus muscle.*

Thigh Radiographic Anatomy and MR Atlas

AXIAL T1 MR, UPPER RIGHT THIGH

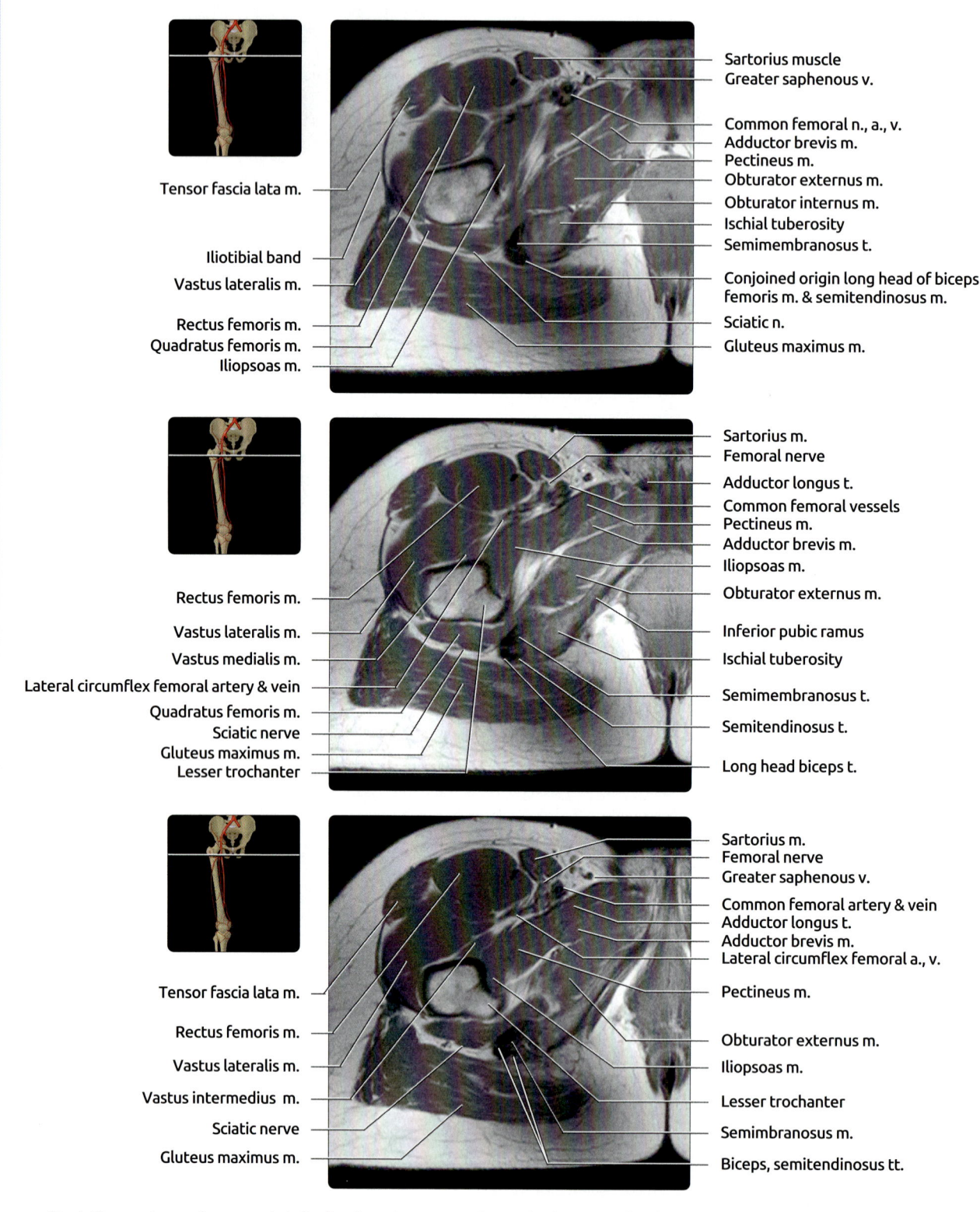

Labels (top image):
- Tensor fascia lata m.
- Iliotibial band
- Vastus lateralis m.
- Rectus femoris m.
- Quadratus femoris m.
- Iliopsoas m.
- Sartorius muscle
- Greater saphenous v.
- Common femoral n., a., v.
- Adductor brevis m.
- Pectineus m.
- Obturator externus m.
- Obturator internus m.
- Ischial tuberosity
- Semimembranosus t.
- Conjoined origin long head of biceps femoris m. & semitendinosus m.
- Sciatic n.
- Gluteus maximus m.

Labels (middle image):
- Rectus femoris m.
- Vastus lateralis m.
- Vastus medialis m.
- Lateral circumflex femoral artery & vein
- Quadratus femoris m.
- Sciatic nerve
- Gluteus maximus m.
- Lesser trochanter
- Sartorius m.
- Femoral nerve
- Adductor longus t.
- Common femoral vessels
- Pectineus m.
- Adductor brevis m.
- Iliopsoas m.
- Obturator externus m.
- Inferior pubic ramus
- Ischial tuberosity
- Semimembranosus t.
- Semitendinosus t.
- Long head biceps t.

Labels (bottom image):
- Tensor fascia lata m.
- Rectus femoris m.
- Vastus lateralis m.
- Vastus intermedius m.
- Sciatic nerve
- Gluteus maximus m.
- Sartorius m.
- Femoral nerve
- Greater saphenous v.
- Common femoral artery & vein
- Adductor longus t.
- Adductor brevis m.
- Lateral circumflex femoral a., v.
- Pectineus m.
- Obturator externus m.
- Iliopsoas m.
- Lesser trochanter
- Semimbranosus m.
- Biceps, semitendinosus tt.

(Top) The greater saphenous vein is feeding into the common femoral vein. Except for the gluteus maximus muscle, the quadratus femoris muscle is the most inferior of the external rotators of the hip. **(Middle)** Pectineus muscle is medial to iliopsoas muscle and will insert inferior to it on the proximal femoral shaft. Semitendinosis tendon and long head of biceps tendon are starting to diverge at this point. **(Bottom)** The vastus lateralis has the most proximal origin of the vasti muscles. The vastus intermedius muscle is now coming into view. The lateral circumflex femoral artery courses deep to the sartorius and rectus femoris muscles.

Thigh Radiographic Anatomy and MR Atlas

AXIAL T1 MR, UPPER LEFT THIGH

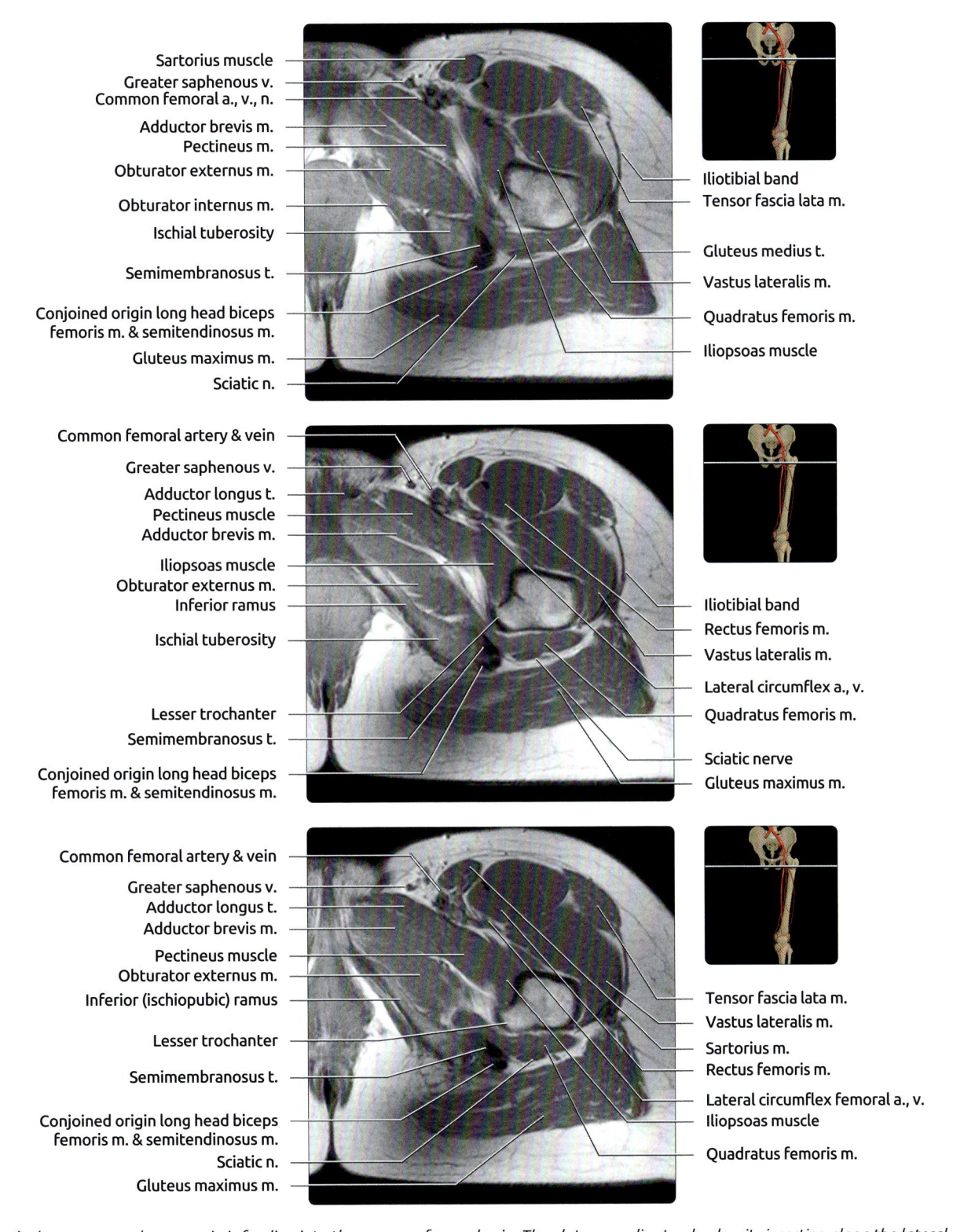

Top image labels (left): Sartorius muscle; Greater saphenous v.; Common femoral a., v., n.; Adductor brevis m.; Pectineus m.; Obturator externus m.; Obturator internus m.; Ischial tuberosity; Semimembranosus t.; Conjoined origin long head biceps femoris m. & semitendinosus m.; Gluteus maximus m.; Sciatic n.

Top image labels (right): Iliotibial band; Tensor fascia lata m.; Gluteus medius t.; Vastus lateralis m.; Quadratus femoris m.; Iliopsoas muscle

Middle image labels (left): Common femoral artery & vein; Greater saphenous v.; Adductor longus t.; Pectineus muscle; Adductor brevis m.; Iliopsoas muscle; Obturator externus m.; Inferior ramus; Ischial tuberosity; Lesser trochanter; Semimembranosus t.; Conjoined origin long head biceps femoris m. & semitendinosus m.

Middle image labels (right): Iliotibial band; Rectus femoris m.; Vastus lateralis m.; Lateral circumflex a., v.; Quadratus femoris m.; Sciatic nerve; Gluteus maximus m.

Bottom image labels (left): Common femoral artery & vein; Greater saphenous v.; Adductor longus t.; Adductor brevis m.; Pectineus muscle; Obturator externus m.; Inferior (ischiopubic) ramus; Lesser trochanter; Semimembranosus t.; Conjoined origin long head biceps femoris m. & semitendinosus m.; Sciatic n.; Gluteus maximus m.

Bottom image labels (right): Tensor fascia lata m.; Vastus lateralis m.; Sartorius m.; Rectus femoris m.; Lateral circumflex femoral a., v.; Iliopsoas muscle; Quadratus femoris m.

(Top) The greater saphenous vein is feeding into the common femoral vein. The gluteus medius tendon has its insertion along the lateral facet of the greater trochanter. Except for the gluteus maximus muscle, the quadratus femoris muscle is the most inferior of the external rotators of the hip and is recognized by its horizontal orientation deep to the gluteus maximus muscle. **(Middle)** Pectineus muscle is medial to the iliopsoas muscle and will insert inferior to it on the proximal femoral shaft. Semitendinosus tendon and long head biceps tendon are starting to diverge at this point. **(Bottom)** The vastus lateralis has the most proximal origin of the vasti muscles. The vastus intermedius muscle is now coming into view. The lateral circumflex femoral artery courses deep to the sartorius and rectus femoris muscles.

Thigh Radiographic Anatomy and MR Atlas

AXIAL T1 MR, UPPER RIGHT THIGH

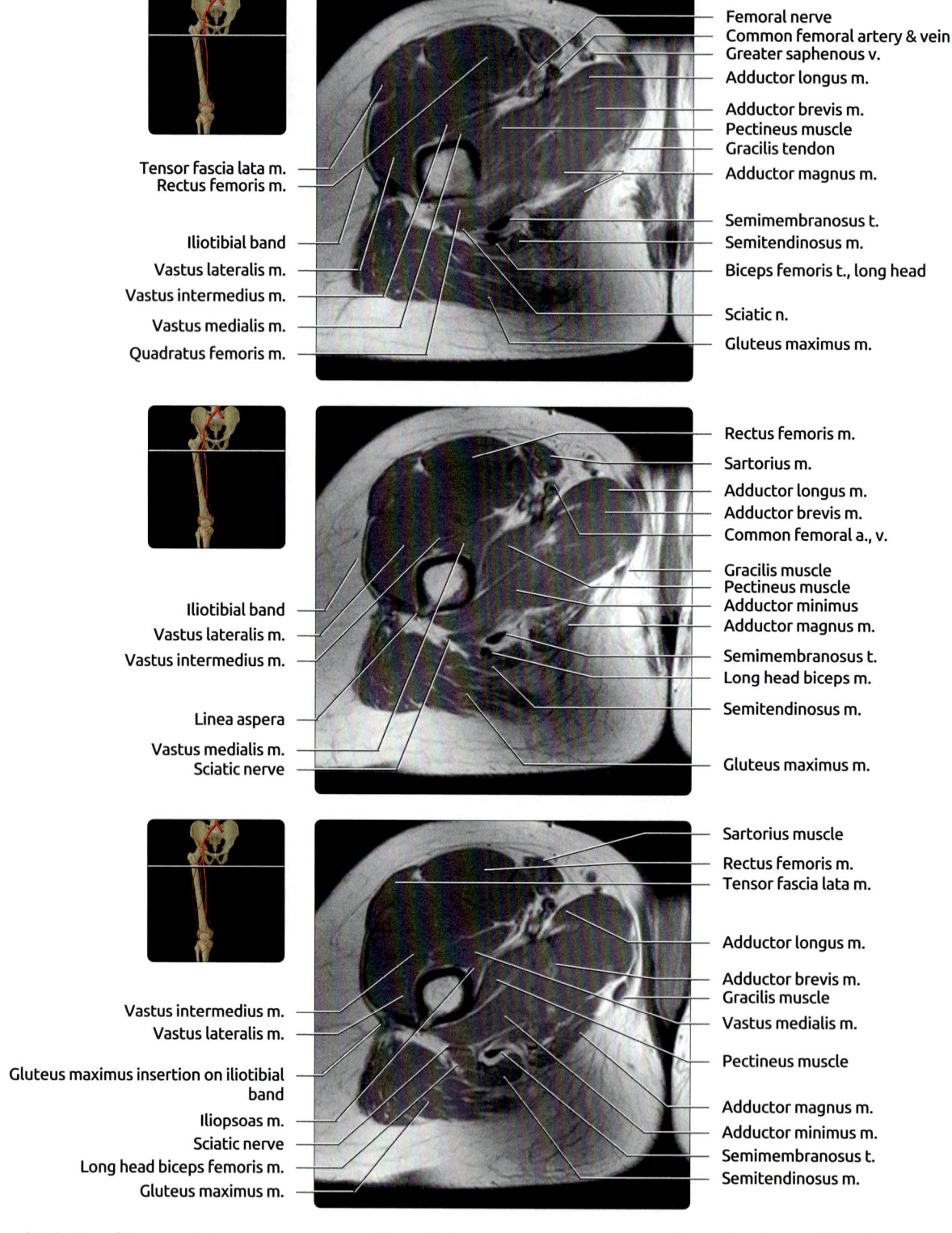

(Top) All 4 of the quadriceps muscles are now visible, with the vastus intermedius and medialis still quite small. This is the most inferior image on which the femoral nerve can be identified. It branches entirely within the femoral triangle. The 2 origins of the adductor magnus muscle are visible. The more anterior adductor portion (a.k.a. adductor minimus) originates from the inferior pubic ramus, and the more posterior portion of the muscle originates from the ischial tuberosity. (Middle) The changing orientation between the semimembranosus and the other hamstring tendons continues. The semimembranosus tendon is now more medially positioned. These are the first images on which the thin gracilis tendon is distinctly visible. It is visually merged with other structures above this level. (Bottom) The gluteus maximus inserts on the iliotibial band and on the gluteal ridge of the femur, the superolateral portion of the linea aspera. The adductor minimus is the most superior portion of the adductor magnus. It inserts adjacent to the gluteus maximus.

Thigh Radiographic Anatomy and MR Atlas

AXIAL T1 MR, UPPER LEFT THIGH

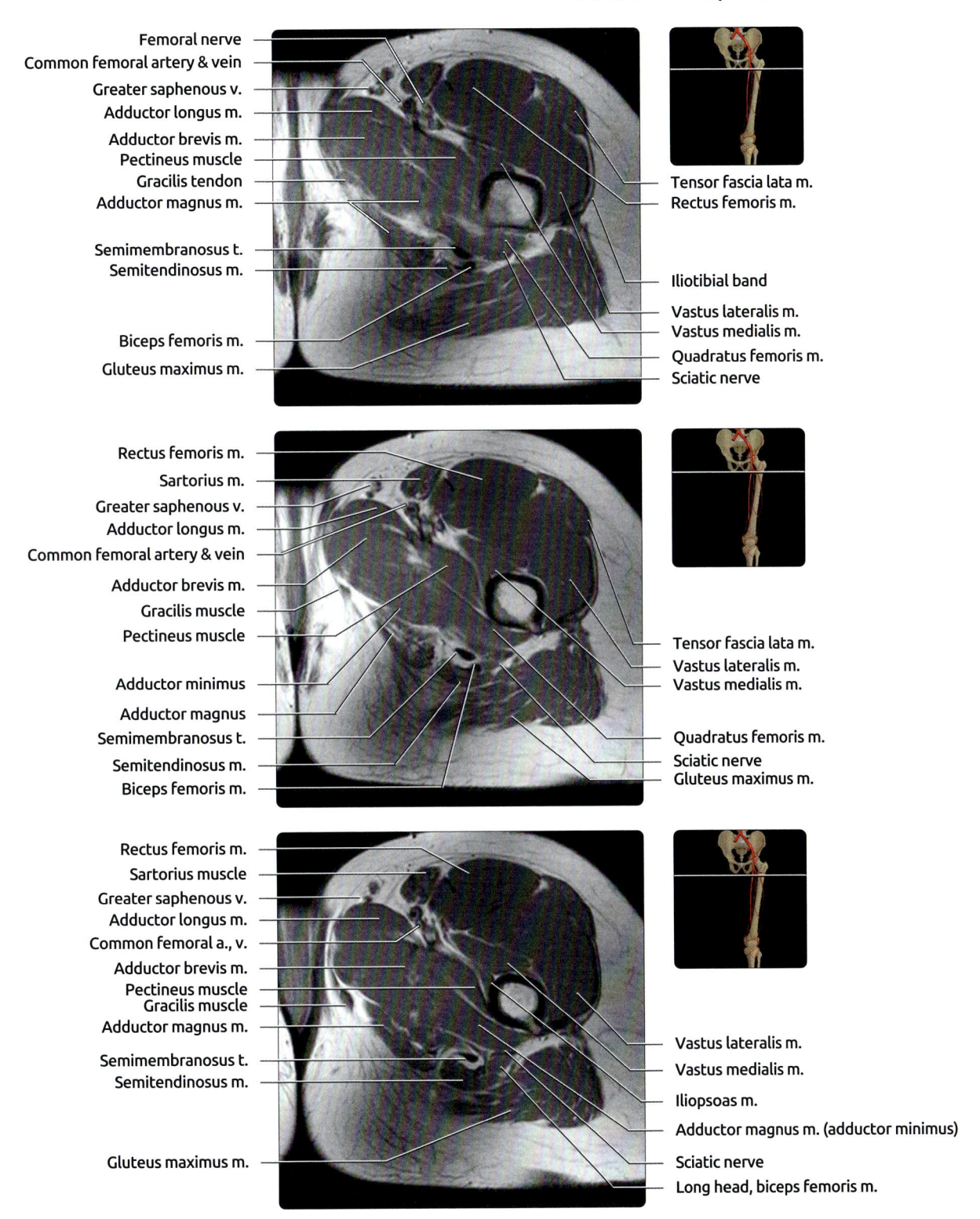

Image 1 labels:
- Femoral nerve
- Common femoral artery & vein
- Greater saphenous v.
- Adductor longus m.
- Adductor brevis m.
- Pectineus muscle
- Gracilis tendon
- Adductor magnus m.
- Semimembranosus t.
- Semitendinosus m.
- Biceps femoris m.
- Gluteus maximus m.
- Tensor fascia lata m.
- Rectus femoris m.
- Iliotibial band
- Vastus lateralis m.
- Vastus medialis m.
- Quadratus femoris m.
- Sciatic nerve

Image 2 labels:
- Rectus femoris m.
- Sartorius m.
- Greater saphenous v.
- Adductor longus m.
- Common femoral artery & vein
- Adductor brevis m.
- Gracilis muscle
- Pectineus muscle
- Adductor minimus
- Adductor magnus
- Semimembranosus t.
- Semitendinosus m.
- Biceps femoris m.
- Tensor fascia lata m.
- Vastus lateralis m.
- Vastus medialis m.
- Quadratus femoris m.
- Sciatic nerve
- Gluteus maximus m.

Image 3 labels:
- Rectus femoris m.
- Sartorius muscle
- Greater saphenous v.
- Adductor longus m.
- Common femoral a., v.
- Adductor brevis m.
- Pectineus muscle
- Gracilis muscle
- Adductor magnus m.
- Semimembranosus t.
- Semitendinosus m.
- Gluteus maximus m.
- Vastus lateralis m.
- Vastus medialis m.
- Iliopsoas m.
- Adductor magnus m. (adductor minimus)
- Sciatic nerve
- Long head, biceps femoris m.

(Top) *All 4 of the quadriceps muscles are now visible, with the vastus intermedius and medialis still quite small. This is the most inferior image on which the femoral nerve can be identified. It branches entirely within the femoral triangle. The 2 origins of the adductor magnus muscle are visible. The more anterior adductor portion (a.k.a. adductor minimus) originates from the inferior pubic ramus, the more posterior portion of the muscle originates from the ischial tuberosity.* **(Middle)** *The changing orientation between the semimembranosus and the other hamstring tendons continues. The semimembranosus tendon is now more medially positioned. These are the first images on which the thin gracilis tendon is distinctly visible. It is visually merged with other structures above this level.* **(Bottom)** *The gluteus maximus inserts on the iliotibial band and on the gluteal ridge of the femur, the superolateral portion of the linea aspera. The adductor minimus is the most superior portion of the adductor magnus. It inserts adjacent to the gluteus maximus.*

Thigh Radiographic Anatomy and MR Atlas

AXIAL T1 MR, UPPER RIGHT THIGH

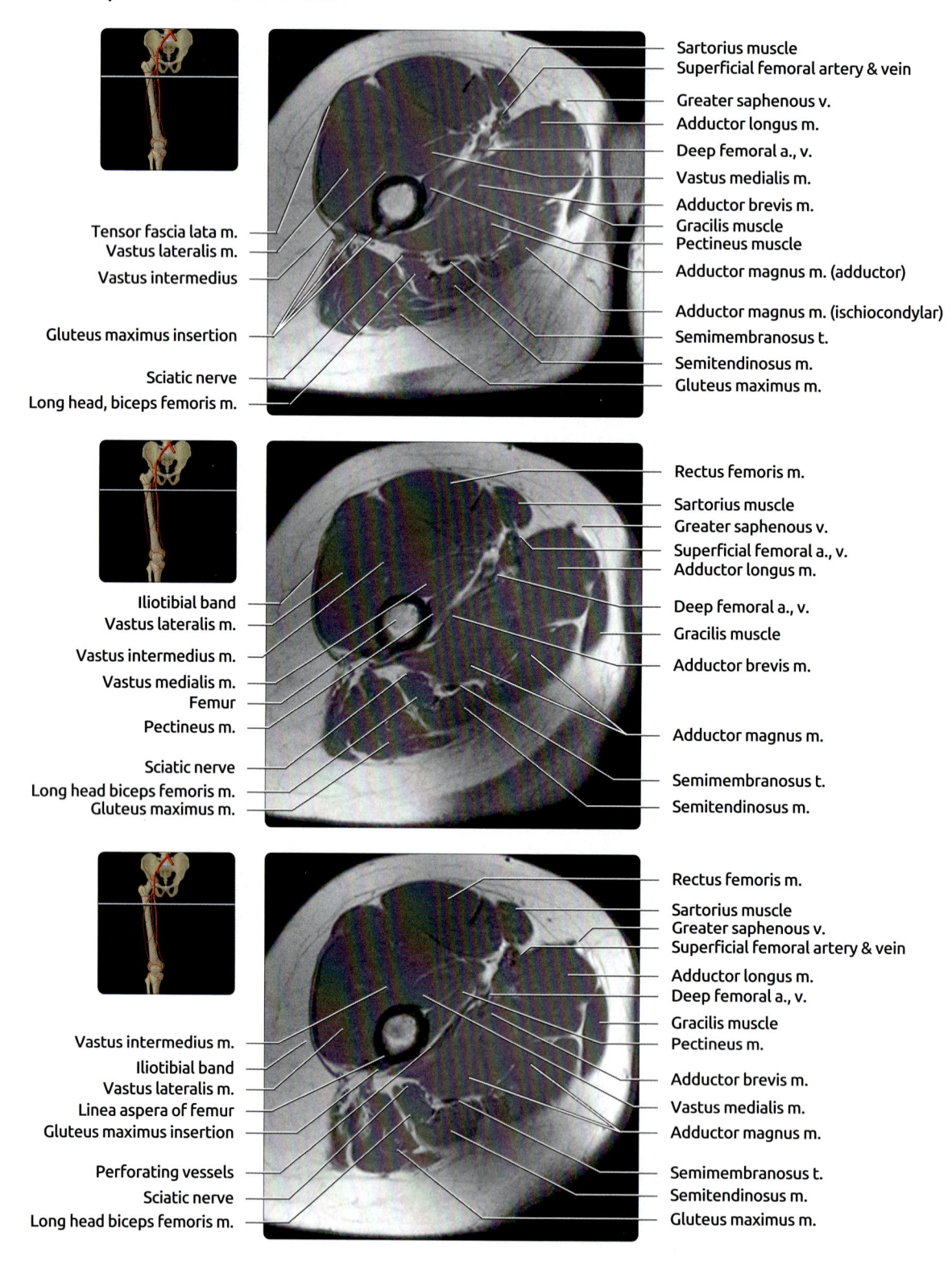

(Top) Labels: Sartorius muscle; Superficial femoral artery & vein; Greater saphenous v.; Adductor longus m.; Deep femoral a., v.; Vastus medialis m.; Adductor brevis m.; Gracilis muscle; Pectineus muscle; Adductor magnus m. (adductor); Adductor magnus m. (ischiocondylar); Semimembranosus t.; Semitendinosus m.; Gluteus maximus m.; Tensor fascia lata m.; Vastus lateralis m.; Vastus intermedius; Gluteus maximus insertion; Sciatic nerve; Long head, biceps femoris m.

(Middle) Labels: Rectus femoris m.; Sartorius muscle; Greater saphenous v.; Superficial femoral a., v.; Adductor longus m.; Deep femoral a., v.; Gracilis muscle; Adductor brevis m.; Adductor magnus m.; Semimembranosus t.; Semitendinosus m.; Iliotibial band; Vastus lateralis m.; Vastus intermedius m.; Vastus medialis m.; Femur; Pectineus m.; Sciatic nerve; Long head biceps femoris m.; Gluteus maximus m.

(Bottom) Labels: Rectus femoris m.; Sartorius muscle; Greater saphenous v.; Superficial femoral artery & vein; Adductor longus m.; Deep femoral a., v.; Gracilis muscle; Pectineus m.; Adductor brevis m.; Vastus medialis m.; Adductor magnus m.; Semimembranosus t.; Semitendinosus m.; Gluteus maximus m.; Vastus intermedius m.; Iliotibial band; Vastus lateralis m.; Linea aspera of femur; Gluteus maximus insertion; Perforating vessels; Sciatic nerve; Long head biceps femoris m.

(Top) *The common femoral vessels have divided into superficial and deep femoral vessels. The gracilis muscle is now visible. The tensor fascia lata muscle has assumed a more flattened profile. The sciatic nerve lies deep to the biceps femoris muscle.* **(Middle)** *The adductor magnus is a large muscle with multiple components. The most medial portion is called the ischiocondylar portion and attaches to the adductor tubercle of the medial femoral epicondyle.* **(Bottom)** *A large perforating artery is visible. It is a branch of the deep femoral artery. The tensor fascia lata muscle has completely inserted onto the iliotibial band. Throughout the thigh, the sciatic nerve resides deep to the biceps femoris muscle.*

Thigh Radiographic Anatomy and MR Atlas

AXIAL T1 MR, UPPER LEFT THIGH

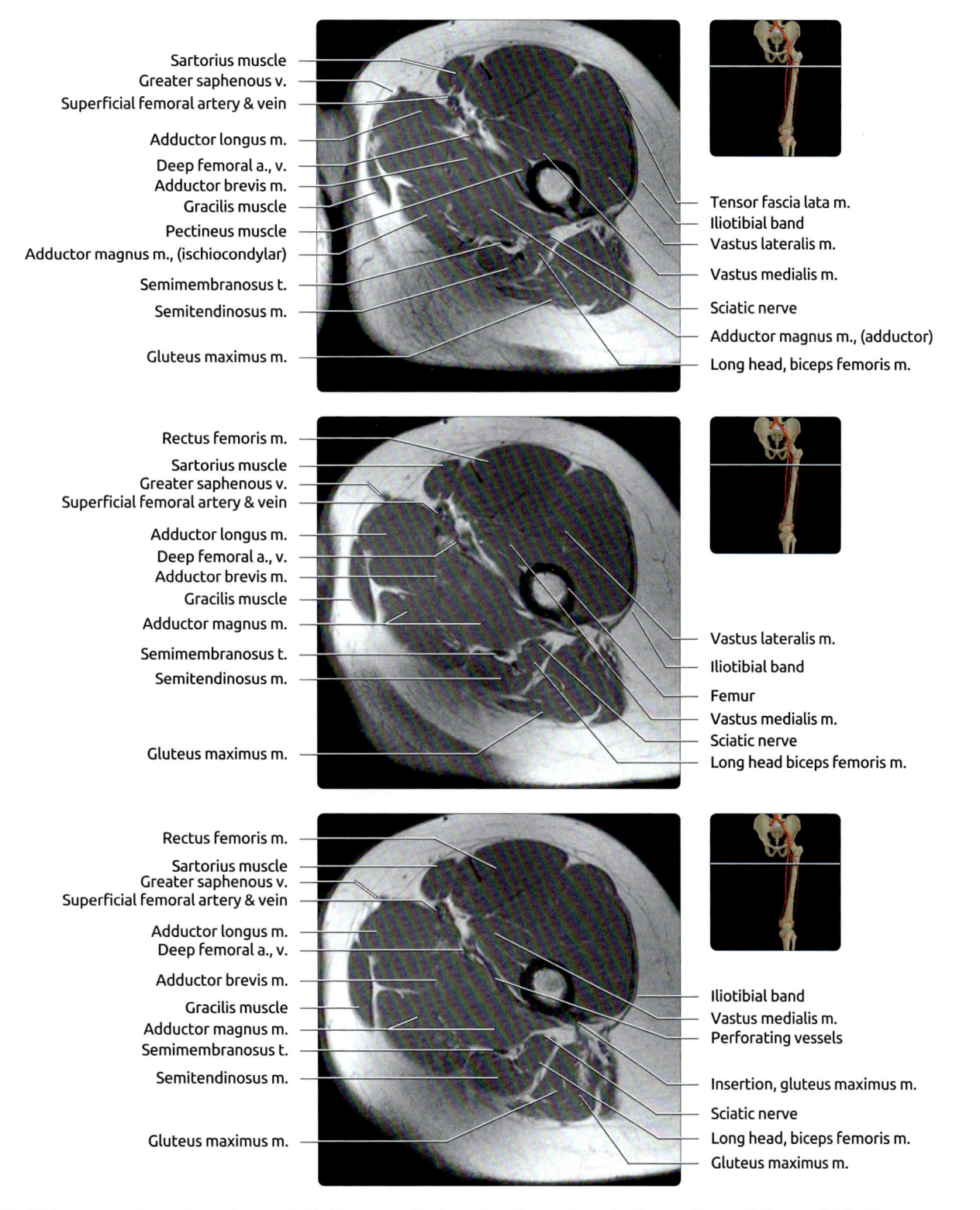

Top image labels (left): Sartorius muscle; Greater saphenous v.; Superficial femoral artery & vein; Adductor longus m.; Deep femoral a., v.; Adductor brevis m.; Gracilis muscle; Pectineus muscle; Adductor magnus m., (ischiocondylar); Semimembranosus t.; Semitendinosus m.; Gluteus maximus m.

Top image labels (right): Tensor fascia lata m.; Iliotibial band; Vastus lateralis m.; Vastus medialis m.; Sciatic nerve; Adductor magnus m., (adductor); Long head, biceps femoris m.

Middle image labels (left): Rectus femoris m.; Sartorius muscle; Greater saphenous v.; Superficial femoral artery & vein; Adductor longus m.; Deep femoral a., v.; Adductor brevis m.; Gracilis muscle; Adductor magnus m.; Semimembranosus t.; Semitendinosus m.; Gluteus maximus m.

Middle image labels (right): Vastus lateralis m.; Iliotibial band; Femur; Vastus medialis m.; Sciatic nerve; Long head biceps femoris m.

Bottom image labels (left): Rectus femoris m.; Sartorius muscle; Greater saphenous v.; Superficial femoral artery & vein; Adductor longus m.; Deep femoral a., v.; Adductor brevis m.; Gracilis muscle; Adductor magnus m.; Semimembranosus t.; Semitendinosus m.; Gluteus maximus m.

Bottom image labels (right): Iliotibial band; Vastus medialis m.; Perforating vessels; Insertion, gluteus maximus m.; Sciatic nerve; Long head, biceps femoris m.; Gluteus maximus m.

(**Top**) *The common femoral vessels have divided into superficial and deep femoral vessels. The gracilis muscle is now visible. The tensor fascia lata muscle has assumed a more flattened profile. Sciatic nerve lies deep to the biceps femoris muscle.* (**Middle**) *The adductor magnus is a large muscle with multiple components. The most medial portion is called the ischiocondylar portion and attaches to the adductor tubercle of the medial femoral epicondyle.* (**Bottom**) *A large perforating artery is visible. It is a branch of the deep femoral artery. The tensor fascia lata muscle has completely inserted onto the iliotibial band. Throughout the thigh, the sciatic nerve resides deep to the biceps femoris muscle.*

Thigh Radiographic Anatomy and MR Atlas

AXIAL T1 MR, RIGHT MID THIGH

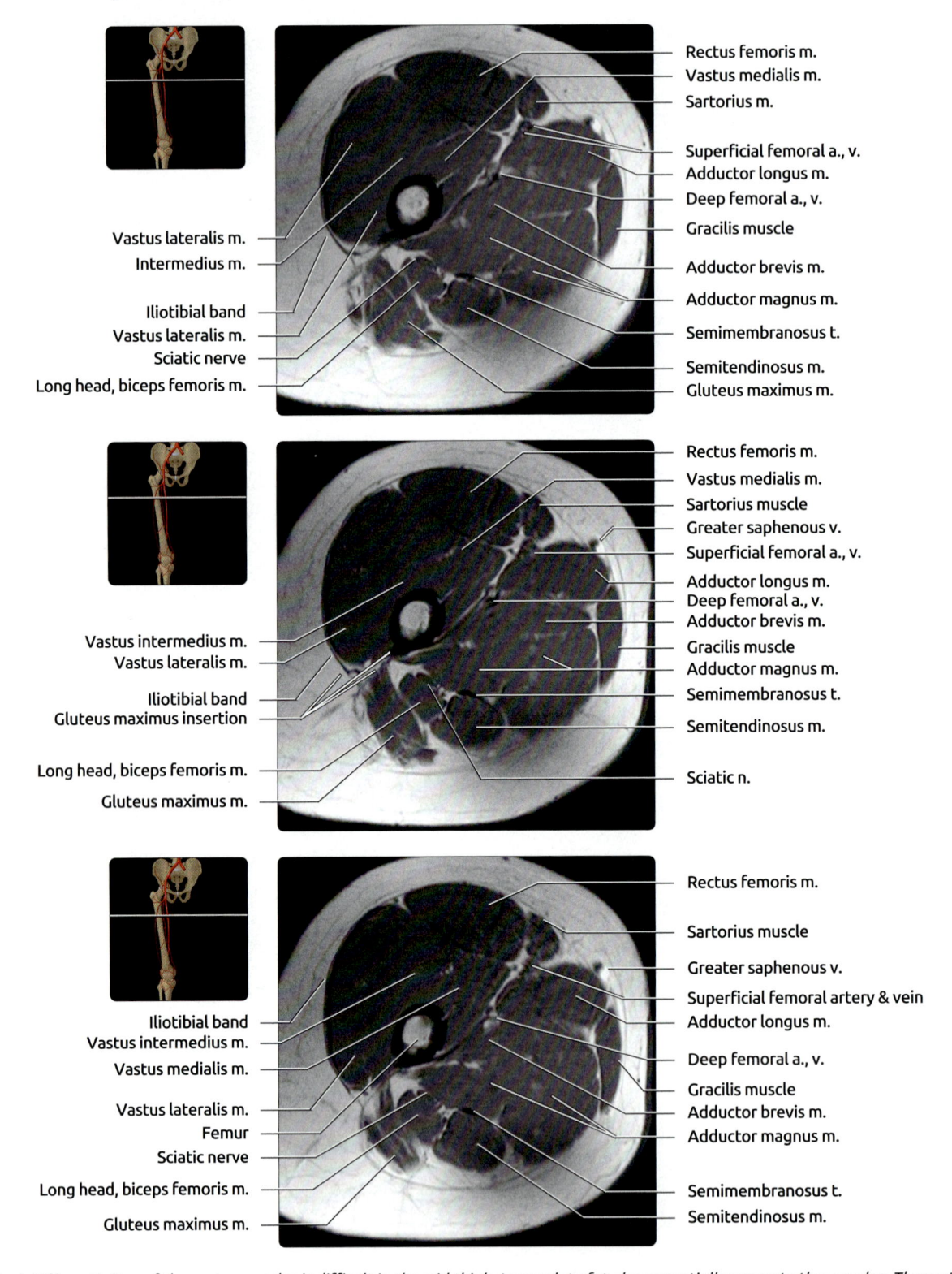

Labels (top image):
- Rectus femoris m.
- Vastus medialis m.
- Sartorius m.
- Superficial femoral a., v.
- Adductor longus m.
- Deep femoral a., v.
- Gracilis muscle
- Adductor brevis m.
- Adductor magnus m.
- Semimembranosus t.
- Semitendinosus m.
- Gluteus maximus m.
- Vastus lateralis m.
- Intermedius m.
- Iliotibial band
- Vastus lateralis m.
- Sciatic nerve
- Long head, biceps femoris m.

Labels (middle image):
- Rectus femoris m.
- Vastus medialis m.
- Sartorius muscle
- Greater saphenous v.
- Superficial femoral a., v.
- Adductor longus m.
- Deep femoral a., v.
- Adductor brevis m.
- Gracilis muscle
- Adductor magnus m.
- Semimembranosus t.
- Semitendinosus m.
- Sciatic n.
- Vastus intermedius m.
- Vastus lateralis m.
- Iliotibial band
- Gluteus maximus insertion
- Long head, biceps femoris m.
- Gluteus maximus m.

Labels (bottom image):
- Rectus femoris m.
- Sartorius muscle
- Greater saphenous v.
- Superficial femoral artery & vein
- Adductor longus m.
- Deep femoral a., v.
- Gracilis muscle
- Adductor brevis m.
- Adductor magnus m.
- Semimembranosus t.
- Semitendinosus m.
- Iliotibial band
- Vastus intermedius m.
- Vastus medialis m.
- Vastus lateralis m.
- Femur
- Sciatic nerve
- Long head, biceps femoris m.
- Gluteus maximus m.

(Top) Differentiation of the vastus muscles is difficult in the mid thigh. Incomplete fat planes partially separate the muscles. The vastus lateralis wraps around the anterior margin of the vastus intermedius. (Middle) The gluteus maximus has a broad insertion on the iliotibial band and the gluteal tuberosity, a prominence at the superolateral aspect of the linea aspera of the femur. (Bottom) The semitendinosus muscle belly enlarges through the mid thigh. The muscle bellies of the semimembranosus and semitendinosus muscle share a reciprocal relationship. As the semitendinosus muscle becomes smaller along its inferior extent, the semimembranosus muscle becomes larger.

Thigh Radiographic Anatomy and MR Atlas

AXIAL T1 MR, LEFT MID THIGH

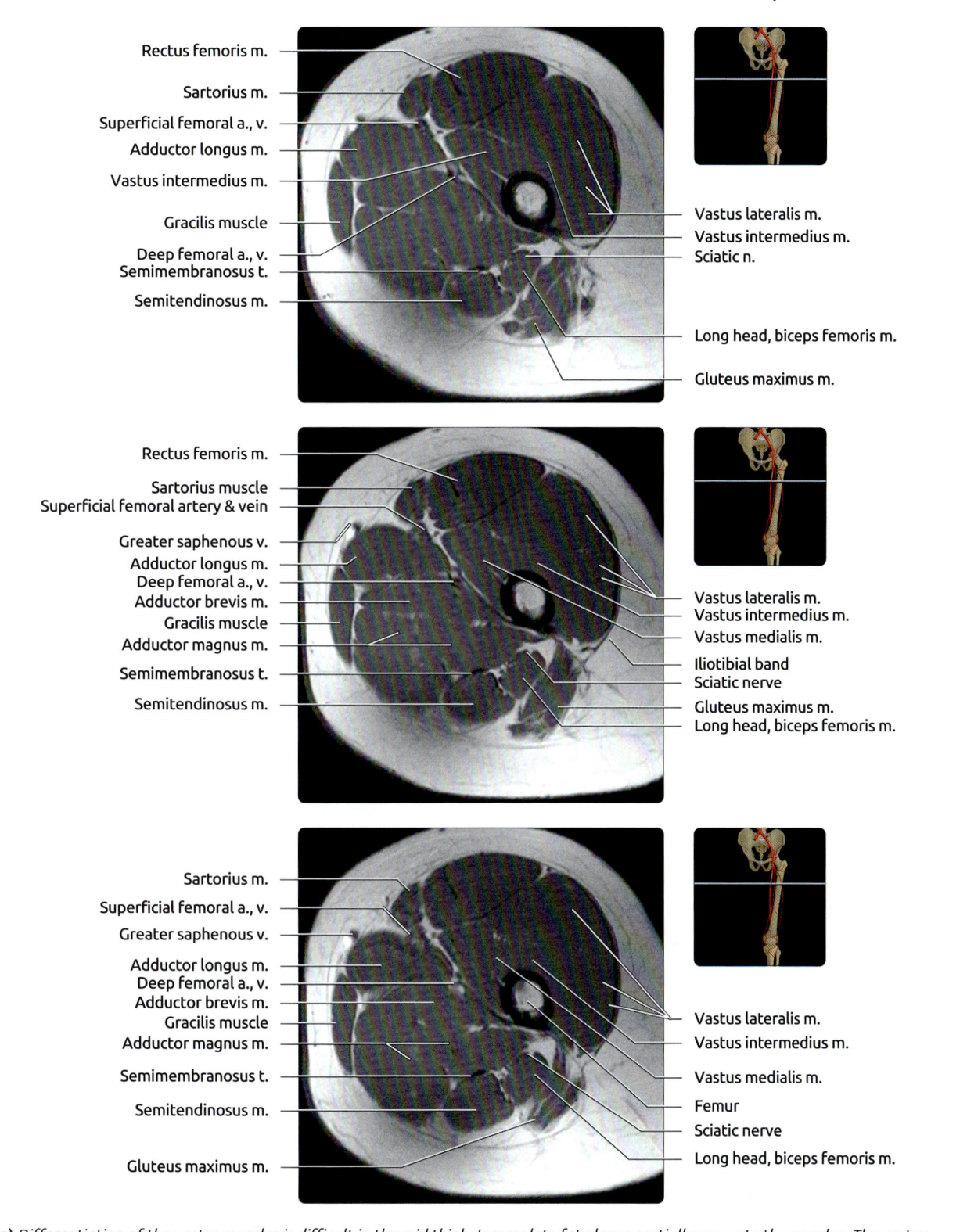

Top image labels:
- Rectus femoris m.
- Sartorius m.
- Superficial femoral a., v.
- Adductor longus m.
- Vastus intermedius m.
- Gracilis muscle
- Deep femoral a., v.
- Semimembranosus t.
- Semitendinosus m.
- Vastus lateralis m.
- Vastus intermedius m.
- Sciatic n.
- Long head, biceps femoris m.
- Gluteus maximus m.

Middle image labels:
- Rectus femoris m.
- Sartorius muscle
- Superficial femoral artery & vein
- Greater saphenous v.
- Adductor longus m.
- Deep femoral a., v.
- Adductor brevis m.
- Gracilis muscle
- Adductor magnus m.
- Semimembranosus t.
- Semitendinosus m.
- Vastus lateralis m.
- Vastus intermedius m.
- Vastus medialis m.
- Iliotibial band
- Sciatic nerve
- Gluteus maximus m.
- Long head, biceps femoris m.

Bottom image labels:
- Sartorius m.
- Superficial femoral a., v.
- Greater saphenous v.
- Adductor longus m.
- Deep femoral a., v.
- Adductor brevis m.
- Gracilis muscle
- Adductor magnus m.
- Semimembranosus t.
- Semitendinosus m.
- Gluteus maximus m.
- Vastus lateralis m.
- Vastus intermedius m.
- Vastus medialis m.
- Femur
- Sciatic nerve
- Long head, biceps femoris m.

(Top) Differentiation of the vastus muscles is difficult in the mid thigh. Incomplete fat planes partially separate the muscles. The vastus lateralis wraps around the anterior margin of the vastus intermedius. **(Middle)** The gluteus maximus has a broad insertion on the iliotibial band and the gluteal tuberosity, a prominence at the superolateral aspect of the linea aspera of the femur. **(Bottom)** The semitendinosus muscle belly enlarges through the mid thigh. The muscle bellies of the semimembranosus and semitendinosus muscle share a reciprocal relationship. As the semitendinosus muscle becomes smaller along its inferior extent, the semimembranosus muscle becomes larger.

Thigh Radiographic Anatomy and MR Atlas

AXIAL T1 MR, RIGHT MID THIGH

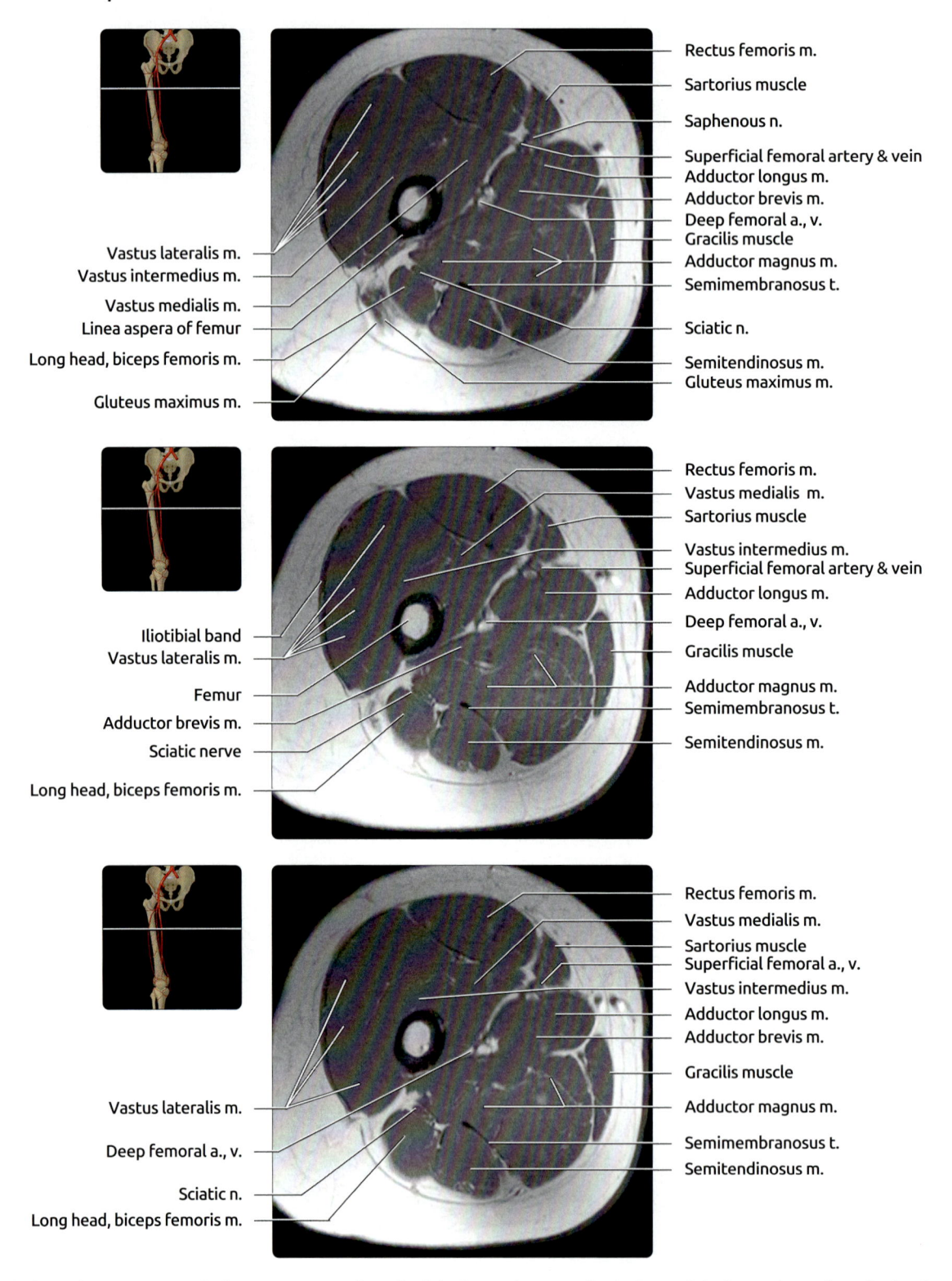

Labels (top image):
- Rectus femoris m.
- Sartorius muscle
- Saphenous n.
- Superficial femoral artery & vein
- Adductor longus m.
- Adductor brevis m.
- Deep femoral a., v.
- Gracilis muscle
- Adductor magnus m.
- Semimembranosus t.
- Sciatic n.
- Semitendinosus m.
- Gluteus maximus m.
- Vastus lateralis m.
- Vastus intermedius m.
- Vastus medialis m.
- Linea aspera of femur
- Long head, biceps femoris m.
- Gluteus maximus m.

Labels (middle image):
- Rectus femoris m.
- Vastus medialis m.
- Sartorius muscle
- Vastus intermedius m.
- Superficial femoral artery & vein
- Adductor longus m.
- Deep femoral a., v.
- Gracilis muscle
- Adductor magnus m.
- Semimembranosus t.
- Semitendinosus m.
- Iliotibial band
- Vastus lateralis m.
- Femur
- Adductor brevis m.
- Sciatic nerve
- Long head, biceps femoris m.

Labels (bottom image):
- Rectus femoris m.
- Vastus medialis m.
- Sartorius muscle
- Superficial femoral a., v.
- Vastus intermedius m.
- Adductor longus m.
- Adductor brevis m.
- Gracilis muscle
- Adductor magnus m.
- Semimembranosus t.
- Semitendinosus m.
- Vastus lateralis m.
- Deep femoral a., v.
- Sciatic n.
- Long head, biceps femoris m.

(Top) *The saphenous nerve is the largest cutaneous branch of the femoral nerve. It lies in front of the femoral vessels at this level; more inferiorly, it moves medially and becomes subcutaneous, accompanying the saphenous vein.* **(Middle)** *The vastus lateralis is broad and covers the vastus intermedius. The gracilis muscle has a band-like configuration and moves slightly posteriorly as it descends caudally.* **(Bottom)** *The adductor magnus is the largest mid-thigh muscle. The semimembranosus tendon is thin and starting to course medially. Although its tendon originates anterior and lateral to the semitendinosus tendon, the semimembranosus muscle will lie medial to the semitendinosus muscle in the mid thigh. It returns anterior to the semitendinosus tendon in the distal thigh.*

Thigh Radiographic Anatomy and MR Atlas

AXIAL T1 MR, LEFT MID THIGH

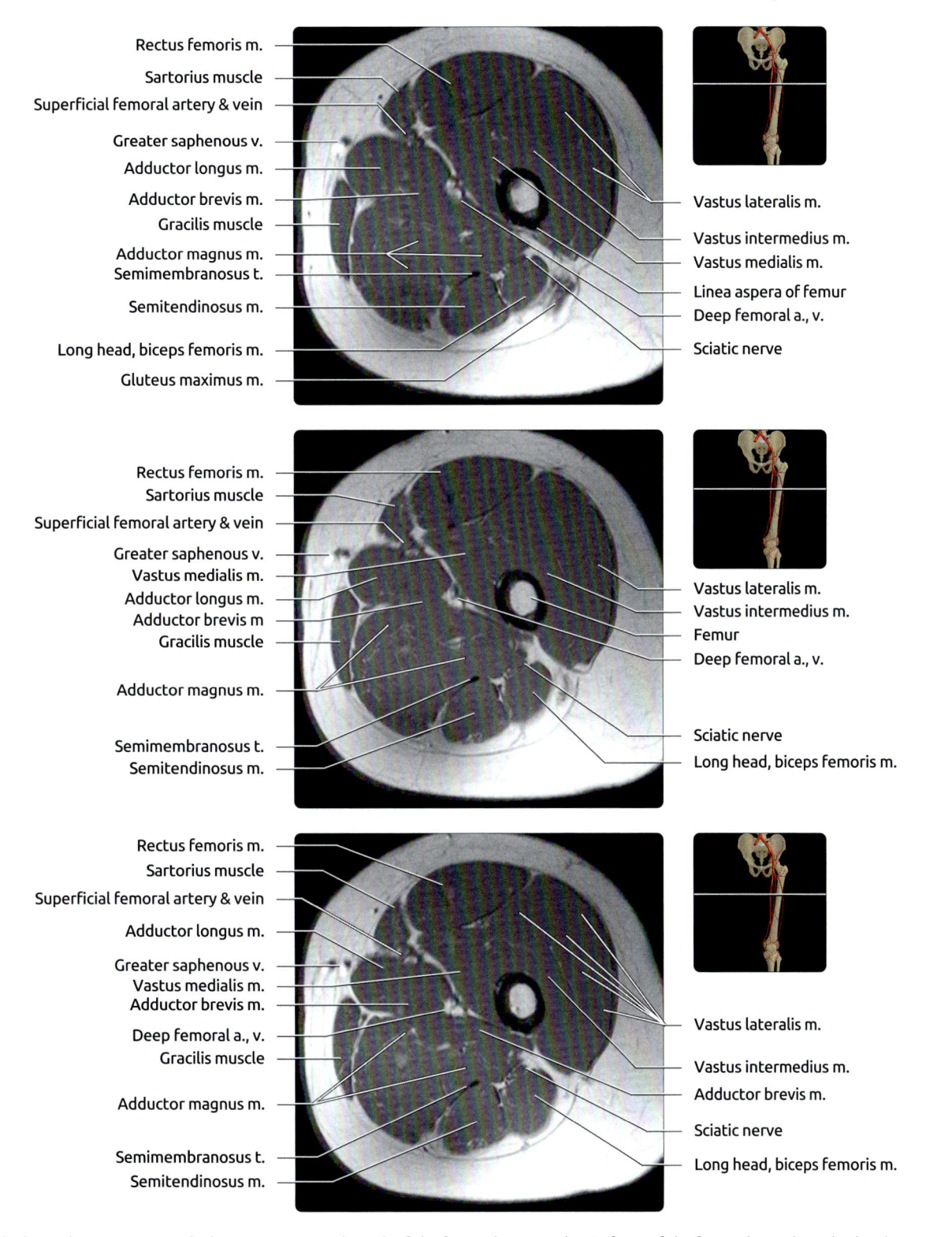

(Top) The saphenous nerve is the largest cutaneous branch of the femoral nerve. It lies in front of the femoral vessels at this level; more inferiorly, it moves medially and becomes subcutaneous, accompanying the saphenous vein. **(Middle)** The vastus lateralis is broad and covers the vastus intermedius. The gracilis muscle has a band-like configuration and moves slightly posteriorly as it descends caudally. **(Bottom)** The adductor magnus is the largest mid-thigh muscle. The semimembranosus tendon is thin and starting to course medially. Although its tendon originates anterior and lateral to the semitendinosus tendon, the semimembranosus muscle will lie medial to the semitendinosus muscle in the mid thigh. It returns anterior to the semitendinosus tendon in the distal thigh.

Thigh Radiographic Anatomy and MR Atlas

AXIAL T1 MR, RIGHT MID THIGH

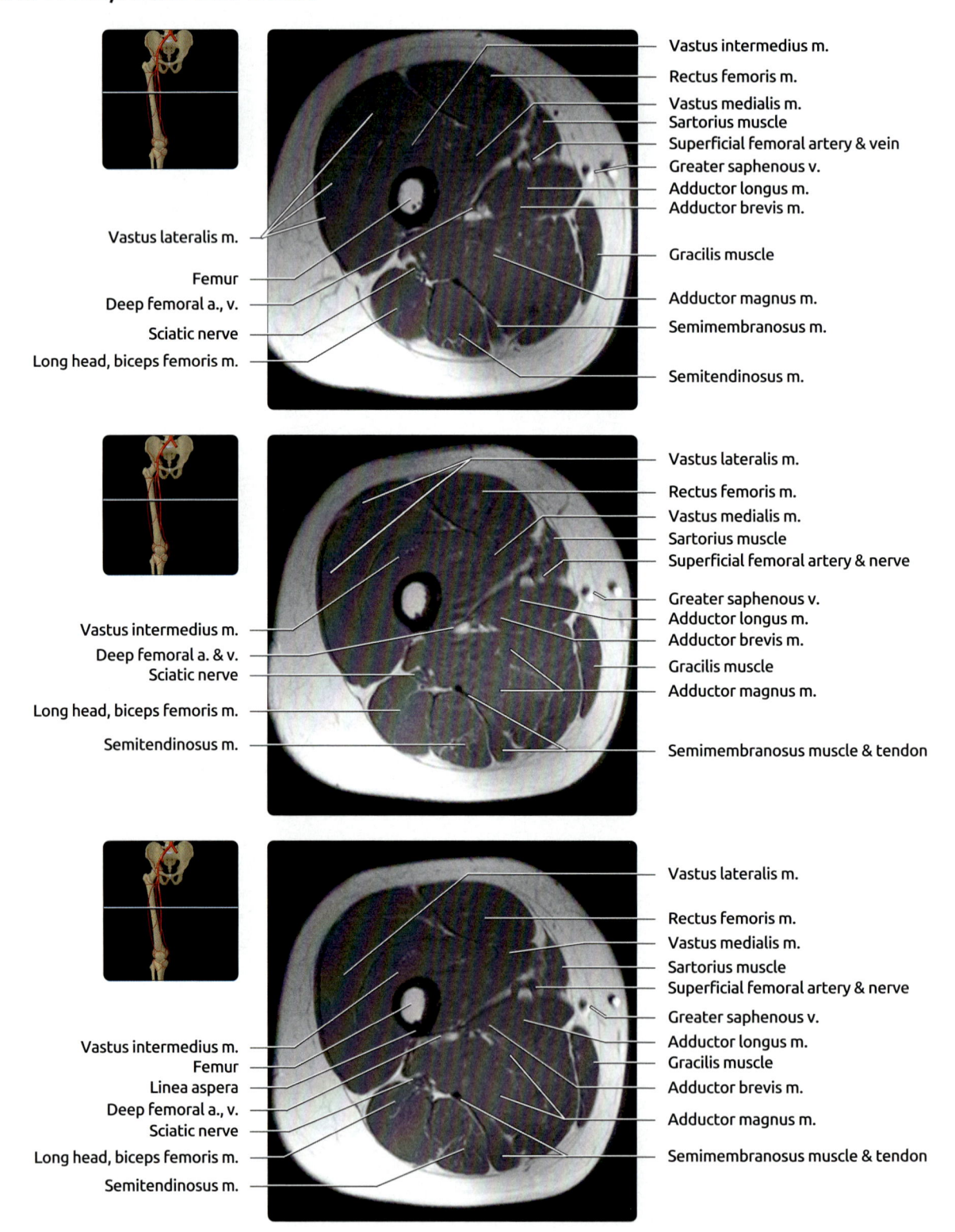

(Top) The fat plane separating the vastus lateralis muscle from the vastus medialis muscle deep to it is clearly defined at this level and below. The semimembranosus muscle is starting to form medial to its tendon and is medial to the semitendinosus muscle. **(Middle)** The sartorius muscle continues its medial and now posterior course. It will eventually reside immediately anterior to the gracilis muscle. The relative position of the sartorius muscle is a guide to the approximate location of an axial image through the thigh. **(Bottom)** The semimembranosus muscle continues to enlarge. The long head of the biceps femoris muscle is at its largest mid thigh. The short head of the biceps is not yet present. Adductor brevis is inserting on the femoral shaft.

Thigh Radiographic Anatomy and MR Atlas

AXIAL T1 MR, LEFT MID THIGH

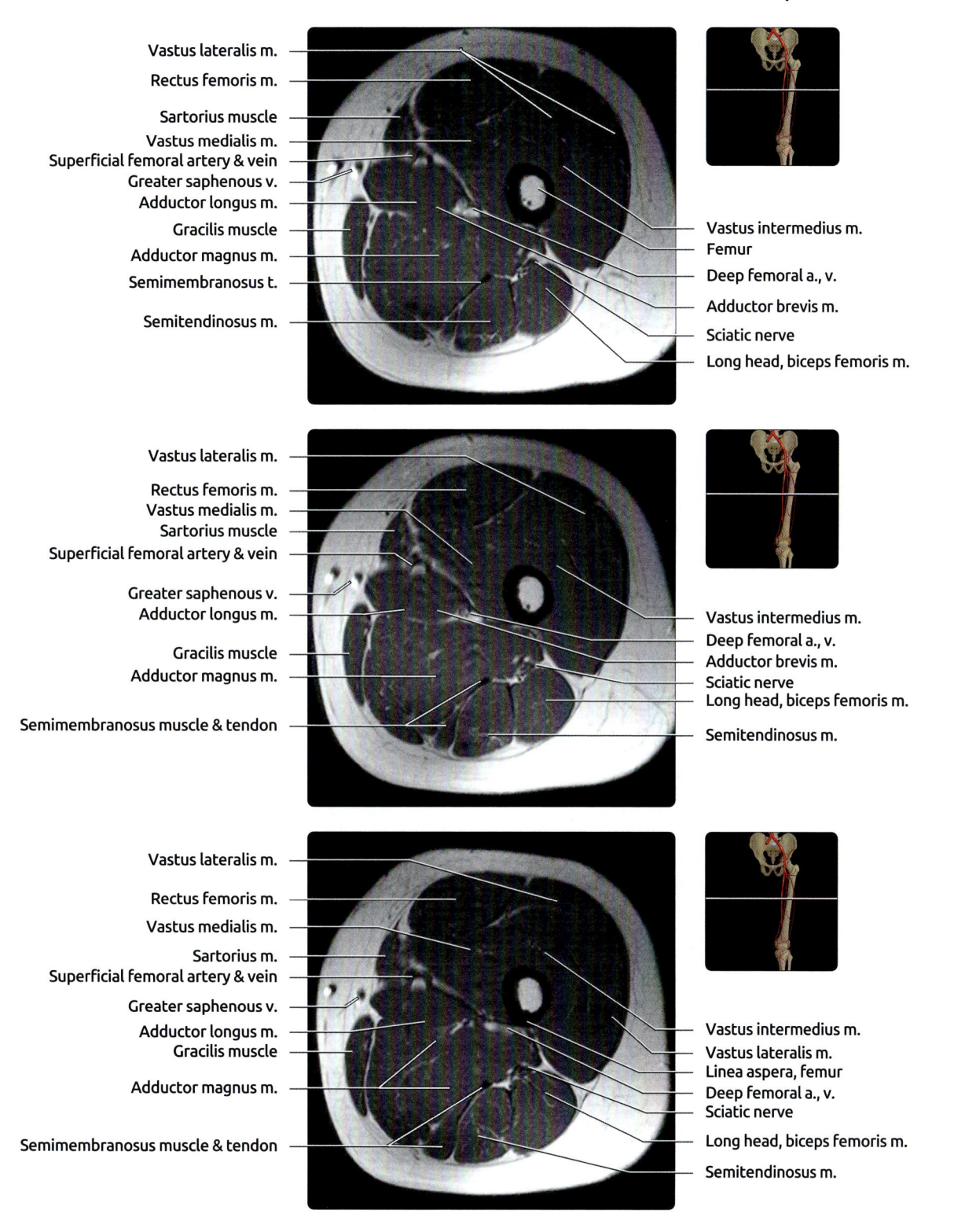

(Top) The fat plane separating the vastus lateralis muscle from the vastus medialis muscle deep to it is clearly defined at this level and below. The semimembranosus muscle is starting to form medial to its tendon and is medial to the semitendinosus muscle. (Middle) The sartorius muscle continues its medial and now posterior course. It will eventually reside immediately anterior to the gracilis muscle. The relative position of the sartorius muscle is a guide to the approximate location of an axial image through the thigh. (Bottom) The semimembranosus muscle continues to enlarge. The long head of the biceps femoris muscle is at its largest mid thigh. The short head of the biceps is not yet present. Adductor brevis is inserting on the femoral shaft.

Thigh Radiographic Anatomy and MR Atlas

AXIAL T1 MR, RIGHT MID THIGH

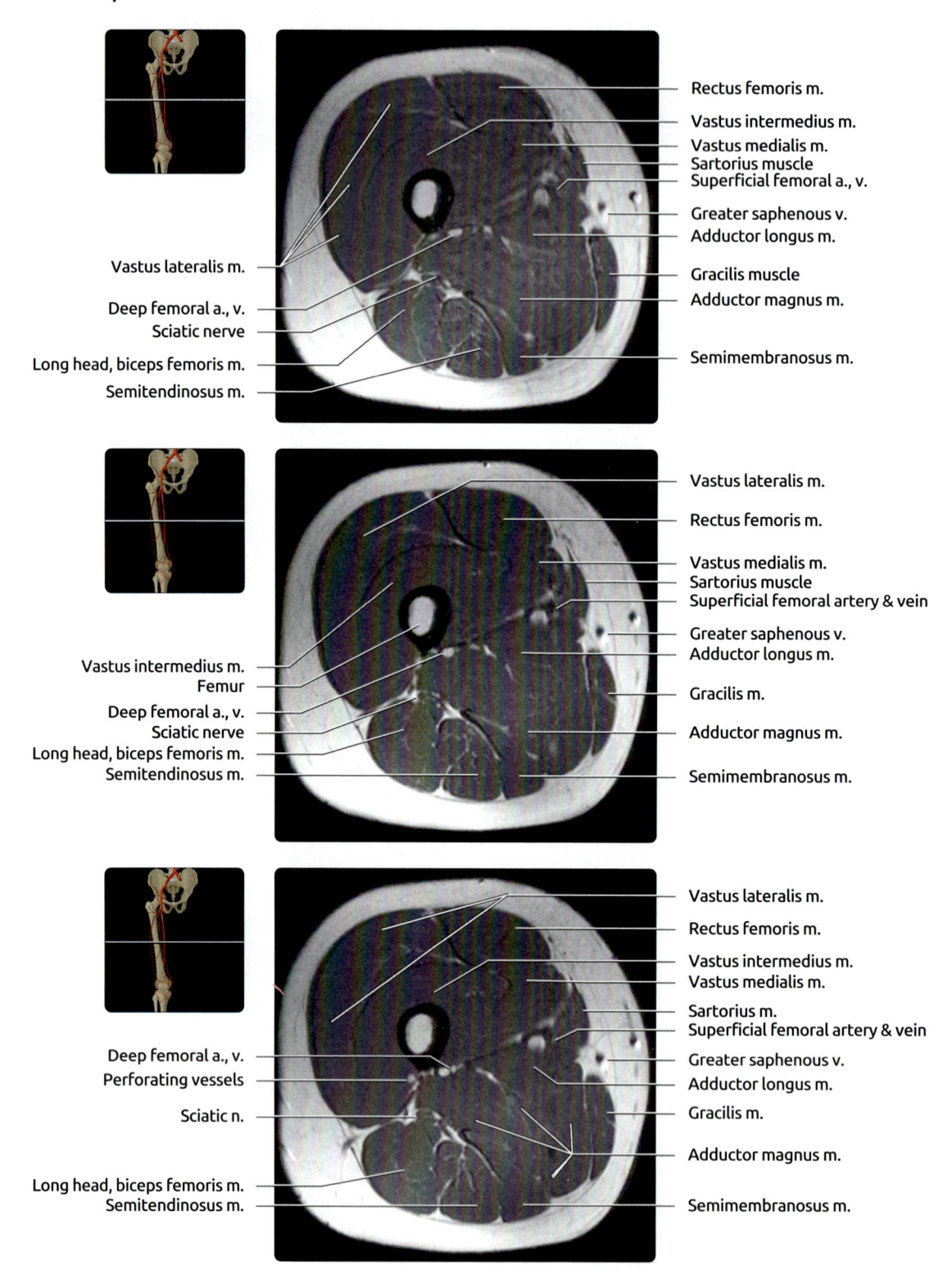

Top image labels:
- Rectus femoris m.
- Vastus intermedius m.
- Vastus medialis m.
- Sartorius muscle
- Superficial femoral a., v.
- Greater saphenous v.
- Adductor longus m.
- Gracilis muscle
- Adductor magnus m.
- Semimembranosus m.
- Vastus lateralis m.
- Deep femoral a., v.
- Sciatic nerve
- Long head, biceps femoris m.
- Semitendinosus m.

Middle image labels:
- Vastus lateralis m.
- Rectus femoris m.
- Vastus medialis m.
- Sartorius muscle
- Superficial femoral artery & vein
- Greater saphenous v.
- Adductor longus m.
- Gracilis m.
- Adductor magnus m.
- Semimembranosus m.
- Vastus intermedius m.
- Femur
- Deep femoral a., v.
- Sciatic nerve
- Long head, biceps femoris m.
- Semitendinosus m.

Bottom image labels:
- Vastus lateralis m.
- Rectus femoris m.
- Vastus intermedius m.
- Vastus medialis m.
- Sartorius m.
- Superficial femoral artery & vein
- Greater saphenous v.
- Adductor longus m.
- Gracilis m.
- Adductor magnus m.
- Semimembranosus m.
- Deep femoral a., v.
- Perforating vessels
- Sciatic n.
- Long head, biceps femoris m.
- Semitendinosus m.

(**Top**) *The gracilis muscle continues its posterior course. The sartorius muscle moves closer to the gracilis muscle.* (**Middle**) *The semimembranosus muscle belly increases in size as the semitendinosus muscle belly decreases in size. The adductor longus muscle lies anterior to the adductor magnus muscle throughout the thigh.* (**Bottom**) *Because of its oblique course and its own separate fascial covering, the sartorius muscle is often considered a separate compartment. Superior to this level, the muscle is not in direct continuity with the other muscles of the anterior compartment.*

Thigh Radiographic Anatomy and MR Atlas

AXIAL T1 MR, LEFT MID THIGH

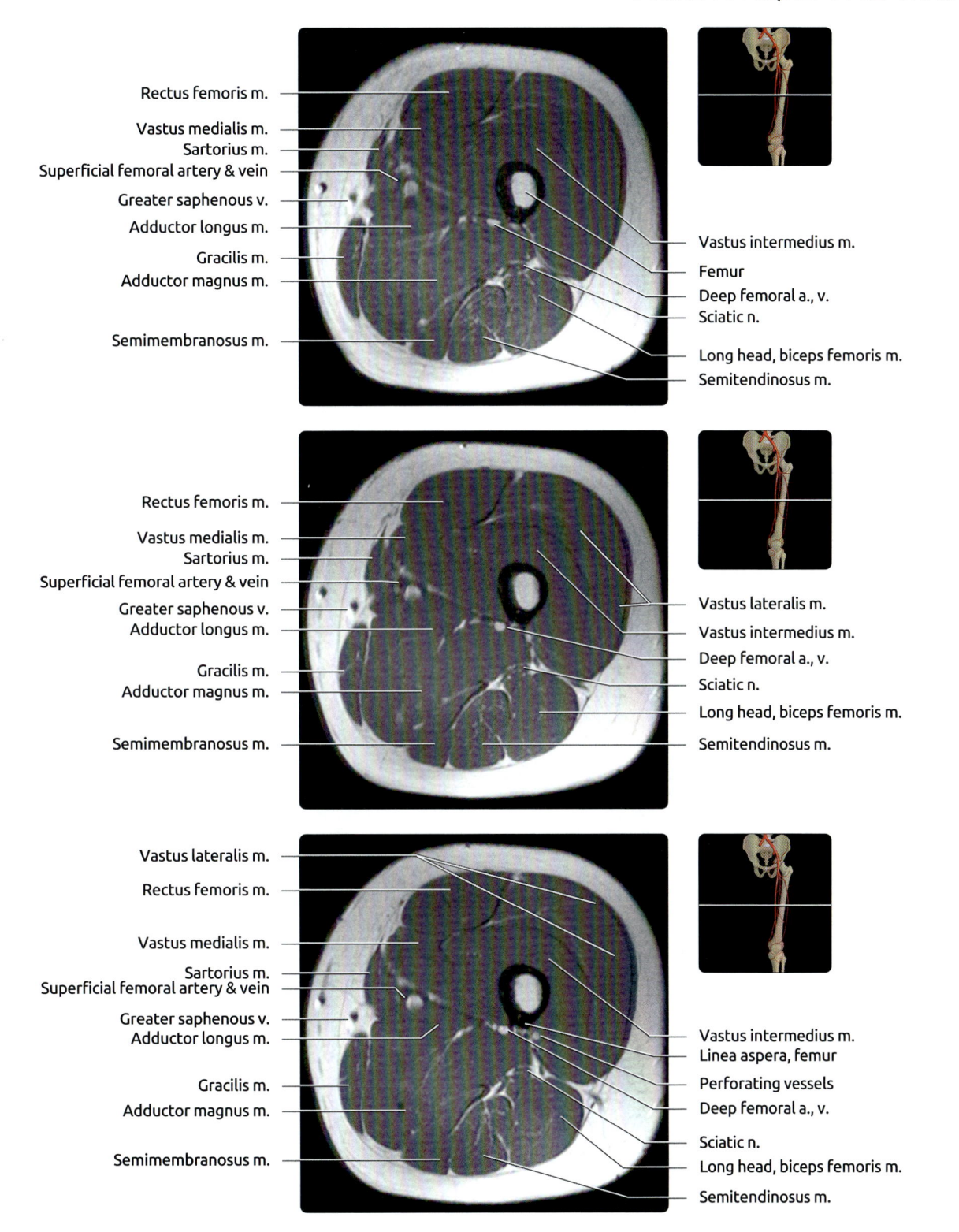

Labels (Top image):
- Rectus femoris m.
- Vastus medialis m.
- Sartorius m.
- Superficial femoral artery & vein
- Greater saphenous v.
- Adductor longus m.
- Gracilis m.
- Adductor magnus m.
- Semimembranosus m.
- Vastus intermedius m.
- Femur
- Deep femoral a., v.
- Sciatic n.
- Long head, biceps femoris m.
- Semitendinosus m.

Labels (Middle image):
- Rectus femoris m.
- Vastus medialis m.
- Sartorius m.
- Superficial femoral artery & vein
- Greater saphenous v.
- Adductor longus m.
- Gracilis m.
- Adductor magnus m.
- Semimembranosus m.
- Vastus lateralis m.
- Vastus intermedius m.
- Deep femoral a., v.
- Sciatic n.
- Long head, biceps femoris m.
- Semitendinosus m.

Labels (Bottom image):
- Vastus lateralis m.
- Rectus femoris m.
- Vastus medialis m.
- Sartorius m.
- Superficial femoral artery & vein
- Greater saphenous v.
- Adductor longus m.
- Gracilis m.
- Adductor magnus m.
- Semimembranosus m.
- Vastus intermedius m.
- Linea aspera, femur
- Perforating vessels
- Deep femoral a., v.
- Sciatic n.
- Long head, biceps femoris m.
- Semitendinosus m.

(Top) The gracilis m. continues its posterior course. The sartorius muscle moves closer to the gracilis muscle. (Middle) The semimembranosus muscle belly increases in size as the semitendinosus muscle belly decreases in size. The adductor longus muscle lies anterior to the adductor magnus muscle throughout the thigh. (Bottom) Because of its oblique course and its own separate fascial covering, the sartorius muscle is often considered a separate compartment. Superior to this level, the muscle is not in direct continuity with the other muscles of the anterior compartment.

Thigh Radiographic Anatomy and MR Atlas

AXIAL T1 MR, RIGHT MID THIGH

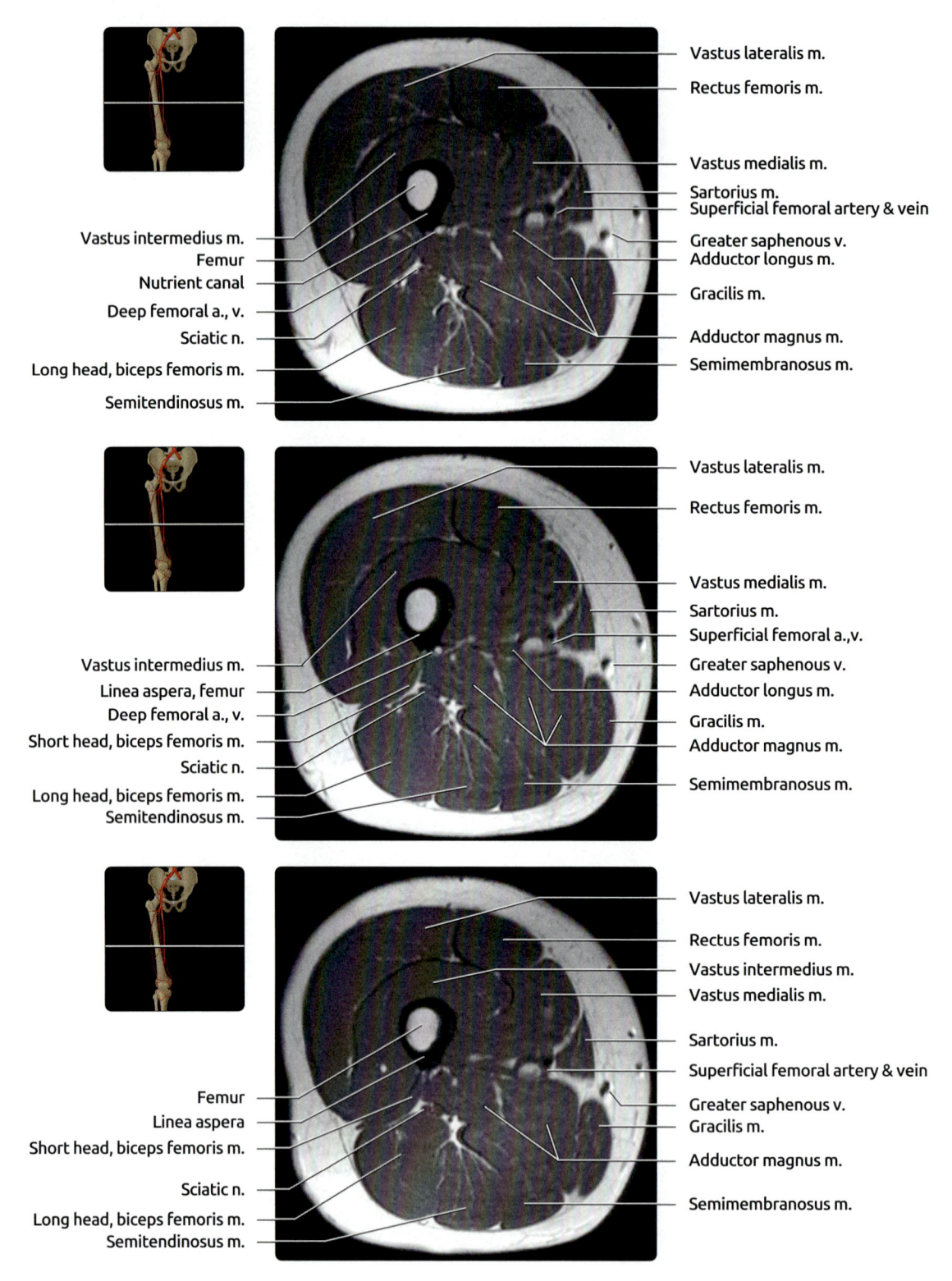

Labels (top image):
- Vastus lateralis m.
- Rectus femoris m.
- Vastus medialis m.
- Sartorius m.
- Superficial femoral artery & vein
- Greater saphenous v.
- Adductor longus m.
- Gracilis m.
- Adductor magnus m.
- Semimembranosus m.
- Vastus intermedius m.
- Femur
- Nutrient canal
- Deep femoral a., v.
- Sciatic n.
- Long head, biceps femoris m.
- Semitendinosus m.

Labels (middle image):
- Vastus lateralis m.
- Rectus femoris m.
- Vastus medialis m.
- Sartorius m.
- Superficial femoral a., v.
- Greater saphenous v.
- Adductor longus m.
- Gracilis m.
- Adductor magnus m.
- Semimembranosus m.
- Vastus intermedius m.
- Linea aspera, femur
- Deep femoral a., v.
- Short head, biceps femoris m.
- Sciatic n.
- Long head, biceps femoris m.
- Semitendinosus m.

Labels (bottom image):
- Vastus lateralis m.
- Rectus femoris m.
- Vastus intermedius m.
- Vastus medialis m.
- Sartorius m.
- Superficial femoral artery & vein
- Greater saphenous v.
- Gracilis m.
- Adductor magnus m.
- Semimembranosus m.
- Femur
- Linea aspera
- Short head, biceps femoris m.
- Sciatic n.
- Long head, biceps femoris m.
- Semitendinosus m.

(Top) The deep femoral vessels have followed an inferior and lateral course from their point of branching in the upper thigh. They now course posterior to the femur. The inferior-most aspect of the adductor longus muscle is visible. The adductor magnus, gracilis, and sartorius muscles are the only medial compartment muscles to continue into the distal thigh. **(Middle)** The short head of the biceps femoris arises between the adductor magnus and the vastus lateralis from the lateral margin of the linea aspera in the mid thigh. **(Bottom)** The rectus femoris muscle is now nestled between the vastus medialis and lateralis muscles. The deep femoral vessels terminate in the mid thigh.

Thigh Radiographic Anatomy and MR Atlas

AXIAL T1 MR, LEFT MID THIGH

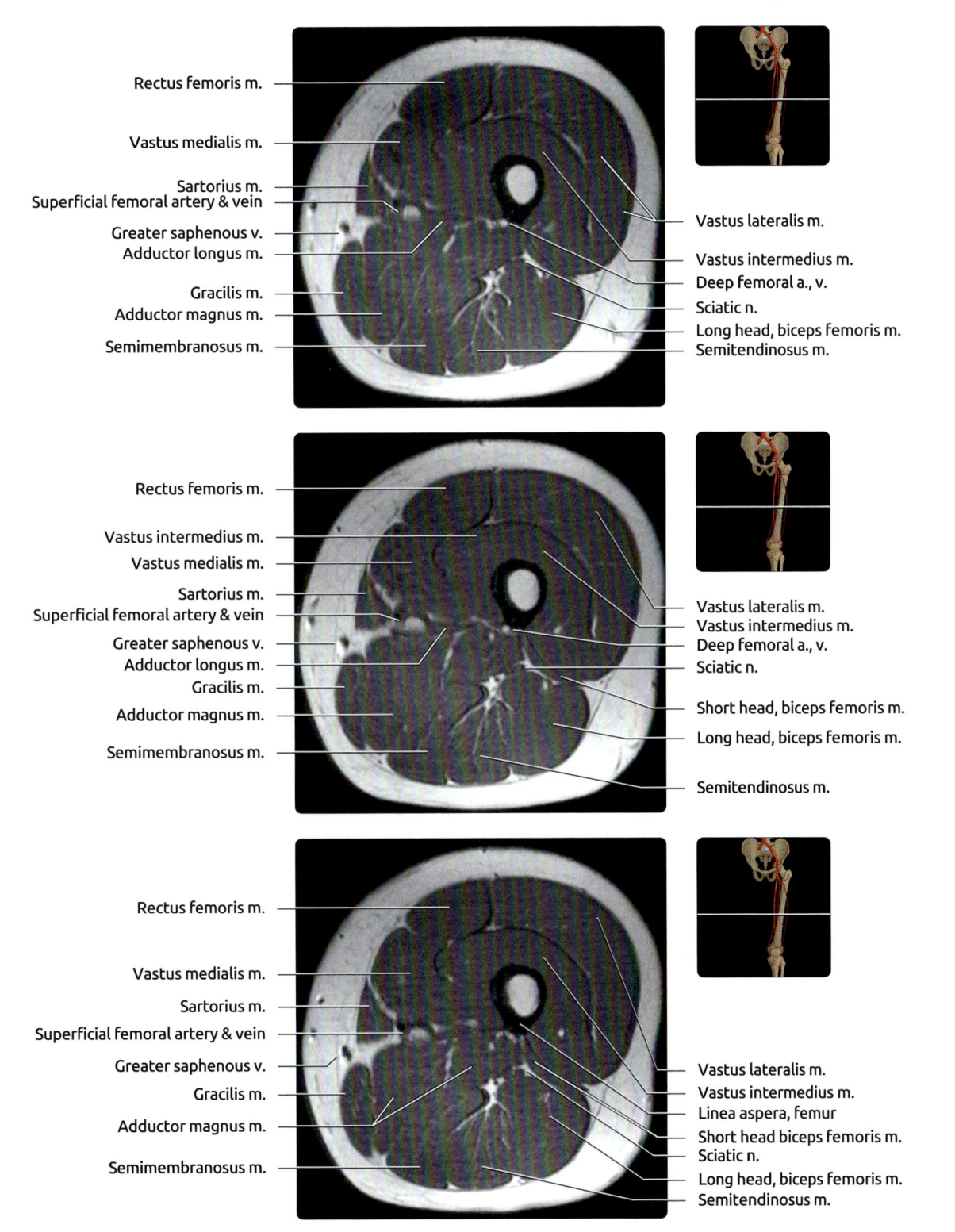

Top image labels:
- Rectus femoris m.
- Vastus medialis m.
- Sartorius m.
- Superficial femoral artery & vein
- Greater saphenous v.
- Adductor longus m.
- Gracilis m.
- Adductor magnus m.
- Semimembranosus m.
- Vastus lateralis m.
- Vastus intermedius m.
- Deep femoral a., v.
- Sciatic n.
- Long head, biceps femoris m.
- Semitendinosus m.

Middle image labels:
- Rectus femoris m.
- Vastus intermedius m.
- Vastus medialis m.
- Sartorius m.
- Superficial femoral artery & vein
- Greater saphenous v.
- Adductor longus m.
- Gracilis m.
- Adductor magnus m.
- Semimembranosus m.
- Vastus lateralis m.
- Vastus intermedius m.
- Deep femoral a., v.
- Sciatic n.
- Short head, biceps femoris m.
- Long head, biceps femoris m.
- Semitendinosus m.

Bottom image labels:
- Rectus femoris m.
- Vastus medialis m.
- Sartorius m.
- Superficial femoral artery & vein
- Greater saphenous v.
- Gracilis m.
- Adductor magnus m.
- Semimembranosus m.
- Vastus lateralis m.
- Vastus intermedius m.
- Linea aspera, femur
- Short head biceps femoris m.
- Sciatic n.
- Long head, biceps femoris m.
- Semitendinosus m.

(Top) The deep femoral vessels have followed an inferior and lateral course from their point of branching in the upper thigh. They now course posterior to the femur. The inferior-most aspect of the adductor longus muscle is visible. The adductor magnus, gracilis, and sartorius muscles are the only medial compartment muscles to continue into the distal thigh. **(Middle)** The short head of the biceps femoris arises between the adductor magnus and the vastus lateralis from the lateral margin of the linea aspera in the mid thigh. **(Bottom)** The rectus femoris muscle is now nestled between the vastus medialis and lateralis muscles. The deep femoral vessels terminate in the mid thigh.

Thigh Radiographic Anatomy and MR Atlas

AXIAL T1 MR, RIGHT MID THIGH

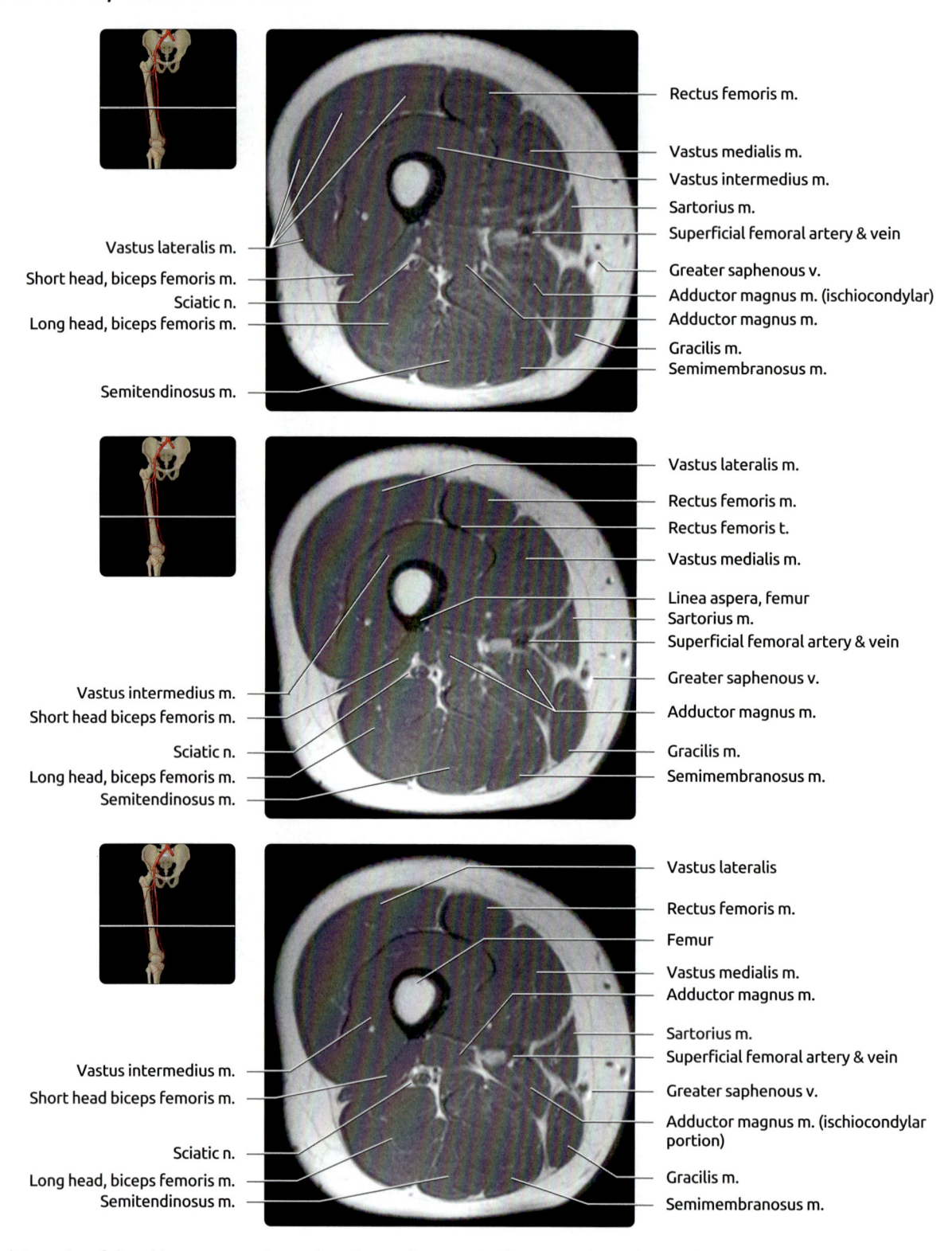

(Top) Labels: Rectus femoris m.; Vastus medialis m.; Vastus intermedius m.; Sartorius m.; Superficial femoral artery & vein; Greater saphenous v.; Adductor magnus m. (ischiocondylar); Adductor magnus m.; Gracilis m.; Semimembranosus m.; Vastus lateralis m.; Short head, biceps femoris m.; Sciatic n.; Long head, biceps femoris m.; Semitendinosus m.

(Middle) Labels: Vastus lateralis m.; Rectus femoris m.; Rectus femoris t.; Vastus medialis m.; Linea aspera, femur; Sartorius m.; Superficial femoral artery & vein; Greater saphenous v.; Adductor magnus m.; Gracilis m.; Semimembranosus m.; Vastus intermedius m.; Short head biceps femoris m.; Sciatic n.; Long head, biceps femoris m.; Semitendinosus m.

(Bottom) Labels: Vastus lateralis; Rectus femoris m.; Femur; Vastus medialis m.; Adductor magnus m.; Sartorius m.; Superficial femoral artery & vein; Greater saphenous v.; Adductor magnus m. (ischiocondylar portion); Gracilis m.; Semimembranosus m.; Vastus intermedius m.; Short head biceps femoris m.; Sciatic n.; Long head, biceps femoris m.; Semitendinosus m.

(Top) *A portion of the adductor magnus is seen inserting on the posterior femur, separating from ischiocondylar muscle fibers that continue caudad. Muscular insertions of the adductor magnus are quite broad.* **(Middle)** *The tendon of the rectus femoris muscle is now located along the deep surface of the muscle. The origin of the short head of biceps and insertion of portions of the adductor magnus muscle on linea aspera of femur are well seen.* **(Bottom)** *The muscle bellies of the rectus femoris and semitendinosus both decrease in size in the distal thigh. The short head of the biceps femoris muscle has a long origin from the linea aspera of the posterior femur.*

Thigh Radiographic Anatomy and MR Atlas

AXIAL T1 MR, LEFT MID THIGH

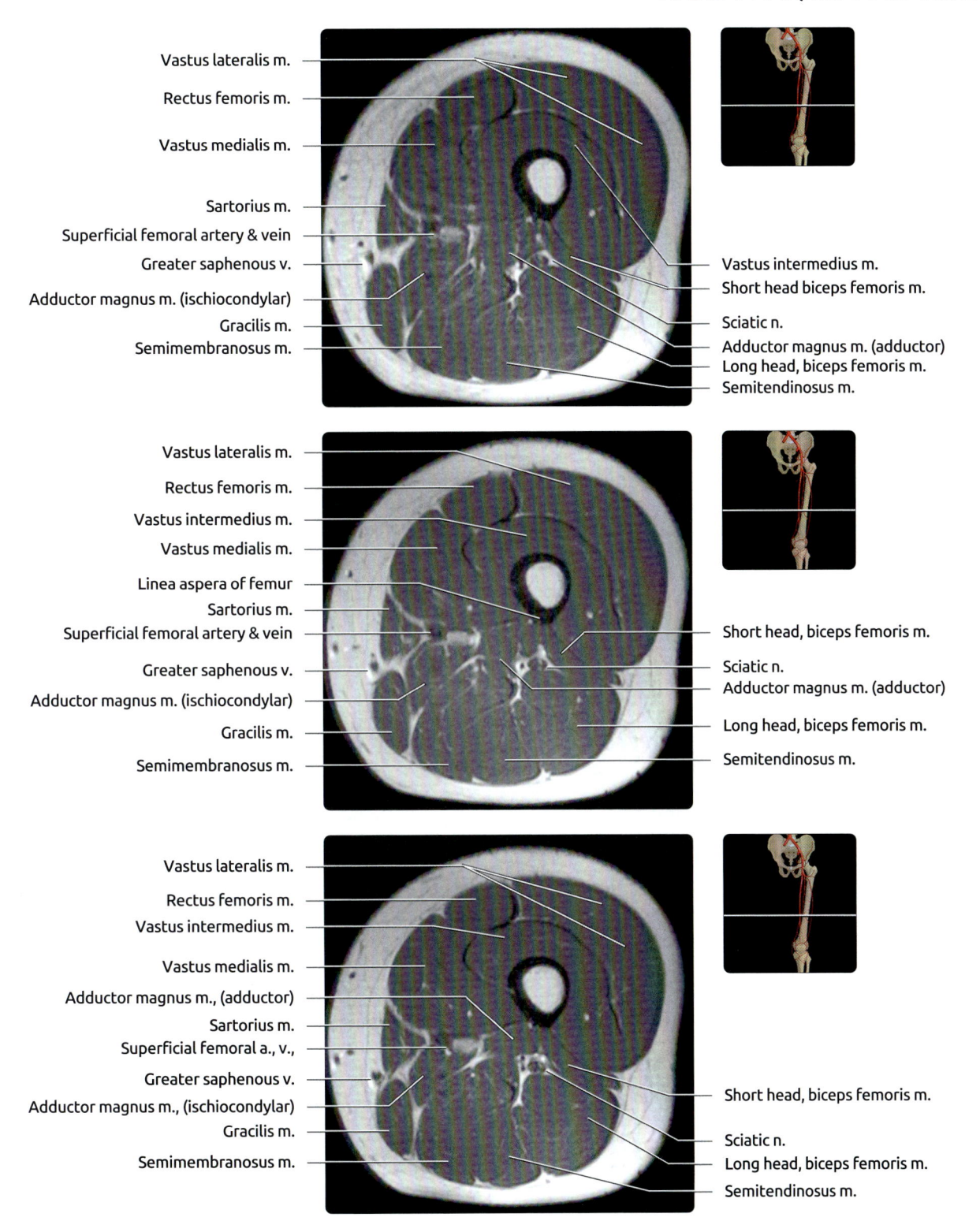

(Top) A portion of the adductor magnus is seen inserting on posterior femur, separating from ischiocondylar muscle fibers that continue caudad. Muscular insertions of the adductor magnus are quite broad. (Middle) The tendon of the rectus femoris muscle is now located along the deep surface of the muscle. The origin of the short head of biceps and insertion of portions of adductor magnus muscle on the linea aspera of femur are well seen. (Bottom) The muscle bellies of the rectus femoris and semitendinosus both decrease in size in the distal thigh. The short head of the biceps femoris muscle has a long origin from the linea aspera of the posterior femur.

Thigh Radiographic Anatomy and MR Atlas

AXIAL T1 MR, RIGHT MID THIGH

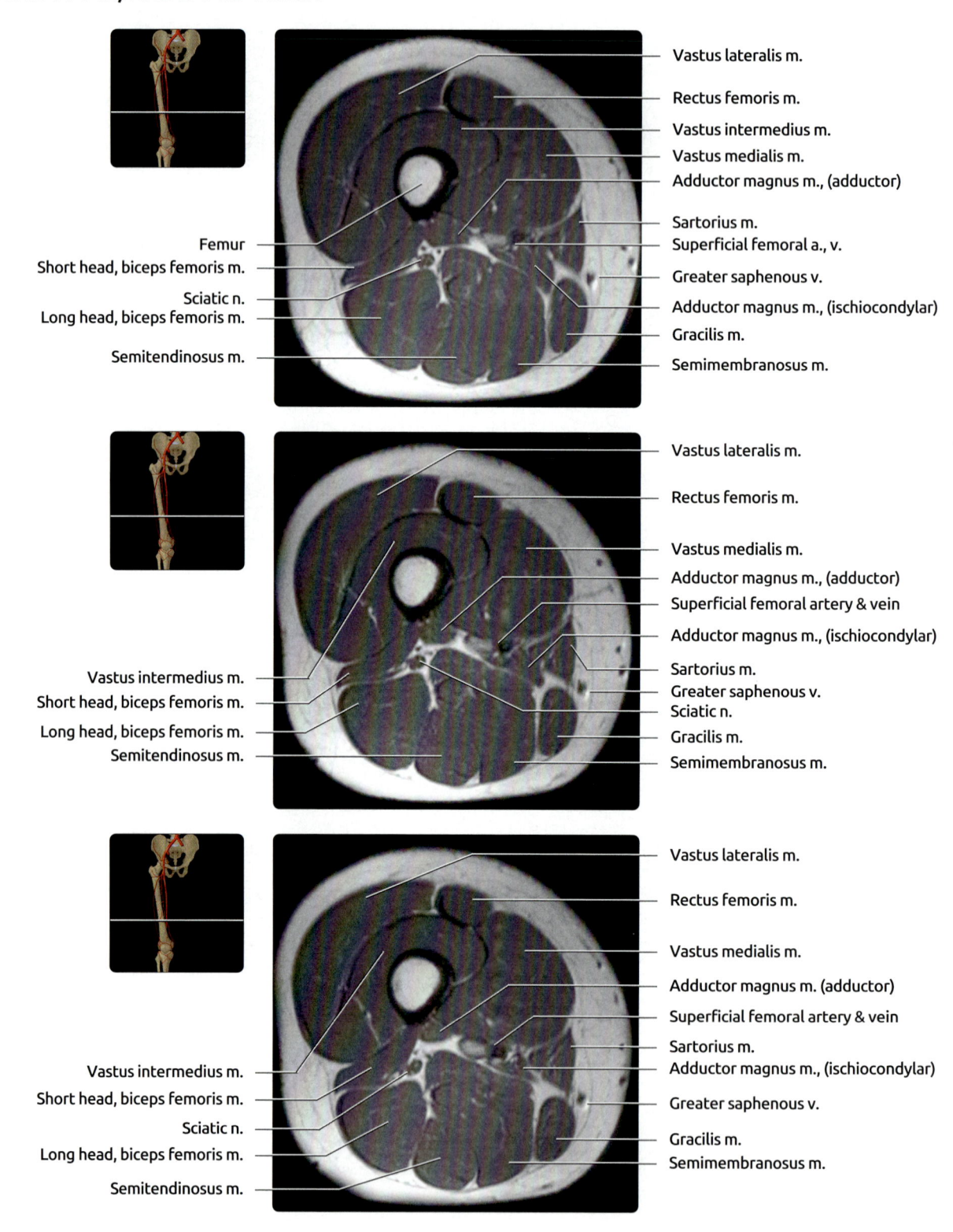

(Top) The vastus medialis muscle enlarges relative to the remainder of the quadriceps in the distal thigh. The sciatic nerve continues to reside along the deep surface of the long head of the biceps femoris muscle. **(Middle)** The sartorius and gracilis muscles are now within the posterior 1/2 of the medial aspect of the thigh. The semitendinosus muscle is becoming quite small. **(Bottom)** The separation of the adductor and ischiocondylar portions of the adductor magnus muscle forms the adductor hiatus. The superficial femoral vessels pass through the adductor hiatus to enter the popliteal fossa. Upon passing through the hiatus, they become the popliteal vessels.

Thigh Radiographic Anatomy and MR Atlas

AXIAL T1 MR, LEFT MID THIGH

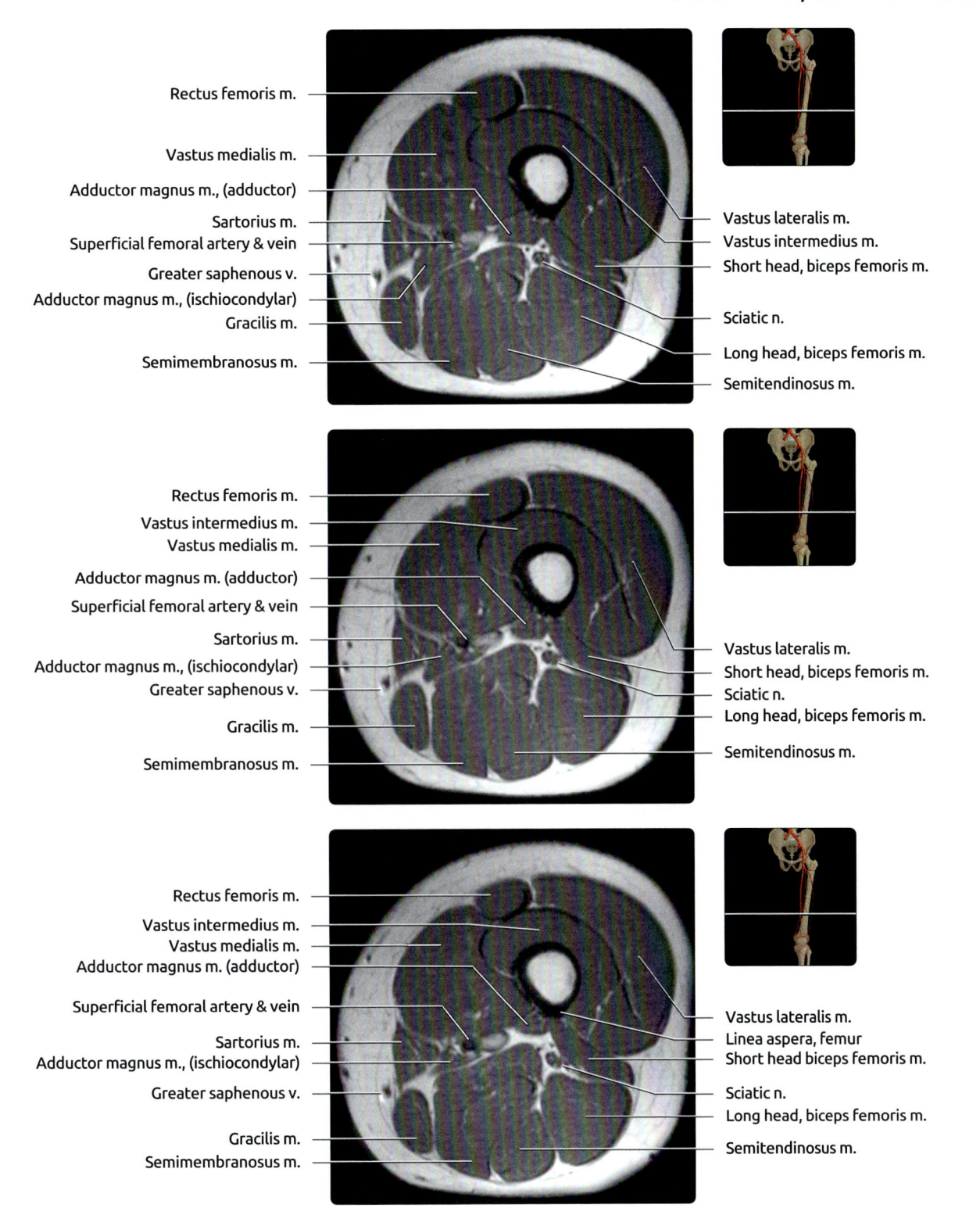

(Top) The vastus medialis muscle enlarges relative to the remainder of the quadriceps in the distal thigh. The sciatic nerve continues to reside along the deep surface of the long head of the biceps femoris muscle. (Middle) The sartorius and gracilis muscles are now within the posterior 1/2 of the medial aspect of the thigh. The semitendinosus muscle is becoming quite small. (Bottom) The separation of the adductor and ischiocondylar portions of the adductor magnus muscle forms the adductor hiatus. The superficial femoral vessels pass through the adductor hiatus to enter the popliteal fossa. Upon passing through the hiatus, they become the popliteal vessels.

639

Thigh Radiographic Anatomy and MR Atlas

AXIAL T1 MR, RIGHT MID THIGH

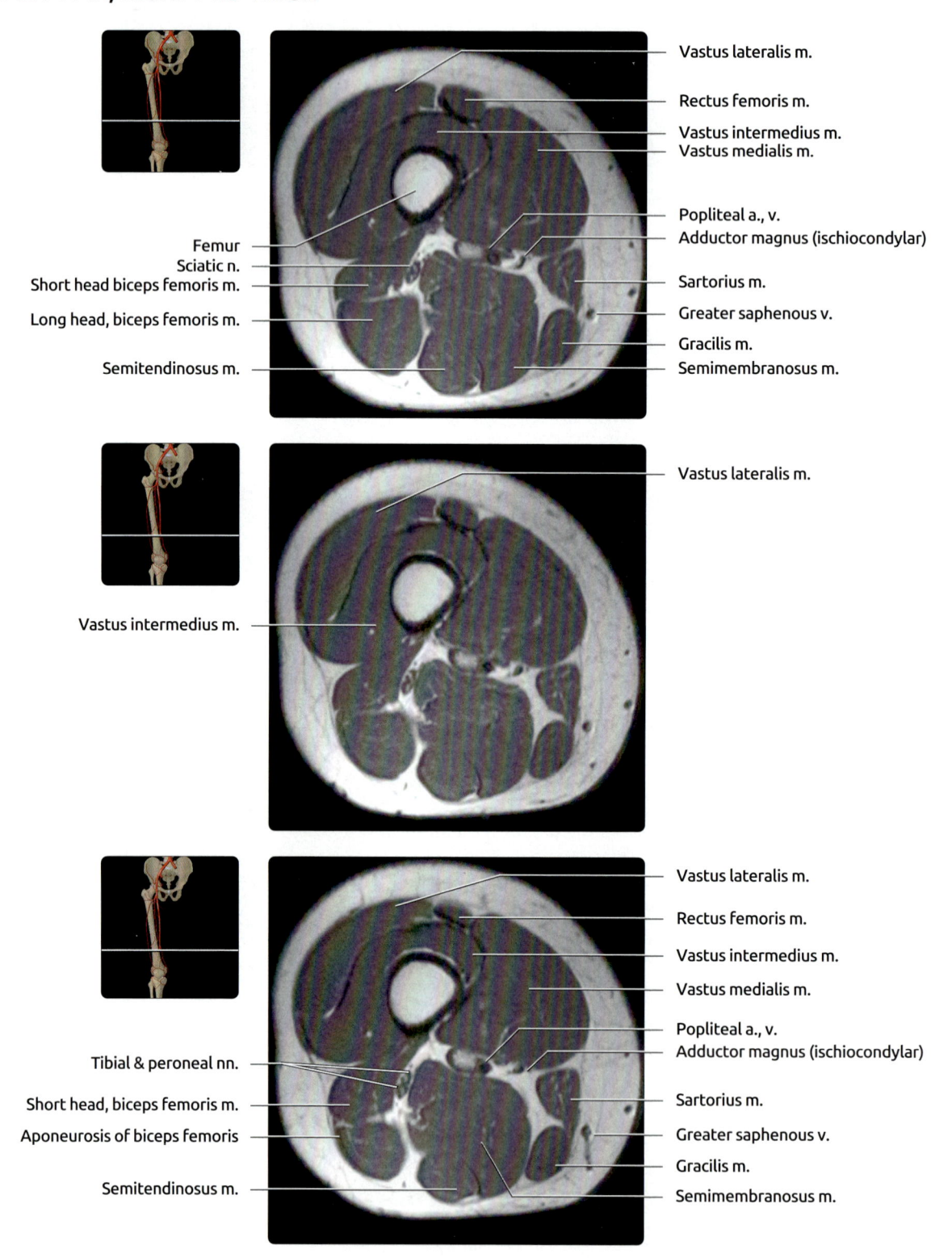

Top image labels:
- Vastus lateralis m.
- Rectus femoris m.
- Vastus intermedius m.
- Vastus medialis m.
- Popliteal a., v.
- Adductor magnus (ischiocondylar)
- Sartorius m.
- Greater saphenous v.
- Gracilis m.
- Semimembranosus m.
- Femur
- Sciatic n.
- Short head biceps femoris m.
- Long head, biceps femoris m.
- Semitendinosus m.

Middle image labels:
- Vastus lateralis m.
- Vastus intermedius m.

Bottom image labels:
- Vastus lateralis m.
- Rectus femoris m.
- Vastus intermedius m.
- Vastus medialis m.
- Popliteal a., v.
- Adductor magnus (ischiocondylar)
- Sartorius m.
- Greater saphenous v.
- Gracilis m.
- Semimembranosus m.
- Tibial & peroneal nn.
- Short head, biceps femoris m.
- Aponeurosis of biceps femoris
- Semitendinosus m.

(Top) Rectus femoris tendon is enlarging, and there is only a small portion of muscle still present. Tendon of vastus intermedius forms a layer along the superficial margin of the muscle. The ischiocondylar portion of adductor magnus forms a long tendon extending to the adductor tubercle of the medial femoral condyle. It lies posterior to the vastus medialis. **(Middle)** The long head of biceps femoris forms a posterior aponeurosis on which the fibers of the short head insert. The sciatic nerve has moved medial to the biceps femoris muscle. **(Bottom)** The tibial and peroneal nerves are distinct within the sciatic nerve from the nerve origin. In the distal thigh, they start to diverge, with the peroneal nerve coursing laterally.

Thigh Radiographic Anatomy and MR Atlas

AXIAL T1 MR, LEFT MID THIGH

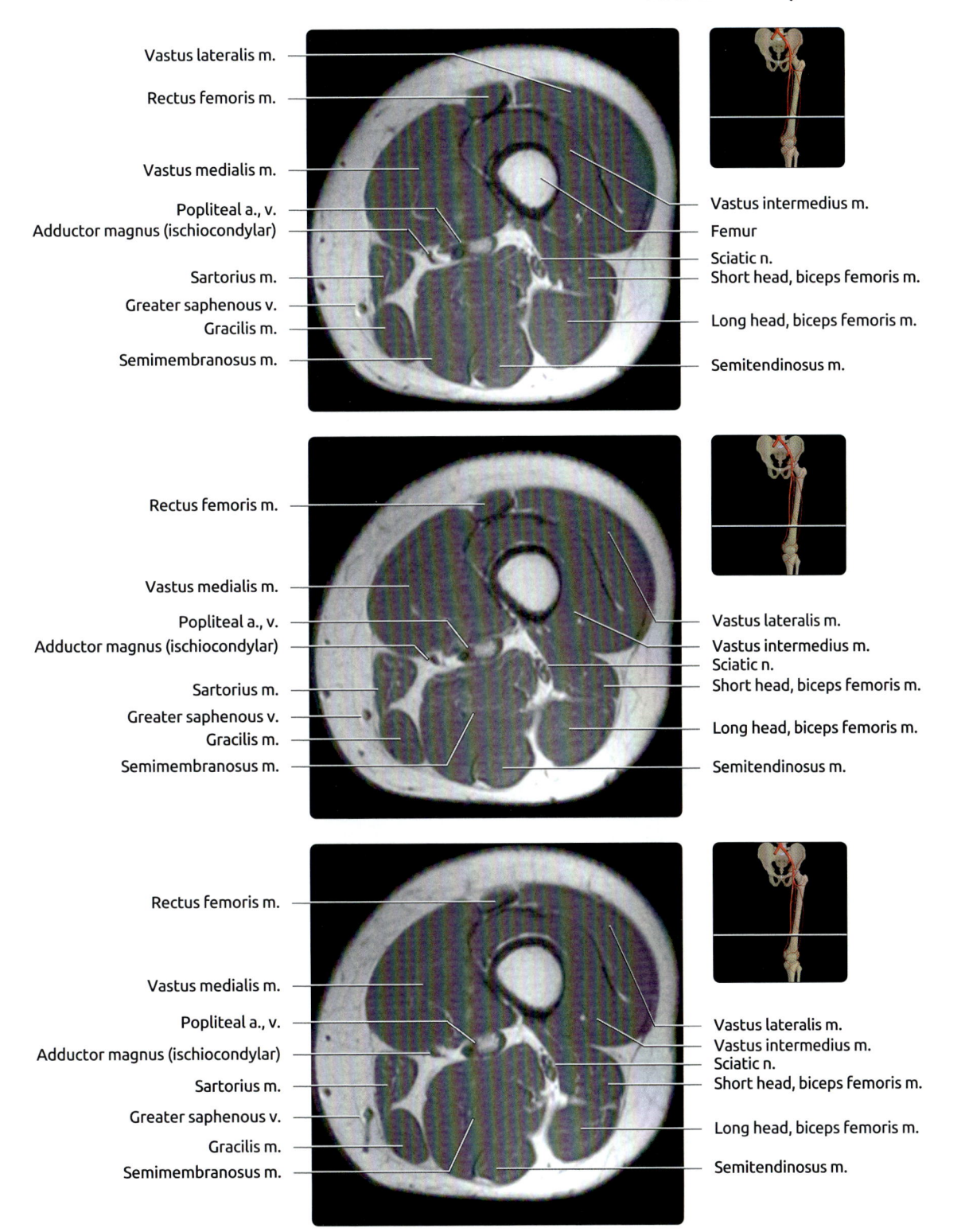

(Top) Rectus femoris tendon is enlarging, and there is only a small portion of muscle still present. Tendon of vastus intermedius forms a layer along the superficial margin of the muscle. Ischiocondylar portion of adductor magnus forms a long tendon extending to the adductor tubercle of the medial femoral condyle. It lies posterior to the vastus medialis. (Middle) The long head of biceps femoris forms a posterior aponeurosis on which the fibers of the short head insert. The sciatic nerve has moved medial to the biceps femoris muscle. (Bottom) The tibial and peroneal nerves are distinct within the sciatic nerve from the nerve origin. In the distal thigh, they start to diverge, with the peroneal nerve coursing laterally.

Thigh Radiographic Anatomy and MR Atlas

AXIAL T1 MR, RIGHT DISTAL THIGH

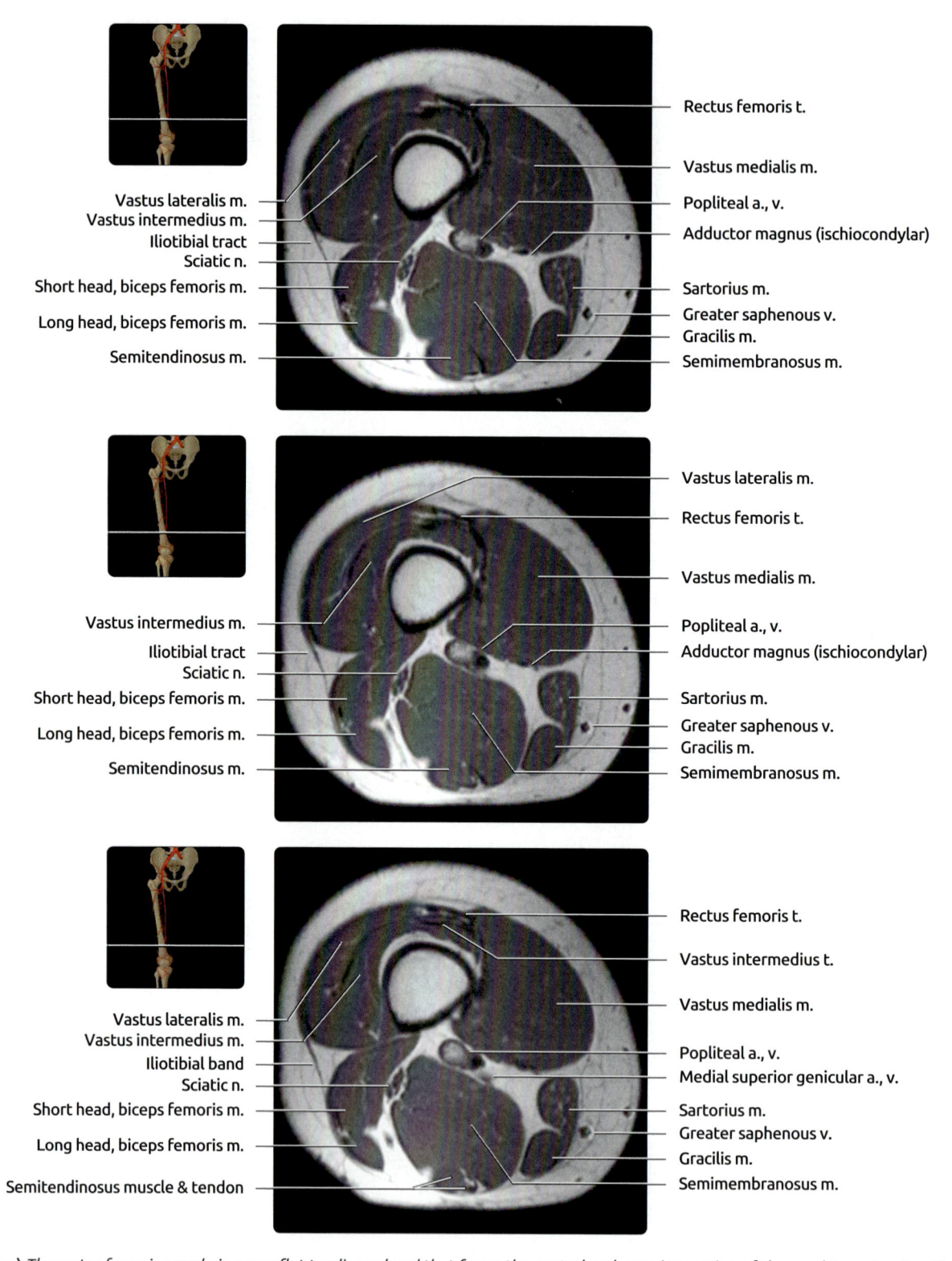

Top image labels (left): Vastus lateralis m.; Vastus intermedius m.; Iliotibial tract; Sciatic n.; Short head, biceps femoris m.; Long head, biceps femoris m.; Semitendinosus m.

Top image labels (right): Rectus femoris t.; Vastus medialis m.; Popliteal a., v.; Adductor magnus (ischiocondylar); Sartorius m.; Greater saphenous v.; Gracilis m.; Semimembranosus m.

Middle image labels (left): Vastus intermedius m.; Iliotibial tract; Sciatic n.; Short head, biceps femoris m.; Long head, biceps femoris m.; Semitendinosus m.

Middle image labels (right): Vastus lateralis m.; Rectus femoris t.; Vastus medialis m.; Popliteal a., v.; Adductor magnus (ischiocondylar); Sartorius m.; Greater saphenous v.; Gracilis m.; Semimembranosus m.

Bottom image labels (left): Vastus lateralis m.; Vastus intermedius m.; Iliotibial band; Sciatic n.; Short head, biceps femoris m.; Long head, biceps femoris m.; Semitendinosus muscle & tendon

Bottom image labels (right): Rectus femoris t.; Vastus intermedius t.; Vastus medialis m.; Popliteal a., v.; Medial superior genicular a., v.; Sartorius m.; Greater saphenous v.; Gracilis m.; Semimembranosus m.

(Top) The rectus femoris muscle is now a flat tendinous band that forms the central and anterior portion of the quadriceps tendon. The vastus medialis obliquus muscle is not a well-defined structure, but simply the most inferior medial portion of the vastus medialis; it has a more horizontal course than the remainder of the muscle. **(Middle)** The sciatic nerve has assumed a bilobed appearance as the common peroneal and tibial nerves separate. On this image, the popliteal vein is lateral to the popliteal artery. The veins and arteries can be identified because a vein will always be larger than its companion artery. The more typical position of the artery is deep to the vein. **(Bottom)** The semitendinosus is tendinous through the distal thigh. Here the tendon is seen along the medial aspect of the residual muscle belly. The long and short heads of the biceps are united via a long aponeurosis.

Thigh Radiographic Anatomy and MR Atlas

AXIAL T1 MR, LEFT DISTAL THIGH

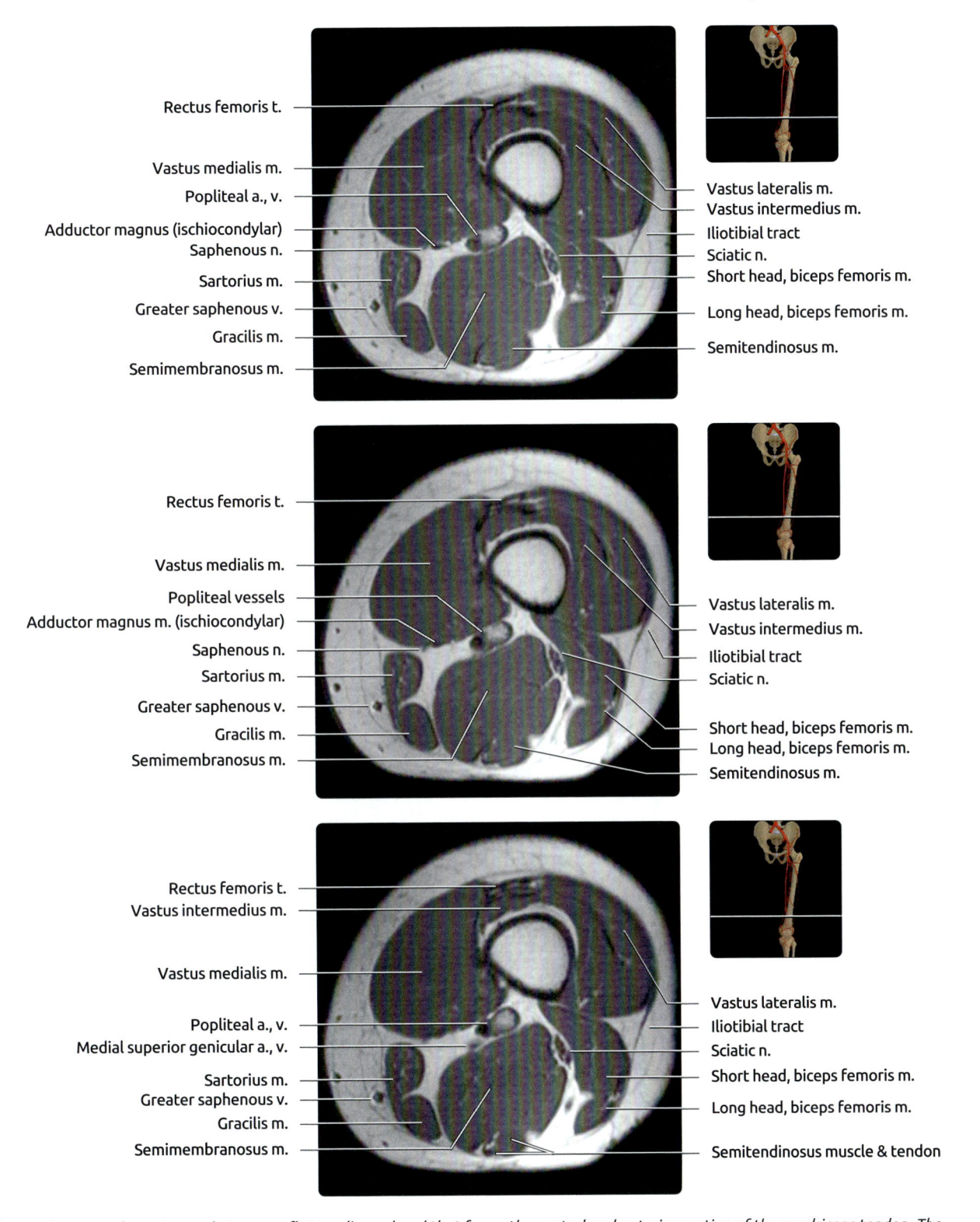

(Top) The rectus femoris muscle is now a flat tendinous band that forms the central and anterior portion of the quadriceps tendon. The vastus medialis obliquus muscle is not a well-defined structure, but simply the most inferior medial portion of the vastus medialis; it has a more horizontal course than the remainder of the muscle. (Middle) The sciatic nerve has assumed a bilobed appearance as the common peroneal and tibial nerves separate. On this image, the popliteal vein is lateral to the popliteal artery. The veins and arteries can be identified because a vein will always be larger than its companion artery. The more typical position of the artery is deep to the vein. (Bottom) The semitendinosus is tendinous through the distal thigh. Here the tendon is seen along the medial aspect of the residual muscle belly. The long and short heads of the biceps are united via a long aponeurosis.

Thigh Radiographic Anatomy and MR Atlas

AXIAL T1 MR, RIGHT DISTAL THIGH

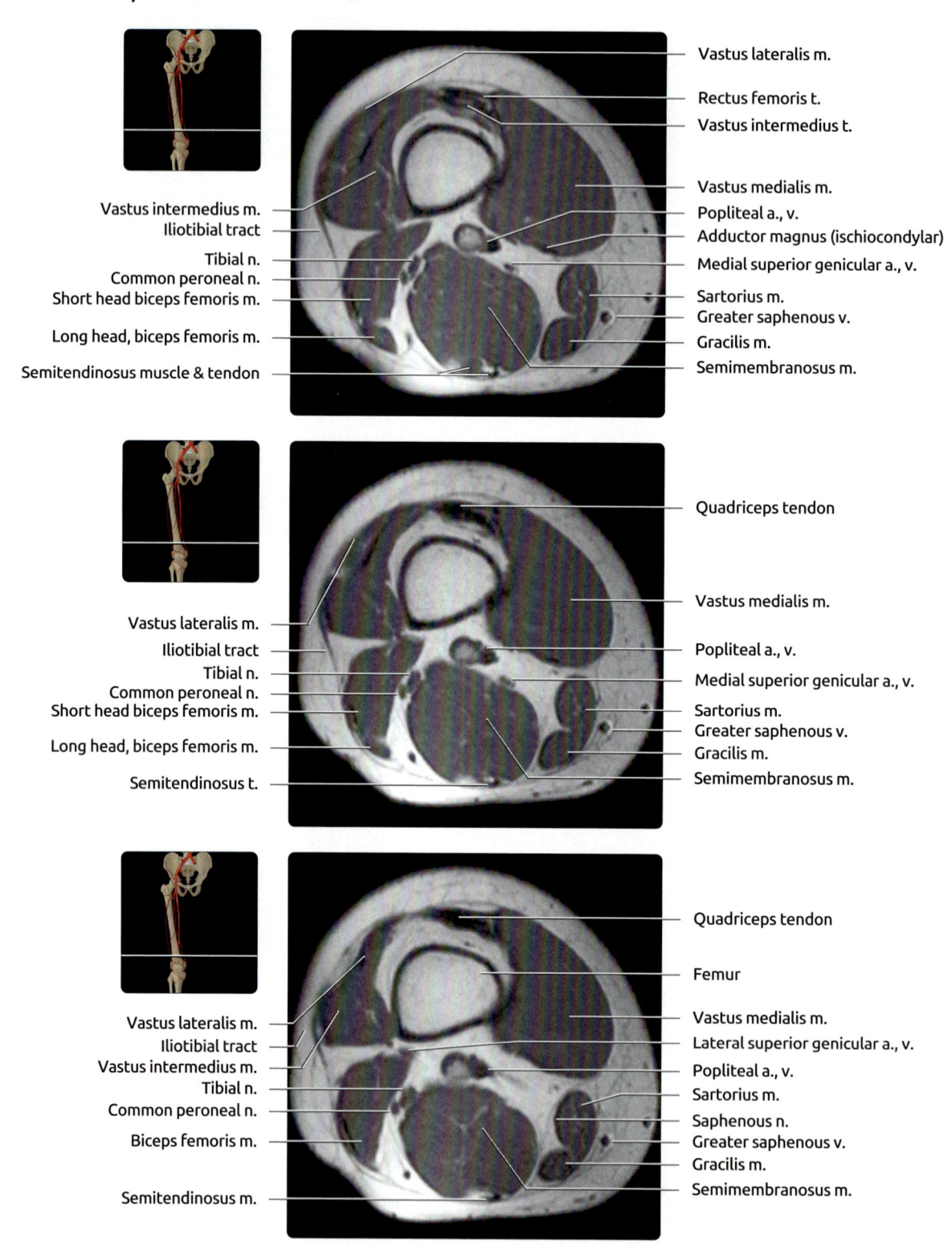

(Top) The sartorius muscle begins to wrap around the gracilis muscle. The medial superior genicular vessels are visible; they are branches of the popliteal vessels. The 2 divisions of the sciatic nerve are now distinct. **(Middle)** Through the distal thigh, the semitendinosus tendon resides along the superficial surface of the semimembranosus muscle. **(Bottom)** Slips from tendons of the vastus medialis, lateralis, intermedius, and rectus femoris muscles join to form the quadriceps tendon. The lateral superior genicular vessels, branches of the popliteal vessels, are present. Saphenous nerve lies deep to sartorius muscle.

Thigh Radiographic Anatomy and MR Atlas

AXIAL T1 MR, LEFT DISTAL THIGH

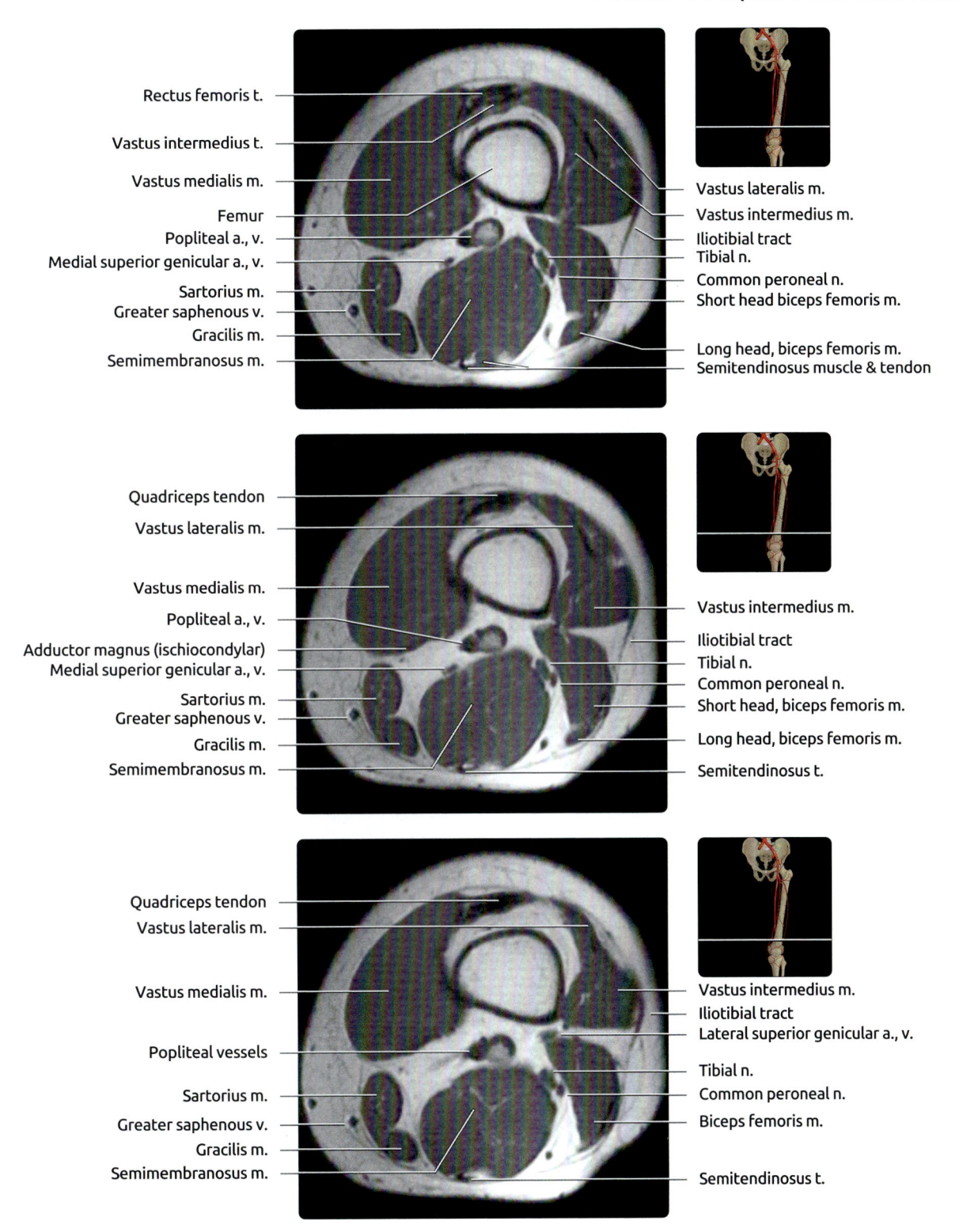

(Top) The sartorius muscle begins to wrap around the gracilis muscle. The medial superior genicular vessels are visible; they are branches of the popliteal vessels. The 2 divisions of the sciatic nerve are now distinct. (Middle) Through the distal thigh, the semitendinosus tendon resides along the superficial surface of the semimembranosus muscle. (Bottom) Slips from tendons of the vastus medialis, lateralis, intermedius, and rectus femoris muscles join to form the quadriceps tendon. The lateral superior genicular vessels, branches of the popliteal vessels, are present. Saphenous nerve lies deep to sartorius muscle.

Thigh Radiographic Anatomy and MR Atlas

AXIAL T1 MR, RIGHT DISTAL THIGH

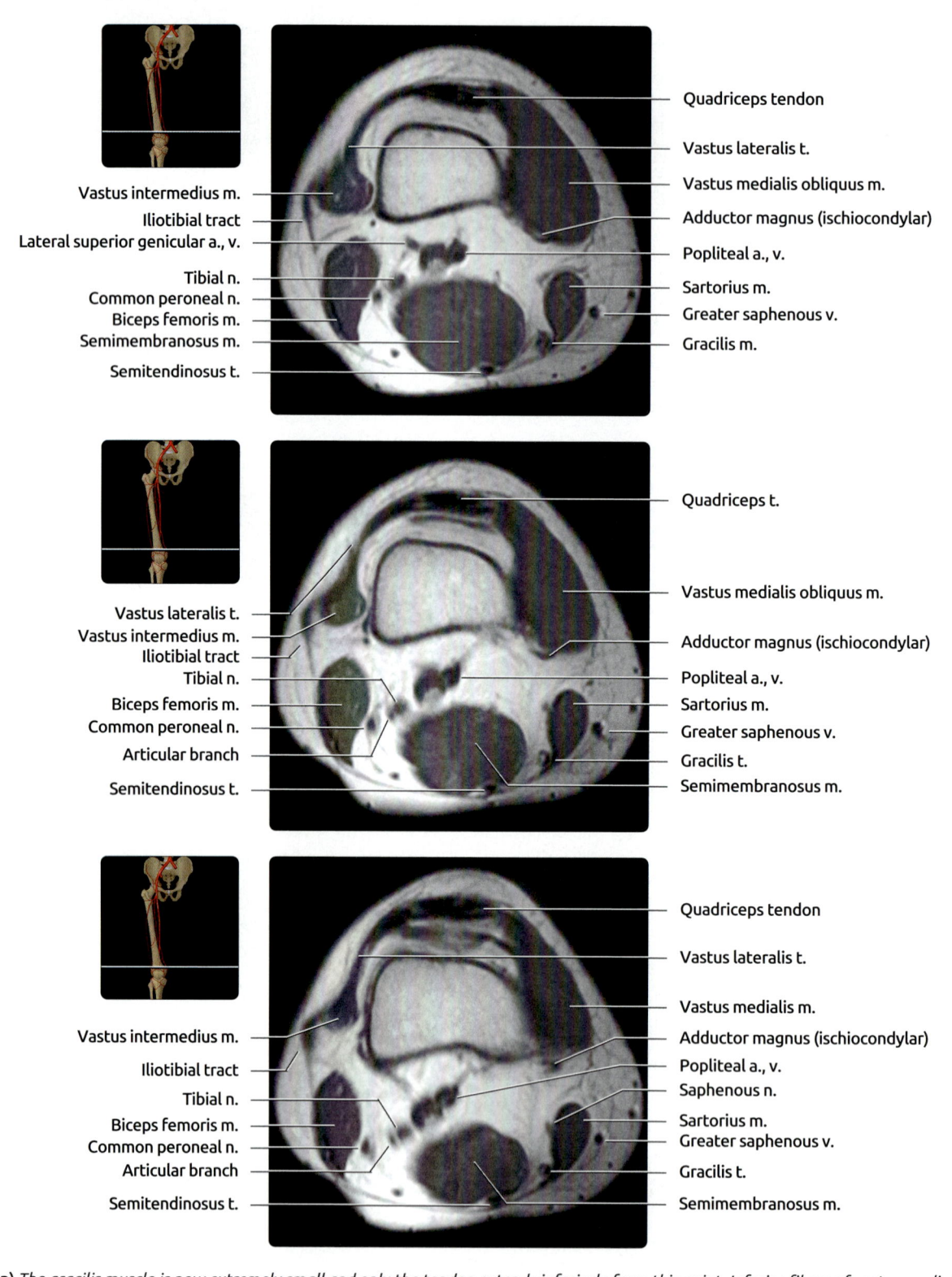

Top image labels:
- Vastus intermedius m.
- Iliotibial tract
- Lateral superior genicular a., v.
- Tibial n.
- Common peroneal n.
- Biceps femoris m.
- Semimembranosus m.
- Semitendinosus t.
- Quadriceps tendon
- Vastus lateralis t.
- Vastus medialis obliquus m.
- Adductor magnus (ischiocondylar)
- Popliteal a., v.
- Sartorius m.
- Greater saphenous v.
- Gracilis m.

Middle image labels:
- Vastus lateralis t.
- Vastus intermedius m.
- Iliotibial tract
- Tibial n.
- Biceps femoris m.
- Common peroneal n.
- Articular branch
- Semitendinosus t.
- Quadriceps t.
- Vastus medialis obliquus m.
- Adductor magnus (ischiocondylar)
- Popliteal a., v.
- Sartorius m.
- Greater saphenous v.
- Gracilis t.
- Semimembranosus m.

Bottom image labels:
- Vastus intermedius m.
- Iliotibial tract
- Tibial n.
- Biceps femoris m.
- Common peroneal n.
- Articular branch
- Semitendinosus t.
- Quadriceps tendon
- Vastus lateralis t.
- Vastus medialis m.
- Adductor magnus (ischiocondylar)
- Popliteal a., v.
- Saphenous n.
- Sartorius m.
- Greater saphenous v.
- Gracilis t.
- Semimembranosus m.

(Top) The gracilis muscle is now extremely small and only the tendon extends inferiorly from this point. Inferior fibers of vastus medialis are known as vastus medialis obliquus muscle. They are not clearly distinct from the remainder of the vastus medialis muscle. **(Middle)** The distance between the semimembranosus and biceps femoris muscles increases in this image through the upper popliteal fossa. An articular branch is seen arising from the tibial nerve. **(Bottom)** The common peroneal nerve is moving lateral along the medial border of the biceps femoris muscle. It will follow this muscle around the fibular head. Note the presence of an articular branch from the tibial nerve. The tibial nerve moves medially and will course through the center of the popliteal fossa. Ischiocondylar portion of adductor magnus is near its insertion on the adductor tubercle of the femur, posterior to the vastus medialis obliquus.

Thigh Radiographic Anatomy and MR Atlas

AXIAL T1 MR, LEFT DISTAL THIGH

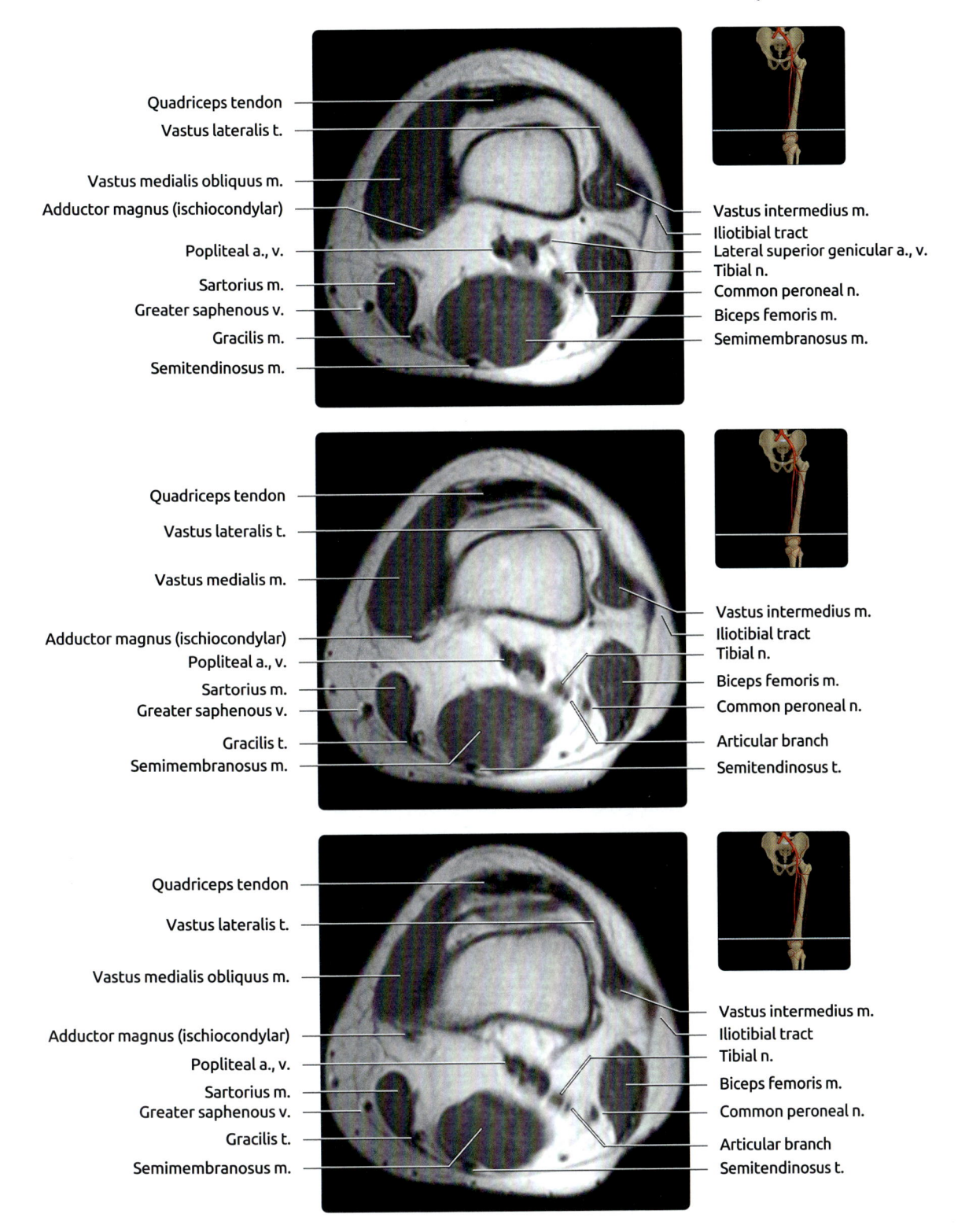

(Top) The gracilis muscle is now extremely small and only the tendon extends inferiorly from this point. Inferior fibers of vastus medialis are known as vastus medialis obliquus muscle. They are not clearly distinct from the remainder of the vastus medialis muscle. *(Middle)* The distance between the semimembranosus and biceps femoris muscles increases in this image through the upper popliteal fossa. An articular branch is seen arising from the tibial nerve. *(Bottom)* The common peroneal nerve is moving laterally along the medial border of the biceps femoris muscle. It will follow this muscle around the fibular head. Note the presence of an articular branch from the tibial nerve. The tibial nerve moves medially and will course through the center of the popliteal fossa. Ischiocondylar portion of adductor magnus is near its insertion on the adductor tubercle of the femur, posterior to the vastus medialis obliquus.

Thigh Radiographic Anatomy and MR Atlas

CORONAL T1 MR, POSTERIOR THIGH

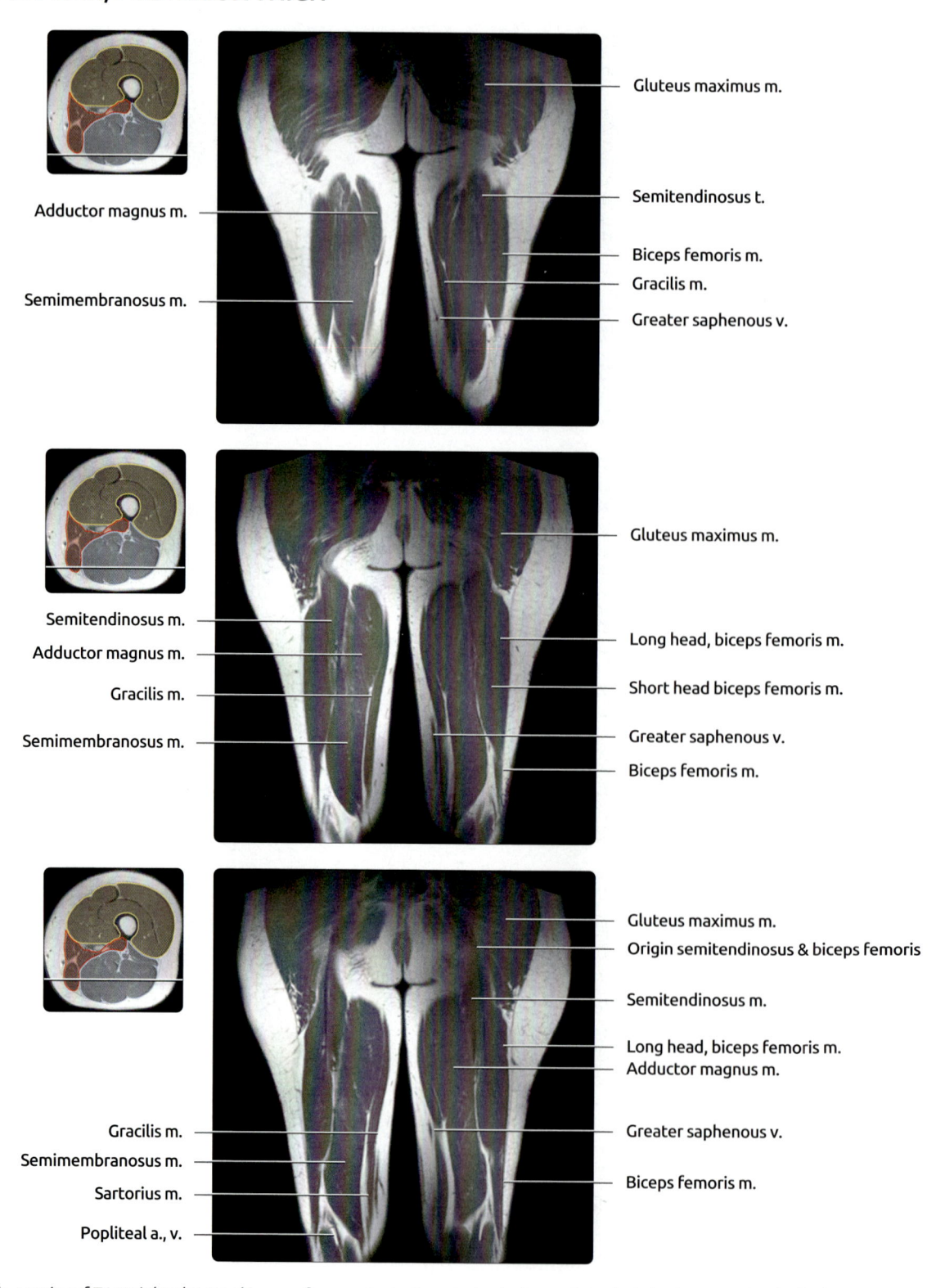

Labels (top image): Adductor magnus m.; Semimembranosus m.; Gluteus maximus m.; Semitendinosus t.; Biceps femoris m.; Gracilis m.; Greater saphenous v.

Labels (middle image): Semitendinosus m.; Adductor magnus m.; Gracilis m.; Semimembranosus m.; Gluteus maximus m.; Long head, biceps femoris m.; Short head biceps femoris m.; Greater saphenous v.; Biceps femoris m.

Labels (bottom image): Gracilis m.; Semimembranosus m.; Sartorius m.; Popliteal a., v.; Gluteus maximus m.; Origin semitendinosus & biceps femoris; Semitendinosus m.; Long head, biceps femoris m.; Adductor magnus m.; Greater saphenous v.; Biceps femoris m.

(Top) First in a series of T1-weighted coronal images from posterior to anterior is shown. Superiorly in the posterior thigh, the semitendinosus muscle is more prominent, whereas inferiorly the semimembranosus muscle is larger and more prominent. (Middle) In this plane, the adductor magnus and semimembranosus muscles are difficult to separate. They can be identified by following their courses more anteriorly. The adductor muscle is more prominent superiorly, the semimembranosus more inferiorly. The greater saphenous vein is the most superficial structure in the medial thigh. (Bottom) The conjoined origin of the biceps and semitendinosus is seen. Semitendinosus courses toward the posteromedial knee, whereas the biceps course posterolaterally.

Thigh Radiographic Anatomy and MR Atlas

CORONAL T1 MR, POSTERIOR THIGH

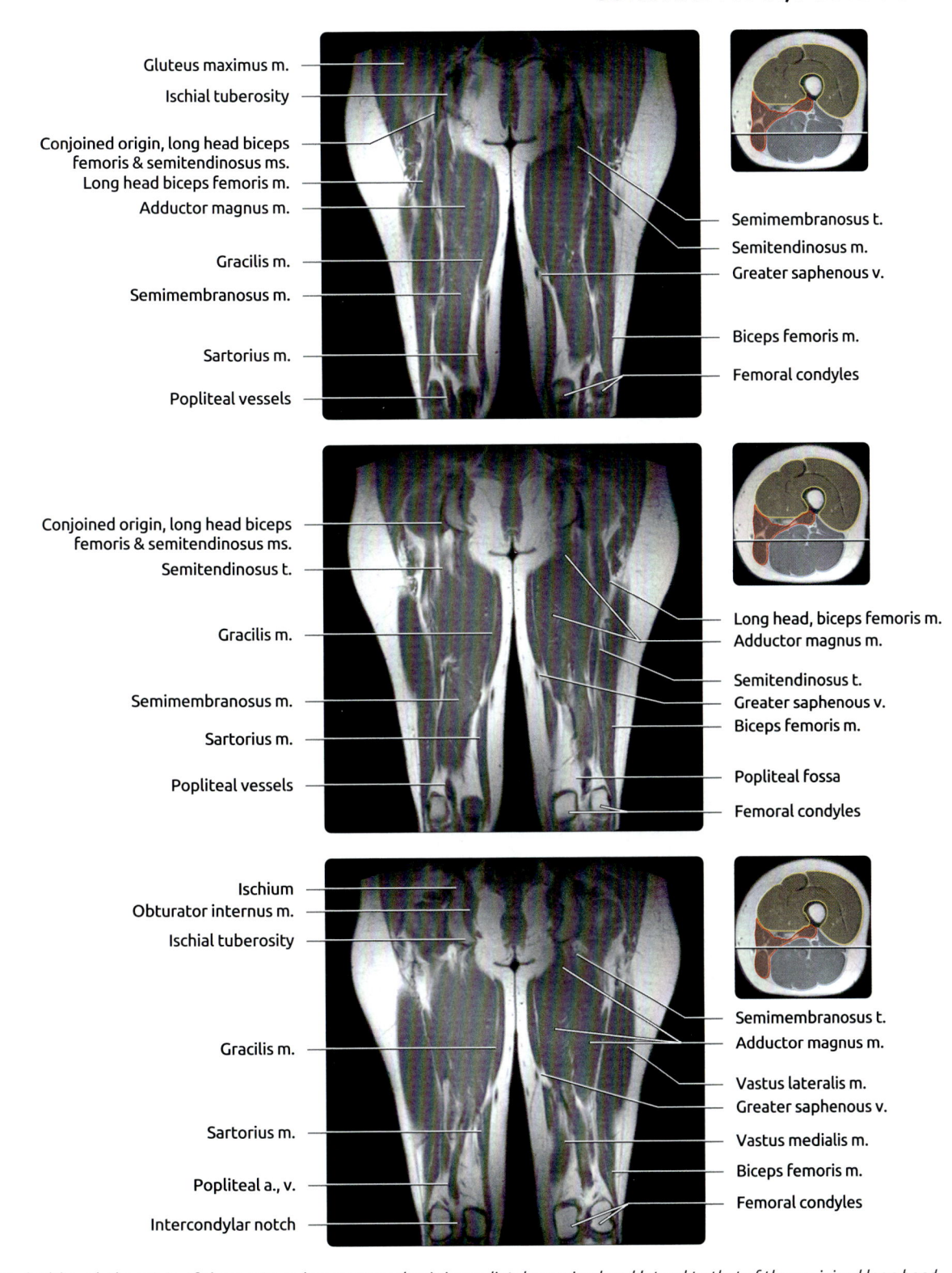

Labels (top image):
- Gluteus maximus m.
- Ischial tuberosity
- Conjoined origin, long head biceps femoris & semitendinosus ms.
- Long head biceps femoris m.
- Adductor magnus m.
- Gracilis m.
- Semimembranosus m.
- Sartorius m.
- Popliteal vessels
- Semimembranosus t.
- Semitendinosus m.
- Greater saphenous v.
- Biceps femoris m.
- Femoral condyles

Labels (middle image):
- Conjoined origin, long head biceps femoris & semitendinosus ms.
- Semitendinosus t.
- Gracilis m.
- Semimembranosus m.
- Sartorius m.
- Popliteal vessels
- Long head, biceps femoris m.
- Adductor magnus m.
- Semitendinosus t.
- Greater saphenous v.
- Biceps femoris m.
- Popliteal fossa
- Femoral condyles

Labels (bottom image):
- Ischium
- Obturator internus m.
- Ischial tuberosity
- Gracilis m.
- Sartorius m.
- Popliteal a., v.
- Intercondylar notch
- Semimembranosus t.
- Adductor magnus m.
- Vastus lateralis m.
- Greater saphenous v.
- Vastus medialis m.
- Biceps femoris m.
- Femoral condyles

(Top) Although the origin of the semimembranosus tendon is immediately proximal and lateral to that of the conjoined long head biceps and semitendinosus tendons, the semimembranosus fairly immediately moves to a more anterior and then medial position relative to the conjoined tendon. The labeled semimembranosus in this image is of the membranous portion, seen just medial to the conjoined origin of the long head of the biceps femoris and semitendinosus muscles. **(Middle)** The origin of the ischiocondylar portion of the adductor magnus muscle from the ischial tuberosity is visible. This muscle is the most medial hamstring. Due to the obliquity of the thigh, portions of both the gracilis and the sartorius muscles are visible. Sartorius remains anterior to gracilis throughout their courses. **(Bottom)** The adductor magnus forms the bulk of the musculature at this level. The vastus lateralis is seen wrapping around the lateral side of the thigh.

Thigh Radiographic Anatomy and MR Atlas

CORONAL T1 MR, MID THIGH

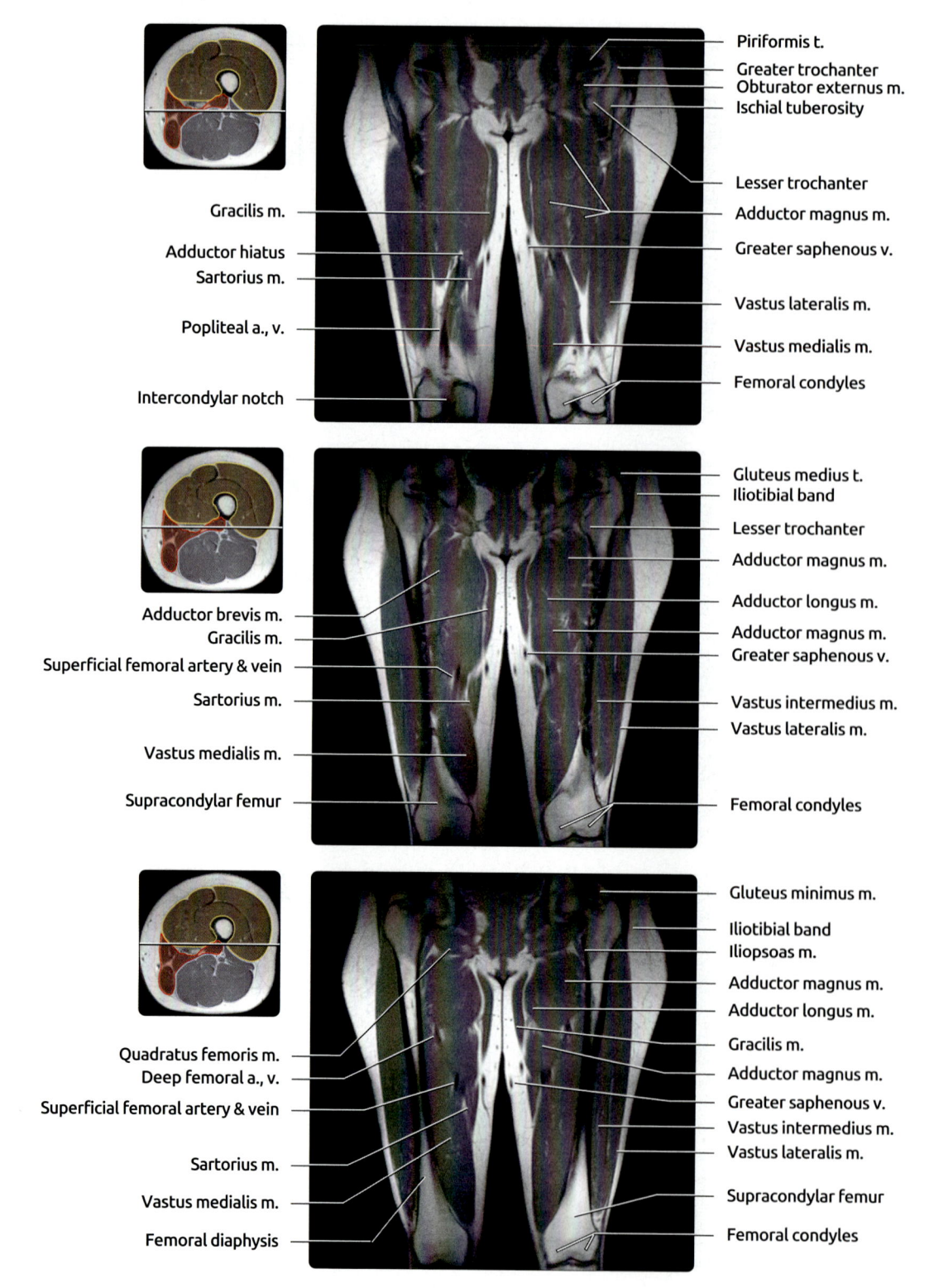

Labels (top image):
- Piriformis t.
- Greater trochanter
- Obturator externus m.
- Ischial tuberosity
- Lesser trochanter
- Adductor magnus m.
- Greater saphenous v.
- Vastus lateralis m.
- Vastus medialis m.
- Femoral condyles
- Gracilis m.
- Adductor hiatus
- Sartorius m.
- Popliteal a., v.
- Intercondylar notch

Labels (middle image):
- Gluteus medius t.
- Iliotibial band
- Lesser trochanter
- Adductor magnus m.
- Adductor longus m.
- Adductor magnus m.
- Greater saphenous v.
- Vastus intermedius m.
- Vastus lateralis m.
- Femoral condyles
- Adductor brevis m.
- Gracilis m.
- Superficial femoral artery & vein
- Sartorius m.
- Vastus medialis m.
- Supracondylar femur

Labels (bottom image):
- Gluteus minimus m.
- Iliotibial band
- Iliopsoas m.
- Adductor magnus m.
- Adductor longus m.
- Gracilis m.
- Adductor magnus m.
- Greater saphenous v.
- Vastus intermedius m.
- Vastus lateralis m.
- Supracondylar femur
- Femoral condyles
- Quadratus femoris m.
- Deep femoral a., v.
- Superficial femoral artery & vein
- Sartorius m.
- Vastus medialis m.
- Femoral diaphysis

(Top) *The separation of the adductor and ischiocondylar portions of the adductor magnus muscle creates the adductor hiatus. The superficial femoral vessels transition to popliteal vessels at this point. Inferior to the adductor hiatus, the ischiocondylar portion of the adductor magnus continues as a thin tendon along the posterior margin of the vastus medialis.* **(Middle)** *Adductor origins from the ischium are visible, and they can be identified by their diverging courses.* **(Bottom)** *The deep and superficial femoral vessels are visualized. The obturator internus and externus muscles are visible on either side of the obturator membrane. The adductor longus muscle is difficult to separate from the adductor magnus muscle.*

Thigh Radiographic Anatomy and MR Atlas

CORONAL T1 MR, MID THIGH

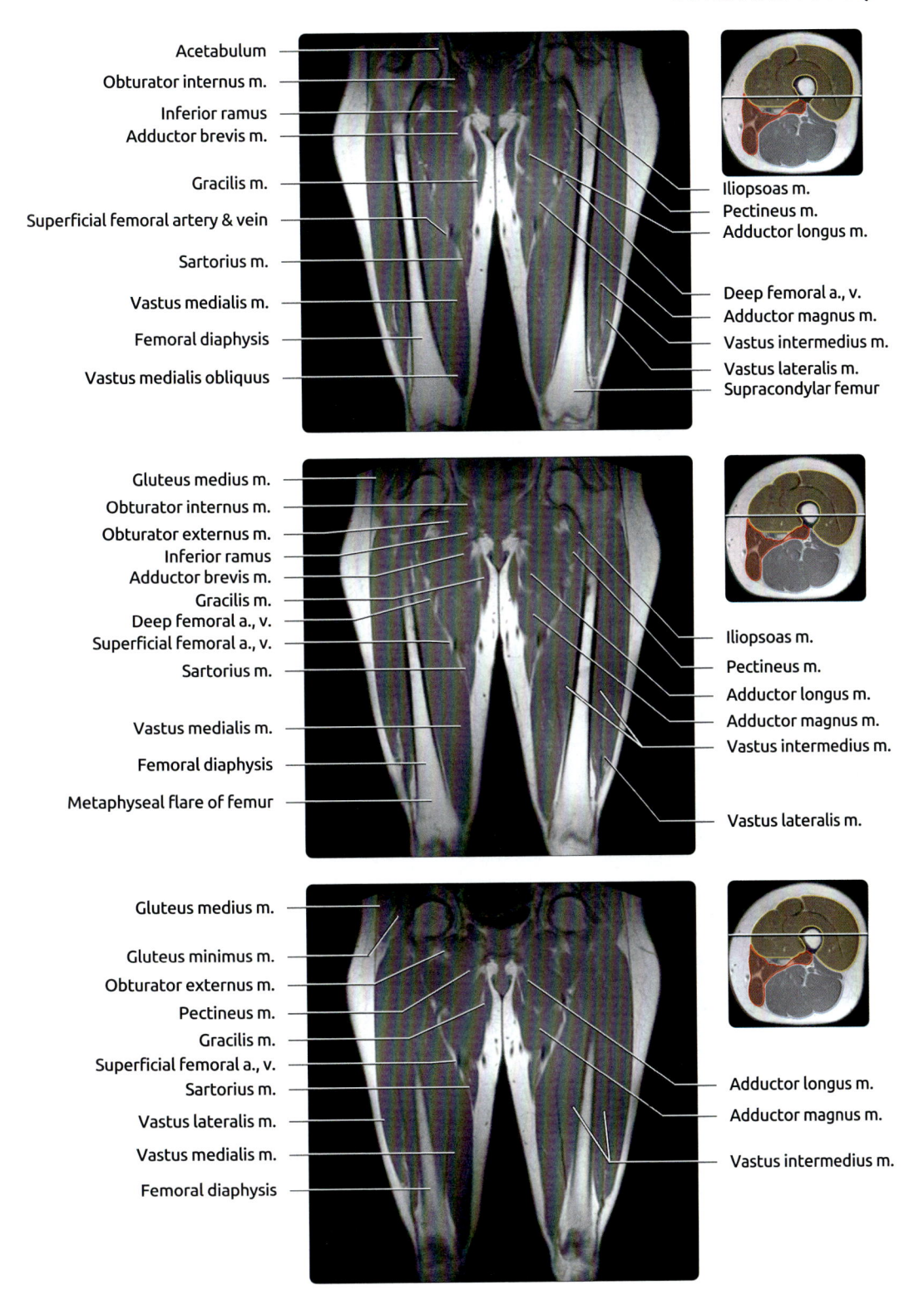

Top image labels (left): Acetabulum; Obturator internus m.; Inferior ramus; Adductor brevis m.; Gracilis m.; Superficial femoral artery & vein; Sartorius m.; Vastus medialis m.; Femoral diaphysis; Vastus medialis obliquus

Top image labels (right): Iliopsoas m.; Pectineus m.; Adductor longus m.; Deep femoral a., v.; Adductor magnus m.; Vastus intermedius m.; Vastus lateralis m.; Supracondylar femur

Middle image labels (left): Gluteus medius m.; Obturator internus m.; Obturator externus m.; Inferior ramus; Adductor brevis m.; Gracilis m.; Deep femoral a., v.; Superficial femoral a., v.; Sartorius m.; Vastus medialis m.; Femoral diaphysis; Metaphyseal flare of femur

Middle image labels (right): Iliopsoas m.; Pectineus m.; Adductor longus m.; Adductor magnus m.; Vastus intermedius m.; Vastus lateralis m.

Bottom image labels (left): Gluteus medius m.; Gluteus minimus m.; Obturator externus m.; Pectineus m.; Gracilis m.; Superficial femoral a., v.; Sartorius m.; Vastus lateralis m.; Vastus medialis m.; Femoral diaphysis

Bottom image labels (right): Adductor longus m.; Adductor magnus m.; Vastus intermedius m.

(**Top**) *The vastus lateralis and medialis are seen wrapping around the femur. The most inferior fibers of the vastus medialis are often called the vastus medialis obliquus but are not separable on MR from the remainder of the muscle.* (**Middle**) *The iliopsoas muscle hugs the medial aspect of the joint as it nears its insertion onto the lesser trochanter. Pectineus will insert on the posterior femur immediately distal to the iliopsoas muscle.* (**Bottom**) *The pectineus and adductor longus muscles are seen in the same coronal plane, and the adductor longus is the more inferior muscle.*

Thigh Radiographic Anatomy and MR Atlas

CORONAL T1 MR, ANTERIOR THIGH

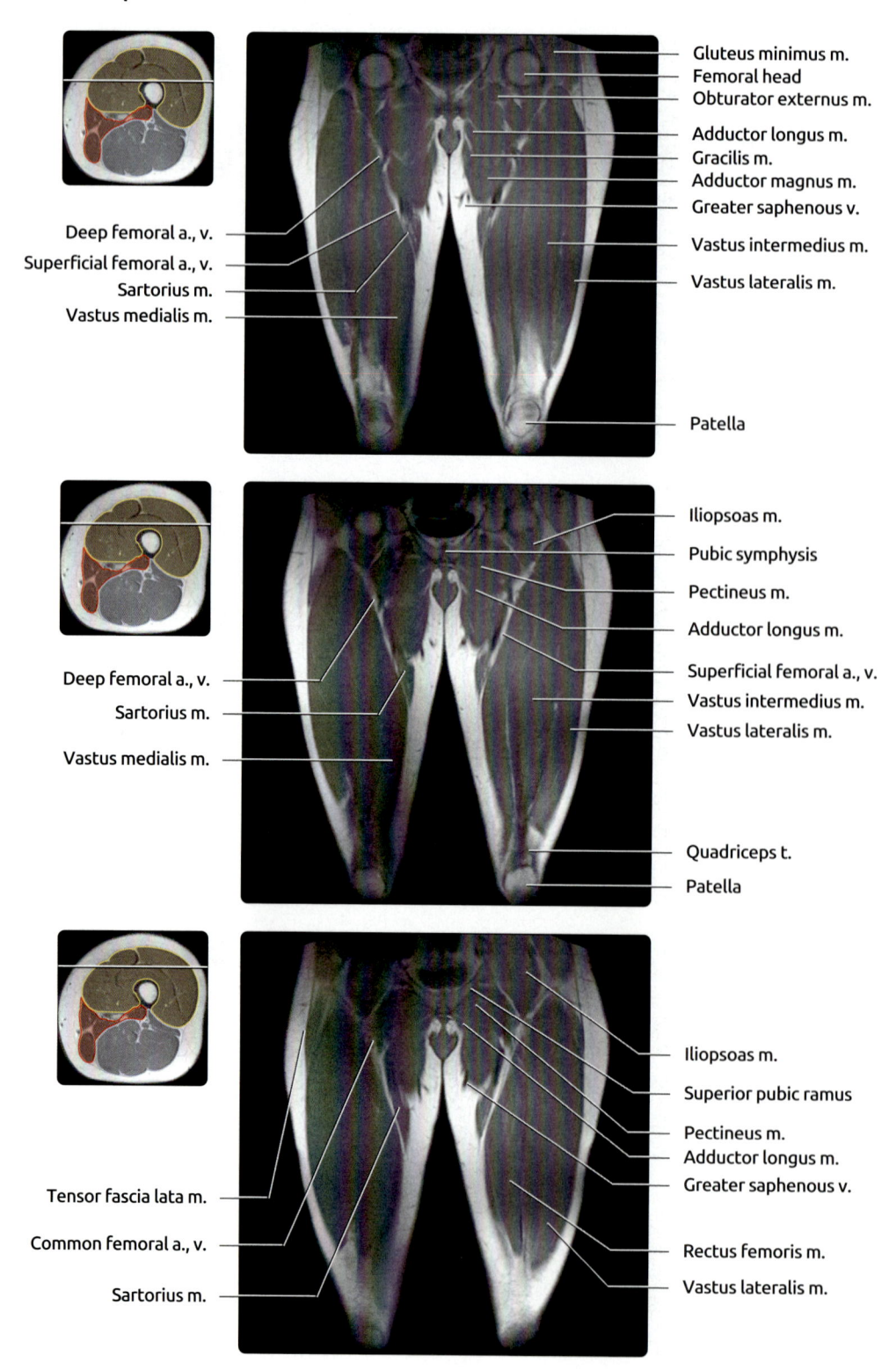

Top image labels:
- Gluteus minimus m.
- Femoral head
- Obturator externus m.
- Adductor longus m.
- Gracilis m.
- Adductor magnus m.
- Greater saphenous v.
- Vastus intermedius m.
- Vastus lateralis m.
- Patella
- Deep femoral a., v.
- Superficial femoral a., v.
- Sartorius m.
- Vastus medialis m.

Middle image labels:
- Iliopsoas m.
- Pubic symphysis
- Pectineus m.
- Adductor longus m.
- Superficial femoral a., v.
- Vastus intermedius m.
- Vastus lateralis m.
- Quadriceps t.
- Patella
- Deep femoral a., v.
- Sartorius m.
- Vastus medialis m.

Bottom image labels:
- Iliopsoas m.
- Superior pubic ramus
- Pectineus m.
- Adductor longus m.
- Greater saphenous v.
- Rectus femoris m.
- Vastus lateralis m.
- Tensor fascia lata m.
- Common femoral a., v.
- Sartorius m.

(Top) The vastus intermedius is immediately anterior to femur, flanked by vastus lateralis and medialis. **(Middle)** The rectus femoris tendon and the tendon of the vastus intermedius tendon blend together in the distal thigh in the plane between the 2 muscles. More distally, with the addition of tendons from the vastus medialis and vastus lateralis muscle, the quadriceps tendon is formed. It maintains a multilaminar structure. **(Bottom)** The iliopsoas muscle is seen as it travels from the pelvis to the lower extremity over the iliopectineal eminence.

Thigh Radiographic Anatomy and MR Atlas

CORONAL T1 MR, ANTERIOR THIGH

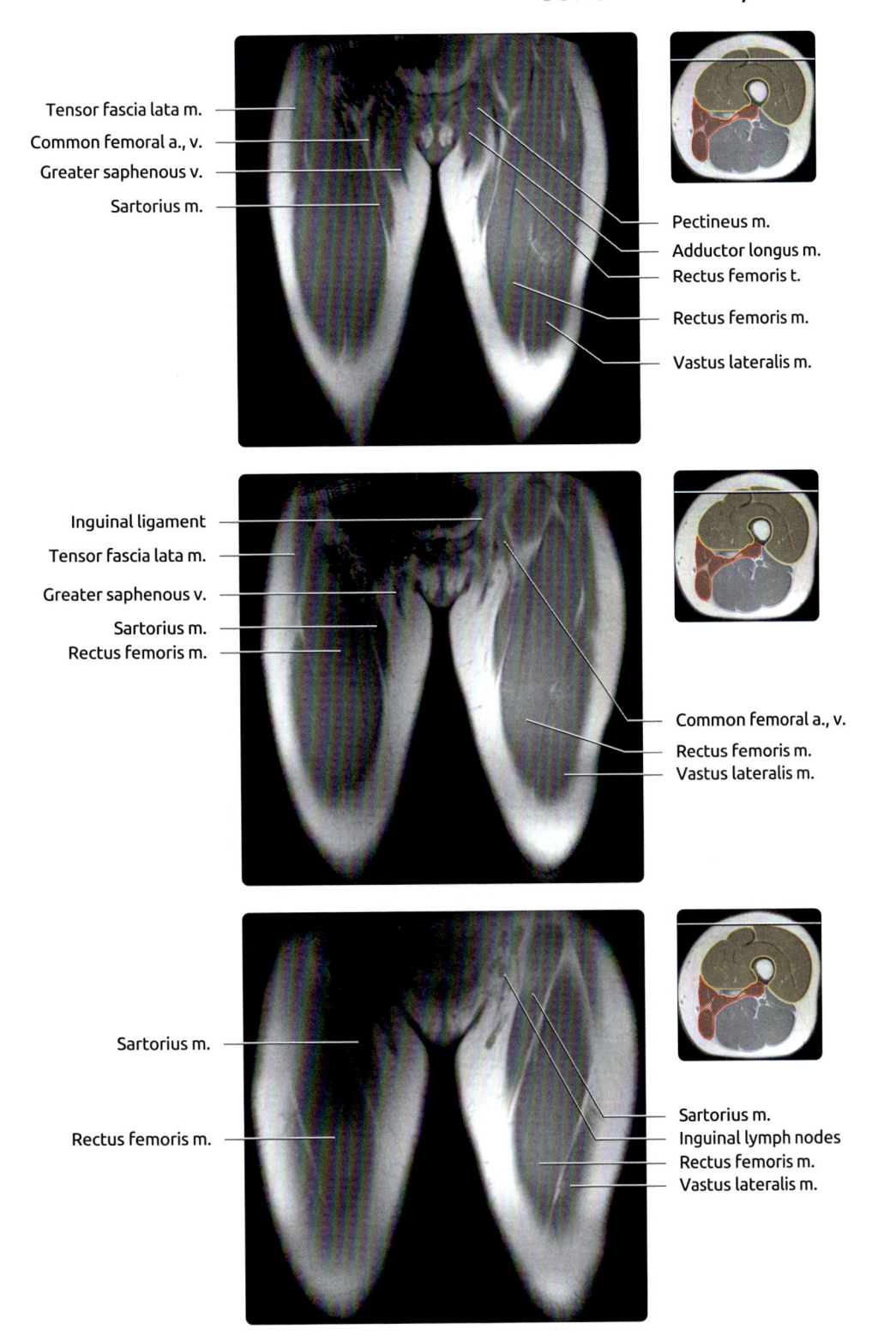

Tensor fascia lata m.
Common femoral a., v.
Greater saphenous v.
Sartorius m.

Pectineus m.
Adductor longus m.
Rectus femoris t.
Rectus femoris m.
Vastus lateralis m.

Inguinal ligament
Tensor fascia lata m.
Greater saphenous v.
Sartorius m.
Rectus femoris m.

Common femoral a., v.
Rectus femoris m.
Vastus lateralis m.

Sartorius m.
Rectus femoris m.

Sartorius m.
Inguinal lymph nodes
Rectus femoris m.
Vastus lateralis m.

(Top) *In the upper thigh, the tendon of the rectus femoris muscle is located along the anterior aspect of the muscle belly. Note that the rectus femoris has a slightly oblique course, paralleling the axis of the femur.* **(Middle)** *The medial edge of the inguinal ligament is nicely seen. The passage of the vessels deep to the ligaments can be visualized.* **(Bottom)** *The lymphatics of the inguinal region are well demonstrated, with a series of lymphatic channels traversing between normal-sized lymph nodes. The anterior-most muscles of the thigh are the sartorius, rectus femoris, and vastus lateralis muscles.*

Thigh Radiographic Anatomy and MR Atlas

SAGITTAL T1 MR, MEDIAL THIGH

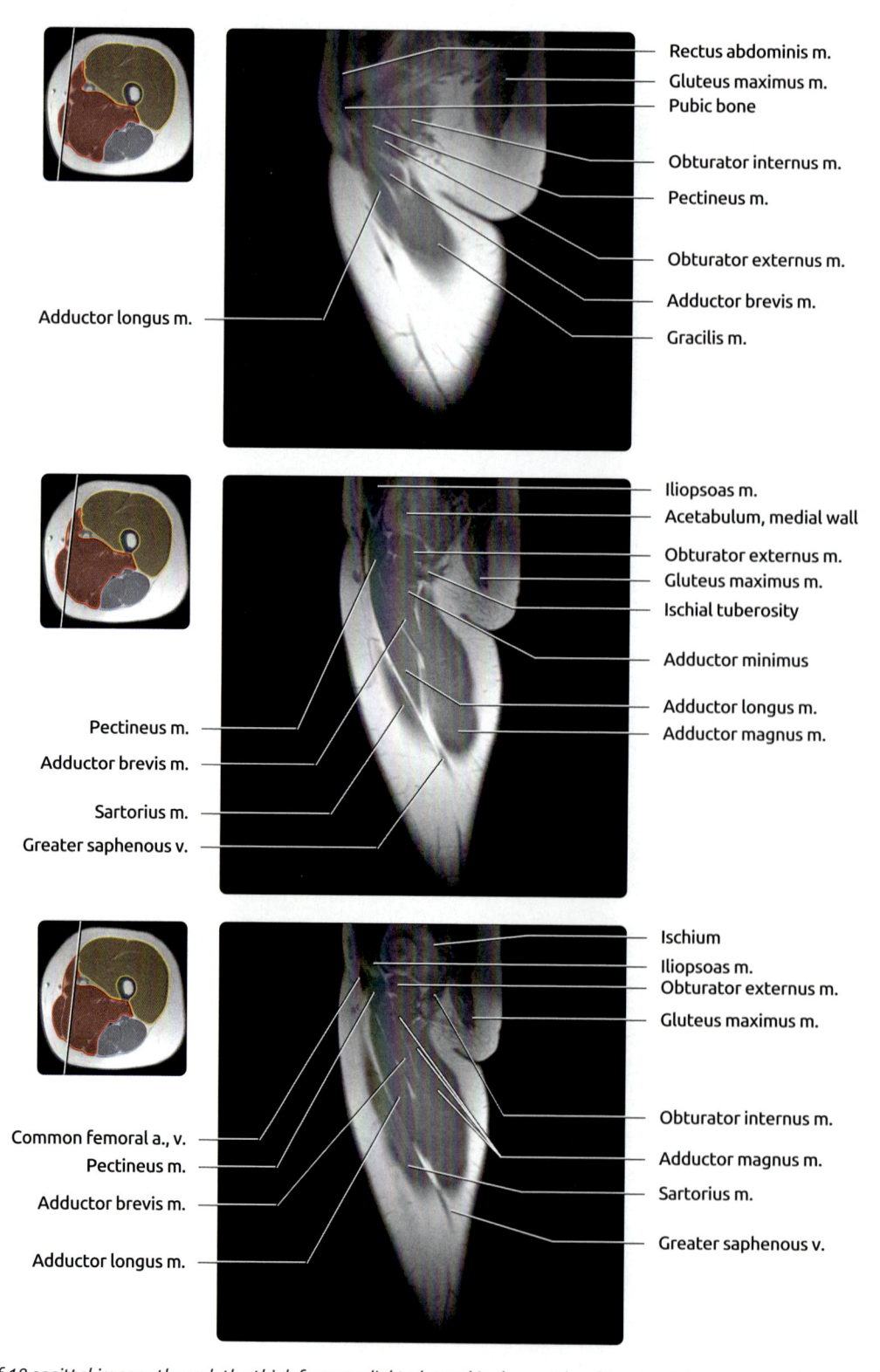

Rectus abdominis m.
Gluteus maximus m.
Pubic bone
Obturator internus m.
Pectineus m.
Obturator externus m.
Adductor brevis m.
Gracilis m.

Adductor longus m.

Iliopsoas m.
Acetabulum, medial wall
Obturator externus m.
Gluteus maximus m.
Ischial tuberosity
Adductor minimus
Adductor longus m.
Adductor magnus m.

Pectineus m.
Adductor brevis m.
Sartorius m.
Greater saphenous v.

Ischium
Iliopsoas m.
Obturator externus m.
Gluteus maximus m.
Obturator internus m.
Adductor magnus m.
Sartorius m.
Greater saphenous v.

Common femoral a., v.
Pectineus m.
Adductor brevis m.
Adductor longus m.

(Top) *First of 18 sagittal images through the thigh from medial to lateral is shown. The obturator internus muscle is seen en face. The long tendinous origin of the adductor longus muscle is well depicted on this image. The adductor brevis muscle is deep to the adductor longus muscle.* **(Middle)** *The relative positions of the adductor muscles are well seen on this image. The short, horizontal fibers of the adductor magnus are often called the adductor minimus.* **(Bottom)** *A long segment of the sartorius muscle is seen on the anterior aspect of this medial image. As it courses from its origin on the anterior superior iliac spine to its insertion as part of the pes anserinus on the medial tibia, it crosses a number of muscles and occupies a separate fascial compartment. The iliopsoas muscle travels from the pelvis to the thigh over the iliopectineal junction.*

Thigh Radiographic Anatomy and MR Atlas

SAGITTAL T1 MR, MEDIAL THIGH

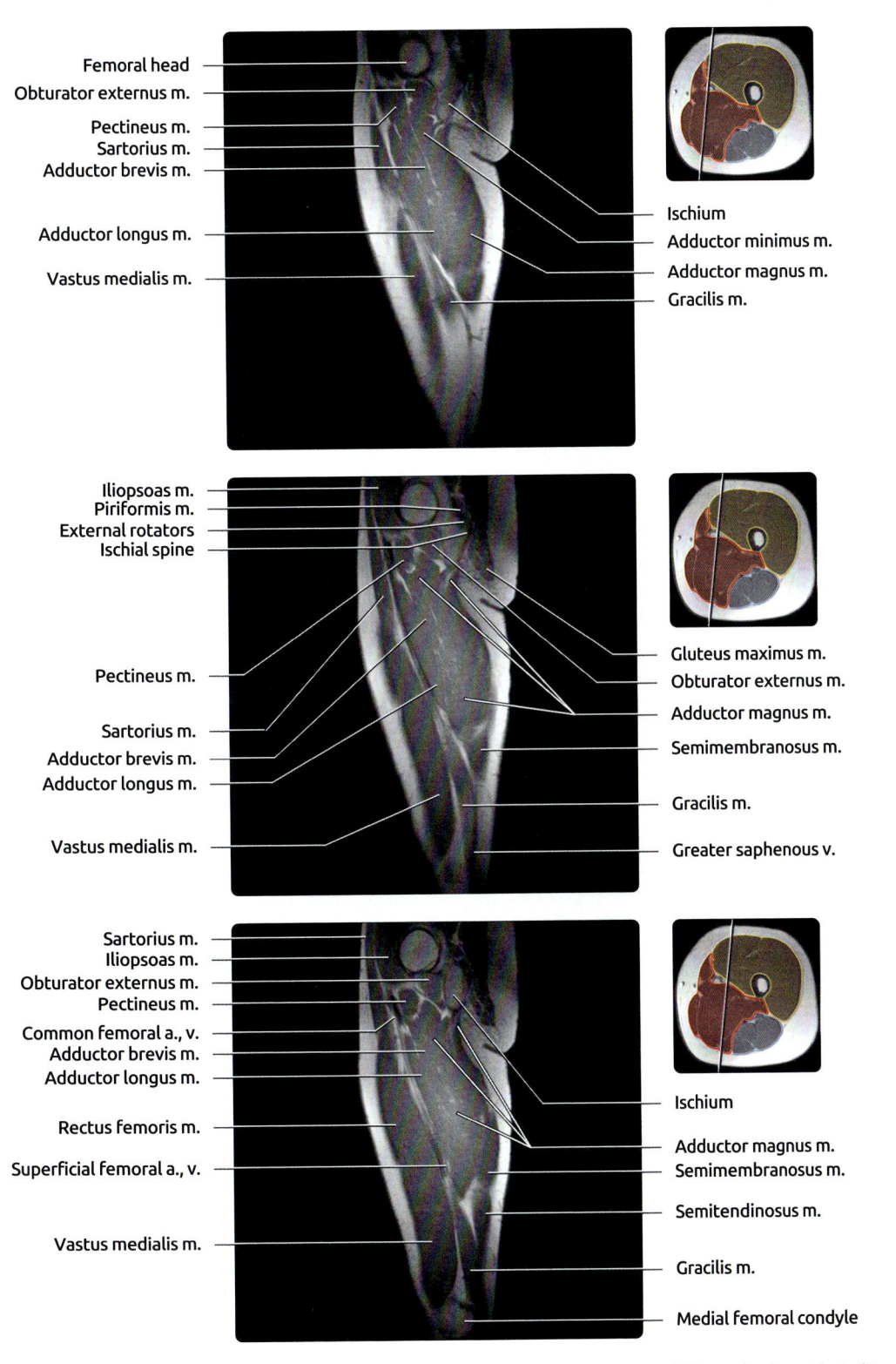

Labels (top image):
- Femoral head
- Obturator externus m.
- Pectineus m.
- Sartorius m.
- Adductor brevis m.
- Adductor longus m.
- Vastus medialis m.
- Ischium
- Adductor minimus m.
- Adductor magnus m.
- Gracilis m.

Labels (middle image):
- Iliopsoas m.
- Piriformis m.
- External rotators
- Ischial spine
- Pectineus m.
- Sartorius m.
- Adductor brevis m.
- Adductor longus m.
- Vastus medialis m.
- Gluteus maximus m.
- Obturator externus m.
- Adductor magnus m.
- Semimembranosus m.
- Gracilis m.
- Greater saphenous v.

Labels (bottom image):
- Sartorius m.
- Iliopsoas m.
- Obturator externus m.
- Pectineus m.
- Common femoral a., v.
- Adductor brevis m.
- Adductor longus m.
- Rectus femoris m.
- Superficial femoral a., v.
- Vastus medialis m.
- Ischium
- Adductor magnus m.
- Semimembranosus m.
- Semitendinosus m.
- Gracilis m.
- Medial femoral condyle

(Top) The adductor magnus muscle occupies a large portion of the medial thigh. The short, horizontal fibers arise from the ischiopubic ramus and are often called the adductor minimus. They lie inferior to the obturator externus. **(Middle)** The 2 origins of the adductor magnus muscle are visible. The ischiocondylar portion arises from the ischial tuberosity, whereas the adductor portion (a.k.a. the adductor minimus) of the muscle originates from the ischiopubic ramus. The vastus medialis muscle is also a large muscle along the medial thigh. **(Bottom)** The inferior course of the gracilis muscle is seen as it nears its insertion onto the tibia. The course of the superficial femoral vessels in the mid thigh is easily appreciated.

Thigh Radiographic Anatomy and MR Atlas

SAGITTAL T1 MR, CENTRAL THIGH

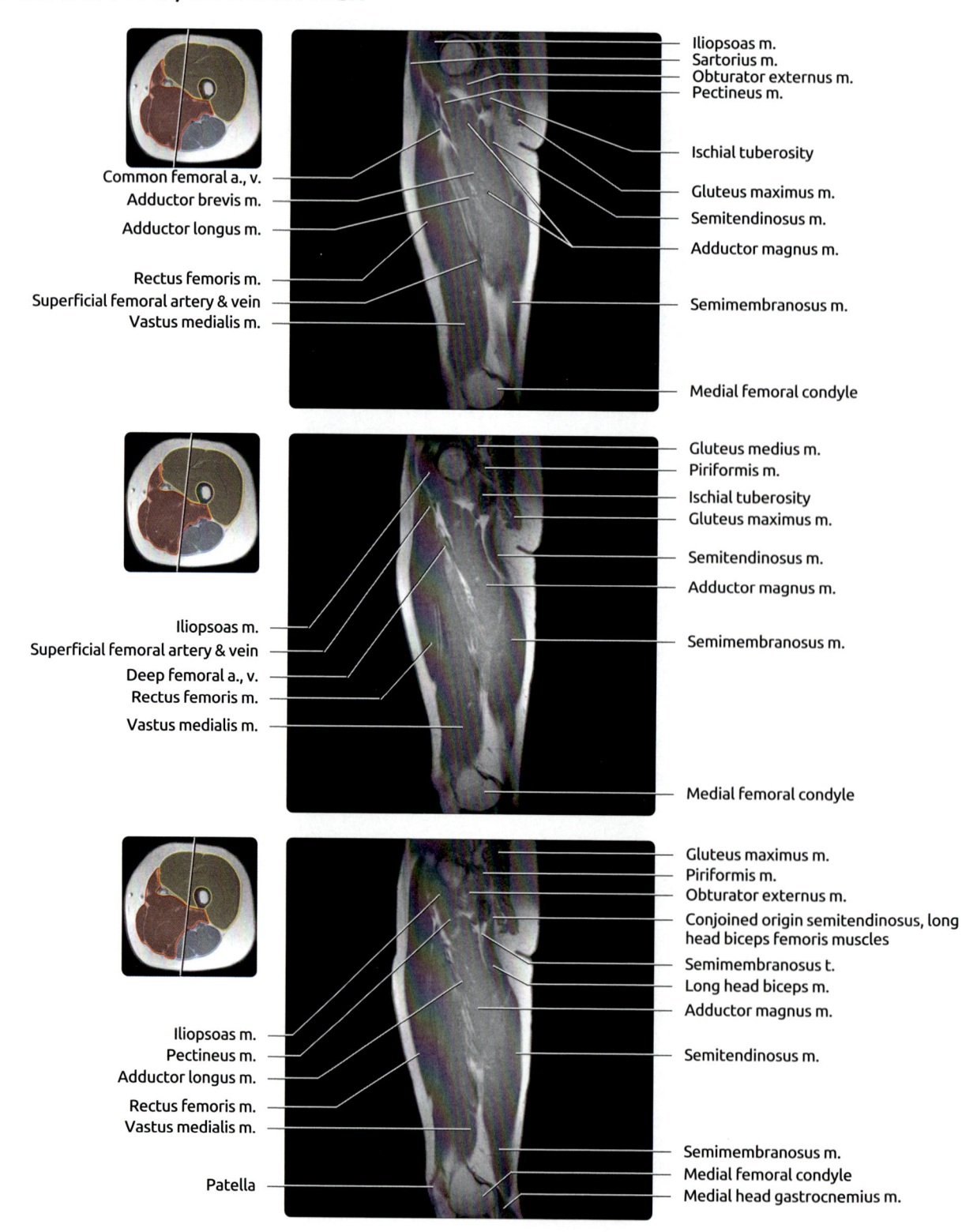

Labels (top image):
- Common femoral a., v.
- Adductor brevis m.
- Adductor longus m.
- Rectus femoris m.
- Superficial femoral artery & vein
- Vastus medialis m.
- Iliopsoas m.
- Sartorius m.
- Obturator externus m.
- Pectineus m.
- Ischial tuberosity
- Gluteus maximus m.
- Semitendinosus m.
- Adductor magnus m.
- Semimembranosus m.
- Medial femoral condyle

Labels (middle image):
- Iliopsoas m.
- Superficial femoral artery & vein
- Deep femoral a., v.
- Rectus femoris m.
- Vastus medialis m.
- Gluteus medius m.
- Piriformis m.
- Ischial tuberosity
- Gluteus maximus m.
- Semitendinosus m.
- Adductor magnus m.
- Semimembranosus m.
- Medial femoral condyle

Labels (bottom image):
- Iliopsoas m.
- Pectineus m.
- Adductor longus m.
- Rectus femoris m.
- Vastus medialis m.
- Patella
- Gluteus maximus m.
- Piriformis m.
- Obturator externus m.
- Conjoined origin semitendinosus, long head biceps femoris muscles
- Semimembranosus t.
- Long head biceps m.
- Adductor magnus m.
- Semitendinosus m.
- Semimembranosus m.
- Medial femoral condyle
- Medial head gastrocnemius m.

(Top) *The semimembranosus has a thin, membranous origin and forms a large muscle that lies medial to the semitendinosus in the mid thigh and anterior to the semitendinosus tendon in the distal thigh. In the mid thigh, they are difficult to distinguish on sagittal images but easily separated on axial images.* **(Middle)** *The common femoral vessels have divided into superficial and deep femoral vessels. The superficial vessels course medially, whereas the deep femoral vessels are seen on this image as they head more laterally.* **(Bottom)** *The rectus femoris muscle occupies the anterior aspect of the thigh. The relationship between the origins of the semimembranosus tendon and the conjoint origin of the semitendinosus and long head biceps femoris tendon is well shown on this image.*

Thigh Radiographic Anatomy and MR Atlas

SAGITTAL T1 MR, CENTRAL THIGH

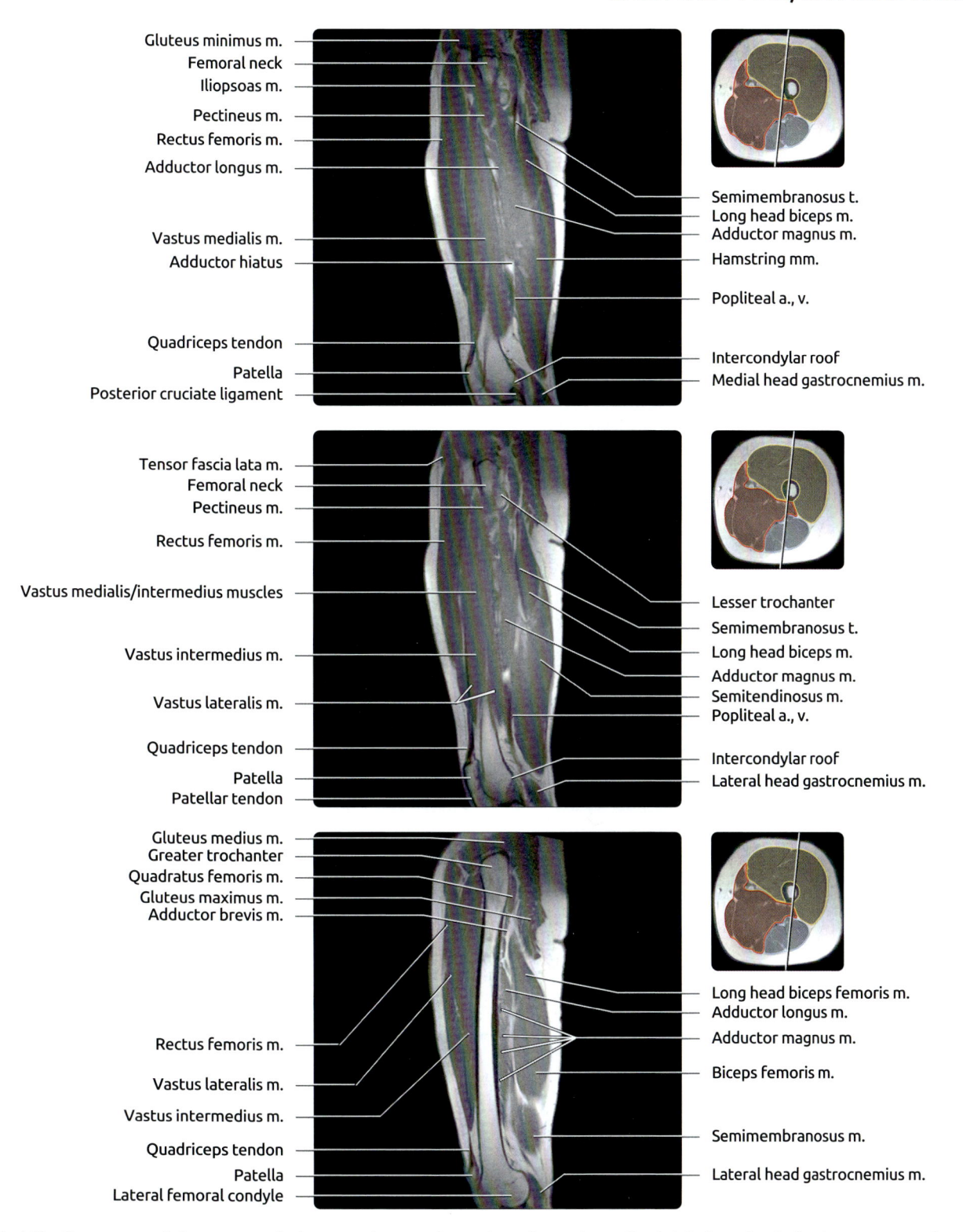

Labels (Top image):
- Gluteus minimus m.
- Femoral neck
- Iliopsoas m.
- Pectineus m.
- Rectus femoris m.
- Adductor longus m.
- Vastus medialis m.
- Adductor hiatus
- Quadriceps tendon
- Patella
- Posterior cruciate ligament
- Semimembranosus t.
- Long head biceps m.
- Adductor magnus m.
- Hamstring mm.
- Popliteal a., v.
- Intercondylar roof
- Medial head gastrocnemius m.

Labels (Middle image):
- Tensor fascia lata m.
- Femoral neck
- Pectineus m.
- Rectus femoris m.
- Vastus medialis/intermedius muscles
- Vastus intermedius m.
- Vastus lateralis m.
- Quadriceps tendon
- Patella
- Patellar tendon
- Lesser trochanter
- Semimembranosus t.
- Long head biceps m.
- Adductor magnus m.
- Semitendinosus m.
- Popliteal a., v.
- Intercondylar roof
- Lateral head gastrocnemius m.

Labels (Bottom image):
- Gluteus medius m.
- Greater trochanter
- Quadratus femoris m.
- Gluteus maximus m.
- Adductor brevis m.
- Rectus femoris m.
- Vastus lateralis m.
- Vastus intermedius m.
- Quadriceps tendon
- Patella
- Lateral femoral condyle
- Long head biceps femoris m.
- Adductor longus m.
- Adductor magnus m.
- Biceps femoris m.
- Semimembranosus m.
- Lateral head gastrocnemius m.

(Top) The iliopsoas muscle inserts onto the lesser trochanter. The pectineus inserts immediately inferior to it. The laminar structure of the quadriceps tendon as it receives contributions from the rectus femoris, vastus medialis, vastus lateralis, and vastus intermedius is well seen. (Middle) The transition from vastus medialis to vastus intermedius is difficult to appreciate and is mostly recognized by anatomic position. The vastus intermedius originates from the anterior surface of the mid to distal femur. The junction of the membranous portion of the semimembranous muscle and its muscle belly is well seen on this image. (Bottom) The sciatic nerve is present along the deep surface of the long head of the biceps femoris muscle. Semimembranosus, semitendinosus, and biceps femoris muscles are adjacent to each other and not readily separable in the sagittal plane, except by relative position.

Thigh Radiographic Anatomy and MR Atlas

SAGITTAL T1 MR, CENTRAL THIGH

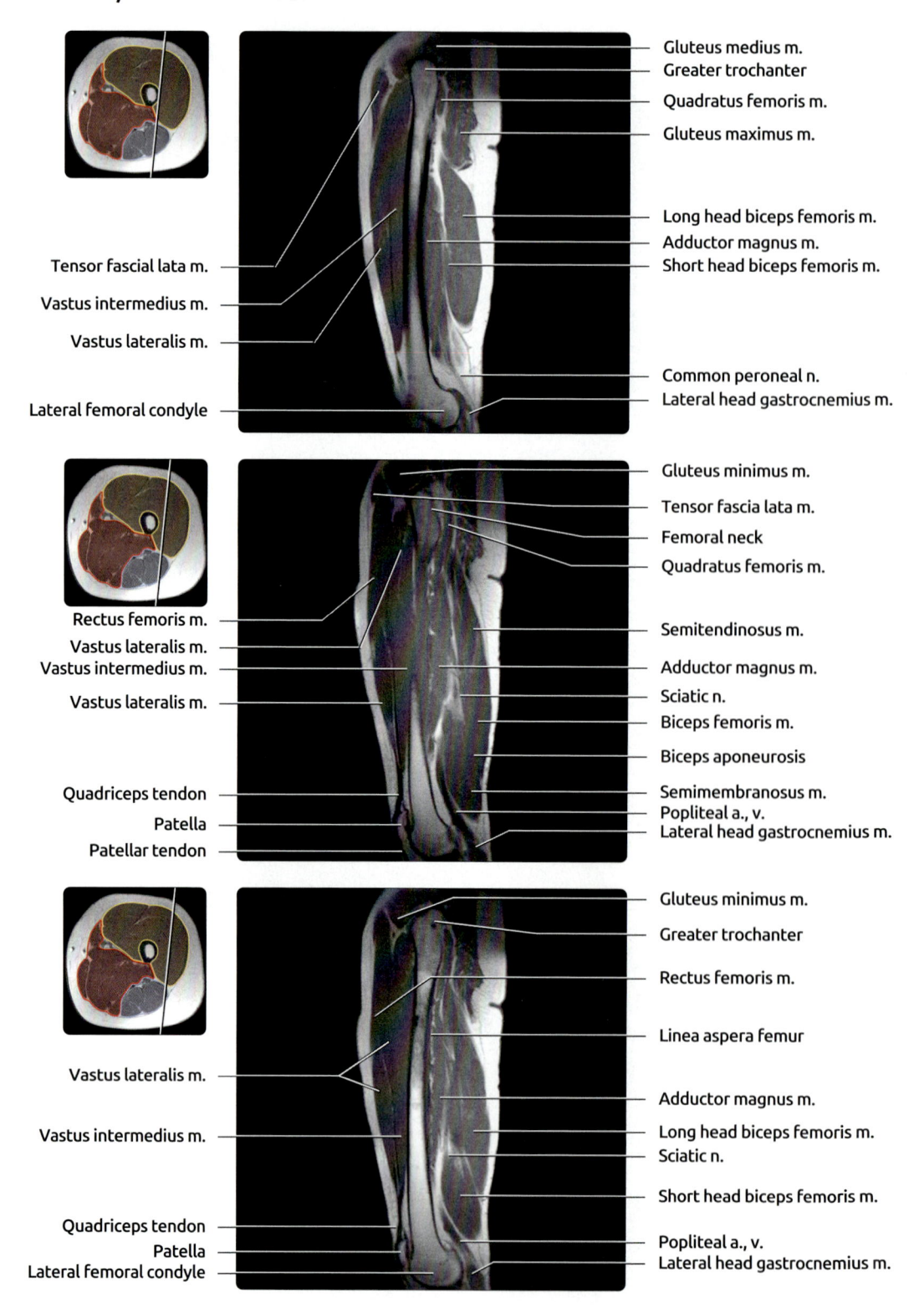

Labels (top image):
- Gluteus medius m.
- Greater trochanter
- Quadratus femoris m.
- Gluteus maximus m.
- Long head biceps femoris m.
- Adductor magnus m.
- Short head biceps femoris m.
- Common peroneal n.
- Lateral head gastrocnemius m.
- Tensor fascial lata m.
- Vastus intermedius m.
- Vastus lateralis m.
- Lateral femoral condyle

Labels (middle image):
- Gluteus minimus m.
- Tensor fascia lata m.
- Femoral neck
- Quadratus femoris m.
- Semitendinosus m.
- Adductor magnus m.
- Sciatic n.
- Biceps femoris m.
- Biceps aponeurosis
- Semimembranosus m.
- Popliteal a., v.
- Lateral head gastrocnemius m.
- Rectus femoris m.
- Vastus lateralis m.
- Vastus intermedius m.
- Vastus lateralis m.
- Quadriceps tendon
- Patella
- Patellar tendon

Labels (bottom image):
- Gluteus minimus m.
- Greater trochanter
- Rectus femoris m.
- Linea aspera femur
- Adductor magnus m.
- Long head biceps femoris m.
- Sciatic n.
- Short head biceps femoris m.
- Popliteal a., v.
- Lateral head gastrocnemius m.
- Vastus lateralis m.
- Vastus intermedius m.
- Quadriceps tendon
- Patella
- Lateral femoral condyle

(**Top**) *The short head of biceps femoris muscle arises in the mid femur. The sciatic nerve is seen bisecting the popliteal fossa.* (**Middle**) *The sciatic nerve lies anterior to biceps femoris muscle.* (**Bottom**) *The long head of the biceps femoris muscle can be seen adjacent to the short head. The long head terminates in an aponeurosis, into which the short head inserts. The aponeurosis then forms the rounded biceps tendon, which will insert on the lateral margin of the fibular head and on the lateral condyle of the tibia.*

Thigh Radiographic Anatomy and MR Atlas

SAGITTAL T1 MR, LATERAL THIGH

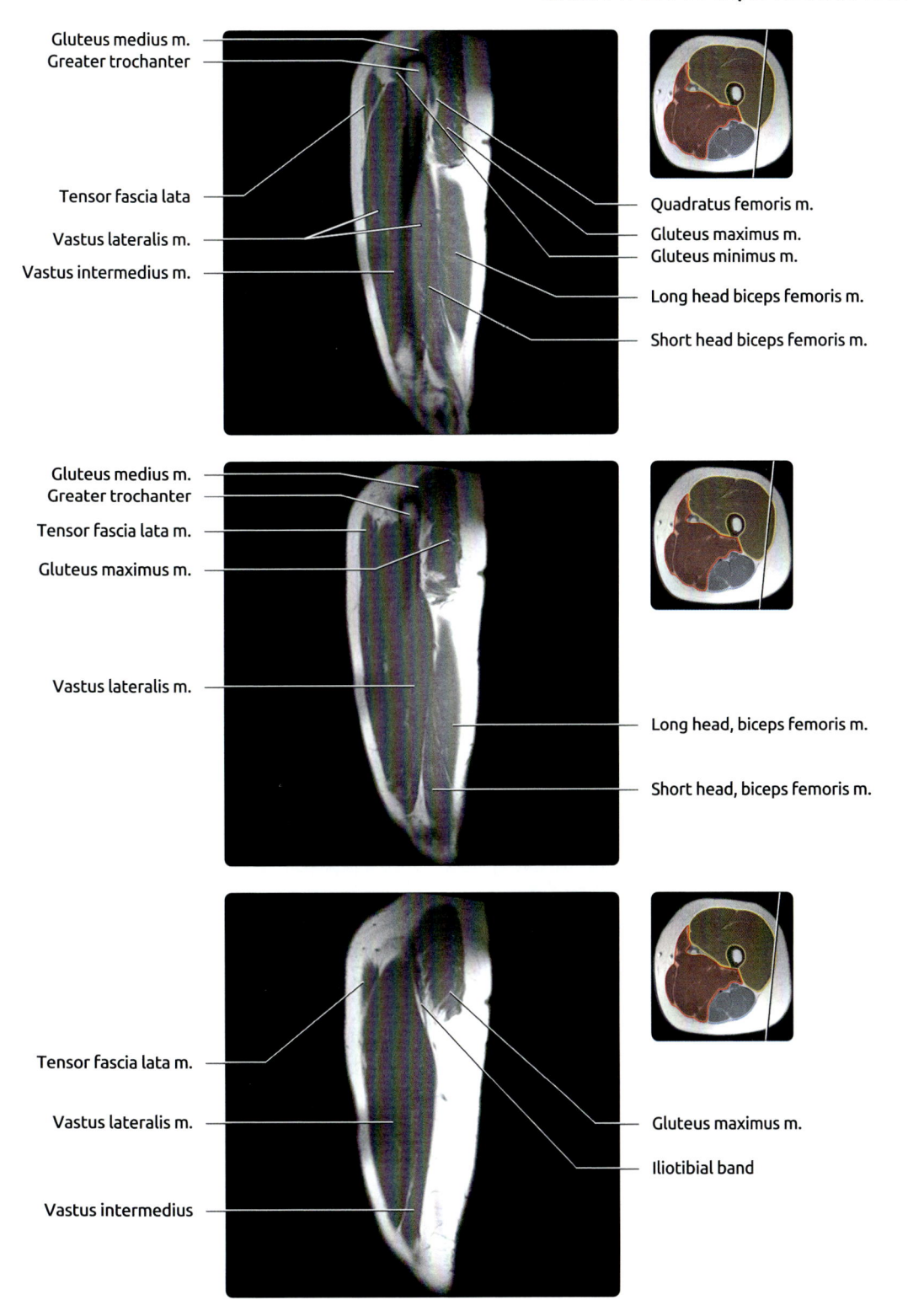

Top image labels:
- Gluteus medius m.
- Greater trochanter
- Tensor fascia lata
- Vastus lateralis m.
- Vastus intermedius m.
- Quadratus femoris m.
- Gluteus maximus m.
- Gluteus minimus m.
- Long head biceps femoris m.
- Short head biceps femoris m.

Middle image labels:
- Gluteus medius m.
- Greater trochanter
- Tensor fascia lata m.
- Gluteus maximus m.
- Vastus lateralis m.
- Long head, biceps femoris m.
- Short head, biceps femoris m.

Bottom image labels:
- Tensor fascia lata m.
- Vastus lateralis m.
- Vastus intermedius
- Gluteus maximus m.
- Iliotibial band

(Top) *The origin of the vastus lateralis muscle from the superior-most aspect of the femoral diaphysis can be easily seen on this image. The vastus lateralis wraps around the lateral side of the femur.* **(Middle)** *The broad insertion of the gluteus medius muscle onto the lateral aspect of the superior greater trochanter is easily appreciated. Gluteus maximus sweeps past the greater trochanter and will insert on the iliotibial band and the superior portion of the linea aspera, the gluteal tuberosity.* **(Bottom)** *Vastus lateralis and gluteus maximus muscles are the most prominent muscles of the lateral thigh. Distally, the vastus intermedius muscle continues inferior to the muscle fibers of the vastus lateralis.*

SECTION 9
Knee

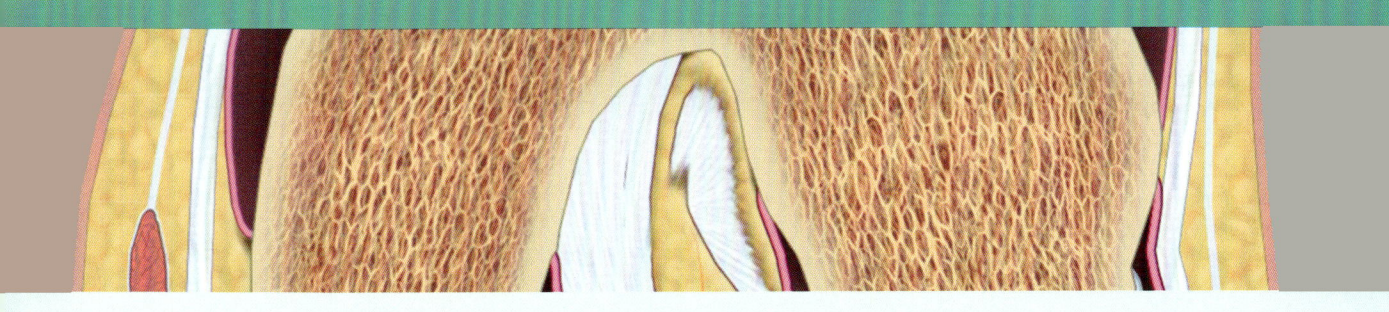

Knee Overview	**662**
Knee Radiographic and Arthrographic Anatomy	**670**
Knee MR Atlas	**686**
Knee Extensor Mechanism and Retinacula	**734**
Menisci	**742**
Cruciate Ligaments/Posterior Capsule	**768**
Knee Medial Supporting Structures	**786**
Knee Lateral Supporting Structures	**796**
Knee and Leg Normal Variants and Imaging Pitfalls	**812**
Knee and Leg Measurements and Lines	**858**

Knee Overview

GROSS ANATOMY

Overview

- Largest and most complex joint
  - Hinge joint throughout its greatest range of motion
  - In all positions, femur in contact with tibia, with large areas of contact
  - In all positions, patella in contact with femur
  - Bones do not interlock; stability maintained by ligaments, tendons, capsule, and menisci
- **Motion** of knee and relationship of osseous structures
  - In full flexion
    - Posterior surfaces of femoral condyles articulate with posterior tibial condyles
    - Lateral facet of patella in contact with lateral femoral condyle
    - Supporting ligaments are not taut, and rotation of leg is allowed
  - During motion of extension
    - Patella slides upwards on femur, passing 1st on to its middle facet and then its lower facets
    - Femoral condyles roll forward on tibial condyles and menisci
    - Lateral femoral condyle shorter anteroposteriorly than medial and reaches full extension earlier
    - Medial femoral condyle continues to slide after lateral stops, rotates slightly medially on tibia and medial meniscus ("screwing it home"), tightens anterior cruciate ligament (ACL), collateral ligaments, and posterior capsular ligaments, turning knee into rigid pillar
  - Initiating flexion from fully extended knee
    - Requires slight medial rotation of tibia, produced by popliteus
    - "Unlocks" joint, allowing remainder of motion to take place
- **Muscles acting on knee joint: Extensors (4 parts of quadriceps femoris)**
  - Rectus femoris
    - Origin straight head: Anterior inferior iliac spine; origin reflected head: Groove immediately superior to acetabulum
    - Insertion: Patella and continuation to inferior patellar tendon
    - Action: Crosses both hip and knee joints, flexing hip and extending knee
    - Innervation: Femoral nerve
    - Vascular supply: Lateral circumflex femoral artery
  - Vastus lateralis
    - Origin: Superior portion of intertrochanteric line, anterior and inferior borders of greater trochanter, superior portion of lateral lip of linea aspera, and lateral portion of gluteal tuberosity of femur
    - Insertion: Lateral base and border of patella; also forms lateral patellar retinaculum and lateral side of quadriceps femoris tendon
    - Action: Extends knee
    - Innervation: Femoral nerve
    - Vascular supply: Lateral circumflex femoral artery
  - Vastus medialis
    - Origin: Inferior portion of intertrochanteric line, spiral line, medial lip of linea aspera, superior part of medial supracondylar ridge of femur, and medial intermuscular septum
    - Insertion: Medial base and border of patella; also forms medial patellar retinaculum and medial side of quadriceps femoris tendon
    - Action: Extends knee
    - Innervation: Femoral nerve
    - Vascular supply: Femoral artery, profunda femoris artery, and superior medial genicular branch of popliteal artery
  - Vastus intermedius
    - Origin: Superior 2/3 of anterior and lateral surfaces of femur; also from lateral intermuscular septum of thigh
    - Insertion: Lateral border of patella; also forms deep portion of quadriceps tendon
    - Action: Extends knee
    - Innervation: Femoral nerve
    - Vascular supply: Lateral circumflex femoral artery
- **Muscles acting on knee joint: Flexors**
  - Biceps femoris
    - Origin: Long head, common tendon with semitendinosus from superior medial quadrant of posterior portion of ischial tuberosity; short head, lateral lip of linea aspera, lateral supracondylar ridge of femur, and lateral intermuscular septum of thigh
    - Insertion: Primarily on fibular head; also on lateral collateral ligament (LCL) and lateral tibial condyle
    - Action: Flexes knee and also rotates tibia laterally; long head also extends hip joint
    - Innervation: Long head, tibial nerve; short head, common peroneal nerve
    - Vascular supply: Perforating branches of profunda femoris artery, inferior gluteal artery, and superior muscular branches of popliteal artery
  - Sartorius
    - Origin: Anterior superior iliac spine
    - Insertion: Anteromedial tibial metaphysis near tibial tuberosity
    - Action: Crosses both hip and knee joints, flexes both hip and knee joints, rotating thigh laterally to bring limbs into position adopted by cross-legged tailor
    - Innervation: Femoral nerve
    - Vascular supply: Muscular branches of femoral artery
  - Gracilis
    - Origin: Inferior margin of pubic symphysis, inferior ramus of pubis, and adjacent ramus of ischium
    - Insertion: Medial tibial metaphysis, just posterior to sartorius
    - Action: Adducts thigh, flexes knee, and rotates flexed leg medially)
    - Innervation: Anterior division of obturator nerve
    - Vascular supply: Obturator artery, medial circumflex femoral artery, and muscular branches of profunda femoris artery
  - Semitendinosus
    - Origin: From common tendon with long head of biceps femoris from superior medial quadrant of posterior portion of ischial tuberosity

Knee Overview

- Insertion: Medial tibial metaphysis, just posterior to gracilis
- Action: Crosses both hip and knee joints, extends hip, flexes knee, medially rotates flexed leg
- Innervation: Tibial nerve
- Vascular supply: Perforating branches of profunda femoris artery, inferior gluteal artery, and superior muscular branches of popliteal artery
  - Semimembranosus
    - Origin: Superior lateral quadrant ischial tuberosity
    - Insertion: Wide insertion posterior and medial tibial condyle
    - Action: Crosses both hip and knee joints, extends hip, flexes knee, medially rotates flexed knee
    - Innervation: Tibial nerve
    - Vascular supply: Perforating branches of profunda femoris artery, inferior gluteal artery, and superior muscular branches of popliteal artery
  - Popliteus
    - Origin: Anterior part of popliteal groove on lateral surface of lateral femoral condyle
    - Insertion: Posterior surface of tibia in fan-like fashion, just superior to popliteal line
    - Action: Flexes knee and medially rotates tibia at beginning of flexion
    - Innervation: Tibial nerve
    - Vascular supply: Medial inferior genicular branch of popliteal artery and muscular branch of posterior tibial artery
- **Muscles acting on knee joint: Superficial flexors of knee**
  - Gastrocnemius
    - Origin: Medial head from posterior nonarticular surface of medial femoral condyle; lateral head from posterior edge of lateral epicondyle; heads unite to form main bulk of muscle
    - Insertion: Unites with deep tendon of soleus to form Achilles tendon, inserting on middle 1/3 of posterior calcaneal surface
    - Action: Flexes knee and plantar flexes ankle
    - Innervation: Tibial nerve
    - Vascular supply: Sural branch of popliteal artery
  - Plantaris
    - Origin: Superior and medial to lateral head of gastrocnemius origin, as well as from oblique popliteal ligament
    - Insertion: Middle 1/3 of posterior calcaneal surface, just medial to Achilles tendon
    - Action: Flexes knee and plantarflexes ankle
    - Innervation: Tibial nerve
    - Vascular supply: Sural arteries
    - Note: Absent in 7-10% of population
- **Muscles acting on knee joint: Internal rotators of leg**
  - Popliteus, gracilis, sartorius, semitendinosus, semimembranosus
- **Muscles acting on knee joint: External rotator of leg**
  - Biceps femoris
- **Extensor mechanism**
  - Quadriceps tendon and retinacula converge to inferior patellar tendon
- **Internal structures**
  - Menisci
    - Cushion lubricate and stabilize knee
  - Cruciate ligaments
    - Major stabilizing structures to anteroposterior motion
  - Medial supporting structures
    - 3 layers, including pes anserinus, medial collateral ligament, capsular layers, and posterior oblique ligament
  - Lateral supporting structures
    - 3 layers, including iliotibial band, biceps femoris, quadriceps retinaculum, fibular collateral ligament, arcuate ligament, and several small inconstant posterolateral structures
- **Nerves** of knee joint
  - **Femoral nerve** supplies
    - 3 branches, 1 to each of vasti and to anterosuperior part of joint
    - Largest is nerve to vastus medialis, which accompanies descending genicular artery
  - **Common peroneal nerve** supplies
    - Superior lateral genicular nerve descends into popliteal fossa and supplies superolateral part of joint, passing deep to biceps, through lateral intermuscular septum above femoral condyle
    - Inferior lateral genicular nerve: Small and sometimes absent; arises with superior lateral genicular nerve and curves downwards and forwards over lateral head of gastrocnemius, passing between capsule and fibular collateral ligament
    - Recurrent genicular nerve: Small twigs reaching anteroinferior part of joint
  - **Tibial nerve** supplies
    - Superior medial genicular nerve: Runs medially around femur above medial condyle, deep to adductor magnus, then through vastus medialis to superomedial part of joint
    - Middle genicular nerve: Runs forward through fibrous capsule to cruciate ligaments
    - Inferior medial genicular nerve: Largest, running along upper border of popliteus, passing forward between shaft of tibia and medial collateral ligament (MCL), curving superiorly to inferomedial part of capsule
  - **Obturator nerve**: Sends genicular branch through adductor magnus to join popliteal artery, running to posterior aspect of joint
- **Vessels** of knee joint: 8 arteries supply large anastomosis
  - **Popliteal** artery supplies 5 genicular branches
  - **Anterior tibial** artery supplies 2 recurrent branches
  - **Femoral** artery supplies descending genicular branch
  - **Lateral circumflex** artery supplies descending genicular branch

Knee Overview

3D CT SHOWING ORIGINS & INSERTIONS (LATERAL, ANTEROLATERAL)

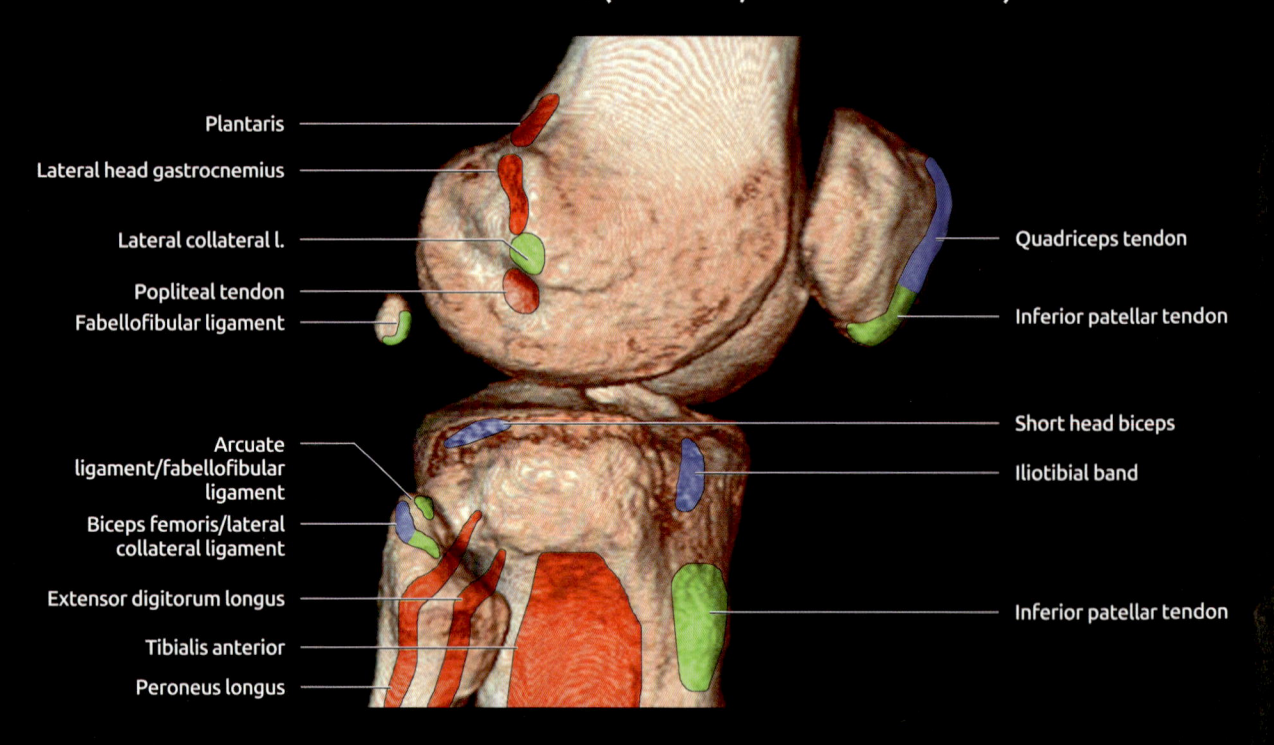

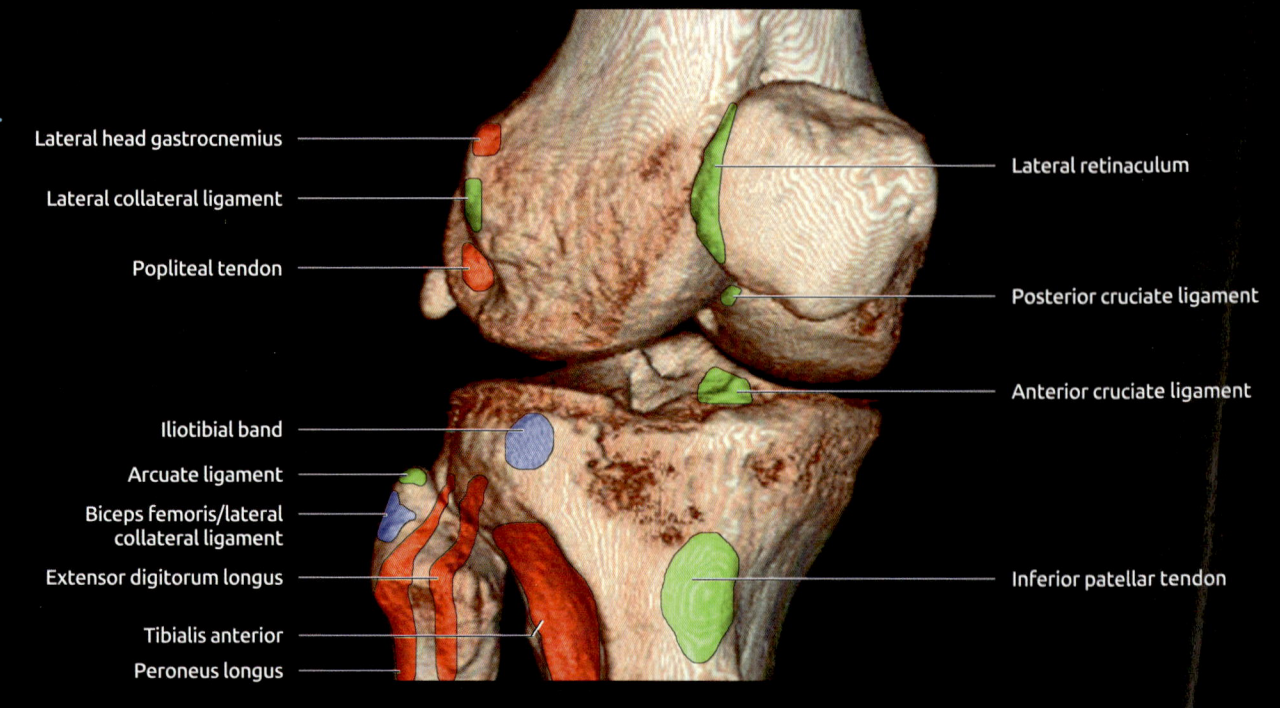

Labels (top image):
- Plantaris
- Lateral head gastrocnemius
- Lateral collateral l.
- Popliteal tendon
- Fabellofibular ligament
- Arcuate ligament/fabellofibular ligament
- Biceps femoris/lateral collateral ligament
- Extensor digitorum longus
- Tibialis anterior
- Peroneus longus
- Quadriceps tendon
- Inferior patellar tendon
- Short head biceps
- Iliotibial band
- Inferior patellar tendon

Labels (bottom image):
- Lateral head gastrocnemius
- Lateral collateral ligament
- Popliteal tendon
- Iliotibial band
- Arcuate ligament
- Biceps femoris/lateral collateral ligament
- Extensor digitorum longus
- Tibialis anterior
- Peroneus longus
- Lateral retinaculum
- Posterior cruciate ligament
- Anterior cruciate ligament
- Inferior patellar tendon

(**Top**) *Lateral view of the knee shows lateral stabilizing structures. Origins of anterior and lateral leg muscles are seen as well.* (**Bottom**) *This slightly anterolateral view shows the lateral stabilizers of the knee and patella. These consist primarily of lateral collateral ligament, arcuate ligament, popliteal tendon, iliotibial band, and biceps femoris. Origins of several leg muscles are seen. The tibialis anterior, extensor digitorum longus, and peroneus longus origins extend several centimeters distally beyond the regions indicated here.*

Knee Overview

3D CT SHOWING ORIGINS & INSERTIONS (ANTEROMEDIAL)

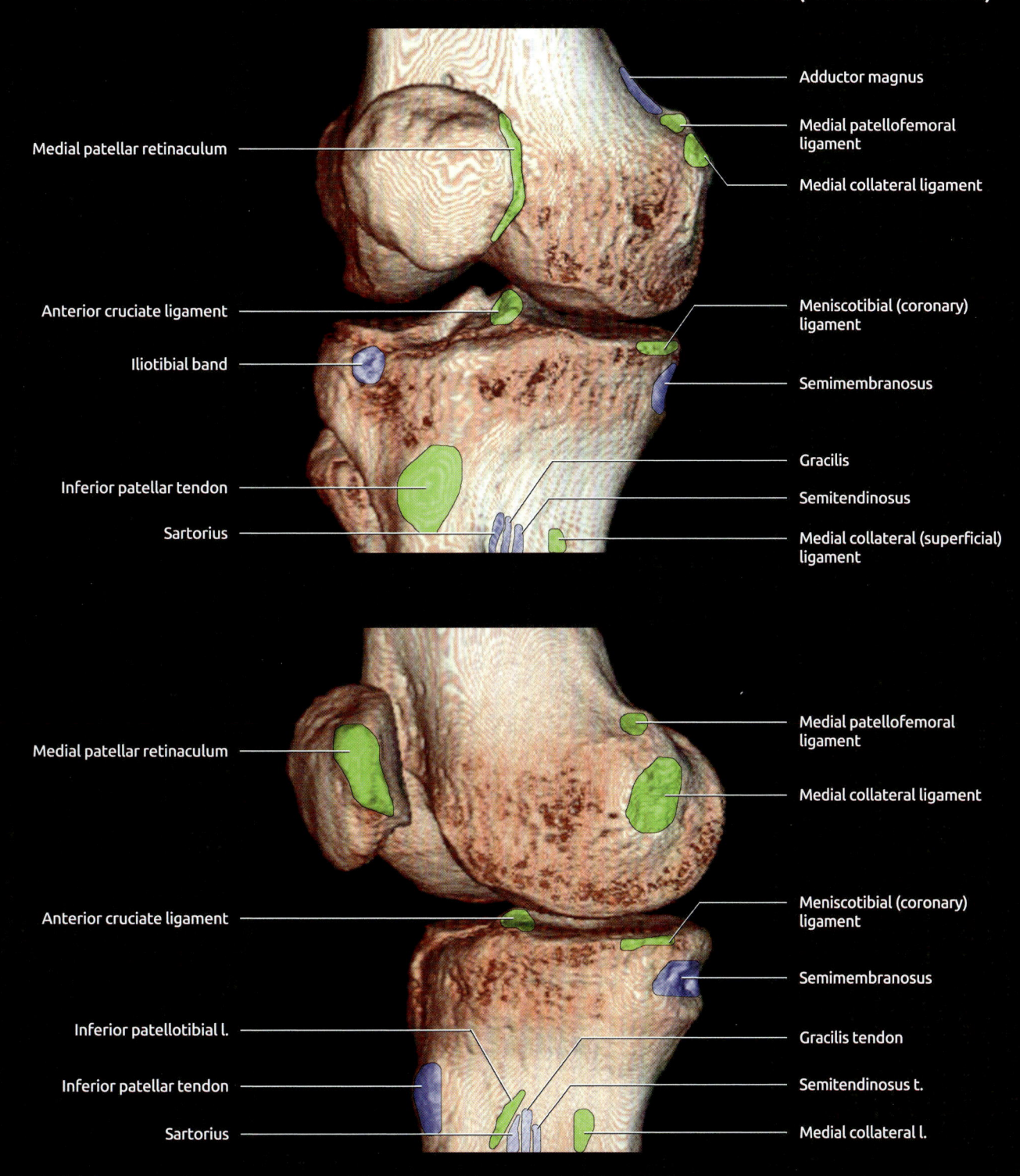

Labels (top image):
- Medial patellar retinaculum
- Anterior cruciate ligament
- Iliotibial band
- Inferior patellar tendon
- Sartorius
- Adductor magnus
- Medial patellofemoral ligament
- Medial collateral ligament
- Meniscotibial (coronary) ligament
- Semimembranosus
- Gracilis
- Semitendinosus
- Medial collateral (superficial) ligament

Labels (bottom image):
- Medial patellar retinaculum
- Anterior cruciate ligament
- Inferior patellotibial l.
- Inferior patellar tendon
- Sartorius
- Medial patellofemoral ligament
- Medial collateral ligament
- Meniscotibial (coronary) ligament
- Semimembranosus
- Gracilis tendon
- Semitendinosus t.
- Medial collateral l.

(Top) Slightly anteromedial view shows the medial stabilizers of the knee and patella. Note that only the uppermost portion of the insertions of the pes anserinus (sartorius, gracilis, and semitendinosus), as well as superficial medial collateral ligament, are shown. These insertions actually extend several cm distally on the tibia. (Bottom) Anteromedial knee, shows medial stabilizers of knee (primarily medial collateral ligament, superficial and deep fibers, secondarily pes anserinus), as well as medial stabilizers of patella (superiorly medial patellofemoral ligament, mid medial retinaculum, inferiorly patellotibial ligament).

Knee Overview

3D CT SHOWING ORIGINS & INSERTIONS (MEDIAL, POSTEROMEDIAL)

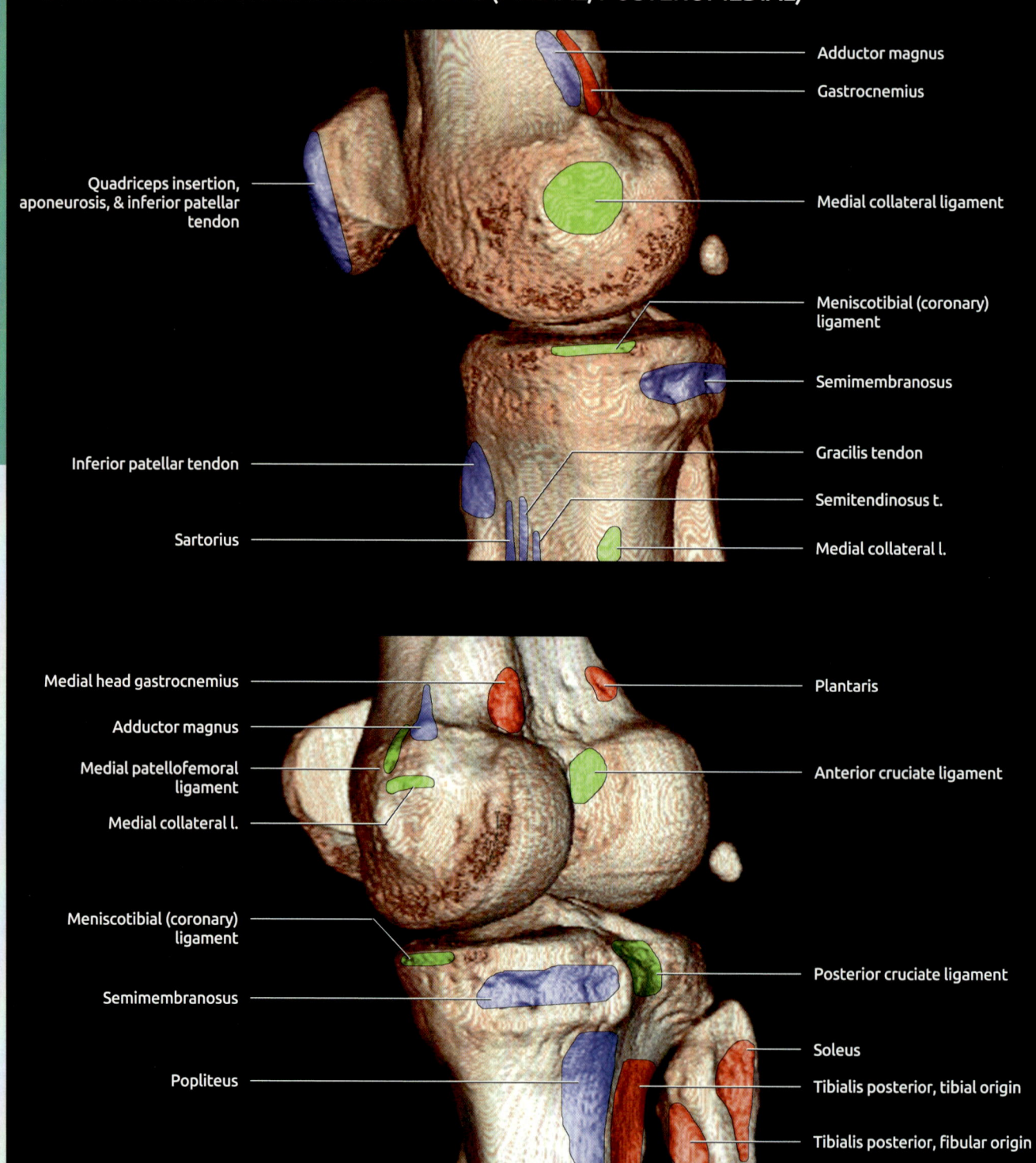

Labels (top image):
- Adductor magnus
- Gastrocnemius
- Quadriceps insertion, aponeurosis, & inferior patellar tendon
- Medial collateral ligament
- Meniscotibial (coronary) ligament
- Semimembranosus
- Inferior patellar tendon
- Gracilis tendon
- Semitendinosus t.
- Sartorius
- Medial collateral l.

Labels (bottom image):
- Medial head gastrocnemius
- Plantaris
- Adductor magnus
- Medial patellofemoral ligament
- Anterior cruciate ligament
- Medial collateral l.
- Meniscotibial (coronary) ligament
- Posterior cruciate ligament
- Semimembranosus
- Soleus
- Popliteus
- Tibialis posterior, tibial origin
- Tibialis posterior, fibular origin

(Top) First of 8 volume-rendered topographic CT images is shown. Image shows the medial aspect of the knee, with associated muscle, tendon, and ligament origins/insertions. *(Bottom)* Posterior CT, oblique to medial, is shown. Note the extensive insertions of both semimembranosus and popliteus on the posteromedial tibia.

Knee Overview

3D CT SHOWING ORIGINS & INSERTIONS (POSTERIOR, POSTEROLATERAL)

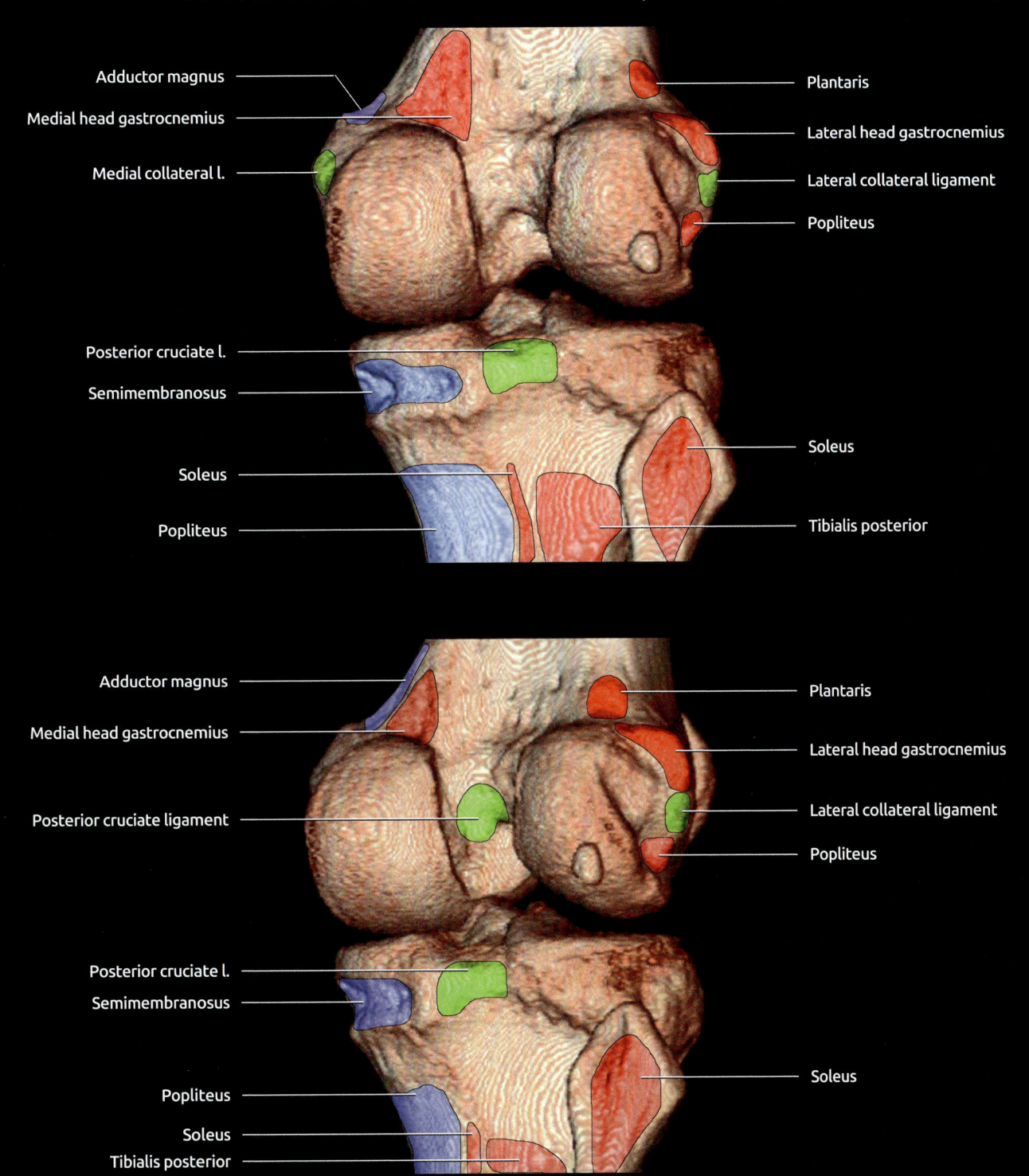

(Top) Direct posterior view shows that posterior cruciate ligament insertion is extraarticular on the posterior central tibia. (Bottom) Posterior (slightly oblique) view of the knee shows the attachments of the posterior structures. Note that fibular origin of soleus is more proximal than tibial origin.

Knee Overview

GRAPHICS, POSTERIOR SUPERFICIAL AND DEEP MUSCLES & NERVES

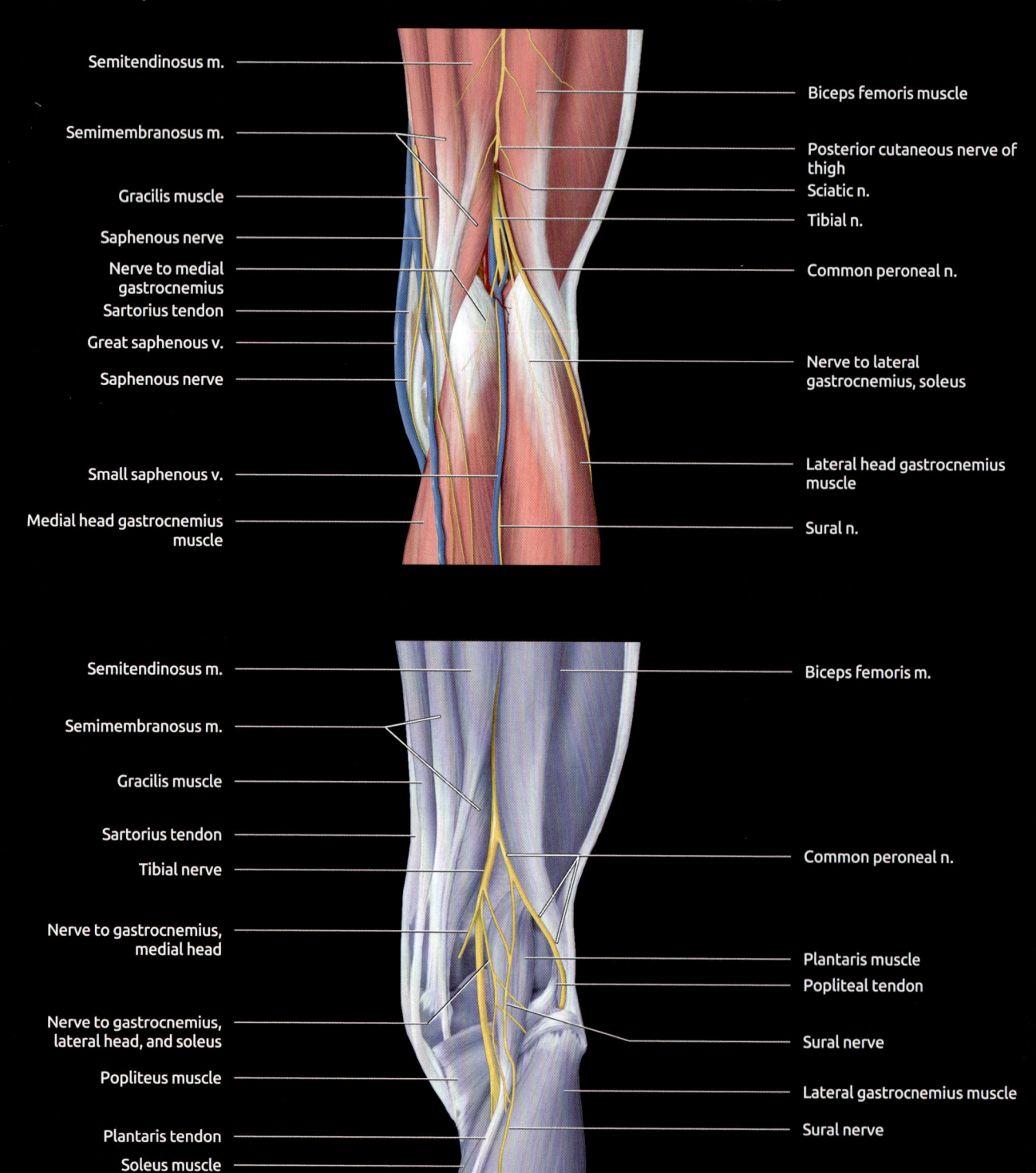

(Top) Graphic shows the superficial posterior muscles and nerves. Note that the common peroneal nerve is part of the deeper nerve system, but travels more superficially, following the posterior biceps femoris muscle and tendon until it wraps around the fibular neck. (Bottom) Graphic shows the relationship of the common peroneal nerve to the posterior biceps femoris tendon. It also shows the tibial nerve with the numerous muscular branches. Note the plantaris muscle coursing over the popliteus (and popliteal vessels, not shown) and becoming tendinous at the level of the popliteus/soleus muscle junction. The plantaris tendon then courses downward and slightly medially between soleus and medial head gastrocnemius (not shown). The sural nerve arises from branches of both common peroneal and tibial nerves, and courses down superficial to the junction of the 2 gastrocnemius heads. The tibial nerve travels downward in a deeper position, just posterior to the posterior tibial vessels.

Knee Overview

GRAPHICS, VESSELS AND ANASTOMOTIC NETWORK

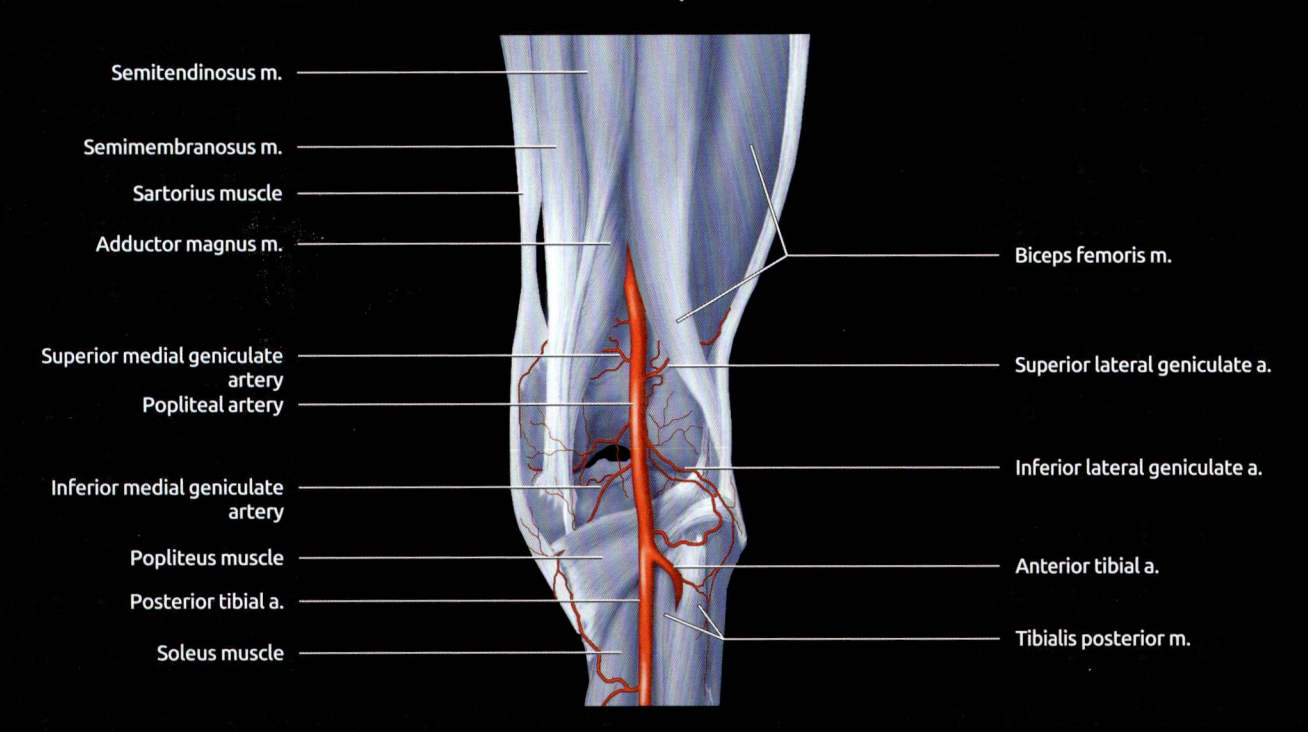

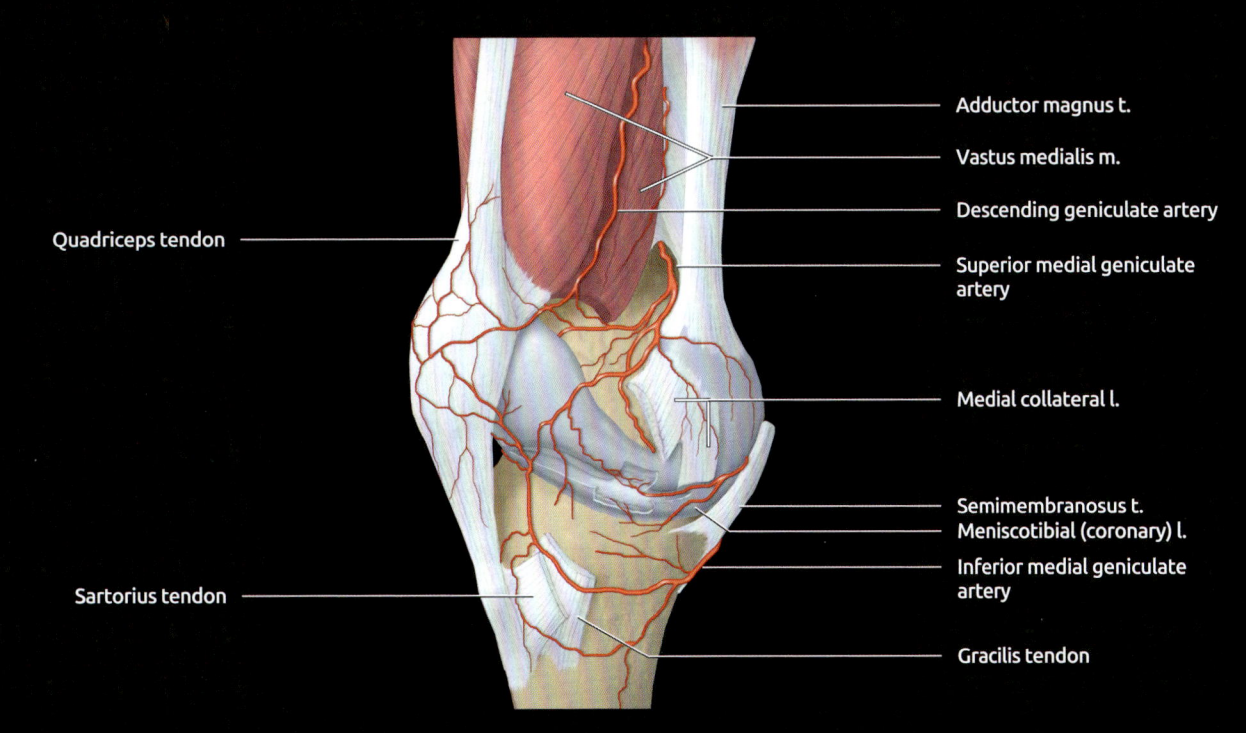

Labels (top image):
- Semitendinosus m.
- Semimembranosus m.
- Sartorius muscle
- Adductor magnus m.
- Superior medial geniculate artery
- Popliteal artery
- Inferior medial geniculate artery
- Popliteus muscle
- Posterior tibial a.
- Soleus muscle
- Biceps femoris m.
- Superior lateral geniculate a.
- Inferior lateral geniculate a.
- Anterior tibial a.
- Tibialis posterior m.

Labels (bottom image):
- Quadriceps tendon
- Sartorius tendon
- Adductor magnus t.
- Vastus medialis m.
- Descending geniculate artery
- Superior medial geniculate artery
- Medial collateral l.
- Semimembranosus t.
- Meniscotibial (coronary) l.
- Inferior medial geniculate artery
- Gracilis tendon

(**Top**) *Graphic shows the anastomoses around the knee, posteriorly. The popliteal artery is seen throughout its course, from the hiatus in adductor magnus proximally to the lower border of popliteus distally. At this point, the popliteal artery bifurcates into anterior and posterior tibial arteries. The anterior tibial is the smaller branch that extends through a slit in tibialis posterior and on through the interosseous membrane to descend along the interosseous membrane down the anterior compartment. There are 4 named geniculate branches, a superior and inferior both medially and laterally.* (**Bottom**) *Graphic of the anteromedial knee shows the rich anastomotic vascular network around the knee. There are 2 named geniculate branches of the popliteal artery in each side (superior and inferior). Additionally, there are 2 supplementary arteries. The descending geniculate artery (a branch of the femoral artery) descends superomedially. There is also an anterior recurrent branch of the anterior tibial artery that runs inferolaterally, not shown here.*

Knee Radiographic and Arthrographic Anatomy

IMAGING ANATOMY

Overview

- Radiographic anatomy
  o Distal femur osseous features
    - Distal femoral metaphysis flares into medial and lateral epicondyles
    - Osseous irregularity may be seen at posteromedial femoral metaphysis; considered to be "tug" at adductor or medial gastrocnemius insertion, oddly termed "cortical desmoid"
    - Medial femoral condyle larger than lateral
    - Lateral femoral condyle has slight concavity in its anterior weight-bearing surface (termed lateral femoral recess or sulcus); normal depth < 2 mm
    - Intercondylar notch cruciate ligaments; visualized as Blumensaat line on lateral radiograph
    - Anteriorly, trochlear groove patella and is generally V-shaped
  o Possible sites of avulsion from femur
    - Posterolateral intercondylar notch (anterior cruciate ligament [ACL] origin)
    - Midmedial intercondylar notch (posterior cruciate ligament [PCL] origin)
    - Medial epicondyle (medial collateral ligament [MCL] origin)
  o Proximal tibia osseous features
    - Posterior tilt of tibial surface by 10°
    - Tibial tubercle (apophysis anterior and slightly lateral on metaphysis, several centimeters distal to joint line)
  o Possible sites of avulsion from tibia
    - Tibial spine (ACL insertion)
    - Posterior midtibia at joint line (PCL insertion)
    - Medial joint line (coronary ligament insertion)
    - Lateral joint line (anterolateral ligament and capsular insertion; termed Segond fracture)
    - Gerdy tubercle (iliotibial band insertion)
    - Tibial apophysis (patellar tendon insertion; usually seen in skeletally immature patients)
  o Proximal fibula osseous features
    - Posterolaterally located relative to tibia
    - Proximal point termed fibular styloid process
  o Possible sites of avulsion from proximal fibula
    - Lateral fibular head/neck (insertion of conjoint tendon)
    - Fibular styloid process (insertion of arcuate, fabellofibular, and popliteofibular ligaments)
  o Patellar osseous features
    - Triangular sesamoid
    - Wider at base superiorly than at apex inferiorly
    - Articular surface divided by vertical ridge into lateral and medial facets
    - Lateral facet elongated and has shallow angle
    - Medial facet short and more strongly angulated
    - Several other facets described but not of imaging importance
    - Lower 25% nonarticular
    - Nonarticular outer surface may develop prominent enthesopathy where quadriceps tendon insertion blends into origin of inferior patellar tendon

- Internal contents
  o **Menisci**: Cushion, lubricate, and stabilize knee
    - Composed of fibrocartilage, triangular in cross section
    - Only peripheral 1/3 is vascularized
    - Each meniscus divided into anterior horn, body, and posterior horn
    - Meniscal roots: Central portions of anterior and posterior horns, anchored to tibia
    - Transverse ligament extends between anterior horns
    - Medial meniscus: Posterior horn larger than anterior horn
    - Menisci tightly attached to medial joint capsule; small perimeniscal recesses
    - Lateral meniscus: Posterior and anterior horns equal in size
    - Loose capsular attachments of lateral meniscus allow rotational motion; large perimeniscal recesses
    - Popliteus tendon passes by body and posterior horn lateral meniscus; popliteomeniscal fascicles extend from posterior horn to popliteus sheath
  o **Cruciate ligaments**
    - Intraarticular but extrasynovial
    - ACL prevents anterior translation of tibia
    - ACL originates at posterolateral intercondylar notch, extends anteromedially, inserts at interspinous tibia and medial tibial spine
    - ACL consists of 2 bundles: Anteromedial and posterolateral
    - PCL prevents posterior translation of tibia
    - PCL originates at medial aspect of intercondylar notch, extends posterolaterally, inserts extraarticularly on posterior cortex of proximal tibia
  o **Meniscofemoral ligaments**: Extend from posterior horn lateral meniscus to medial femoral condyle adjacent to PCL origin at intercondylar notch
    - Ligament of Humphrey: Passes anterior to PCL
    - Ligament of Wrisberg: Passes posterior to PCL
  o **Medial collateral ligament**
    - Superficial portion: Thick, extends from femoral condyle to proximal tibia
    - Deep portion: Meniscofemoral (coronary) and meniscotibial ligament
    - Stabilizes to valgus stress
  o **Lateral collateral ligament complex**
    - Iliotibial band: Distal extension of tensor fascia lata, inserts on Gerdy tubercle of anterolateral tibia; anterolateral stabilizer
    - Lateral (fibular) collateral ligament (LCL): Femoral condyle to fibula
    - Anterolateral ligament: Arises immediately anterior to lateral collateral ligament, crosses obliquely and anteriorly to attach at lateral tibial condyle between Gerdy tubercle and fibular head
    - Biceps femoris: Complex insertions on fibula and tibia; often forms conjoint tendon distally with fibular collateral ligament
    - Posterolateral corner: LCL, biceps, popliteus; fabellofibular/arcuate/popliteofibular ligaments
  o **Extensor mechanism**
    - Quadriceps tendon: Inserts on anterosuperior margin of patella

Knee Radiographic and Arthrographic Anatomy

- Patellar tendon: Continuation of quadriceps tendon, extends from anteroinferior margin of patella to tibial tubercle
- Patella: Medial and lateral articular facets divided by median ridge (apex)
- Hoffa fat pad: Triangle-shaped, vascularized fat pad posterior to patellar tendon
○ Hyaline cartilage surfaces
- Patella has thickest cartilage in body; can be up to 7 mm
- Patella articulates with wedge-shaped trochlear groove of femur
- Bipartite patella: Superolateral accessory ossicle, intact cartilage over junction with patella
- Medial tibiofemoral compartment normally has thinner cartilage width than lateral compartment
- Lateral tibiofemoral compartment has thin cartilage at lateral femoral sulcus
- Tibial cartilage gradually thins near periphery; tibial spines, anteriorly
○ Joint capsule, recesses
- Suprapatellar recess: Large recess, communicates freely with remainder of joint
- Perimeniscal recesses: Larger laterally than medially
- Popliteus tendon sheath: Communicates with joint
- Capsule may extend into/through origin of medial or lateral gastrocnemius
- Popliteal cyst ("Baker cyst"): Fluid extends through weak point in capsule between semimembranosus tendon and medial head of gastrocnemius
- Plicae: Remnants of tissue between developing compartments
- Superior patellar plica: Curves through suprapatellar recess medial to lateral (not commonly symptomatic)
- Infrapatellar plica: Extends from origin adjacent to ACL into Hoffa fat pad; parallels ACL
- Medial patellar plica: Vertically oriented in medial patellofemoral recess (can result in snapping on flexion/extension and medial patellofemoral cartilage wear)
- Extraarticular bursae
○ Prepatellar bursa: Anterior to patella
○ Infrapatellar bursa: Within Hoffa fat pad, adjacent to tibial tubercle, deep to patellar tendon

ANATOMY IMAGING ISSUES

Imaging Approaches
- Radiographs
○ Standard includes AP standing, lateral in slight flexion, and axial patella with 20° flexion
○ Evaluation for arthritis or total knee arthroplasty often also employs standing PA flexion (notch) view
- Emphasizes cartilage width in posterior weight-bearing portion of joint
- Arthrography procedure: Needle placement
○ No need for fluoroscopic or ultrasound guidance in most cases
○ Patient supine with knee slightly flexed over pillow, quadriceps relaxed
○ Either lateral or medial approach; palpate patellofemoral joint line
- Inject at or below equator of patella; more cephalad placement may result in embedding the needle in prefemoral fat pad and sequestering of contrast at that site
- If 20-g needle is used, generally get return of joint fluid, proving intraarticular location
- Aspirate as much effusion fluid as possible to improve crispness of contrast at imaging
- Arthrography procedure: Expected contrast flow
○ Contrast freely flows away from needle in joint; often collects in suprapatellar recess
- CT arthrogram: Useful if MR arthrography is contraindicated
○ Technique: Inject 40 cc dilute contrast of choice 50/50 with bacteriostatic saline
○ Acquire submillimeter sections; reformat
- MR arthrogram
○ Useful for postsurgical evaluation or searching for osteochondral defect if no effusion is present
○ Technique: Inject volume of 40 cc gadolinium diluted 1:200 in saline
- Indirect MR arthrogram
○ Useful for postsurgical evaluation or searching for osteochondral defect if no effusion is present
○ Technique: Exercise following IV injection; image 20-30 minutes later

Imaging Pitfalls
- Radiographic pitfalls
○ Malpositioning
- AP radiograph: Flexion obscures joint space
- Axial patella radiograph: Flexion > 20° may reduce subluxation or tilt
○ Bipartite (multipartite) patella
- Always upper outer quadrant
- Osseous fragments may not appear to "match," but cartilage is continuous over osseous defect
○ Other osseous variants: Dorsal defect of patella, meniscal ossicle
- MR/CT arthrogram pitfalls
○ Positioning for oblique coronal or sagittal MR imaging
- Incorrect alignment can either obscure or exaggerate anatomical landmarks
○ Attachment of structures to menisci can simulate tear
- Transverse ligament: Attaches to both anterior meniscal horns
- Meniscofemoral ligament: Attaches to posterior horn, lateral meniscus
○ Popliteus tendon sheath may mimic tear of posterior horn, lateral meniscus
○ Normal meniscal vascularity in young patients can appear hyperintense on MR
○ Anterior horn of lateral meniscus separates into fascicles at insertion, can simulate tear

Knee Radiographic and Arthrographic Anatomy

STANDARD RADIOGRAPHS OF KNEE

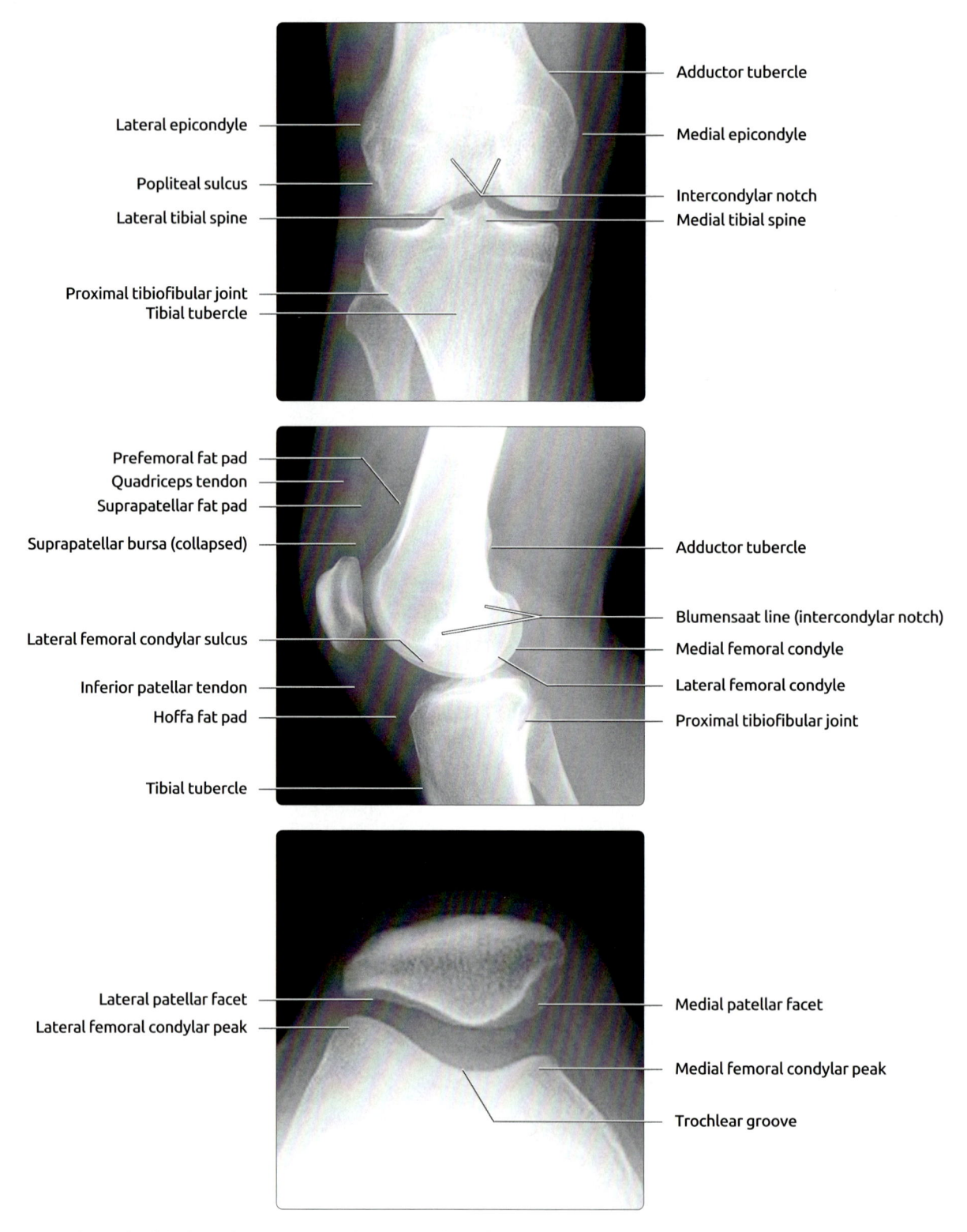

(Top) AP radiograph of the knee shows its osseous features, with the fibular head slightly posterolateral to the lateral tibial condyle. **(Middle)** Lateral radiograph shows the intercondylar notch to be delineated by Blumensaat line. The medial femoral condyle is slightly larger than the lateral; the lateral femoral condyle can also be identified by the presence of the lateral femoral sulcus at its anterior weight-bearing portion. The medial femoral condyle is slightly larger than the lateral. The lateral radiograph is generally obtained in slight flexion; note the posterior tilt of the tibial surface that should approximate 10 degrees. **(Bottom)** Axial radiograph shows the knee, obtained with the knee flexed 20 degrees (allows maximal subluxation of the patella). Note that the lateral facet of the patella is elongated and less sharply angled than the medial. There are numerous described facets of the patella, but the medial and lateral hold the greatest clinical importance.

Knee Radiographic and Arthrographic Anatomy

NEEDLE PLACEMENT FOR ARTHROGRAPHY OR INJECTION

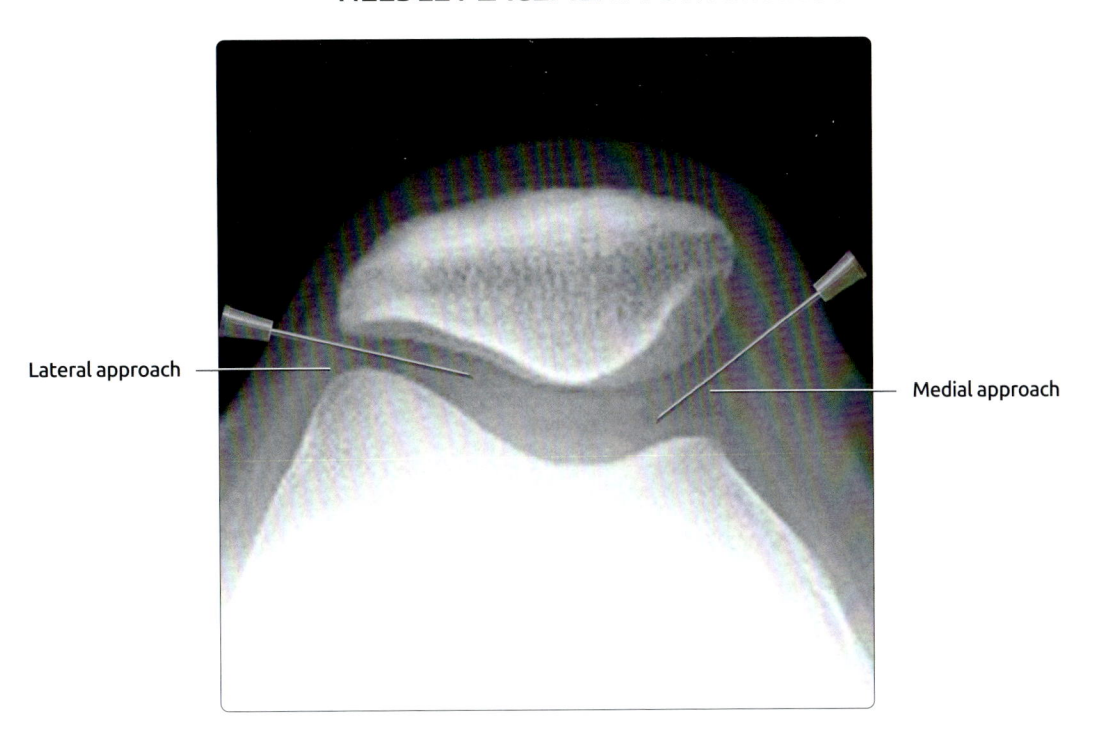

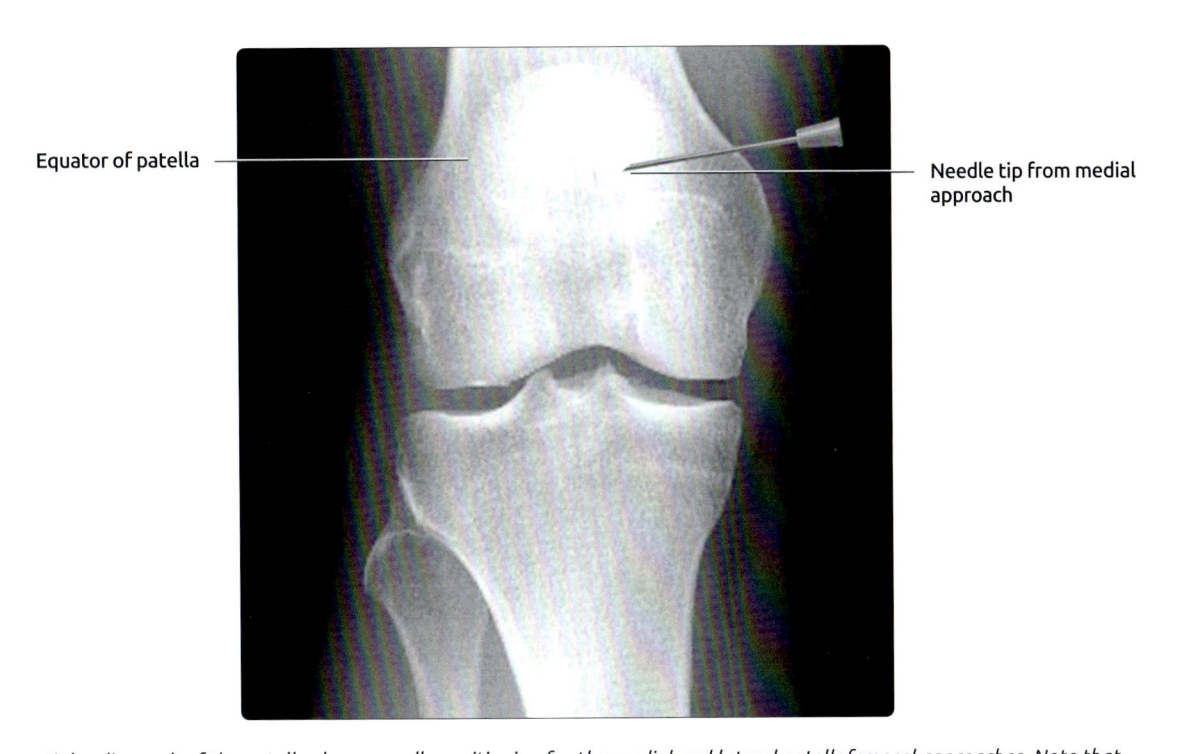

- Lateral approach
- Medial approach
- Equator of patella
- Needle tip from medial approach

(Top) Tangential radiograph of the patella shows needle positioning for the medial and lateral patellofemoral approaches. Note that there is more room for access at the medial aspect of the knee joint. The angle of the needle entry is more steep for the medial than for the lateral approach. (From DI: Procedures.) *(Bottom)* Frontal knee radiograph with the patient supine shows proper positioning for placement of a needle into the medial patellofemoral joint. Note that the needle tip is below the equator of the patella. If the tip ends up in a more cephalad position, it may embed in the prefemoral fat pad, resulting in a sequestered injection. Stabilization of the patella with the hand that is not holding the needle aids in needle placement. (From DI: Procedures.)

Knee Radiographic and Arthrographic Anatomy

AXIAL KNEE ANATOMY

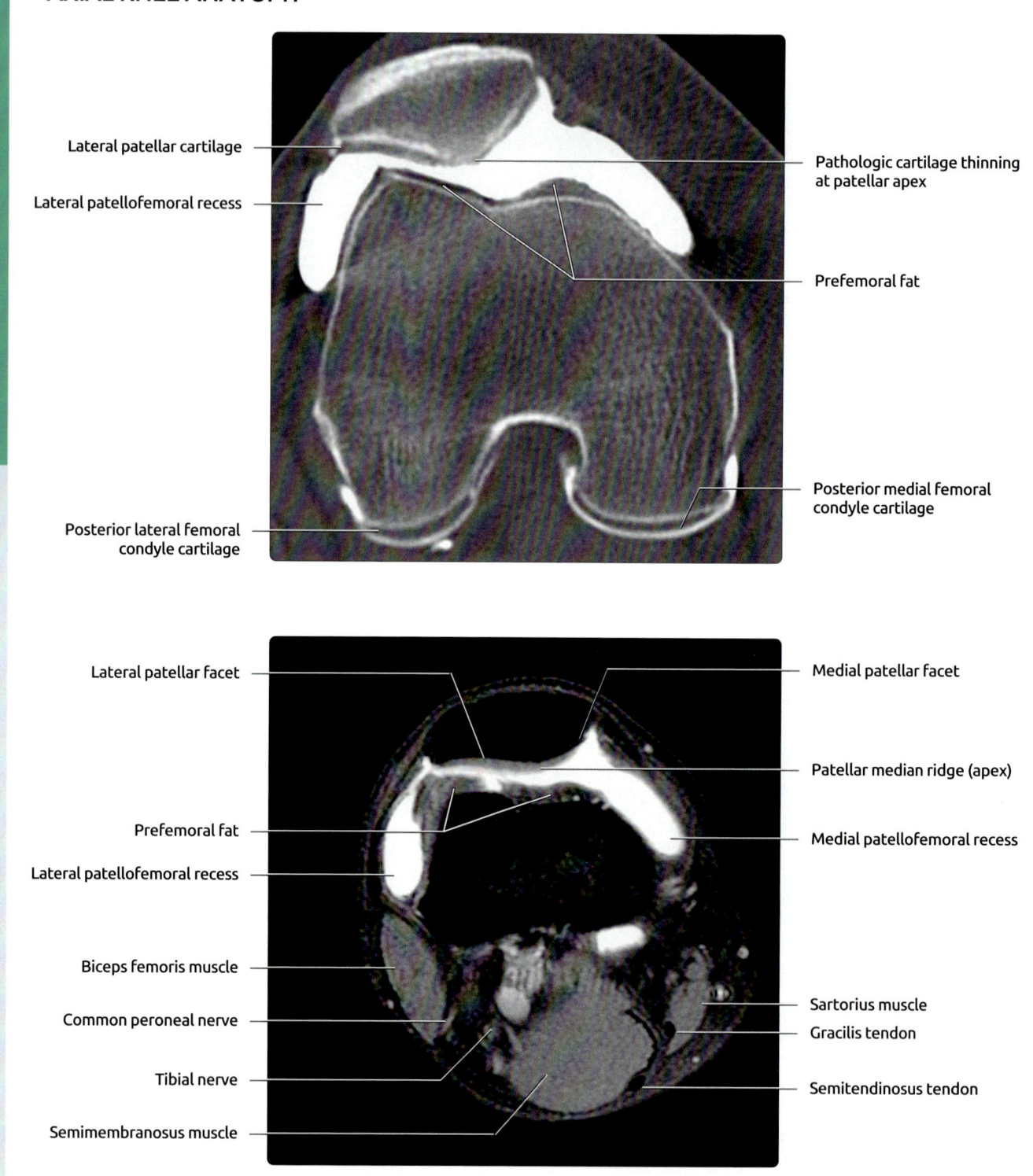

- Lateral patellar cartilage
- Lateral patellofemoral recess
- Posterior lateral femoral condyle cartilage
- Pathologic cartilage thinning at patellar apex
- Prefemoral fat
- Posterior medial femoral condyle cartilage

- Lateral patellar facet
- Prefemoral fat
- Lateral patellofemoral recess
- Biceps femoris muscle
- Common peroneal nerve
- Tibial nerve
- Semimembranosus muscle
- Medial patellar facet
- Patellar median ridge (apex)
- Medial patellofemoral recess
- Sartorius muscle
- Gracilis tendon
- Semitendinosus tendon

(**Top**) In the 1st of 4 axial images from superior to inferior, axial CT arthrogram image through the femoral condyles shows contrast outlining cartilage. The patella appears slightly subluxated laterally, but this is normal in the fully extended knee. (**Bottom**) Axial MR PD FS arthrogram through the patella shows intact cartilage. When the knee is fully extended, the apex of the patella and the trochlear articular surface of femur are at the same axial level. Undulation of the prefemoral fat above the trochlea should not be confused with cartilage defects.

Knee Radiographic and Arthrographic Anatomy

AXIAL KNEE ANATOMY

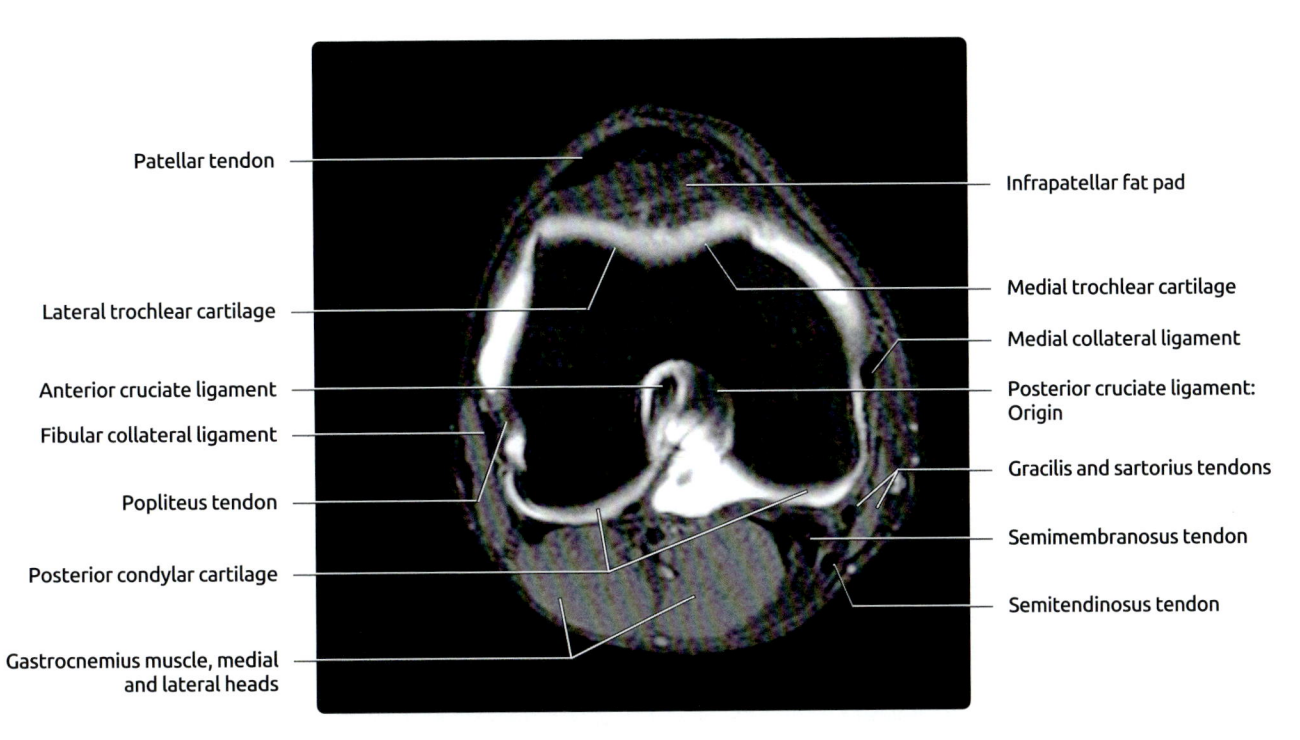

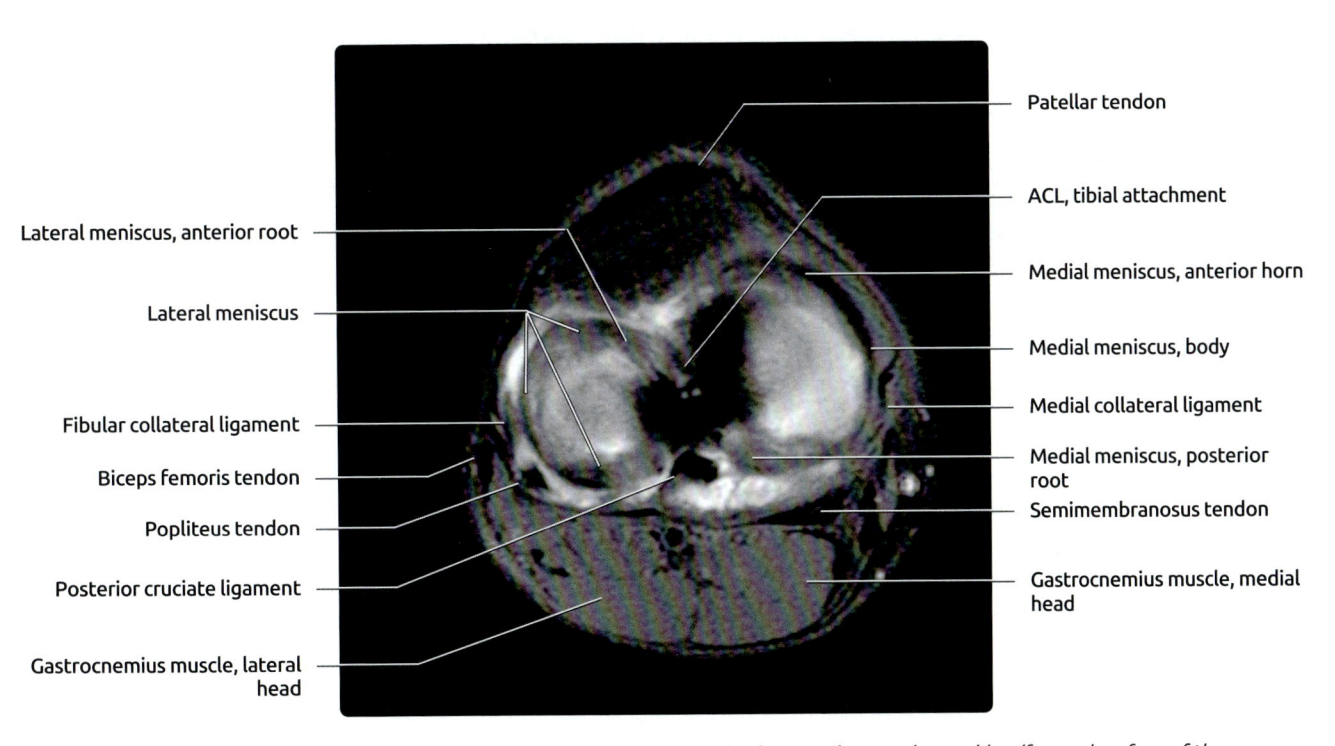

(Top) Axial MR PD FS arthrogram image through the femoral condyles shows hyaline cartilage at the trochlea (femoral surface of the patellofemoral joint) and posterior femoral condyles, as well as the anterior and posterior cruciate ligaments within the intercondylar notch. (Bottom) Axial PD FS MR arthrogram image through the menisci is shown. The medial meniscus has an open C shape, while the lateral meniscus approaches a circle. The anterior root of the lateral meniscus divides into thin fascicles, which may be mistaken for a tear when seen in cross section on sagittal or coronal images.

Knee Radiographic and Arthrographic Anatomy

GRAPHICS: AXIAL KNEE ANATOMY

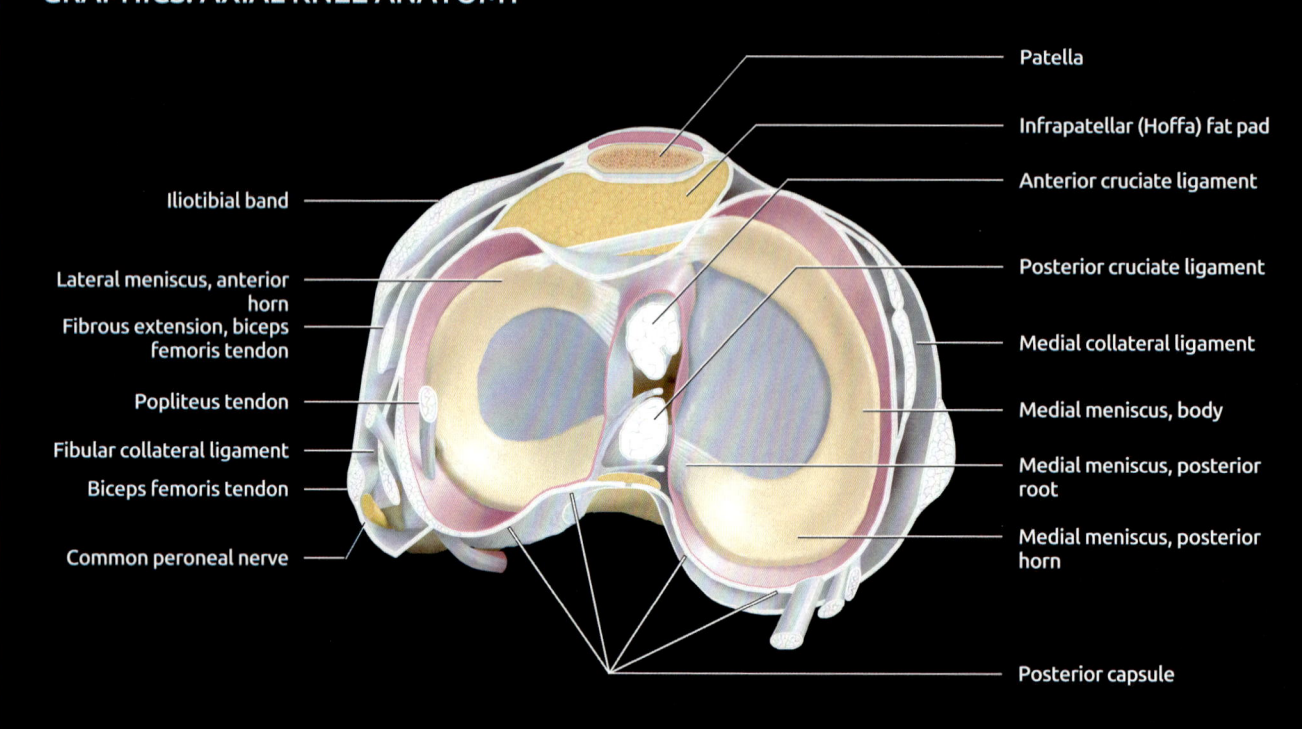

Labels (top figure):
- Patella
- Infrapatellar (Hoffa) fat pad
- Anterior cruciate ligament
- Posterior cruciate ligament
- Medial collateral ligament
- Medial meniscus, body
- Medial meniscus, posterior root
- Medial meniscus, posterior horn
- Posterior capsule
- Iliotibial band
- Lateral meniscus, anterior horn
- Fibrous extension, biceps femoris tendon
- Popliteus tendon
- Fibular collateral ligament
- Biceps femoris tendon
- Common peroneal nerve

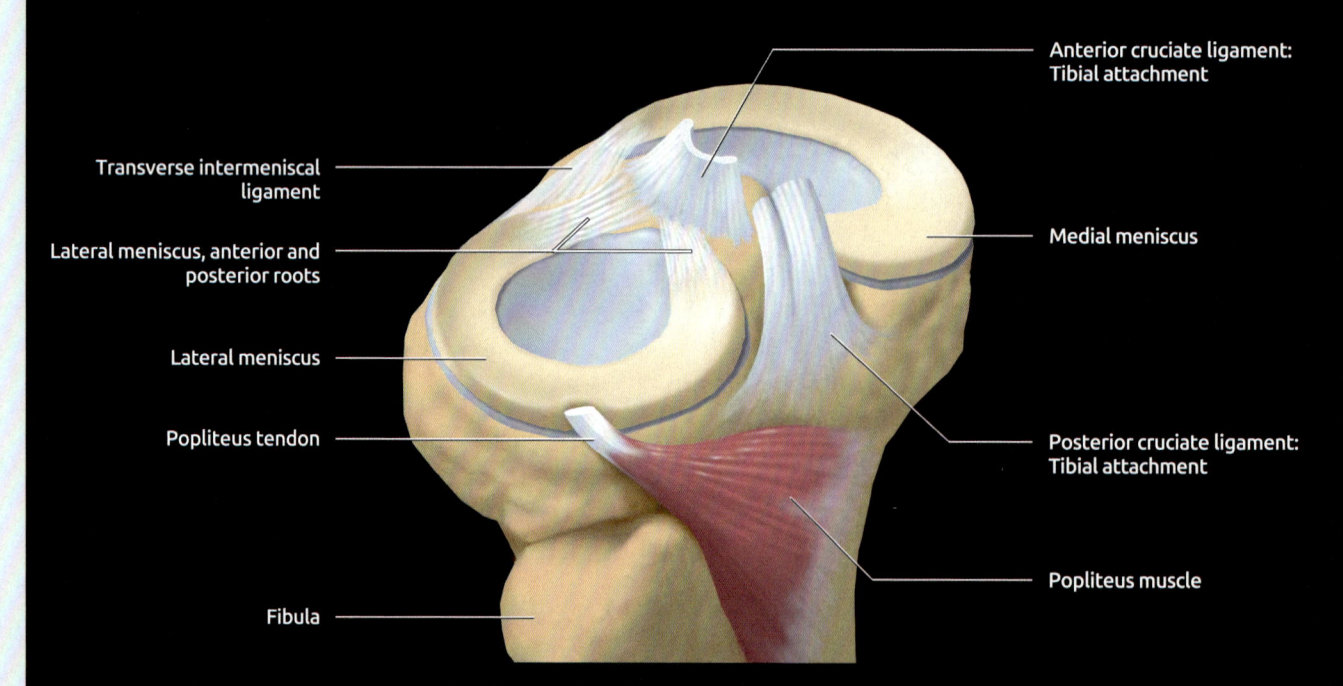

Labels (bottom figure):
- Anterior cruciate ligament: Tibial attachment
- Medial meniscus
- Posterior cruciate ligament: Tibial attachment
- Popliteus muscle
- Transverse intermeniscal ligament
- Lateral meniscus, anterior and posterior roots
- Lateral meniscus
- Popliteus tendon
- Fibula

(**Top**) *Axial graphic through the joint line corresponding to the previous MR arthrogram image shows that the posterolateral stabilizing structures are well seen.* (**Bottom**) *Graphic shows the tibial surface of the joint from a posterolateral perspective. The relationship of the popliteus tendon to the posterolateral corner of the lateral meniscus is well seen.*

Knee Radiographic and Arthrographic Anatomy

SAGITTAL KNEE ANATOMY: MEDIAL

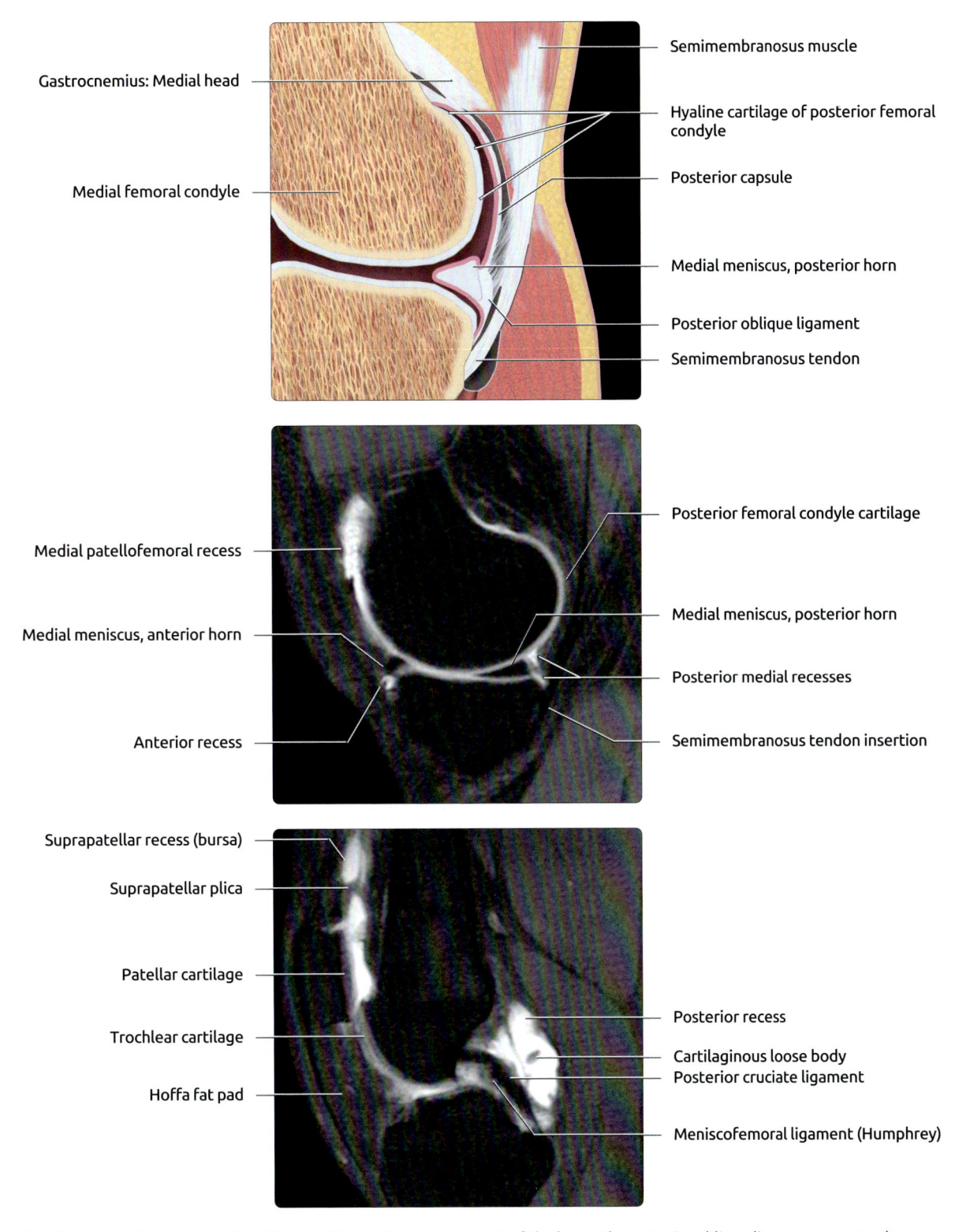

Labels (Top graphic):
- Gastrocnemius: Medial head
- Medial femoral condyle
- Semimembranosus muscle
- Hyaline cartilage of posterior femoral condyle
- Posterior capsule
- Medial meniscus, posterior horn
- Posterior oblique ligament
- Semimembranosus tendon

Labels (Middle):
- Medial patellofemoral recess
- Medial meniscus, anterior horn
- Anterior recess
- Posterior femoral condyle cartilage
- Medial meniscus, posterior horn
- Posterior medial recesses
- Semimembranosus tendon insertion

Labels (Bottom):
- Suprapatellar recess (bursa)
- Suprapatellar plica
- Patellar cartilage
- Trochlear cartilage
- Hoffa fat pad
- Posterior recess
- Cartilaginous loose body
- Posterior cruciate ligament
- Meniscofemoral ligament (Humphrey)

(**Top**) *Graphic shows a sagittal cross section through the medial compartment of the knee. The posterior oblique ligament courses along the capsular margin, reinforcing the joint against posterior tibial translation. Hyaline cartilage extends to the most superior margin of the posterior femoral condyles.* (**Middle**) *Sagittal T1W FS MR arthrogram image through the medial compartment of the joint shows contrast in small recesses around the medial meniscus. Hyaline cartilage is intermediate signal intensity on T1WI FS.* (**Bottom**) *Sagittal T1W FS MR arthrogram image through the medial portion of intercondylar notch shows the posterior cruciate ligament (PCL) with anterior meniscofemoral ligament in cross section at its anterior margin. Cartilage loose body is seen posteriorly; MR arthrography is more sensitive in detection of loose bodies than noncontrast MR.*

Knee Radiographic and Arthrographic Anatomy

SAGITTAL KNEE ANATOMY: LATERAL

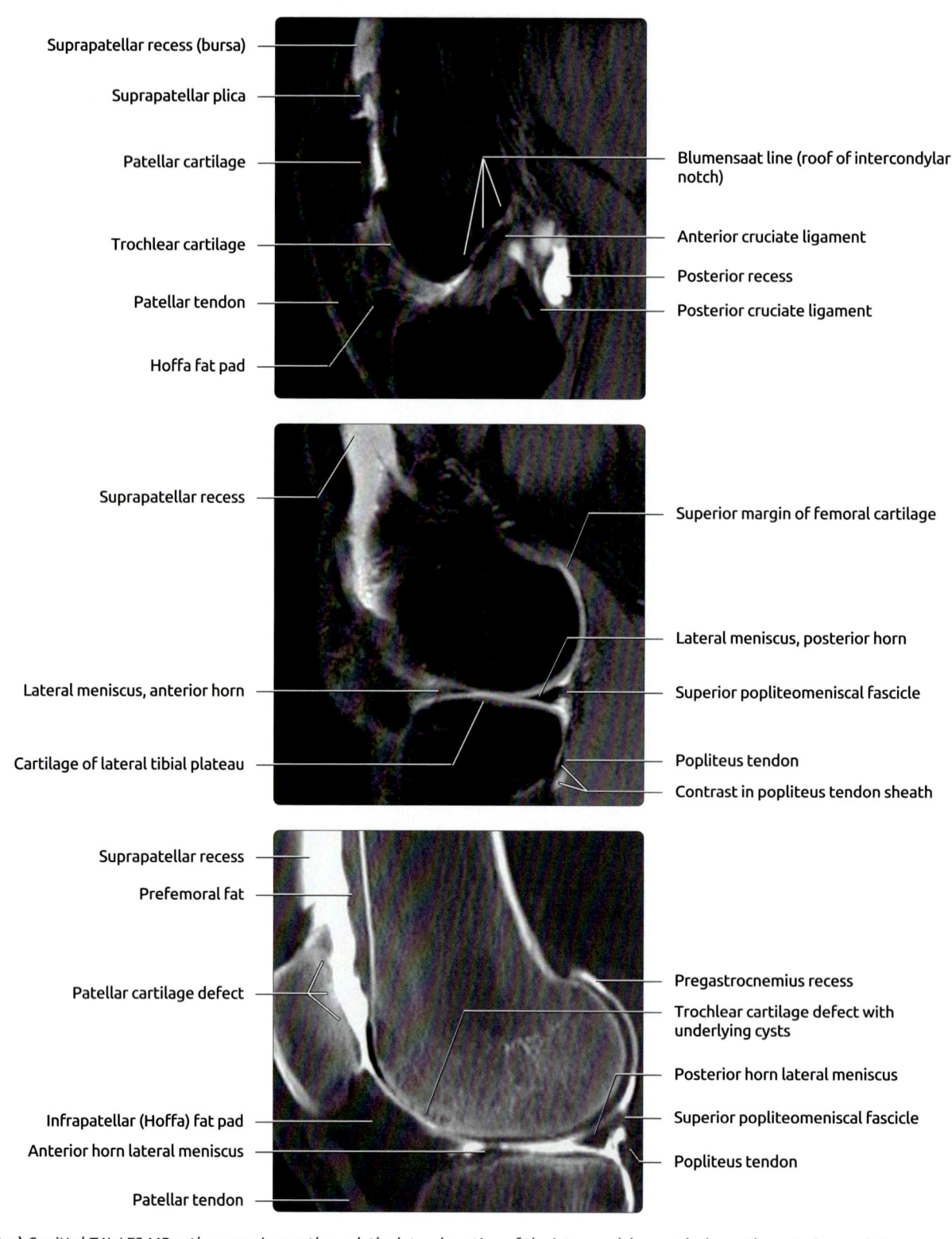

Labels (top image):
- Suprapatellar recess (bursa)
- Suprapatellar plica
- Patellar cartilage
- Trochlear cartilage
- Patellar tendon
- Hoffa fat pad
- Blumensaat line (roof of intercondylar notch)
- Anterior cruciate ligament
- Posterior recess
- Posterior cruciate ligament

Labels (middle image):
- Suprapatellar recess
- Lateral meniscus, anterior horn
- Cartilage of lateral tibial plateau
- Superior margin of femoral cartilage
- Lateral meniscus, posterior horn
- Superior popliteomeniscal fascicle
- Popliteus tendon
- Contrast in popliteus tendon sheath

Labels (bottom image):
- Suprapatellar recess
- Prefemoral fat
- Patellar cartilage defect
- Infrapatellar (Hoffa) fat pad
- Anterior horn lateral meniscus
- Patellar tendon
- Pregastrocnemius recess
- Trochlear cartilage defect with underlying cysts
- Posterior horn lateral meniscus
- Superior popliteomeniscal fascicle
- Popliteus tendon

(Top) *Sagittal T1W FS MR arthrogram image through the lateral portion of the intercondylar notch shows the anterior cruciate ligament, which characteristically contains intermediate signal intensity synovial folds extending longitudinally between its loosely connected bundles.* (Middle) *Sagittal T1W FS MR arthrogram image through midportion of lateral compartment shows contrast outlining the lateral meniscus. Note that the popliteus sheath communicates with the posterolateral joint and thereby contains contrast on this image.* (Bottom) *Sagittal CT arthrogram image through the midportion of the lateral compartment is shown. The patient has osteoarthritis, and cartilage loss is seen in multiple areas. The lateral meniscus is outlined by contrast. The superior fascicle of posterior horn is well seen, as is the popliteal tendon in its hiatus.*

Knee Radiographic and Arthrographic Anatomy

SAGITTAL KNEE ANATOMY: LATERAL

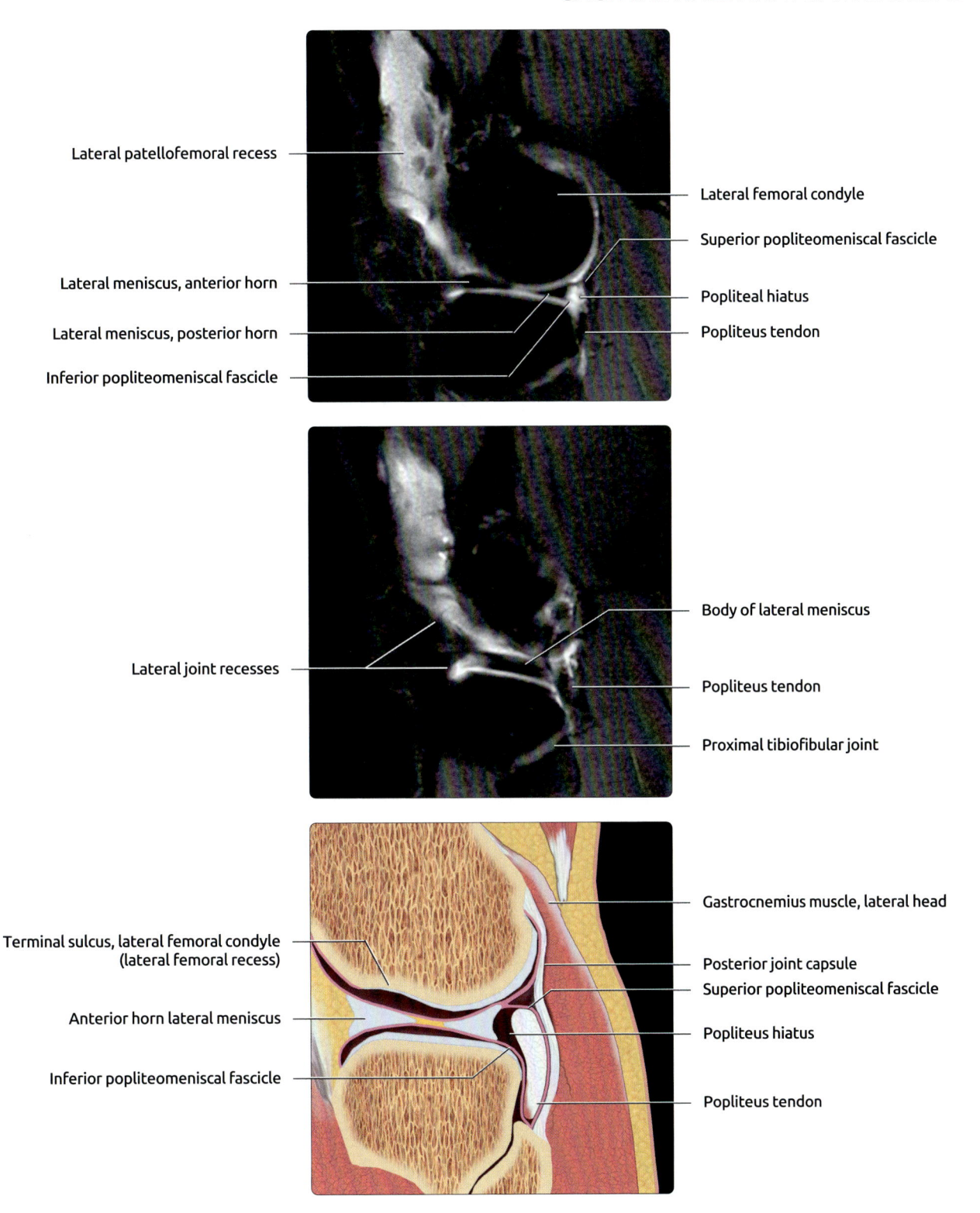

(Top) Sagittal T1W FS MR arthrogram image through the lateral portion of the lateral compartment shows the popliteus tendon passing inferiorly by the lateral meniscus. The popliteal hiatus is the opening in the capsule through which the tendon enters. Note that the inferior popliteomeniscal fascicle appears incomplete, a normal finding at the hiatus. *(Middle)* Sagittal T1W FS MR arthrogram image through the far lateral portion of the lateral compartment shows the body of the lateral meniscus, with the popliteus tendon posterior to it. *(Bottom)* Sagittal graphic shows the popliteus tendon passing through the posterolateral margin of the joint. The tendon is contained within a sheath that communicates with the joint and is connected to the posterior horn of the lateral meniscus by the popliteomeniscal fascicles.

Knee Radiographic and Arthrographic Anatomy

CORONAL KNEE ANATOMY

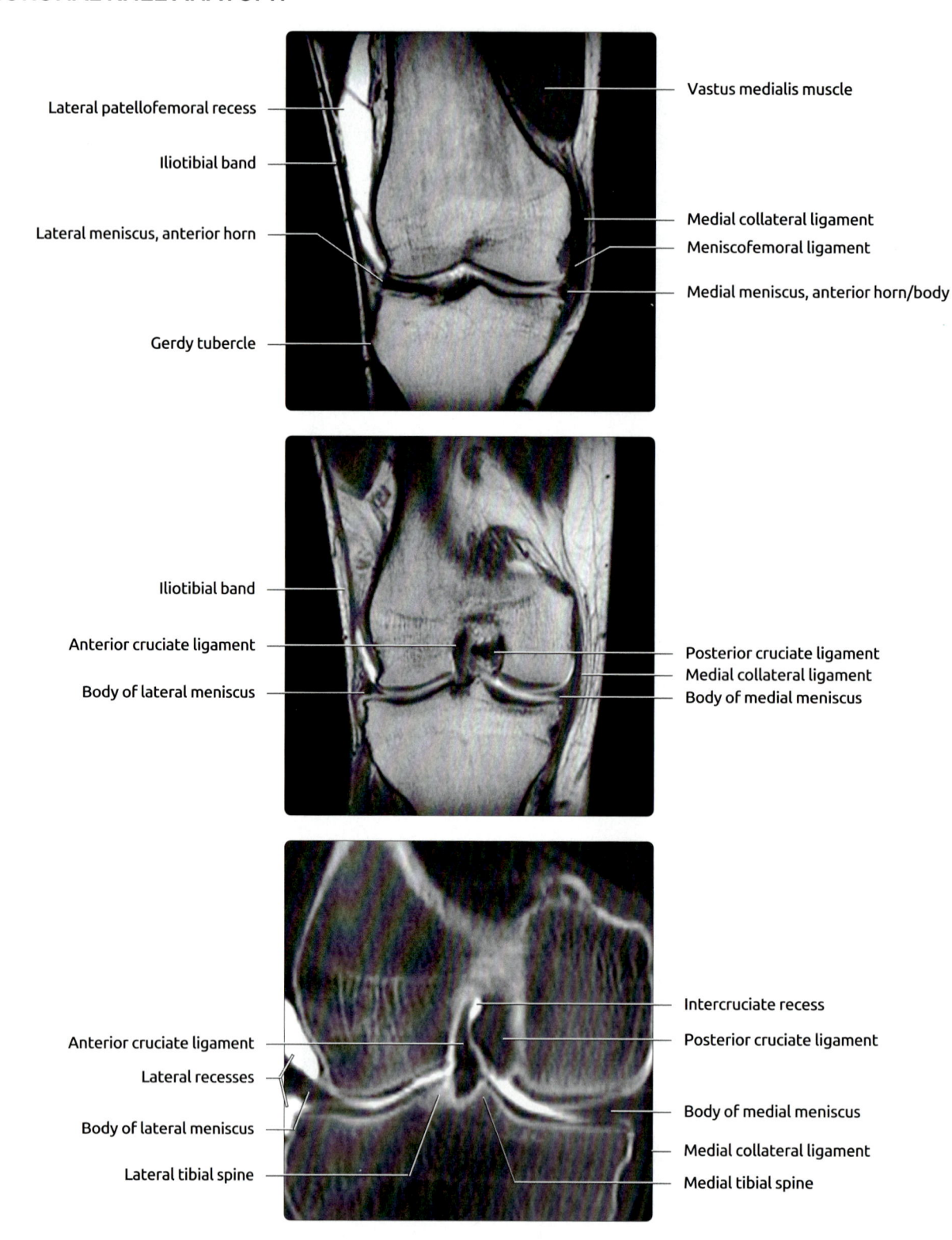

Labels (top image): Lateral patellofemoral recess; Iliotibial band; Lateral meniscus, anterior horn; Gerdy tubercle; Vastus medialis muscle; Medial collateral ligament; Meniscofemoral ligament; Medial meniscus, anterior horn/body

Labels (middle image): Iliotibial band; Anterior cruciate ligament; Body of lateral meniscus; Posterior cruciate ligament; Medial collateral ligament; Body of medial meniscus

Labels (bottom image): Anterior cruciate ligament; Lateral recesses; Body of lateral meniscus; Lateral tibial spine; Intercruciate recess; Posterior cruciate ligament; Body of medial meniscus; Medial collateral ligament; Medial tibial spine

(Top) Coronal T1W MR arthrogram image through the anterior portion of the femorotibial articulations shows the iliotibial band inserting on the tibia at Gerdy tubercle. In this example, the medial collateral ligament is thickened from prior injury. (Middle) Coronal T1W MR arthrogram image posterior to prior image shows the body of the medial and lateral meniscus, as well as the anterior and posterior cruciate ligaments within the intercondylar notch. (Bottom) Coronal CT arthrogram image is through the intercondylar notch, at approximately the same position as the prior MR image. This section outlines the bodies of the menisci, as well as the cruciate ligaments. Note normal capacious recesses around the lateral meniscus, compared to only minimal fluid extending above and below the medial meniscus.

Knee Radiographic and Arthrographic Anatomy

CORONAL KNEE ANATOMY

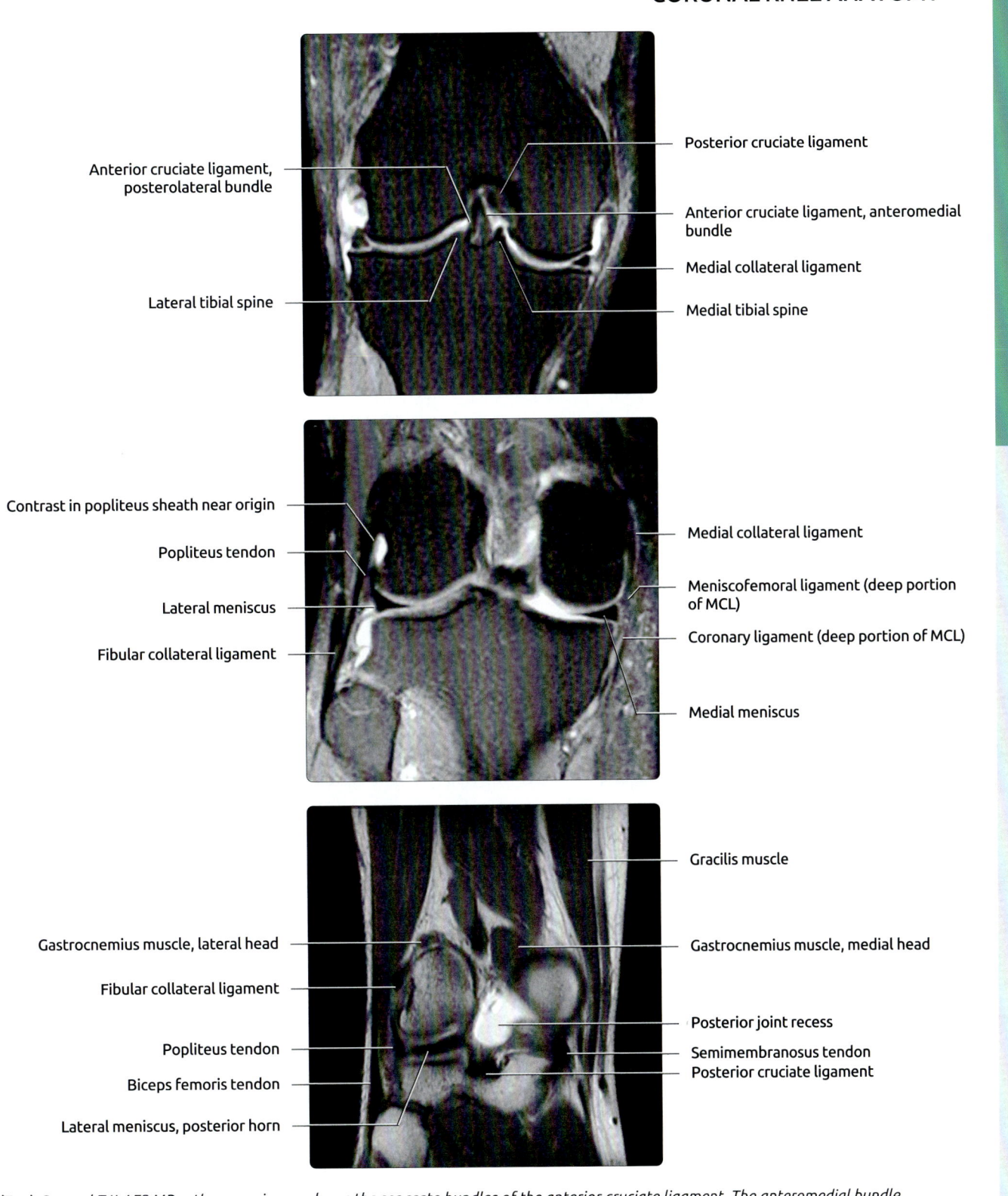

(Top) Coronal T1W FS MR arthrogram image shows the separate bundles of the anterior cruciate ligament. The anteromedial bundle inserts on the medial tibial spine, and the posterolateral bundle inserts near the lateral tibial spine. (Middle) Coronal T1W FS MR arthrogram image shows the medial and lateral joint recesses. The medial meniscus has tight attachments to the femur and tibia (meniscofemoral and coronary ligaments, respectively), resulting in small medial recesses. These meniscal-capsular ligaments comprise the deep portion of the medial collateral ligament. The lateral meniscal Attachments are relatively loose, resulting in large recesses. (Bottom) Coronal T1W MR arthrogram image through the posterior joint margin shows the insertion of the posterior cruciate ligament on the posterior surface of the tibia.

Knee Radiographic and Arthrographic Anatomy

POPLITEAL (BAKER) CYST

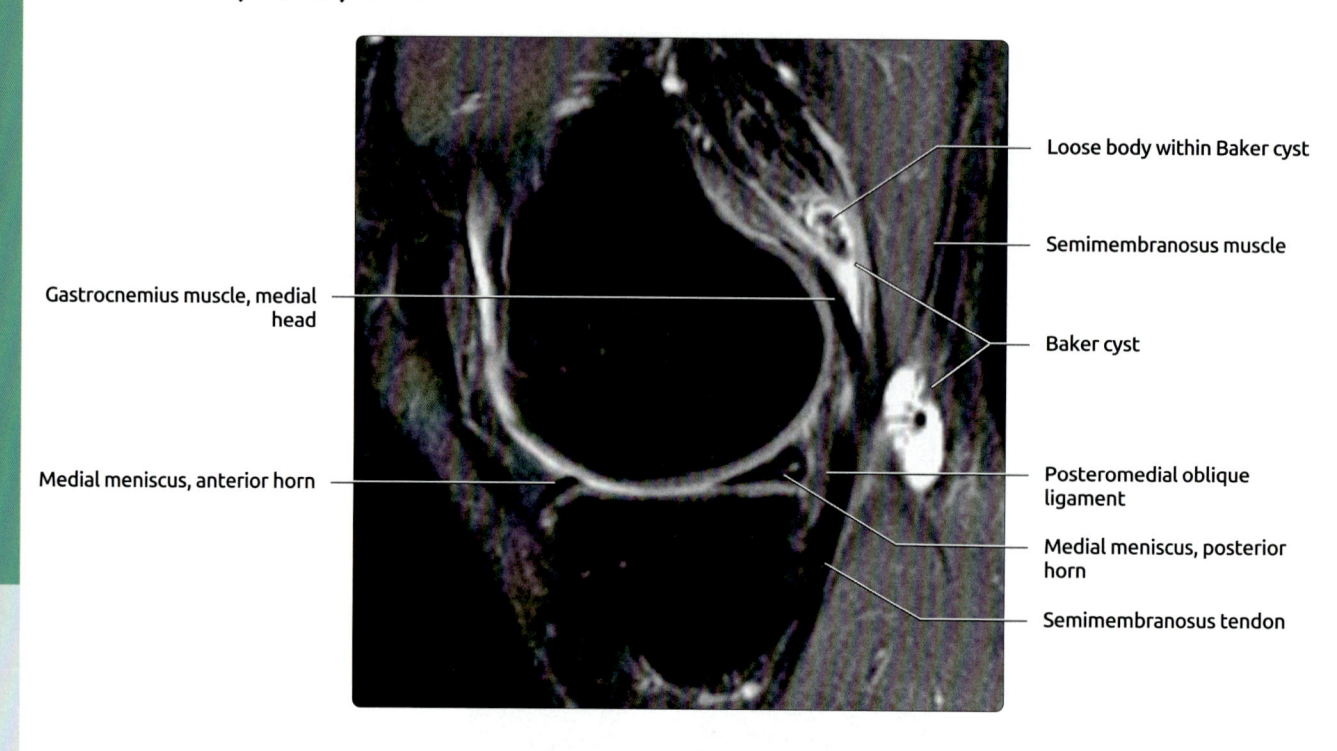

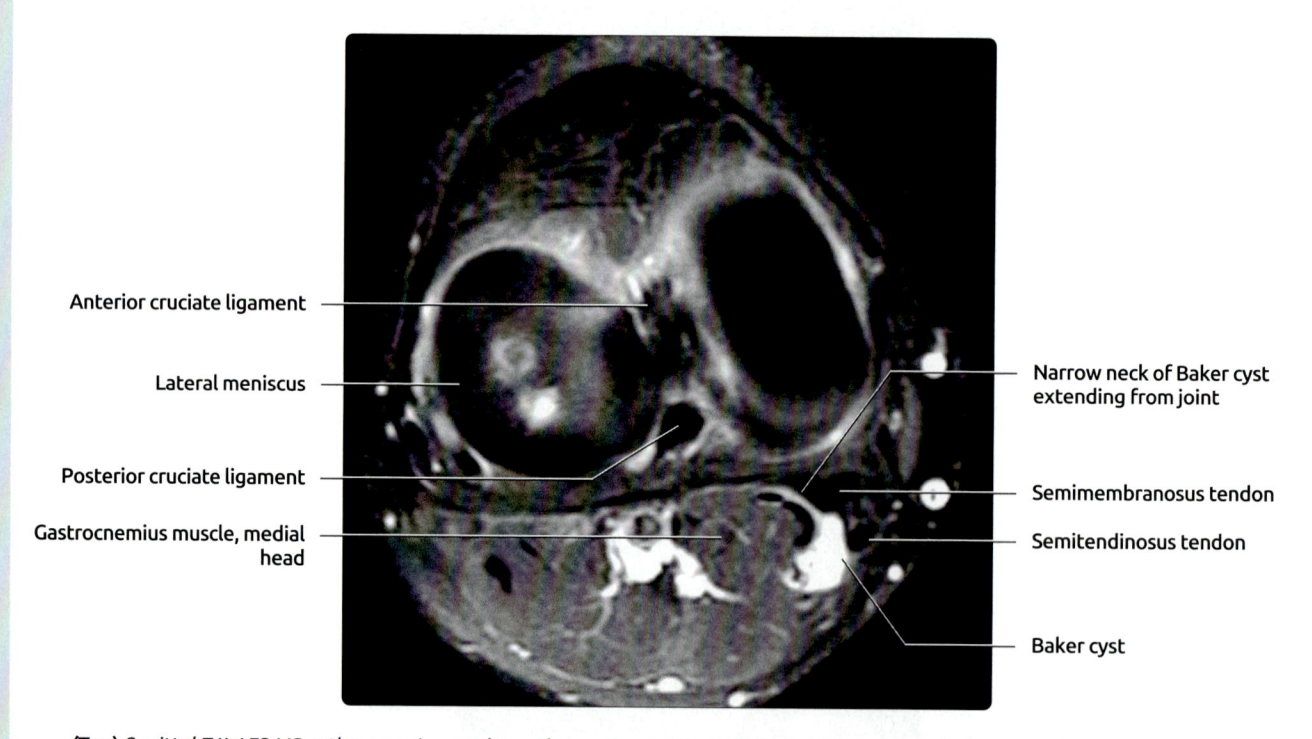

Labels (top image): Gastrocnemius muscle, medial head; Medial meniscus, anterior horn; Loose body within Baker cyst; Semimembranosus muscle; Baker cyst; Posteromedial oblique ligament; Medial meniscus, posterior horn; Semimembranosus tendon

Labels (bottom image): Anterior cruciate ligament; Lateral meniscus; Posterior cruciate ligament; Gastrocnemius muscle, medial head; Narrow neck of Baker cyst extending from joint; Semimembranosus tendon; Semitendinosus tendon; Baker cyst

(Top) Sagittal T1W FS MR arthrogram image shows that contrast, injected into the joint anteriorly, has extended into a Baker cyst through the posteromedial joint capsule. (Bottom) Axial T1W FS MR arthrogram image shows a Baker cyst posteromedially with a characteristic narrow neck extending between the medial head of the gastrocnemius and the semimembranosus tendon. If a fluid-filled structure in the soft tissues does not demonstrate communication with the joint, it cannot be assumed to be a Baker or popliteal cyst.

Knee Radiographic and Arthrographic Anatomy

POSTEROLATERAL CORNER STRUCTURES

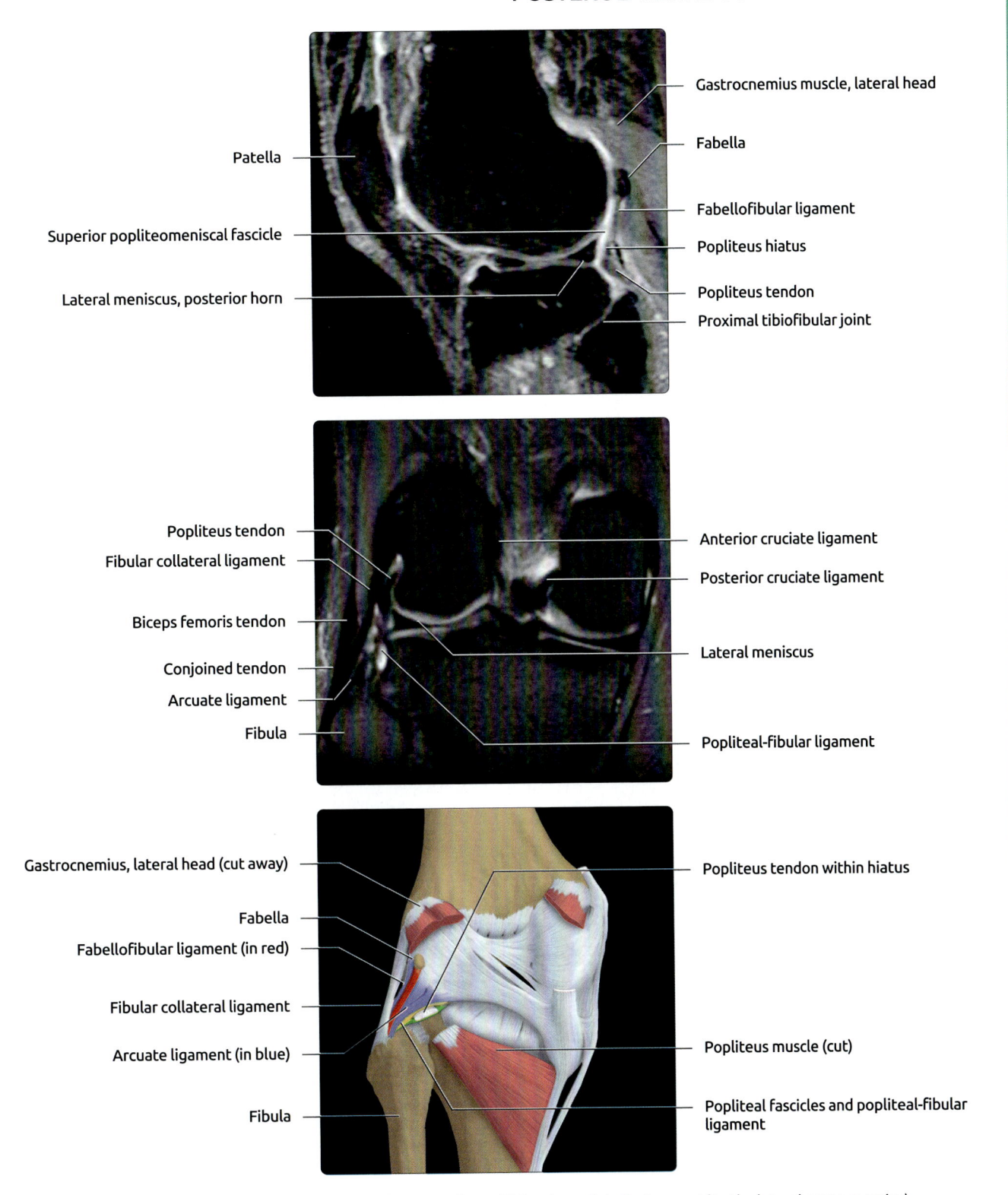

(Top) Sagittal T1W FS MR arthrogram image through the posterolateral joint shows fabella (sesamoid in the lateral gastrocnemius) with the fabellofibular ligament extending inferiorly. This ligament (and associated fabella) are often absent. (Middle) Coronal T1W FS MR arthrogram image through the posterior joint shows posterolateral structures including the fibular collateral ligament and biceps femoris (together forming the conjoined tendon inserting on the fibula), the arcuate ligament, the popliteal-fibular ligament, and the popliteus tendon. (Bottom) Graphic of the posterior joint seen from behind shows diagrammatic representation of posterolateral joint ligaments.

Knee Radiographic and Arthrographic Anatomy

MENISCAL LIGAMENTS

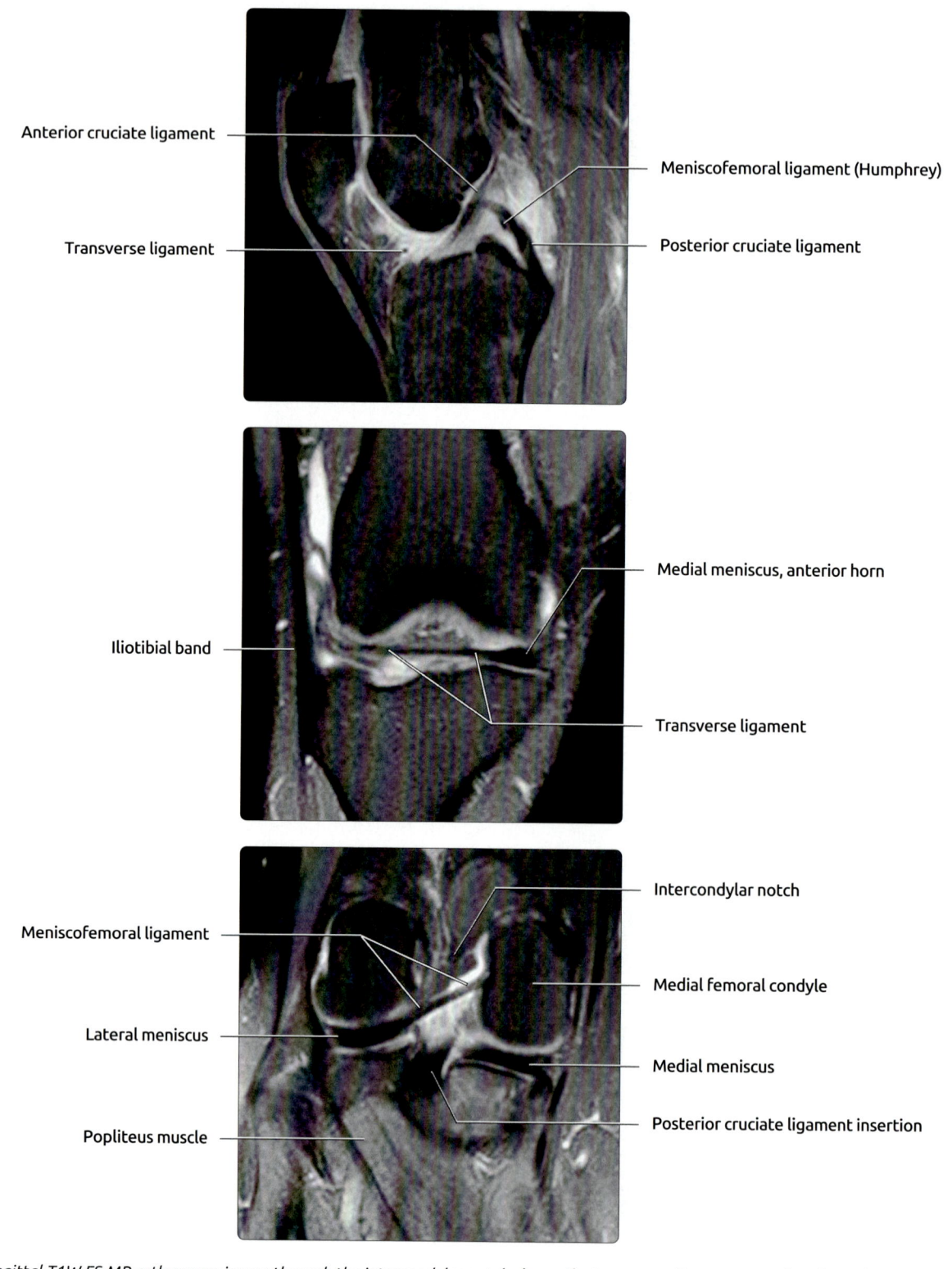

(Top) Sagittal T1W FS MR arthrogram image through the intercondylar notch shows the transverse ligament coursing through the anterior joint from medial to lateral meniscus, seen in cross section as a round focus of low signal intensity. (Middle) Coronal T1W FS MR arthrogram image through the anterior joint shows the transverse ligament in plane, extending from the anterior horn of the medial meniscus to the anterior horn of the lateral meniscus. (Bottom) Coronal T1W FS MR arthrogram image through the posterior joint shows the meniscofemoral ligament, which originates from the posterior horn of the lateral meniscus, medially and superiorly to the medial femoral condyle at the intercondylar notch. The ligament is variably present and may be anterior to the PCL (Humphrey ligament) &/or posterior to the PCL (Wrisberg ligament).

Knee Radiographic and Arthrographic Anatomy

PLICAE

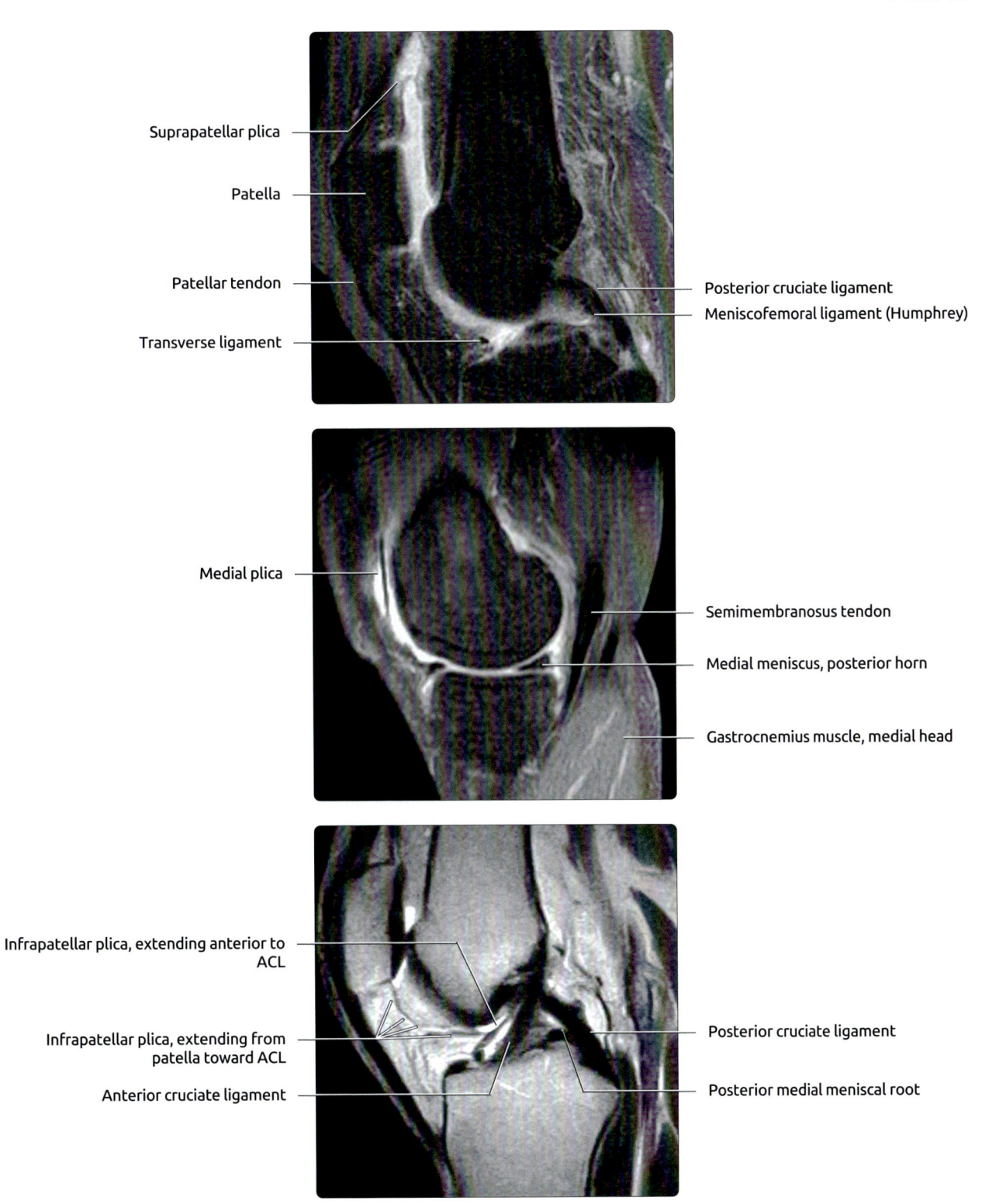

(Top) Sagittal T1W FS MR arthrogram image shows a suprapatellar plica. A suprapatellar plica rarely can become symptomatic if it is thickened and obstructs the suprapatellar recess, leading to entrapment of fluid and synovial tissue above the plica. *(Middle)* Sagittal T1W FS MR arthrogram image through the medial joint shows a medial plica, which is the most commonly symptomatic type of plica. The plica extends vertically through the medial patellofemoral joint and can cause a snapping sensation on flexion/extension as it rubs across the femoral condyle. It may contribute to trochlear or patellar cartilage wear. *(Bottom)* Sagittal T1W FS MR arthrogram image shows an infrapatellar plica, which extends from Hoffa fat pad to the intercondylar notch anterior to the ACL. It is not thought to cause symptoms. Fluid may dissect along the plica into Hoffa fat.

Knee MR Atlas

TERMINOLOGY

Abbreviations
- Anterior cruciate ligament (ACL)
- Posterior cruciate ligament (PCL)
- Medial (tibial) collateral ligament (MCL)
- Lateral (fibular) collateral ligament (LCL)

IMAGING ANATOMY

Overview
- Multiple specific anatomic relationships must be maintained in order to assure stability and full function

Distal Femur
- **Possible sites of avulsion**
  - Posterolateral intercondylar notch (ACL origin)
  - Medial epicondyle (MCL origin)
- **Cartilage**
  - Thicker over posterior condyles than normal weight-bearing surface
  - Focally thin at lateral femoral condylar recess

Proximal Tibia
- **Possible sites of avulsion**
  - Tibial spine (ACL insertion)
  - Posterior mid tibial joint line (PCL insertion)
  - Medial joint line (coronary ligament insertion)
  - Lateral joint line (anterolateral ligament and capsular insertion; may avulse with valgus twist): Segond fracture
  - Gerdy tubercle (iliotibial band)
  - Tibial apophysis (patellar tendon insertion): In skeletally immature patient
- **Cartilage**: Uniformly thin

Proximal Fibula
- **Possible sites of avulsion**
  - Lateral fibular head/neck (insertion of conjoint tendon)
  - Thin, fragment styloid process (insertion of arcuate, fabellofibular, popliteofibular ligaments)

Tibiofibular Joint
- True synovial joint; subject to any arthritic process
- Connects to knee joint in 20%

Patella
- **Cartilage**
  - Thickest cartilage in body (3-4 mm)
  - Uniform thickness
  - May have dorsal patellar defect or bipartite/multipartite patella as normal variant but with normal overlying cartilage

Articular Capsule
- Highly complex, noncontiguous structure
- Contributions from multiple muscles, tendons, and ligaments
- Some structures may be intraarticular but extrasynovial

Extensor Mechanism
- Quadriceps tendon converges on patella
- Fibers of rectus femoris course over patella to form inferior patellar tendon
- Fibers of vastus lateralis and medialis contribute to lateral and medial retinacula, respectively

Internal Structures
- **Menisci**
  - Cushion, lubricate, and stabilize knee
  - Fibrocartilage
  - Only peripheral portion vascularized
  - Attached by anterior and posterior roots to tibial surface
  - Medial attached to capsule throughout extent
  - Lateral attached to capsule at anterior horn and far posteriorly, but by fascicles to popliteus/capsule at body and posterior horn
  - Lateral has constant size and shape
  - Medial has elongated posterior horn and small body
- **Cruciate ligaments**
  - Intraarticular but extrasynovial
  - Major stabilizing structures to anteroposterior motion
  - ACL originates at posterolateral intercondylar notch, crosses anteromedially, and inserts at medial tibial spine/tibial surface
  - PCL originates at mid medial intercondylar notch, crosses posteriorly and slightly laterally, and inserts extraarticularly at posterior center of tibia below joint line
  - Injury generally intrasubstance, but avulsions may indicate injury (origin and insertion, respectively)
    - ACL: Posterolateral Blumensaat line or medial tibial spine
    - PCL: Mid medial intercondylar notch or posterior central tibia
  - Normal variants could possibly be confusing
    - ACL: Infrapatellar plica, meniscocruciate ligament, meniscomeniscal ligament
    - PCL: Meniscofemoral ligaments

Medial Supporting Structures
- **Superficial (layer 1)**
  - Pes anserinus: Anteromedial tibial insertion
    - Sartorius embedded in crural fascia
    - Gracilis immediately deep to sartorius
    - Semitendinosus immediately deep to gracilis
- **Middle (layer 2)**
  - Superficial medial collateral ligament (longitudinal and oblique components)
    - Origin is medial epicondyle; runs slightly anteromedially to insert on tibia, 5 cm distal to joint line
    - Anteriorly, longitudinal component fascia blends with layer 1
    - Posteriorly, oblique component blends with layer 3 as posterior oblique ligament
- **Deep (layer 3)**
  - Capsular layers (sometimes termed deep fibers of MCL) at mid portion of knee
    - Meniscofemoral ligament
    - Meniscotibial (coronary) ligament
  - More posteriorly, superficial MCL blends with capsular layers of MCL
  - Posterior oblique ligament arises from superficial MCL
    - Blends with posteromedial meniscus

- Receives fibers from semimembranosus tendon
- Envelops posterior aspect femoral condyle, termed oblique popliteal ligament

Lateral Supporting Structures
- Superficial (layer 1)
  o Iliotibial band anteriorly, inserting on Gerdy tubercle
  o Superficial portion of biceps femoris posterolaterally, inserting on fibular styloid
- Middle (layer 2)
  o Quadriceps retinaculum anteriorly
  o Posteriorly, 2 ligamentous thickenings, which originate from lateral patella
    - Proximal one terminates at lateral intermuscular septum on femur
    - Distal one terminates at femoral insertion of posterolateral capsule and lateral head of gastrocnemius
- Deep (layer 3): Several thickenings in lateral part of capsule function as discrete structures
  o Lateral (fibular) collateral ligament originates from lateral femoral epicondyle, extends posterolaterally to insert on lateral fibular head
  o Anterolateral ligament originates from lateral femoral epicondyle just anterior to lateral collateral ligament (may have connecting fibers), interdigitates with lateral meniscus, and extends obliquely and anteriorly to insert on anterolateral tibia posterior to Gerdy tubercle
  o Arcuate ligament originates from styloid process fibular head, interdigitates with popliteus, and inserts into posterior capsule near oblique popliteal ligament
  o Several other small and inconstant structures located posterolaterally, which are difficult to differentiate by imaging

ANATOMY IMAGING ISSUES

Imaging Recommendations
- MR
  o T1 in 1 plane to evaluate marrow and anatomy
  o PD (± fat saturation) is most accurate sequence to evaluate menisci
  o Fluid-sensitive sequence to evaluate location and tracking of fluid collections

Imaging Pitfalls
- Variants: Multiple osseous and soft tissue normal variants
- Loose bodies on MR: Easily missed
- Partial voluming over convex surfaces: Morphology of trochlea, femoral condyles, and patella makes them particularly difficult to evaluate in 3 standard planes
- Imaging cartilage
  o T2 underestimates cartilage thickness since cortex and cartilage have similar signal
  o PD may have similar signal for cartilage and adjacent joint fluid, obscuring defects; fat saturation solves this

CLINICAL IMPLICATIONS

Denervation Syndromes Related to Knee Anatomy
- Tibial nerve denervation
  o Tibial nerve branches from sciatic nerve in popliteal fossa
    - Relatively protected, so compression fairly rare
    - Provides motor innervation to gastrocnemius, plantaris, popliteus, soleus, tibialis posterior, flexor digitorum longus, and flexor hallucis longus
  o Proximal tibial neuropathy symptoms
    - Sensory change on bottom of foot
    - Weakness of plantar flexor and inverter muscles
    - Weakness of intrinsic muscles of foot
  o Common causes of proximal tibial neuropathy
    - Significant fracture
    - Compression by Baker cyst
    - Nerve sheath tumor
    - Vasculitis-related neuropathy (diabetes mellitus or polyarteritis nodosa)
- Common peroneal nerve denervation
  o Most common mononeuropathy of lower extremity
  o At greatest risk for direct compression/trauma, as it winds around outer fibular neck
    - Superficial position with only subcutaneous fat and skin coverage puts nerve at risk for direct trauma
    - Nerve then pierces the anterior fascia to enter anterior compartment, between tendinous origins of peroneus longus muscle; tethering may occur, making nerve susceptible to stretch injury
    - Trifurcation into recurrent articular branch, superficial peroneal nerve, and deep peroneal nerve
  o Innervation
    - Deep peroneal nerve provides innervation to extensor muscles in anterior compartment of lower leg (tibialis anterior, extensor hallucis longus, extensor digitorum longus)
    - Superficial peroneal branch innervates peroneus longus and peroneus brevis
  o Common peroneal neuropathy symptoms
    - Footdrop
    - Pain in lower lateral 2/3 of leg
  o Common causes of common peroneal neuropathy
    - Direct trauma
    - Fibular neck fracture or knee dislocation
    - Knee arthroplasty in patient with prior significant valgus deformity
    - Tight cast
    - Ganglia/mass lesions
    - Variations in distal and posterior extent of distal biceps muscle in up to 23% of population may create tunnel with entrapment of nerve

Knee MR Atlas

AXIAL T1 MR, RIGHT KNEE

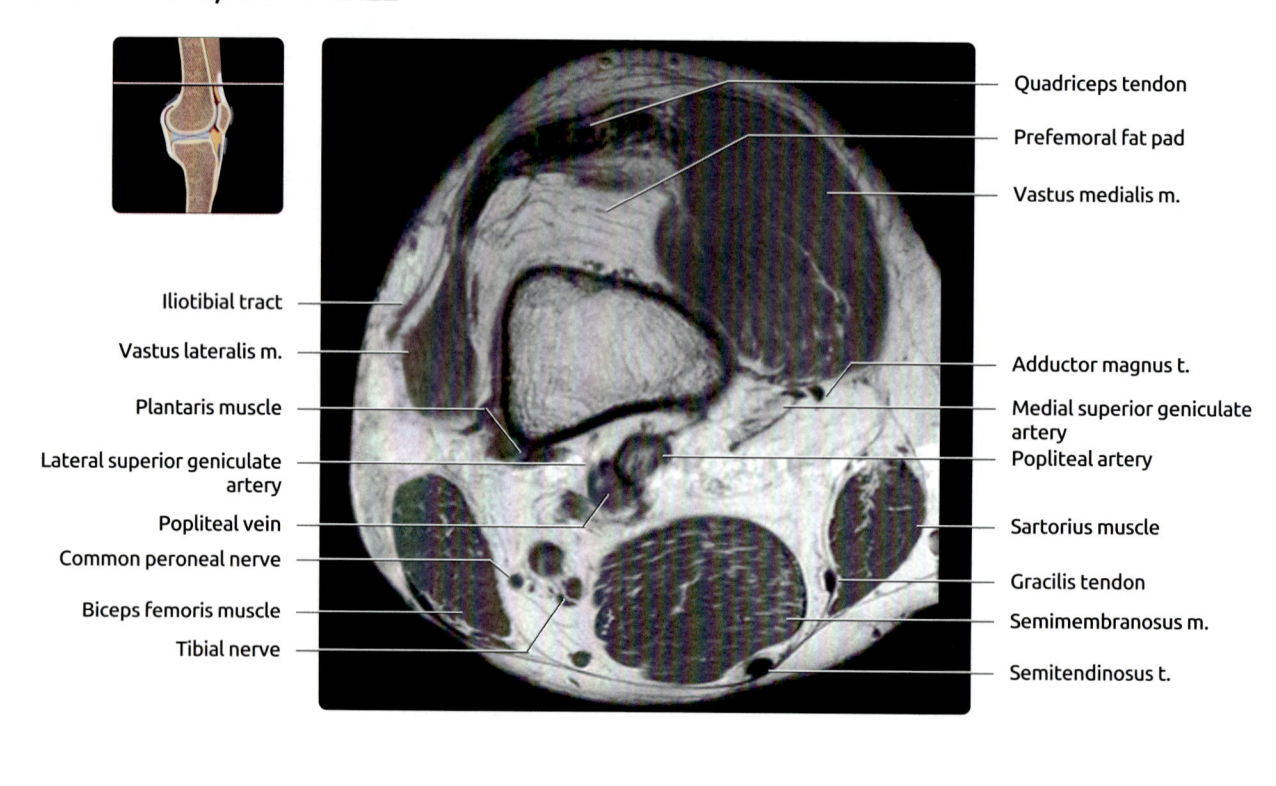

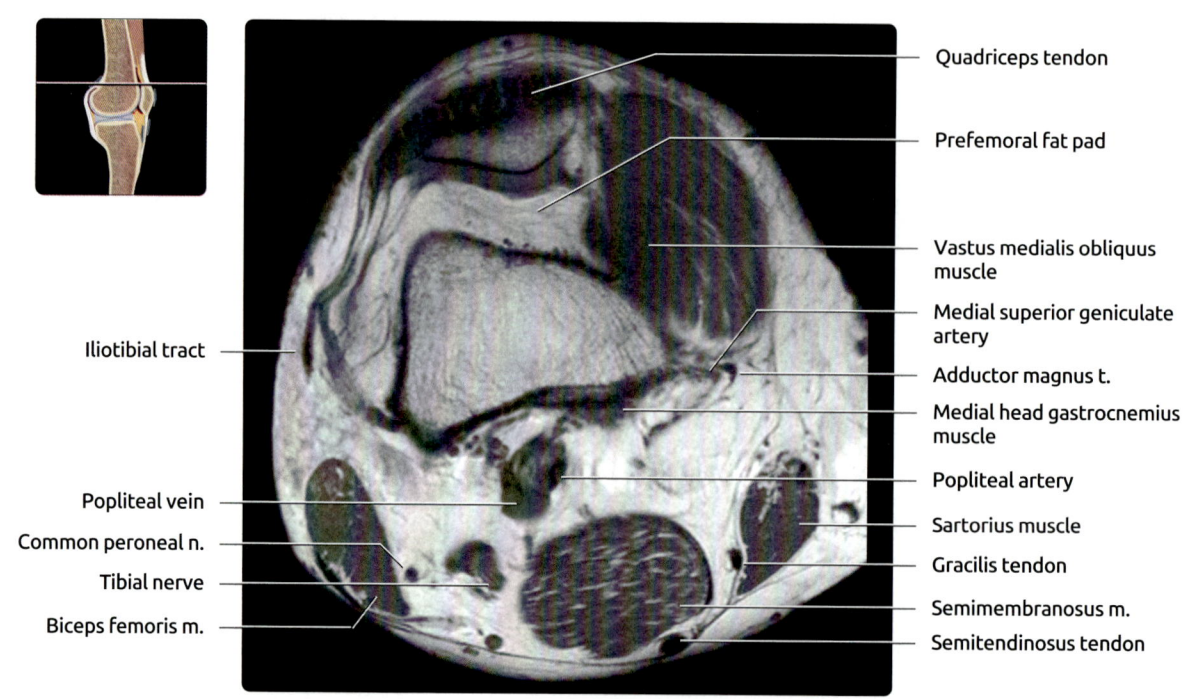

Labels (top image):
- Quadriceps tendon
- Prefemoral fat pad
- Vastus medialis m.
- Iliotibial tract
- Vastus lateralis m.
- Plantaris muscle
- Lateral superior geniculate artery
- Popliteal vein
- Common peroneal nerve
- Biceps femoris muscle
- Tibial nerve
- Adductor magnus t.
- Medial superior geniculate artery
- Popliteal artery
- Sartorius muscle
- Gracilis tendon
- Semimembranosus m.
- Semitendinosus t.

Labels (bottom image):
- Quadriceps tendon
- Prefemoral fat pad
- Vastus medialis obliquus muscle
- Medial superior geniculate artery
- Adductor magnus t.
- Medial head gastrocnemius muscle
- Popliteal artery
- Sartorius muscle
- Gracilis tendon
- Semimembranosus m.
- Semitendinosus tendon
- Iliotibial tract
- Popliteal vein
- Common peroneal n.
- Tibial nerve
- Biceps femoris m.

(Top) The 1st in a series of axial T1 MR images of the right knee shows that the cut is above the patella and at the proximal portion of the femoral metaphysis. At this level, the origin of the plantaris muscle is seen, but it is still proximal to the adductor tubercle. **(Bottom)** This cut is immediately above the adductor tubercle. The vastus medialis obliquus is seen, serving as medial support for the superior portion of the patella.

Knee MR Atlas

AXIAL T1 MR, LEFT KNEE

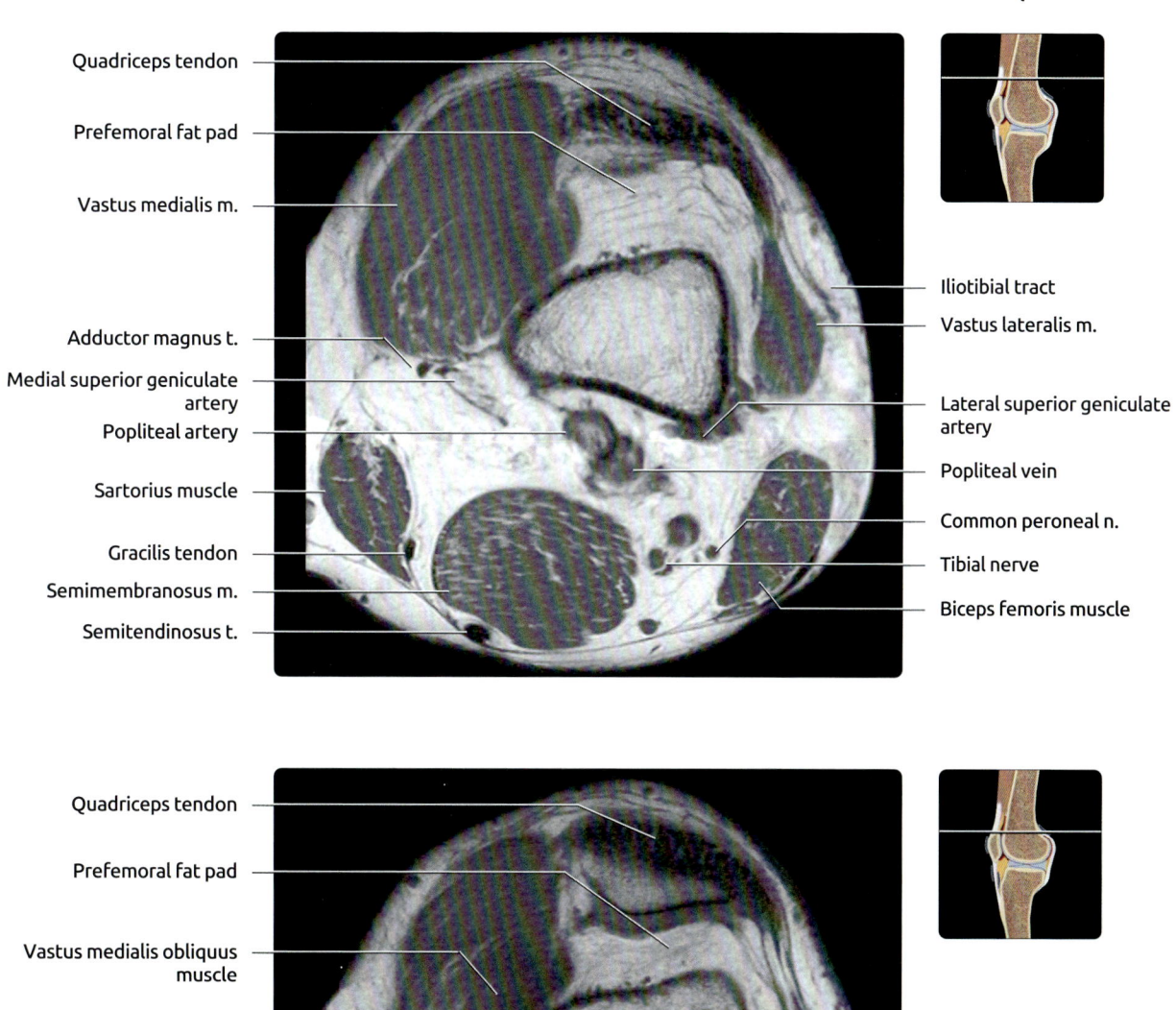

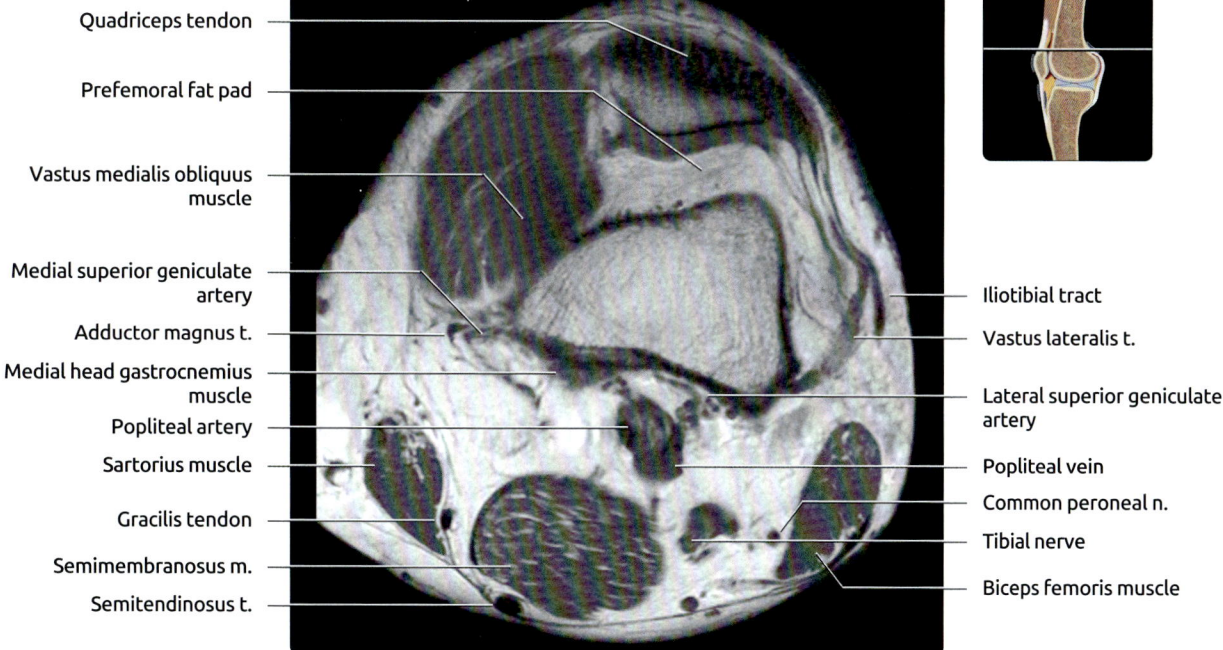

Labels (top image), left side:
- Quadriceps tendon
- Prefemoral fat pad
- Vastus medialis m.
- Adductor magnus t.
- Medial superior geniculate artery
- Popliteal artery
- Sartorius muscle
- Gracilis tendon
- Semimembranosus m.
- Semitendinosus t.

Labels (top image), right side:
- Iliotibial tract
- Vastus lateralis m.
- Lateral superior geniculate artery
- Popliteal vein
- Common peroneal n.
- Tibial nerve
- Biceps femoris muscle

Labels (bottom image), left side:
- Quadriceps tendon
- Prefemoral fat pad
- Vastus medialis obliquus muscle
- Medial superior geniculate artery
- Adductor magnus t.
- Medial head gastrocnemius muscle
- Popliteal artery
- Sartorius muscle
- Gracilis tendon
- Semimembranosus m.
- Semitendinosus t.

Labels (bottom image), right side:
- Iliotibial tract
- Vastus lateralis t.
- Lateral superior geniculate artery
- Popliteal vein
- Common peroneal n.
- Tibial nerve
- Biceps femoris muscle

(Top) The 1st in a series of axial T1 MR images of the left knee shows that the cut is above the patella and at the proximal portion of the femoral metaphysis. At this level, the origin of plantaris muscle is seen, but it is still proximal to the adductor tubercle. **(Bottom)** This cut is immediately above the adductor tubercle. The vastus medialis obliquus is seen, serving as medial support for the superior portion of the patella.

Knee MR Atlas

AXIAL T1 MR, RIGHT KNEE

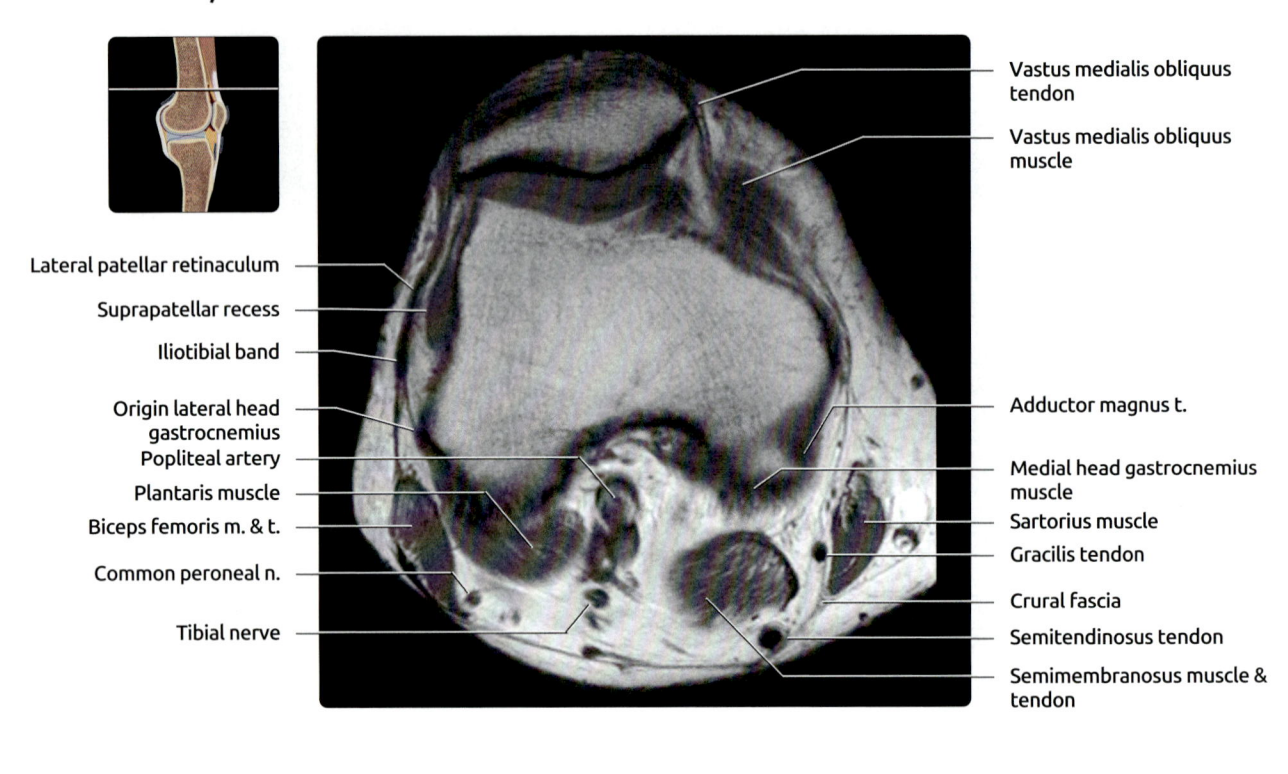

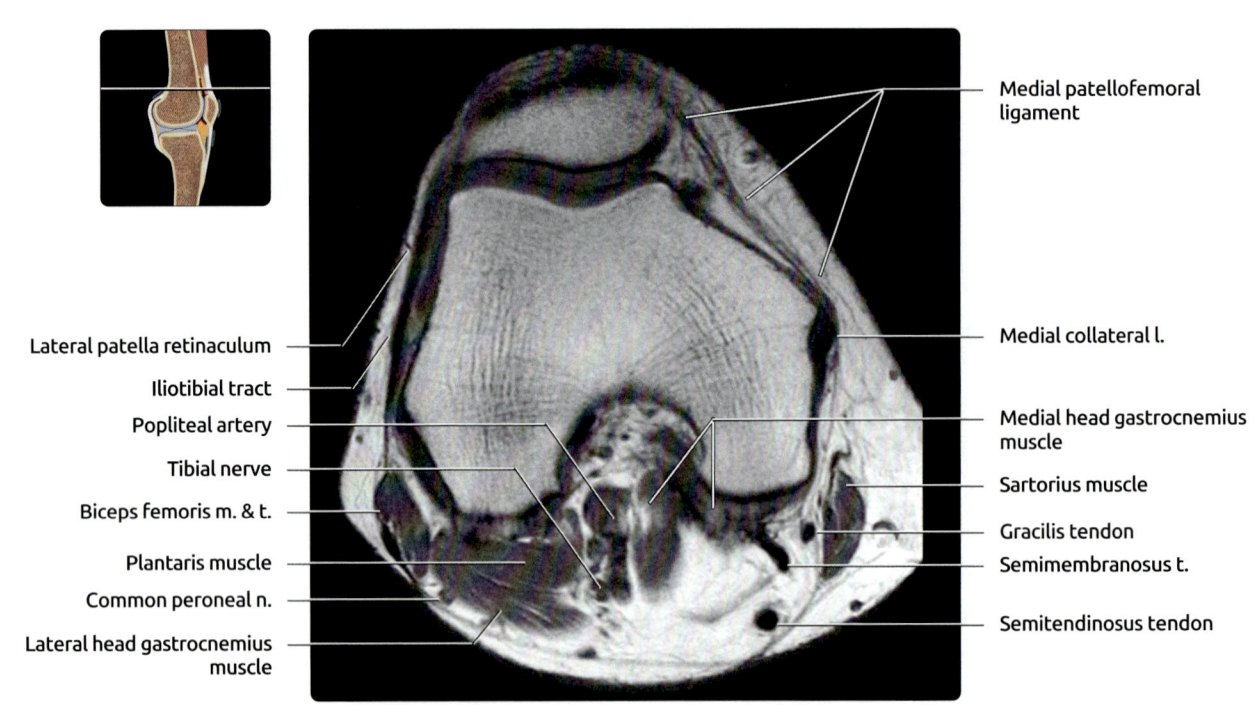

Labels (top image):
- Vastus medialis obliquus tendon
- Vastus medialis obliquus muscle
- Lateral patellar retinaculum
- Suprapatellar recess
- Iliotibial band
- Origin lateral head gastrocnemius
- Popliteal artery
- Plantaris muscle
- Biceps femoris m. & t.
- Common peroneal n.
- Tibial nerve
- Adductor magnus t.
- Medial head gastrocnemius muscle
- Sartorius muscle
- Gracilis tendon
- Crural fascia
- Semitendinosus tendon
- Semimembranosus muscle & tendon

Labels (bottom image):
- Medial patellofemoral ligament
- Lateral patella retinaculum
- Iliotibial tract
- Popliteal artery
- Tibial nerve
- Biceps femoris m. & t.
- Plantaris muscle
- Common peroneal n.
- Lateral head gastrocnemius muscle
- Medial collateral l.
- Medial head gastrocnemius muscle
- Sartorius muscle
- Gracilis tendon
- Semimembranosus t.
- Semitendinosus tendon

(Top) This cut is at the level of the adductor tubercle, which serves at its superior aspect as the insertion site of the adductor magnus tendon. The superior portion of the medial patella is stabilized by the tendinous attachment of the vastus medialis obliquus. Note that the structures comprising the pes anserinus are aligning themselves. **(Bottom)** Slightly distal, the inferior aspect of the adductor tubercle serves as the site of origin of the medial patellofemoral ligament, which inserts on the upper 2/3 of the medial patella and is an important patellar stabilizer. It also serves as the site of origin of the superficial medial collateral ligament fibers.

Knee MR Atlas

AXIAL T1 MR, LEFT KNEE

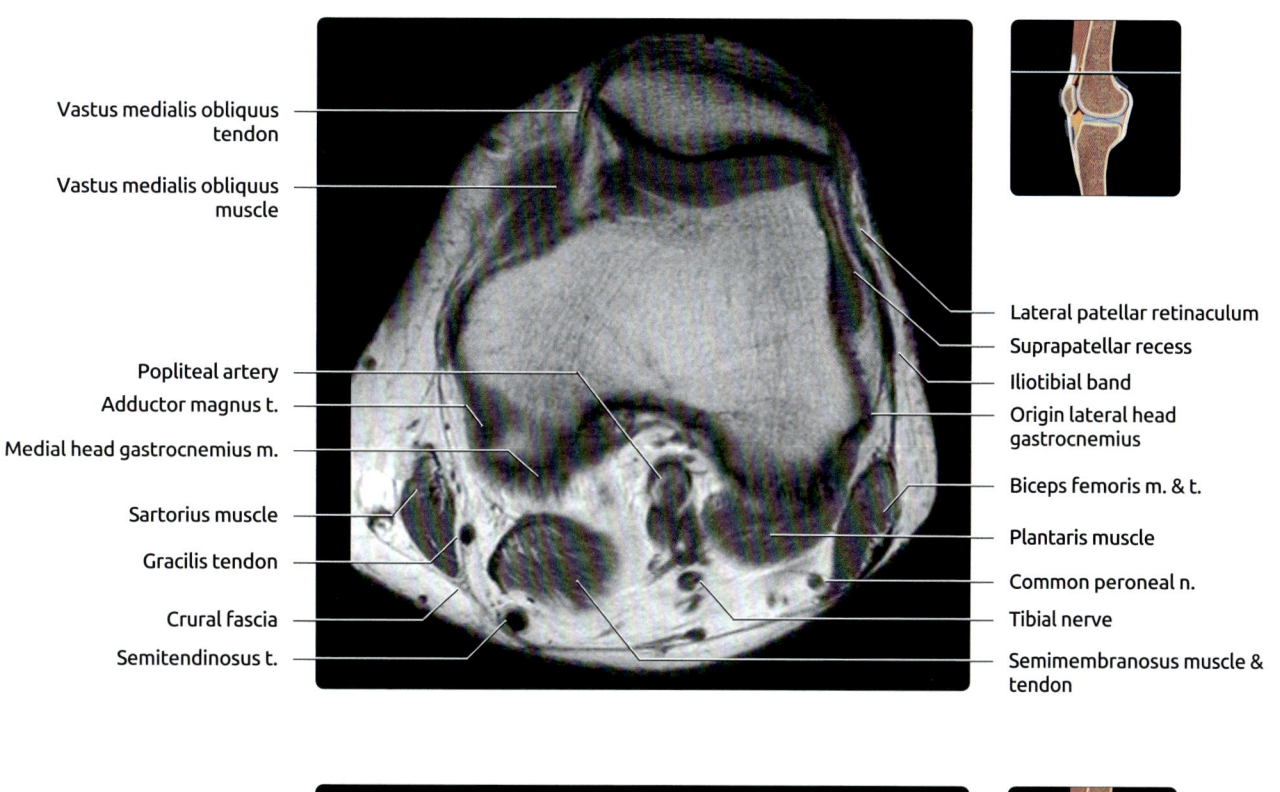

Top image labels (left side):
- Vastus medialis obliquus tendon
- Vastus medialis obliquus muscle
- Popliteal artery
- Adductor magnus t.
- Medial head gastrocnemius m.
- Sartorius muscle
- Gracilis tendon
- Crural fascia
- Semitendinosus t.

Top image labels (right side):
- Lateral patellar retinaculum
- Suprapatellar recess
- Iliotibial band
- Origin lateral head gastrocnemius
- Biceps femoris m. & t.
- Plantaris muscle
- Common peroneal n.
- Tibial nerve
- Semimembranosus muscle & tendon

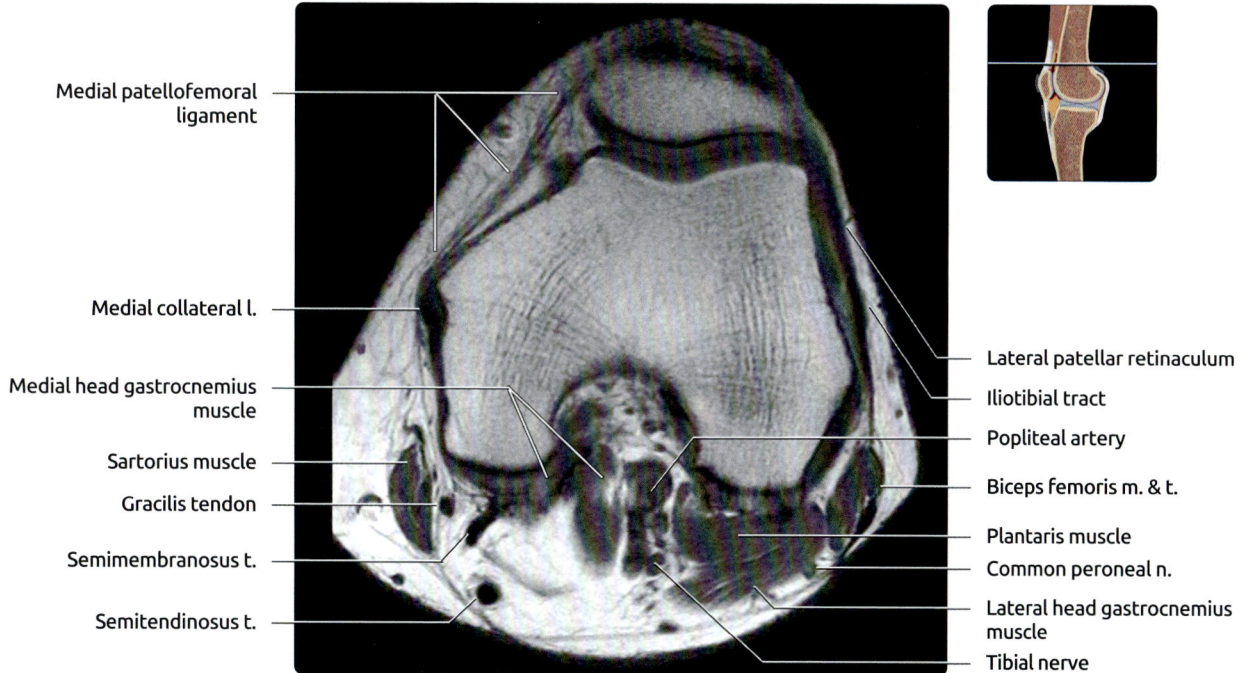

Bottom image labels (left side):
- Medial patellofemoral ligament
- Medial collateral l.
- Medial head gastrocnemius muscle
- Sartorius muscle
- Gracilis tendon
- Semimembranosus t.
- Semitendinosus t.

Bottom image labels (right side):
- Lateral patellar retinaculum
- Iliotibial tract
- Popliteal artery
- Biceps femoris m. & t.
- Plantaris muscle
- Common peroneal n.
- Lateral head gastrocnemius muscle
- Tibial nerve

(Top) This cut is at the level of the adductor tubercle, which serves at its superior aspect as the insertion site of the adductor magnus tendon. The superior portion of the medial patella is stabilized by the tendinous attachment of the vastus medialis obliquus. Note that the structures comprising the pes anserinus are aligning themselves. **(Bottom)** Slightly distal, the inferior aspect of the adductor tubercle serves as the site of origin of the medial patellofemoral ligament, which inserts on the upper 2/3 of the medial patella and is an important patellar stabilizer. It also serves as the site of origin of the superficial medial collateral ligament fibers.

Knee MR Atlas

AXIAL T1 MR, RIGHT KNEE

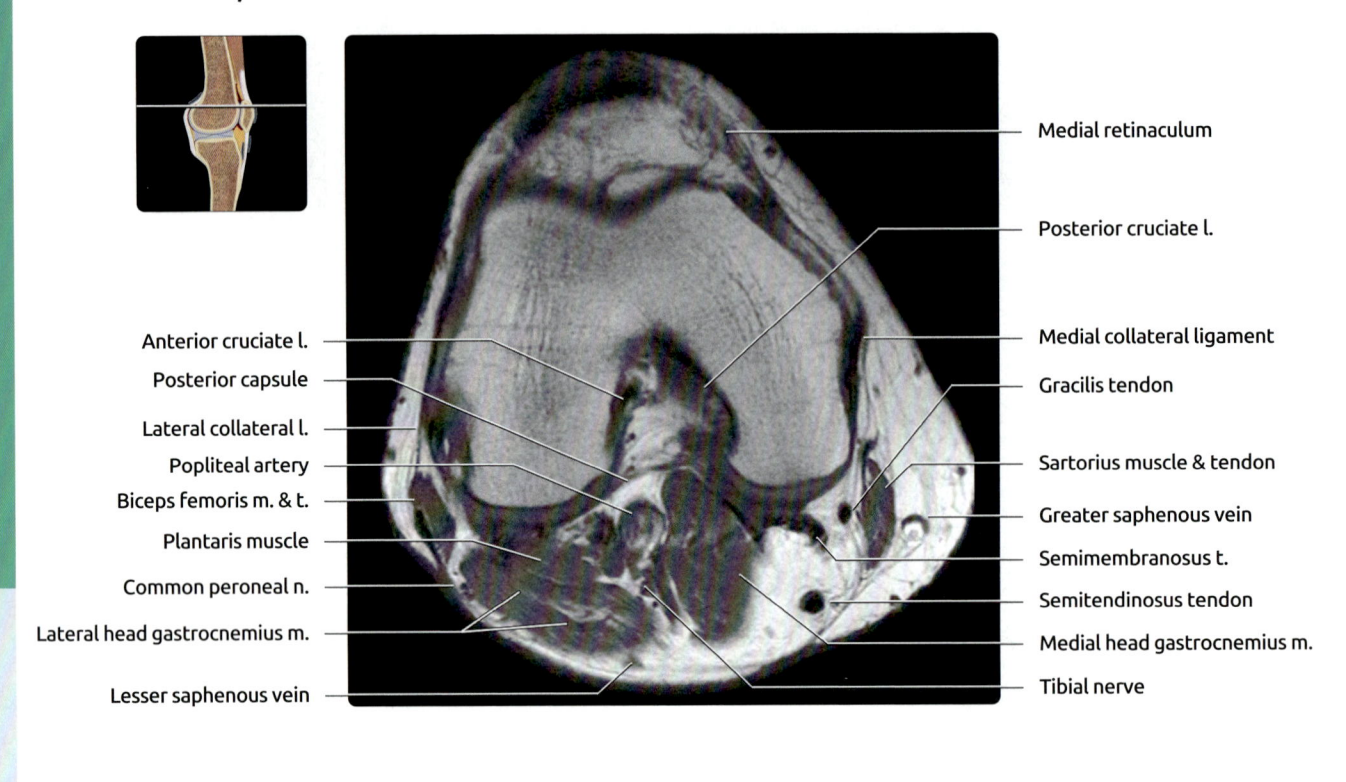

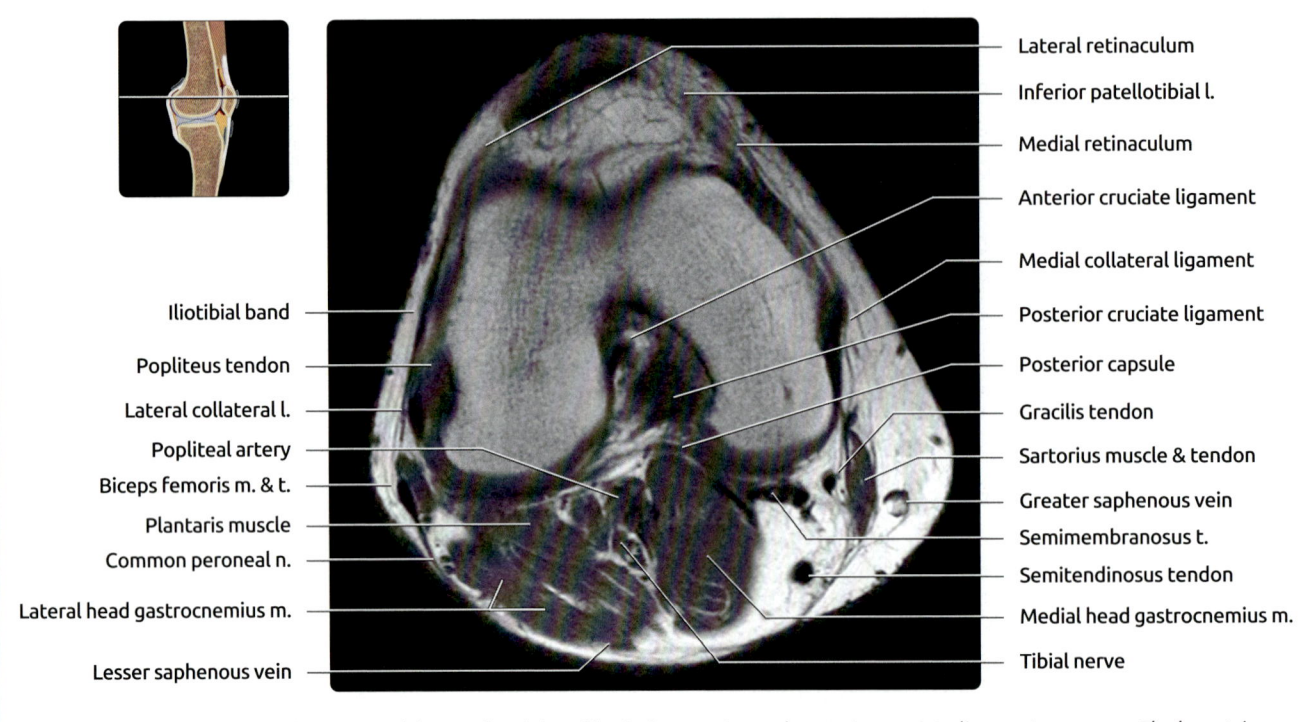

Top image labels (left side):
- Anterior cruciate l.
- Posterior capsule
- Lateral collateral l.
- Popliteal artery
- Biceps femoris m. & t.
- Plantaris muscle
- Common peroneal n.
- Lateral head gastrocnemius m.
- Lesser saphenous vein

Top image labels (right side):
- Medial retinaculum
- Posterior cruciate l.
- Medial collateral ligament
- Gracilis tendon
- Sartorius muscle & tendon
- Greater saphenous vein
- Semimembranosus t.
- Semitendinosus tendon
- Medial head gastrocnemius m.
- Tibial nerve

Bottom image labels (left side):
- Iliotibial band
- Popliteus tendon
- Lateral collateral l.
- Popliteal artery
- Biceps femoris m. & t.
- Plantaris muscle
- Common peroneal n.
- Lateral head gastrocnemius m.
- Lesser saphenous vein

Bottom image labels (right side):
- Lateral retinaculum
- Inferior patellotibial l.
- Medial retinaculum
- Anterior cruciate ligament
- Medial collateral ligament
- Posterior cruciate ligament
- Posterior capsule
- Gracilis tendon
- Sartorius muscle & tendon
- Greater saphenous vein
- Semimembranosus t.
- Semitendinosus tendon
- Medial head gastrocnemius m.
- Tibial nerve

(Top) This cut is through the intercondylar notch; origins of both the anterior and posterior cruciate ligaments are seen. The hamstrings are nearly completely tendinous, about to cross medially to the knee joint. The origins of both collateral ligaments are now seen. **(Bottom)** At the lower end of the patella, the medial support is from the inferior patellotibial ligament. The C-shaped semimembranosus tendon is distinctly different from the elements of pes anserinus (sartorius, gracilis, semitendinosus). The biceps femoris and lateral collateral ligament begin to approach one another as they extend to their insertion on the fibular head; the popliteus tendon arises from its sulcus on the lateral femoral condyle.

Knee MR Atlas

AXIAL T1 MR, LEFT KNEE

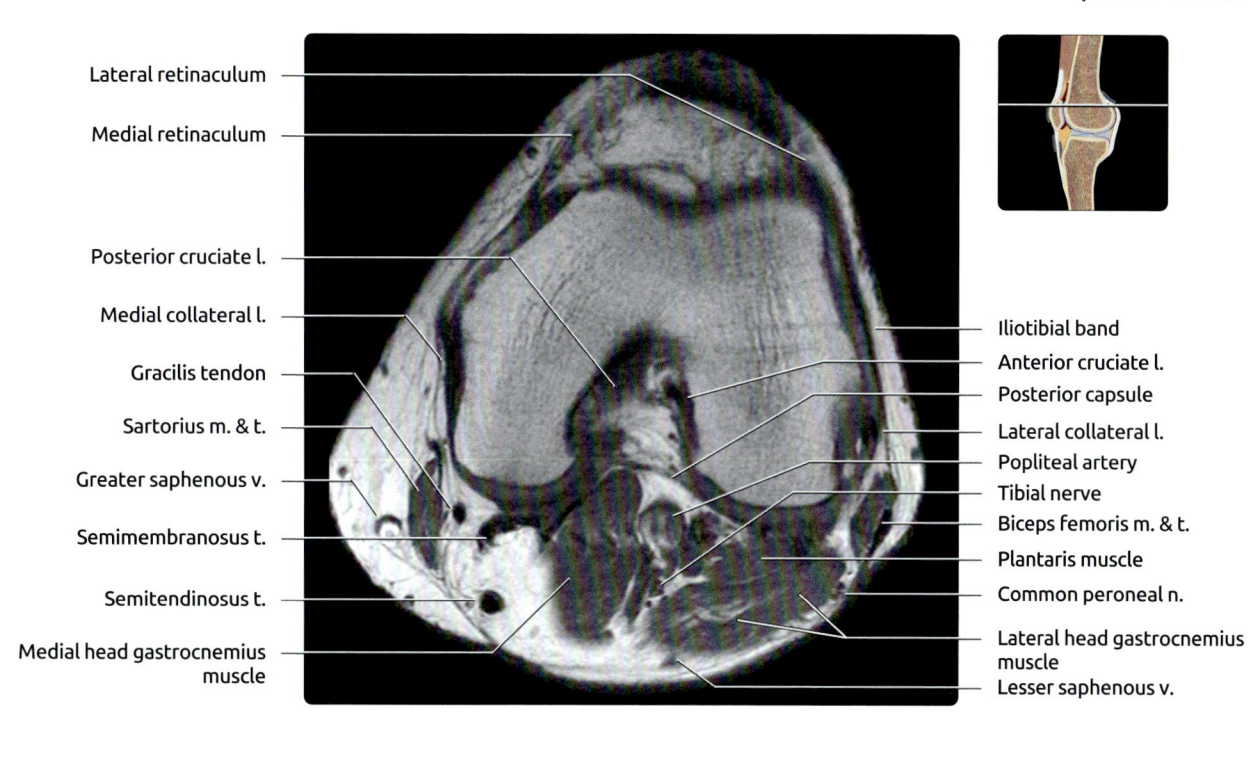

Top image labels (left):
- Lateral retinaculum
- Medial retinaculum
- Posterior cruciate l.
- Medial collateral l.
- Gracilis tendon
- Sartorius m. & t.
- Greater saphenous v.
- Semimembranosus t.
- Semitendinosus t.
- Medial head gastrocnemius muscle

Top image labels (right):
- Iliotibial band
- Anterior cruciate l.
- Posterior capsule
- Lateral collateral l.
- Popliteal artery
- Tibial nerve
- Biceps femoris m. & t.
- Plantaris muscle
- Common peroneal n.
- Lateral head gastrocnemius muscle
- Lesser saphenous v.

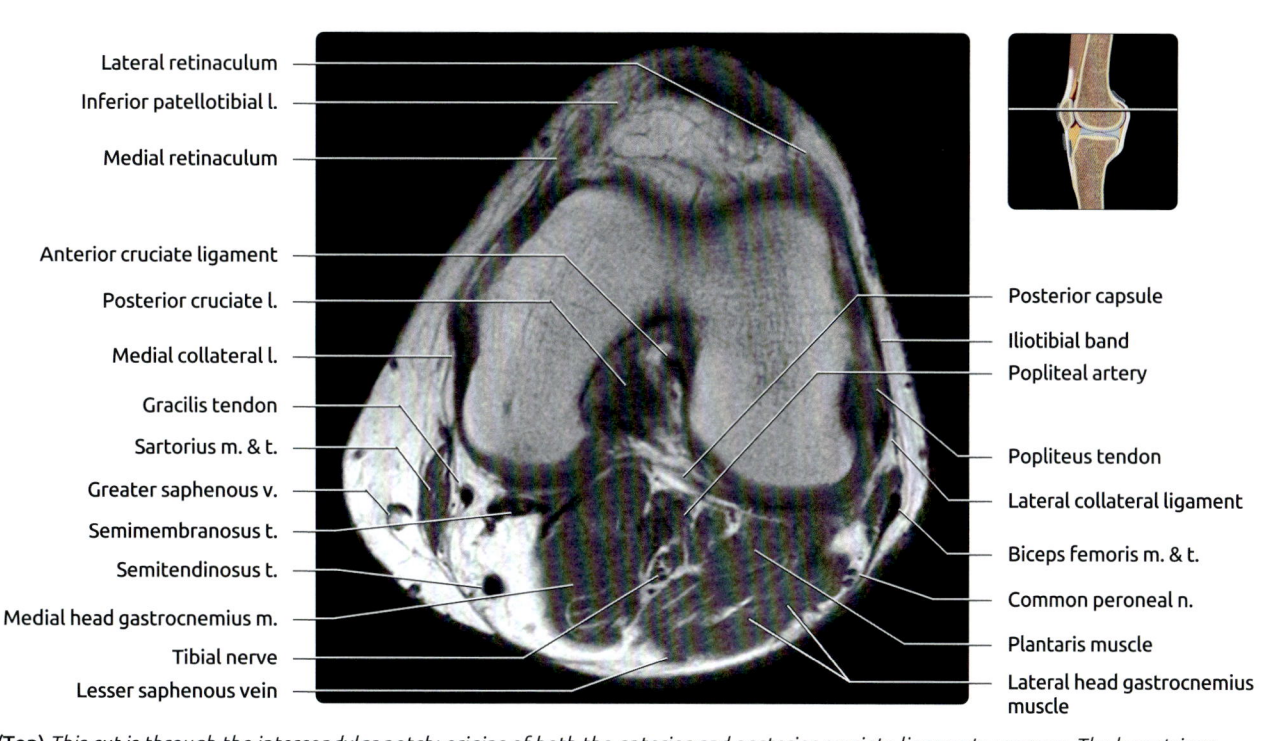

Bottom image labels (left):
- Lateral retinaculum
- Inferior patellotibial l.
- Medial retinaculum
- Anterior cruciate ligament
- Posterior cruciate l.
- Medial collateral l.
- Gracilis tendon
- Sartorius m. & t.
- Greater saphenous v.
- Semimembranosus t.
- Semitendinosus t.
- Medial head gastrocnemius m.
- Tibial nerve
- Lesser saphenous vein

Bottom image labels (right):
- Posterior capsule
- Iliotibial band
- Popliteal artery
- Popliteus tendon
- Lateral collateral ligament
- Biceps femoris m. & t.
- Common peroneal n.
- Plantaris muscle
- Lateral head gastrocnemius muscle

(Top) This cut is through the intercondylar notch; origins of both the anterior and posterior cruciate ligaments are seen. The hamstrings are nearly completely tendinous, about to cross medial to the knee joint. The origins of both collateral ligaments are now seen.
(Bottom) At the lower end of the patella, the medial support is from the inferior patellotibial ligament. The C-shaped semimembranosus tendon is distinctly different from the elements of the pes anserinus (sartorius, gracilis, semitendinosus). The biceps femoris and lateral collateral ligament begin to approach one another as they extend to their insertion on the fibular head; the popliteus tendon arises from its sulcus on the lateral femoral condyle.

Knee MR Atlas

AXIAL T1 MR, RIGHT KNEE

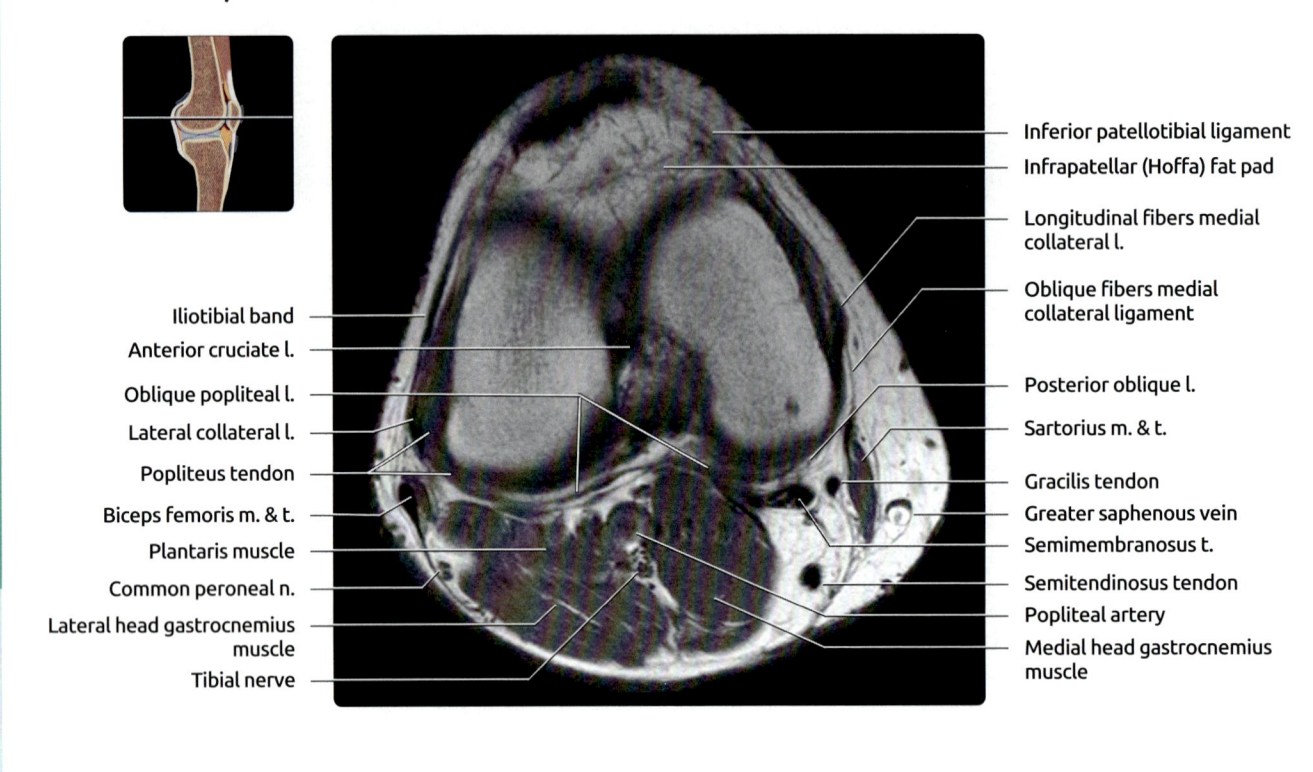

Top image labels (left):
- Iliotibial band
- Anterior cruciate l.
- Oblique popliteal l.
- Lateral collateral l.
- Popliteus tendon
- Biceps femoris m. & t.
- Plantaris muscle
- Common peroneal n.
- Lateral head gastrocnemius muscle
- Tibial nerve

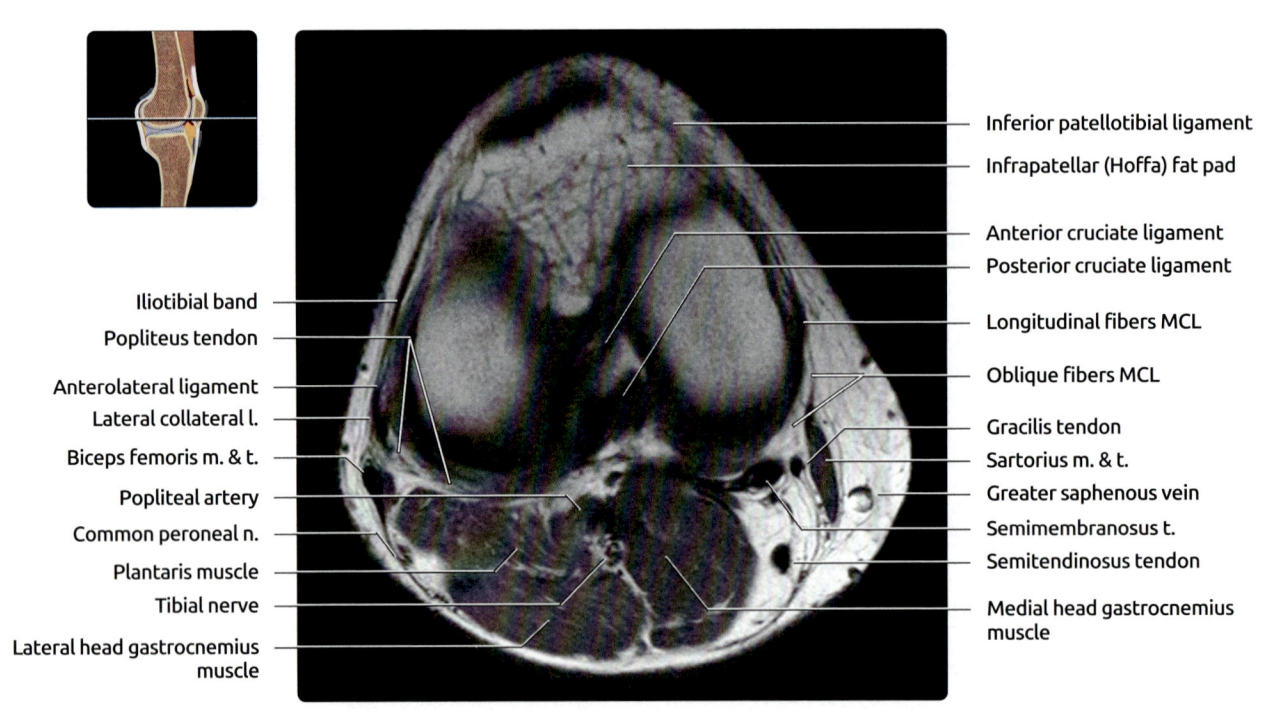

Top image labels (right):
- Inferior patellotibial ligament
- Infrapatellar (Hoffa) fat pad
- Longitudinal fibers medial collateral l.
- Oblique fibers medial collateral ligament
- Posterior oblique l.
- Sartorius m. & t.
- Gracilis tendon
- Greater saphenous vein
- Semimembranosus t.
- Semitendinosus tendon
- Popliteal artery
- Medial head gastrocnemius muscle

Bottom image labels (left):
- Iliotibial band
- Popliteus tendon
- Anterolateral ligament
- Lateral collateral l.
- Biceps femoris m. & t.
- Popliteal artery
- Common peroneal n.
- Plantaris muscle
- Tibial nerve
- Lateral head gastrocnemius muscle

Bottom image labels (right):
- Inferior patellotibial ligament
- Infrapatellar (Hoffa) fat pad
- Anterior cruciate ligament
- Posterior cruciate ligament
- Longitudinal fibers MCL
- Oblique fibers MCL
- Gracilis tendon
- Sartorius m. & t.
- Greater saphenous vein
- Semimembranosus t.
- Semitendinosus tendon
- Medial head gastrocnemius muscle

(Top) This cut is 1.5 cm above the knee joint. The posterolateral structures now include the popliteus tendon, extending posteromedially around the lateral femoral condyle within the popliteal hiatus. Additionally, the posterior oblique ligament, arising from fibers of the medial collateral ligament, joins fibers from the semimembranosus to supplement the posterior capsule as the oblique popliteal ligament. **(Bottom)** This cut is immediately above the knee joint. The posterior cruciate is approaching its insertion on the posterior tibia and the anterior cruciate spreads out towards its insertion on the plateau.

Knee MR Atlas

AXIAL T1 MR, LEFT KNEE

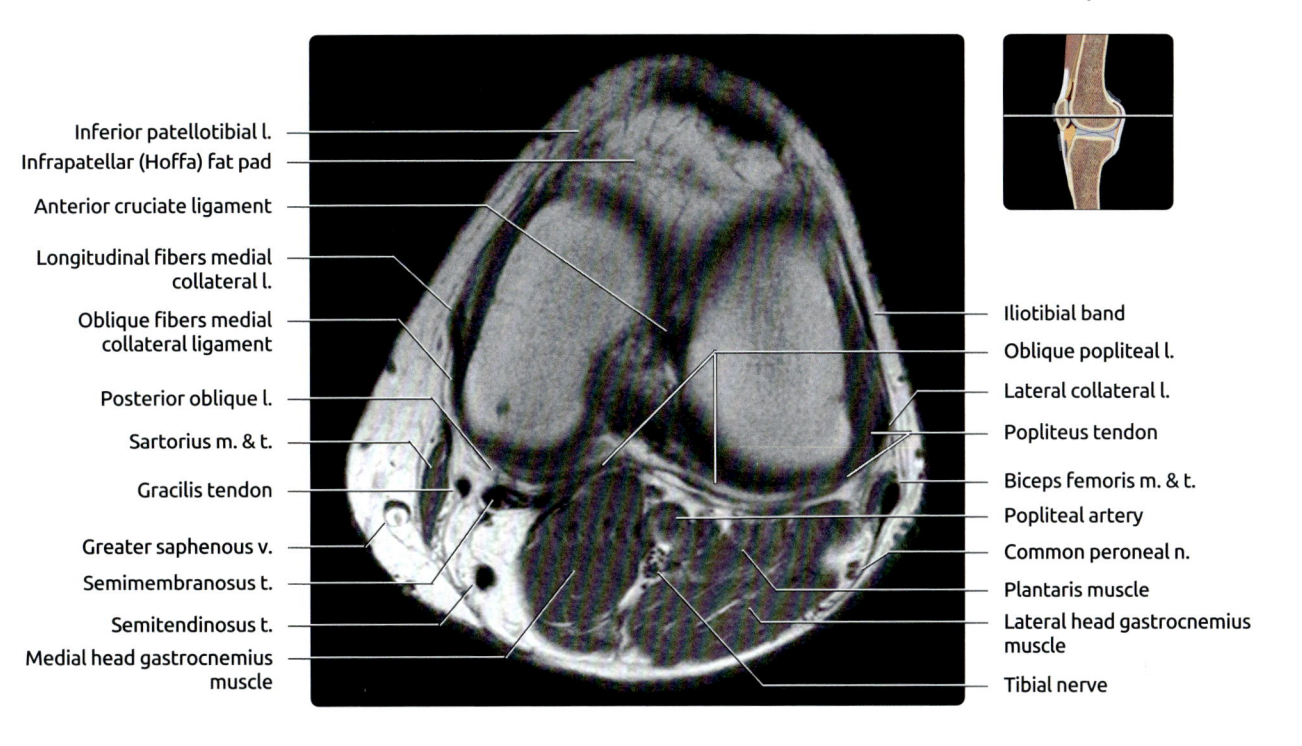

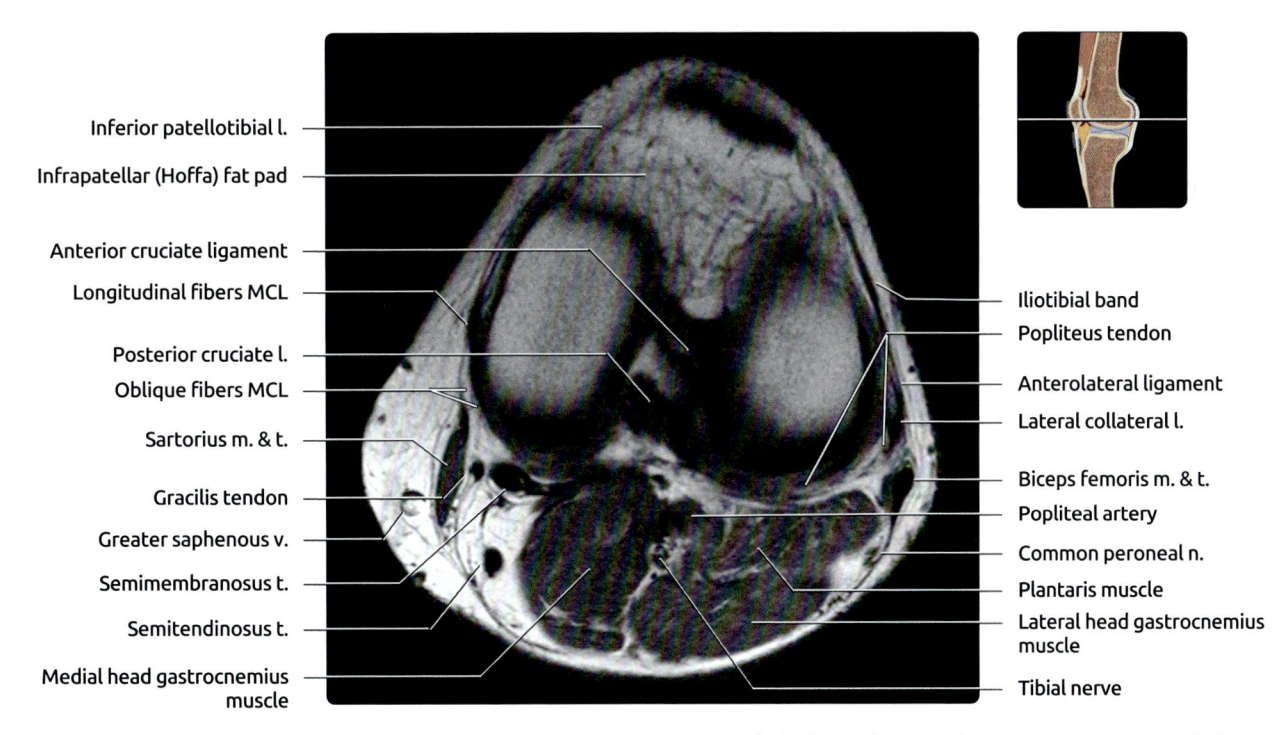

Top image labels (left side):
- Inferior patellotibial l.
- Infrapatellar (Hoffa) fat pad
- Anterior cruciate ligament
- Longitudinal fibers medial collateral l.
- Oblique fibers medial collateral ligament
- Posterior oblique l.
- Sartorius m. & t.
- Gracilis tendon
- Greater saphenous v.
- Semimembranosus t.
- Semitendinosus t.
- Medial head gastrocnemius muscle

Top image labels (right side):
- Iliotibial band
- Oblique popliteal l.
- Lateral collateral l.
- Popliteus tendon
- Biceps femoris m. & t.
- Popliteal artery
- Common peroneal n.
- Plantaris muscle
- Lateral head gastrocnemius muscle
- Tibial nerve

Bottom image labels (left side):
- Inferior patellotibial l.
- Infrapatellar (Hoffa) fat pad
- Anterior cruciate ligament
- Longitudinal fibers MCL
- Posterior cruciate l.
- Oblique fibers MCL
- Sartorius m. & t.
- Gracilis tendon
- Greater saphenous v.
- Semimembranosus t.
- Semitendinosus t.
- Medial head gastrocnemius muscle

Bottom image labels (right side):
- Iliotibial band
- Popliteus tendon
- Anterolateral ligament
- Lateral collateral l.
- Biceps femoris m. & t.
- Popliteal artery
- Common peroneal n.
- Plantaris muscle
- Lateral head gastrocnemius muscle
- Tibial nerve

(Top) This cut is 1.5 cm above the knee joint. The posterolateral structures now include the popliteus tendon, extending posteromedially around the lateral femoral condyle within the popliteal hiatus. Additionally, the posterior oblique ligament, arising from fibers of the medial collateral ligament, joins fibers from the semimembranosus to supplement the posterior capsule as the oblique popliteal ligament. **(Bottom)** This cut is immediately above the knee joint. The posterior cruciate is approaching its insertion on the posterior tibia and the anterior cruciate spreads out towards its insertion on the plateau.

Knee MR Atlas

AXIAL T1 MR, RIGHT KNEE

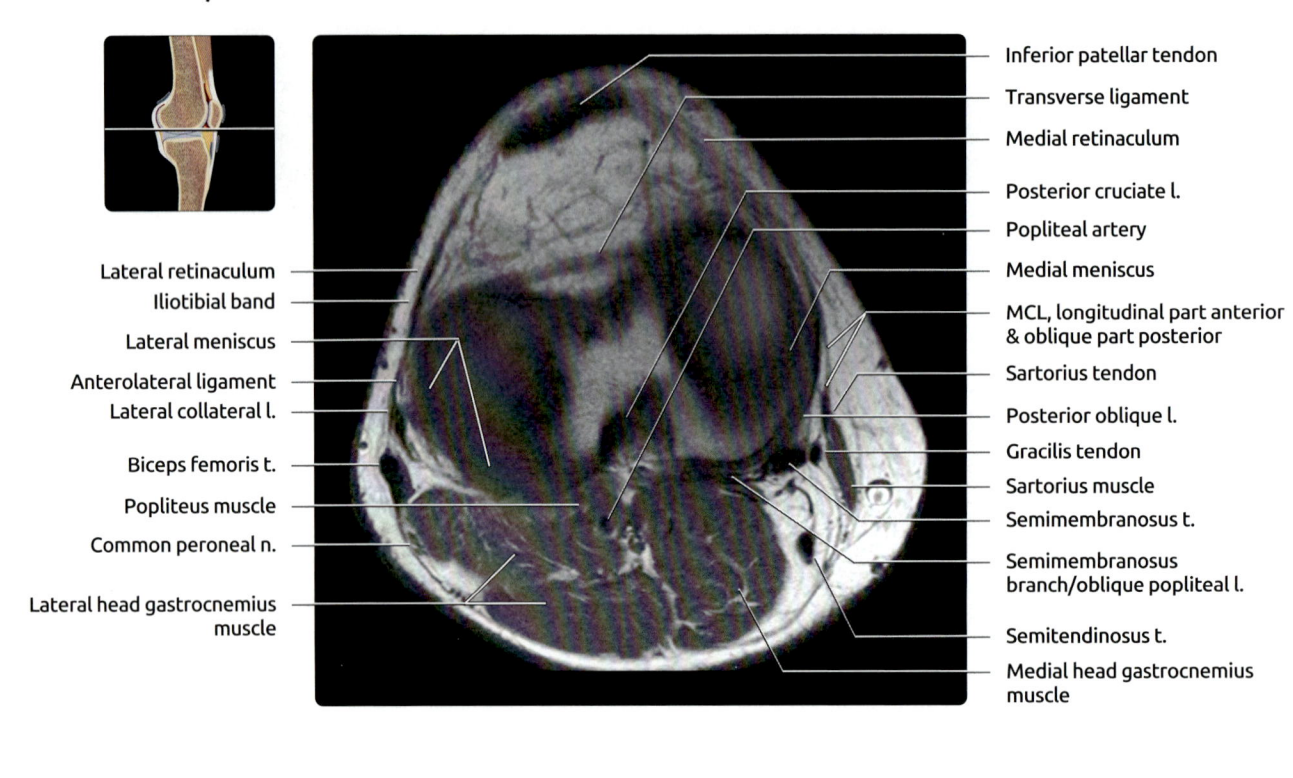

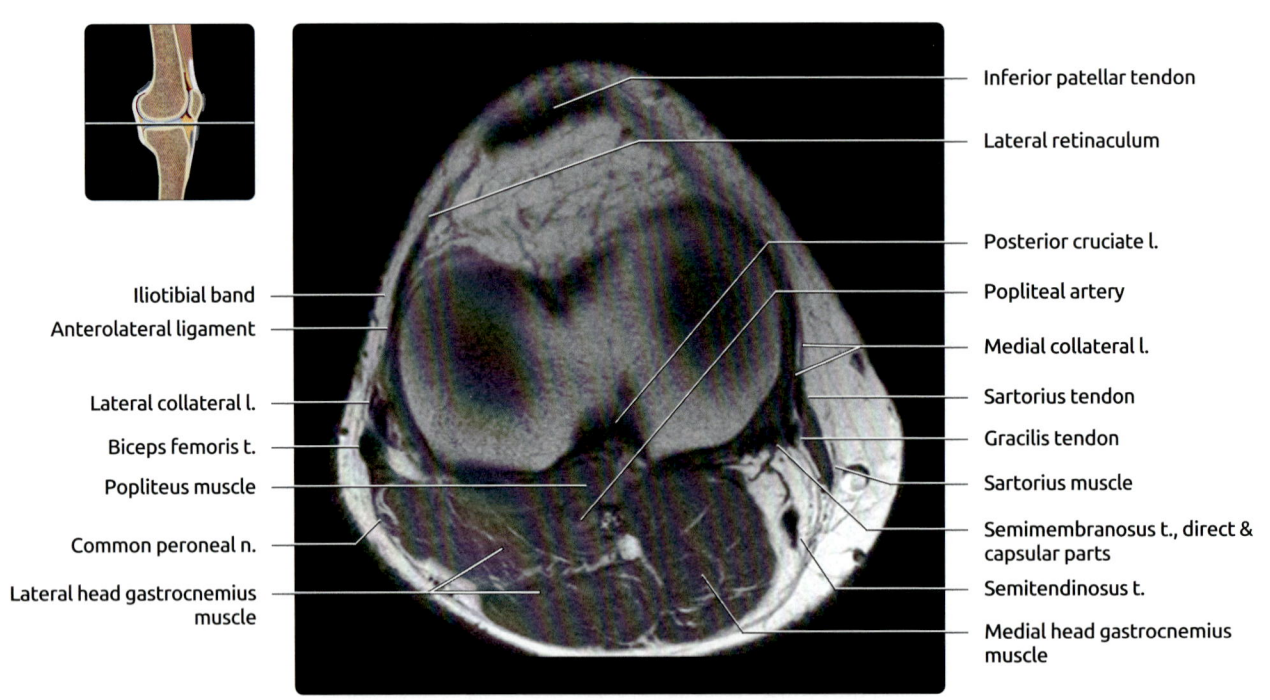

Labels (top image):
- Inferior patellar tendon
- Transverse ligament
- Medial retinaculum
- Posterior cruciate l.
- Popliteal artery
- Medial meniscus
- MCL, longitudinal part anterior & oblique part posterior
- Sartorius tendon
- Posterior oblique l.
- Gracilis tendon
- Sartorius muscle
- Semimembranosus t.
- Semimembranosus branch/oblique popliteal l.
- Semitendinosus t.
- Medial head gastrocnemius muscle
- Lateral retinaculum
- Iliotibial band
- Lateral meniscus
- Anterolateral ligament
- Lateral collateral l.
- Biceps femoris t.
- Popliteus muscle
- Common peroneal n.
- Lateral head gastrocnemius muscle

Labels (bottom image):
- Inferior patellar tendon
- Lateral retinaculum
- Posterior cruciate l.
- Popliteal artery
- Medial collateral l.
- Sartorius tendon
- Gracilis tendon
- Sartorius muscle
- Semimembranosus t., direct & capsular parts
- Semitendinosus t.
- Medial head gastrocnemius muscle
- Iliotibial band
- Anterolateral ligament
- Lateral collateral l.
- Biceps femoris t.
- Popliteus muscle
- Common peroneal n.
- Lateral head gastrocnemius muscle

(Top) This cut is through the knee joint. The menisci are seen, along with the transverse ligament extending between the anterior horns. The anterior cruciate ligament has inserted adjacent to the tibial spines and the posterior cruciate ligament is heading posterior to its insertion on the tibia in an extraarticular position. **(Bottom)** This cut is immediately distal to the menisci within the joint. The semimembranosus begins to attach to the posteromedial tibia and the popliteus muscle broadens to its insertion on the posterior tibia as well.

Knee MR Atlas

AXIAL T1 MR, LEFT KNEE

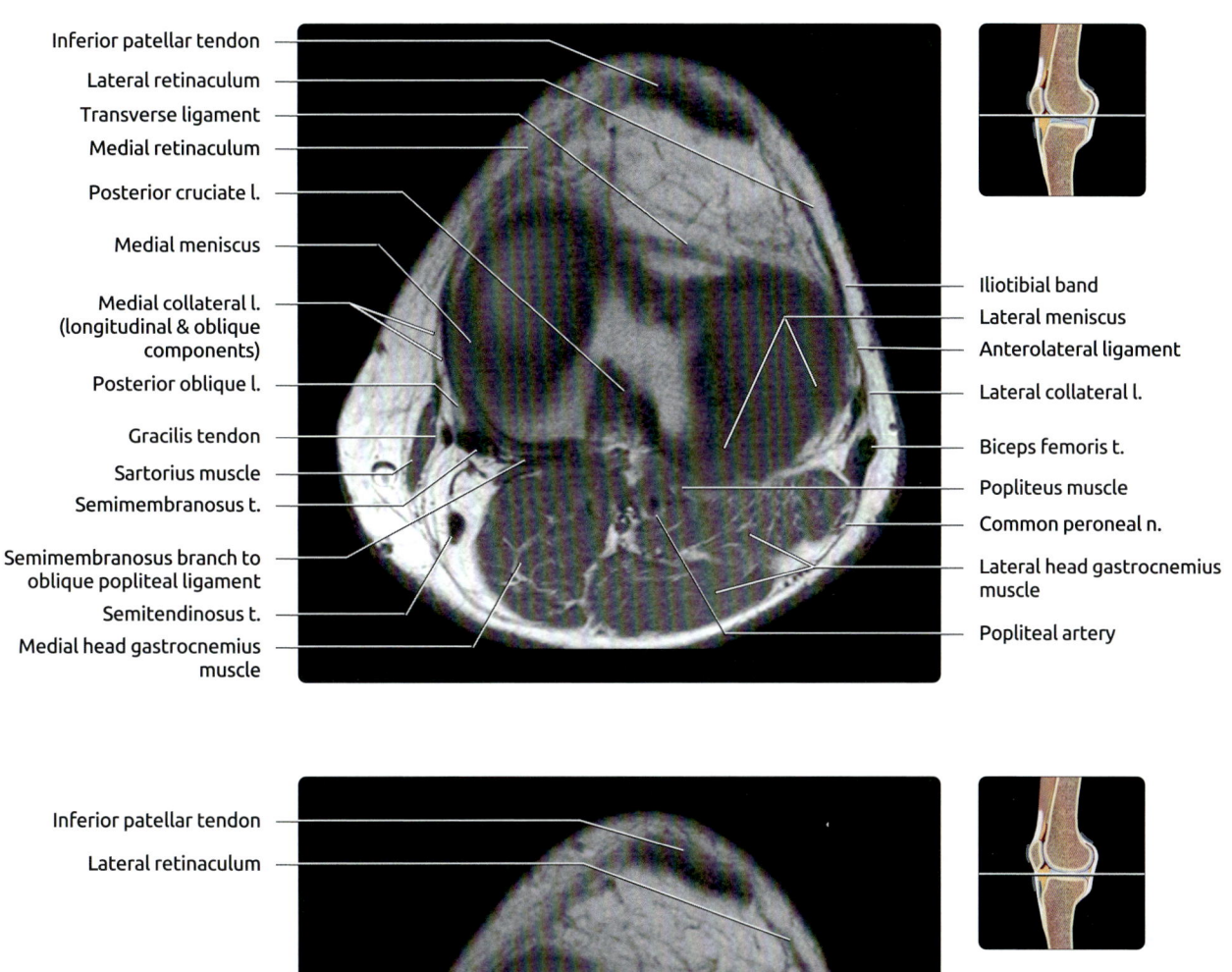

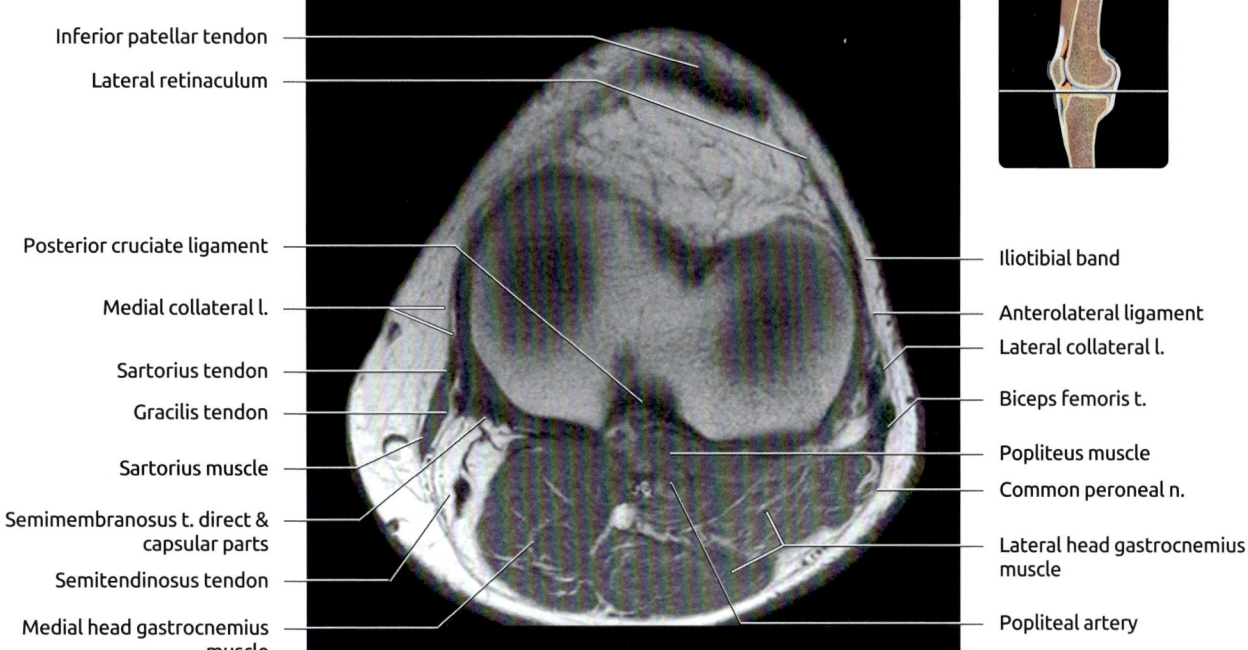

Top image labels (left):
- Inferior patellar tendon
- Lateral retinaculum
- Transverse ligament
- Medial retinaculum
- Posterior cruciate l.
- Medial meniscus
- Medial collateral l. (longitudinal & oblique components)
- Posterior oblique l.
- Gracilis tendon
- Sartorius muscle
- Semimembranosus t.
- Semimembranosus branch to oblique popliteal ligament
- Semitendinosus t.
- Medial head gastrocnemius muscle

Top image labels (right):
- Iliotibial band
- Lateral meniscus
- Anterolateral ligament
- Lateral collateral l.
- Biceps femoris t.
- Popliteus muscle
- Common peroneal n.
- Lateral head gastrocnemius muscle
- Popliteal artery

Bottom image labels (left):
- Inferior patellar tendon
- Lateral retinaculum
- Posterior cruciate ligament
- Medial collateral l.
- Sartorius tendon
- Gracilis tendon
- Sartorius muscle
- Semimembranosus t. direct & capsular parts
- Semitendinosus tendon
- Medial head gastrocnemius muscle

Bottom image labels (right):
- Iliotibial band
- Anterolateral ligament
- Lateral collateral l.
- Biceps femoris t.
- Popliteus muscle
- Common peroneal n.
- Lateral head gastrocnemius muscle
- Popliteal artery

(**Top**) *This cut is through the knee joint. The menisci are seen, along with the transverse ligament extending between the anterior horns. The anterior cruciate ligament has inserted adjacent to the tibial spines and the posterior cruciate ligament is heading posterior to its insertion on the tibia in an extraarticular position.* (**Bottom**) *This cut is immediately distal to the menisci within the joint. The semimembranosus begins to attach to the posteromedial tibia and the popliteus muscle broadens to its insertion on the posterior tibia as well.*

Knee MR Atlas

AXIAL T1 MR, RIGHT KNEE

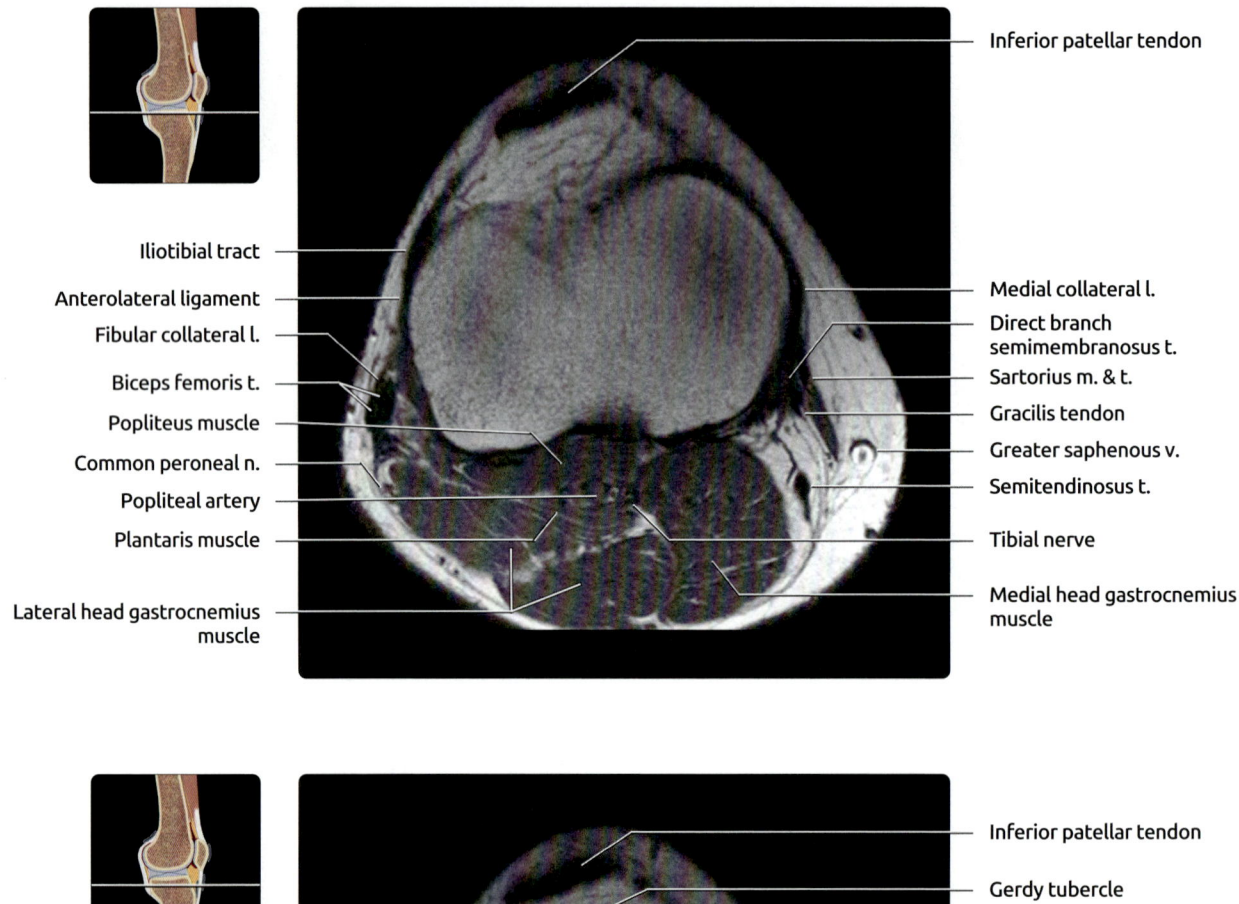

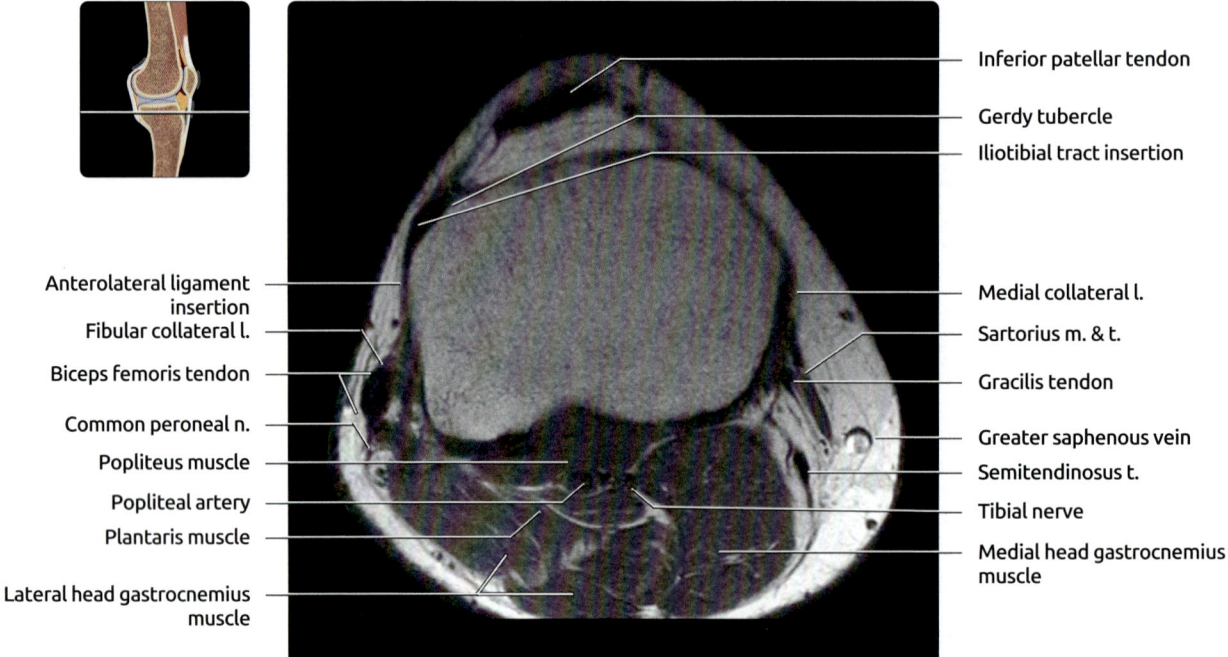

Labels (top image):
- Inferior patellar tendon
- Iliotibial tract
- Anterolateral ligament
- Fibular collateral l.
- Biceps femoris t.
- Popliteus muscle
- Common peroneal n.
- Popliteal artery
- Plantaris muscle
- Lateral head gastrocnemius muscle
- Medial collateral l.
- Direct branch semimembranosus t.
- Sartorius m. & t.
- Gracilis tendon
- Greater saphenous v.
- Semitendinosus t.
- Tibial nerve
- Medial head gastrocnemius muscle

Labels (bottom image):
- Inferior patellar tendon
- Gerdy tubercle
- Iliotibial tract insertion
- Anterolateral ligament insertion
- Fibular collateral l.
- Biceps femoris tendon
- Common peroneal n.
- Popliteus muscle
- Popliteal artery
- Plantaris muscle
- Lateral head gastrocnemius muscle
- Medial collateral l.
- Sartorius m. & t.
- Gracilis tendon
- Greater saphenous vein
- Semitendinosus t.
- Tibial nerve
- Medial head gastrocnemius muscle

(Top) This cut is through the tibial plateau. The tendons of pes anserinus (sartorius, gracilis, and semitendinosus) are lining up, extending towards their insertion on the anteromedial tibia. The popliteus muscle is still broad, with the tibial nerve and popliteal vessels interposed between it and the superficial muscles of the leg. **(Bottom)** This cut is through the lower portion of the tibial plateau, immediately proximal to the fibular head. Note the common peroneal nerve, located posterior to the biceps femoris tendon.

Knee MR Atlas

AXIAL T1 MR, LEFT KNEE

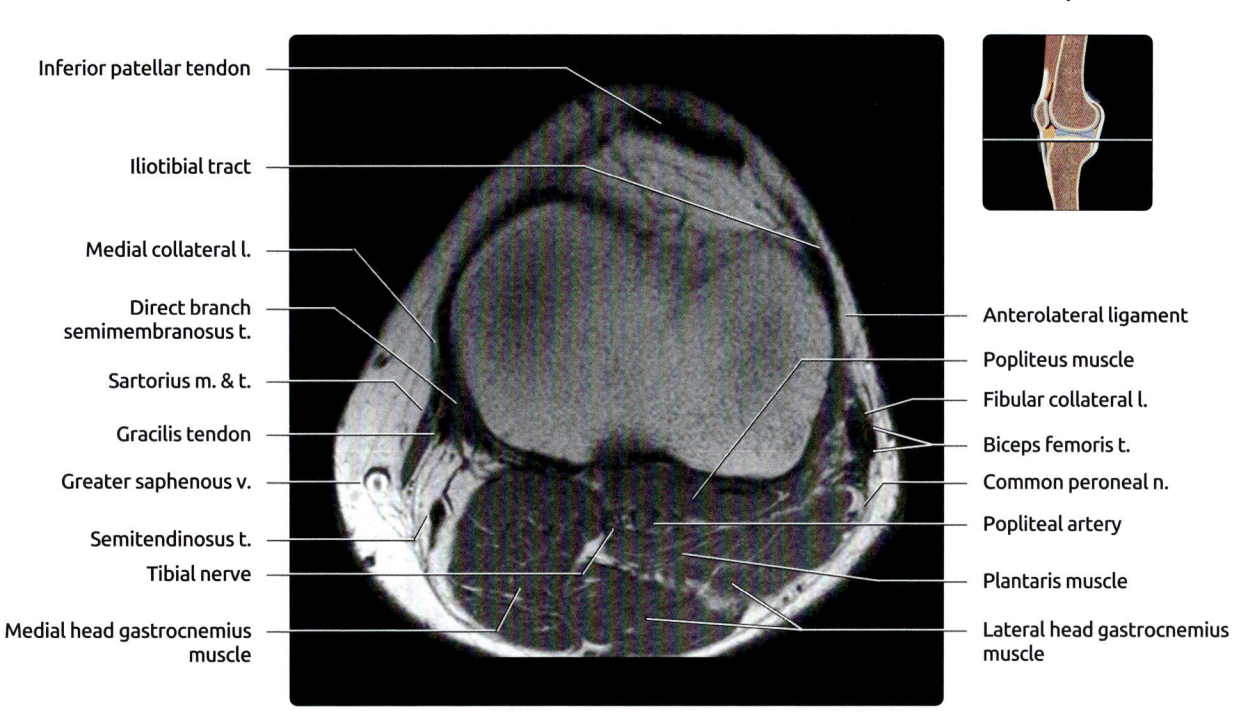

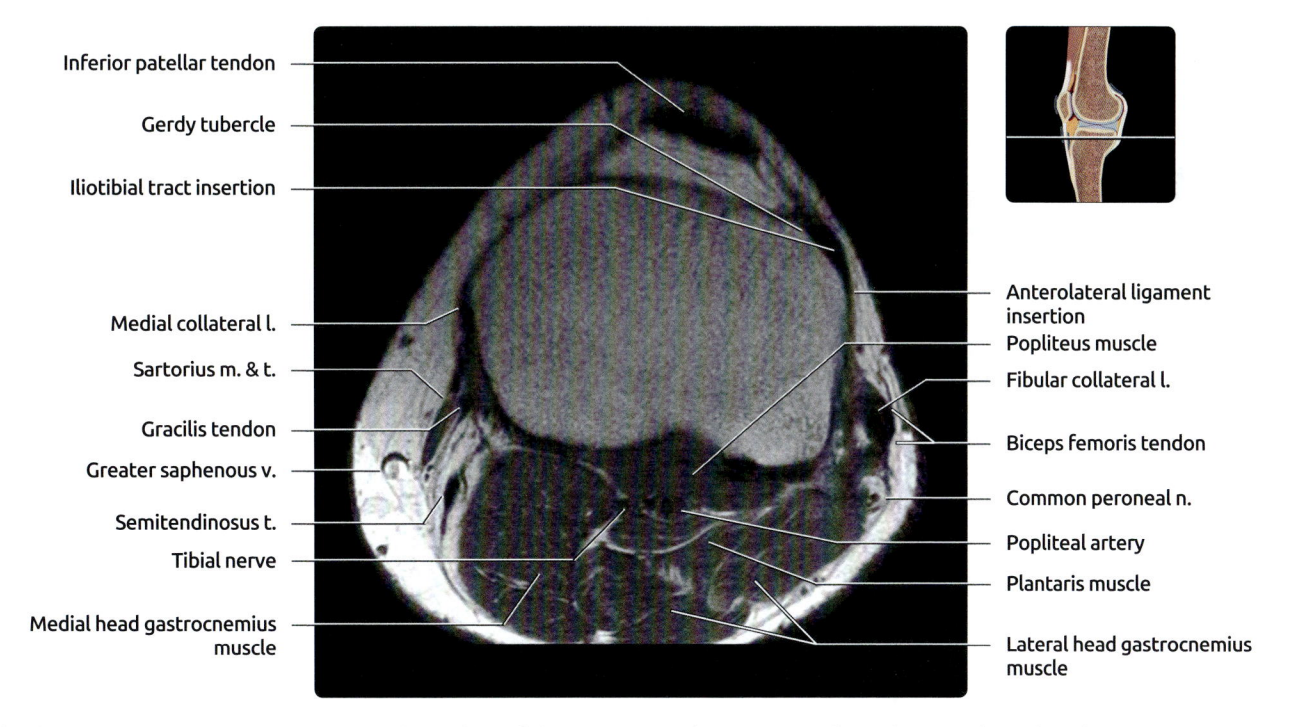

Labels (top image):
- Inferior patellar tendon
- Iliotibial tract
- Medial collateral l.
- Direct branch semimembranosus t.
- Sartorius m. & t.
- Gracilis tendon
- Greater saphenous v.
- Semitendinosus t.
- Tibial nerve
- Medial head gastrocnemius muscle
- Anterolateral ligament
- Popliteus muscle
- Fibular collateral l.
- Biceps femoris t.
- Common peroneal n.
- Popliteal artery
- Plantaris muscle
- Lateral head gastrocnemius muscle

Labels (bottom image):
- Inferior patellar tendon
- Gerdy tubercle
- Iliotibial tract insertion
- Medial collateral l.
- Sartorius m. & t.
- Gracilis tendon
- Greater saphenous v.
- Semitendinosus t.
- Tibial nerve
- Medial head gastrocnemius muscle
- Anterolateral ligament insertion
- Popliteus muscle
- Fibular collateral l.
- Biceps femoris tendon
- Common peroneal n.
- Popliteal artery
- Plantaris muscle
- Lateral head gastrocnemius muscle

(**Top**) *This cut is through the tibial plateau. The tendons of the pes anserinus (sartorius, gracilis, and semitendinosus) are lining up, extending towards their insertion on the anteromedial tibia. The popliteus muscle is still broad, with the tibial nerve and popliteal vessels interposed between it and the superficial muscles of the leg.* (**Bottom**) *This cut is through the lower portion of the tibial plateau, immediately proximal to the fibular head. Note the common peroneal nerve, located posterior to the biceps femoris tendon.*

Knee MR Atlas

AXIAL T1 MR, RIGHT KNEE

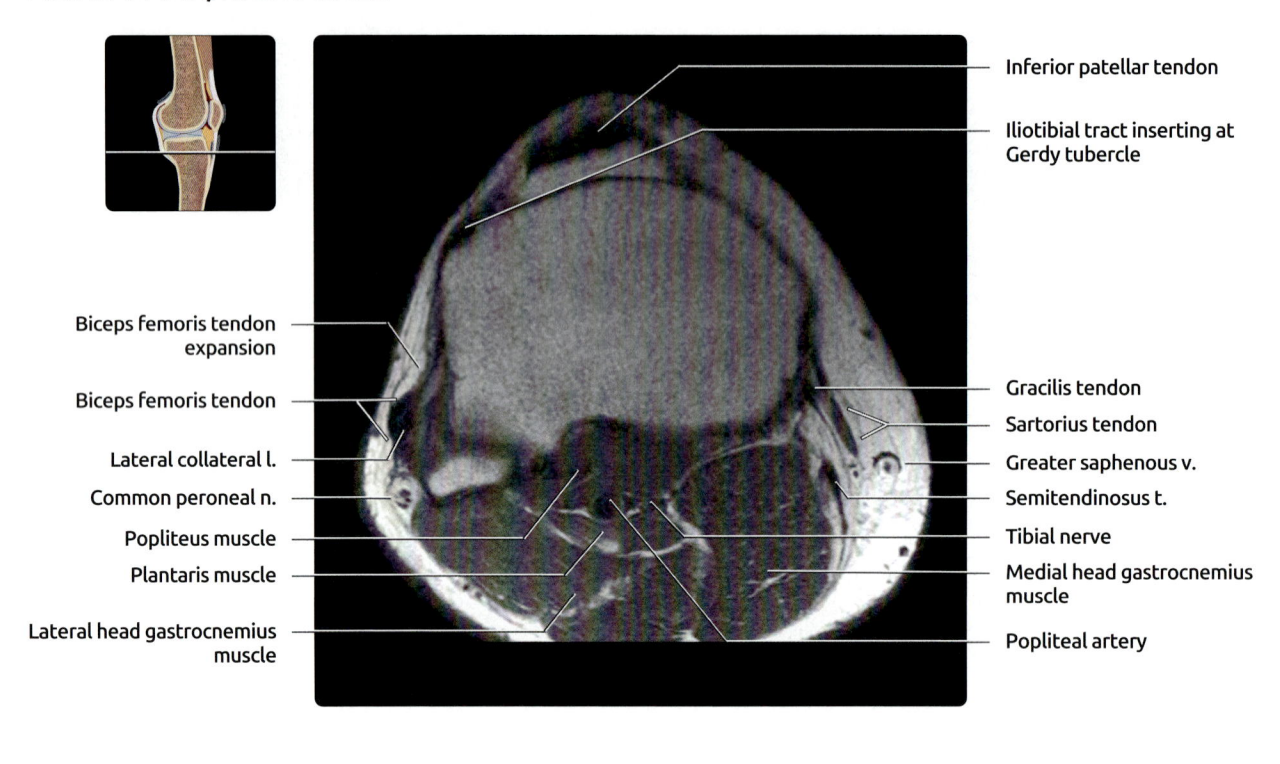

Labels (top image):
- Inferior patellar tendon
- Iliotibial tract inserting at Gerdy tubercle
- Biceps femoris tendon expansion
- Biceps femoris tendon
- Lateral collateral l.
- Common peroneal n.
- Popliteus muscle
- Plantaris muscle
- Lateral head gastrocnemius muscle
- Gracilis tendon
- Sartorius tendon
- Greater saphenous v.
- Semitendinosus t.
- Tibial nerve
- Medial head gastrocnemius muscle
- Popliteal artery

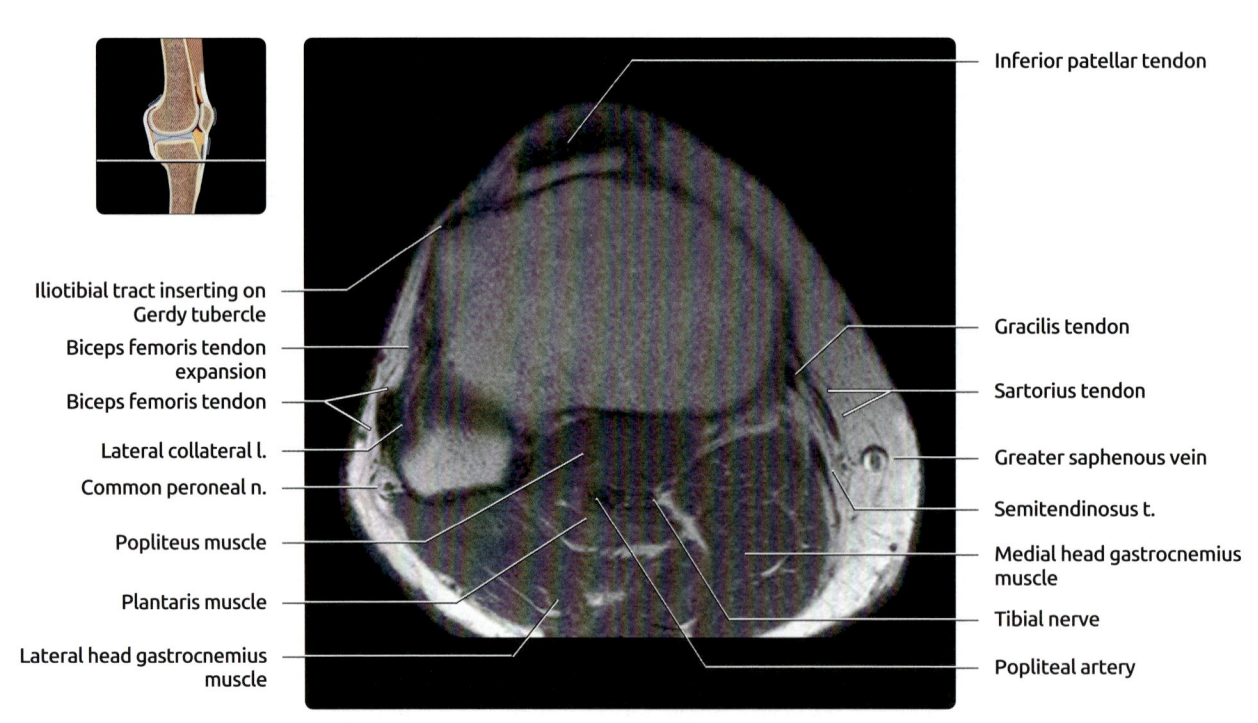

Labels (bottom image):
- Inferior patellar tendon
- Iliotibial tract inserting on Gerdy tubercle
- Biceps femoris tendon expansion
- Biceps femoris tendon
- Lateral collateral l.
- Common peroneal n.
- Popliteus muscle
- Plantaris muscle
- Lateral head gastrocnemius muscle
- Gracilis tendon
- Sartorius tendon
- Greater saphenous vein
- Semitendinosus t.
- Medial head gastrocnemius muscle
- Tibial nerve
- Popliteal artery

(Top) At the level of the apex of the fibular head, the pes anserinus is wrapping around the tibial metaphysis to its insertion anteromedially. The biceps femoris tendon expands around the lateral collateral ligament as both course towards their insertion on the fibular head. (Bottom) This cut is at the level of the fibular head and shows the insertion of the biceps femoris and lateral collateral ligament anterolaterally on the head. The short head of the biceps femoris has a thin anterior expansion that extends to the anterolateral tibia.

Knee MR Atlas

AXIAL T1 MR, LEFT KNEE

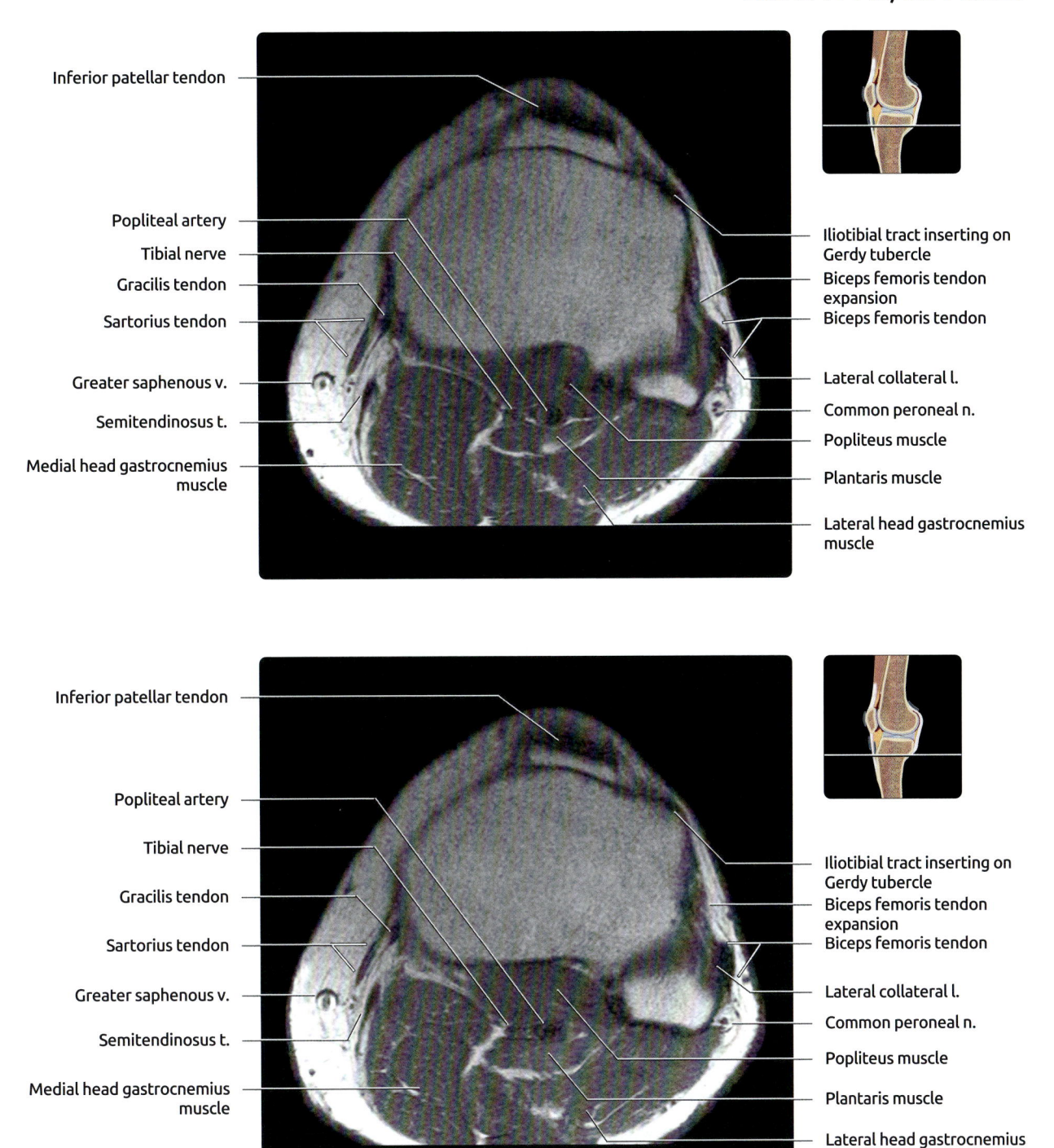

(Top) At the level of the apex of the fibular head, the pes anserinus is wrapping around the tibial metaphysis to its insertion anteromedially. The biceps femoris tendon expands around the lateral collateral ligament as both course towards their insertion on the fibular head. **(Bottom)** This cut is at the level of the fibular head and shows the insertion of the biceps femoris and lateral collateral ligament anterolaterally on the head. The short head of the biceps femoris has a thin anterior expansion that extends to the anterolateral tibia.

Knee MR Atlas

CORONAL T1 MR, RIGHT KNEE

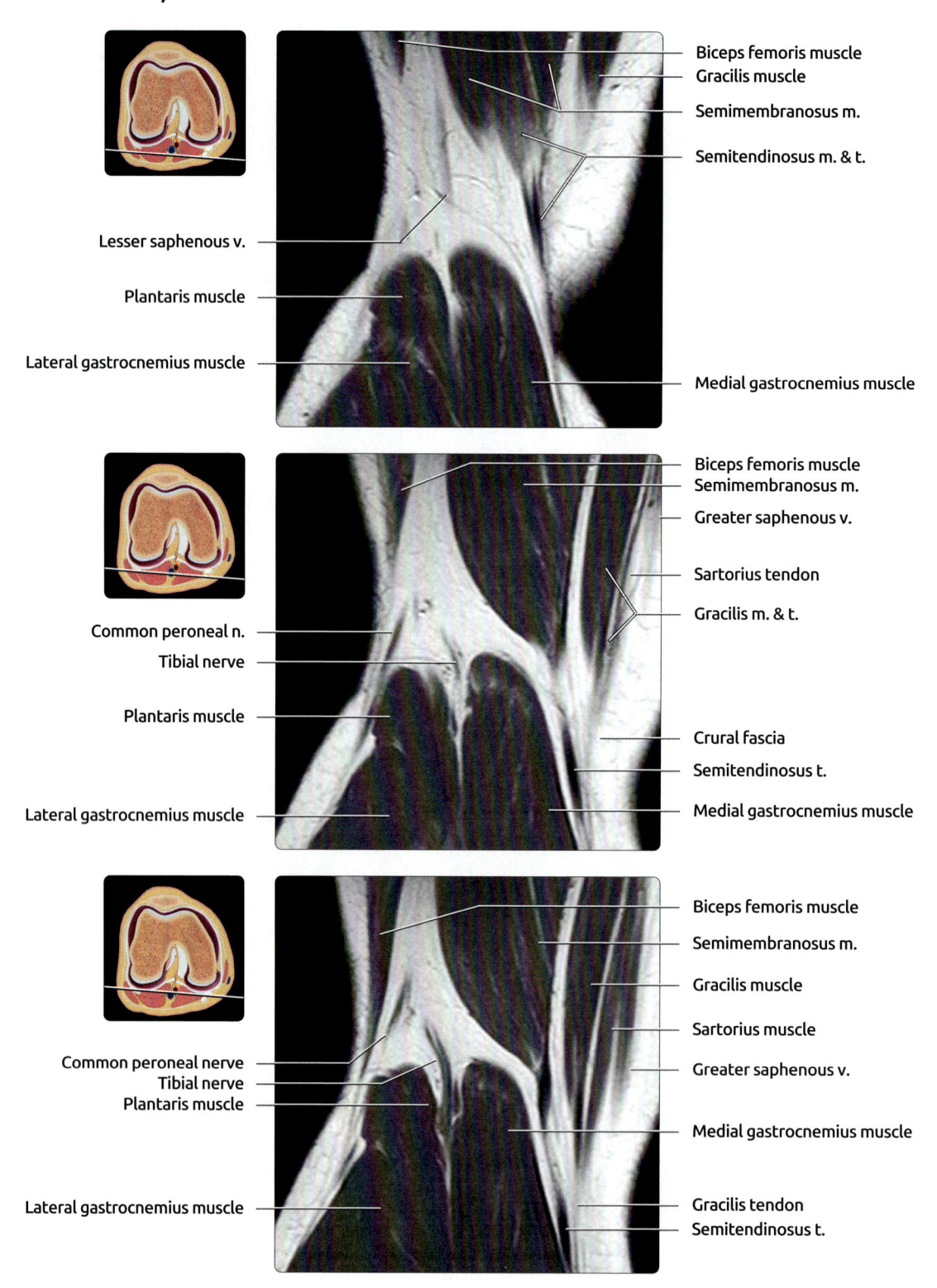

(Top) The 1st in a series of coronal posterior T1 MR images of the right knee, displayed from posterior to anterior, shows the semitendinosus muscle as well as tendon. The image is posterior enough to also see the lesser saphenous vein. More distally in the leg, the sural nerve accompanies this structure. (Middle) Slightly more anterior, courses of the common peroneal and tibial nerves can be seen. The semitendinosus tendon is distinctly seen as the posterior portion of the pes anserinus. (Bottom) In this slightly more anterior cut, the course of common peroneal nerve is seen following the posterior biceps femoris tendon. The elements of the pes anserinus are distinctly seen, with the gracilis and sartorius muscles in this plane posterior to their tendons (seen in slightly more anterior cuts). The semitendinosus tendon, the most posterior of the 3 elements of the pes, is seen in this section; however, its muscle fibers are in a more posterior section.

Knee MR Atlas

CORONAL T1 MR, LEFT KNEE

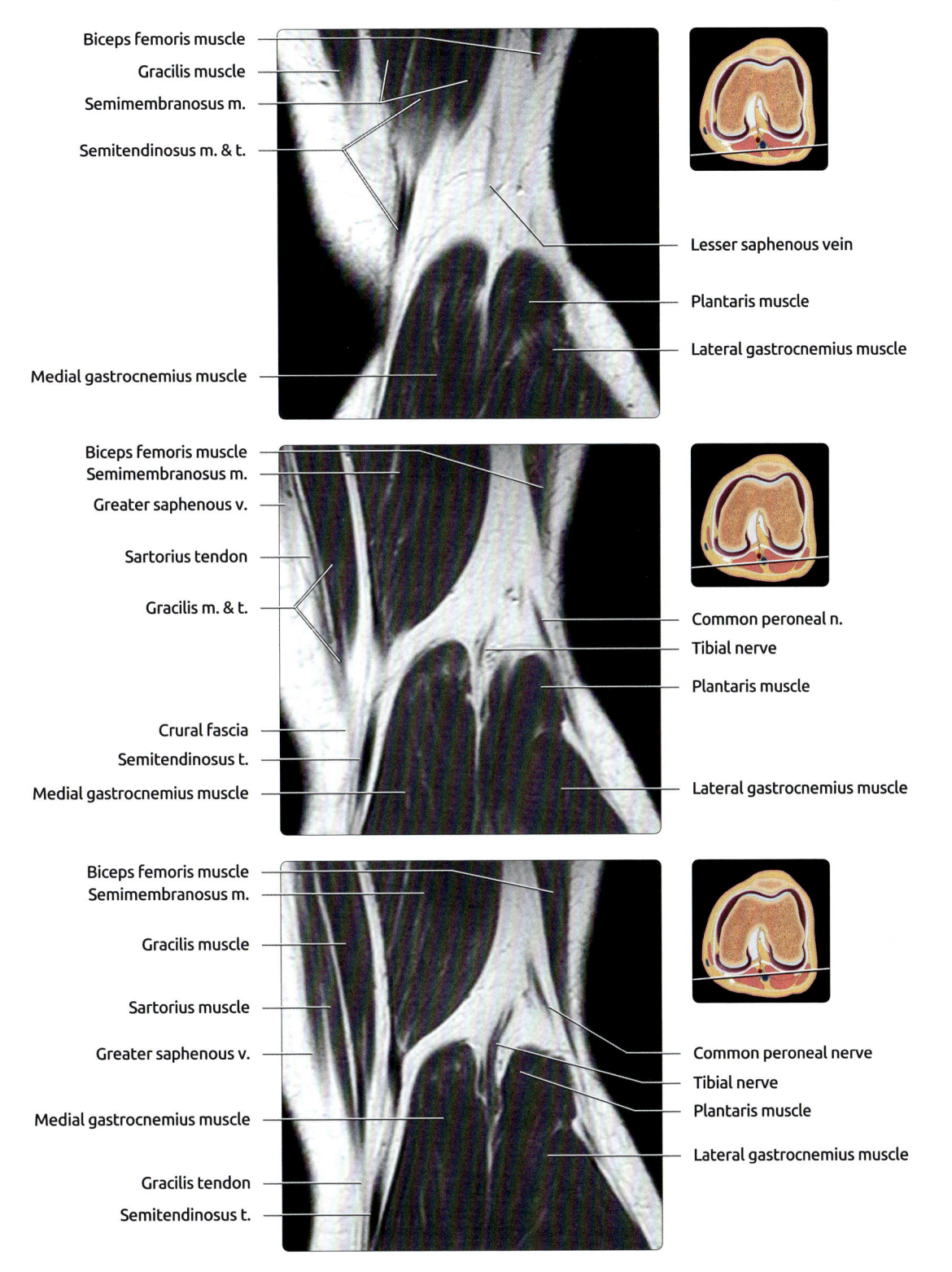

Labels (Top image): Biceps femoris muscle; Gracilis muscle; Semimembranosus m.; Semitendinosus m. & t.; Medial gastrocnemius muscle; Lesser saphenous vein; Plantaris muscle; Lateral gastrocnemius muscle

Labels (Middle image): Biceps femoris muscle; Semimembranosus m.; Greater saphenous v.; Sartorius tendon; Gracilis m. & t.; Crural fascia; Semitendinosus t.; Medial gastrocnemius muscle; Common peroneal n.; Tibial nerve; Plantaris muscle; Lateral gastrocnemius muscle

Labels (Bottom image): Biceps femoris muscle; Semimembranosus m.; Gracilis muscle; Sartorius muscle; Greater saphenous v.; Medial gastrocnemius muscle; Gracilis tendon; Semitendinosus t.; Common peroneal nerve; Tibial nerve; Plantaris muscle; Lateral gastrocnemius muscle

(Top) The 1st in a series of posterior coronal T1 MR images of the left knee, displayed from posterior to anterior, shows the semitendinosus muscle and tendon. The images are posterior enough to also see the lesser saphenous vein. More distally in the leg, the sural nerve accompanies this structure. **(Middle)** Slightly more anterior, courses of the common peroneal and tibial nerves can be seen. The semitendinosus tendon is distinctly seen as the posterior portion of the pes anserinus. **(Bottom)** In this slightly more anterior cut, the course of the common peroneal nerve is seen following the posterior biceps femoris tendon. The elements of the pes anserinus are distinctly seen, with the gracilis and sartorius muscles in this plane posterior to their tendons (seen in slightly more anterior cuts). The semitendinosus tendon, the most posterior of the 3 elements of the pes, is seen in this section; however, its muscle fibers are in a more posterior section.

Knee MR Atlas

CORONAL T1 MR, RIGHT KNEE

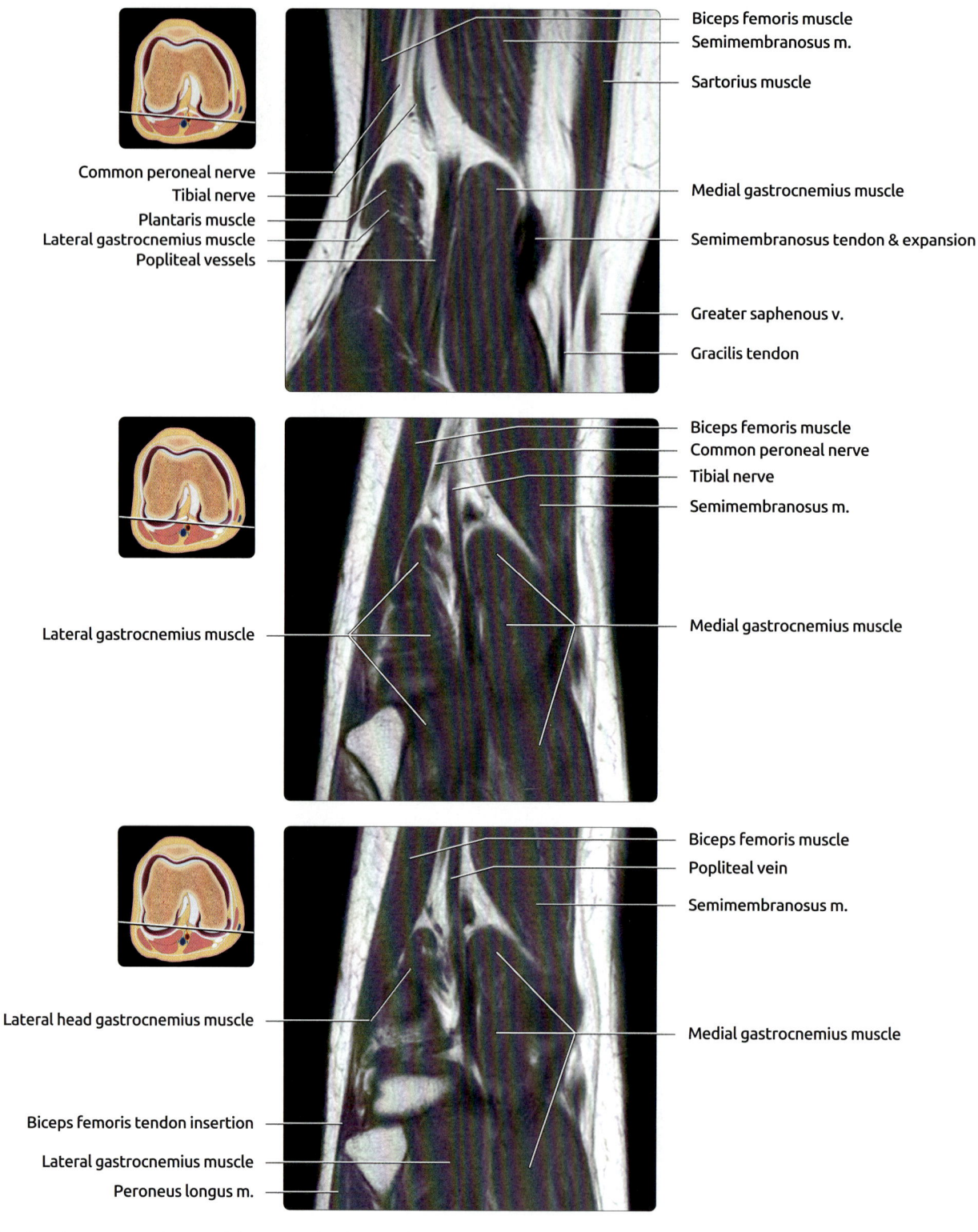

Labels (top image):
- Common peroneal nerve
- Tibial nerve
- Plantaris muscle
- Lateral gastrocnemius muscle
- Popliteal vessels
- Biceps femoris muscle
- Semimembranosus m.
- Sartorius muscle
- Medial gastrocnemius muscle
- Semimembranosus tendon & expansion
- Greater saphenous v.
- Gracilis tendon

Labels (middle image):
- Lateral gastrocnemius muscle
- Biceps femoris muscle
- Common peroneal nerve
- Tibial nerve
- Semimembranosus m.
- Medial gastrocnemius muscle

Labels (bottom image):
- Lateral head gastrocnemius muscle
- Biceps femoris tendon insertion
- Lateral gastrocnemius muscle
- Peroneus longus m.
- Biceps femoris muscle
- Popliteal vein
- Semimembranosus m.
- Medial gastrocnemius muscle

(Top) In the most anterior cut of this series, the division of the tibial and common peroneal nerves can be seen as well as the separate components of the pes anserinus. *(Middle)* The 1st in a series of coronal T1 MR images of the right knee is shown. This series is in a slightly different obliquity than the prior series, allowing slightly different combinations of structures to be seen in a single cut. The series is shown from posterior to anterior. The tibial nerve and common peroneal nerve are seen in this cut, as they lie more posterior than the popliteal vessels. *(Bottom)* In this slightly more anterior image, the gastrocnemius muscles predominate in the posterior portion of the lower knee; the deeper muscles are smaller at this point. Laterally, the origin of the peroneus longus muscle is seen at the fibula.

Knee MR Atlas

CORONAL T1 MR, LEFT KNEE

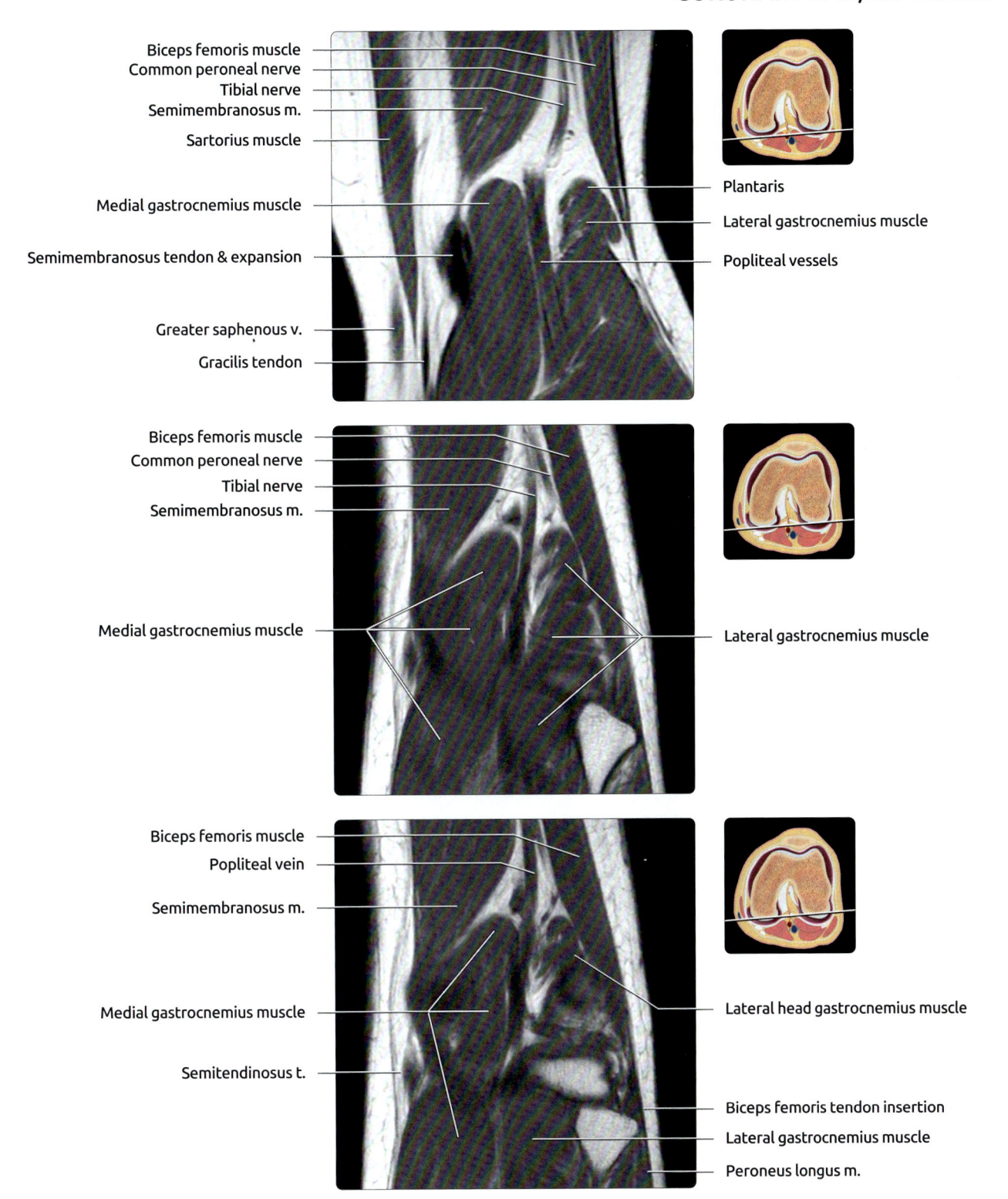

(Top) In this most anterior cut of this series, we see the division of the tibial and common peroneal nerves as well as the separate components of the pes anserinus. **(Middle)** This is the 1st in a series of T1 MR images of the left knee. This series is in a slightly different obliquity than the prior series, allowing slightly different combinations of structures to be seen in a single cut. The series is shown from posterior to anterior. The tibial nerve and common peroneal nerve are seen in this cut, as they lie more posterior than the popliteal vessels. **(Bottom)** In this slightly more anterior image, the gastrocnemius muscles predominate in the posterior portion of the lower knee; the deeper muscles are smaller at this point. Laterally, the origin of the peroneus longus muscle is seen at the fibula.

Knee MR Atlas

CORONAL T1 MR, RIGHT KNEE

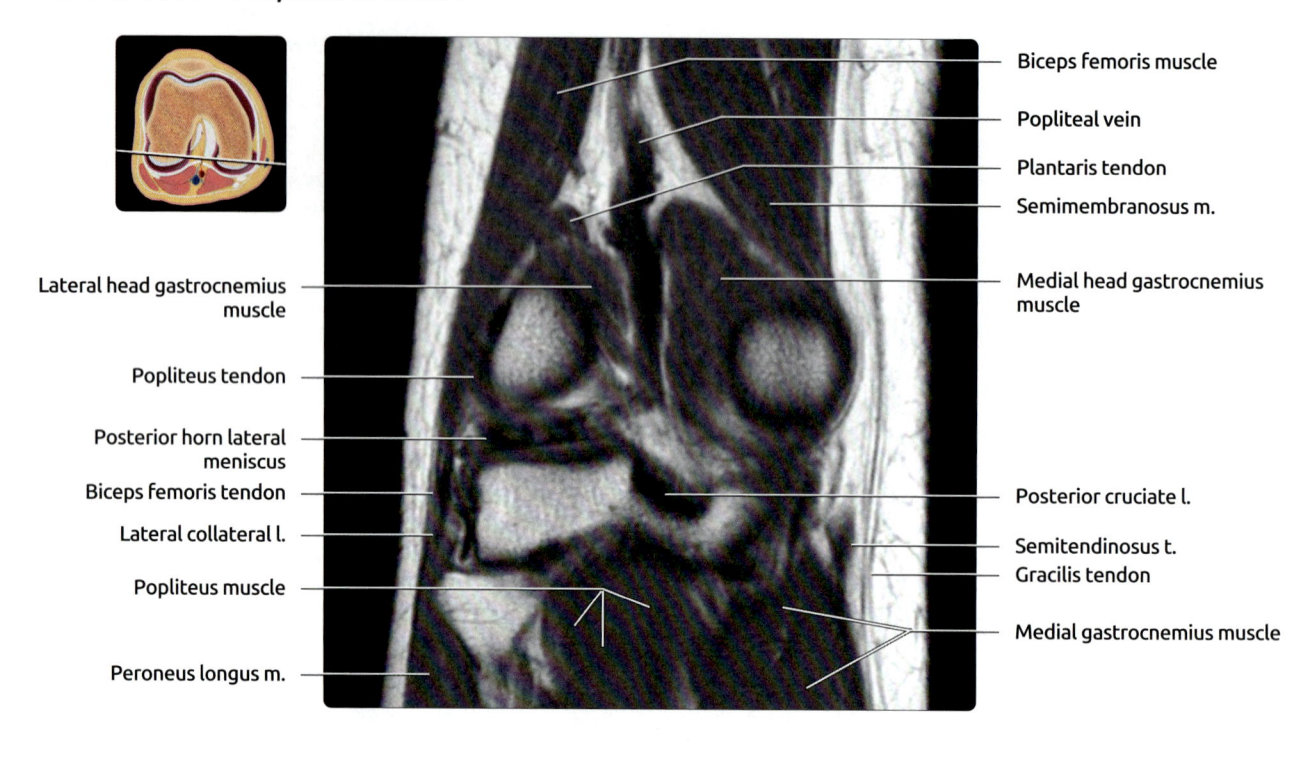

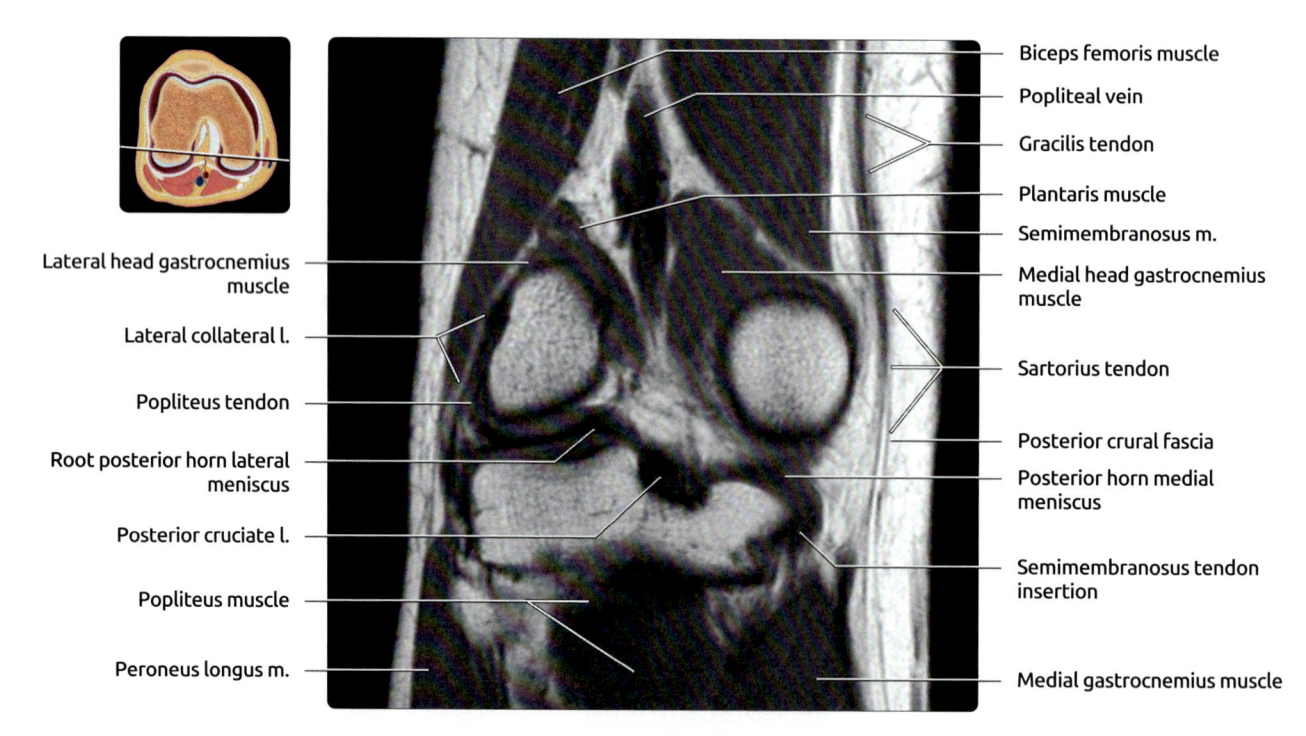

Labels (top image, left): Lateral head gastrocnemius muscle; Popliteus tendon; Posterior horn lateral meniscus; Biceps femoris tendon; Lateral collateral l.; Popliteus muscle; Peroneus longus m.

Labels (top image, right): Biceps femoris muscle; Popliteal vein; Plantaris tendon; Semimembranosus m.; Medial head gastrocnemius muscle; Posterior cruciate l.; Semitendinosus t.; Gracilis tendon; Medial gastrocnemius muscle

Labels (bottom image, left): Lateral head gastrocnemius muscle; Lateral collateral l.; Popliteus tendon; Root posterior horn lateral meniscus; Posterior cruciate l.; Popliteus muscle; Peroneus longus m.

Labels (bottom image, right): Biceps femoris muscle; Popliteal vein; Gracilis tendon; Plantaris muscle; Semimembranosus m.; Medial head gastrocnemius muscle; Sartorius tendon; Posterior crural fascia; Posterior horn medial meniscus; Semimembranosus tendon insertion; Medial gastrocnemius muscle

(Top) *Slightly more anterior, and deep to the majority of the gastrocnemius muscle mass, the popliteus tendon is seen arising from its notch on the lateral femoral condyle, extending posteriorly and inferiorly to the popliteal hiatus. The individual structures in the posterolateral corner are generally better seen on a fluid-sensitive sequence because of the fluid in the popliteal hiatus.* **(Bottom)** *The lateral collateral ligament can now be seen arising from lateral femoral condyle, coursing towards its insertion, along with the biceps femoris, on the fibular styloid process.*

Knee MR Atlas

CORONAL T1 MR, LEFT KNEE

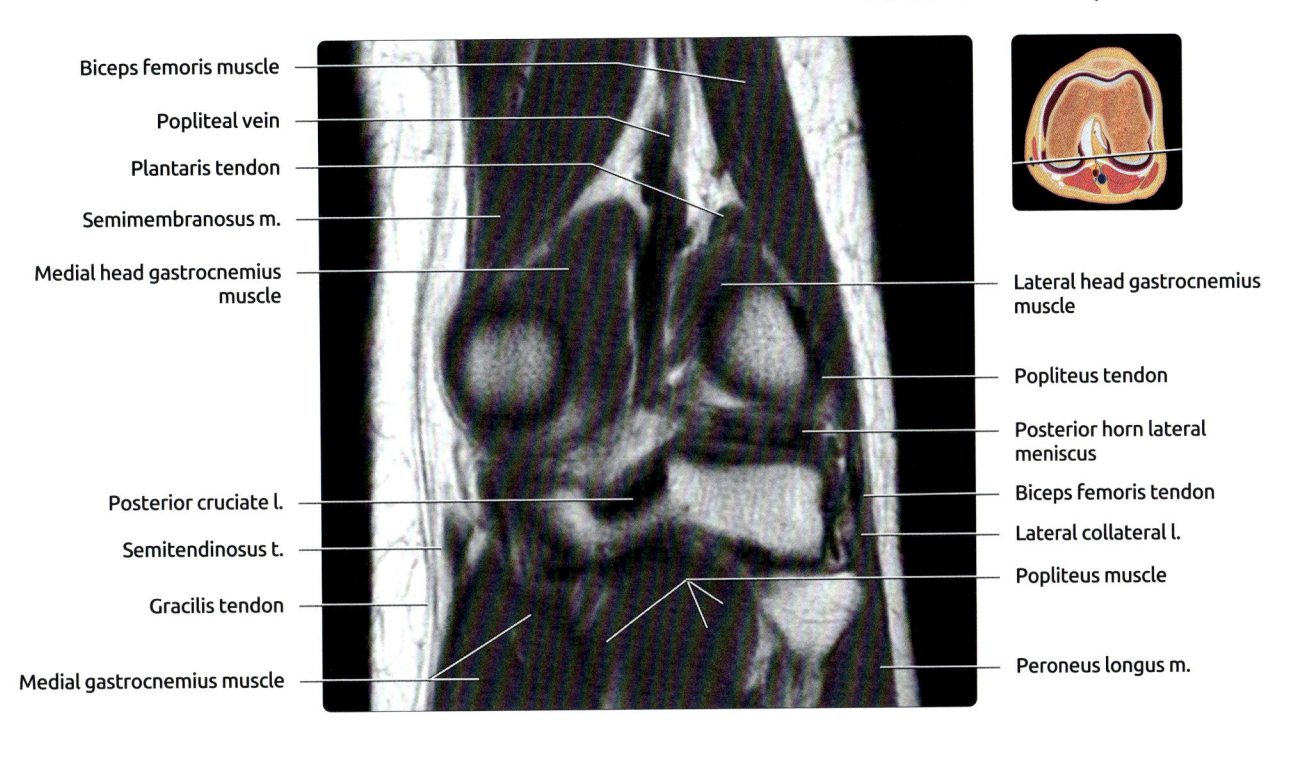

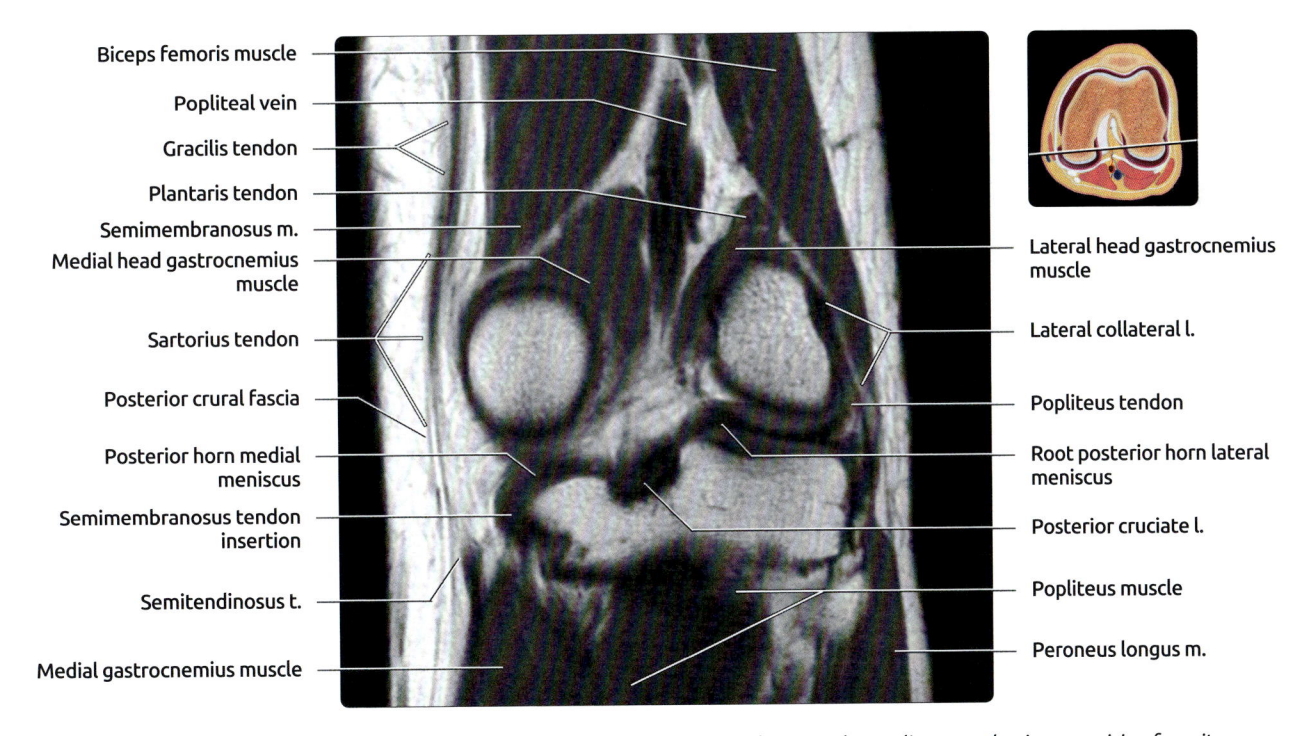

Top image labels (left):
- Biceps femoris muscle
- Popliteal vein
- Plantaris tendon
- Semimembranosus m.
- Medial head gastrocnemius muscle
- Posterior cruciate l.
- Semitendinosus t.
- Gracilis tendon
- Medial gastrocnemius muscle

Top image labels (right):
- Lateral head gastrocnemius muscle
- Popliteus tendon
- Posterior horn lateral meniscus
- Biceps femoris tendon
- Lateral collateral l.
- Popliteus muscle
- Peroneus longus m.

Bottom image labels (left):
- Biceps femoris muscle
- Popliteal vein
- Gracilis tendon
- Plantaris tendon
- Semimembranosus m.
- Medial head gastrocnemius muscle
- Sartorius tendon
- Posterior crural fascia
- Posterior horn medial meniscus
- Semimembranosus tendon insertion
- Semitendinosus t.
- Medial gastrocnemius muscle

Bottom image labels (right):
- Lateral head gastrocnemius muscle
- Lateral collateral l.
- Popliteus tendon
- Root posterior horn lateral meniscus
- Posterior cruciate l.
- Popliteus muscle
- Peroneus longus m.

(Top) Slightly more anterior, and deep to the majority of the gastrocnemius muscle mass, the popliteus tendon is seen arising from its notch on the lateral femoral condyle, extending posteriorly and inferiorly to the popliteal hiatus. The individual structures in the posterolateral corner are generally better seen on a fluid-sensitive sequence because of the fluid in the popliteal hiatus. **(Bottom)** The lateral collateral ligament can now be seen arising from lateral femoral condyle, coursing towards its insertion, along with the biceps femoris, on the fibular styloid process.

Knee MR Atlas

CORONAL T1 MR, RIGHT KNEE

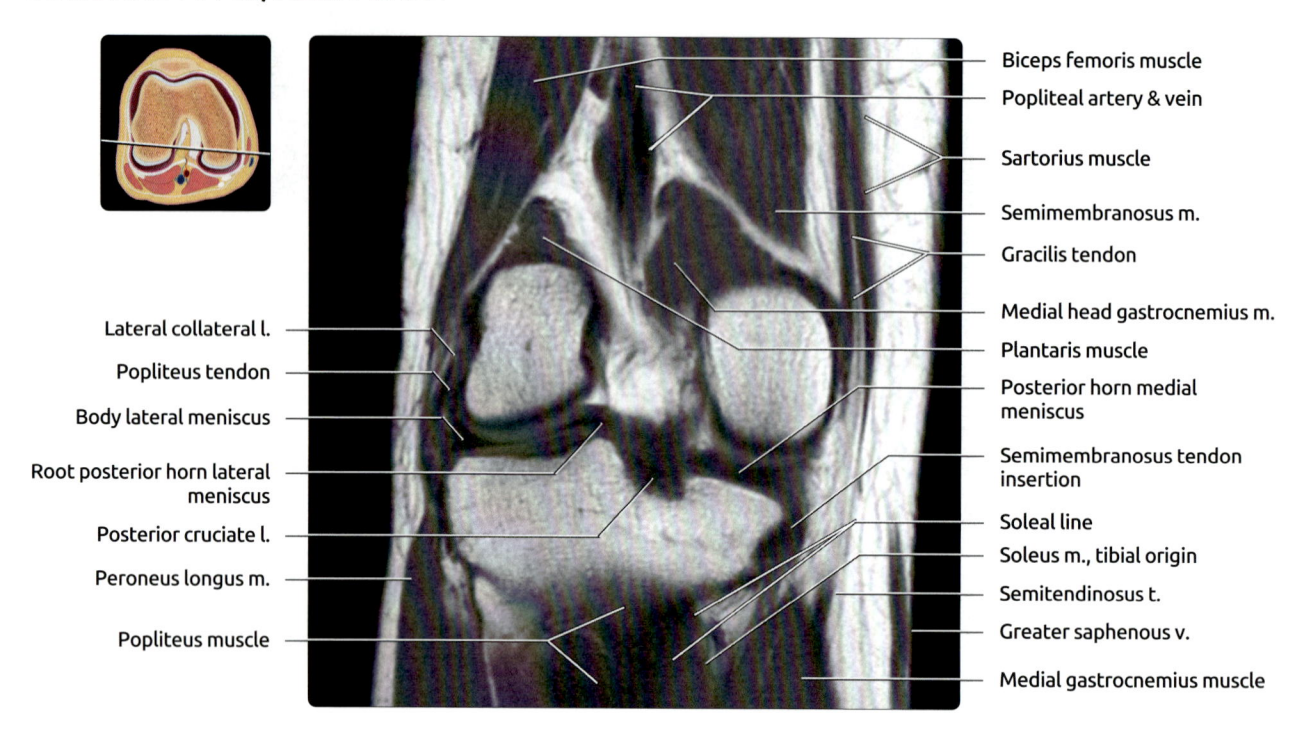

Labels (top image):
- Biceps femoris muscle
- Popliteal artery & vein
- Sartorius muscle
- Semimembranosus m.
- Gracilis tendon
- Medial head gastrocnemius m.
- Plantaris muscle
- Posterior horn medial meniscus
- Semimembranosus tendon insertion
- Soleal line
- Soleus m., tibial origin
- Semitendinosus t.
- Greater saphenous v.
- Medial gastrocnemius muscle
- Lateral collateral l.
- Popliteus tendon
- Body lateral meniscus
- Root posterior horn lateral meniscus
- Posterior cruciate l.
- Peroneus longus m.
- Popliteus muscle

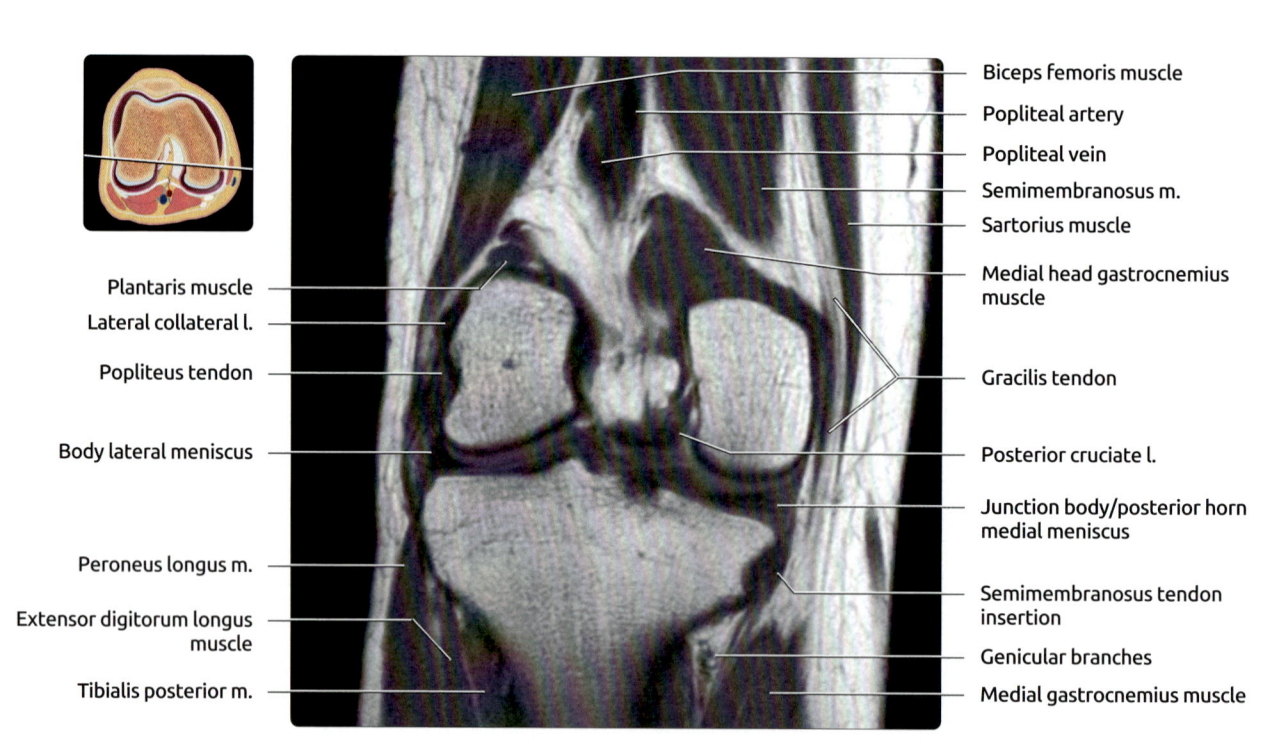

Labels (bottom image):
- Biceps femoris muscle
- Popliteal artery
- Popliteal vein
- Semimembranosus m.
- Sartorius muscle
- Medial head gastrocnemius muscle
- Gracilis tendon
- Posterior cruciate l.
- Junction body/posterior horn medial meniscus
- Semimembranosus tendon insertion
- Genicular branches
- Medial gastrocnemius muscle
- Plantaris muscle
- Lateral collateral l.
- Popliteus tendon
- Body lateral meniscus
- Peroneus longus m.
- Extensor digitorum longus muscle
- Tibialis posterior m.

(**Top**) *More anteriorly, note the large expanse of insertion of the popliteus muscle on the posterior tibia. The medial soleus origin arises at its distal edge, along the soleal line. The fibular origin of the soleus occurs more proximally.* (**Bottom**) *This is an image of the posterior portion of the knee joint, which is more complex than the anterior. The gastrocnemius and posterior vessels are still seen as well as the hamstring muscles. Inferolaterally, the muscles can be confusing on coronal imaging since in a single plane such as this, muscles from the lateral compartment (peroneus), anterior compartment (extensor digitorum longus), and posterior compartment (tibialis posterior) can be seen. This is because the cut extends obliquely across the interosseous membrane between the tibia and fibula.*

Knee MR Atlas

CORONAL T1 MR, LEFT KNEE

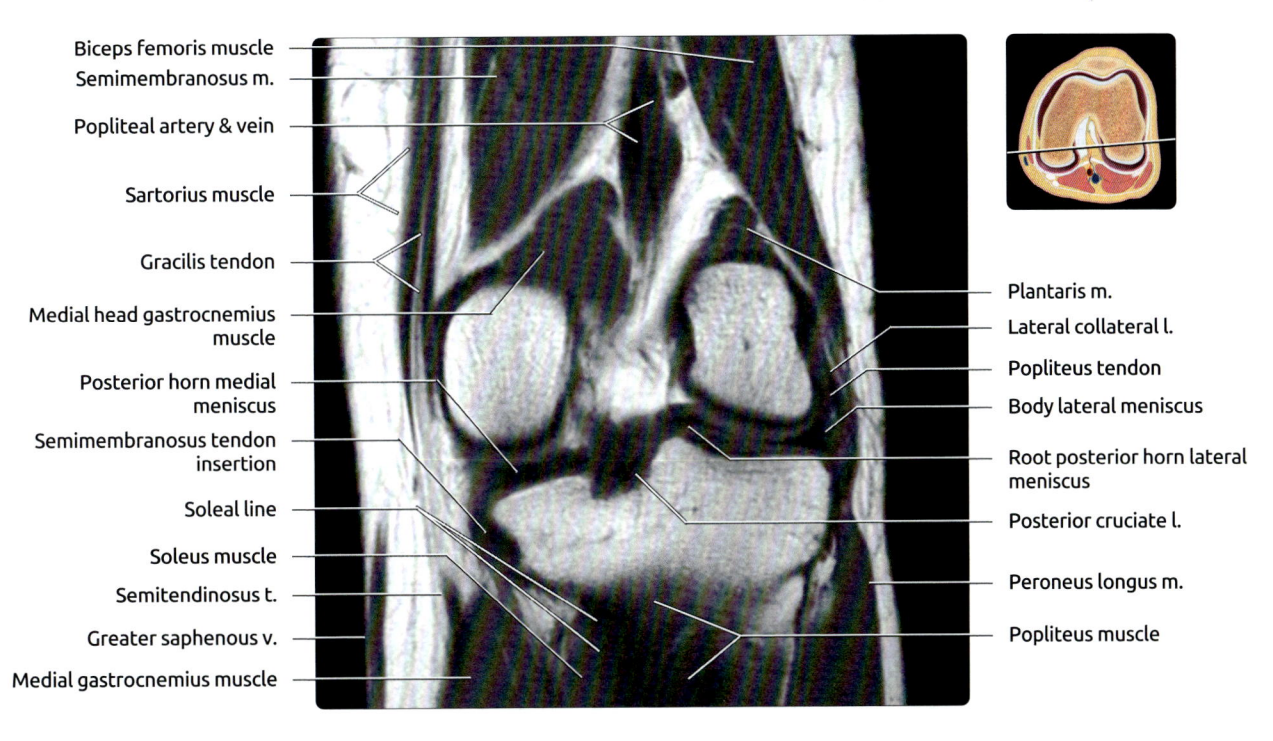

Labels (top image):
- Biceps femoris muscle
- Semimembranosus m.
- Popliteal artery & vein
- Sartorius muscle
- Gracilis tendon
- Medial head gastrocnemius muscle
- Posterior horn medial meniscus
- Semimembranosus tendon insertion
- Soleal line
- Soleus muscle
- Semitendinosus t.
- Greater saphenous v.
- Medial gastrocnemius muscle
- Plantaris m.
- Lateral collateral l.
- Popliteus tendon
- Body lateral meniscus
- Root posterior horn lateral meniscus
- Posterior cruciate l.
- Peroneus longus m.
- Popliteus muscle

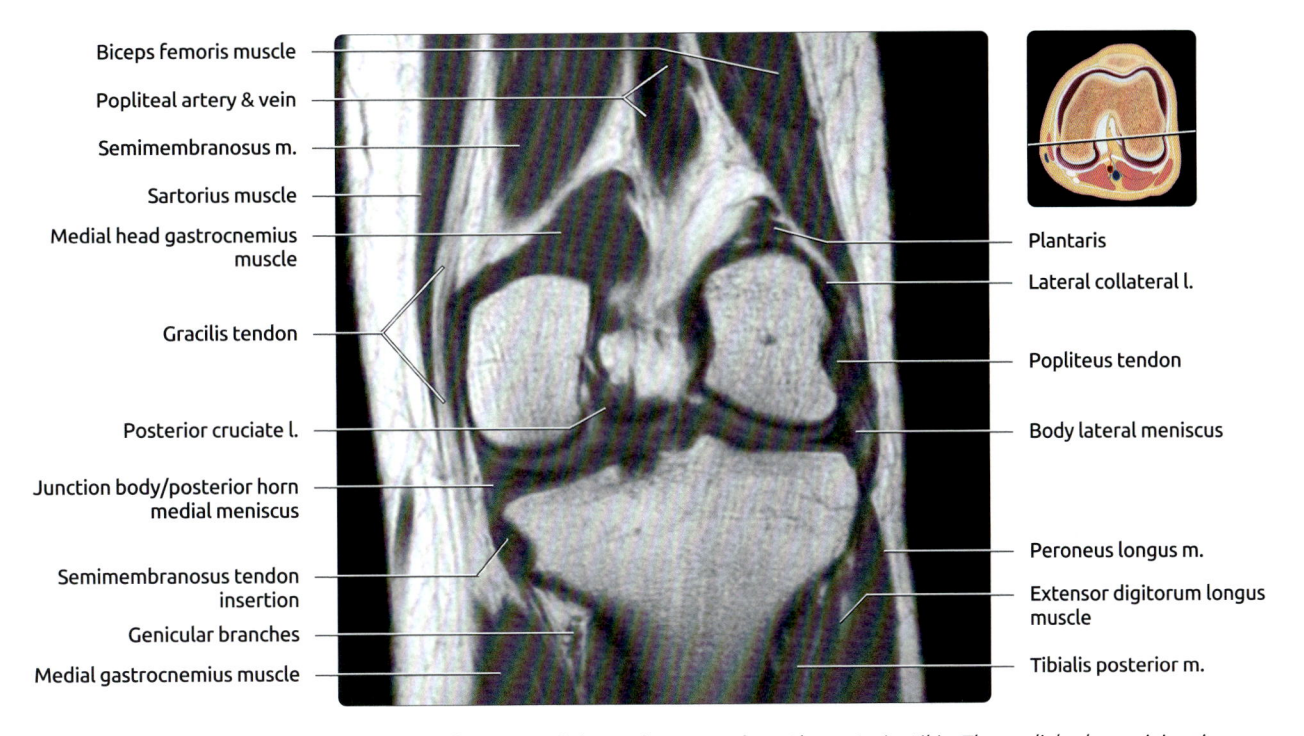

Labels (bottom image):
- Biceps femoris muscle
- Popliteal artery & vein
- Semimembranosus m.
- Sartorius muscle
- Medial head gastrocnemius muscle
- Gracilis tendon
- Posterior cruciate l.
- Junction body/posterior horn medial meniscus
- Semimembranosus tendon insertion
- Genicular branches
- Medial gastrocnemius muscle
- Plantaris
- Lateral collateral l.
- Popliteus tendon
- Body lateral meniscus
- Peroneus longus m.
- Extensor digitorum longus muscle
- Tibialis posterior m.

(Top) *More anteriorly, note the large expanse of insertion of the popliteus muscle on the posterior tibia. The medial soleus origin arises at its distal edge, along the soleal line. The fibular origin of the soleus occurs more proximally.* (Bottom) *This is an image of the posterior portion of the knee joint, which is more complex than the anterior. The gastrocnemius and posterior vessels are still seen as well as the hamstring muscles. Inferolaterally, the muscles can be confusing on coronal imaging since in a single plane such as this, muscles from the lateral compartment (peroneus), anterior compartment (extensor digitorum longus), and posterior compartment (tibialis posterior) can be seen. This is because the cut extends obliquely across the interosseous membrane between tibia and fibula.*

Knee MR Atlas

CORONAL T1 MR, RIGHT KNEE

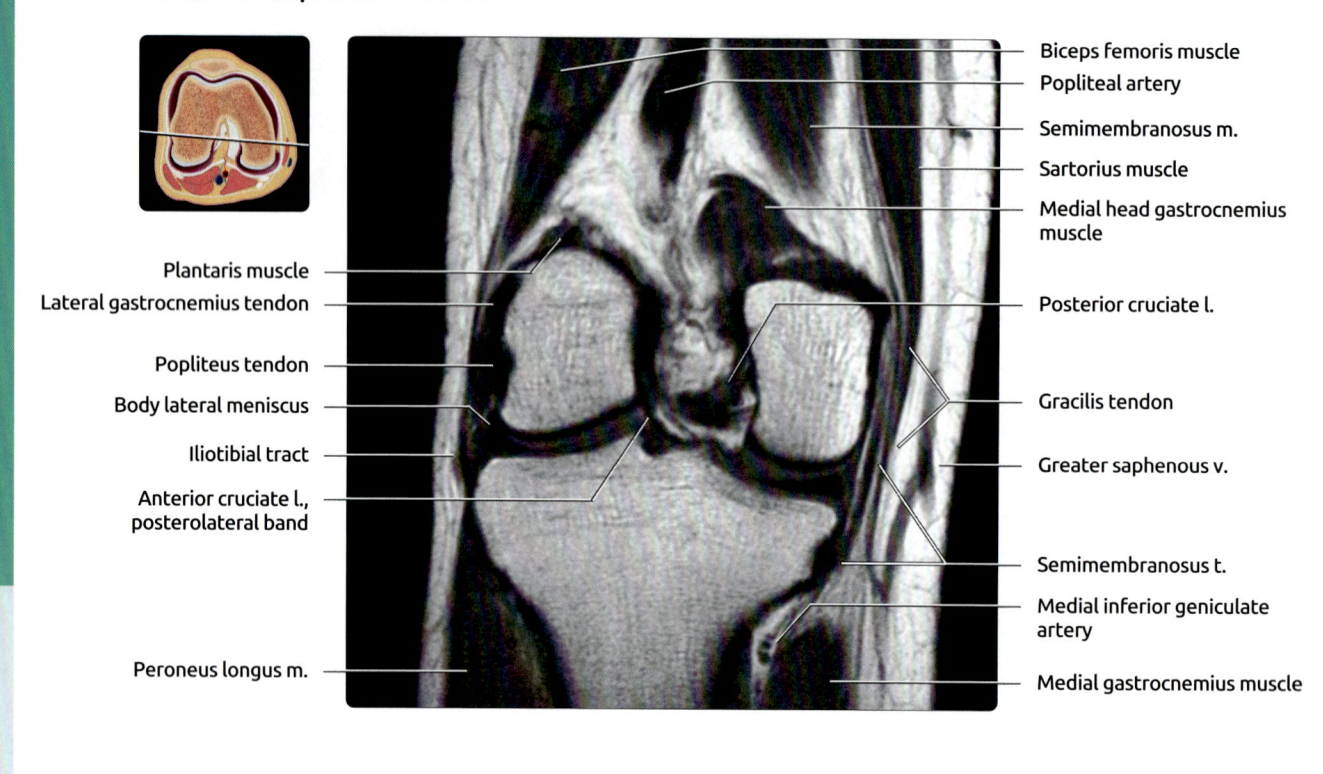

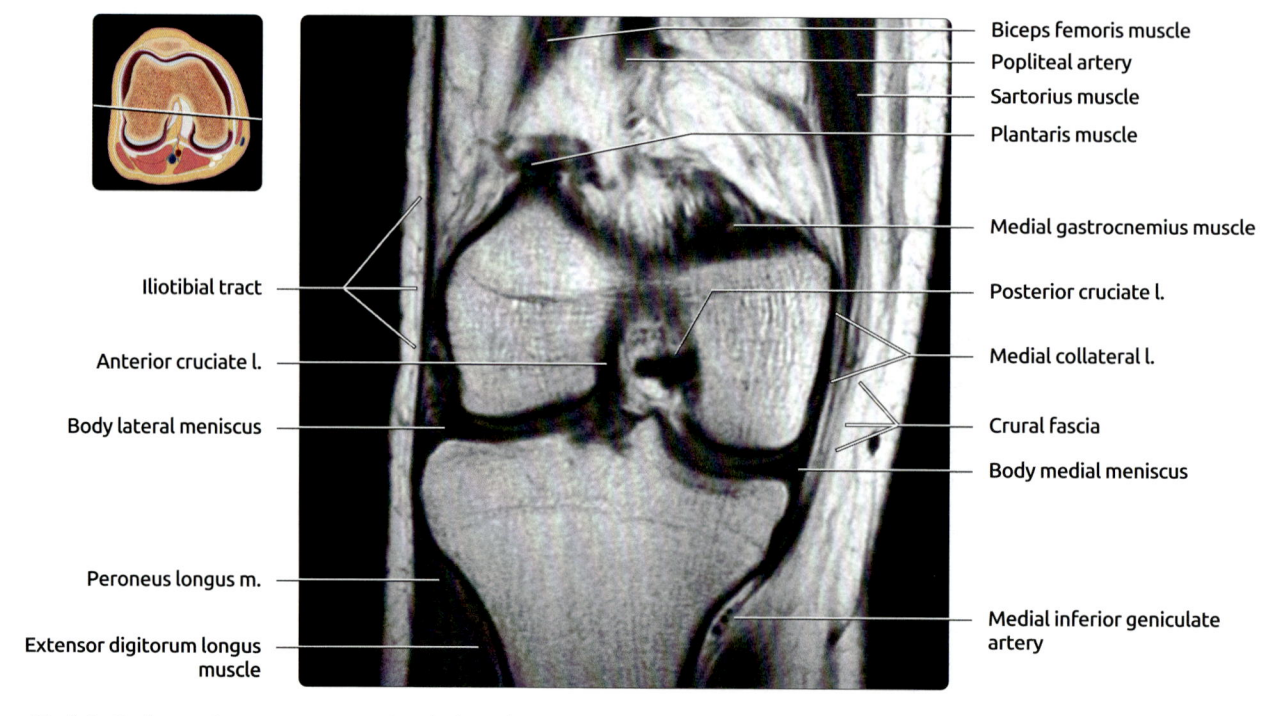

Labels (top image):
- Plantaris muscle
- Lateral gastrocnemius tendon
- Popliteus tendon
- Body lateral meniscus
- Iliotibial tract
- Anterior cruciate l., posterolateral band
- Peroneus longus m.
- Biceps femoris muscle
- Popliteal artery
- Semimembranosus m.
- Sartorius muscle
- Medial head gastrocnemius muscle
- Posterior cruciate l.
- Gracilis tendon
- Greater saphenous v.
- Semimembranosus t.
- Medial inferior geniculate artery
- Medial gastrocnemius muscle

Labels (bottom image):
- Iliotibial tract
- Anterior cruciate l.
- Body lateral meniscus
- Peroneus longus m.
- Extensor digitorum longus muscle
- Biceps femoris muscle
- Popliteal artery
- Sartorius muscle
- Plantaris muscle
- Medial gastrocnemius muscle
- Posterior cruciate l.
- Medial collateral l.
- Crural fascia
- Body medial meniscus
- Medial inferior geniculate artery

(**Top**) *As the images become more anterior, the last elements of the pes anserinus can be seen. The sartorius and gracilis are shown in this image located more anteriorly at the joint line than the 3rd element of the pes and semitendinosus. The most posterior fibers of the anterior cruciate ligament are seen as well.* (**Bottom**) *More anteriorly within the notch, the entire anterior cruciate ligament is seen in its oblique route from the lateral femoral condyle to the insertion adjacent to the medial spines. Note that the deep and superficial fibers of medial collateral ligament are not separable on these T1 images. For more definition of these medial structures.*

Knee MR Atlas

CORONAL T1 MR, LEFT KNEE

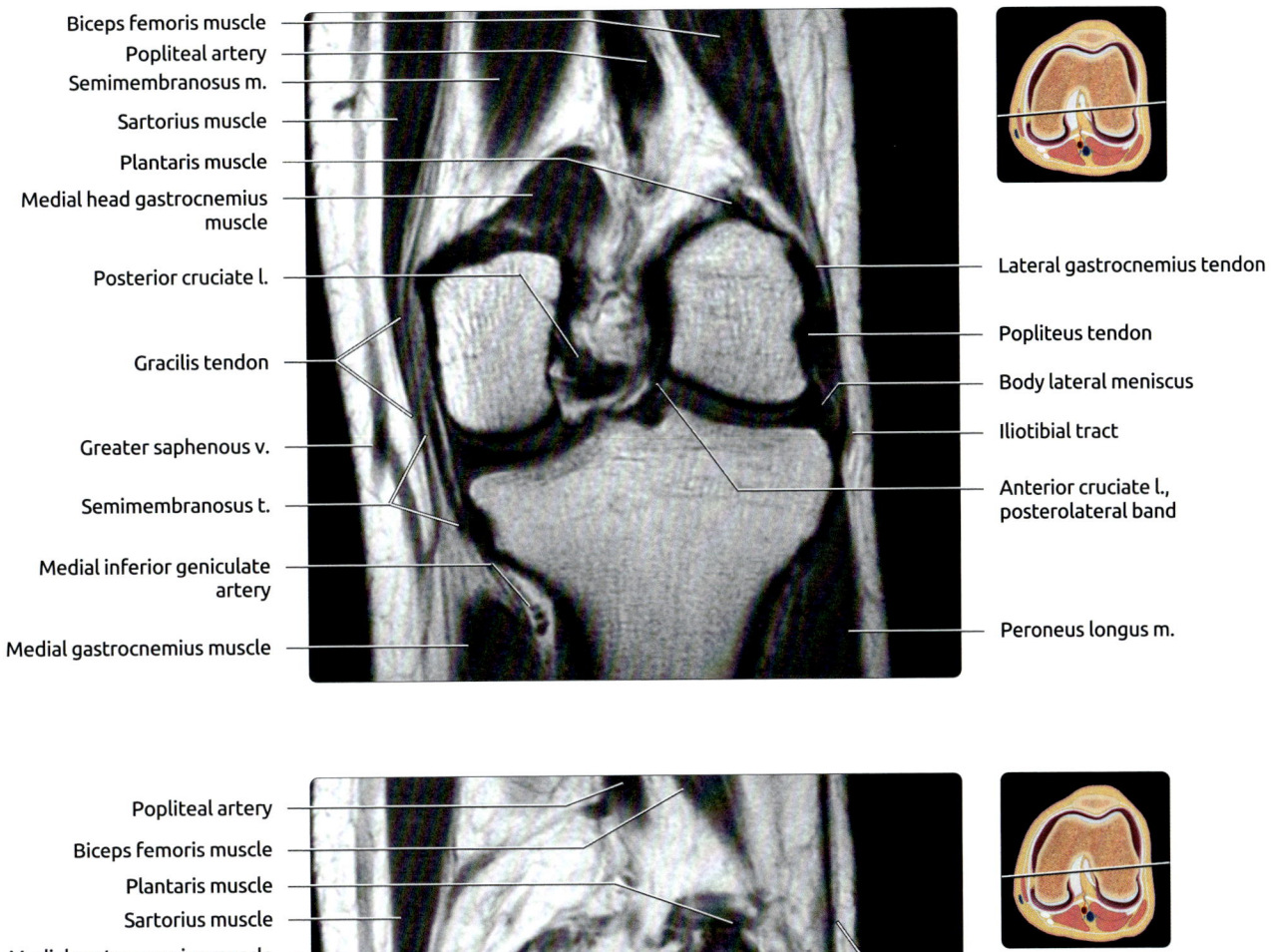

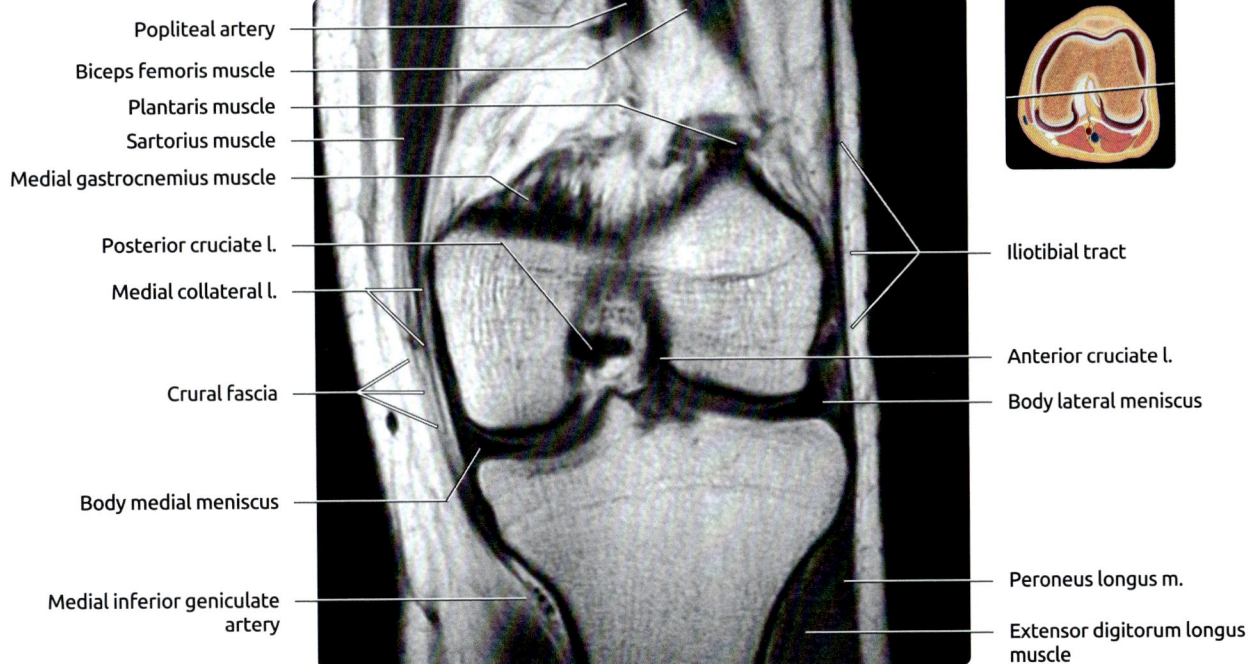

(Top) *As the images become more anterior, the last elements of the pes anserinus can be seen. The sartorius and gracilis are shown in this image located more anteriorly at the joint line than the 3rd element of the pes and semitendinosus. The most posterior fibers of the anterior cruciate ligament are seen as well.* **(Bottom)** *More anteriorly within the notch, the entire anterior cruciate ligament is seen in its oblique route from the lateral femoral condyle to the insertion adjacent to the medial spines. Note that the deep and superficial fibers of the medial collateral ligament are not separable on these T1 images.*

CORONAL T1 MR, RIGHT KNEE

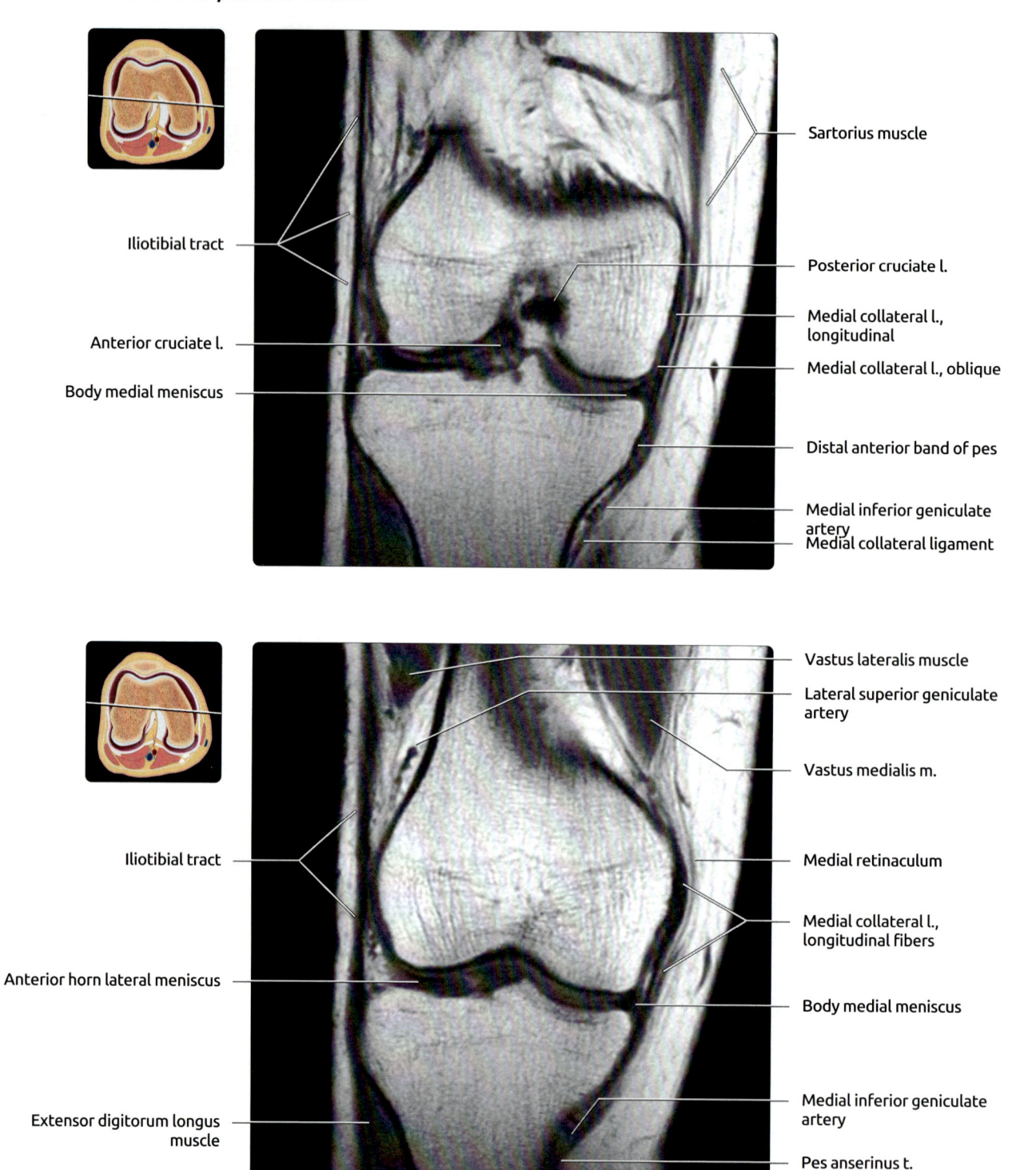

Labels (top image):
- Iliotibial tract
- Anterior cruciate l.
- Body medial meniscus
- Sartorius muscle
- Posterior cruciate l.
- Medial collateral l., longitudinal
- Medial collateral l., oblique
- Distal anterior band of pes
- Medial inferior geniculate artery
- Medial collateral ligament

Labels (bottom image):
- Iliotibial tract
- Anterior horn lateral meniscus
- Extensor digitorum longus muscle
- Vastus lateralis muscle
- Lateral superior geniculate artery
- Vastus medialis m.
- Medial retinaculum
- Medial collateral l., longitudinal fibers
- Body medial meniscus
- Medial inferior geniculate artery
- Pes anserinus t.

(Top) *Note the length of the medial collateral ligament in this image. The origin is intimately associated with the origin of the medial patellofemoral ligament, immediately distal to the adductor tubercle. The insertion is about 5 cm distal to the knee joint and is usually not entirely included in standard knee MR exams. The medial inferior geniculate arterial branches are seen in cross section between the superficial medial collateral ligament and the tibial cortex.* **(Bottom)** *The anterior cut is through the anterior midportion of the joint. Because these are T1 images, there is little contrast between the hyaline cartilage and menisci.*

Knee MR Atlas

CORONAL T1 MR, LEFT KNEE

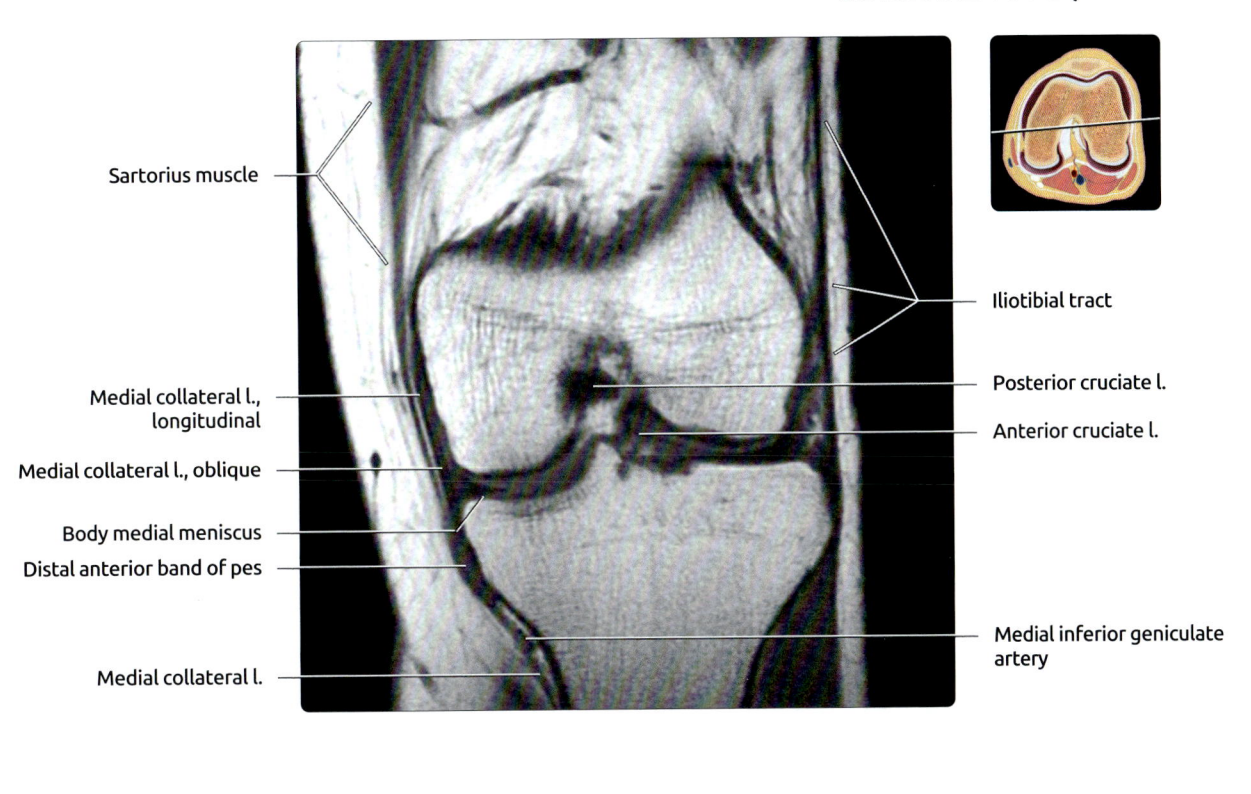

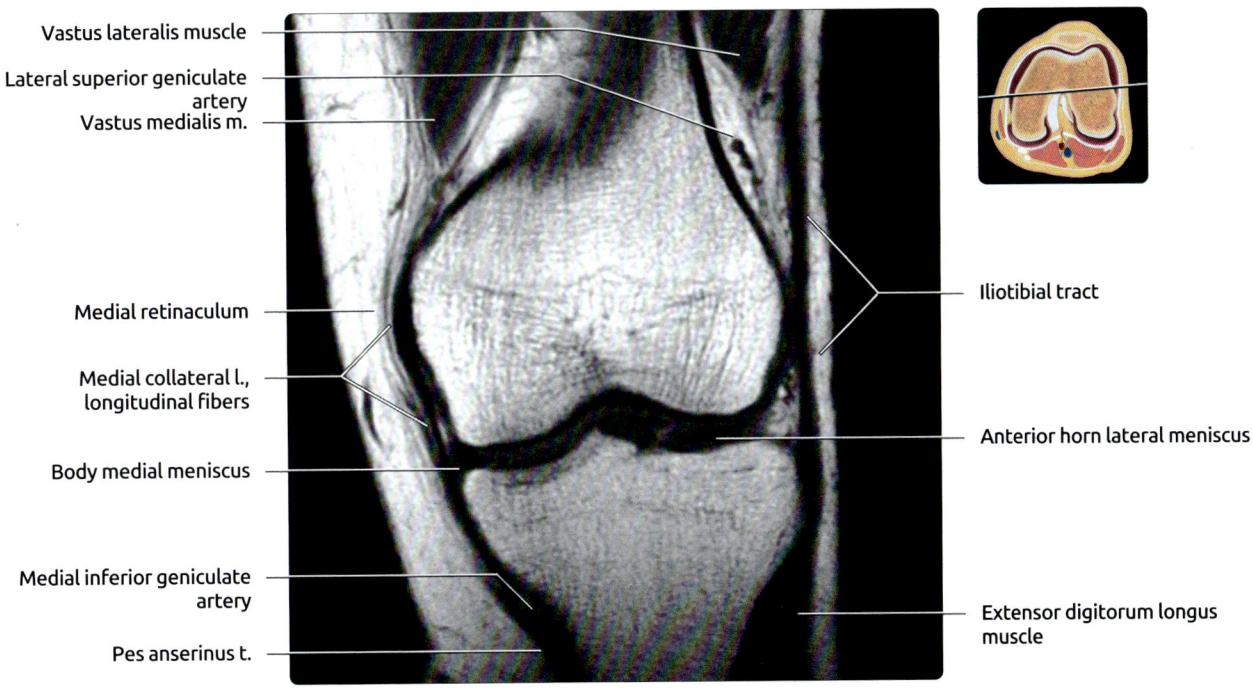

Labels (top image):
- Sartorius muscle
- Medial collateral l., longitudinal
- Medial collateral l., oblique
- Body medial meniscus
- Distal anterior band of pes
- Medial collateral l.
- Iliotibial tract
- Posterior cruciate l.
- Anterior cruciate l.
- Medial inferior geniculate artery

Labels (bottom image):
- Vastus lateralis muscle
- Lateral superior geniculate artery
- Vastus medialis m.
- Medial retinaculum
- Medial collateral l., longitudinal fibers
- Body medial meniscus
- Medial inferior geniculate artery
- Pes anserinus t.
- Iliotibial tract
- Anterior horn lateral meniscus
- Extensor digitorum longus muscle

(**Top**) *Note the length of the medial collateral ligament in this image. The origin is intimately associated with the origin of the medial patellofemoral ligament, immediately distal to the adductor tubercle. The insertion is about 5 cm distal to the knee joint and is usually not entirely included in standard knee MR exams. The medial inferior geniculate arterial branches are seen in cross section between the superficial medial collateral ligament and the tibial cortex.* (**Bottom**) *The anterior cut is through the anterior midportion of the joint. Because these are T1 images, there is little contrast between the hyaline cartilage and menisci.*

Knee MR Atlas

CORONAL T1 MR, RIGHT KNEE

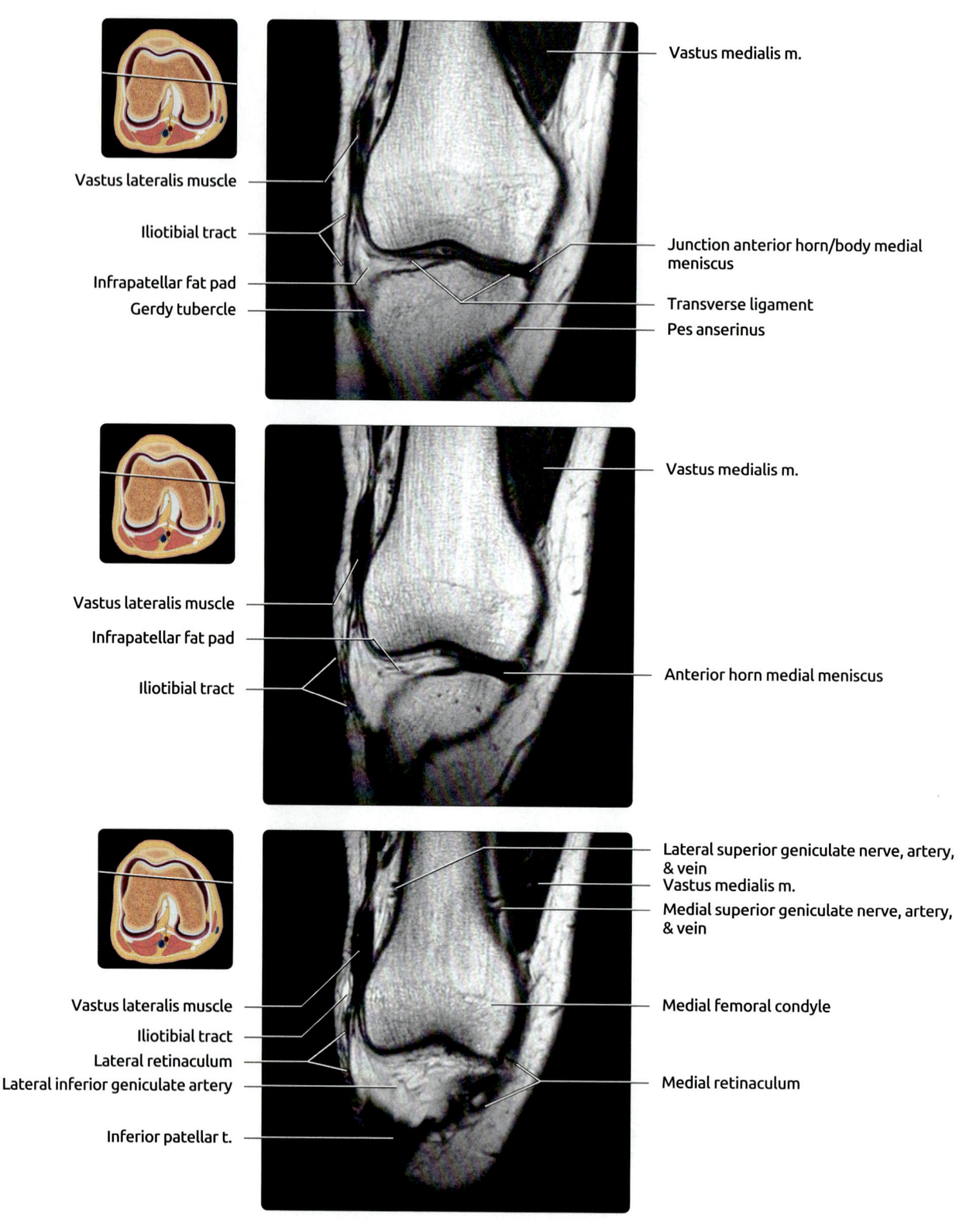

- Vastus lateralis muscle
- Iliotibial tract
- Infrapatellar fat pad
- Gerdy tubercle
- Vastus medialis m.
- Junction anterior horn/body medial meniscus
- Transverse ligament
- Pes anserinus

- Vastus lateralis muscle
- Infrapatellar fat pad
- Iliotibial tract
- Vastus medialis m.
- Anterior horn medial meniscus

- Vastus lateralis muscle
- Iliotibial tract
- Lateral retinaculum
- Lateral inferior geniculate artery
- Inferior patellar t.
- Lateral superior geniculate nerve, artery, & vein
- Vastus medialis m.
- Medial superior geniculate nerve, artery, & vein
- Medial femoral condyle
- Medial retinaculum

(**Top**) In this far anterior image, the transverse ligament is seen crossing the anterior joint from the anterior horn medial meniscus towards the anterior horn lateral meniscus. The iliotibial tract is seen inserting on the Gerdy tubercle. (**Middle**) In this far anterior cut through the joint space, note that because of the slightly oblique angle at which coronal knee MR images are obtained, the anterior horn medial meniscus is visualized in the far anterior coronal cuts without any portion of the lateral meniscus. (**Bottom**) A coronal cut through the anterior femoral shaft shows that the joint is fairly featureless, consisting mostly of fat pads and anastomosing vascular structures.

Knee MR Atlas

CORONAL T1 MR, LEFT KNEE

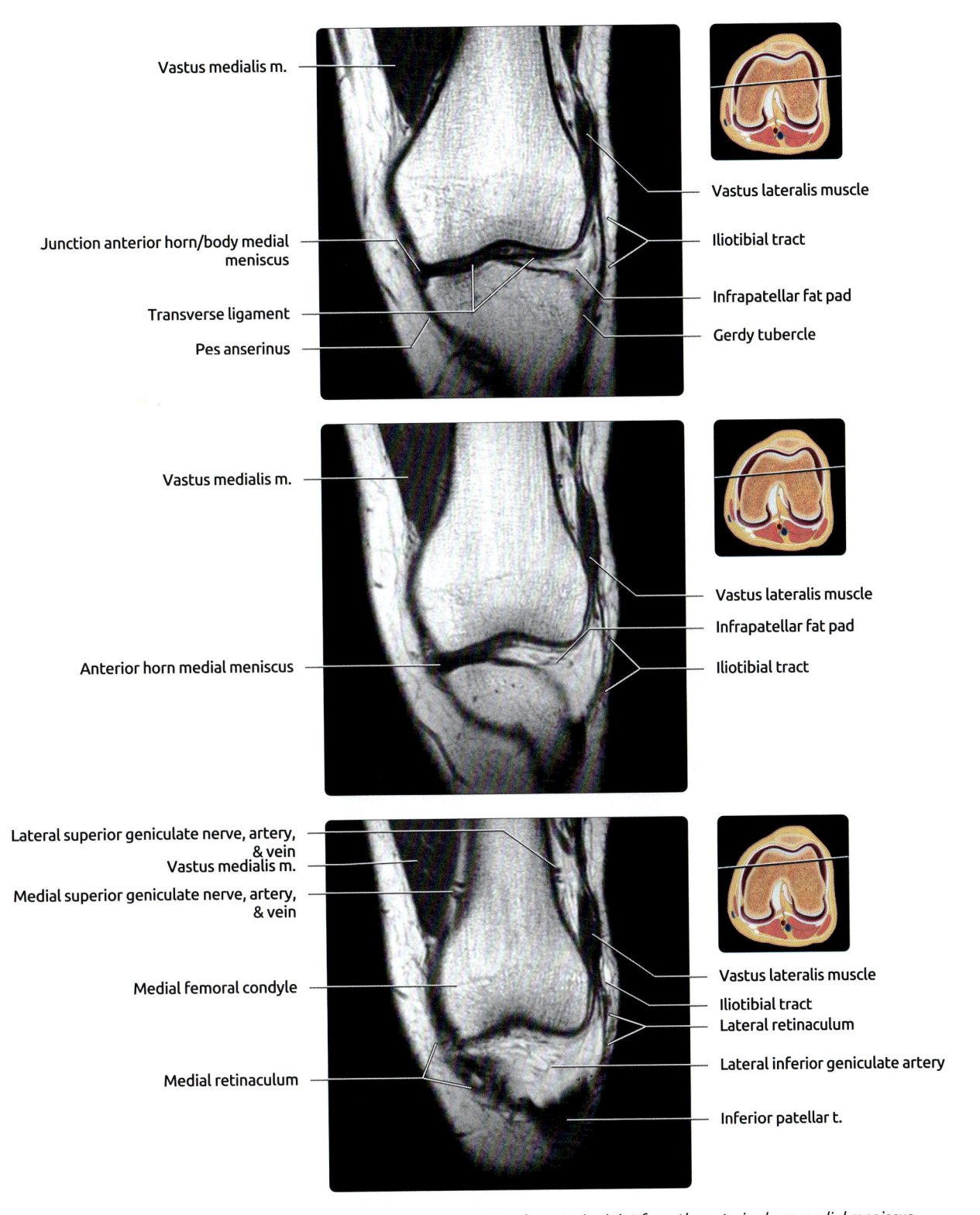

Top image labels:
- Vastus medialis m.
- Junction anterior horn/body medial meniscus
- Transverse ligament
- Pes anserinus
- Vastus lateralis muscle
- Iliotibial tract
- Infrapatellar fat pad
- Gerdy tubercle

Middle image labels:
- Vastus medialis m.
- Anterior horn medial meniscus
- Vastus lateralis muscle
- Infrapatellar fat pad
- Iliotibial tract

Bottom image labels:
- Lateral superior geniculate nerve, artery, & vein
- Vastus medialis m.
- Medial superior geniculate nerve, artery, & vein
- Medial femoral condyle
- Medial retinaculum
- Vastus lateralis muscle
- Iliotibial tract
- Lateral retinaculum
- Lateral inferior geniculate artery
- Inferior patellar t.

(Top) In this far anterior image, the transverse ligament is seen crossing the anterior joint from the anterior horn medial meniscus towards the anterior horn lateral meniscus. The iliotibial tract is seen inserting on the Gerdy tubercle. **(Middle)** In this far anterior cut through the joint space, note that because of the slightly oblique angle at which the coronal knee MR images are obtained, the anterior horn medial meniscus is visualized in far anterior coronal cuts without any portion of the lateral meniscus. **(Bottom)** Coronal cut through the anterior femoral shaft shows that the joint is fairly featureless, consisting mostly of fat pads and anastomosing vascular structures.

Knee MR Atlas

CORONAL T1 MR, RIGHT KNEE

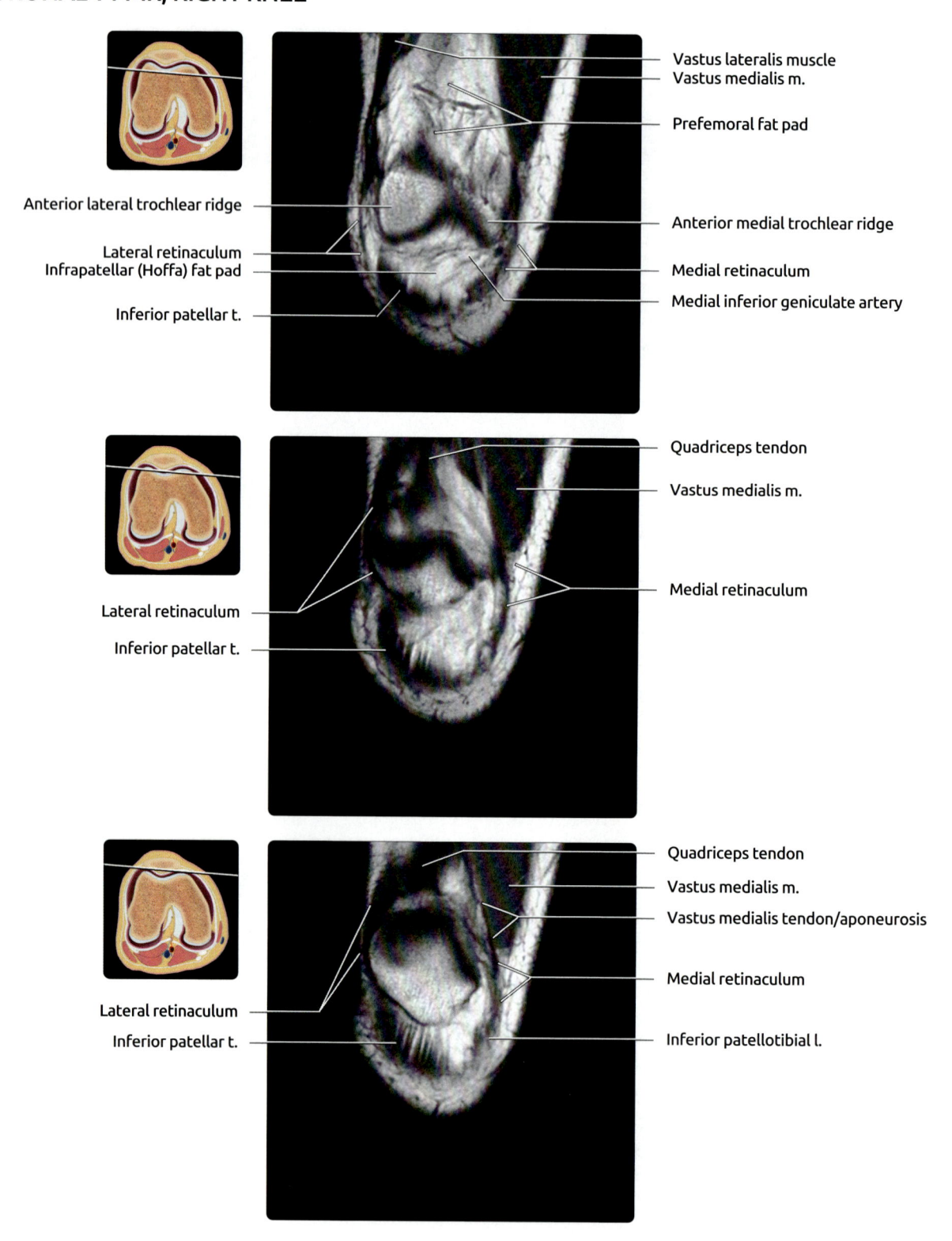

Anterior lateral trochlear ridge
Lateral retinaculum
Infrapatellar (Hoffa) fat pad
Inferior patellar t.

Vastus lateralis muscle
Vastus medialis m.
Prefemoral fat pad
Anterior medial trochlear ridge
Medial retinaculum
Medial inferior geniculate artery

Lateral retinaculum
Inferior patellar t.

Quadriceps tendon
Vastus medialis m.
Medial retinaculum

Lateral retinaculum
Inferior patellar t.

Quadriceps tendon
Vastus medialis m.
Vastus medialis tendon/aponeurosis
Medial retinaculum
Inferior patellotibial l.

(Top) The cut is through the anterior femoral condyles. Fat pads, both prefemoral and infrapatellar, predominate in the anterior joint. The retinacula are seen as well. Note the multiple geniculate and collateral arteries supplying the knee joint. **(Middle)** This is a coronal cut through the posterior patella. Note the large size of the vastus medialis. This can help identify the medial side of the knee on coronal or axial planes. **(Bottom)** This anterior-most image of the series shows the medial and lateral supporting structures of the patella as well as the quadriceps and inferior patellar tendons. Both the quadriceps and inferior patellar tendons are fairly broad, as are the medial and lateral retinacula, effectively surrounding the patella.

Knee MR Atlas

CORONAL T1 MR, LEFT KNEE

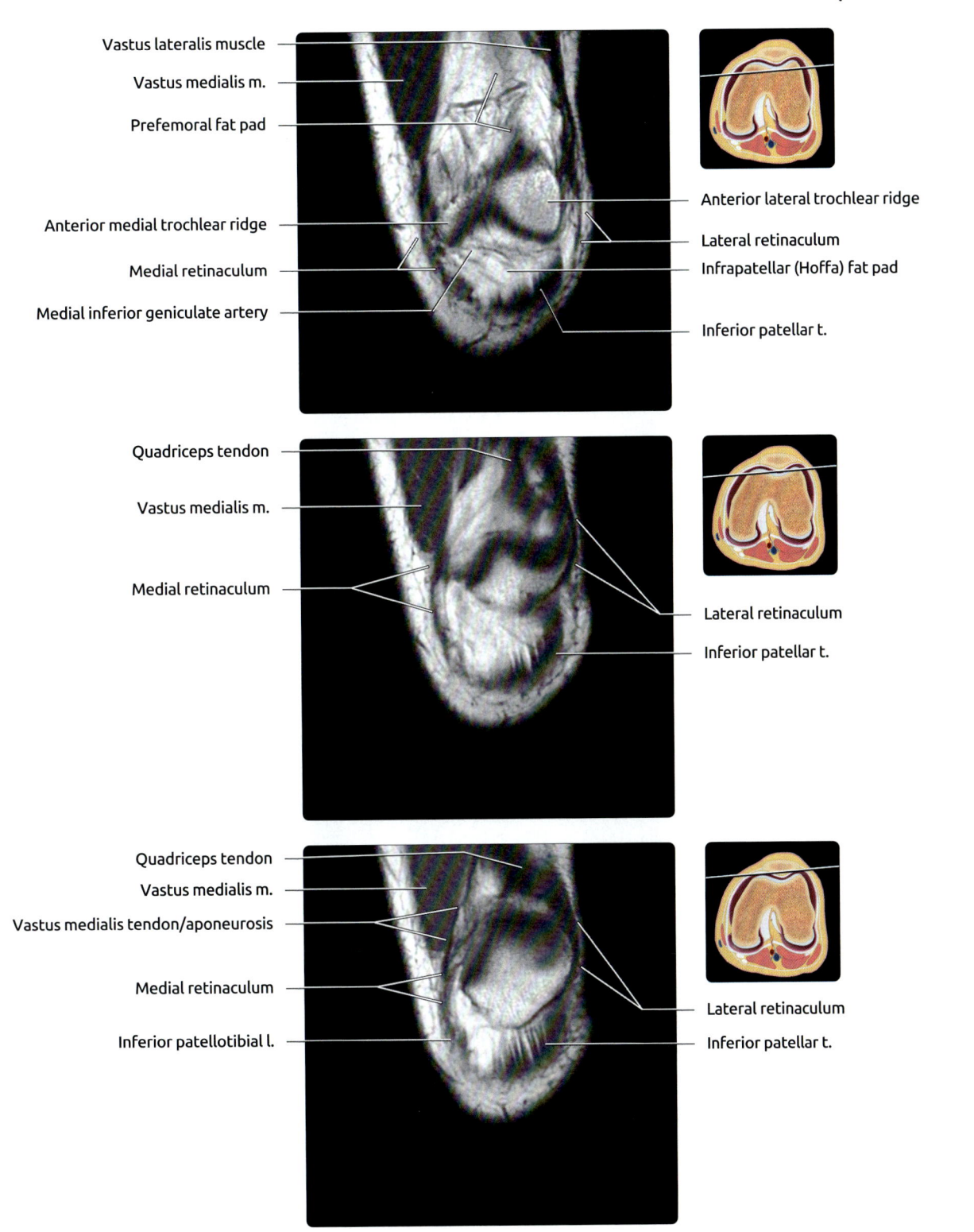

Top image labels:
- Vastus lateralis muscle
- Vastus medialis m.
- Prefemoral fat pad
- Anterior medial trochlear ridge
- Medial retinaculum
- Medial inferior geniculate artery
- Anterior lateral trochlear ridge
- Lateral retinaculum
- Infrapatellar (Hoffa) fat pad
- Inferior patellar t.

Middle image labels:
- Quadriceps tendon
- Vastus medialis m.
- Medial retinaculum
- Lateral retinaculum
- Inferior patellar t.

Bottom image labels:
- Quadriceps tendon
- Vastus medialis m.
- Vastus medialis tendon/aponeurosis
- Medial retinaculum
- Inferior patellotibial l.
- Lateral retinaculum
- Inferior patellar t.

(**Top**) The cut is through the anterior femoral condyles. Fat pads, both prefemoral and infrapatellar, predominate in the anterior joint. The retinacula are seen as well. Note the multiple geniculate and collateral arteries supplying the knee joint. (**Middle**) This is a coronal cut through posterior patella. Note the large size of the vastus medialis. This can help identify the medial side of the knee on coronal or axial planes. (**Bottom**) This anterior-most image of the series shows the medial and lateral supporting structures of the patella as well as the quadriceps and inferior patellar tendons. Both the quadriceps and inferior patellar tendons are fairly broad, as are the medial and lateral retinacula, effectively surrounding the patella.

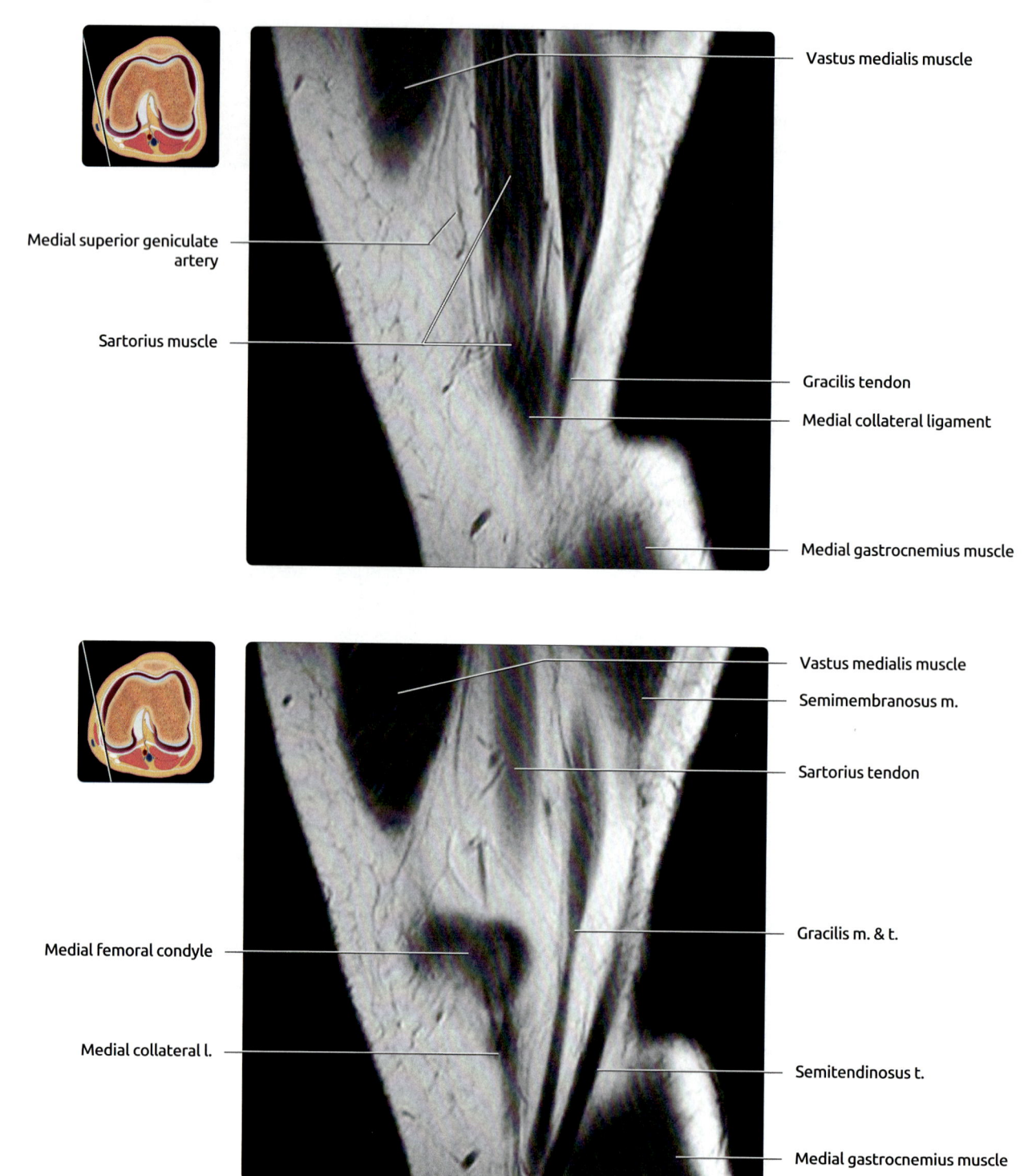

SAGITTAL T1 MR, KNEE

- Vastus medialis muscle
- Medial superior geniculate artery
- Sartorius muscle
- Gracilis tendon
- Medial collateral ligament
- Medial gastrocnemius muscle

- Vastus medialis muscle
- Semimembranosus m.
- Sartorius tendon
- Medial femoral condyle
- Gracilis m. & t.
- Medial collateral l.
- Semitendinosus t.
- Medial gastrocnemius muscle

(Top) The 1st of 20 sagittal T1 MR images of the knee shows a far medial cut. Note the sartorius muscle and tendon, with the gracilis muscle and tendon extending immediately posterior to it. (Bottom) This cut is barely through the medial femoral condyle, so only a thin remnant of the sartorius is seen. The gracilis and semitendinosus tendons are seen extending posteriorly, forming with the sartorius and the 3 tendons of the pes anserinus.

Knee MR Atlas

SAGITTAL T1 MR, KNEE

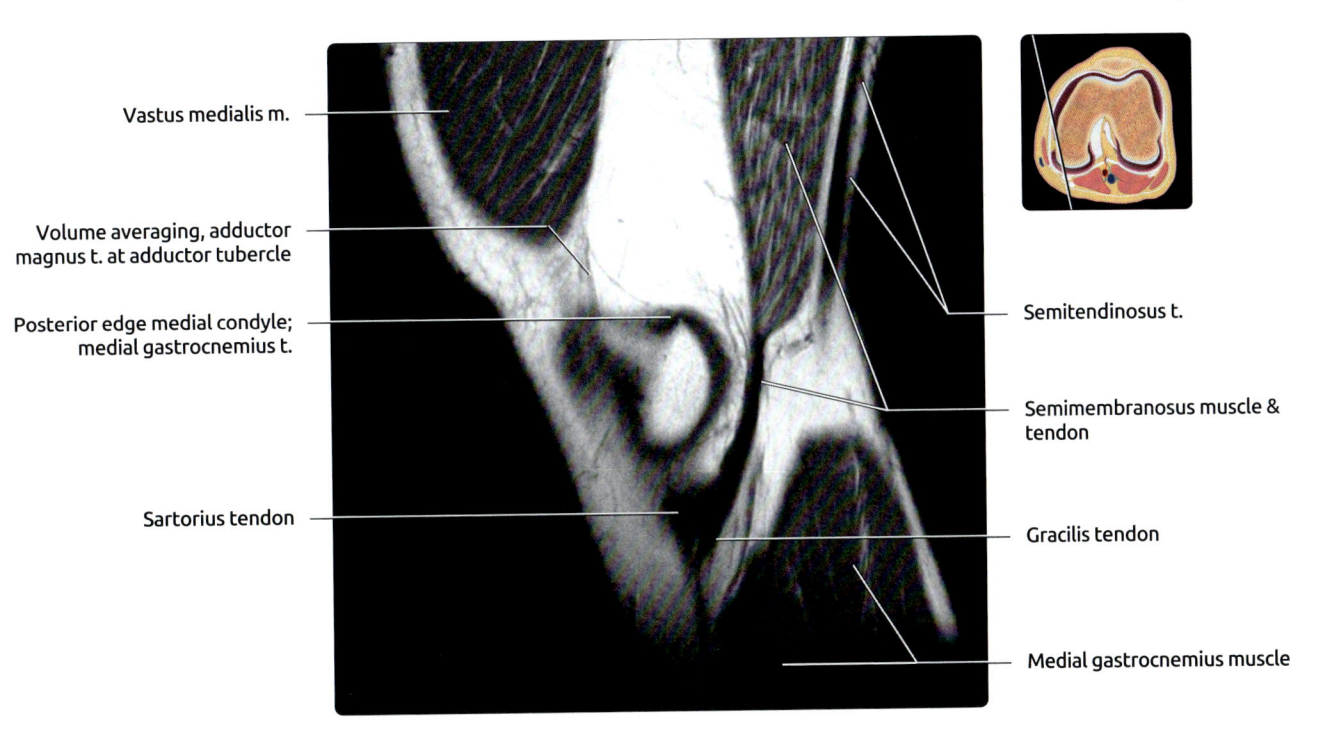

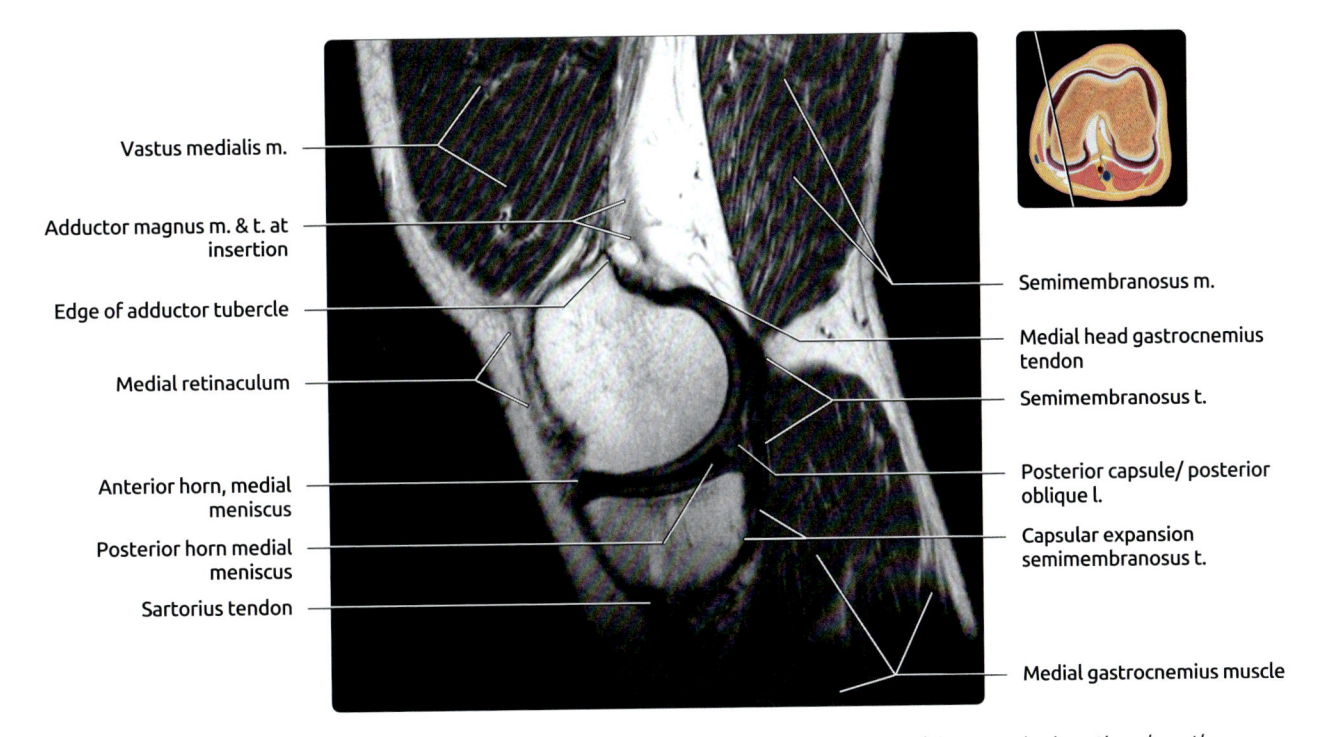

Top image labels (left):
- Vastus medialis m.
- Volume averaging, adductor magnus t. at adductor tubercle
- Posterior edge medial condyle; medial gastrocnemius t.
- Sartorius tendon

Top image labels (right):
- Semitendinosus t.
- Semimembranosus muscle & tendon
- Gracilis tendon
- Medial gastrocnemius muscle

Bottom image labels (left):
- Vastus medialis m.
- Adductor magnus m. & t. at insertion
- Edge of adductor tubercle
- Medial retinaculum
- Anterior horn, medial meniscus
- Posterior horn medial meniscus
- Sartorius tendon

Bottom image labels (right):
- Semimembranosus m.
- Medial head gastrocnemius tendon
- Semimembranosus t.
- Posterior capsule/ posterior oblique l.
- Capsular expansion semimembranosus t.
- Medial gastrocnemius muscle

(Top) *This is a medial cut through the femoral condyle. Note the large semimembranosus tendon with its extensive insertion along the posteromedial tibia.* **(Bottom)** *This cut goes through the medial compartment, near the central edge of the body of the medial meniscus. This is still slightly a "bow tie" configuration of the meniscus.*

Knee MR Atlas

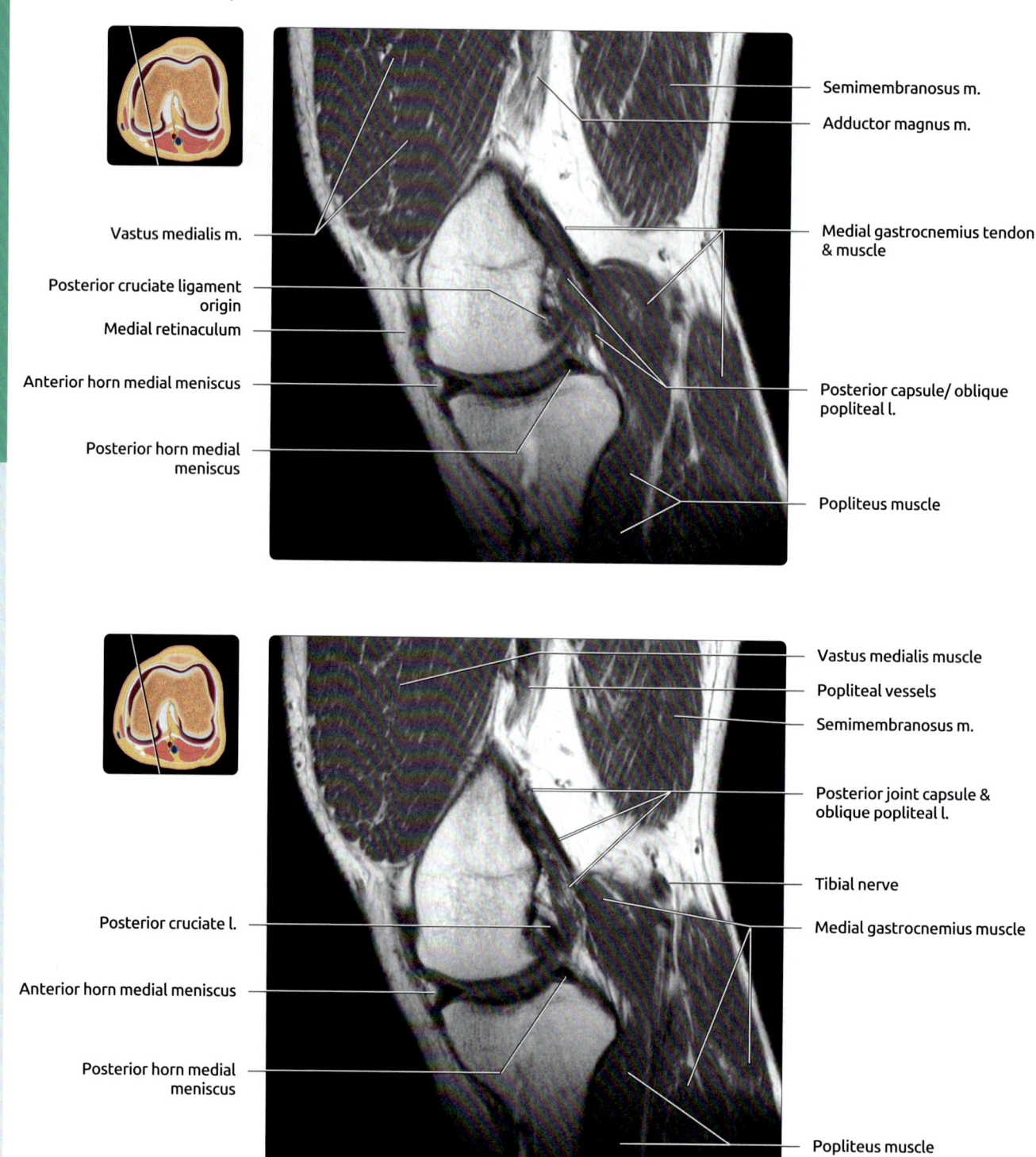

SAGITTAL T1 MR, KNEE

Labels (top image):
- Semimembranosus m.
- Adductor magnus m.
- Medial gastrocnemius tendon & muscle
- Posterior capsule/ oblique popliteal l.
- Popliteus muscle
- Vastus medialis m.
- Posterior cruciate ligament origin
- Medial retinaculum
- Anterior horn medial meniscus
- Posterior horn medial meniscus

Labels (bottom image):
- Vastus medialis muscle
- Popliteal vessels
- Semimembranosus m.
- Posterior joint capsule & oblique popliteal l.
- Tibial nerve
- Medial gastrocnemius muscle
- Popliteus muscle
- Posterior cruciate l.
- Anterior horn medial meniscus
- Posterior horn medial meniscus

(**Top**) *This cut is through the medial compartment, approaching the intercondylar notch. The posterior aspect of the medial femoral condyle is only partially seen. The oblique popliteal ligament contributes to the posterior capsule at this point.* (**Bottom**) *This cut is at the medial-most aspect of the intercondylar notch, where the origin of the posterior cruciate ligament is 1st seen. Note that by this point, the oblique popliteal ligament contributes more fully to the posterior joint capsule.*

Knee MR Atlas

SAGITTAL T1 MR, KNEE

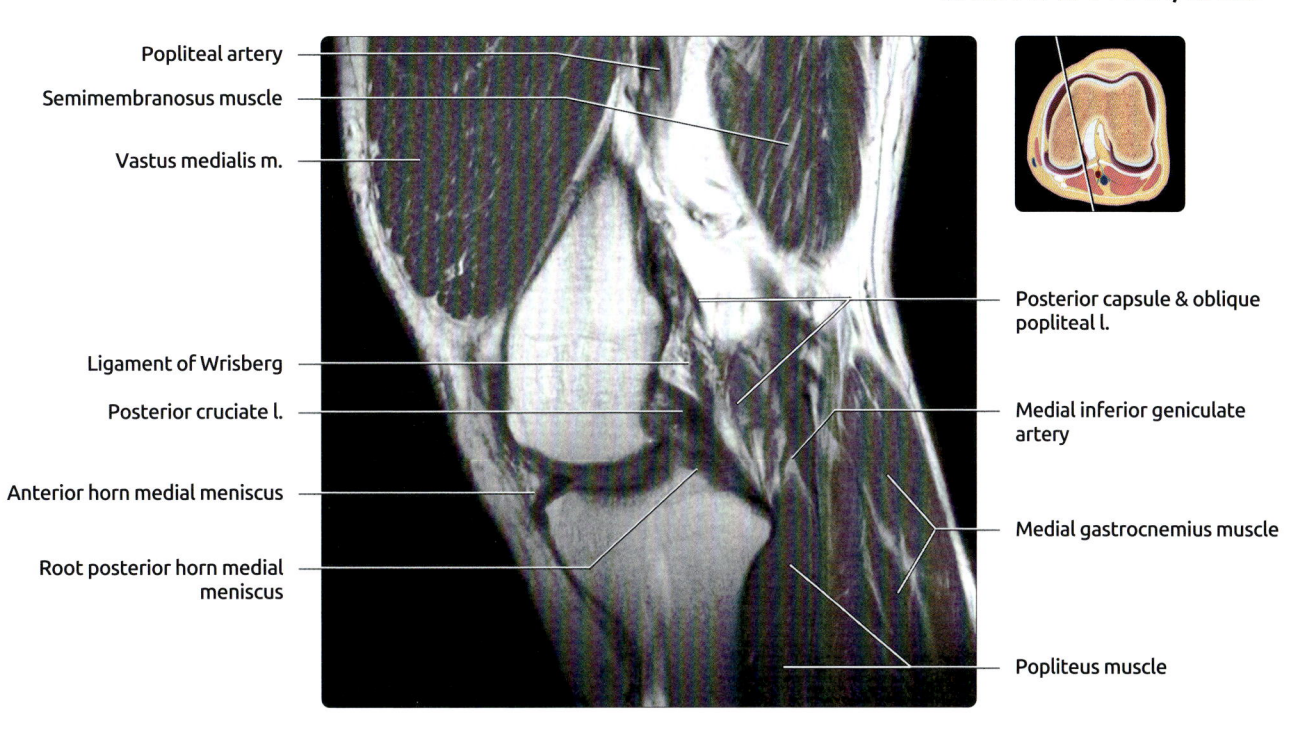

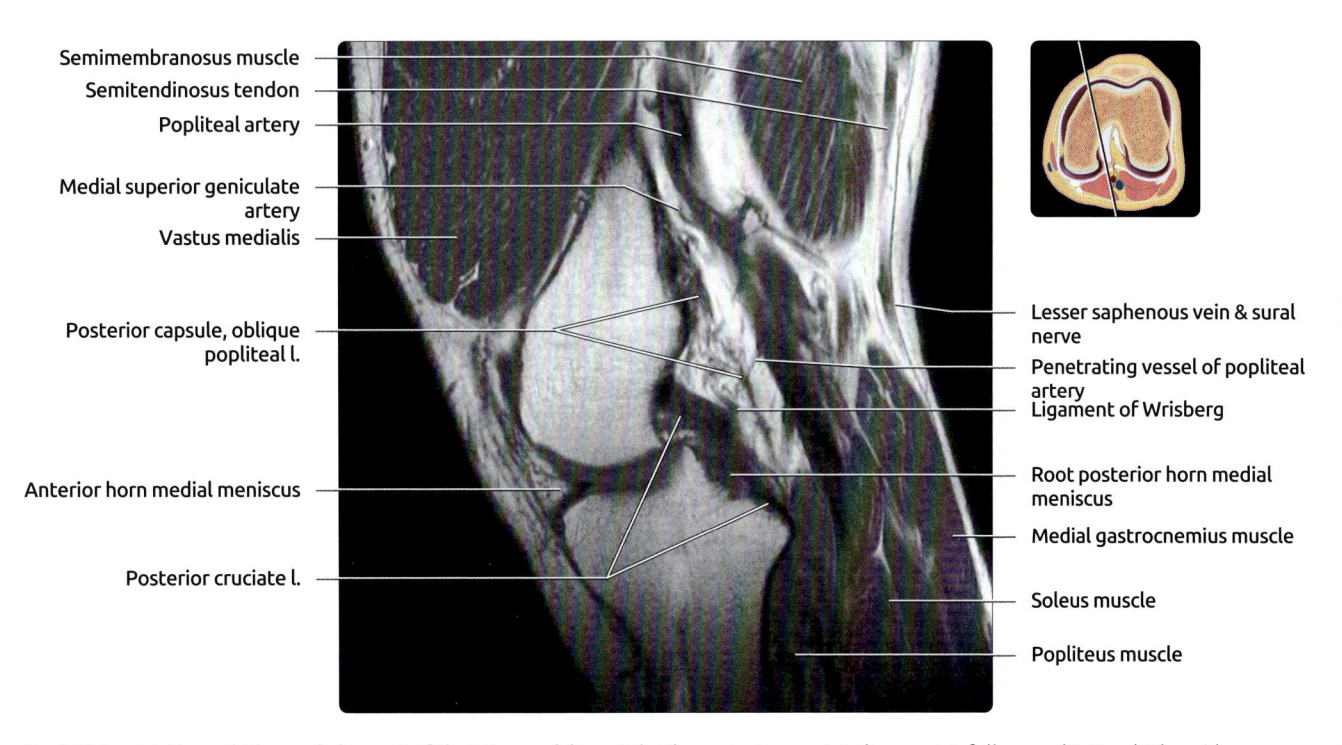

Top image labels (left):
- Popliteal artery
- Semimembranosus muscle
- Vastus medialis m.
- Ligament of Wrisberg
- Posterior cruciate l.
- Anterior horn medial meniscus
- Root posterior horn medial meniscus

Top image labels (right):
- Posterior capsule & oblique popliteal l.
- Medial inferior geniculate artery
- Medial gastrocnemius muscle
- Popliteus muscle

Bottom image labels (left):
- Semimembranosus muscle
- Semitendinosus tendon
- Popliteal artery
- Medial superior geniculate artery
- Vastus medialis
- Posterior capsule, oblique popliteal l.
- Anterior horn medial meniscus
- Posterior cruciate l.

Bottom image labels (right):
- Lesser saphenous vein & sural nerve
- Penetrating vessel of popliteal artery
- Ligament of Wrisberg
- Root posterior horn medial meniscus
- Medial gastrocnemius muscle
- Soleus muscle
- Popliteus muscle

(**Top**) *This cut is through the medial aspect of the intercondylar notch. The posterior cruciate ligament is fully seen.* (**Bottom**) *The mid intercondylar notch is shown. Note that at the posterior intercondylar notch, the posterior capsule is penetrated by vessels from the popliteal artery. The capsule is therefore incomplete posteriorly.*

Knee MR Atlas

SAGITTAL T1 MR, KNEE

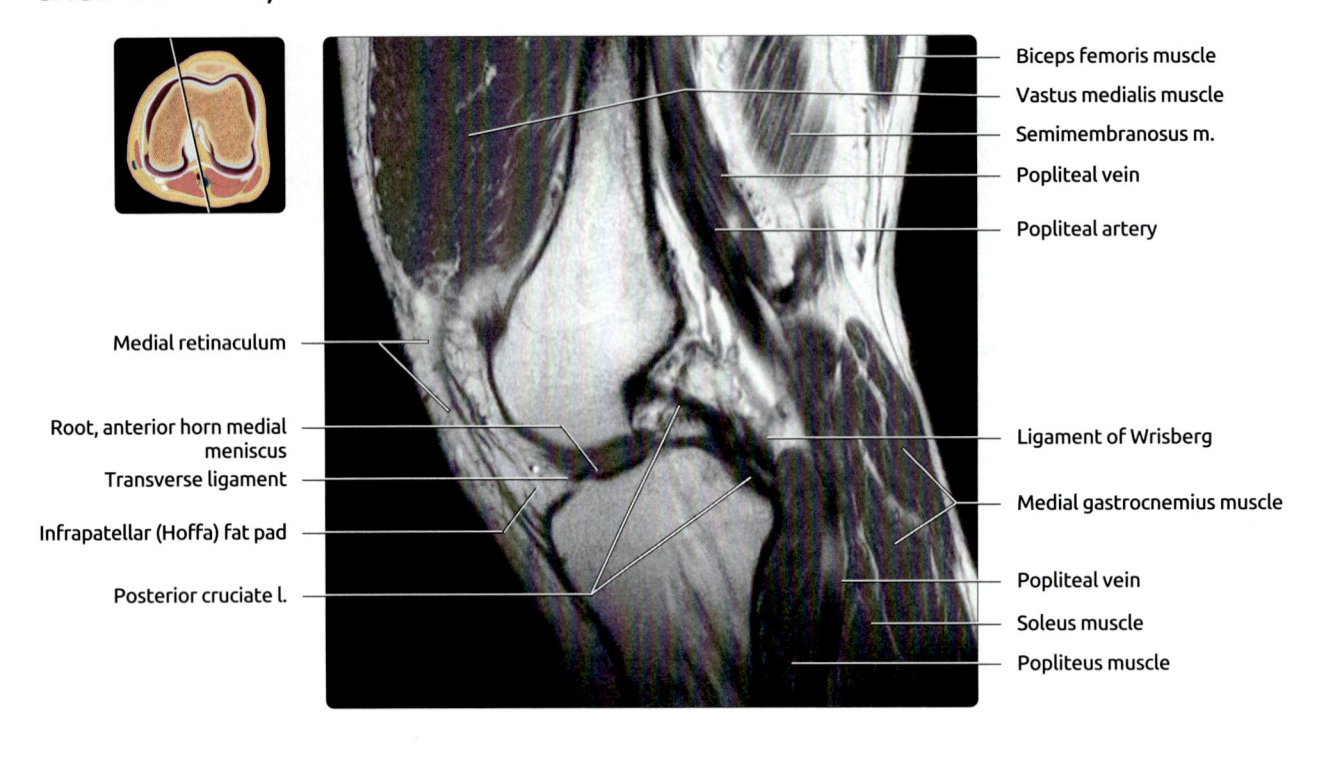

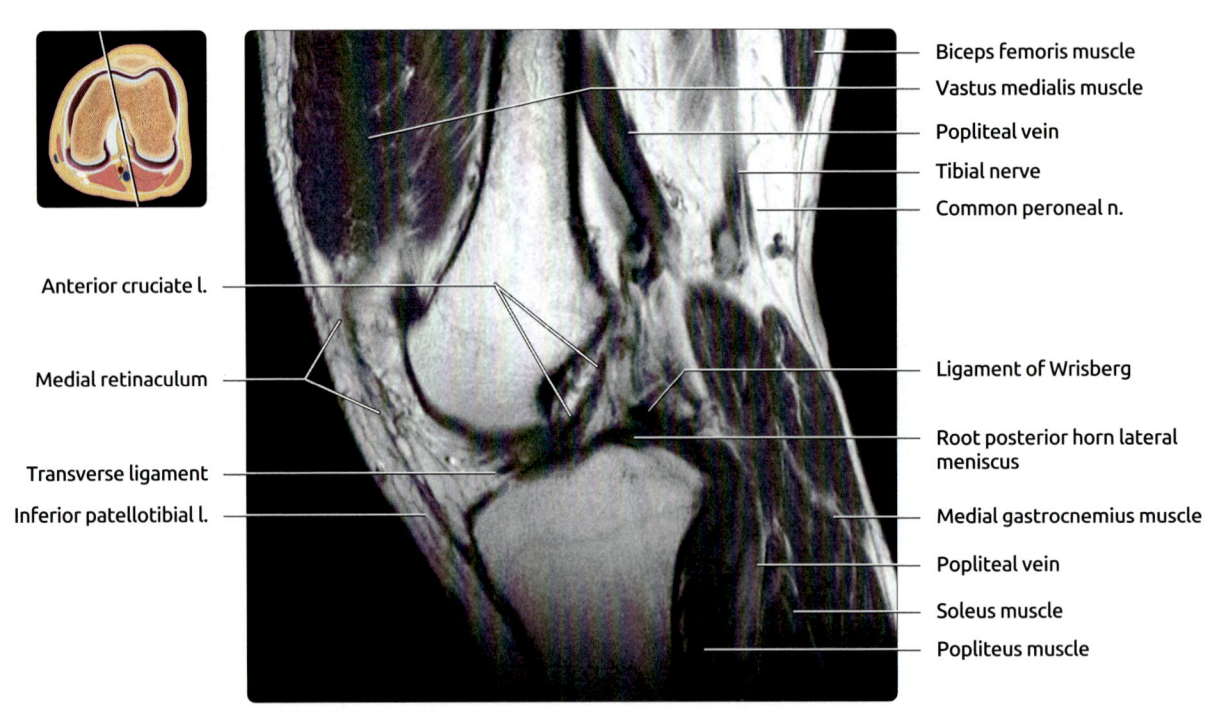

Labels (top image):
- Biceps femoris muscle
- Vastus medialis muscle
- Semimembranosus m.
- Popliteal vein
- Popliteal artery
- Medial retinaculum
- Root, anterior horn medial meniscus
- Transverse ligament
- Infrapatellar (Hoffa) fat pad
- Posterior cruciate l.
- Ligament of Wrisberg
- Medial gastrocnemius muscle
- Popliteal vein
- Soleus muscle
- Popliteus muscle

Labels (bottom image):
- Biceps femoris muscle
- Vastus medialis muscle
- Popliteal vein
- Tibial nerve
- Common peroneal n.
- Anterior cruciate l.
- Medial retinaculum
- Transverse ligament
- Inferior patellotibial l.
- Ligament of Wrisberg
- Root posterior horn lateral meniscus
- Medial gastrocnemius muscle
- Popliteal vein
- Soleus muscle
- Popliteus muscle

(Top) *The cut on this image is at the mid intercondylar notch, transitioning from the posterior to anterior cruciate ligament. The posterior capsule is still incomplete due to penetrating vessels.* **(Bottom)** *Slightly laterally within the intercondylar notch, the anterior cruciate ligament is most fully seen. Note the pathway of the ligament of Wrisberg (posterior meniscofemoral ligament), arising from the medial aspect of the intercondylar notch, traversing posterior and superior to the posterior cruciate ligament, and inserting on the superior aspect of the root of the posterior horn lateral meniscus.*

Knee MR Atlas

SAGITTAL T1 MR, KNEE

Top image labels:
- Biceps femoris muscle
- Tibial & common peroneal nerve
- Vastus medialis m.
- Medial patella
- Medial retinaculum
- Transverse ligament
- Anterior cruciate l.
- Root, posterior horn lateral meniscus
- Posterior capsule & oblique popliteal l.
- Plantaris muscle
- Lateral head gastrocnemius m.
- Popliteus muscle
- Soleus muscle

Bottom image labels:
- Biceps femoris muscle
- Vastus medialis m.
- Rectus femoris muscle
- Tibial nerve
- Common peroneal nerve
- Medial patella
- Inferior patellar t./medial retinaculum
- Transverse ligament
- Root anterior horn lateral meniscus
- Plantaris muscle
- Posterior horn lateral meniscus
- Lateral gastrocnemius muscle
- Popliteus m. & t.
- Soleus muscle

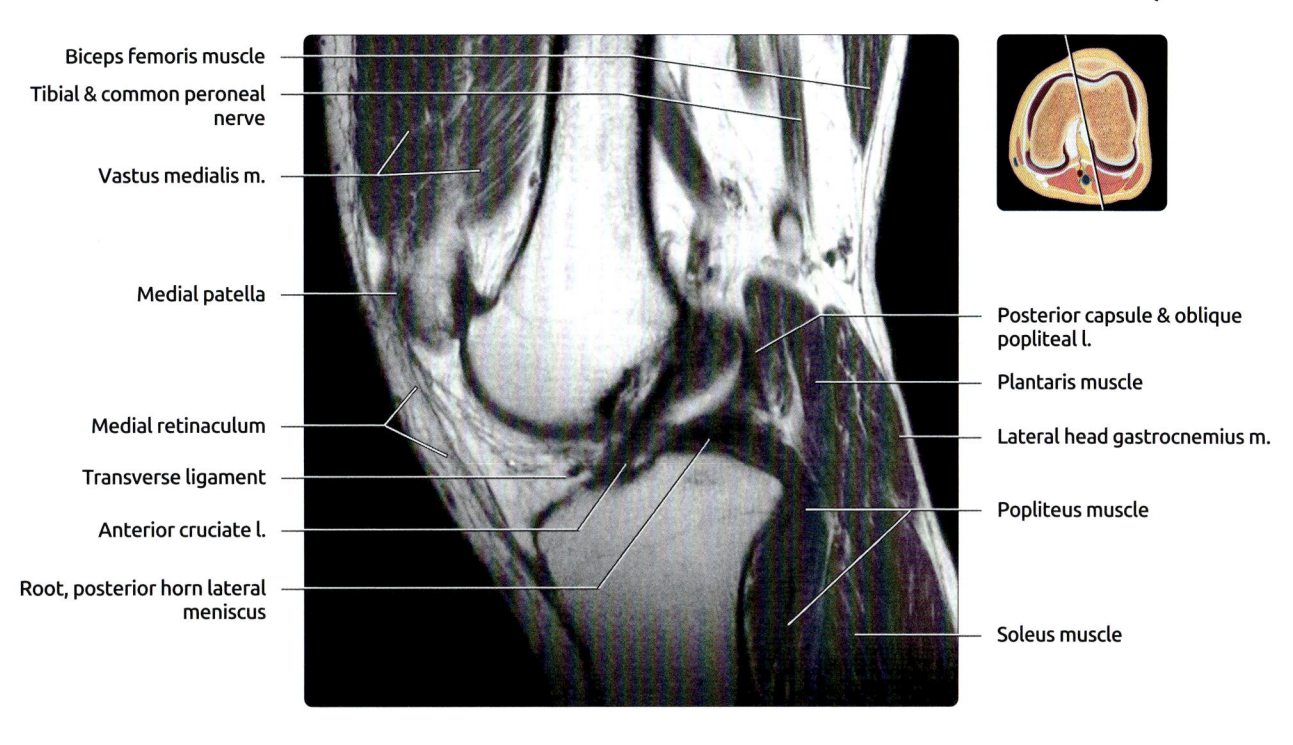

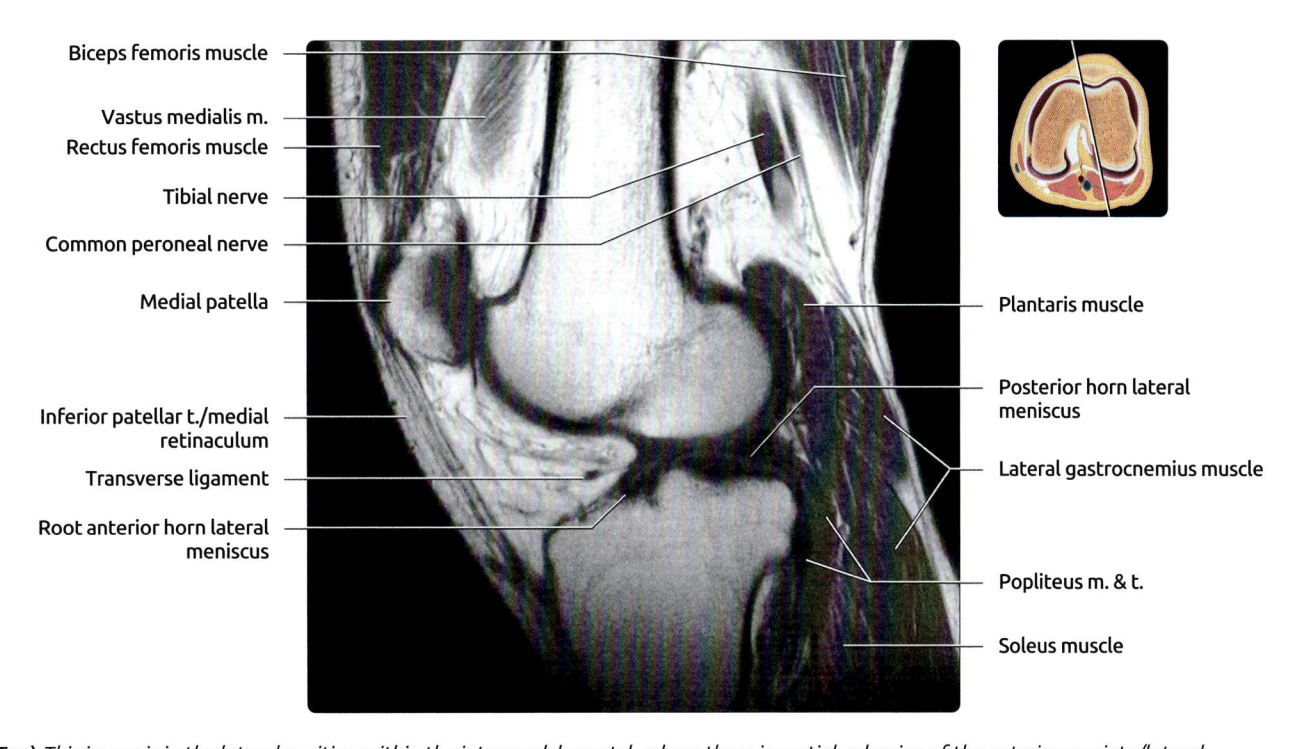

(**Top**) *This image is in the lateral position within the intercondylar notch where there is partial voluming of the anterior cruciate/lateral femoral condyle at the ACL insertion. Note the transverse ligament, seen in cross section, extending across in front of the anterior cruciate ligament towards the root of the anterior horn lateral meniscus. The anterior horn is not yet seen.* (**Bottom**) *This cut shows the beginning of the lateral compartment, immediately adjacent to the intercondylar notch. Note the musculotendinous junction of the popliteus.*

Knee MR Atlas

SAGITTAL T1 MR, KNEE

Top image labels (left):
- Quadriceps tendon
- Inferior patellar t.
- Transverse ligament
- Infrapatellar (Hoffa) fat pad
- Root anterior horn lateral meniscus

Top image labels (right):
- Rectus femoris muscle
- Biceps femoris muscle
- Common peroneal n.
- Plantaris muscle
- Lateral gastrocnemius muscle
- Arcuate popliteal ligament & capsule
- Posterior horn lateral meniscus
- Popliteus m. & t.
- Soleus muscle

Bottom image labels (left):
- Vastus intermedius t.
- Infrapatellar (Hoffa) fat pad
- Inferior patellar t.
- Transverse ligament
- Anterior horn lateral meniscus

Bottom image labels (right):
- Rectus femoris muscle
- Rectus femoris tendon
- Vastus medialis & lateralis tendon
- Biceps femoris muscle
- Common peroneal n.
- Plantaris muscle
- Arcuate popliteal ligament & capsule
- Lateral head gastrocnemius m.
- Popliteus tendon
- Posterior horn lateral meniscus
- Soleus muscle
- Extensor digitorum longus muscle

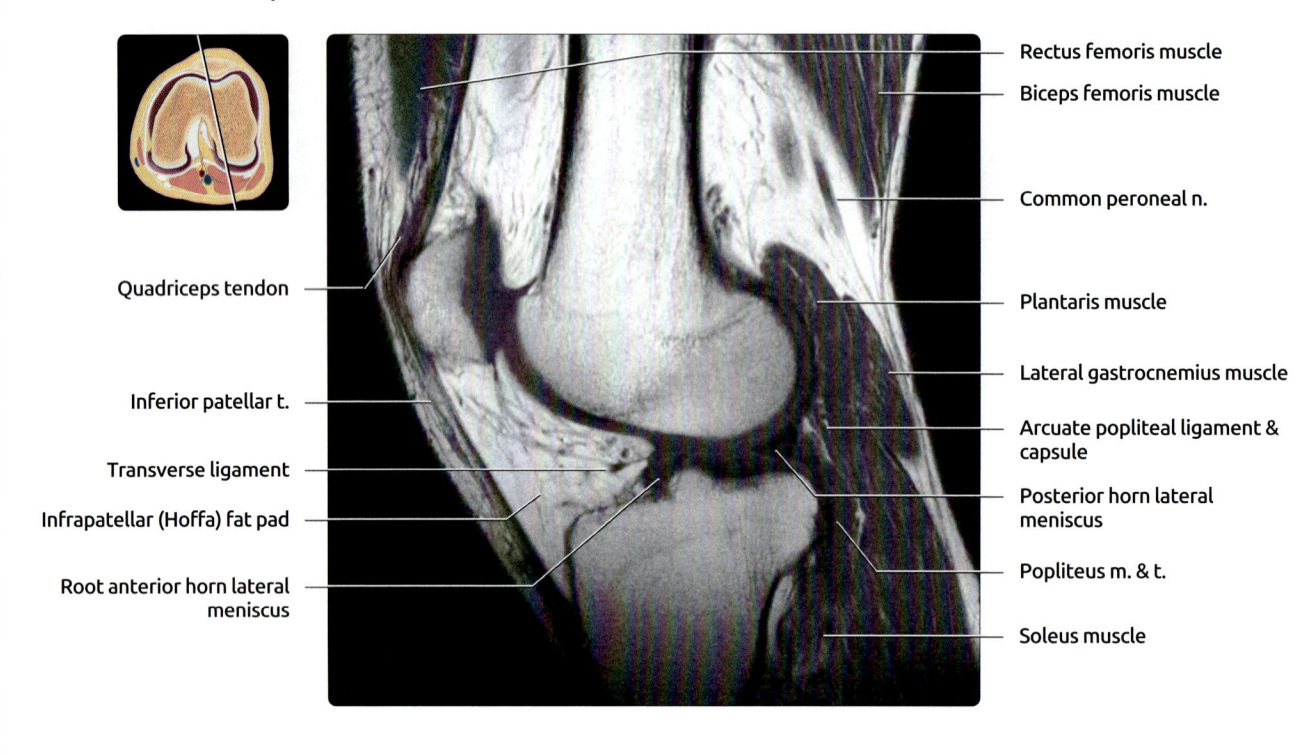

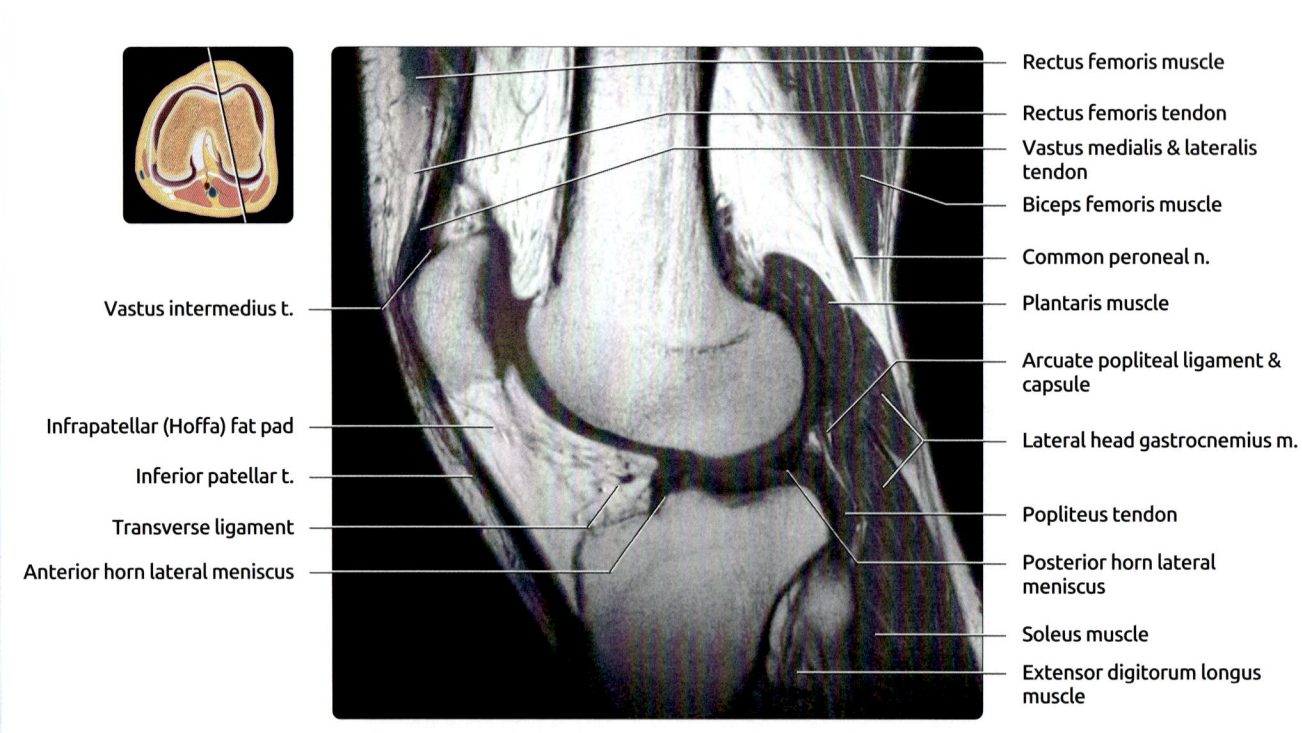

(**Top**) *The lateral compartment is shown. Note the path of the common peroneal nerve, anteromedial to the bulk of the biceps femoris muscle. The plantaris muscle is seen, arising on the lateral femoral condyle, just medial to the lateral head of gastrocnemius.* (**Bottom**) *Because of the obliquity with which sagittal images are obtained, the extensor complex is seen in the more lateral sagittal images. The trilaminate nature of the quadriceps tendon is demonstrated here. The transverse ligament has not yet contacted the anterior horn lateral meniscus. Note the popliteus tendon. Although it is within the popliteal hiatus, it is difficult to distinguish from fluid in the hiatus as well as the lateral meniscus. This region is better imaged with fluid-sensitive sequences.*

Knee MR Atlas

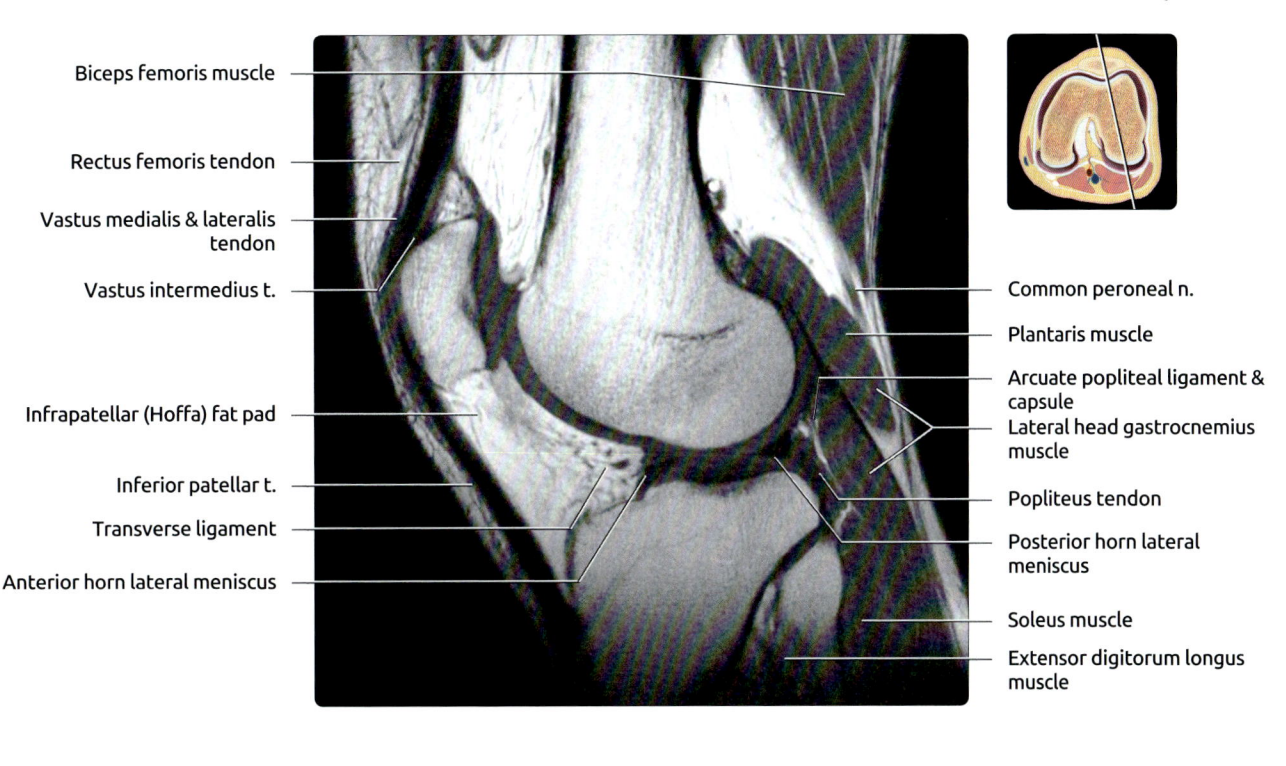

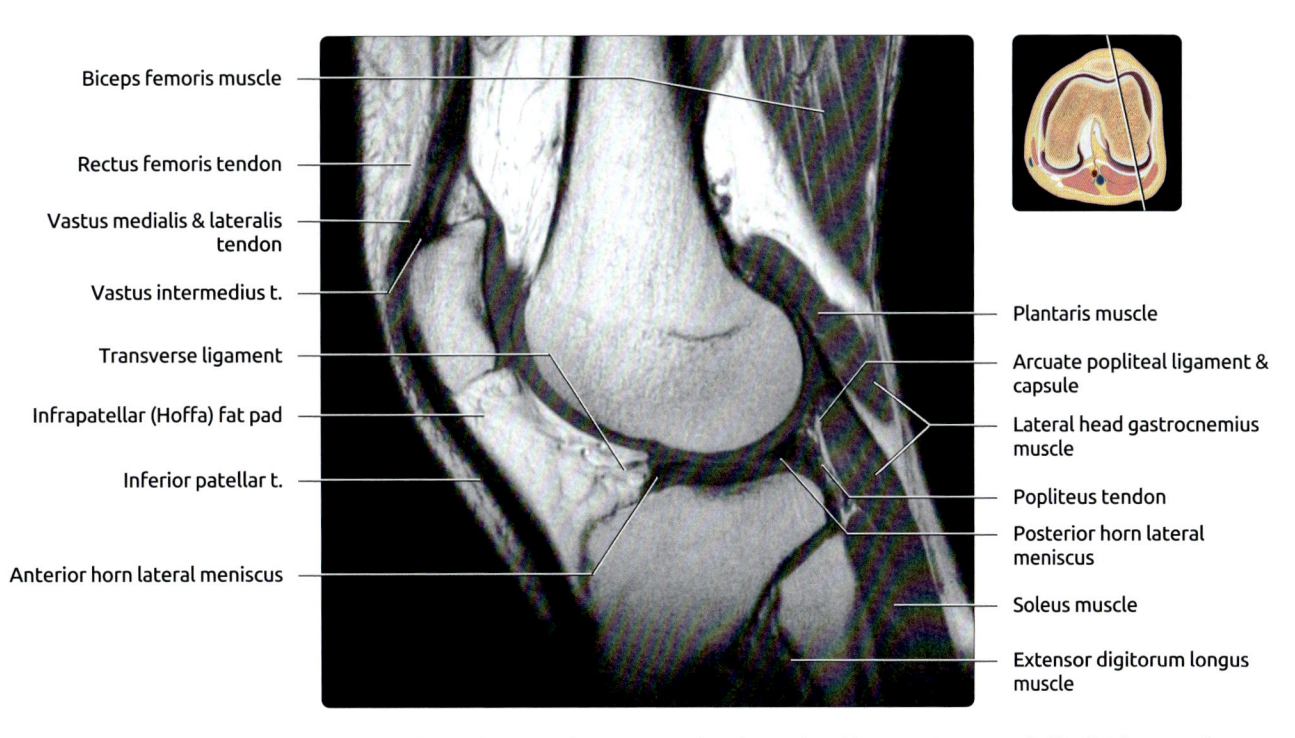

SAGITTAL T1 MR, KNEE

Top image labels:
- Biceps femoris muscle
- Rectus femoris tendon
- Vastus medialis & lateralis tendon
- Vastus intermedius t.
- Infrapatellar (Hoffa) fat pad
- Inferior patellar t.
- Transverse ligament
- Anterior horn lateral meniscus
- Common peroneal n.
- Plantaris muscle
- Arcuate popliteal ligament & capsule
- Lateral head gastrocnemius muscle
- Popliteus tendon
- Posterior horn lateral meniscus
- Soleus muscle
- Extensor digitorum longus muscle

Bottom image labels:
- Biceps femoris muscle
- Rectus femoris tendon
- Vastus medialis & lateralis tendon
- Vastus intermedius t.
- Transverse ligament
- Infrapatellar (Hoffa) fat pad
- Inferior patellar t.
- Anterior horn lateral meniscus
- Plantaris muscle
- Arcuate popliteal ligament & capsule
- Lateral head gastrocnemius muscle
- Popliteus tendon
- Posterior horn lateral meniscus
- Soleus muscle
- Extensor digitorum longus muscle

(Top) *In the lateral portion of the knee joint, the popliteus tendon is seen within the popliteal hiatus. It is surrounded by fluid, not easily distinguished on a T1 sequence. Similarly, the fascicles (or popliteomeniscal ligaments) connecting the posterior horn lateral meniscus with popliteus tendon are not easily seen as separate structures.* **(Bottom)** *As shown here, the transverse ligament approaches its insertion site on the anterior horn lateral meniscus. The muscles arising from the anterior fibula and anterolateral tibia are seen but not easily distinguished from one another.*

Knee MR Atlas

SAGITTAL T1 MR, KNEE

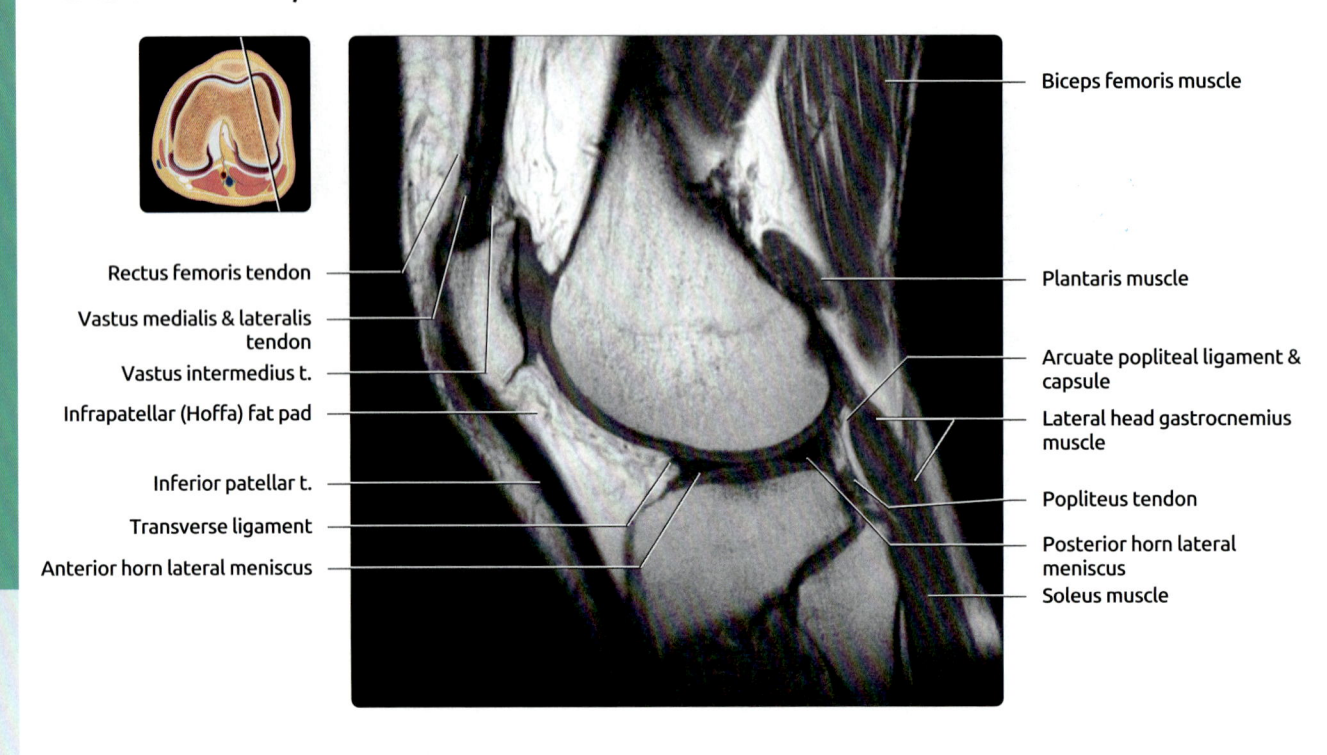

Labels (top image):
- Rectus femoris tendon
- Vastus medialis & lateralis tendon
- Vastus intermedius t.
- Infrapatellar (Hoffa) fat pad
- Inferior patellar t.
- Transverse ligament
- Anterior horn lateral meniscus
- Biceps femoris muscle
- Plantaris muscle
- Arcuate popliteal ligament & capsule
- Lateral head gastrocnemius muscle
- Popliteus tendon
- Posterior horn lateral meniscus
- Soleus muscle

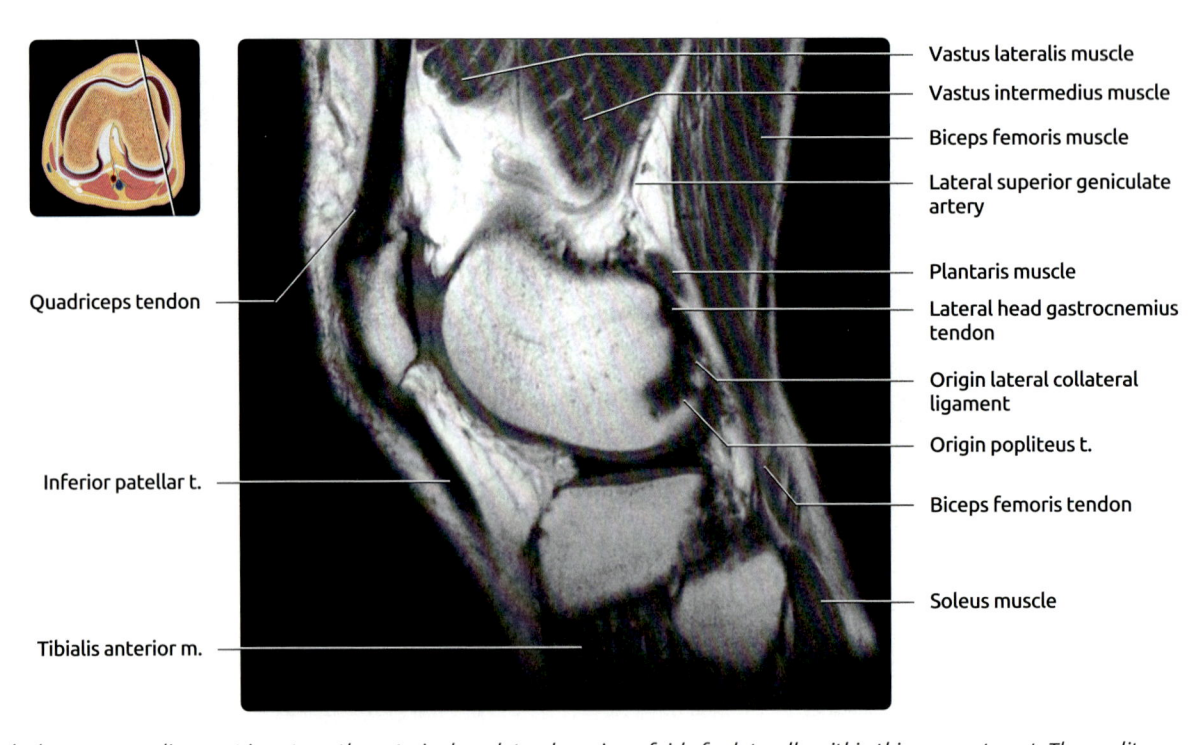

Labels (bottom image):
- Quadriceps tendon
- Inferior patellar t.
- Tibialis anterior m.
- Vastus lateralis muscle
- Vastus intermedius muscle
- Biceps femoris muscle
- Lateral superior geniculate artery
- Plantaris muscle
- Lateral head gastrocnemius tendon
- Origin lateral collateral ligament
- Origin popliteus t.
- Biceps femoris tendon
- Soleus muscle

(Top) The transverse ligament inserts on the anterior horn lateral meniscus fairly far laterally within this compartment. The popliteus tendon just enters the popliteal hiatus at this posterolateral corner. **(Bottom)** At the lateral aspect of the lateral femoral condyle, one sees the origin of the lateral head of the gastrocnemius from the lateral femoral epicondyle as well as the lateral collateral ligament and the popliteal tendon.

Knee MR Atlas

SAGITTAL T1 MR, KNEE

Top image labels:
- Biceps femoris muscle
- Vastus lateralis m.
- Lateral superior geniculate artery
- Quadriceps tendon
- "Bow tie" lateral meniscus
- Lateral head gastrocnemius muscle
- Popliteal tendon
- Lateral collateral l.
- Biceps femoris tendon

Bottom image labels:
- Vastus lateralis m.
- Quadriceps tendon
- Lateral retinaculum
- Gerdy tubercle (iliotibial tract insertion)
- Tibialis anterior m.
- Iliotibial tract
- Lateral collateral l.
- Biceps femoris t.
- Head of fibula
- Peroneus longus m.

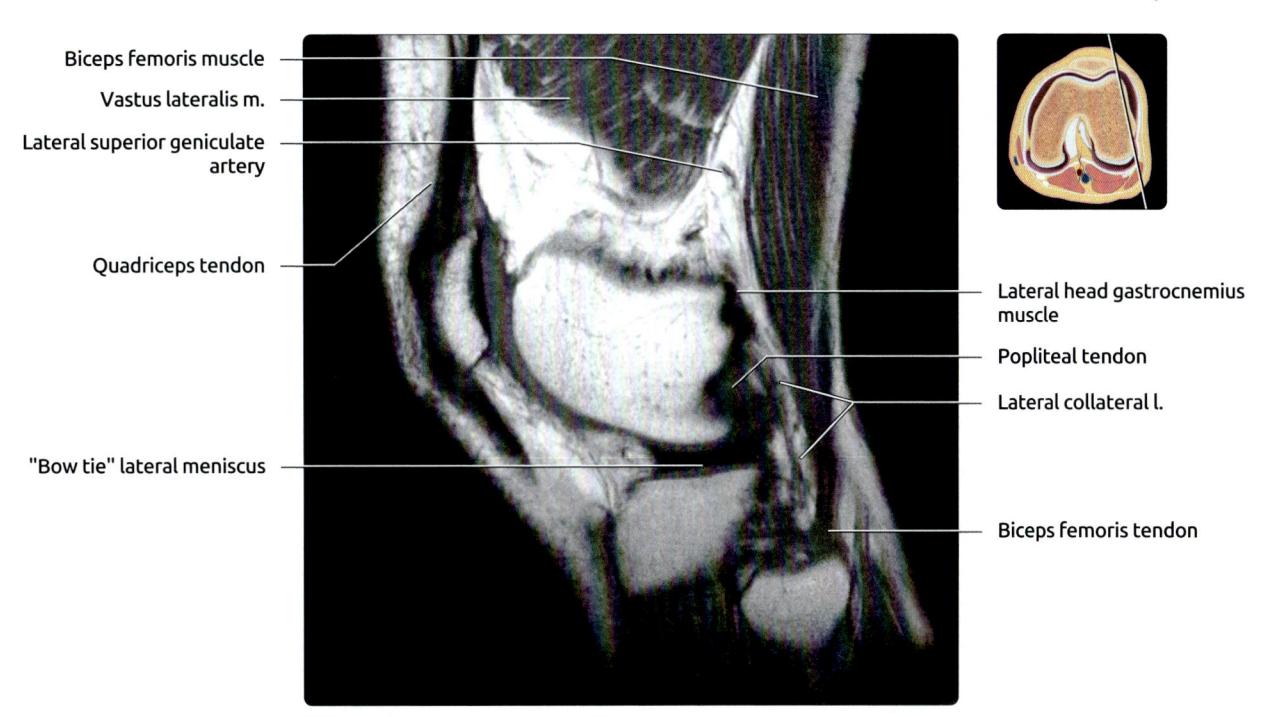

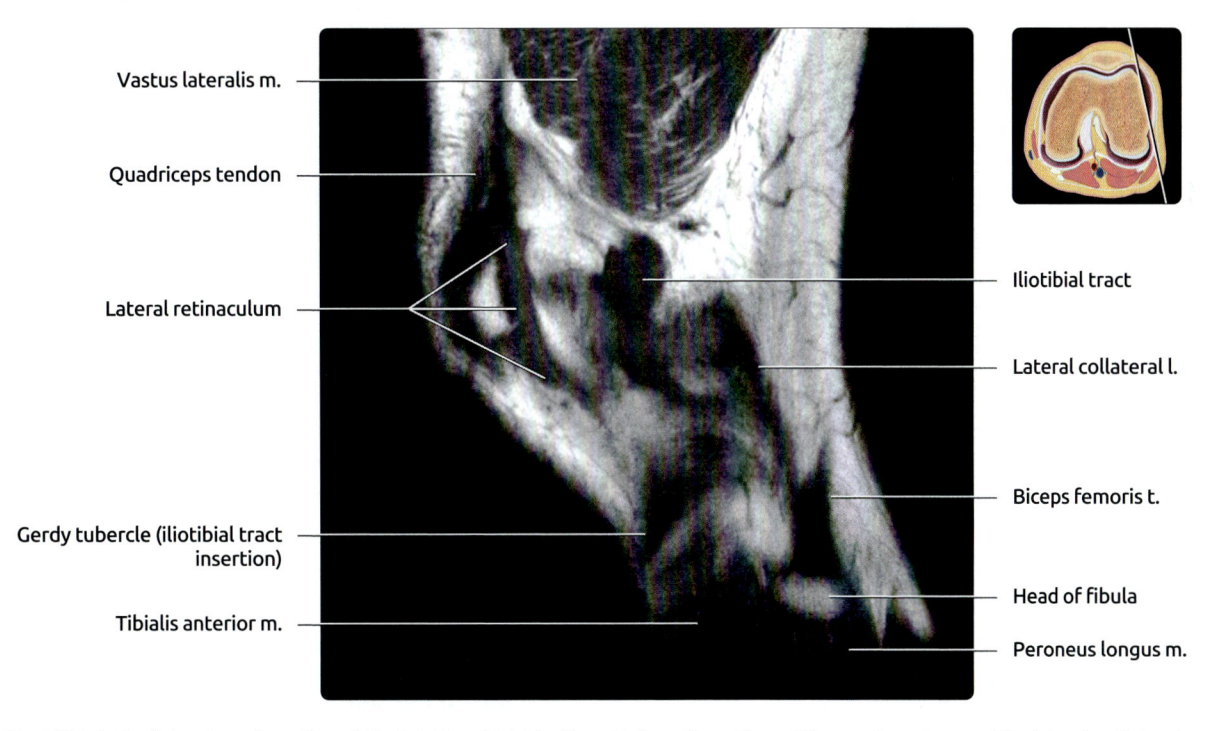

(Top) This is the lateral-most portion of the joint in which the "bow tie" configuration of the meniscus is seen. The lateral collateral ligament is also seen extending posteroinferiorly towards its insertion on the fibular head, adjacent to the insertion of the biceps femoris tendon. (Bottom) Far lateral in the knee, the lateral collateral ligament and biceps femoris tendon insert adjacent to one another on the head of the fibula. Only portions of other lateral stabilizing structures (iliotibial tract, lateral retinaculum) are seen on this image.

Knee MR Atlas

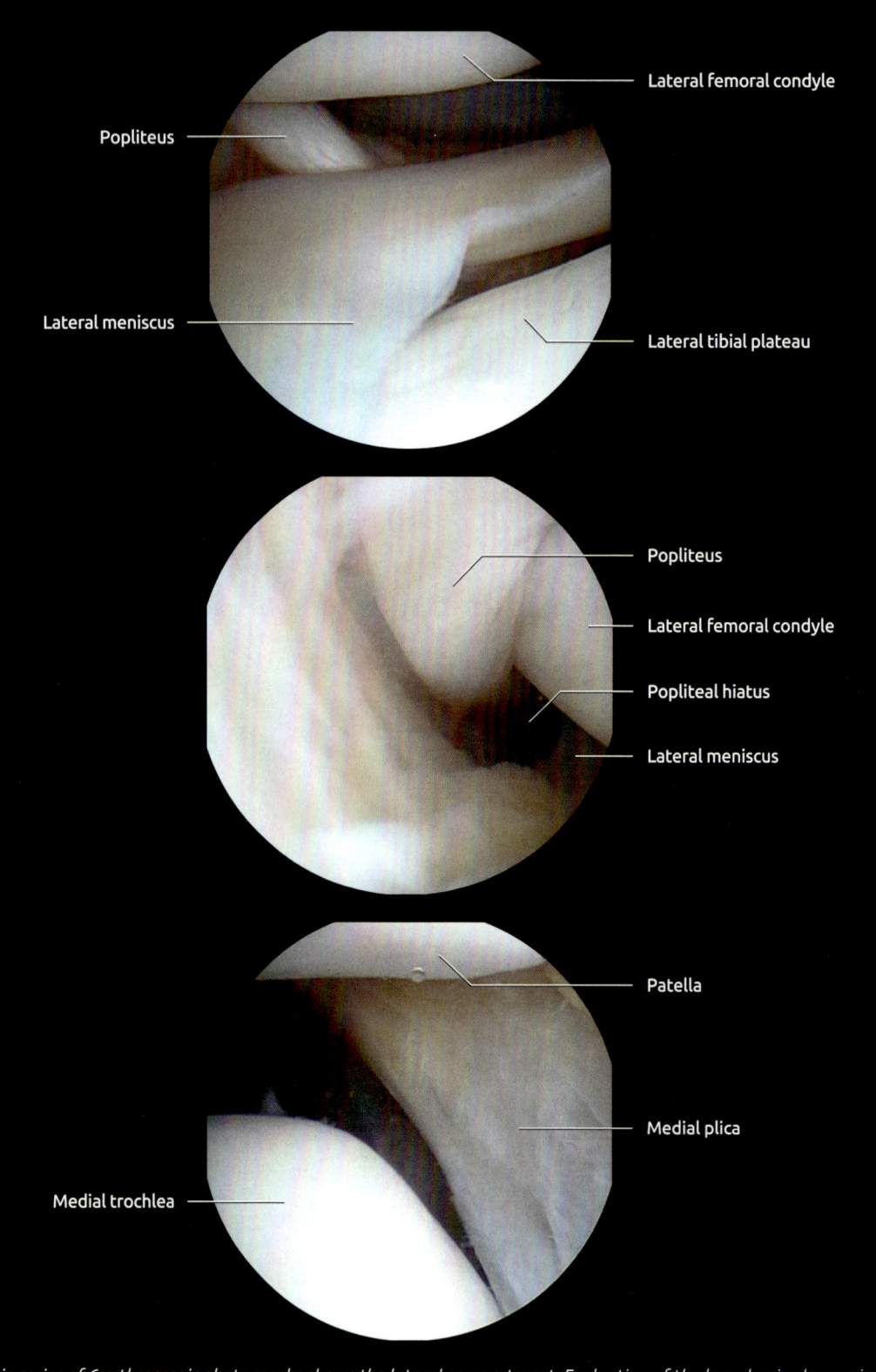

ARTHROSCOPIC PHOTOGRAPHS

Lateral femoral condyle
Popliteus
Lateral meniscus
Lateral tibial plateau

Popliteus
Lateral femoral condyle
Popliteal hiatus
Lateral meniscus

Patella
Medial plica
Medial trochlea

(Top) The 1st in series of 6 arthroscopic photographs shows the lateral compartment. Evaluation of the knee begins by moving the arthroscope into the lateral recess and performing a sweep of the lateral gutter down to the popliteal hiatus. (Middle) Arthroscopic photo of the lateral gutter is shown. The superior and inferior fascicles of the lateral meniscus are viewed from the popliteal hiatus. (Bottom) After evaluating the lateral recess, the arthroscope is moved into the medial recess and proximally into the suprapatellar pouch. A normal suprapatellar plica is seen in 80-90% of knees. The suprapatellar plica may cross the suprapatellar pouch to the lateral sidewall and, rarely, may compartmentalize the suprapatellar pouch. The patellofemoral joint is inspected.

Knee MR Atlas

ARTHROSCOPIC PHOTOGRAPHS

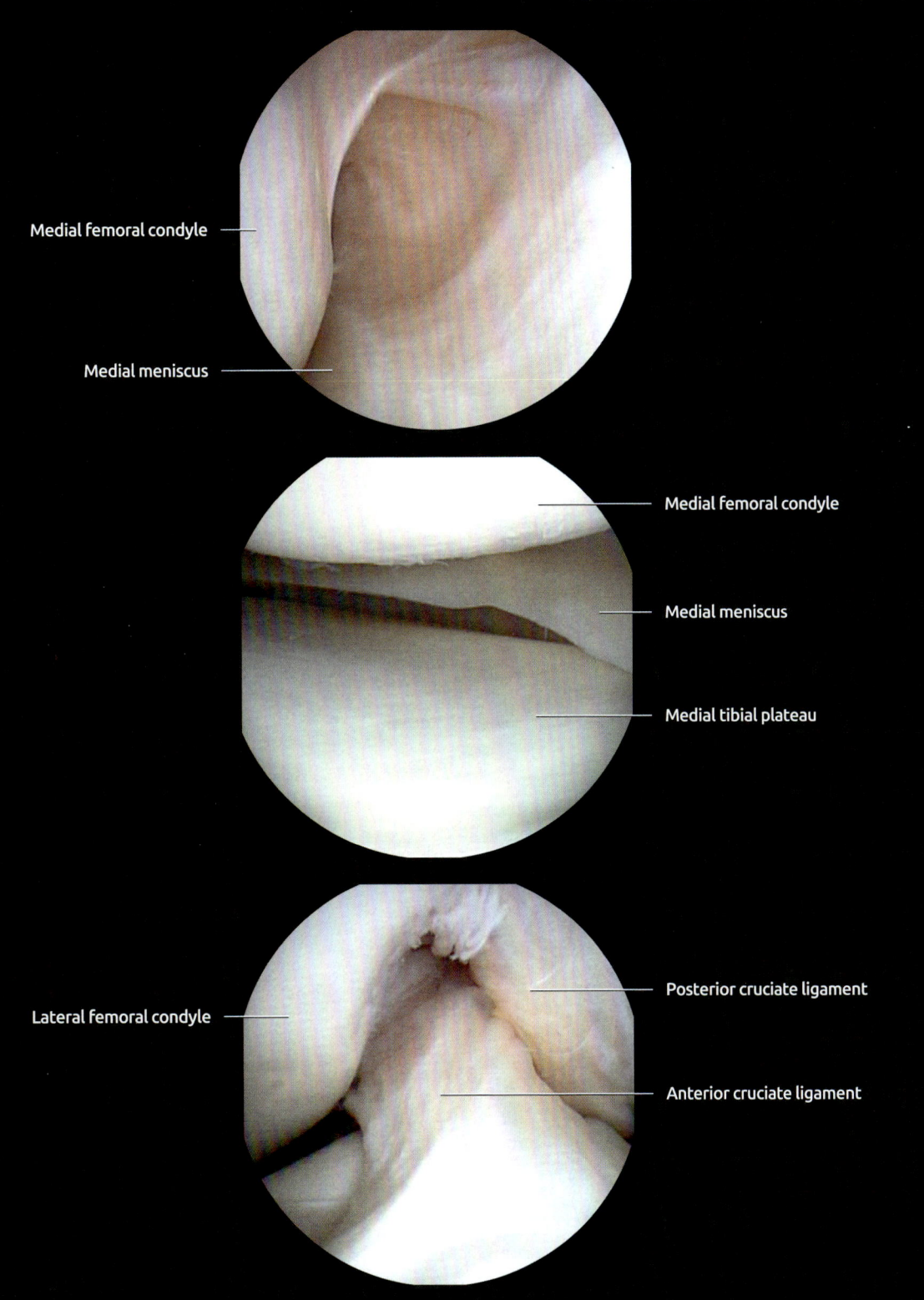

Medial femoral condyle

Medial meniscus

Medial femoral condyle

Medial meniscus

Medial tibial plateau

Lateral femoral condyle

Posterior cruciate ligament

Anterior cruciate ligament

(Top) The arthroscope is then moved to the medial compartment, inspecting the posterior horn and sweeping to the anterior horn. The articular cartilage of the medial femoral condyle and medial tibial plateau is assessed. **(Middle)** The articular cartilage is followed from the medial edge of the intercondylar notch upward and over the ligamentum mucosum, which attaches at the top of the intercondylar notch. The medial meniscus is further evaluated by pulling the anterior horn anteriorly to generate circumferential hoop stresses. **(Bottom)** In this image, the anterior and posterior cruciate ligaments are probed.

Knee MR Atlas

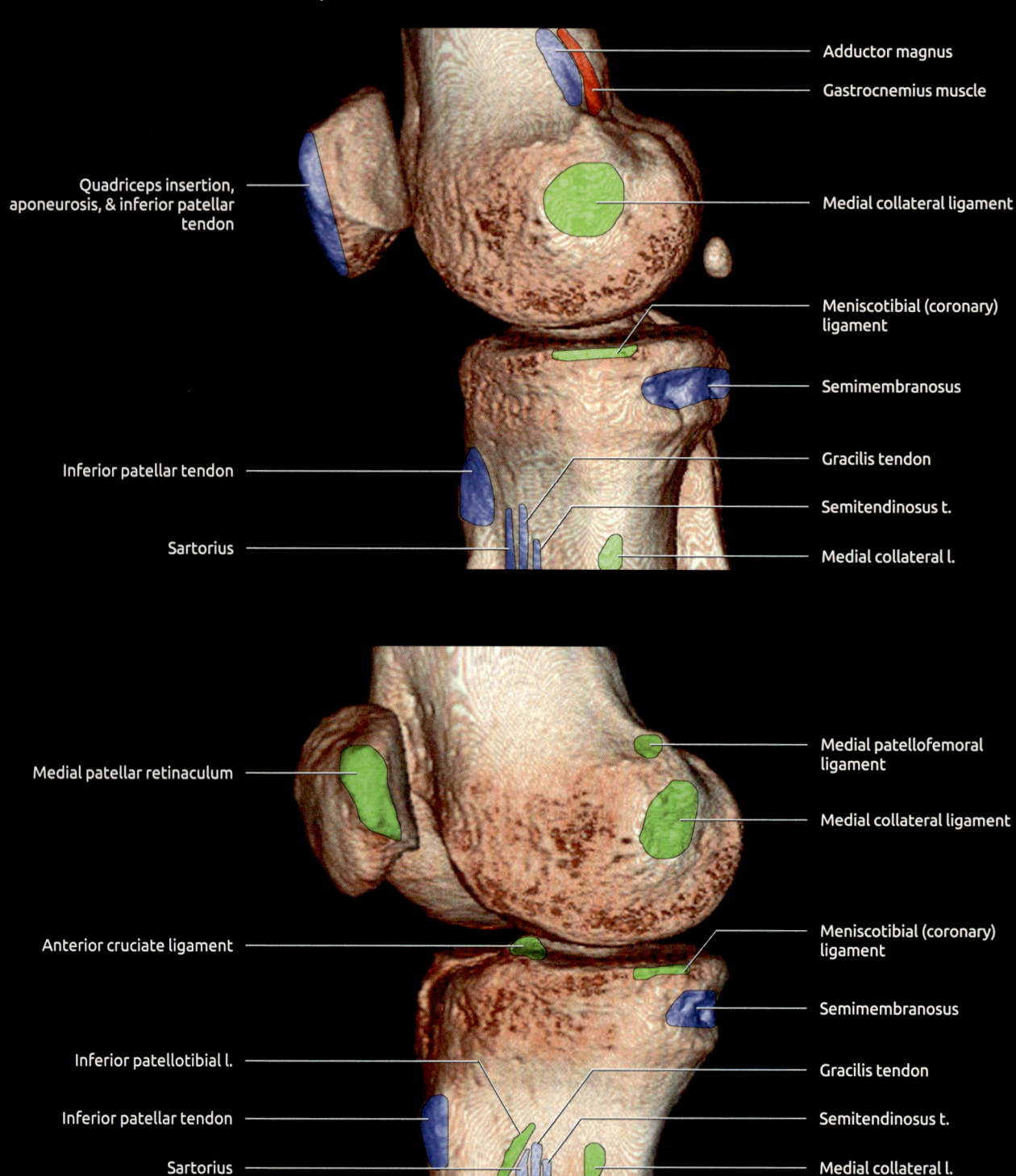

3D RECONSTRUCTION CT, ORIGINS & INSERTIONS

Top labels:
- Adductor magnus
- Gastrocnemius muscle
- Quadriceps insertion, aponeurosis, & inferior patellar tendon
- Medial collateral ligament
- Meniscotibial (coronary) ligament
- Semimembranosus
- Inferior patellar tendon
- Gracilis tendon
- Semitendinosus t.
- Sartorius
- Medial collateral l.

Bottom labels:
- Medial patellofemoral ligament
- Medial patellar retinaculum
- Medial collateral ligament
- Anterior cruciate ligament
- Meniscotibial (coronary) ligament
- Semimembranosus
- Inferior patellotibial l.
- Gracilis tendon
- Inferior patellar tendon
- Semitendinosus t.
- Sartorius
- Medial collateral l.

(**Top**) *This is the 1st of 8 volume-rendered topographic CT images. This image shows the medial aspect of the knee, with associated muscle, tendon, and ligament origins/insertions.* (**Bottom**) *This image of the anteromedial knee shows medial stabilizers of the knee (primarily medial collateral ligament, superficial and deep fibers, secondarily pes anserinus), as well as medial stabilizers of the patella (superiorly, medial patellofemoral ligament, mid medial retinaculum, inferiorly, patellotibial ligament).*

Knee MR Atlas

3D RECONSTRUCTION CT, ORIGINS & INSERTIONS

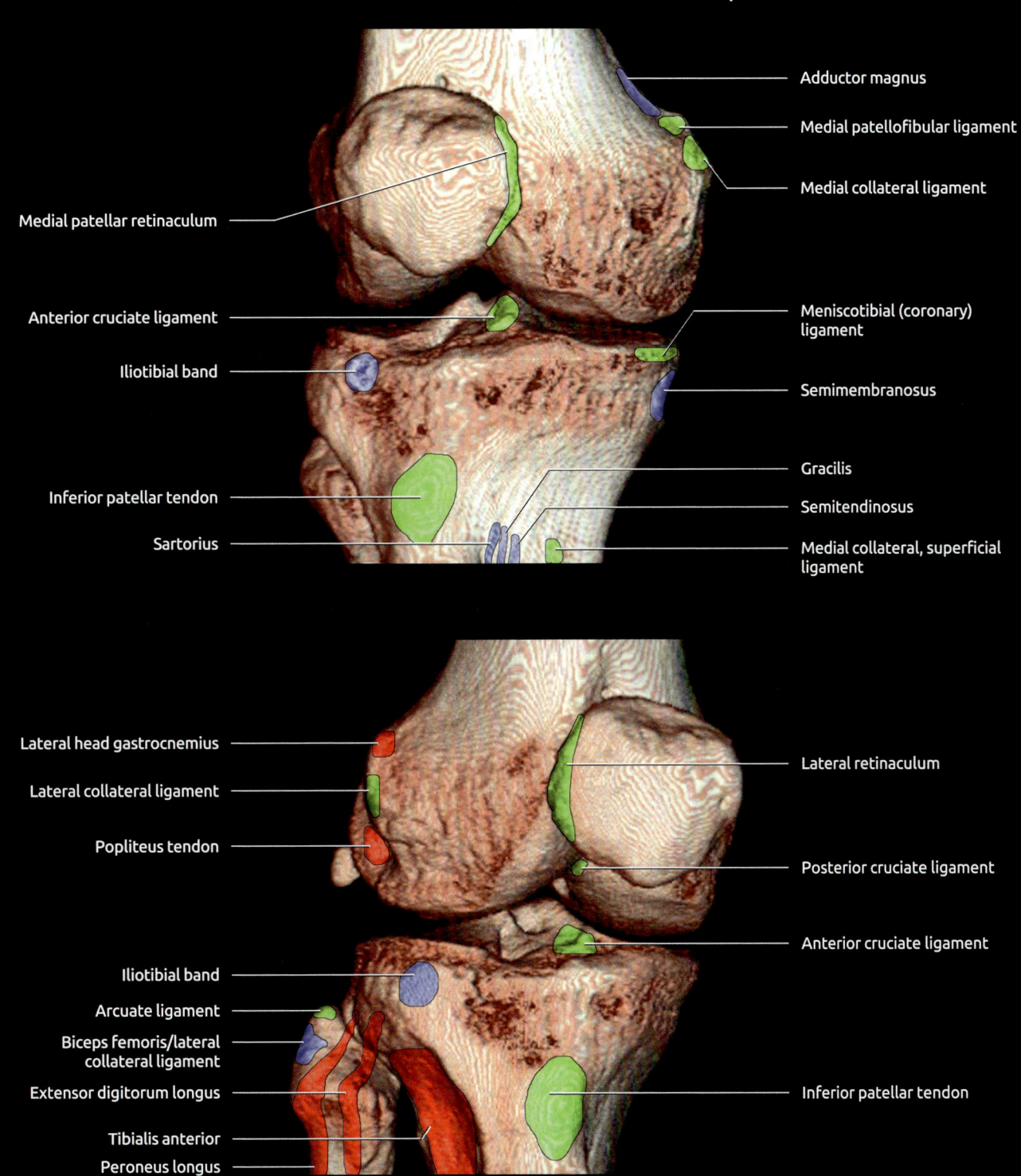

(Top) A slightly anteromedial view shows the medial stabilizers of the knee and patella. Note that only the uppermost portion of the insertions of the pes anserinus (sartorius, gracilis, and semitendinosus) as well as superficial medial collateral ligament are shown; these insertions actually extend several cm distally on the tibia. (Bottom) A slightly anterolateral view shows the lateral stabilizers of the knee and patella. These consist primarily of lateral collateral ligament, arcuate ligament, popliteal tendon, iliotibial band, and biceps femoris. Origins of several leg muscles are seen; the tibialis anterior, extensor digitorum longus, and peroneus longus origins extend several cm distally beyond the regions indicated here.

Knee MR Atlas

3D RECONSTRUCTION CT, ORIGINS & INSERTIONS

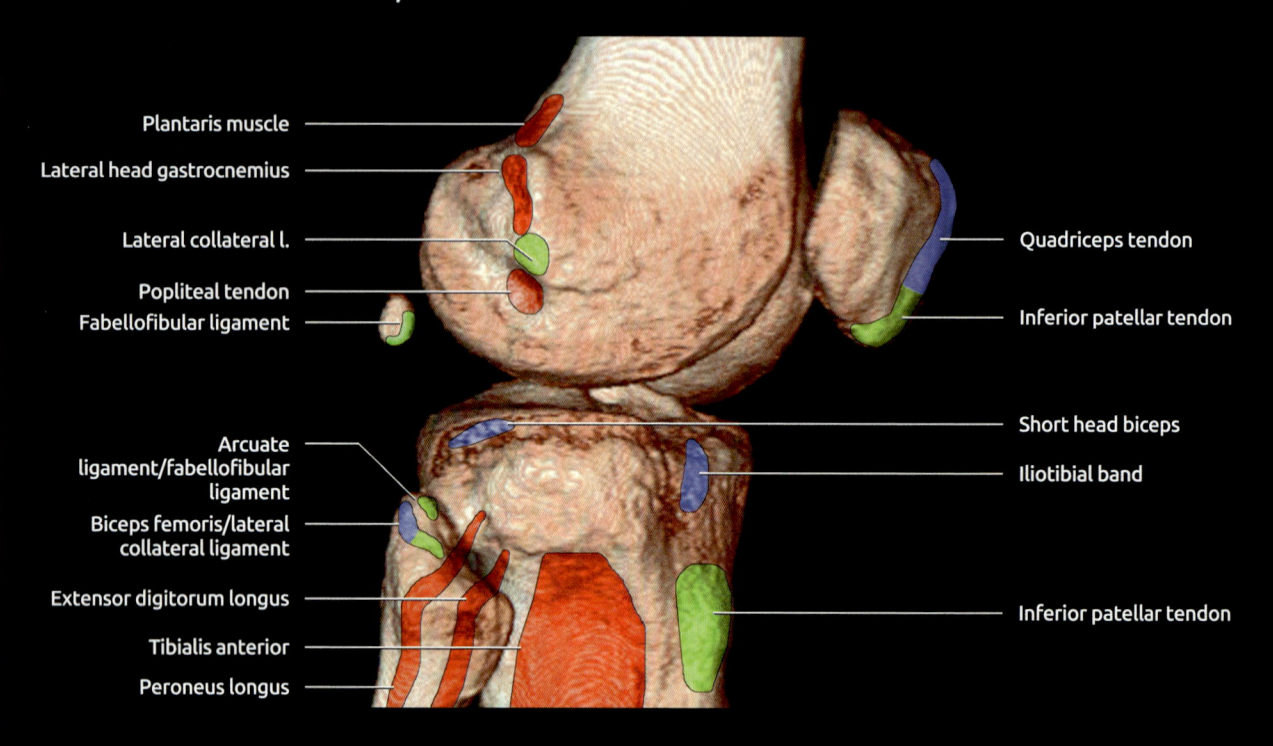

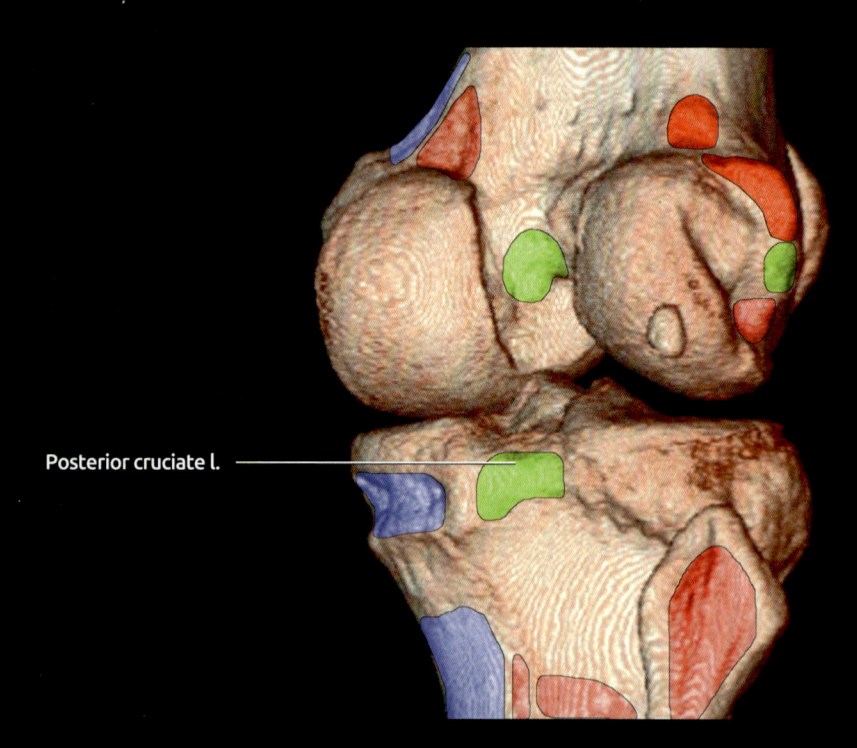

Plantaris muscle
Lateral head gastrocnemius
Lateral collateral l.
Popliteal tendon
Fabellofibular ligament
Arcuate ligament/fabellofibular ligament
Biceps femoris/lateral collateral ligament
Extensor digitorum longus
Tibialis anterior
Peroneus longus

Quadriceps tendon
Inferior patellar tendon
Short head biceps
Iliotibial band
Inferior patellar tendon

Posterior cruciate l.

(Top) A lateral view of the knee shows lateral stabilizing structures. Origins of anterior and lateral leg muscles are seen as well. (Bottom) A posterior (slightly oblique) view of the knee shows the attachments of the posterior structures. Note that the fibular origin of the soleus is more proximal than the tibial origin.

Knee MR Atlas

3D RECONSTRUCTION CT, ORIGINS & INSERTIONS

Adductor magnus
Medial head gastrocnemius
Medial collateral l.
Posterior cruciate l.
Semimembranosus
Soleus
Popliteus

Plantaris muscle
Lateral head gastrocnemius
Lateral collateral ligament
Popliteus
Soleus
Tibialis posterior

Medial head gastrocnemius
Adductor magnus
Medial patellofemoral ligament
Medial collateral l.
Meniscotibial (coronary) ligament
Semimembranosus
Popliteus

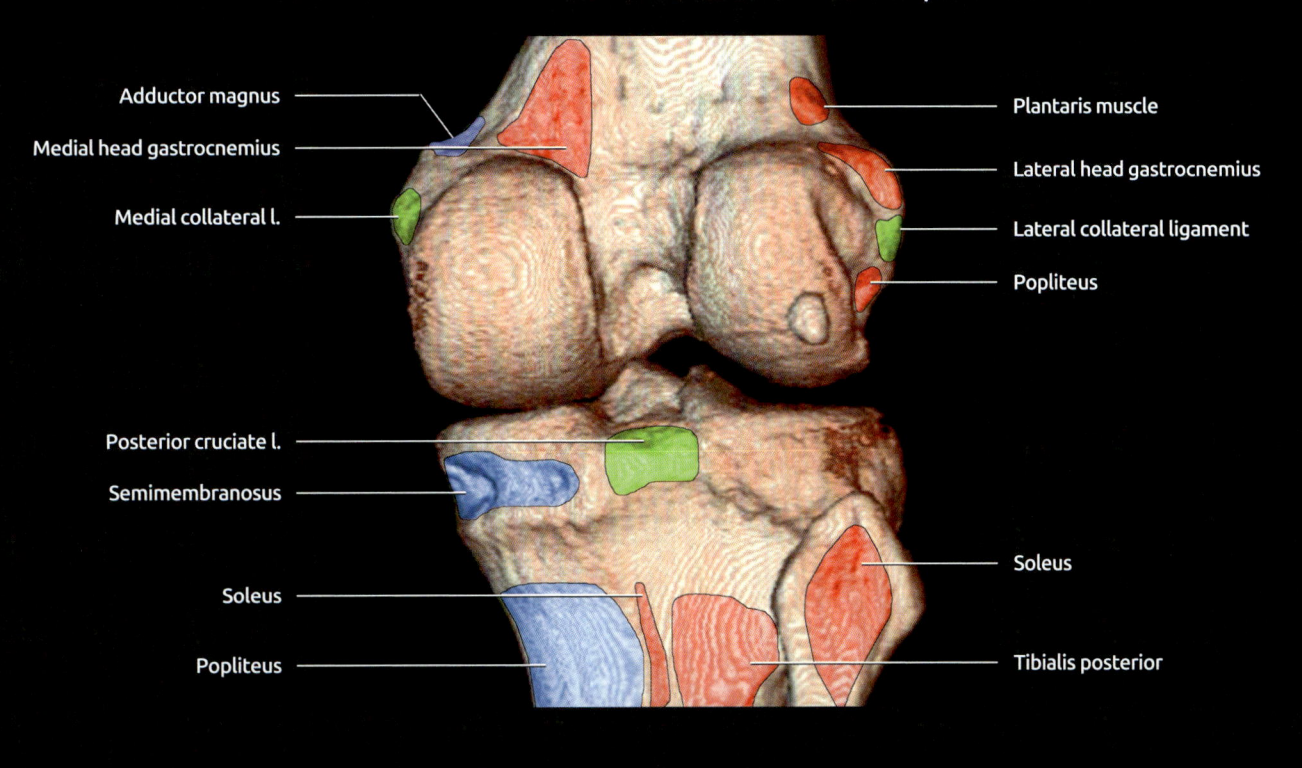

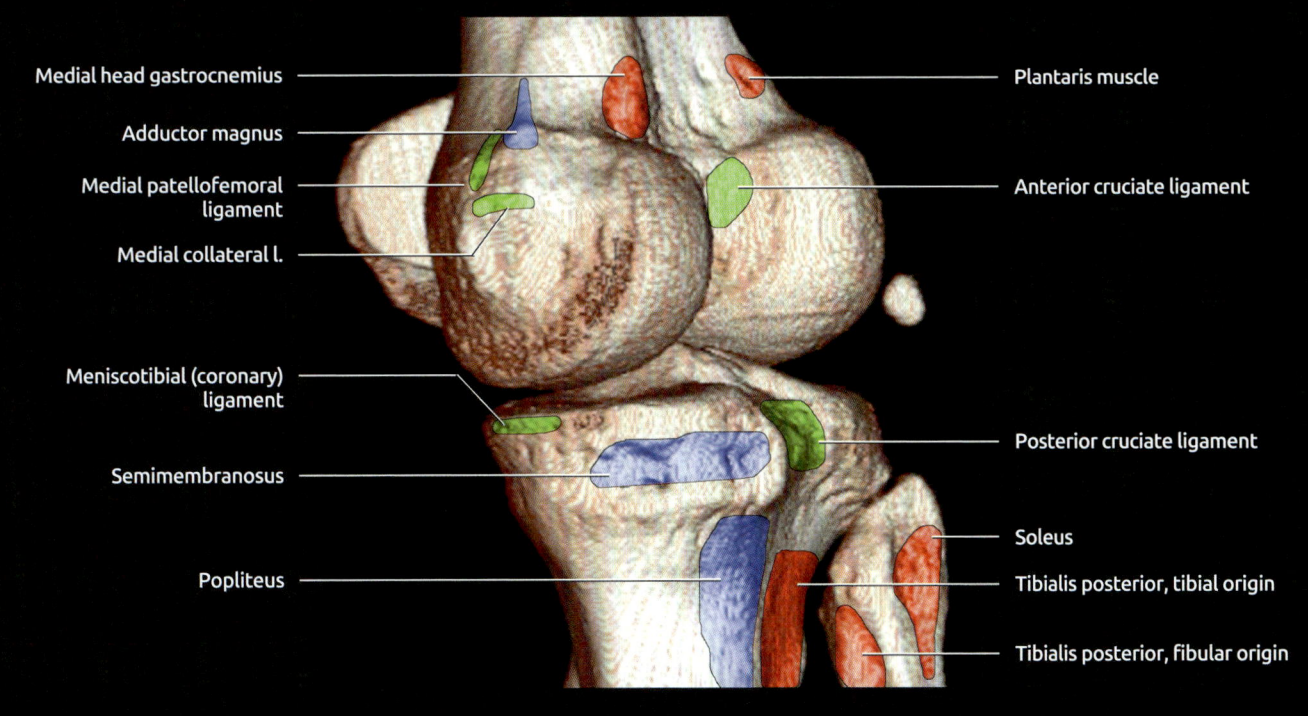

Plantaris muscle
Anterior cruciate ligament
Posterior cruciate ligament
Soleus
Tibialis posterior, tibial origin
Tibialis posterior, fibular origin

(Top) *In this direct posterior view, note that PCL insertion is extraarticular on the posterior central tibia.* (Bottom) *On this posterior (oblique to medial) view, note the extensive insertions of both the semimembranosus tendon and popliteus vein on the posteromedial tibia.*

Knee Extensor Mechanism and Retinacula

IMAGING ANATOMY

Overview
- Extensor mechanism: Quadriceps muscle and tendon, patella, patellar tendon, and patellar retinacula

Quadriceps
- **Muscles**: Rectus femoris, vastus lateralis, vastus medialis, vastus intermedius
- **Quadriceps tendon**
  - Trilaminar configuration (generally): Fascia of component muscles with interposed fat
    - Superficial (anterior on sagittal): Rectus femoris
    - Middle: Vastus lateralis and vastus medialis
    - Deep (posterior on sagittal): Vastus intermedius
  - May appear as 2 or 4 layers: Medial and lateral components of middle layer merge in different combinations or remain discrete
  - Tendon inserts on nonarticular (anterior) patella

Patellar Tendon
- Mainly composed of rectus femoris fibers that course over patella forming the prepatellar quadriceps seam of fibrocartilage connecting to inferior patellar tendon
- Extends from inferior pole of patella to tibial tuberosity
- Length ~ 5 cm
  - Length about equal to height of patella
  - Variation by > 20% of craniocaudal length of patella results in patella alta or baja
- 3 cm wide superiorly to 2 cm inferiorly; 5-6 mm thick

Medial Retinaculum Complex
- Medial stabilizer of patellofemoral joint
- Extends from patella to vastus medialis
- Medial retinacular complex divided into superior, mid, and inferior portions that blend into one another
  - **Superior: Vastus medialis obliquus (VMO) and medial patellofemoral ligament (MPFL)**
    - VMO: Muscular slip of vastus medialis; arises either from adductor magnus tendon or from adductor tubercle
    - VMO inserts at superior medial border of patella
    - VMO aponeurosis tightly adherent to underlying MPFL
    - MPFL: Arises from adductor tubercle adjacent to MCL origin and inserts at medial border of patella
  - **Midportion**: Thin fibers of superficial MCL fascia
  - **Inferior**
    - Patellotibial ligament arises from tibia at level of insertion of gracilis and semitendinosus and inserts on inferior aspect patella and patellar tendon
    - Medial patellomeniscal ligament lies deep to patellotibial ligament

Lateral Retinaculum
- Lateral stabilizer of patellofemoral joint
- Extends from patella to vastus lateralis
- 3 layers
  - **I (superficial)**: Iliotibial tract (band) and its anterior expansion, supplemented posteriorly by superficial portion of biceps femoris and its anterior expansion
  - **II (mid)**: Retinaculum of quadriceps (vastus lateralis)
  - **III (deep)**: Lateral part of joint capsule

Anterior Fat Pads
- Each interposed between joint capsule externally and synovium-lined joint cavity (intracapsular but extrasynovial)
- Suprapatellar bursa outlined by anterior (quadriceps) and posterior (prefemoral) suprapatellar fat pads
- Infrapatellar (Hoffa fat pad)
  - Bordered by
    - Inferior pole patella (superior)
    - Joint capsule and patellar tendon (anterior)
    - Proximal tibia and deep infrapatellar bursa (inferior)
    - Synovial-lined joint capsule (posterior)
  - Can be tethered posteriorly at apex by infrapatellar plica
  - Attached to anterior horns of menisci inferiorly and to tibial periosteum
  - Transverse ligament courses within fat pad
  - Interface between posterior aspect of fat pad and joint space consists of several synovial recesses
  - Anastomotic vessels course through fat pad, seen in cross section on sagittal images

Plica
- Synovial folds; persistent embryonic remnants
- **Superior** (suprapatellar, superomedial): Common
  - Medial suprapatellar pouch, 2 cm superior to patella
  - Seen as fold or complete septum
  - Runs obliquely downward from synovium at anterior aspect of femoral metaphysis to posterior aspect of quadriceps tendon
  - Inserts above patella; best seen on sagittal
- **Medial** (plica synovialis, patellar shelf, medial intraarticular band)
  - Arises from medial wall of synovial pouch or under medial retinaculum and extends obliquely downward to insert on synovium covering infrapatellar fat pad
  - Inserts on synovium covering infrapatellar fat pad, at medial edge of patella; seen on sagittal or axial
  - If large, can impinge on medial facet of trochlea or under medial facet of patella
- **Inferior** (infrapatellar plica/fold/septum, ligamentum mucosa): Common
  - Extends from Hoffa fat pad in intercondylar notch, paralleling and anterior to ACL; best seen on sagittal
  - May be split or fenestrated; dimensions vary
- **Lateral**: Rare
  - Originates from lateral wall superior to popliteal hiatus and extends to infrapatellar fat pad
  - Oblique coronal orientation; 1-2 cm lateral to patella
- Size and morphologic features of given plica do not reliably indicate whether it is clinically significant

SELECTED REFERENCES
1. Wangwinyuvirat M et al: Prepatellar quadriceps continuation: MRI of cadavers with gross anatomic and histologic correlation. AJR Am J Roentgenol. 192(3):W111-6, 2009

Knee Extensor Mechanism and Retinacula

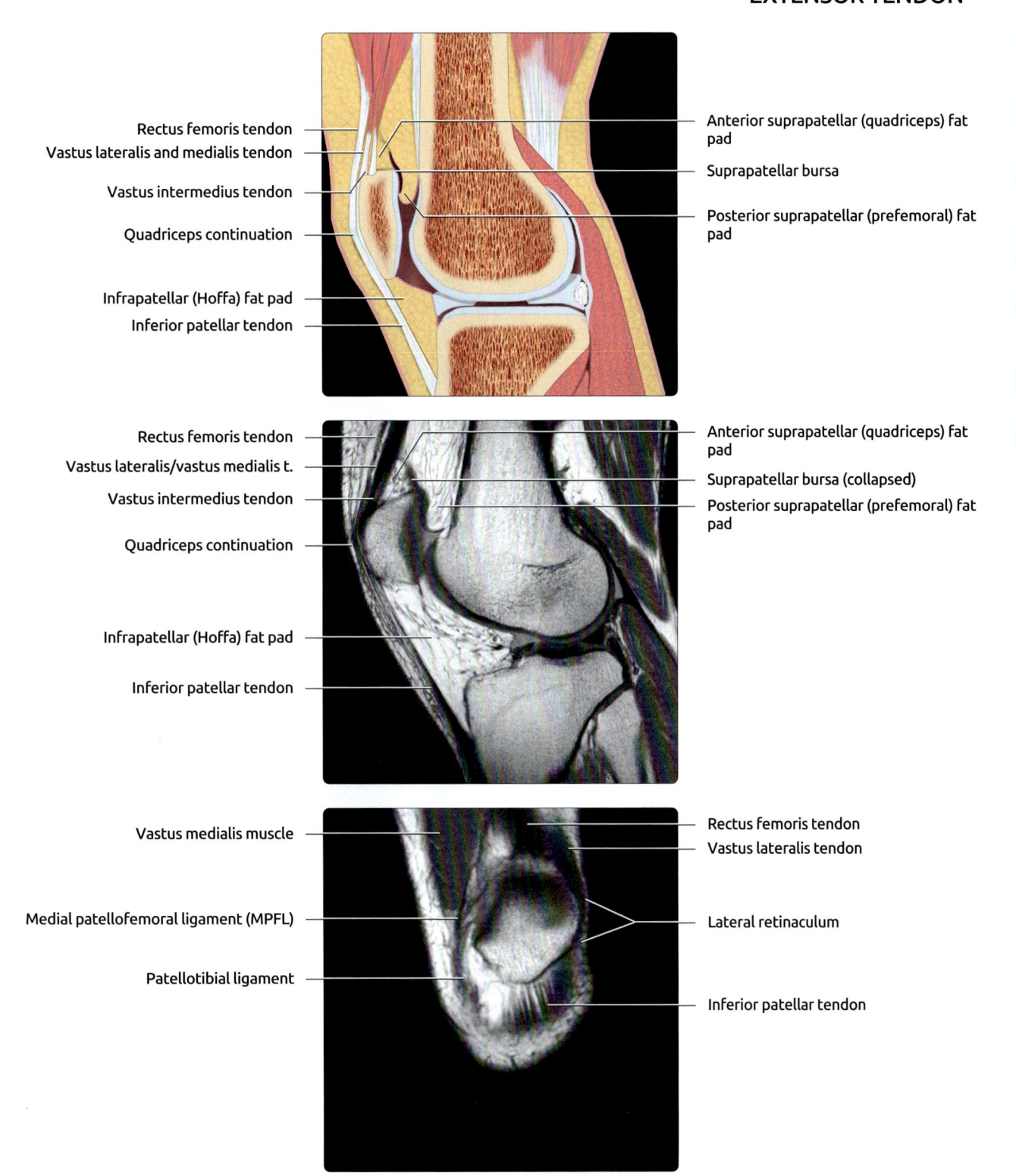

EXTENSOR TENDON

Labels (Top graphic):
- Rectus femoris tendon
- Vastus lateralis and medialis tendon
- Vastus intermedius tendon
- Quadriceps continuation
- Infrapatellar (Hoffa) fat pad
- Inferior patellar tendon
- Anterior suprapatellar (quadriceps) fat pad
- Suprapatellar bursa
- Posterior suprapatellar (prefemoral) fat pad

Labels (Middle MR):
- Rectus femoris tendon
- Vastus lateralis/vastus medialis t.
- Vastus intermedius tendon
- Quadriceps continuation
- Infrapatellar (Hoffa) fat pad
- Inferior patellar tendon
- Anterior suprapatellar (quadriceps) fat pad
- Suprapatellar bursa (collapsed)
- Posterior suprapatellar (prefemoral) fat pad

Labels (Bottom MR):
- Vastus medialis muscle
- Medial patellofemoral ligament (MPFL)
- Patellotibial ligament
- Rectus femoris tendon
- Vastus lateralis tendon
- Lateral retinaculum
- Inferior patellar tendon

(**Top**) *Graphic shows trilaminar configuration of the quadriceps tendon. The superficial portion is rectus femoris, the middle portion is the aponeurosis of vastus medialis and lateralis, and the deep portion is vastus intermedius tendon.* (**Middle**) *Sagittal PD MR shows the trilaminate character of the extensor tendon. The suprapatellar bursa is not distended. The surrounding fat pads are well demonstrated. The infrapatellar fat pad, with anastomosing joint vessels coursing through it, is also seen.* (**Bottom**) *Anterior coronal T1 MR shows components of patellar attachments. The quadriceps and inferior patellar tendons attach superiorly and inferiorly, respectively. The lateral retinaculum attaches along the entire lateral edge of patella. Vastus medialis obliquus (VMO), medial patellofemoral, and inferior patellotibial ligaments contribute to medial retinaculum from superior to inferior.*

Knee Extensor Mechanism and Retinacula

PATELLAR STABILIZERS

Labels (top graphic):
- Vastus medialis m.
- Quadriceps tendon
- Vastus medialis obliquus
- Adductor magnus m.
- Medial patellofemoral ligament
- Adductor tubercle
- Medial patellomeniscal ligament
- Deep fibers medial collateral (coronary) l.
- Patellotibial ligament
- Superficial fibers medial collateral l.
- Inferior patellar tendon

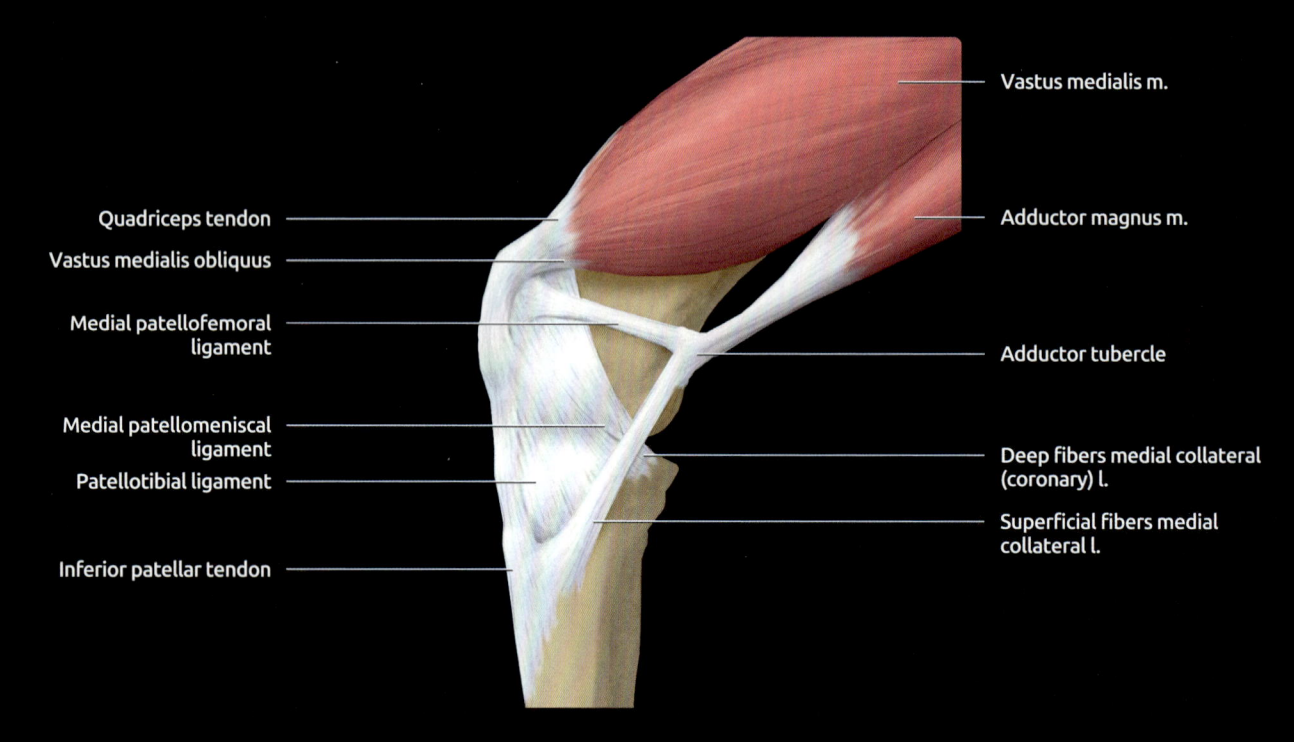

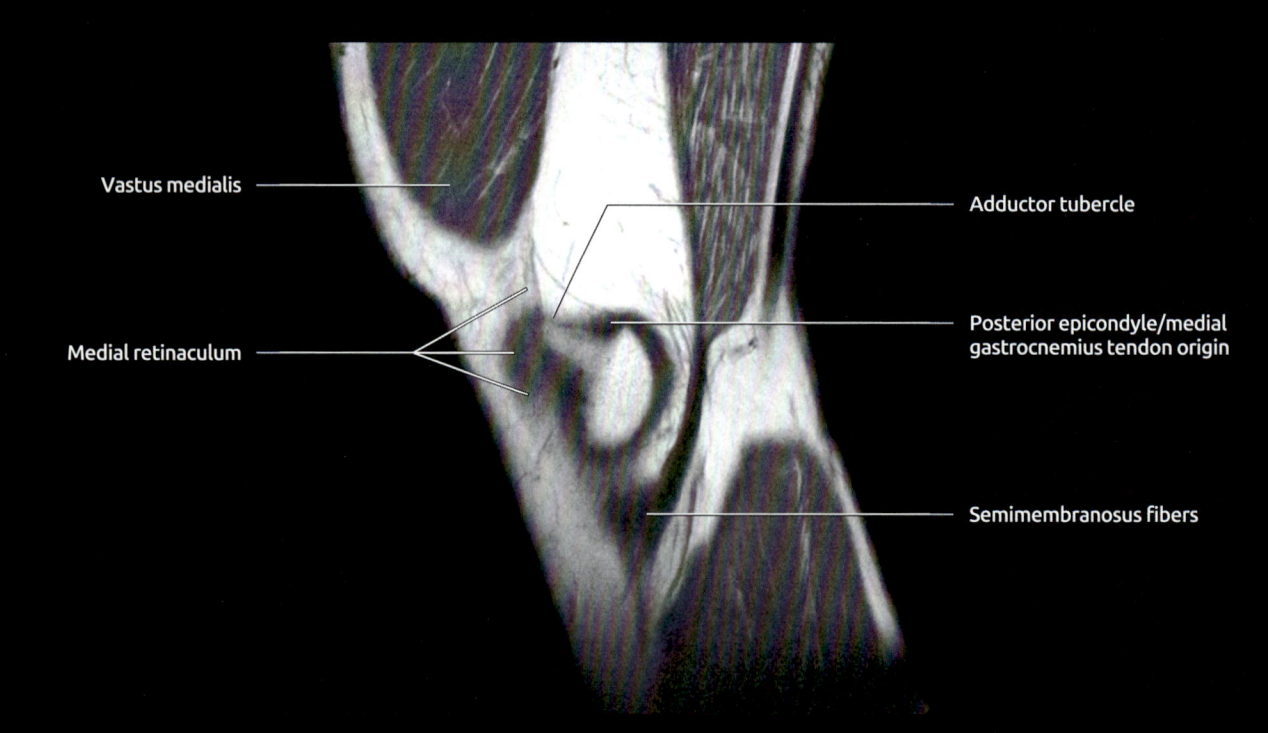

Labels (bottom MR):
- Vastus medialis
- Adductor tubercle
- Posterior epicondyle/medial gastrocnemius tendon origin
- Medial retinaculum
- Semimembranosus fibers

(Top) Graphic shows medial patellar stabilizers. Vastus medialis obliquus arises from adductor magnus tendon. Medial patellofemoral ligament arises from adductor tubercle; both insert along superior 1/3 of medial patella. The patellotibial ligament originates on tibia at the level of insertion of the pes anserinus; it inserts on inferior 2/3 of patella and on patellar tendon. The medial patellomeniscal ligament is deep in relation to patellotibial ligament. Fibers from superficial MCL also contribute to medial retinaculum. (Bottom) Sagittal PD MR shows that the individual components of medial retinaculum are rarely seen in this plane. The semimembranosus contributes thin fibers to superficial MCL, which in turn contributes to medial retinaculum. The fibers labeled medial retinaculum are contributed from VMO, MPFL, patellotibial ligament, and patellomeniscal ligament.

Knee Extensor Mechanism and Retinacula

PATELLAR STABILIZERS

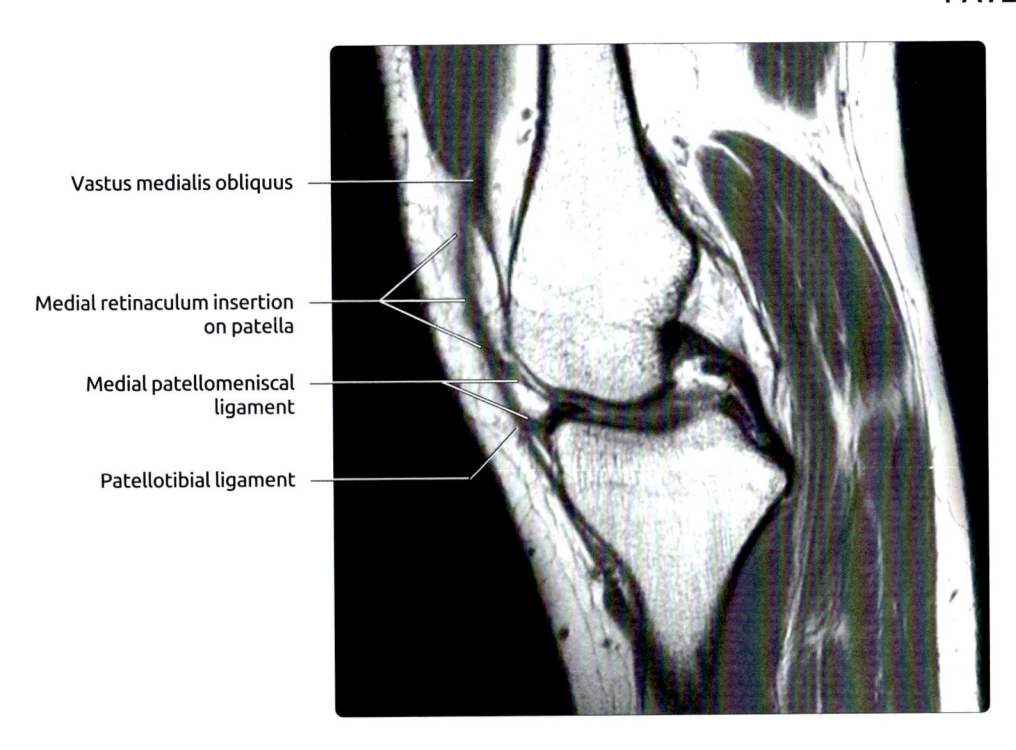

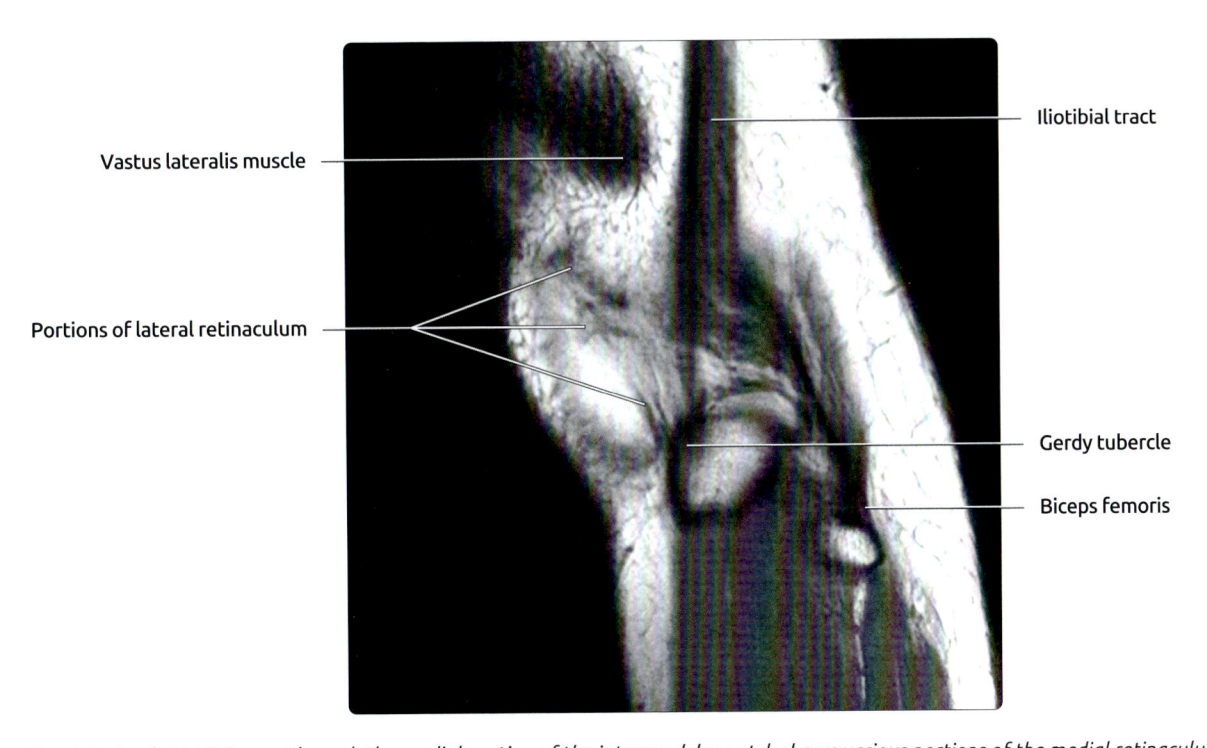

(Top) Sagittal PD MR image through the medial portion of the intercondylar notch shows various portions of the medial retinaculum, including VMO, the medial patellomeniscal ligament, and the patellotibial ligament. These, along with the medial patellofemoral ligament, blend together to form the medial retinaculum. (Bottom) Sagittal PD MR image, far lateral, shows portions of the lateral retinaculum. Contributions come from the vastus lateralis, anterior expansion iliotibial tract, anterior expansion superficial biceps femoris, and joint capsule.

Knee Extensor Mechanism and Retinacula

PATELLAR STABILIZERS

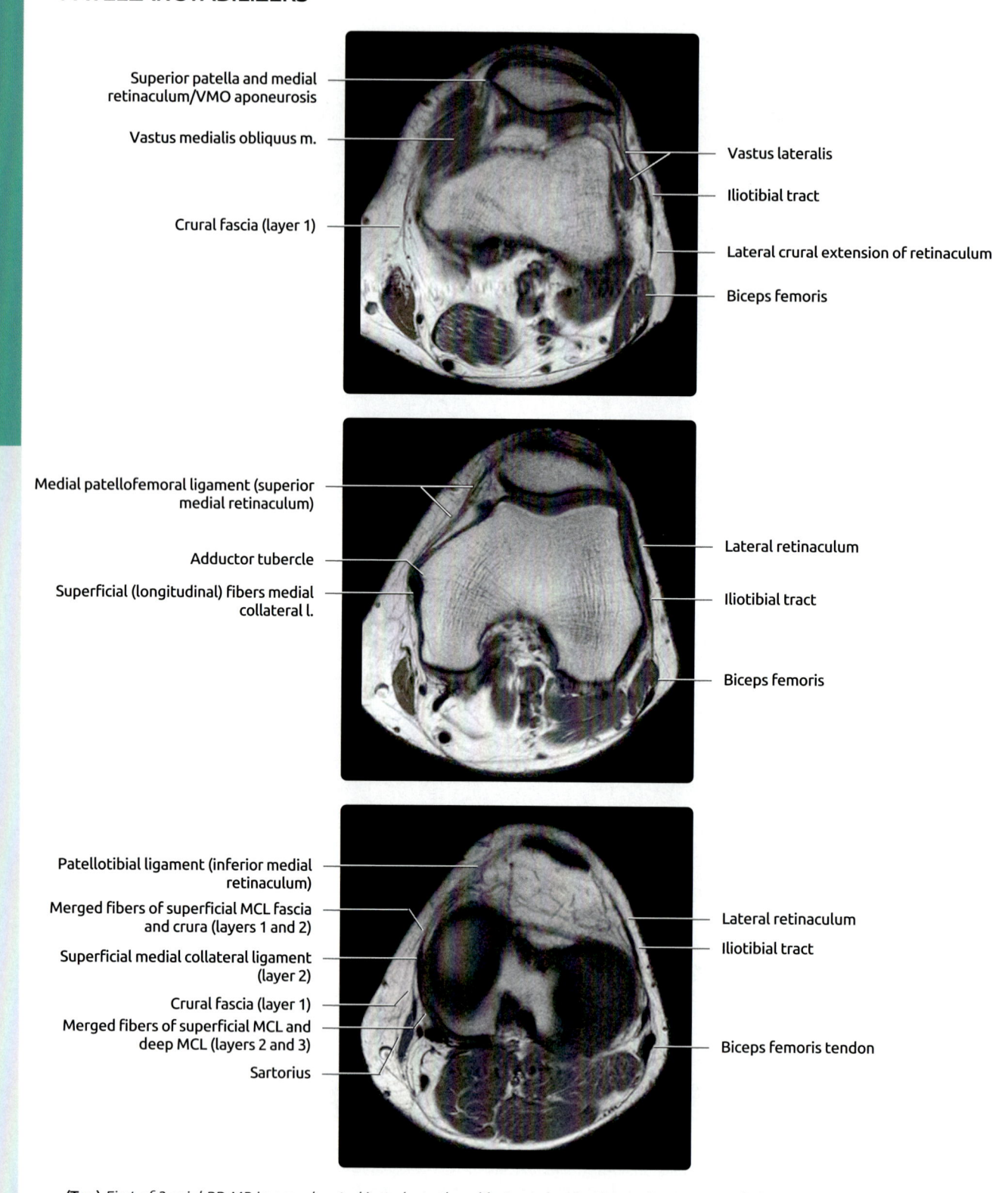

Labels (top image):
- Superior patella and medial retinaculum/VMO aponeurosis
- Vastus medialis obliquus m.
- Crural fascia (layer 1)
- Vastus lateralis
- Iliotibial tract
- Lateral crural extension of retinaculum
- Biceps femoris

Labels (middle image):
- Medial patellofemoral ligament (superior medial retinaculum)
- Adductor tubercle
- Superficial (longitudinal) fibers medial collateral l.
- Lateral retinaculum
- Iliotibial tract
- Biceps femoris

Labels (bottom image):
- Patellotibial ligament (inferior medial retinaculum)
- Merged fibers of superficial MCL fascia and crura (layers 1 and 2)
- Superficial medial collateral ligament (layer 2)
- Crural fascia (layer 1)
- Merged fibers of superficial MCL and deep MCL (layers 2 and 3)
- Sartorius
- Lateral retinaculum
- Iliotibial tract
- Biceps femoris tendon

(Top) *First of 3 axial PD MR images, located just above the adductor tubercle, shows the vastus medialis obliquus contributing to the superior portion of the medial retinaculum. The lateral retinaculum receives fibers from the anterior expansions of both the iliotibial tract and the biceps femoris.* (Middle) *At the level of the adductor tubercle, the superficial fibers of MCL and the medial patellofemoral ligament are seen at their origin. The MPFL extends to the patella as the superior portion of the medial retinaculum at this level.* (Bottom) *At the level of the joint line, the medial retinaculum receives a contribution from the merged fibers of the superficial MCL fascia and its overlying crura. The patellotibial ligament is also a major contributor at this level.*

Knee Extensor Mechanism and Retinacula

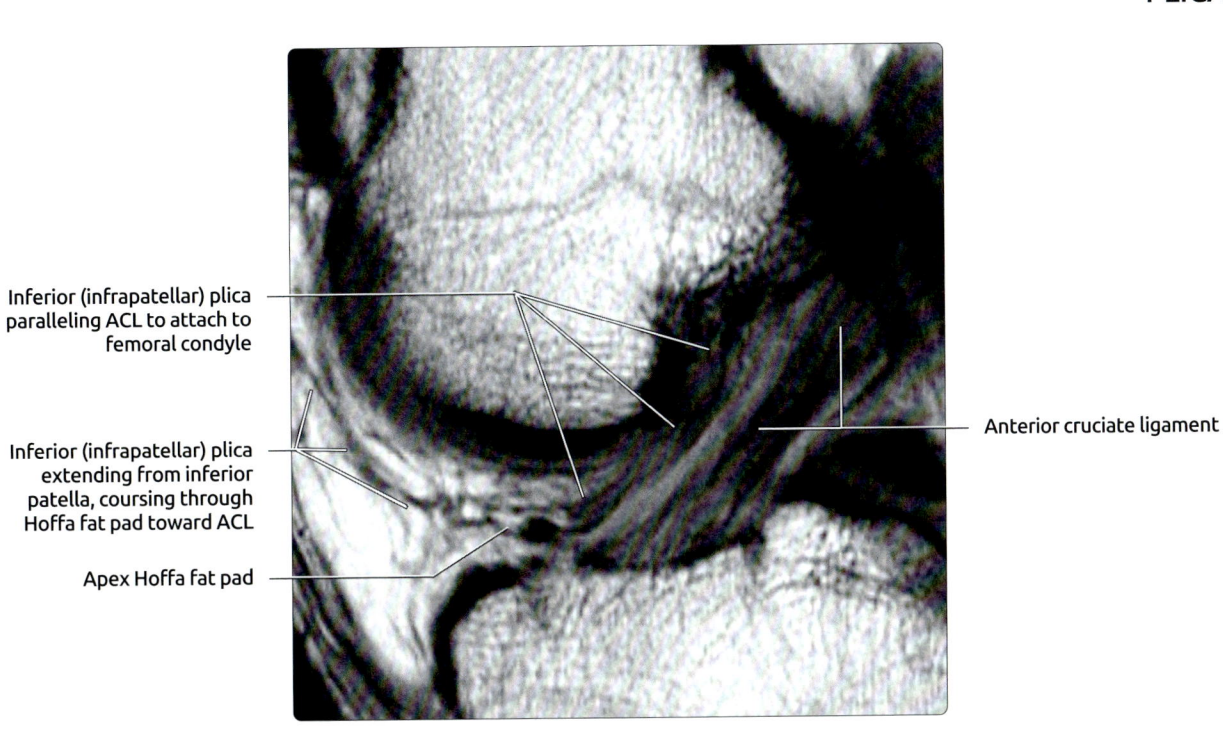

PLICA

- Inferior (infrapatellar) plica paralleling ACL to attach to femoral condyle
- Anterior cruciate ligament
- Inferior (infrapatellar) plica extending from inferior patella, coursing through Hoffa fat pad toward ACL
- Apex Hoffa fat pad

- Superior (suprapatellar) plica
- Vastus medialis

(Top) Sagittal PD MR image through the intercondylar notch shows a typical inferior (infrapatellar) plica. This normal variant extends from the inferior pole of the patella, through the Hoffa fat pad, parallels the ACL, and attaches to the femoral condyle at the intercondylar notch. It may simulate a meniscocruciate ligament, but the anterior sites of origin are distinctly different. (Bottom) Axial T2 MR image at the level of the distal femur shows a synovial fold extending across the medial side of the suprapatellar pouch. This is a common form of plica, seen particularly well because of the large effusion. It is termed the superior, or suprapatellar, plica.

Knee Extensor Mechanism and Retinacula

PLICA

Superior (suprapatellar) plica
Patella
Anterior cruciate ligament

Superior (suprapatellar) plica
Posterior cruciate ligament

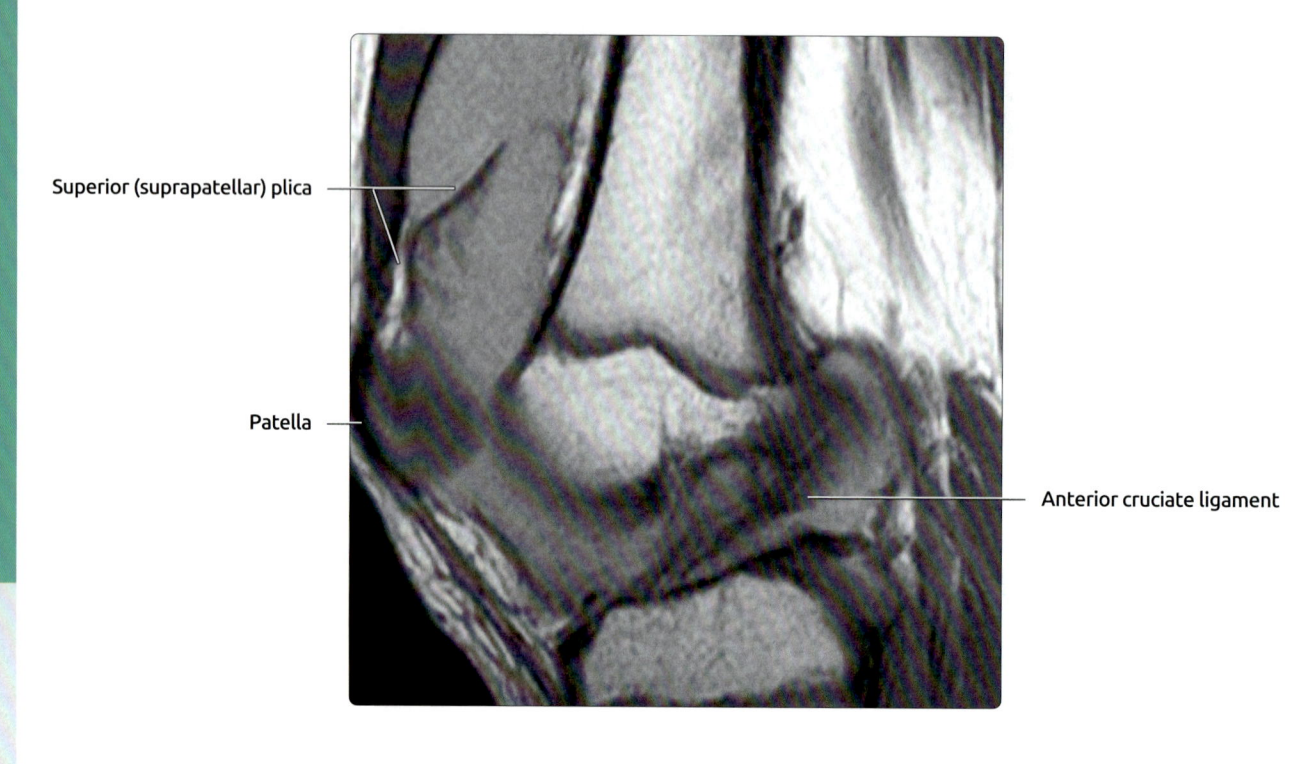

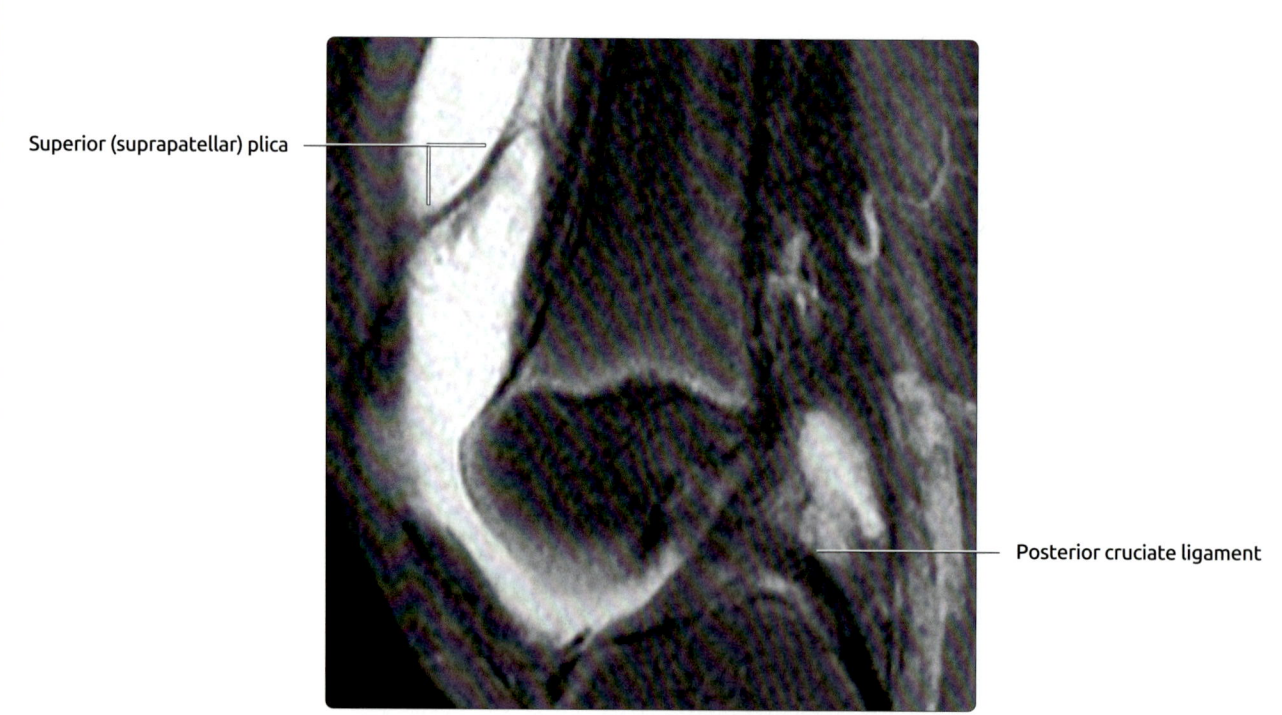

(Top) *Sagittal PD MR through the intercondylar notch of the same patient shows a superior (suprapatellar) plica. The plica extends from just superior to the patella, medially through the suprapatellar pouch.* **(Bottom)** *Sagittal PD FS MR image (note the posterior cruciate ligament) shows the plica extending further superomedially. This is a common variant, which does not have clinical consequences.*

PLICA

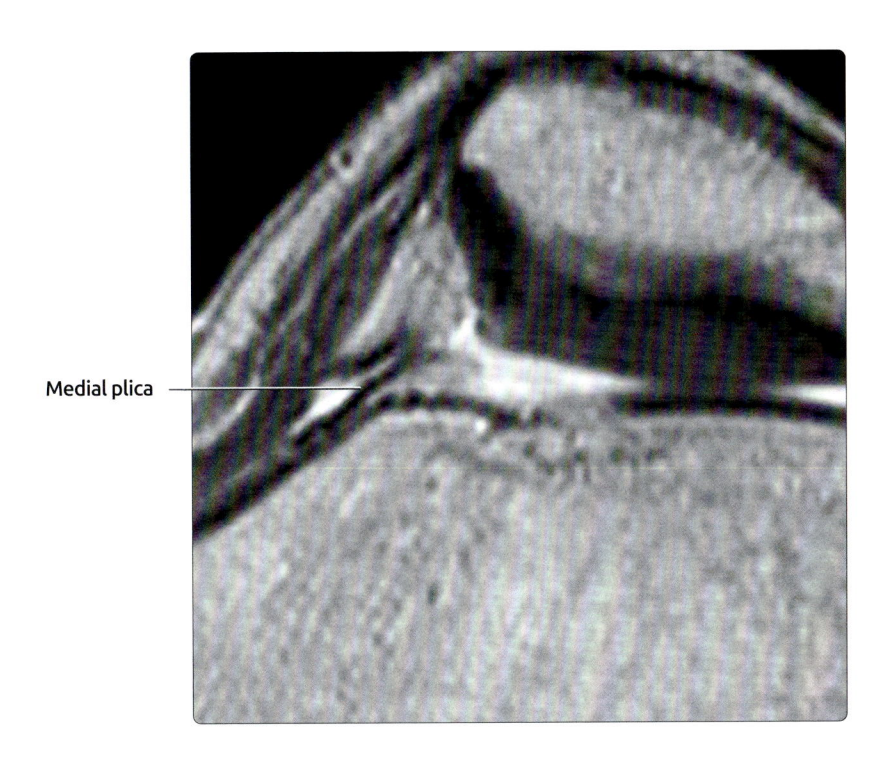

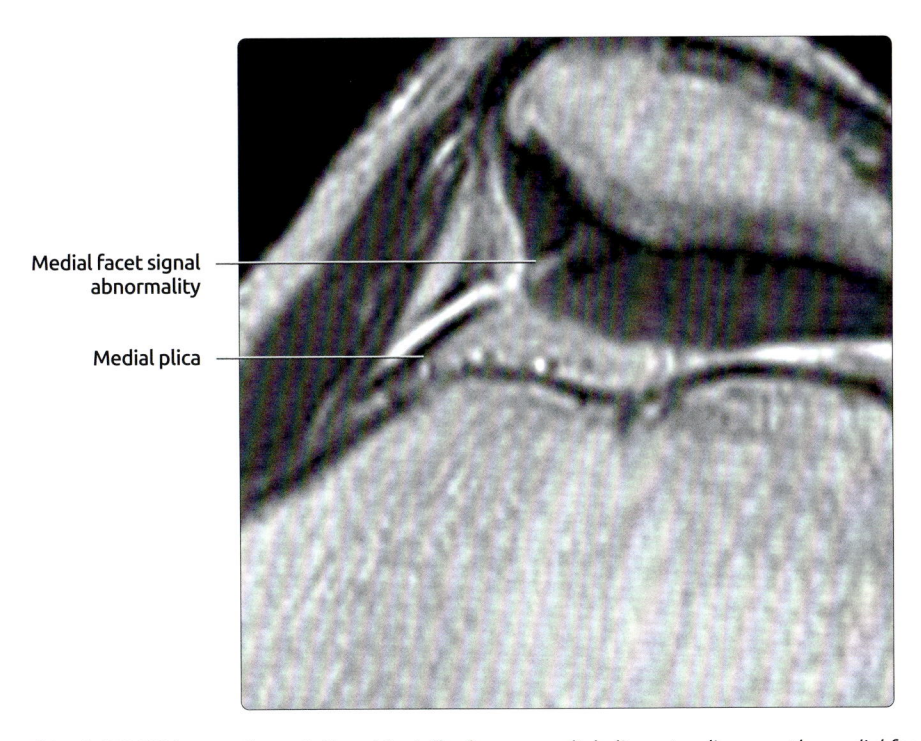

Medial plica

Medial facet signal abnormality
Medial plica

(Top) First of 2 axial T2 MR images through the midpatella shows a medial plica extending over the medial facet of the trochlea and under the medial facet of the patella. (Bottom) Slightly distal image shows the medial plica, with signal abnormality, approaching the medial facet of the patella, which also shows signal abnormality. The medial plica is more likely to result in symptomatic damage (either at the medial patellar facet or medial trochlea) than the other plicae.

Menisci

TERMINOLOGY

Abbreviations
- Anterior/posterior cruciate ligament (ACL/PCL)
- Lateral/medial meniscus (LM/MM)
- Medial collateral ligament (MCL)

IMAGING ANATOMY

Overview
- Menisci evaluated by morphology, signal, and attachments
- All portions taper from height of 3-5 mm peripherally to sharp, thin, central (free) edge
- Normally specific and predictable size/shape
- Morphology variance indicates tear or variant which is at increased risk for tear

Morphology
- **Lateral meniscus**
  - Overall configuration: **Semicircular**
  - **Shape: Uniform**, minimally and gradually enlarging from anterior to posterior
  - Normal recess: Peripheral, inferior at anterior horn
- **Medial meniscus**
  - Overall configuration: **Semilunar (C-shaped)**
  - **Shape nonuniform**: Anterior horn similar in size & shape to LM but midbody is small, approximating an equilateral triangle; MM posterior horn is largest portion of MM, nearly 2x as long as anterior horn
  - Normal recess: Peripheral, superior at posterior horn
- **Meniscal "flounce"**: Buckling of a portion of meniscus, perhaps related to femorotibial subluxation

Signal
- Generally **uniformly low signal** throughout
- Exceptions
  - Children and adolescents may have normal increased intrameniscal signal that does not extend to surface (due to rich vascular supply)
  - Adults may develop central degenerative changes seen as linear or globular signal that does not extend to surface and does not represent a tear
  - Various high signal clefts and dots can normally be seen in anterior horn LM at and near its root attachment, due to immediate adjacency of origin of ACL and divergence of longitudinal fibers at root; do not misinterpret as tear
  - Peripheral portion of meniscus is quite vascular
    - Outer meniscal margin as seen by MR is usually not true periphery of structure: Meniscus signal in its peripheral vascular portion (10-30%) blends in with gray signal of the capsule
  - "Magic angle" may affect signal in posterior horn of LM in region of intercondylar notch

Meniscal Attachments
- **Osseous attachments**: Both menisci are firmly attached to tibia at their roots
  - **LM roots**: Located near center of tibial plateau
    - Anterior horn attaches immediately lateral to origin of ACL
    - Posterior horn attaches just posterior to ACL and anterior to PCL as PCL extends behind tibial plateau to its insertion on posterior tibia
    - Root of posterior horn LM also is anterior to root of posterior horn MM
  - **MM roots**: MM is more semilunar in shape than semicircular LM, so its roots are located at center of tibial plateau, but more anteriorly and posteriorly for anterior horn and posterior horn, respectively, than those of LM
    - Root anterior horn MM anterior to origin of ACL
    - Root posterior horn MM immediately anterior to PCL but posterior to root of posterior horn LM
- **Capsular attachments**
  - **MM entirely attached to joint capsule** with exception of small interruption at MCL
    - MM serves as origin of meniscofemoral ligament portion of deep fibers of MCL; this ligament either inserts on adjacent femur or superficial MCL
    - MM also serves as origin of meniscotibial ligament (coronary ligament) portion of deep fibers of the MCL, which inserts on the adjacent tibia
    - Fibrofatty tissue as well as MCL bursa separate MM and deep fibers of MCL from superficial MCL
  - **LM entirely attached to joint capsule only in anterior and far posterior portions, with attachment being interrupted at body and much of posterior horn by popliteal hiatus**
    - After origination from lateral femoral condyle, popliteus tendon penetrates capsule and takes intra-articular course
    - Intraarticularly, popliteus tendon extends distally in posteromedial direction
    - Popliteus tendon separates LM from its capsular insertion along body & majority of posterior horn
    - Superior and inferior fascicles serve as attachments between LM and popliteal tendon and, in turn, capsule
    - Inferior popliteomeniscal fascicle extends from lateral edge of body of meniscus to inferior portion of popliteus paratenon, forming floor of popliteal hiatus
    - Inferior fascicle complete at level of body of LM, but not posterior horn
    - Superior popliteomeniscal fascicle extends from body/posterior horn LM to superior portion popliteal paratenon and on to capsule, forming ceiling of popliteal hiatus
    - Superior fascicle incomplete at body, but complete at body/posterior horn LM

Meniscal Variants
- **Transverse ligament**: Connects menisci anteriorly
  - Oblique insertion on LM anterior horn may simulate a tear; may be absent
- **Meniscofemoral ligaments**: Extend from posterior medial femoral condyle to posterior horn LM
  - At insertion on LM, may simulate a tear
  - Ligament of Wrisberg passes posterior to PCL
  - Ligament of Humphrey passes anterior to PCL
- **Oblique menisco-meniscal ligaments**: Cross from anterior horn of one to posterior horn of other meniscus, passing between ACL and PCL

Menisci

GRAPHICS: MEDIAL MENISCUS

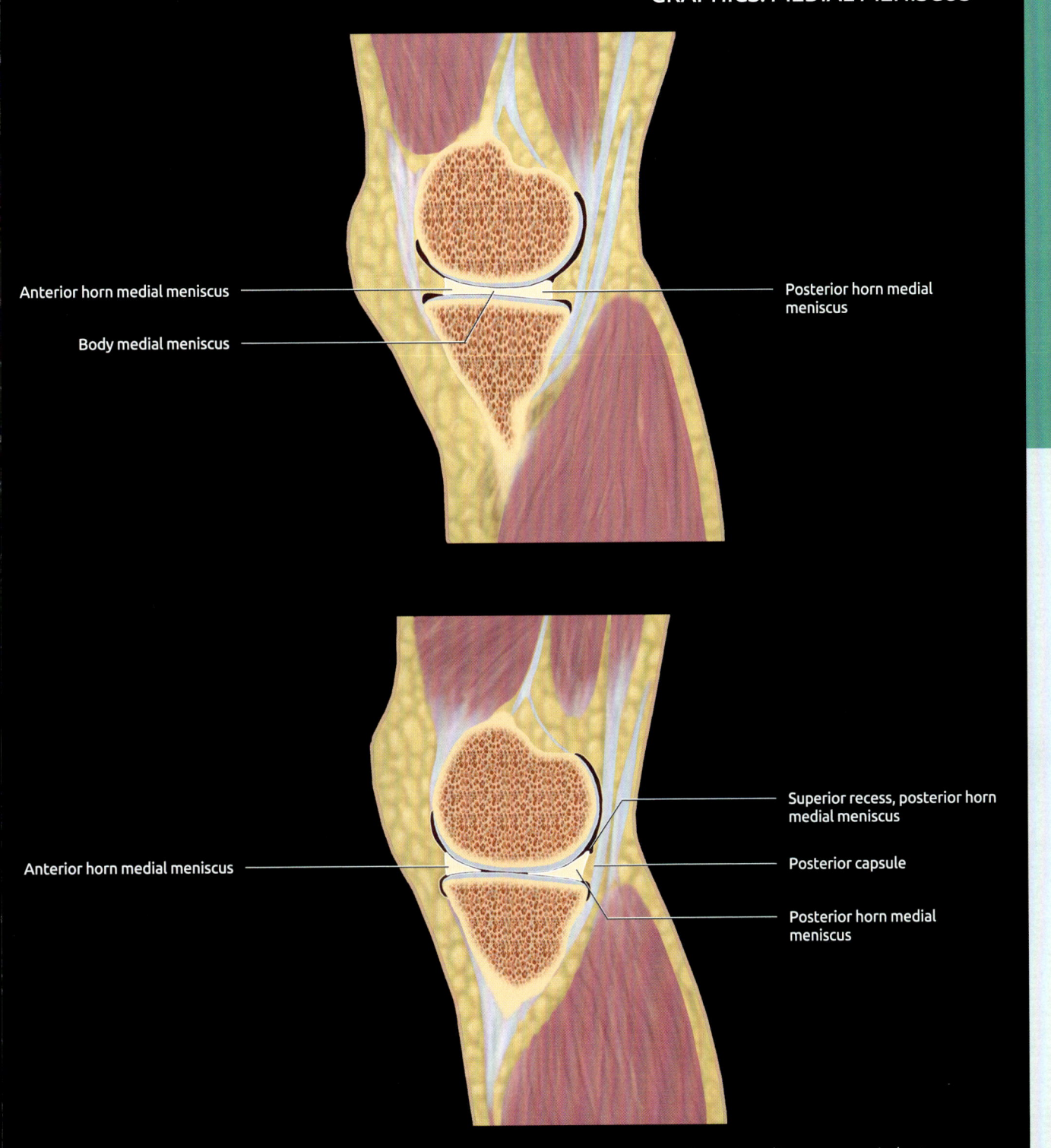

Anterior horn medial meniscus

Body medial meniscus

Posterior horn medial meniscus

Anterior horn medial meniscus

Superior recess, posterior horn medial meniscus

Posterior capsule

Posterior horn medial meniscus

(Top) Sagittal cut through the medial-most aspect of the medial meniscus, shows the bowtie configuration. This appearance is due to the cut extending across the full thickness of both the anterior and posterior horns but across only the thinner mid portion of the body. **(Bottom)** Sagittal cut through the mid portion of the medial meniscus, shows the triangular anterior and posterior horns. The posterior horn of the medial meniscus is normally elongated and larger than the anterior horn. There may be a superior recess at the meniscocapsular junction of the posterior horn.

Menisci

SAGITTAL PD MR, MEDIAL MENISCUS

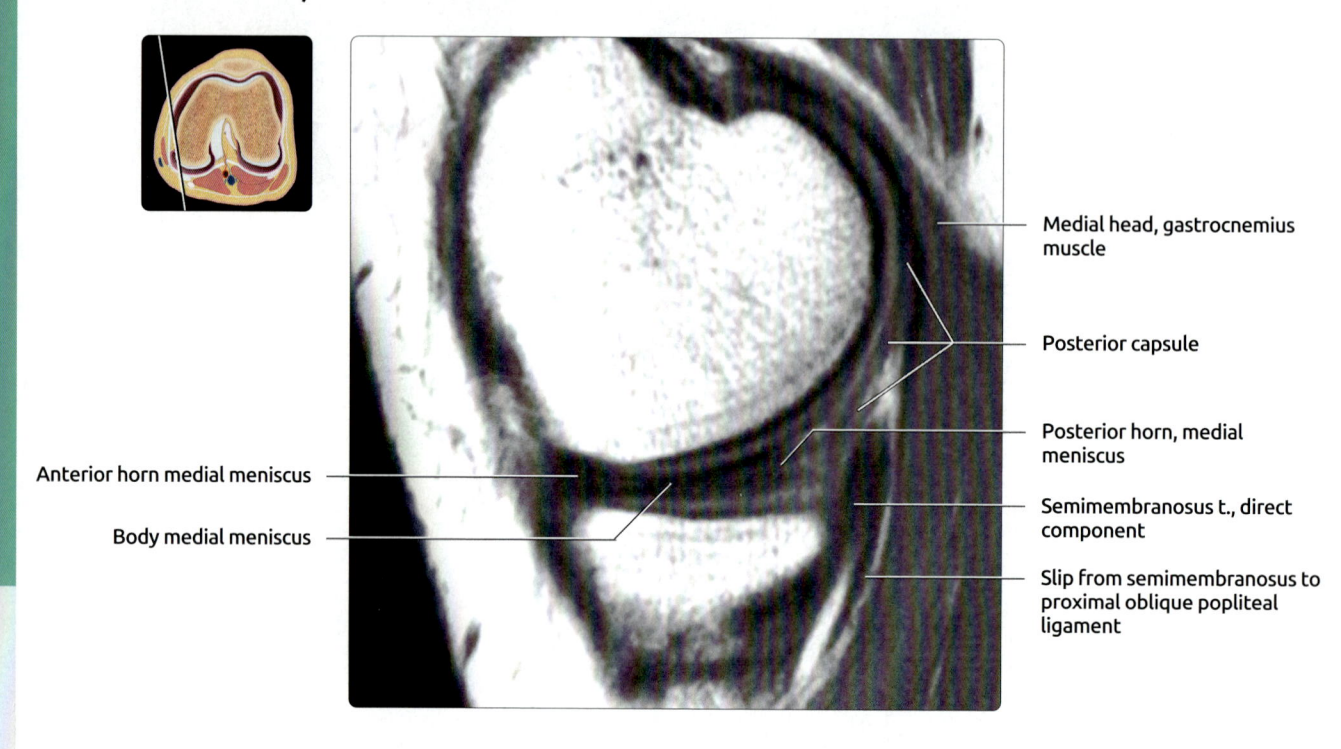

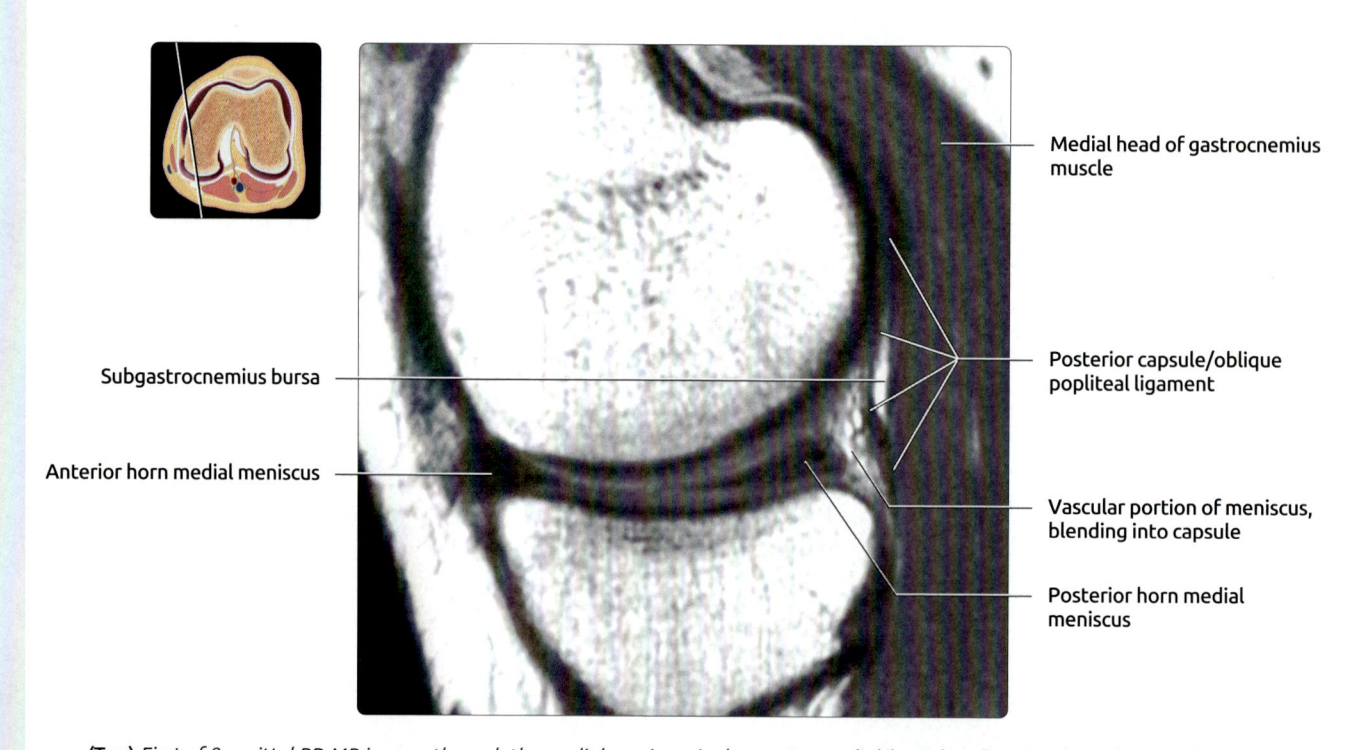

Labels (top image):
- Medial head, gastrocnemius muscle
- Posterior capsule
- Posterior horn, medial meniscus
- Semimembranosus t., direct component
- Slip from semimembranosus to proximal oblique popliteal ligament
- Anterior horn medial meniscus
- Body medial meniscus

Labels (bottom image):
- Medial head of gastrocnemius muscle
- Posterior capsule/oblique popliteal ligament
- Vascular portion of meniscus, blending into capsule
- Posterior horn medial meniscus
- Subgastrocnemius bursa
- Anterior horn medial meniscus

(**Top**) *First of 8 sagittal PD MR images through the medial meniscus is shown. Far medial (peripheral) sagittal cut through the medial meniscus shows the bowtie configuration encompassing portions of the anterior horn, body, and posterior horn of the medial meniscus.* (**Bottom**) *Mid sagittal cut through the medial meniscus shows the differential size and shape of the anterior and posterior horns. This image and the previous image show the low signal meniscus blending indistinctly into the gray vascular portion of the meniscus, which in turn blends into the capsule.*

Menisci

SAGITTAL PD MR, MEDIAL MENISCUS

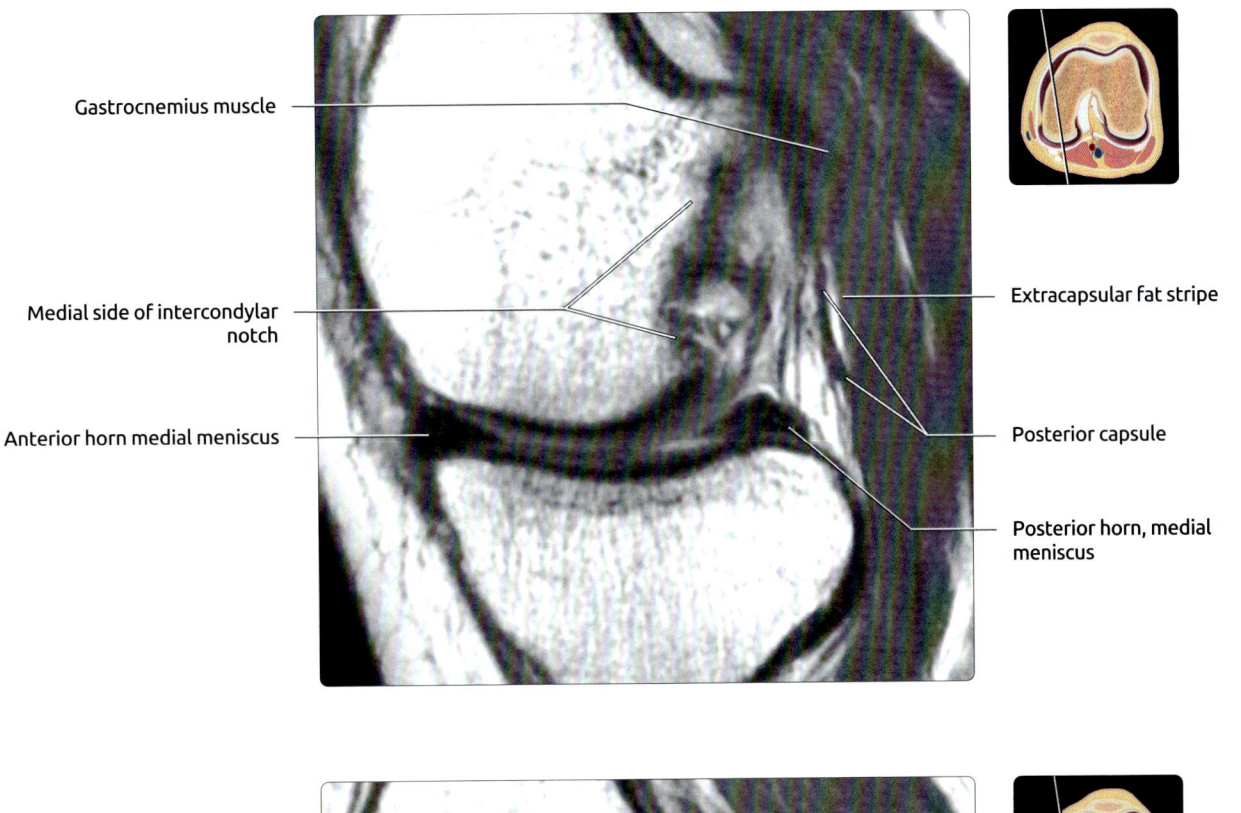

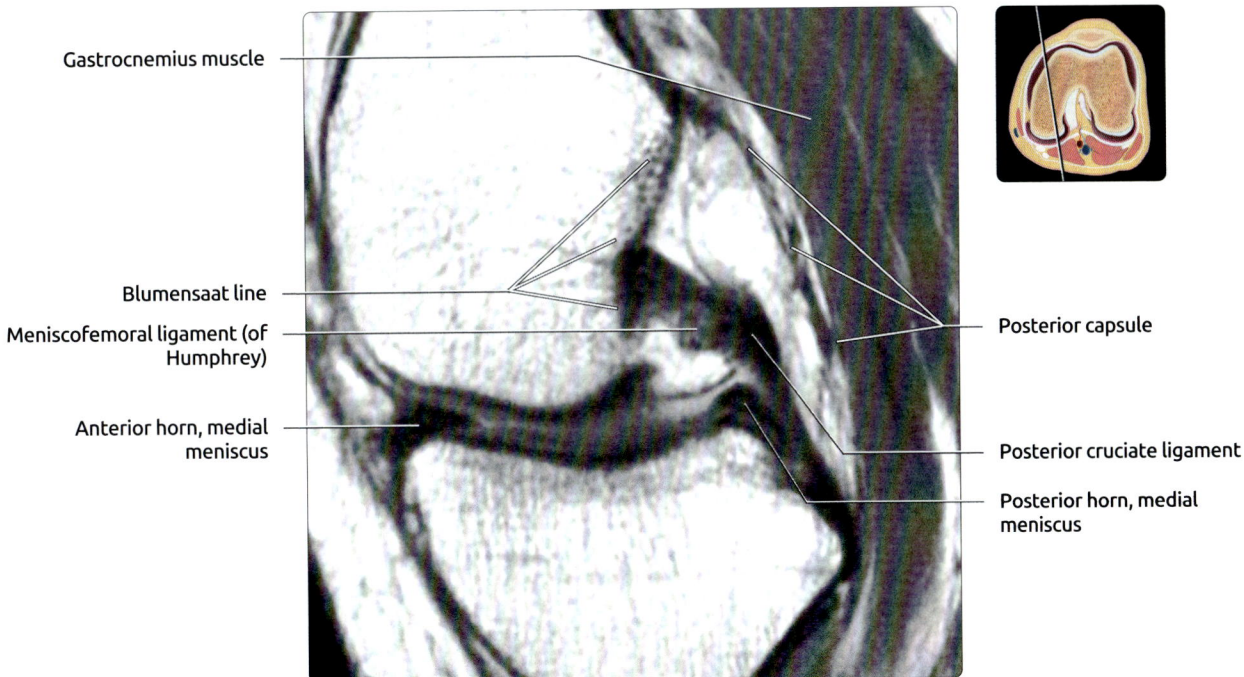

Top image labels:
- Gastrocnemius muscle
- Medial side of intercondylar notch
- Anterior horn medial meniscus
- Extracapsular fat stripe
- Posterior capsule
- Posterior horn, medial meniscus

Bottom image labels:
- Gastrocnemius muscle
- Blumensaat line
- Meniscofemoral ligament (of Humphrey)
- Anterior horn, medial meniscus
- Posterior capsule
- Posterior cruciate ligament
- Posterior horn, medial meniscus

(Top) Image shows cut through the medial meniscus, approaching the intercondylar notch. The anterior and posterior horns retain their differential size and shape. (Bottom) Cut through the medial meniscus as it enters the medial portion of the intercondylar notch is demonstrated. The posterior cruciate ligament is seen, arising from the mid portion of Blumensaat line along the medial femoral condyle. The anteroinferior meniscofemoral ligament (of Humphrey) is seen in cross section beneath the posterior cruciate ligament. The posterior horn of the medial meniscus is beginning to change its shape as it approaches its root attachment to the tibial plateau. Because of the obliquity at which the knee is scanned for the sagittal images, the anterior horn is not yet approaching its root, but retains its triangular shape.

Menisci

SAGITTAL PD MR, MEDIAL MENISCUS

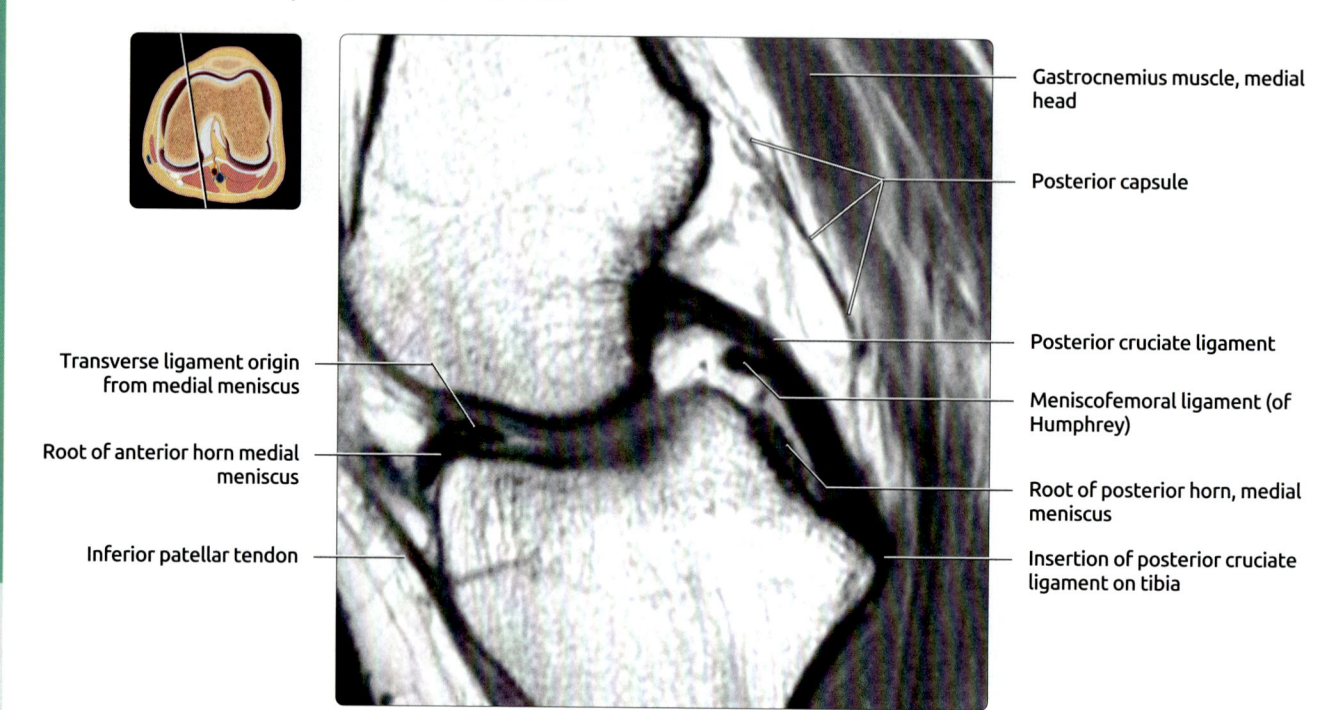

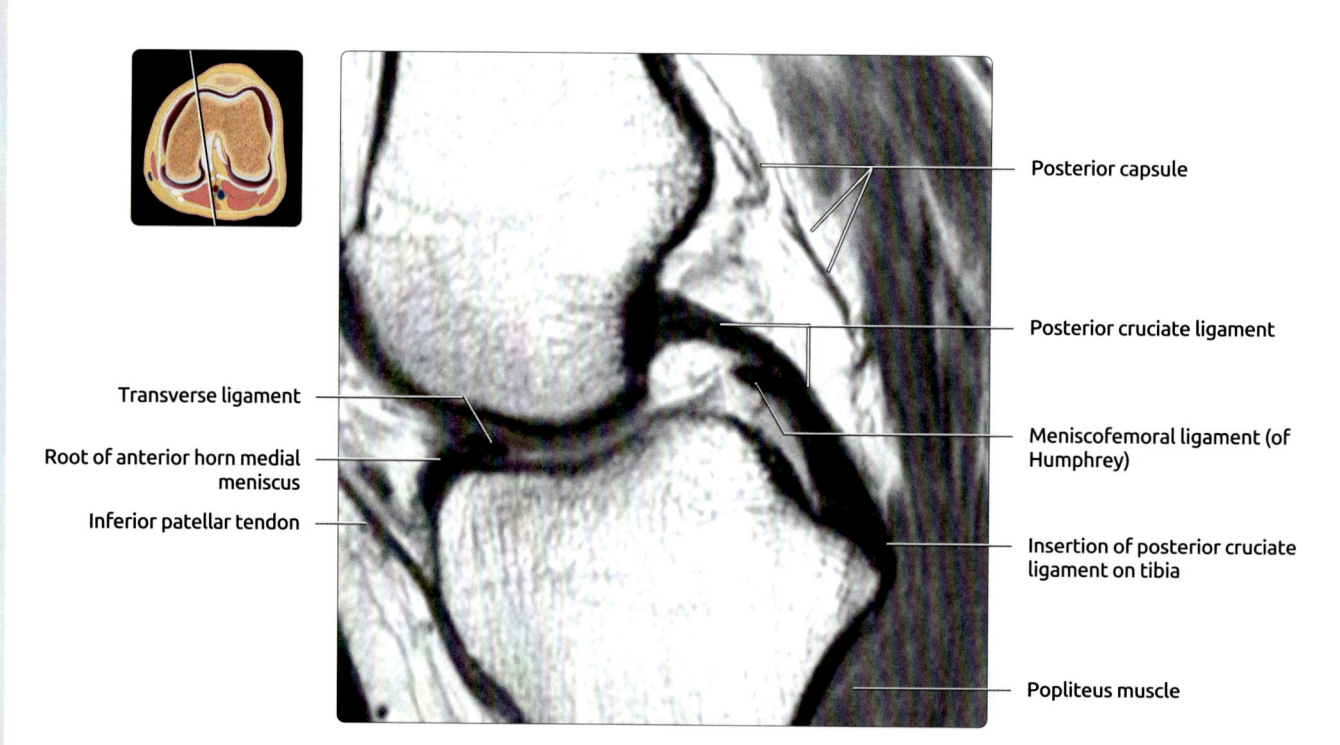

Top image labels:
- Gastrocnemius muscle, medial head
- Posterior capsule
- Posterior cruciate ligament
- Meniscofemoral ligament (of Humphrey)
- Root of posterior horn, medial meniscus
- Insertion of posterior cruciate ligament on tibia
- Transverse ligament origin from medial meniscus
- Root of anterior horn medial meniscus
- Inferior patellar tendon

Bottom image labels:
- Posterior capsule
- Posterior cruciate ligament
- Meniscofemoral ligament (of Humphrey)
- Insertion of posterior cruciate ligament on tibia
- Popliteus muscle
- Transverse ligament
- Root of anterior horn medial meniscus
- Inferior patellar tendon

(**Top**) This cut shows the roots of both the anterior and posterior horns of the medial meniscus. The root of the posterior horn of medial meniscus terminates immediately in front of the posterior cruciate insertion on the tibia. (**Bottom**) The adjacent image shows the anterior horn of the medial meniscus terminating in its root; the transverse ligament arises at this point. Both the transverse and meniscofemoral ligaments are seen in cross section.

Menisci

SAGITTAL PD MR, MEDIAL MENISCUS

Labels (top image):
- Posterior capsule
- Transverse ligament
- Infrapatellar (Hoffa) fat pad
- Inferior patellar tendon
- Popliteal artery
- Meniscofemoral ligament (of Humphrey)
- Insertion of posterior cruciate ligament on tibia
- Popliteus muscle

Labels (bottom image):
- Posterior capsule
- Anterior cruciate ligament
- Transverse ligament
- Inferior patellar fat pad
- Intracapsular fatty tissue
- Meniscofemoral ligament (of Humphrey)

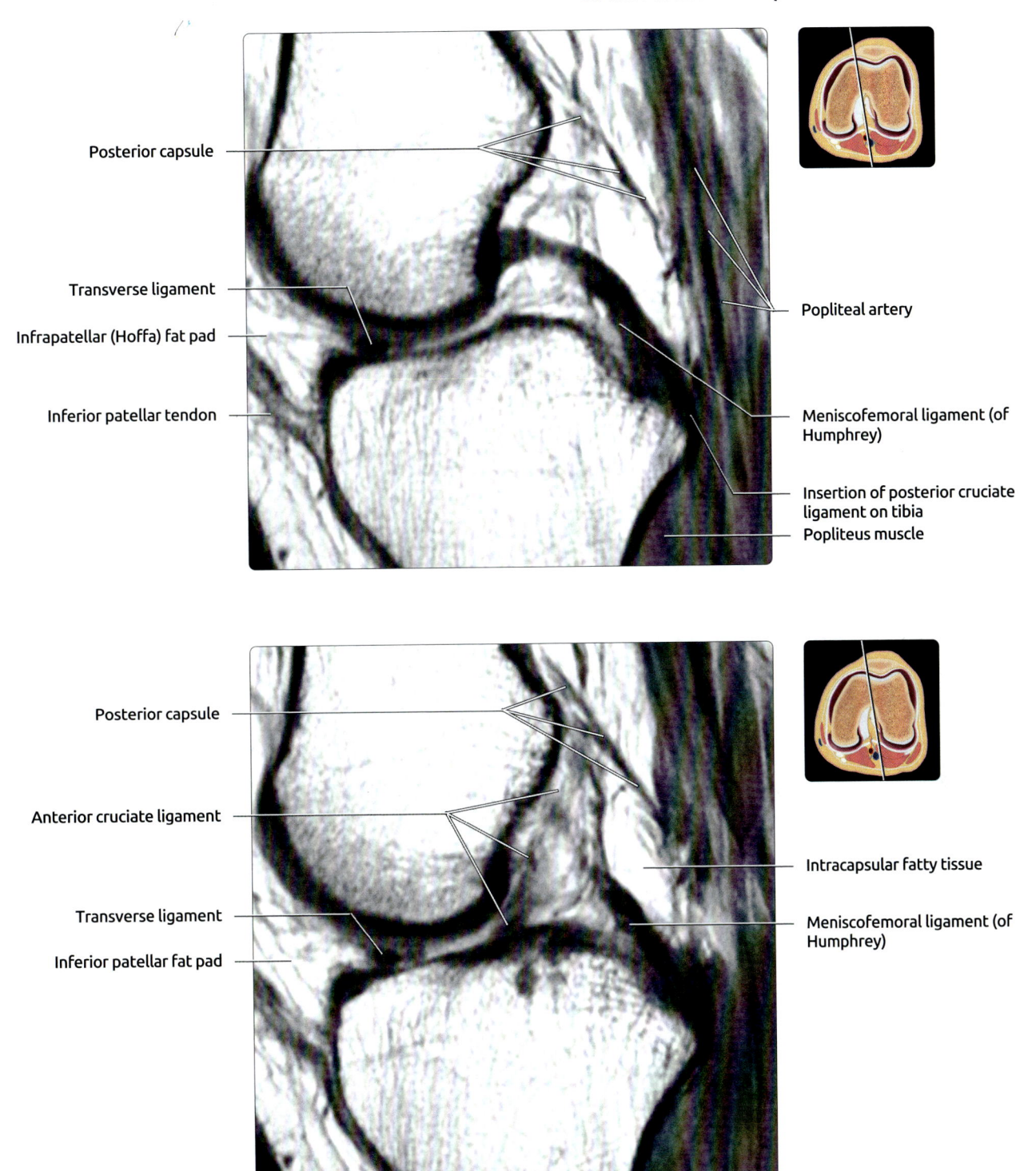

(Top) This cut shows no menisci; the meniscofemoral ligament is beginning to elongate and parallel the posterior cruciate ligament. Note that the posterior capsule is interrupted, allowing neurovascular structures to enter the joint. **(Bottom)** Cut between the cruciate ligaments shows the transverse ligament in cross section, continuing across the anterior joint space. The meniscofemoral ligament elongates towards its insertion on the posterior horn of the lateral meniscus; the latter structure is not seen until the next cut towards the lateral side.

Menisci

GRAPHICS: MENISCAL ROOTS & MORPHOLOGY

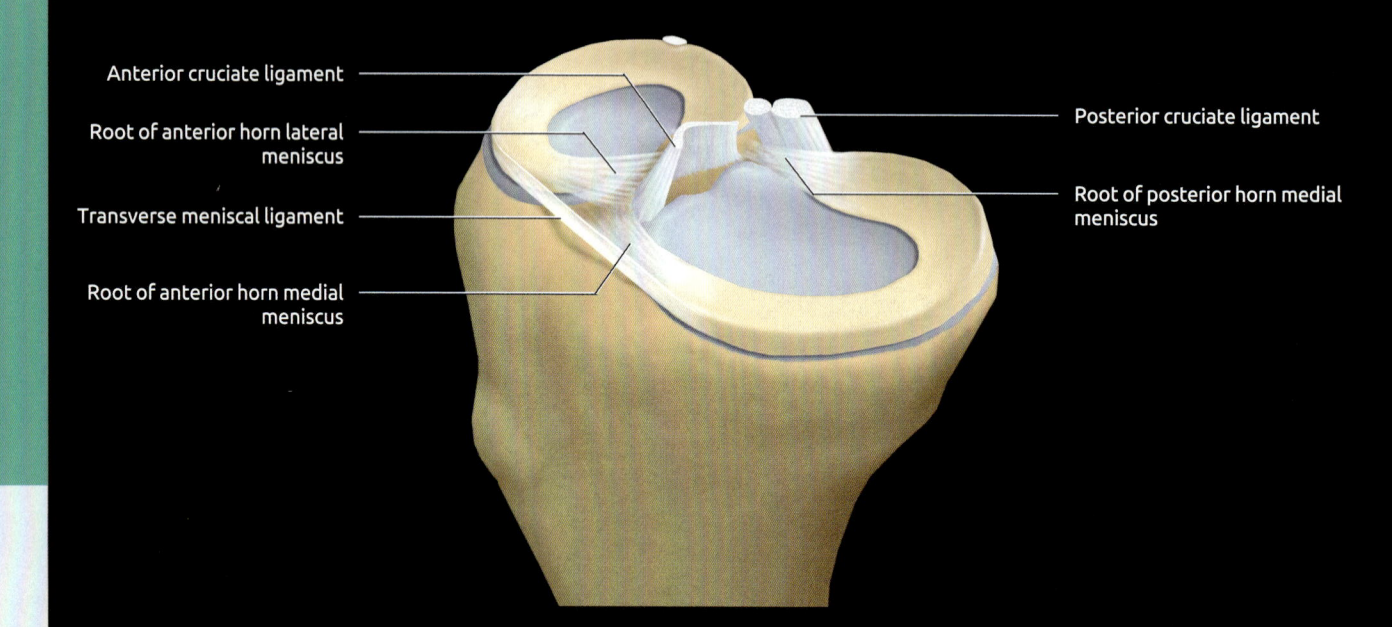

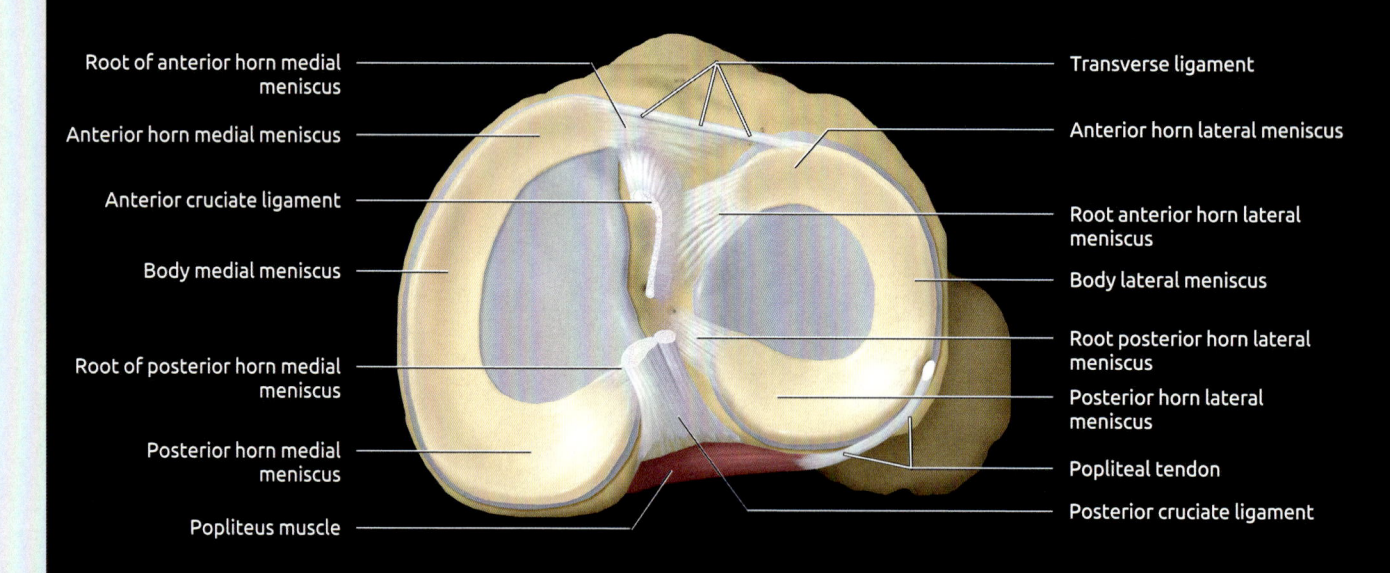

Anterior cruciate ligament
Root of anterior horn lateral meniscus
Transverse meniscal ligament
Root of anterior horn medial meniscus
Posterior cruciate ligament
Root of posterior horn medial meniscus

Root of anterior horn medial meniscus
Anterior horn medial meniscus
Anterior cruciate ligament
Body medial meniscus
Root of posterior horn medial meniscus
Posterior horn medial meniscus
Popliteus muscle
Transverse ligament
Anterior horn lateral meniscus
Root anterior horn lateral meniscus
Body lateral meniscus
Root posterior horn lateral meniscus
Posterior horn lateral meniscus
Popliteal tendon
Posterior cruciate ligament

(**Top**) Oblique axial graphic shows the tibial surface of the knee joint in an external oblique position. It highlights the semilunar medial meniscus, with its anterior and posterior roots located anterior to the ACL and PCL, respectively. The transverse ligament is seen coursing between the anterior horns of the medial and lateral menisci. (**Bottom**) Graphic is an axial view through the joint line. It shows the semilunar MM, with its wider C-shape compared to the more circular LM. The position of the meniscal roots is seen relative to one another as well as to the ACL and PCL. The transverse ligament and popliteal tendon are shown in relation to the menisci. Note also the different sizes of the various parts of the menisci.

Menisci

AXIAL PD FS MR, MENISCI

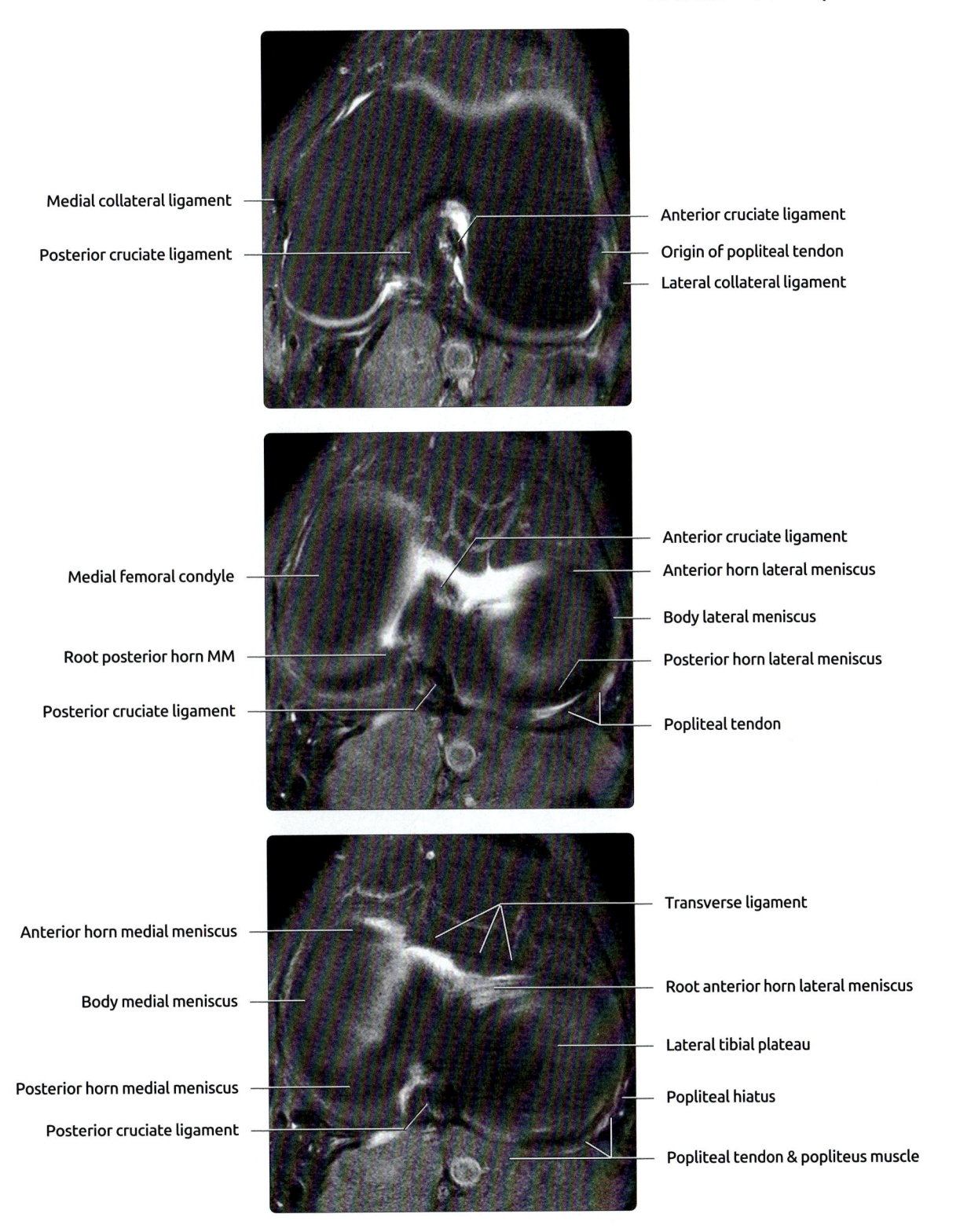

Labels (top image): Medial collateral ligament; Posterior cruciate ligament; Anterior cruciate ligament; Origin of popliteal tendon; Lateral collateral ligament

Labels (middle image): Medial femoral condyle; Root posterior horn MM; Posterior cruciate ligament; Anterior cruciate ligament; Anterior horn lateral meniscus; Body lateral meniscus; Posterior horn lateral meniscus; Popliteal tendon

Labels (bottom image): Anterior horn medial meniscus; Body medial meniscus; Posterior horn medial meniscus; Posterior cruciate ligament; Transverse ligament; Root anterior horn lateral meniscus; Lateral tibial plateau; Popliteal hiatus; Popliteal tendon & popliteus muscle

(**Top**) First of 3 axial PD FS MR images through the joint line. Image located immediately above the knee joint line. The cruciate ligaments as well as the origins of the medial and lateral collateral ligaments are seen. (**Middle**) Image through the knee joint line shows parts of the menisci as well as the course of the popliteal tendon through the popliteal hiatus. (**Bottom**) Image through the tibial plateau at the joint line shows parts of the menisci and their roots. The popliteal tendon is also seen extending to the popliteus muscle. The transverse meniscal ligament bridges between the 2 anterior horns.

Menisci

GRAPHICS: POPLITEAL TENDON, HIATUS, & FASCICLES

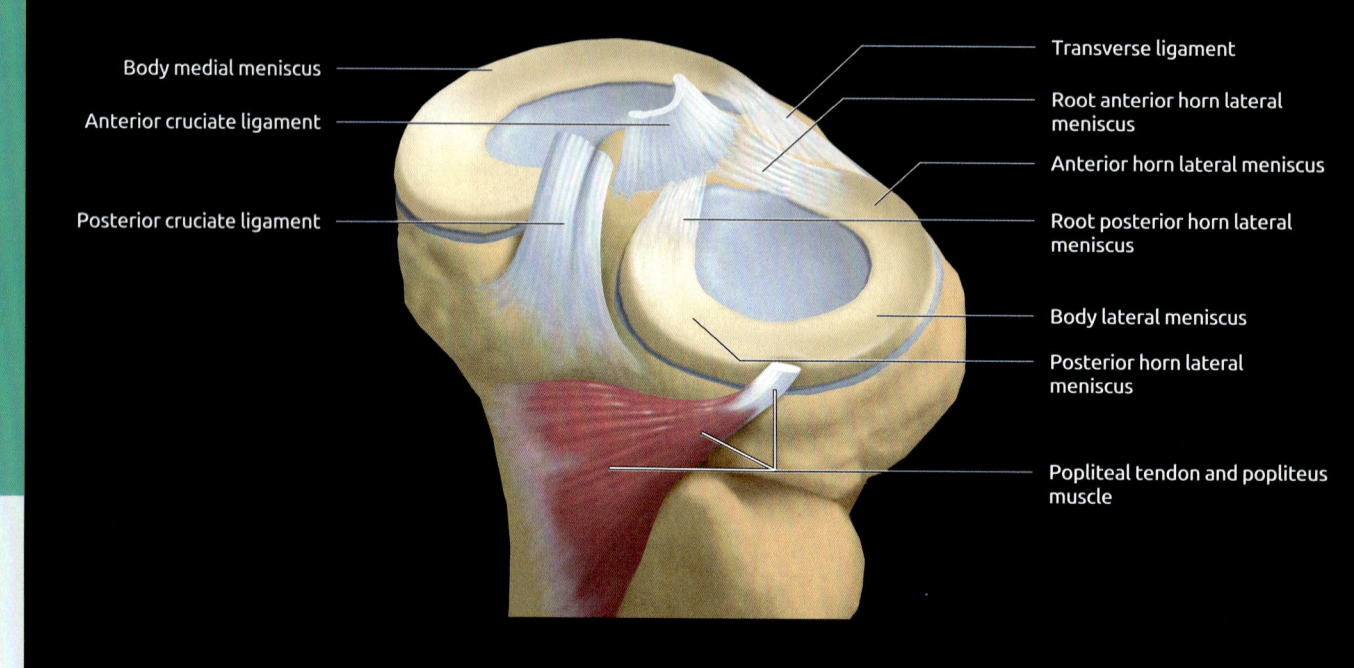

Labels (top image):
- Body medial meniscus
- Anterior cruciate ligament
- Posterior cruciate ligament
- Transverse ligament
- Root anterior horn lateral meniscus
- Anterior horn lateral meniscus
- Root posterior horn lateral meniscus
- Body lateral meniscus
- Posterior horn lateral meniscus
- Popliteal tendon and popliteus muscle

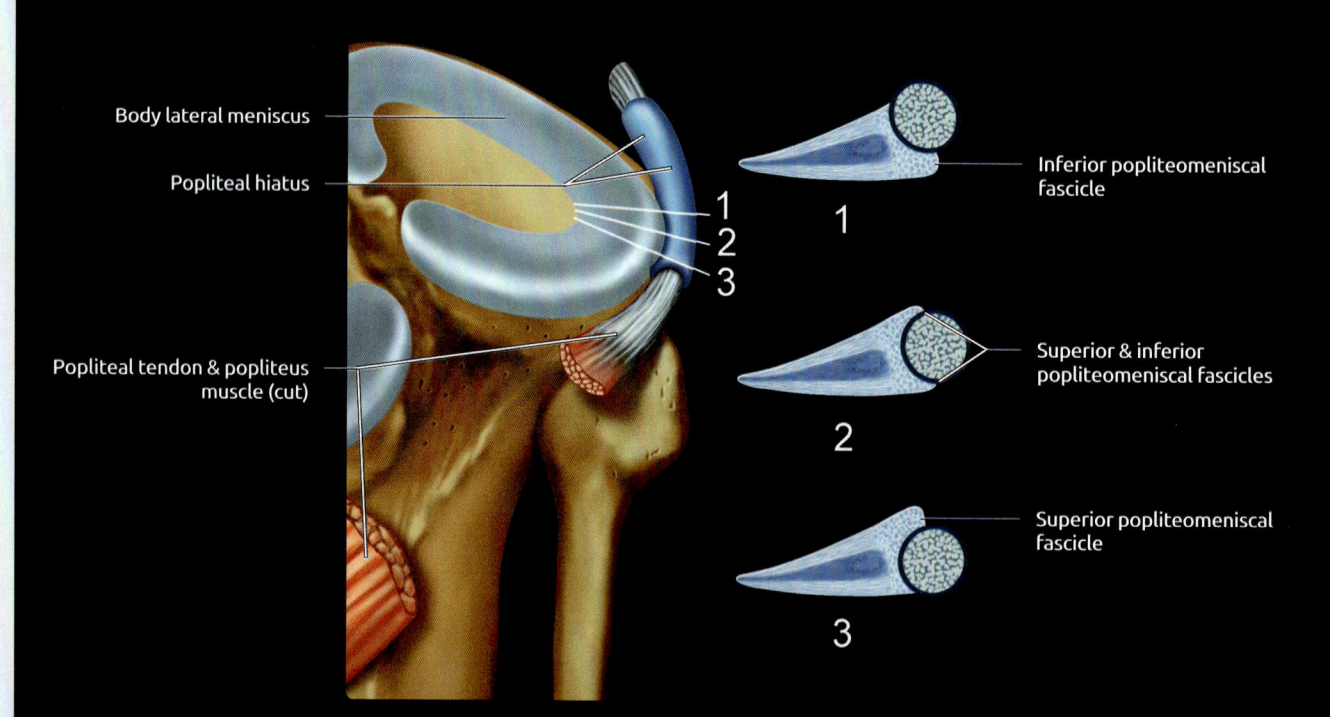

Labels (bottom image):
- Body lateral meniscus
- Popliteal hiatus
- Popliteal tendon & popliteus muscle (cut)
- 1 — Inferior popliteomeniscal fascicle
- 2 — Superior & inferior popliteomeniscal fascicles
- 3 — Superior popliteomeniscal fascicle

(Top) Posterolateral oblique view of the knee joint line shows the semicircular lateral meniscus, with its roots located immediately lateral to the anterior cruciate ligament. The popliteal tendon is shown curving around the lateral meniscus. (Bottom) Oblique axial graphic shows the course of the popliteal tendon through the knee joint. After the popliteal tendon originates from the lateral femoral condyle, it enters the joint space, interrupting the capsular attachment of the body of the lateral meniscus. It travels posteriorly and downward, curving around the body and posterior horns of the LM. It is bathed in synovial fluid within this space (termed the popliteal hiatus). Note the inferior fascicle which forms the floor of the hiatus at the body of the LM, and the superior fascicle which forms the roof of the hiatus at the LM body/posterior horn. Different combinations of the superior and inferior fascicles are visualized as the popliteal tendon proceeds through the hiatus from the level of the body to posterior horn of lateral meniscus.

Menisci

GRAPHICS, LATERAL MENISCUS

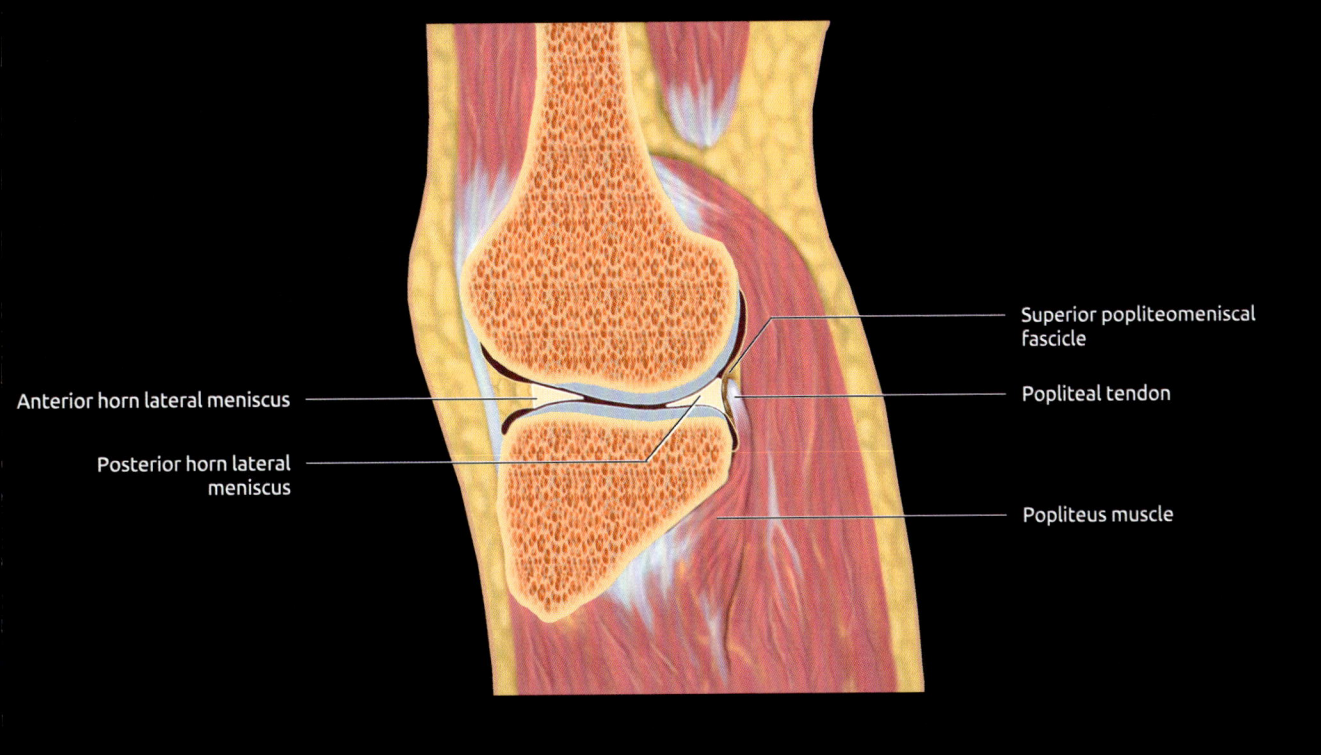

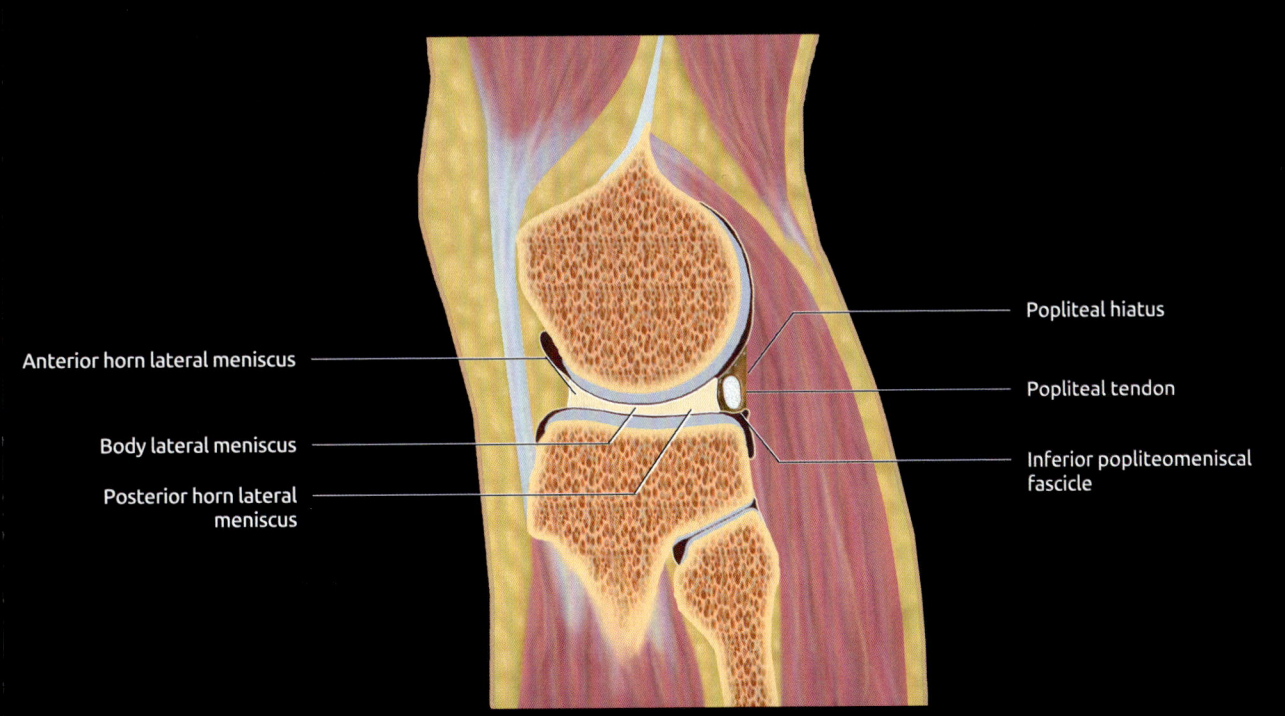

Anterior horn lateral meniscus

Posterior horn lateral meniscus

Superior popliteomeniscal fascicle

Popliteal tendon

Popliteus muscle

Anterior horn lateral meniscus

Body lateral meniscus

Posterior horn lateral meniscus

Popliteal hiatus

Popliteal tendon

Inferior popliteomeniscal fascicle

(Top) In the mid portion of the lateral compartment, the anterior and posterior horns of the LM are nearly equal in size and shape. The popliteal tendon extends into the popliteus muscle. The superior fascicle can be seen extending from the superior portion of the posterior horn to the superior edge of the popliteal tendon (paratenon), continuing to the capsule and forming the roof of the popliteal hiatus. The inferior fascicle is not continuous at this level since it is interrupted by passage of the popliteal tendon inferolaterally through the hiatus. (Bottom) Sagittal graphic located far laterally in the joint shows the bowtie configuration of the anterior horn, body, and posterior horn of the LM. The popliteal tendon is seen in the hiatus; at this junction of body and posterior horn of LM, the inferior fascicle can be seen extending from the meniscus towards (but not connecting to) the popliteal tendon. It forms the floor of the popliteal hiatus. At this site, the superior fascicle is interrupted by the popliteal tendon.

Menisci

SAGITTAL PD MR, LATERAL MENISCUS

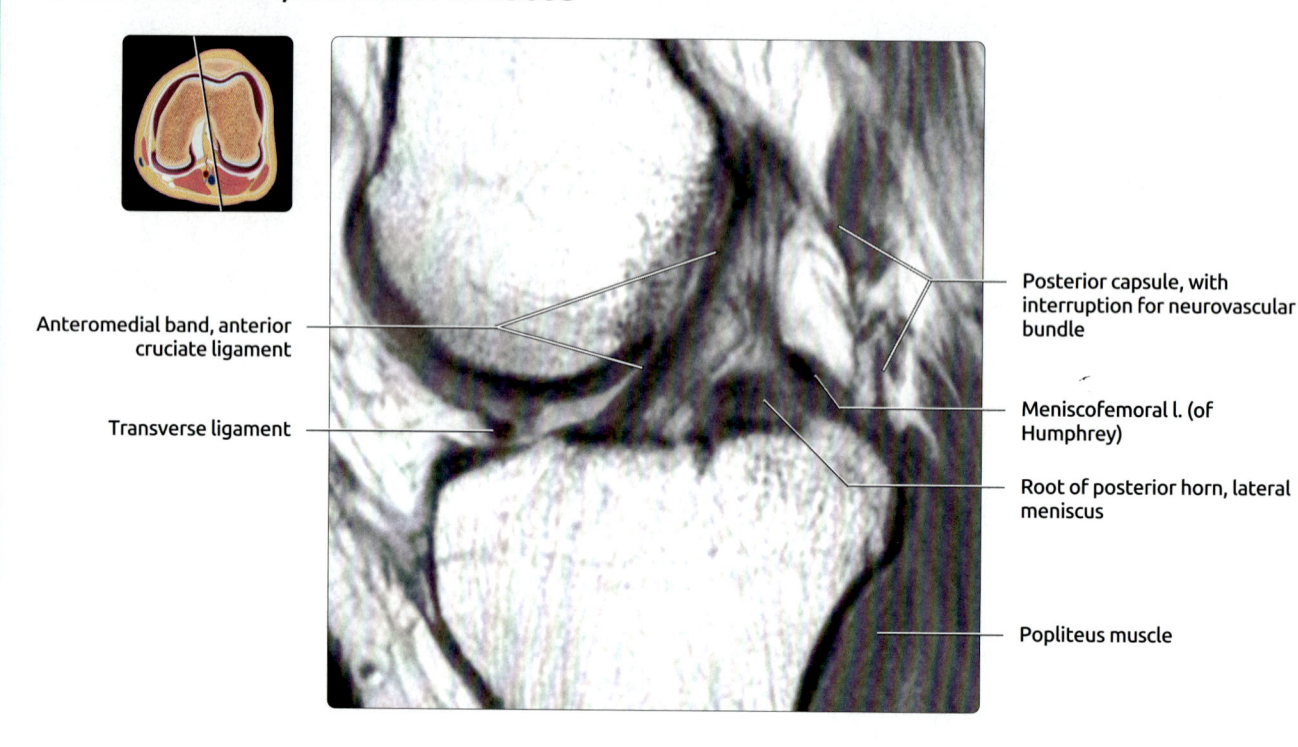

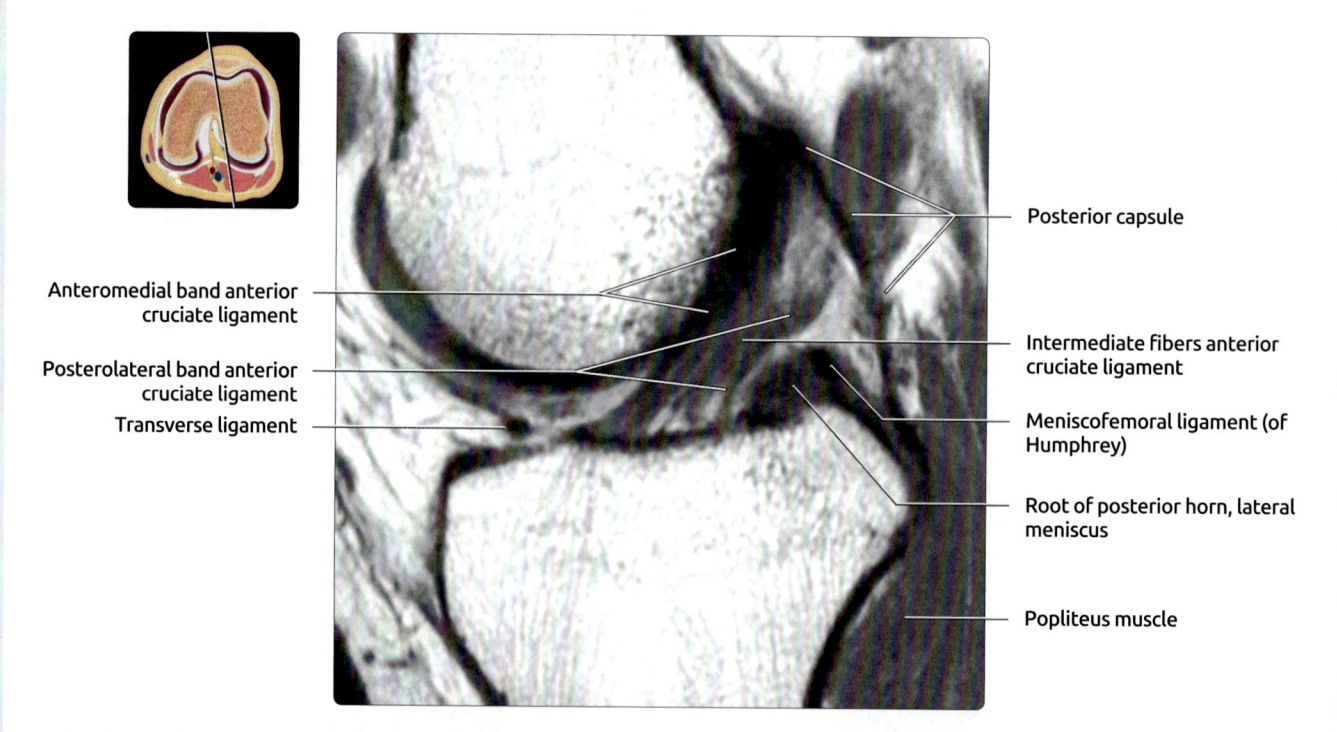

Top image labels:
- Anteromedial band, anterior cruciate ligament
- Transverse ligament
- Posterior capsule, with interruption for neurovascular bundle
- Meniscofemoral l. (of Humphrey)
- Root of posterior horn, lateral meniscus
- Popliteus muscle

Bottom image labels:
- Anteromedial band anterior cruciate ligament
- Posterolateral band anterior cruciate ligament
- Transverse ligament
- Posterior capsule
- Intermediate fibers anterior cruciate ligament
- Meniscofemoral ligament (of Humphrey)
- Root of posterior horn, lateral meniscus
- Popliteus muscle

(Top) First of 8 sagittal PD MR images through the lateral compartment shows the mid portion of the intercondylar notch. Note the meniscofemoral ligament approaching the posterior horn lateral meniscus. **(Bottom)** At the lateral aspect of intercondylar notch, the meniscofemoral ligament joins the posterior horn lateral meniscus near its root. This attachment may be misinterpreted as a torn meniscus. Note that, due to the obliquity with which sagittal sequences are routinely obtained, it is not uncommon to see the transverse ligament anteriorly as well as the root of the posterior horn for several cuts before the root of the anterior horn of the lateral meniscus is seen. The root of the lateral meniscal anterior horn arises lateral to the origin of the anterior cruciate ligament from the tibia; therefore we should not expect to see it in these images.

Menisci

SAGITTAL PD MR, LATERAL MENISCUS

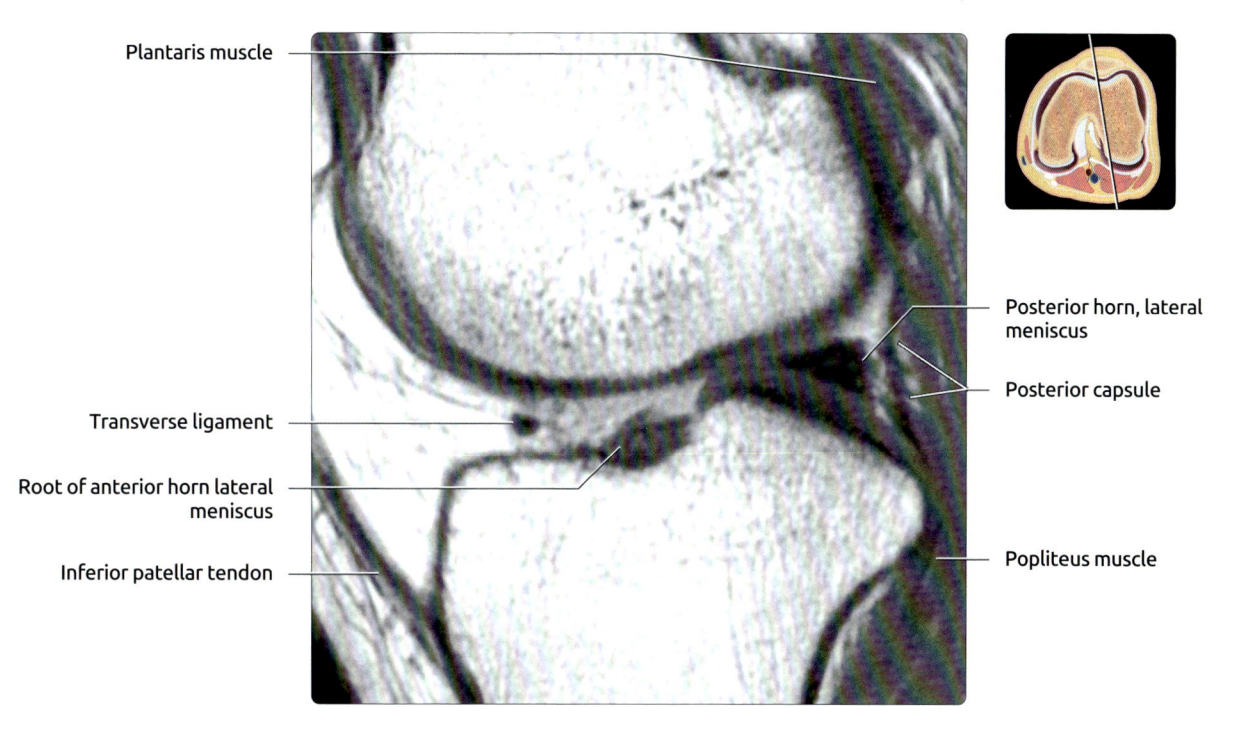

Top image labels:
- Plantaris muscle
- Transverse ligament
- Root of anterior horn lateral meniscus
- Inferior patellar tendon
- Posterior horn, lateral meniscus
- Posterior capsule
- Popliteus muscle

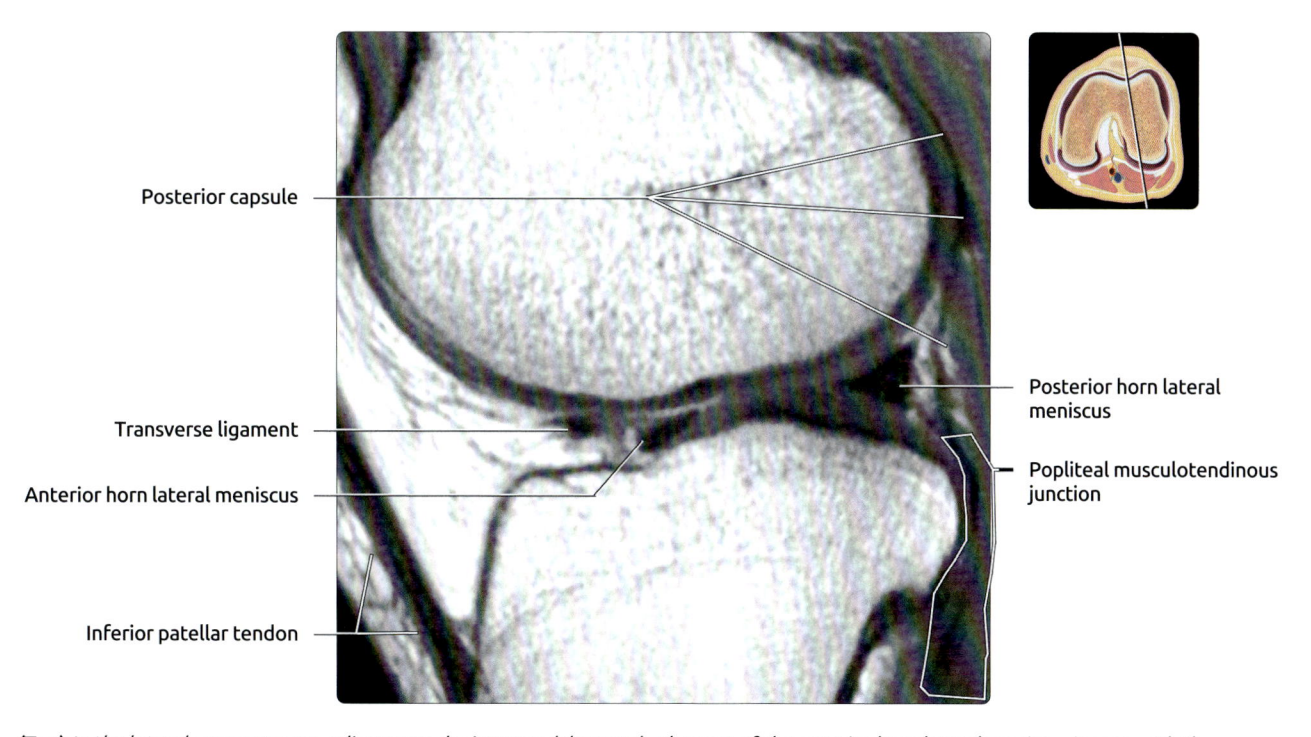

Bottom image labels:
- Posterior capsule
- Transverse ligament
- Anterior horn lateral meniscus
- Inferior patellar tendon
- Posterior horn lateral meniscus
- Popliteal musculotendinous junction

(Top) In the lateral compartment, adjacent to the intercondylar notch, the root of the anterior horn lateral meniscus is seen with the transverse ligament approaching it. (Bottom) In the adjacent, slightly more lateral, image, the transverse ligament more closely approaches the anterior horn of lateral meniscus. Note that in both of these cuts, the posterior horn of the lateral meniscus blends in directly to the posterior capsule. In these cuts the popliteus muscle (top) and popliteal musculotendinous junction (bottom) are extra-articular. This far posterior region is the only portion of the lateral meniscus which directly attaches to the posterior capsule and is not interrupted by the popliteal hiatus.

Menisci

SAGITTAL PD MR, LATERAL MENISCUS

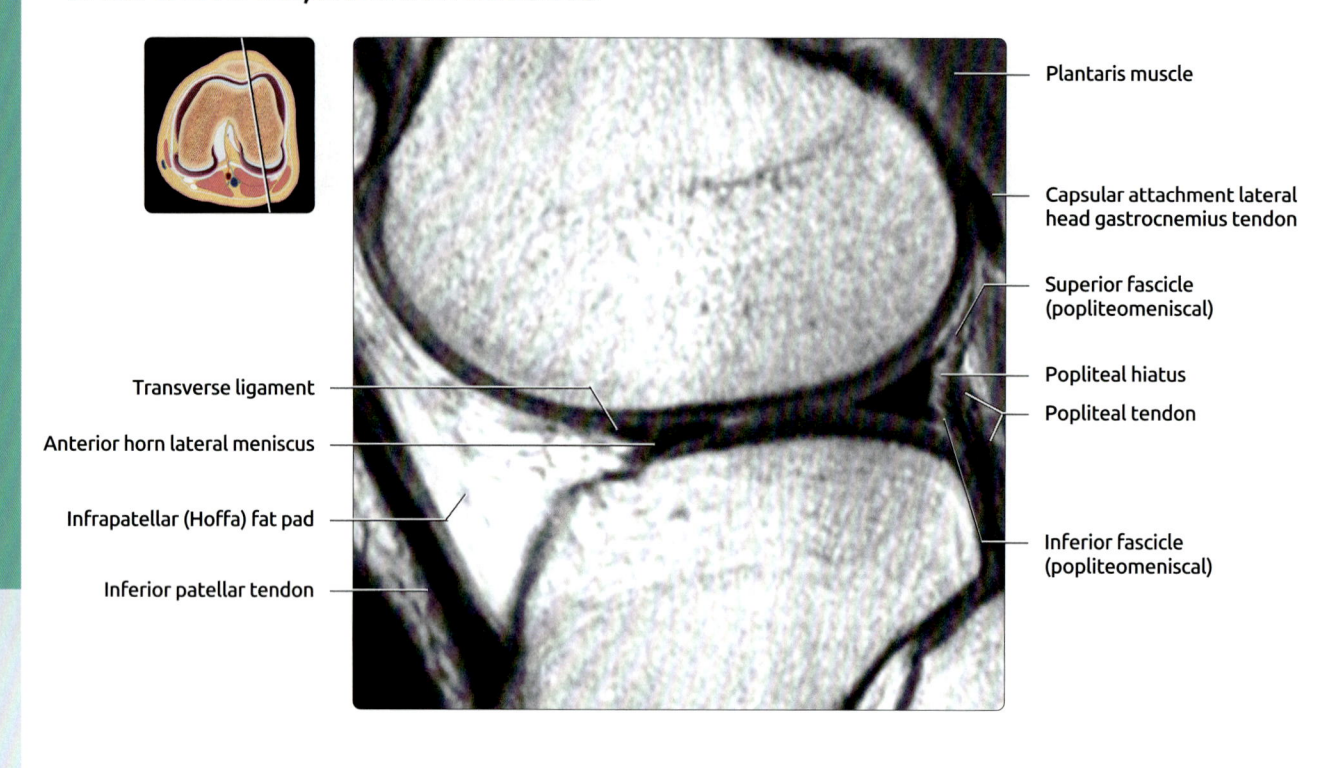

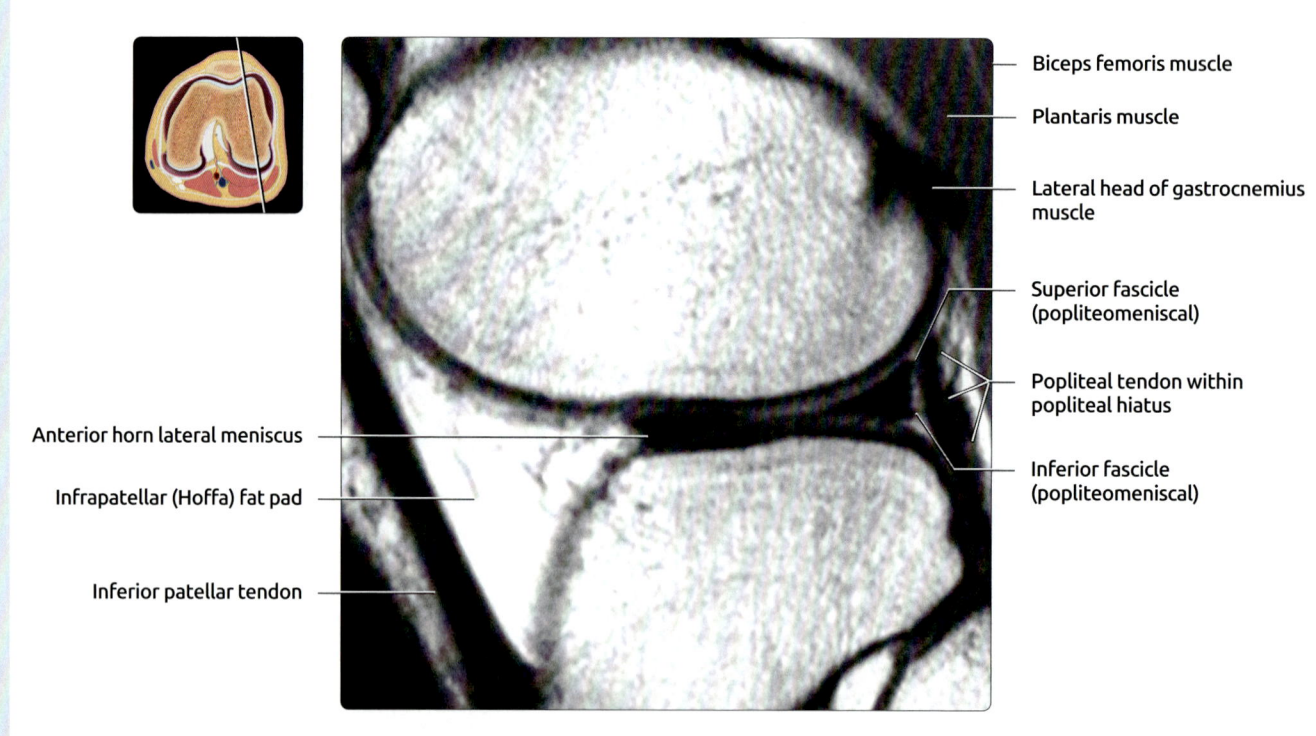

Labels (top image): Plantaris muscle; Capsular attachment lateral head gastrocnemius tendon; Superior fascicle (popliteomeniscal); Popliteal hiatus; Popliteal tendon; Inferior fascicle (popliteomeniscal); Transverse ligament; Anterior horn lateral meniscus; Infrapatellar (Hoffa) fat pad; Inferior patellar tendon

Labels (bottom image): Biceps femoris muscle; Plantaris muscle; Lateral head of gastrocnemius muscle; Superior fascicle (popliteomeniscal); Popliteal tendon within popliteal hiatus; Inferior fascicle (popliteomeniscal); Anterior horn lateral meniscus; Infrapatellar (Hoffa) fat pad; Inferior patellar tendon

(Top) *Image through the lateral compartment shows the transverse ligament joining the anterior horn lateral meniscus. Posteriorly, the popliteal tendon is seen within the popliteal hiatus. This structure is intraarticular but extrasynovial. The superior fascicle extends from the superior aspect of the posterior horn lateral meniscus to the paratenon of the popliteal tendon and on to the capsule, forming the roof of the popliteal hiatus. The inferior fascicle extends from the inferior aspect of the posterior horn lateral meniscus towards the popliteal tendon but is interrupted by the tendon's passage into the extraarticular position of the musculotendinous junction.* (Bottom) *The adjacent more lateral cut shows a similar relationship of the fascicles, with the superior extending to the popliteal tendon and capsule, and the inferior fascicle being interrupted.*

Menisci

SAGITTAL PD MR, LATERAL MENISCUS

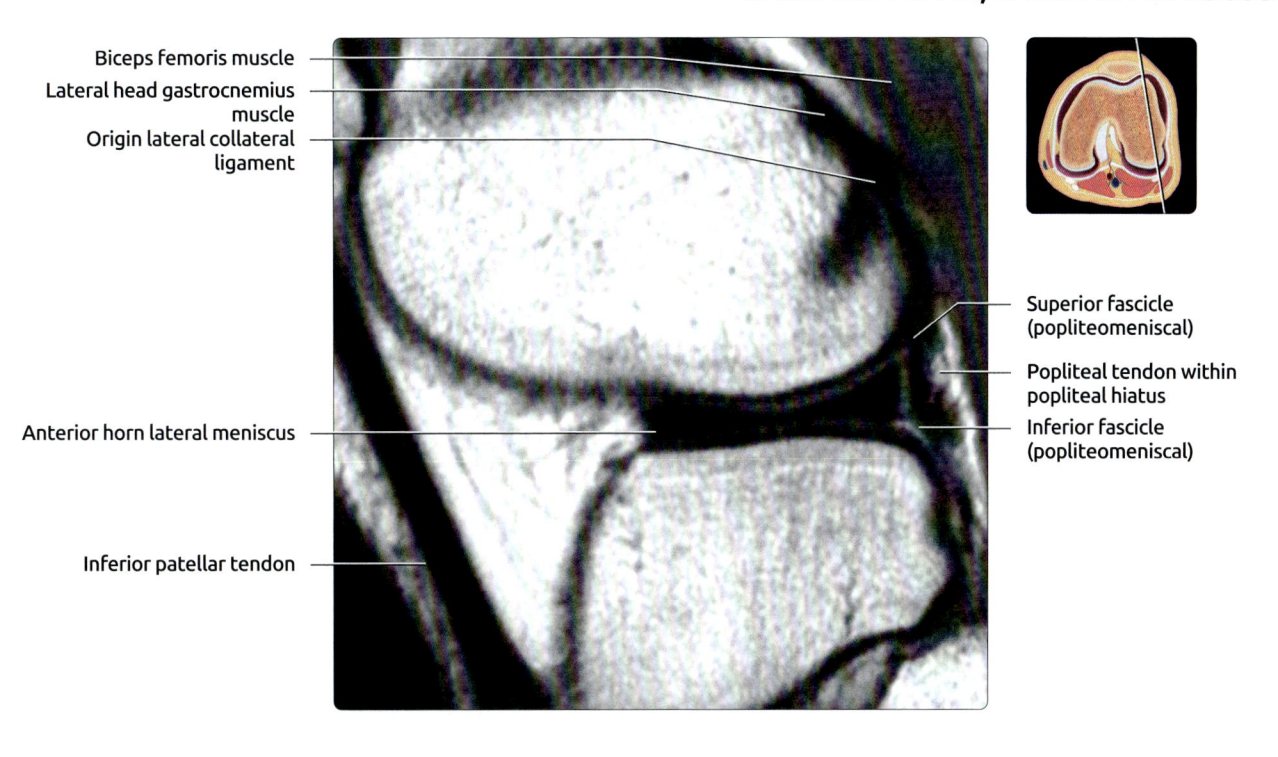

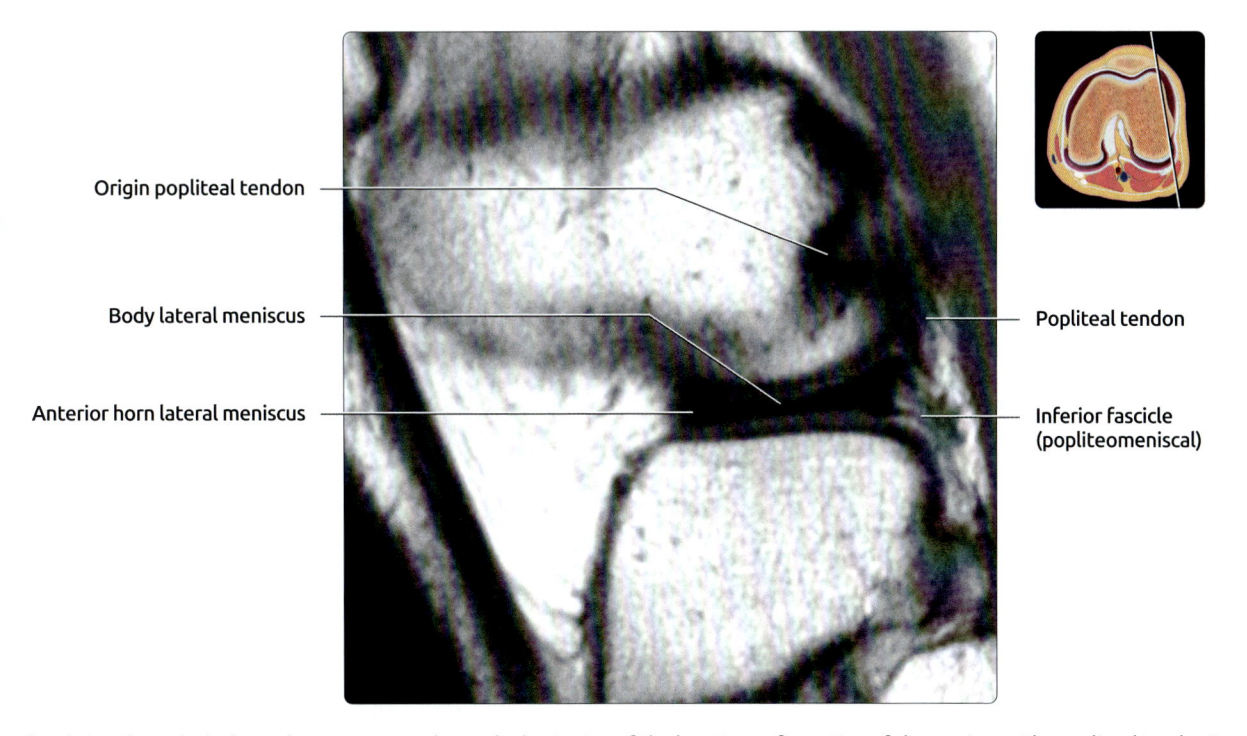

(Top) Cut through the lateral compartment shows the beginning of the bowtie configuration of the meniscus. The popliteal tendon is within the hiatus, outlined superiorly by the superior popliteomeniscal fascicle and inferiorly by the inferior popliteomeniscal fascicle. *(Bottom)* Farther laterally, the bowtie configuration of the lateral meniscus is complete. The origin of the popliteus tendon (located just anteriorly and inferiorly to the origin of the lateral collateral ligament on the lateral femoral condyle) is seen. A portion of the popliteal tendon is seen coursing towards its intraarticular position in the popliteal hiatus. The superior popliteomeniscal fascicle has not yet formed as the popliteal tendon passes the superior portion of the posterior horn but the inferior popliteomeniscal fascicle clearly forms the floor of the hiatus.

Menisci

GRAPHICS, CORONAL MENISCI

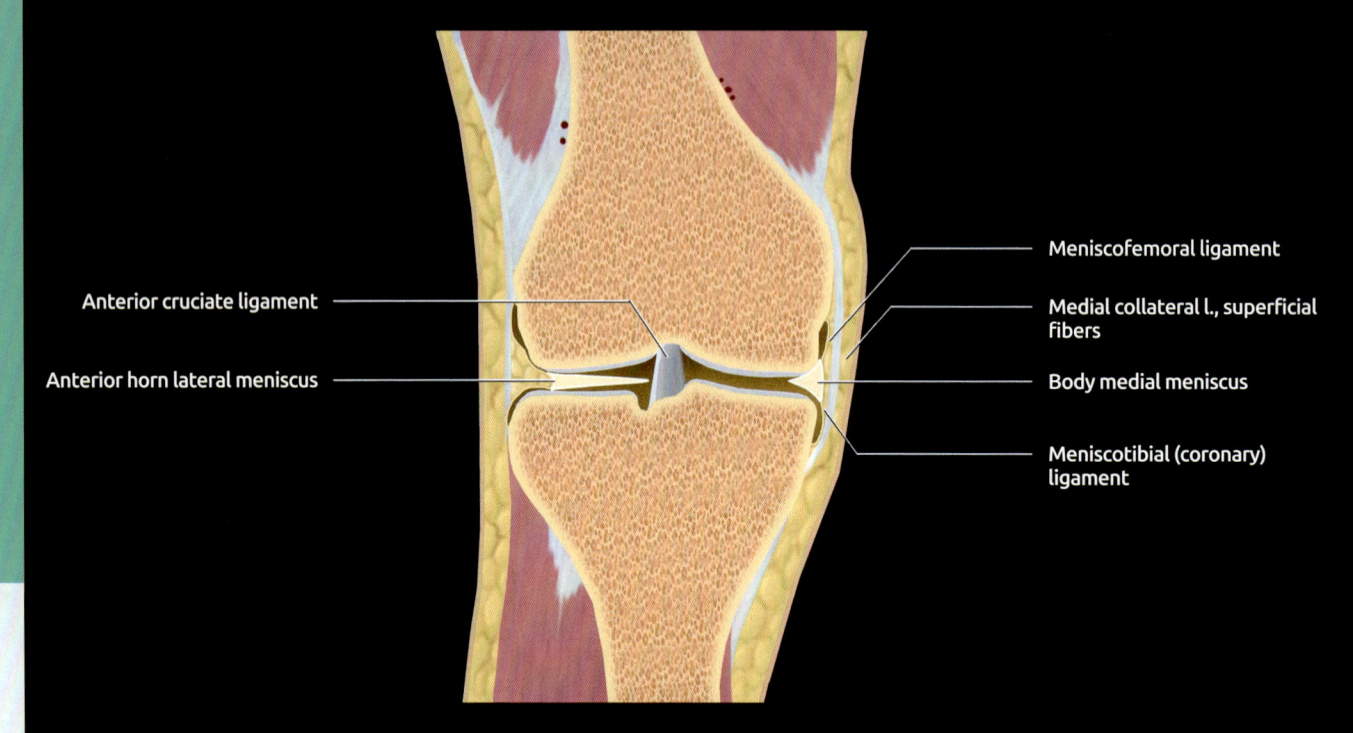

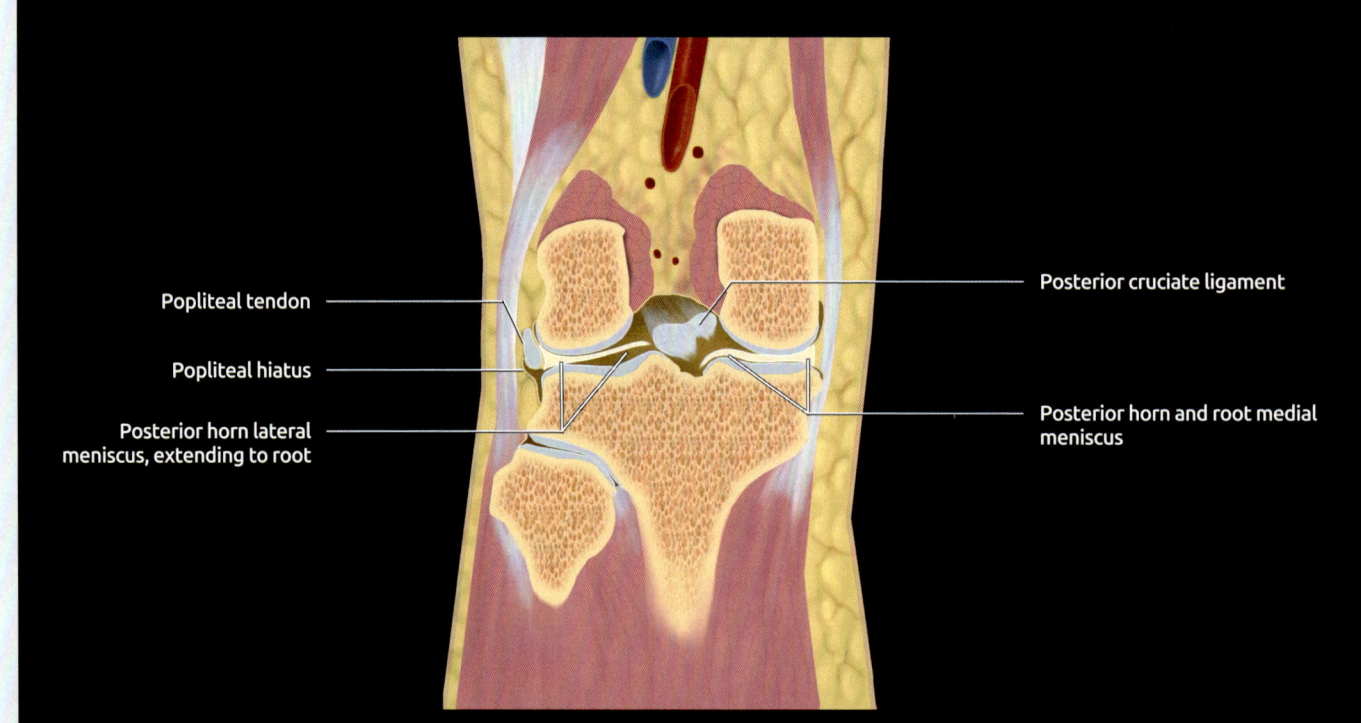

Anterior cruciate ligament

Anterior horn lateral meniscus

Meniscofemoral ligament

Medial collateral l., superficial fibers

Body medial meniscus

Meniscotibial (coronary) ligament

Popliteal tendon

Popliteal hiatus

Posterior horn lateral meniscus, extending to root

Posterior cruciate ligament

Posterior horn and root medial meniscus

(Top) Coronal graphic through the anterior/mid knee joint, shows the anterior horn near the root of the LM. The same cut shows the body of the MM, which is short and shaped as an equilateral triangle. The deep fibers of the medial collateral ligament arise from the body of the MM; the meniscofemoral ligament inserts either on the femoral condyle or the superficial medial collateral ligament while the meniscotibial (coronary) ligament inserts on the tibia. (Bottom) Coronal graphic more posteriorly shows the roots of the posterior horns of both the medial and lateral menisci. The popliteal tendon is also seen coursing through the hiatus adjacent to the body/posterior horn of the LM.

Menisci

CORONAL T2 FS MR, MENISCI

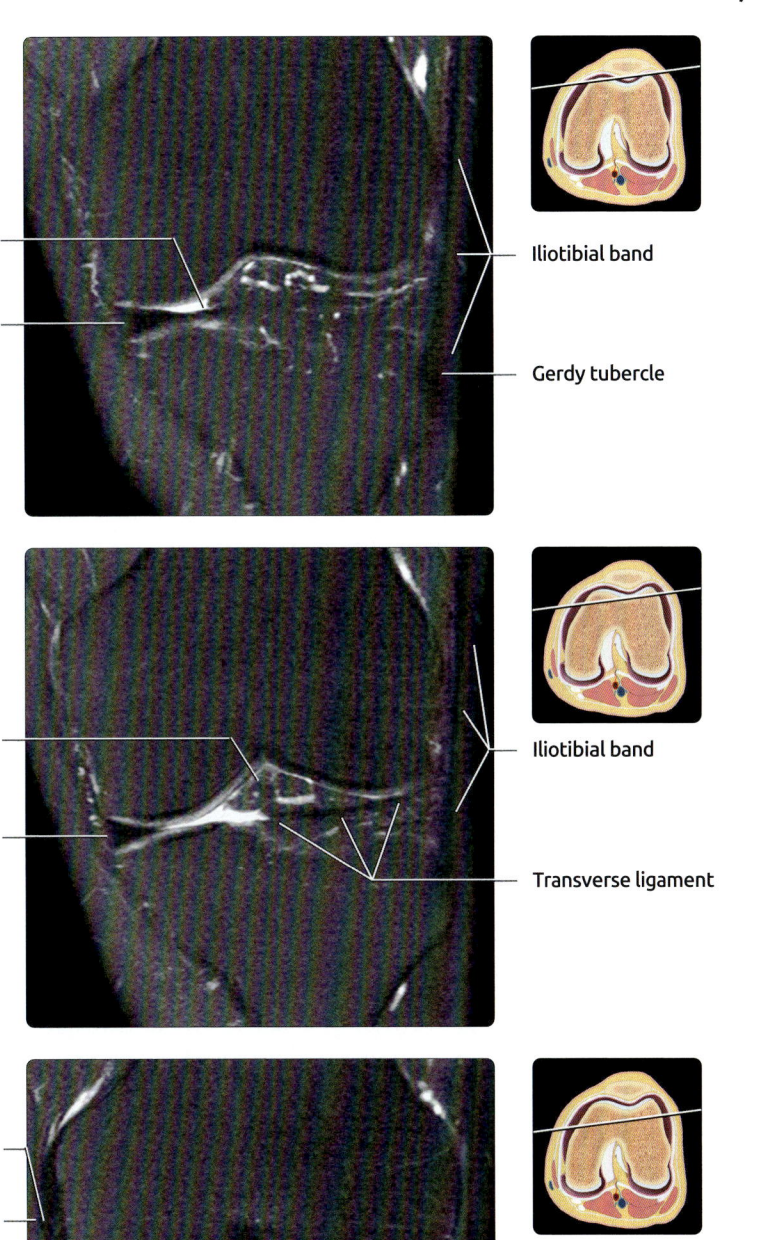

Root, anterior horn medial meniscus, extending into transverse ligament

Anterior horn, medial meniscus

Iliotibial band

Gerdy tubercle

Infrapatellar fat pad

Anterior horn, medial meniscus

Iliotibial band

Transverse ligament

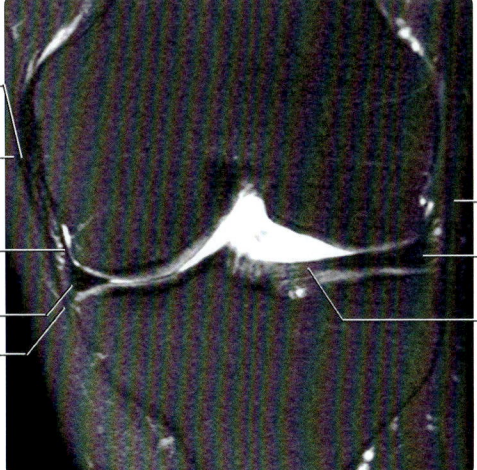

Superficial fibers, medial collateral l. (layer 2 of medial complex)

Medial patellofemoral l./retinaculum (layer 1 of medial complex)

Meniscofemoral ligament (medial collateral ligament, deep fibers)

Body medial meniscus

Meniscotibial ligament (coronary ligament, medial collateral ligament deep fibers)

Iliotibial band

Anterior horn lateral meniscus

Root, anterior horn lateral meniscus

(Top) First of 9 coronal T2 FS MR images presented from anterior to posterior. Anterior cut shows that anterior horn medial meniscus is located anterior to anterior horn lateral meniscus. This appearance is due to the obliquity of the coronal images. Transverse ligament extends from anterior horn medial meniscus towards anterior horn lateral meniscus. (Middle) Transverse ligament is seen extending towards anterior horn LM which itself is not yet visible due to the obliquity of the image. (Bottom) Root of anterior horn lateral meniscus is several mm posterior to that of medial meniscus. By this cut, medial meniscus is transforming from anterior horn to body. One can see that in the mid portion of knee there is separation between layer 2 and 3 of medial supporting structures (superficial and deep fibers of medial collateral ligament, respectively). Deep fibers consist of the meniscofemoral ligament, extending from the body of the meniscus to the superficial medial collateral ligament, and meniscotibial (coronary) ligament.

Menisci

CORONAL T2 FS MR, MENISCI

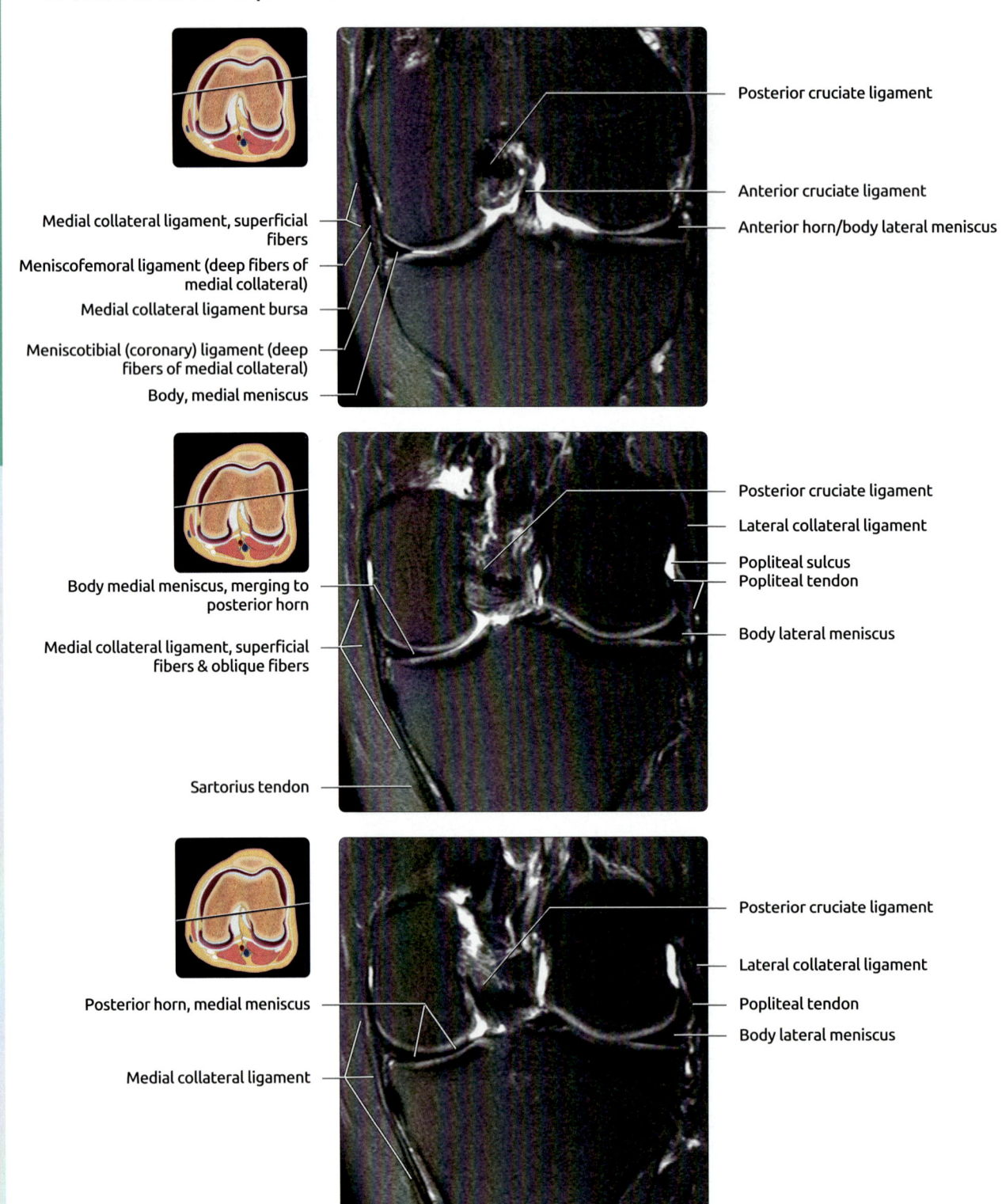

Labels (top image):
- Medial collateral ligament, superficial fibers
- Meniscofemoral ligament (deep fibers of medial collateral)
- Medial collateral ligament bursa
- Meniscotibial (coronary) ligament (deep fibers of medial collateral)
- Body, medial meniscus
- Posterior cruciate ligament
- Anterior cruciate ligament
- Anterior horn/body lateral meniscus

Labels (middle image):
- Body medial meniscus, merging to posterior horn
- Medial collateral ligament, superficial fibers & oblique fibers
- Sartorius tendon
- Posterior cruciate ligament
- Lateral collateral ligament
- Popliteal sulcus
- Popliteal tendon
- Body lateral meniscus

Labels (bottom image):
- Posterior horn, medial meniscus
- Medial collateral ligament
- Posterior cruciate ligament
- Lateral collateral ligament
- Popliteal tendon
- Body lateral meniscus

(**Top**) *Coronal cut through the mid joint shows the body of the medial meniscus to be the smallest, approaching an equilateral triangle in shape. The anterior cruciate ligament is reliably seen in this mid cut, as are both the deep and superficial layers of the medial collateral ligament.* (**Middle**) *In a cut that is slightly more posterior, note the deep and superficial layers of the medial collateral ligament merge together. On the lateral side, the popliteal tendon is seen at its origin, extending towards the joint line. The body of the lateral meniscus is still firmly attached to the capsule.* (**Bottom**) *Even more posteriorly, the medial meniscus is transforming to its posterior horn. On the lateral side, the popliteal tendon is seen entering the joint superiorly to the body of the lateral meniscus, at the beginning of the popliteal hiatus.*

Menisci

CORONAL T2 FS MR, MENISCI

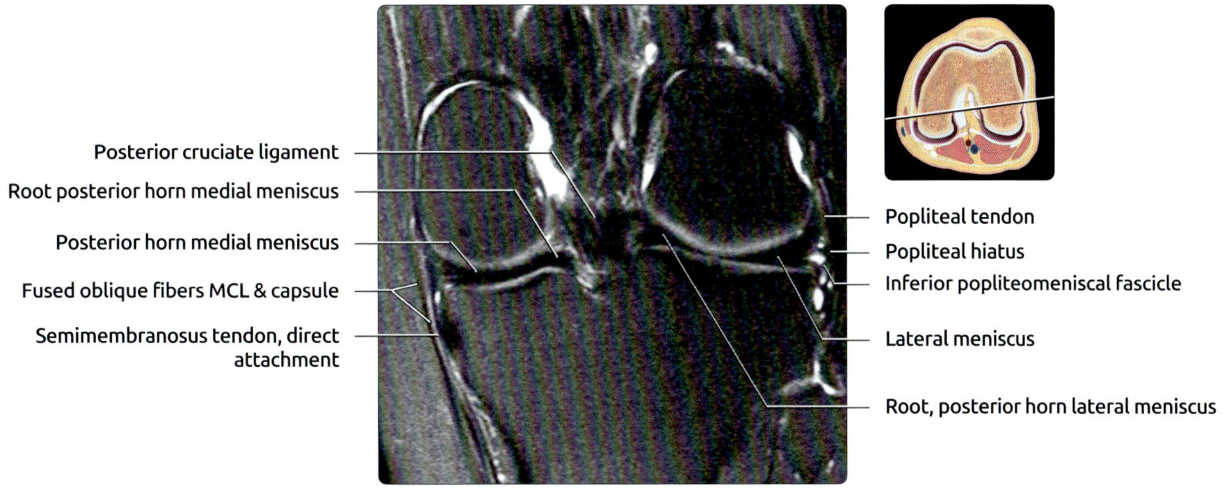

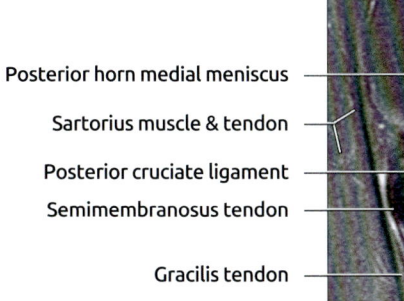

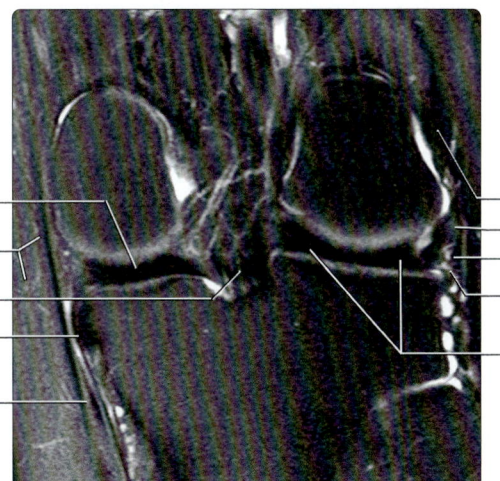

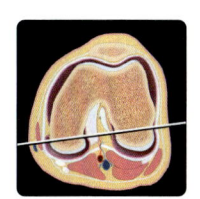

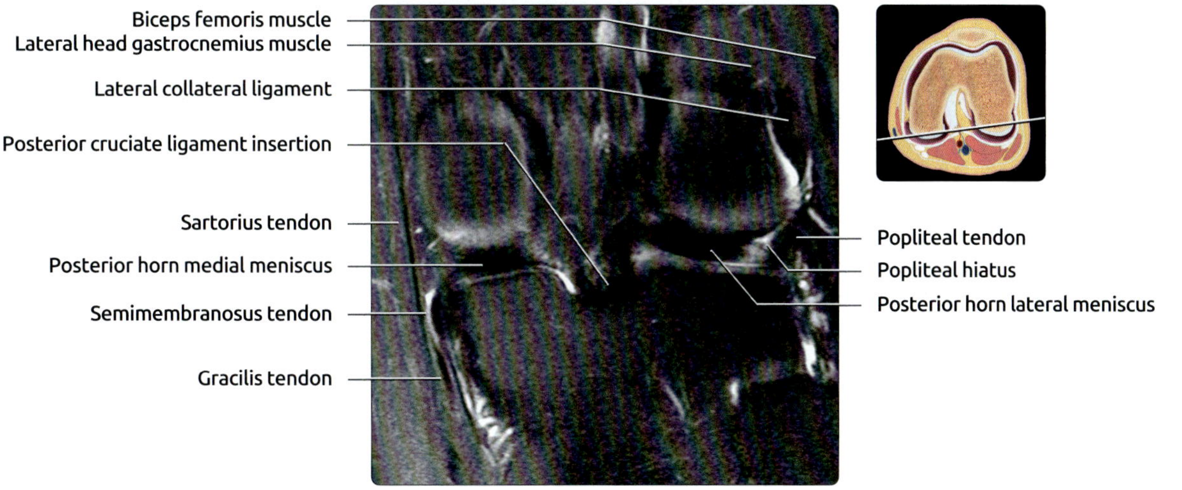

Posterior cruciate ligament
Root posterior horn medial meniscus
Posterior horn medial meniscus
Fused oblique fibers MCL & capsule
Semimembranosus tendon, direct attachment

Popliteal tendon
Popliteal hiatus
Inferior popliteomeniscal fascicle
Lateral meniscus
Root, posterior horn lateral meniscus

Posterior horn medial meniscus
Sartorius muscle & tendon
Posterior cruciate ligament
Semimembranosus tendon
Gracilis tendon

Lateral collateral ligament
Popliteal tendon
Popliteal hiatus
Inferior popliteomeniscal fascicle
Posterior horn lateral meniscus

Biceps femoris muscle
Lateral head gastrocnemius muscle
Lateral collateral ligament
Posterior cruciate ligament insertion
Sartorius tendon
Posterior horn medial meniscus
Semimembranosus tendon
Gracilis tendon

Popliteal tendon
Popliteal hiatus
Posterior horn lateral meniscus

(Top) *Posteriorly in the joint, but anterior to the posterior cruciate ligament nearing its insertion, the posterior meniscal roots are found. Medially, the medial collateral ligament has merged with the capsule. Laterally, the popliteal tendon enters the articular space by way of the popliteal hiatus.* **(Middle)** *The popliteal hiatus becomes more prominent as the tendon extends posteriorly and downward. The inferior popliteomeniscal fascicle forms the floor of the popliteal hiatus at this point.* **(Bottom)** *At the posterior extent of the intraarticular portion of the knee joint, the popliteal tendon crosses in its downward and posterior course to its musculotendinous junction. The hiatus is prominent here, and must not be mistaken for a tear in the posterior horn lateral meniscus. Both posterior horns are seen this far posteriorly, beyond their roots (which are located more anteriorly).*

Menisci

VARIANT: DISCOID MENISCUS

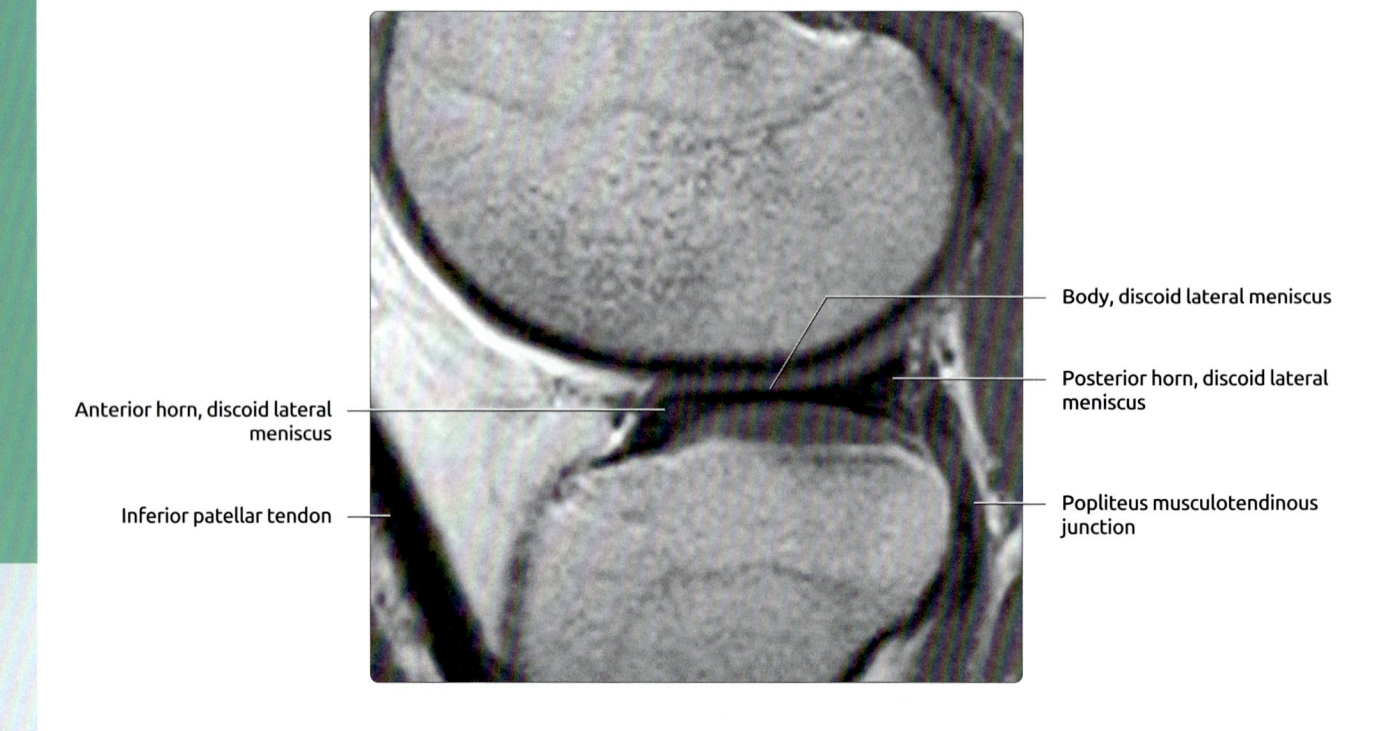

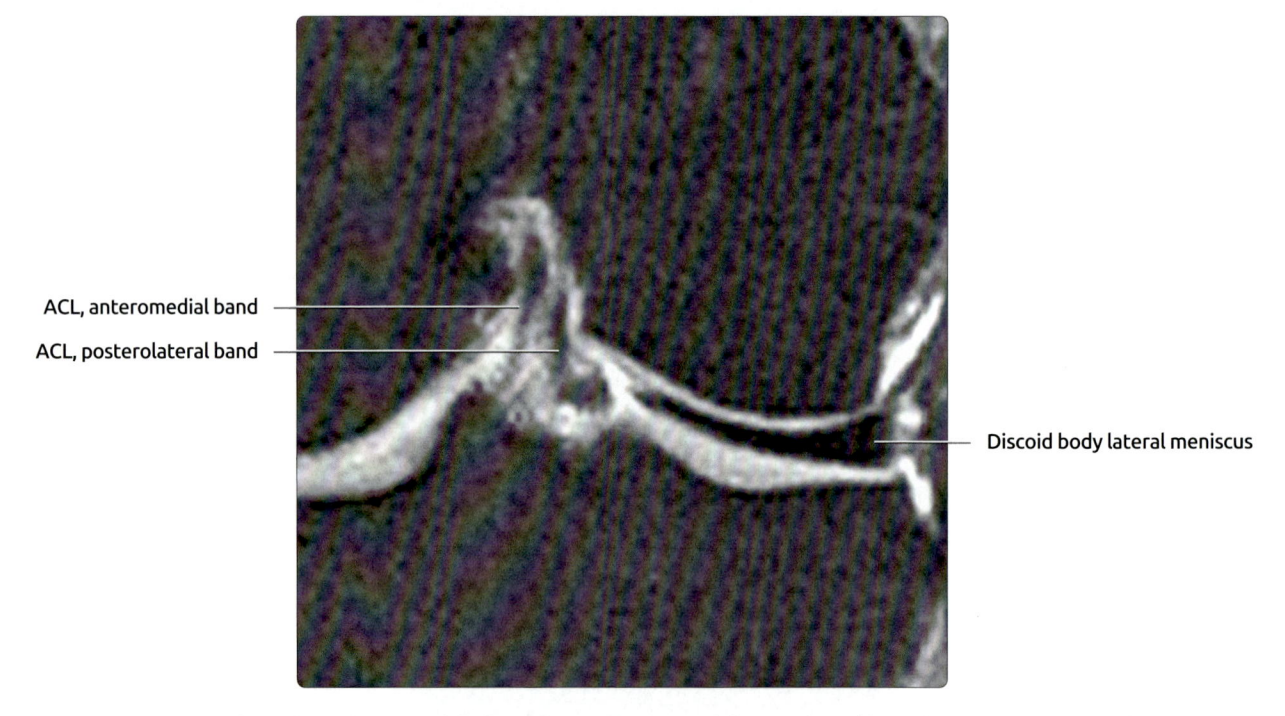

Body, discoid lateral meniscus

Posterior horn, discoid lateral meniscus

Anterior horn, discoid lateral meniscus

Popliteus musculotendinous junction

Inferior patellar tendon

ACL, anteromedial band

ACL, posterolateral band

Discoid body lateral meniscus

(Top) Sagittal image is from the mid portion of the lateral compartment, and shows a discoid lateral meniscus. Note that the meniscus is seen with all 3 portions, the anterior horn, body, and posterior horn. This bowtie appearance should be seen only in the outer portion of the joint. The fact that the fibula is not seen, as well as that the popliteus musculotendinous junction (rather than just the popliteus tendon) and patellar tendon are both in this image indicates that the location is far too interior in the joint for a normal body of meniscus to be seen. Thus, the body of the meniscus is too large, indicating the discoid variant. (Bottom) Coronal image through the mid portion of the joint (as indicated by the morphology and presence of the ACL) shows the body of the lateral meniscus to be too large, confirming that it is discoid.

Menisci

ARTHROGRAM: DISTENDED JOINT SHOWING POSTERIOR MENISCAL ATTACHMENTS

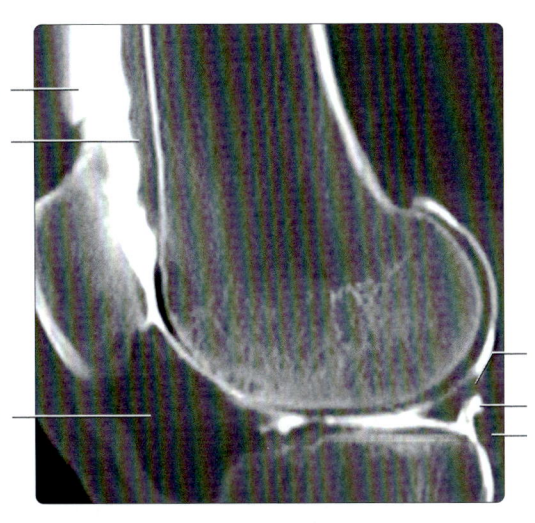

Labels (top image): Suprapatellar bursa; Posterior suprapatellar (prefemoral) fat pad; Infrapatellar (Hoffa) fat pad; Superior popliteomeniscal fascicle; Popliteal hiatus; Popliteal tendon.

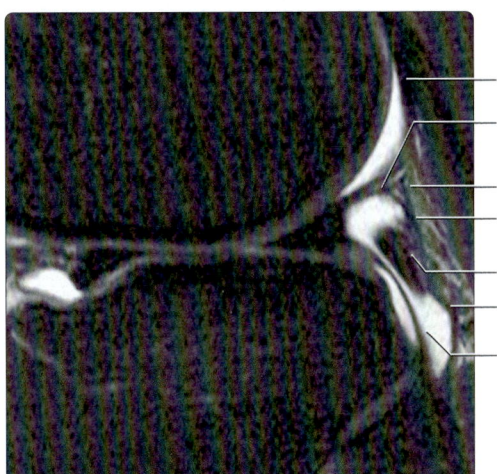

Labels (middle image): Posterior capsule; Meniscocapsular portion superior fascicle; Oblique (medial) arcuate l.; Superior fascicle (meniscopopliteal ligament); Popliteal tendon; Popliteofibular ligament; Inferior fascicle (popliteomeniscal ligament).

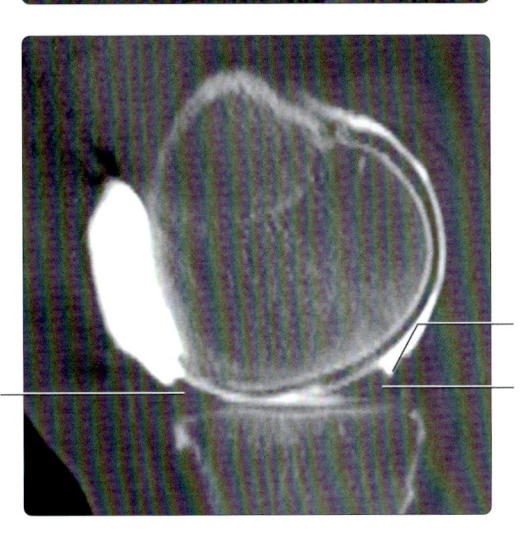

Labels (bottom image): Anterior horn medial meniscus; Superior recess posterior horn medial meniscus; Posterior horn medial meniscus.

(Top) Reformatted sagittal image through the lateral compartment in a CT arthrogram. Note that with distension of the joint by contrast, continuum of the joint fluid with the popliteal hiatus is readily seen. The superior popliteomeniscal fascicle, extending between the posterior horn lateral meniscus and the popliteal paratenon, is outlined by fluid. (Middle) MR arthrogram shows distended popliteal hiatus and outlines both the superior and inferior meniscopopliteal fascicles (struts) as well as the popliteal tendon. The popliteofibular and arcuate ligaments are seen well. (Bottom) Reformatted sagittal image through medial compartment in a CT arthrogram shows the superior recess of the posterior horn medial meniscus. This should not be mistaken for a peripheral meniscal tear or meniscocapsular separation. Note that cartilage width varies over the femoral condyle (thicker posteriorly).

Menisci

MENISCOFEMORAL LIGAMENT

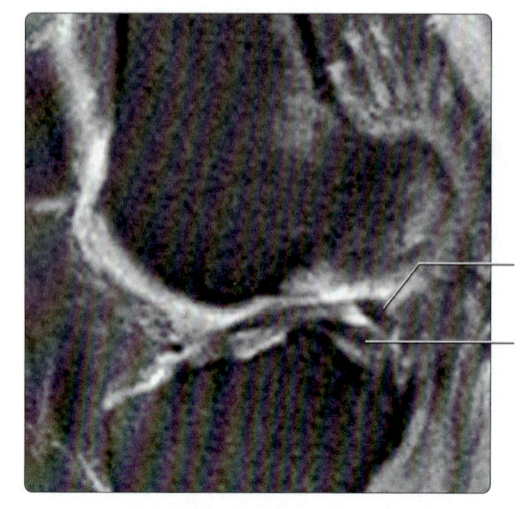

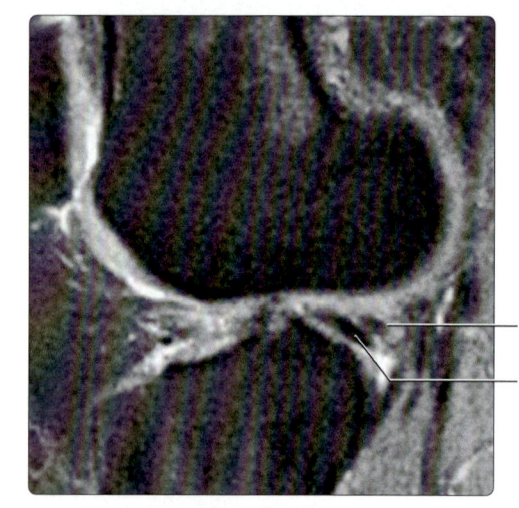

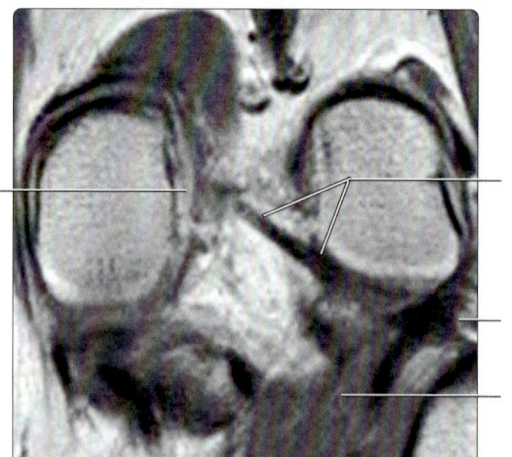

(Top) First of 3 images depicting the meniscofemoral ligament of Wrisberg. This sagittal image is slightly lateral to the intercondylar notch and the root of posterior horn lateral meniscus. The meniscofemoral ligament is distinctly separate from meniscus. (Middle) Approaching the intercondylar notch and the root of posterior horn lateral meniscus, the meniscofemoral ligament more closely approaches the lateral meniscus to merge with it. It is at this point that a tear of the posterior horn could be mistakenly diagnosed. (Bottom) Coronal image located posteriorly in the joint shows the meniscofemoral ligament of Wrisberg over nearly its entire extent, originating at the medial femoral condyle in the intertrochanteric notch and merging with the posterior horn lateral meniscus.

Menisci

VARIANTS: LARGE TRANSVERSE LIGAMENT & MENISCOCRUCIATE LIGAMENT

Transverse ligament
Anterior horn lateral meniscus

Anterior cruciate ligament
Anterior lateral meniscocruciate l.
Anterior root lateral meniscus

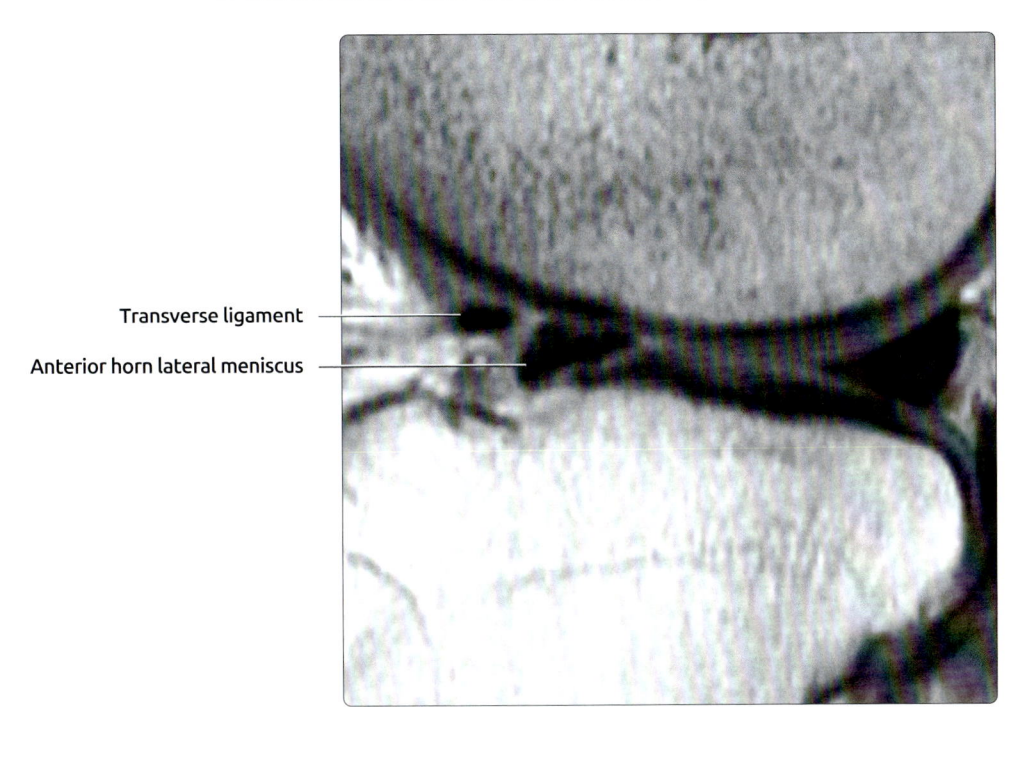

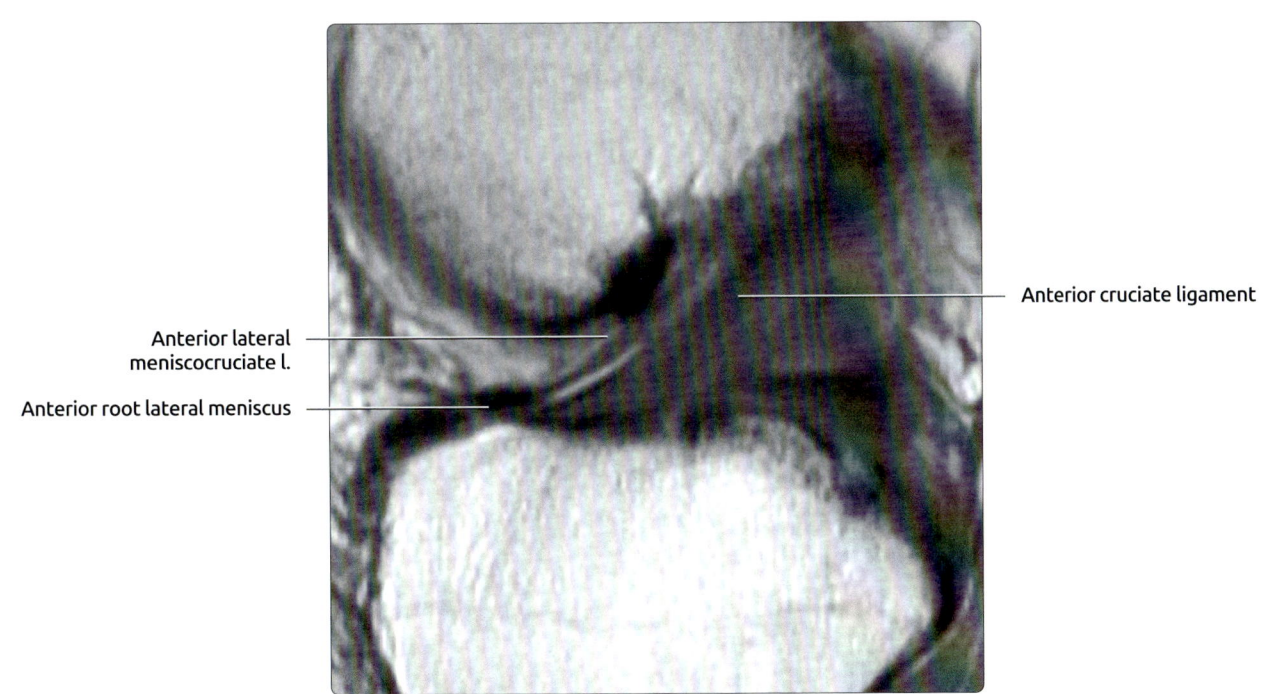

(Top) First of 2 sagittal PD MR images near the intercondylar notch, lateral to medial, shows a large transverse ligament. This ligament connects the 2 anterior meniscal horns and is seen in cross section on sagittal images. It could possibly be confused for a meniscal tear as it merges with the lateral meniscus, closer to the notch. The ligament is generally smaller than this, or may be absent. (Bottom) Image through the lateral portion of the intercondylar notch shows a discrete structure which parallels the anterior cruciate ligament and extends from the root of the anterior horn lateral meniscus to the lateral femoral condyle. This represents the normal variant, anterior lateral meniscocruciate ligament. It is distinguished from the infrapatellar plica (which can also parallel the ACL in the same manner) by its site of origin at the meniscus rather than the patella.

Menisci

VARIANT: MENISCOCRUCIATE LIGAMENT

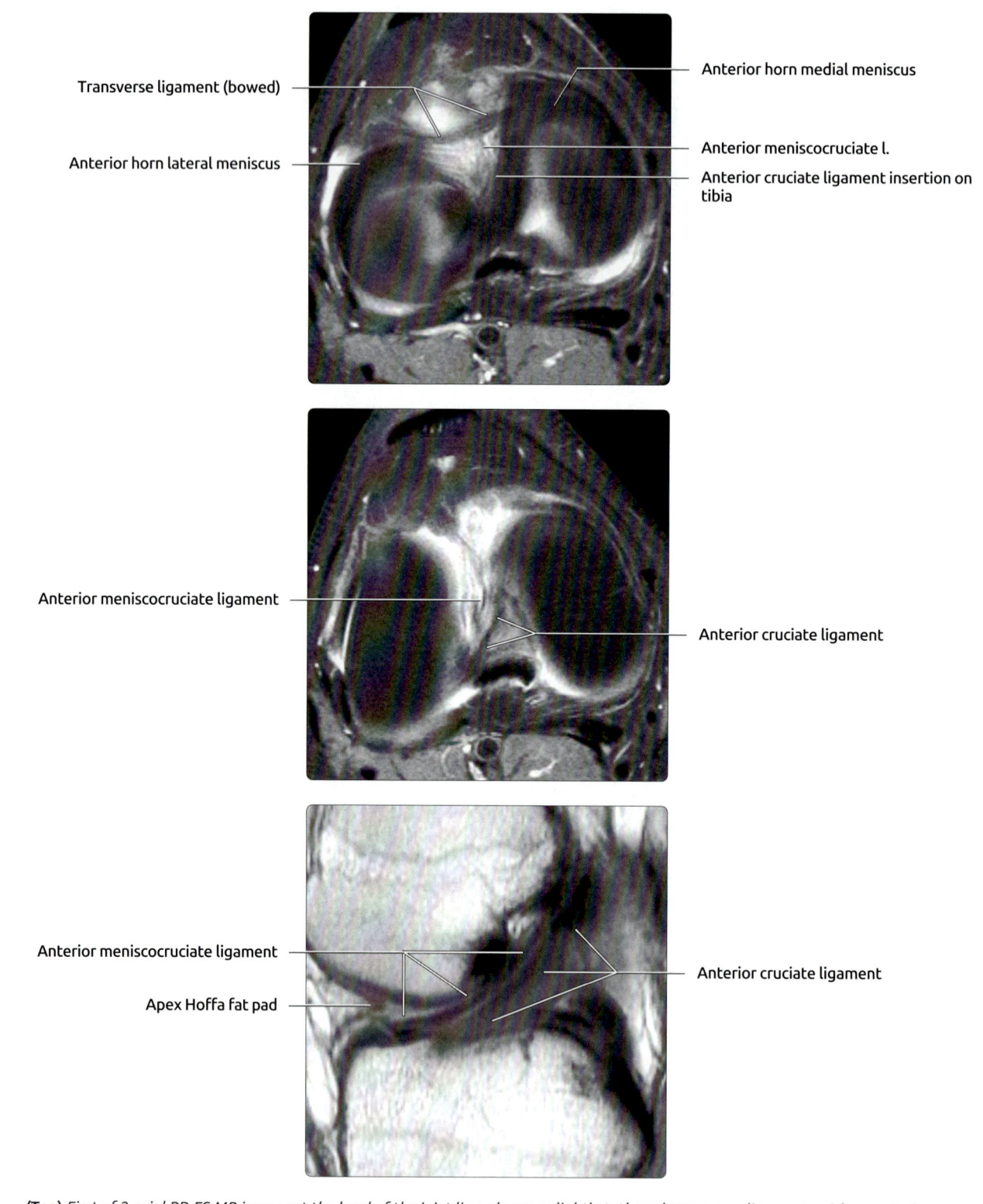

Labels (top image): Transverse ligament (bowed); Anterior horn lateral meniscus; Anterior horn medial meniscus; Anterior meniscocruciate l.; Anterior cruciate ligament insertion on tibia

Labels (middle image): Anterior meniscocruciate ligament; Anterior cruciate ligament

Labels (bottom image): Anterior meniscocruciate ligament; Apex Hoffa fat pad; Anterior cruciate ligament

(Top) *First of 2 axial PD FS MR images at the level of the joint line, shows a slightly tethered transverse ligament, with an anterior meniscocruciate ligament arising from it. Note that the ligament is anterior to the anterior cruciate ligament.* **(Middle)** *This image is slightly higher than the previous image, in the intercondylar notch. The anterior meniscocruciate ligament parallels the anterior cruciate ligament throughout the notch.* **(Bottom)** *Sagittal PD MR image shows the length of the anterior meniscocruciate ligament, paralleling the anterior cruciate ligament. This normal variant should not be mistaken for an intrasubstance tear of the anterior cruciate. Note that the apex of Hoffa fat pad is free of this ligament (not attached as in an infrapatellar plica).*

Menisci

VARIANT: MENISCOCRUCIATE FASCICLES

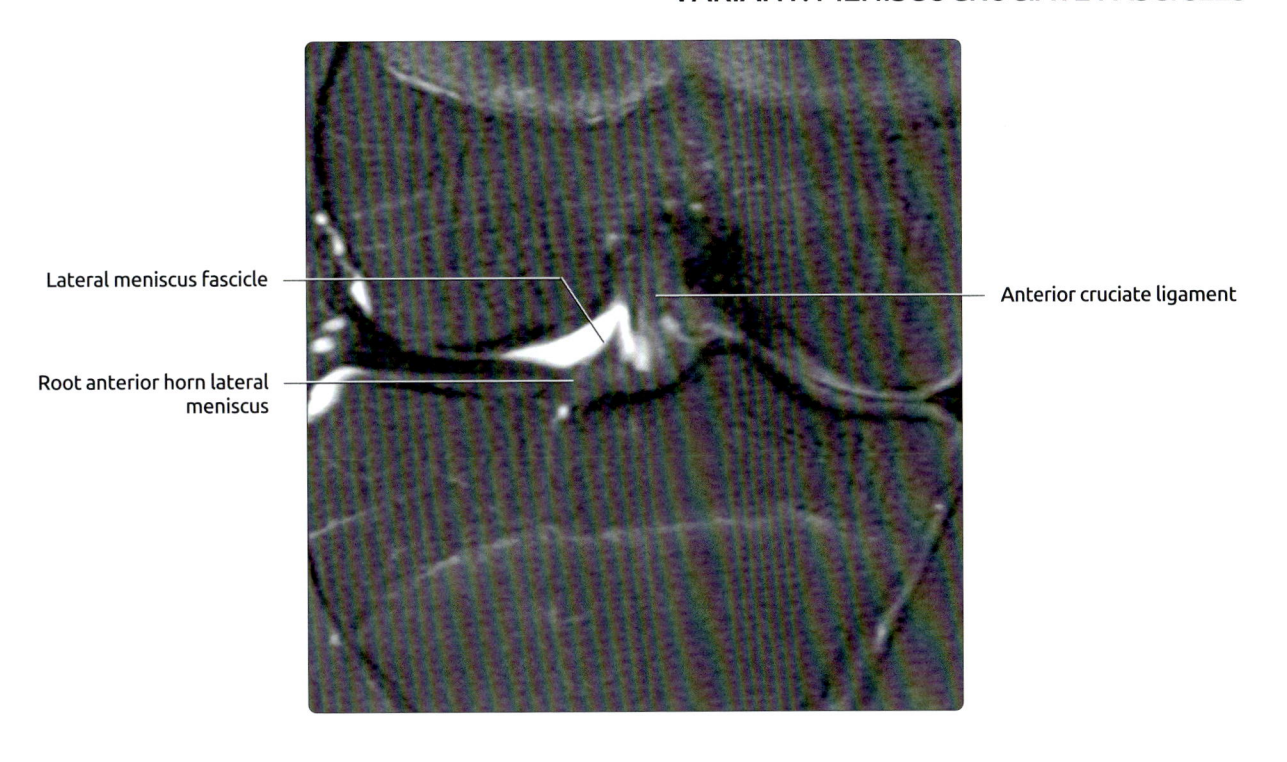

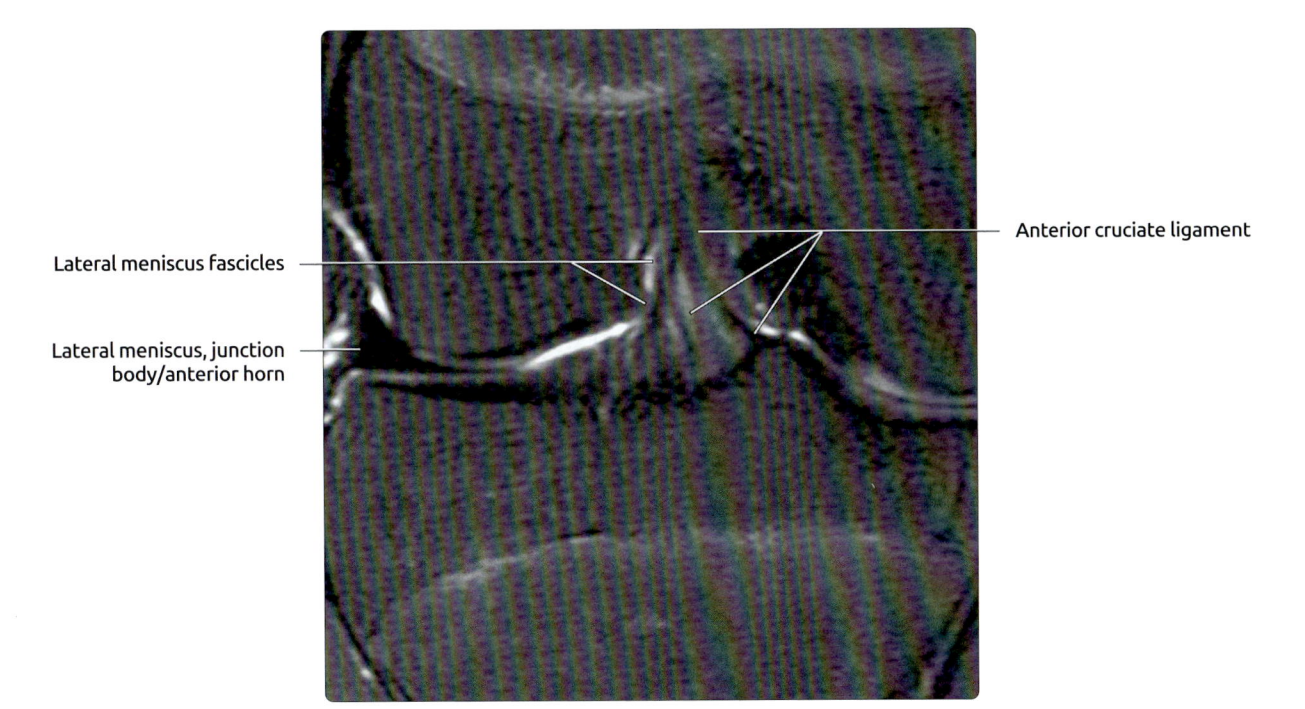

Lateral meniscus fascicle

Root anterior horn lateral meniscus

Anterior cruciate ligament

Lateral meniscus fascicles

Lateral meniscus, junction body/anterior horn

Anterior cruciate ligament

(Top) First of 2 coronal PD FS MR images in the anterior portion of the joint. The transverse ligament in this patient was absent (more anterior cut not shown). The fibers of the anterior horn lateral meniscus, which normally blend into the transverse ligament, instead form discrete lateral meniscal fascicles which ascend towards the anterior cruciate ligament. (Bottom) Coronal image slightly posterior to the previous image shows the lateral meniscal fascicles ascending to intersect the anterior cruciate ligament. These fibers clearly are not part of the anterior cruciate ligament since they ascend at a different angle. This normal variant should not be mistaken for pathology such as a disrupted ACL or a meniscal fragment from a bucket handle tear.

Menisci

VARIANT: MENISCOMENISCAL LIGAMENT

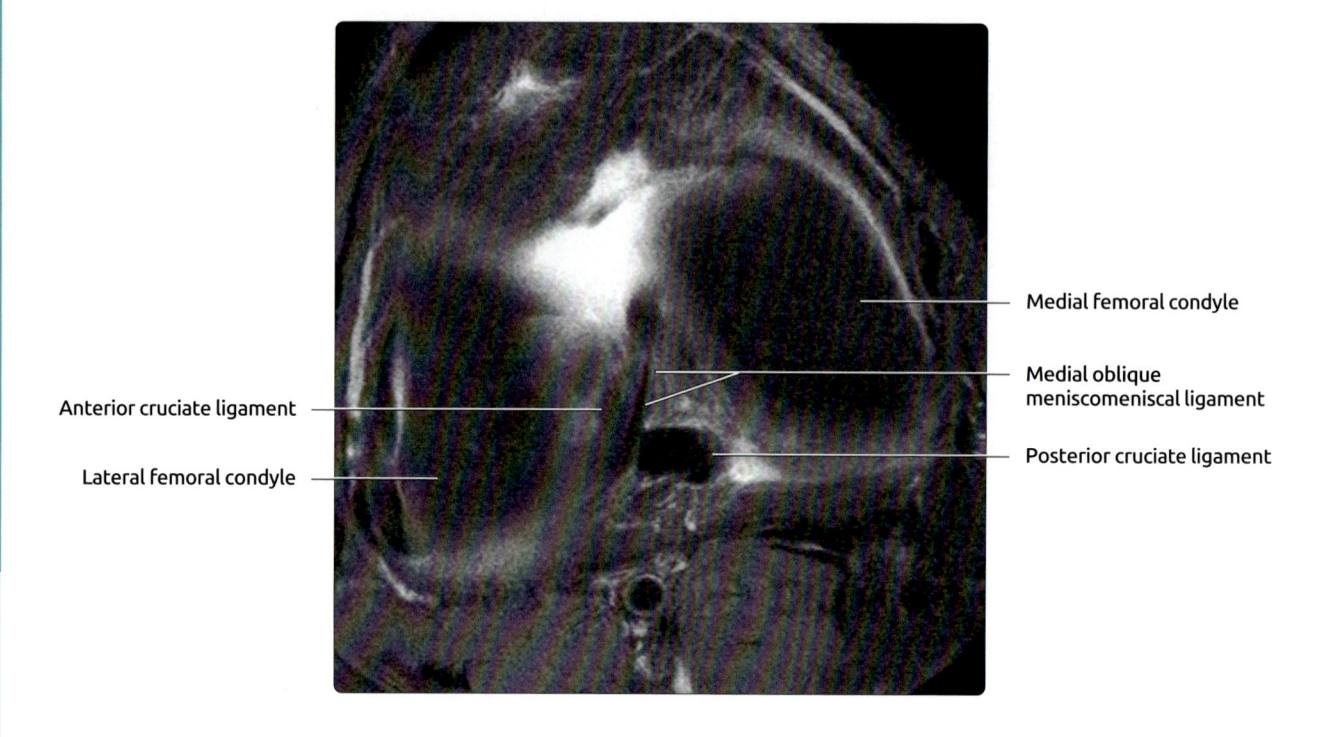

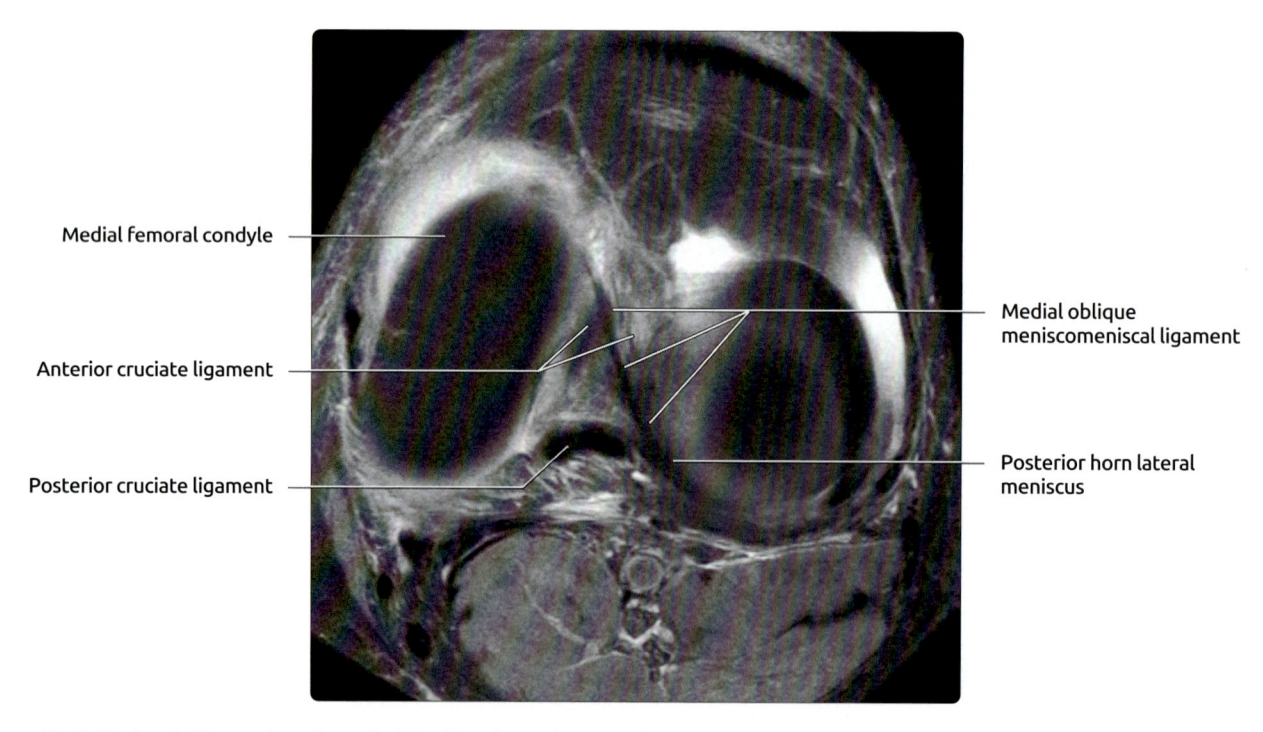

(Top) *Single axial image, just above the joint line, shows the normal variant medial oblique meniscomeniscal ligament. It arises from the anterior horn medial meniscus and inserts on the posterior horn lateral meniscus, threading its way between the ACL and PCL.* (Bottom) *First of 3 images in a different patient, axial PD FS MR through the joint line, shows a normal variant, the medial oblique meniscomeniscal ligament. The ligament extends from the anterior horn medial meniscus across the intercondylar notch to insert on posterior horn lateral meniscus. At this level of the menisci, the variant ligament appears to split the ACL at its insertion on the tibia. It normally extends between the ACL and PCL. The mirror image variant, lateral meniscomeniscal ligament, extends from anterior horn lateral meniscus to posterior horn medial meniscus (not shown here).*

Menisci

VARIANT: MENISCOMENISCAL LIGAMENT

Medial femoral condyle — Lateral femoral condyle

Medial meniscomeniscal ligament — Anterior cruciate ligament

Medial femoral condyle — Lateral femoral condyle

Medial meniscomeniscal ligament — Anterior cruciate ligament

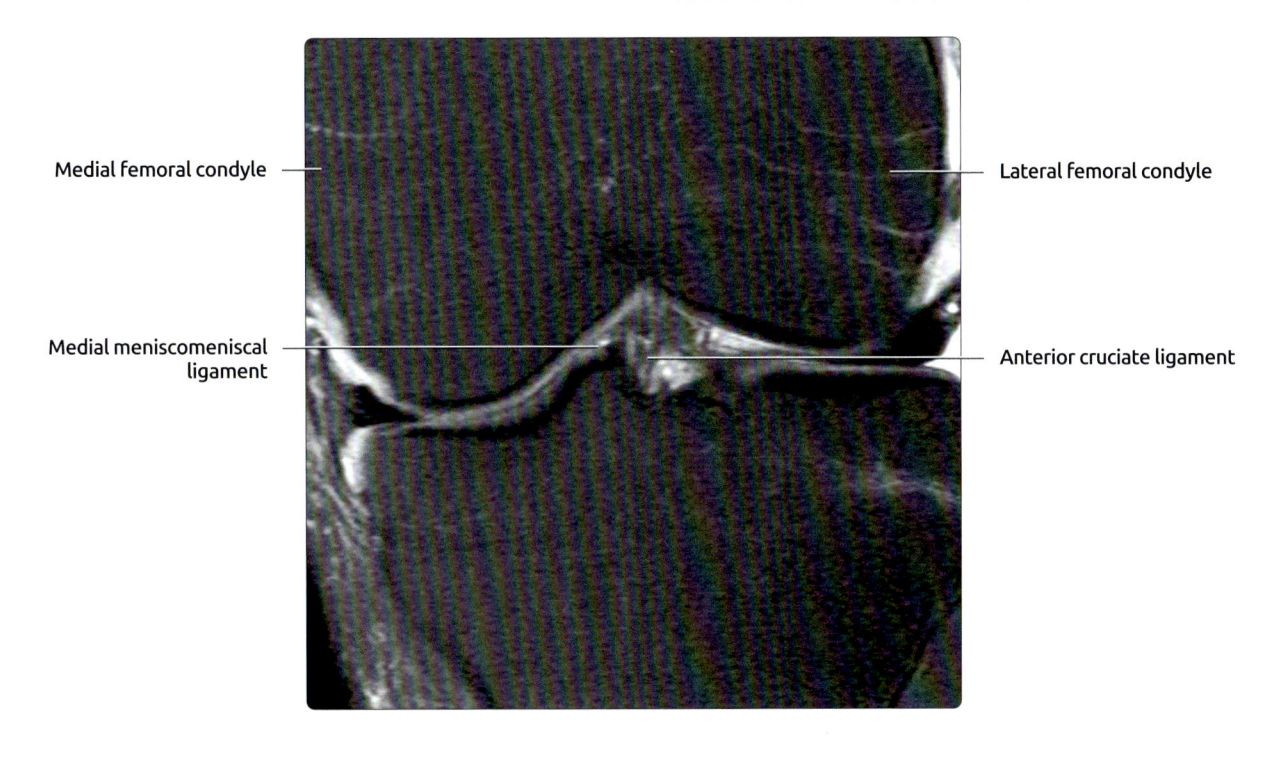

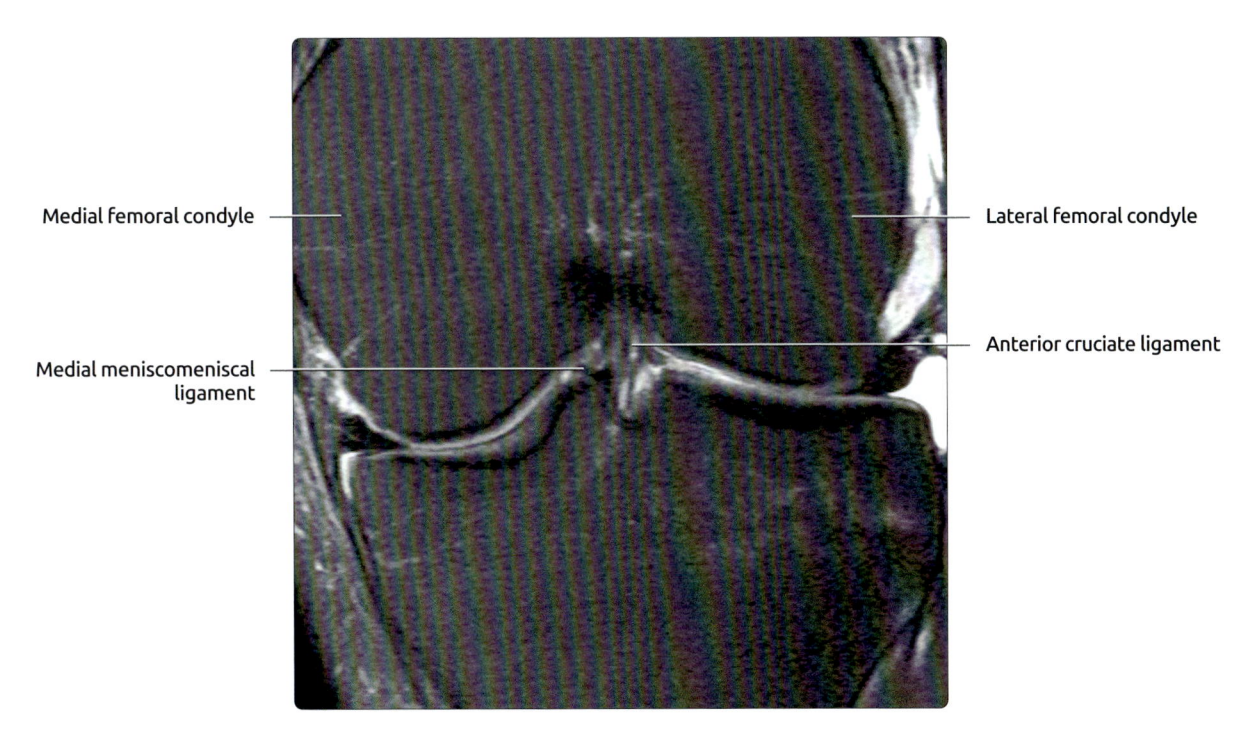

(Top) First of 2 coronal MR images, at the anterior portion of mid-joint, shows the tiny medial meniscomeniscal ligament in cross section adjacent to the anterior cruciate ligament. This is the same patient as shown on the immediate previous axial image. (Bottom) Second coronal image, 3 mm posterior, shows the meniscomeniscal ligament giving the appearance of a loose body or fragment adjacent to the ACL. The location and low signal of this normal variant ligament may be misdiagnosed as a meniscal fragment or bucket handle fragment. It is important to correlate it with the appearance on either axial or sagittal images, where the ligament will be seen as a longitudinal structure placed between the ACL and PCL, and angling obliquely across the notch between the 2 menisci.

Cruciate Ligaments/Posterior Capsule

TERMINOLOGY

Abbreviations
- Anterior cruciate ligament (ACL)
- Posterior cruciate ligament (PCL)

IMAGING ANATOMY

Overview
- Cruciate ligaments are in **extrasynovial but intracapsular** location
  - Fatty tissue lies between the cruciates
  - Synovial membrane surrounds anterior, medial, and lateral portions of cruciates but is reflected posteriorly from PCL to adjoining parts of joint capsule

ACL
- **Multiple separate fascicles**, which spiral laterally from femur to tibia (fibers rotate externally 90°); fatty tissue is seen between fibers
  - Continuum of fibers allows variable tension, with some taut throughout knee range of motion
  - **Anteromedial bundle**: Tight in flexion, lax in extension
  - **Posterolateral bundle**: Tight in extension, lax in flexion
- **Origin of ACL**: Posteriorly from lateral femoral condyle at intercondylar notch (seen on radiograph as junction of posterior femoral cortex and Blumensaat line)
- **Insertion of ACL**: Anteromedial tibial spine and adjacent plateau; bundles fan out at tibial attachment, forming "foot"
- **Function**
  - Primary restraint to anterior tibial translation
  - Major secondary restraint to internal rotation; minor secondary restraint to external rotation
  - Minor secondary restraint to varus/valgus at full extension
- **MR imaging**: Seen well in all 3 planes, low signal with fat interspersed between bundles
- Blood supply: Middle geniculate artery (pierces posterior capsule from popliteal); lesser supply from fat pad (inferior medial and lateral geniculates)
- Nerve: Posterior articular (branch of posterior tibial)

PCL
- **Appears as single round ligament** but consists of 2 major parts; rotates 90° from anteroposterior alignment at femoral origin to medial-lateral alignment at insertion on posterior tibia
  - **Anterolateral bundle**: Bulk of ligament, taut in flexion, lax in extension
  - **Posteromedial (oblique) bundle**: Taut in extension, lax in flexion
- **Origin of PCL**: Mid portion of medial femoral condyle at intercondylar notch
- **Insertion of PCL**: Mid posterior tibia, 1 cm below joint line, where it blends in with posterior capsule
- **Function**: Primary restraint against posterior translation
- **Meniscofemoral ligaments**
  - Both arise from posterior horn lateral meniscus and insert on medial femoral condyle; at least 1 present 70% of time
  - **Posterior (Wrisberg)** lies posterior to PCL
  - **Anterior (Humphrey)** lies anterior to PCL; intact ligament of Humphrey may mimic intact PCL in the setting of complete PCL tear
  - May play a role in secondary restraint to posterior instability; may stabilize lateral meniscus during flexion
- **MR imaging**: Seen well in all 3 planes, solid low signal throughout
- Blood supply: Middle geniculate artery proximal and middle thirds; geniculate and popliteal artery base; capsular vessels through entire length

Posterior Capsule
- **Complex fibrous structure:** Augmented by extensions of adjacent tendons
- **Incomplete:** Pierced centrally by neurovascular structures
- **Proximal attachment**: Vertical fibers attached to posterior margins of femoral condyles and intercondylar fossae
- **Distal attachment** is to posterior margins of tibial condyles and intercondylar areas
- **Tendons/ligaments:** Attach to posterior capsule to provide reinforcement
  - **Proximally** (medially and laterally): Tendinous heads of gastrocnemius
  - **Posteromedial corner**: Semimembranosus and posterior oblique ligament
  - **Posterolateral corner**: Arcuate ligament and iliotibial tract
  - **Posterior central**: Oblique popliteal ligament

Spaces Within Cruciate/Posterior Capsule
- Synovial membrane surrounds anterior, medial, and lateral portions of cruciates but is reflected posteriorly from PCL to adjoining parts of joint capsule
- Results in potential space (**PCL bursa or recess**)
  - Seen only when fluid-filled; best on coronal and sagittal planes
  - Seen posterior to PCL and adjacent to lateral aspect of medial femoral condyle
  - No contact between PCL recess and proximal 1/3 of PCL (fat is interposed)
  - Communicates with medial (femorotibial) compartment of knee
  - Does not communicate with lateral compartment
  - If ligament of Wrisberg is present, it lies posterosuperior to PCL recess
- **Intercruciate recess**
  - Localized potential fluid collection between ACL and PCL; best seen on sagittal and axial planes
  - Communicates with either lateral or medial (femorotibial) compartments

SELECTED REFERENCES

1. De Maeseneer M et al: Normal anatomy and pathology of the posterior capsular area of the knee: findings in cadaveric specimens and in patients. AJR Am J Roentgenol. 182(4):955-62, 2004
2. Delgado GJ et al: Tennis leg: Clinical US study of 141 patients and anatomic investigation of four cadavers with MR imaging and US. Radiology 224(1):112-9, 2002

Cruciate Ligaments/Posterior Capsule

CRUCIATE LIGAMENTS: SAGITTAL

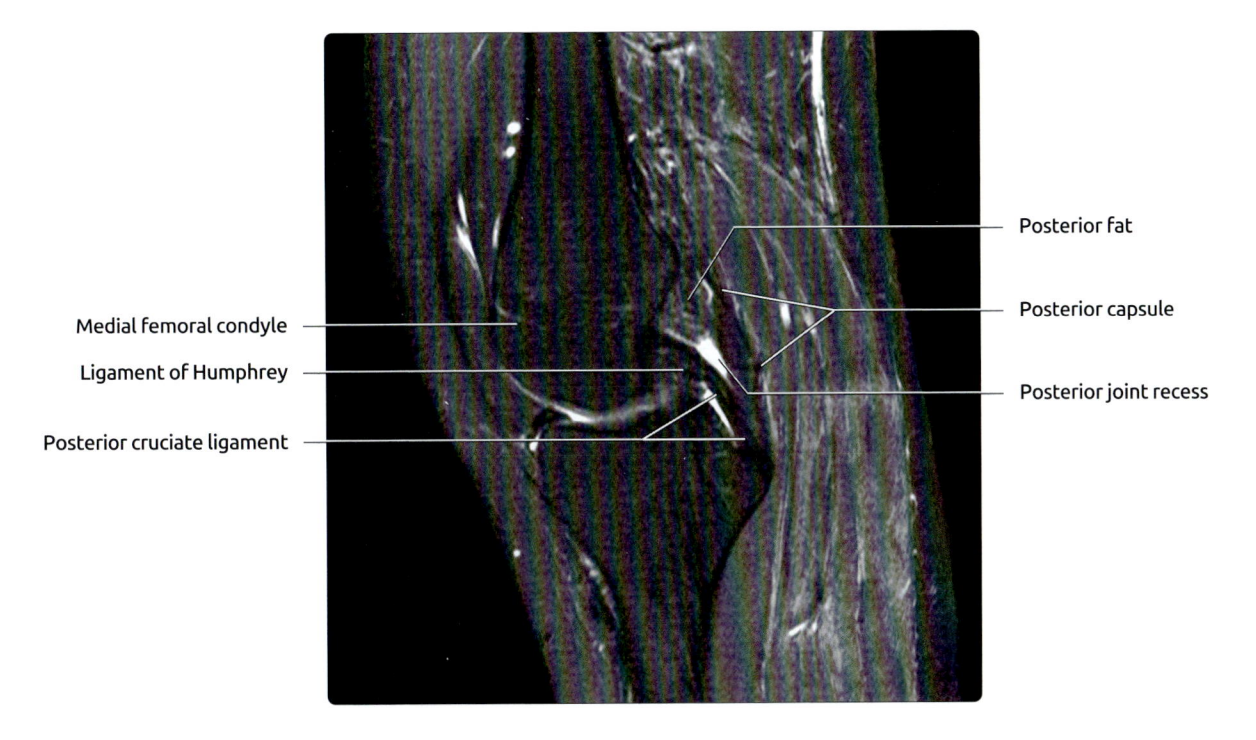

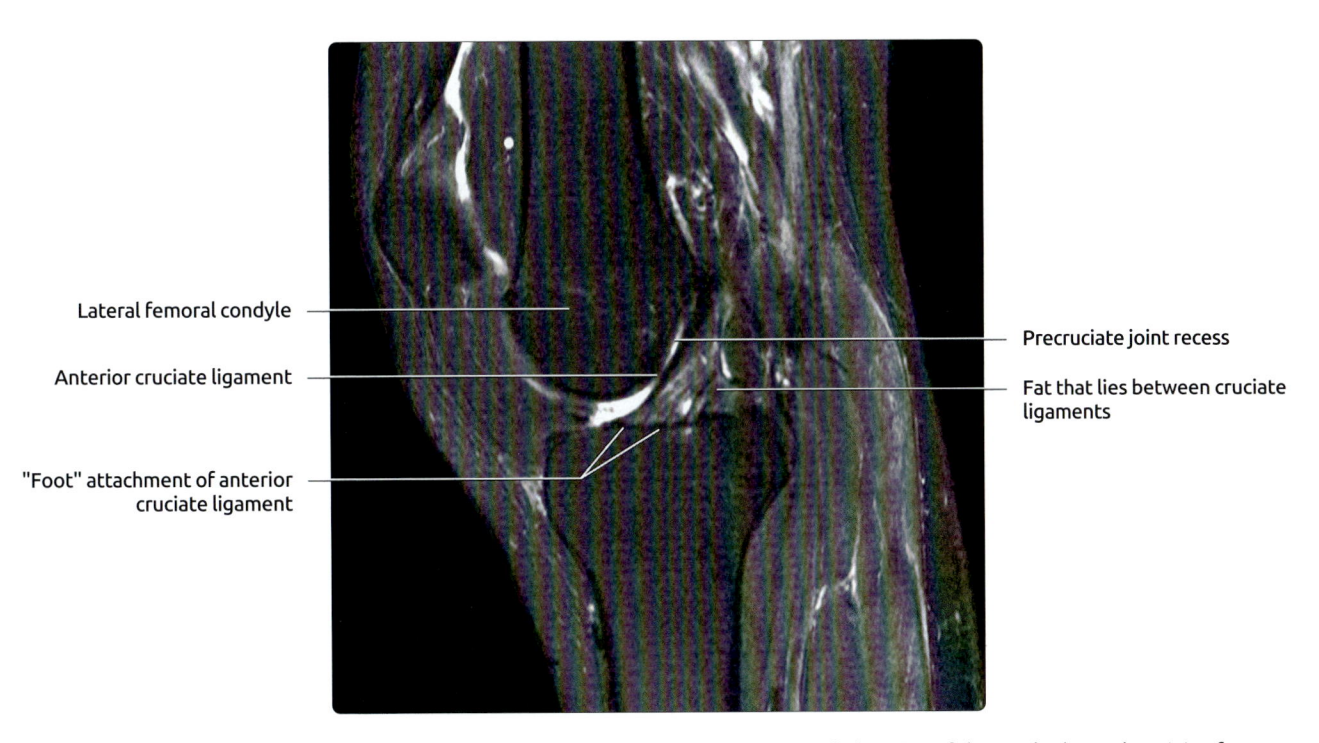

Medial femoral condyle
Ligament of Humphrey
Posterior cruciate ligament
Posterior fat
Posterior capsule
Posterior joint recess

Lateral femoral condyle
Anterior cruciate ligament
"Foot" attachment of anterior cruciate ligament
Precruciate joint recess
Fat that lies between cruciate ligaments

(Top) *First of 2 sagittal T2 FS MR images, through the intercondylar notch in the more medial portion of the notch, shows the origin of the PCL from the anterior portion of the medial notch, as well as the insertion posteriorly on the tibia, 1 cm below the joint line. The PCL appears as a thick single band, usually in at least two adjacent images. There is fat located immediately posterior to the proximal portion of the PCL. More distally, the posterior joint recess abuts the PCL. The posterior capsule lies behind this fat and the recess. In this case, the meniscofemoral ligament of Humphrey is present; the ligament of Wrisberg is absent.* (Bottom) *This image is located slightly laterally to the previous image, within the intercondylar notch. The anterior cruciate ligament arises from the posterior lateral femoral condyle within the notch; the broad insertion on the tibial plateau is seen.*

Cruciate Ligaments/Posterior Capsule

CRUCIATE LIGAMENTS: CORONAL

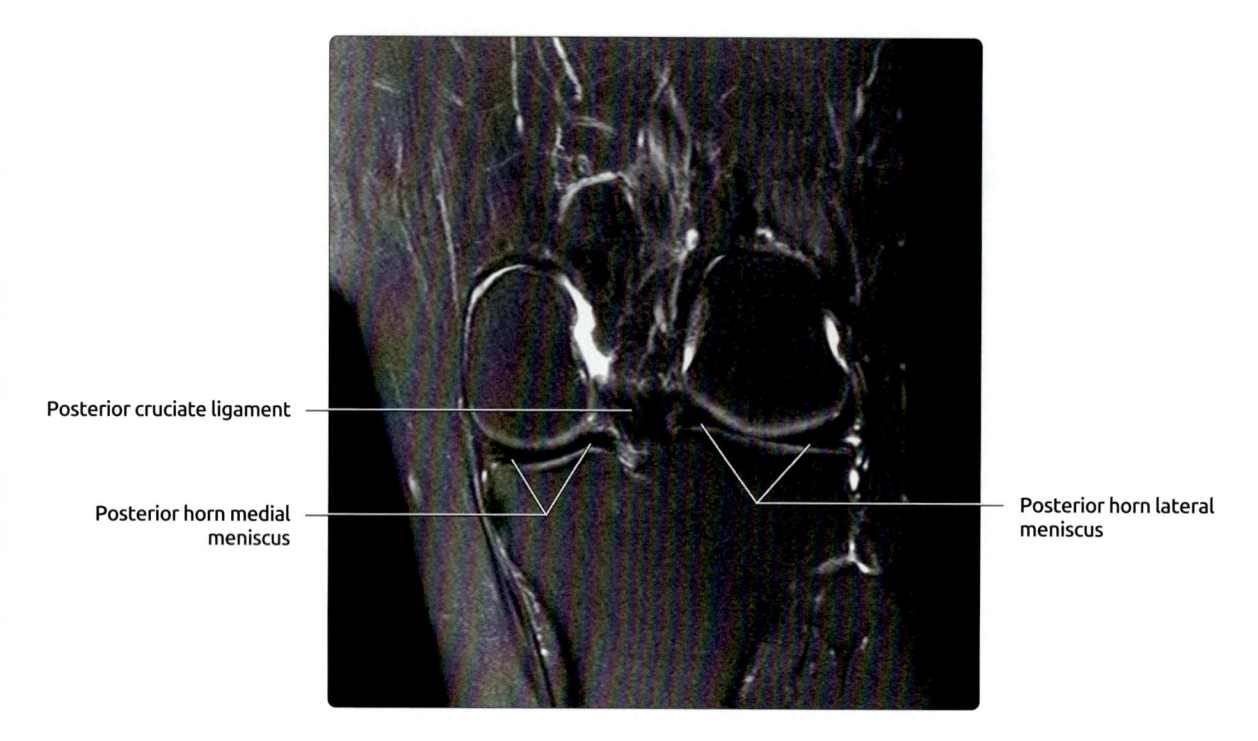

Posterior cruciate ligament

Posterior horn medial meniscus

Posterior horn lateral meniscus

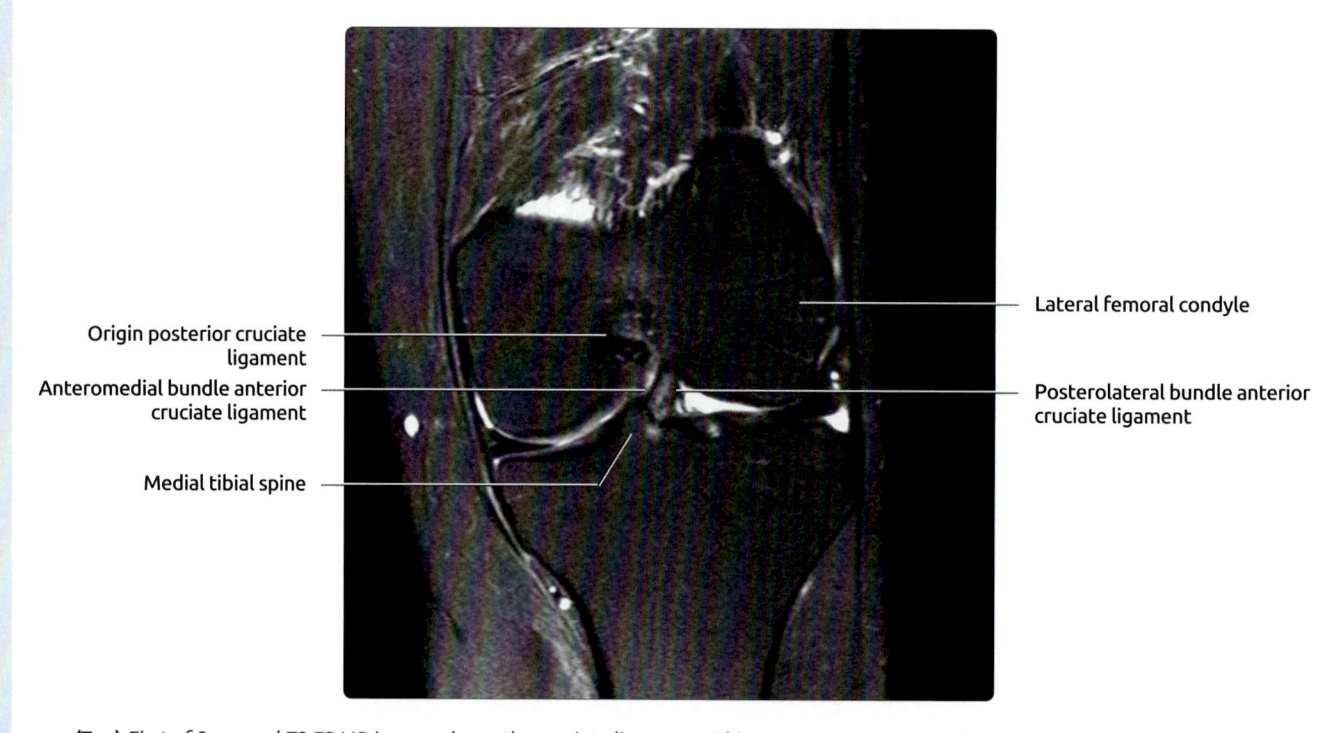

Origin posterior cruciate ligament

Anteromedial bundle anterior cruciate ligament

Medial tibial spine

Lateral femoral condyle

Posterolateral bundle anterior cruciate ligament

(Top) *First of 2 coronal T2 FS MR images shows the cruciate ligaments. This more posterior image shows the posterior cruciate ligament approaching its insertion on the posterior aspect of the tibial plateau. No portion of the anterior cruciate is seen. Note that while we expect to see the ACL as a complete band on coronal images located more anteriorly, the PCL is incompletely seen on coronal images.* **(Bottom)** *This more anterior image also shows the cruciate ligaments. The anteromedial bundle and posterolateral bundle of the ACL are seen arising from the lateral femoral condyle and inserting on the tibial plateau adjacent to the medial tibial spine. Both are seen on the same cut because of the obliquity at which coronal images are obtained. Because the leg is in extension, the posterolateral bundle is taut.*

Cruciate Ligaments/Posterior Capsule

CRUCIATE LIGAMENTS: AXIAL

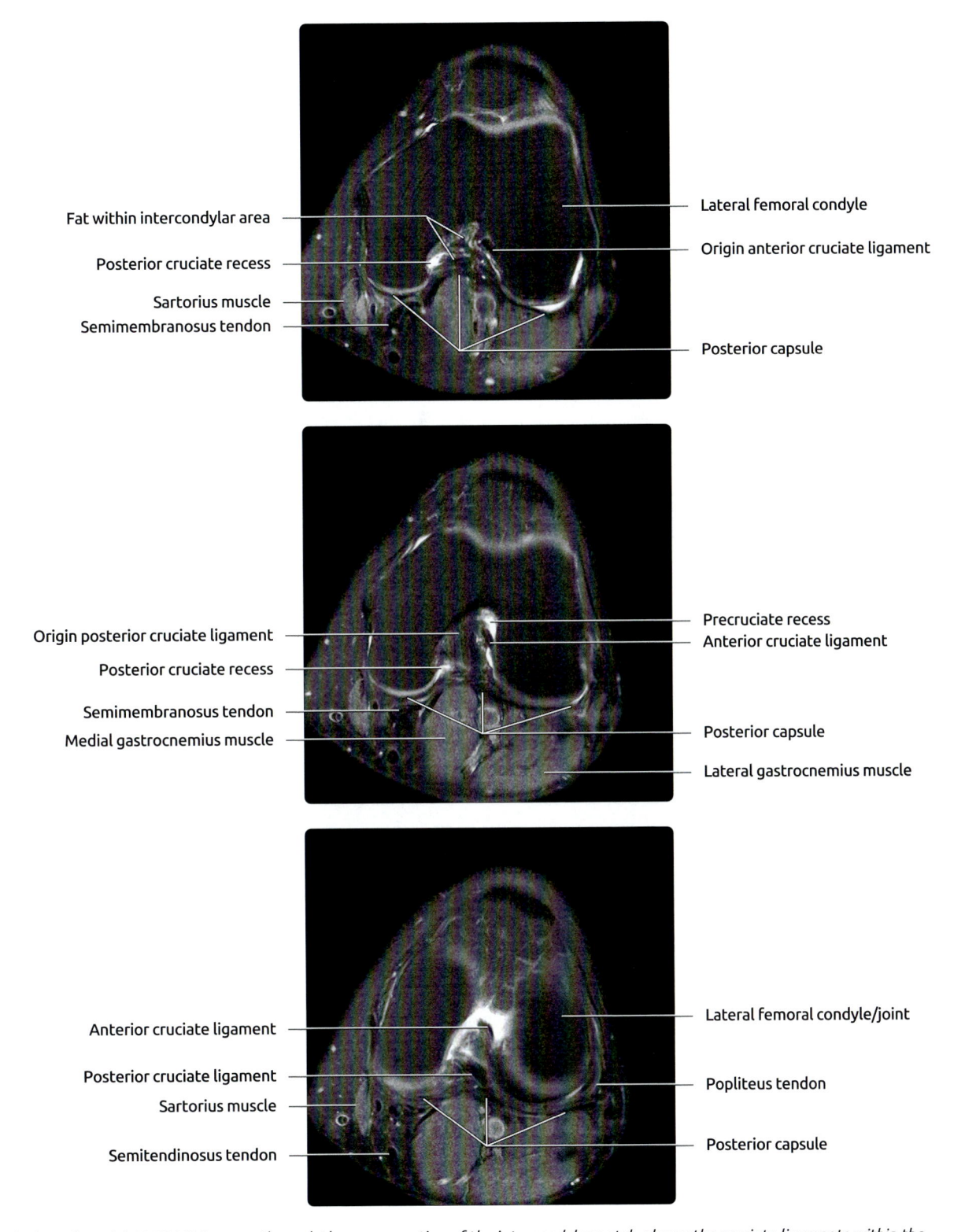

- Fat within intercondylar area
- Posterior cruciate recess
- Sartorius muscle
- Semimembranosus tendon
- Lateral femoral condyle
- Origin anterior cruciate ligament
- Posterior capsule

- Origin posterior cruciate ligament
- Posterior cruciate recess
- Semimembranosus tendon
- Medial gastrocnemius muscle
- Precruciate recess
- Anterior cruciate ligament
- Posterior capsule
- Lateral gastrocnemius muscle

- Anterior cruciate ligament
- Posterior cruciate ligament
- Sartorius muscle
- Semitendinosus tendon
- Lateral femoral condyle/joint
- Popliteus tendon
- Posterior capsule

(Top) First of 3 axial T2 FS MR images, through the upper portion of the intercondylar notch, shows the cruciate ligaments within the intercondylar notch. In the upper portion of the notch, the ACL is seen arising from the posterior aspect of the lateral femoral condyle within the notch. The remainder of the notch is filled with fat and is a potential space (posterior cruciate bursa). **(Middle)** Axial cut through the mid portion of the intercondylar notch is shown. The ACL extends obliquely toward its insertion on the tibial plateau. The origin of PCL is seen at the anterior medial femoral condyle within the notch. Fluid-filled recesses are seen anterior to the ACL and posteromedial to the PCL. **(Bottom)** The inferior portion of the intercondylar notch shows the ACL as it approaches insertion on the tibial plateau. The PCL is still within the capsule, but beginning to blend with it as it approaches insertion on the posterior tibia. The cruciates are well seen axially.

Cruciate Ligaments/Posterior Capsule

VARIANTS: MENISCOMENISCAL LIGAMENT AND INFRAPATELLAR PLICA

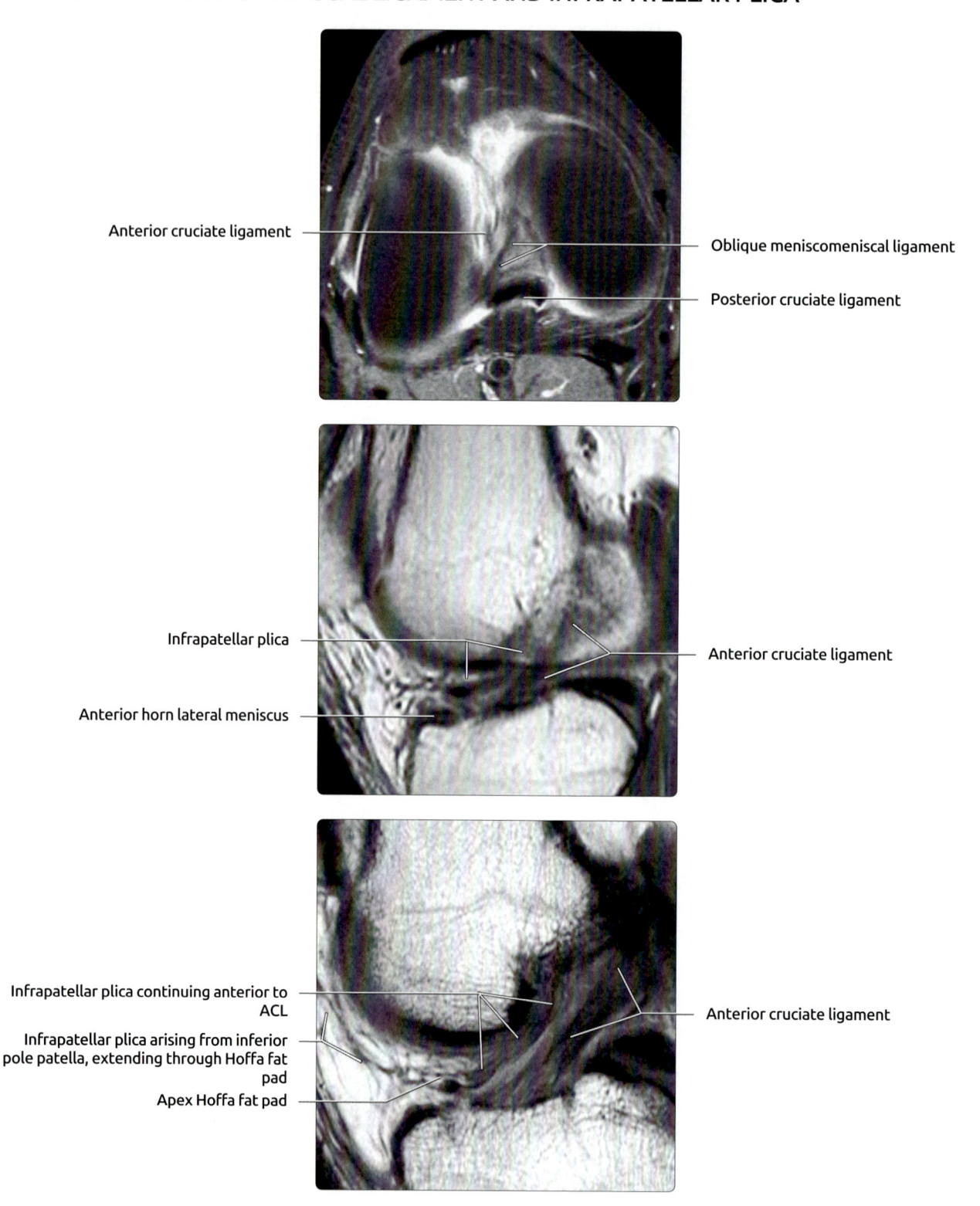

(Top) Axial PD FS MR through the femoral condyles shows an oblique meniscomeniscal ligament. This uncommon variant connects the anterior horn of one meniscus with the posterior horn of the contralateral meniscus. It runs between the anterior and posterior cruciate ligaments. *(Middle)* Sagittal PD MR image through the intercondylar notch shows the variant infrapatellar plica. This plica arises from the patella, extends across the Hoffa fat pad, and along the anterior surface of the anterior cruciate ligament. It should not be mistaken for a longitudinal split in the ACL. *(Bottom)* Sagittal PD MR through the intercondylar notch shows an infrapatellar plica. The plica is seen extending through the Hoffa fat pad, paralleling the curvature of the femoral condyle, and then paralleling the anterior cruciate ligament.

Cruciate Ligaments/Posterior Capsule

VARIANT: MENISCOCRUCIATE LIGAMENT

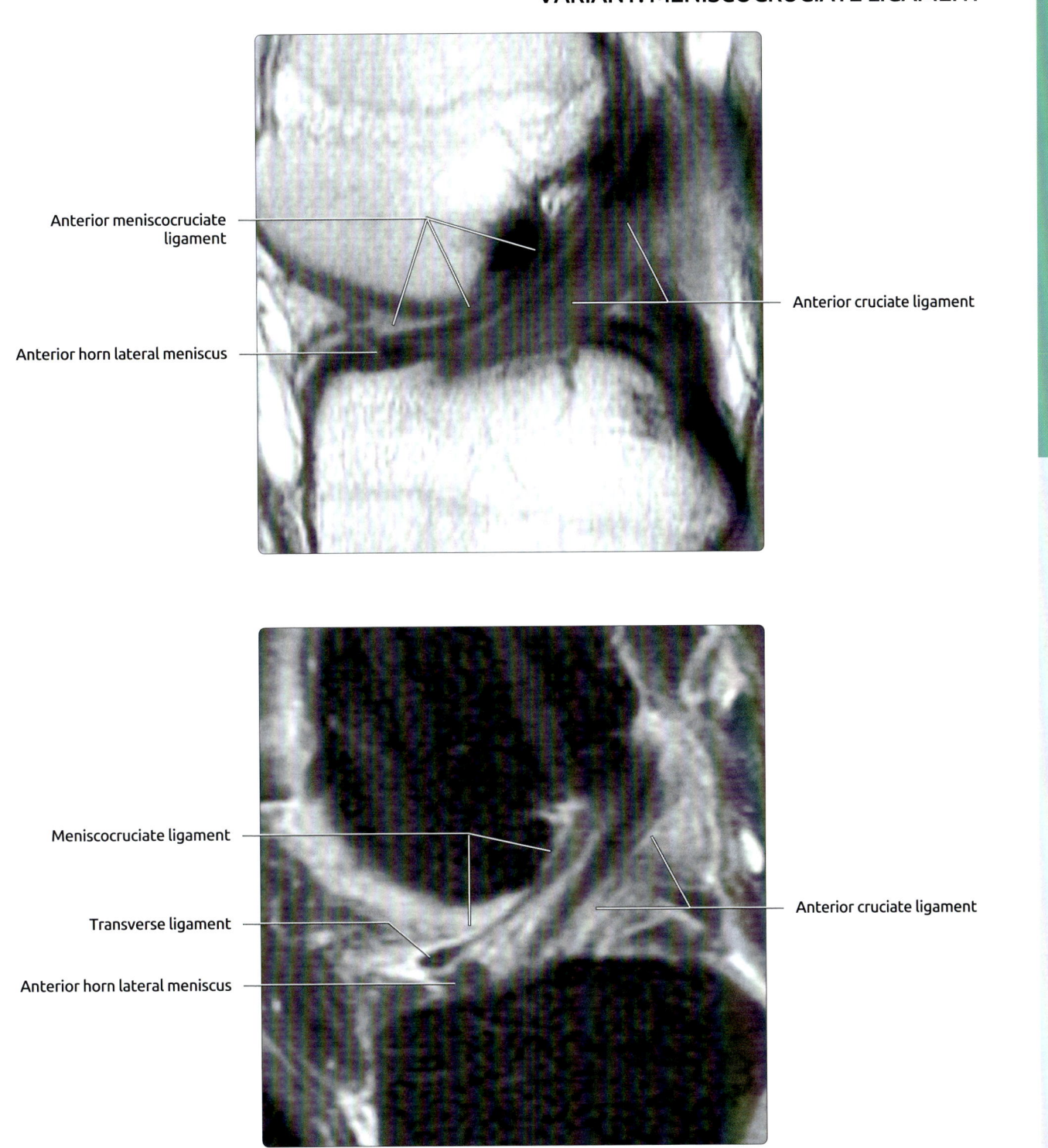

Labels (top image): Anterior meniscocruciate ligament; Anterior horn lateral meniscus; Anterior cruciate ligament

Labels (bottom image): Meniscocruciate ligament; Transverse ligament; Anterior horn lateral meniscus; Anterior cruciate ligament

(Top) *Sagittal PD MR through the intercondylar notch shows a meniscocruciate ligament. The ligament arises from the anterior horn medial meniscus and extends along the anterior surface of the anterior cruciate ligament to the femoral condyle. It could possibly be mistaken for a longitudinal tear in the anterior cruciate.* **(Bottom)** *Sagittal PD FS MR shows another variant meniscocruciate ligament. This ligament is arising from the transverse ligament; as it extends parallel to and anterior to the anterior cruciate ligament, it could simulate a longitudinal or partial tear in this cruciate.*

Cruciate Ligaments/Posterior Capsule

VARIANT: MENISCAL FASCICLE

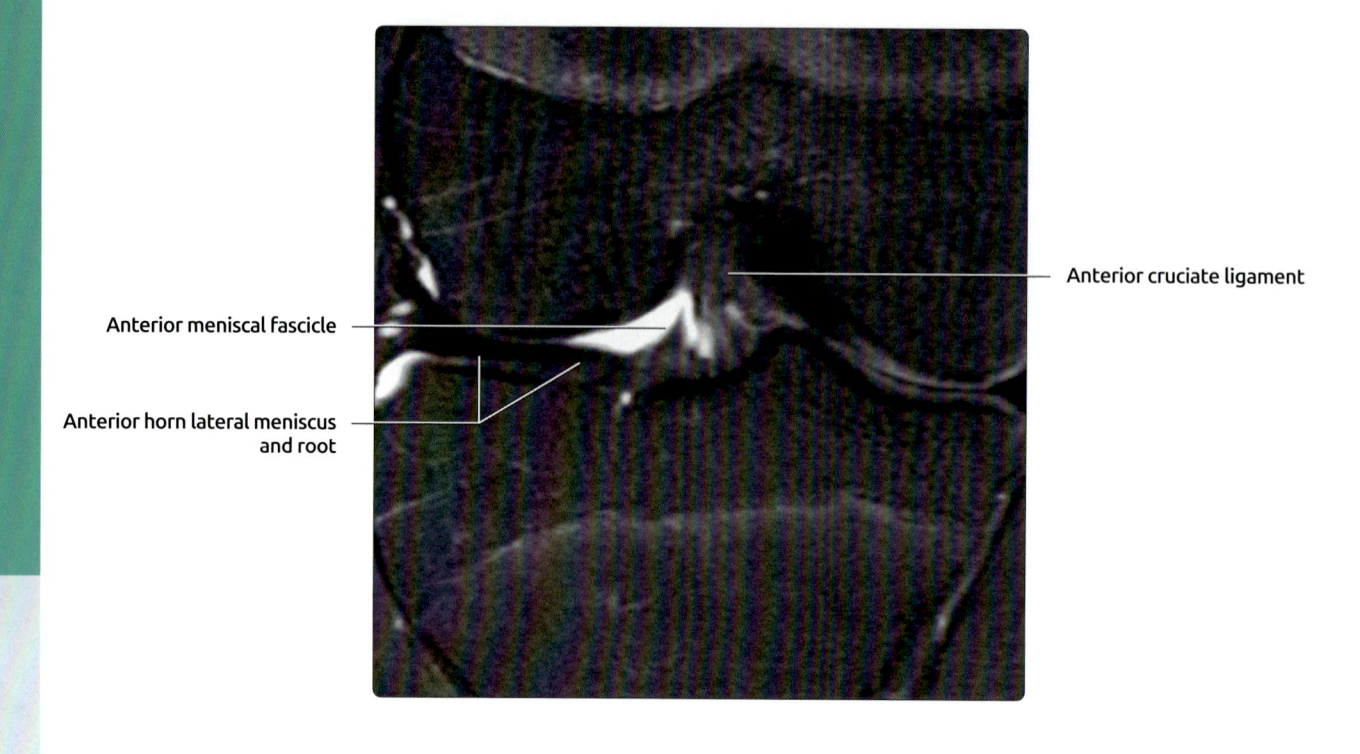

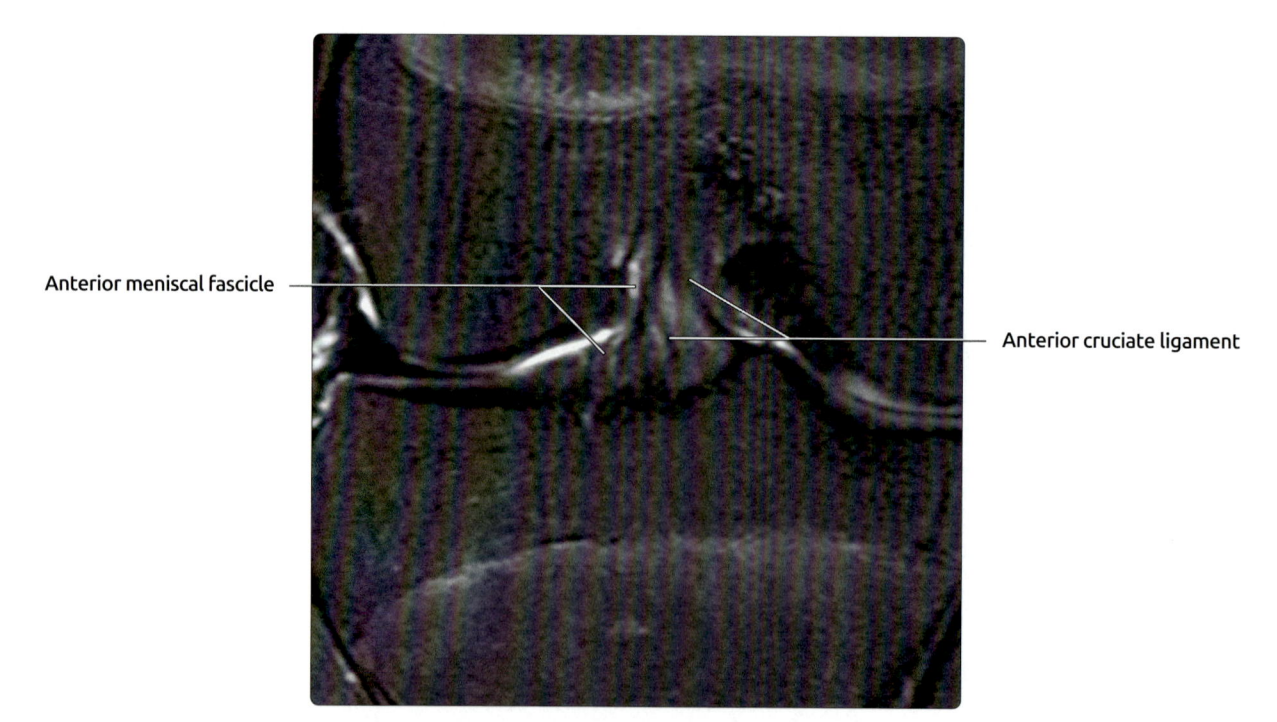

(Top) First of 2 coronal PD FS MR images shows a variant anterior meniscal fascicle extending to the anterior cruciate ligament. The fascicle arises from the anterior horn lateral meniscus and its root. It then extends upward to merge with the synovium over the anterior cruciate ligament. In this anterior slice, the fascicle appears as a separate fiber. The anterior cruciate is in its normal position, extending from the lateral femoral condyle to its insertion adjacent to the medial tibial spine. (Bottom) Image is located slightly posterior to the previous image. The meniscal fascicle is seen extending from inferolateral to superomedial, an opposite angulation relative to the anterior cruciate. This is a potentially confusing appearance and should not be confused with cruciate pathology.

Cruciate Ligaments/Posterior Capsule

MENISCOFEMORAL LIGAMENT OF WRISBERG

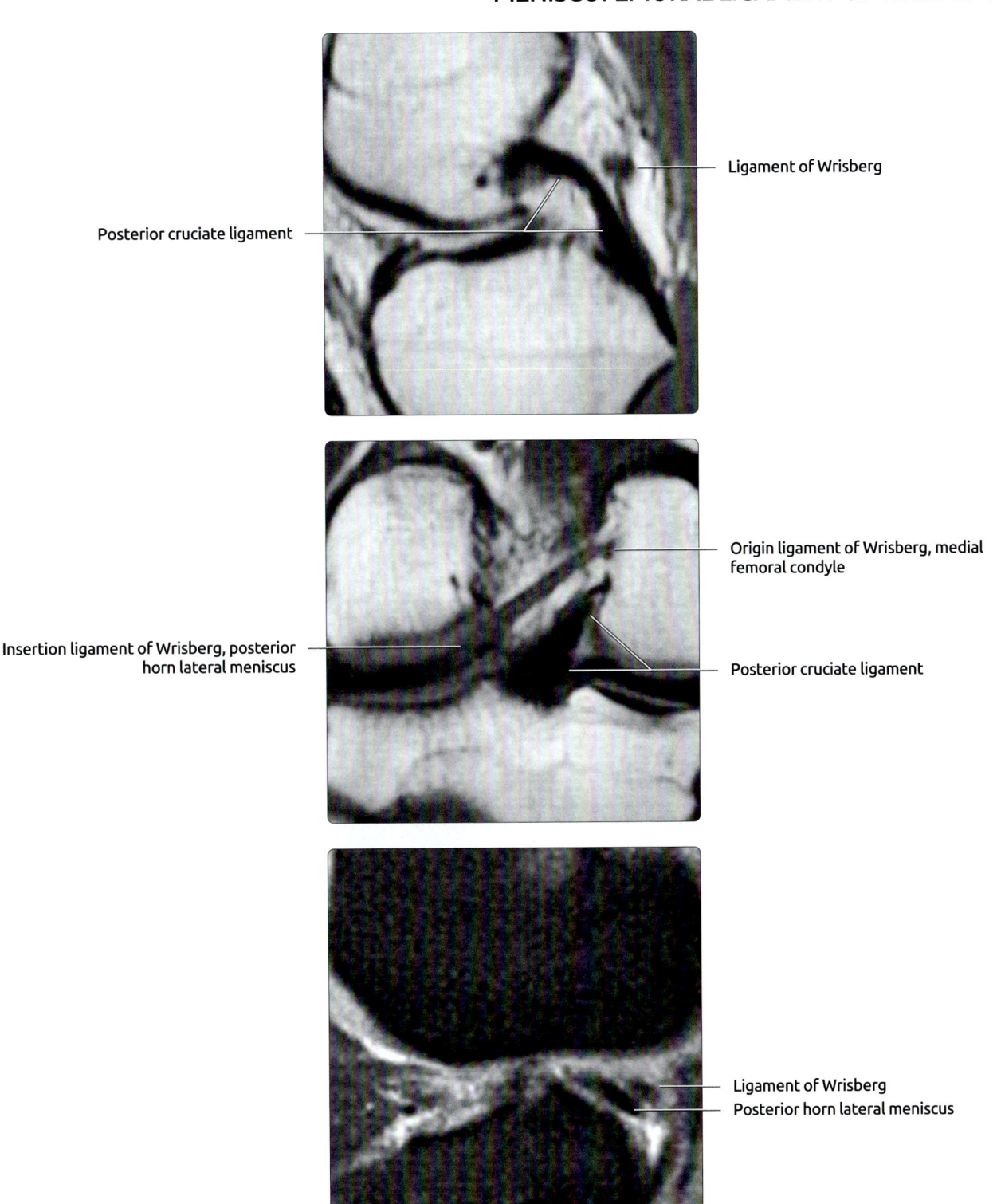

Posterior cruciate ligament — Ligament of Wrisberg

Insertion ligament of Wrisberg, posterior horn lateral meniscus — Origin ligament of Wrisberg, medial femoral condyle — Posterior cruciate ligament

Ligament of Wrisberg — Posterior horn lateral meniscus

(Top) First of 3 images shows the posterior cruciate ligament and the associated posterior meniscofemoral ligament (Wrisberg). Sagittal image through the posterior cruciate shows the ligament of Wrisberg in cross section as it extends from the medial femoral condyle toward the posterior horn lateral meniscus. (Middle) Coronal PD MR image located posteriorly in the joint in the same patient shows the ligament of Wrisberg paralleling the posterior cruciate ligament in its path from the medial femoral condyle to the posterior horn lateral meniscus. (Bottom) Sagittal PD FS MR image located in the lateral compartment immediately adjacent to the intercondylar notch at the root of posterior horn lateral meniscus is shown. The ligament of Wrisberg inserts at this point; just prior to the insertion, this appearance could give a false impression of meniscal tear.

Cruciate Ligaments/Posterior Capsule

MENISCOFEMORAL LIGAMENT OF HUMPHREY

Meniscofemoral ligament of Humphrey

Posterior cruciate ligament

Lateral femoral condyle

Medial femoral condyle

Meniscofemoral ligament of Humphrey

Anterior cruciate ligament

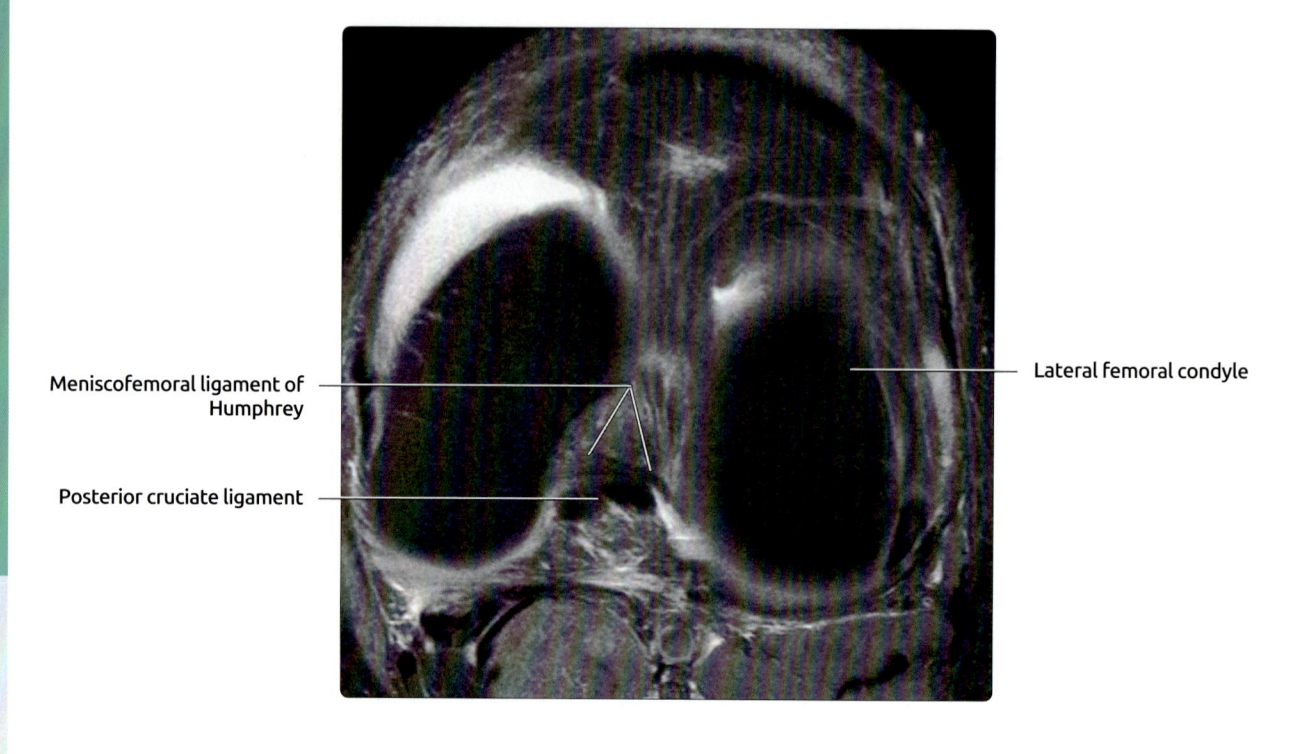

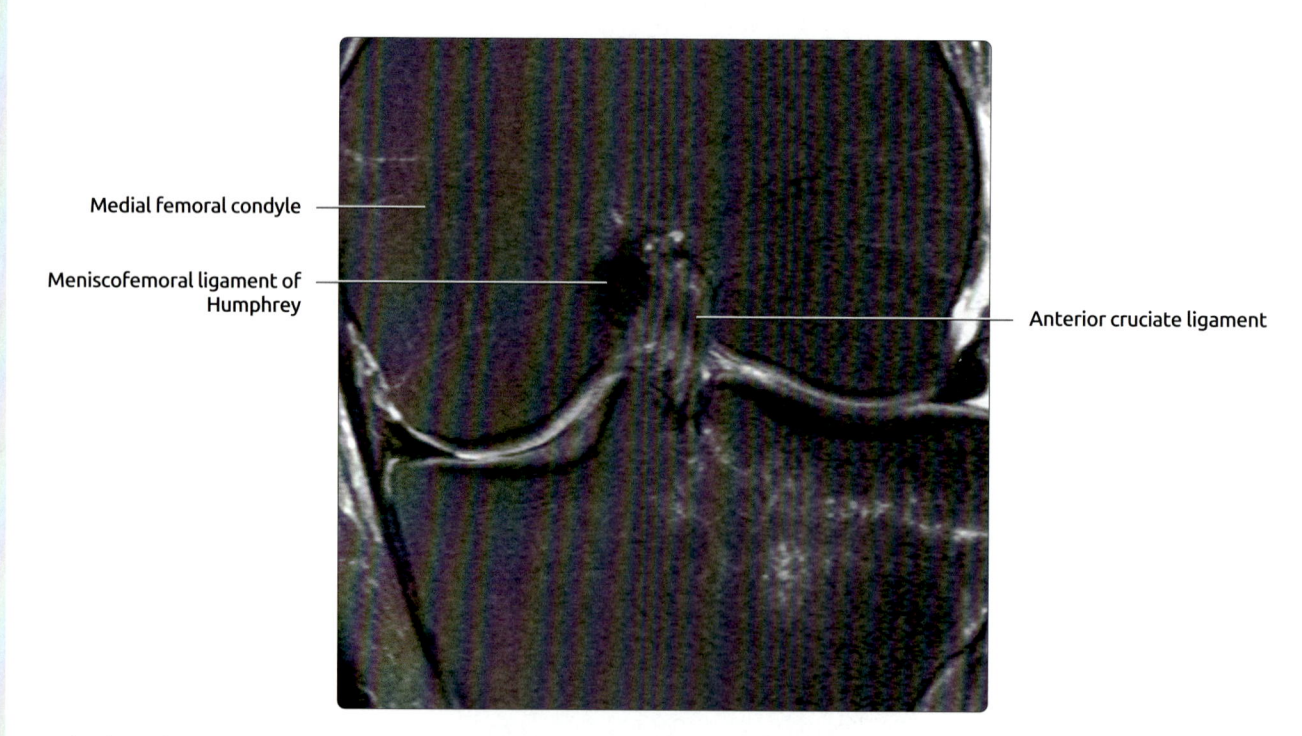

(Top) Axial PD FS MR through the femoral condyles and intercondylar notch is shown. The meniscofemoral ligament of Humphrey extends from the medial femoral condyle across in front of the posterior cruciate ligament toward its insertion on the posterior horn lateral meniscus. *(Bottom)* First of 3 coronal PD FS MR images shows the anterior cruciate ligament extending from the lateral femoral condyle toward the tibial spine. At the same level, there is a ligamentous structure arising from the medial femoral condyle. This is located slightly anterior to the origin of the posterior cruciate ligament and is the meniscofemoral ligament of Humphrey.

Cruciate Ligaments/Posterior Capsule

MENISCOFEMORAL LIGAMENT OF HUMPHREY

Posterior cruciate ligament

Meniscofemoral ligament of Humphrey

Lateral femoral condyle

Anterior cruciate ligament

Posterior cruciate ligament

Meniscofemoral ligament of Humphrey

Lateral femoral condyle

Root posterior horn lateral meniscus

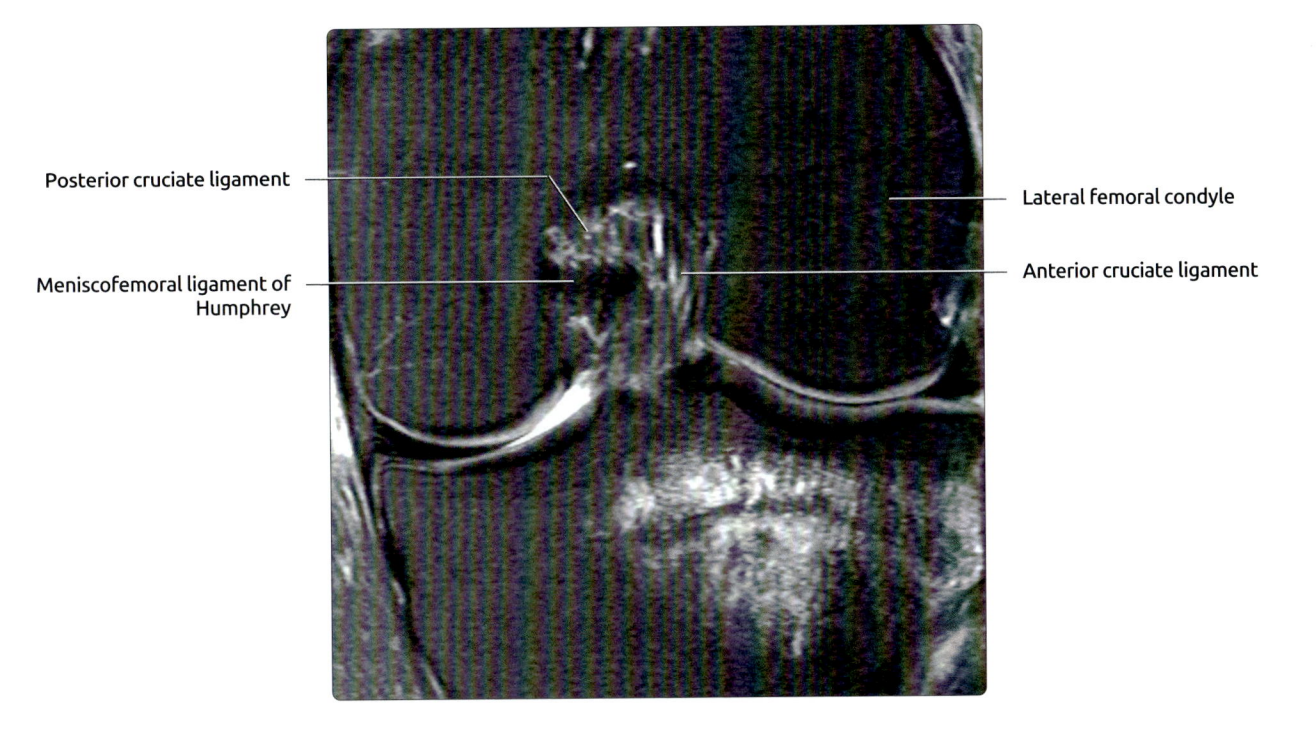

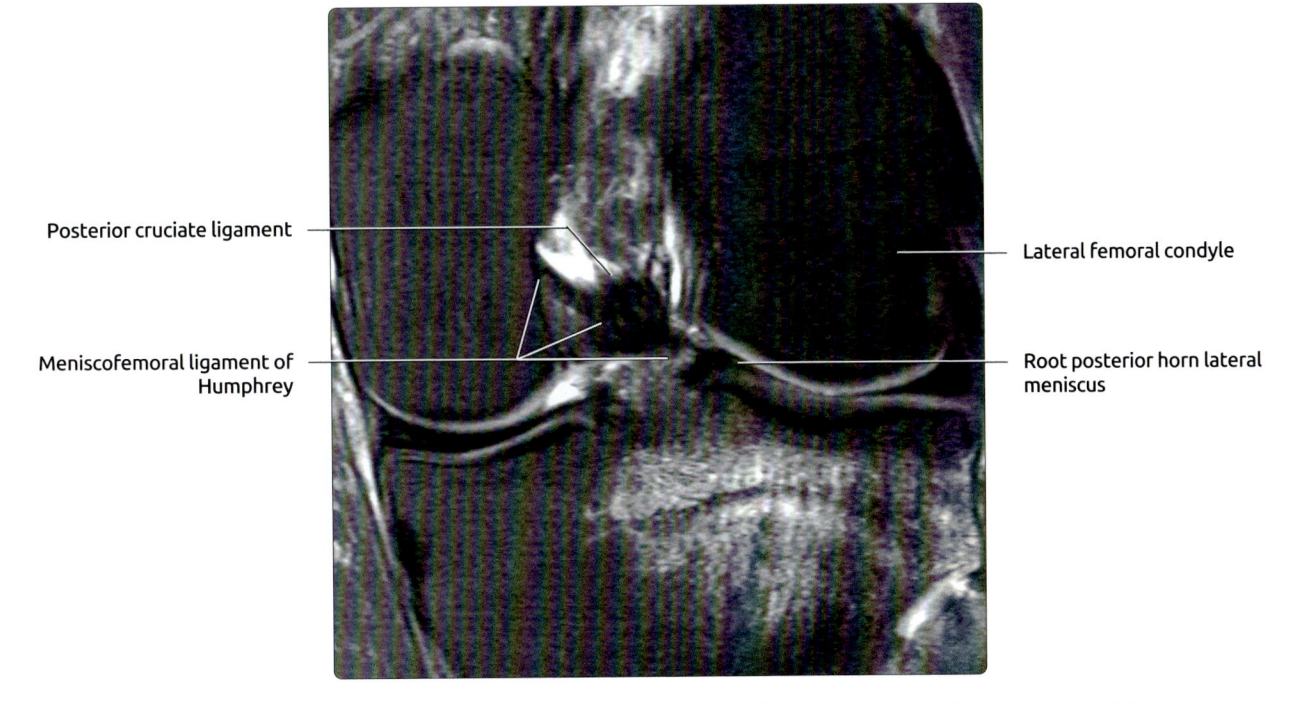

(Top) Coronal PD FS MR image located slightly posterior to the previous image is shown. The intercondylar notch is quite full, containing the normally positioned anterior cruciate ligament as well as the origin of posterior cruciate ligament. The origin of the meniscofemoral ligament of Humphrey is noted immediately anterior and inferior to that of posterior cruciate. **(Bottom)** Coronal image is located further posteriorly, showing the meniscofemoral ligament of Humphrey crossing from the medial femoral condyle to insert on the root of the posterior horn lateral meniscus. It crosses directly in front of the posterior cruciate ligament. It is somewhat unusual to see it in its entirety on a single coronal image. Bone bruise on the lateral tibial plateau is incidentally seen in this example.

Cruciate Ligaments/Posterior Capsule

MENISCOFEMORAL LIGAMENT OF HUMPHREY

Origin, ligament of Humphrey

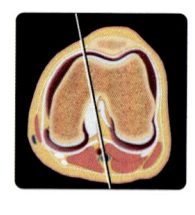

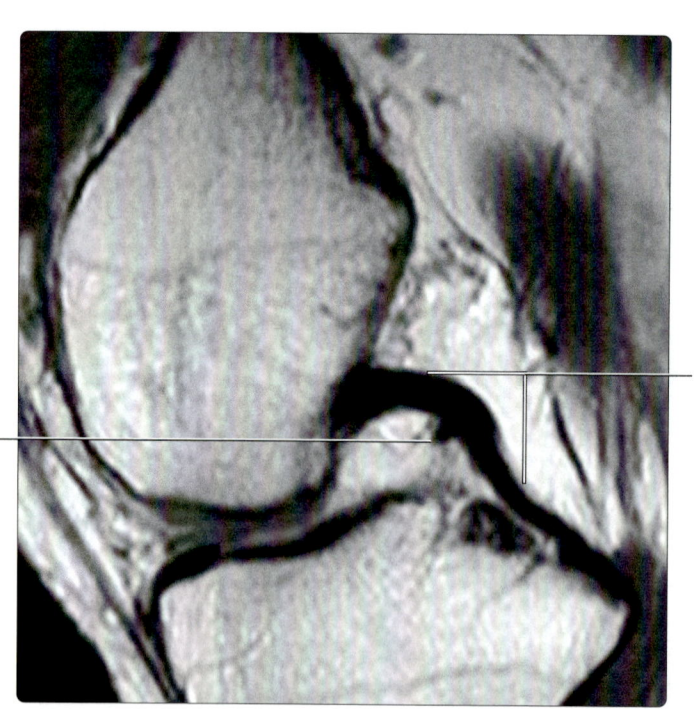

Posterior cruciate ligament

Mid portion, ligament of Humphrey

Posterior cruciate ligament

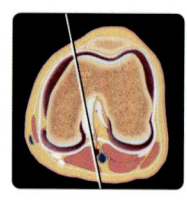

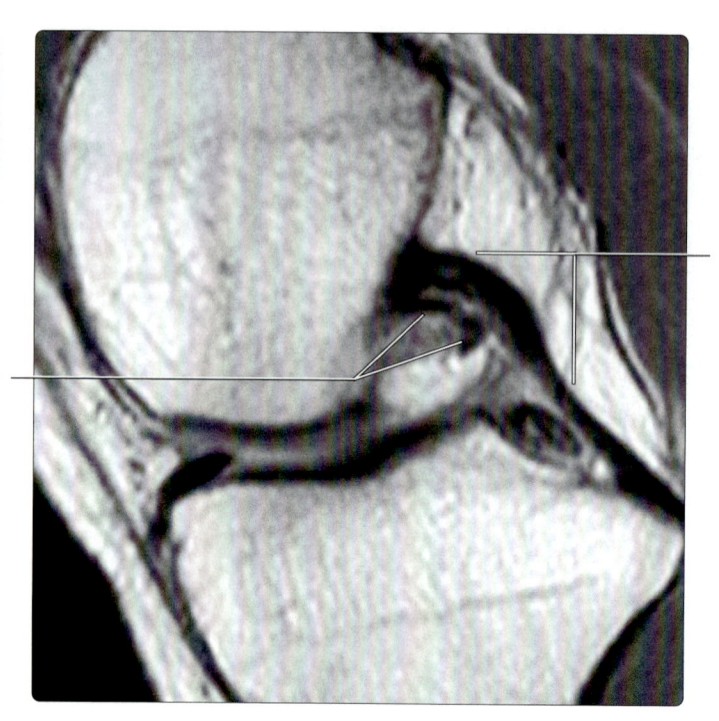

(Top) First of 4 sagittal PD MR images shows the meniscofemoral ligament of Humphrey. Image is medial within the intercondylar notch, at the level of the posterior cruciate ligament. The ligament of Humphrey is seen originating from the medial intercondylar notch, immediately inferior and anterior to the posterior cruciate ligament. *(Bottom)* This image, minimally lateral to the previous image, shows the ligament of Humphrey in cross section, immediately inferior to the posterior cruciate ligament.

Cruciate Ligaments/Posterior Capsule

MENISCOFEMORAL LIGAMENT OF HUMPHREY

Anterior cruciate ligament

Ligament of Humphrey

Posterior cruciate ligament

Anterior cruciate ligament

Insertion ligament of Humphrey

Root posterior horn lateral meniscus

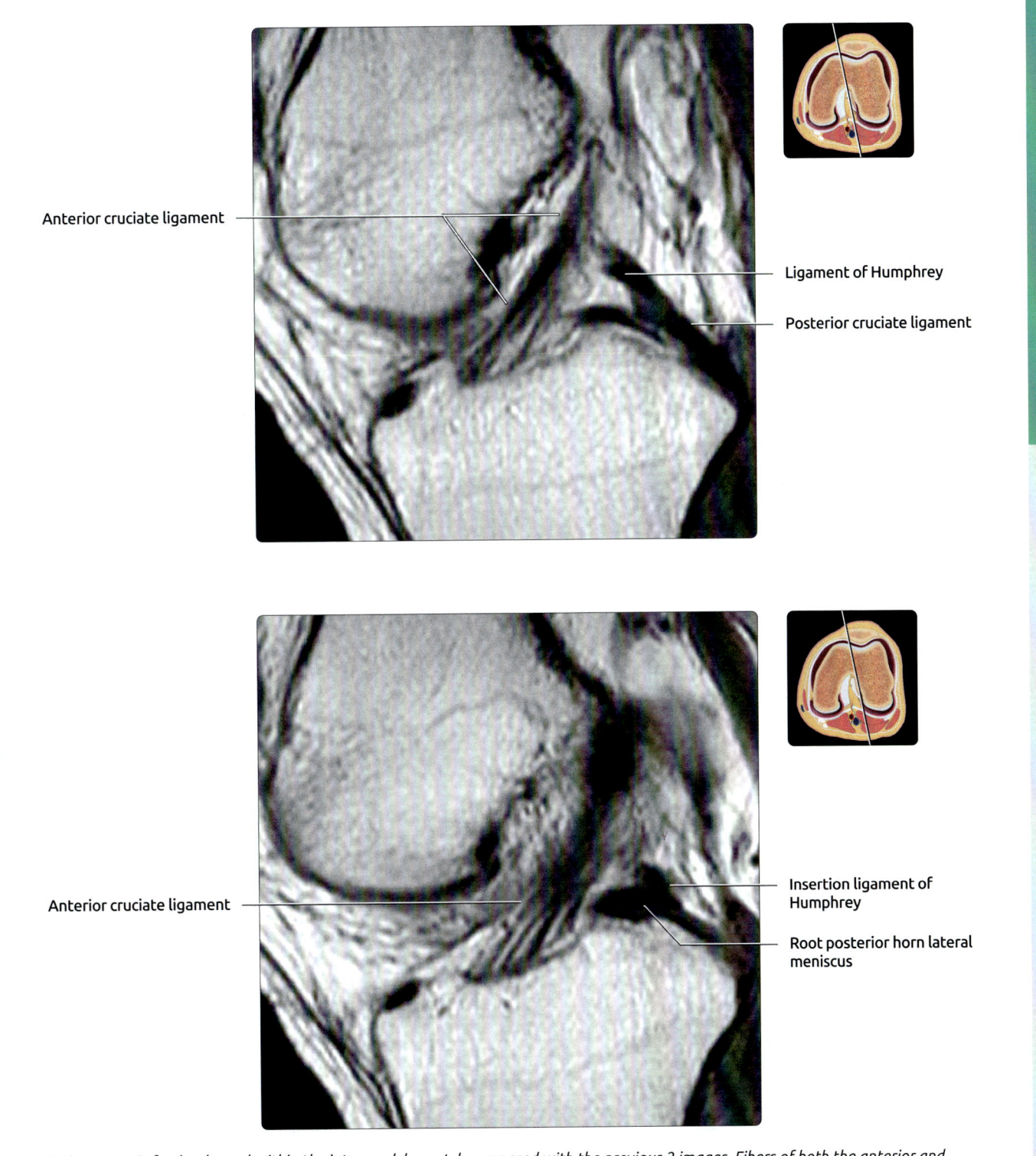

(Top) This image is further lateral within the intercondylar notch compared with the previous 2 images. Fibers of both the anterior and posterior cruciate ligament are seen. The ligament of Humphrey is still located anteroinferior to the posterior cruciate, extending toward the root of the posterior horn lateral meniscus. (Bottom) Further lateral within the intercondylar notch, this image shows the termination of the ligament of Humphrey as it inserts on the posterior horn lateral meniscus at its root. This insertion may be mistaken for a loose body, meniscal fragment, or other abnormality if it is not correctly identified.

Cruciate Ligaments/Posterior Capsule

POSTERIOR CAPSULE

Labels (top graphic): Retrocondylar bursa; Medial femoral condyle; Subgastrocnemius bursa; Posterior horn medial meniscus; Posterior capsule; Semimembranosus m.; Gastrocnemius tendon; Posterior capsule; Posterior oblique l.; Semimembranosus t.; Deep & superficial semimembranosus bursae

Labels (bottom MR): Posterior horn medial meniscus; Semimembranosus m.; Gastrocnemius tendon/capsular junction; Posterior capsule; Posterior oblique l.; Insertion direct band of semimembranosus t.; Medial gastrocnemius muscle

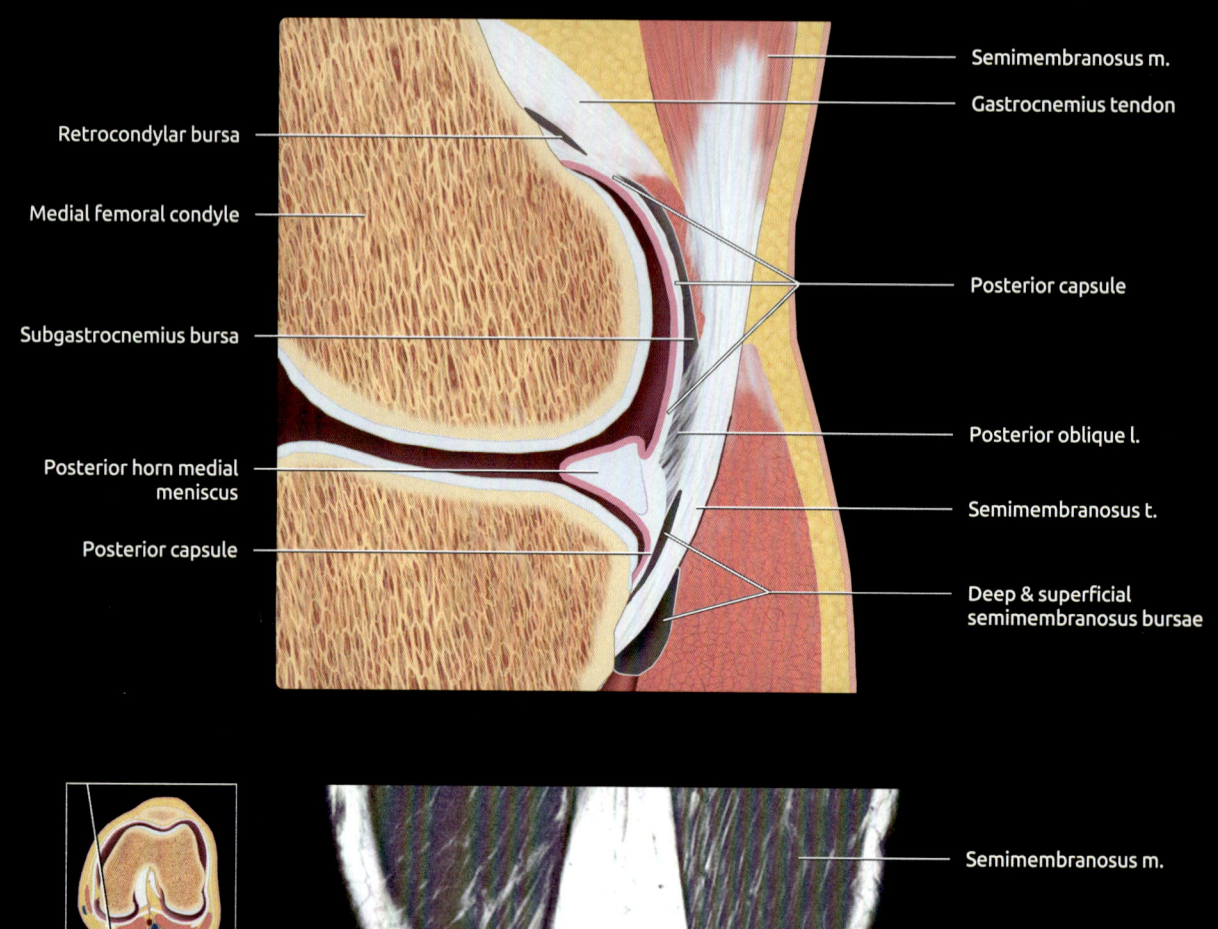

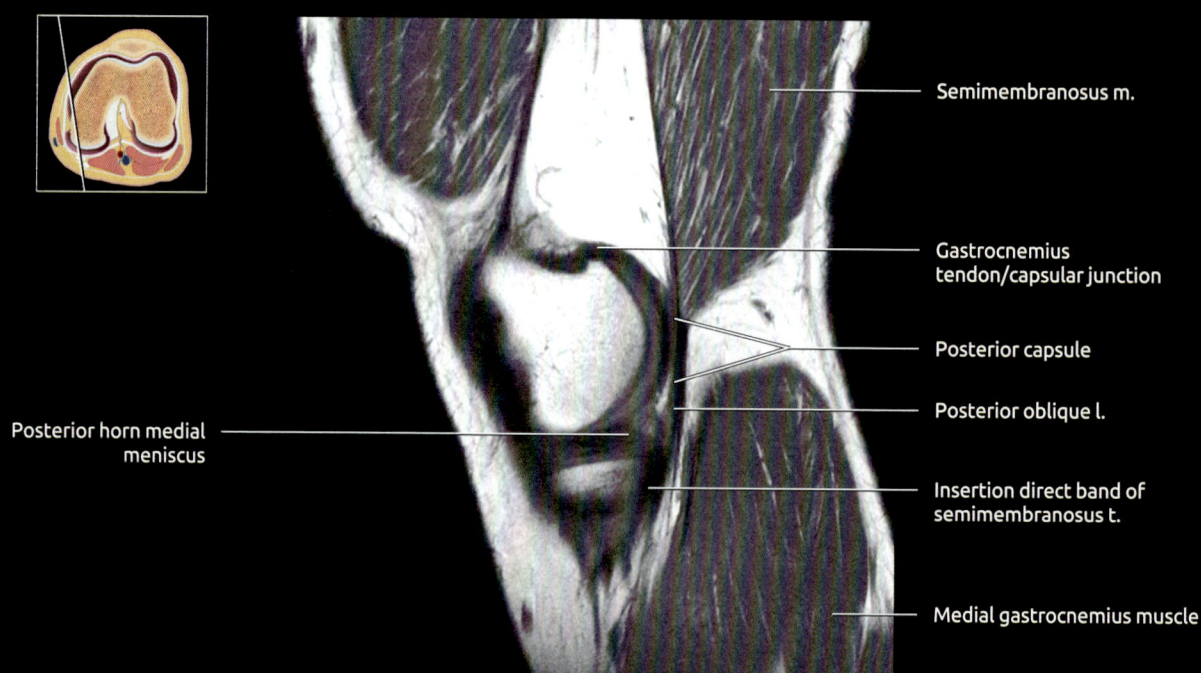

(**Top**) *Graphic shows the far medial portion of the posterior capsule. The capsule proper is complete, and the posterior horn of the meniscus attaches to it. Superiorly, the capsule attaches to the cortex of the posterior femoral condyle and then fuses with fibers of the medial gastrocnemius. A portion of the distal semimembranosus tendon contributes fibers to the oblique popliteal ligament; these continue as the posterior oblique ligament, contributing to the posterior capsule. Possible fluid collections in this area include the retrocondylar bursa superiorly, the subgastrocnemius bursa, and deep/superficial bursae on either side of semimembranosus tendon as it inserts on tibia.* (**Bottom**) *Sagittal PD MR image, located far medially, shows the contribution made by the semimembranosus tendon to the posterior capsule. Note that the posterior horn medial meniscus blends directly into the posterior capsule.*

Cruciate Ligaments/Posterior Capsule

POSTERIOR CAPSULE

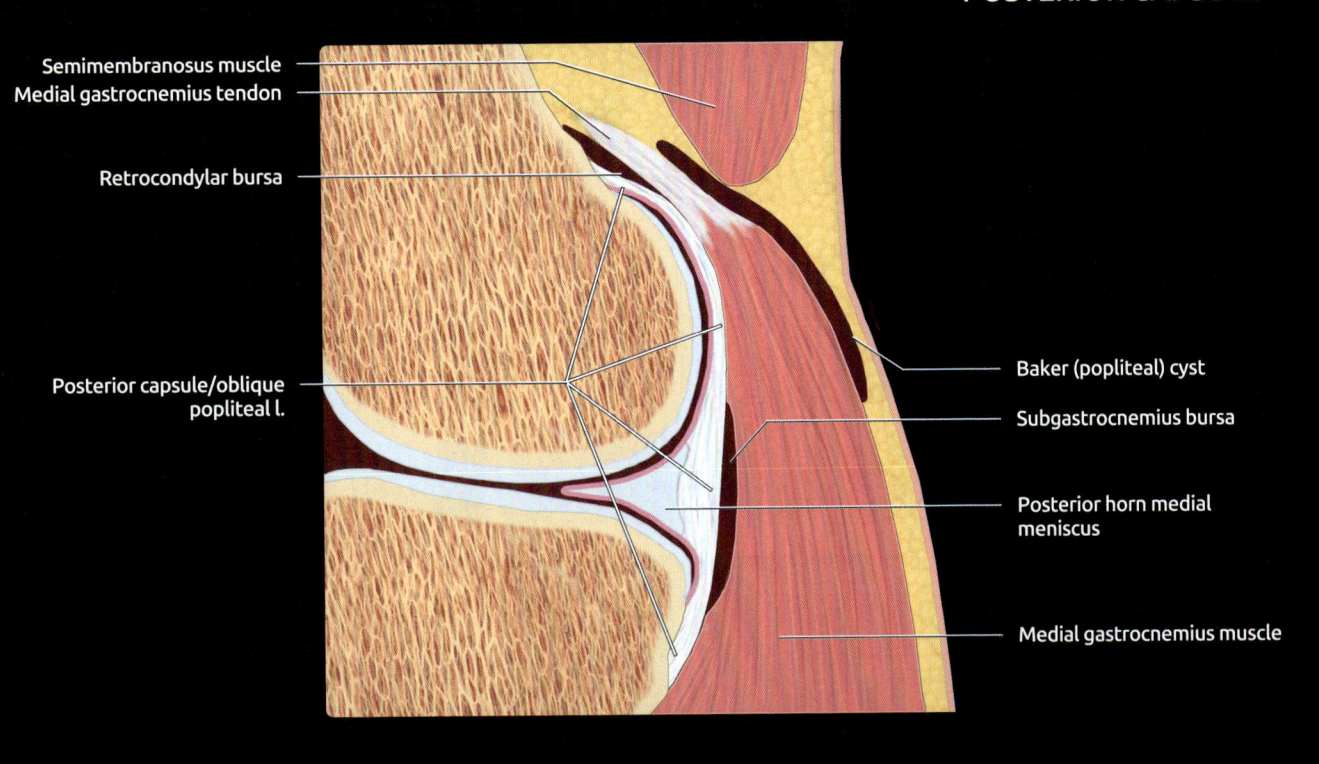

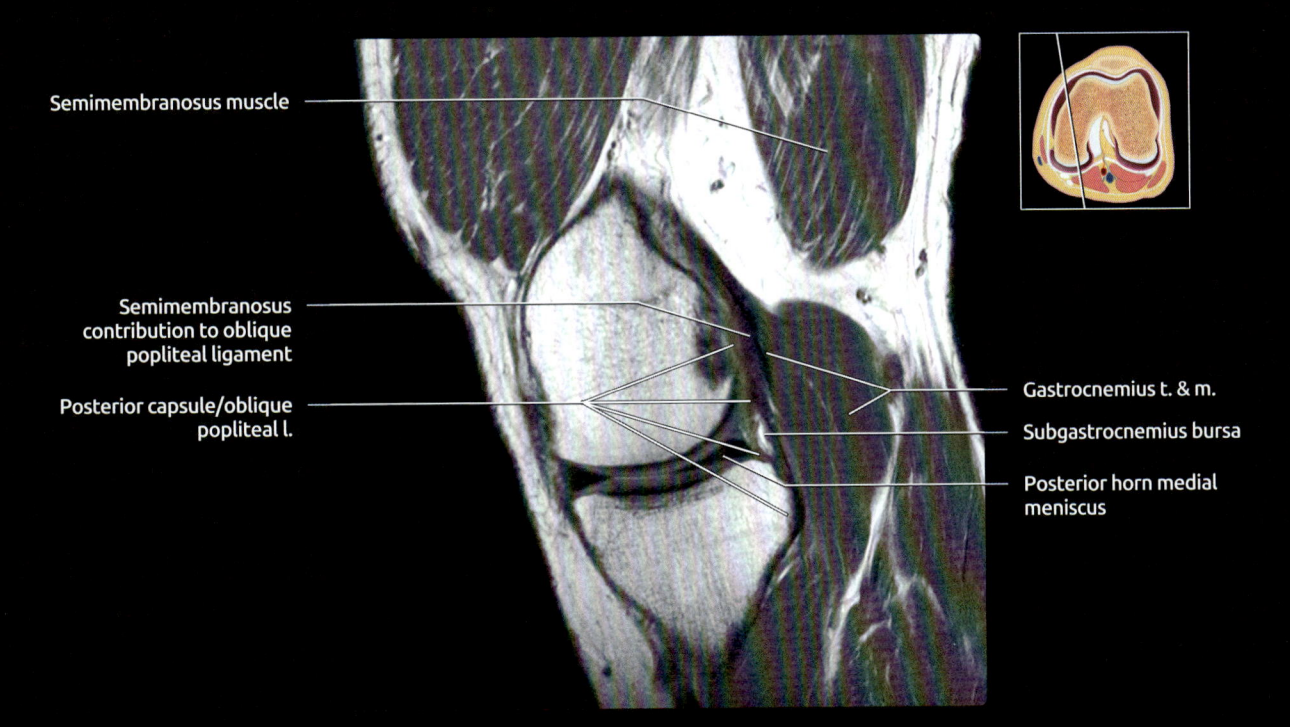

(Top) Sagittal graphic medially in the joint is shown. The capsule is fused superiorly with gastrocnemius tendon. A Baker (popliteal) cyst is shown at the gastrocnemius-semimembranosus bursa. The posterior horn medial meniscus is attached to the posterior capsule, reinforced by the oblique popliteal ligament. A small subgastrocnemius bursa is between the capsule and gastrocnemius muscle; another bursa is more superior between joint capsule and gastrocnemius tendon, the retrocondylar bursa. **(Bottom)** Sagittal image shows the posterior capsule to be inseparable from the medial gastrocnemius tendon proximally. Behind the meniscal attachment to the capsule; however, there is a subgastrocnemius bursa separating the capsule and gastrocnemius muscle. This case does not show a Baker (popliteal) cyst, but if it were present, it would lie between the semimembranosus and gastrocnemius muscle bellies.

781

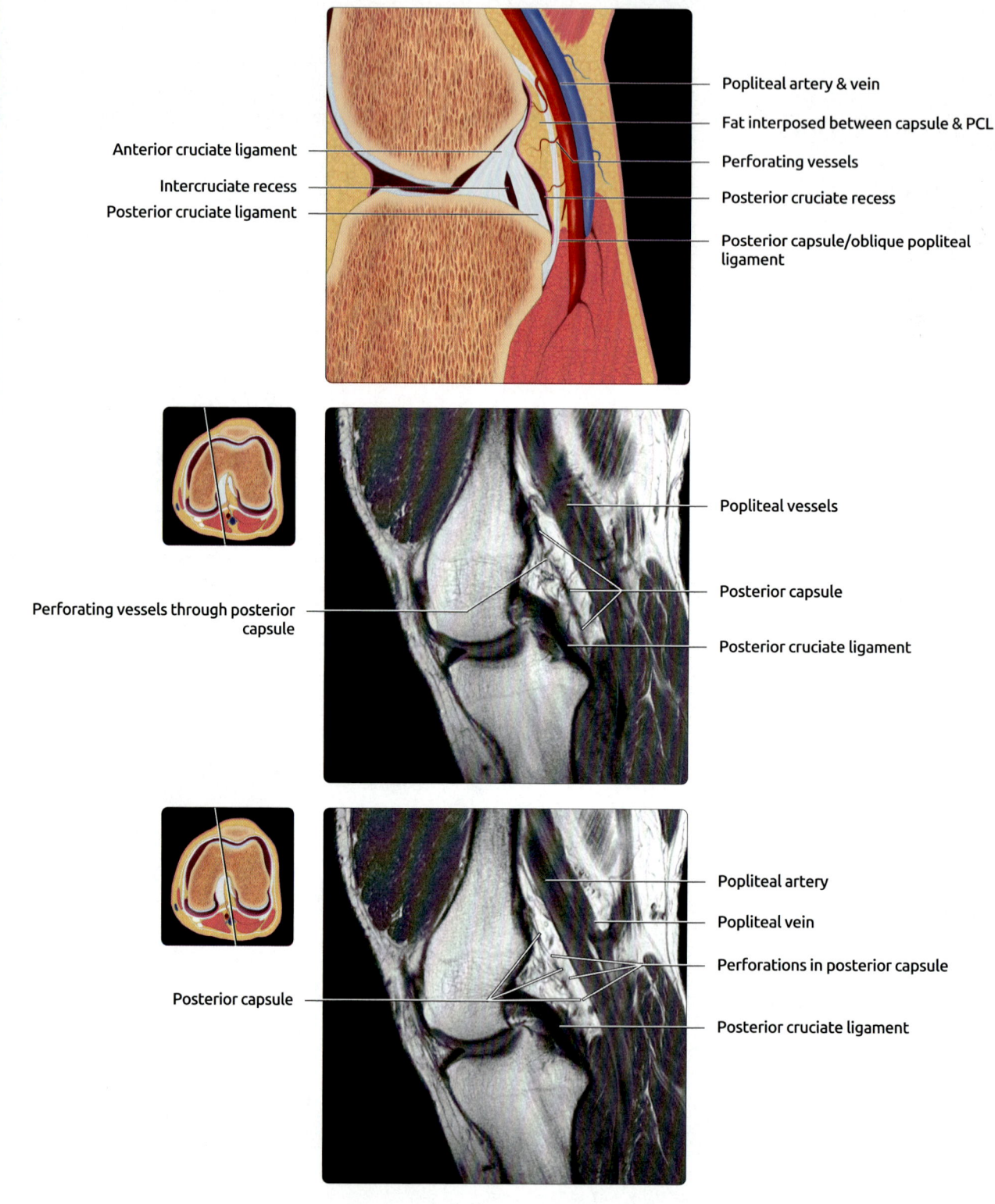

Cruciate Ligaments/Posterior Capsule

POSTERIOR CAPSULE

Labels (top graphic):
- Anterior cruciate ligament
- Intercruciate recess
- Posterior cruciate ligament
- Popliteal artery & vein
- Fat interposed between capsule & PCL
- Perforating vessels
- Posterior cruciate recess
- Posterior capsule/oblique popliteal ligament

Labels (middle):
- Perforating vessels through posterior capsule
- Popliteal vessels
- Posterior capsule
- Posterior cruciate ligament

Labels (bottom):
- Posterior capsule
- Popliteal artery
- Popliteal vein
- Perforations in posterior capsule
- Posterior cruciate ligament

(Top) *Graphic at the level of cruciate ligaments is shown. The capsule, strengthened by the oblique popliteal ligament, extends from the posterior margin of femoral condyles to the intercondylar fossa at the tibia. It is incomplete, with several small perforations at its mid portion for vessels extending from the popliteal vessels to the joint. The posterior cruciate recess is found between the capsule and the lower 2/3 of the PCL. There may be a small amount of fluid in the intercruciate recess.* **(Middle)** *Sagittal image through posterior cruciate shows posterior capsule with only a small perforation for a vessel; the majority of the capsule appears complete.* **(Bottom)** *Immediately adjacent, slightly lateral sagittal image shows several more perforations in posterior capsule for vessels. The capsule is incomplete at this point but is surrounded both anteriorly and posteriorly by fat.*

Cruciate Ligaments/Posterior Capsule

POSTERIOR CAPSULE

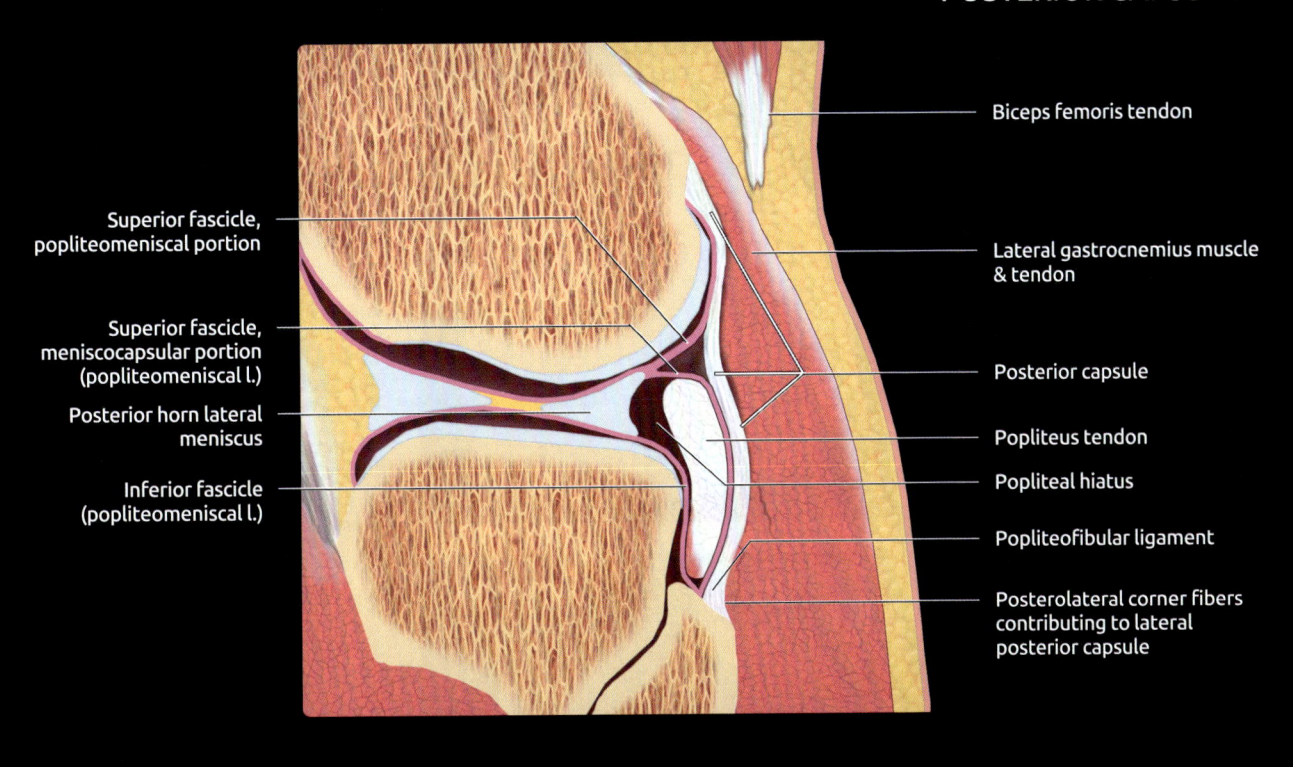

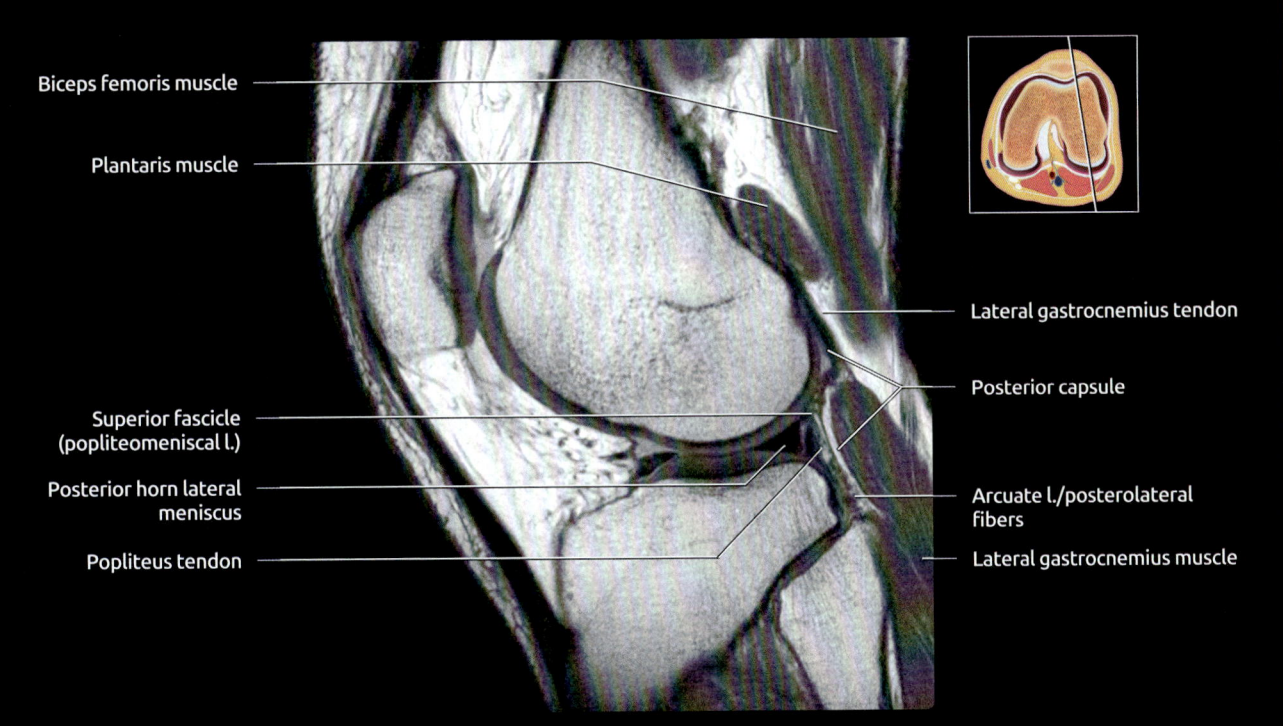

(Top) Graphic of the lateral part of posterior capsule shows that it is intimately attached to the lateral gastrocnemius muscle. The popliteus tendon is intraarticular but extrasynovial and is attached to the capsule. Fibers from the posterolateral corner and arcuate ligament originating from the fibular head contribute to the lateral portion of the posterior capsule. (Bottom) Sagittal MR image shows the gastrocnemius tendon contributing to the posterior capsule as well as the arcuate ligament (and fibers from other posterolateral structures). The popliteus tendon and superior fascicle (popliteomeniscal ligament) attach to the capsule as well.

Cruciate Ligaments/Posterior Capsule

SPACES WITHIN POSTERIOR CAPSULE REGION: AXIAL

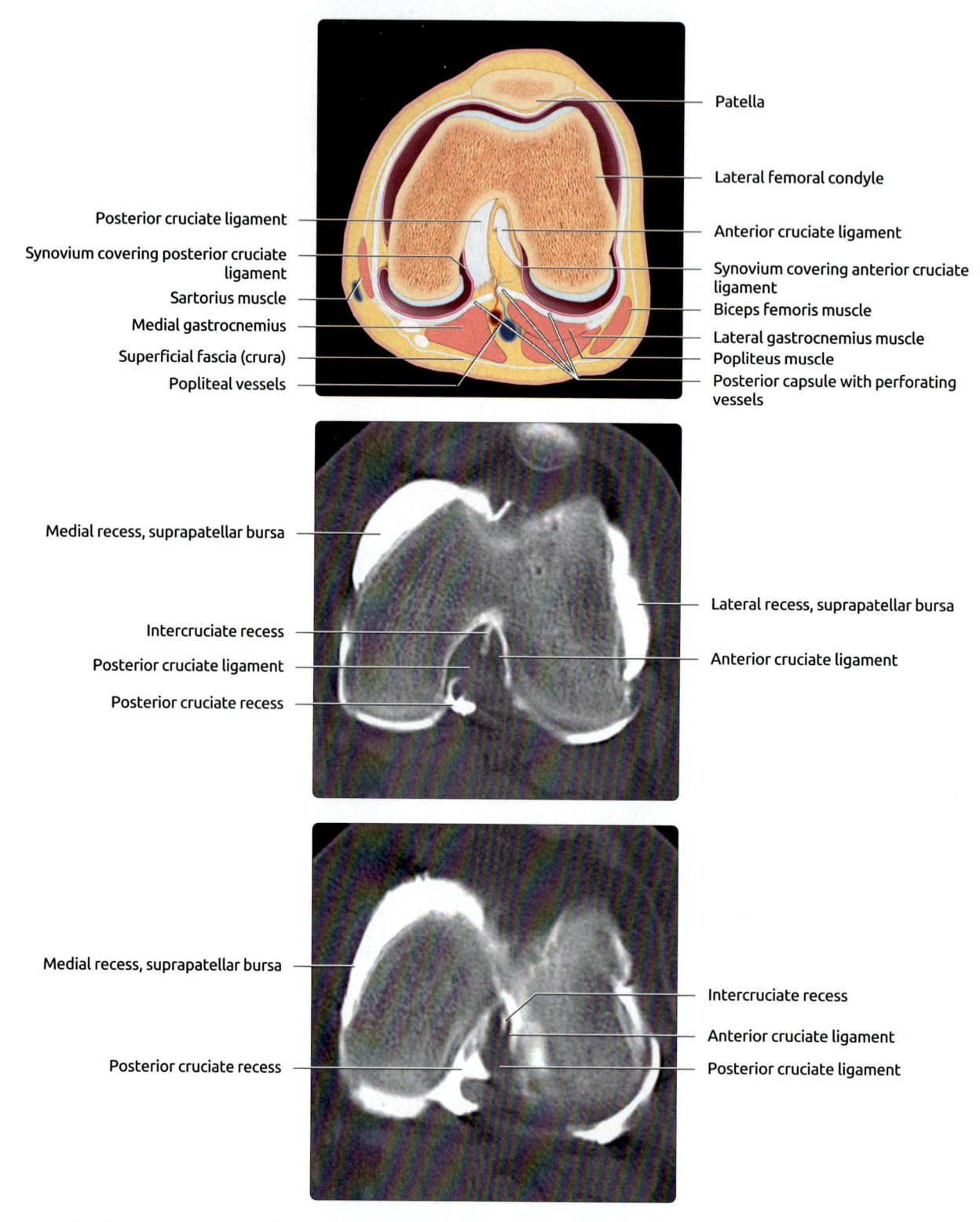

Top image labels:
- Patella
- Lateral femoral condyle
- Posterior cruciate ligament
- Anterior cruciate ligament
- Synovium covering posterior cruciate ligament
- Synovium covering anterior cruciate ligament
- Sartorius muscle
- Biceps femoris muscle
- Medial gastrocnemius
- Lateral gastrocnemius muscle
- Superficial fascia (crura)
- Popliteus muscle
- Popliteal vessels
- Posterior capsule with perforating vessels

Middle image labels:
- Medial recess, suprapatellar bursa
- Lateral recess, suprapatellar bursa
- Intercruciate recess
- Anterior cruciate ligament
- Posterior cruciate ligament
- Posterior cruciate recess

Bottom image labels:
- Medial recess, suprapatellar bursa
- Intercruciate recess
- Anterior cruciate ligament
- Posterior cruciate recess
- Posterior cruciate ligament

(**Top**) *Graphic shows the relationships of the posterior capsule. The most superficial layer is the crural fascia, which envelops the sartorius and otherwise confines all the structures. The posterior capsule (white) is continuous with the synovium (pink, next to purple synovial fluid) both posteromedially and posterolaterally. However, at the intercondylar area, the synovium separates from the capsule and covers the cruciate ligaments. It is this feature that allows us to outline the cruciates with injected fluid; they are intraarticular but extrasynovial. Thus, at this intercondylar area, the posterior capsule has no synovial covering. The capsule continues across the posterior aspect of the joint, anterior to the popliteal vessels, and is interrupted by perforating vessels.* (**Middle**) *CT arthrogram shows fluid-filled spaces.* (**Bottom**) *Here, the spaces are seen more distally.*

Cruciate Ligaments/Posterior Capsule

SPACES WITHIN POSTERIOR CAPSULE REGION: CORONAL

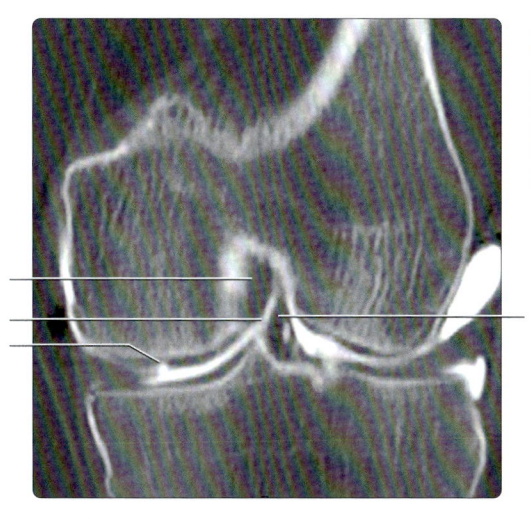

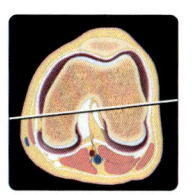

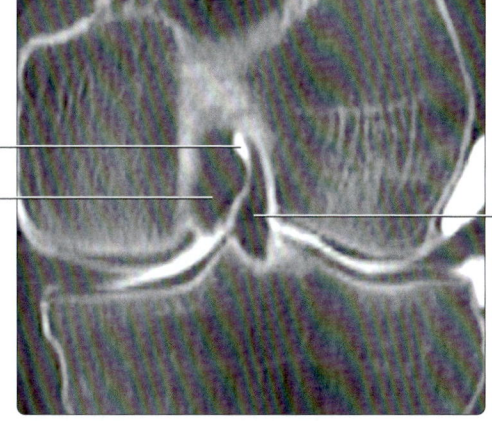

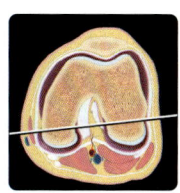

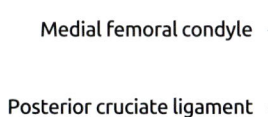

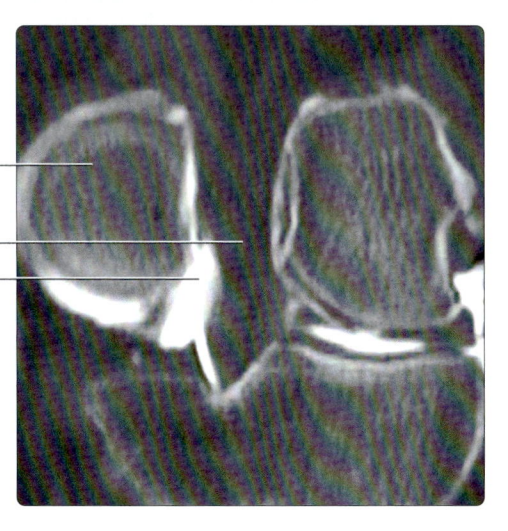

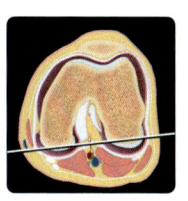

Origin posterior cruciate ligament
Intercruciate recess
Focal cartilage defect
Anteromedial band anterior cruciate ligament

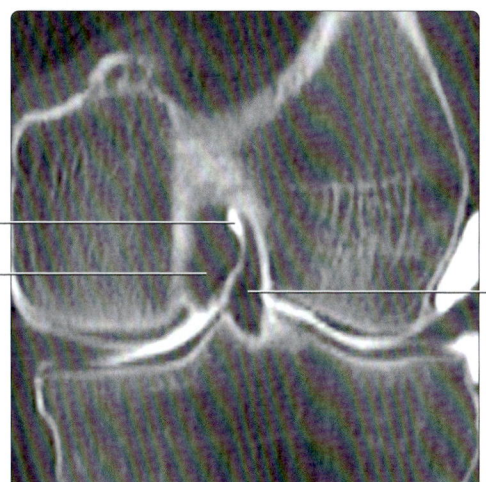

Intercruciate recess
Posterior cruciate ligament
Posterolateral band anterior cruciate ligament

Medial femoral condyle
Posterior cruciate ligament
Posterior cruciate recess

(Top) First of 3 coronal reformatted images from CT arthrogram is shown. With joint distension, the synovial-lined surfaces of the cruciate ligaments are outlined. In this more anterior cut, the anteromedial band of the ACL is primarily seen; only the origin of the PCL is seen at the medial femoral condylar portion of the notch. There is an intercruciate recess that fills with joint distension. Incidental note is made of a focal cartilage defect in the medial femoral weight-bearing surface. (Middle) Slightly more posteriorly, both the posterolateral band of the ACL and a larger portion of the PCL are seen. The menisci are well outlined, and the intercruciate recess is again noted. (Bottom) More posteriorly, the PCL is seen approaching its posterior tibial insertion. The posterior cruciate recess contacts the distal 2/3 of the PCL and flows into the medial (not lateral) compartment of the knee.

Knee Medial Supporting Structures

TERMINOLOGY

Abbreviations
- Medial (tibial) collateral ligament (MCL)
- Vastus medialis obliquus (VMO)
- Medial patellofemoral ligament (MPFL)

IMAGING ANATOMY

Overview
- Medial capsuloligamentous complex has **3 layers** that vary from anterior to mid to posterior; highly complex, with layers merging at different sites
- Primary stabilizers of femorotibial joint in valgus motion; secondary stabilizers to rotation
- Primary stabilizer against lateral subluxation/dislocation of patella

Superficial Layer (Layer 1)
- Primarily consists of **crural fascia**
- Anteriorly and superiorly, this crural fascia is continuous with fascia overlying vastus medialis
- **Sartorius** muscle/tendon enveloped by this fascia and is part of superficial layer
- Semimembranosus, semitendinosus, and gracilis are immediately deep to sartorius and superficial fascia
- Tendons of semitendinosus and gracilis blend with fascia of layer 1 and fibers of MCL as they insert distally on tibia
    - This means semitendinosus and gracilis cross just superficial to MCL (layer 2) and are between layers 1 and 2
    - Sartorius, semitendinosus, and gracilis together form pes anserinus at their insertion on anteromedial tibia, approximately 5 cm below joint line
        - Sartorius crosses medial knee joint anterior to gracilis, which in turn is anterior to semitendinosus
        - Sartorius has the broadest and most anterior insertion on tibia
        - Gracilis inserts directly adjacent to sartorius, with semitendinosus directly posterior and slightly inferior to gracilis

Middle Layer (Layer 2)
- **Anteriorly**, superficial (longitudinal) fibers of MCL (layer 2) merge with crural fascia (layer 1)
- **Mid knee**: Superficial fibers of MCL form layer 2
    - Vertical fibers
    - 12 cm long
    - 1-2 cm wide
    - 2-4 mm thick
    - Origin: Medial epicondyle
    - Courses slightly anteriorly to insert on tibia approximately 5 cm below joint line
    - Layer of fat containing medial inferior genicular artery lies between superficial MCL and tibia
- **Posteriorly**, superficial MCL has a posterior oblique component
    - Oblique fibers extend from layer 2 posteriorly and fuse with layer 3
    - Attaches closely to posteromedial portion of meniscus; this conjoined structure is termed posterior oblique ligament

Semimembranosus
- Complex insertion, involving both middle and deep layers
- Main portion inserts on posteromedial tibial plateau
- Other attachments
    - Tibia beneath MCL
    - Posteromedial capsule
    - Oblique popliteal ligament
    - Superficial fibers of MCL

Deep Layer (Layer 3)
- **Anterior**
    - Continuous with capsule along suprapatellar recess
    - Patellomeniscal ligament extends anteriorly from meniscus to patella margin
- **Mid knee**: Capsular layer, sometimes termed deep fibers of MCL
    - Capsule thickens to form these two ligaments
    - **Meniscofemoral**
        - 1-2 cm long
        - Extends from outer superior aspect of body of medial meniscus obliquely and cephalad
        - Attaches to either superficial MCL or femur
    - **Meniscotibial (coronary ligament)**
        - Short (1 cm)
        - Extends from outer inferior aspect of body of medial meniscus to tibia just distal to joint line
        - Slightly more posterior than meniscofemoral
    - Capsular layers fuse posteriorly with oblique fibers of superficial MCL (no fat interposed) to form posterior oblique ligament
- **Posteriorly**, primarily capsule, but receives fibers from
    - Semimembranosus
    - Oblique fibers of superficial MCL (in form of **posterior oblique ligament**)
    - **Oblique popliteal ligament**
        - Receives fibers from semimembranosus, superficial MCL (posterior oblique ligament), and synovial sheath
        - Envelops posterior aspect of femoral condyle to become a posterior structure

Bursae
- Variable amounts of fat between layers 1, 2, and 3
- May see small bursa (MCL bursa) between superficial and deep layers of MCL
    - Requires fluid (distension) to be seen on MR
    - Bursa can extend to distal extent of superficial MCL, though usually is smaller, lying just over body of meniscus and deep fibers of MCL
    - Delineated anteriorly by anterior margin of superficial MCL
    - Delineated posteriorly by merger of superficial and deep fibers of MCL
- Another bursa separates semimembranosus tendon from posterior capsule

Medial Stabilizers of Patella
- Loosely termed medial retinaculum
    - Extends from vastus medialis superiorly to tibia inferiorly
    - Inserts along medial edge of patella
- Highly complex, with **3 layers** which differ in superior, mid, and inferior portions

Knee Medial Supporting Structures

- **Layer 1** is most superficial, just deep to subcutaneous tissues
  - Deep crural fascia
  - Anterosuperiorly, continuous with fascia overlying vastus medialis
- **Layer 2** is just deep to layer 1, and just superficial to layer 3 (joint capsule)
- Within layers 2 and 3, condensations of fibers form ligaments of **medial retinacular complex**
- Within layer 2, medial retinacular complex ligaments form an inverted triangle in sagittal plane, with a central split which defines 3 separate ligaments
  - MPFL: Superior aspect of triangle
  - Superficial MCL: Posterior aspect of triangle
  - Patellotibial ligament: Anteroinferior aspect of triangle
- **Layer 3**: Joint capsule
- **Superior portion** of medial patellar stabilizers
  - **Vastus medialis obliquus**
    - Inferior portion of vastus medialis
    - Acts as dynamic stabilizer, neutralizing lateralizing forces on patella exerted by vastus lateralis during quadriceps contraction
    - Arises from adductor magnus tendon, medial intermuscular septum, or adductor tubercle
    - Merges with MPFL and inserts on superior 2/3 of medial patella
  - **Medial patellofemoral ligament**
    - Major ligamentous restraint preventing lateral patellar subluxation (50-60% total restraining force)
    - Origin is variable: Adductor tubercle, medial epicondyle, or superficial MCL
    - Runs forward and slightly inferiorly, just deep to VMO, fuses with aponeurosis of VMO
    - Inserts on superior 2/3 of medial patella; seen as distinct structure at insertion
    - 4.5-6 cm in length
    - < 0.5 cm thick
    - Width: 1-2 cm at femur, 2-3 cm at patella
    - Merges with layer 2 (medial retinaculum) inferiorly
- **Mid portion** of medial patellar stabilizers
  - Superficial MCL (layer 2), fuses with crural fascia (layer 1) to form medial retinaculum (proper) anteriorly
  - Merges with VMO fascia anteriorly
  - Inserts into medial margin of patella
- **Inferior portion** of medial patellar stabilizers
  - Patellotibial ligament
    - Originates on tibia at level of insertion of gracilis and semitendinosus
    - Joins layer 1 and extends obliquely proximally to insert on inferior aspect of patella and on patellar tendon
  - Medial patellomeniscal ligament
    - Deep in relation to patellotibial ligament (anatomically in layer 3)

Posteromedial Capsule

- **Medial side of posterior capsule**: Fibers from several structures merge with and contribute to capsule
  - Fibers from distal semimembranosus tendon, forming oblique popliteal ligament
  - Fibers from superficial MCL, forming posterior oblique ligament, which also contribute to oblique popliteal ligament
  - Capsule attaches to posterior femoral cortex a few cm above level of most superior aspect of cartilage
  - Capsule attaches inferiorly to tibia 1-2 cm below joint line
  - Bursa separates capsule and semimembranosus tendon
  - A little more towards center of knee, semimembranosus is replaced by medial gastrocnemius
  - Superiorly, capsule joins gastrocnemius tendon
- **Mid portion of posterior capsule**
  - Capsule is incomplete posteriorly
  - Therefore, intraarticular space is not completely separate from extraarticular fat
  - Popliteal artery and vein course behind capsule
    - Perforating vessels extend from these through posterior capsule
    - Perforating nerves accompany vessels

ANATOMY IMAGING ISSUES

Imaging Recommendations

- Superficial MCL: Coronal and axial
- Capsular layers (deep MCL): Coronal
- MPFL and VMO best seen on axials immediately inferior to adductor tubercle
  - MPFL seen at its origin in 80%
  - MPFL seen at patellar insertion in 100%
- Medial retinaculum seen just inferior to MPFL/VMO, also on axials
  - Medial retinaculum seen at midsubstance and patellar insertion in 100%
- Patellotibial and medial patellomeniscal meniscal ligaments seen at level of knee joint, on axials
- Oblique popliteal ligament envelops posterior aspect of femoral condyle, best seen on axials
  - Seen 100% on axial MR

SELECTED REFERENCES

1. Elias DA et al: Acute lateral patellar dislocation at MR imaging: injury patterns of medial patellar soft-tissue restraints and osteochondral injuries of the inferomedial patella. Radiology. 225(3):736-43, 2002
2. De Maeseneer M et al: Three layers of the medial capsular and supporting structures of the knee: MR imaging-anatomic correlation. Radiographics. 20 Spec No:S83-9, 2000
3. Spritzer CE et al: Medial retinacular complex injury in acute patellar dislocation: MR findings and surgical implications. AJR Am J Roentgenol. 168(1):117-22, 1997

Knee Medial Supporting Structures

PES ANSERINUS: SAGITTAL

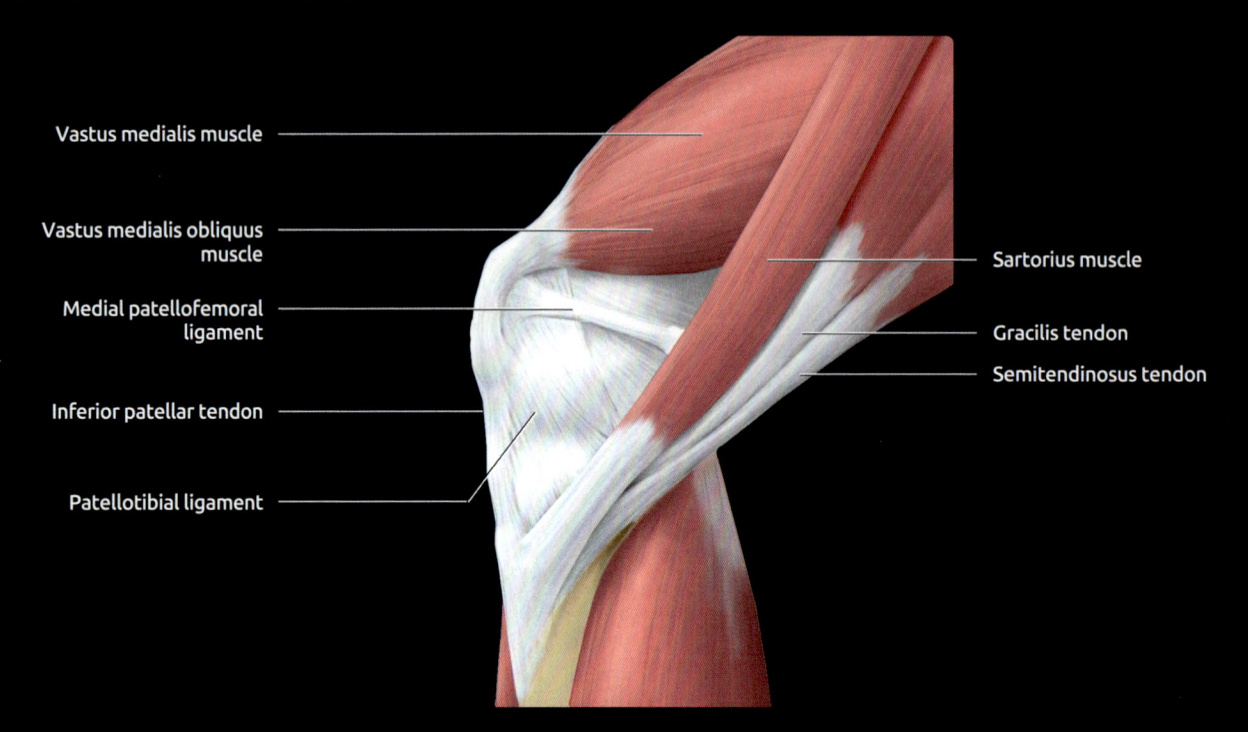

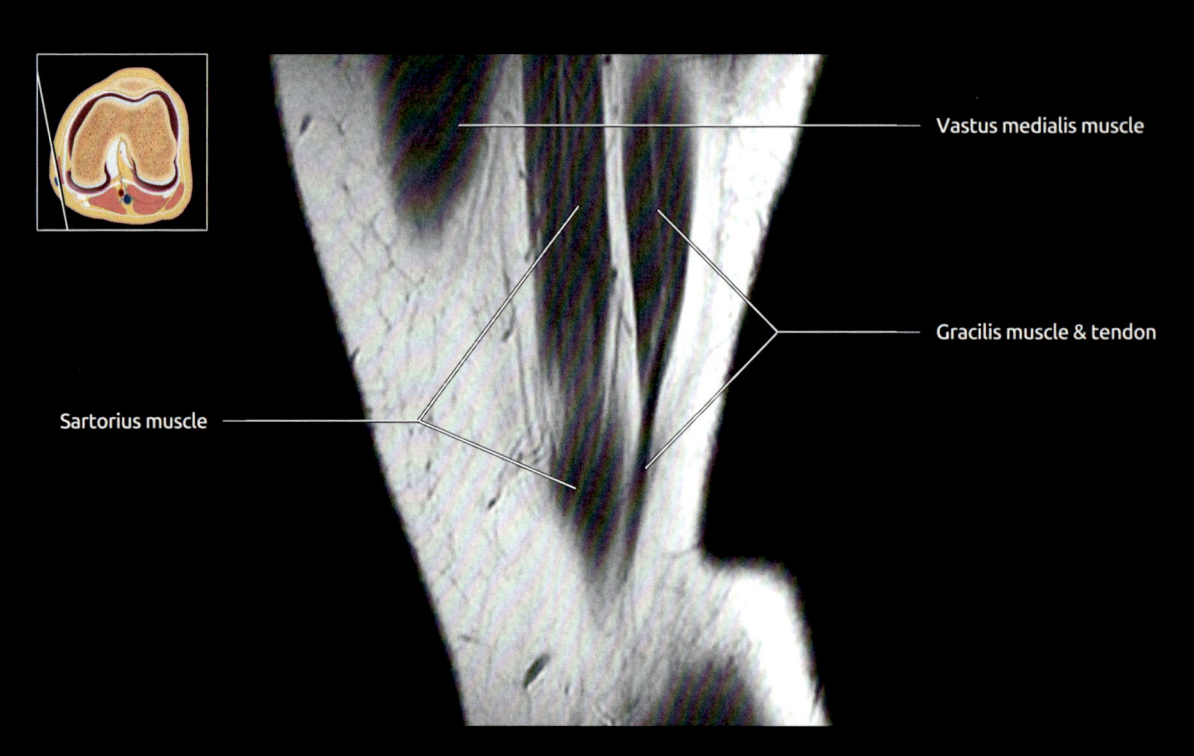

- Vastus medialis muscle
- Vastus medialis obliquus muscle
- Medial patellofemoral ligament
- Inferior patellar tendon
- Patellotibial ligament
- Sartorius muscle
- Gracilis tendon
- Semitendinosus tendon

- Vastus medialis muscle
- Gracilis muscle & tendon
- Sartorius muscle

(Top) Graphic shows the anteromedial attachment of the pes anserinus tendons. Sartorius is the most anterior & superficial. Gracilis inserts directly adjacent & deep to sartorius & semitendinosus inserts directly posterior & slightly inferior to gracilis. These tendons & their crural fascia comprise the superficial layer of the medial capsuloligamentous complex. (Bottom) First of 4 sagittal T1 MR images, starting far medially, shows the components of pes anserinus. The sartorius has a straight course above the knee joint, directly medial to the knee. Sartorius is invested by the crural fascia to form layer 1 of the medial capsuloligamentous complex. Gracilis maintains its position slightly posterior and deep to sartorius.

Knee Medial Supporting Structures

PES ANSERINUS: SAGITTAL

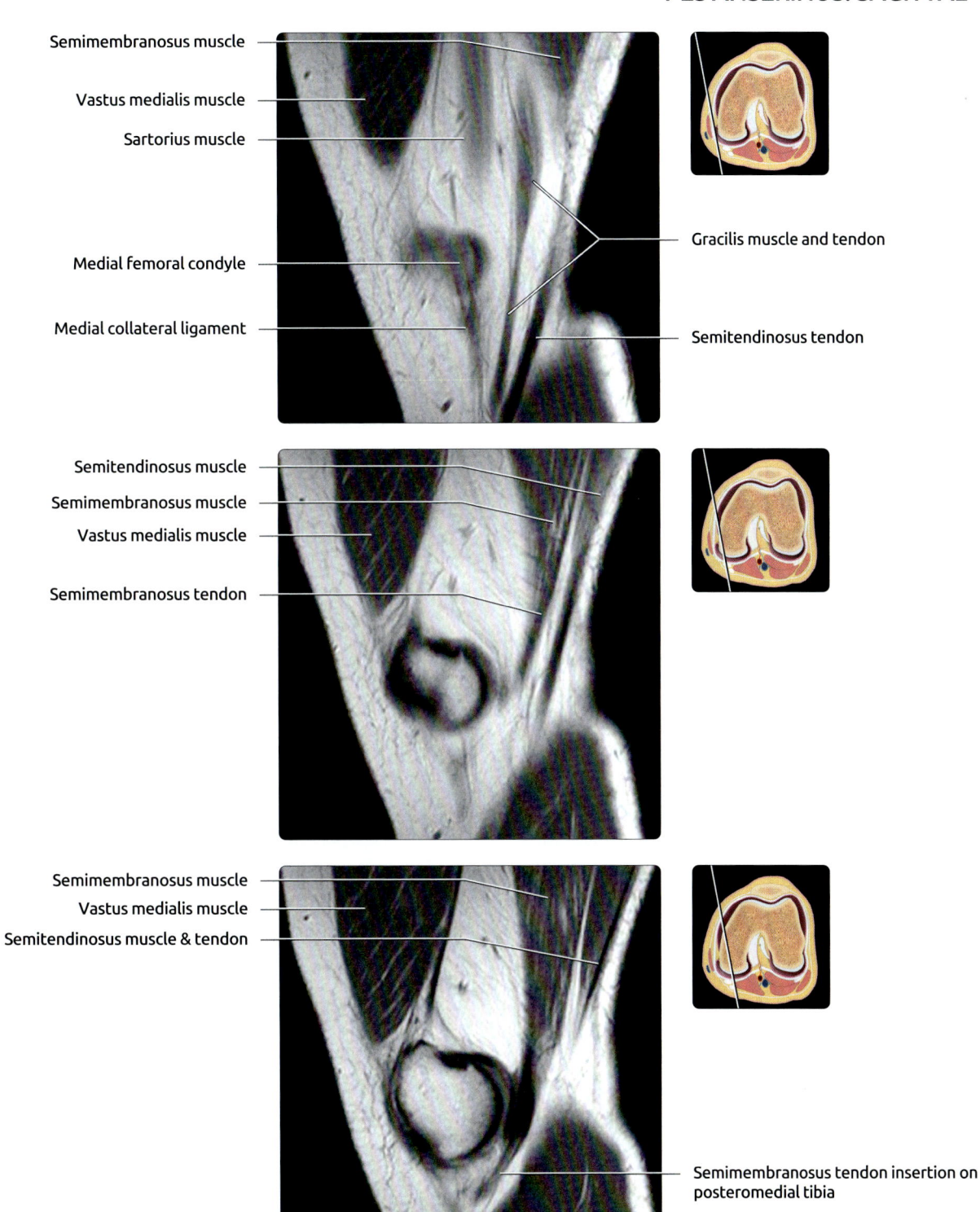

Labels (Top): Semimembranosus muscle; Vastus medialis muscle; Sartorius muscle; Medial femoral condyle; Medial collateral ligament; Gracilis muscle and tendon; Semitendinosus tendon

Labels (Middle): Semitendinosus muscle; Semimembranosus muscle; Vastus medialis muscle; Semimembranosus tendon

Labels (Bottom): Semimembranosus muscle; Vastus medialis muscle; Semitendinosus muscle & tendon; Semimembranosus tendon insertion on posteromedial tibia

(**Top**) *Slightly more lateral cut (toward the intercondylar notch) shows a remnant of sartorius. The gracilis tendon is immediately posterior and deep to sartorius. The semitendinosus tendon follows even more posteriorly and medially. The MCL is barely seen arising from the medial femoral condyle.* (**Middle**) *More laterally, the semimembranosus muscle and tendon are seen, with semitendinosus muscle and tendon remaining behind them. While the semitendinosus continues its course, following gracilis toward its anteromedial tibial insertion, semimembranosus inserts at the proximal tibia posteriorly and medially.* (**Bottom**) *Approaching the tibia with a more lateral section, semimembranosus is seen to broaden at its tendinous insertion on the posterior as well as medial tibia, immediately below the joint line. The slips from semimembranosus to medial collateral ligament and posterior capsule via the posterior oblique ligament are not seen as separate structures here.*

Knee Medial Supporting Structures

PES ANSERINUS: CORONAL

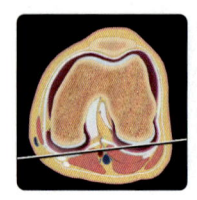

Sartorius muscle
Semimembranosus insertion
Sartorius tendon moving anteriorly out of plane
Gracilis tendon

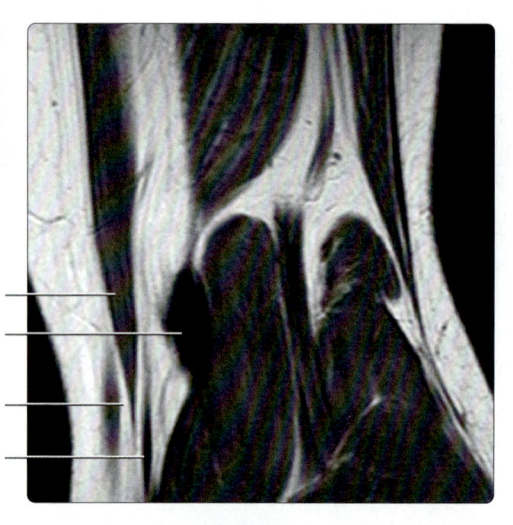

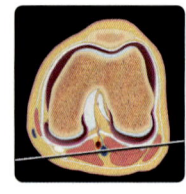

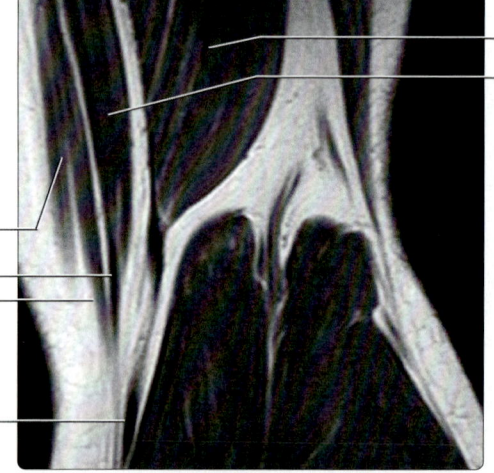

Semimembranosus muscle
Gracilis muscle
Sartorius muscle
Gracilis tendon
Sartorius tendon
Semitendinosus tendon

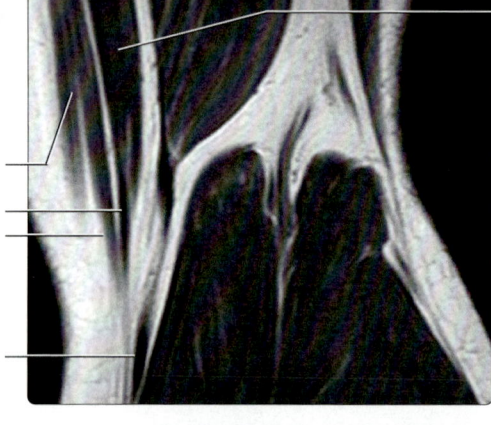

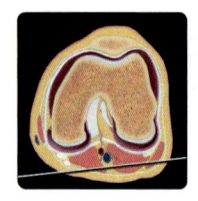

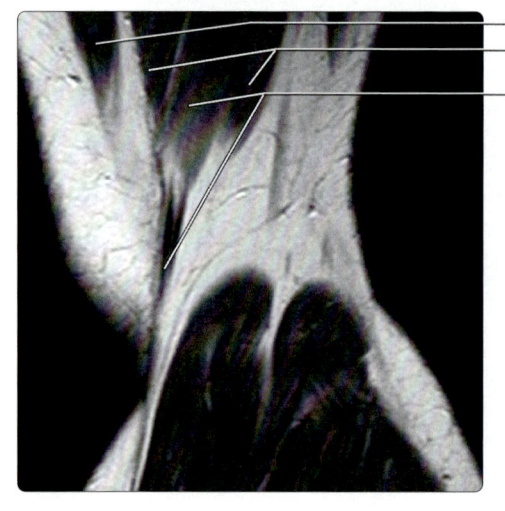

Gracilis muscle
Semimembranosus muscle
Semitendinosus muscle & tendon

(Top) First of 3 coronal T1 MR images, through the posterior portion of the joint, shows the medial-lateral relationships of the tendons comprising the pes anserinus. At the level of the popliteal vessels, just posterior to the tibia, the semimembranosus spreads out into its insertion, which is wide at the posterior as well as posteromedial tibia. The sartorius muscle is seen at this level, with its tendon curving anteriorly out of the plane. A portion of the gracilis tendon is seen paralleling and deep to the sartorius tendon. (Middle) Shown slightly more posteriorly, a remnant of sartorius muscle and tendon is seen, but the gracilis muscle & tendon are more completely seen. A very small portion of the semitendinosus tendon is seen distally, behind & medial to gracilis. Semitendinosus muscle is more proximal and posterior, and out of plane. (Bottom) Even more posteriorly, the semitendinosus muscle & tendon are shown posterior to the muscle belly of semimembranosus.

Knee Medial Supporting Structures

PES ANSERINUS: AXIAL

Labels (Top image): Vastus medialis obliquus m.; Anterior medial crural fascia; Origin, medial patellofemoral ligament & medial collateral l.; Sartorius tendon; Sartorius muscle; Gracilis tendon; Crural fascia; Semitendinosus tendon; Semimembranosus muscle

Labels (Middle image): Medial patellofemoral ligament; Medial collateral ligament; Sartorius tendon; Sartorius muscle; Gracilis tendon; Semimembranosus tendon; Semitendinosus tendon; Crural fascia

Labels (Bottom image): Medial retinaculum; Medial collateral ligament, longitudinal portion; Medial collateral ligament, oblique portion; Sartorius tendon; Gracilis tendon; Semitendinosus tendon; Posterior oblique ligamentous extension of oblique fibers MCL; Semimembranosus t.

(**Top**) First of 3 axial T1 MR images shows the anatomy of pes anserinus. Sartorius is the most superficial. It is invested by crural fascia to form layer 1. The gracilis tendon is medial to sartorius and follows its tendon in a slightly posterior position. Semitendinosus is posterior to semimembranosus, and distinctly posterior and lateral (towards the intercondylar notch) relative to the gracilis tendon. (**Middle**) Superficial MCL arises distal to adductor tubercle and forms layer 2. (**Bottom**) At the level of the joint line, the elements of the pes line up in order of their insertion (sartorius, gracilis, semitendinosus) on the anteromedial tibia. Anteriorly, layers 1 (sartorius) and 2 (superficial MCL) merge to contribute to medial retinaculum. Gracilis & semitendinosus lie between layers 1 & 2. Posteriorly, layers 2 & 3 (superficial & deep MCL, respectively) merge to form the posterior oblique ligament, contributing to capsule.

Knee Medial Supporting Structures

POSTEROMEDIAL STRUCTURES

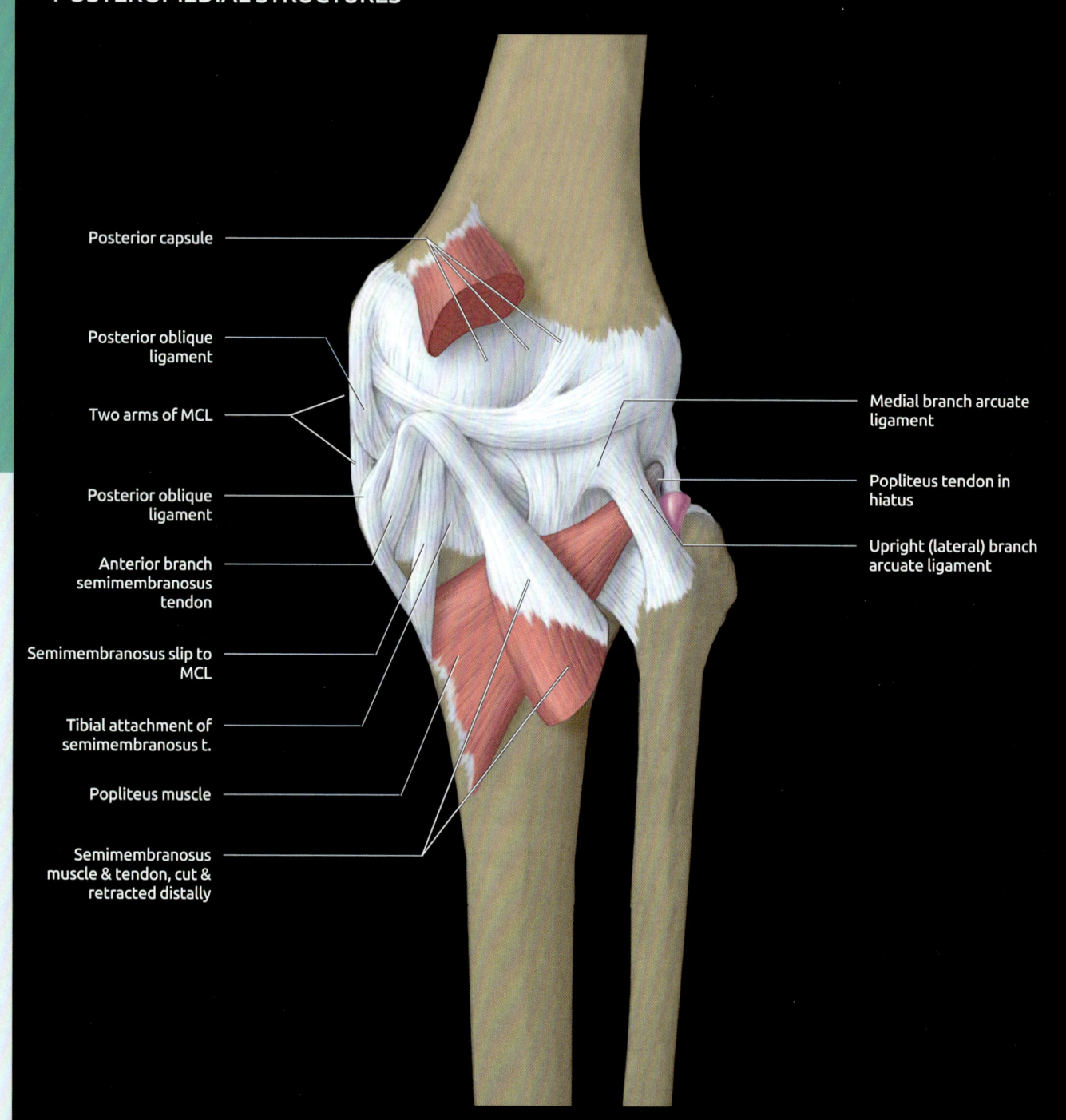

- Posterior capsule
- Posterior oblique ligament
- Two arms of MCL
- Posterior oblique ligament
- Anterior branch semimembranosus tendon
- Semimembranosus slip to MCL
- Tibial attachment of semimembranosus t.
- Popliteus muscle
- Semimembranosus muscle & tendon, cut & retracted distally
- Medial branch arcuate ligament
- Popliteus tendon in hiatus
- Upright (lateral) branch arcuate ligament

The semimembranosus tendon has a complex insertion, both at the posteromedial tibia and more anteriorly at the medial tibia. Semimembranosus also provides slips to the posterior aspect of MCL, as well as providing an expansion to the oblique popliteal ligament. The posterior oblique ligament arises from several arms of the superficial MCL, both superiorly and inferiorly, as well as from the posterior aspect of the deep MCL (therefore both layers 2 and 3 contribute to it). The posterior oblique ligament then extends from its posteromedial position to contribute to the oblique popliteal ligament, which in turn strengthens the posterior capsule. On the lateral side, fibers from the arcuate ligament blend into and contribute to the oblique popliteal ligament as well.

Knee Medial Supporting Structures

POSTEROMEDIAL STRUCTURES: SEMIMEMBRANOSUS

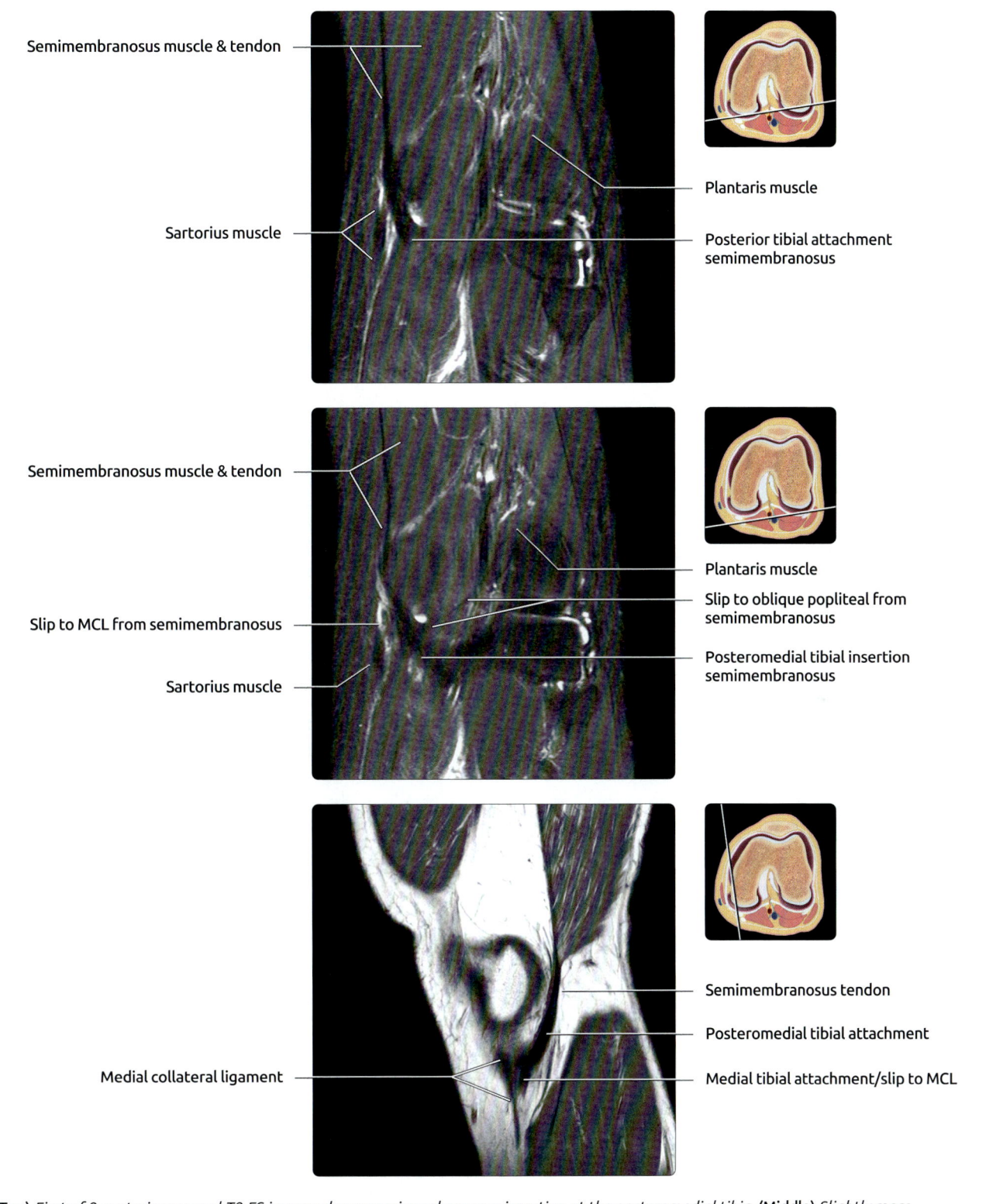

Labels (Top): Semimembranosus muscle & tendon; Sartorius muscle; Plantaris muscle; Posterior tibial attachment semimembranosus

Labels (Middle): Semimembranosus muscle & tendon; Slip to MCL from semimembranosus; Sartorius muscle; Plantaris muscle; Slip to oblique popliteal from semimembranosus; Posteromedial tibial insertion semimembranosus

Labels (Bottom): Medial collateral ligament; Semimembranosus tendon; Posteromedial tibial attachment; Medial tibial attachment/slip to MCL

(Top) First of 2 posterior coronal T2 FS images shows semimembranosus insertion at the posteromedial tibia. (Middle) Slightly more anterior cut shows the multiple slips of semimembranosus. These include insertions at the posteromedial tibia, and another more directly medially. Additionally, there are slips extending from semimembranosus to the oblique popliteal and medial collateral ligaments. (Bottom) Sagittal PD MR image shows semimembranosus insertion on the posteromedial tibia, along with its slip extending to the medial collateral ligament.

Knee Medial Supporting Structures

MEDIAL CAPSULOLIGAMENTOUS COMPLEX

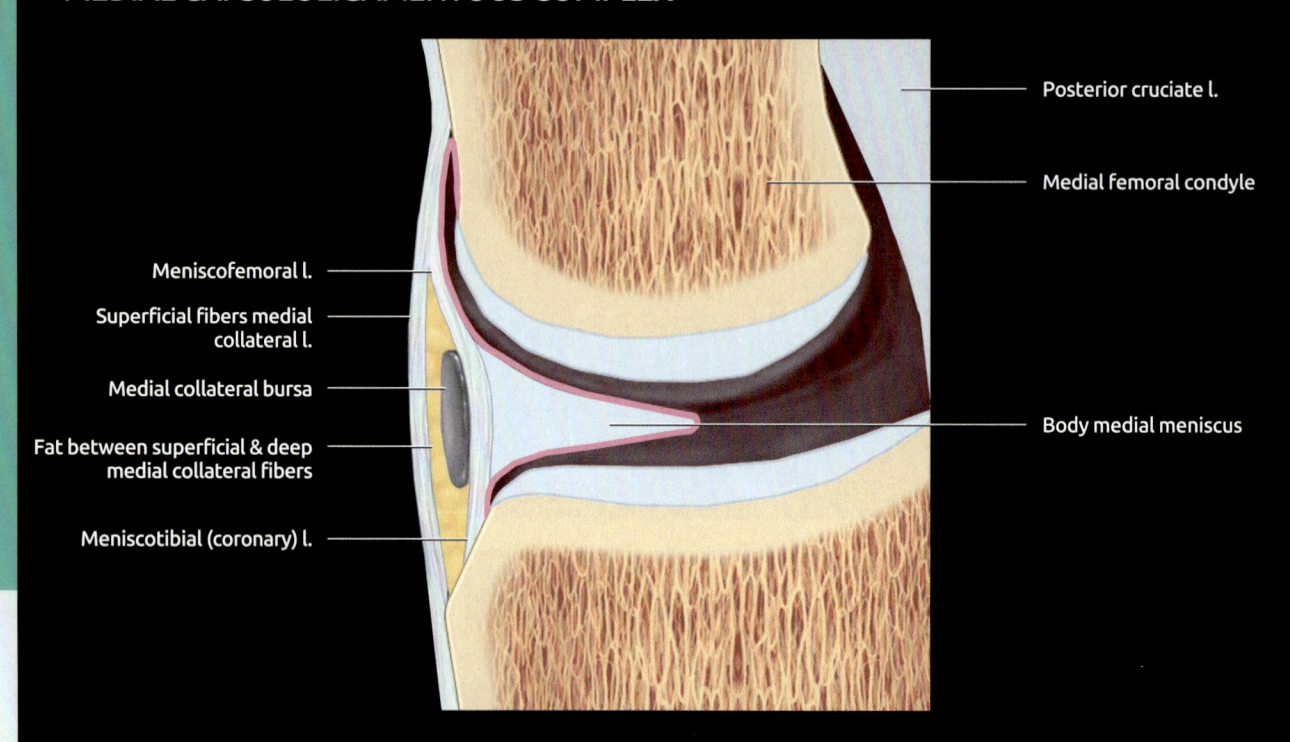

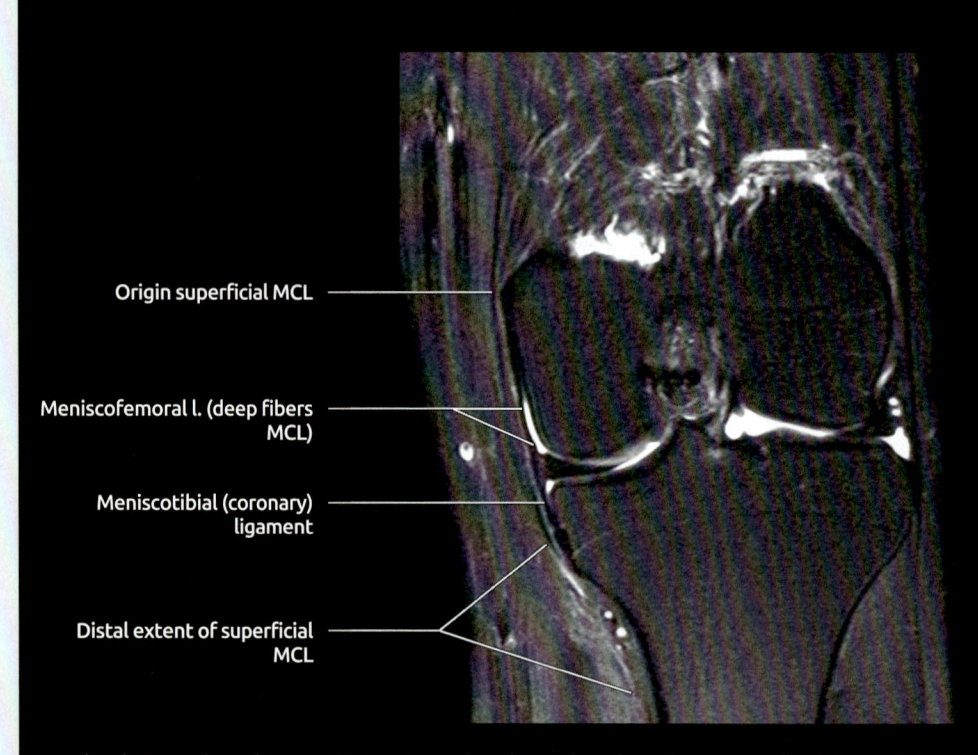

Labels (top graphic):
- Meniscofemoral l.
- Superficial fibers medial collateral l.
- Medial collateral bursa
- Fat between superficial & deep medial collateral fibers
- Meniscotibial (coronary) l.
- Posterior cruciate l.
- Medial femoral condyle
- Body medial meniscus

Labels (bottom MRI):
- Origin superficial MCL
- Meniscofemoral l. (deep fibers MCL)
- Meniscotibial (coronary) ligament
- Distal extent of superficial MCL

(Top) Coronal graphic at mid joint, shows the relationship of the deep & superficial fibers of the medial collateral ligament. Superficial fibers extend from adjacent to the adductor tubercle to approximately 5 cm distal to the joint line. Deep fibers are much shorter: The meniscotibial (coronary) ligament extends from meniscus to tibia adjacent to the joint line & the meniscofemoral ligament extends from meniscus to either femur or superficial MCL. A variable amount of fat and a small bursa may be seen between deep & superficial fibers. (Bottom) Coronal view shows the deep medial collateral fibers, outlined by joint fluid. The meniscofemoral ligament inserts on the femur in this case; it may also normally insert on the superficial MCL at the same level above the joint. The short coronary (meniscotibial) ligament is seen. Superficial MCL is only faintly seen due to the fat-saturation. There is no bursal fluid present to separate the deep and superficial layers of the MCL.

Knee Medial Supporting Structures

MEDIAL CAPSULOLIGAMENTOUS COMPLEX

Labels (top graphic):
- Layers 1 & 2 merge: Medial retinaculum
- Superficial MCL (longitudinal)
- Superficial MCL (oblique)
- Deep MCL fibers/capsular layer
- Posterior oblique l.
- Sartorius muscle
- Crural fascia
- Gracilis tendon
- Semitendinosus tendon
- Anterior cruciate l.
- Meniscofemoral l. (Humphrey)
- Posterior cruciate ligament
- Meniscofemoral l. (Wrisberg)
- Posterior capsule
- Semimembranosus tendon

Labels (bottom MR):
- Retinaculum: Merger of layers 1 & 2
- Meniscocapsular junction
- Superficial MCL
- Sartorius muscle
- Gracilis tendon
- Semimembranosus tendon
- Semitendinosus tendon
- Layers 2 & 3 merge: Posterior oblique ligament
- Posterior capsule, with slips from posterior oblique
- Slip to posterior capsule from semimembranosus

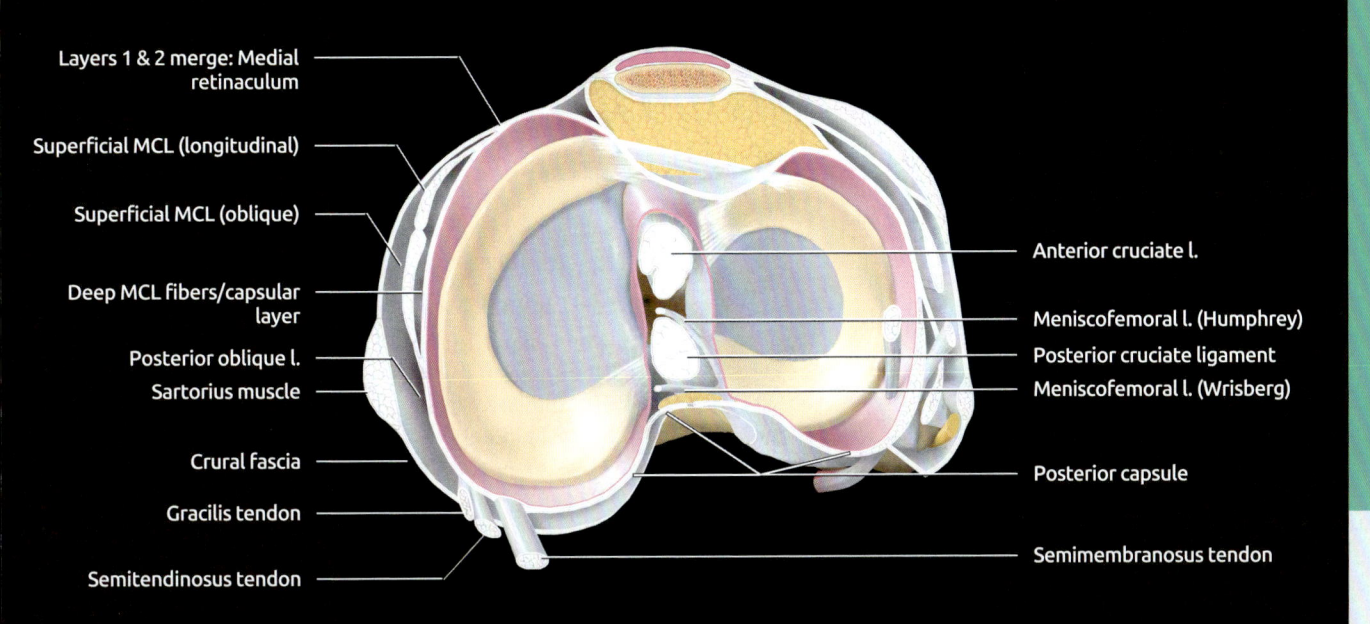

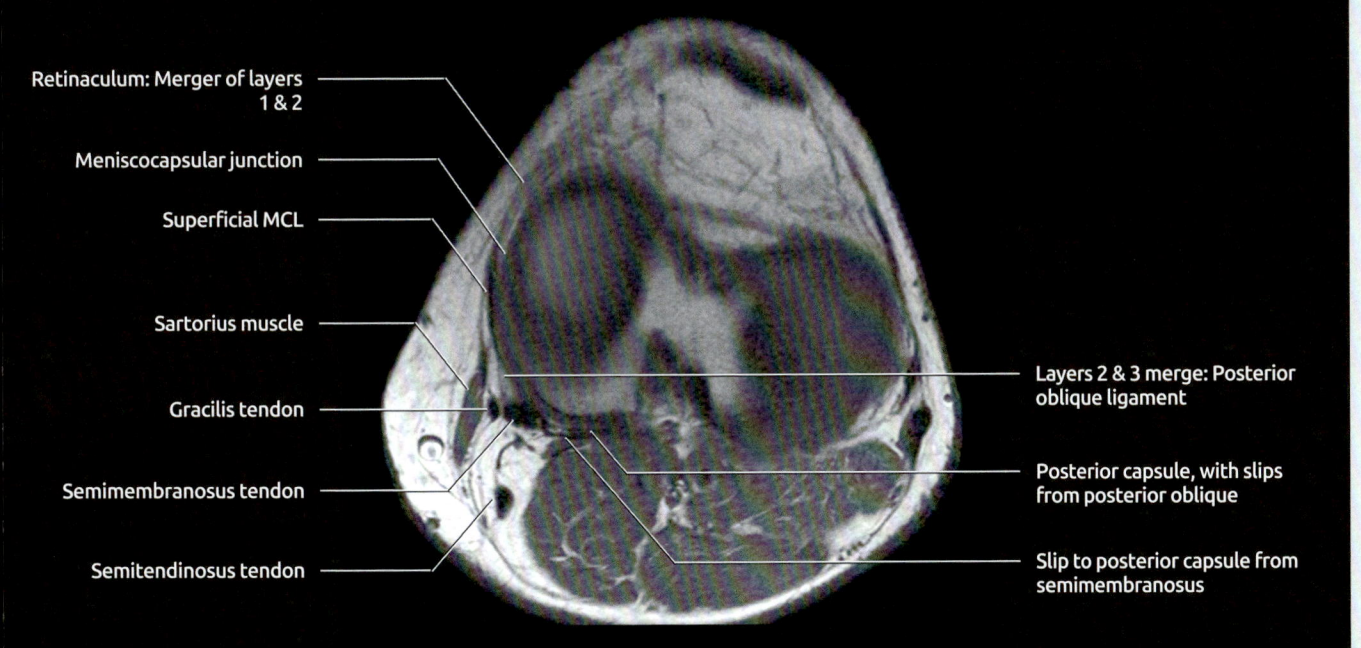

(Top) Graphic shows 3 layers of medial capsuloligamentous complex. Layer 1 consists of crural fascia, which envelops sartorius. Superficial fibers of MCL form layer 2. Layers 1 & 2 merge anteriorly to contribute to medial retinaculum. Gracilis & semitendinosus lie between layers 1 & 2. Posteriorly, superficial MCL fibers (layer 2) fuse with deep MCL fibers (layer 3) to form the posterior oblique ligament; this ligament contributes to the posterior capsule at its posteromedial aspect. (Bottom) Axial T1 MR shows some of the complexity of the posteromedial structures, including the elements of the pes anserinus as well as the various attachments and slips of the semimembranosus tendon. Note in this example the slip from semimembranosus extending to the posterior oblique ligament & posterior capsule.

Knee Lateral Supporting Structures

TERMINOLOGY

Abbreviations
- Iliotibial (IT) tract
- Lateral (fibular) collateral ligament (LCL)

Synonyms
- Popliteofibular = short external lateral ligament = fibular origin of popliteus = popliteofibular fascicles

IMAGING ANATOMY

Overview
- Combination of muscles, tendons, and ligaments that contribute to lateral stability of knee

Muscles Contributing to Lateral Stability
- **Iliotibial tract**
  - **Origin**: Strong band of deep fascia composed of fusion of aponeurotic coverings of
    - Tensor fascia lata
    - Gluteus maximus
    - Gluteus minimus
  - Above knee, IT tract has insertion arms to
    - Supracondylar tubercle of lateral femoral condyle
    - Blends with intermuscular septum
  - Main insertion
    - Gerdy tubercle (anterolateral tibia near plateau)
    - Small other attachments to patella and patellar ligament
- **Biceps femoris**
  - Long head joined by short head above knee
  - **Main insertion** site is head and styloid process fibula
  - Several tendinous and fascial insertional components, including a portion that inserts on posterior edge of IT tract
  - Anterior oblique fibers of conjoined tendon arise from anterior bundle of short head biceps and insert on tibia
- **Popliteus**
  - Tendinous attachment at **popliteal sulcus** of lateral femoral condyle
    - Inferior and deep to origin of LCL
  - Extends posteromedially through **popliteal hiatus** (runs deep to fabellofibular and arcuate ligaments)
  - **Superior popliteomeniscal fascicle** extends from posterior horn lateral meniscus to paratenon tissues of popliteus tendon
    - Superior popliteomeniscal fascicle and arcuate ligament form **roof of popliteal hiatus**
  - **Inferior popliteomeniscal fascicle** extends from posterior horn lateral meniscus to paratenon tissues of popliteus tendon
    - Inferior popliteomeniscal fascicle forms **floor of popliteal hiatus**
  - Superior and inferior fascicles join and insert on fibular styloid as **popliteofibular ligament**
  - **Popliteus muscle** attaches to posteromedial aspect of proximal tibial metaphysis
  - **Function** of popliteus muscle
    - Assist with flexion of knee
    - Internally rotates tibia on femur (at initiation of flexion of knee)
    - Protects posterior horn lateral meniscus by withdrawing it from joint space during flexion and rotation
    - Stabilizes posterolateral corner from rotatory instability

Posterolateral Capsule
- Arcuate ligament fibers contribute to capsule laterally
- Popliteal tendon (intraarticular but extrasynovial) firmly attached to posterior capsule
- Popliteal recess may extend deeply behind tibia (in front of capsule); may have continuity with proximal tibiofibular joint
- Lateral gastrocnemius muscle contributes fibers to capsule

Lateral Support System Consists of 3 Layers
- **Layer 1 (superficial)**
  - Anteriorly, IT tract
  - Posterolaterally, superficial portion of biceps
- **Layer 2 (middle)**
  - Anteriorly, lateral retinaculum
  - 2 ligamentous thickenings originate from lateral patella
    - Proximal one terminates at lateral intermuscular septum
    - Distal one terminates at femoral insertion of posterolateral capsule and lateral head of gastrocnemius tendon
- **Layer 3 (deep)**
  - Forms lateral part of capsule
  - Contains several thickenings that function as discrete structures
    - Anterolateral ligament (originates immediately anterior to LCL, extends obliquely and anteriorly to insert on tibia midway between Gerdy tubercle and fibular head; firm attachment to lateral meniscus
    - Lateral (fibular) collateral ligament
    - Arcuate complex, consisting of multiple ligaments
  - Posterolateral corner ligament anatomy is extremely complex

Posterolateral Corner Structures
- All insert on fibular head and provide posterolateral support
- Not all are seen with equal reliability on imaging
- Posterolateral corner structures may be divided into superficial and deep
  - Superficial: Long and short heads of biceps femoris, and LCL
  - Deep: Posterolateral reinforcements of fibrous capsule, including fabellofibular, arcuate, oblique popliteal, and popliteofibular ligaments
- **Long head of biceps femoris**
  - 2 major tendinous components
    - Direct arm inserts on fibular head
    - Anterior arm inserts just anterior to direct arm on fibular head and continues distally as anterior aponeurosis that extends anterolaterally around leg
- **Short head of biceps femoris**
  - 2 tendinous components
    - Direct arm inserts on fibular head anterior to styloid process and medial to long head biceps

Knee Lateral Supporting Structures

- Anterior arm passes medial to lateral collateral ligament and inserts into superolateral edge of lateral tibial condyle, approaching Gerdy tubercle
- **Lateral collateral ligament**
  - Proximal attachment at distal femur just proximal and posterior to lateral epicondyle
  - Proximal attachment is slightly proximal and anterior to sulcus for origin of popliteus tendon
  - LCL extends posterolaterally to insert on upper facet of fibular head
    - Anterolateral to attachment of fabellofibular and arcuate ligaments
- **Fabellofibular ligament**
  - Originates at fabella (or proximal to it)
  - Inserts at lateral aspect of apex of fibular head (styloid process)
  - Inserts just anterolateral to insertion of popliteofibular ligament on fibular head
  - Fabellofibular ligament may be dominant when arcuate is diminutive
- **Arcuate ligament**
  - Y shaped
  - Arises from fibular styloid process, just deep to fabellofibular ligament
  - Lateral limb courses straight upward along lateral knee capsule to reach lateral femoral condyle
  - Medial limb crosses over posterior surface of popliteal tendon and attaches to posterior knee capsule
    - Medial limb, along with superior popliteomeniscal fascicle, forms bowed roof of popliteal hiatus
    - At insertion on posterior knee capsule, medial limb arcuate merges with fibers from oblique popliteal ligament
  - Arcuate may be dominant when fabellofibular is absent (or may contain fibers of fabellofibular ligament)
  - Inferior lateral geniculate artery passes anterior relative to arcuate
- **Oblique popliteal ligament**
  - Arises medially from slips of semimembranosus and medial tibial condyle, courses superolaterally
  - Joins arcuate ligament posterolaterally at its femoral insertion (margin of intercondylar fossa and posterior surface of lateral femoral condyle)
- **Popliteofibular ligament**
  - Arises from confluence of superior and inferior fascicles
  - Inserts on fibular head
  - Popliteofibular ligament may be dominant, with neither arcuate or fabellofibular ligaments present

ANATOMY IMAGING ISSUES

Imaging Recommendations

- Crucial posterolateral structures seen on axial and routine oblique sagittal imaging (generally prescribed on axial, oblique along course of anterior cruciate ligament [l.])
- **Coronal oblique** suggested to increase probability of visualizing posterolateral structures
  - Prescribed off sagittal image
  - Obliquity runs anterosuperior to posteroinferior, generally parallel to popliteal tendon as seen on sagittals

Imaging Sweet Spots

- Statistics below based on 1.5T MR imaging
- Biceps seen well in all 3 planes, 100%
  - Individual components may be seen separately on axials near fibular attachment
    - Short head biceps, direct arm 70%
    - Long head biceps, direct and anterior arms 70%
- LCL seen well in all 3 planes, 100%
- Superior popliteomeniscal fascicle seen best on sagittal fluid sensitive sequence, at level of posterior horn lateral meniscus; 100%
- Inferior popliteomeniscal fascicle seen best on coronal fluid sensitive sequence, at level of body lateral meniscus; 100%
- Arcuate ligament
  - In cadaver study, at least 1 limb seen in 70% on sagittal or coronal MR
    - Lateral limb arcuate seen 57% (better when fabella absent)
    - Medial limb arcuate seen 57% (better when fabella present)
  - Coronal oblique MR may increase likelihood
- Fabellofibular ligament rarely seen as separate entity (coronal or sagittal)
- Popliteofibular ligament
  - In cadaver study, seen 57% using coronal oblique (38% with standard planes)
- Oblique popliteal ligament 100%, axial

Avulsion Fractures at Posterolateral Corner

- **Arcuate sign**
  - Thin sliver avulsion at posterosuperior portion of fibular styloid
  - Site of (near) common insertion of fabellofibular, popliteofibular, and arcuate ligaments
  - Marrow edema may also indicate injury at this site
  - Posterior cruciate ligament injury is often associated
- **Anterolateral fibular head avulsion** (not fibular styloid)
  - LCL/biceps avulsion

CLINICAL IMPLICATIONS

Clinical Importance

- Posterolateral structures act primarily as static constraints to varus angulation and external rotation of knee
- Secondary restraint against posterior translation of tibia

Biomechanical Selective Cutting Study

- Major structures preventing posterolateral instability are LCL and popliteus tendon
- Popliteofibular ligament also important in providing static stability
- Surgery primarily focuses on restoring these ligaments
- Identifying popliteofibular on MR is variable (even with coronal oblique)
  - Limitation in assessing posterolateral corner injuries

Knee Lateral Supporting Structures

POSTEROLATERAL CORNER

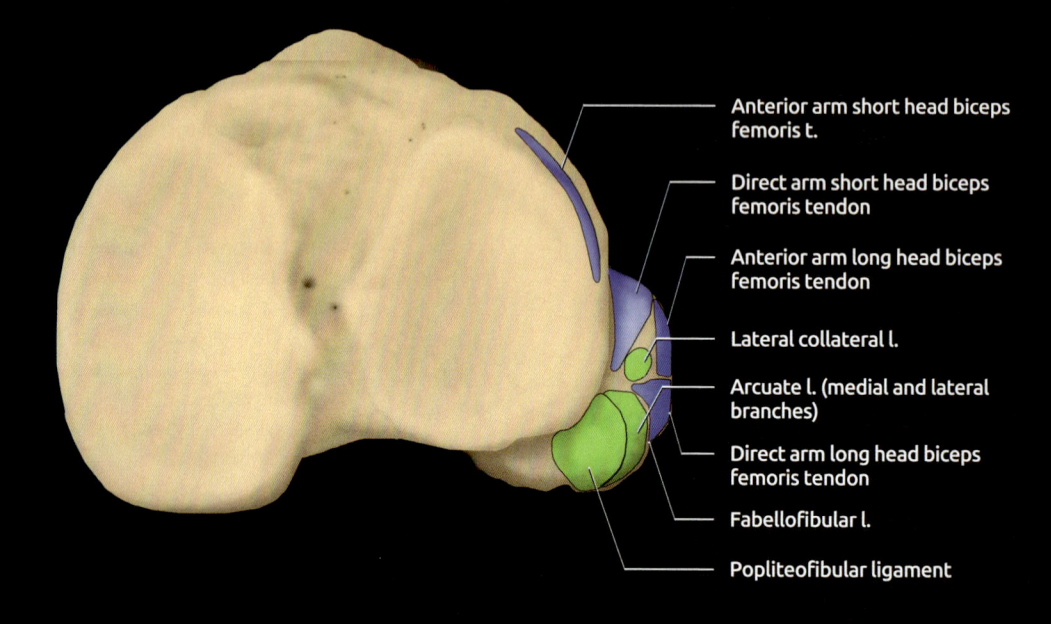

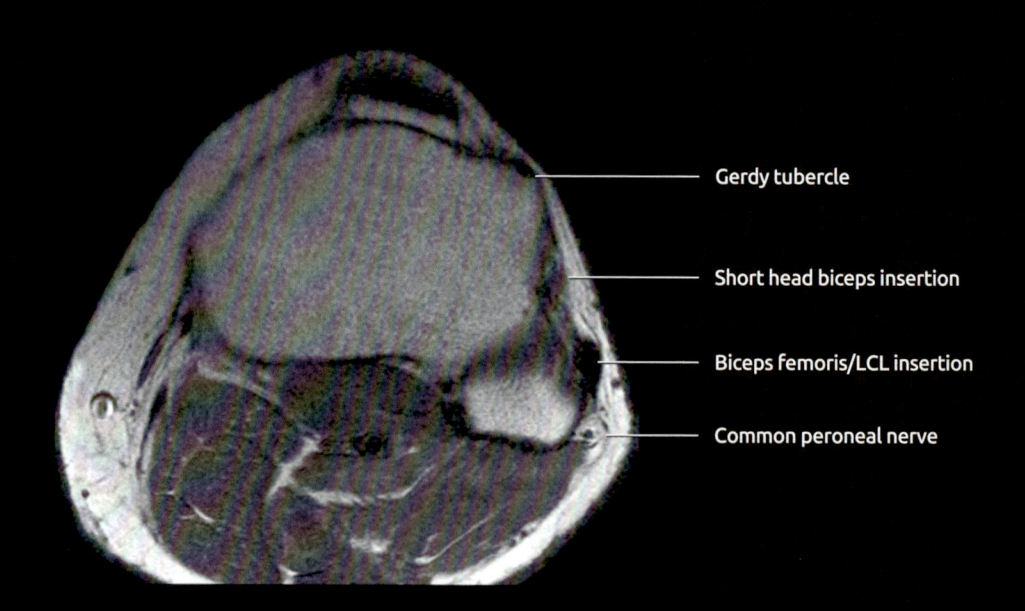

- Anterior arm short head biceps femoris t.
- Direct arm short head biceps femoris tendon
- Anterior arm long head biceps femoris tendon
- Lateral collateral l.
- Arcuate l. (medial and lateral branches)
- Direct arm long head biceps femoris tendon
- Fabellofibular l.
- Popliteofibular ligament

- Gerdy tubercle
- Short head biceps insertion
- Biceps femoris/LCL insertion
- Common peroneal nerve

(Top) Graphic shows the insertion sites of posterolateral structures on the proximal fibula. Note that the 2 heads of the short head biceps femoris insert most anteriorly, with the lateral collateral ligament and 2 heads of the long head biceps femoris directly posterior to that. The arcuate, fabellofibular, and popliteofibular ligaments insert more posteriorly at the apex of the fibular head (fibular styloid process). (Bottom) Axial T1 MR at the head of the fibula, biceps femoris/LCL tendon insert laterally. The arcuate and popliteofibular ligaments have already inserted on the fibular styloid apex slightly more proximally (not shown).

Knee Lateral Supporting Structures

POSTEROLATERAL CORNER

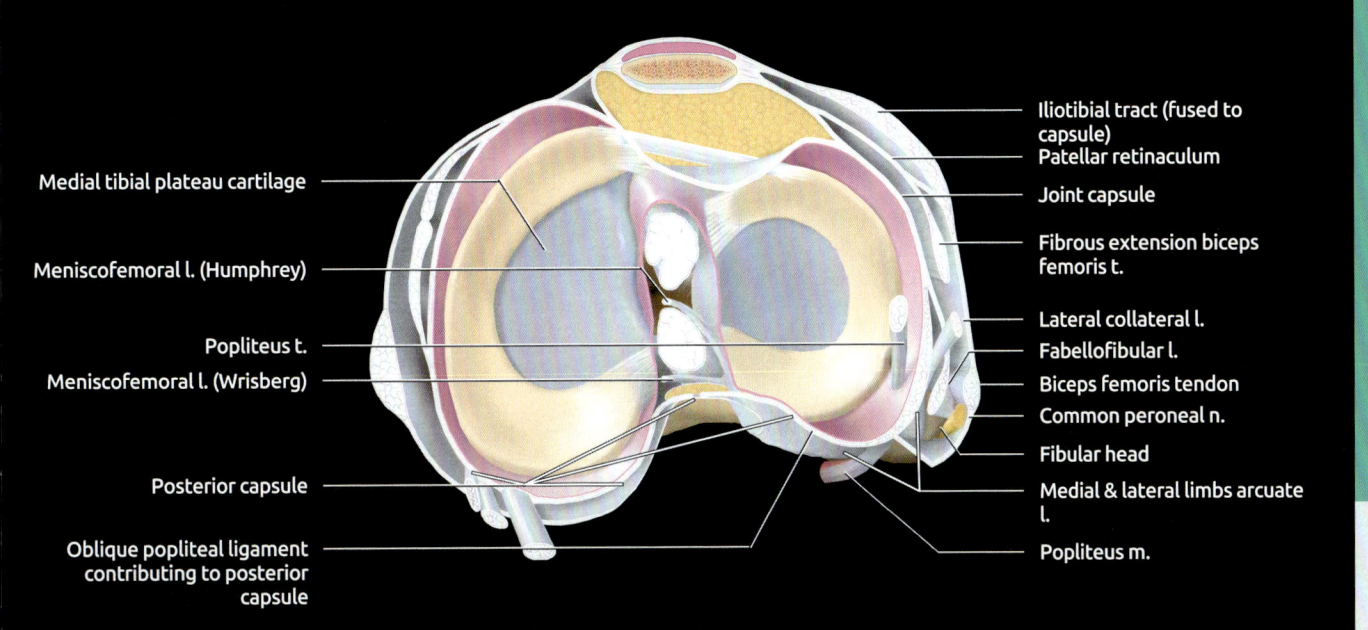

Labels (top, axial graphic):
- Medial tibial plateau cartilage
- Meniscofemoral l. (Humphrey)
- Popliteus t.
- Meniscofemoral l. (Wrisberg)
- Posterior capsule
- Oblique popliteal ligament contributing to posterior capsule
- Iliotibial tract (fused to capsule)
- Patellar retinaculum
- Joint capsule
- Fibrous extension biceps femoris t.
- Lateral collateral l.
- Fabellofibular l.
- Biceps femoris tendon
- Common peroneal n.
- Fibular head
- Medial & lateral limbs arcuate l.
- Popliteus m.

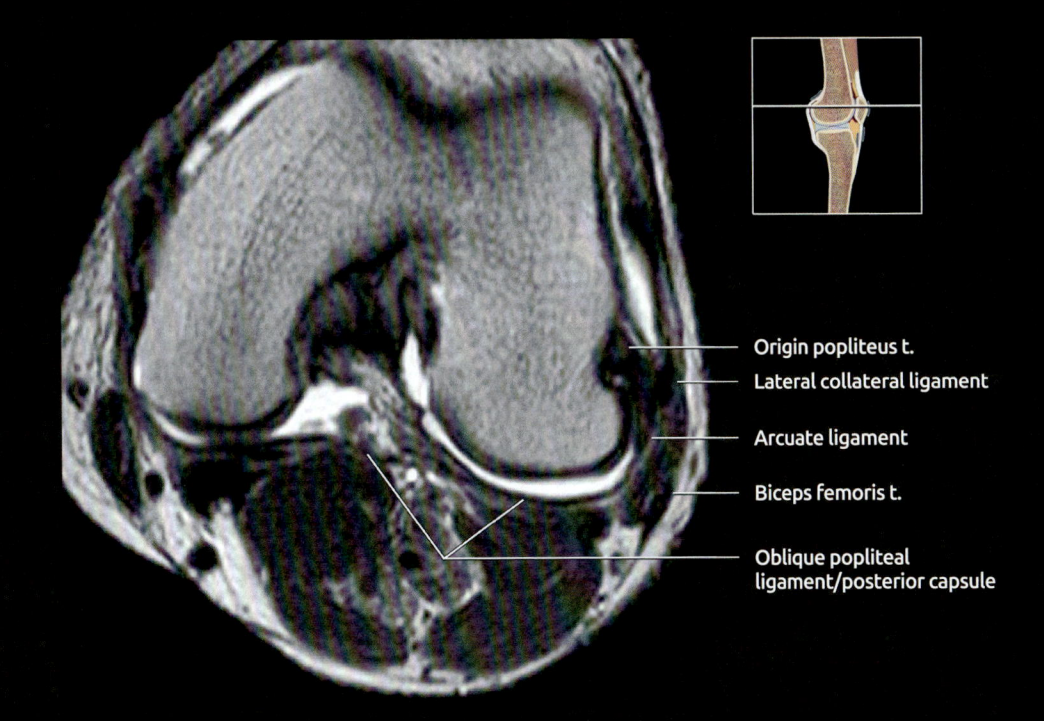

Labels (bottom, axial T2 MR):
- Origin popliteus t.
- Lateral collateral ligament
- Arcuate ligament
- Biceps femoris t.
- Oblique popliteal ligament/posterior capsule

(Top) *Axial graphic through the joint line shows the lateral capsuloligamentous complex. Superficial posterolateral structures include long and short heads biceps femoris and lateral collateral ligament. Deep posterolateral structures include the fabellofibular, arcuate, oblique popliteal, and popliteofibular ligaments. The oblique popliteal is not pictured here as a separate structure, but the medial arcuate ligament joins it posterior to the popliteal hiatus to help strengthen the posterior capsule.* **(Bottom)** *First of 5 axial T2 MR images, at the level of intercondylar notch, shows the popliteus tendon originating from its sulcus at the lateral femoral condyle. The posterior capsule, strengthened by the oblique popliteal ligament, is seen. The lateral (oblique) arm of the arcuate ligament contributes, as well. The LCL approaches the biceps tendon.*

Knee Lateral Supporting Structures

POSTEROLATERAL STRUCTURES

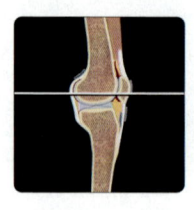

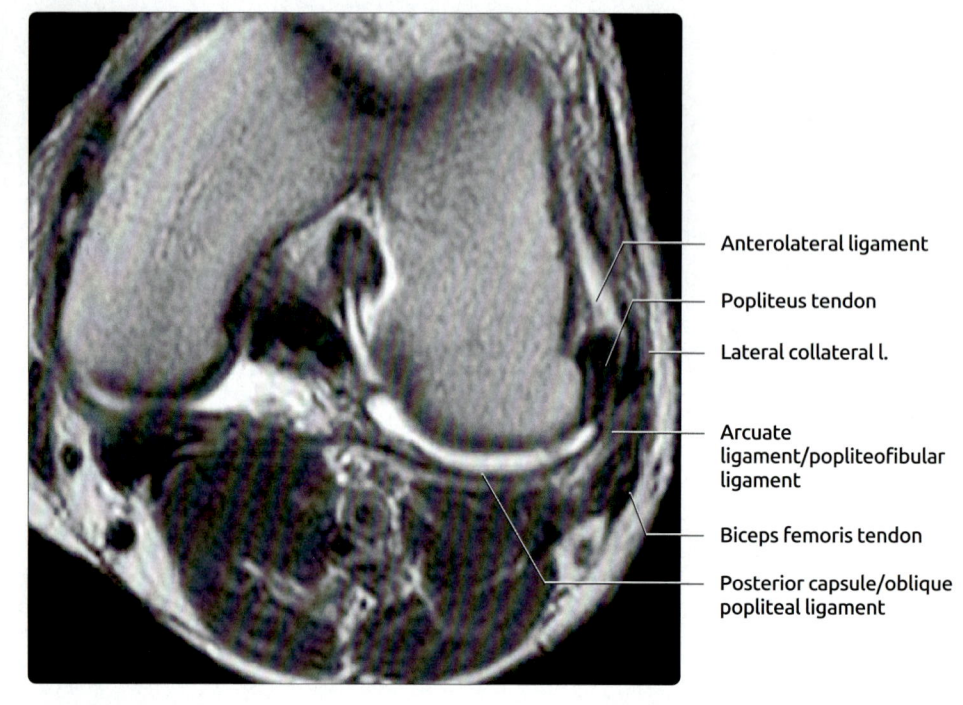

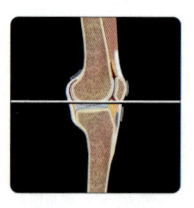

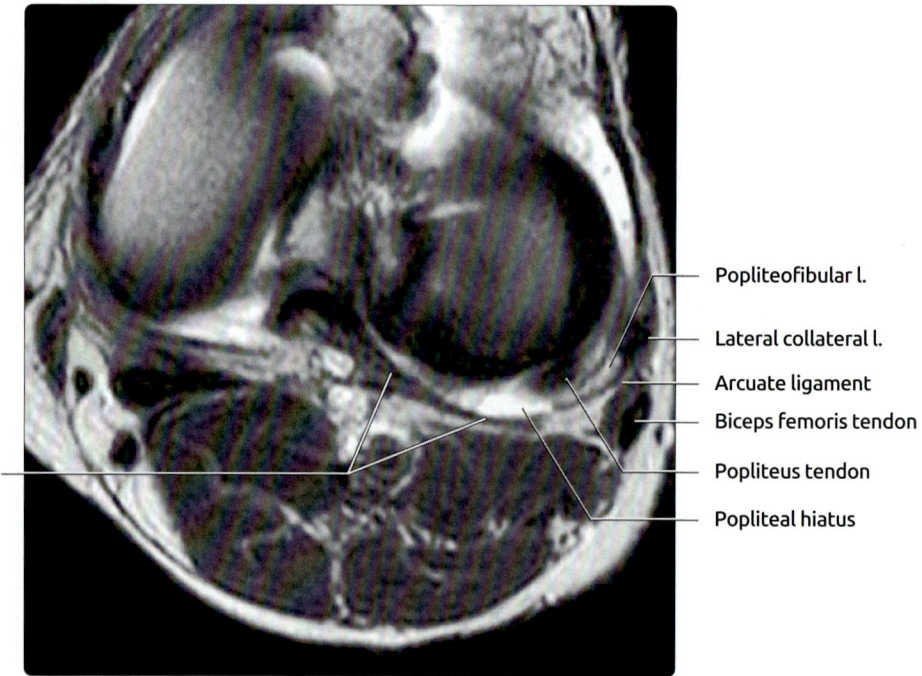

- Anterolateral ligament
- Popliteus tendon
- Lateral collateral l.
- Arcuate ligament/popliteofibular ligament
- Biceps femoris tendon
- Posterior capsule/oblique popliteal ligament

- Posterior capsule/oblique popliteal ligament
- Popliteofibular l.
- Lateral collateral l.
- Arcuate ligament
- Biceps femoris tendon
- Popliteus tendon
- Popliteal hiatus

(Top) Slightly distally, the popliteus tendon enters the popliteal hiatus as it travels posteriorly and inferiorly around the lateral femoral condyle towards the joint line. (Bottom) Approaching the joint line, the popliteus tendon curves posteriorly within the popliteal hiatus. Both the arcuate and popliteofibular ligaments are seen extending from their origin at the fibular styloid process proximally to contribute to the posterior capsule and popliteus paratenon, respectively. More superficially, the lateral collateral ligament approaches the biceps femoris as they head towards their insertion on the lateral fibular head.

Knee Lateral Supporting Structures

POSTEROLATERAL STRUCTURES

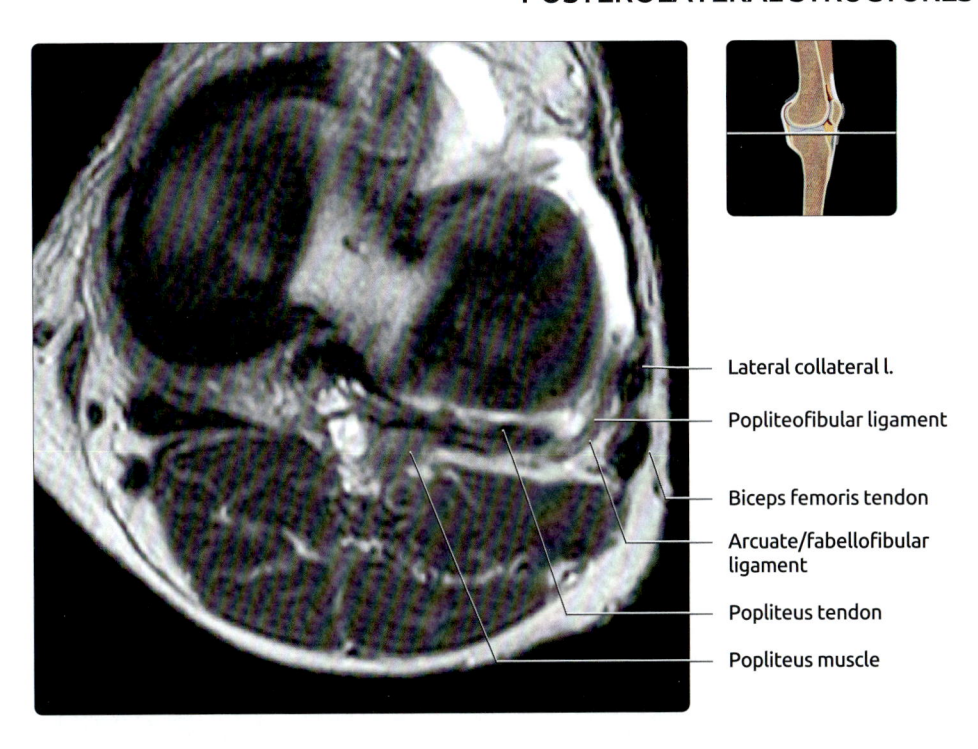

- Lateral collateral l.
- Popliteofibular ligament
- Biceps femoris tendon
- Arcuate/fabellofibular ligament
- Popliteus tendon
- Popliteus muscle

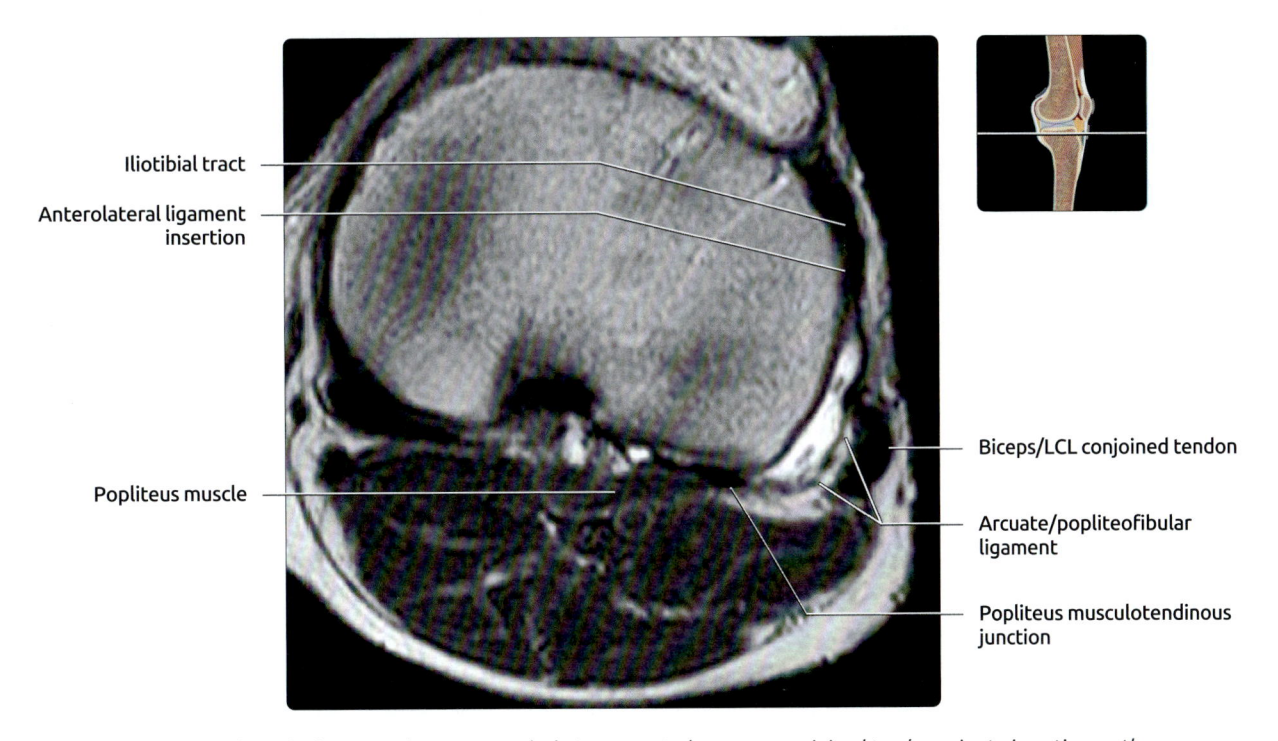

- Iliotibial tract
- Anterolateral ligament insertion
- Popliteus muscle
- Biceps/LCL conjoined tendon
- Arcuate/popliteofibular ligament
- Popliteus musculotendinous junction

(Top) At the level of the joint line, the biceps and LCL approach their merger to become a conjoined tendon prior to insertion on the fibular head; this occurs fairly often. The tissue lying between the conjoined tendon and posterolateral tibia consists of the popliteofibular ligament (deep) and the arcuate and fabellofibular ligaments (more superficial). The popliteus continues in the hiatus towards its musculotendinous junction. (Bottom) Approaching the fibular head, the same relationships maintain except that popliteus tendon now reaches the musculotendinous junction and popliteus muscle is seen posterior to the tibia. Anterolaterally, the iliotibial band approaches its insertion on Gerdy tubercle.

Knee Lateral Supporting Structures

POSTEROLATERAL STRUCTURES

Labels (top graphic):
- Superior fascicle (popliteomeniscal ligament)
- Oblique popliteal ligament
- Posterior capsule
- Inferior fascicle (popliteomeniscal ligament)
- Lateral collateral l.
- Fabella and fabellofibular ligament
- Lateral arm arcuate l.
- Medial arm arcuate l.
- Popliteus tendon
- Popliteofibular ligament
- Proximal tibiofibular ligament
- Cut popliteus musculotendinous junction

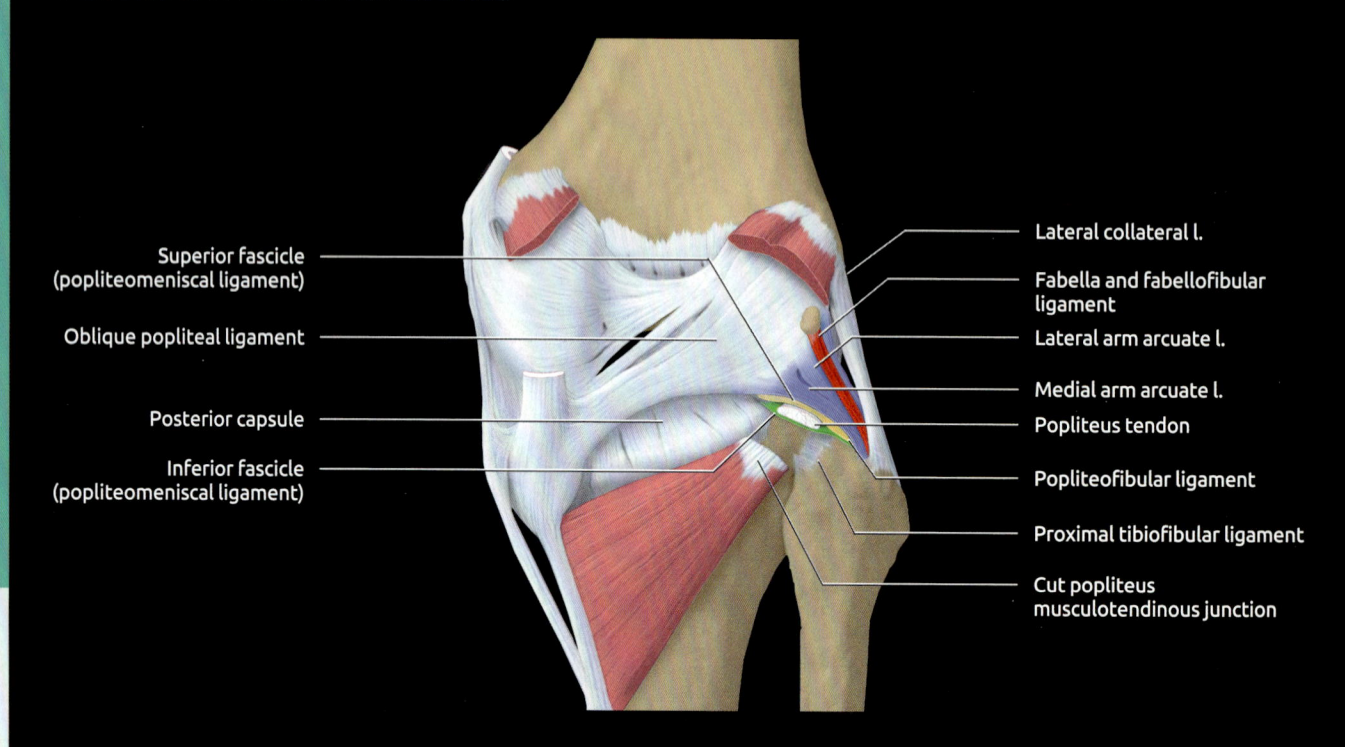

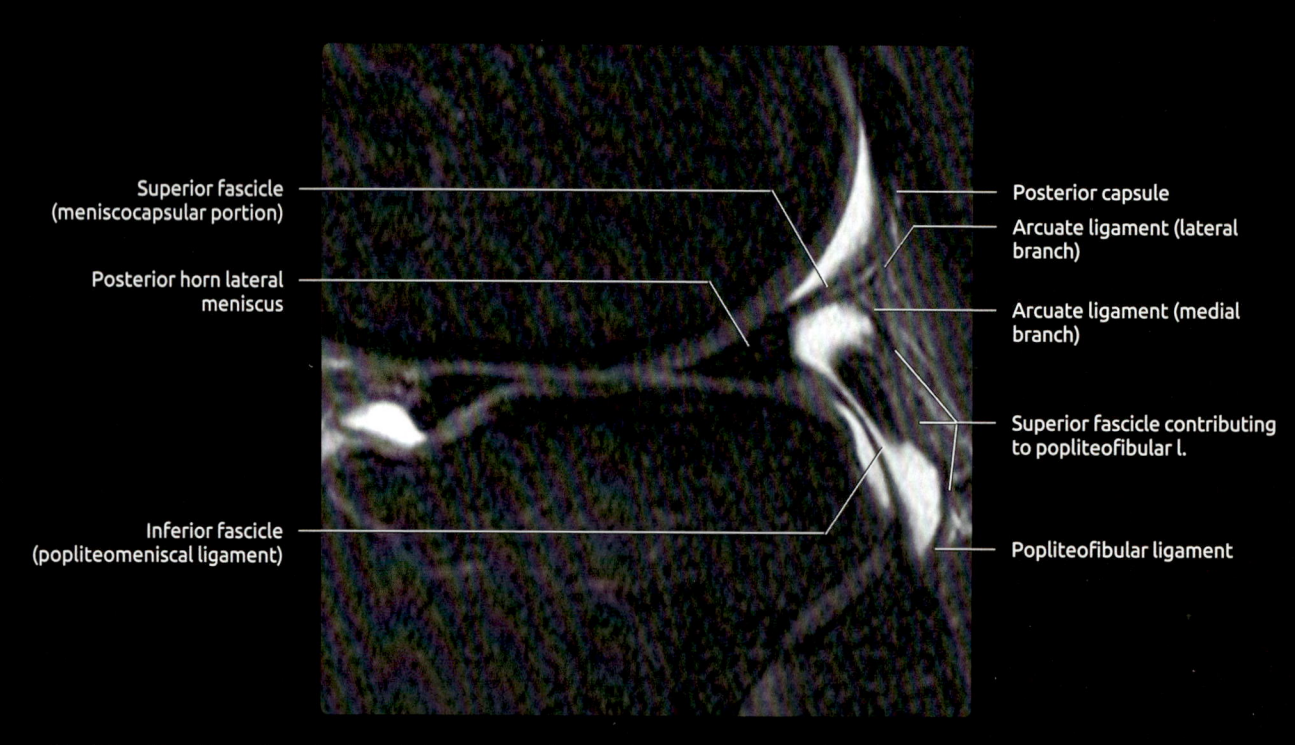

Labels (bottom MR image):
- Superior fascicle (meniscocapsular portion)
- Posterior horn lateral meniscus
- Inferior fascicle (popliteomeniscal ligament)
- Posterior capsule
- Arcuate ligament (lateral branch)
- Arcuate ligament (medial branch)
- Superior fascicle contributing to popliteofibular l.
- Popliteofibular ligament

(Top) Graphic with popliteus tendon cut shows its complex attachments. The superior fascicle extends from posterior horn meniscus over the popliteus tendon to attach to its paratenon and capsule. Medial (oblique) arcuate joins this to form the roof of popliteal hiatus. Inferior fascicle forms the floor of hiatus; the convergence of the superior and inferior fascicles attach on the fibula form the popliteofibular ligament. (Bottom) The distension in this image demonstrates the posterolateral structures about the popliteus tendon. The superior and inferior fascicles extend from the paratenon of popliteus to the meniscus. Medial branch of arcuate ligament is seen joining the superior fascicle to form the roof of popliteal hiatus. Lateral branch of arcuate ligament contributes to posterior capsule. Popliteofibular ligament is formed by convergence of fascicles on the fibula.

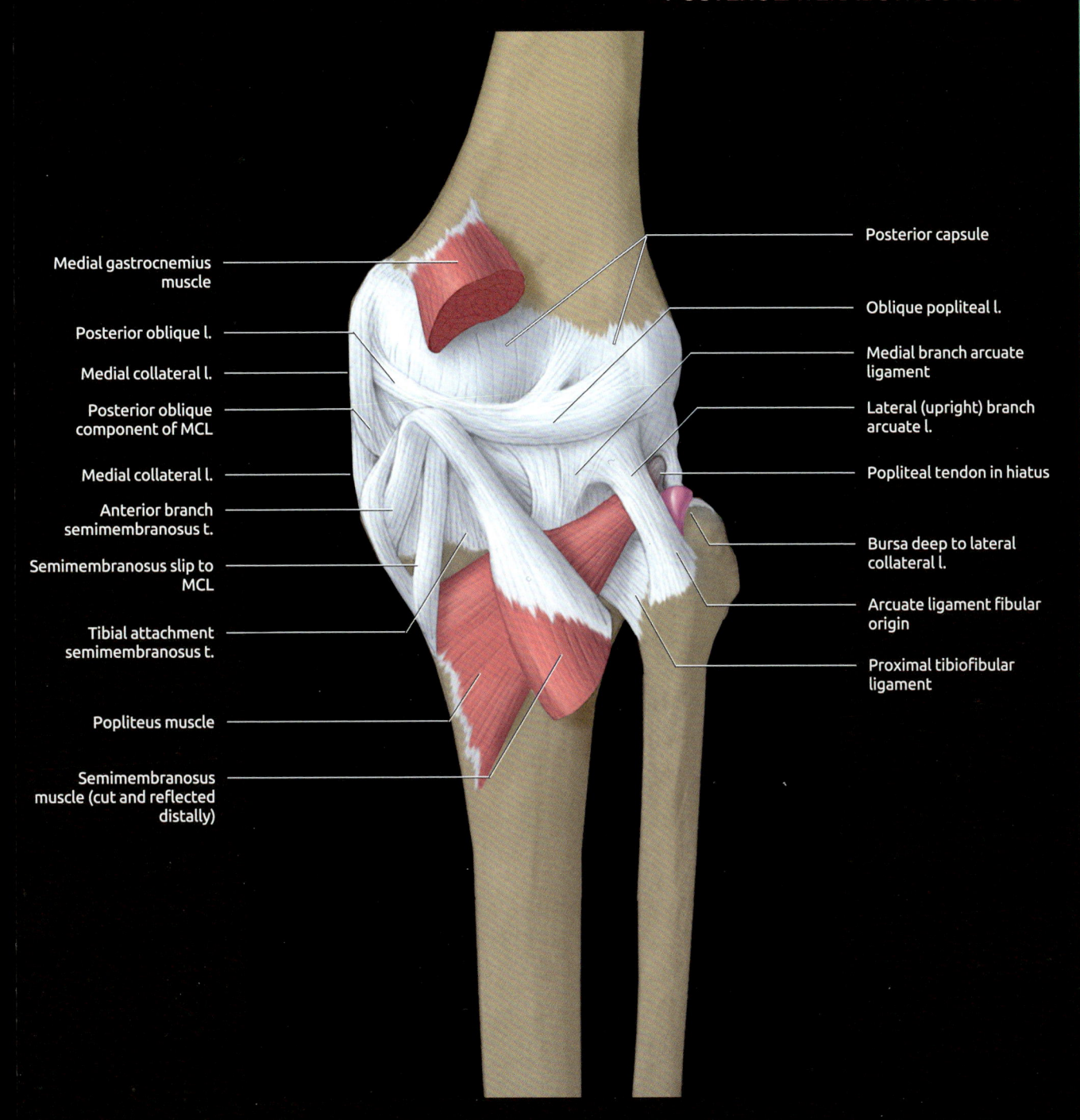

POSTEROLATERAL STRUCTURES

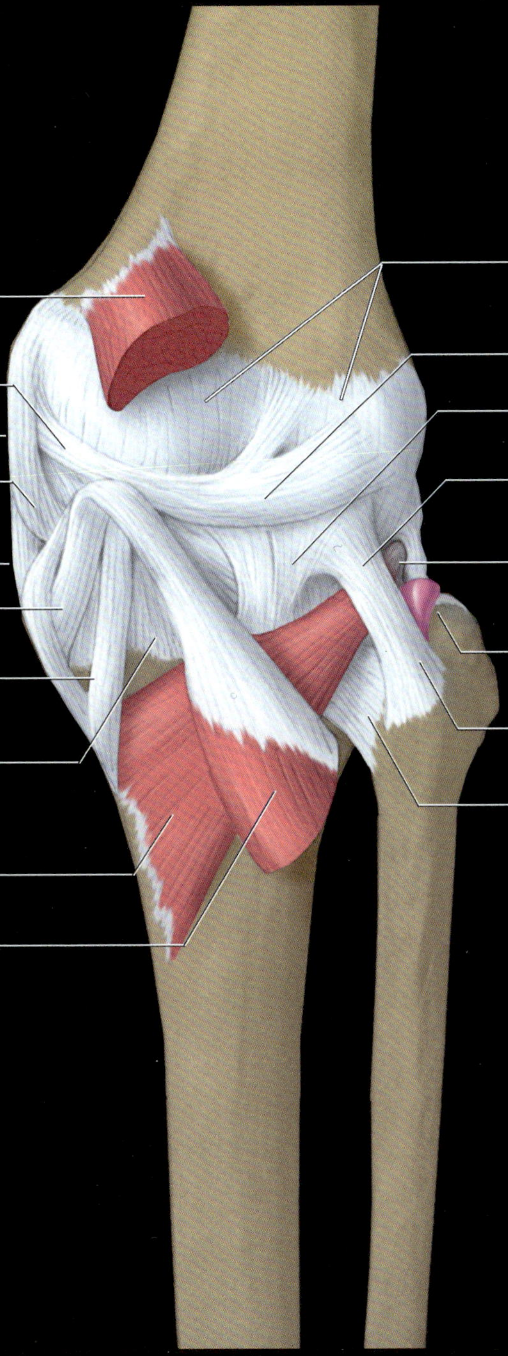
Medial gastrocnemius muscle
Posterior oblique l.
Medial collateral l.
Posterior oblique component of MCL
Medial collateral l.
Anterior branch semimembranosus t.
Semimembranosus slip to MCL
Tibial attachment semimembranosus t.
Popliteus muscle
Semimembranosus muscle (cut and reflected distally)
Posterior capsule
Oblique popliteal l.
Medial branch arcuate ligament
Lateral (upright) branch arcuate l.
Popliteal tendon in hiatus
Bursa deep to lateral collateral l.
Arcuate ligament fibular origin
Proximal tibiofibular ligament

Graphic shows the posterior stabilizing structures of the knee. Posterolateral structures include the popliteus tendon and muscle, with the fascicles' insertion on the fibular head (popliteofibular ligament). The arcuate ligament arises from the posterior fibular head; both the lateral and medial branches contribute to the oblique popliteal ligament, which strengthens the posterior capsule. The semimembranosus insertion is complex and does not have such distinct structures as are shown in the graphic. These attachments include posteromedial tibial plateau, anterior branch to tibia beneath medial collateral ligament (MCL), posteromedial capsule (not shown as separate structure), and slips to oblique popliteal ligament (not shown as separate structure). The posterior oblique ligament, originating from posterior fibers of MCL, blends posteriorly into the capsule and the oblique popliteal ligament.

Knee Lateral Supporting Structures

POSTEROLATERAL STRUCTURES: FABELLOFIBULAR LIGAMENT

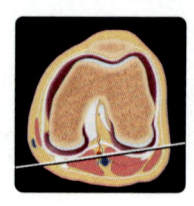

Image labels (top, coronal): Semimembranosus muscle; Biceps femoris muscle; Lateral head gastrocnemius muscle; Fabella; Fabellofibular ligament; Biceps femoris tendon; Head of fibula; Medial head of gastrocnemius muscle

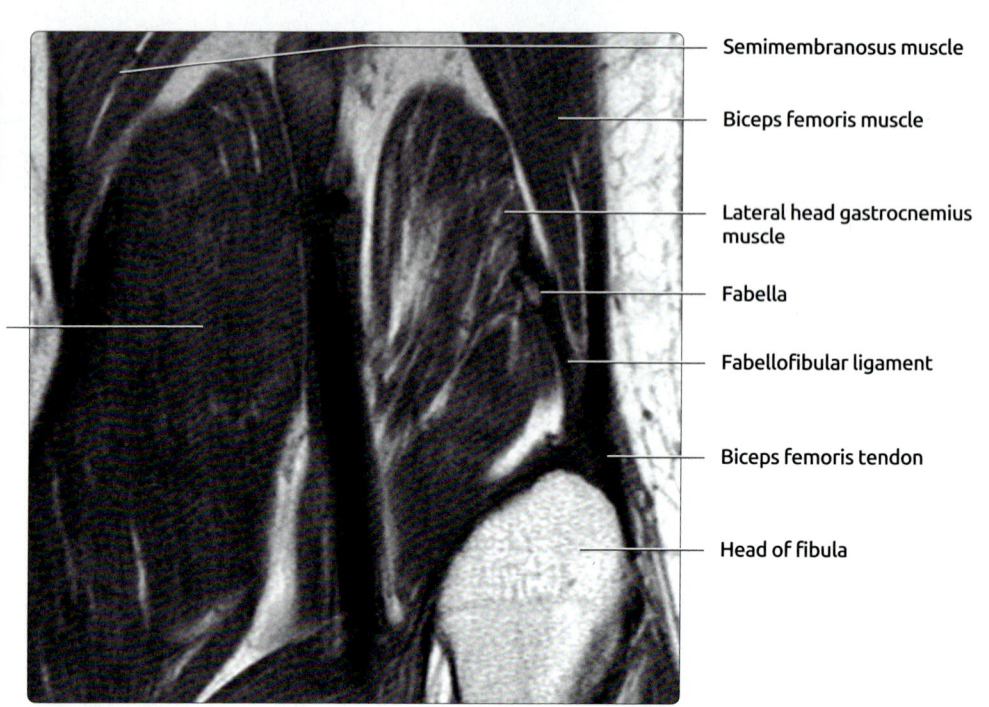

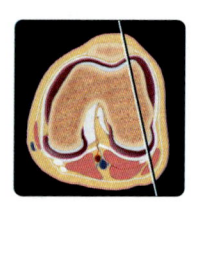

Image labels (bottom, sagittal): Lateral head gastrocnemius muscle; Biceps femoris muscle; Fabella; Superior fascicle; Fabellofibular ligament; Popliteofibular ligament; Insertion fabellofibular ligament on fibular head; Posterior horn lateral meniscus; Popliteus tendon

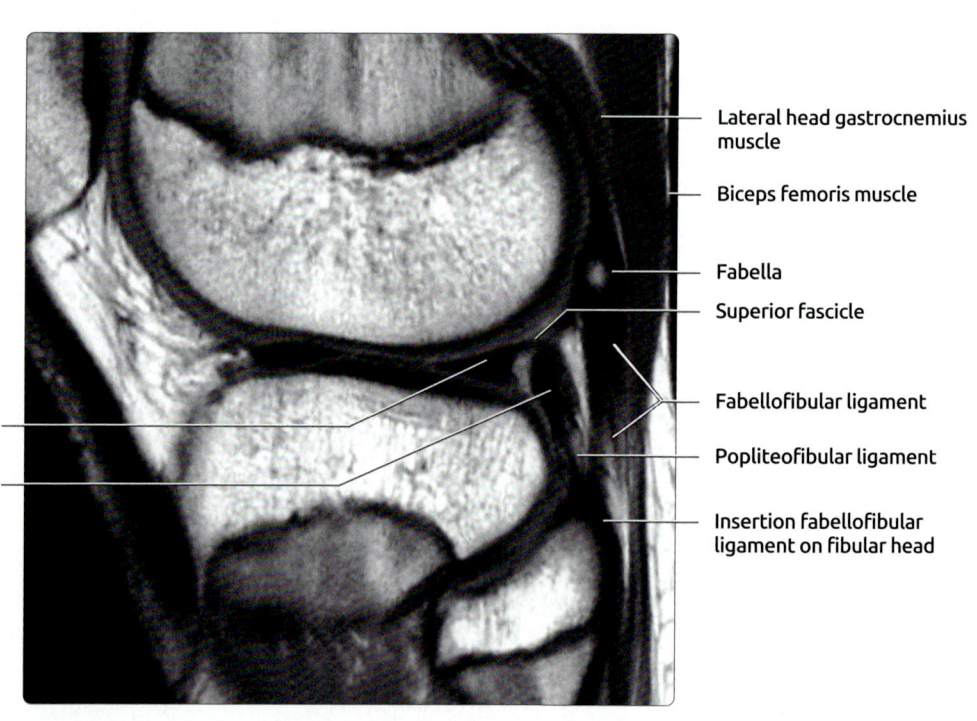

(**Top**) *This far posterior coronal cut shows a fabella within the lateral head of the gastrocnemius. There is a prominent fabellofibular ligament, extending from the fabella to the posterior aspect of the head of the fibula, immediately posteromedial to the long head biceps tendon insertion. This ligament is hypertrophied; it is not usually seen this well.* (**Bottom**) *Sagittal cut located laterally shows the hypertrophied fabellofibular ligament in the same patient. The fabella is distinctly seen with the fabellofibular ligament investing it and extending to the apex of fibular styloid. The popliteus tendon is within the popliteal hiatus; the superior fascicle extends from posterior horn lateral meniscus to the superior paratenon of popliteus. The thin popliteofibular ligament is seen extending from fibular head to popliteus, as well.*

Knee Lateral Supporting Structures

POSTEROLATERAL STRUCTURES: BICEPS FEMORIS, FABELLOFIBULAR, ARCUATE

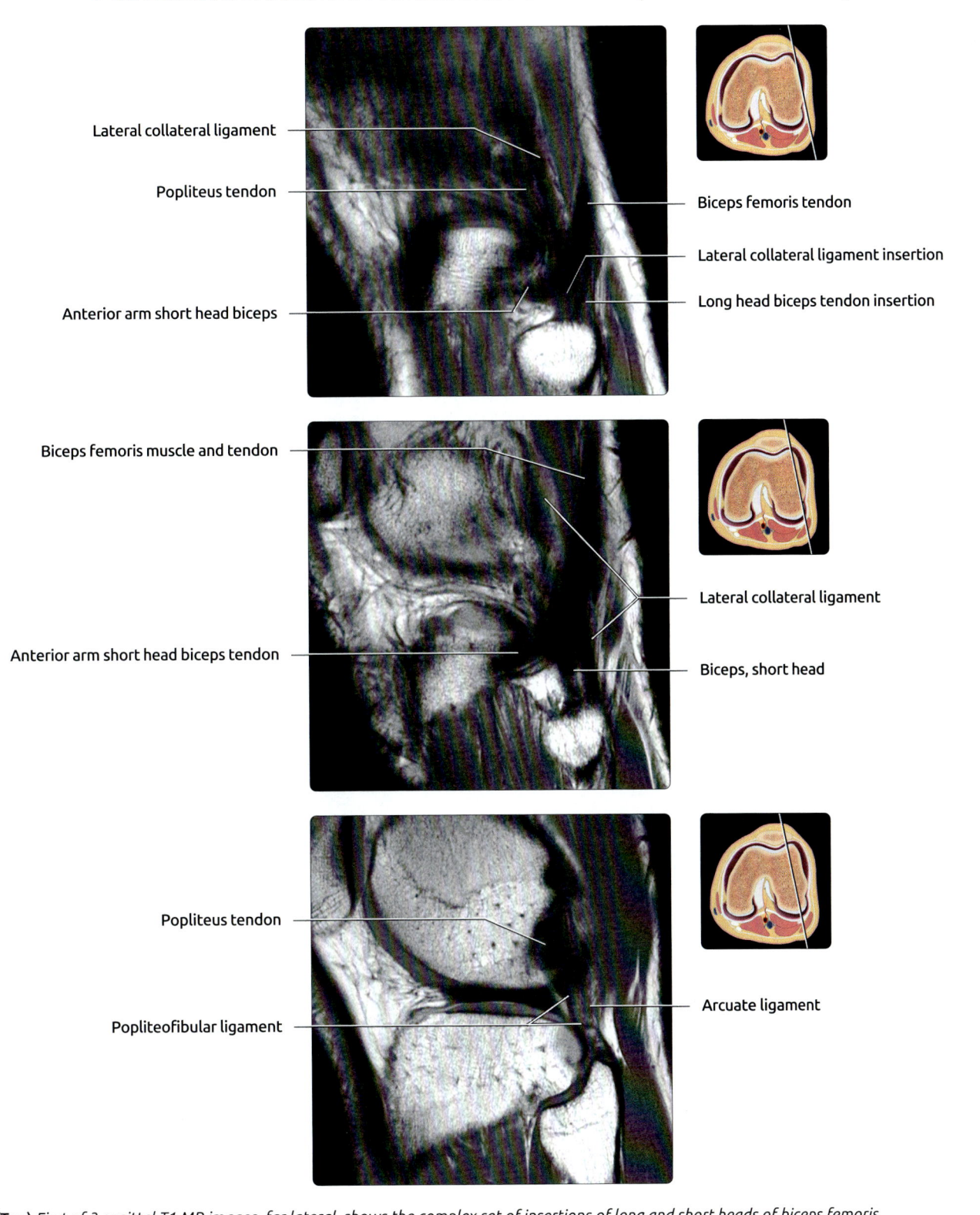

(Top) First of 3 sagittal T1 MR images, far lateral, shows the complex set of insertions of long and short heads of biceps femoris. Although they are not often discerned as separate on MR imaging, the long head of biceps has 2 insertions on the posterolateral portion of fibular head. The short head of biceps has 1 insertion on the fibular head immediately anterior to the long head and a 2nd broad insertion on anterolateral tibia. The LCL inserts immediately medial to long head biceps. (Middle) Slightly medial, one sees partial volumning of the lateral collateral ligament. Short head of biceps is still seen inserting on the anterolateral tibia with a branch inserting on fibular head. (Bottom) Image at the level of bow tie of meniscus shows popliteus tendon extending to hiatus, the popliteofibular ligament extending from paratenon to fibula and posteriorly, the arcuate ligament.

SAGITTAL PD MR, POPLITEUS TENDON

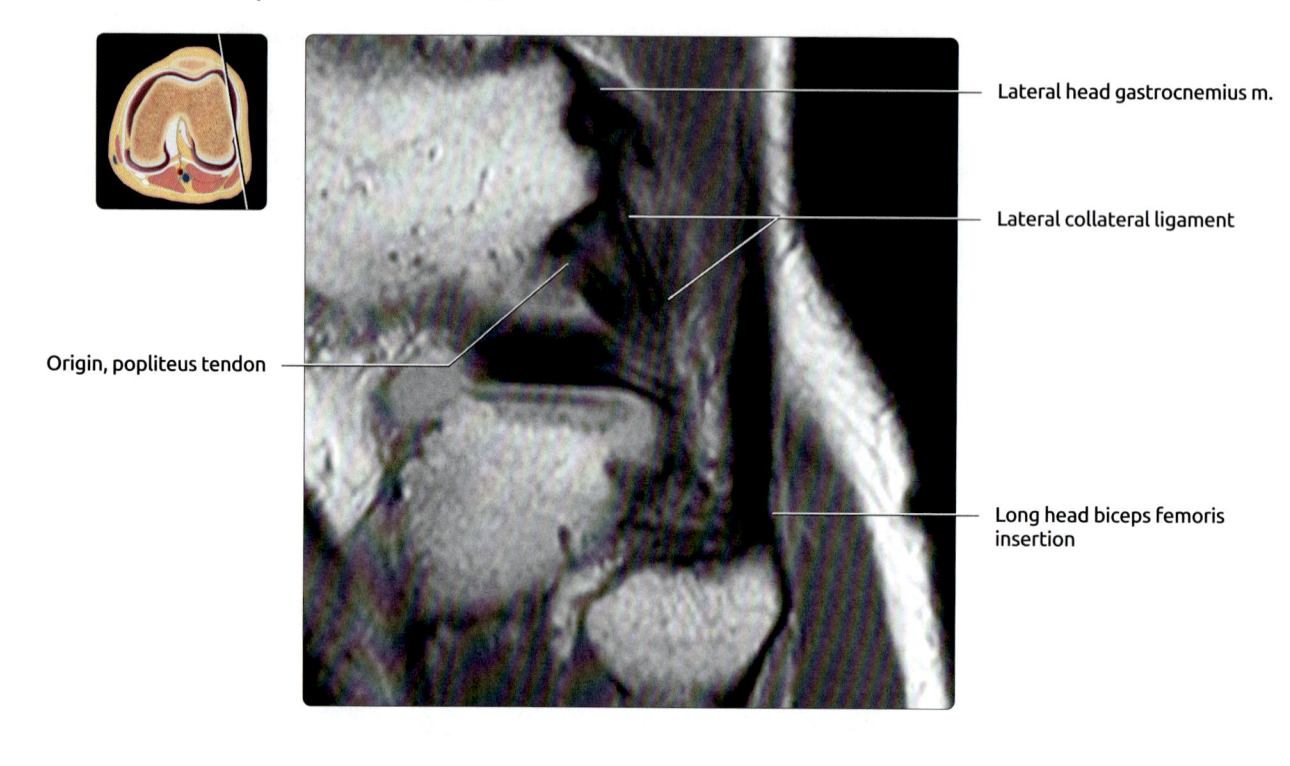

- Lateral head gastrocnemius m.
- Lateral collateral ligament
- Origin, popliteus tendon
- Long head biceps femoris insertion

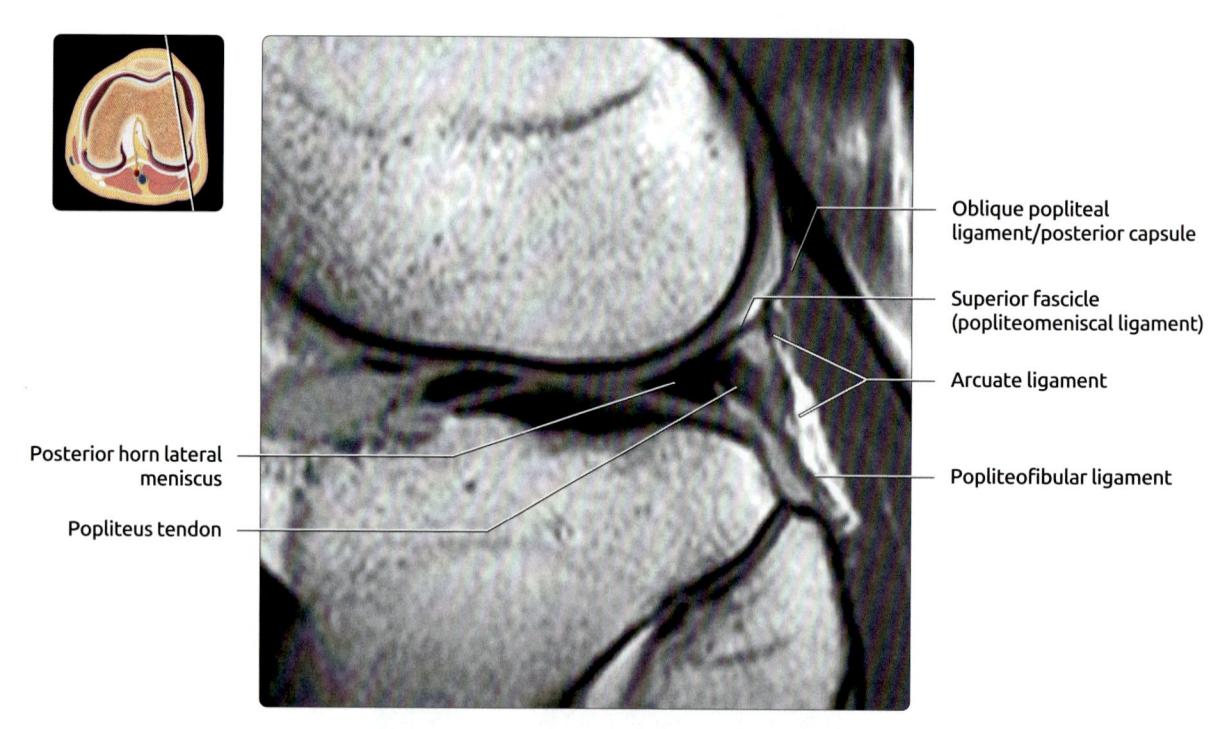

- Oblique popliteal ligament/posterior capsule
- Superior fascicle (popliteomeniscal ligament)
- Arcuate ligament
- Posterior horn lateral meniscus
- Popliteofibular ligament
- Popliteus tendon

(Top) This is the 1st of 5 sagittal PD MR images following the course of the popliteus tendon. In this far lateral image, the biceps femoris is seen inserting on fibular head. A hint of origin of popliteus tendon in its sulcus in lateral femoral condyle is seen, along with the origin of lateral collateral ligament. (Bottom) Slightly medially, the popliteus tendon enters the joint and its hiatus. The lateral (oblique) head of arcuate ligament is seen arising along with popliteofibular ligament from the fibular styloid; the arcuate ligament continues toward the oblique popliteal ligament and capsule of the joint.

Knee Lateral Supporting Structures

SAGITTAL PD MR, POPLITEUS TENDON

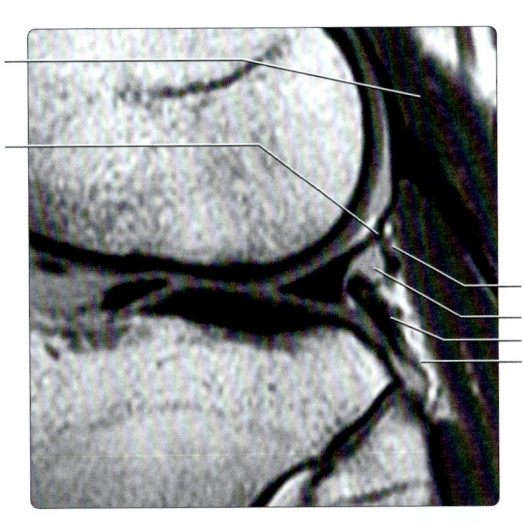

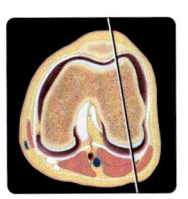

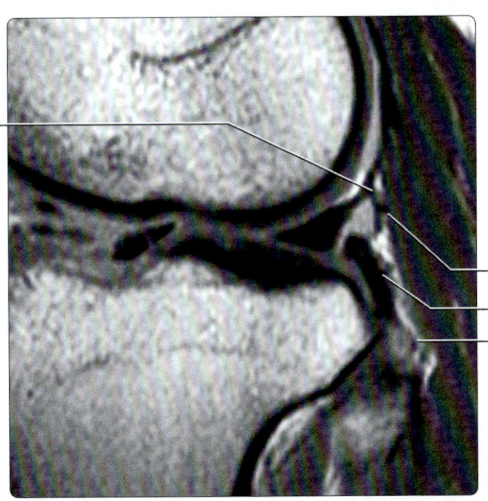

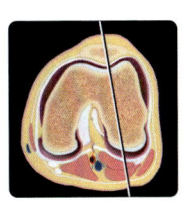

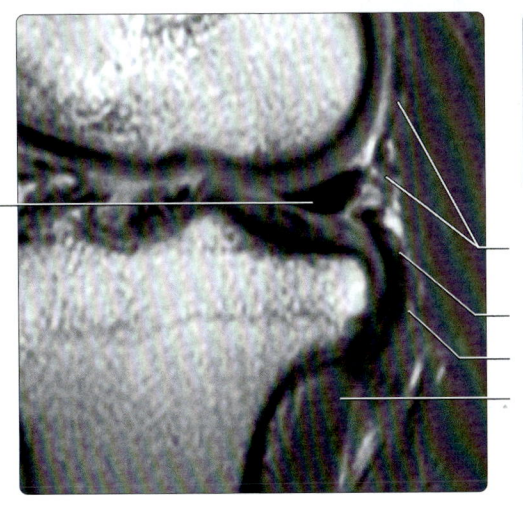

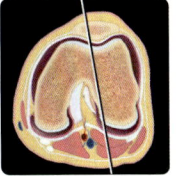

Top image labels:
- Lateral head gastrocnemius m.
- Superior fascicle/medial arcuate ligament
- Medial branch arcuate ligament
- Popliteal hiatus
- Popliteus tendon
- Popliteofibular ligament

Middle image labels:
- Superior fascicle/medial arcuate ligament: Roof of popliteal hiatus
- Medial branch arcuate ligament
- Popliteus tendon
- Popliteofibular ligament

Bottom image labels:
- Posterior horn lateral meniscus
- Posterior capsule
- Popliteus tendon
- Popliteus musculotendinous junction
- Popliteus muscle

(Top) Slightly more medially, the popliteus elongates downward; the popliteofibular ligament merges with its paratenon. By this point, the medial branch of arcuate ligament has joined the superior fascicle to form the roof of the popliteal hiatus. (Middle) The popliteus tendon approaches its musculotendinous junction. Note the arched roof of popliteal hiatus formed by the superior fascicle and the medial branch of the arcuate ligament. (Bottom) Approaching, but not yet in the intercondylar notch, the popliteus tendon is at its musculotendinous junction. The muscle can be seen extending distally toward its insertion on posterior tibia. By this point, the posterior horn lateral meniscus has rejoined the posterior capsule.

Knee Lateral Supporting Structures

CORONAL MR, POSTEROLATERAL STRUCTURES

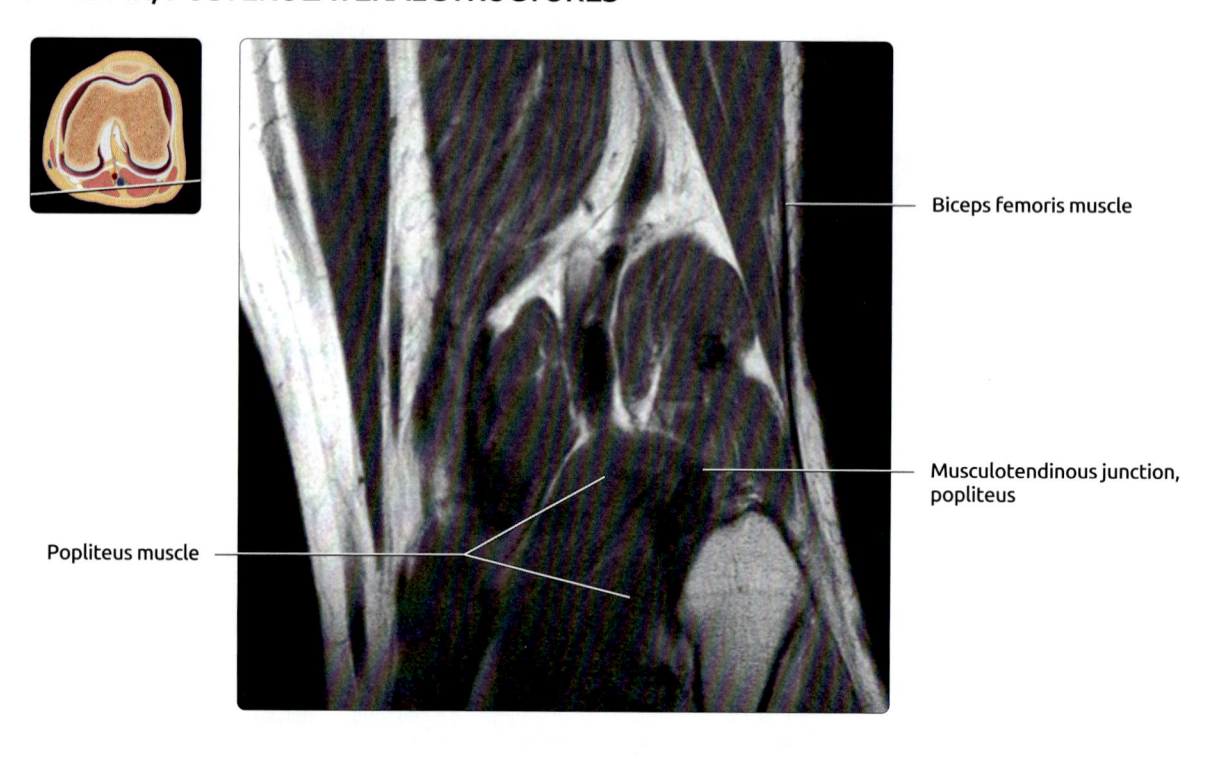

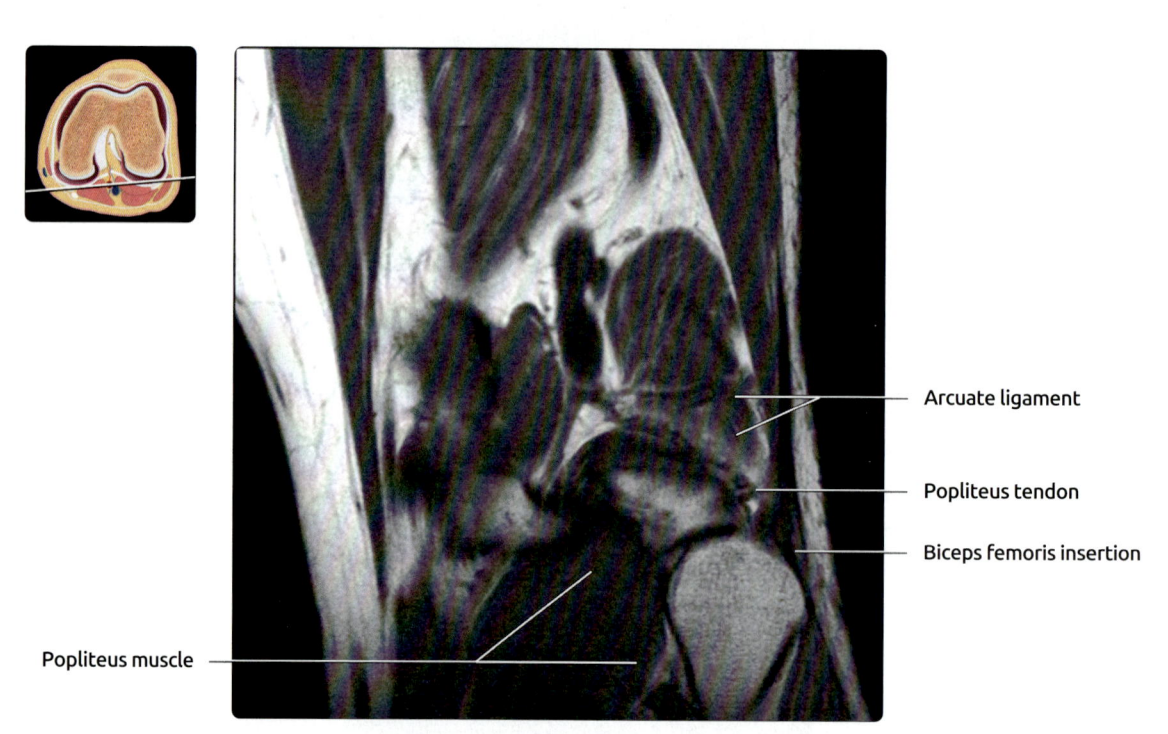

Biceps femoris muscle

Musculotendinous junction, popliteus

Popliteus muscle

Arcuate ligament

Popliteus tendon

Biceps femoris insertion

Popliteus muscle

(Top) First of 2 coronal T1 MR images, far posterior, shows structures in the posteriormost aspect of posterolateral corner. The musculotendinous junction of popliteus is seen, extending into popliteus muscle. (Bottom) Slightly more anteriorly, the long head of biceps femoris inserts on the outer aspect of fibular head. A corner of popliteus tendon is seen extending around the posterolateral tibia towards its musculotendinous junction. Arcuate ligament is seen joining posterior capsule.

Knee Lateral Supporting Structures

CORONAL MR, POSTEROLATERAL STRUCTURES

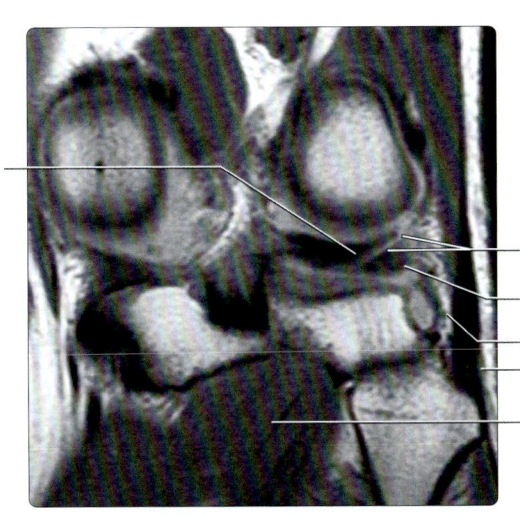

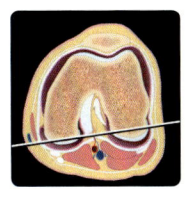

Posterior horn, lateral meniscus

Fluid in popliteal hiatus
Popliteus tendon
Popliteofibular ligament
Biceps femoris tendon
Popliteus muscle

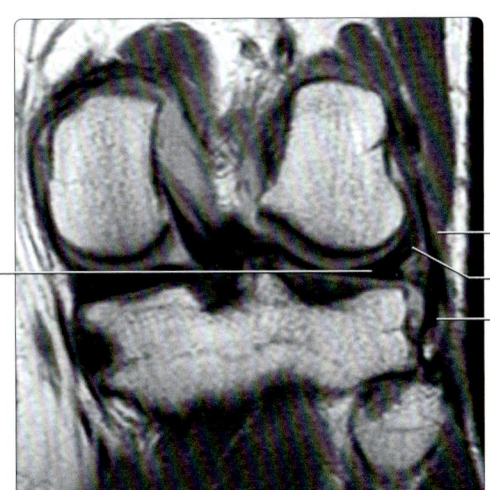

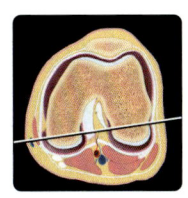

Body/posterior horn lateral meniscus

Lateral collateral ligament
Popliteus tendon
Popliteofibular/lateral arm arcuate ligaments

Biceps femoris muscle
Origin lateral collateral ligament
Origin popliteus tendon

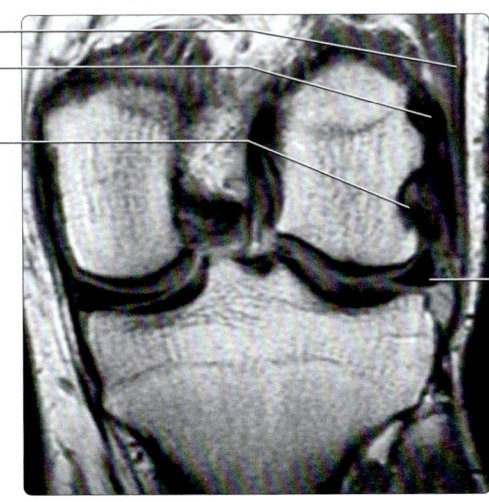

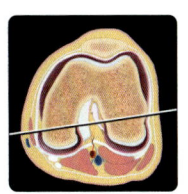

Body lateral meniscus

(Top) This is the 1st of 3 coronal PD MR images, following the popliteus tendon, outlined by fluid within the popliteal hiatus. This more posterior of the 3 shows the popliteus muscle, as well as the popliteus tendon as it traverses the hiatus, with fluid separating the tendon from the posterior horn lateral meniscus. Biceps femoris tendon inserts laterally on fibular head. (Middle) Slightly more anteriorly, the midportion of lateral collateral ligament is seen extending towards its insertion on the lateral femoral head. Popliteus tendon is just entering the hiatus at the level of junction posterior horn/body of lateral meniscus. (Bottom) At a midcoronal cut, the origins of both the lateral collateral ligament and popliteus tendon are seen. At this point, the body of lateral meniscus is directly attached to capsule since popliteus has not yet entered the hiatus.

Knee Lateral Supporting Structures

CORONAL OBLIQUE T1 MR, POSTEROLATERAL STRUCTURES

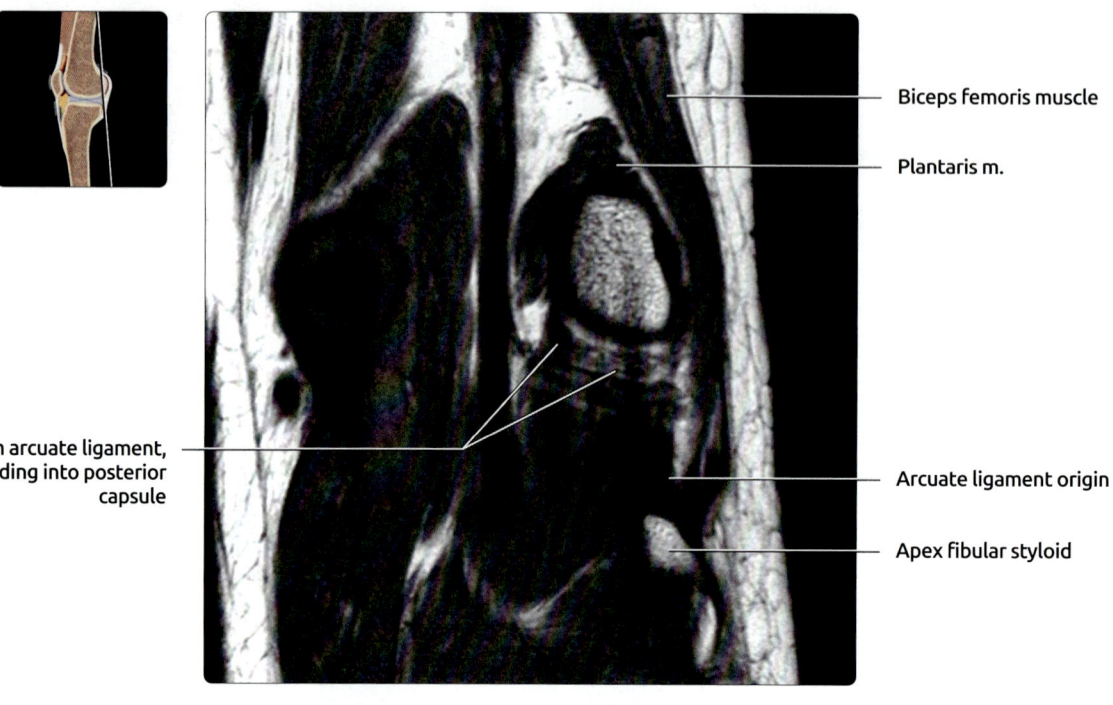

Labels (top image): Biceps femoris muscle; Plantaris m.; Arcuate ligament origin; Apex fibular styloid; Medial arm arcuate ligament, blending into posterior capsule

Labels (bottom image): Biceps femoris muscle; Popliteus tendon origin; Popliteus tendon within hiatus; Popliteus musculotendinous junction; Fibular origin popliteofibular ligament; Lateral geniculate nerve and vein

(**Top**) First of 4 coronal oblique T1 MR images of posterolateral structures is seen. The images are prescribed off a sagittal, angling from anterosuperior to posteroinferior, following the popliteus tendon. Thus, in this image we see more of the lateral femoral condyle than fibula. It allows visualization of oblique posterior structures, such as the fabellofibular ligament and arcuate ligament. This image is too far posterior to include much popliteus tendon. (**Bottom**) Slightly anterior to the previous image, this lays the popliteus tendon out such that it is seen from its origin to the musculotendinous junction. The fibular origin of the popliteofibular ligament is seen, with fibers stretching up to meet the popliteal paratenon. Portions of the arcuate ligament may be present but are not well seen. Since we are at the apex of the fibula, the biceps has not yet inserted.

Knee Lateral Supporting Structures

CORONAL OBLIQUE T1 MR, POSTEROLATERAL

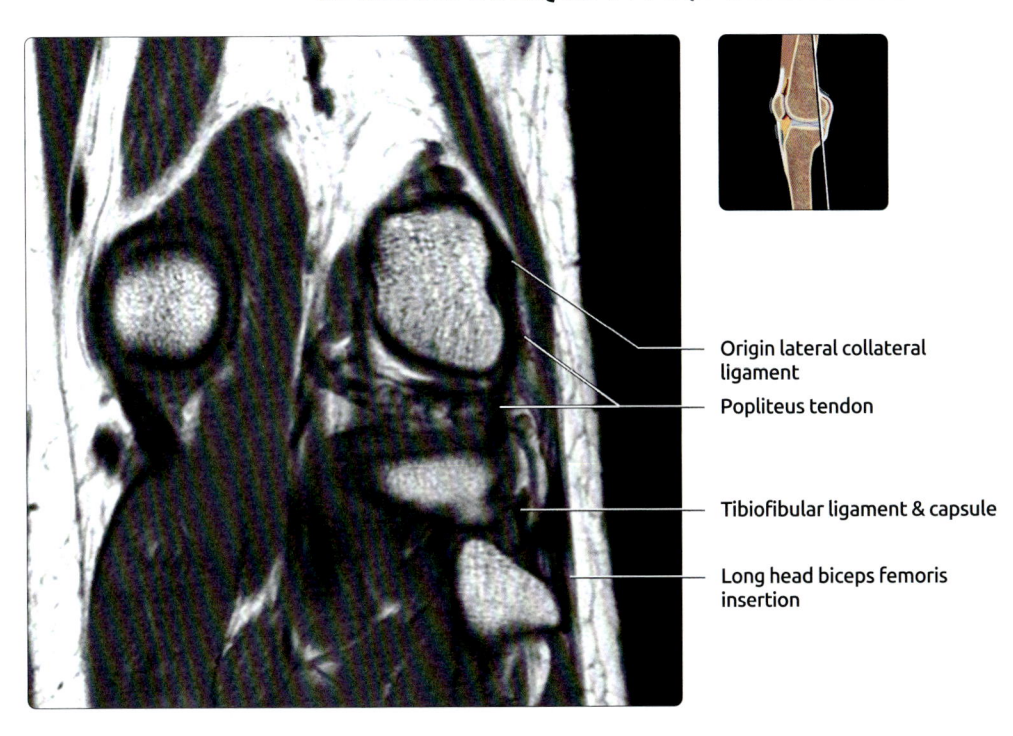

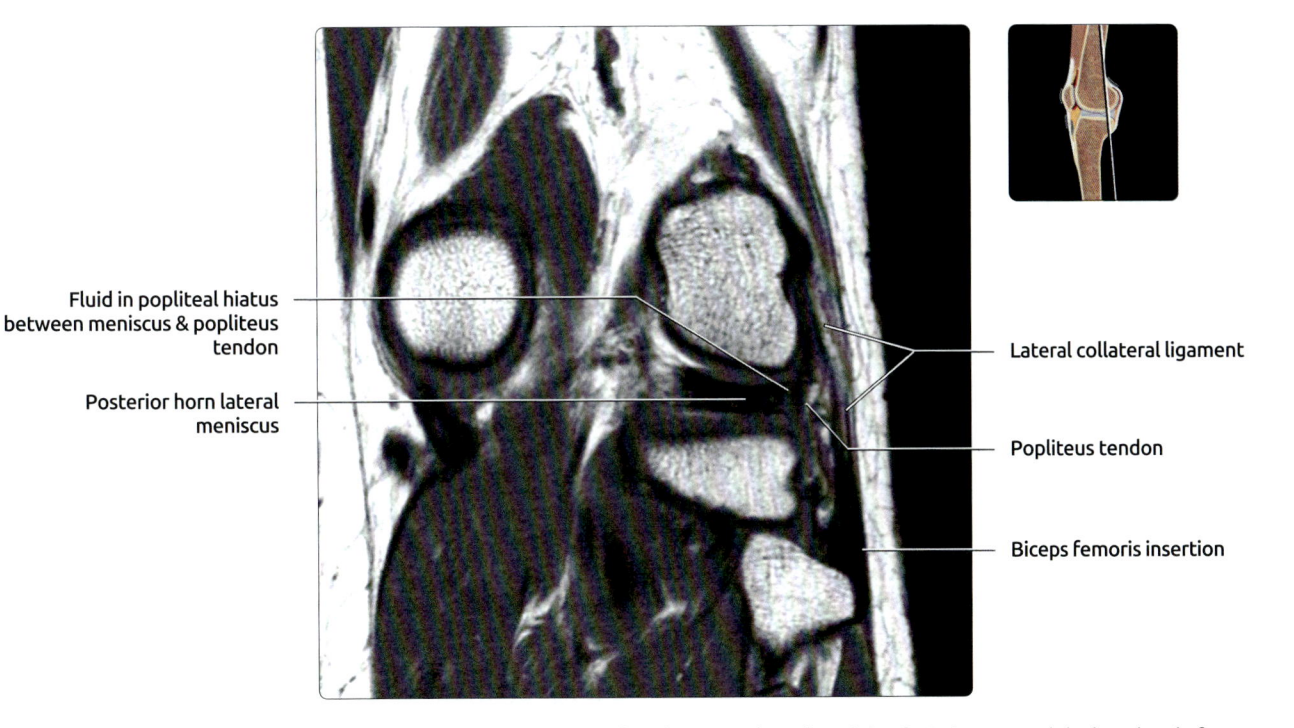

- Origin lateral collateral ligament
- Popliteus tendon
- Tibiofibular ligament & capsule
- Long head biceps femoris insertion

- Fluid in popliteal hiatus between meniscus & popliteus tendon
- Posterior horn lateral meniscus
- Lateral collateral ligament
- Popliteus tendon
- Biceps femoris insertion

(Top) Slightly anterior image continues to show more of the origin of popliteus tendon. The origin of LCL is seen, and the long head of biceps femoris inserts on the midportion of the fibula laterally. (Bottom) More anteriorly, the popliteus tendon is seen separated from posterior horn lateral meniscus by fluid in the popliteal hiatus. The biceps more fully inserts on the fibula, with the lateral collateral ligament inserting immediately medial to it.

Knee and Leg Normal Variants and Imaging Pitfalls

NORMAL VARIANTS

Muscle Variants

- Many minor variations of muscle size, insertion, and origin exist
  - Most are clinically nonconsequential
  - Absence of plantaris muscle is 1 of the more frequent of these
- Biceps femoris muscle hypertrophy
  - Common peroneal nerve follows biceps femoris to fibular head insertion of muscle
  - If biceps femoris is hypertrophied, it can entrap common peroneal nerve; may be symptomatic
  - Other morphologic abnormalities which may affect nerve at this site: Hypertrophy of lateral head of gastrocnemius or fatty hypertrophy (often secondary to diabetes)
- Gastrocnemius muscle origin variants and popliteal artery entrapment (prevalence estimated at 0.16%)
  - Popliteal artery is normally adjacent and lateral to medial head of gastrocnemius muscle
    - Popliteal artery may take abnormal course medial to attachment of medial gastrocnemius
    - Numerous anomalous popliteal fossa relationships can result in entrapment
  - Several gastrocnemius anomalies described that may entrap popliteal vessels
    - Origin lateral head gastrocnemius from medial femoral condyle
    - Origin medial head gastrocnemius from lateral femoral condyle
    - 3rd head gastrocnemius (seen in 1.9% knee MR exams)
    - Fibrous bands
  - Clinical association
    - Many variants are not symptomatic
    - May produce symptoms of claudication
    - Rarely, repetitive insult can cause arterial aneurysm or thrombosis
    - Anomalous structure usually splits vessels in symptomatic cases
- Accessory muscles at ankle
  - Multiple accessory muscles are described; will be more fully described in ankle section
- Articularis genus muscle
  - Originates distal femur, deep to vastus intermedius, inserts on superior knee joint capsule
  - Pulls suprapatellar recess superiorly during knee extension

Osseous Variants

- Fabella: Sesamoid in lateral head of gastrocnemius
  - To qualify as fabella, rounded ossific density must be located both posteriorly and laterally, at expected site of lateral gastrocnemius
  - Fabella may be absent; then fabellofibular ligament is also absent and arcuate ligament enlarged
  - Fabella may be bipartite or multipartite
- Bipartite patella (prevalence about 2%)
  - 40% bilateral; male:female = 9:1
  - Separate ossification site, usually superior and lateral to main patella
  - May be bipartite or multipartite
  - Fragments appear rounded, but may not appear to "fit" perfectly together
  - Overlying cartilage is smooth, uniting the parts
  - Rarely may be symptomatic
  - Debated whether it is anomaly of ossification or stress related
- Dorsal defect of patella (prevalence < 1%)
  - Well-defined lucent lesion, usually in superolateral quadrant of patella
  - Should not be confused with osteochondral defect
  - Defect may become smaller and sclerotic over time
  - Overlying cartilage is normal
  - Debated whether it is anomaly of ossification or stress related
- Posterior femoral condylar irregularity
  - Seen in adolescents (girls < 10 years of age, boys < 12 years of age)
  - Distinctly located in posterior 1/3 of weight-bearing portion of femoral condyle; seen well on lateral view
  - Because of posterior location, better seen on notch view than AP
  - No extension to intercondylar notch
  - Overlying cartilage is normal
  - No significant marrow edema
  - With maturation, ossification becomes smooth and regular
  - Do not confuse with osteochondral defect or injury
  - Does not require reduction of activity or other treatment
- Posteromedial distal femoral metaphyseal cortical defect
  - Variably called "cortical desmoid" or "cortical avulsive tug lesion"
  - Seen in adolescents or teenagers
  - Very specific in location, adjacent to insertion of adductor magnus aponeurosis
  - May appear somewhat aggressive: Cortical indistinctness, mild spiculation, scalloping of bone, small soft tissue mass
  - Debated as to whether it is chronic avulsive lesion or normal growth phenomenon
  - Important to not suggest it is more aggressive lesion as long as it precisely fits this description
- FOPE zone
  - FOPE = focal periphyseal edema
  - Occurs in skeletally immature patients approaching age of physeal fusion at knee
  - Edema signal seen surrounding a central portion of physis
  - Entire physis is open and no other abnormality seen
  - Edema felt to relate to early stages of physiologic physeal closure
  - May be associated with pain when no other MR abnormality is present
  - If characteristic, no further diagnostic procedure or imaging follow-up required
  - No treatment recommended

Ligamentous Variants

- Meniscofemoral ligaments (Wrisberg and Humphrey)

Knee and Leg Normal Variants and Imaging Pitfalls

- Both originate at intercondylar notch of medial femoral condyle and insert on posterior horn lateral meniscus, Humphrey anterior to PCL, and Wrisberg posterior to PCL
- Variable presence: 1 or both are present in 83% of knees
- Seen in profile as round low signal on sagittal; do not mistake for loose body
- May mimic tear as ligament approaches its attachment on posterior horn lateral meniscus
- Transverse ligament
  - Connects 2 anterior meniscal horns; occasionally may be absent or hypertrophied
  - May mimic anterior horn tear at anterior horn lateral meniscus as it inserts
  - May be site of origin of meniscomeniscal or meniscocruciate ligament
- Meniscocruciate ligament
  - Extends from anterior horn lateral meniscus to lateral femoral condyle
  - Rarely originates at transverse ligament
  - Parallels ACL; distinguish from partial ACL tear
- Oblique meniscomeniscal ligament
  - Anterior horn of one meniscus to posterior horn of other; appears to split ACL
  - May mimic loose body

Plica Variant

- Infrapatellar plica
  - Arises from inferior patella, crosses Hoffa fat pad and extends along anterior surface ACL
  - Parallels ACL; must distinguish from partial ACL tear

Meniscal Variants

- Discoid meniscus
  - Extra meniscal material extends towards intercondylar notch, making meniscus discoid rather than C-shaped
    - Generally seen on both coronal and sagittal imaging (occasionally axial)
    - May be partial and seen in only 1 plane
  - Lateral meniscus more commonly discoid than medial
  - Posterolateral knee morphology unusual
    - Posterior horn appears to be "drawn in," leaving large popliteal hiatus and elongated superior and inferior fascicles
  - At greater risk for tear, particularly at young age
- Anterior horn medial meniscus origin
  - Usual origin from tibial plateau, far anteriorly
  - Occasionally originates anterior to this, off edge of plateau
  - Location may mimic extrusion, but meniscus itself is normal with normal surrounding tissue
  - On axial, anterior horn tissue mimics bucket handle tear fragment
- Meniscal ossicle
  - Trabeculated osseous tissue formed within meniscus
  - Almost exclusively located in posterior horn medial meniscus
    - Other locations rarely occur
  - Follows osseous signal throughout (fatty signal on T1, saturates out on fat saturated sequences)
  - Usually associated with meniscal tear, often radial tear at posterior root
  - Uncertain whether it is true normal variant or related to trauma in childhood

IMAGING PITFALLS

Radiographic Positioning

- Axial (tangential) radiographs of patella should be obtained at 20° flexion
  - Over- or under-flexion may reduce subluxating patella, resulting in missed diagnosis

MR Positioning

- Choice of obliquity of sagittal and coronal obliques is crucial
  - Failure to oblique sagittals along ACL results in poor visualization of that structure
  - Over-obliquing sagittals or coronals may give false impression of extrusion of meniscus

Cartilage Thickness

- Posterior weight-bearing femoral cartilage thickness exaggerated
- T2 underestimates cartilage thickness since cortex and cartilage have similar signal
- PD may have similar signal for cartilage and adjacent joint fluid, obscuring defects
  - Fat-saturation on PD solves this issue

Partial Voluming Over Convex Surfaces

- Morphology of trochlea, femoral condyles, and patella makes them difficult to evaluate in 3 standard planes

Truncation Artifact

- Occurs due to approximation errors in Fourier transform analysis
- Seen at boundary between high and low signal structures
- Menisci with adjacent high-signal effusion particularly subject to this
  - Gives false appearance of horizontal tear in meniscus in fat-saturated images
  - Compare non-fat-saturated PD image to fat-saturated ones; the former will not show the "tear"

Motion Mimicking Meniscal Tear

- Slight motion of knee during acquisition of images may give false appearance of horizontal meniscal tear, with slightly convex line crossing meniscus
- Slightly convex lines through adjacent femoral condyle, exactly paralleling line through meniscus, are best hint of situation; use other planes and sequences to determine integrity of meniscus

Vacuum Phenomenon Mimicking Loose Body

- Full extension of knee may result in vacuum-produced air bubble within joint
  - Round low signal of air bubble may mimic loose body or meniscal tear
  - Particularly prominent on gradient-echo imaging in which air bubble "blooms"

Knee and Leg Normal Variants and Imaging Pitfalls

HYPERTROPHIED BICEPS FEMORIS

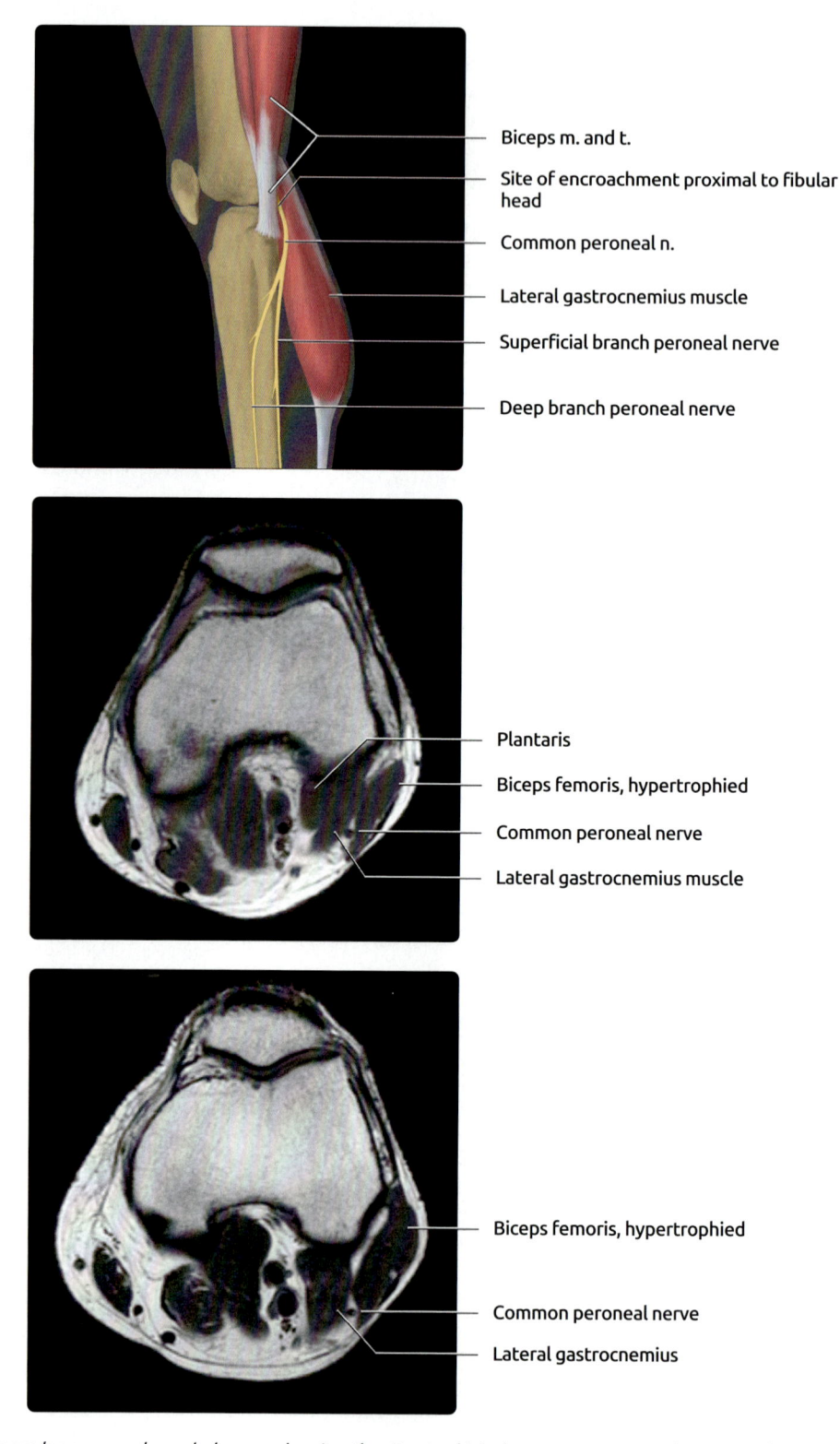

Labels (top graphic): Biceps m. and t.; Site of encroachment proximal to fibular head; Common peroneal n.; Lateral gastrocnemius muscle; Superficial branch peroneal nerve; Deep branch peroneal nerve

Labels (middle MR): Plantaris; Biceps femoris, hypertrophied; Common peroneal nerve; Lateral gastrocnemius muscle

Labels (bottom MR): Biceps femoris, hypertrophied; Common peroneal nerve; Lateral gastrocnemius

(Top) *Lateral graphic shows the peroneus longus muscle peeled away, showing the site at which the common peroneal nerve can be compressed proximal to the fibular head. Compression at this site has been described with hypertrophy of biceps femoris, lateral gastrocnemius, or fat.* **(Middle)** *First of 2 images shows the top of the intercondylar notch. These 2 axial T1 MR images show compression of the common peroneal nerve between a hypertrophied biceps femoris muscle and the lateral gastrocnemius. Normally the biceps are more gracile in this location, with the common peroneal nerve located more posteriorly. This variant may cause nerve compression and may be symptomatic.* **(Bottom)** *Slightly more distal axial T1 MR image shows persistence of the relationship of the hypertrophied biceps, compressing the common peroneal nerve against the gastrocnemius muscle.*

Knee and Leg Normal Variants and Imaging Pitfalls

3RD HEAD GASTROCNEMIUS

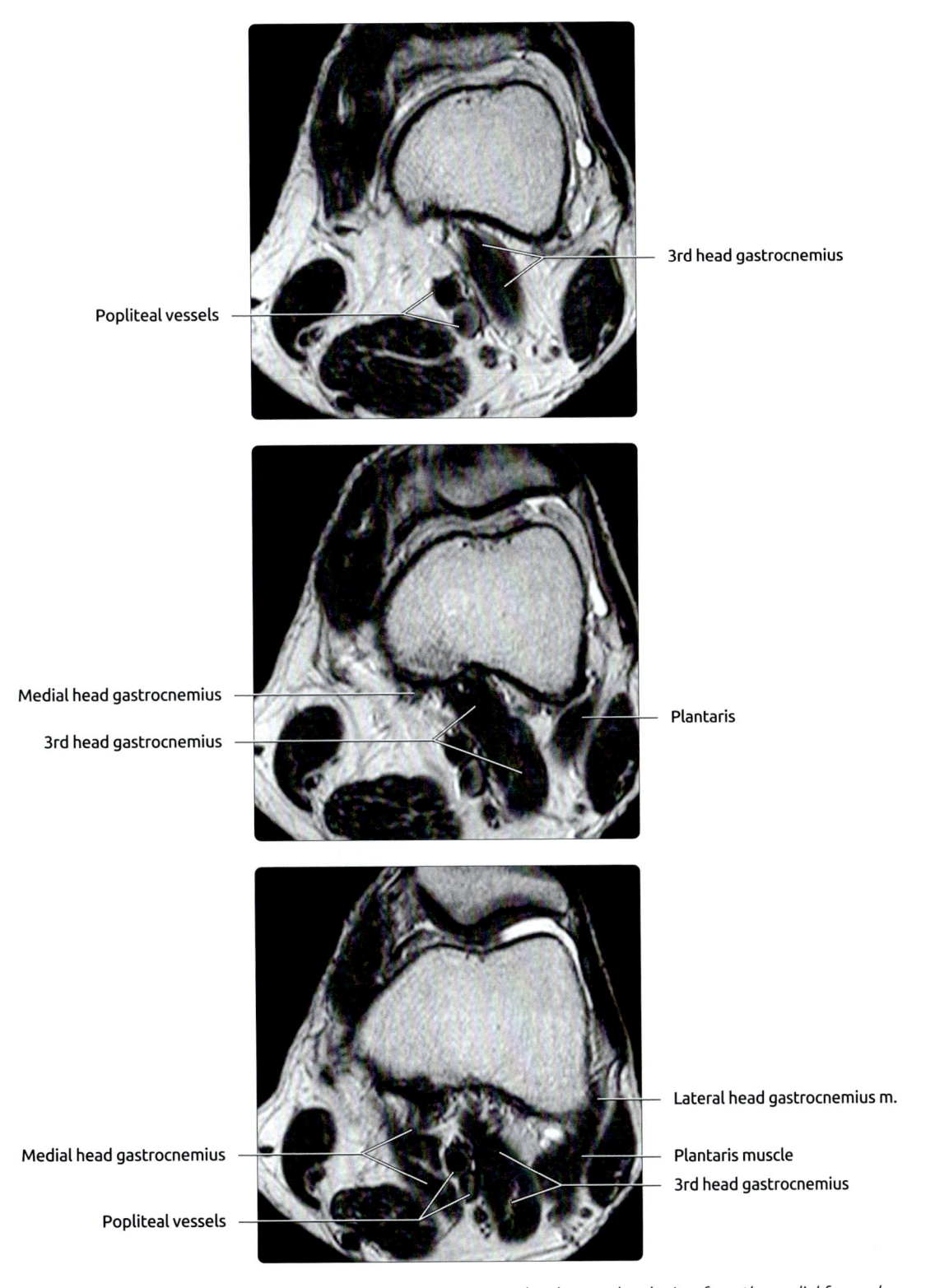

(Top) First of 3 axial T2 MR images shows a variant, 3rd head of gastrocnemius. The aberrant head arises from the medial femoral metaphysis, adjacent to the normal medial head gastrocnemius. However, it deviates laterally, forming a muscular sling around the popliteal vessels. (Middle) Slightly more distal image shows the aberrant 3rd head, as well as the normal medial head of gastrocnemius and plantaris. (Bottom) Slightly more distal image toward the knee joint shows the popliteal vessels surrounded by the normal medial head and the 3rd head of the gastrocnemius. This may result in symptoms of claudication. However, the variant is more likely to cause symptoms if it splits the popliteal artery and vein.

ABERRANT ORIGIN LATERAL HEAD GASTROCNEMIUS

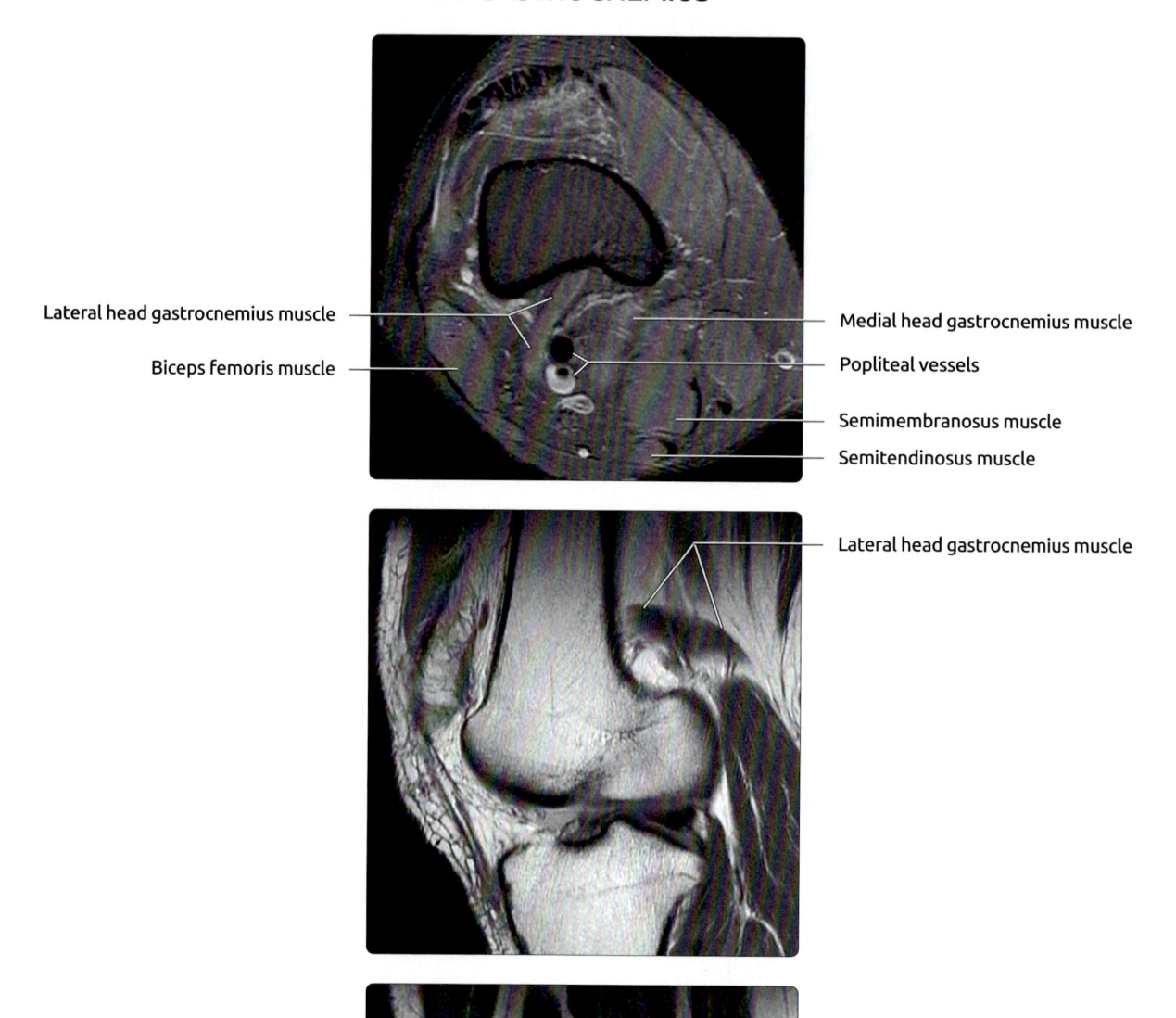

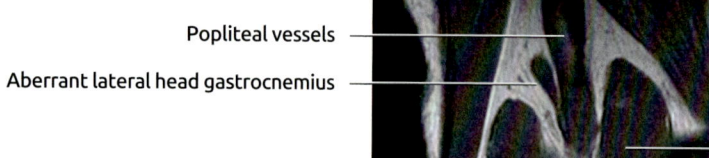

Lateral head gastrocnemius muscle
Biceps femoris muscle
Medial head gastrocnemius muscle
Popliteal vessels
Semimembranosus muscle
Semitendinosus muscle

Lateral head gastrocnemius muscle

Popliteal vessels
Aberrant lateral head gastrocnemius
Medial head gastrocnemius muscle

(Top) Axial PD FS MR demonstrates an aberrant origin of the lateral head of gastrocnemius, encircling the popliteal neurovascular bundle. Although patients with this abnormality may be asymptomatic, others present with symptoms of claudication. **(Middle)** Sagittal PD MR in the same patient shows the aberrant origin of the lateral head of the gastrocnemius. The course of the muscle is more horizontal than normal, which may be the only hint of the abnormal morphology. **(Bottom)** Coronal T1 MR in the same patient shows the aberrant lateral head of gastrocnemius encircling the popliteal vessels. This static image alone is not diagnostic; however, scrolling through the image stack shows this muscle slip originating more medially, corresponding to the morphology seen on the axial view.

Knee and Leg Normal Variants and Imaging Pitfalls

ABERRANT ORIGIN LATERAL HEAD GASTROCNEMIUS

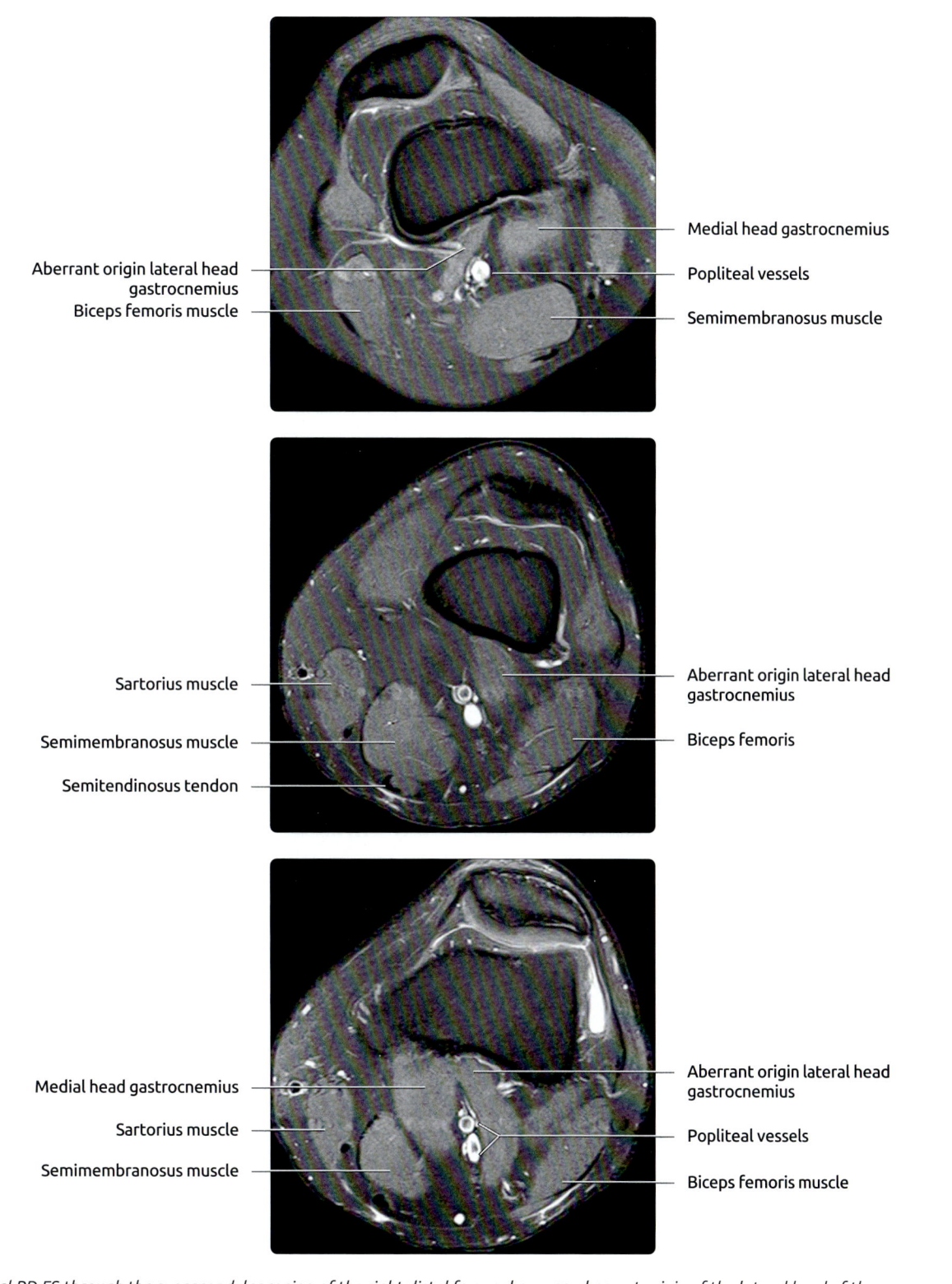

(Top) Axial PD FS through the supracondylar region of the right distal femur shows an aberrant origin of the lateral head of the gastrocnemius. As it heads towards its normal position posterolaterally, it encircles the popliteal vessels, potentially resulting in claudication symptoms. **(Middle)** Axial PD FS MR of the left knee in a different patient shows lateral head of gastrocnemius arising from the central/medial portion of the femoral metaphysis. **(Bottom)** Axial PD FS MR in the same patient, shows the aberrant head of the lateral head of gastrocnemius and the normal medial head of the gastrocnemius encircling the popliteal vessels. This patient had symptoms of claudication secondary to this morphologic anomaly.

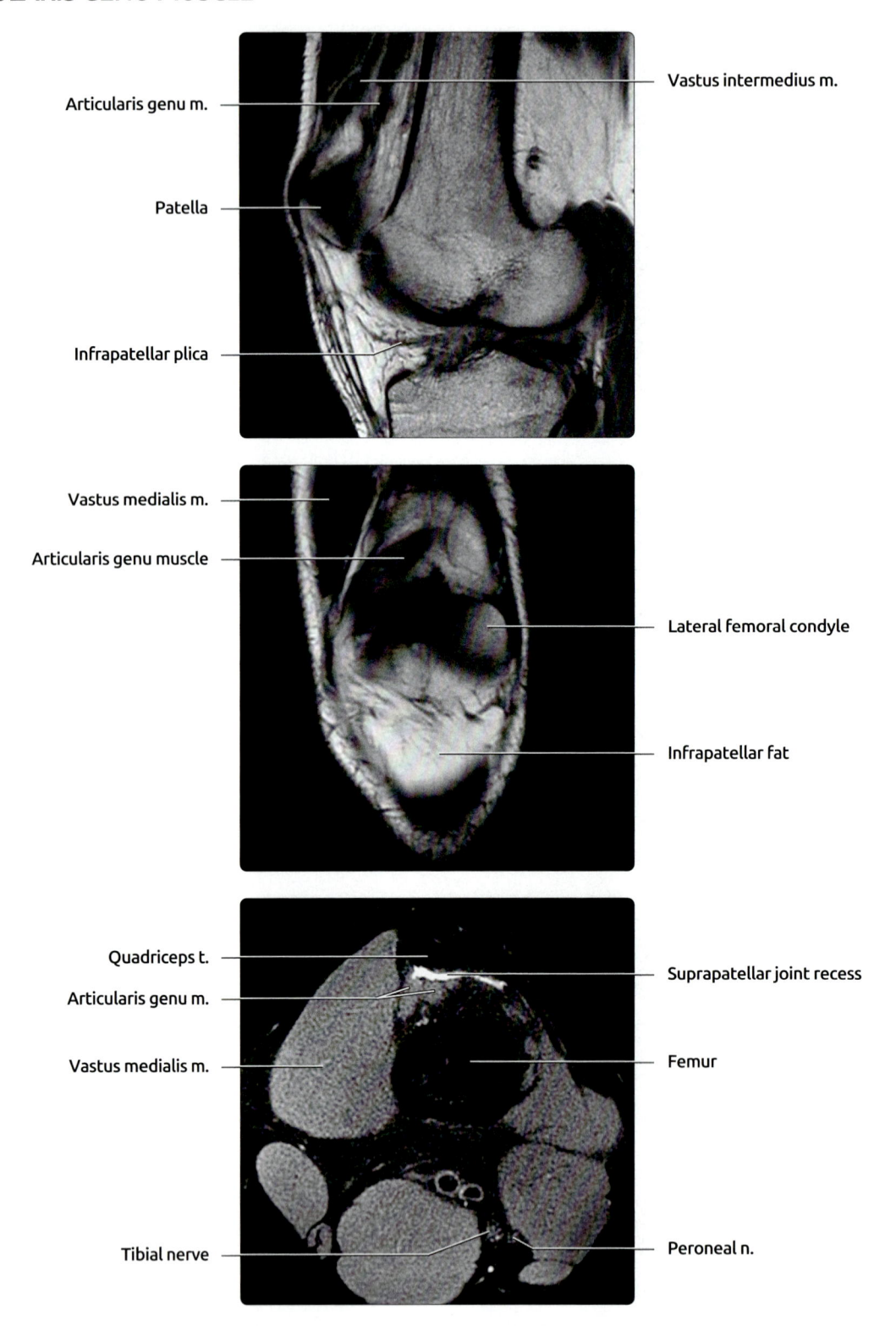

Knee and Leg Normal Variants and Imaging Pitfalls

ARTICULARIS GENU MUSCLE

Labels (top, sagittal PD MR): Articularis genu m.; Patella; Infrapatellar plica; Vastus intermedius m.

Labels (middle, coronal T1 MR): Vastus medialis m.; Articularis genu muscle; Lateral femoral condyle; Infrapatellar fat

Labels (bottom, axial PD FS MR): Quadriceps t.; Articularis genu m.; Vastus medialis m.; Tibial nerve; Suprapatellar joint recess; Femur; Peroneal n.

(Top) Sagittal PD MR shows the articularis genu muscle, which is variably present in the knee. It is sometimes merged with the vastus intermedius muscle. It originates from the distal femur and inserts on the suprapatellar synovium and acts to pull the suprapatellar recess superiorly during knee extension. (Middle) Coronal T1 MR immediately posterior to the patella shows the articularis genus as an ellipsoid, wispy structure. Its appearance is quite variable. It is innervated by the femoral nerve. (Bottom) Axial PD FS MR immediately superior to the patella shows the articularis genu muscle attaching to the synovium of the suprapatellar recess. In this case, 2 separate muscle bundles are seen. The articularis genu may have single or multiple bundles and is variable in appearance.

Knee and Leg Normal Variants and Imaging Pitfalls

ACCESSORY MUSCLE: TENSOR FASCIA SURALIS

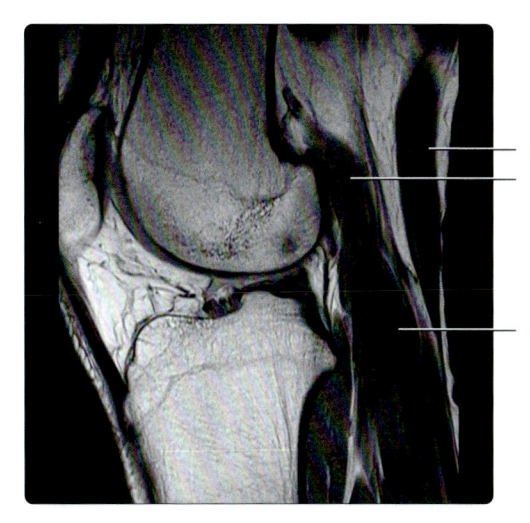

(Top) Sagittal PD MR of the knee through the lateral condyle demonstrates the expected plantaris and gastrocnemius muscles. However, there is an additional longitudinal structure located posterior to the gastrocnemius that displays signal and texture of muscle. (Middle) Sagittal PD MR of knee through the lateral condyle with accessory muscle shaded green. This accessory muscle is termed the tensor fascia suralis. Such accessory muscles may present clinically as a mass, as in this case. (Bottom) Axial PD MR in the same patient shows the accessory muscle (tensor fascia suralis) with nearby normal muscles. It is important to note expected muscles and be certain that there are not "extras" since there is no signal abnormality to alert one to the abnormality. (Courtesy A. Kingzett-Taylor, MD.)

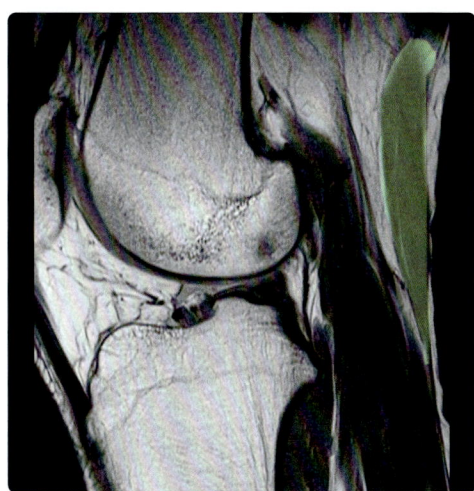

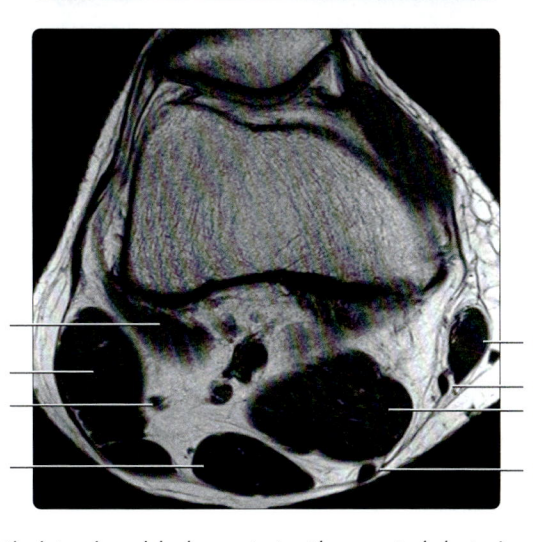

Knee and Leg Normal Variants and Imaging Pitfalls

ACCESSORY SOLEUS MUSCLE

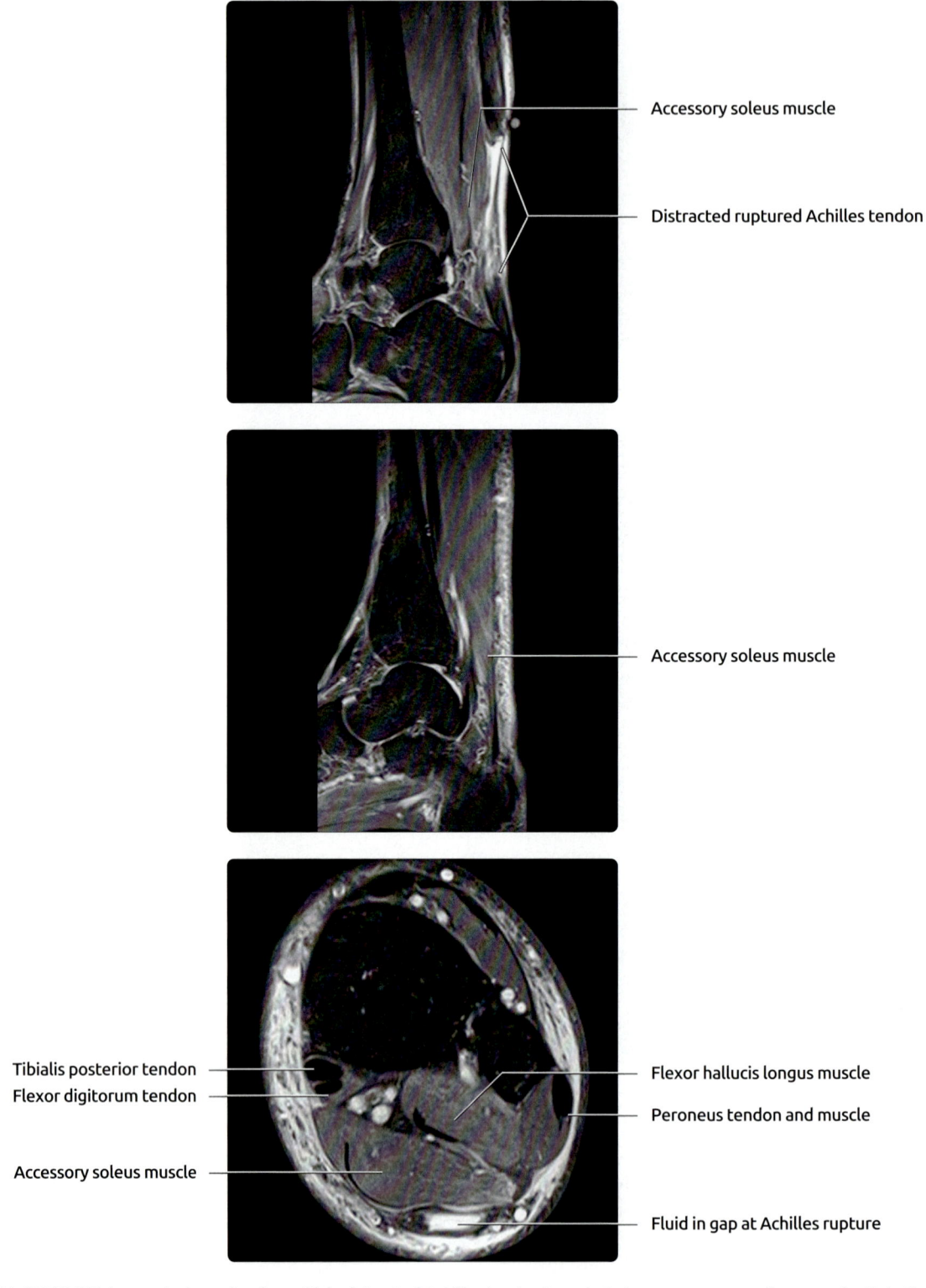

(Top) Sagittal T2FS MR demonstrates not only a widely distracted Achilles tendon tear, but also an accessory soleus muscle. Note the space normally occupied by Kager fat pad. (Middle) Adjacent sagittal cut shows full bulk of accessory soleus muscle. (Bottom) Axial PD FS shows fluid at the gap from the Achilles rupture. However, the space normally occupied by Kager fat pad is filled with a large accessory soleus muscle.

Knee and Leg Normal Variants and Imaging Pitfalls

ACCESSORY FLEXOR HALLUCIS LONGUS

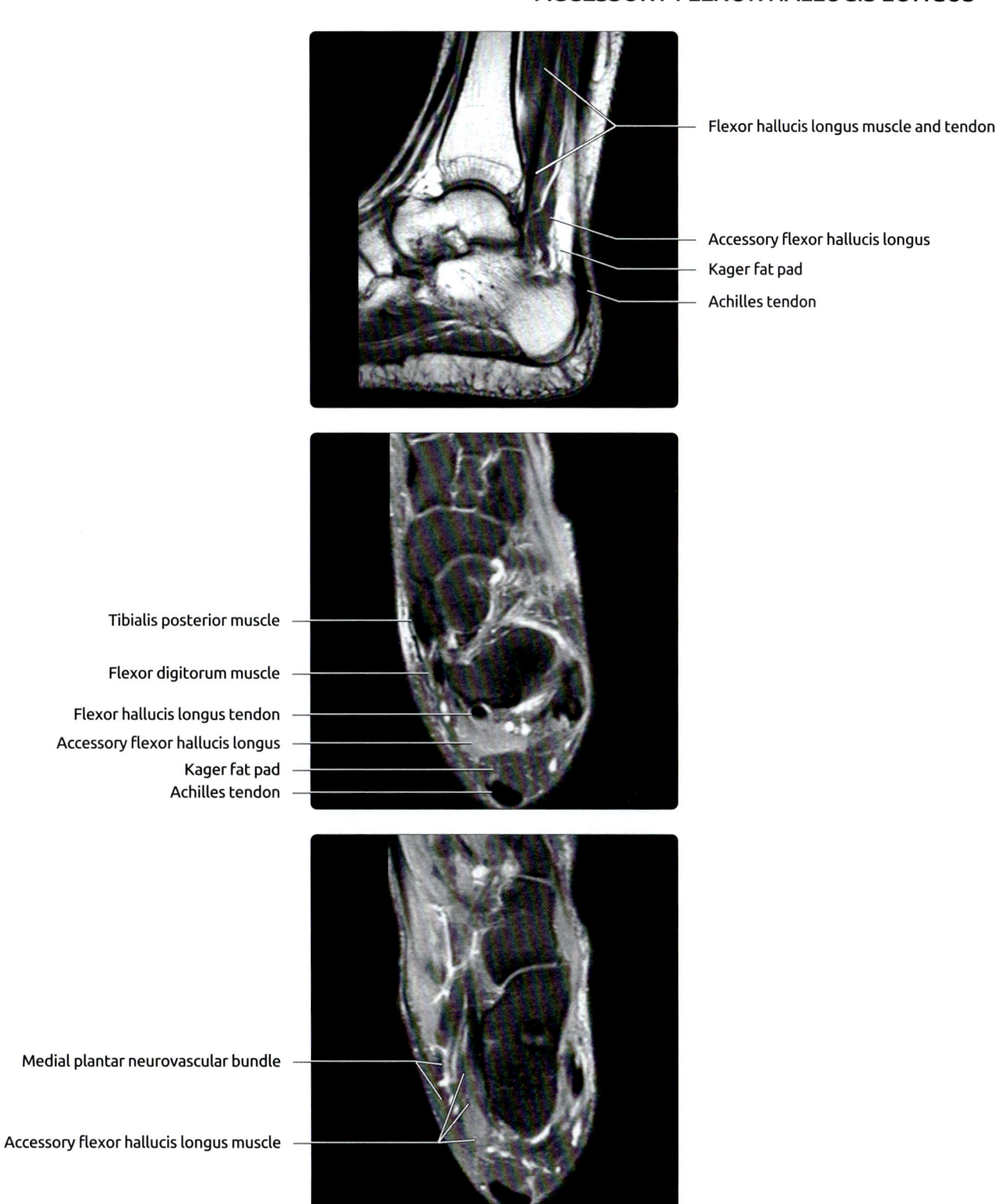

(Top) Sagittal PD MR demonstrates the flexor hallucis longus muscle and tendon with the muscle fibers extending distally to the level of the tibiotalar joint before becoming entirely tendinous. In addition, there is a structure that has signal intensity of muscle located within the Kager fat pad, anterior to the Achilles tendon. In this region, the structure is likely to be an accessory muscle. Axial imaging will prove the origin of this accessory muscle. (Middle) Long-axis PD FS MR in the same patient shows the expected locations of the tibialis posterior, flexor digitorum, and flexor hallucis longus tendons. In addition, there is a mass located posterior to the flexor hallucis longus tendon that has signal intensity of muscle and encroaches upon Kager fat pad. By location, this muscle is the flexor hallucis longus accessory muscle. (Bottom) Long-axis PD FS MR located slightly distal to the prior image shows the muscle fibers of the accessory muscle continue medial to the calcaneus. This space-occupying muscle may compress the medial plantar nerve.

ENLARGED FABELLOFIBULAR LIGAMENT

Fabella
Fabellofibular ligament
Popliteal hiatus
Popliteofibular ligament

Popliteal tendon
Arcuate ligament
Fabellofibular ligament

Fabella
Fabellofibular ligament

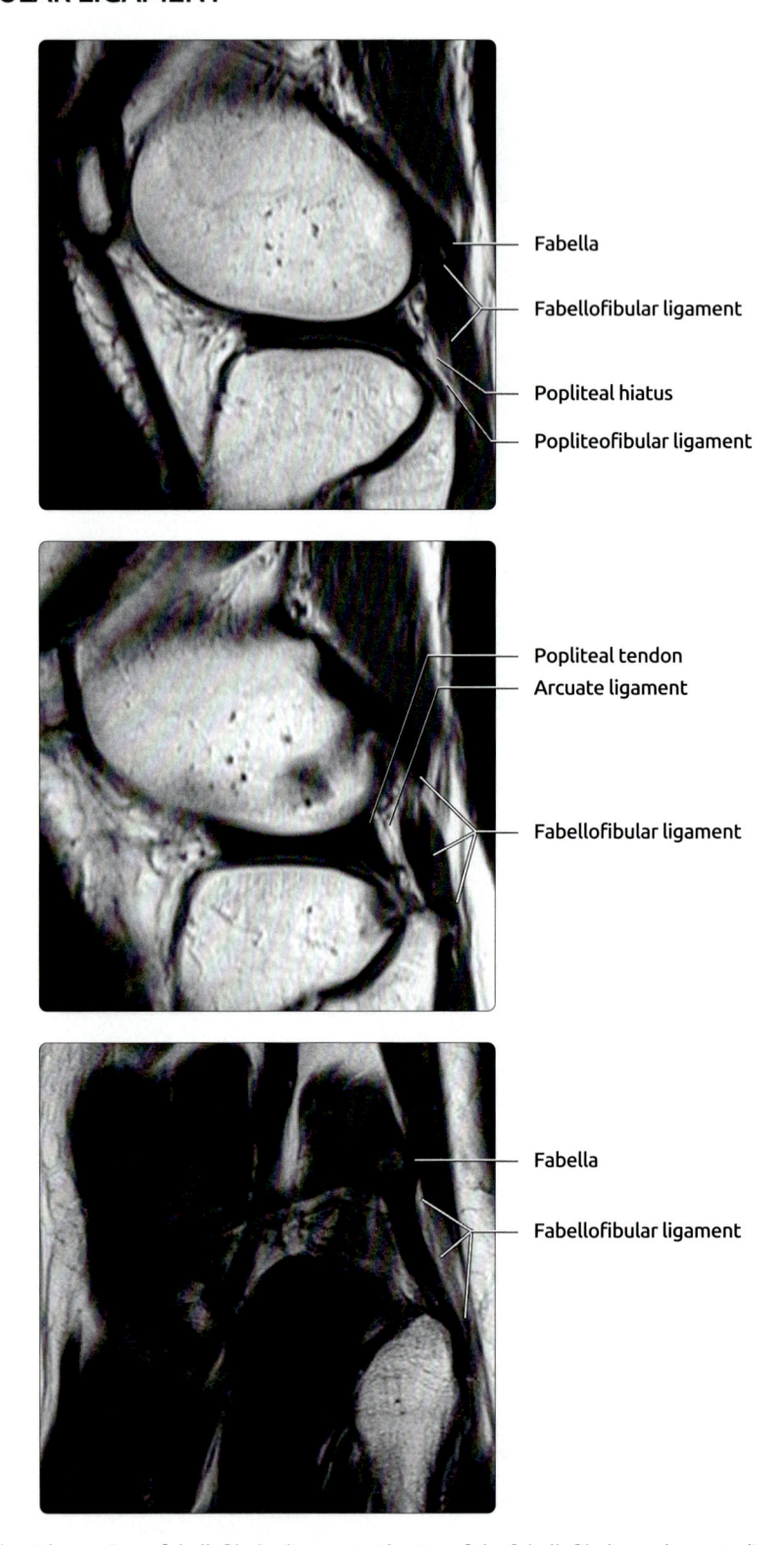

(Top) Sagittal PD MR shows a fabella with prominent fabellofibular ligament. The size of the fabellofibular and arcuate ligaments tends to be inversely related; if there is no fabella (and therefore no fabellofibular ligament) present then the arcuate ligament is well seen. In this patient, there is an enlarged fabellofibular ligament and the arcuate ligament is not visible. **(Middle)** A slightly more lateral image shows the enlarged fabellofibular ligament extending to the fibular styloid insertion. The arcuate ligament is extremely thin. **(Bottom)** Coronal T1 MR, far posterior, shows the enlarged fabellofibular ligament extending from the fabella to its insertion on the fibular styloid process.

Knee and Leg Normal Variants and Imaging Pitfalls

MULTIPARTITE PATELLA

Multipartite patella

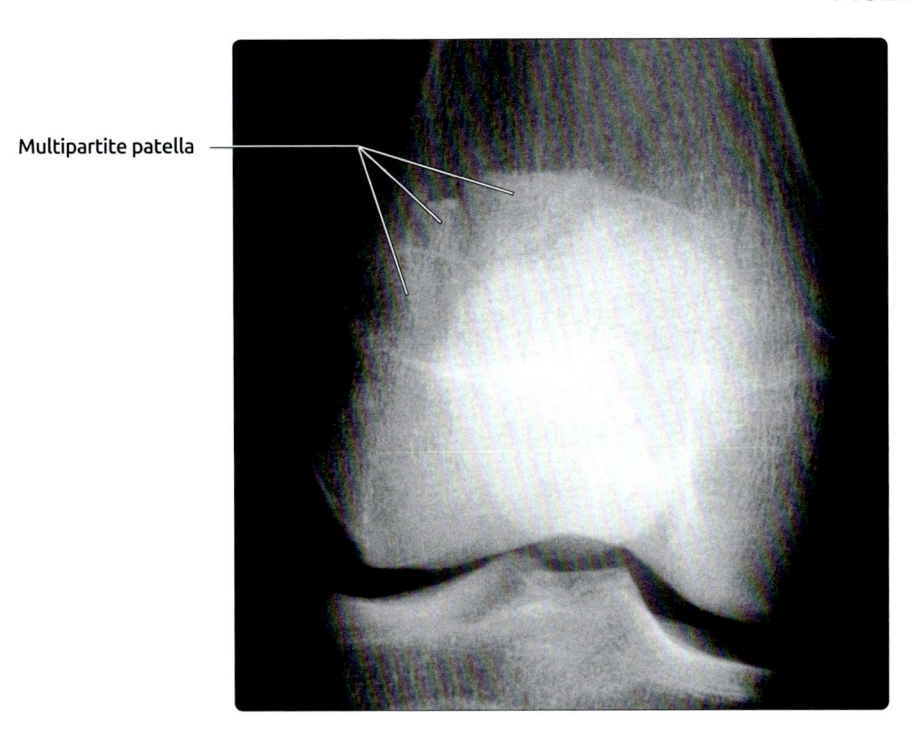

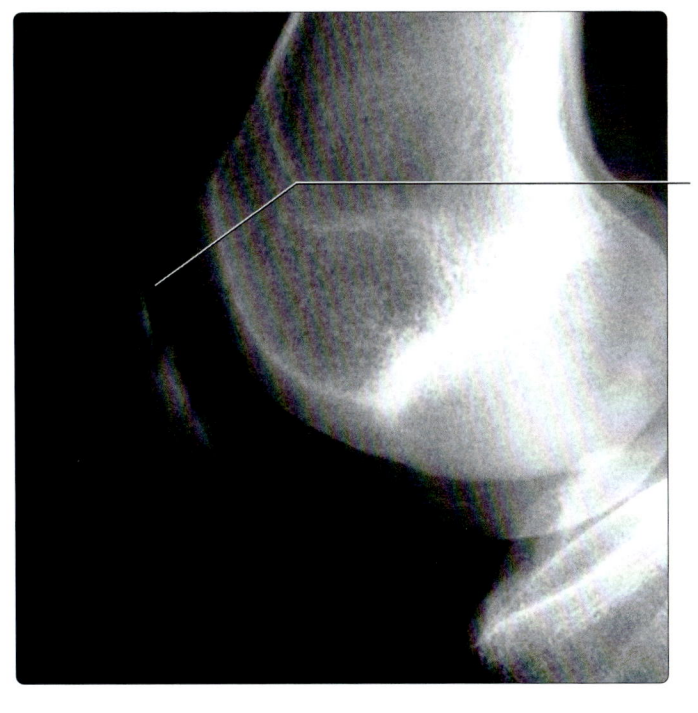

"Malalignment" of bipartite fragment

(Top) The patellar ossification center may be segmented, resulting in a bipartite or multipartite structure. The "fragments" may not appear to fit together perfectly (the pieces do not always correspond perfectly with their underlying fossa). The majority of bipartite or multipartite patella have the fragmentation at the superolateral quadrant, as in this case. **(Bottom)** The lateral view of this patient demonstrates the common feature of the bipartite fragments not aligning perfectly with the adjacent patellar surfaces. Despite this apparent angulation of ossific structures, the overlying cartilage is intact and the abnormality is not symptomatic.

Knee and Leg Normal Variants and Imaging Pitfalls

BIPARTITE PATELLA

Bipartite fragment

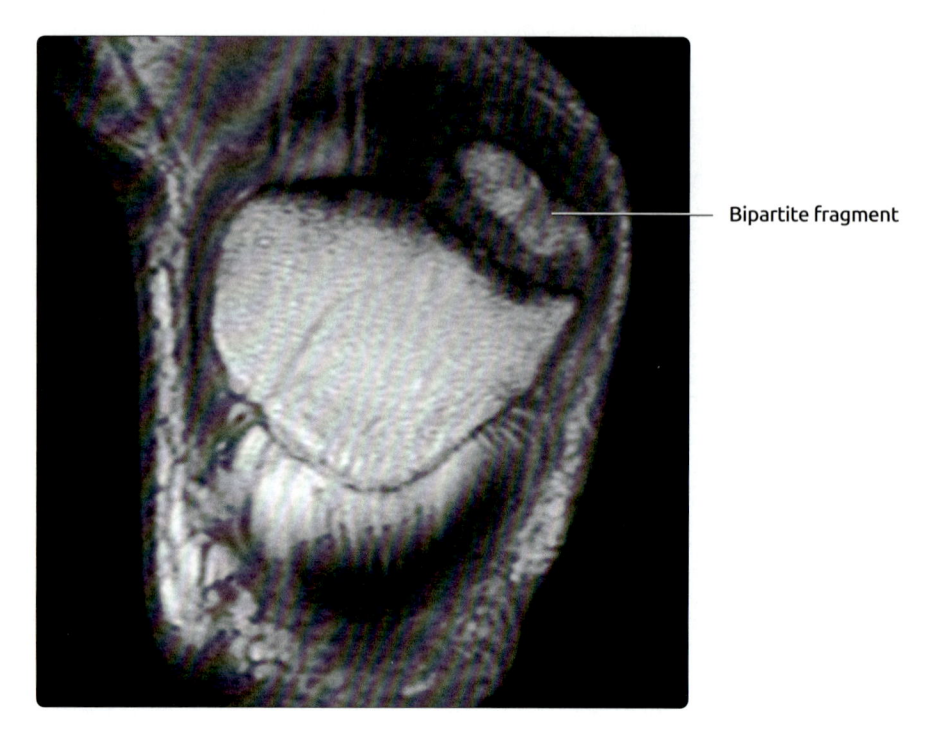

Bipartite ossific center

Normal cartilage outlining bipartite patella

(Top) Coronal T1WI MR located far anteriorly demonstrates a bipartite patella, with the fragment located in the superolateral quadrant. Note the rounded edges of both the fragment and adjacent patella. Additionally, there is no edema present. Both of these findings negate the possibility that this is a fracture. (Bottom) Fat-saturated T2WI axial image through the superior portion of the patella shows the bipartite ossific center adjacent to the remainder of the patella. The small effusion nicely outlines the patellar cartilage. Note that the cartilage is smooth and completely covers the osseous "defect." Normal cartilage coverage of a bipartite or multipartite patella is standard. (Courtesy A. Sonin, MD.)

Knee and Leg Normal Variants and Imaging Pitfalls

DORSAL DEFECT OF THE PATELLA

Dorsal defect of patella

Dorsal defect of patella

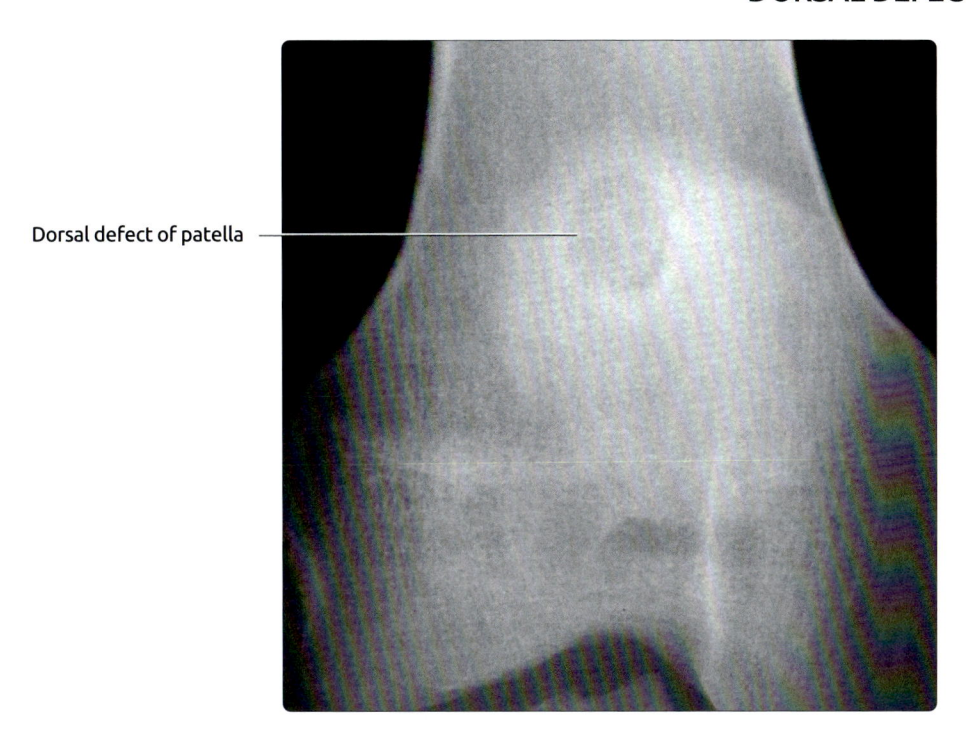

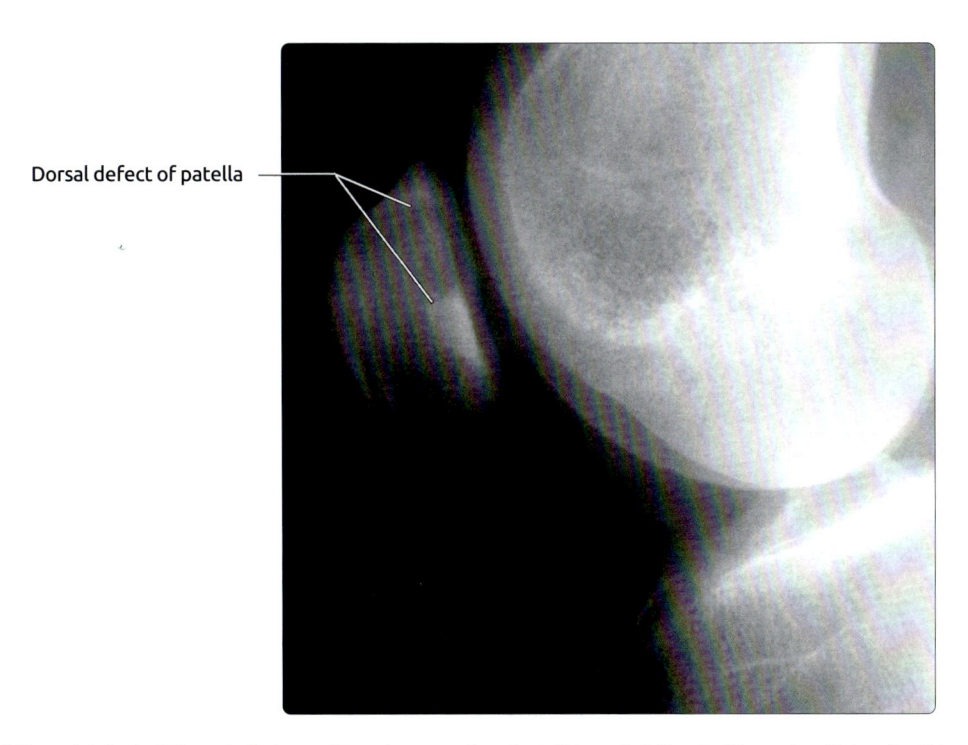

(Top) *Dorsal defect of the patella is considered a normal variant. It is well defined with a sclerotic border. It is usually located within the superolateral quadrant of the patella.* **(Bottom)** *The defect appears less distinct on this lateral view, but the appearance overall is classic for the diagnosis. If a MR was performed, it would show the cartilage to be normal overlying the osseous abnormality. It is important that the abnormality be distinguished from an osteochondral injury.*

Knee and Leg Normal Variants and Imaging Pitfalls

DORSAL DEFECT OF THE PATELLA

Dorsal defect of the patella

Dorsal defect of the patella

Dorsal defect of the patella
Lateral femoral condyle

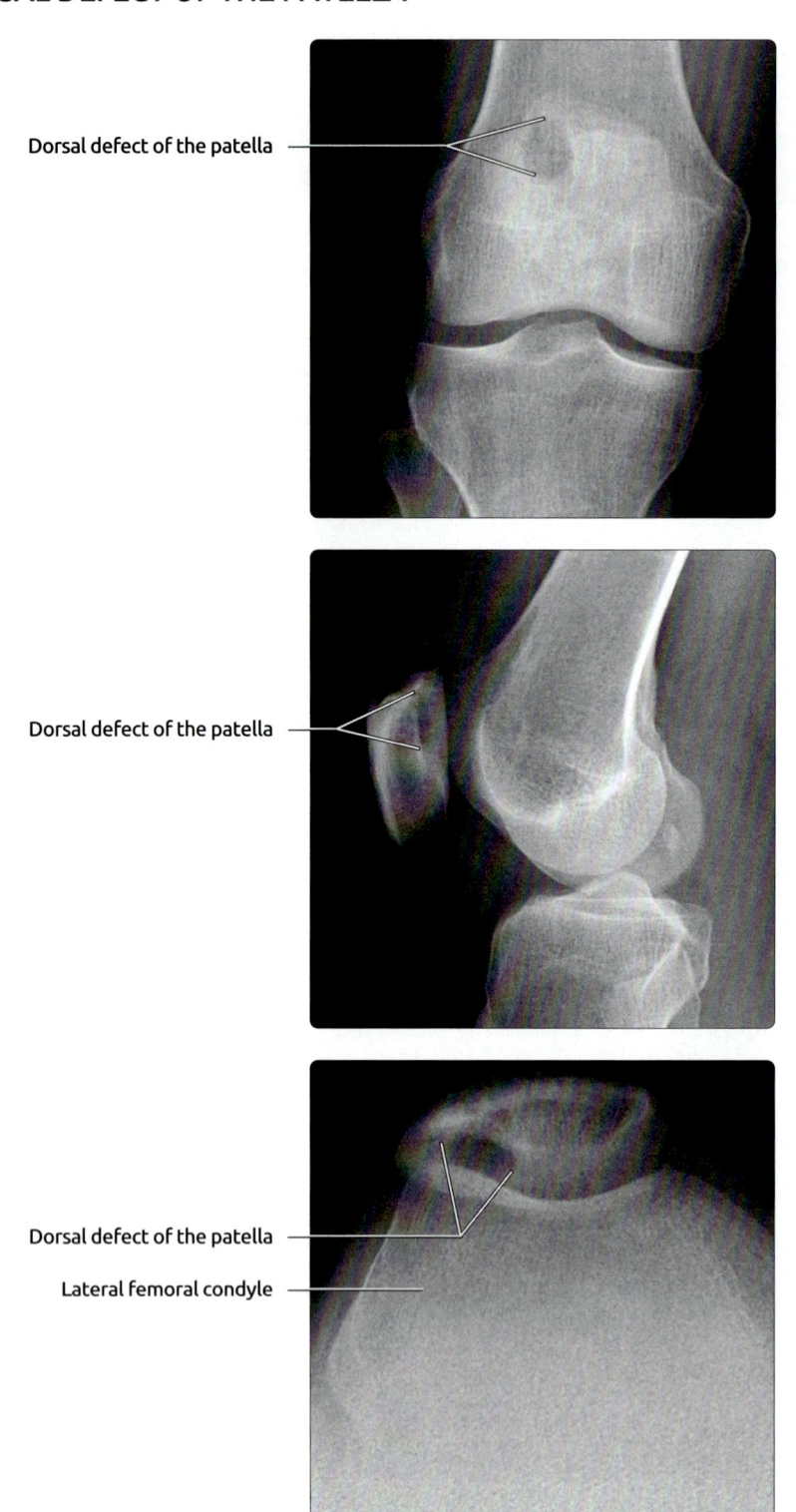

(Top) *AP radiograph shows a rounded lucency superimposed over the upper outer aspect of the patella.* **(Middle)** *Lateral radiograph confirms that the rounded lucency is within the upper aspect of the patella. No other abnormality is seen.* **(Bottom)** *Axial radiograph in the same patient shows the smooth rounded lucency at the upper outer quadrant of the patella. This is the typical appearance and location of dorsal defect of the patella.*

Knee and Leg Normal Variants and Imaging Pitfalls

DORSAL DEFECT OF THE PATELLA

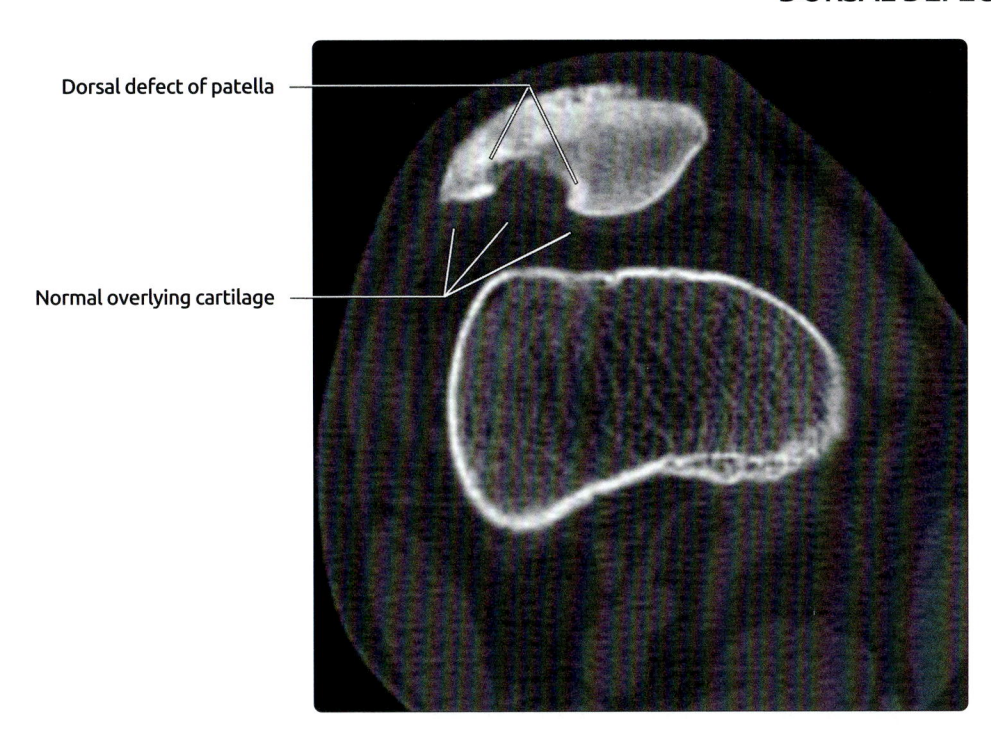

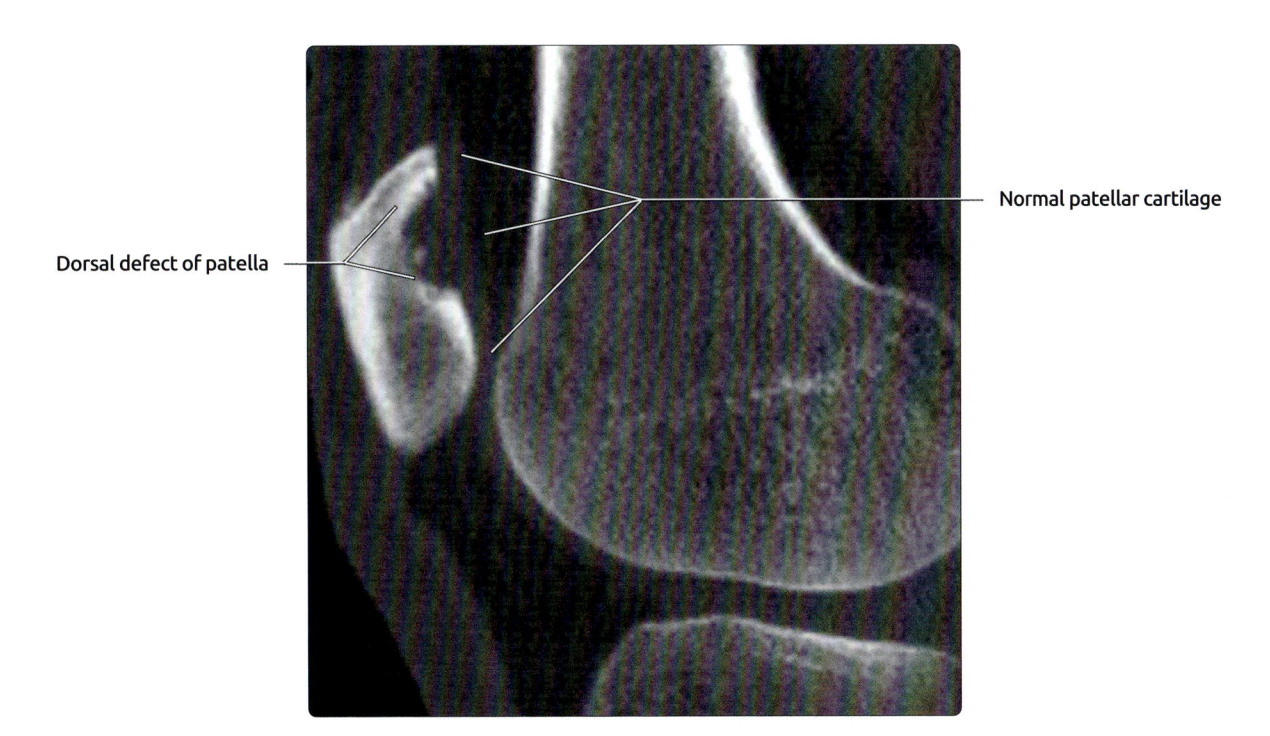

(Top) *Axial CT in the same patient shows the large dorsal defect of the patella. Note the cartilage overlying the defect is completely normal. Given the smooth defect, typical location, and normal overlying cartilage, the diagnosis of dorsal defect is definitive. No further work-up or treatment is needed.* (Bottom) *Sagittal CT reconstruction again shows normal cartilage overlying the dorsal defect.*

Knee and Leg Normal Variants and Imaging Pitfalls

DEVELOPMENTAL VARIATION LATERAL FEMORAL CONDYLE

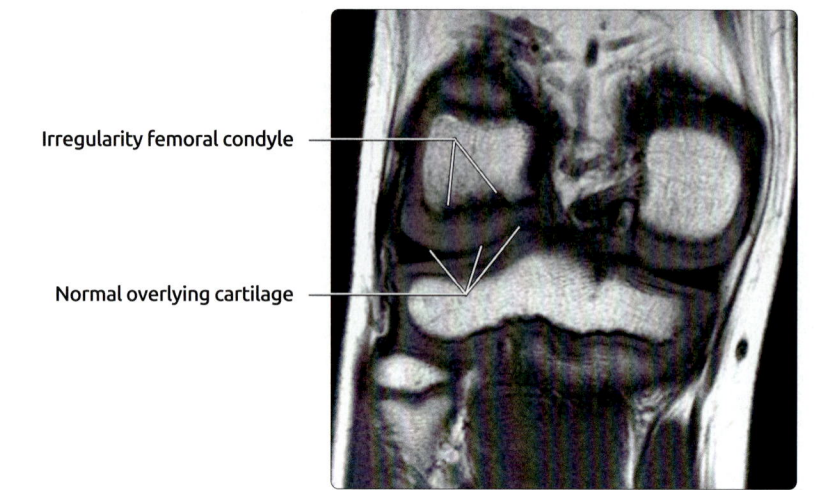

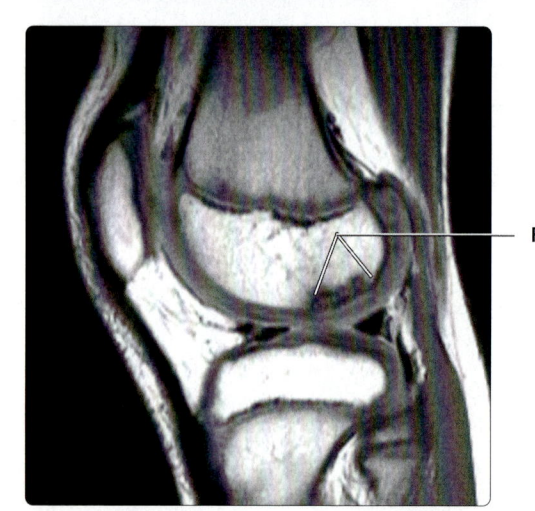

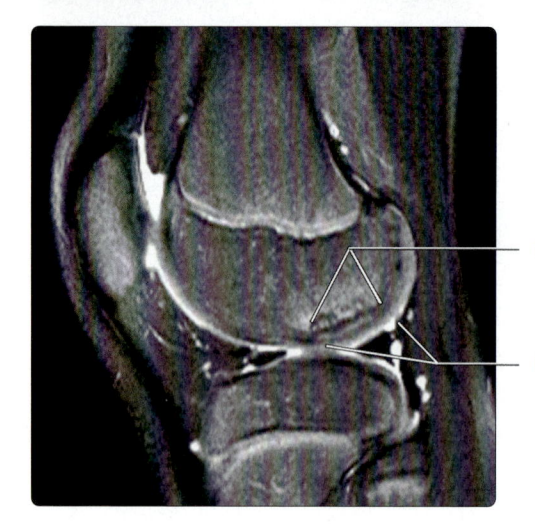

(Top) Coronal T1 MR in the posterior aspect of the joint demonstrates irregularity of the lateral femoral condyle in a 9-year-old girl. The overlying cartilage is thick and normal. The location in the posterior 1/3 of the condyle, without extension to the intercondylar notch, helps to differentiate this normal variant from an osteochondral defect. (Middle) Sagittal T1 MR in the same patient confirms the irregularity is located in the posterior 1/3 of the femoral condyle. (Bottom) Sagittal T2 FS MR in the same patient shows slight hyperintensity at the femoral condylar defect with normal overlying cartilage. This is considered normal in this developmental variant and the patient was given instructions to continue normal activity.

Knee and Leg Normal Variants and Imaging Pitfalls

DEVELOPMENTAL VARIATION LATERAL FEMORAL CONDYLE

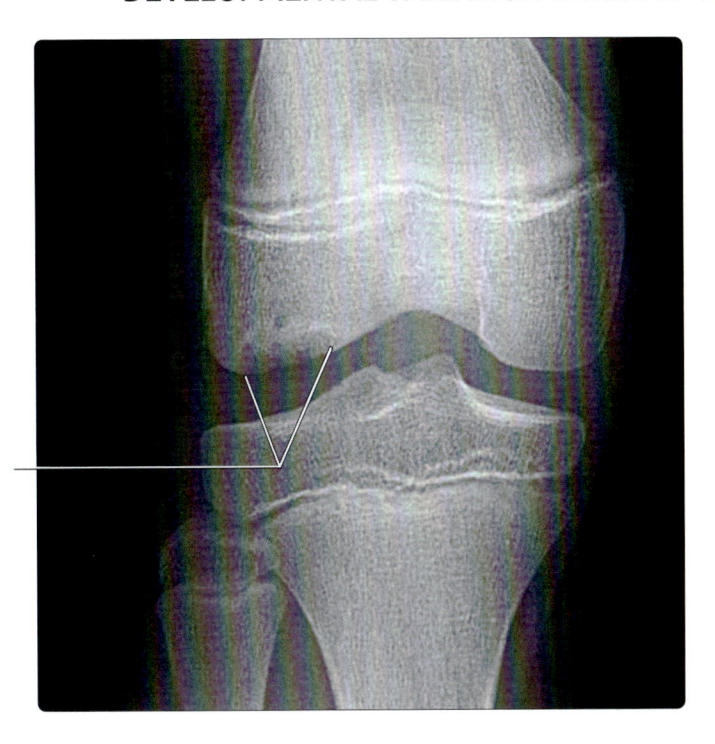

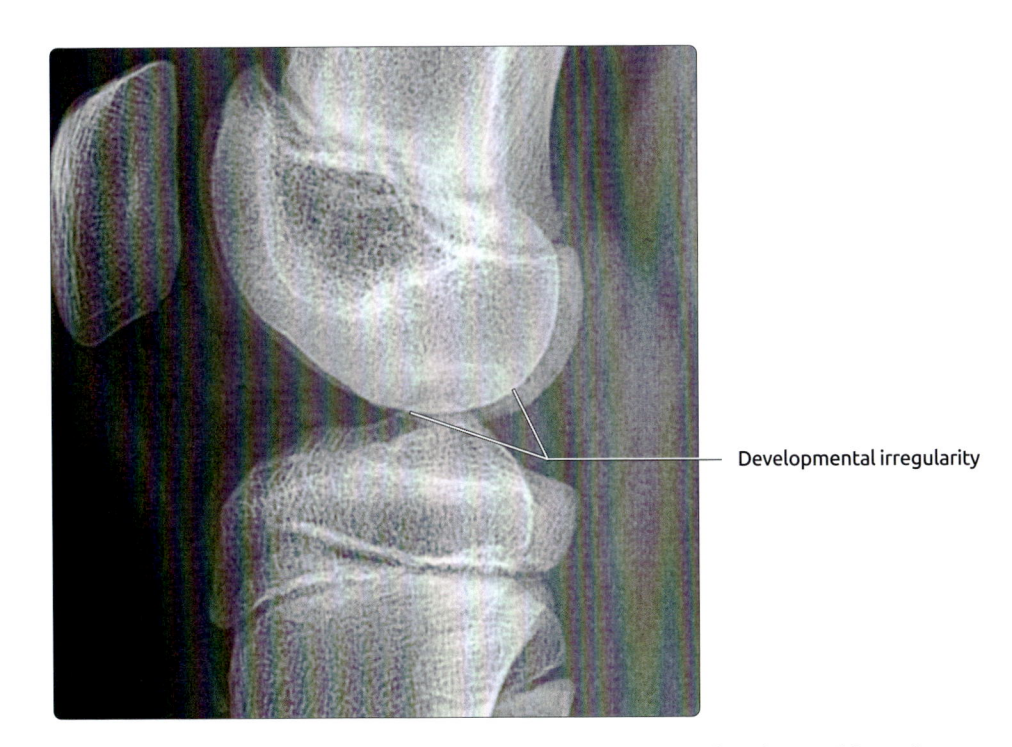

Developmental irregularity

Developmental irregularity

(Top) AP radiograph, obtained 1 year later, of the same patient shows apparent "healing in" or normal growth at the site of femoral condylar irregularity. (Bottom) Lateral radiograph confirms that the developmental irregularity is forming normal bone and that there is no collapse at the site. Remember that the location of the abnormality is restricted to the posterior portion of the condyle and does not extend to the intercondylar notch. The lack of significant marrow edema can help differentiate this normal developmental variant from an osteochondral lesion. Treatment of the 2 is significantly different.

DEVELOPMENTAL VARIATION LATERAL FEMORAL CONDYLE

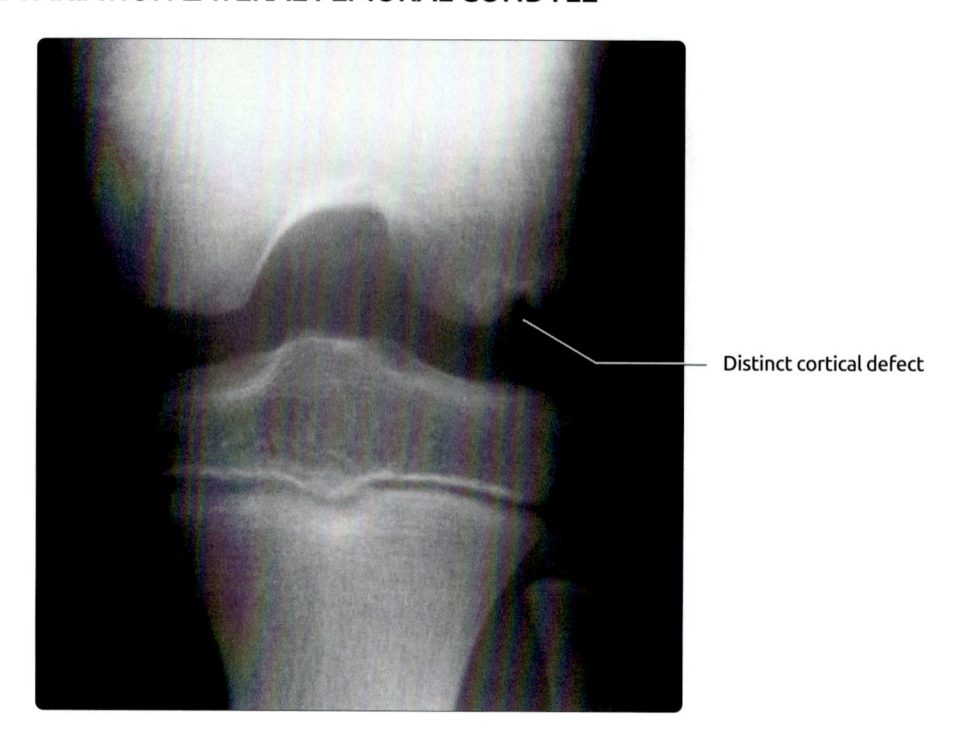

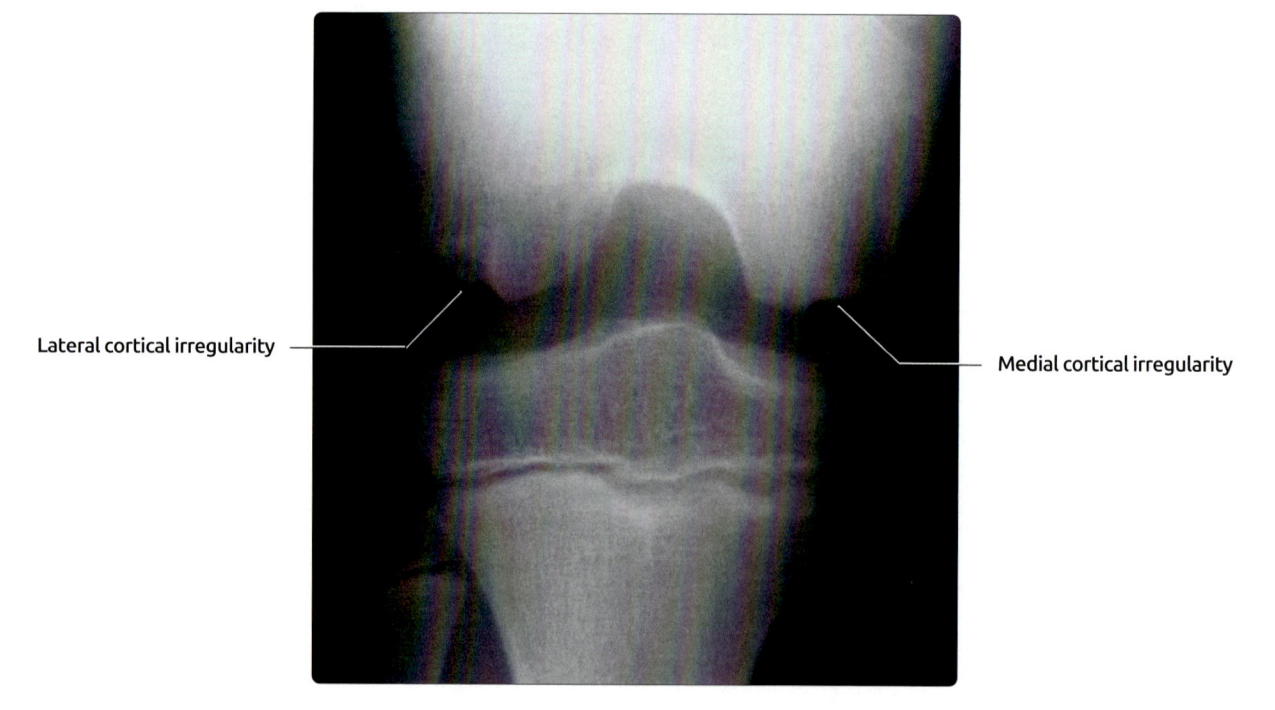

(Top) *This is a notch view of the same patient. Because the notch position brings the posterior portion of the femoral condyle into profile, the cortical irregularity is seen much more distinctly than on either AP or lateral views.* (Bottom) *This image is a notch view of the contralateral knee in the same patient. It shows posterior cortical irregularity on both the medial and lateral femoral condyles. As in this case, the findings may be bilateral, though not necessarily symmetric. The involvement of the lateral femoral condyle is far more common than the medial. This appearance and location is typical in adolescents and must not be mistaken for an osteochondral defect or injury. The overlying cartilage is normal.*

DEVELOPMENTAL VARIATION LATERAL FEMORAL CONDYLE

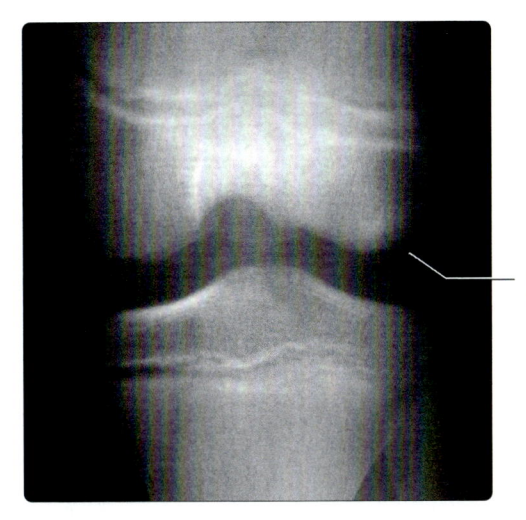

Posterolateral femoral condylar irregularity

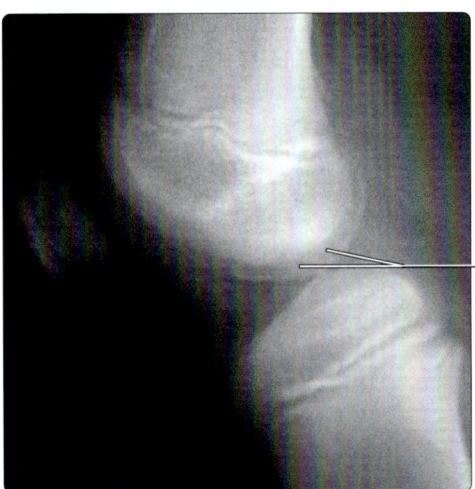

Posterolateral condylar irregularity

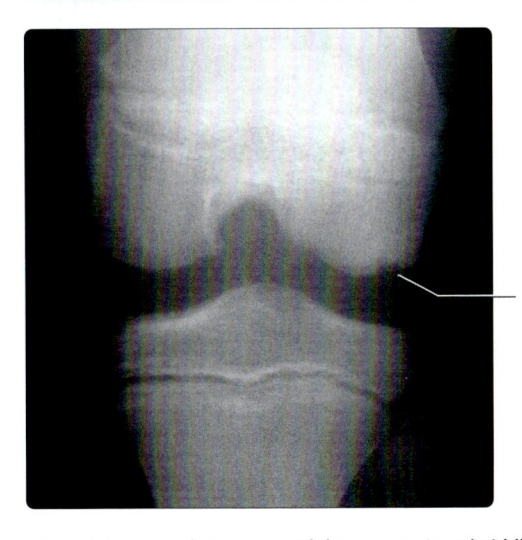

Posterolateral femoral condylar defect

(Top) *This AP view shows a mild lateral femoral condylar irregularity in an adolescent patient.* **(Middle)** *The lateral view confirms the location of the irregularity as being typical for the normal variant.* **(Bottom)** *Notch view of the same patient shows the abnormality more clearly and confirms its posterior location. The radiographs are sufficient to make the diagnosis of normal variant. No further imaging should be required, and since it does not represent an osteochondral injury, no treatment need be instituted.*

DEVELOPMENTAL VARIATION LATERAL FEMORAL CONDYLE

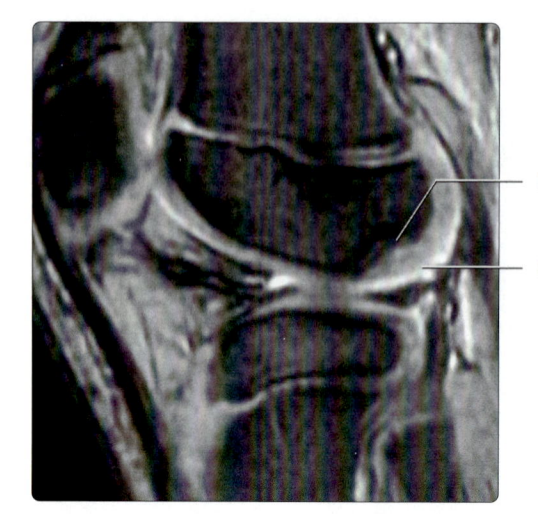

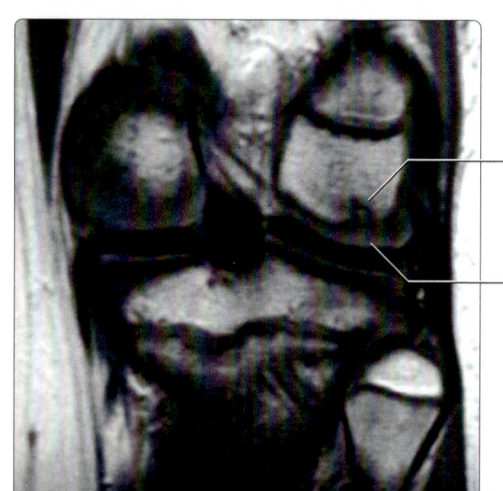

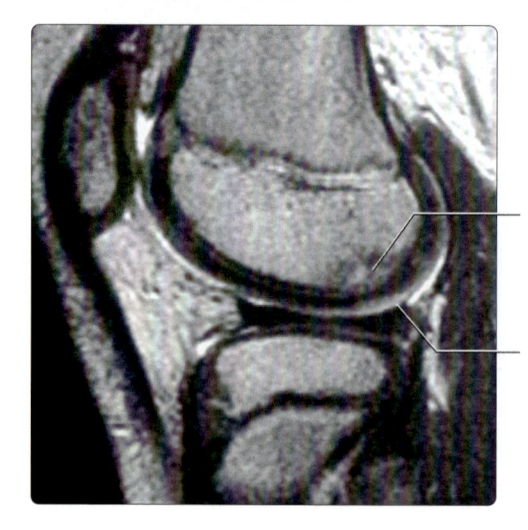

(Top) Gradient-echo sagittal in the same patient shows the osseous defect in the posterior lateral femoral condyle. The overlying cartilage is seen to be normal in thickness and contour, confirming that this is a variant rather than a true osteochondral injury. (Middle) Proton density coronal located posteriorly in the joint shows both the femoral condylar defect and the normal overlying cartilage. (Bottom) T2 weighted sagittal image in the same patient shows both the osseous defect in the typical posterior lateral femoral condylar region and the normal overlying cartilage. There is no marrow edema and no other abnormality. The defect is a normal variant that is seen in adolescents (note the open physes), which routinely ossifies normally. It is not in the usual location to suggest an osteochondral defect.

POSTEROMEDIAL CORTICAL DEFECT

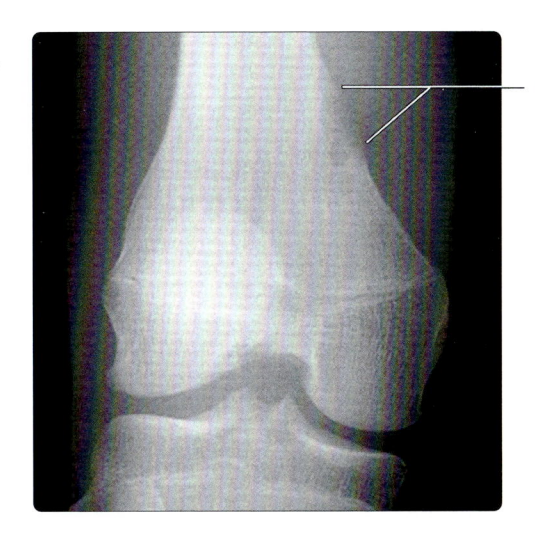

Posteromedial defect

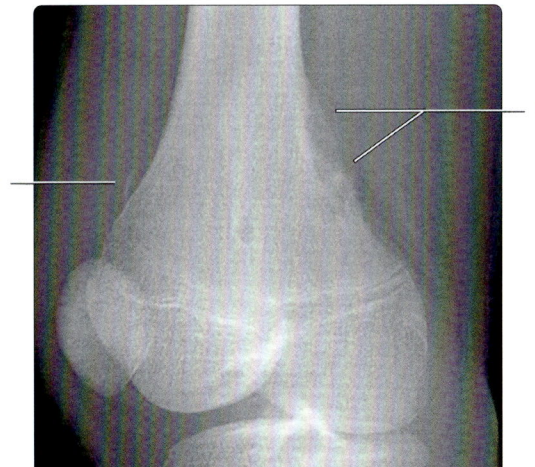

Chip fracture within large effusion — *Posteromedial cortical defect*

Chip fracture within large effusion, unrelated to defect — *Posteromedial cortical defect*

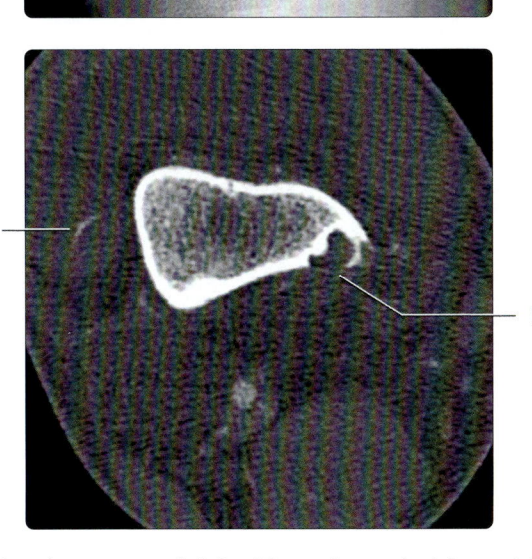

(Top) *This defect seen on the AP radiograph in the posteromedial distal femoral metaphysis has variably been termed "cortical desmoid," "avulsive or tug lesion," or simply a "cortical defect." These authors prefer the latter term. It is site-specific at the posteromedial corner and is anatomically related to the adductor magnus aponeurotic insertion. It is debated as to whether it represents a chronic avulsive injury or is a normal growth phenomenon.* **(Middle)** *External oblique view profiles the cortical defect. Note that the defect may not have overlying cortex; it may sometimes even appear slightly spiculated. Despite that appearance, it is judged by location to be a normal variant rather than something more aggressive. This patient also has a large effusion and chip fracture, unrelated to the defect.* **(Bottom)** *CT confirms location and appearance of posteromedial cortical defect.*

Knee and Leg Normal Variants and Imaging Pitfalls

POSTEROMEDIAL CORTICAL DEFECT

Posteromedial cortical defect

Posteromedial cortical defect

Posteromedial cortical defect

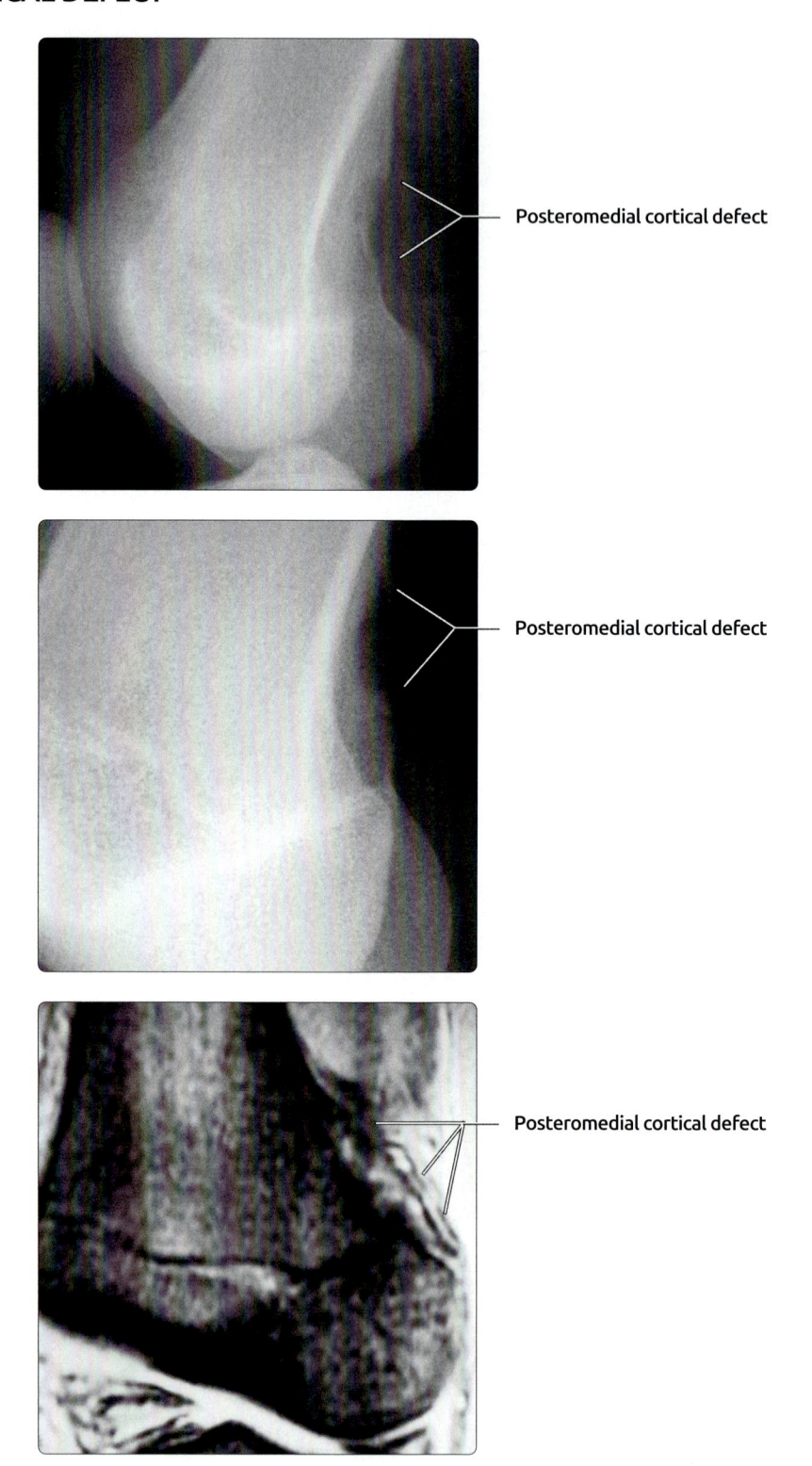

(Top) Slightly obliqued lateral radiograph shows a posteromedial cortical defect with typically slightly aggressive appearance of scalloping and indistinct cortex. *(Middle)* Lateral radiograph shows another posteromedial cortical defect. *(Bottom)* Radial gradient-echo MR image profiles the posteromedial distal femoral cortical defect. Note how indistinct the cortex and scalloped margin are and the suggestion of soft tissue mass. This is typical of the normal variant cortical defect. As long as the location corresponds to the posteromedial distal femoral metaphysis, and appearance shows nothing more aggressive, this can be considered a normal variant.

Knee and Leg Normal Variants and Imaging Pitfalls

FOPE (FOCAL PERIPHYSEAL EDEMA) ZONE

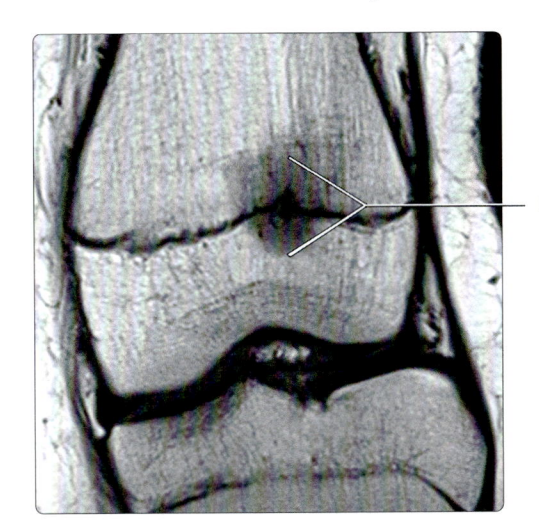

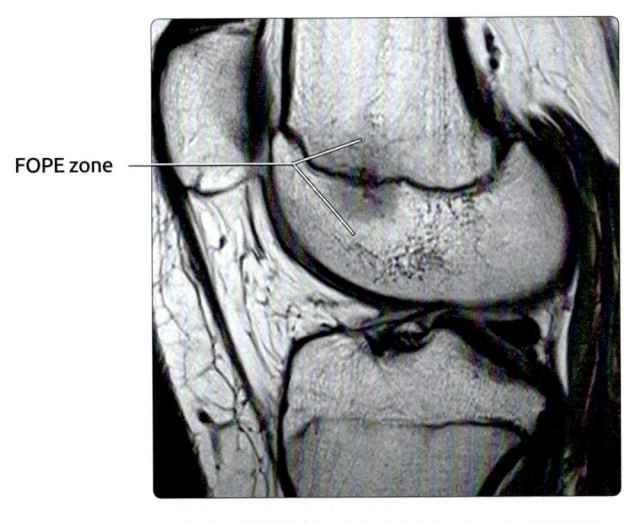

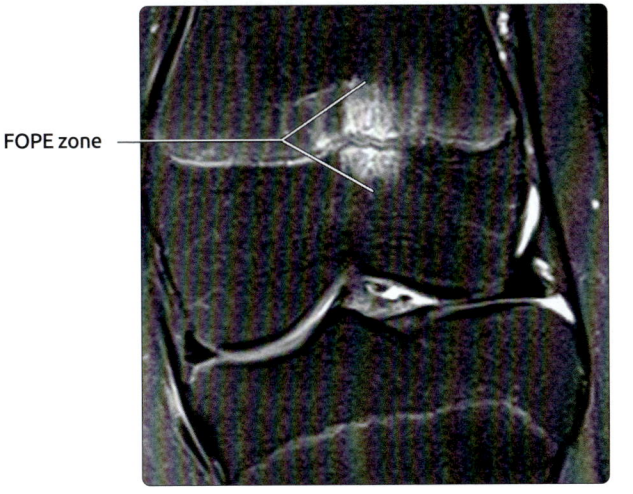

(Top) Coronal T1 MR in a skeletally immature patient demonstrates low signal surrounding a central portion of the femoral physis. The entire physis is open and shows no other abnormality. (Middle) Sagittal PD MR in the same patient confirms that the region of abnormal signal is periphyseal and central. No other abnormality is seen. (Bottom) Coronal PD FS MR shows edema within the bone surrounding the central physis. This edema is felt to relate to the early stages of physiologic physeal closure. It may be associated with pain particularly when no other MR abnormalities are present. When the characteristic appearance of a FOPE zone is observed, as in this case, the patient requires no invasive diagnostic procedure, and does not need imaging follow-up.

MENISCOCRUCIATE LIGAMENT ARISING FROM TRANSVERSE LIGAMENT

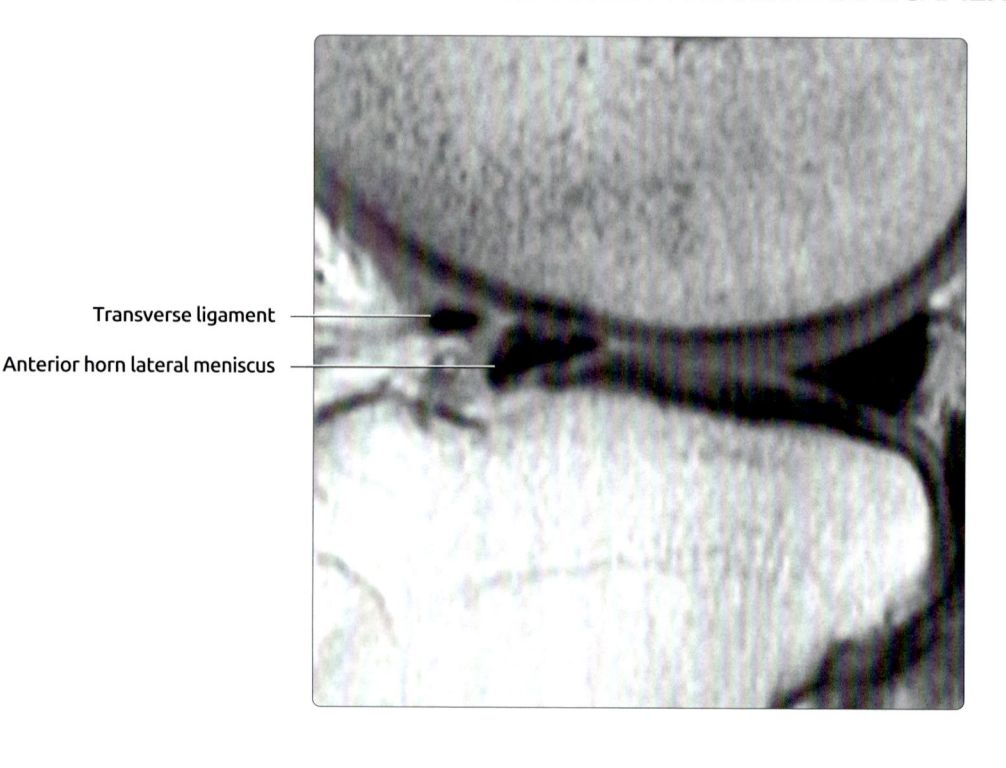

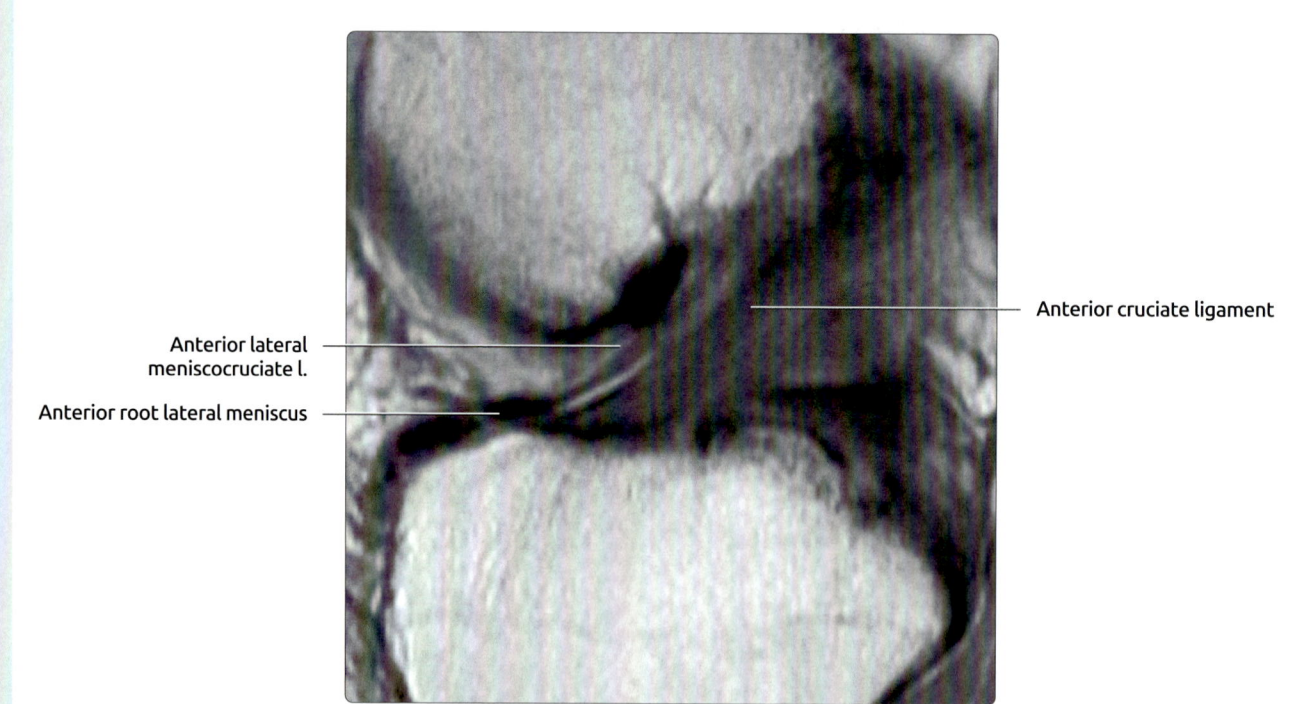

(Top) Sagittal PD MR image near the intercondylar notch, lateral to medial, shows a large transverse ligament. This ligament connects the 2 anterior meniscal horns and is seen in cross section on sagittal images. It could possibly be confused for a meniscal tear as it merges with the lateral meniscus, closer to the notch. The ligament is generally smaller than this, or may be absent. (Bottom) Image through the lateral portion of the intercondylar notch shows a discrete structure that parallels the anterior cruciate ligament and extends from the junction of the transverse ligament and root of the anterior horn lateral meniscus to the lateral femoral condyle. This represents the normal variant, anterior lateral meniscocruciate ligament. It is distinguished from infrapatellar plica (which can also parallel the ACL in the same manner) by its site of origin at the meniscus rather than the patella.

Knee and Leg Normal Variants and Imaging Pitfalls

MENISCOCRUCIATE LIGAMENT ARISING FROM TRANSVERSE LIGAMENT

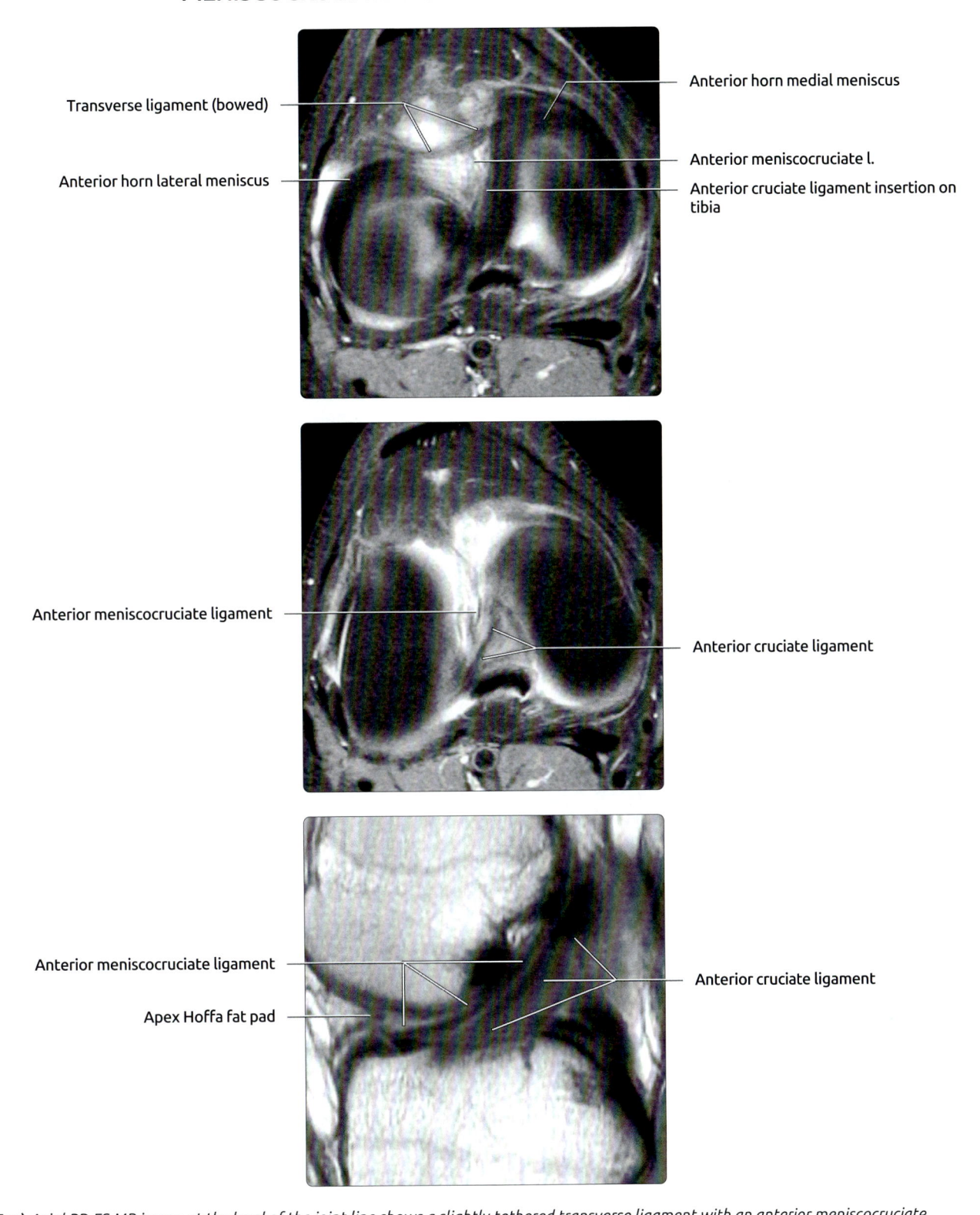

(Top) Axial PD FS MR image at the level of the joint line shows a slightly tethered transverse ligament with an anterior meniscocruciate ligament arising from it. Note that the ligament is anterior to the anterior cruciate ligament. (Middle) Image is slightly higher in the intercondylar notch. The anterior meniscocruciate ligament parallels the anterior cruciate ligament throughout the notch. (Bottom) Sagittal PD MR image shows the length of the anterior meniscocruciate ligament, paralleling the anterior cruciate ligament. This normal variant should not be mistaken for an intrasubstance tear of the anterior cruciate. Note that the apex of Hoffa fat pad is free of this ligament (not attached as in an infrapatellar plica).

MENISCOCRUCIATE LIGAMENT

Anterior meniscocruciate ligament

Anterior cruciate ligament

Anterior horn lateral meniscus

Meniscocruciate ligament

Anterior cruciate ligament

Transverse ligament

Anterior horn lateral meniscus

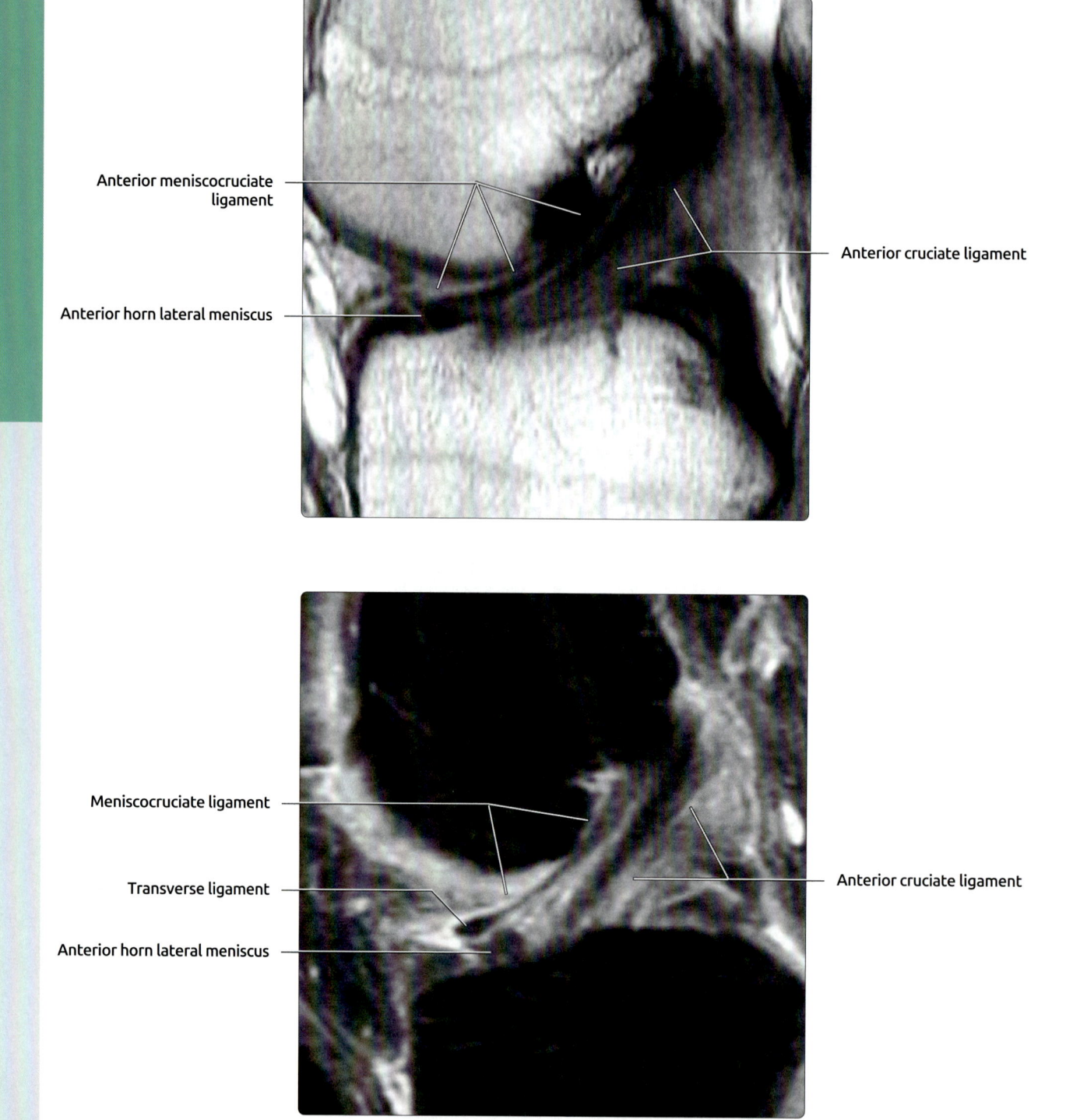

(Top) Sagittal PD MR through the intercondylar notch shows a meniscocruciate ligament. The ligament arises from the anterior horn medial meniscus and extends along the anterior surface of the anterior cruciate ligament to the femoral condyle. It could possibly be mistaken for a longitudinal tear in the anterior cruciate. (Bottom) Sagittal PD FS MR shows another variant meniscocruciate ligament. This ligament is arising from the transverse ligament; as it extends parallel to and anterior to the anterior cruciate ligament, it could simulate a longitudinal or partial tear in this cruciate.

Knee and Leg Normal Variants and Imaging Pitfalls

LATERAL MENISCAL FASCICLES

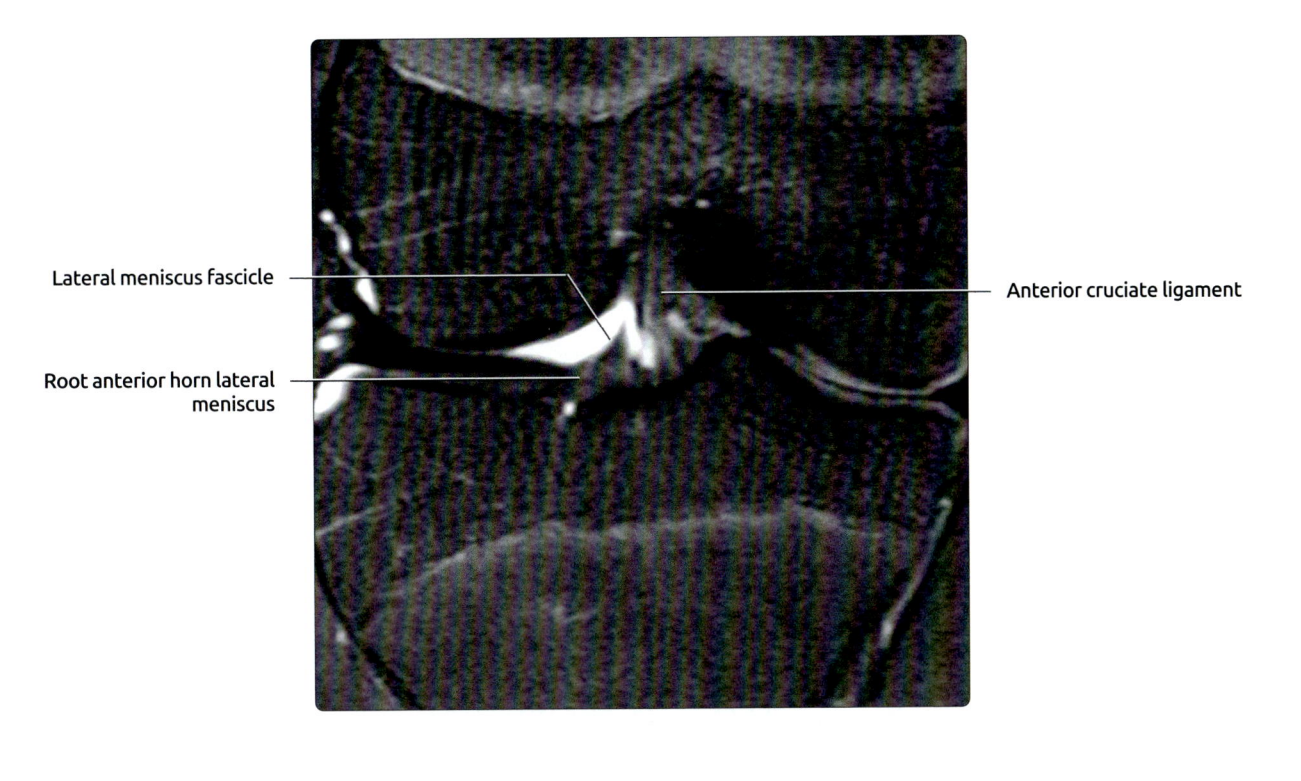

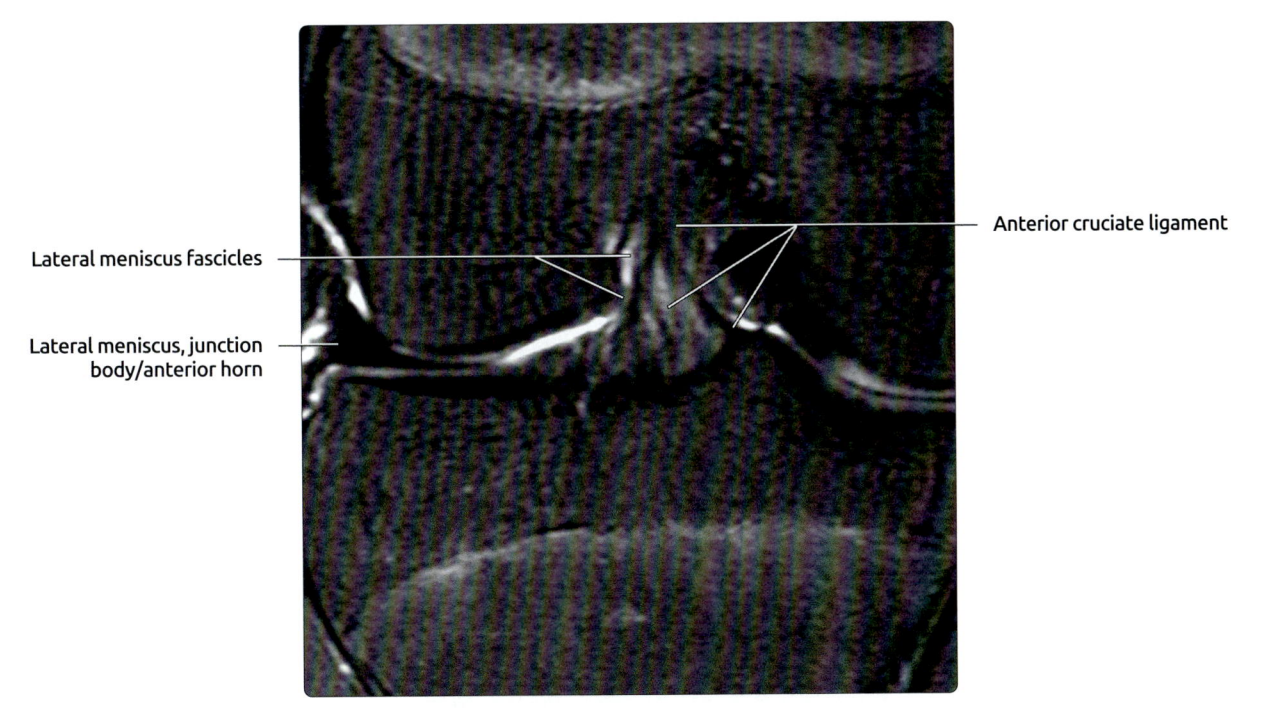

Lateral meniscus fascicle

Root anterior horn lateral meniscus

Anterior cruciate ligament

Lateral meniscus fascicles

Lateral meniscus, junction body/anterior horn

Anterior cruciate ligament

(Top) Coronal PD FS MR image in the anterior portion of the joint shows a patient with an absent transverse ligament (more anterior cut not shown). The fibers of the anterior horn lateral meniscus, which normally blend into the transverse ligament, form discrete lateral meniscal fascicles, which ascend towards the anterior cruciate ligament. **(Bottom)** Coronal image, slightly posterior, shows the lateral meniscal fascicles ascending to intersect the anterior cruciate ligament. These fibers clearly are not part of the anterior cruciate ligament since they ascend at a different angle. This normal variant should not be mistaken for pathology such as a disrupted ACL or a meniscal fragment from a bucket handle tear.

Knee and Leg Normal Variants and Imaging Pitfalls

MENISCOCRUCIATE LIGAMENT MIMICKING MENISCAL TEAR

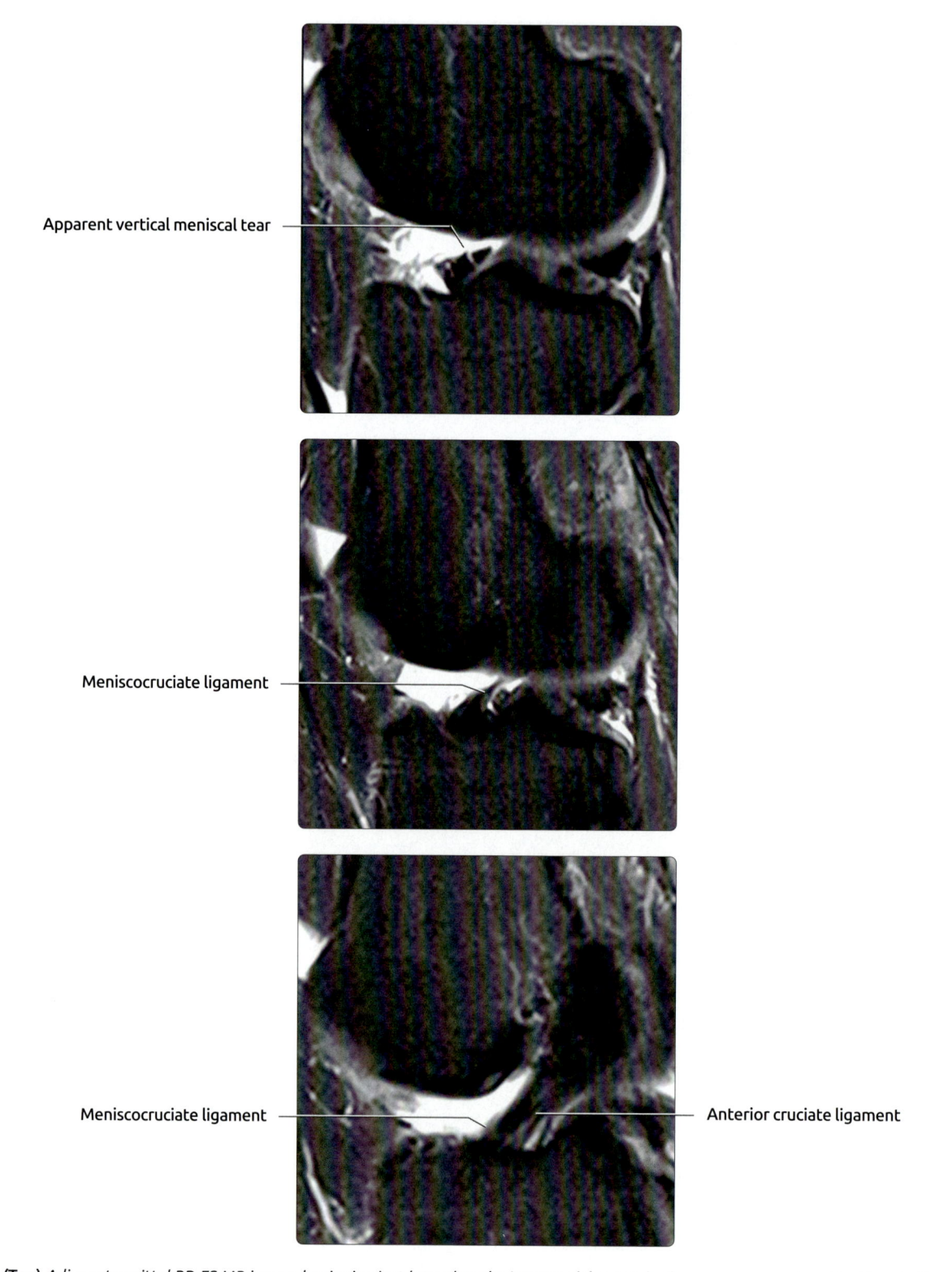

Apparent vertical meniscal tear

Meniscocruciate ligament

Meniscocruciate ligament — Anterior cruciate ligament

(Top) Adjacent sagittal PD FS MR image, beginning just lateral to the intercondylar notch, shows an apparent vertical tear in the anterior horn of the lateral meniscus. **(Middle)** Adjacent sagittal PD FS MR image shows that the apparent meniscal fragment in fact is continuous with a ligamentous structure extending in the direction of the anterior cruciate ligament. **(Bottom)** Adjacent sagittal PD FS MR image, at the level of the intercondylar notch, shows the ligamentous structure to blend into the anterior cruciate ligament. Since the abnormal structure extends from the meniscus to the cruciate ligament, it represents a normal variant meniscocruciate ligament. These may mimic partial cruciate ligament tears or, as in this case, a vertical peripheral meniscal tear.

Knee and Leg Normal Variants and Imaging Pitfalls

MENISCOCRUCIATE LIGAMENT MIMICKING PARTIAL ACL TEAR

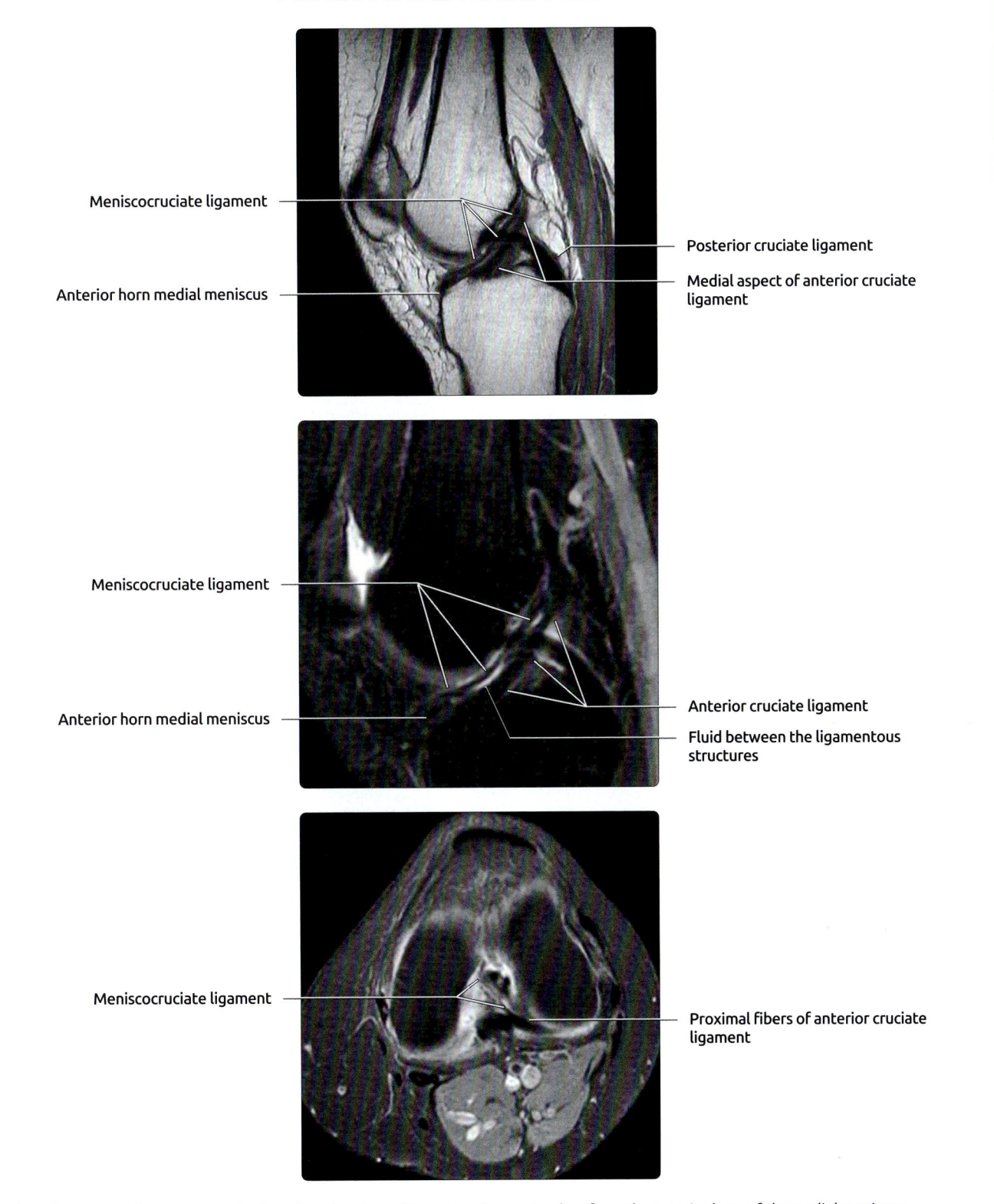

(Top) Sagittal PD MR image demonstrates a low signal curvilinear structure extending from the anterior horn of the medial meniscus along and immediately anterior to the medial fibers of the anterior cruciate ligament. This is a meniscofemoral ligament, seen in its full extent. These normal variants may mimic partial cruciate ligament tears. (Middle) Sagittal T2FS image in the same patient and same level demonstrates synovial fluid between the meniscocruciate ligament and the anterior cruciate ligament. Since the ACL is an extrasynovial structure, a tear should not be bathed in synovial fluid. Therefore the presence of fluid between the 2 structures helps solidify the diagnosis of normal variant meniscocruciate ligament. (Bottom) Axial PD FS image in the same patient demonstrates the intercondylar notch course of the meniscocruciate ligament traveling along the course of and eventually blending in with proximal fibers of the anterior cruciate ligament.

OBLIQUE MENISCOMENISCAL LIGAMENT

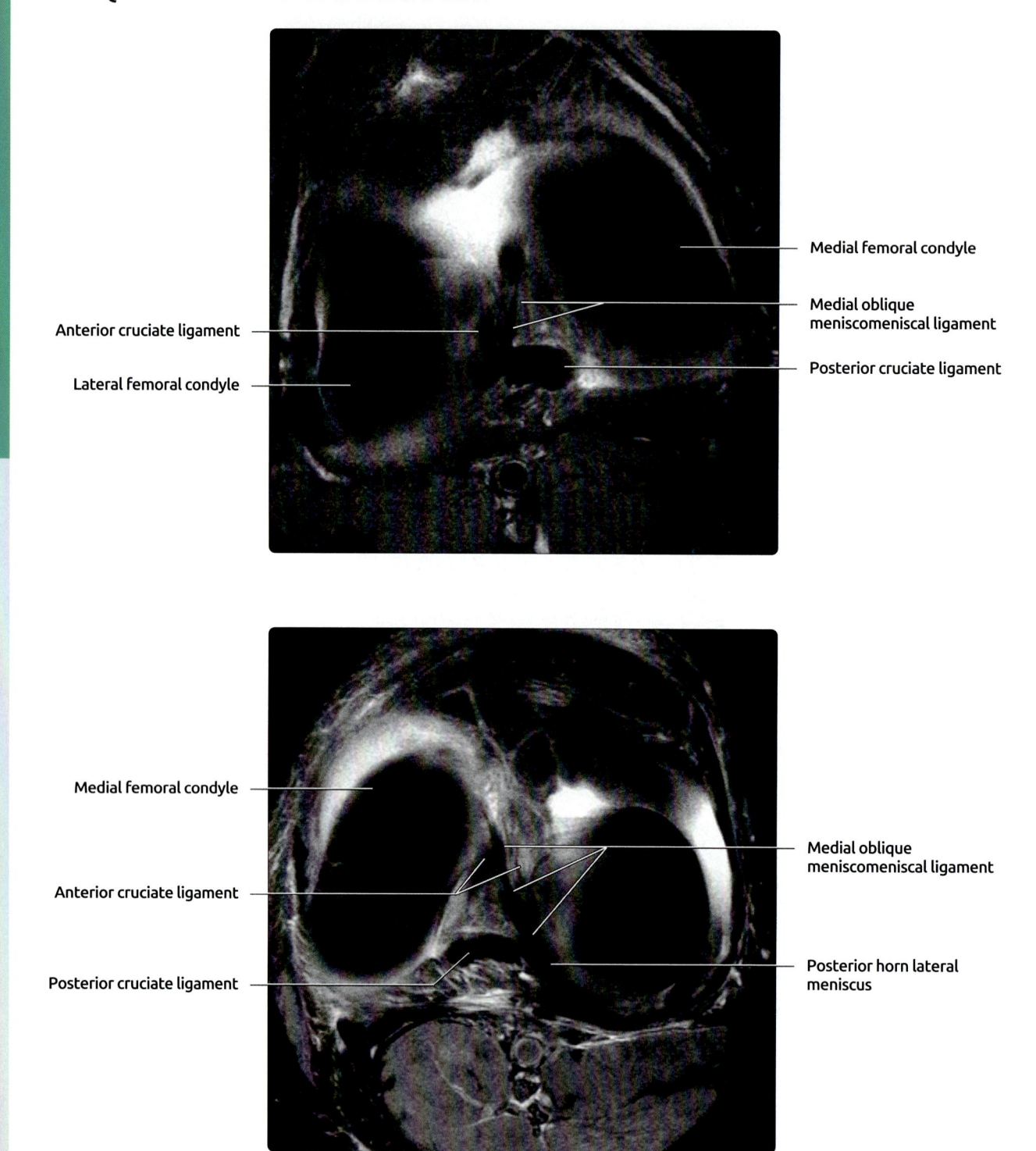

(Top) Single axial image, just above the joint line, shows the normal variant medial oblique meniscomeniscal ligament. It arises from the anterior horn medial meniscus and inserts on the posterior horn lateral meniscus, threading its way between the ACL and PCL. (Bottom) Axial PD FS MR image through the joint line in a different patient shows a normal variant, the medial oblique meniscomeniscal ligament. The ligament extends from the anterior horn medial meniscus across the intercondylar notch to insert on the posterior horn lateral meniscus. At this level of the menisci, the variant ligament appears to split the ACL at its insertion on the tibia. It normally extends between the ACL and PCL. The mirror image variant, lateral meniscomeniscal ligament, extends from the anterior horn lateral meniscus to the posterior horn medial meniscus (not shown here).

Knee and Leg Normal Variants and Imaging Pitfalls

OBLIQUE MENISCOMENISCAL LIGAMENT

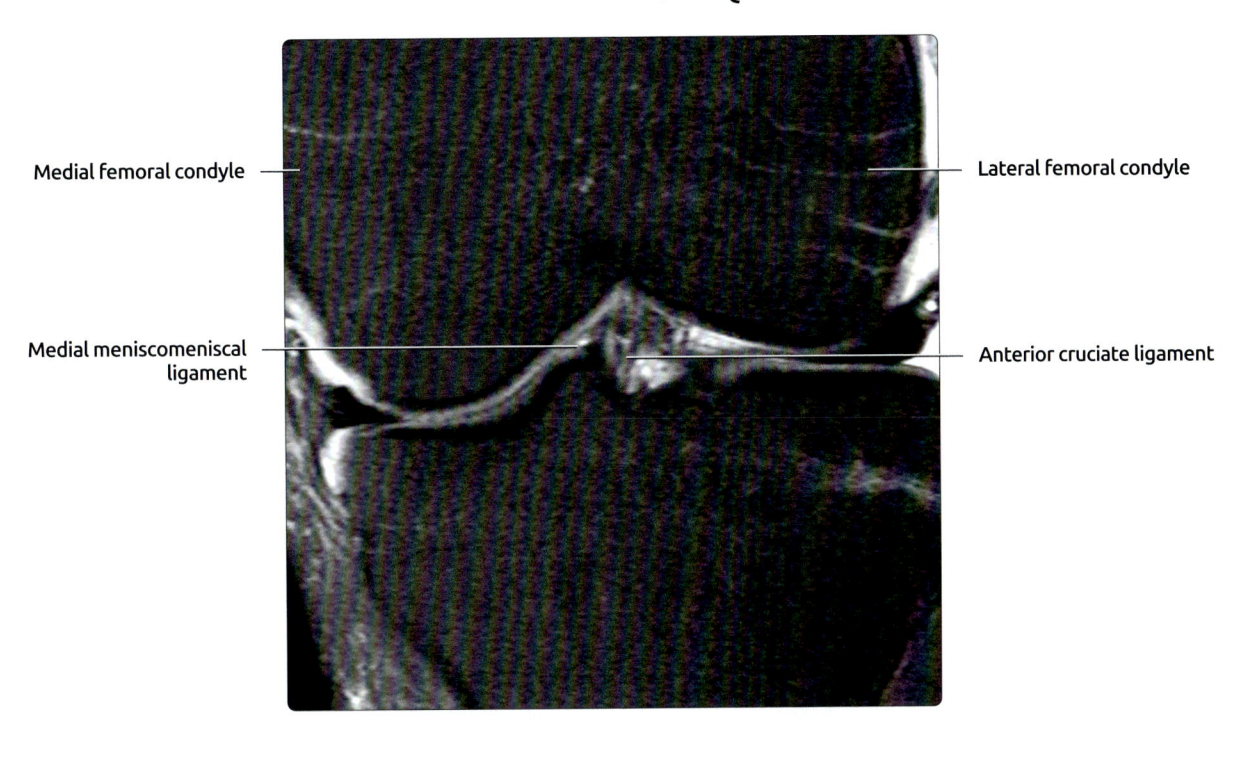

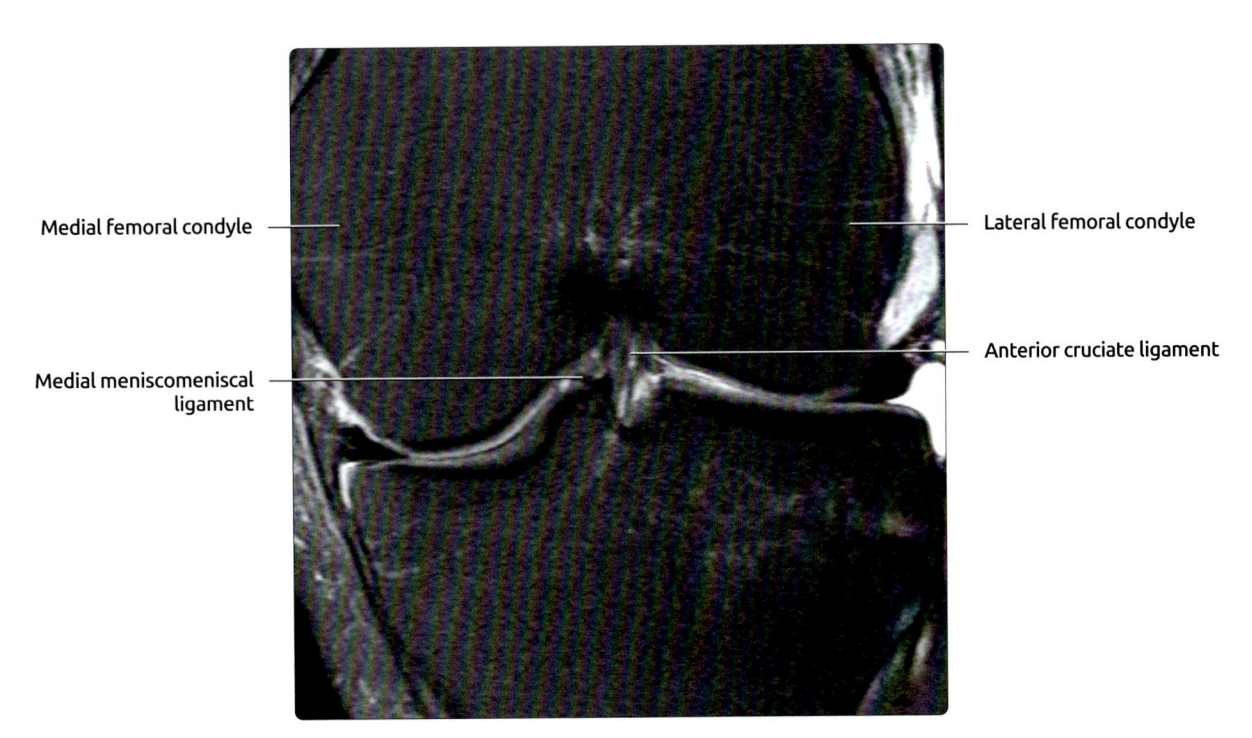

(Top) Coronal MR image, at the anterior portion of midjoint, shows the tiny medial meniscomeniscal ligament in cross section adjacent to the anterior cruciate ligament. **(Bottom)** Coronal image, 3 mm posterior, with the meniscomeniscal ligament giving the appearance of a loose body or fragment adjacent to the ACL. The location and low signal of this normal variant ligament may be misdiagnosed as a meniscal fragment or bucket handle fragment. It is important to correlate it with the appearance on either axial or sagittal images, where the ligament will be seen as a longitudinal structure placed between the ACL and PCL and angling obliquely across the notch between the 2 menisci.

Knee and Leg Normal Variants and Imaging Pitfalls

OBLIQUE MENISCOMENISCAL LIGAMENT; INFRAPATELLAR PLICA

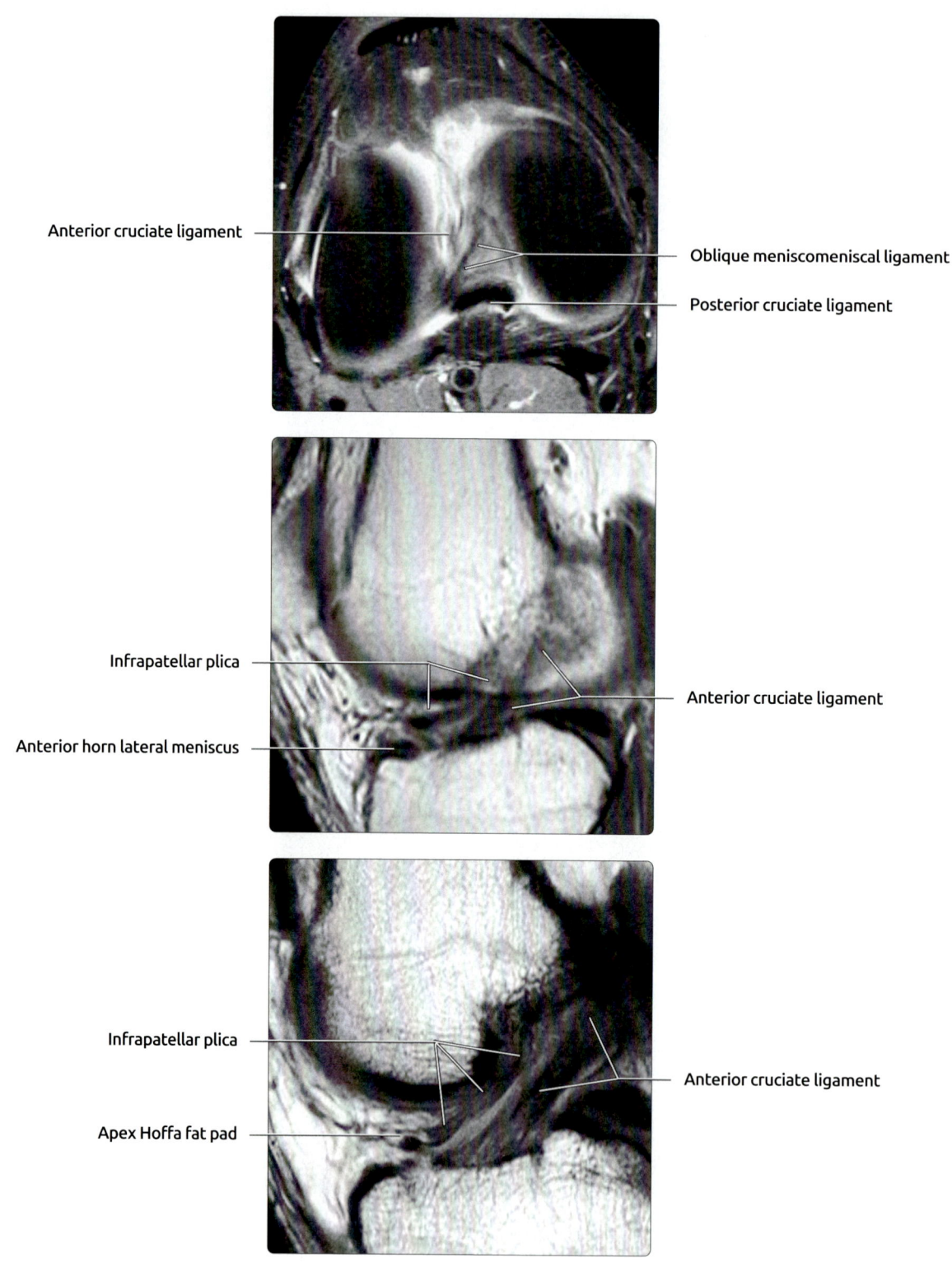

(Top) Axial PD FS MR image through the femoral condyles shows an oblique meniscomeniscal ligament. This uncommon variant connects the anterior horn of 1 meniscus with the posterior horn of the contralateral meniscus. It runs between the anterior and posterior cruciate ligaments. (Middle) Sagittal PD MR image through the intercondylar notch shows the variant infrapatellar plica. This plica arises from the patella, extends across Hoffa fat pad, and along the anterior surface of the anterior cruciate ligament. (Bottom) Sagittal PD MR through the intercondylar notch shows an infrapatellar plica. The plica is seen extending through the Hoffa fat pad, paralleling the curvature of the femoral condyle, and then paralleling the anterior cruciate ligament.

Knee and Leg Normal Variants and Imaging Pitfalls

DISCOID MENISCUS

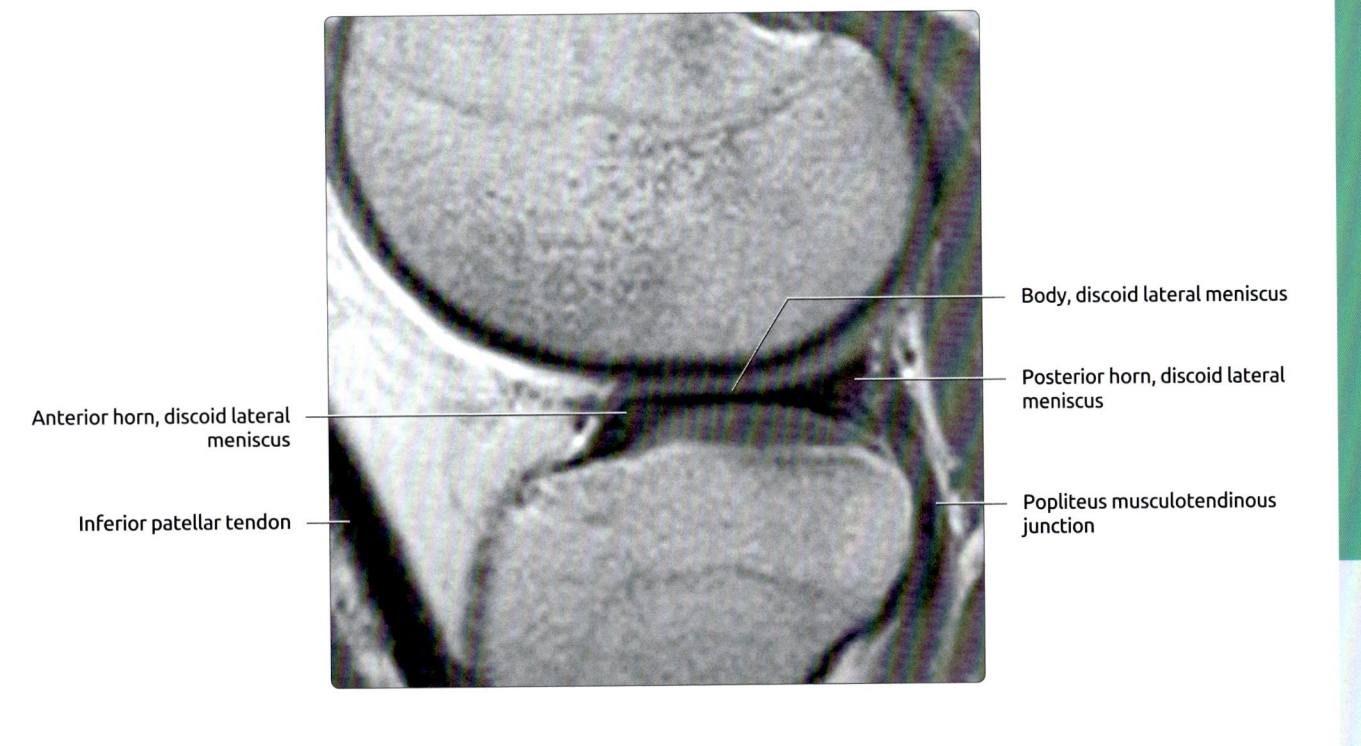

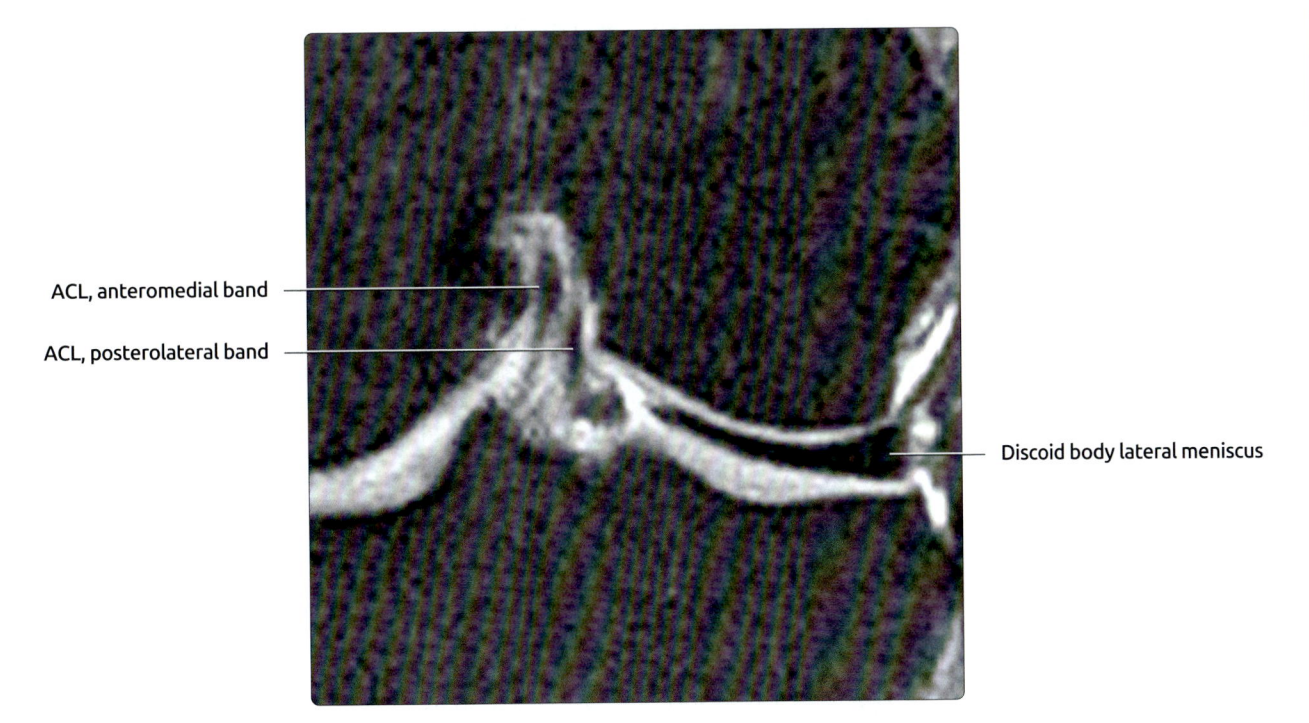

- Anterior horn, discoid lateral meniscus
- Inferior patellar tendon
- Body, discoid lateral meniscus
- Posterior horn, discoid lateral meniscus
- Popliteus musculotendinous junction

- ACL, anteromedial band
- ACL, posterolateral band
- Discoid body lateral meniscus

(Top) Sagittal image is from the midportion of the lateral compartment and shows a discoid lateral meniscus. Note that the meniscus is seen with all 3 portions; the anterior horn, body, and posterior horn. This bow tie appearance should be seen only in the outer portion of the joint. The fact that the fibula is not seen, as well as that the popliteus musculotendinous junction (rather than just the popliteus tendon) and patellar tendon are both in this image, indicates that the location is far too interior in the joint for a normal body of meniscus to be seen. Thus, the body of the meniscus is too large, indicating the discoid variant. (Bottom) Coronal image through the midportion of the joint (as indicated by the morphology and presence of the ACL) shows the body of the lateral meniscus to be too large, confirming that it is discoid.

Knee and Leg Normal Variants and Imaging Pitfalls

DISCOID LATERAL MENISCUS MORPHOLOGY

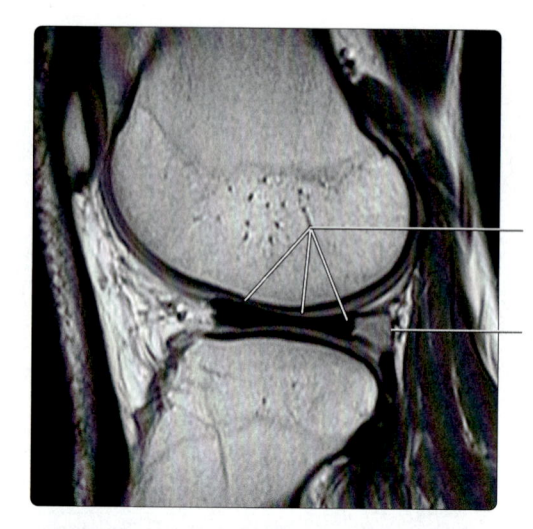

- Discoid lateral meniscus
- Prominent popliteal hiatus

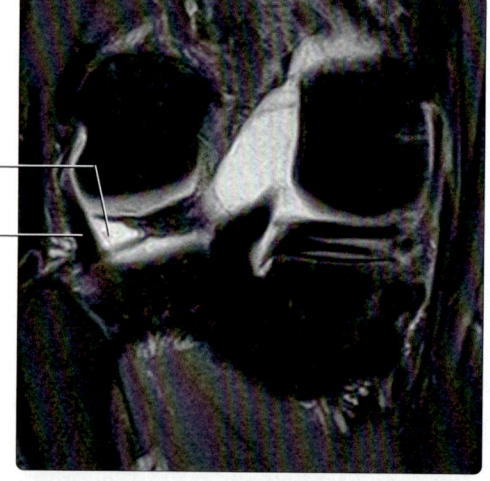

- Enlarged popliteal hiatus with prominent fascicles
- Popliteus tendon

- Discoid lateral meniscus

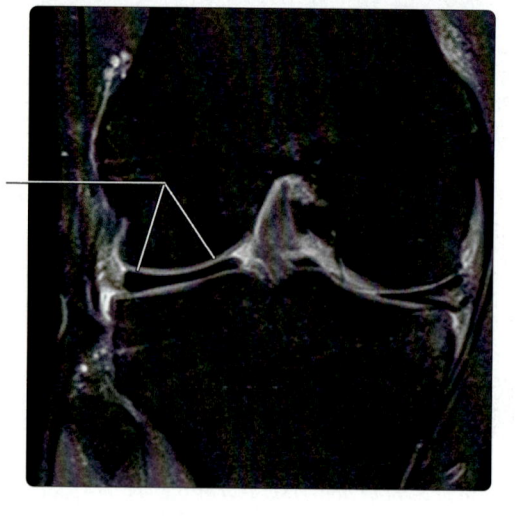

(Top) Sagittal PD MR in the midlateral compartment demonstrates a discoid lateral meniscus. The lateral meniscus is discoid in morphology far more frequently than is the medial. It is interesting that with this variant meniscus the popliteal hiatus is large with prominent fascicles. (Middle) Coronal PD FS image located posteriorly in the joint of the same patient again demonstrates the unusual morphology of the popliteal hiatus in the presence of a discoid meniscus. The hiatus becomes enlarged with thickened fascicles. (Bottom) Coronal PD FS image in the same patient, midjoint, confirms the discoid morphology of the lateral meniscus.

Knee and Leg Normal Variants and Imaging Pitfalls

DISCOID MENISCUS

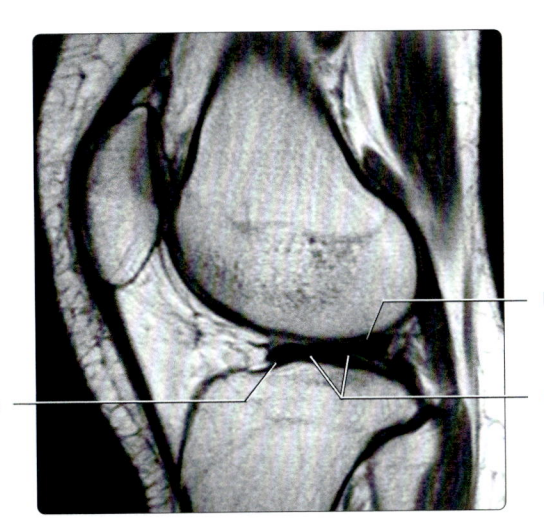

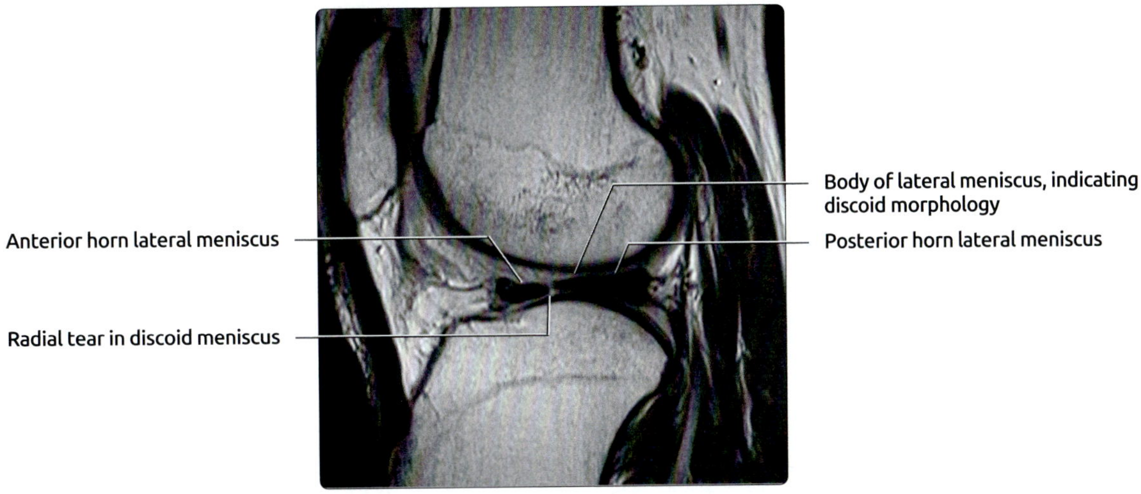

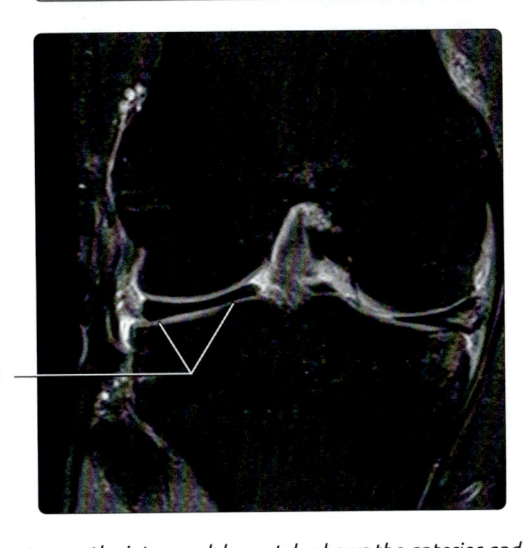

(Top) Sagittal PD in the lateral compartment, near the intercondylar notch, shows the anterior and posterior horns of the lateral meniscus with a thin body of meniscus. This far within the joint, the body of meniscus should not be seen. Therefore, this represents a discoid meniscus. **(Middle)** Sagittal PD 1 cut closer to the intercondylar notch confirms the discoid meniscus with a radial tear at the junction of the anterior horn and body. **(Bottom)** Coronal PD FS MR at midjoint confirms the discoid morphology of the lateral meniscus. The radial tear noted on the sagittal is not seen directly but may be inferred by the blunted edge of the meniscus.

Knee and Leg Normal Variants and Imaging Pitfalls

ANTERIOR HORN MEDIAL MENISCUS ORIGINATING FROM TIBIAL PLATEAU

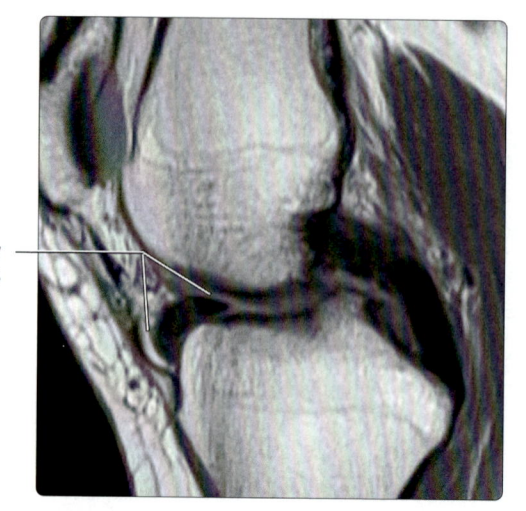

Appearance of enlarged and partially extruded medial meniscus

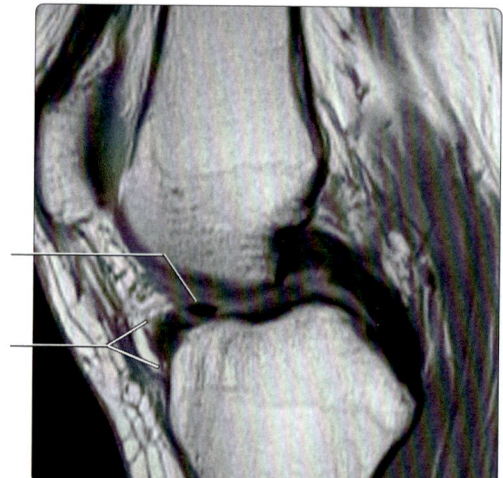

Transverse ligament

Anterior horn medial meniscus arising from anterior tibial plateau

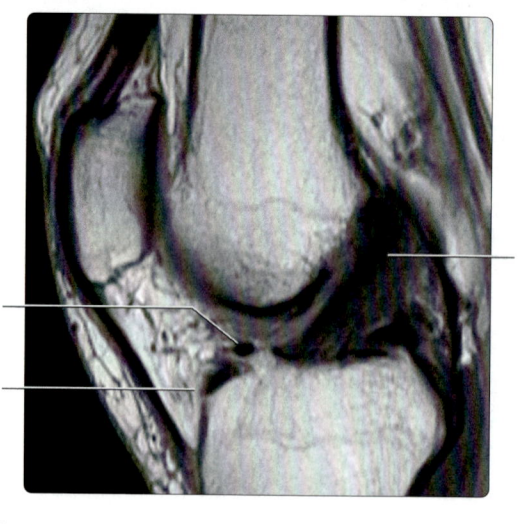

Anterior cruciate ligament

Transverse ligament

Remnant of anterior horn, medial meniscus

(Top) First of 3 contiguous PD sagittal MR images through the intercondylar notch showing both the PCL and the anterior horn medial meniscus. This image suggests an enlarged and partially extruded medial meniscus. In fact, it is a normal anterior horn that is arising in a slightly variant position of the anterior tibial plateau with the attached transverse ligament that has not yet separated. (Middle) Second consecutive image, slightly lateral (towards the ACL), shows an apparent "vertical tear" in the enlarged meniscus. In actuality, this represents the normal anterior horn originating from the anterior tibial plateau with the transverse ligament separating from it. (Bottom) Third contiguous PD MR image in the sequence, now at the level of the ACL, shows the remnant of anterior horn medial meniscus, as well as the prominent transverse ligament.

Knee and Leg Normal Variants and Imaging Pitfalls

ANTERIOR HORN MEDIAL MENISCUS ORIGINATING FROM TIBIAL PLATEAU

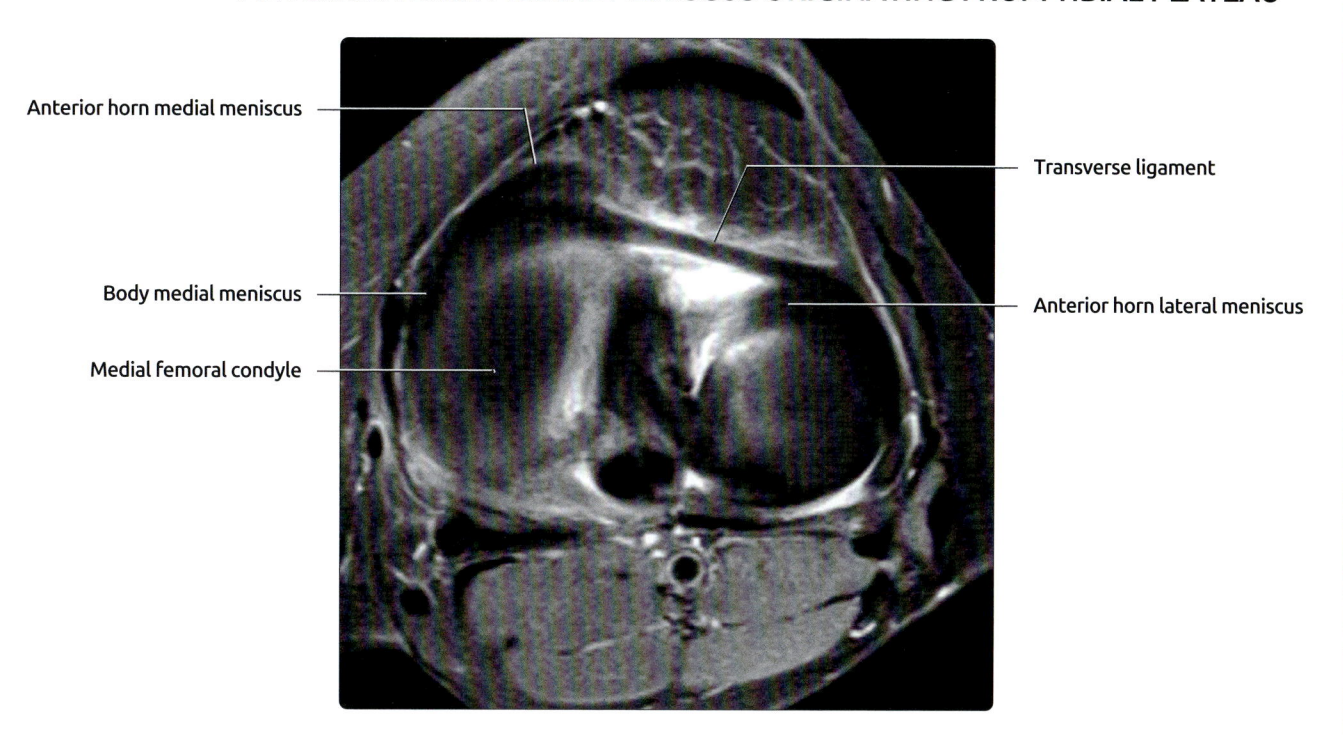

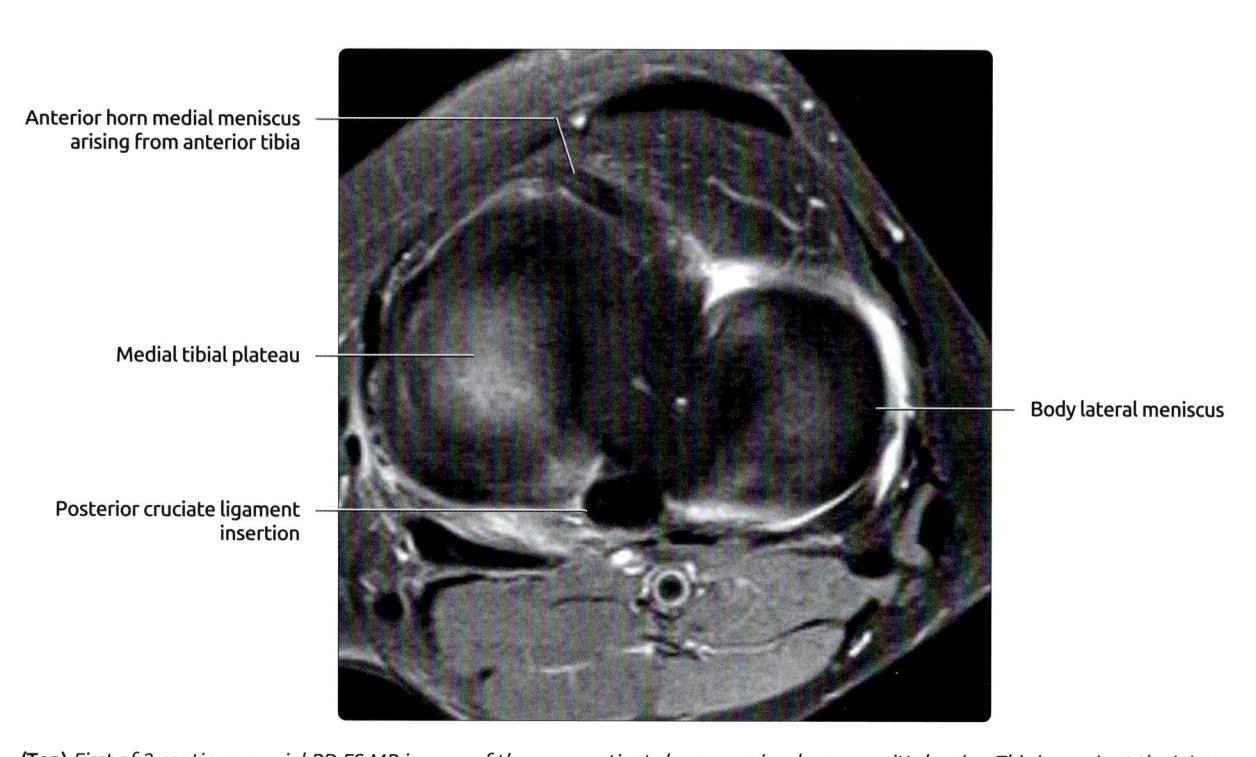

(Top) First of 2 contiguous axial PD FS MR images of the same patient shown previously on a sagittal series. This image is at the joint line and shows both the large transverse ligament and the anterior horn of medial meniscus that arises anterior to the tibial plateau rather than from on top of the plateau. This is a normal variant origin of the anterior horn medial meniscus. (Bottom) Second axial PD FS MR image, at the level of the joint and tibial plateau, shows the anterior horn of medial meniscus still as a prominent structure arising anteriorly from the tibia rather than from the top of the plateau. It is important to not misinterpret this appearance as a bucket handle fragment.

Knee and Leg Normal Variants and Imaging Pitfalls

MENISCAL OSSICLE

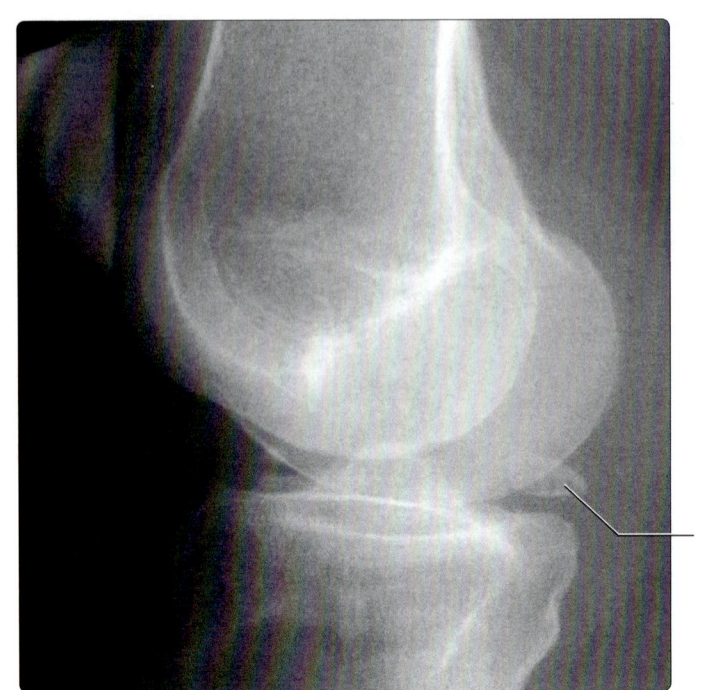

Meniscal ossicle within posterior horn

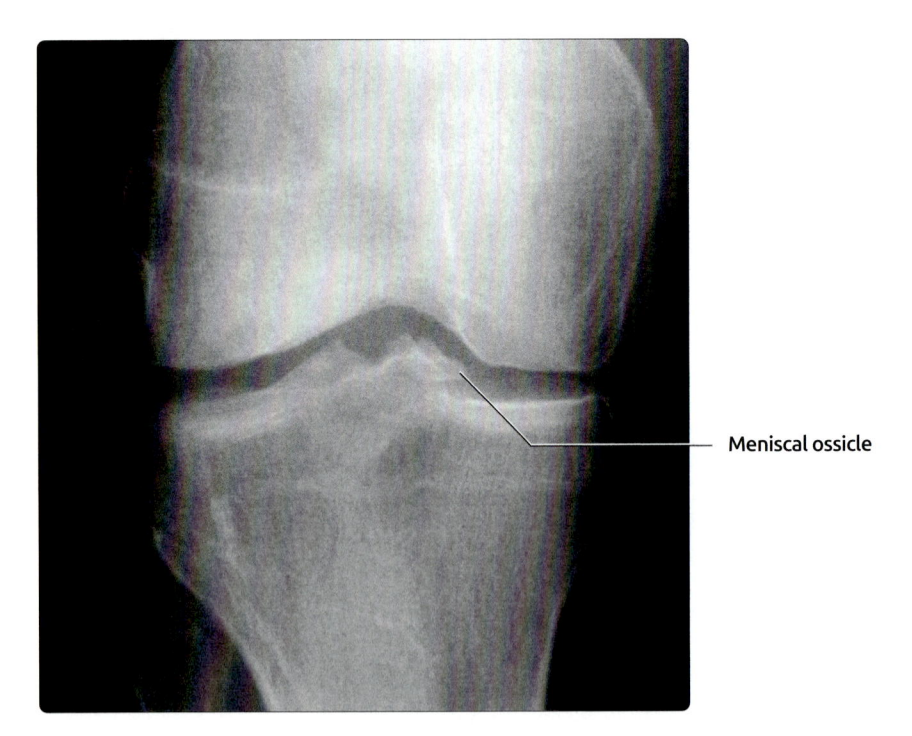

Meniscal ossicle

(Top) Lateral radiograph in a case of meniscal ossicle shows an ossicle located in the region of the posterior horn of meniscus. It is too low and too horizontally oriented to represent a fabella. **(Bottom)** AP radiograph confirms the location of the ossicle to be within the posterior horn of the medial meniscus. It is important to differentiate a meniscal ossicle from a loose body since they are treated differently. Shape and location are both useful parameters in the differentiation. It is also useful to remember that the most common location of a meniscal ossicle is the posterior horn of medial meniscus, as in this case.

Knee and Leg Normal Variants and Imaging Pitfalls

MENISCAL OSSICLE

Meniscal ossicle

Meniscal ossicle

Meniscal ossicle

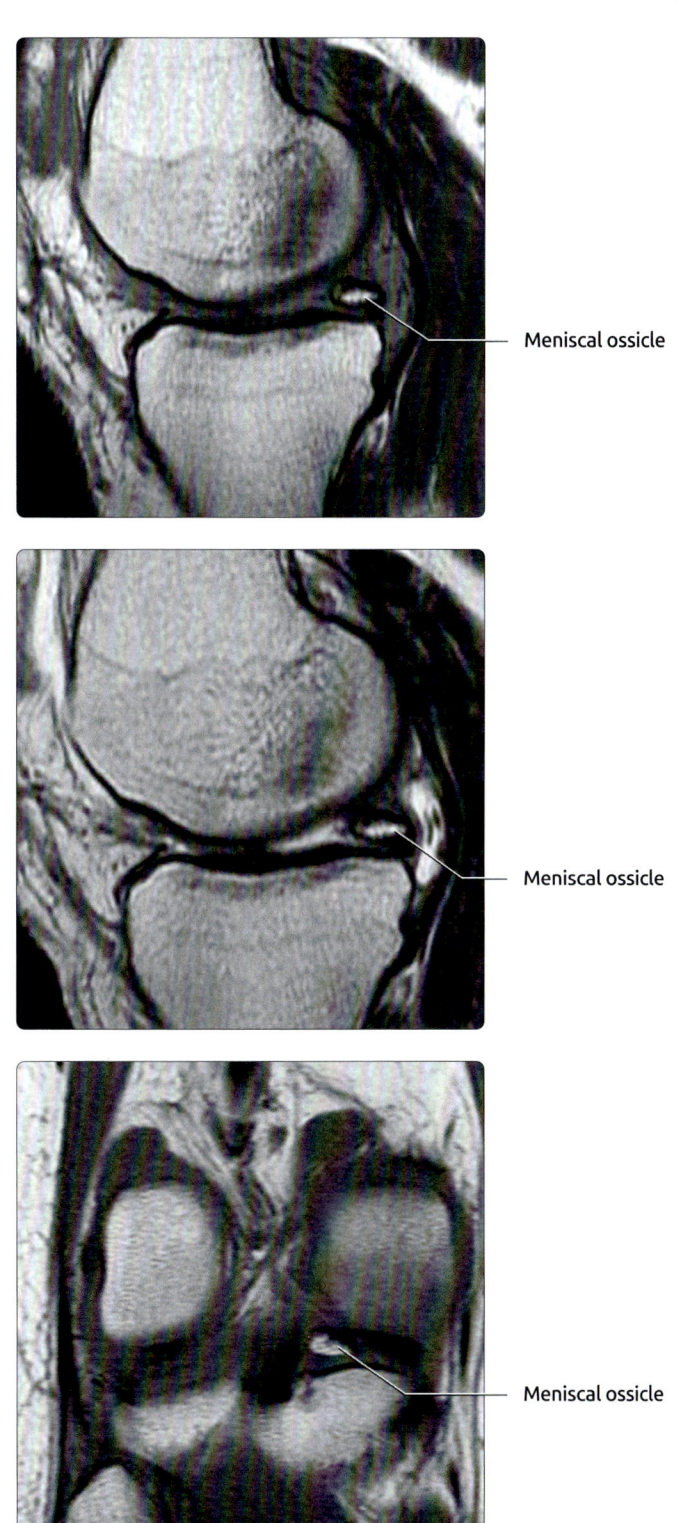

(Top) PD sagittal image shows ossicle (note trabeculae and signal which matches that of bone) within the posterior horn of the medial meniscus. (Middle) T2WI at the same level as the prior image shows the ossicle to occupy the majority of posterior horn. (Bottom) T1WI in the coronal plane, located posteriorly in the joint, shows the meniscal ossicle within the posterior horn medial meniscus. Trabeculae and cortex of the ossicle are seen, and the signal matches that of bone. Meniscal ossicles are uncommon (prevalence 0.15% on one series) and may be symptomatic. (Courtesy A. Sonin, MD.)

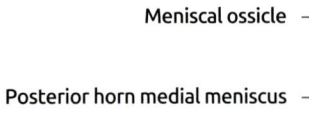

Knee and Leg Normal Variants and Imaging Pitfalls

MENISCAL OSSICLE

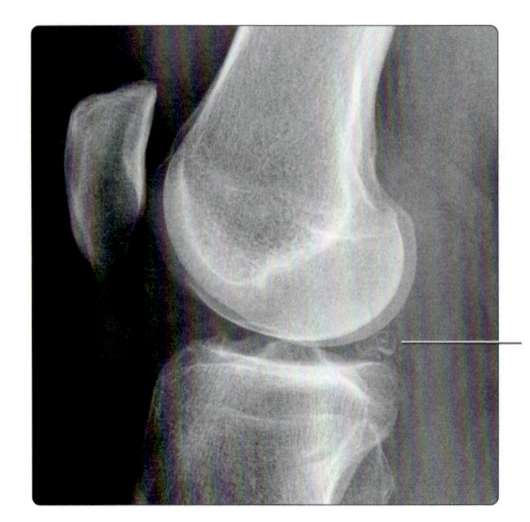

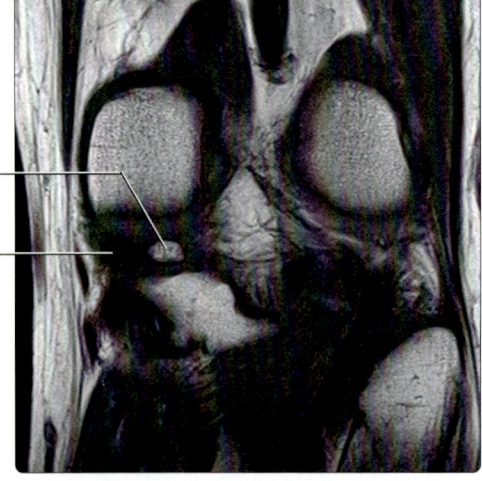

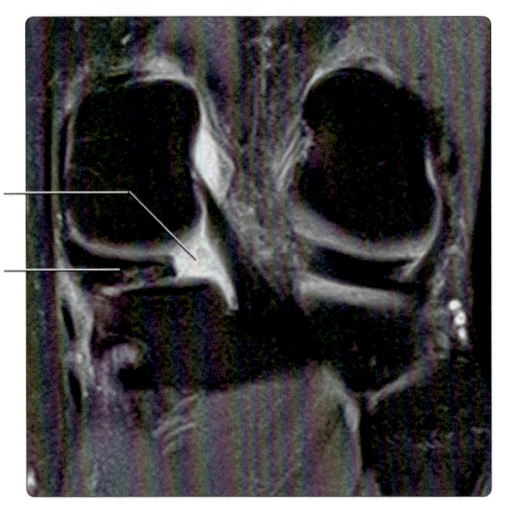

(Top) Lateral radiograph shows an osseous density superimposed over the posterior knee joint space. It is in a typical position of meniscal ossicle. (Middle) Coronal T1 MR located posteriorly in the joint shows that there is a rounded structure located within the posterior horn of the medial meniscus that retains high signal expected of bone. Both the osseous signal and location confirm the diagnosis of meniscal ossicle. (Bottom) Coronal PD FS located in the posterior portion of the knee joint shows there is a radial tear in the root of the posterior horn medial meniscus. This is associated with the meniscal ossicle. This cut is slightly anterior to the previous image, so that the ossicle is out of the plane.

Knee and Leg Normal Variants and Imaging Pitfalls

MENISCAL OSSICLE

Meniscal ossicle

Meniscal ossicle

Meniscal ossicle, fat saturated

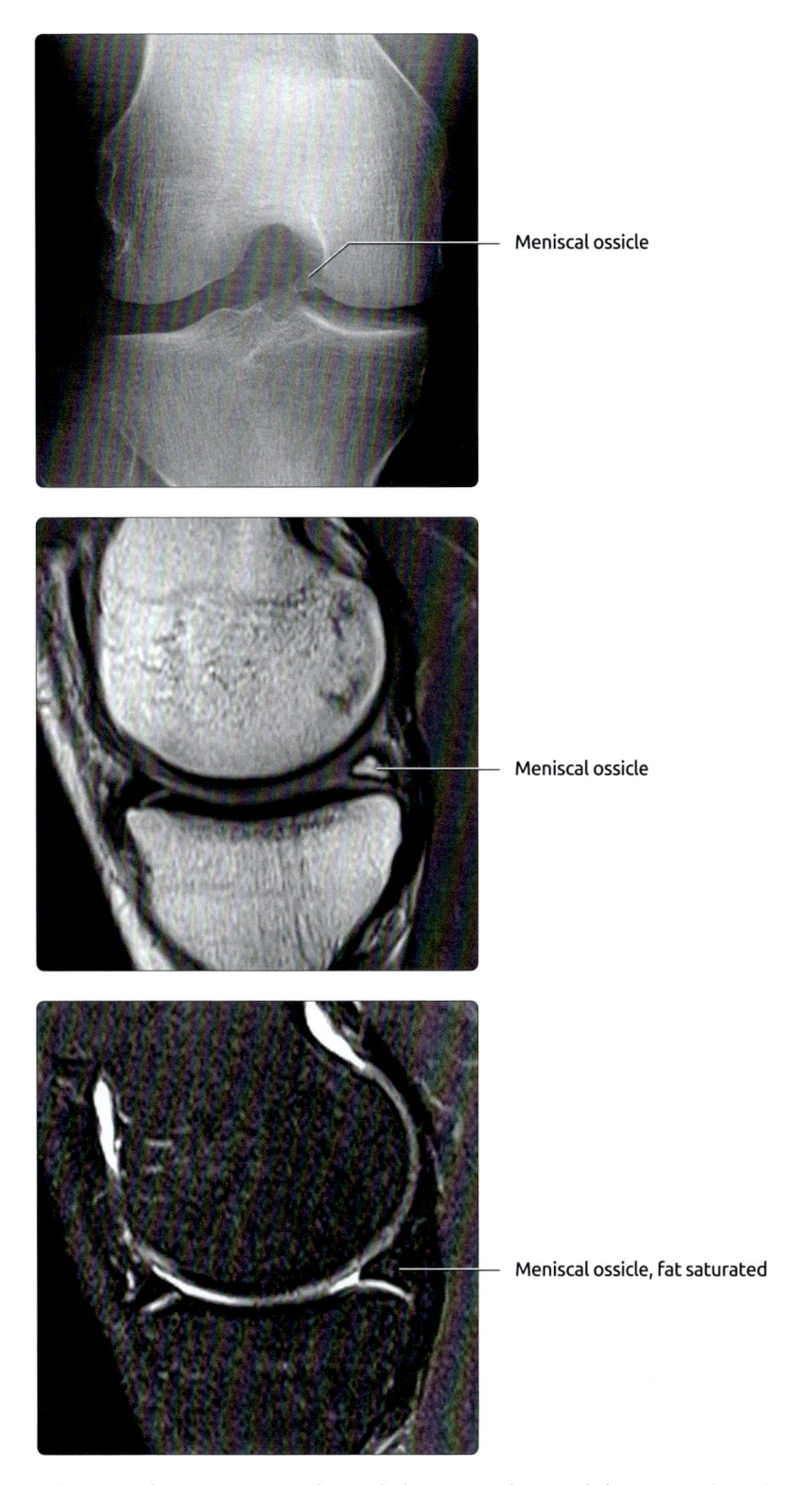

(Top) AP radiograph shows a rounded osseous density in a location corresponding with the posterior horn medial meniscus. This is the typical location of meniscal ossicle. Note that although meniscal ossicle is being treated as a "normal variant" in this discussion, some believe it to be a result of trauma occurring at a young age. Since posterior horn of medial meniscus is an area at high risk for meniscal injury at any age, if trauma is indeed the etiology of meniscal ossicle it is not surprising that the location of an ossicle would most often be within the posterior horn of medial meniscus. (Middle) Sagittal PD MR through the medial condyle shows the posterior horn medial meniscus to be replaced by osseous signal. This corresponds to the location of the meniscal ossicle noted on the previous radiograph. (Bottom) Sagittal T2 FS MR of the same patient in same location shows the fat density of the meniscal ossicle to be saturated out.

MENISCAL OSSICLE

Meniscal ossicle

Meniscal ossicle

Anterior horn medial meniscus

Meniscal ossicle
Radial tear, posterior horn medial meniscus

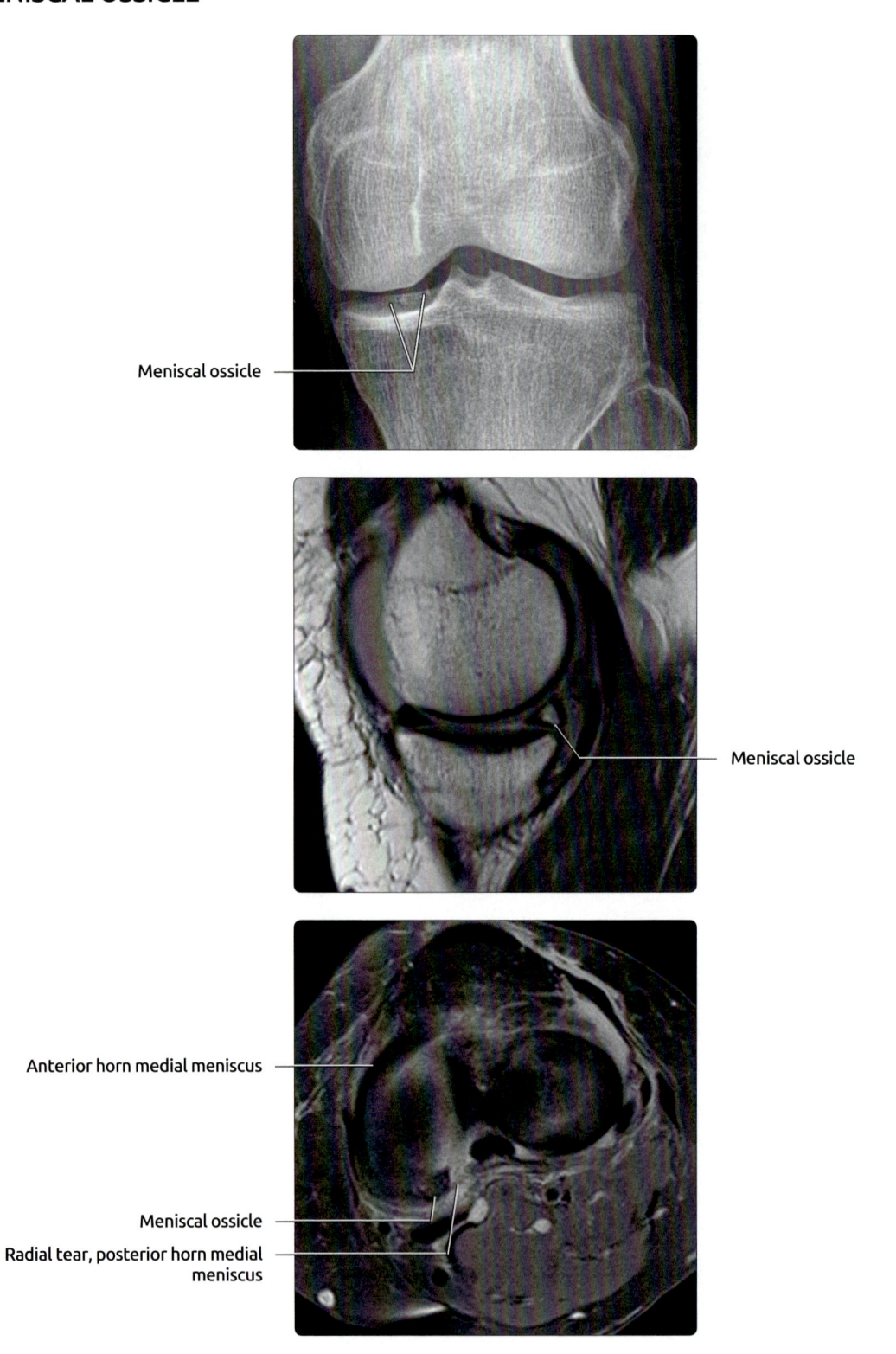

(Top) AP radiograph shows a trabeculated ossicle located at the posterior horn of the medial meniscus (confirmed on lateral radiograph; not shown). By location, this represents a meniscal ossicle rather than a loose body. (Middle) Sagittal PD MR in the same patient confirms the bone marrow signal within the ossicle, which itself is located within the posterior horn of the medial meniscus. (Bottom) Axial PD FS in the same patient, at the level of the joint line, shows the meniscal ossicle (low signal since it is fat saturated). The ossicle is, as expected, within the posterior horn of the medial meniscus. Immediately adjacent to the ossicle there is a gap in the posterior horn representing a large radial tear. It is common to have meniscal tears associated with meniscal ossicle.

Knee and Leg Normal Variants and Imaging Pitfalls

MENISCAL OSSICLE, UNUSUAL LOCATION

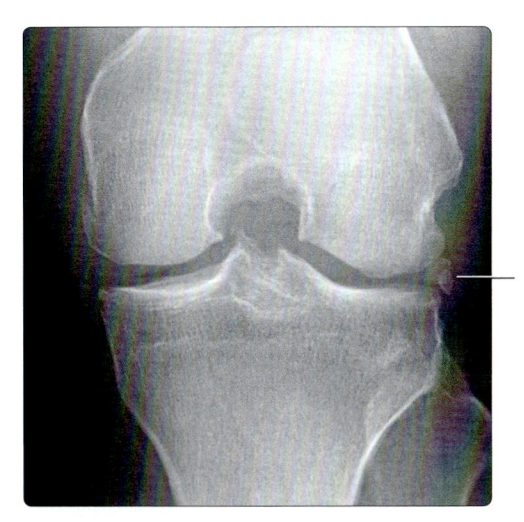

Meniscal ossicle

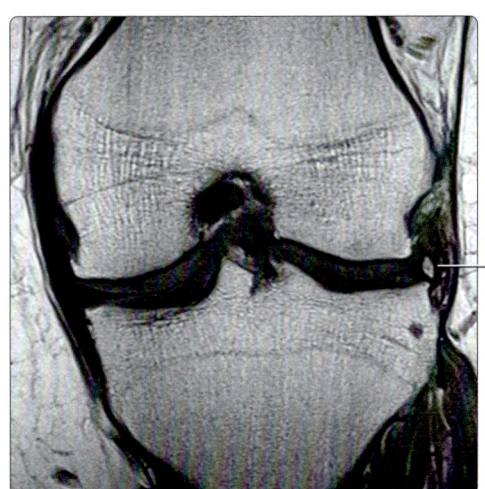

Meniscal ossicle

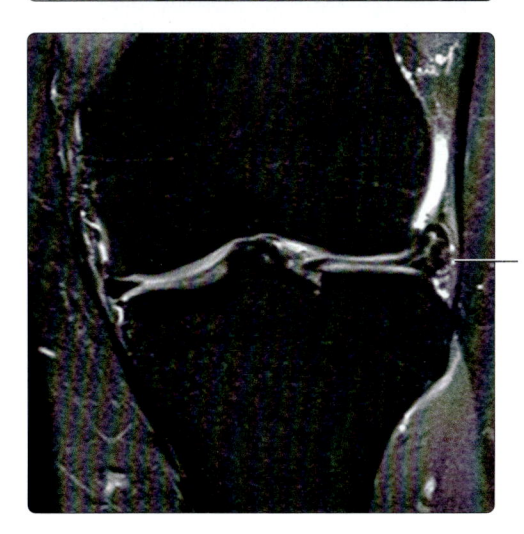

Lateral meniscus body with ossicle saturated out and associated tear

(Top) AP radiograph demonstrates a meniscal ossicle in an unusual location, the body of lateral meniscus. (Middle) Coronal T1 MR in the midjoint shows the bone-signal meniscal ossicle within the body of lateral meniscus. It is unusual for a meniscal ossicle to be found either in the lateral rather than medial meniscus or in the body rather than posterior horn of the meniscus. (Bottom) Coronal PD FS MR at the same level as the prior image shows the ossicle to be fat saturated and an associated tear of the body of lateral meniscus.

TRUNCATION ARTIFACT

Truncation artifact

Truncation artifact mimicking meniscal tear

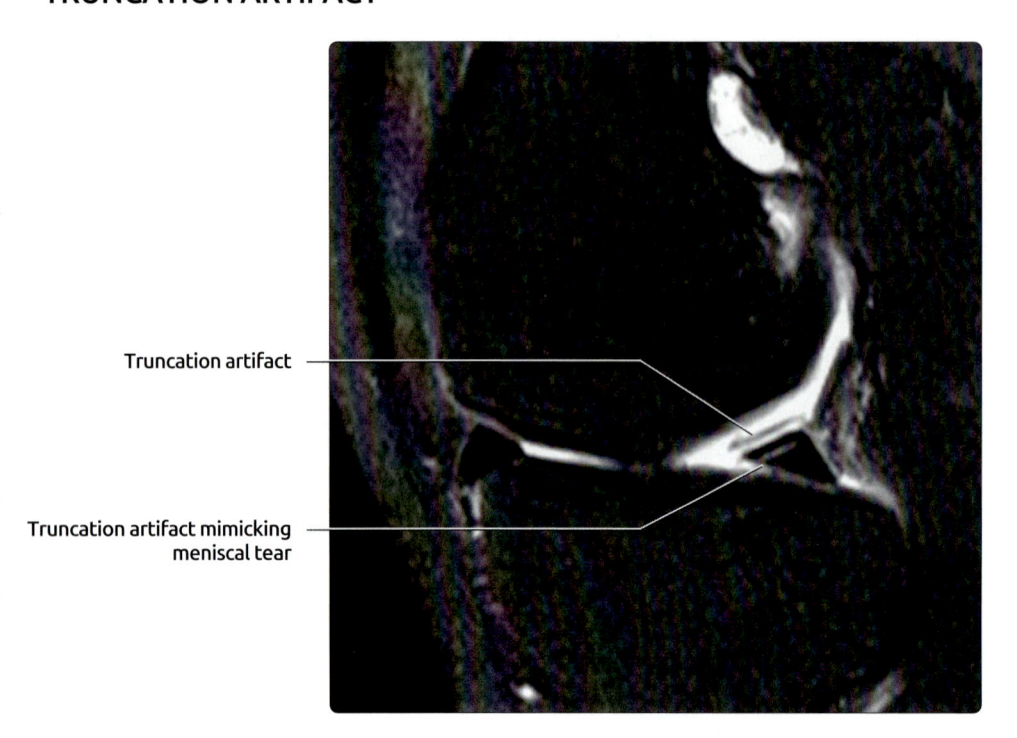

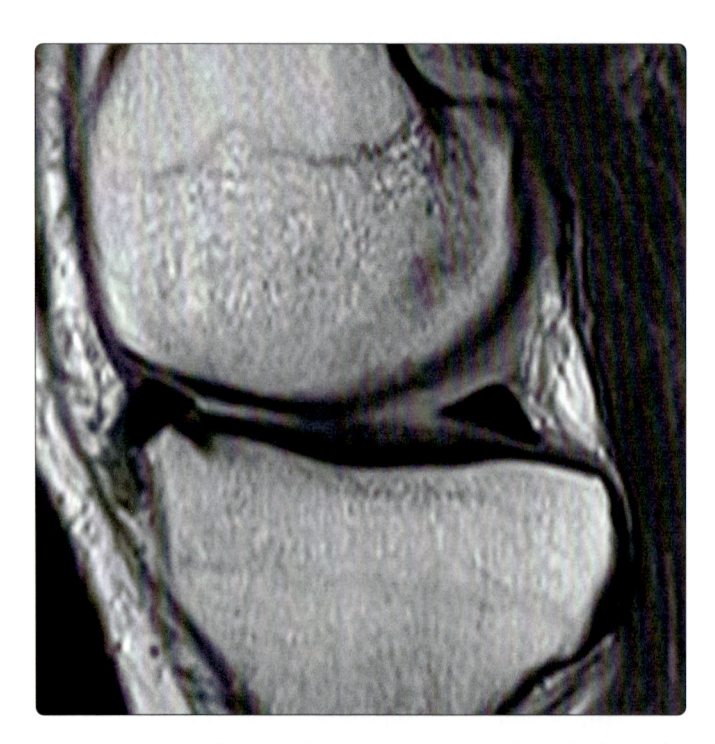

(Top) Sagittal T2FS image demonstrates posterior horn meniscus with an apparent linear high signal extending to the free edge. Although this gives the appearance of an oblique meniscal tear, there is also a low signal linear appearance extending along the superior aspect of the meniscus. This parallel linear signal should cause suspicion that the "tear" is due to truncation artifact. (Bottom) Sagittal PD MR in the same patient, same cut as the previous T2FS image, shows a normal posterior horn with no evidence of tear. PD is the most reliable sequence for evaluating menisci; this image proves that the "tear" seen on the T2FS image is due to truncation artifact, often seen at the boundary between high and low signal structures. These artifacts are caused by approximation errors in Fourier transform analysis.

Knee and Leg Normal Variants and Imaging Pitfalls

MOTION & VACUUM ARTIFACTS

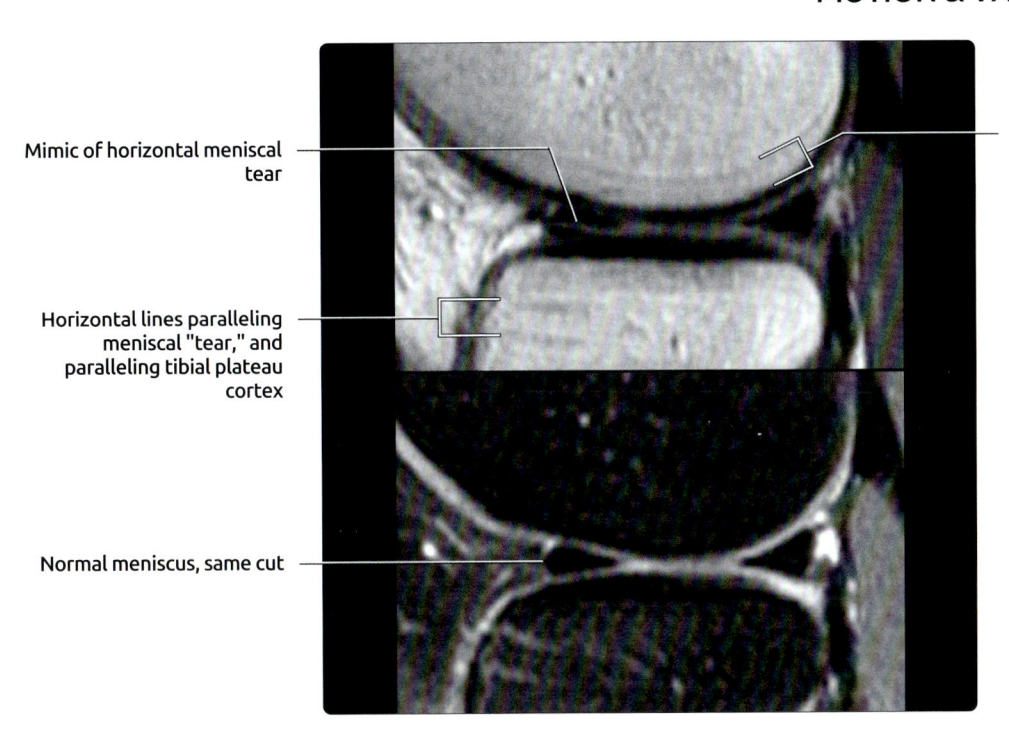

Mimic of horizontal meniscal tear

Concave line paralleling the concavity of the femoral cortex

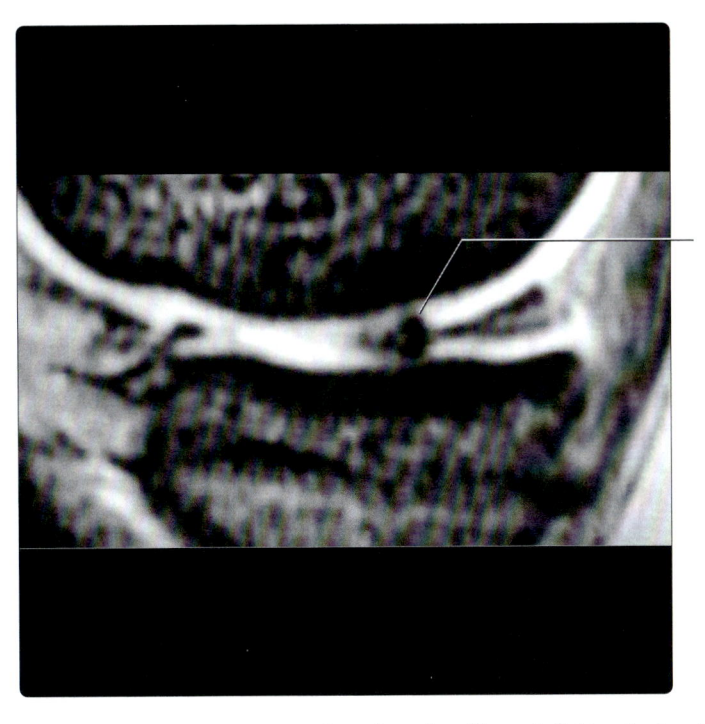

Horizontal lines paralleling meniscal "tear," and paralleling tibial plateau cortex

Normal meniscus, same cut

Air bubble mimicking loose body

(Top) Sagittal PD and sagittal PD FS MR images, same cuts at same time, show the effects of slight patient motion. The PD image shows a horizontal high signal through the anterior horn, suggesting a meniscal tear. However, there are also horizontal lines within the tibia paralleling the meniscal line, as well as the tibial plateau cortex. There are, in addition, concave lines in the femoral condyle paralleling the concavity of the femoral condylar cortex. These paralleling lines indicate motion and that the meniscal "tear" is artifactual.
(Bottom) Sagittal gradient-echo MR demonstrates a low signal round "body" superimposed over the free edge of the posterior horn. This is an air bubble that developed via vacuum phenomenon when the knee was extended in the coil. The air bubble "blooms" on gradient-echo imaging; it would not be as prominent on other sequences, though may be visible.

Knee and Leg Measurements and Lines

IMAGING ANATOMY

Measurement of Patellar Height

- Insall-Salvati method uses sagittal image in 30° flexion
  - Measure maximum diagonal length of patella (A)
  - Measure shortest length of patellar tendon (B)
  - Ratio B:A = 1.0 ± 0.2
  - < 0.8 = patella baja; > 1.2 = patella alta
- Caton method uses sagittal image in full extension
  - Measure length patellar cartilage (A)
  - Measure shortest line between patellar articular surface and tibial plateau (B)
  - Ratio B:A = 1.0 ± 0.2
  - < 0.8 = patella baja; > 1.2 = patella alta

Valgus/Varus on Standing AP View: 2 Methods

- Mechanical axis
  - Line center femoral head to center tibial plafond
  - Should fall through middle of knee
  - Lateral position to center of knee indicates valgus, medial position indicates varus angulation
- Angle described by line bisecting distal femur and line bisecting proximal tibia; normal angle 6° ± 2°

Measurement of Translational Force Exerted on Patella With Contraction of Extensor Mechanism

- Q angle: Standing AP view; angle described by 2 lines
  - 1 line joins center of patella and anterior superior iliac spine (ASIS)
  - 2nd line joins center of patella and tibial tuberosity
  - Normal angle for males: 14° ± 3°, for females 17° ± 3°
- Tibial tubercle-trochlear groove method (TT-TG)
  - Cross sectional method (CT or MR) in extension
  - Axial image through apex of intercondylar notch superimposed on axial image through tibial tubercle
  - Horizontal distance between apex of notch and tibial tubercle measured
  - Normal 1.5 ± 0.4 cm; > 2.0 cm = patellar maltracking

Measurement of Trochlear Inclination

- Knee in either flexion or extension, axial image through apex of intercondylar notch
- Reference line: Posterior transcondylar line
- Angle described by posterior transcondylar line and line extending down lateral facet of trochlea
- Normal trochlear inclination: ≥ 11°

Measurement of Trochlear Facet Asymmetry

- Knee in either flexion or extension, axial image through apex of intercondylar notch
- Ratio of length of medial trochlear facet to length of lateral trochlear facet normal if ≥ 40%

Measurement of Trochlear Depth

- Knee in either flexion or extension, axial image through apex of intercondylar notch
- Reference line: Posterior transcondylar line
- 3 lines drawn perpendicular to reference line showing greatest anteroposterior lengths to (A) lateral trochlear facet, (B) deepest point of trochlear sulcus, and (C) medial trochlear facet
- Trochlear depth = (A + C/2) - B; normal depth > 3 mm

Measurement of Trochlear Sulcus Angle

- Knee in either flexion or extension, axial image through apex of intercondylar notch
- Angle described by line along trochlear medial facet and line along trochlear lateral facet
- Normal trochlear angle: 138° ± 6°; if > 145°, describes trochlear dysplasia

Measurement of Patellar Tilt

- Knee in 20° flexion, axial radiographic view
  - Line drawn across tops of medial and lateral trochlea
  - 2nd line drawn along lateral patellar facet
  - Angle should be "open" laterally
- Patellar tilt angle: Knee in flexion or extension, axial image through equator of patella
  - Draw line across posterior condyles, then auxiliary line at level of trochlea parallel to 1st line
  - Draw line through equator of patella; 2 lines form patellar tilt angle; normal is 2° ± 2°

Measurement of Patellar Congruence to Trochlea

- Knee in 30° flexion, axial image through patellofemoral joint
- Draw A and B, medial and lateral trochlear facet lines
- Draw line C, bisecting trochlear sulcus (angle formed by A and B)
- Draw line D, from patellar apex to trochlear sulcus
- Congruence angle is formed between lines C and D
- Normal ranges from -6° to +6°

Dynamic Assessment of Patellar Congruence

- 4 axial images through patellofemoral joint taken in extension, 15° flexion, 30° flexion, and 30° flexion with contraction of quadriceps
- Check for changing position of patellar tilt and subluxation in these different positions

Measurement of Femoral and Tibial Torsion

- Femoral torsion
  - Measure degree of hip anteversion by superimposing CT through mid femoral head and femoral shaft at level of lesser trochanter
  - Measure degree of femoral torsion by angle formed by hip anteversion relative to line at posterior femoral condyles
  - Distal femur is normally internally rotated relative to hip (femoral anteversion or antetorsion)
- Tibial torsion
  - Superimpose proximal tibial axial cut on distal tibial axial cut
  - Measured by angle formed by transverse axes of these 2 levels
  - Distal tibia is normally externally rotated relative to proximal tibia (average 30° in adults; range 20°-50°)

SELECTED REFERENCES

1. Diederichs G et al: MR imaging of patellar instability: injury patterns and assessment of risk factors. Radiographics. 2010 Jul-Aug;30(4):961-81. Erratum in: Radiographics. 31(2):624, 2011

Knee and Leg Measurements and Lines

MEASUREMENT OF PATELLAR HEIGHT

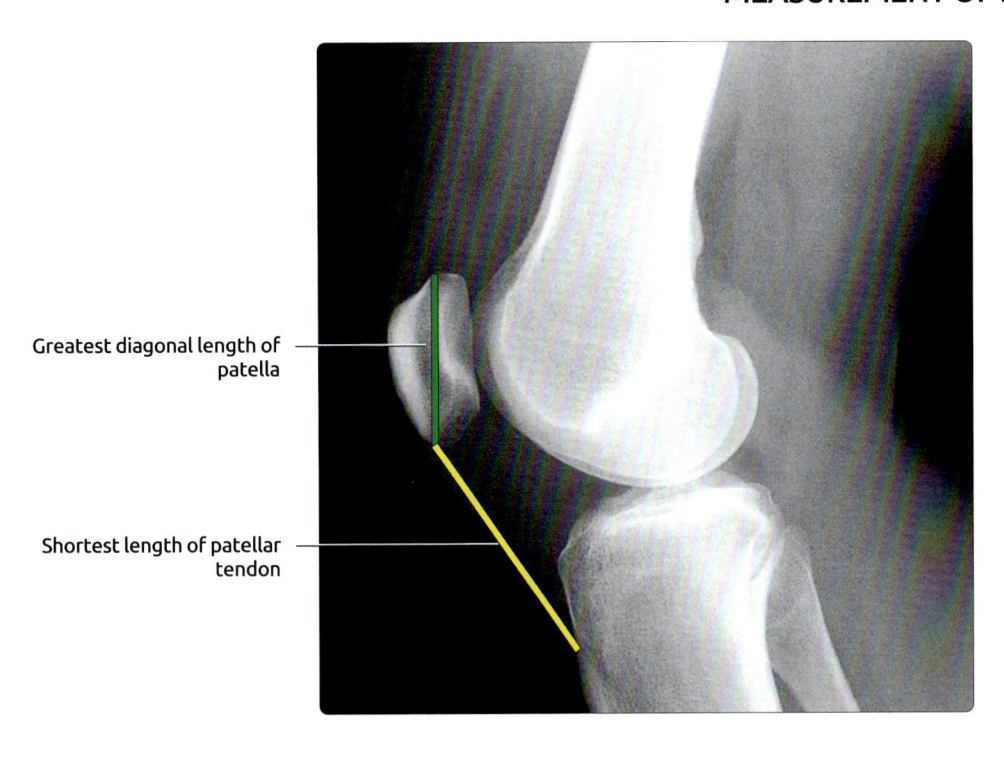

Greatest diagonal length of patella

Shortest length of patellar tendon

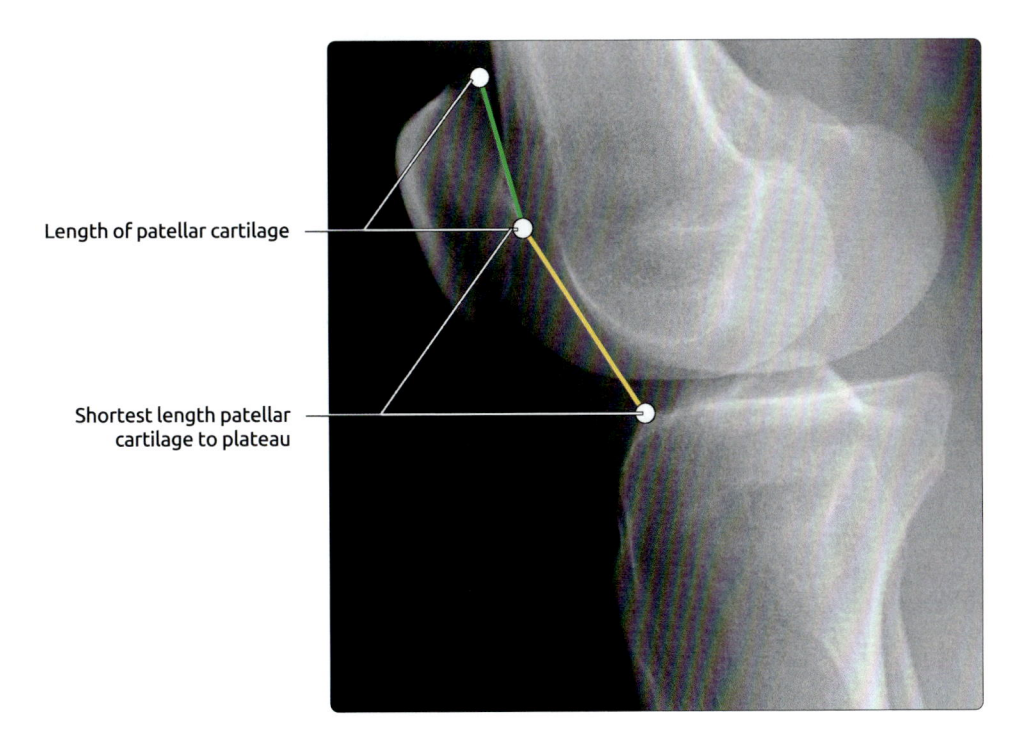

Length of patellar cartilage

Shortest length patellar cartilage to plateau

(Top) Patellar height measurement is shown by the Insall-Salvati method. On lateral radiograph, in 30° flexion, the shortest length of the patellar tendon (yellow line), and the greatest diagonal length of the patella (green line), form a ratio that averages 1.0 ± 0.2 (range 0.8-1.2). If the ratio is < 0.8, it represents patella baja; if the ratio is > 1.2, it is patella alta. **(Bottom)** If the landmarks are not clear for the Insall-Salvati method, the Caton method may be used. It requires a lateral image in full extension. The length of the patellar cartilage is measured (A; green line). The shortest line between the patellar articular surface and tibial plateau is measured (B; yellow line). The ratio of B:A is normally 1.0 ± 0.2. A ratio of < 0.8 indicates patella baja, while a ratio of > 1.2 indicates patella alta.

Knee and Leg Measurements and Lines

MECHANICAL AXIS, KNEE ANGULATION

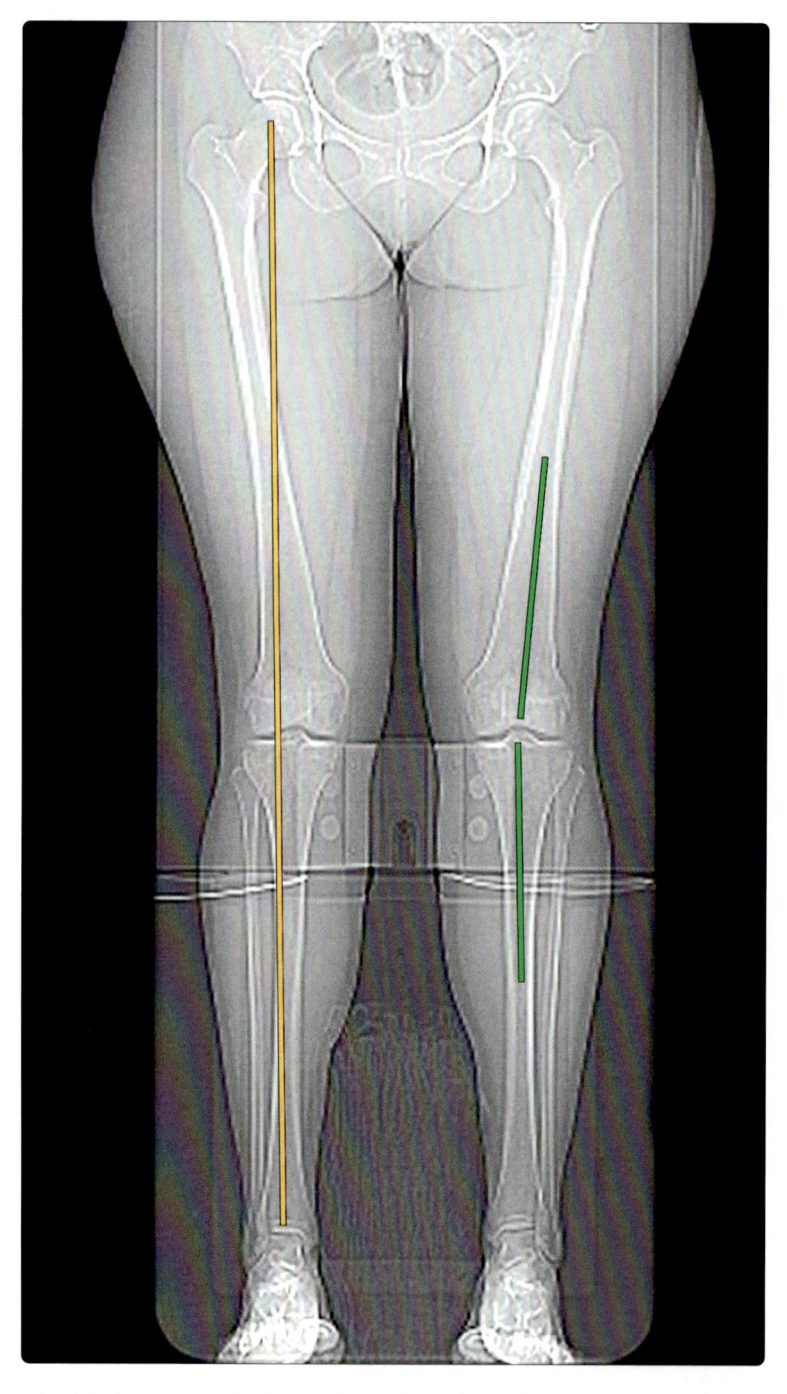

The yellow line drawn on the right lower extremity depicts the mechanical axis drawn from the center of the femoral head to the center of the tibial plafond. The normal mechanical axis traverses the center of the knee joint. The green lines bisecting the distal femur and proximal tibia show the normal valgus angulation of the knee (average 6°).

Knee and Leg Measurements and Lines

Q ANGLE: TRANSLATIONAL FORCE ON PATELLA

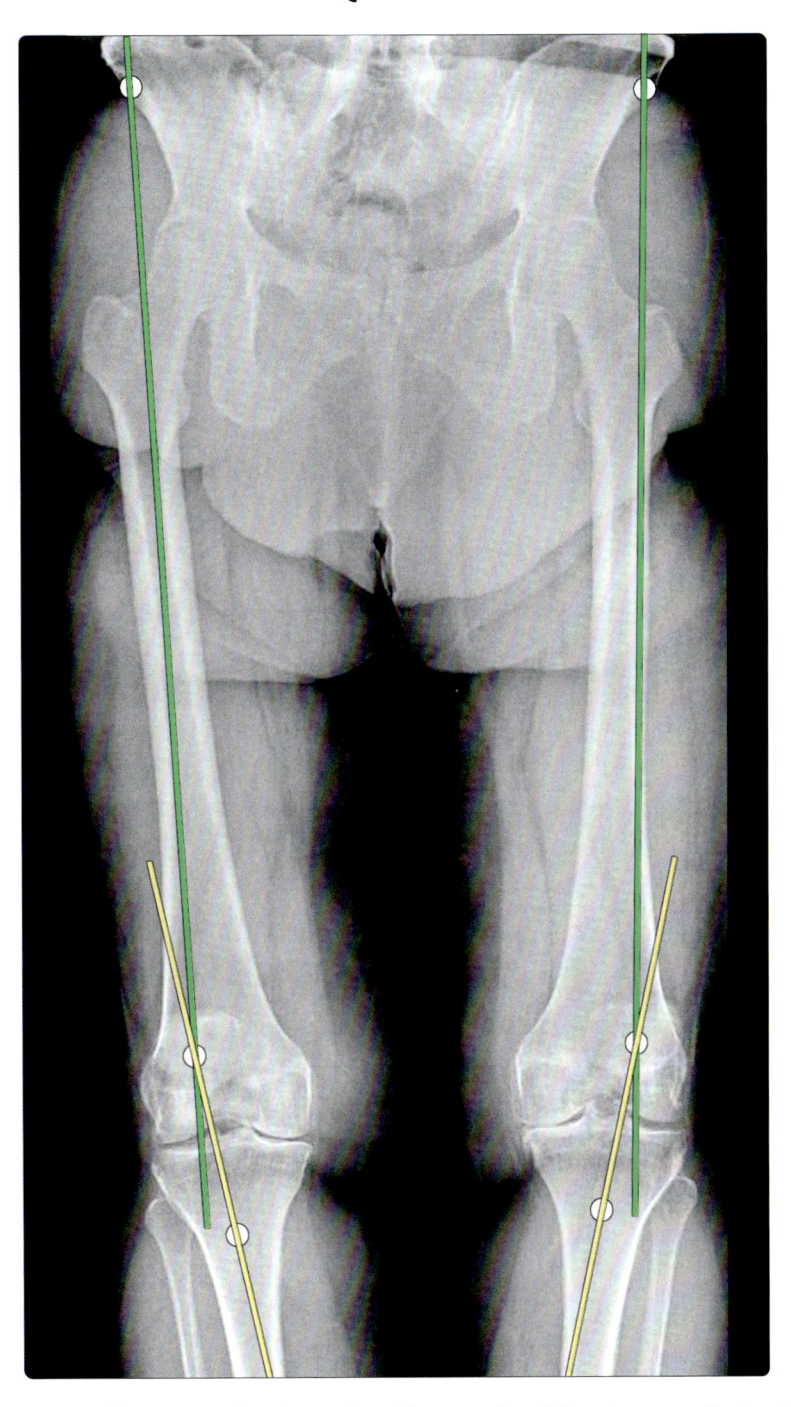

The Q angle measures the translational force exerted on the patella with contraction of the extensor mechanism. A standing AP view is used; the angle is described by 2 lines. The 1st line (green) joins the center of the patella and the anterior superior iliac spine (ASIS). The 2nd line joins the center of patella and tibial tuberosity (yellow). The normal angle is 14° ± 3° in males and 17° ± 3° in females. The Q angle, in this case, is at the upper limits of normal on the right but abnormal on the left.

LATERAL TRANSLATION: TT-TG METHOD FOR CT

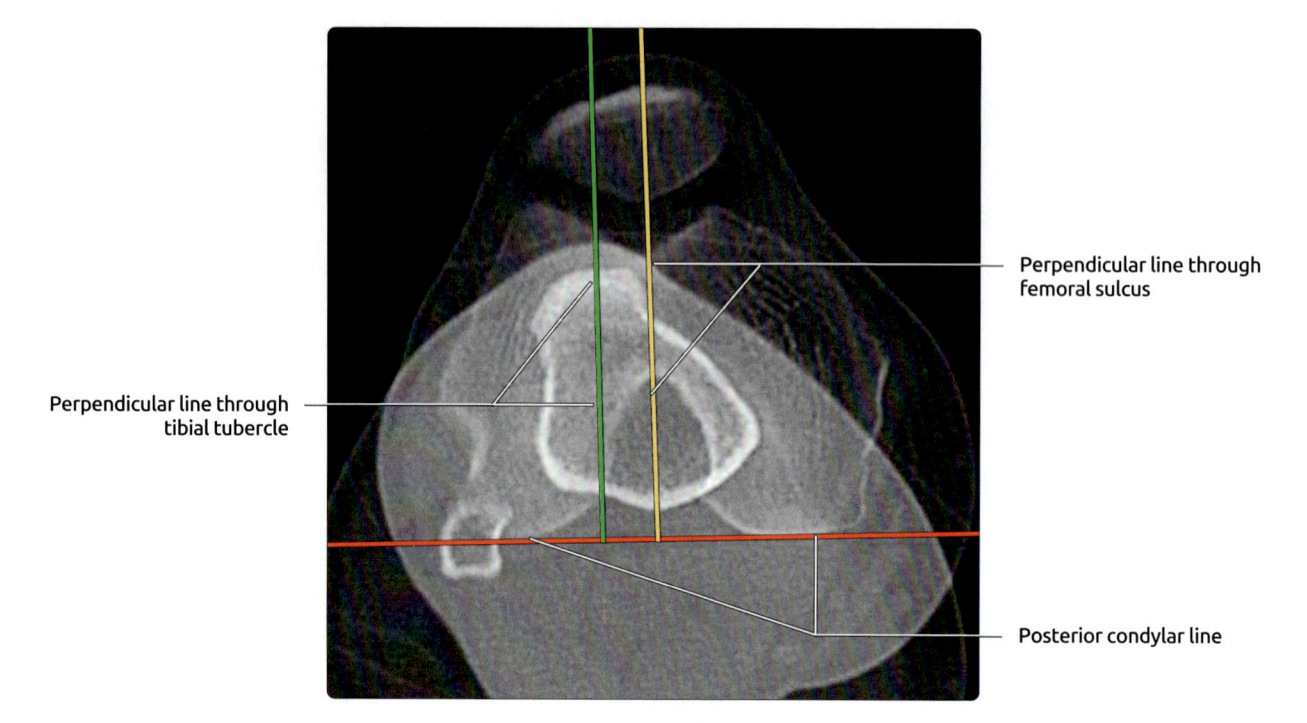

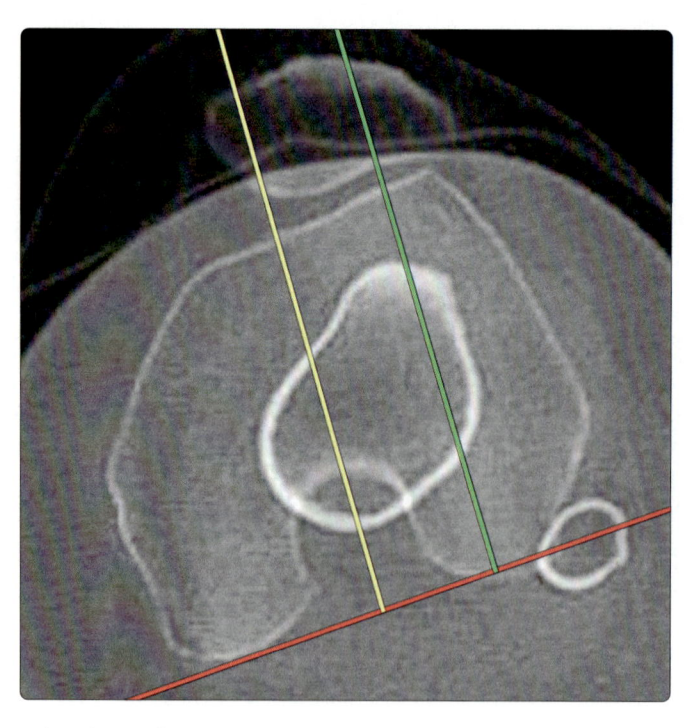

Perpendicular line through femoral sulcus

Perpendicular line through tibial tubercle

Posterior condylar line

(Top) *Translational force exerted on the patella may be measured by the tibial tubercle-trochlear groove (TT-TG) method. This is performed using cross-sectional images (CT or MR) with the knee in extension. An axial image through the apex of the intercondylar notch is superimposed on an axial image through the tibial tubercle. The horizontal distance between the apex of the notch and tibial tubercle is measured in the following manner: Draw the posterior condylar line (red); draw a line perpendicular to the red line through the tibial tubercle (green; this is the TT line); draw a line perpendicular to the red line through the trochlear groove sulcus (yellow; this is the TG line). Normal for the TT-TG distance is 1.5 ± 0.4 cm. In this case, the measurement falls within normal limits.* **(Bottom)** *In this case, the TT-TG distance is greater than 2 cm, indicating patellar maltracking.*

Knee and Leg Measurements and Lines

LATERAL TRANSLATION: TT-TG METHOD FOR MR

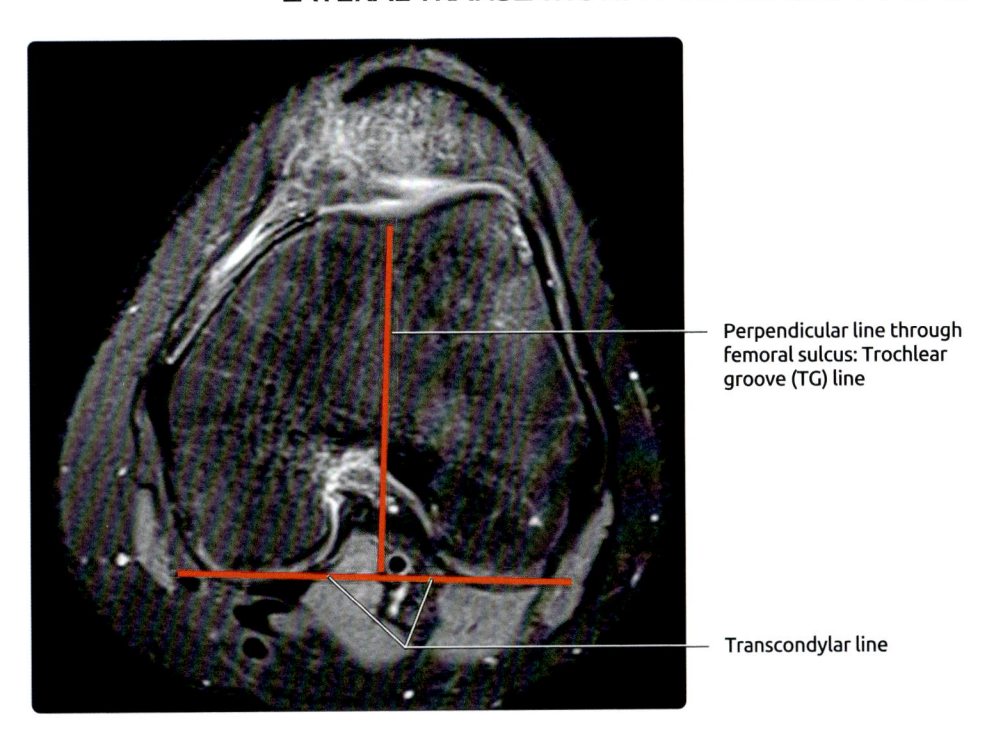

Perpendicular line through femoral sulcus: Trochlear groove (TG) line

Transcondylar line

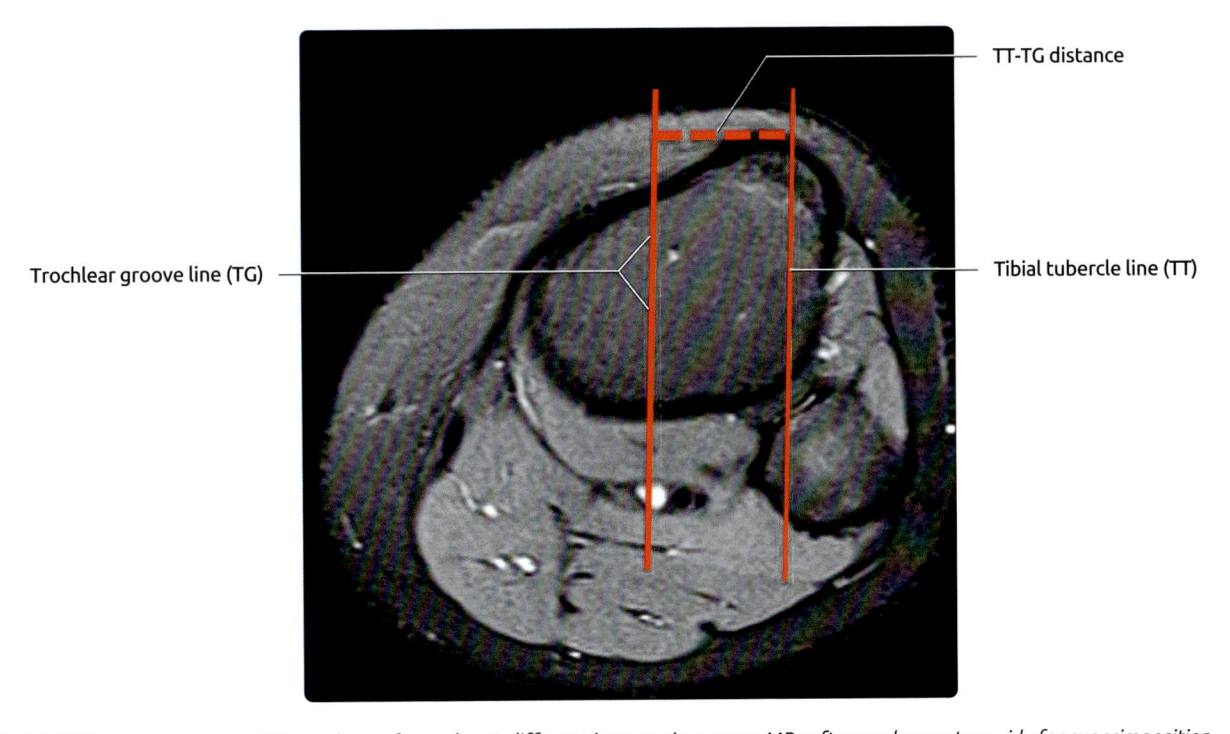

TT-TG distance

Trochlear groove line (TG)

Tibial tubercle line (TT)

(Top) TT-TG measurement on MR may be performed on 2 different images since some MR software does not provide for superimposition of images. The reference line is the posterior transcondylar line; a perpendicular line is drawn through the deepest point of the trochlea. This is the trochlear groove (TG) line. (Bottom) The axial cut shows that the tibial tubercle is chosen. The TG line from the same patient is reproduced. A parallel line extending through the midpoint of the tibial tuberosity (tibial tubercle or TT line) is drawn and the distance between the 2 lines is measured. Normal TT-TG < 1.5 cm. Measurements > 2 cm are specific for patellar maltracking.

Knee and Leg Measurements and Lines

MEASUREMENT OF TROCHLEAR INCLINATION

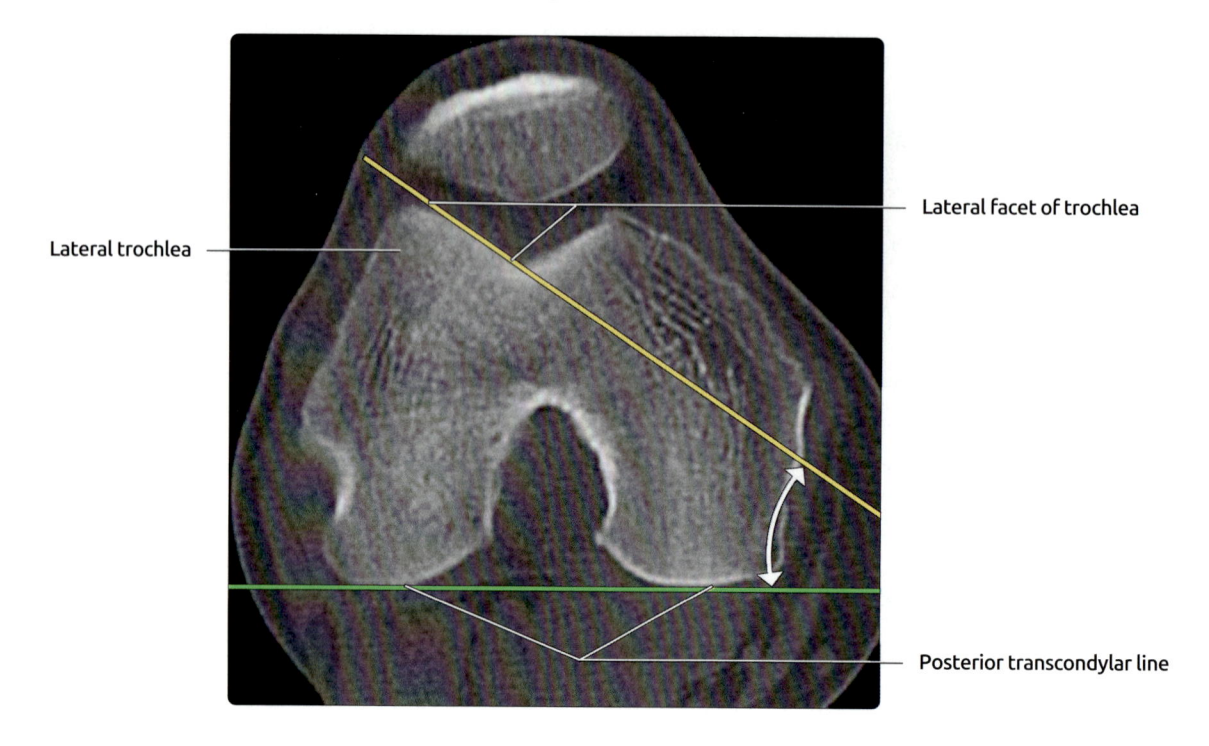

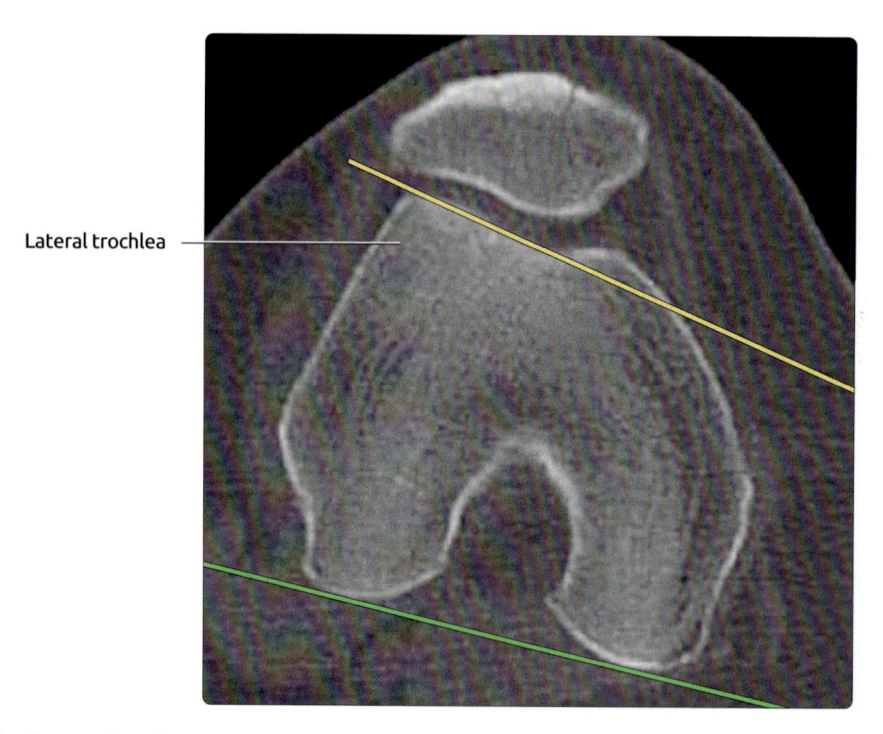

Lateral trochlea

Lateral facet of trochlea

Posterior transcondylar line

Lateral trochlea

(Top) *The degree of trochlear inclination relates to trochlear dysplasia and consequent patellofemoral disorders. The measurement is obtained on an axial image through the apex of the intercondylar notch, with the knee in either flexion or extension. The posterior transcondylar line is drawn as a reference line (green). The angle is described by the posterior transcondylar line and a line extending along the lateral facet of the trochlea (yellow). The normal trochlear inclination is greater than or equal to 11°. If the angle is < 11°, it describes trochlear dysplasia. In this example, the angle is > 11° and there is no dysplasia.* **(Bottom)** *This image shows a trochlear inclination angle that measures less than 11°. This is a case of trochlear dysplasia with a fairly flat trochlear sulcus.*

Knee and Leg Measurements and Lines

MEASUREMENT OF TROCHLEAR FACET ASYMMETRY & TROCHLEAR DEPTH

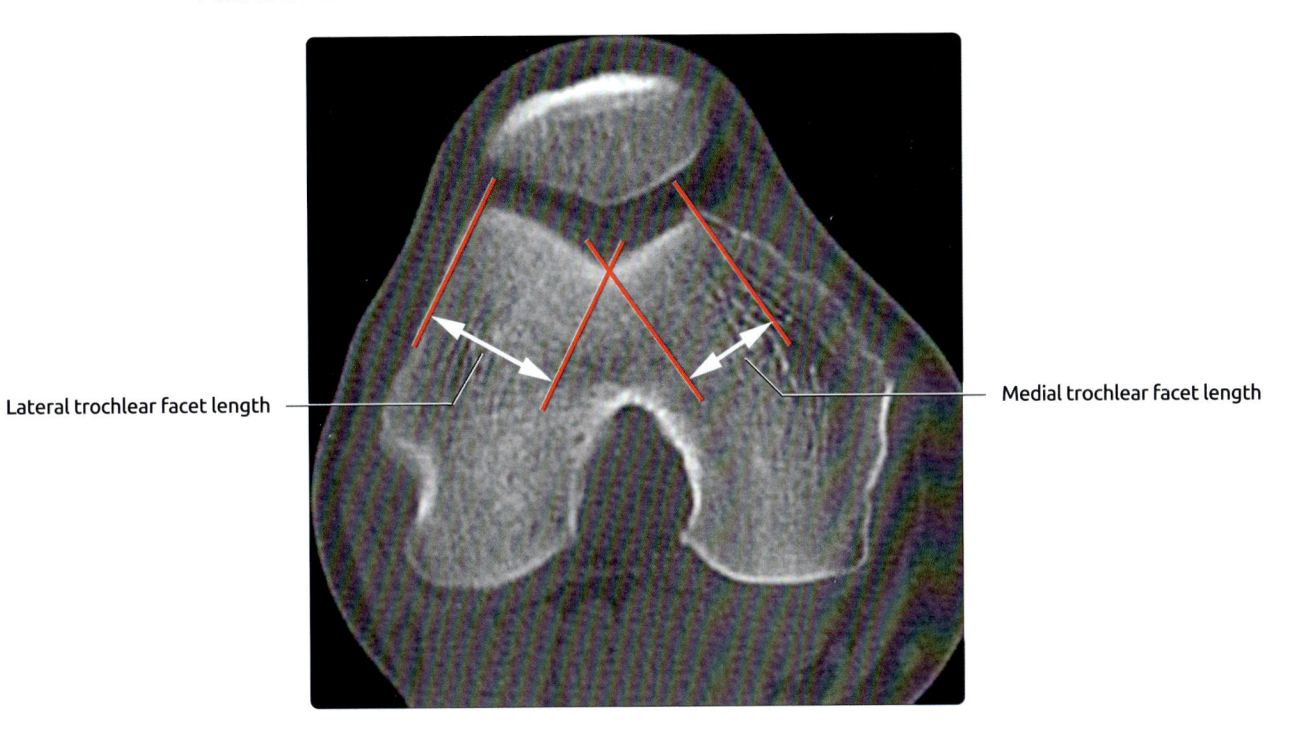

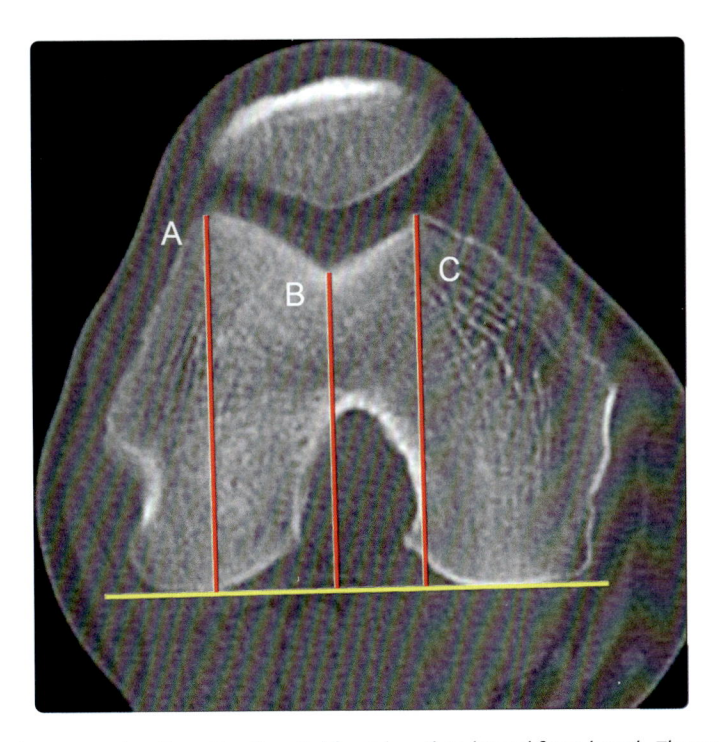

Lateral trochlear facet length

Medial trochlear facet length

(Top) *Trochlear facet asymmetry is measured as the ratio of medial facet length to lateral facet length. The normal measurement is ≥ 40%.* (Bottom) *Measurement of trochlear depth utilizes the transcondylar line as the reference line. Perpendicular lines are drawn to the greatest AP length of the lateral trochlear facet (A), the greatest AP length of the medial trochlear facet (C), and the deepest part of the trochlear sulcus (B). Trochlear depth = (A + C/2) - B. Normal trochlear depth is > 3mm.*

MEASUREMENT OF TROCHLEAR SULCUS ANGLE

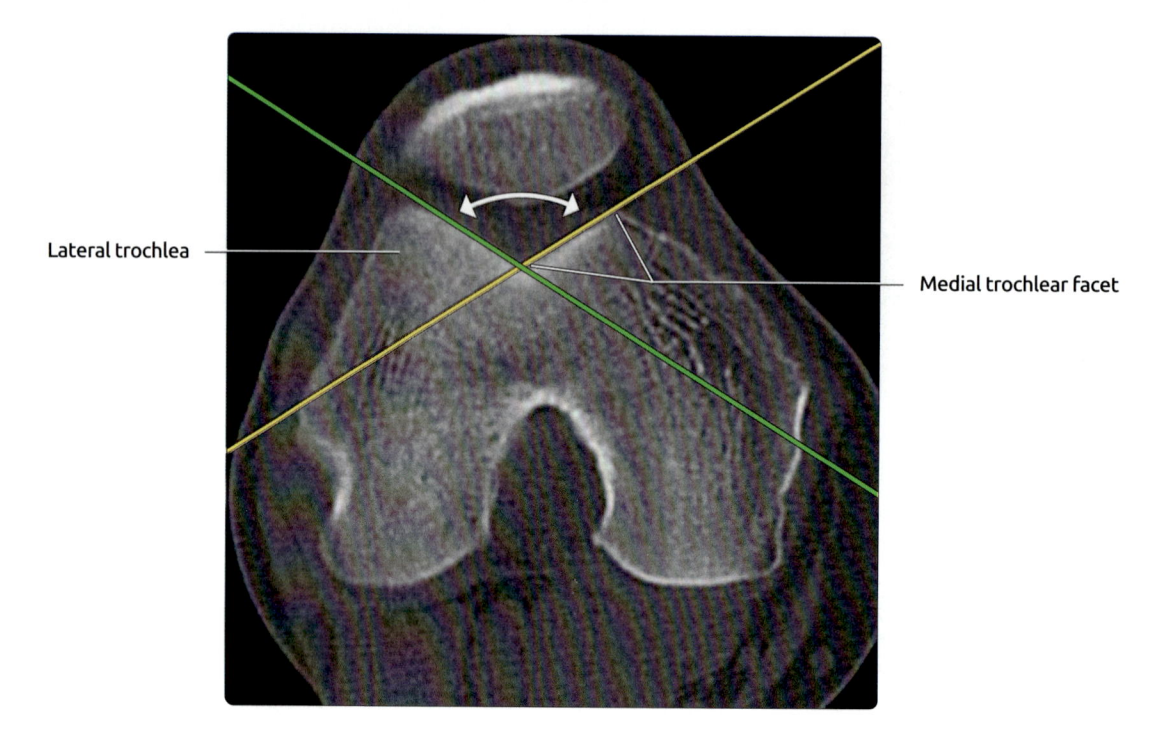

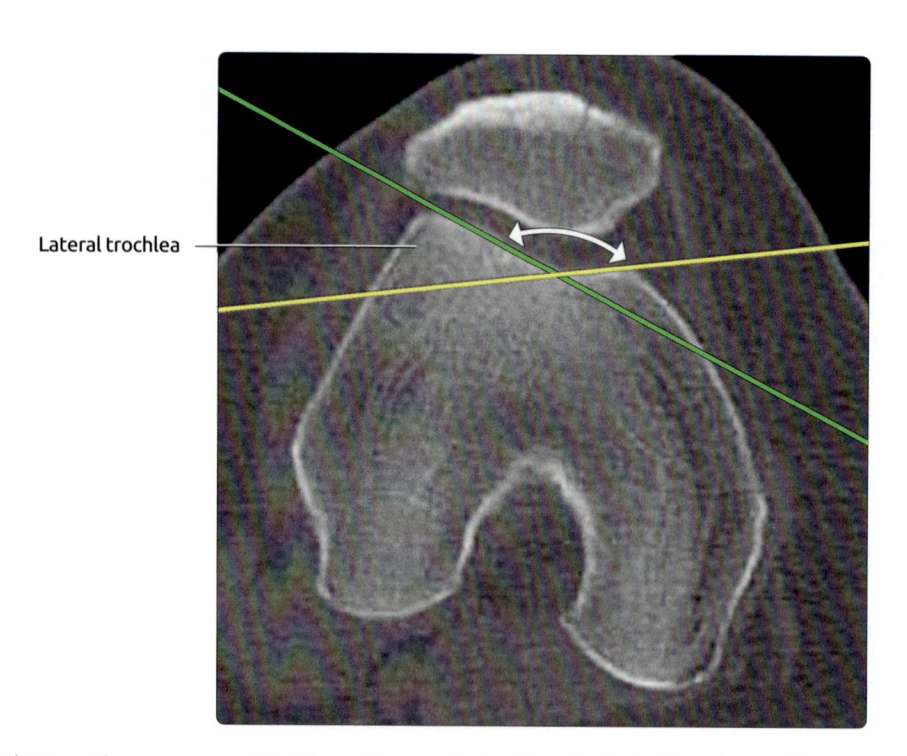

(Top) This is another measurement that is used to evaluate trochlear dysplasia. The sulcus angle is measured on an axial image through the apex of the intercondylar notch, with the knee in either flexion or extension. The angle is described by a line along the trochlear medial facet (yellow) and another line along the trochlear lateral facet (green). The normal trochlear sulcus angle is 138° ± 6°. If the angle is > 145°, it demonstrates trochlear dysplasia. In this case, there is no evidence of dysplasia. (Bottom) In this patient, the trochlear sulcus angle is much greater than 145°. This demonstrates flattening of the trochlear angle in a patient with dysplasia.

Knee and Leg Measurements and Lines

MEASUREMENT OF PATELLAR TILT

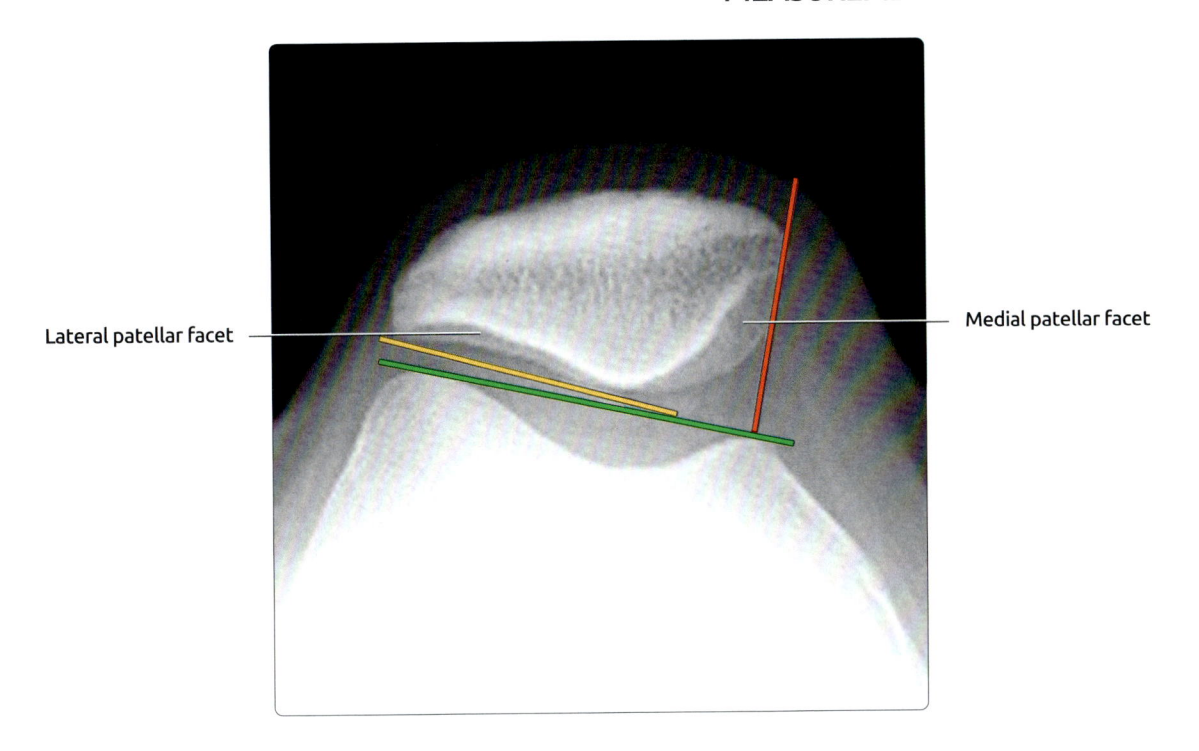

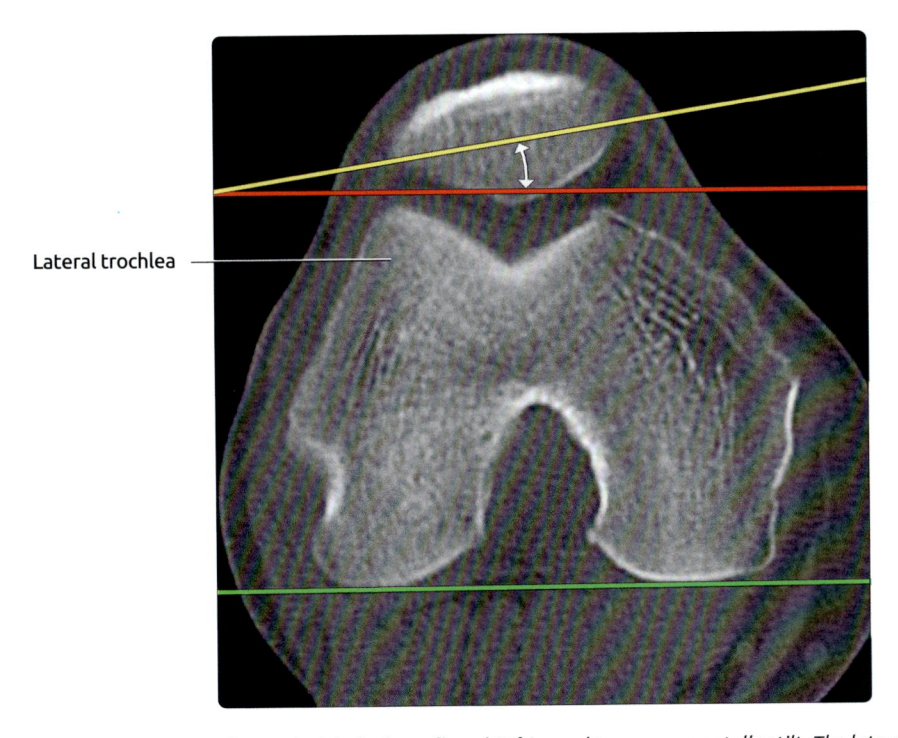

Lateral patellar facet

Medial patellar facet

Lateral trochlea

(Top) Axial radiograph of the knee obtained with the knee flexed 20° is used to measure patellar tilt. The lateral patellar facet is elongated and less sharply angled than the medial. The angle formed by the line through the condylar peaks (green) and lateral patellar facet (yellow) is normally open laterally; reversal of this angle constitutes patellar tilt. A line drawn perpendicular (red) to the condylar peaks line (green), 2 mm lateral to the medial condylar peak, should intersect the patella. If the patella lies lateral to this line, it is laterally subluxed. Both the laterally open angle and the red line evaluating subluxation are normal in this case. (Bottom) Patellar tilt can be measured on an axial image through the equator of the patella. A line is drawn across the posterior condyles (green), then an auxiliary line parallel to it is drawn at the level of the trochlea (red). An angle is formed between that and a line drawn through the equator of the patella (yellow). Normal is 2° ± 2°.

Knee and Leg Measurements and Lines

PATELLAR CONGRUENCE TO TROCHLEA

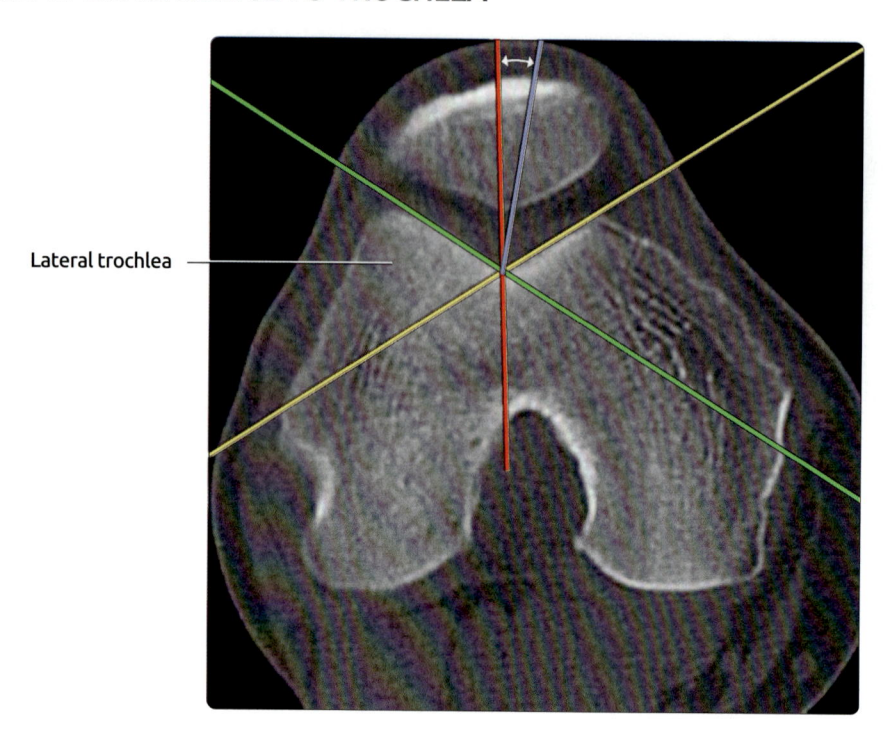

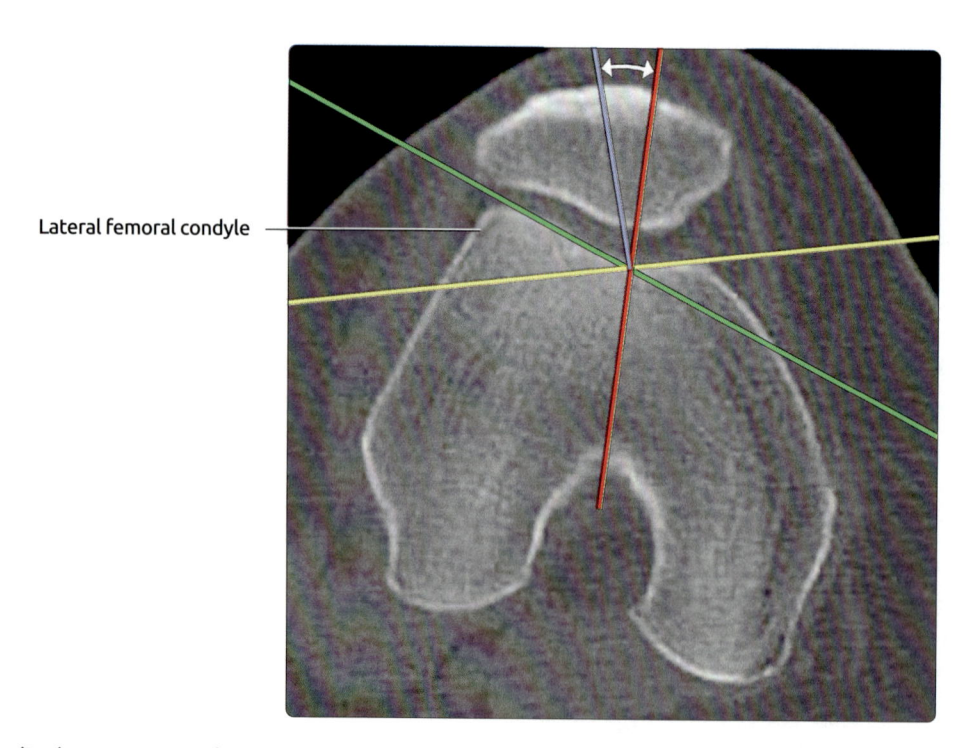

Lateral trochlea

Lateral femoral condyle

(Top) Measurement of the patellar congruence to the trochlea is obtained on an axial image through the patellofemoral joint with the knee in 30° flexion. Draw the medial trochlear facet line (yellow) and lateral facet line (green). The angle formed by these 2 lines is then bisected (red line). A line is then drawn from the patellar apex to trochlear sulcus (blue; this line is termed the congruence line). The angle formed between the red and blue lines measures the patellar congruence. If the congruence angle is lateral to the bisector of the sulcus, the angle is positive. If the congruence angle is medial to the bisector of the sulcus, the angle is negative. The normal average congruence angle is -6° in males and -10° in females. In this case, the congruence angle is negative and within normal measurements. **(Bottom)** In this case, the congruence angle is positive and, therefore, abnormal.

Knee and Leg Measurements and Lines

DYNAMIC ASSESSMENT PATELLAR CONGRUENCE

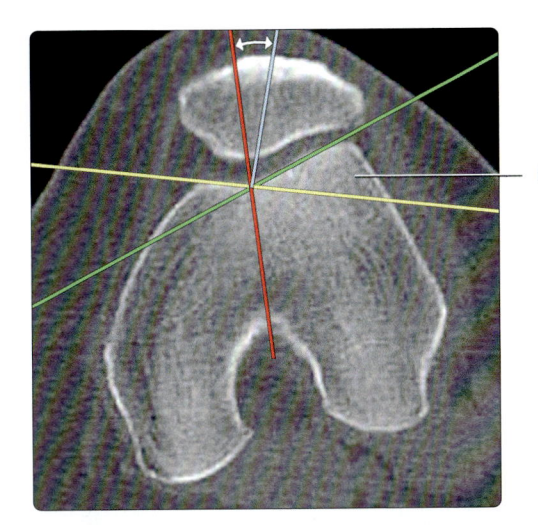

Lateral trochlea, knee in extension

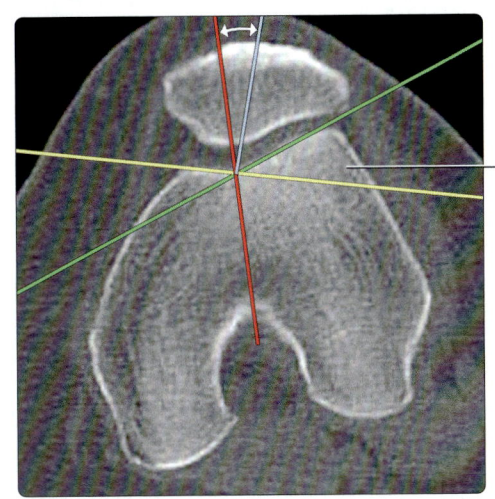

Lateral trochlea, knee in 15° flexion

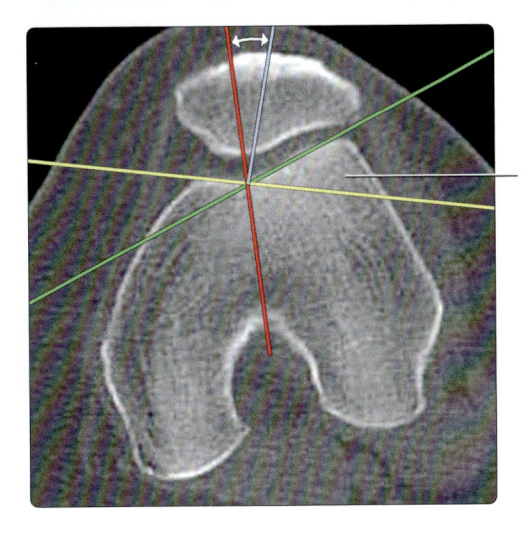

Lateral trochlea, knee in 30° flexion

(Top) Dynamic assessment of the patellar congruence is performed either by axial radiographic imaging or by CT or MR axial imaging. Four axial images are obtained through the patellofemoral joint, 1 each in extension, 15° flexion, 30° flexion, and 30° flexion during contraction of the quadriceps. The congruence angle can be measured on each, and changing position of patellar tilt and subluxation is evaluated in each position. This image is obtained with the knee in extension and shows a positive congruence angle with lateral subluxation of the patella, both of which are abnormal. (Middle) With flexion of 15°, the lateral subluxation of the patella is reduced, but the congruence angle is still positive. (Bottom) With 30° flexion, the congruence angle remains slightly positive, though there is no subluxation or patellar tilt. Note the slightly flattened trochlear dysplasia.

Knee

HIP ANTEVERSION & FEMORAL TORSION

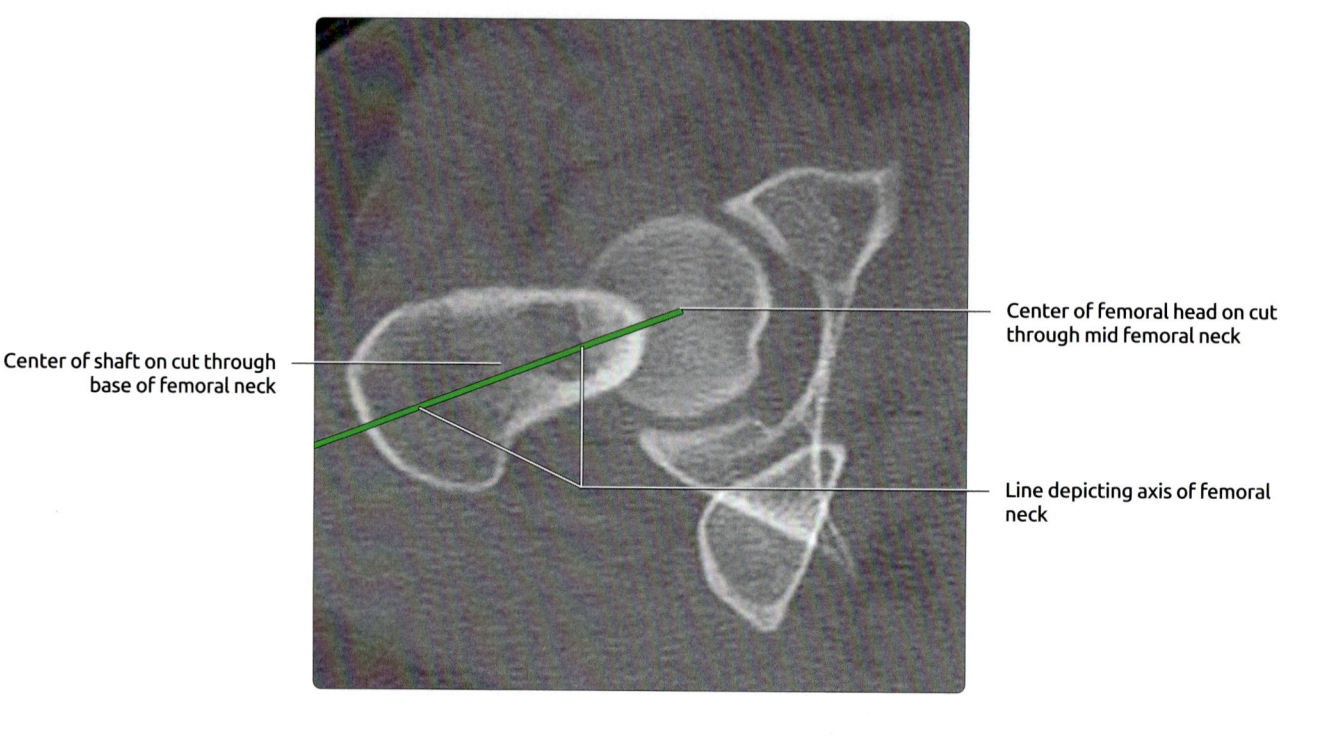

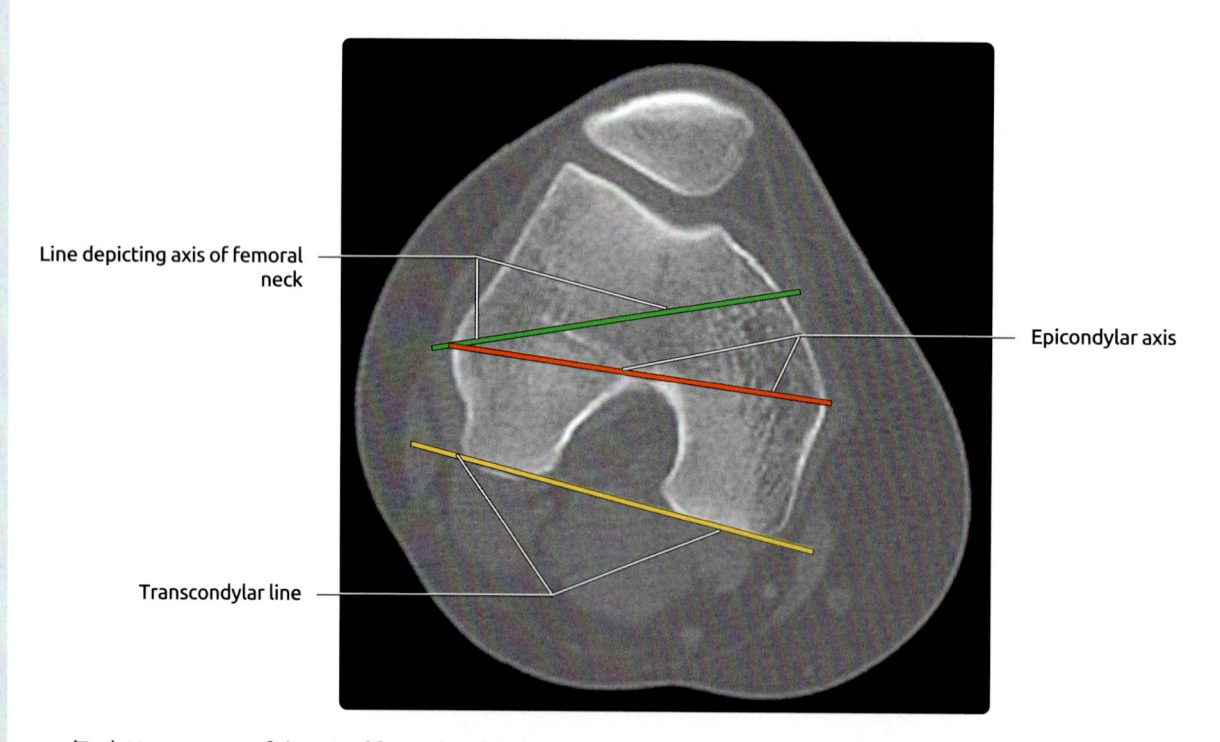

Center of shaft on cut through base of femoral neck

Center of femoral head on cut through mid femoral neck

Line depicting axis of femoral neck

Line depicting axis of femoral neck

Epicondylar axis

Transcondylar line

(Top) Measurement of the axis of femoral neck is determined by superimposed CT scans through the mid femoral neck and base of femoral neck. The line connecting the center of the head in the superior cut and the center of shaft in the lower cut determines the femoral neck axis; this line makes an angle with the transischial line; in this case there is 15° femoral neck anteversion. (Bottom) Method of measurement of femoral torsion is shown by CT. Angle formed by the axis of the femoral neck (green line from previous image) and transcondylar line (yellow) gives the degree of femoral torsion. Normally, the distal femur is internally rotated relative to the femoral neck, which is termed femoral anteversion or antetorsion; different studies show average anteversion to be 15-24° in adults (range: 3-48°). Epicondylar axis (red line) is another useful landmark. The epicondylar/posterior condylar angle should be 5.7 ± 1.7°.

Knee and Leg Measurements and Lines

TIBIAL TORSION

Transcondylar line (distal femur)

Transverse axis of proximal tibia

Transverse axis of proximal tibia

Transverse axis of distal tibia

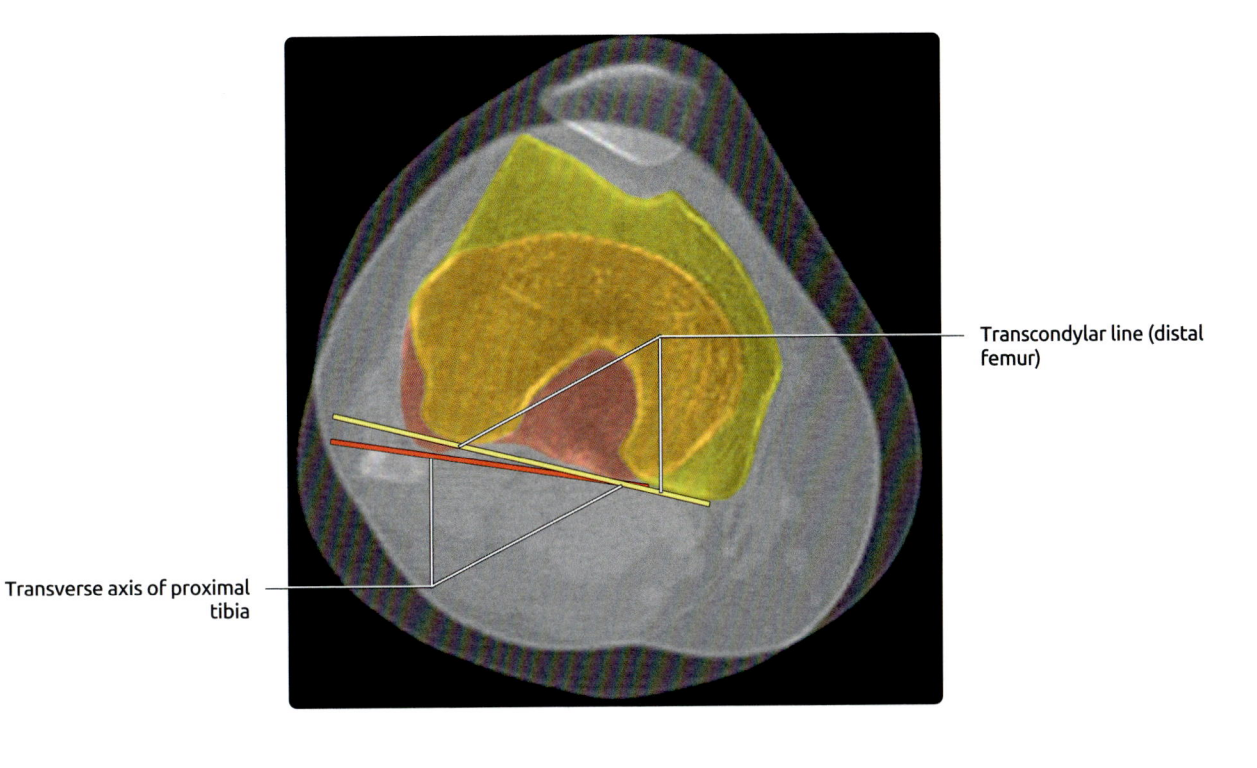

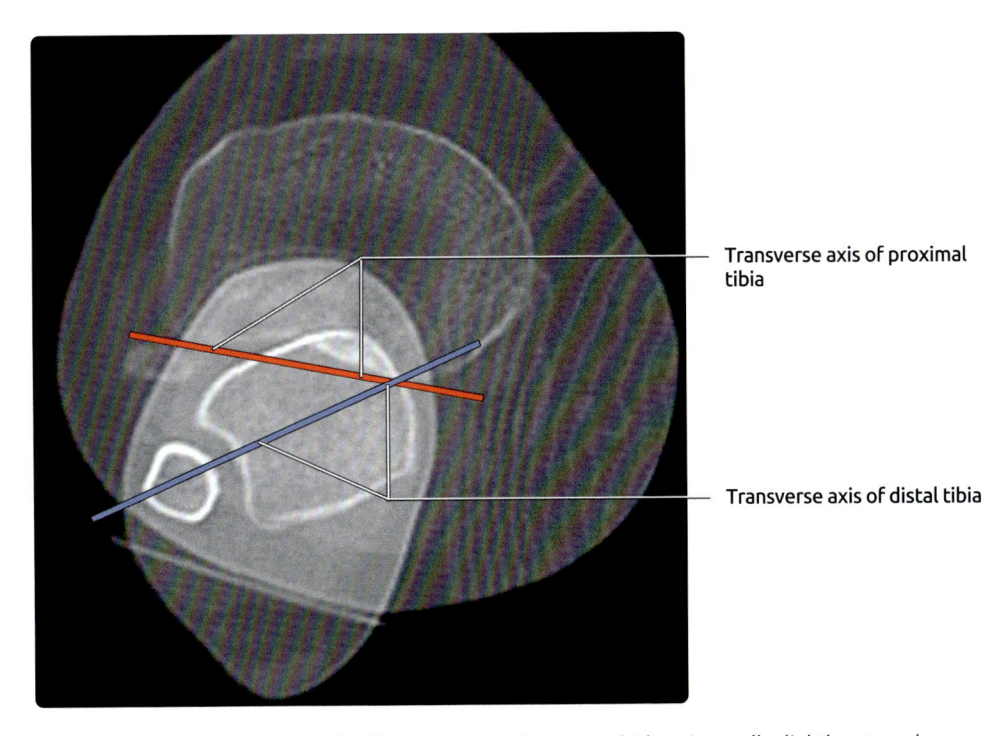

(Top) Occasionally, measuring the rotation of the proximal tibia on the distal femur may be required. There is usually slightly external rotation of the tibia relative to the femur; it is measured by the angle formed by the transcondylar line of the distal femur (yellow) and the transverse axis of the proximal tibia (red line). (Bottom) Tibial torsion is measured by the angle formed by the proximal tibial transverse axis (red line) and distal tibial transverse axis (blue line). There is normal external rotation (torsion) of the distal tibia measuring 30° in adults (range 20-50°), as shown by several CT studies. Tibial torsion greater than 40° shows an increased incidence of adverse patellar mechanics and malalignment syndrome.

Knee and Leg Measurements and Lines

PCL RATIO/ANGLE: 2° SIGNS OF ACL TEAR

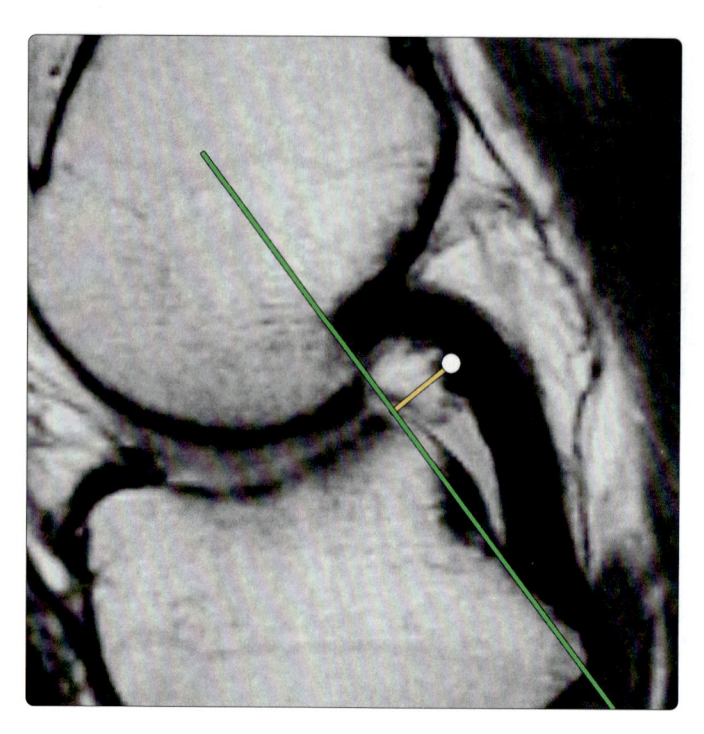

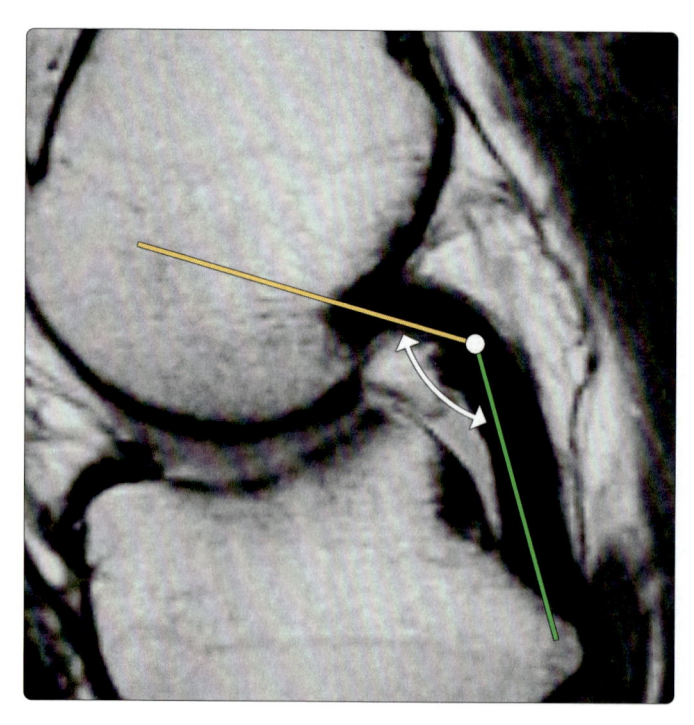

(Top) The PCL is normally mildly concave in an anterior direction. With ACL tear and anterior subluxation of the tibia, the PCL may become "buckled." This may be measured on a sagittal image through the mid PCL. The PCL index is formed by a line drawn between the anterior portions of the femoral and tibial attachments of the PCL (green line) and a line across the maximum perpendicular distance between the green line and the apex of the PCL (yellow line). The normal ratio of yellow:green is 0:19. (Bottom) PCL bowing or buckling can also be assessed by the PCL angle. This is measured by a line drawn through the proximal portion of the PCL (yellow) and another through the distal portion of the PCL (green). The normal PCL angle ranges from 114-123°. An increase in either the PCL ratio or angle suggests ACL tear.

Knee and Leg Measurements and Lines

ACL ANGLE, RELATIVE TO FEMUR AND TIBIA

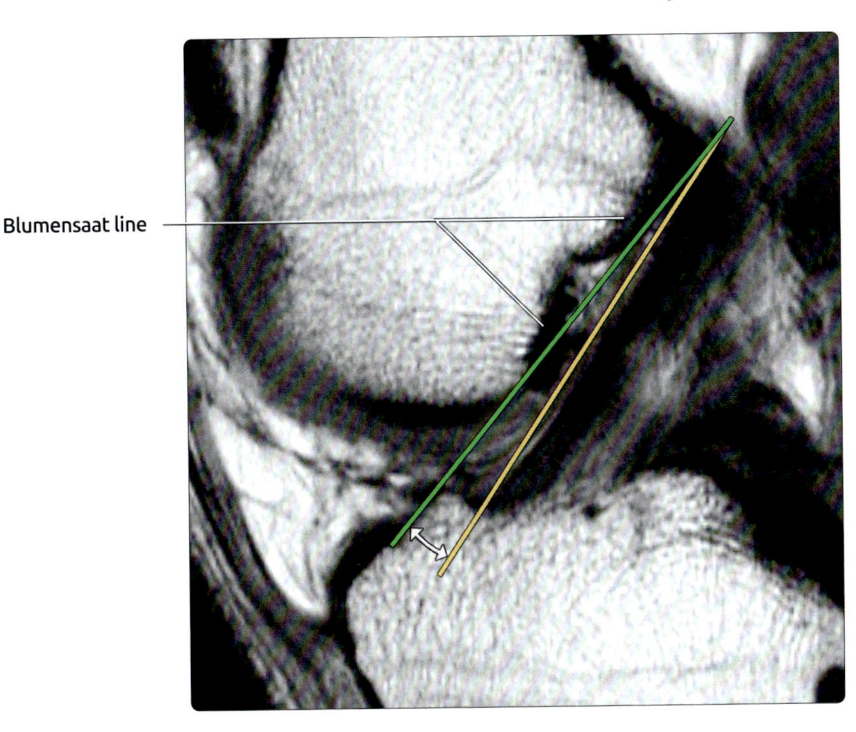

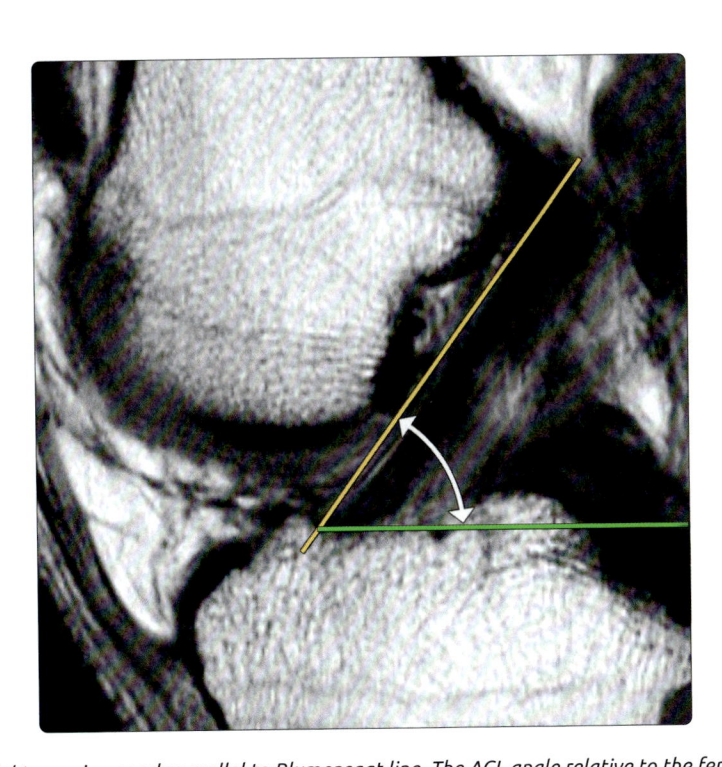

Blumensaat line

(Top) The ACL is normally straight, running nearly parallel to Blumensaat line. The ACL angle relative to the femur can be measured by drawing a line along the anterior margin of the ACL (yellow) and another along Blumensaat line (green). The angle described by these lines averages -1.6°. Abnormal criteria are published ranging from 9-15°. **(Bottom)** The ACL can be evaluated relative to the tibial plateau. The angle is described by a line along the anterior margin of the ACL (yellow) and another along the tibial plateau (green). This angle normally averages 56°; abnormal criteria are published ranging from 45-50°.

Knee and Leg Measurements and Lines

LATERAL FEMORAL SULCUS/LATERAL MENISCAL COVERAGE

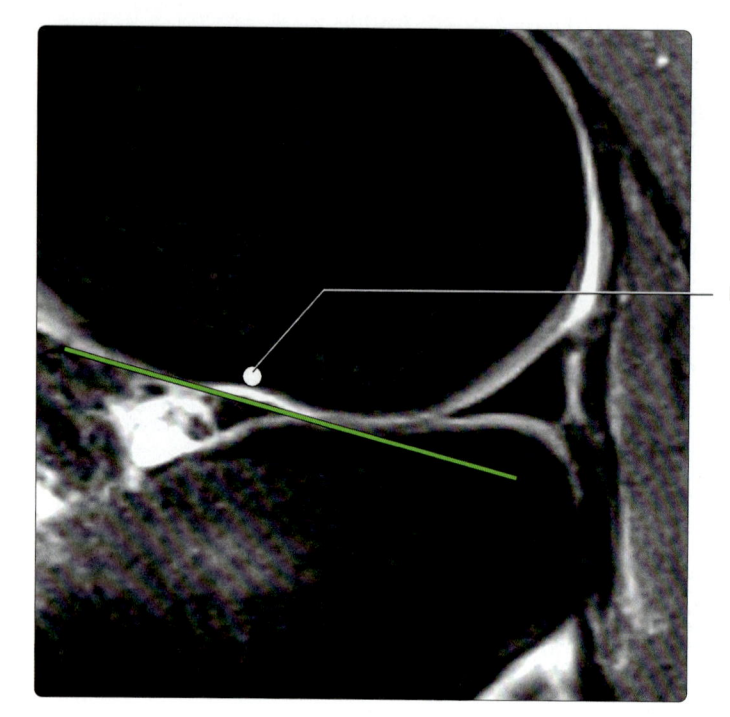

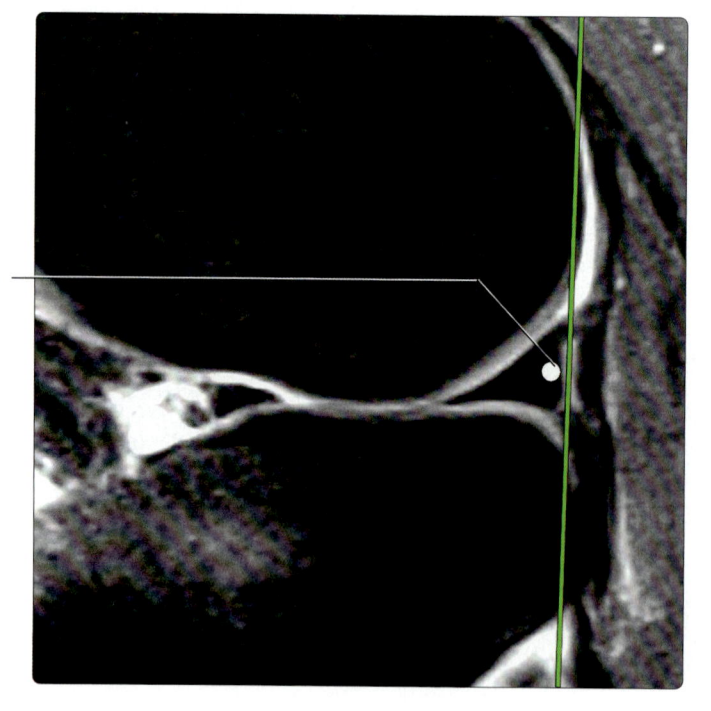

Lateral femoral sulcus

Posterior lateral meniscus

(Top) The lateral femoral sulcus has a normal slight concavity. This sulcus may be impacted with an injury mechanism that often results in ACL tear. The depth of the sulcus can be measured on the lateral image, which maximizes it. A line is drawn across the roof of the notch and the maximal depth is measured. Normal depth averages 0.35 mm. Depth > 2 mm is considered abnormal. (Bottom) Anterior tibial translation can be measured by evaluation of lateral meniscal ""uncovering."" This is measured on the sagittal image midway between the tibial insertion of the PCL and the lateral most portion of the tibial condyle. A line is drawn through the posterior tibia parallel to the long axis of the tibia. The distance of the line from the posterior lateral meniscus is measured (if the meniscus is anterior to the line, it is negative). Average is 2 mm; > 5 mm is abnormal.

Knee and Leg Measurements and Lines

ACL/PCL ISOMETRIC TUNNEL LOCATIONS

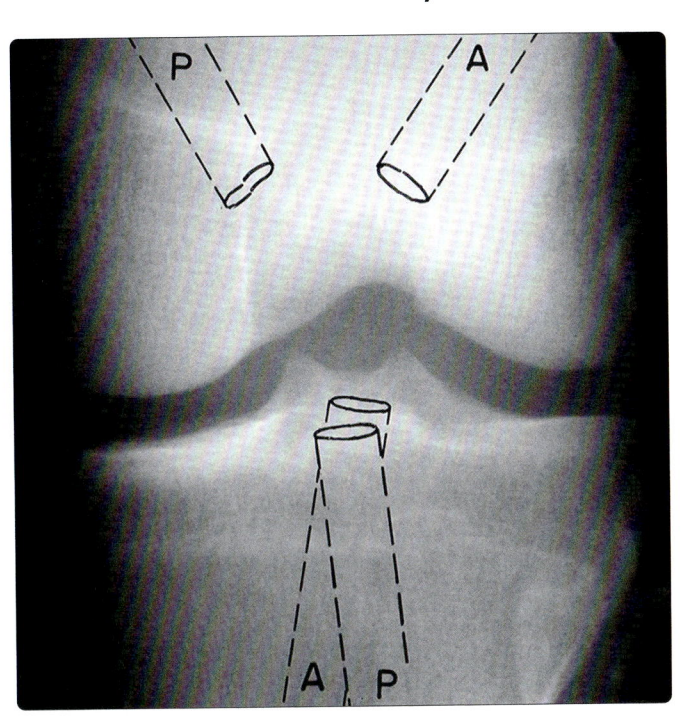

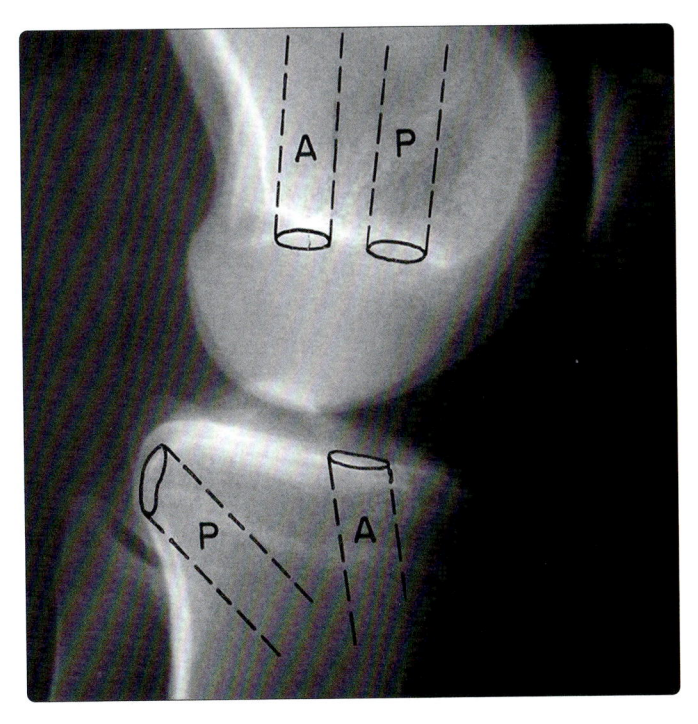

(Top) AP radiograph demonstrates isometric tunnel positions for ACL and PCL reconstruction grafts. In this projection, both the femoral and tibial tunnel openings appear to be at the normal expected positions of the cruciate ligaments. (A = ACL, P = PCL). **(Bottom)** Lateral radiograph depicts isometric tunnel openings for ACL and PCL reconstructions. The femoral tunnel for the ACL should lie at the intersection of the posterior cortex and Blumensaat line. The tibial tunnel for the ACL should lie 2-3 mm posterior to the normal ACL insertion site; the impingement-free zone has the tunnel centered 22-28 mm posterior to the anterior edge of tibia. The femoral PCL tunnel is at the normal origin of the PCL; note the tibial tunnel opening for the PCL is posterior and distal to the tibial articular surface, matching the normal insertion.

SECTION 10
Leg

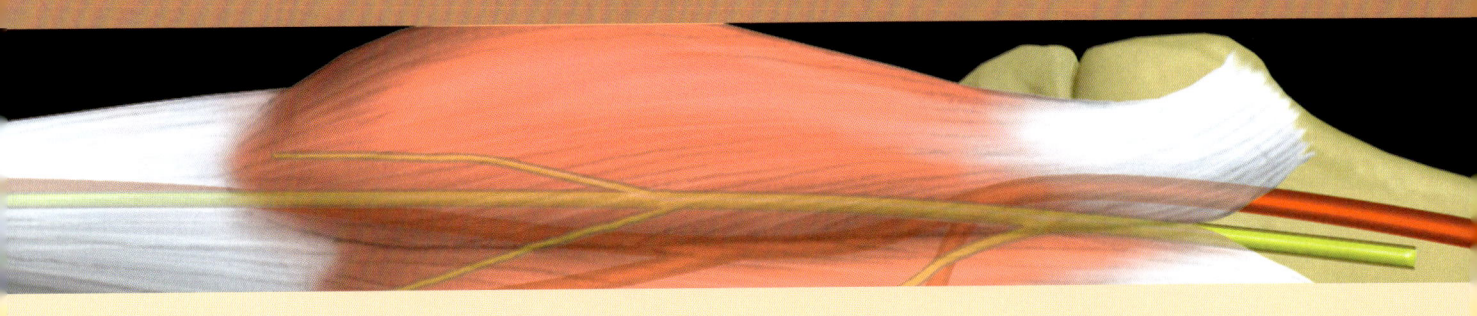

Leg Radiographic Anatomy and MR Atlas — 878

Leg Radiographic Anatomy and MR Atlas

GROSS ANATOMY

Osseous Anatomy

- Tibia
  - Proximal tibiofibular joint
    - Head of fibula and lateral condyle tibia joined by fibrous capsule
    - May communicate with knee joint
    - Posterolaterally located
    - Synovial; at risk for any articular process
  - Anterolateral tibia: Origin of anterior muscles of leg
  - Anterior border (shin): Sharp ridge running from tibial tuberosity proximally to anterior margin of medial malleolus
  - Medial tibial surface
    - Wide and flat
    - Proximally, covered by pes anserinus
    - Remainder is subcutaneous
  - Medial border of tibia: Saphenous nerve and great saphenous vein run along it
  - Posterior tibia: Origin of deep posterior muscles of leg
  - Lateral border of tibia: Ridge for attachment of interosseous membrane
  - Medial malleolus: 2 colliculi, anterior longer than posterior
  - Distal tibiofibular joint
    - Fibula articulates with tibia at fibular notch; joined by interosseous ligament
    - Strengthened by anterior and posterior tibiofibular ligaments
    - Posterolaterally located
- Fibula
  - Anterior fibula
    - Origin of lateral muscles of leg
  - Medial fibula
    - Origin of deep posterior muscles of leg
  - Posterolateral fibula
    - Origin of posterior muscles of leg
  - Lateral malleolus: 1 cm longer than medial malleolus

Interosseous Membrane

- Stretches across interval between tibia and fibula
- Greatly extends surface for origin of muscles
- Strong, oblique fibers run downwards and laterally from tibia to fibula
- In upper part, below lateral condyle of tibia, there is an opening for passage of anterior tibial vessels
- Distally, opening allows passage of perforating branch of peroneal artery
- Tibialis posterior and flexor hallucis longus take partial origin from back of membrane
- Tibialis anterior, long extensors of toes, and peroneus tertius take partial origin from front of membrane

Retinacula

- Superior extensor retinaculum
  - Strong, broad band
  - Stretches across front of leg from tibia to fibula, immediately above ankle joint
  - Ends attached to anterior borders of tibia and fibula
  - Long extensors, peroneus tertius, anterior tibial vessels, and deep peroneal nerve pass behind retinaculum
  - Medial part of retinaculum splits to enclose tendon of tibialis anterior, forming sling for the muscle
- Inferior extensor retinaculum: Distal to ankle joint except for attachment of one band to anterior part of medial malleolus
- Superior peroneal retinaculum
  - Thickened deep fascia securing peroneal tendons to back of lateral malleolus, peroneus longus superficial to brevis
  - Retinaculum attached to back of lateral malleolus and to lateral retrotrochlear tubercle of calcaneus
- Flexor retinaculum: Posteroinferior to medial malleolus

Muscles of Leg

- Compartments separated by deep fascia, which give partial origin to several muscles
- Posterior compartment: Superficial muscles
  - Gastrocnemius
    - Origin: Medial from posterior femoral metaphysis; lateral from posterior edge of lateral epicondyle
    - Heads separated from posterior capsule by bursa
    - 2 heads unite to form main bulk of muscle
    - Join in thin aponeurotic tendon near mid leg
    - Joins soleus aponeurosis to form Achilles tendon; concave in cross section; musculotendinous junction 5 cm above calcaneal insertion
    - Nerve supply: Tibial nerve
    - Action: Plantar flexor of ankle and flexor of knee
  - Plantaris
    - Origin: Superior and medial to lateral head of gastrocnemius origin, as well as from oblique popliteal ligament
    - Continues deep to lateral head gastrocnemius
    - Myotendinous junction at level of origin of soleus (muscle is 5-10 cm long)
    - Tendon then lies between medial head of gastrocnemius and soleus
    - Follows medial side of Achilles to insert either anteromedially on Achilles or on calcaneus
    - Plantaris absent 7-10%
    - Nerve supply: Tibial nerve
    - Action: Acts with gastrocnemius
  - Soleus
    - Origin: Extensive, from back of fibular head and upper 1/3 of posterior surface of shaft of fibula, from soleal line and middle 1/3 of medial border of tibia, and from tendinous arch joining these across popliteal vessels
    - Flat, thick, powerful muscle ends in strong tendon
    - Joins with tendon of gastrocnemius to form Achilles tendon
    - Nerve supply: Tibial nerve
    - Action: Stabilizes ankle in standing, plantarflexes ankle
    - Accessory soleus: Rare variant, arises from anterior surface of soleus or from fibula and soleal line of tibia; inserts into Achilles or onto calcaneus anteromedially to Achilles; presents as mass
- Posterior compartment: Deep muscles
  - Popliteus

Leg Radiographic Anatomy and MR Atlas

- Origin: Tendon from popliteal groove of lateral femoral condyle
- Passes through popliteal hiatus posteriorly and medially, pierces posterior capsule of knee
- Muscle fibers directed medially & downwards to insert on posterior surface of tibia above soleal line
- Nerve supply: Tibial nerve
- Action: Flexes knee and medially rotates leg at onset of flexion (unlocking extension "screwing home" mechanism)
  - Tibialis posterior
    - Origin: Interosseous membrane and adjoining parts of posterior surfaces of tibia and fibula
    - Superior end bifid; anterior tibial vessels pass forward between the 2 attachments
    - Distally it inclines medially, under flexor digitorum longus
    - Grooves and curves around medial malleolus
    - Nerve supply: Tibial nerve
    - Action: Plantarflexes and inverts foot
  - Flexor digitorum longus
    - Origin: Posterior surface of tibia, below popliteus, and medial to vertical ridge
    - Crosses superficial to distal part of tibialis posterior
    - Tendon grooves lower end of tibia lateral to that of tibialis posterior, passes around medial malleolus to foot
    - Nerve supply: Tibial nerve
    - Action: Flexes interphalangeal and metatarsophalangeal joints of lateral 4 toes; plantarflexes and inverts foot
  - Flexor hallucis longus
    - Origin: Posterior surface of fibula, below origin of soleus
    - Passes medially, descends down posterior to mid tibia
    - Associated with os trigonum posterior to talus
    - Tendon occupies deep groove on posterior surface of talus, passes around medial malleolus, to great toe
    - Nerve supply: Tibial nerves
    - Action: Flexes interphalangeal and metatarsophalangeal joints of great toe; plantar flexes foot
- Lateral compartment
  - Peroneals separated from extensors by anterior intermuscular septum and from posterior muscles by posterior septum
  - Peroneus longus
    - Origin upper 2/3 lateral surface of fibula and intermuscular septa and adjacent muscular fascia
    - Becomes tendinous a few cm above lateral malleolus
    - Curves forward behind lateral malleolus, posterior to peroneus brevis
    - Nerve supply: Superficial peroneal
    - Action: Everts foot and secondarily plantarflexes foot
  - Peroneus brevis
    - Origin lower 2/3 lateral surface of fibula and intermuscular septa and adjacent muscular fascia
    - Muscle is medial to peroneus longus at origin but overlaps peroneus longus in middle 1/3
    - Tendon curves forward behind lateral malleolus, in front of peroneus longus tendon
    - Nerve supply: Superficial peroneal
    - Action: Everts foot and secondarily plantarflexes foot
  - Synovial sheath for peroneals begins 5 cm above tip of lateral malleolus and envelopes both tendons; divides into 2 sheaths at level of calcaneus
  - Peroneus tertius (see anterior compartment)
  - **Peroneus quartus**: Accessory muscle with prevalence of 10%; originates from distal leg, frequently from peroneal muscles, with variable insertion sites at foot; at level of malleolus, located medial or posterior to both peroneal tendons
  - **Peroneus digiti minimi**: Accessory with prevalence of 15-36%; extends from peroneus brevis muscle around medial malleolus to foot; tiny tendinous slip
- Anterior compartment
  - Tibialis anterior
    - Origin upper 1/2 of lateral surface of tibia and interosseous membrane
    - Tendon originates in distal 1/3; passes through retinacula
    - Nerve supply: Deep peroneal and recurrent genicular
    - Action: Dorsiflexor and invertor of foot
  - Extensor digitorum longus
    - Origin from upper 3/4 anterior surface fibula
    - Descends behind extensor retinacula to ankle
    - Nerve supply: Deep peroneal
    - Action: Extends IP and MTP joints of lateral 4 toes, dorsiflexes foot
  - Peroneus tertius
    - Small, not always present
    - Origin: Continuous with extensor digitorum longus, arising from distal 1/4 of anterior surface of fibula and interosseous membrane
    - Inserts into dorsal surface base 5th metatarsal
    - Nerve supply: Deep peroneal
    - Action: Dorsiflexes ankle and everts foot
  - Extensor hallucis
    - Thin muscle hidden between tibialis anterior and extensor digitorum longus
    - Origin: Middle 2/4 of anterior surface of fibula and interosseous membrane
    - Tendon passes deep to retinacula to great toe
    - Nerve supply: Deep peroneal
    - Action: Extends phalanges of great toe and dorsiflexes foot

Vessels of Leg

- Popliteal artery
  - Ends at distal border of popliteus in two branches: Anterior and posterior tibial arteries
  - Paired venae comitantes of anterior and posterior tibial arteries join to form popliteal vein
- Anterior tibial artery
  - Smaller of 2 terminal branches of popliteal
  - Origin in back of leg, at distal border of popliteus muscle
  - Passes through upper part of interosseous membrane
  - Straight course down front of leg → dorsalis pedis
  - Muscular branches along length
  - Malleolar branches ramify over malleoli; lateral branch anastomoses with perforating branch of peroneal artery
- **Posterior tibial artery**

Leg Radiographic Anatomy and MR Atlas

- o Larger of 2 terminal branches of popliteal
- o Main blood supply to foot
- o Passes downwards and slightly medially along with tibial nerve to end in space between medial malleolus and calcaneus
- o Divides into lateral and medial plantar arteries
- o Branches
  - Circumflex fibular (may arise from anterior tibial), runs laterally around neck of fibula
  - Nutrient artery to tibia
  - Muscular branches
  - **Peroneal artery**: Largest branch of posterior tibial artery; runs obliquely downwards and laterally beneath soleus to fibula, along which it descends deep to flexor hallucis longus
- **Great saphenous vein**
  - o Begins at medial border of foot
  - o Ascends in front of medial malleolus
  - o Passes obliquely upwards and backwards across medial surface of distal 1/3 of tibia
  - o Passes vertically upward along medial border of tibia to posterior part of medial side of knee
- **Small saphenous vein**
  - o Extends behind lateral malleolus, ascends lateral to Achilles
  - o At midline of calf in lower popliteal region, pierces popliteal fascia and terminates in popliteal vein

Nerves of Leg

- **Common peroneal**
  - o Smaller of 2 terminal divisions of sciatic nerve
  - o Arises mid thigh, runs downward laterally along medial border of biceps femoris
  - o Crosses plantaris and lateral head of gastrocnemius, passes posterior and superficial to head of fibula
  - o This location at fibular head/neck put peroneal nerve at risk in multiple clinical situations
    - Fibular neck fracture may result in foot drop
    - Total knee replacement in a patient who had been in chronic valgus may damage nerve with realignment of knee
  - o Ends between lateral side of neck of fibula and peroneus longus by dividing into 2 terminal branches
  - o **Deep peroneal nerve**: 1st of 2 terminal branches
    - Arises lateral to neck of fibula, under peroneus longus
    - Pierces anterior intermuscular septum and extensor digitorum longus to enter anterior compartment
    - Extends down to ankle between tibialis anterior and long extensors
    - Near ankle, crossed by extensor hallucis and passes to ankle midway between malleoli
    - Muscular branches to anterior compartment and articular twig to ankle joint
    - Medial terminal branch to dorsum of foot
    - Lateral terminal branch to lateral dorsum of ankle
  - o **Superficial peroneal nerve**: 2nd of 2 terminal branches
    - Descends in substance of peroneus longus until it reaches peroneus brevis
    - Passes obliquely over anterior border of brevis and descends in groove between peroneus brevis and extensor digitorum longus
    - In distal 1/3 of leg, pierces deep fascia and divides into medial and lateral branches to foot
- **Tibial nerve**
  - o Descends under fascial septum that separates deep and superficial posterior muscle compartments
  - o In upper 2/3, lies on fascia of tibialis posterior and on flexor digitorum longus
  - o In lower 1/3, located midway between Achilles tendon and medial border of tibia
  - o Crosses posterior surfaces of tibia and ankle joint
  - o Posterior tibial vessels run with it, crossing in front of it from lateral to medial side
  - o At ankle, under flexor retinaculum, divides into lateral and medial plantar nerves
- **Saphenous nerve**
  - o Longest branch of femoral nerve, arising 2 cm below inguinal ligament and descending via adductor canal
  - o Passes posterior to sartorius, descends posteromedial to knee where it pierces deep fascia
  - o In leg, accompanies great saphenous vein
- **Sural nerve**
  - o Arises in popliteal fossa from tibial nerve
  - o Descends between 2 heads of gastrocnemius
  - o Pierces deep fascia midway between knee and ankle
  - o Accompanies small saphenous vein to lateral foot border

IMAGING ANATOMY

Anatomy Relationships

- Critical variant: 3rd head of gastrocnemius
  - o Muscular anomalies of gastrocnemius are numerous
  - o 2% show anomalous 3rd head of gastrocnemius
    - Originate from posterior distal femoral metaphysis either medially or at mid portion
    - Courses laterally to join lateral head of gastrocnemius
    - Popliteal vessels located between 3rd head and medial head of gastrocnemius
  - o These anomalies have potential for causing popliteal compression, and should be sought (axial images), but may be asymptomatic
- Critical variant: Hypertrophy of short head biceps
  - o May cause encroachment on fat surrounding common peroneal nerve
  - o Abnormalities which may cause peroneal neuropathy
    - Hypertrophied short head biceps
    - Distal extension of long head of biceps
    - Prominent lateral head of gastrocnemius
    - Diabetics may accumulate excess fat around peroneal nerve at fibular neck

Leg Radiographic Anatomy and MR Atlas

GRAPHICS: MUSCLE ATTACHMENTS

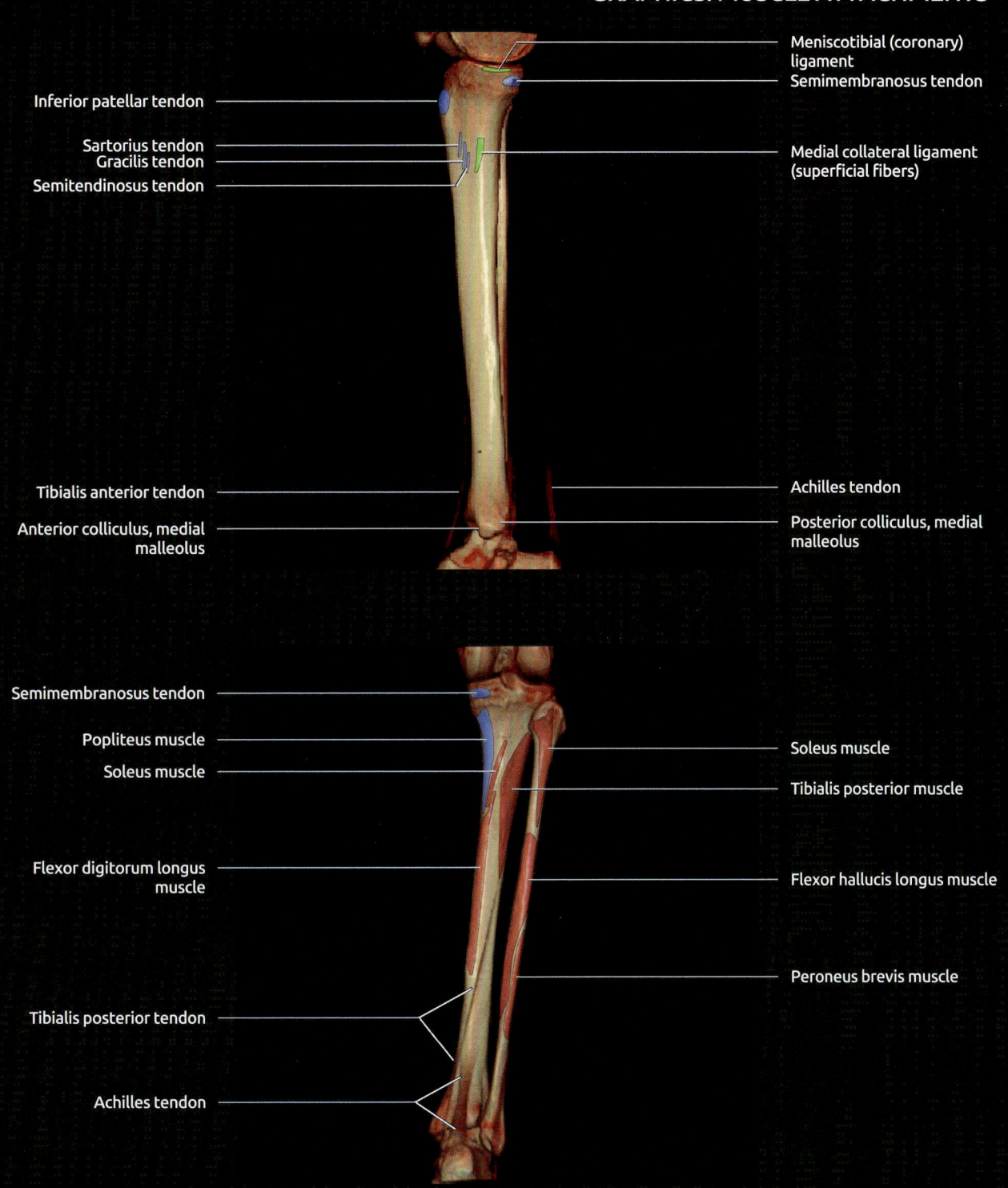

- Inferior patellar tendon
- Sartorius tendon
- Gracilis tendon
- Semitendinosus tendon
- Tibialis anterior tendon
- Anterior colliculus, medial malleolus
- Meniscotibial (coronary) ligament
- Semimembranosus tendon
- Medial collateral ligament (superficial fibers)
- Achilles tendon
- Posterior colliculus, medial malleolus

- Semimembranosus tendon
- Popliteus muscle
- Soleus muscle
- Flexor digitorum longus muscle
- Tibialis posterior tendon
- Achilles tendon
- Soleus muscle
- Tibialis posterior muscle
- Flexor hallucis longus muscle
- Peroneus brevis muscle

(**Top**) *View of the medial leg is shown. Other than insertions of the pes anserinus and medial collateral ligament proximally, the medial tibial surface is subcutaneous.* (**Bottom**) *Posterior view of the leg is shown. Note the large surface area that serves as origin of muscles from the tibia and fibula. The interosseous septum extends this surface area.*

Leg Radiographic Anatomy and MR Atlas

GRAPHICS: MUSCLE ATTACHMENTS

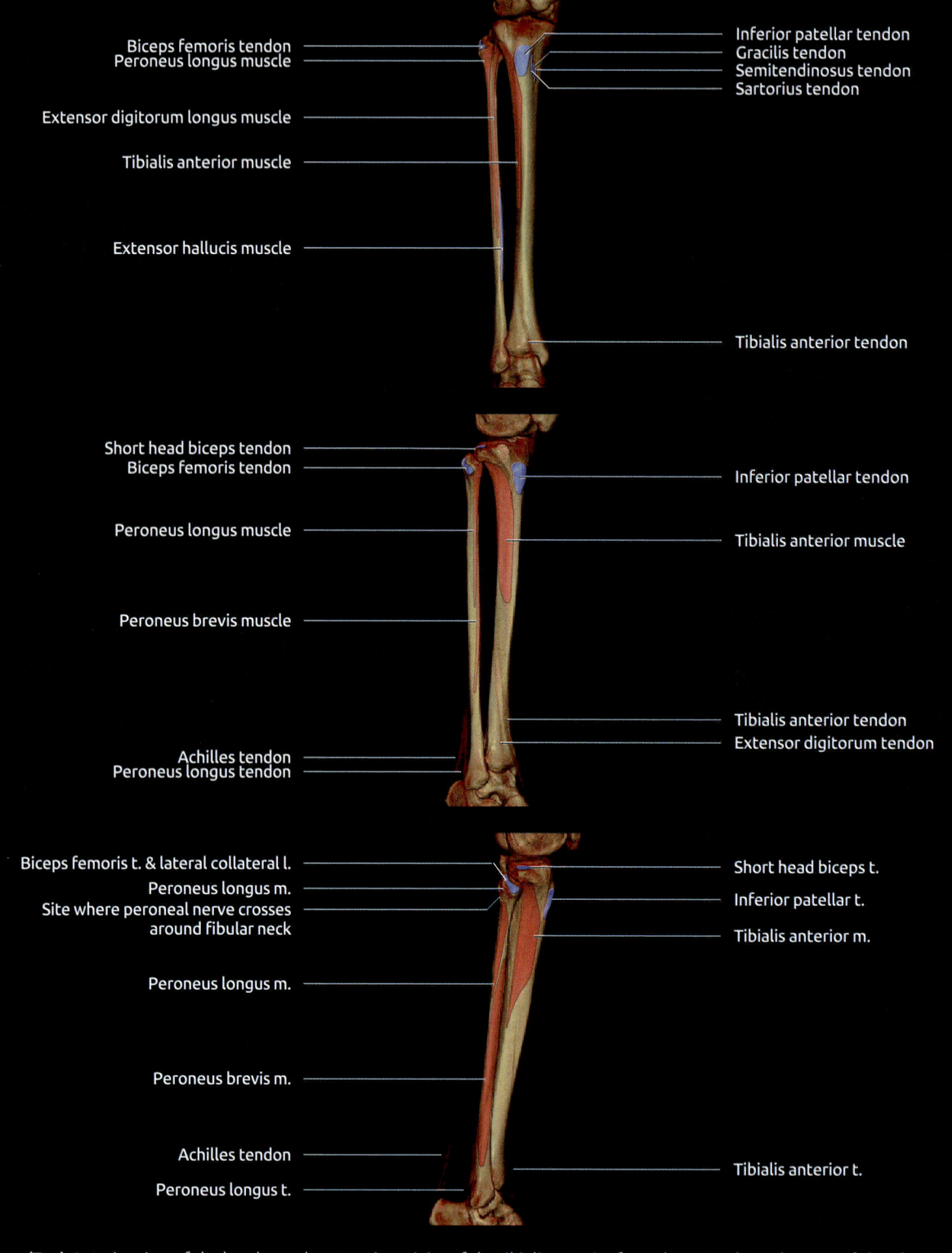

Labels (top, anterior view): Biceps femoris tendon; Peroneus longus muscle; Extensor digitorum longus muscle; Tibialis anterior muscle; Extensor hallucis muscle; Inferior patellar tendon; Gracilis tendon; Semitendinosus tendon; Sartorius tendon; Tibialis anterior tendon.

Labels (middle, anterior view internally rotated): Short head biceps tendon; Biceps femoris tendon; Peroneus longus muscle; Peroneus brevis muscle; Achilles tendon; Peroneus longus tendon; Inferior patellar tendon; Tibialis anterior muscle; Tibialis anterior tendon; Extensor digitorum tendon.

Labels (bottom, lateral view): Biceps femoris t. & lateral collateral l.; Peroneus longus m.; Site where peroneal nerve crosses around fibular neck; Peroneus longus m.; Peroneus brevis m.; Achilles tendon; Peroneus longus t.; Short head biceps t.; Inferior patellar t.; Tibialis anterior m.; Tibialis anterior t.

(Top) *Anterior view of the leg shows the extensive origins of the tibialis anterior from the anterolateral aspect of the tibia and the long origins of the peroneus longus, extensor hallucis, and extensor digitorum longus from the fibula. These muscles also all have extensive origin from the interosseous membrane.* **(Middle)** *Anterior view of leg, internally rotated, shows the extensive origins of tibialis anterior, peroneus longus, and peroneus brevis.* **(Bottom)** *Lateral view of the leg is shown. Note that the peroneus longus is shown as having 2 separate origins, so that the site of passage of the common peroneal nerve around the neck of the fibula is seen. Also note that there is some overlap of sites of origin of the peroneus longus and brevis from the anterolateral fibula, with peroneus longus originating in the upper 2/3 and brevis in the lower 2/3 of the bone.*

Leg Radiographic Anatomy and MR Atlas

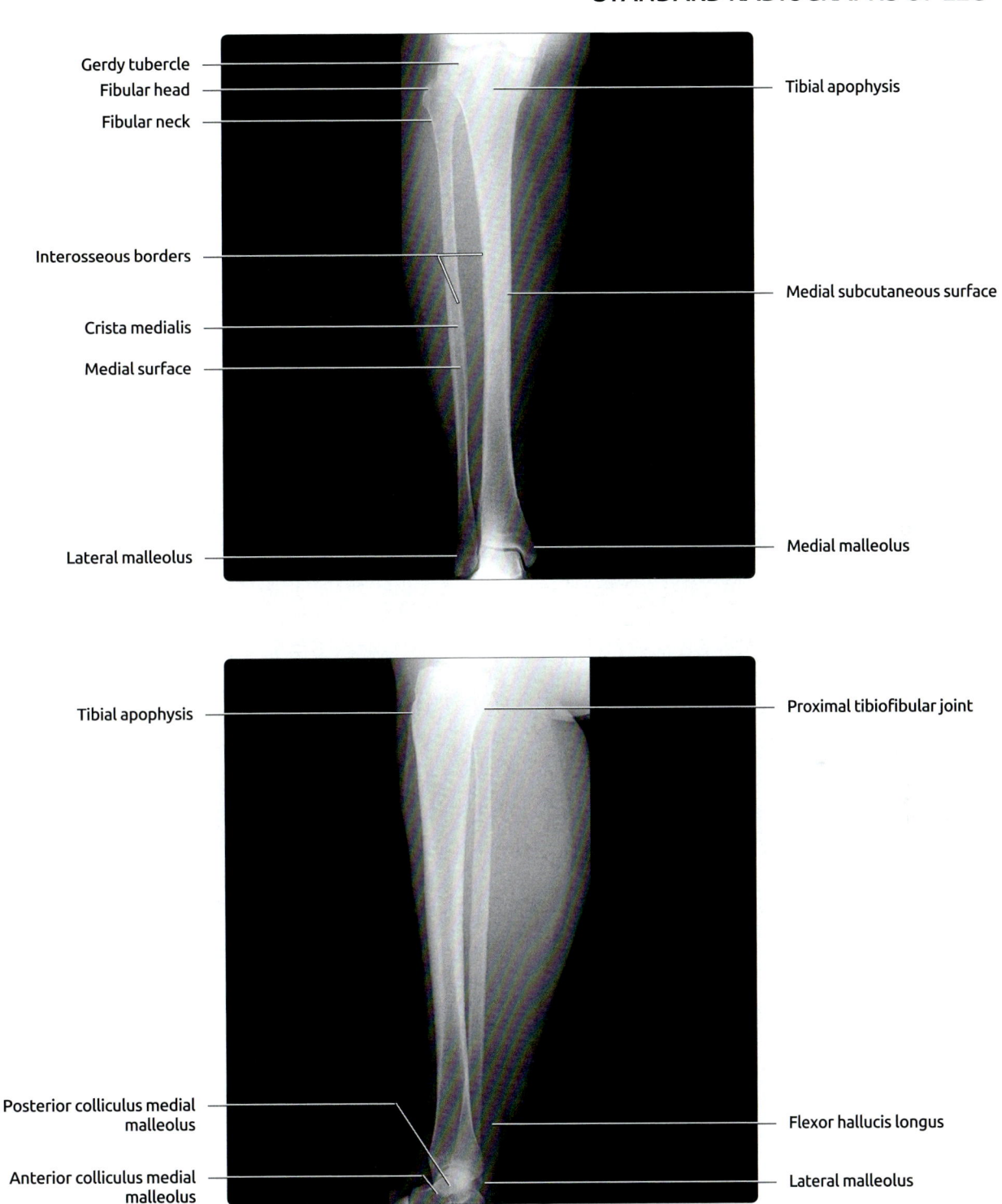

STANDARD RADIOGRAPHS OF LEG

Labels (top image): Gerdy tubercle; Fibular head; Fibular neck; Interosseous borders; Crista medialis; Medial surface; Lateral malleolus; Tibial apophysis; Medial subcutaneous surface; Medial malleolus

Labels (bottom image): Tibial apophysis; Posterior colliculus medial malleolus; Anterior colliculus medial malleolus; Proximal tibiofibular joint; Flexor hallucis longus; Lateral malleolus

(Top) Anteroposterior radiograph shows the leg. Note that the fibula is slightly posterolateral to the tibia, and that there is expected overlap at both the proximal and distal tibiofibular joints. The interosseous borders of both long bones are often irregular; this relates to the insertion of the strong interosseous membrane and is not periosteal reaction. The lateral malleolus extends 1 cm farther distal than the medial malleolus. **(Bottom)** Lateral radiograph shows the leg. As on the anteroposterior view, there is overlap of the bones at both the proximal and distal tibiofibular joints. At the ankle, both the colliculi of the medial malleolus can be seen, along with the slightly longer lateral malleolus.

Leg Radiographic Anatomy and MR Atlas

GRAPHICS: POSTERIOR SUPERFICIAL MUSCLES

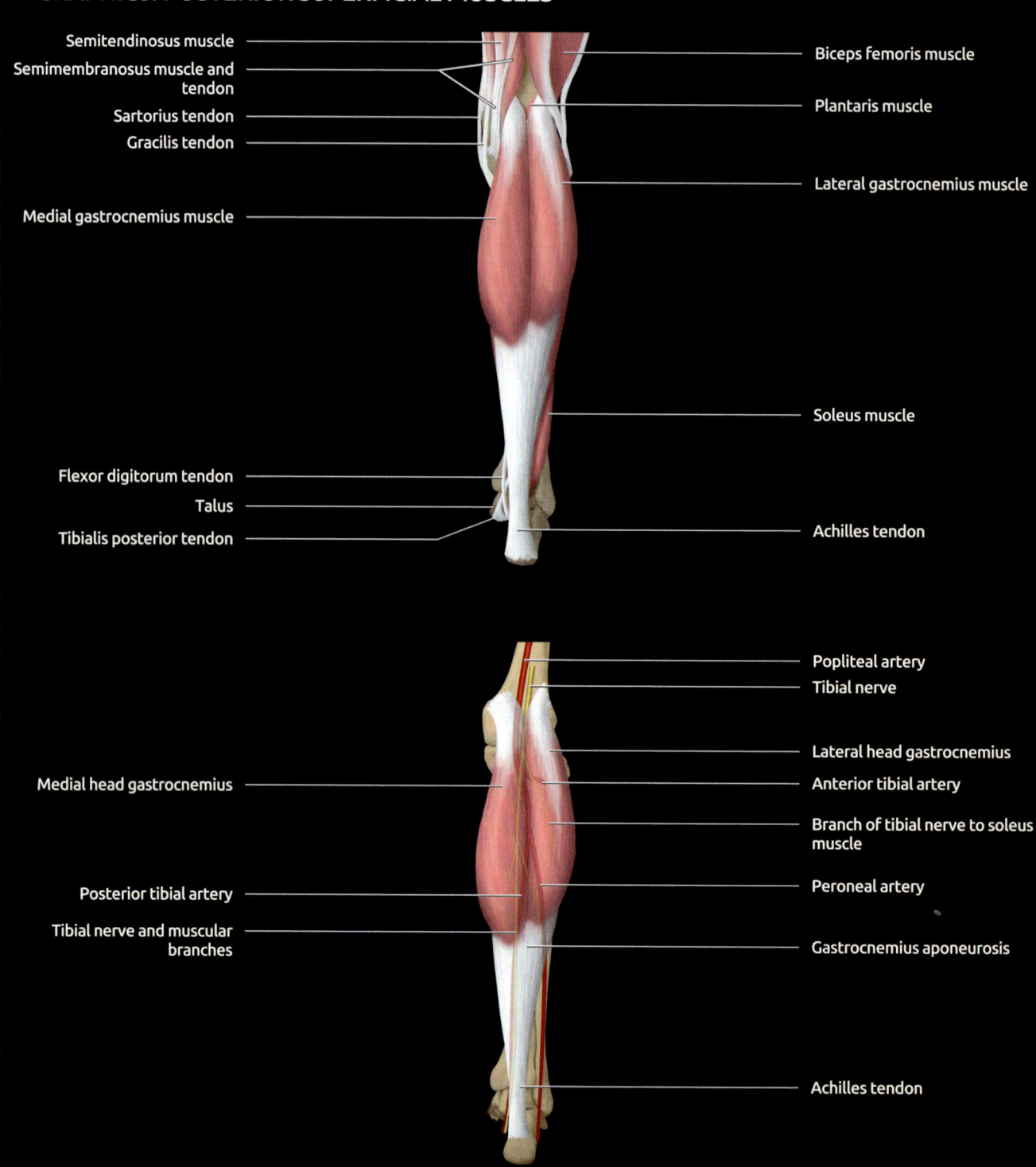

(Top) Posterior view of superficial muscles and tendons of the leg. The gastrocnemius muscles are bulky in the proximal half of the leg and taper to an aponeurosis that blends with the soleus more distally to become the Achilles tendon. (Bottom) Posterior view shows the gastrocnemius muscles, with the plantaris and proximal muscles removed. The medial head arises from the posterior femoral metaphysis, and the lateral head arises from the posterior edge of the lateral epicondyle (just lateral to the origin of plantaris muscle). The 2 heads unite to form the main bulk of muscle that extends as far as mid leg. The muscles then form a thin aponeurotic tendon at mid leg and extend distally. After the soleus joins the aponeurotic tendon of the gastrocnemius at the distal leg (~ 10 cm proximal to the calcaneus), the strong Achilles continues to its attachment at the posterior tuberosity of the calcaneus.

Leg Radiographic Anatomy and MR Atlas

GRAPHICS: SOLEUS, PLANTARIS, NEUROVASCULAR STRUCTURES

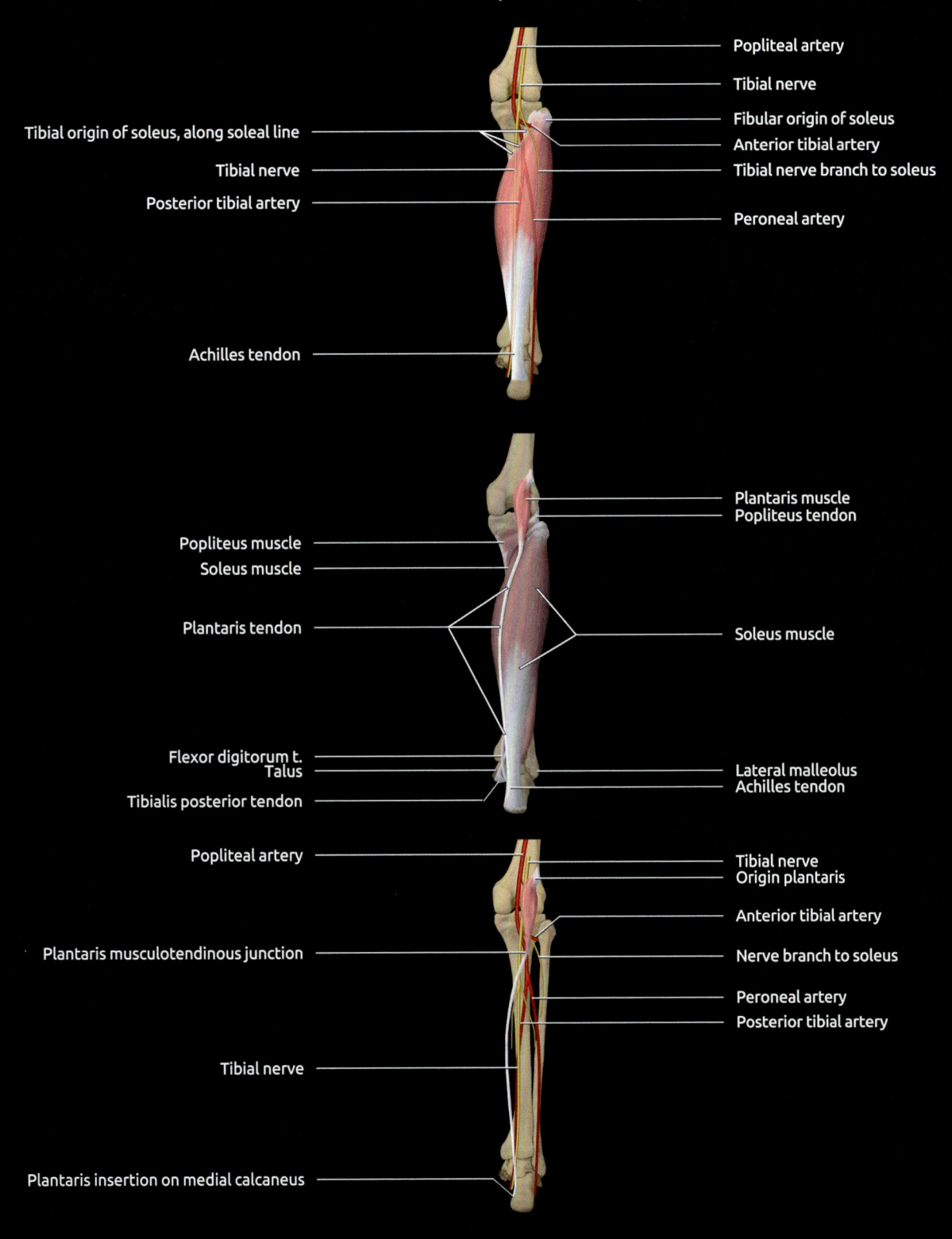

(Top) Posterior view of the soleus shows its extensive lateral origin from the back of the fibular head and the upper 1/3 of its shaft. The medial portion originates from the medial border of the tibia and the soleal line on the posterior tibia. There is a thick tendinous arch joining the medial and lateral origins of the soleus across the popliteal vessels. Distal to this arch, the neurovascular bundle lies deep to the soleus. (Middle) Graphic shows the course of the plantaris muscle and tendon. The origin of the plantaris is superficial, adjacent to the origin of the lateral gastrocnemius. The muscle is fleshy over a short distance. The tendon then continues to course distally, located between the soleus (anterior to plantaris) and medial gastrocnemius (posterior to plantaris). The plantaris tendon moves slightly medially over this course. It becomes superficial once the soleus joins the Achilles tendon, and inserts either on the Achilles or the calcaneus, medial to the Achilles. (Bottom) Graphic shows a posterior view of the plantaris with all other muscle structures deleted.

Leg Radiographic Anatomy and MR Atlas

GRAPHIC AND MR: POPLITEUS

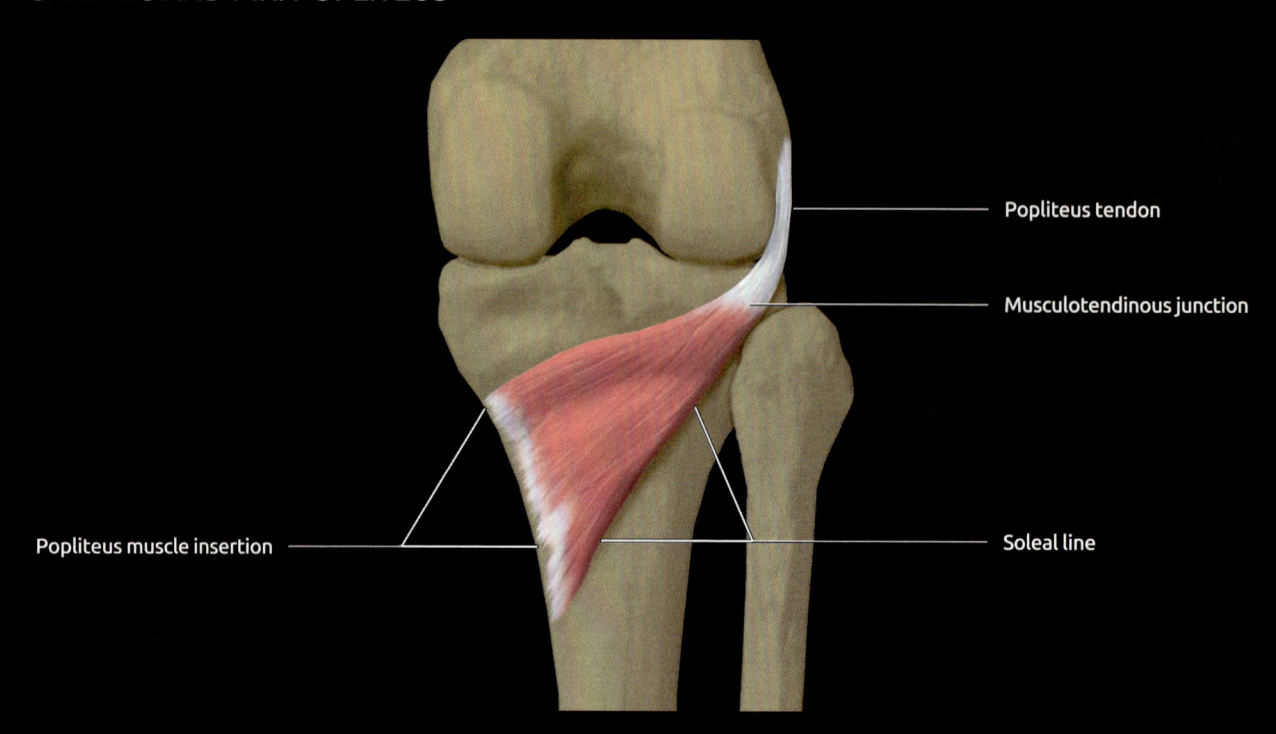

- Popliteus tendon
- Musculotendinous junction
- Popliteus muscle insertion
- Soleal line

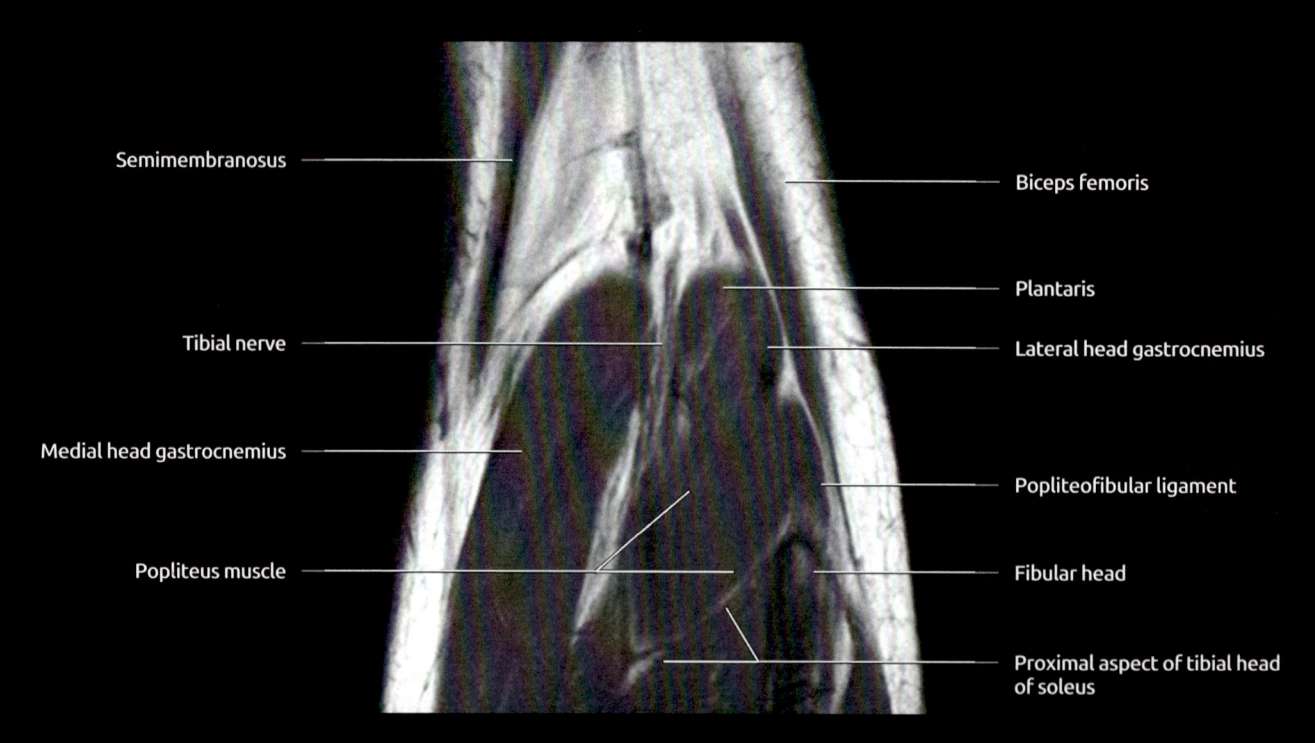

- Semimembranosus
- Biceps femoris
- Plantaris
- Tibial nerve
- Lateral head gastrocnemius
- Medial head gastrocnemius
- Popliteofibular ligament
- Popliteus muscle
- Fibular head
- Proximal aspect of tibial head of soleus

(**Top**) *Graphic shows the complicated path of the popliteus tendon and muscle. After the popliteus tendon arises from the sulcus at the lateral femoral condyle, it passes through the popliteal hiatus and then expands to the musculotendinous junction. The muscle broadens over a large area of the proximal posterior tibia to insert at the posteromedial tibia, immediately proximal to the tibial origin of the tibial head of the soleus.* (**Bottom**) *Posterior coronal T1 MR image shows the large popliteus muscle, which is found deep to the popliteal vessels and gastrocnemius muscles. Note that in this example the popliteus muscle fibers are oriented superolateral to inferomedial, as opposed to the portion of gastrocnemius seen which runs superoinferior. The proximal aspect of the tibial head of soleus is located at the distal aspect of the popliteus insertion on the tibia.*

Leg Radiographic Anatomy and MR Atlas

GRAPHICS: POSTERIOR DEEP MUSCLES OF LEG

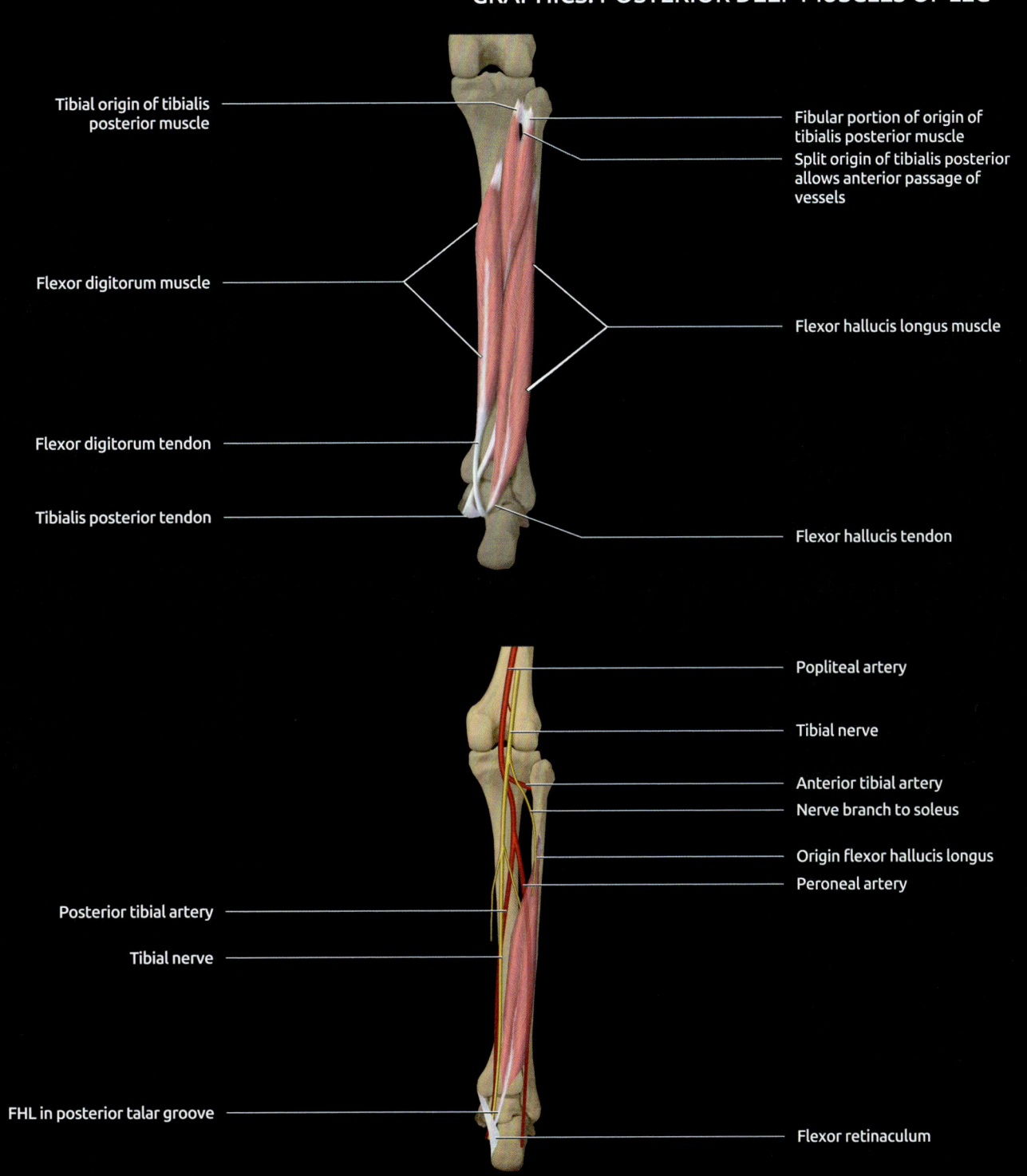

- Tibial origin of tibialis posterior muscle
- Flexor digitorum muscle
- Flexor digitorum tendon
- Tibialis posterior tendon
- Fibular portion of origin of tibialis posterior muscle
- Split origin of tibialis posterior allows anterior passage of vessels
- Flexor hallucis longus muscle
- Flexor hallucis tendon

- Posterior tibial artery
- Tibial nerve
- FHL in posterior talar groove
- Popliteal artery
- Tibial nerve
- Anterior tibial artery
- Nerve branch to soleus
- Origin flexor hallucis longus
- Peroneal artery
- Flexor retinaculum

(Top) Graphic shows the deep muscles of the leg. Flexor hallucis longus is the largest of the muscles; its muscular portion extends far distal to the others, becoming tendinous at the level of the talus. The tibialis posterior originates from the interosseous membrane and adjoining parts of the posterior surfaces of the tibia and fibula; its tendon crosses anteriorly to the tendon of flexor digitorum longus, so that it is the most medial of the 3 tendons coursing around the medial malleolus. (Bottom) Graphic of the flexor hallucis longus (FHL) which originates from the posterior surface of the fibula, below the origin of the soleus. It passes medially and descends distally posterior to the peroneal artery. It passes through 3 fibro-osseous tunnels. The 1st is between the medial and lateral talar tubercles on the posterior talus. The 2nd is in a groove under the sustentaculum tali. The 3rd is between the medial and lateral sesamoids of the great toe to its insertion on the base of the distal phalanx.

Leg Radiographic Anatomy and MR Atlas

GRAPHICS: FLEXOR DIGITORUM LONGUS & TIBIALIS POSTERIOR

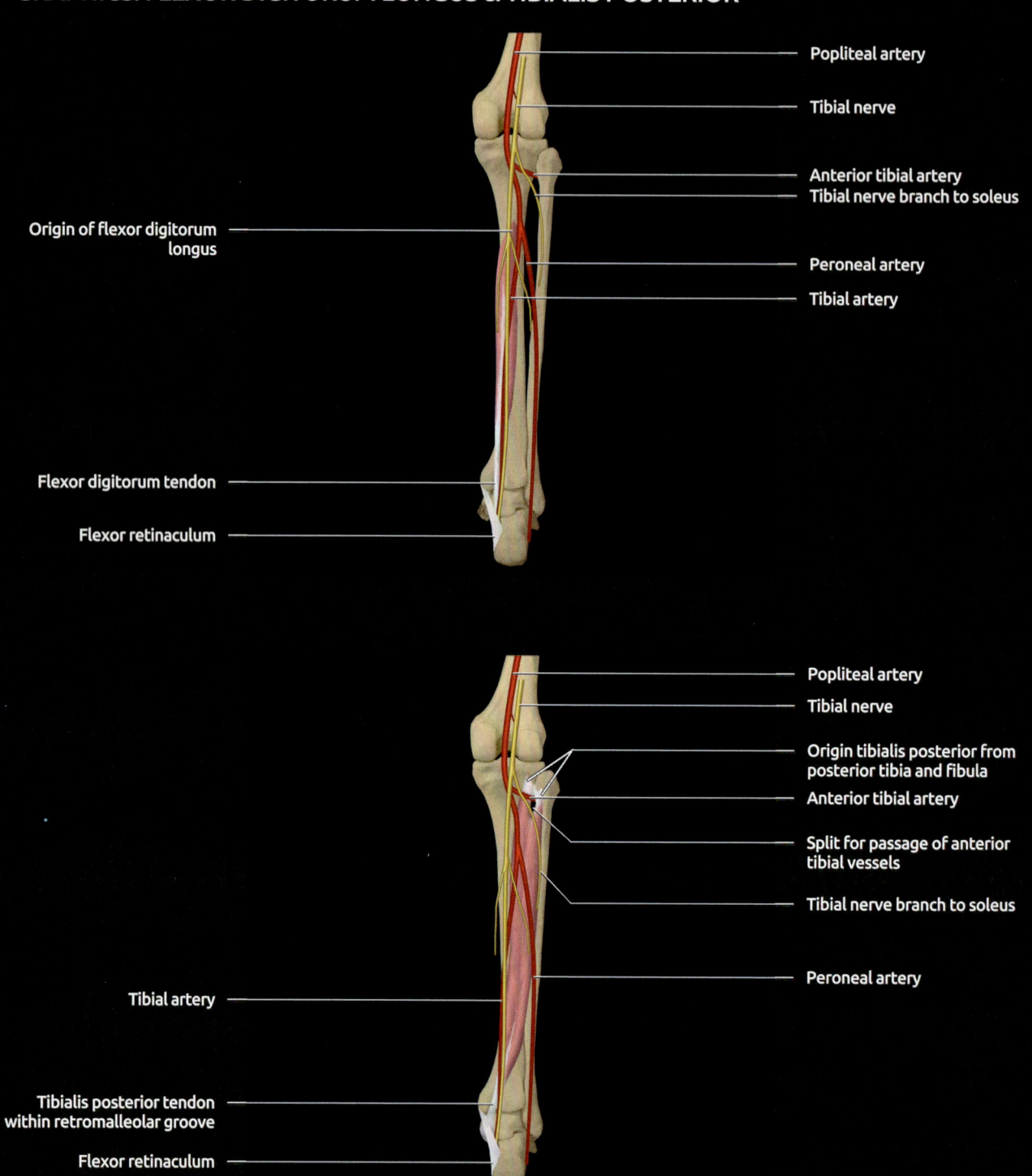

Labels (top graphic):
- Popliteal artery
- Tibial nerve
- Anterior tibial artery
- Tibial nerve branch to soleus
- Origin of flexor digitorum longus
- Peroneal artery
- Tibial artery
- Flexor digitorum tendon
- Flexor retinaculum

Labels (bottom graphic):
- Popliteal artery
- Tibial nerve
- Origin tibialis posterior from posterior tibia and fibula
- Anterior tibial artery
- Split for passage of anterior tibial vessels
- Tibial nerve branch to soleus
- Peroneal artery
- Tibial artery
- Tibialis posterior tendon within retromalleolar groove
- Flexor retinaculum

(**Top**) *Graphic of the flexor digitorum longus shows the origin at the posterior surface of the tibia, below the popliteus. It crosses superficial to the distal part of the tibialis posterior to become tendinous at the level of the distal leg. The tendon passes in a groove at the lower end of the tibia, lateral to the tibialis posterior tendon and passes around the medial malleolus. It crosses the flexor hallucis longus tendon at the master knot of Henry and proceeds to its insertions on the bases of digits 2-5.* (**Bottom**) *Graphic of the tibialis posterior shows its origin from adjacent areas of the posterior fibula, tibia, and interosseous membrane. The superior aspect is bifid, allowing anterior passage of the anterior tibial vessels. Distally, the muscle inclines medially, beneath the flexor digitorum longus. The tendon passes in a groove around the medial malleolus, medial to the tendon of flexor digitorum longus. There are multiple sites of insertion, including the navicular tuberosity, cuneiforms, sustentaculum tali and bases of the 2nd through 4th metatarsals.*

Leg Radiographic Anatomy and MR Atlas

GRAPHICS: ANTERIOR LEG MUSCLES

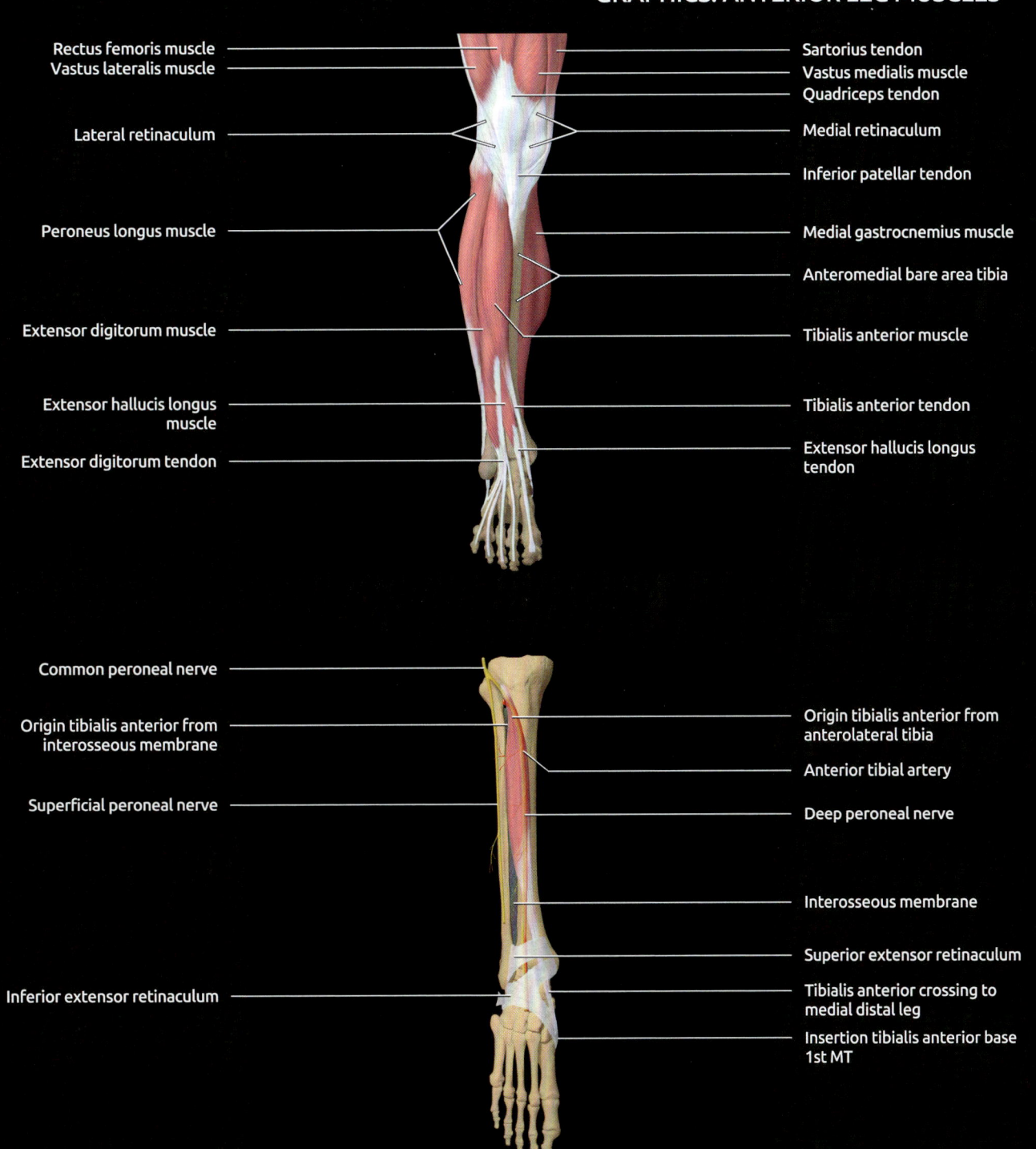

(Top) Graphic shows the anterior leg muscles. Note that nearly the entire anteromedial tibia is bare of muscle; it is thus poorly vascularized, resulting in slow fracture healing. The tibialis anterior has an extensive origin from both tibia and interosseous membrane and is the most substantial muscle of the anterior compartment. The extensor digitorum originates from the fibula. The extensor hallucis longus originates between the tibialis anterior and extensor digitorum, from the fibula and interosseous membrane. These 3 muscles retain the same orientation as they become tendinous, anterior to the ankle. (Bottom) Graphic of the tibialis anterior shows its origin from the upper half of the lateral surface of the tibia and the interosseous membrane. The tendon originates at the distal third and passes beneath the flexor retinacula. The tibialis anterior is the most medial and largest tendon in the anterior compartment. It inserts on the medial and plantar surface of the medial cuneiform and the base of the 1st metatarsal.

Leg Radiographic Anatomy and MR Atlas

GRAPHICS: EXTENSOR DIGITORUM MUSCLE & EXTENSOR HALLUCIS LONGUS

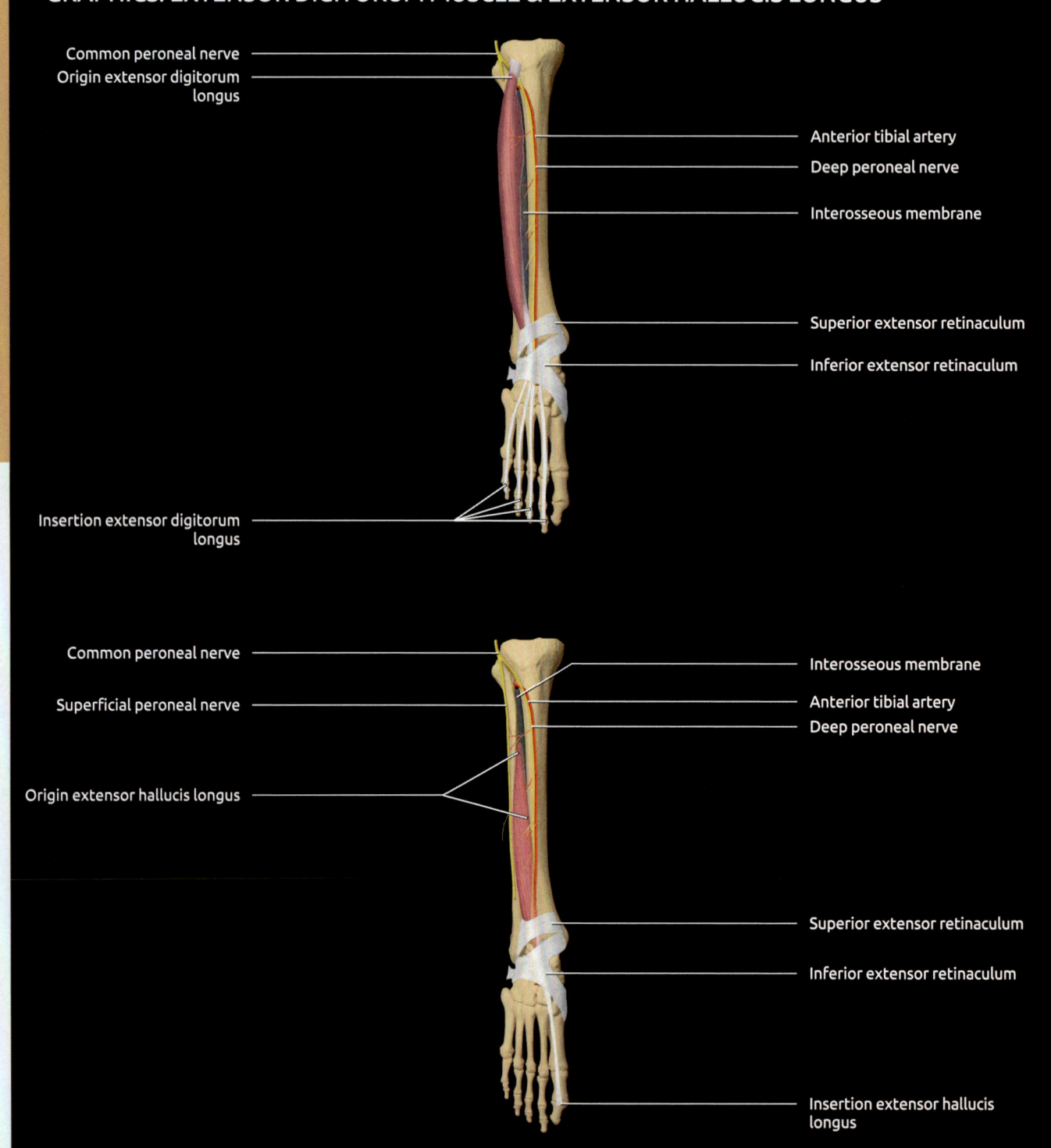

(Top) Graphic of the extensor digitorum longus shows the origin from the lateral aspect of the tibial condyle, the anteromedial aspect of the proximal fibula and the interosseous membrane. It passes beneath the extensor retinacula where it divides into 4 slips. These slips receive tendinous contributions from the extensor digitorum brevis, the lumbricals, and the interosseous muscles. Each slip accepts slips from the extensor digitorum brevis, which insert at the base of middle phalanges, with the tendon continuing to its terminal insertion on the bases of distal phalanges 2-5. *(Bottom)* Graphic shows the extensor hallucis longus, with tibialis anterior, flexor digitorum longus, and lateral compartment muscles peeled away. The extensor hallucis longus originates from the anterior aspect of the mid fibula (over its middle 2/4) and the adjacent interosseous membrane. It passes beneath the extensor retinacula to insert on the dorsal base of the distal phalanx of the great toe.

Leg Radiographic Anatomy and MR Atlas

GRAPHICS: PERONEUS TERTIUS AND LATERAL LEG MUSCLES

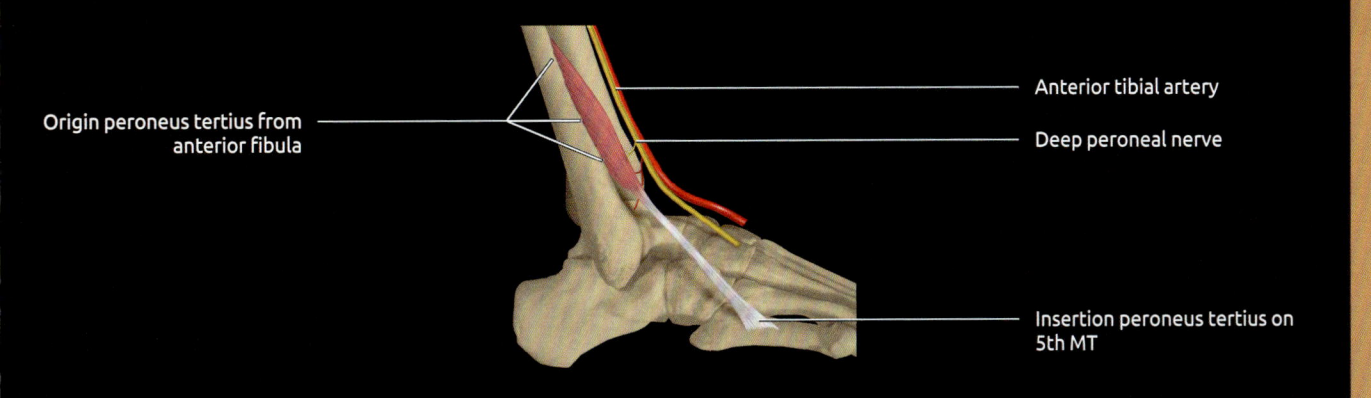

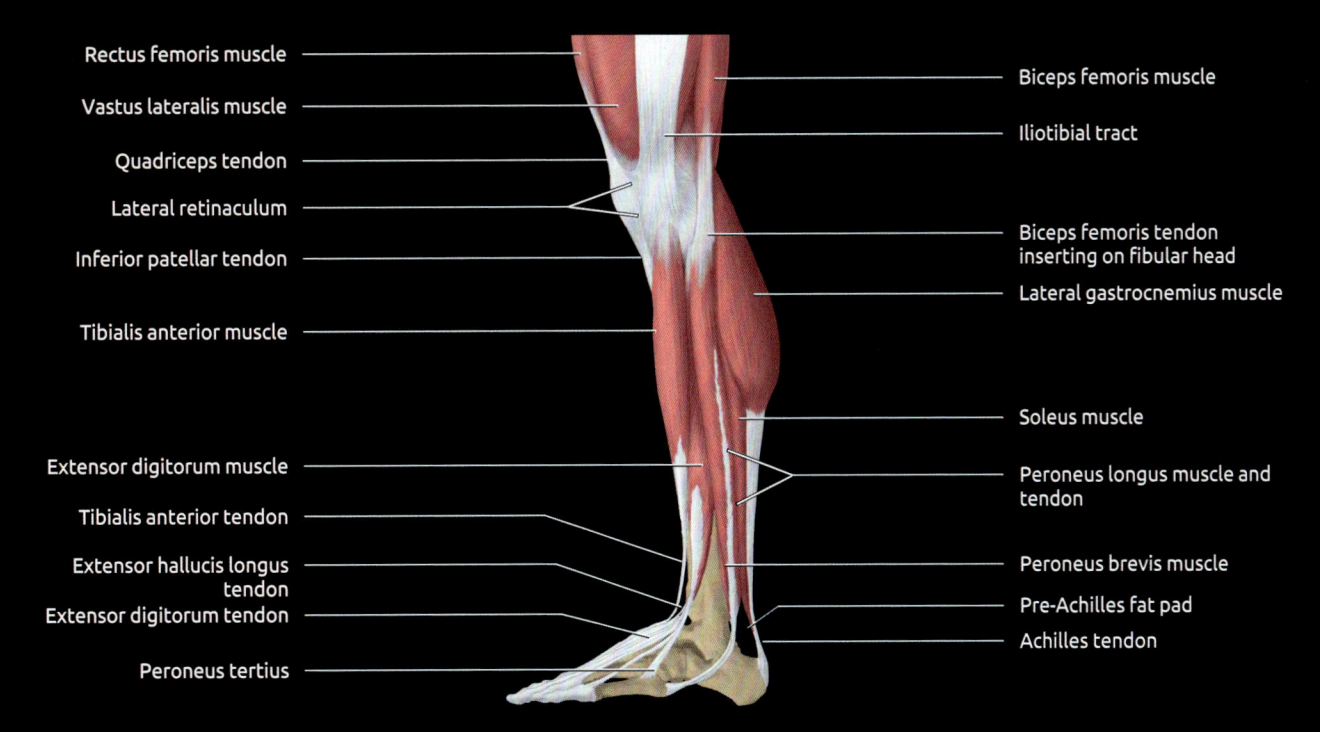

(Top) Graphic of the peroneus tertius, with all other extensors and lateral compartment muscles peeled away. The peroneus tertius is a lateral slip of the extensor digitorum longus. Its origin is along the anterior aspect of the distal fibula. It inserts on the dorsal aspect of the proximal shaft of the 5th metatarsal. (Bottom) Graphic of the lateral leg shows the anterior compartment (extensors), lateral compartment (peroneals), and superficial muscles of the posterior compartment.

Leg Radiographic Anatomy and MR Atlas

GRAPHICS: PERONEUS LONGUS & PERONEUS BREVIS MUSCLES

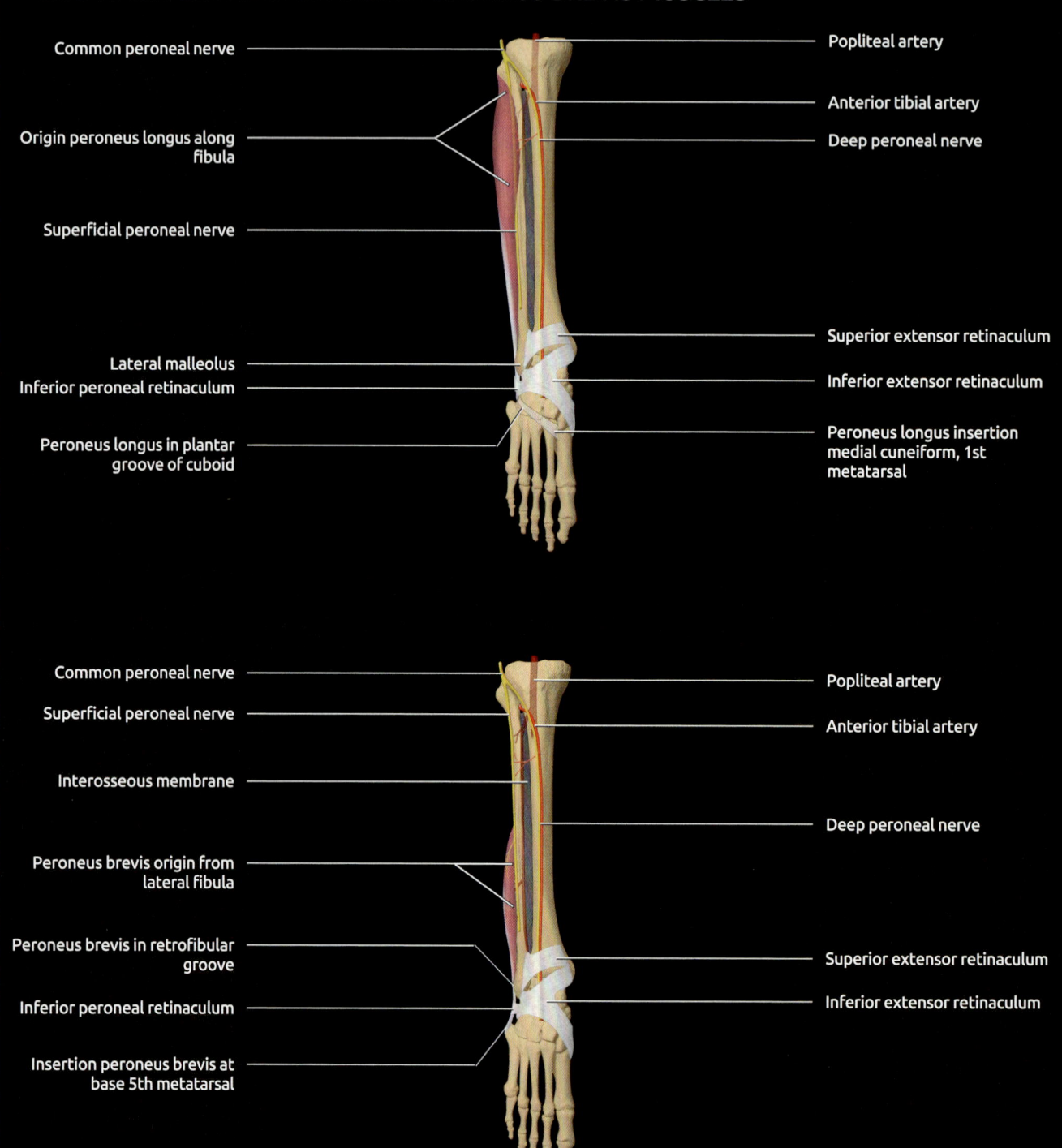

Common peroneal nerve

Origin peroneus longus along fibula

Superficial peroneal nerve

Lateral malleolus
Inferior peroneal retinaculum

Peroneus longus in plantar groove of cuboid

Popliteal artery

Anterior tibial artery

Deep peroneal nerve

Superior extensor retinaculum

Inferior extensor retinaculum

Peroneus longus insertion medial cuneiform, 1st metatarsal

Common peroneal nerve
Superficial peroneal nerve

Interosseous membrane

Peroneus brevis origin from lateral fibula

Peroneus brevis in retrofibular groove

Inferior peroneal retinaculum

Insertion peroneus brevis at base 5th metatarsal

Popliteal artery

Anterior tibial artery

Deep peroneal nerve

Superior extensor retinaculum

Inferior extensor retinaculum

(**Top**) Graphic of the peroneus longus (PL) shows its origin from the upper 2/3 of the lateral fibula and the adjacent intermuscular septa/fascia. It extends distally and becomes tendinous a few centimeters above the lateral malleolus. It curves forward around the lateral malleolus, posterolateral to the peroneus brevis (PB) tendon within the retrofibular groove. It passes deep to the superior retinaculum, then crosses the lateral calcaneus behind the peroneal tubercle, deep to the inferior peroneal retinaculum, and curves under the cuboid to insert on the bases of the medial cuneiform and 1st metatarsal. (**Bottom**) Graphic of the PB shows its origin from the inferior 2/3 of the lateral aspect of the fibula and the adjacent intermuscular septa/fascia. It lies medial to the PL at its origin but overlaps the PL in its middle 1/3, then lies anteromedial to the PL in the retrofibular groove, deep to the superior peroneal retinaculum. It descends anterior to the calcaneal peroneal tubercle to insert at the base of the 5th metatarsal.

Leg Radiographic Anatomy and MR Atlas

GRAPHICS: LEG VESSELS & NERVES

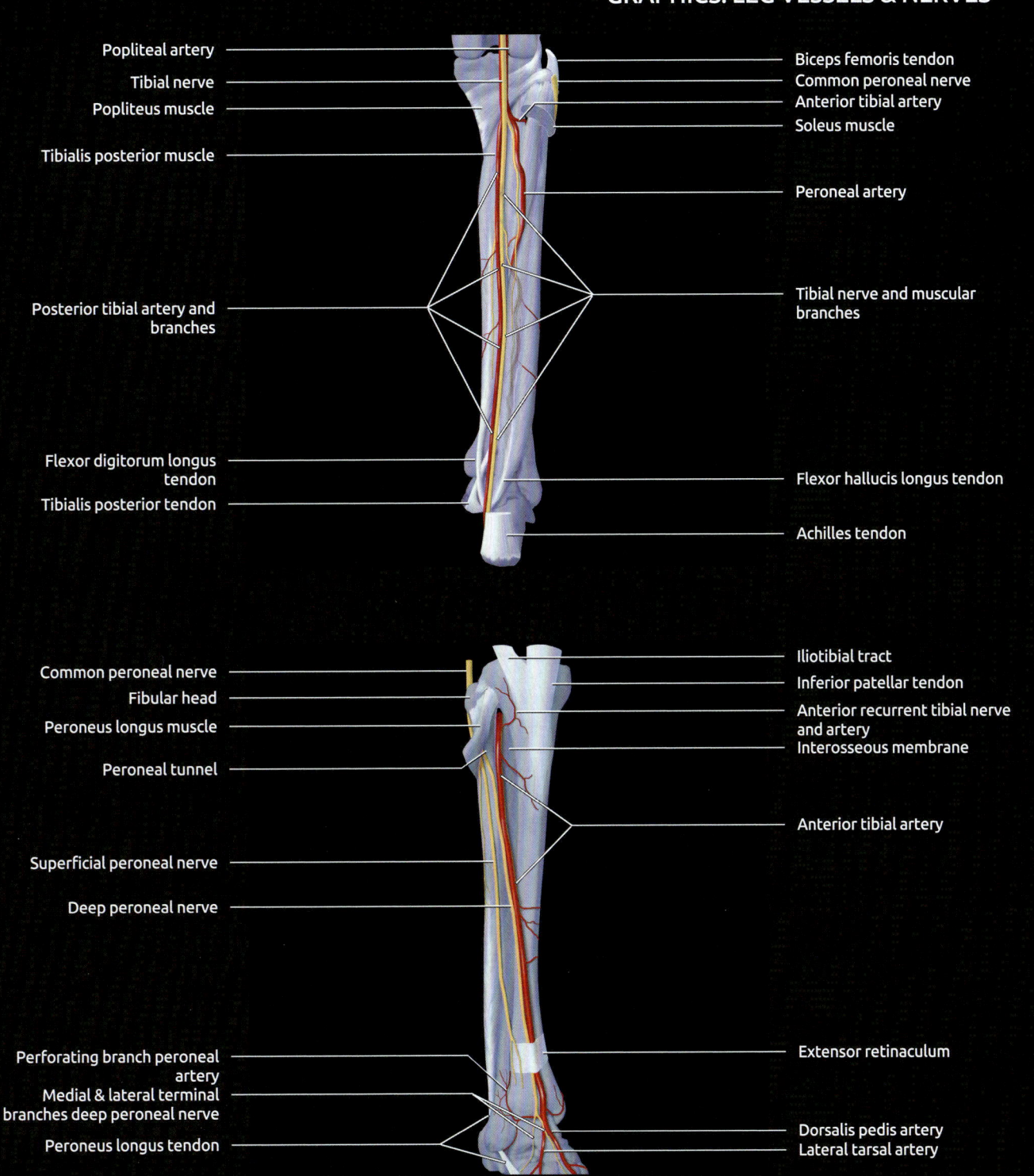

Popliteal artery
Tibial nerve
Popliteus muscle
Tibialis posterior muscle

Posterior tibial artery and branches

Flexor digitorum longus tendon
Tibialis posterior tendon

Biceps femoris tendon
Common peroneal nerve
Anterior tibial artery
Soleus muscle

Peroneal artery

Tibial nerve and muscular branches

Flexor hallucis longus tendon

Achilles tendon

Common peroneal nerve
Fibular head
Peroneus longus muscle
Peroneal tunnel

Superficial peroneal nerve
Deep peroneal nerve

Perforating branch peroneal artery
Medial & lateral terminal branches deep peroneal nerve
Peroneus longus tendon

Iliotibial tract
Inferior patellar tendon
Anterior recurrent tibial nerve and artery
Interosseous membrane

Anterior tibial artery

Extensor retinaculum

Dorsalis pedis artery
Lateral tarsal artery

(Top) Graphic shows the anterior tibial artery passing through a slit in the tibialis posterior muscle and interosseous membrane to the anterior compartment. The posterior tibial artery passes downwards and slightly medially, adjacent to the tibial nerve. The largest branch of the posterior tibial artery is the peroneal, which runs obliquely downwards and laterally beneath the soleus to the fibula. The common peroneal nerve follows posterior to the biceps and around the lateral fibular neck. The tibial nerve descends between the deep and superficial posterior leg muscles, paralleling the posterior tibial artery. (Bottom) Graphic of the anterior leg shows the anterior tibial artery perforating the interosseous septum proximally and descending along this membrane down the front of the leg to terminate as the dorsalis pedis. The common peroneal nerve is seen extending through the peroneal tunnel, branching into deep and superficial components. The deep peroneal nerve parallels the anterior tibial artery and terminates in medial and lateral branches.

Leg Radiographic Anatomy and MR Atlas

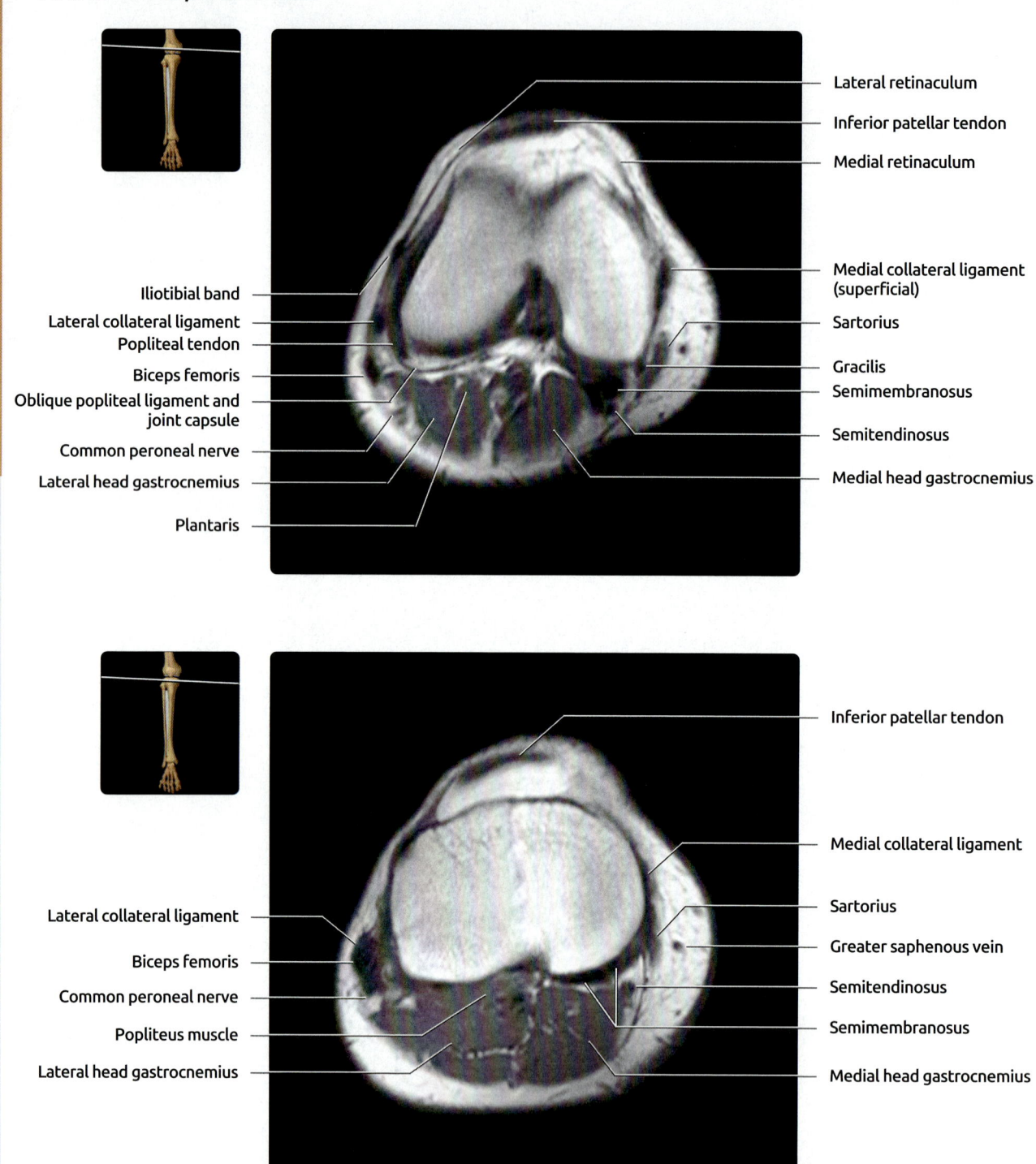

AXIAL T1 MR, RIGHT LEG

Labels (top image):
- Lateral retinaculum
- Inferior patellar tendon
- Medial retinaculum
- Medial collateral ligament (superficial)
- Sartorius
- Gracilis
- Semimembranosus
- Semitendinosus
- Medial head gastrocnemius
- Iliotibial band
- Lateral collateral ligament
- Popliteal tendon
- Biceps femoris
- Oblique popliteal ligament and joint capsule
- Common peroneal nerve
- Lateral head gastrocnemius
- Plantaris

Labels (bottom image):
- Inferior patellar tendon
- Medial collateral ligament
- Sartorius
- Greater saphenous vein
- Semitendinosus
- Semimembranosus
- Medial head gastrocnemius
- Lateral collateral ligament
- Biceps femoris
- Common peroneal nerve
- Popliteus muscle
- Lateral head gastrocnemius

(Top) *First in a series of axial T1 MR images of the right leg; this is just above the knee joint, included for continuity of structures.*
(Bottom) *Axial T1 MR image shows the right leg, just below the knee joint.*

Leg Radiographic Anatomy and MR Atlas

AXIAL T1 MR, LEFT LEG

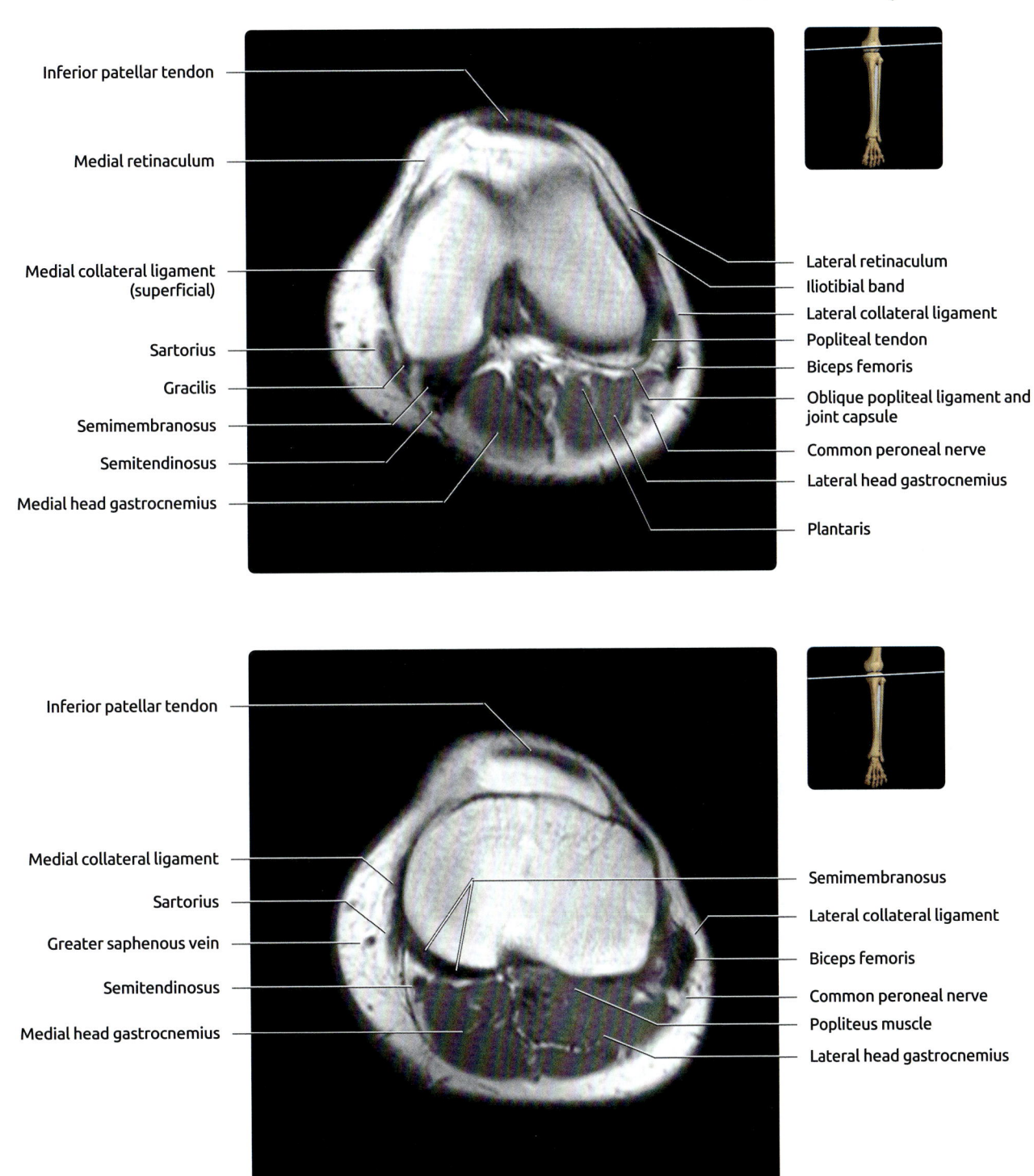

Top image labels (left side):
- Inferior patellar tendon
- Medial retinaculum
- Medial collateral ligament (superficial)
- Sartorius
- Gracilis
- Semimembranosus
- Semitendinosus
- Medial head gastrocnemius

Top image labels (right side):
- Lateral retinaculum
- Iliotibial band
- Lateral collateral ligament
- Popliteal tendon
- Biceps femoris
- Oblique popliteal ligament and joint capsule
- Common peroneal nerve
- Lateral head gastrocnemius
- Plantaris

Bottom image labels (left side):
- Inferior patellar tendon
- Medial collateral ligament
- Sartorius
- Greater saphenous vein
- Semitendinosus
- Medial head gastrocnemius

Bottom image labels (right side):
- Semimembranosus
- Lateral collateral ligament
- Biceps femoris
- Common peroneal nerve
- Popliteus muscle
- Lateral head gastrocnemius

(Top) *First in series of axial T1 MR images of the left leg; this is just above the knee joint, included for continuity of structures* (Bottom) *Axial MR image shows the left leg, just below the knee joint.*

Leg Radiographic Anatomy and MR Atlas

AXIAL T1 MR, RIGHT LEG

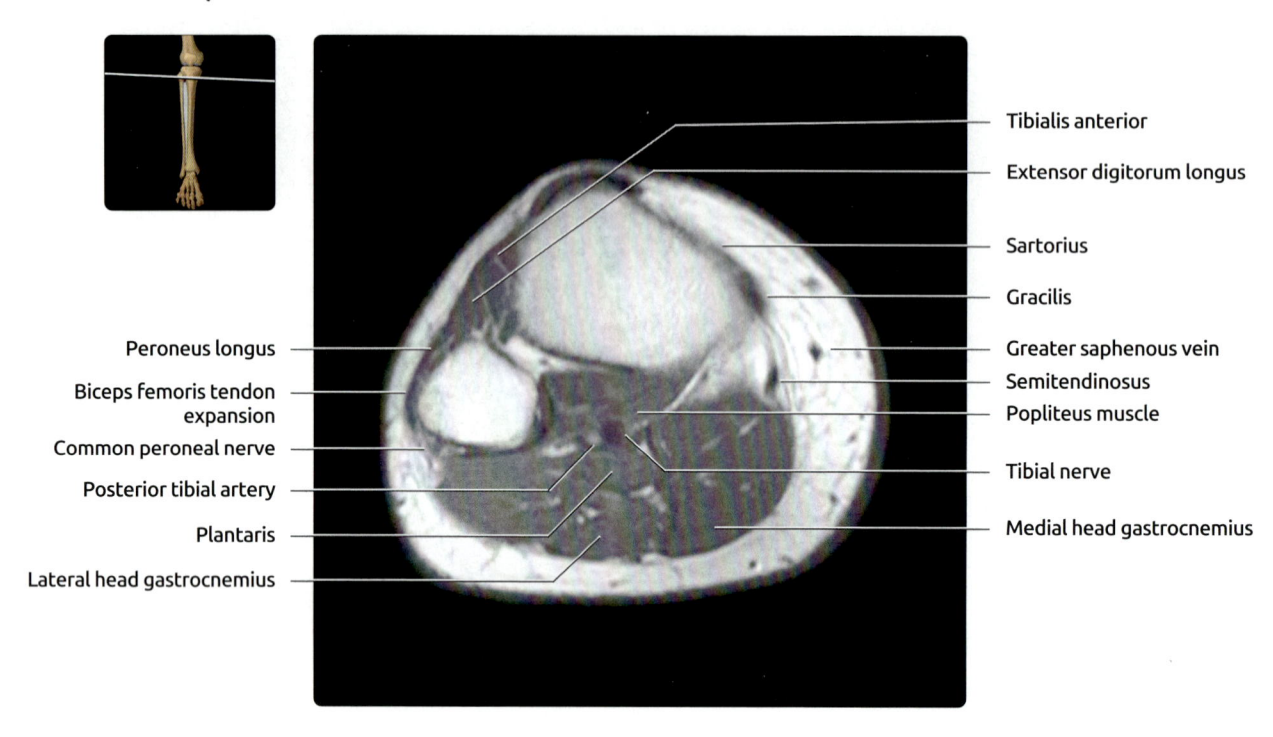

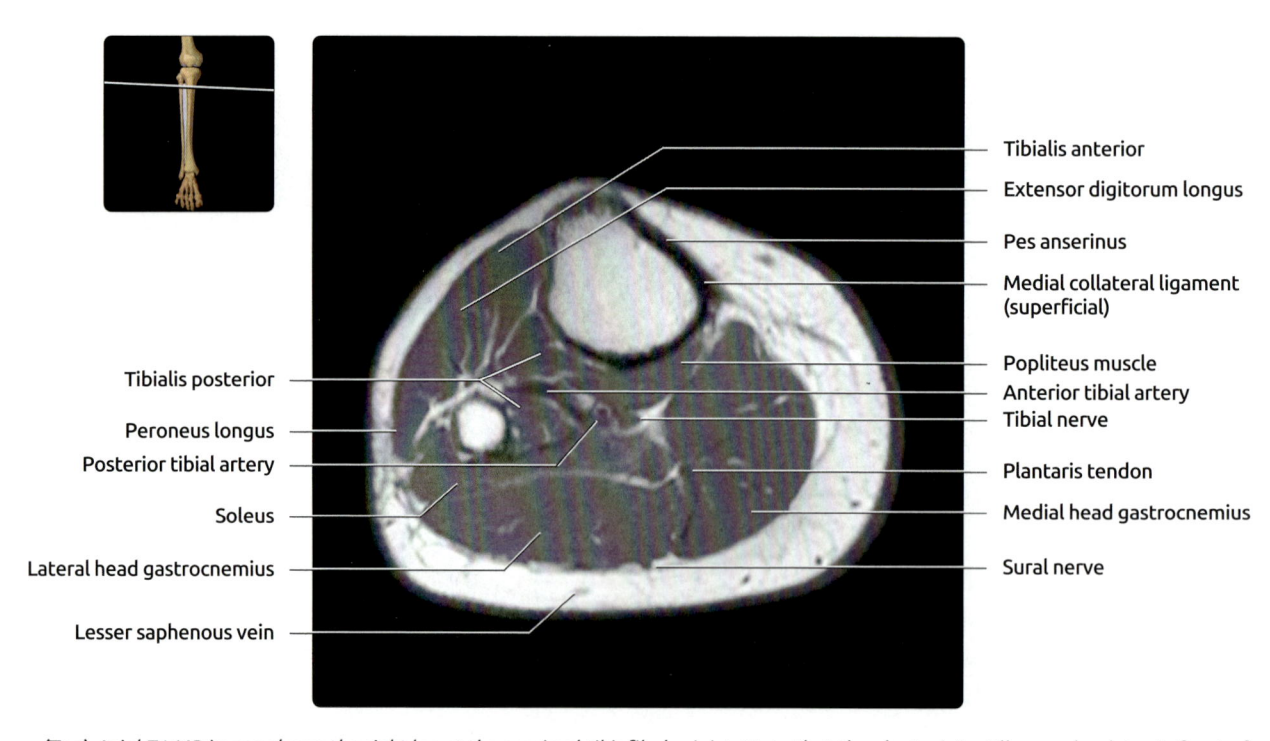

Labels (top image):
- Tibialis anterior
- Extensor digitorum longus
- Sartorius
- Gracilis
- Greater saphenous vein
- Semitendinosus
- Popliteus muscle
- Tibial nerve
- Medial head gastrocnemius
- Peroneus longus
- Biceps femoris tendon expansion
- Common peroneal nerve
- Posterior tibial artery
- Plantaris
- Lateral head gastrocnemius

Labels (bottom image):
- Tibialis anterior
- Extensor digitorum longus
- Pes anserinus
- Medial collateral ligament (superficial)
- Popliteus muscle
- Anterior tibial artery
- Tibial nerve
- Plantaris tendon
- Medial head gastrocnemius
- Sural nerve
- Tibialis posterior
- Peroneus longus
- Posterior tibial artery
- Soleus
- Lateral head gastrocnemius
- Lesser saphenous vein

(Top) Axial T1 MR image shows the right leg at the proximal tibiofibular joint. Note that the plantaris is still muscular, lying in front of the lateral head of the gastrocnemius. (Bottom) Axial T1 MR image of the right leg at the proximal metaphysis. By this point, the soleus has arisen from the fibula; the section is too proximal to see the tibial origin of the soleus since the popliteal muscle is still present. The plantaris is now tendinous, lying between the soleus and the medial head of gastrocnemius. At this level, one sees the tibialis posterior arising as a bifid structure from both tibia and fibula; the anterior tibial vessels are seen coursing forward towards the anterior compartment, between these two attachments.

Leg Radiographic Anatomy and MR Atlas

AXIAL T1 MR, LEFT LEG

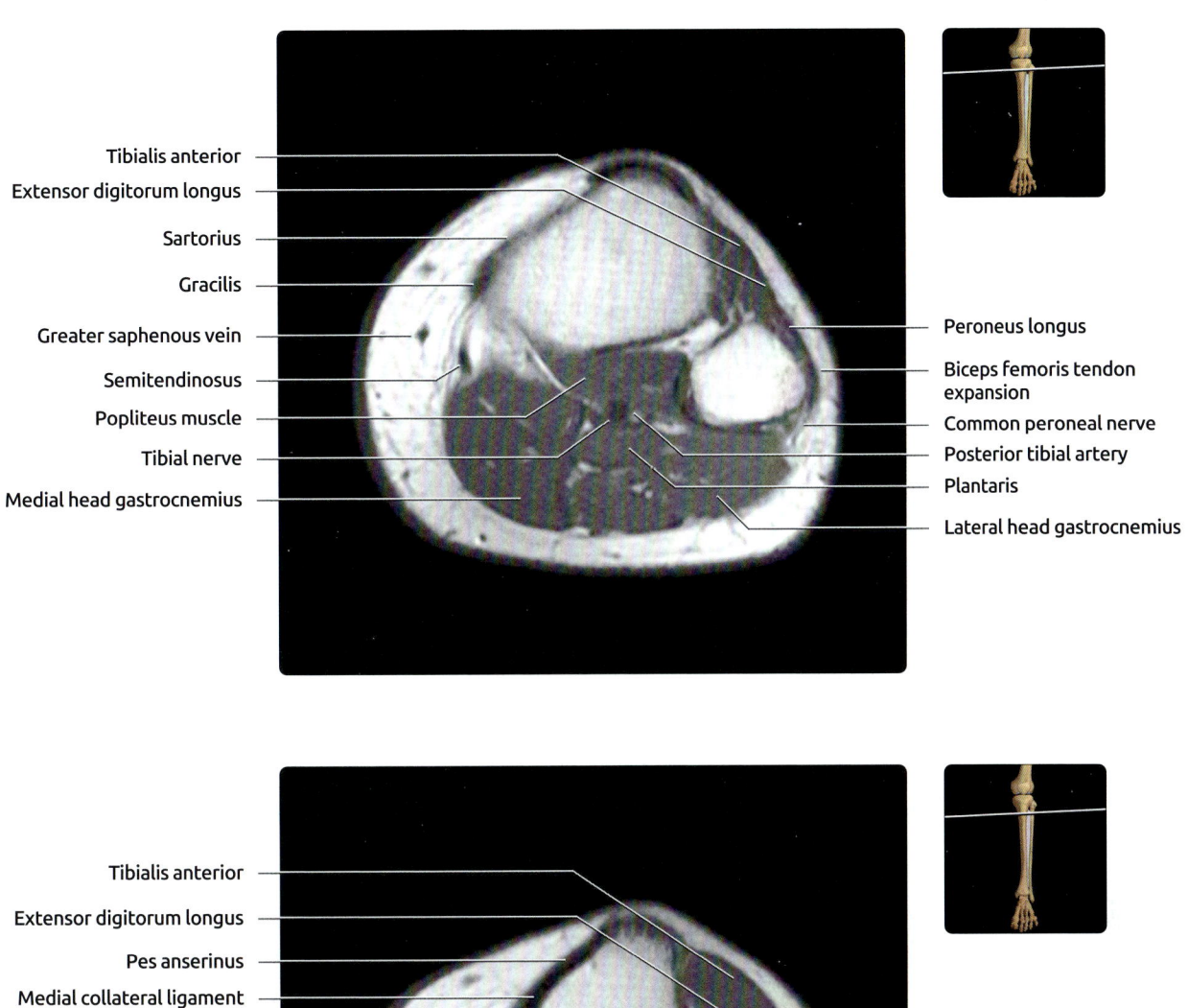

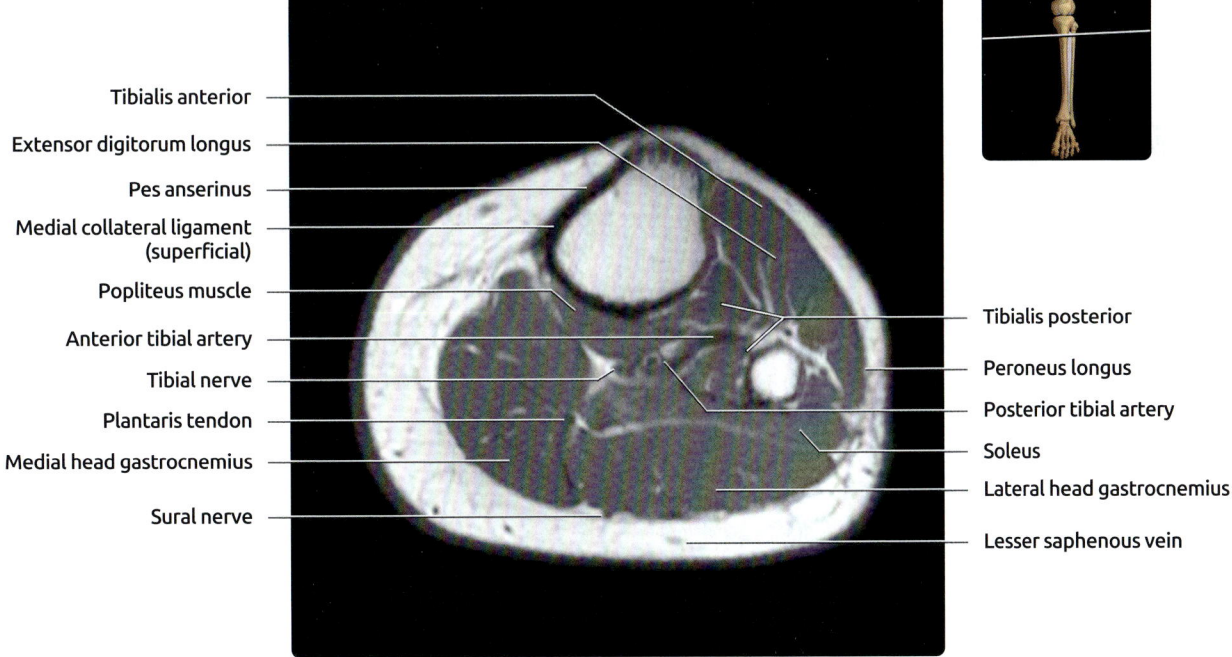

Top image labels: Tibialis anterior; Extensor digitorum longus; Sartorius; Gracilis; Greater saphenous vein; Semitendinosus; Popliteus muscle; Tibial nerve; Medial head gastrocnemius; Peroneus longus; Biceps femoris tendon expansion; Common peroneal nerve; Posterior tibial artery; Plantaris; Lateral head gastrocnemius.

Bottom image labels: Tibialis anterior; Extensor digitorum longus; Pes anserinus; Medial collateral ligament (superficial); Popliteus muscle; Anterior tibial artery; Tibial nerve; Plantaris tendon; Medial head gastrocnemius; Sural nerve; Tibialis posterior; Peroneus longus; Posterior tibial artery; Soleus; Lateral head gastrocnemius; Lesser saphenous vein.

(Top) Axial T1 MR image shows the left leg at the proximal tibiofemoral joint. Note that the plantaris is still muscular, lying in front of the lateral head of the gastrocnemius. **(Bottom)** Axial T1 MR image of the left leg at the proximal metaphysis. By this point, the soleus has arisen from the fibula; the section is too proximal to see the tibial origin of the soleus since the popliteus muscle is still present. The plantaris is now tendinous, lying between the soleus and the medial head of gastrocnemius. At this level, one sees the tibialis posterior arising as a bifid structure from both tibia and fibula; the anterior tibial vessels are seen coursing forward towards the anterior compartment, between these 2 attachments.

Leg Radiographic Anatomy and MR Atlas

AXIAL T1 MR, RIGHT LEG

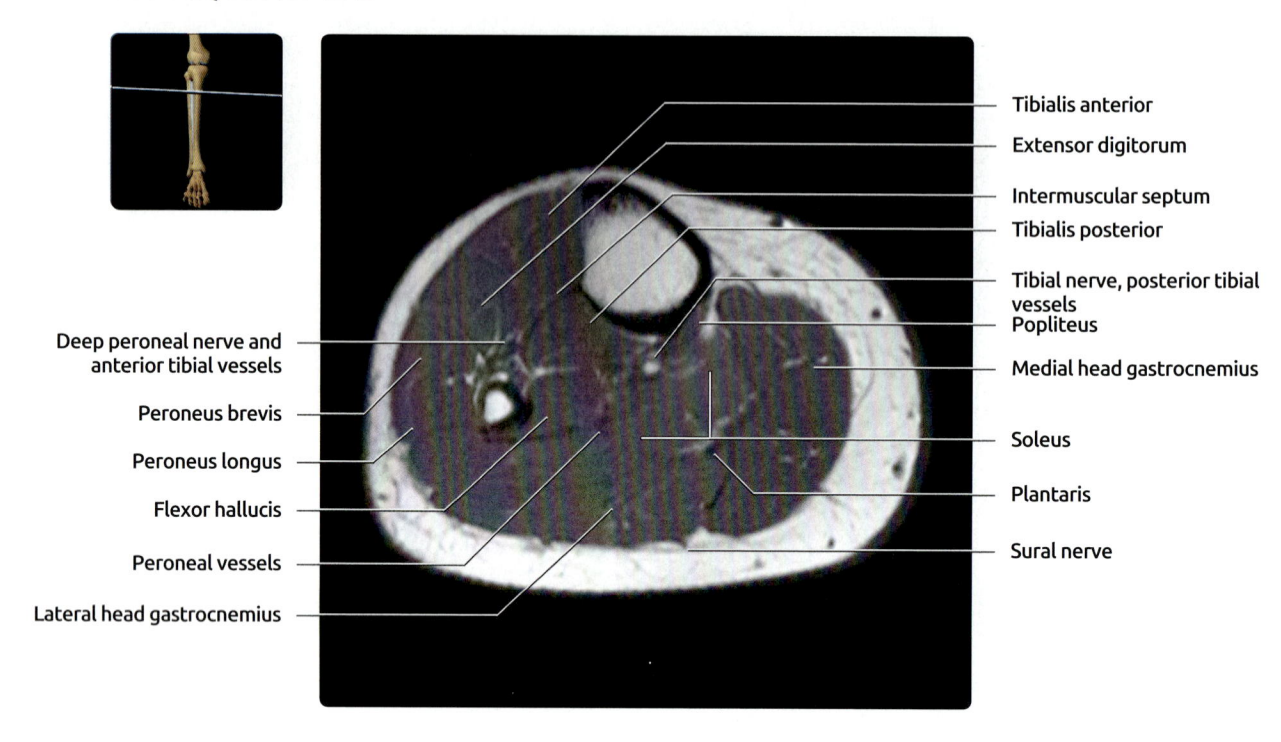

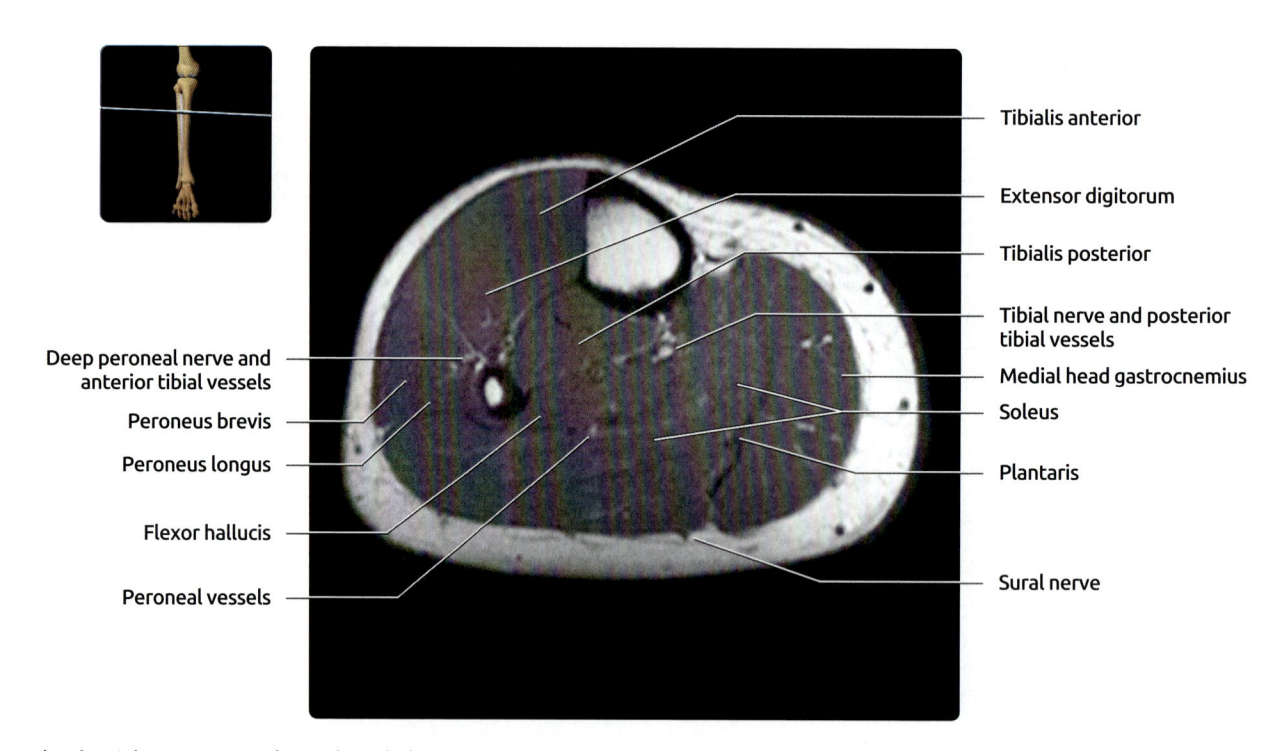

Labels (top image):
- Tibialis anterior
- Extensor digitorum
- Intermuscular septum
- Tibialis posterior
- Tibial nerve, posterior tibial vessels
- Popliteus
- Medial head gastrocnemius
- Soleus
- Plantaris
- Sural nerve
- Deep peroneal nerve and anterior tibial vessels
- Peroneus brevis
- Peroneus longus
- Flexor hallucis
- Peroneal vessels
- Lateral head gastrocnemius

Labels (bottom image):
- Tibialis anterior
- Extensor digitorum
- Tibialis posterior
- Tibial nerve and posterior tibial vessels
- Medial head gastrocnemius
- Soleus
- Plantaris
- Sural nerve
- Deep peroneal nerve and anterior tibial vessels
- Peroneus brevis
- Peroneus longus
- Flexor hallucis
- Peroneal vessels

(**Top**) *Axial T1 MR image shows the right leg at the proximal diaphysis. Note that by this point, the peroneus brevis and flexor hallucis begin to originate from the fibula. There remains a slip of popliteus at the posterior tibia. The major vessels of the leg have trifurcated.* (**Bottom**) *Axial T1 MR image of the right leg, slightly distal. Note that the popliteus insertion on the tibia has ended, and the soleus gains its tibial origin. The lateral head of gastrocnemius has become entirely tendinous.*

Leg Radiographic Anatomy and MR Atlas

AXIAL T1 MR, LEFT LEG

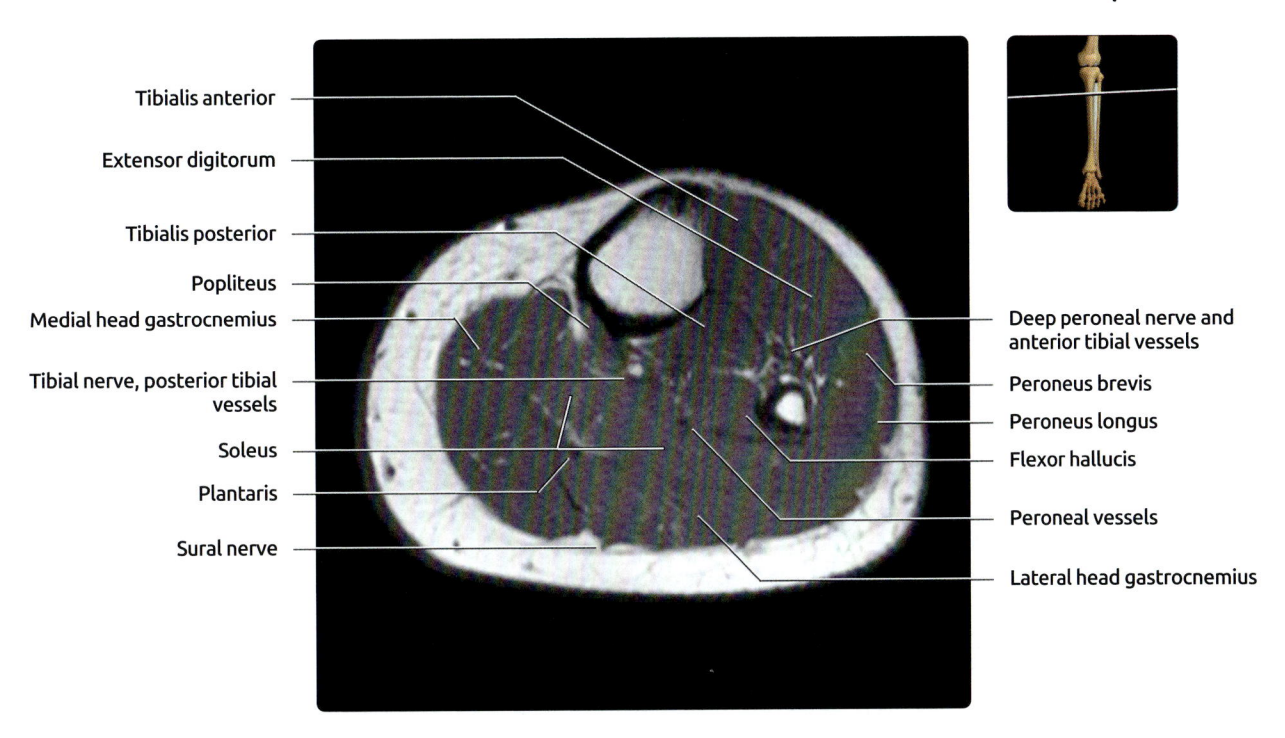

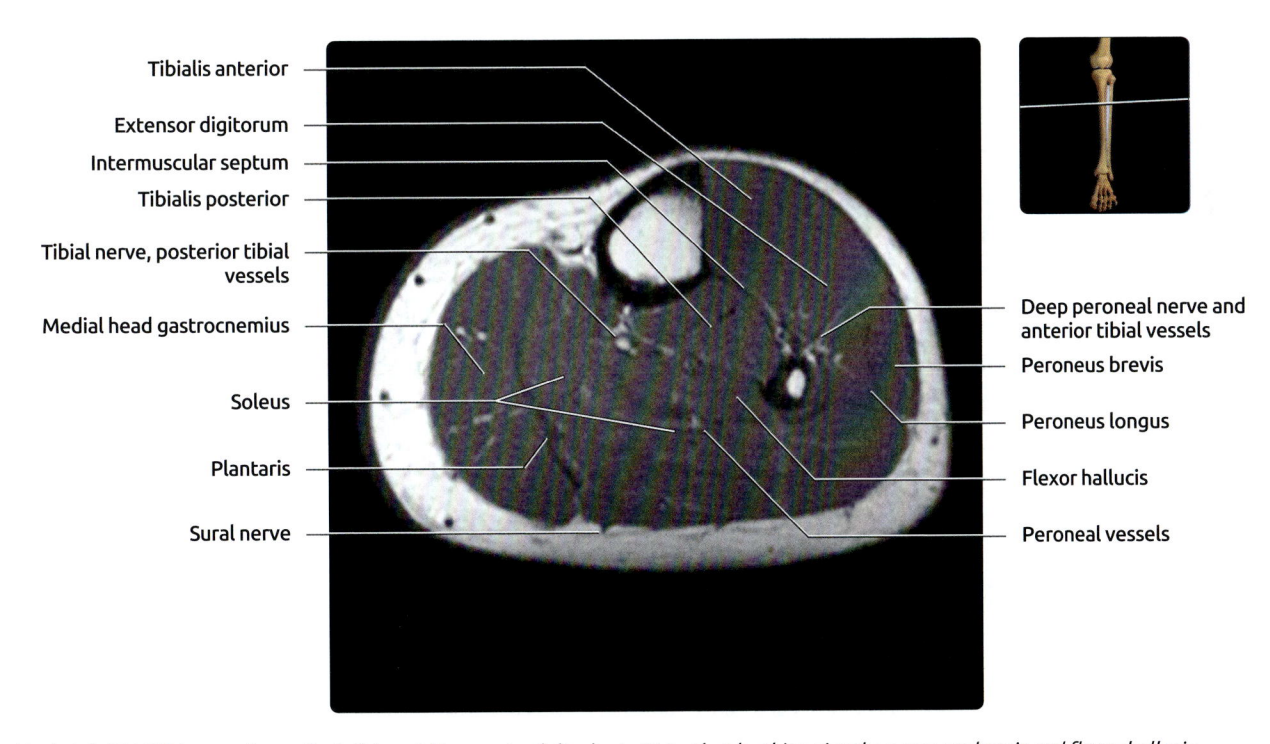

(Top) Axial T1 MR image shows the left leg at the proximal diaphysis. Note that by this point the peroneus brevis and flexor hallucis begin to originate from the fibula. There remains a slip of popliteus at the posterior tibia. The major vessels of the leg have trifurcated.
(Bottom) Axial T1 MR image shows the left leg, slightly distal. Note that the popliteus insertion on the tibia has ended, and the soleus gains its tibial origin. The lateral head of gastrocnemius has become entirely tendinous.

Leg Radiographic Anatomy and MR Atlas

AXIAL T1 MR, RIGHT LEG

Top image labels:
- Tibialis anterior
- Extensor digitorum longus
- Extensor hallucis longus
- Tibialis posterior
- Flexor digitorum longus
- Tibial nerve and posterior tibial vessels
- Soleus
- Plantaris tendon
- Medial head gastrocnemius
- Sural nerve
- Deep peroneal nerve and anterior tibial vessels
- Peroneus longus
- Peroneus brevis
- Peroneal vessels
- Flexor hallucis longus

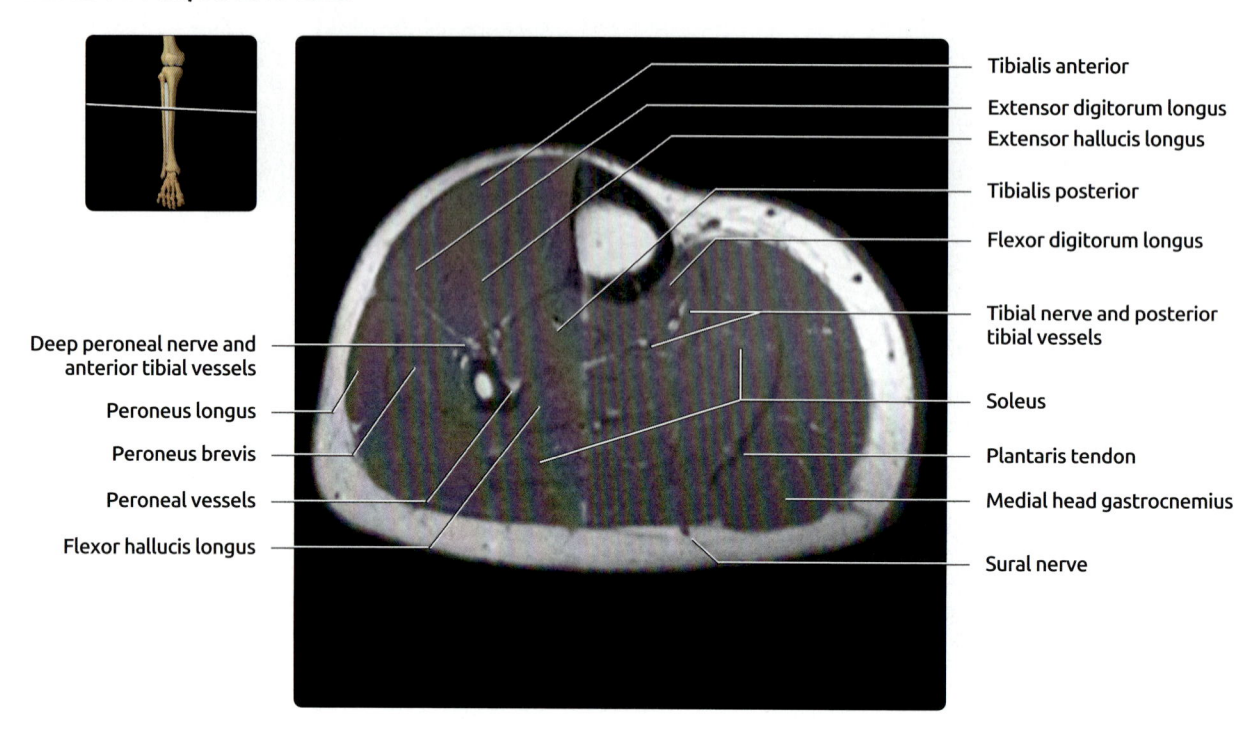

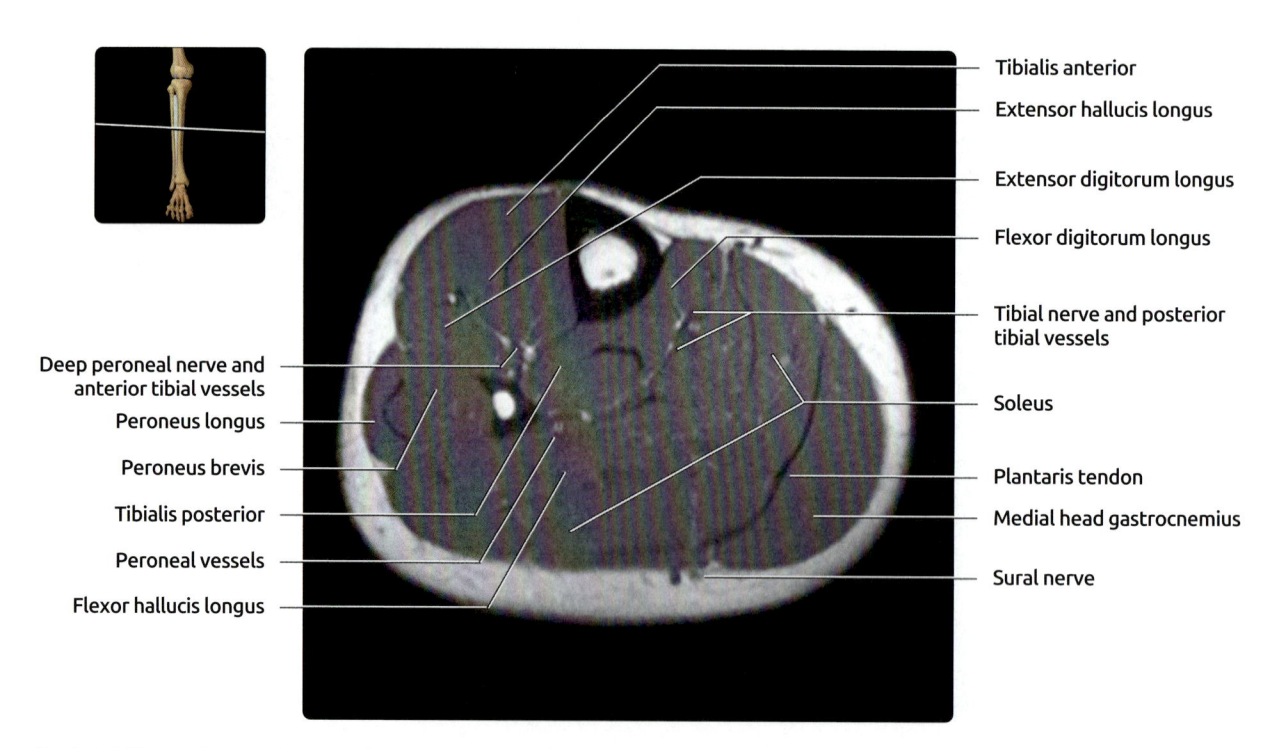

Bottom image labels:
- Tibialis anterior
- Extensor hallucis longus
- Extensor digitorum longus
- Flexor digitorum longus
- Tibial nerve and posterior tibial vessels
- Soleus
- Plantaris tendon
- Medial head gastrocnemius
- Sural nerve
- Deep peroneal nerve and anterior tibial vessels
- Peroneus longus
- Peroneus brevis
- Tibialis posterior
- Peroneal vessels
- Flexor hallucis longus

(Top) Axial T1 MR image of the right leg at the junction of proximal and middle thirds. At this point, the extensor hallucis longus makes its appearance, arising from the anterior fibula and interosseous membrane. Flexor digitorum longus also is now seen, arising from the posterior tibia. The lateral head of gastrocnemius has become tendinous, with the soleus making up the bulk of the posterior muscles. **(Bottom)** Slightly distal axial T1 MR image shows the right leg. At this point, the extensor hallucis longus is located between the tibialis anterior and extensor digitorum longus and is not easily distinguished from them. Similarly, the peroneal muscle/tendons are not easily distinguished because of poorly visualized fat planes in the leg. Note also that the plantaris tendon still lies between the medial head of gastrocnemius and the soleus, but is tracking medially.

Leg Radiographic Anatomy and MR Atlas

AXIAL T1 MR, LEFT LEG

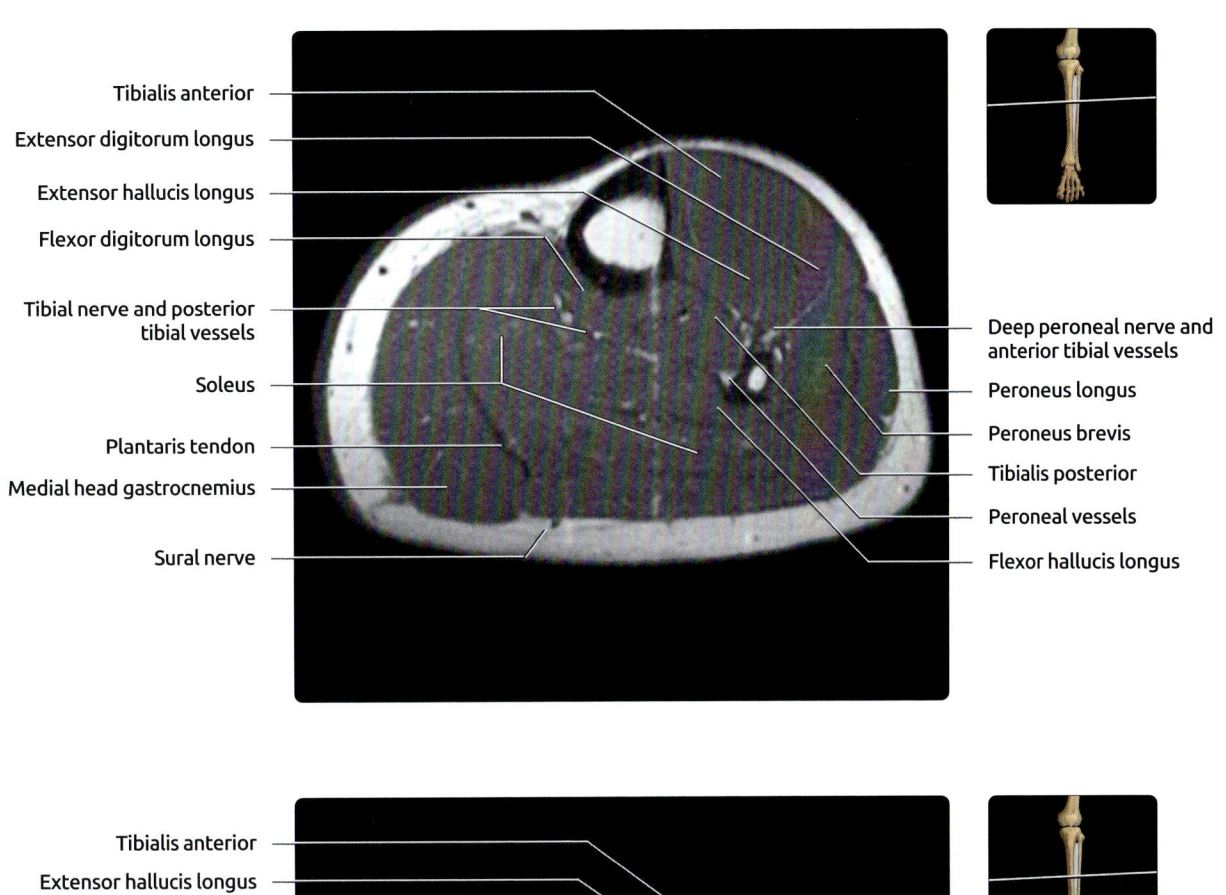

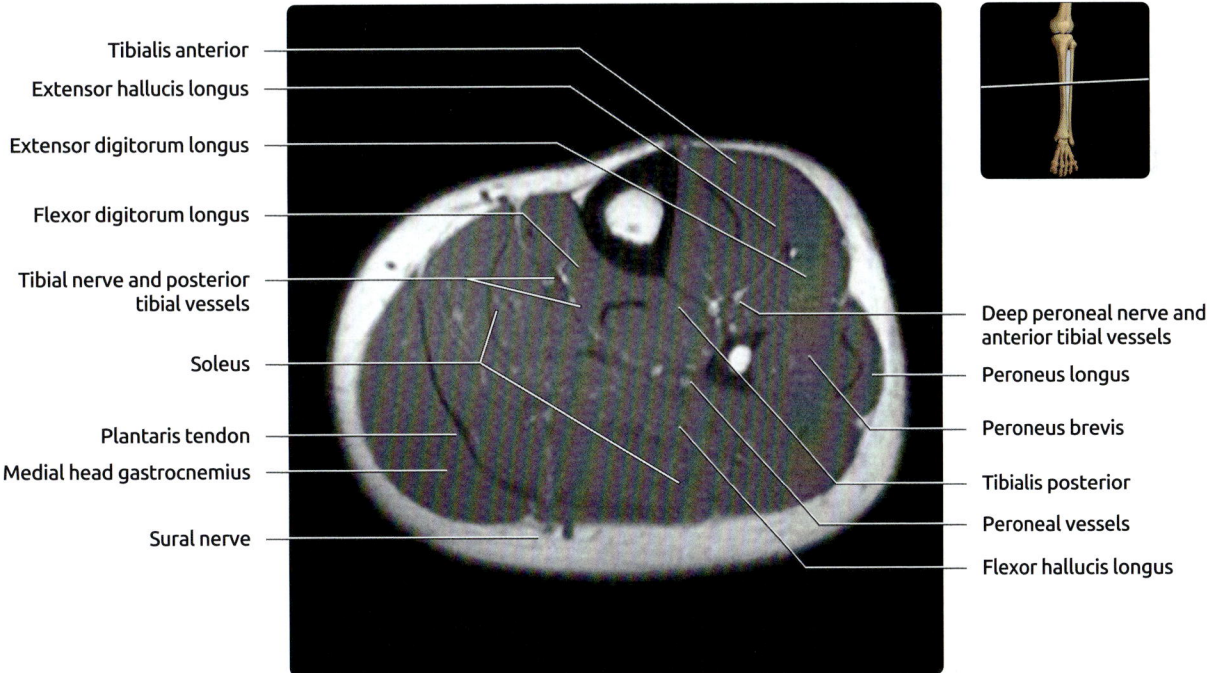

(Top) Axial T1 MR image shows the left leg at the junction of proximal and middle thirds. At this point, the extensor hallucis longus makes its appearance, arising from the anterior fibula and interosseous membrane. The flexor digitorum longus also is now seen, arising from the posterior tibia. The lateral head of gastrocnemius has become tendinous, with the soleus making up the bulk of the posterior muscles. (Bottom) Slightly distal axial T1 MR image shows the left leg. At this point, the extensor hallucis longus is located between the tibialis anterior and extensor digitorum longus and is not easily distinguished from them. Similarly, the peroneal muscle/tendons are not easily distinguished because of poorly visualized fat planes in the leg. Note also that the plantaris tendon still lies between the medial head of gastrocnemius and soleus, but is tracking medially.

AXIAL T1 MR, RIGHT LEG

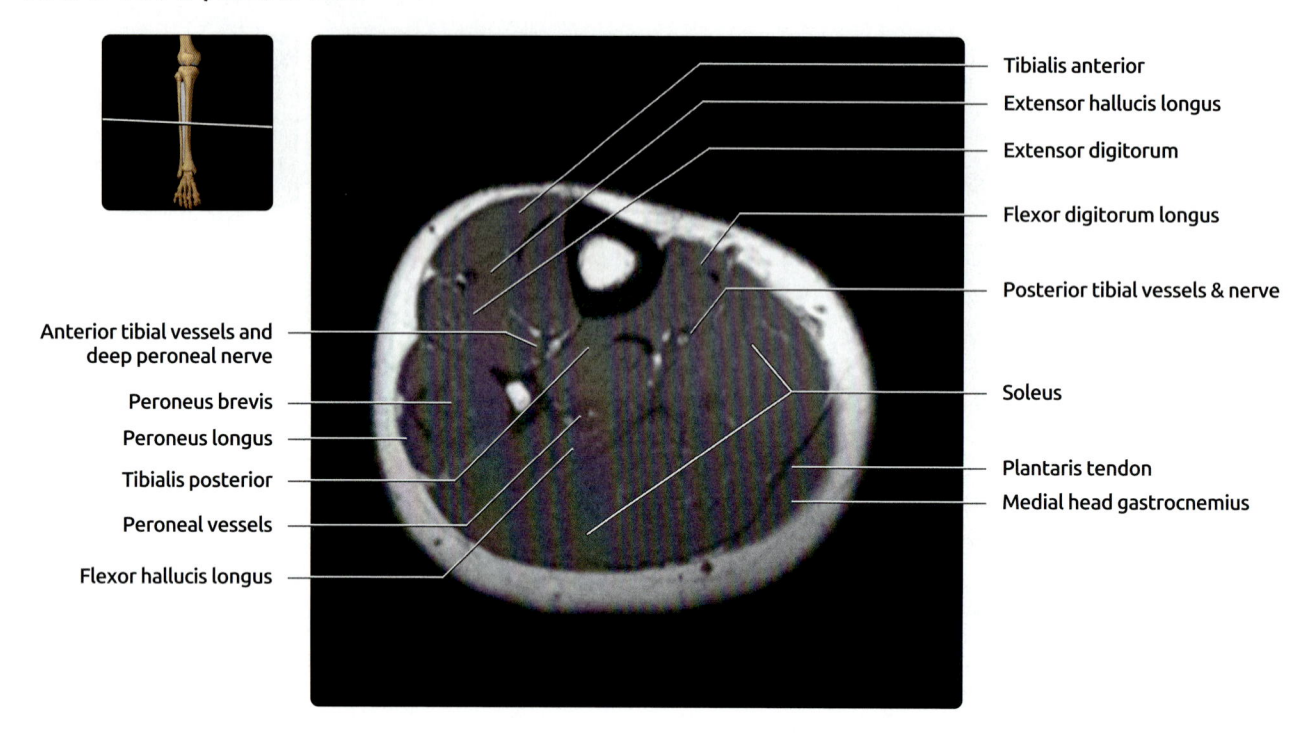

Tibialis anterior
Extensor hallucis longus
Extensor digitorum
Flexor digitorum longus
Posterior tibial vessels & nerve
Soleus
Plantaris tendon
Medial head gastrocnemius

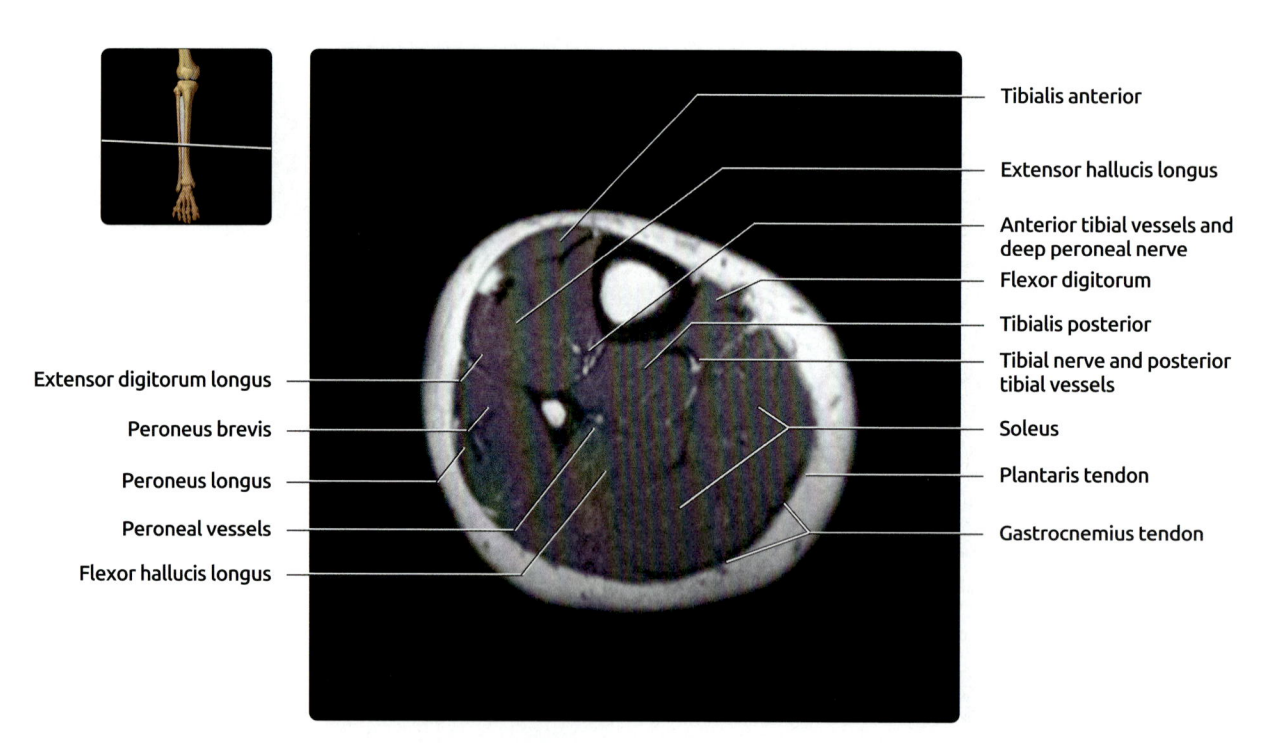

Anterior tibial vessels and deep peroneal nerve
Peroneus brevis
Peroneus longus
Tibialis posterior
Peroneal vessels
Flexor hallucis longus

Tibialis anterior
Extensor hallucis longus
Anterior tibial vessels and deep peroneal nerve
Flexor digitorum
Tibialis posterior
Tibial nerve and posterior tibial vessels
Soleus
Plantaris tendon
Gastrocnemius tendon

Extensor digitorum longus
Peroneus brevis
Peroneus longus
Peroneal vessels
Flexor hallucis longus

(Top) Axial T1 MR image shows the right leg at the mid diaphysis. At this point in the mid leg the gastrocnemius muscle has become nearly completely tendinous. (Bottom) Slightly distal axial T1 MR image shows the right leg. The gastrocnemius is now entirely tendinous, and the plantaris tendon lies subcutaneously adjacent to the medial aspect of the gastrocnemius tendon.

Leg Radiographic Anatomy and MR Atlas

AXIAL T1 MR, LEFT LEG

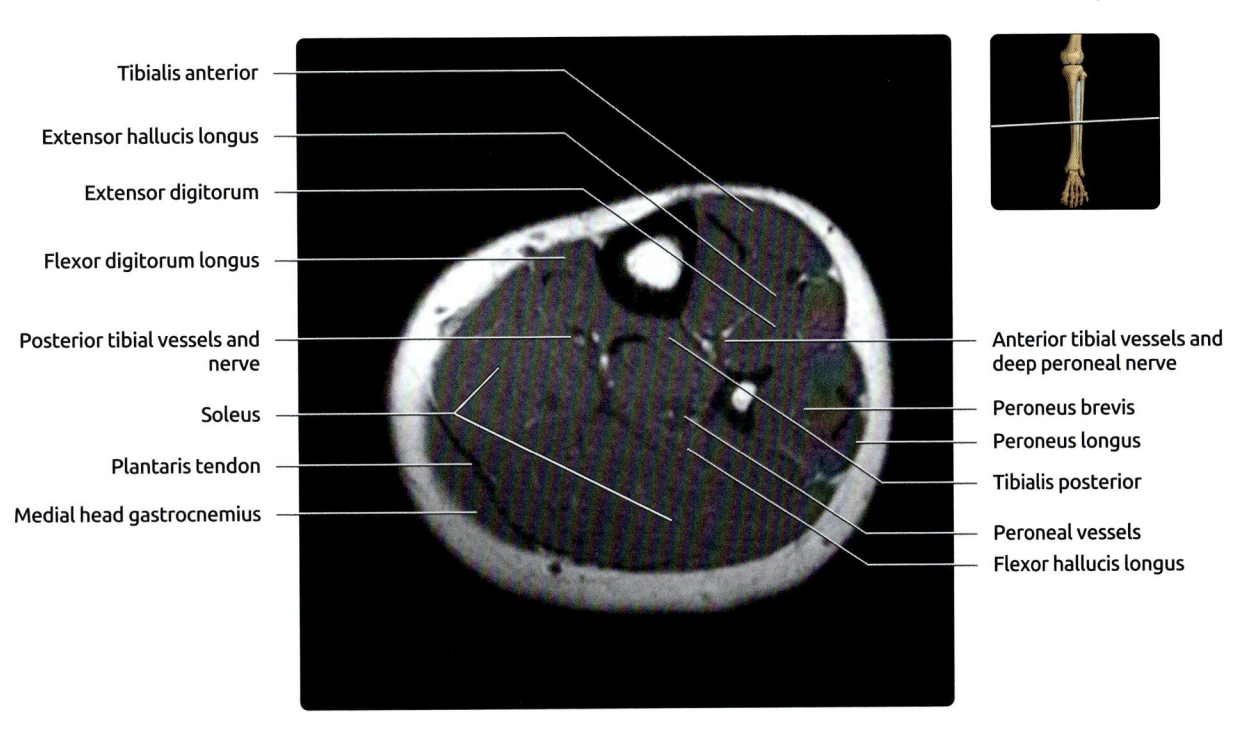

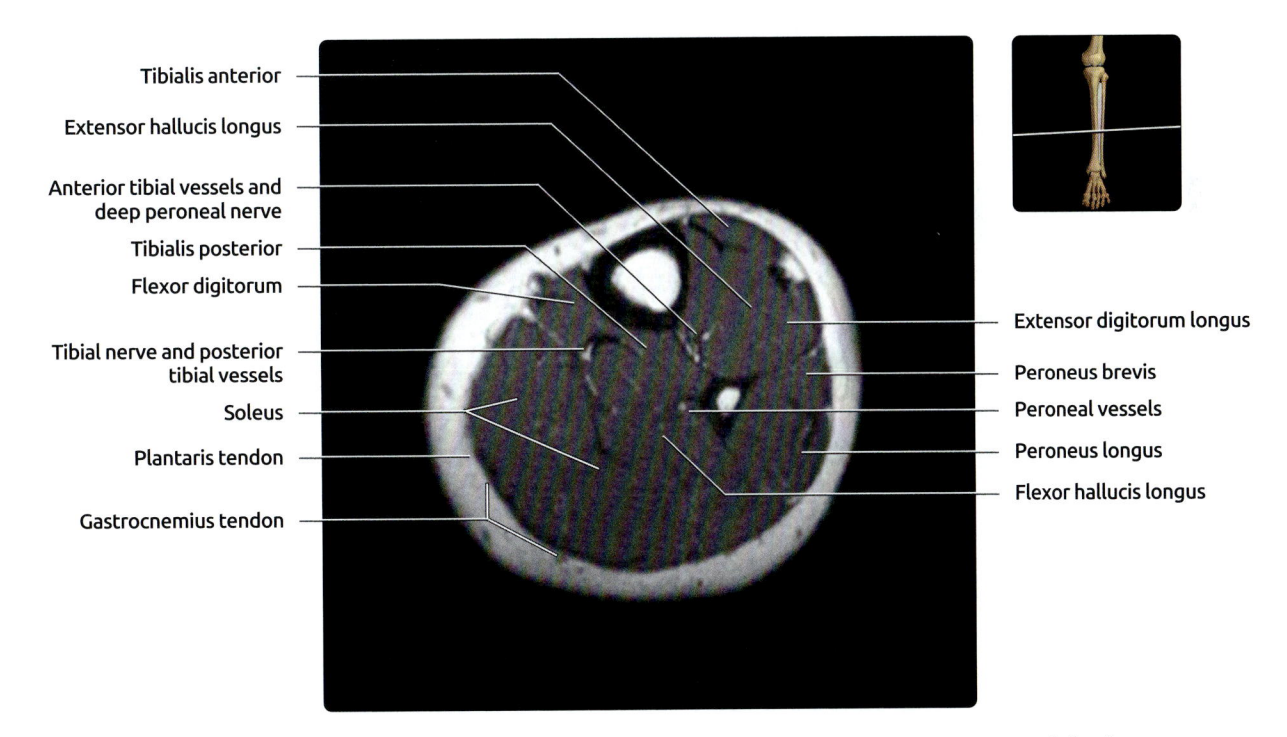

Labels (Top image):
- Tibialis anterior
- Extensor hallucis longus
- Extensor digitorum
- Flexor digitorum longus
- Posterior tibial vessels and nerve
- Soleus
- Plantaris tendon
- Medial head gastrocnemius
- Anterior tibial vessels and deep peroneal nerve
- Peroneus brevis
- Peroneus longus
- Tibialis posterior
- Peroneal vessels
- Flexor hallucis longus

Labels (Bottom image):
- Tibialis anterior
- Extensor hallucis longus
- Anterior tibial vessels and deep peroneal nerve
- Tibialis posterior
- Flexor digitorum
- Tibial nerve and posterior tibial vessels
- Soleus
- Plantaris tendon
- Gastrocnemius tendon
- Extensor digitorum longus
- Peroneus brevis
- Peroneal vessels
- Peroneus longus
- Flexor hallucis longus

(Top) Axial T1 MR image shows the left leg at the mid diaphysis. At this point in the mid leg the gastrocnemius muscle has become nearly completely tendinous. **(Bottom)** Slightly distal axial T1 MR image shows the left leg. The gastrocnemius is now entirely tendinous and the plantaris tendon lies subcutaneously adjacent to the medial aspect of the gastrocnemius tendon.

AXIAL T1 MR, RIGHT LEG

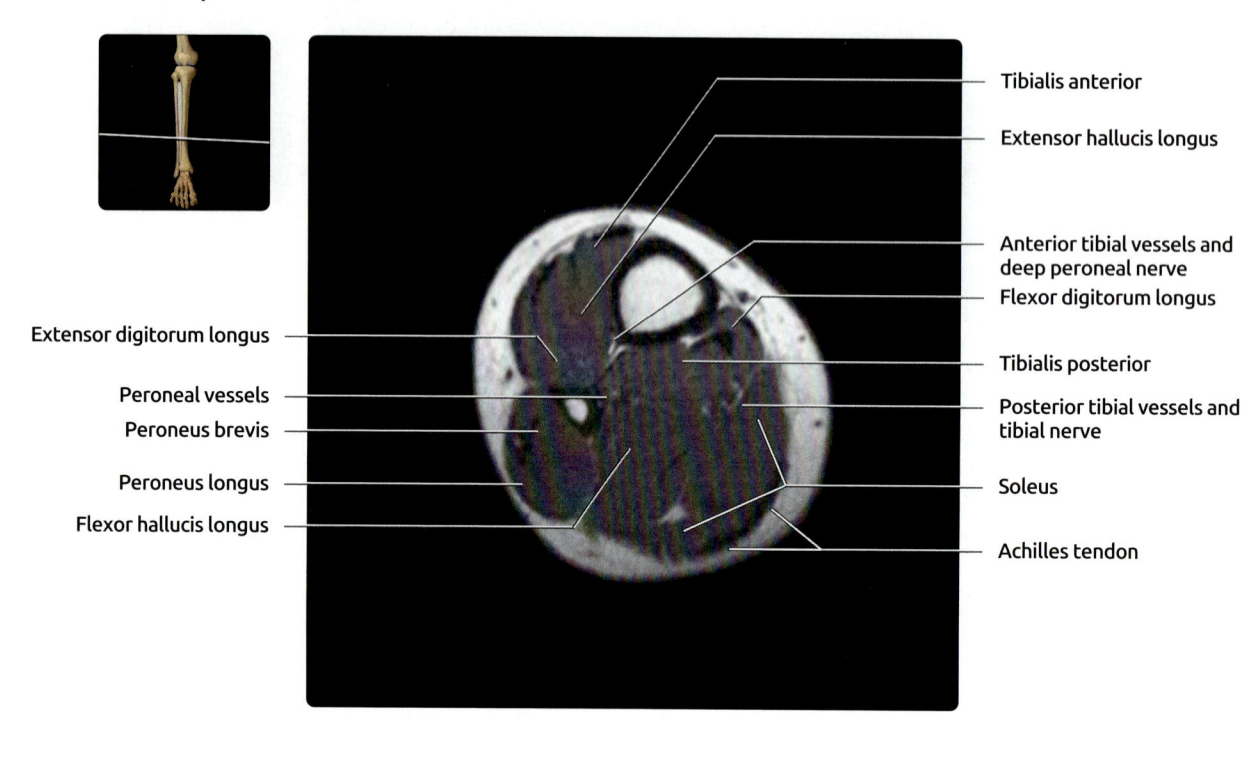

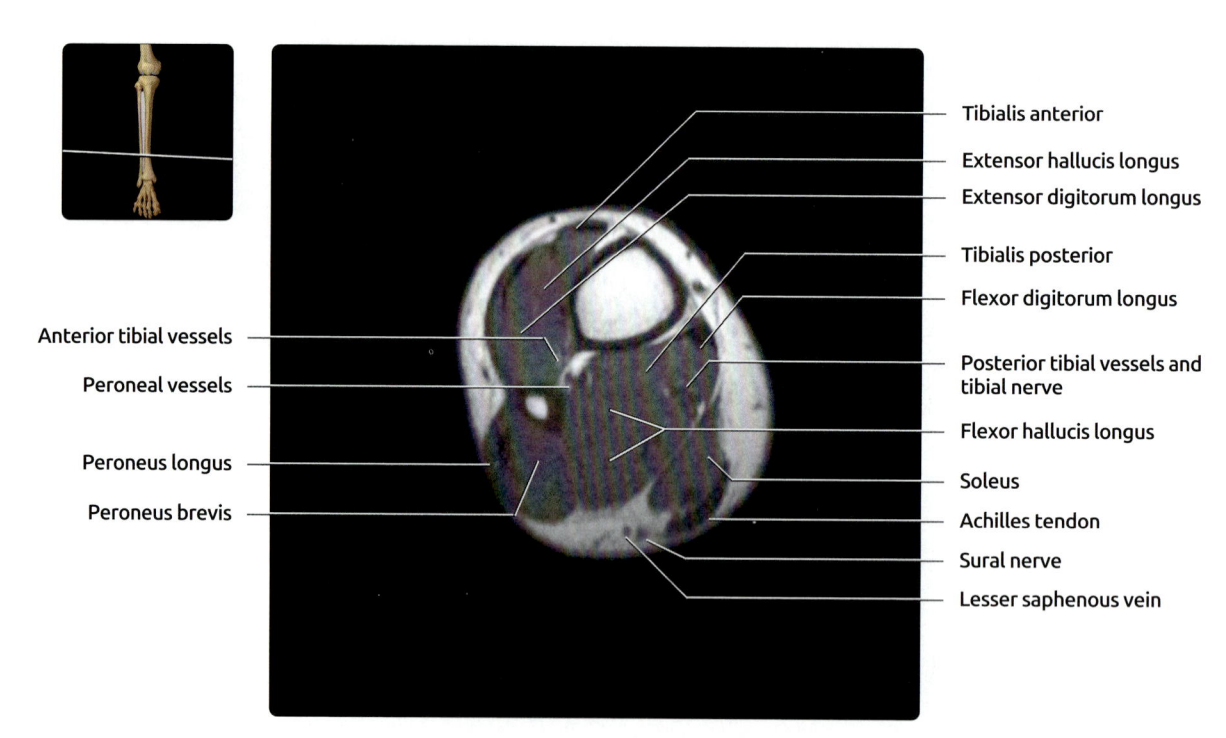

Tibialis anterior
Extensor hallucis longus
Anterior tibial vessels and deep peroneal nerve
Flexor digitorum longus
Tibialis posterior
Posterior tibial vessels and tibial nerve
Soleus
Achilles tendon

Extensor digitorum longus
Peroneal vessels
Peroneus brevis
Peroneus longus
Flexor hallucis longus

Tibialis anterior
Extensor hallucis longus
Extensor digitorum longus
Tibialis posterior
Flexor digitorum longus
Posterior tibial vessels and tibial nerve
Flexor hallucis longus
Soleus
Achilles tendon
Sural nerve
Lesser saphenous vein

Anterior tibial vessels
Peroneal vessels
Peroneus longus
Peroneus brevis

(Top) Axial T1 MR image shows the right leg at the junction of middle and distal thirds. The deep muscles of the posterior compartment are now more prominent than the superficial. (Bottom) Slightly distal axial T1 MR images show the right leg with the compartments more distinctly seen.

Leg Radiographic Anatomy and MR Atlas

AXIAL T1 MR, LEFT LEG

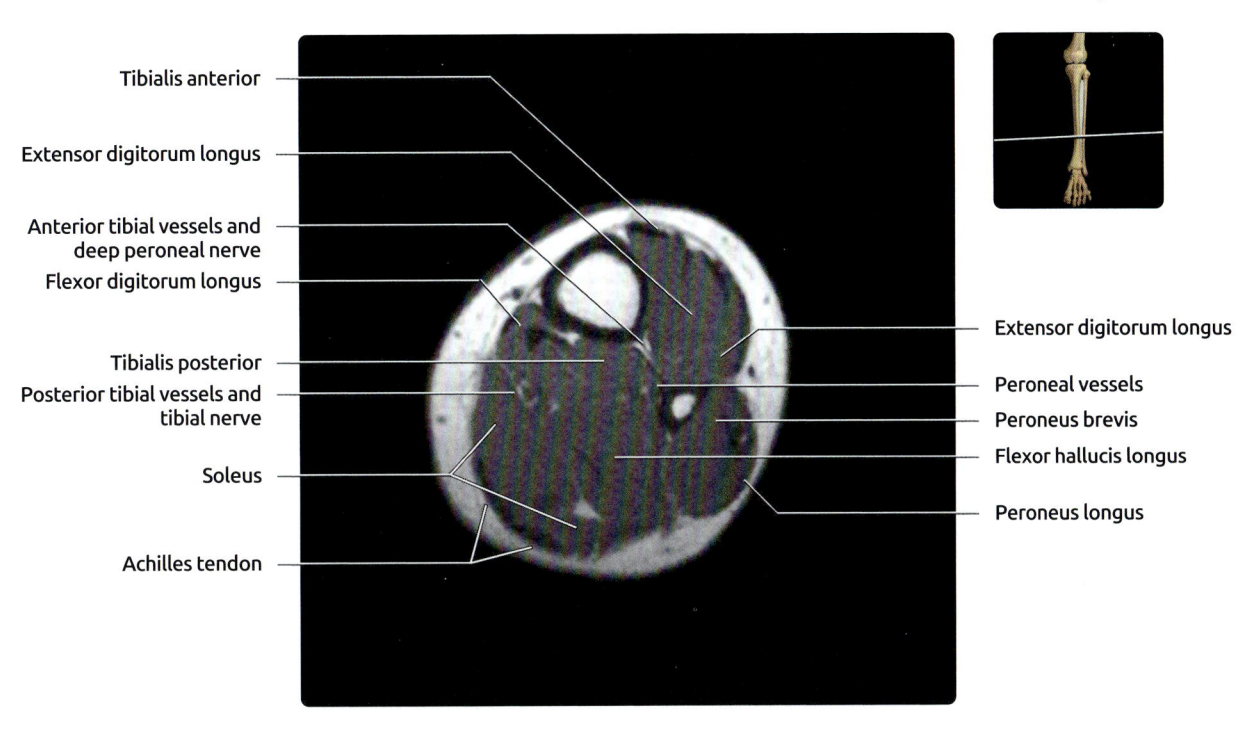

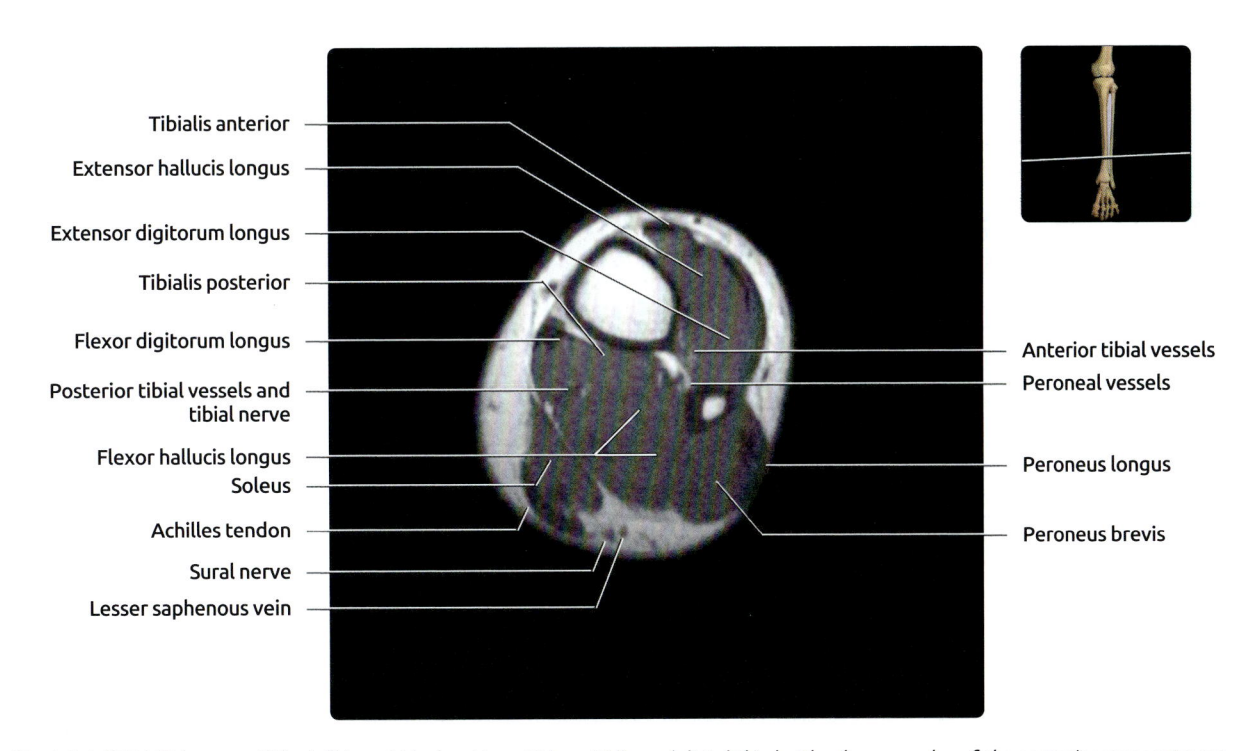

(Top) Axial T1 MR images of the left leg at the junction of the middle and distal thirds. The deep muscles of the posterior compartment are now more prominent than the superficial. *(Bottom)* Slightly distal axial T1 MR image shows the left leg with the compartments more distinctly seen.

Leg Radiographic Anatomy and MR Atlas

AXIAL T1 MR, RIGHT LEG

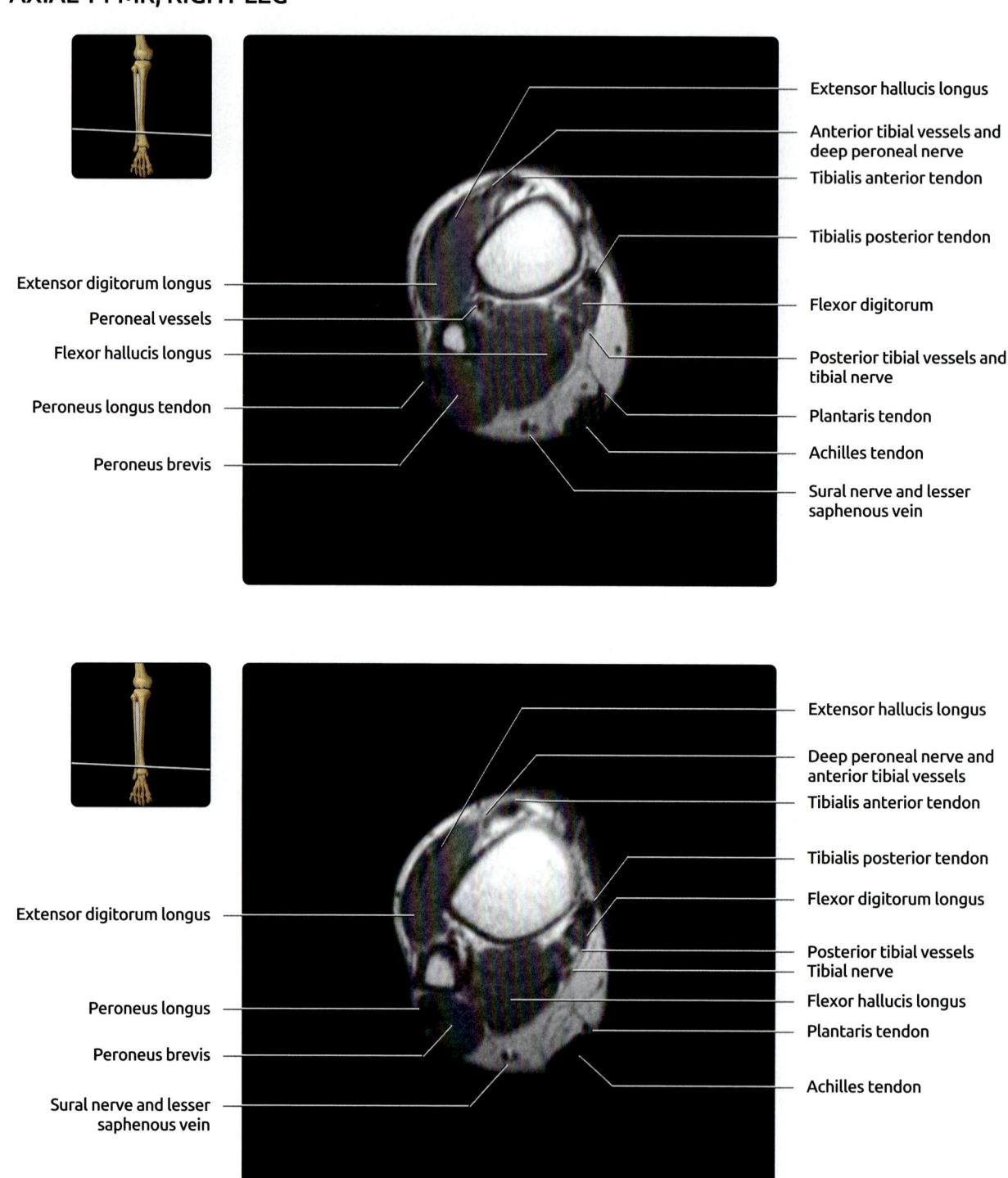

(Top) Axial T1 MR image shows the right leg approaching the distal metaphysis. The anterior and posterior tibialis tendons are now defined, as is the Achilles tendon. *(Bottom)* Axial T1 MR image shows the right leg at the distal metaphysis. The major tendons of the leg are becoming more distinct.

Leg Radiographic Anatomy and MR Atlas

AXIAL T1 MR, LEFT LEG

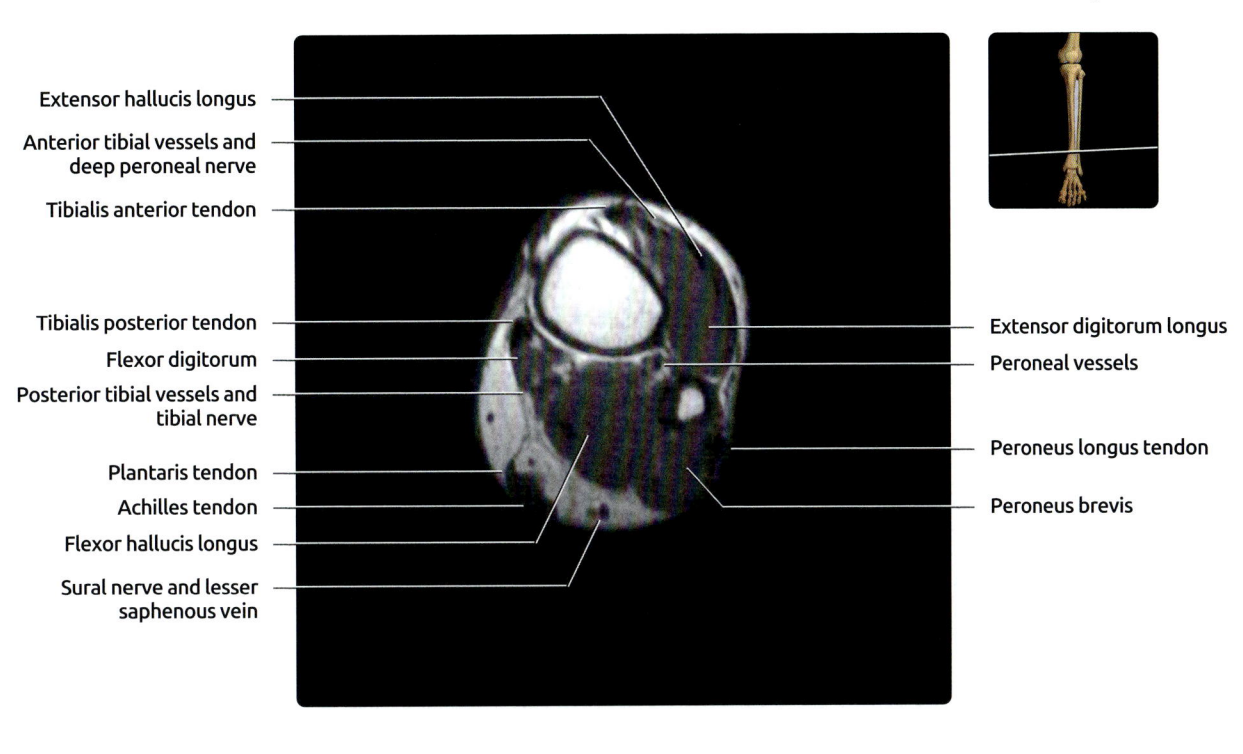

Top image labels:
- Extensor hallucis longus
- Anterior tibial vessels and deep peroneal nerve
- Tibialis anterior tendon
- Tibialis posterior tendon
- Flexor digitorum
- Posterior tibial vessels and tibial nerve
- Plantaris tendon
- Achilles tendon
- Flexor hallucis longus
- Sural nerve and lesser saphenous vein
- Extensor digitorum longus
- Peroneal vessels
- Peroneus longus tendon
- Peroneus brevis

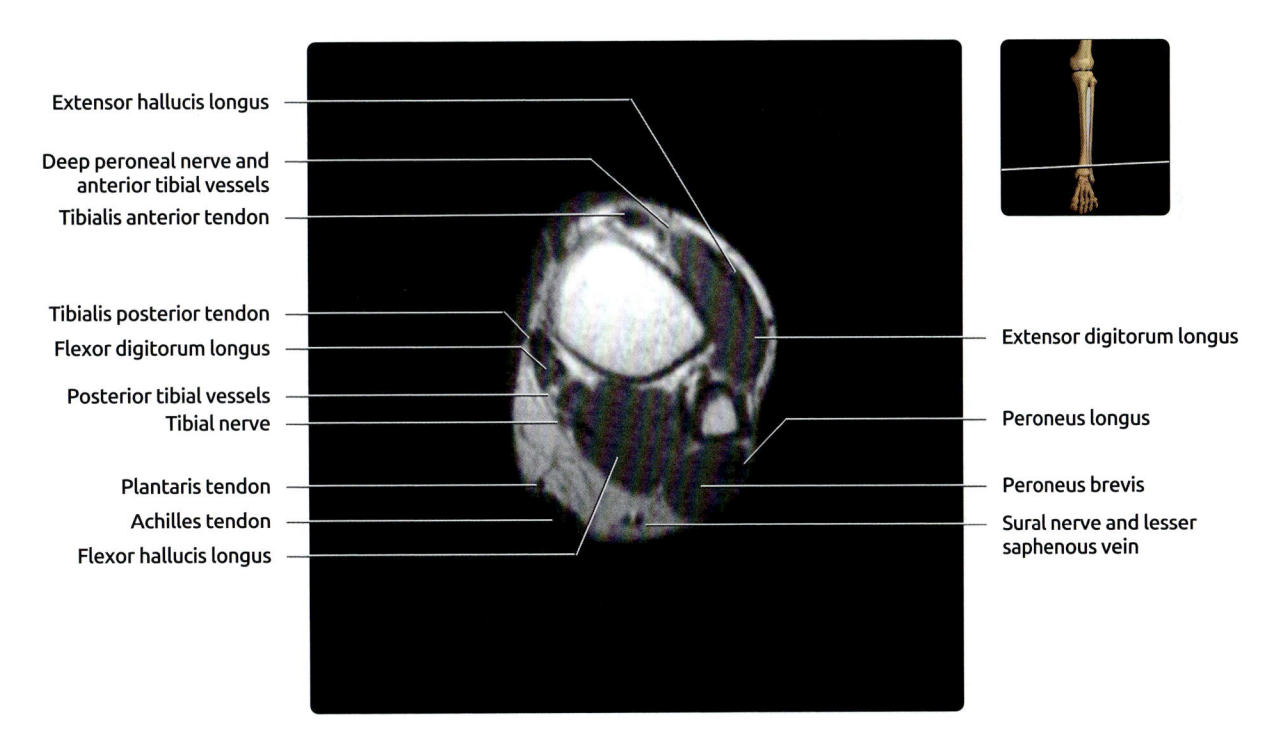

Bottom image labels:
- Extensor hallucis longus
- Deep peroneal nerve and anterior tibial vessels
- Tibialis anterior tendon
- Tibialis posterior tendon
- Flexor digitorum longus
- Posterior tibial vessels
- Tibial nerve
- Plantaris tendon
- Achilles tendon
- Flexor hallucis longus
- Extensor digitorum longus
- Peroneus longus
- Peroneus brevis
- Sural nerve and lesser saphenous vein

(**Top**) Axial T1 MR image shows the left leg approaching the distal metaphysis. The anterior and posterior tibialis tendons are now defined, as is the Achilles tendon. (**Bottom**) Axial T1 MR image shows the left leg at the distal metaphysis. The major tendons of the leg are becoming more distinct.

Leg Radiographic Anatomy and MR Atlas

AXIAL T1 MR, RIGHT LEG

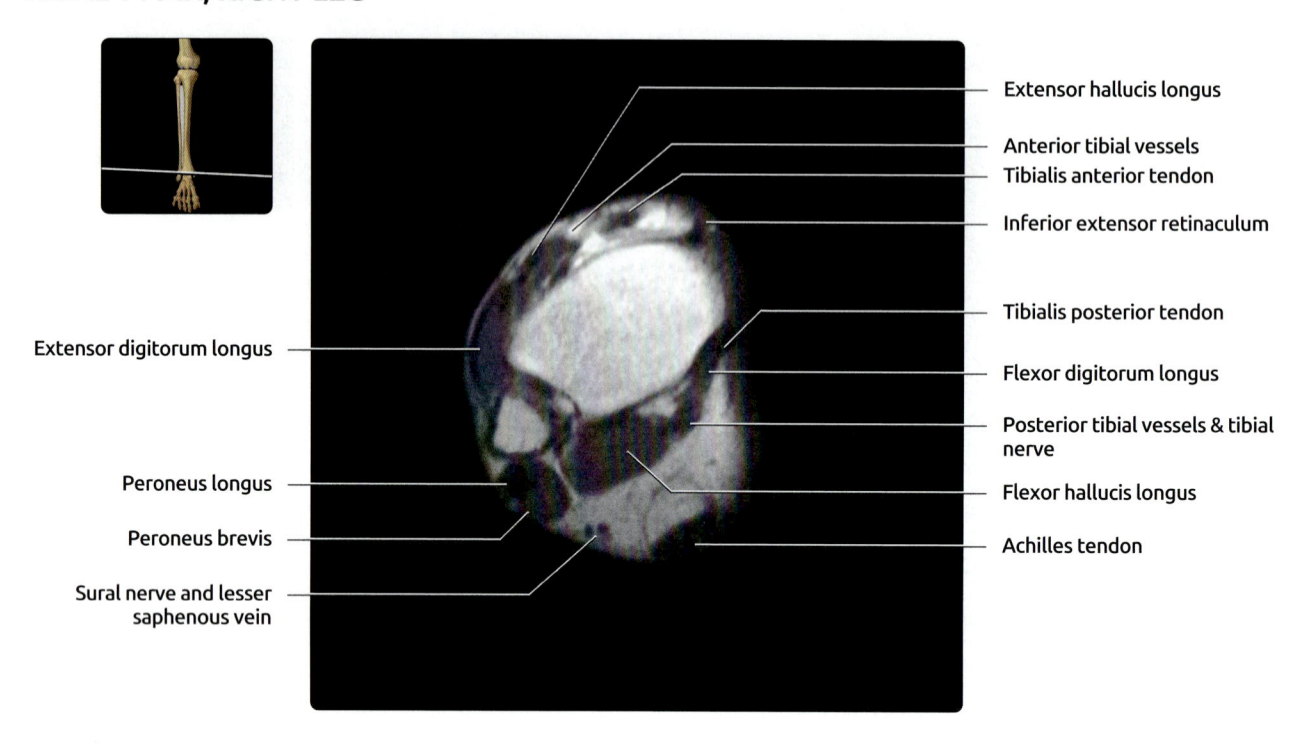

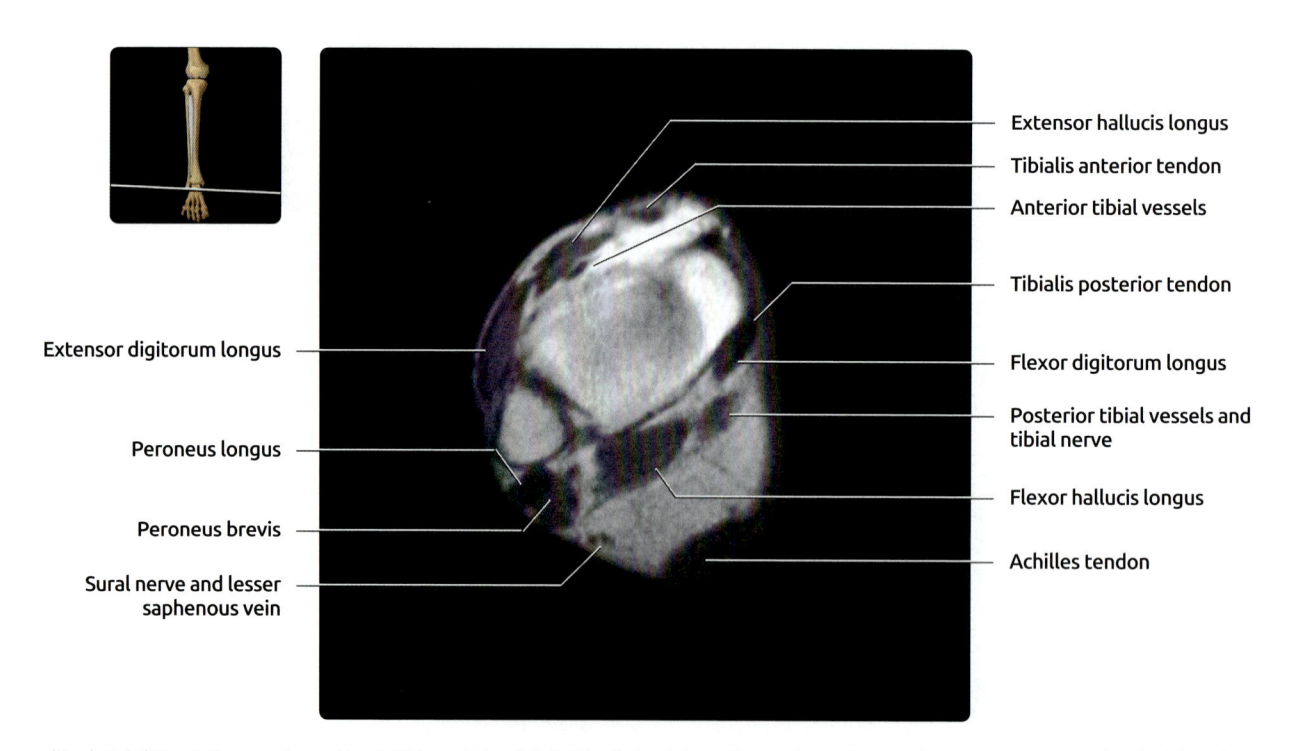

Top image labels:
- Extensor hallucis longus
- Anterior tibial vessels
- Tibialis anterior tendon
- Inferior extensor retinaculum
- Tibialis posterior tendon
- Flexor digitorum longus
- Posterior tibial vessels & tibial nerve
- Flexor hallucis longus
- Achilles tendon
- Extensor digitorum longus
- Peroneus longus
- Peroneus brevis
- Sural nerve and lesser saphenous vein

Bottom image labels:
- Extensor hallucis longus
- Tibialis anterior tendon
- Anterior tibial vessels
- Tibialis posterior tendon
- Flexor digitorum longus
- Posterior tibial vessels and tibial nerve
- Flexor hallucis longus
- Achilles tendon
- Extensor digitorum longus
- Peroneus longus
- Peroneus brevis
- Sural nerve and lesser saphenous vein

(**Top**) Axial T1 MR image shows the right leg at the distal tibiofibular joint. The tendons of the ankle are much more clearly defined, though the flexor hallucis longus is still highly muscular. (**Bottom**) Axial T1 MR image shows the right leg at the ankle joint.

Leg Radiographic Anatomy and MR Atlas

AXIAL T1 MR, LEFT LEG

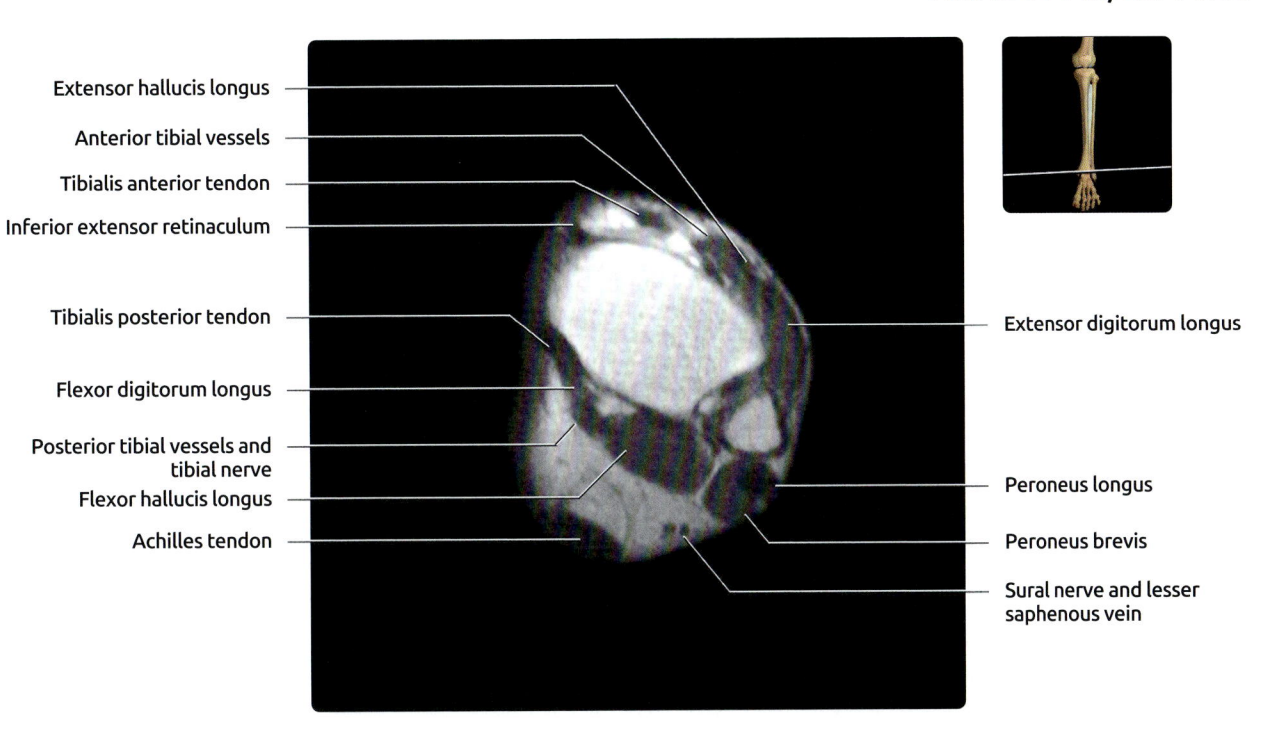

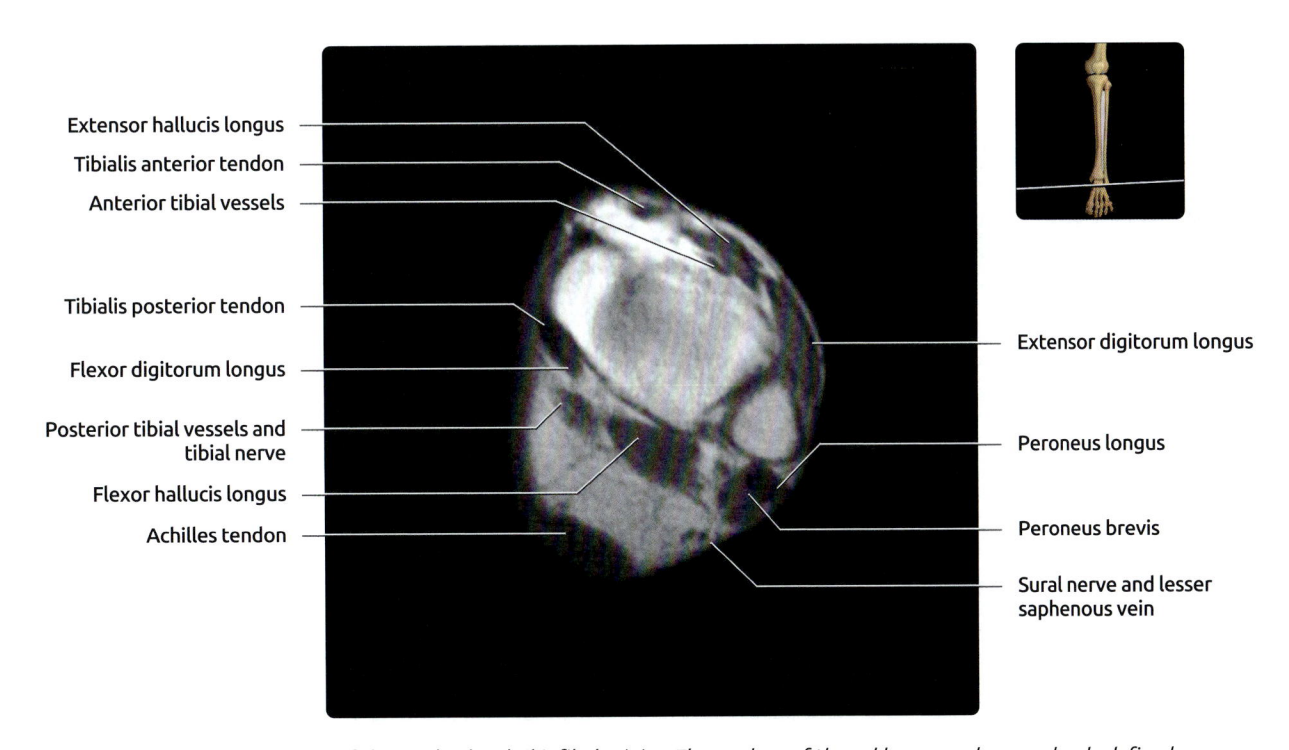

Labels (top image):
- Extensor hallucis longus
- Anterior tibial vessels
- Tibialis anterior tendon
- Inferior extensor retinaculum
- Tibialis posterior tendon
- Flexor digitorum longus
- Posterior tibial vessels and tibial nerve
- Flexor hallucis longus
- Achilles tendon
- Extensor digitorum longus
- Peroneus longus
- Peroneus brevis
- Sural nerve and lesser saphenous vein

Labels (bottom image):
- Extensor hallucis longus
- Tibialis anterior tendon
- Anterior tibial vessels
- Tibialis posterior tendon
- Flexor digitorum longus
- Posterior tibial vessels and tibial nerve
- Flexor hallucis longus
- Achilles tendon
- Extensor digitorum longus
- Peroneus longus
- Peroneus brevis
- Sural nerve and lesser saphenous vein

(Top) Axial T1 MR image shows the left leg at the distal tibiofibular joint. The tendons of the ankle are much more clearly defined, though the flexor hallucis longus is still highly muscular. (Bottom) Axial T1 MR image shows the left leg at the ankle joint.

CORONAL T1 MR

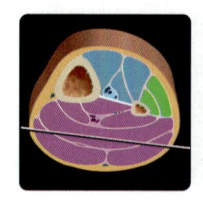

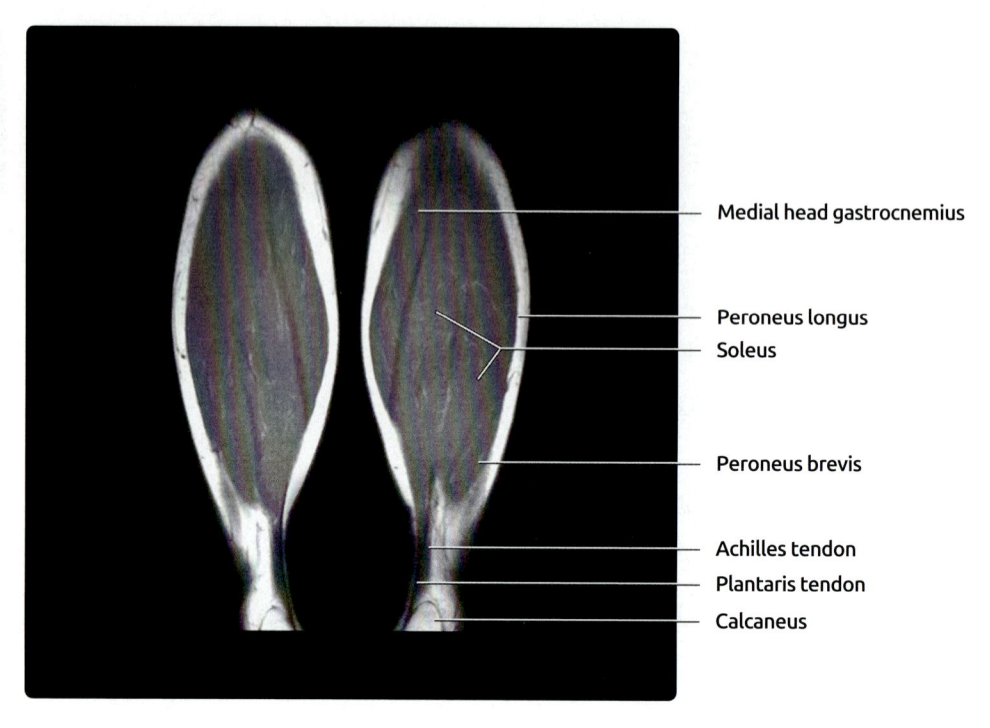

Medial head gastrocnemius
Peroneus longus
Soleus
Peroneus brevis
Achilles tendon
Plantaris tendon
Calcaneus

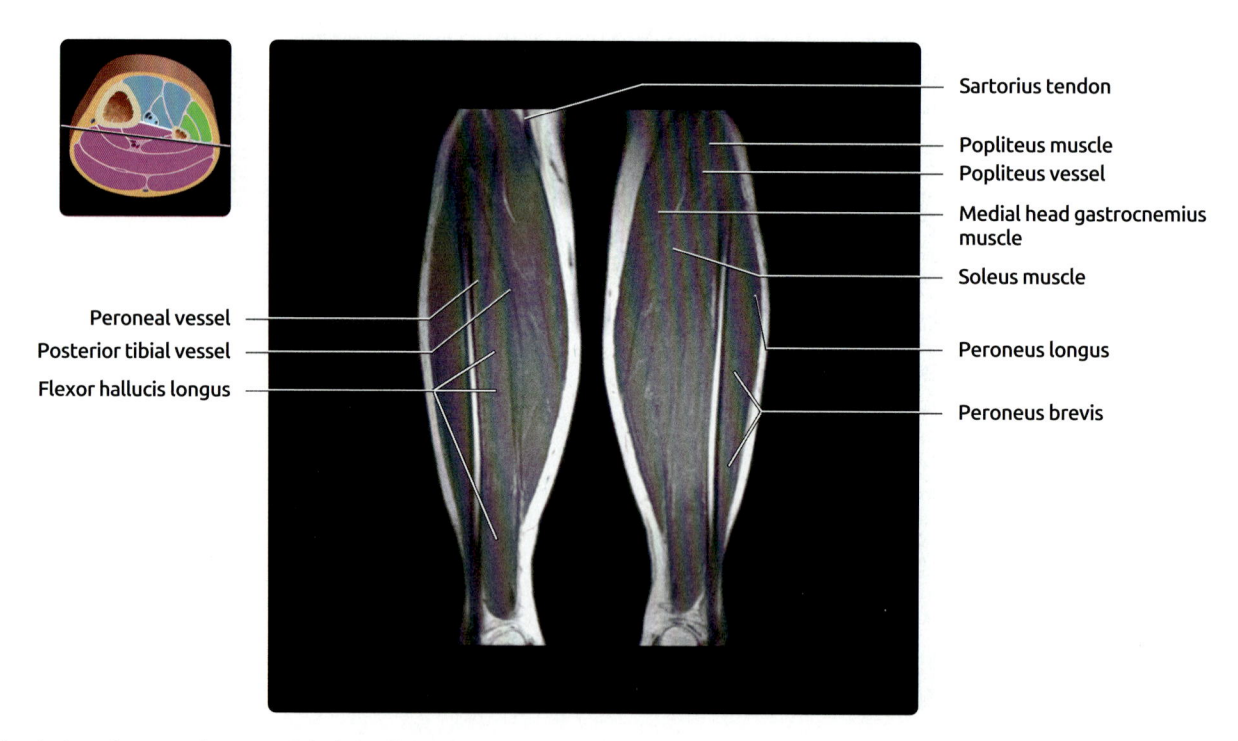

Peroneal vessel
Posterior tibial vessel
Flexor hallucis longus

Sartorius tendon
Popliteus muscle
Popliteus vessel
Medial head gastrocnemius muscle
Soleus muscle
Peroneus longus
Peroneus brevis

(Top) *First of 4 coronal images of the legs. This is the most posterior image, largely through the posterior superficial muscles. Note the plantaris tendon, which is seen well in the left leg, traveling and inserting medially to the Achilles tendon.* **(Bottom)** *Slightly more anterior coronal image shows the legs, located posteriorly, through the fibula. Portions of the deep and superficial posterior compartment are seen, along with the lateral compartment.*

Leg Radiographic Anatomy and MR Atlas

CORONAL T1 MR

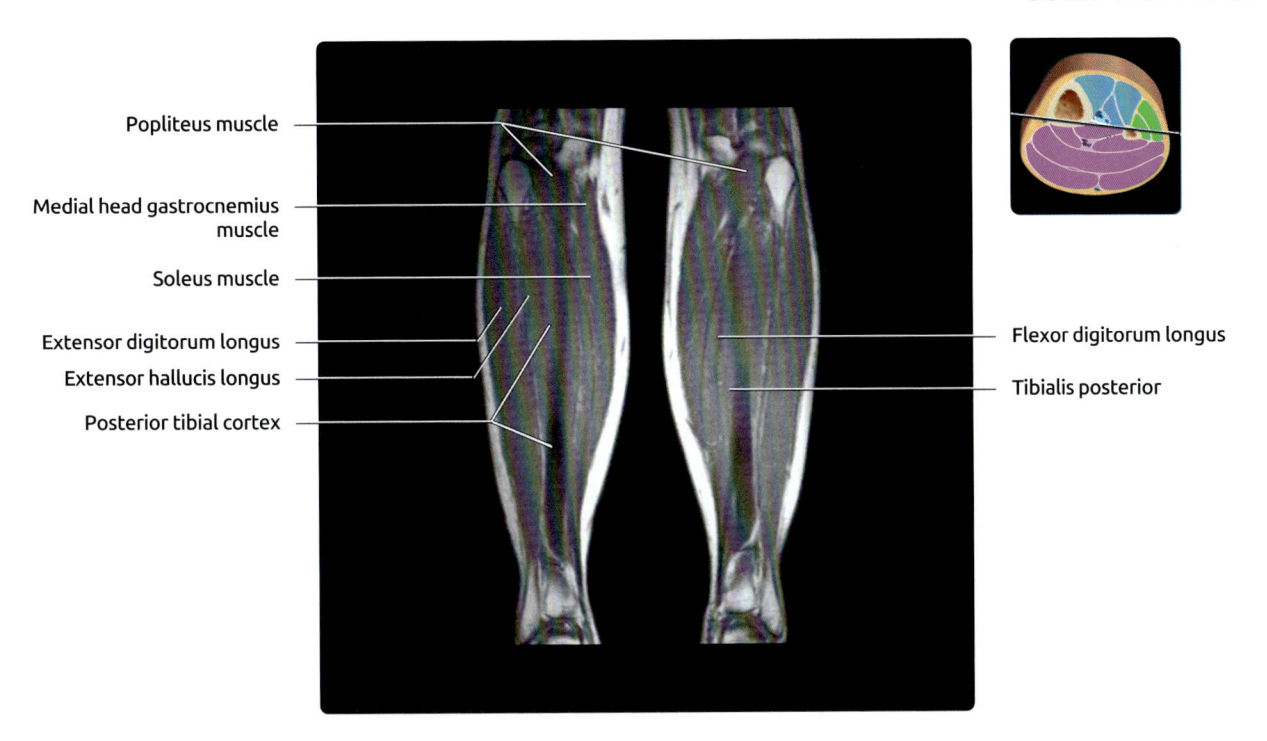

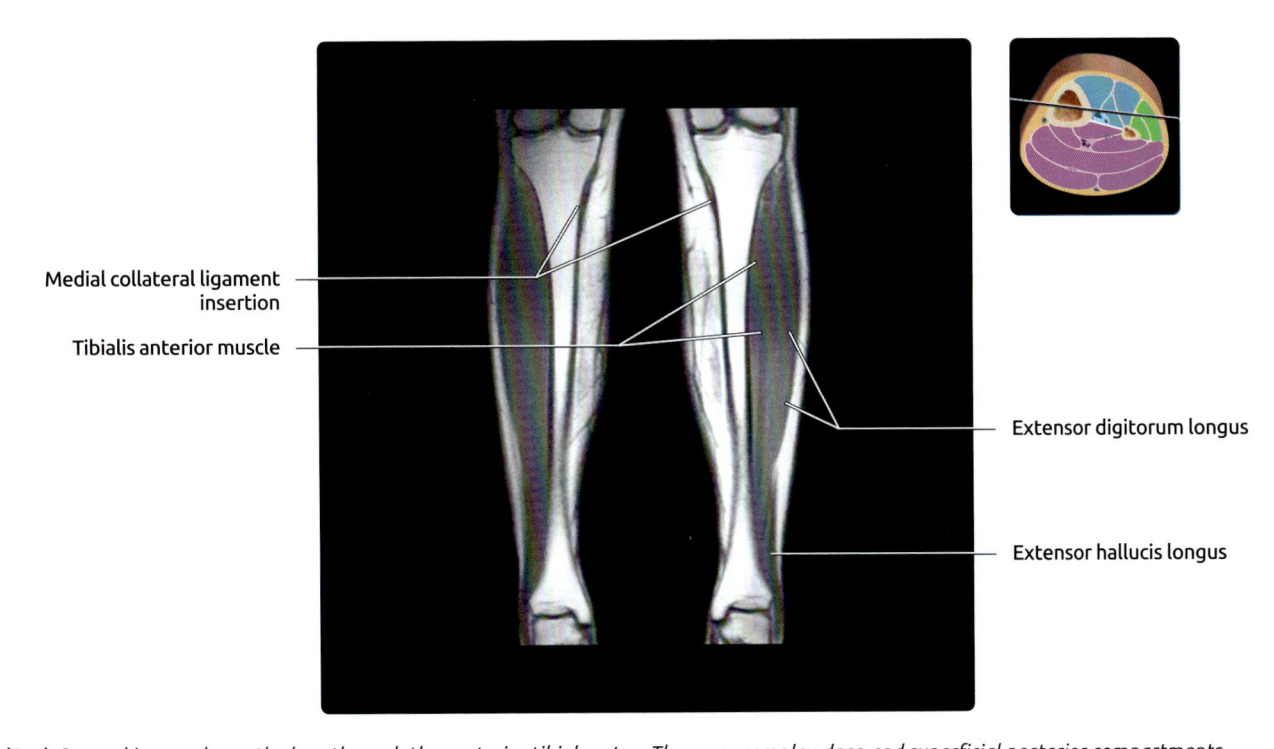

Popliteus muscle

Medial head gastrocnemius muscle

Soleus muscle

Extensor digitorum longus

Extensor hallucis longus

Posterior tibial cortex

Flexor digitorum longus

Tibialis posterior

Medial collateral ligament insertion

Tibialis anterior muscle

Extensor digitorum longus

Extensor hallucis longus

(Top) *Coronal image shows the legs through the posterior tibial cortex. The more complex deep and superficial posterior compartments are partially seen.* (Bottom) *Coronal image shows the legs, located anteriorly. Note the bare anteromedial aspect of the tibia. Because there is no overlying muscle, the blood supply is easily compromised when the tibia is fractured.*

Leg Radiographic Anatomy and MR Atlas

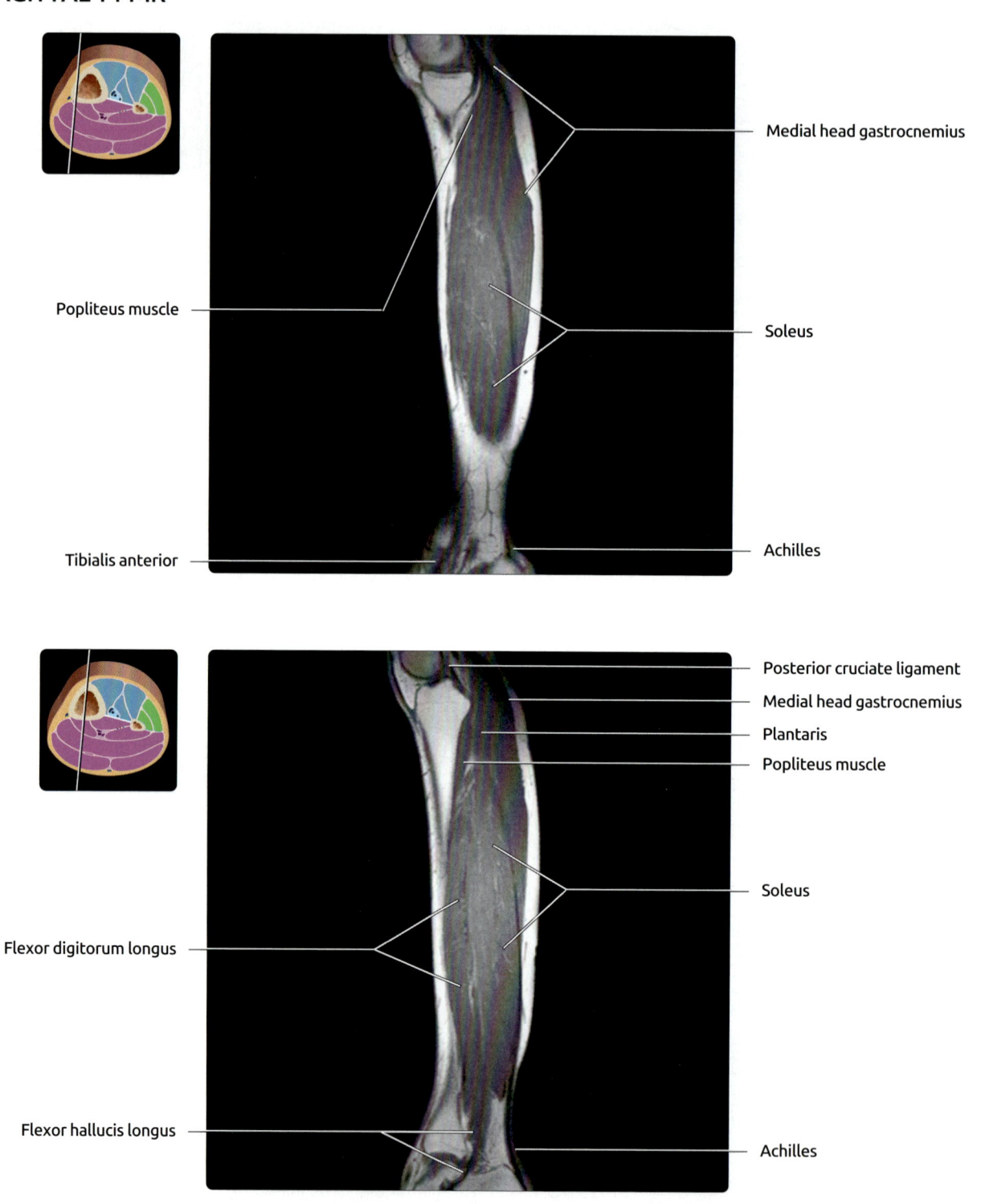

SAGITTAL T1 MR

Top image labels:
- Medial head gastrocnemius
- Soleus
- Achilles
- Popliteus muscle
- Tibialis anterior

Bottom image labels:
- Posterior cruciate ligament
- Medial head gastrocnemius
- Plantaris
- Popliteus muscle
- Soleus
- Achilles
- Flexor digitorum longus
- Flexor hallucis longus

(Top) First of 6 sagittal T1 MR images of the leg, starting medially. The bulk of the muscle here is the medial superficial posterior muscles, soleus, and gastrocnemius. **(Bottom)** Sagittal T1 MR image shows the medial leg. A portion of the deep posterior muscles is now seen, including the distal tendon of flexor hallucis longus. Note the distal extent of popliteus muscle, and the fact that the tibial origin of the soleus is from the soleal line, along the distal site of insertion of the popliteus.

Leg Radiographic Anatomy and MR Atlas

SAGITTAL T1 MR

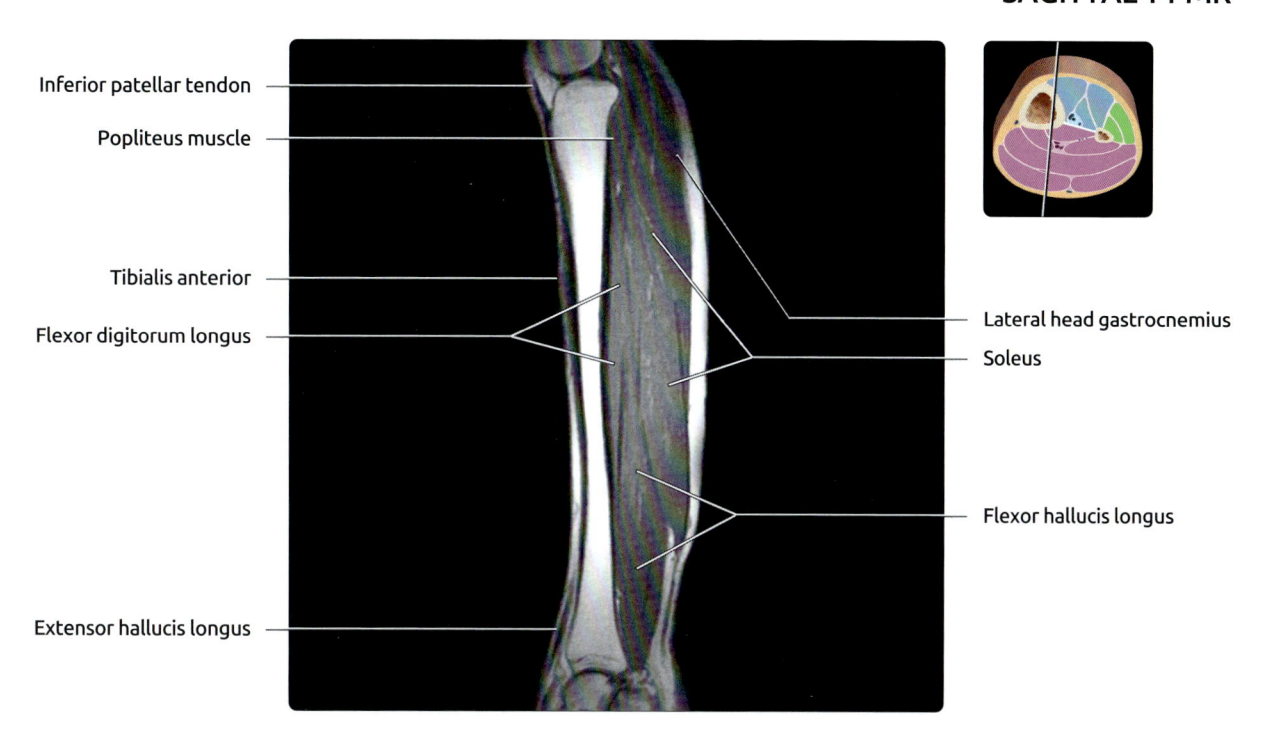

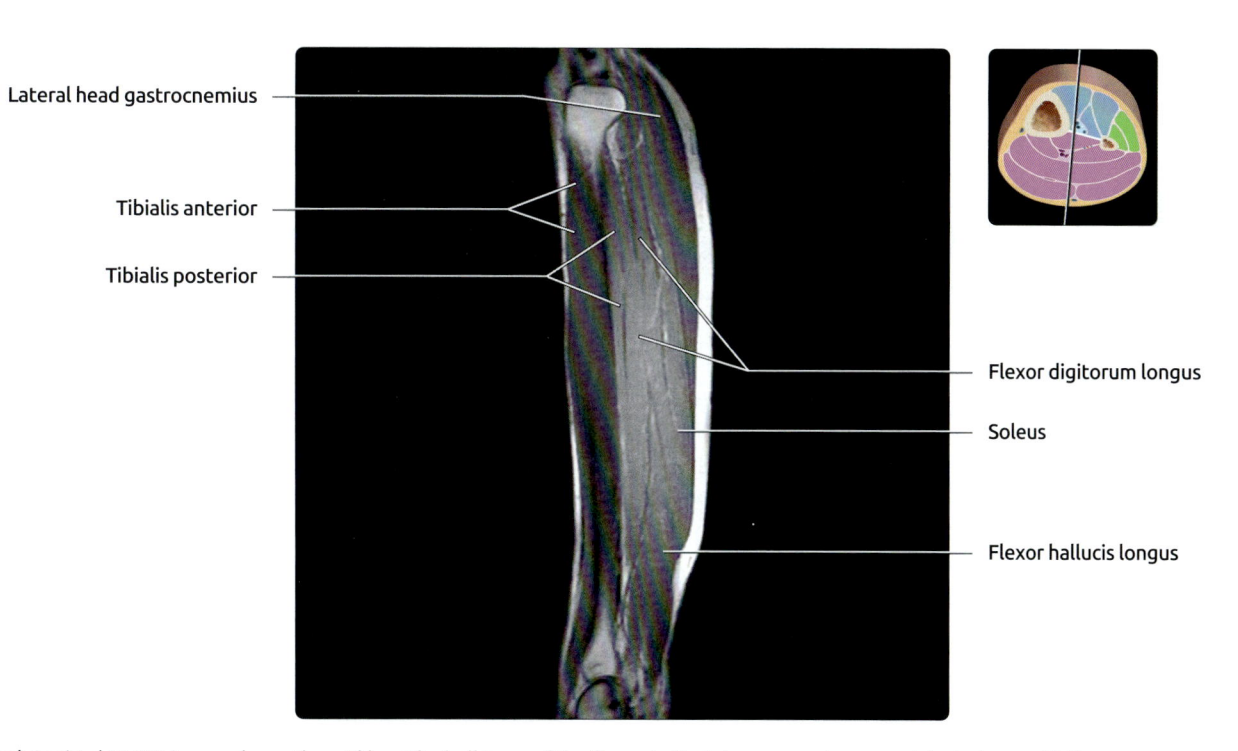

- Inferior patellar tendon
- Popliteus muscle
- Tibialis anterior
- Flexor digitorum longus
- Extensor hallucis longus
- Lateral head gastrocnemius
- Soleus
- Flexor hallucis longus

- Lateral head gastrocnemius
- Tibialis anterior
- Tibialis posterior
- Flexor digitorum longus
- Soleus
- Flexor hallucis longus

(Top) Sagittal T1 MR image shows the mid leg. The bulkiness of the flexor hallucis longus can be appreciated, along with the pre-Achilles fat pad separating it from the Achilles tendon. Note also the bare medial aspect of the shaft of the tibia. (Bottom) Sagittal T1 MR image, slightly lateral in the leg, is shown. The tibialis anterior is seen arising from the lateral aspect of the shaft of the tibia.

Leg Radiographic Anatomy and MR Atlas

SAGITTAL T1 MR

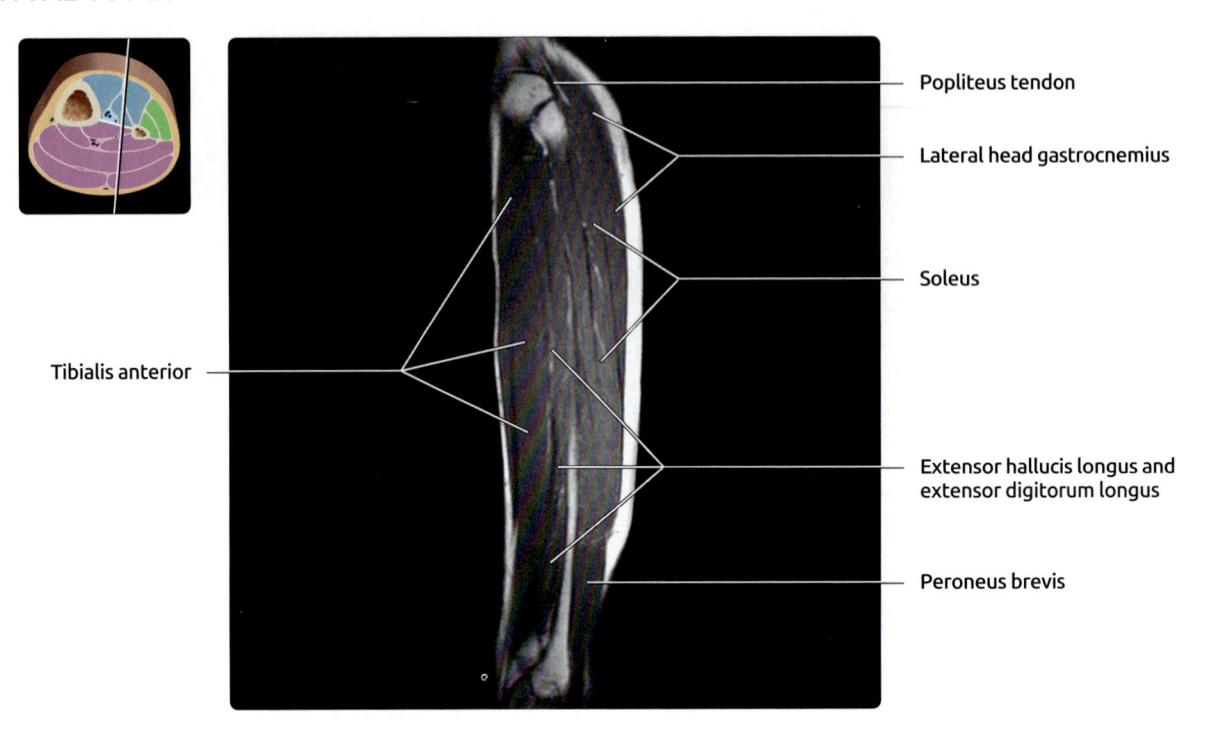

- Popliteus tendon
- Lateral head gastrocnemius
- Soleus
- Tibialis anterior
- Extensor hallucis longus and extensor digitorum longus
- Peroneus brevis

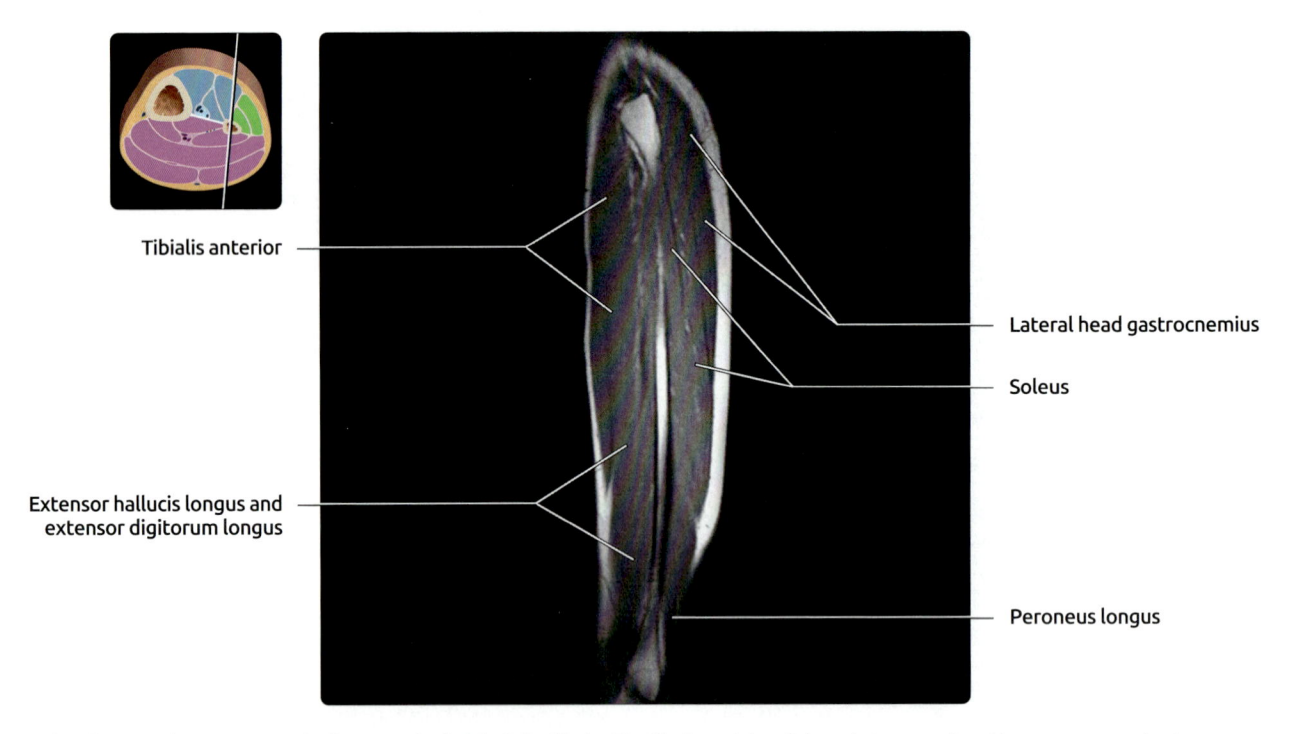

- Tibialis anterior
- Lateral head gastrocnemius
- Soleus
- Extensor hallucis longus and extensor digitorum longus
- Peroneus longus

(Top) Sagittal T1 MR image is shown at the level of the fibula. The fibular origin of the soleus, as well as the peroneus and extensor digitorum, are seen. (Bottom) Sagittal T1 MR image is shown at the level of the fibula. Given the bulky muscles arising from the fibula, it is not surprising that the fibular surface is irregular. This should not be mistaken for periosteal reaction.

Leg Radiographic Anatomy and MR Atlas

GRAPHICS: PERONEAL NERVE

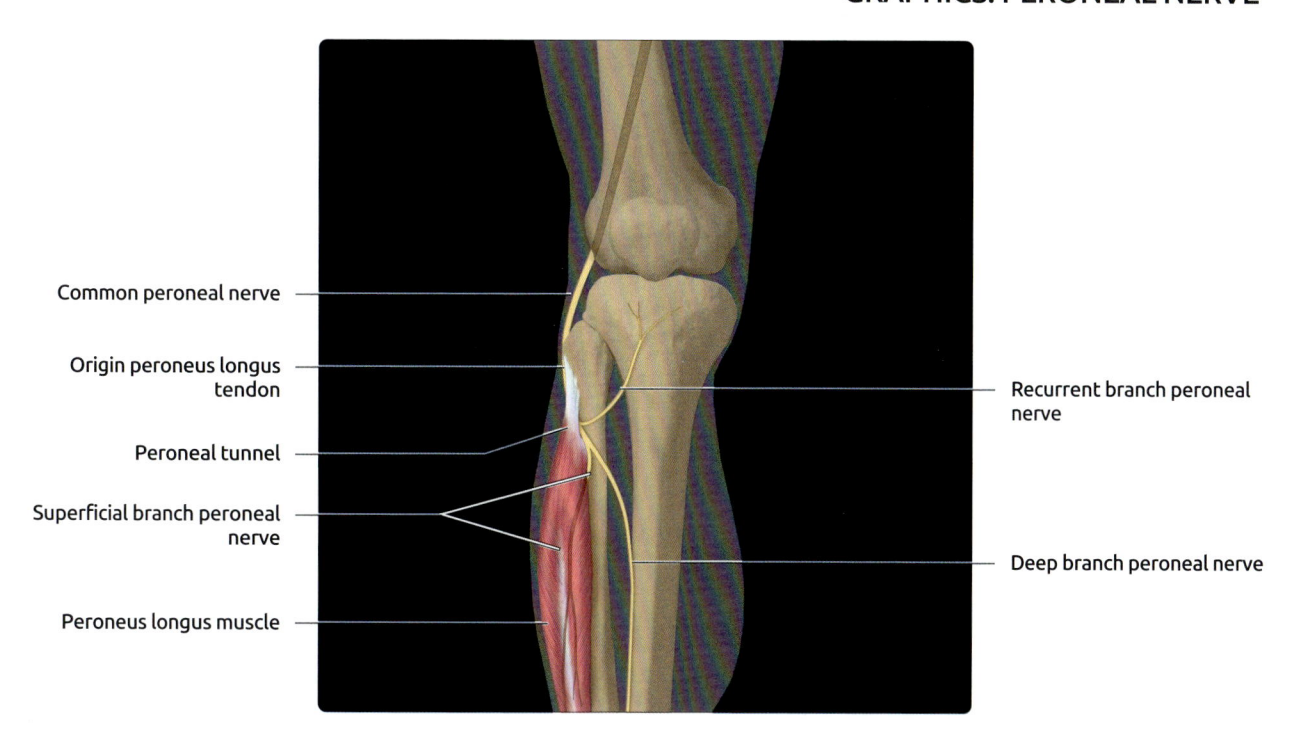

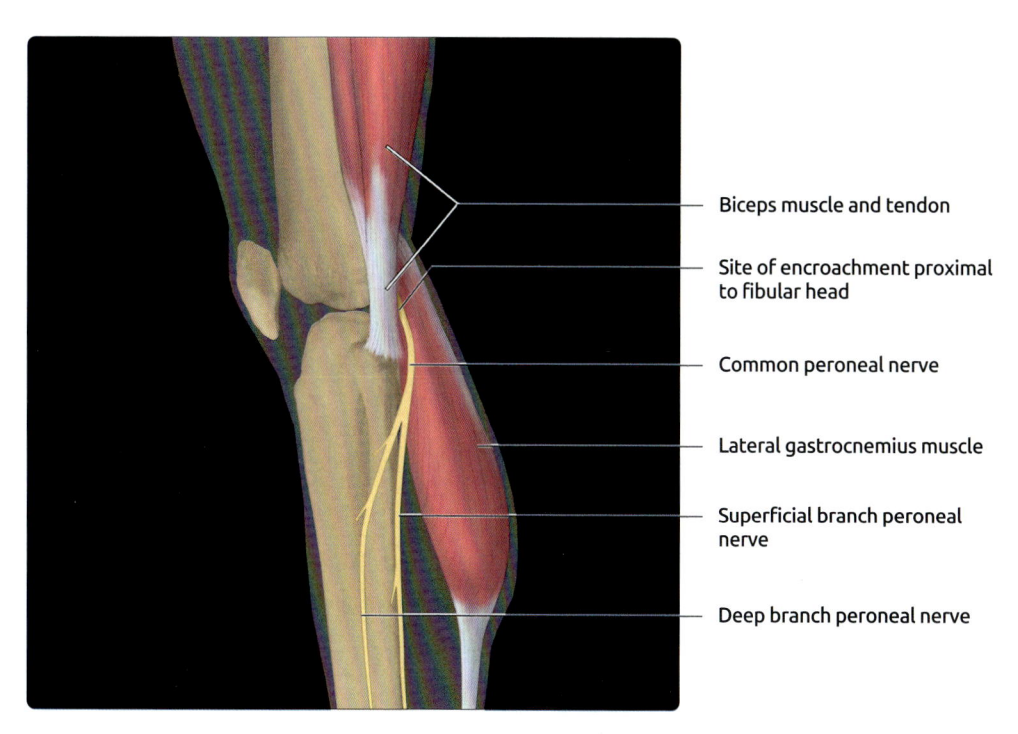

Labels (top image): Common peroneal nerve; Origin peroneus longus tendon; Peroneal tunnel; Superficial branch peroneal nerve; Peroneus longus muscle; Recurrent branch peroneal nerve; Deep branch peroneal nerve

Labels (bottom image): Biceps muscle and tendon; Site of encroachment proximal to fibular head; Common peroneal nerve; Lateral gastrocnemius muscle; Superficial branch peroneal nerve; Deep branch peroneal nerve

(**Top**) *The common peroneal nerve branches from the sciatic nerve. It courses anterolaterally, posterior to the biceps femoris muscle, and winds around fibular head. As it curves around the anterior surface of the fibula, the nerve enters the peroneal (fibular) tunnel, where it runs deep to the tendinous origin of peroneus longus and rests against the surface of the fibular neck. Peroneal nerve compression may occur at the peroneal tunnel, either from repetitive activity involving inversion or pronation of the foot, fibular neck fracture, or total knee arthroplasty with correction of a significant valgus angulation of the knee. Fat hypertrophy within the tunnel has been reported to relate to the peroneal nerve compression in diabetic patients.* (**Bottom**) *Lateral graphic with the peroneus longus muscle peeled away, showing the site at which the common peroneal nerve can be compressed proximal to the fibular head. Biceps muscle variants or hypertrophy may be the culprit.*

SECTION 11
Ankle

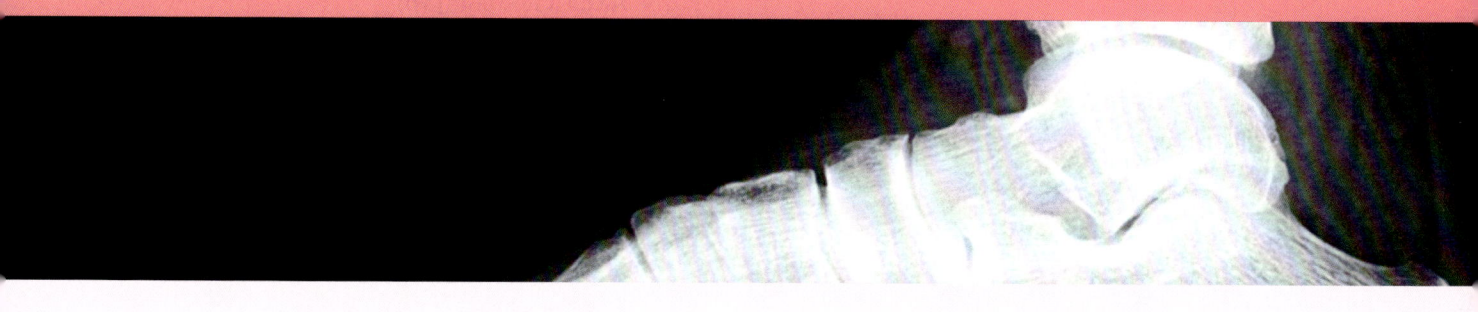

Ankle Overview	**918**
Ankle Radiographic and Arthrographic Anatomy	**934**
Ankle MR Atlas	**946**
Ankle Tendons	**980**
Ankle Ligaments	**1004**

Ankle Overview

TERMINOLOGY

Definitions
- Hindfoot: General term for ankle and subtalar joints, talus and calcaneus
- Midfoot: General term for remaining tarsal bones and their articulations
  - Navicular, cuboid, cuneiforms
- Forefoot: General term for metatarsals and phalanges

GROSS ANATOMY

Osseous Structures
- **Tibia**
  - Plafond articulates with talar body
    - Slightly convex from medial to lateral, concave anterior to posterior
  - Medial malleolus articulates with medial surface of talar body
    - Forms anterior and posterior colliculi
    - Anterior colliculus extends further inferiorly than posterior colliculus
  - Posterior malleolus is broad posterior margin of tibia
- **Fibula**
  - Articulates with tibia via distal tibiofibular joint
  - Lateral malleolus articulates with lateral surface of talar body
- **Talus**
  - Articulates with tibia, fibula, calcaneus, and navicular
    - 2/3 covered by articular cartilage
    - No muscle attachments
  - Divided into body, neck, and head
  - Trochlea of body articulates with tibia
    - Term "talar dome" is a misnomer
    - Slightly concave from medial to lateral, rounded convexity anterior to posterior
    - Trochlea is broader anteriorly than posteriorly
  - Posterior process projects posteriorly from body
    - Divided into medial and lateral tubercles, between which passes flexor hallucis longus tendon
    - Separate center of ossification, often remains a separate ossicle in adulthood (os trigonum)
  - Lateral process projects laterally from body
    - Articulates with lateral malleolus superiorly, posterior subtalar joint inferiorly
  - Neck forms superomedial boundary of tarsal sinus
    - Major blood supply to talar body enters via neck
  - Head articulates with navicular and calcaneus
- **Calcaneus**
  - Articulates with talus (3 facets) and cuboid
  - Weightbearing, springboard for locomotion
  - Divided into posterior process, body, sustentaculum tali, anterior process

Articulations
- **Inferior tibiofibular joint**
  - Primarily a fibrous joint
    - Synovial recess from ankle joint extends at least 1 cm into syndesmosis
    - May have articular cartilage at inferior portion
  - Close apposition of tibia and fibula is maintained by syndesmotic ligaments
  - Motion: Minimal superior-inferior motion and external rotation
- **Ankle (talocrural) joint**
  - Synovial joint between tibia, fibula, and talus
  - Inferior tibiofibular joint unites tibia and fibula into mortise
  - Talus is tenon within mortise of tibia + fibula
  - Motion: Hinge joint: Extension (dorsiflexion) and flexion (plantar flexion)
    - Dynamic shift of axis of rotation during dorsi and plantar flexion
  - Supported by lateral and medial collateral ligaments
- **Subtalar joint**
  - Synovial joints between talus and calcaneus
  - 3 facets: Posterior, middle, and anterior
  - Posterior facet has separate joint capsule
    - 15% communicate with ankle joint
    - 50% of weightbearing occurs through posterior subtalar joint
    - Motion: Inversion, eversion, and anteroposterior gliding
  - Middle and anterior facets communicate with each other and talonavicular joint
  - Motions: Inversion, eversion, adduction, abduction

Ligaments
- 3 sets stabilize ankle: Distal tibiofibular syndesmotic complex, lateral collateral, and deltoid ligaments
- **4 tibiofibular syndesmotic ligaments**
  - Maintain width of ankle mortise, stabilize against eversion
  - **Anterior and posterior inferior tibiofibular ligaments**
  - **Inferior transverse ligament**: Distal to main posterior tibiofibular ligament
  - **Interosseous ligament**: Distal thickening of syndesmotic membrane
- **3 lateral collateral ligaments**: Stabilize ankle against inversion and anterior, posterior subluxation
  - **Anterior talofibular ligament**
    - Originates 1 cm proximal to lateral malleolar tip, inserts on talar neck
    - Stabilizes talus against anterior displacement, internal rotation, and inversion
    - Weakest and first to tear
    - Isolated tear is common and may not result in clinical ankle instability
  - **Calcaneofibular ligament**
    - Originates from lateral malleolar tip, inserts on calcaneal trochlear eminence
    - Deep to peroneal tendons
    - Lateral restraint of subtalar joint, often tears with anterior talofibular ligament
  - **Posterior talofibular ligament**
    - Extends from lateral malleolar fossa to lateral talar tubercle
    - Strongest, rarely tears
- **Medial collateral ligament = deltoid ligament**
  - Divided into superficial and deep components

Ankle Overview

- Superficial: From medial (superficial) margin of medial malleolus
  - Fibers merge with flexor retinaculum along posteromedial margin of medial malleolus
  - Multiple, variable bands, named for sites of attachment
  - Anterior tibiotalar, tibiospring, and tibionavicular, deep to posterior tibial tendon
    - Tibiocalcaneal is strongest band
  - Posterior tibiotalar and tibiocalcaneal
  - Provide rotational stability
- Deep: Posterior and anterior tibiotalar
  - Posterior tibiotalar: Thick, striated, nearly horizontal in orientation, from posterior colliculus medial malleolus to medial fossa of talar body, prevent joint eversion
  - Anterior tibiotalar: Thin, from anterior colliculus to junction talar body and neck
- **Spring ligament (plantar calcaneonavicular ligament)**
  - Binds calcaneus to navicular, 3 components
  - Superomedial **origin:** Sustentaculum tali; **insertion:** Superomedial navicular, tibiospring band of deltoid
  - Medioplantar oblique **origin:** Calcaneal coronoid fossa; **insertion:** Plantar navicular
  - Inferoplantar longitudinal **origin:** Coronoid fossa; **insertion:** Navicular beak

Retinacula

- Focal thickening of deep fascia
- Maintain tendons in position when they change orientation
- **Superior extensor retinaculum**
  - A few cm above ankle joint
  - Attaches to anterior fibula laterally, tibia medially
  - Distally attaches to inferior extensor retinaculum
  - Prevents bowstringing of anterior compartment muscles
- **Inferior extensor retinaculum**
  - At ankle joint, Y-shaped, stem laterally, proximal, and distal bands medially
  - Stem attaches laterally to upper calcaneus
    - Loops around extensor tendons
    - Roots extend into sinus tarsi
  - Proximal medial band has deep and superficial layers, loop around extensor hallus longus tendon and occasionally tibialis anterior tendon
  - Distal medial band superficial to extensor hallucis longus and tibialis anterior tendons
    - Attaches to plantar aponeurosis
  - Dorsalis pedis vessels, deep peroneal nerve: Deep to all layers of inferior extensor retinaculum
- **Flexor retinaculum**
  - Attaches to tubercle at posteromedial corner of medial malleolus
    - Continuous with periosteum and origin of superficial deltoid ligament
  - Proximally continuous with deep fascia of leg
  - Distally continuous with plantar aponeurosis
  - Abductor hallucis partly attached to it
  - Maintains position of extrinsic flexor tendons as they pass from leg into foot
  - Lateral border of tarsal tunnel
- **Superior peroneal retinaculum**
  - Origin: Lateral malleolus, insertions vary, most commonly to deep fascia of leg and calcaneus
  - Maintains position of peroneal tendons posterior to fibula
- **Inferior peroneal retinaculum**
  - Continuous with inferior extensor retinaculum
  - Inserts on lateral calcaneus, peroneal tubercle (trochlea)
  - Maintains position of peroneal tendons adjacent to calcaneus

Tendons

- **Anterior (extensor) compartment:** Tendons listed from medial to lateral
  - **Anterior tibial (tibialis anterior) tendon**
    - Dorsiflexes ankle, inverts foot, tightens plantar aponeurosis
    - Inserts on medial cuneiform, base of 1st metatarsal
    - Supports medial longitudinal arch during walking
  - **Extensor hallucis longus tendon**
    - Extends 1st phalanges, dorsiflexes foot and great toe
    - Inserts on dorsal base of 1st distal phalanx
  - **Extensor digitorum longus tendon**
    - Dorsiflexes ankle, extends toes, tightens plantar aponeurosis
    - Divides into 4 slips on dorsum of foot
    - Slips receive tendinous contributions from extensor digitorum brevis, lumbricals and interosseous muscles
    - Each slip divides into 3: Central one inserts on dorsal base of middle phalanx and 2 collateral ones which reunite and insert on bases of 2nd-5th distal phalanges
  - **Peroneus tertius tendon**
    - Typically part of extensor digitorum longus tendon
    - Inserts on dorsal base of 5th metatarsal
    - Variably present
- **Lateral compartment**
  - **Peroneus longus tendon**
    - Plantarflexes ankle, everts foot, supports longitudinal and transverse arches during walking
    - Posterolateral to peroneus brevis tendon in retrofibular groove, deep to superior peroneal retinaculum
    - Descends behind peroneal tubercle, deep to inferior peroneal retinaculum
    - Curves under cuboid sulcus, deep to long plantar ligament
    - Inserts on plantar base of 1st metatarsal, medial cuneiform
    - Os peroneum always present, ossified in about 20% of individuals
  - **Peroneus brevis tendon**
    - Everts foot, limits foot inversion
    - Anteromedial to peroneus longus tendon in retrofibular groove, deep to superior peroneal retinaculum
    - Descends anterior to peroneal tubercle of calcaneus, deep to inferior peroneal retinaculum
    - Inserts into base of 5th metatarsal
- **Superficial posterior compartment**
  - **Achilles tendon**
    - Main plantar flexor of ankle, foot

Ankle Overview

- Largest and strongest tendon in body
- Conjoined tendon of medial and lateral gastrocnemius and soleus muscles
- Approximately 15 cm long
- Lacks tendon sheath, enclosed by paratenon
- Inserts on posterior calcaneal tuberosity
- Retrocalcaneal bursa between distal tendon and calcaneal tuberosity

- **Plantaris tendon**
  - Vestigial, slender tendon, medial to Achilles tendon
  - Inserts on, or medial to, Achilles tendon on calcaneus
- **Deep posterior (flexor) compartment**
  - Posterior tibial (tibialis posterior) tendon
    - Crosses flexor digitorum longus tendon above ankle joint to become most posteromedial tendon
    - Shares tibial groove with flexor digitorum longus tendon
    - Inserts on navicular tuberosity, cuneiforms, sustentaculum tali, bases of 2nd-4th metatarsals
    - Main invertor of foot, aids in plantar flexion
    - Supports medial longitudinal arch
  - Flexor digitorum longus tendon
    - Lateral to tibialis posterior tendon in tibial groove
    - Crosses flexor hallucis longus tendon at master knot of Henry
    - Divides into 4 slips that give origin to lumbricals
    - Slips pass through openings in corresponding tendons of flexor digitorum brevis
    - Slips insert on bases of 2nd-5th distal phalanges
    - Flexes distal phalanges, assists in plantar flexion of ankle
  - Flexor hallucis longus tendon
    - Passes 3 fibro-osseous tunnels: 1) between medial and lateral talar tubercles, 2) under sustentaculum tali, 3) between 1st medial and lateral sesamoids
    - Crosses and sends slip to flexor digitorum longus at master knot of Henry
    - Inserts on base of 1st distal phalanx
    - When foot is on ground: Maintains pad of 1st toe on ground
    - When foot is off ground: Plantar flexes 1st phalanges, aids in maintaining medial longitudinal arch
    - Weak plantar flexor of ankle

Vessels

- **Anterior tibial artery** becomes **dorsalis pedis** at ankle joint
- **Posterior tibial artery** divides into medial and lateral plantar arteries in tarsal tunnel

Nerves

- **Tibial nerve**
  - Largest, medial terminal branch of sciatic nerve
  - May be called posterior tibial nerve in ankle
  - Curves around medial malleolus, travels in tarsal tunnel under flexor retinaculum
  - Divides in, or proximal to, tarsal tunnel
    - Medial calcaneal nerve: Sensory medial heel
    - Medial plantar nerve: Sensory to medial 2/3 plantar foot, motor to abductor hallucis, flexor digitorum brevis, flexor hallucis brevis, 1st lumbrical
    - Lateral plantar nerve: Sensory to lateral 1/3 of plantar foot, motor to abductor digiti minimi, quadratus plantae, adductor hallucis, flexor digiti minimi, 2nd-4th lumbricals, all interossei
  - Vulnerable to impingement in tarsal tunnel
- **Common peroneal nerve**
  - Smaller, lateral, terminal branch of sciatic nerve, divides below knee into deep and superficial peroneal nerves
- **Deep peroneal nerve**
  - Deep to extensor retinacula, in anterior tarsal tunnel
  - Predominantly motor
  - Divides just above ankle into medial (mainly sensory), lateral (mainly motor) branches
    - **Medial branch** continues dorsal to talonavicular joint, middle cuneiform and in between 1st and 2nd metatarsals
    - **Lateral branch** ends at extensor digitorum brevis
  - In leg: Motor to anterior tibial, extensor digitorum longus, extensor hallucis longus, peroneus tertius
  - In foot: Motor to extensor digitorum brevis, sensory (and sometimes motor) to 1st web space
- **Superficial peroneal nerve**
  - Exits deep fascia 10-15 cm above ankle joint
  - Subcutaneous 6 cm above ankle, divides into subcutaneous branches
  - In leg: Motor to peroneus brevis and peroneus longus tendons, sensory to distal 2/3 lateral leg
  - In foot: Sensory to dorsal foot
- **Sural nerve**
  - Formed by medial sural branch of tibial nerve and peroneal (sural) communicating branch of common peroneal nerve
  - Purely sensory to lateral ankle and foot, up to 5th toe base
  - Subcutaneous along posterolateral ankle
- **Saphenous nerve** (branch of femoral nerve)
  - Subcutaneous, lateral to greater saphenous vein

Spaces of Ankle

- **Tarsal sinus (sinus tarsi)**
  - Lateral, funnel-shaped space between talar neck and calcaneus
  - Contains insertions of 3 bands of inferior extensor retinaculum
  - Contains cervical ligament between talar neck and calcaneus
  - Artery of tarsal sinus courses retrograde through sinus to supply talar body
- **Tarsal tunnel**
  - Roof: Flexor retinaculum
  - Floor: Medial tibia, talus, calcaneus
  - Contains tibialis posterior, flexor digitorum and flexor hallucis tendons
  - Contains posterior tibial neurovascular bundle
    - Tibial nerve divides in tunnel into branches to calcaneus, plus medial and lateral plantar nerves
- **Tarsal canal**
  - Between talus and calcaneus, posteromedial extent of tarsal sinus
  - Contains interosseous ligament

Ankle Overview

GRAPHICS: TALUS

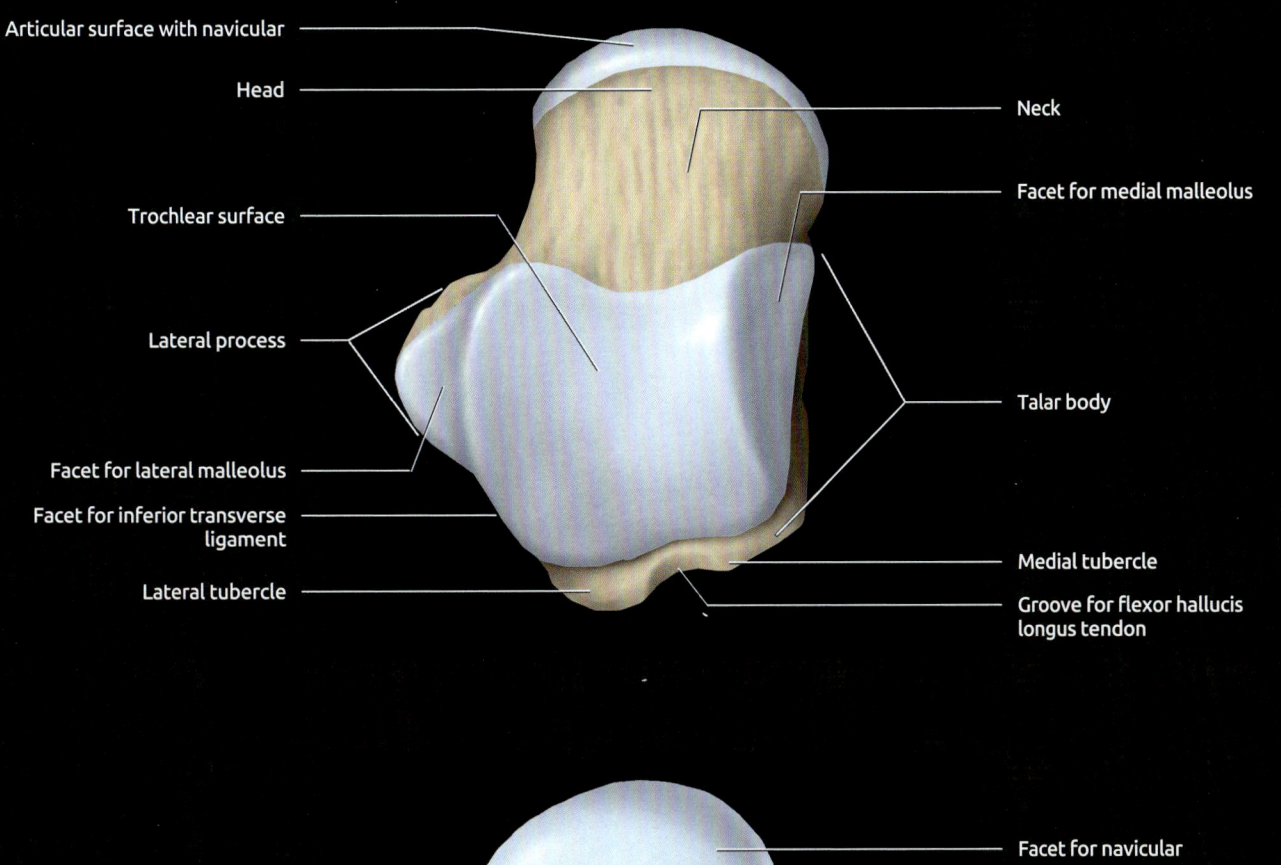

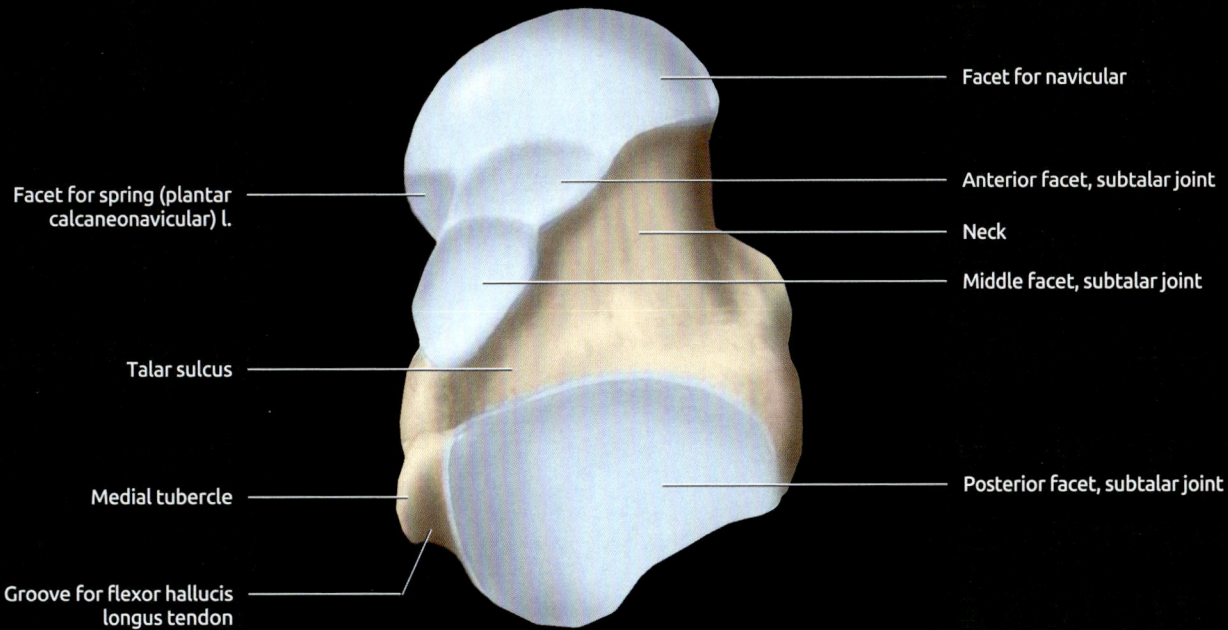

Labels (top view):
- Articular surface with navicular
- Head
- Trochlear surface
- Lateral process
- Facet for lateral malleolus
- Facet for inferior transverse ligament
- Lateral tubercle
- Neck
- Facet for medial malleolus
- Talar body
- Medial tubercle
- Groove for flexor hallucis longus tendon

Labels (plantar view):
- Facet for spring (plantar calcaneonavicular) l.
- Talar sulcus
- Medial tubercle
- Groove for flexor hallucis longus tendon
- Facet for navicular
- Anterior facet, subtalar joint
- Neck
- Middle facet, subtalar joint
- Posterior facet, subtalar joint

(Top) *View of the talus from above is shown. The tibia transmits body weight to the talus, which then redistributes it to the calcaneus and navicular. The talus is subdivided into body, neck, and head. The body contains the trochlea, which forms the talocrural joint with the tibia. The trochlear surface is narrower posteriorly than anteriorly. The flexor hallucis longus tendon traverses in a groove between the medial and lateral tubercles of the posterior talar process.* (Bottom) *Plantar view of the talus shows the articular facets for the subtalar joint and the talonavicular joint. The cervical and interosseous ligaments insert into the plantar talar neck. The talar sulcus and calcaneal sulcus together form the tarsal canal and sinus tarsi space.*

Ankle Overview

GRAPHICS: TALUS

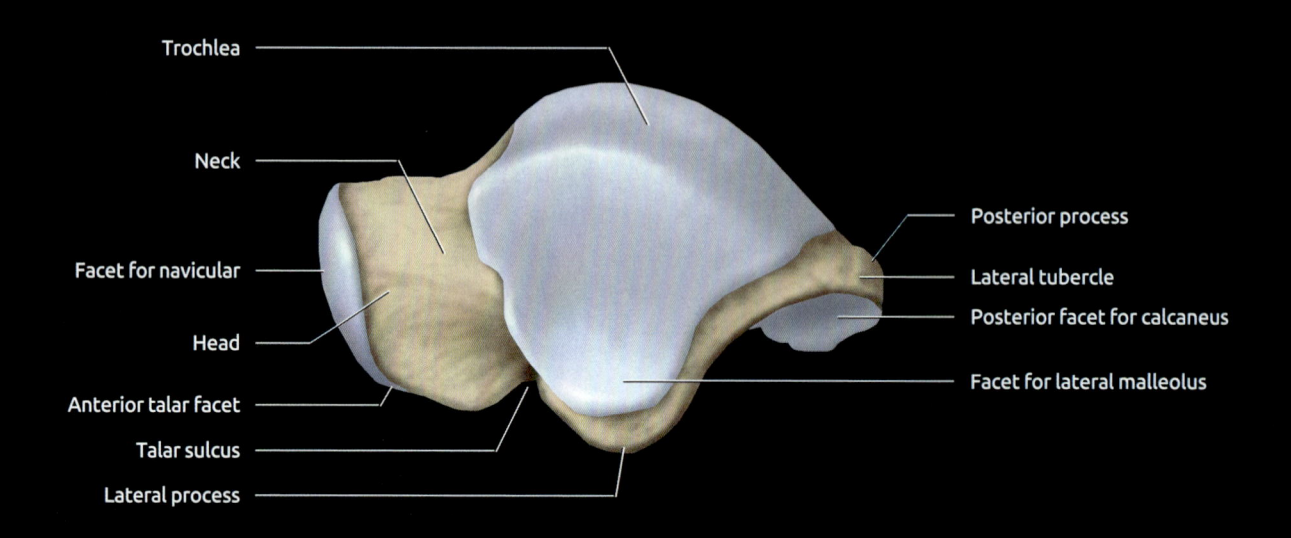

Labels (top, lateral view): Trochlea, Neck, Facet for navicular, Head, Anterior talar facet, Talar sulcus, Lateral process, Posterior process, Lateral tubercle, Posterior facet for calcaneus, Facet for lateral malleolus

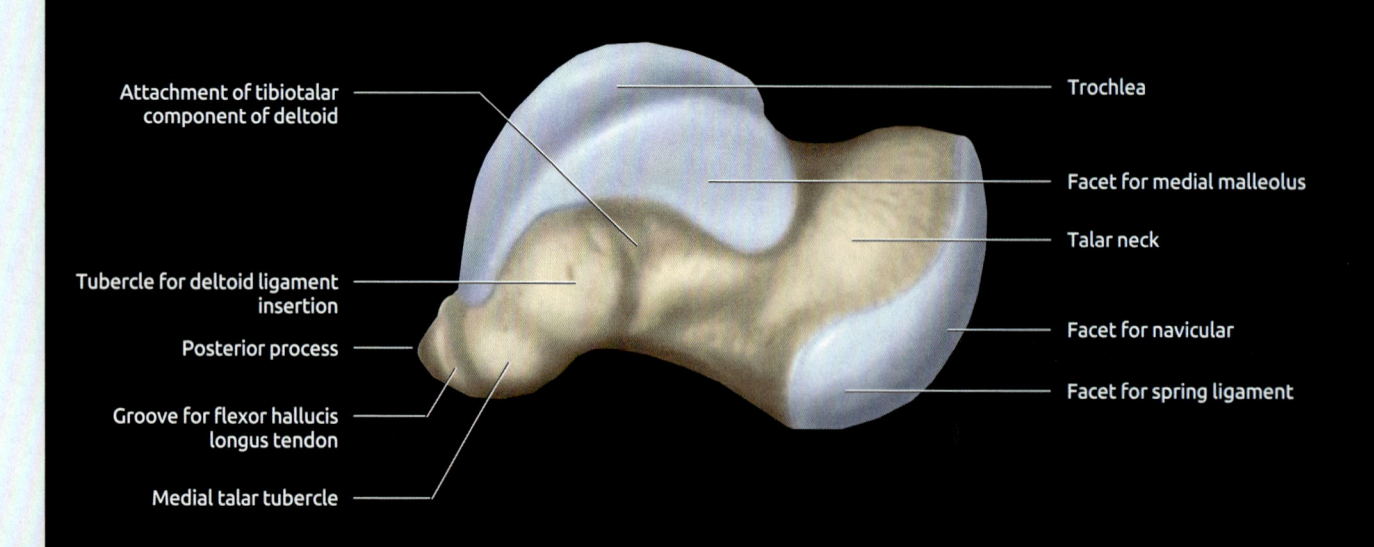

Labels (bottom, medial view): Attachment of tibiotalar component of deltoid, Tubercle for deltoid ligament insertion, Posterior process, Groove for flexor hallucis longus tendon, Medial talar tubercle, Trochlea, Facet for medial malleolus, Talar neck, Facet for navicular, Facet for spring ligament

(**Top**) *A lateral view of the talus is shown. The talar facet for the lateral malleolus is quite large and covers most of the lateral process of the talus. The lateral facet is obliquely oriented. It is also larger and extends more posteriorly than the medial facet. When elongated, the lateral tubercle is termed a Stieda process. An os trigonum is an unfused lateral talar tubercle which forms a synchondrosis with the posterior process of talus. The talus has no muscles or tendons attaching to it & 2/3 of its surface is covered with cartilage (blue).* (**Bottom**) *Medial view of the talus shows the short facet for the medial malleolus. The deltoid ligament inserts onto the fovea of the talus below the facet. The trochlea has a central indentation that increases and stabilizes the articular contact with the tibia.*

Ankle Overview

GRAPHICS: CALCANEUS

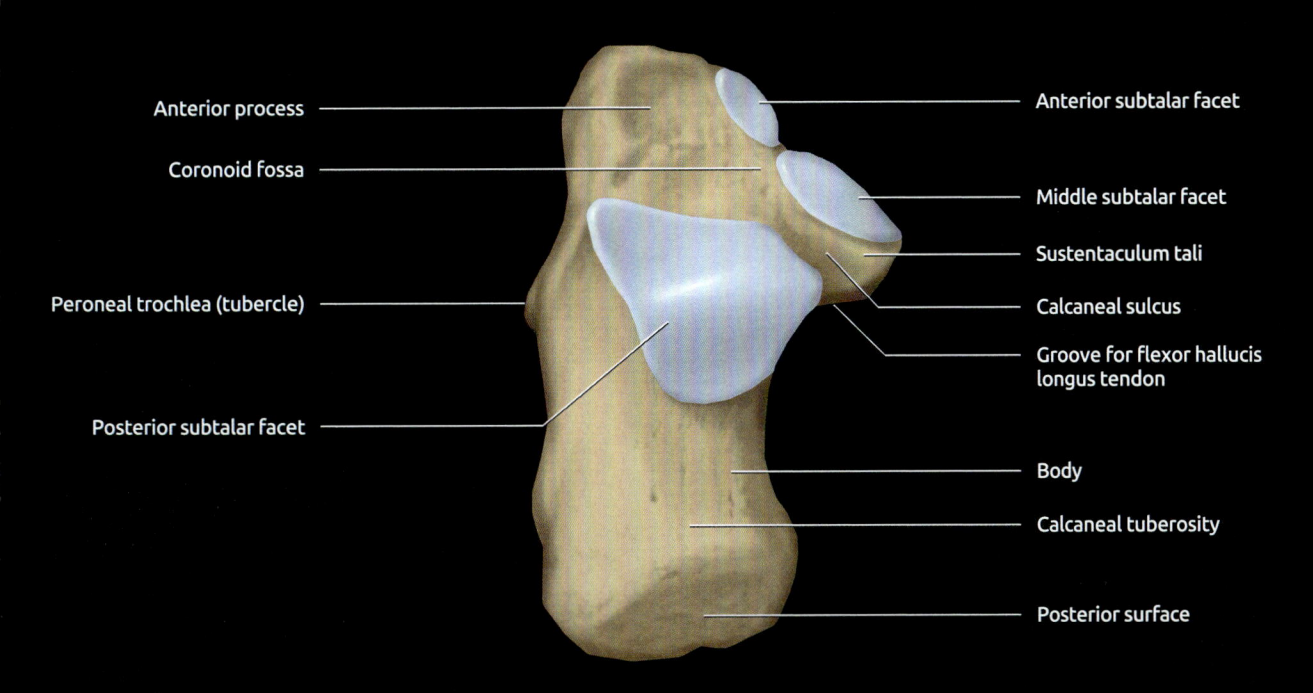

Anterior process — Coronoid fossa — Peroneal trochlea (tubercle) — Posterior subtalar facet — Anterior subtalar facet — Middle subtalar facet — Sustentaculum tali — Calcaneal sulcus — Groove for flexor hallucis longus tendon — Body — Calcaneal tuberosity — Posterior surface

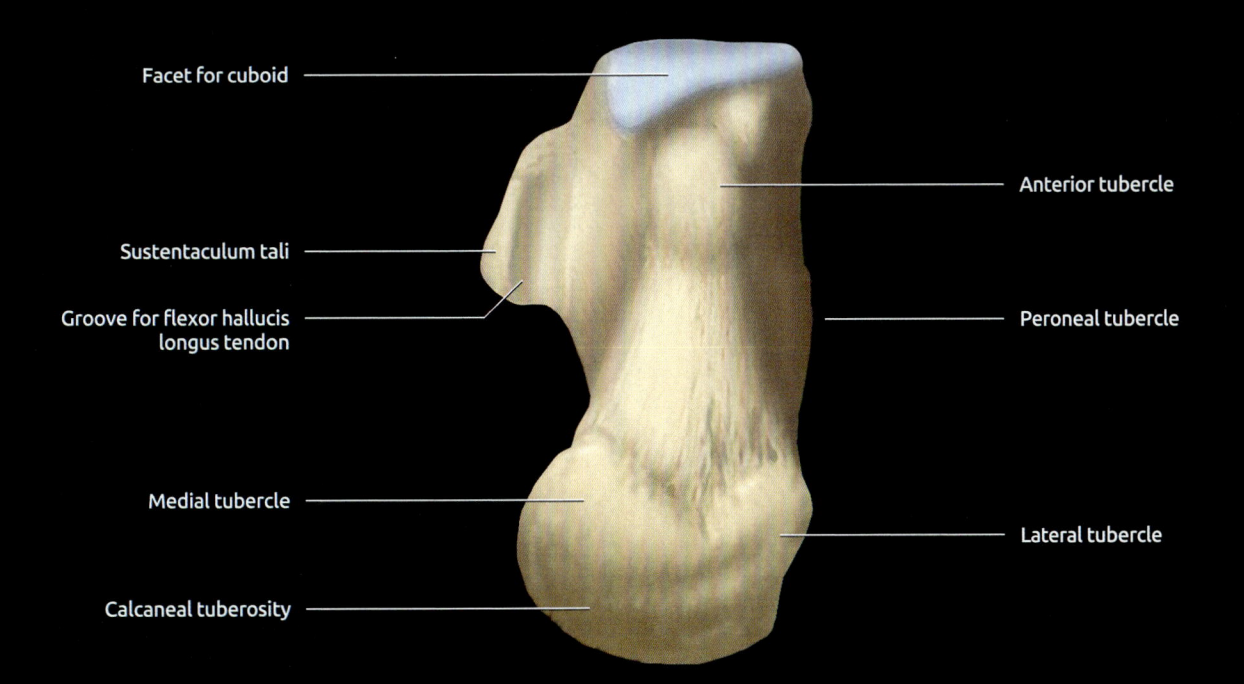

Facet for cuboid — Sustentaculum tali — Groove for flexor hallucis longus tendon — Medial tubercle — Calcaneal tuberosity — Anterior tubercle — Peroneal tubercle — Lateral tubercle

(Top) View of the calcaneus from above is shown. The calcaneus is subdivided into anterior process, body, and tuberosity. The calcaneus articulates with the talus via 3 facets: Anterior, middle, and posterior. The anterior and middle facets are often confluent. The anterior process of the calcaneus is the site of origin of the bifurcate ligament, which inserts on the navicular and cuboid.. (Bottom) Plantar view of the calcaneus is shown. The plantar calcaneus has a rough surface, especially proximally. It gives origins to the lateral, medial and anterior tubercle (processes). These serve as attachments for the superficial layer of foot muscles and plantar ligaments. The medial tubercle is broader than the lateral tubercle. The anterior tubercle marks the distal attachment of the long plantar ligament. The flexor hallucis longus traverses in a groove along the plantar surface of the sustentaculum tali.

Ankle Overview

GRAPHICS: CALCANEUS

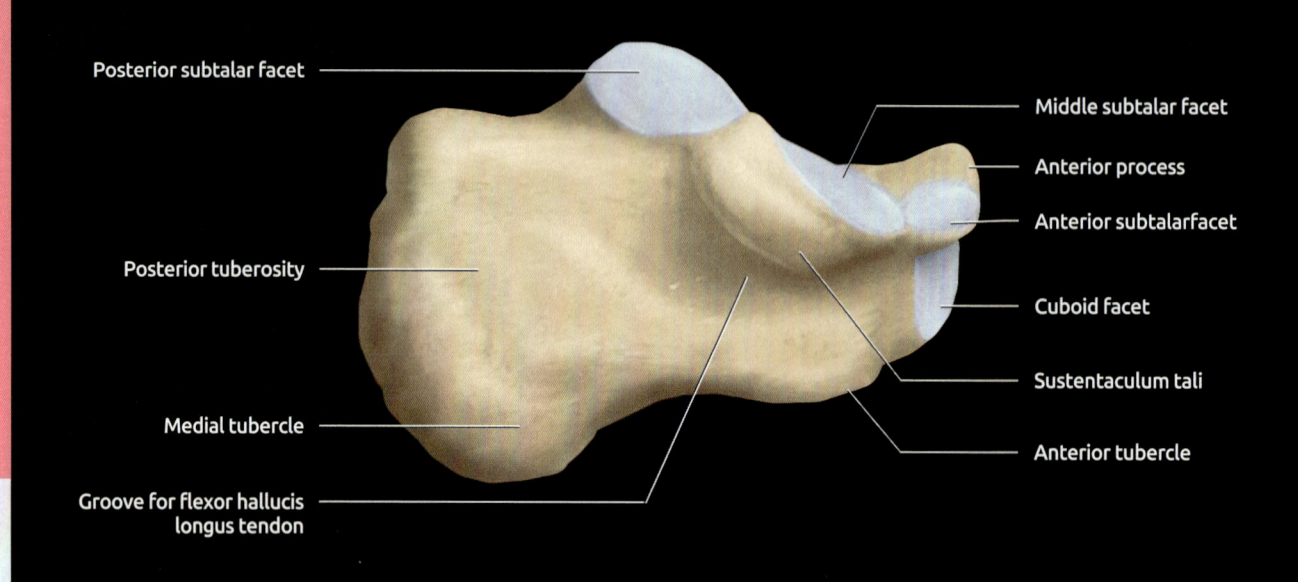

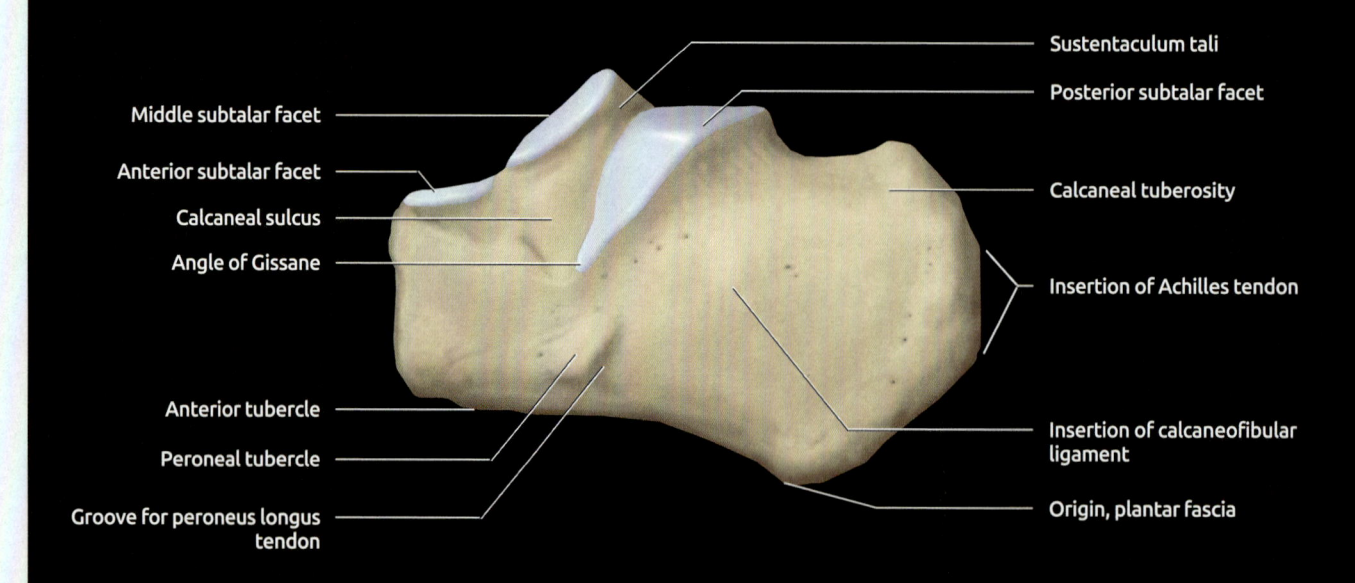

Posterior subtalar facet

Middle subtalar facet

Anterior process

Anterior subtalar facet

Posterior tuberosity

Cuboid facet

Sustentaculum tali

Medial tubercle

Anterior tubercle

Groove for flexor hallucis longus tendon

Sustentaculum tali

Posterior subtalar facet

Middle subtalar facet

Anterior subtalar facet

Calcaneal tuberosity

Calcaneal sulcus

Angle of Gissane

Insertion of Achilles tendon

Anterior tubercle

Insertion of calcaneofibular ligament

Peroneal tubercle

Groove for peroneus longus tendon

Origin, plantar fascia

(Top) *Medial view of calcaneus is shown. The calcaneus has a medial, shelf-like process termed sustentaculum tali, which projects medially and superiorly from the upper border of the distal calcaneus. The sustentaculum tali provides medial support to the talus and has a plantar groove for the flexor hallucis longus and, less frequently, for the flexor digitorum longus tendons.* **(Bottom)** *A lateral view of the calcaneus is shown. The Achilles and plantaris tendons insert into the calcaneus at the posterior calcaneal tuberosity. The peroneal tendons descend along the lateral aspect of the calcaneus, separated from one another by the peroneal tubercle (present in 40% of people) and inferior peroneal retinaculum.*

Ankle Overview

GRAPHICS: MUSCLE ATTACHMENTS TO HINDFOOT

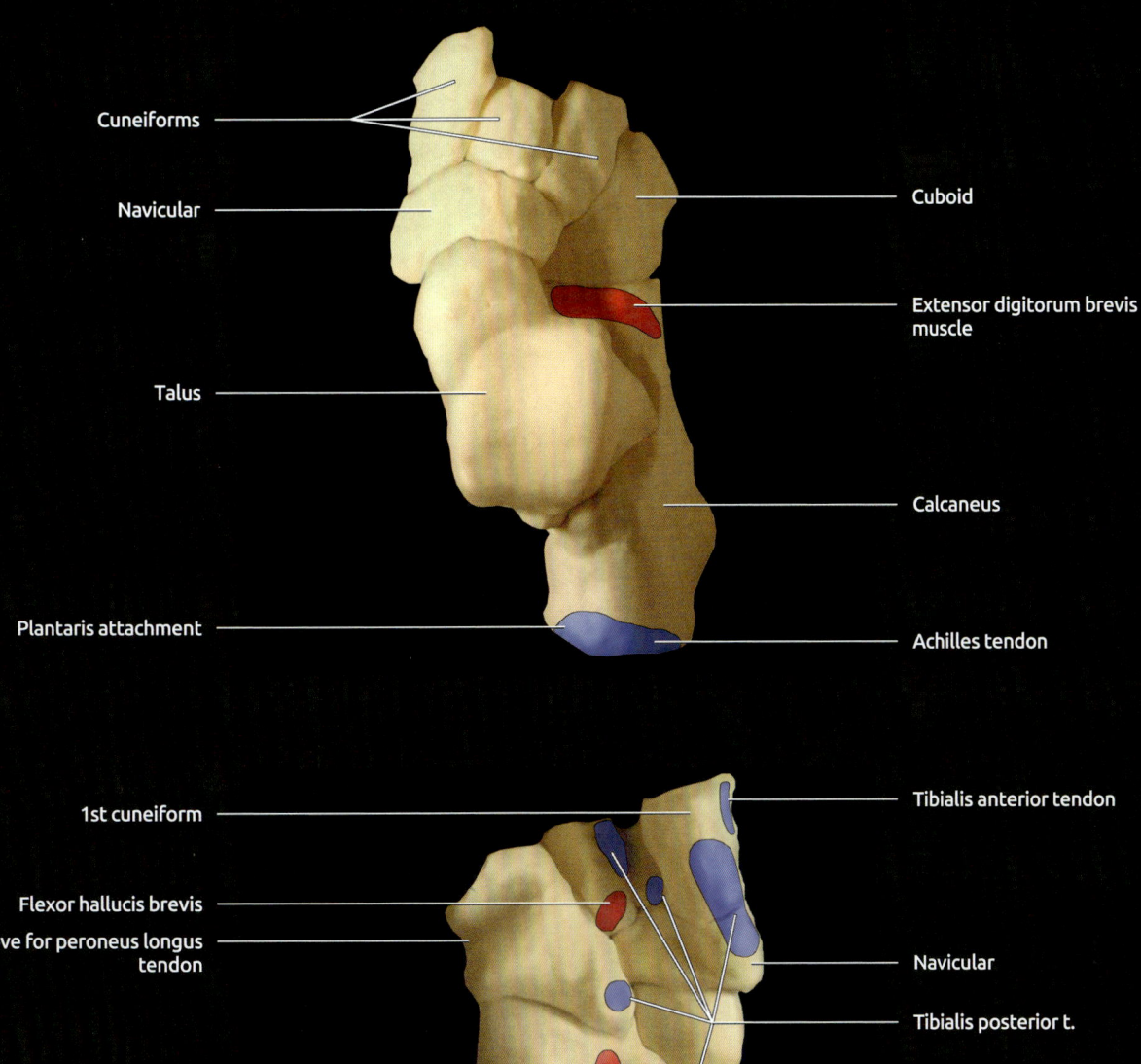

Cuneiforms

Navicular

Talus

Plantaris attachment

Cuboid

Extensor digitorum brevis muscle

Calcaneus

Achilles tendon

1st cuneiform

Flexor hallucis brevis

Groove for peroneus longus tendon

Calcaneus

Abductor digiti minimi

Lateral tubercle

Flexor digitorum brevis

Tibialis anterior tendon

Navicular

Tibialis posterior t.

Talus

Sustentaculum tali

Quadratus plantae

Abductor hallucis

Medial tubercle

(Top) Dorsal muscle attachments are shown. The posterior tuberosity of calcaneus has a broad ridge, inferior to its superior posterior margin, for Achilles and plantaris tendon attachments. A retrocalcaneal bursa is interposed between the Achilles tendon and calcaneus above insertion. The extensor digitorum brevis originates from the dorsolateral aspect of the anterior process of calcaneus, just distal to the calcaneal articulation with the talus. Note that the talus has no dorsal muscular attachments. (Bottom) Plantar muscle attachments are shown. Four muscles originate from the calcaneus: Abductor hallucis from the medial tubercle, flexor digitorum brevis from the medial tubercle, and abductor digiti minimi from the medial and lateral tubercles. The quadratus plantae originates more distally via 2 heads from the medial and lateral plantar calcaneal surfaces. Note again that the talus has no muscular insertions.

Ankle Overview

GRAPHICS: HINDFOOT LIGAMENTS

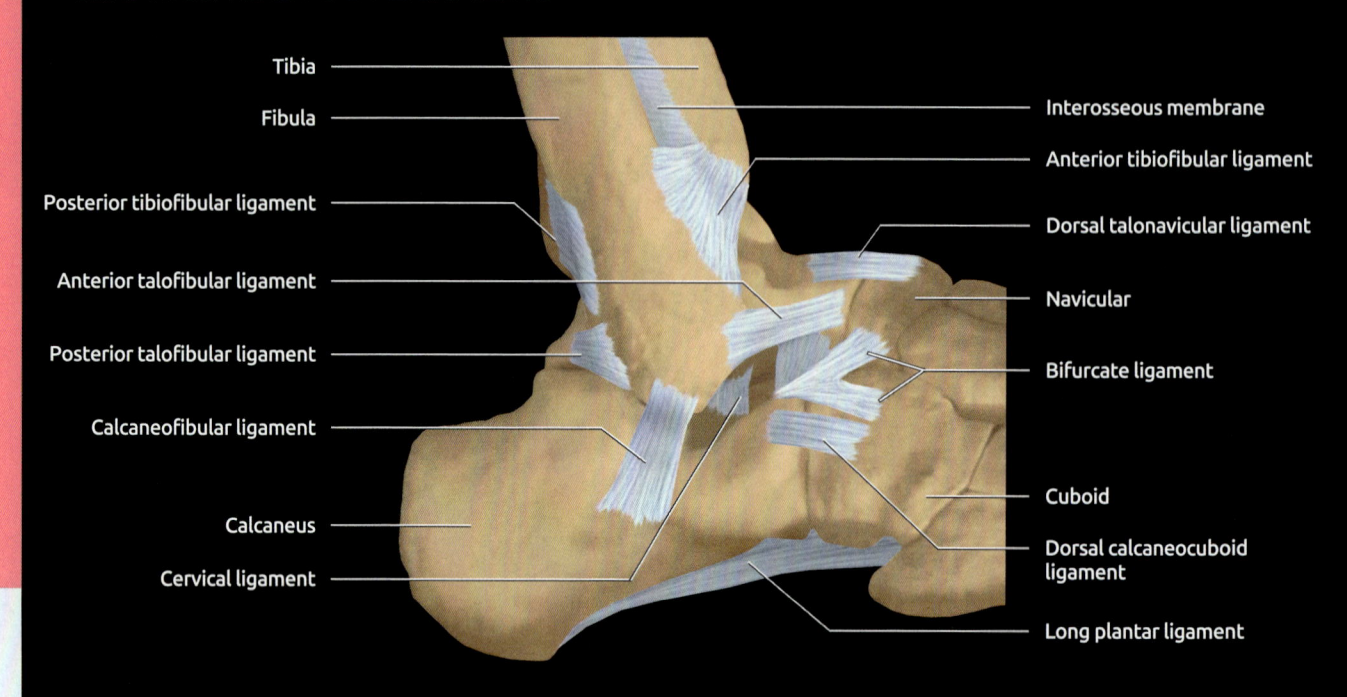

Labels (top, lateral view): Tibia, Fibula, Posterior tibiofibular ligament, Anterior talofibular ligament, Posterior talofibular ligament, Calcaneofibular ligament, Calcaneus, Cervical ligament, Interosseous membrane, Anterior tibiofibular ligament, Dorsal talonavicular ligament, Navicular, Bifurcate ligament, Cuboid, Dorsal calcaneocuboid ligament, Long plantar ligament.

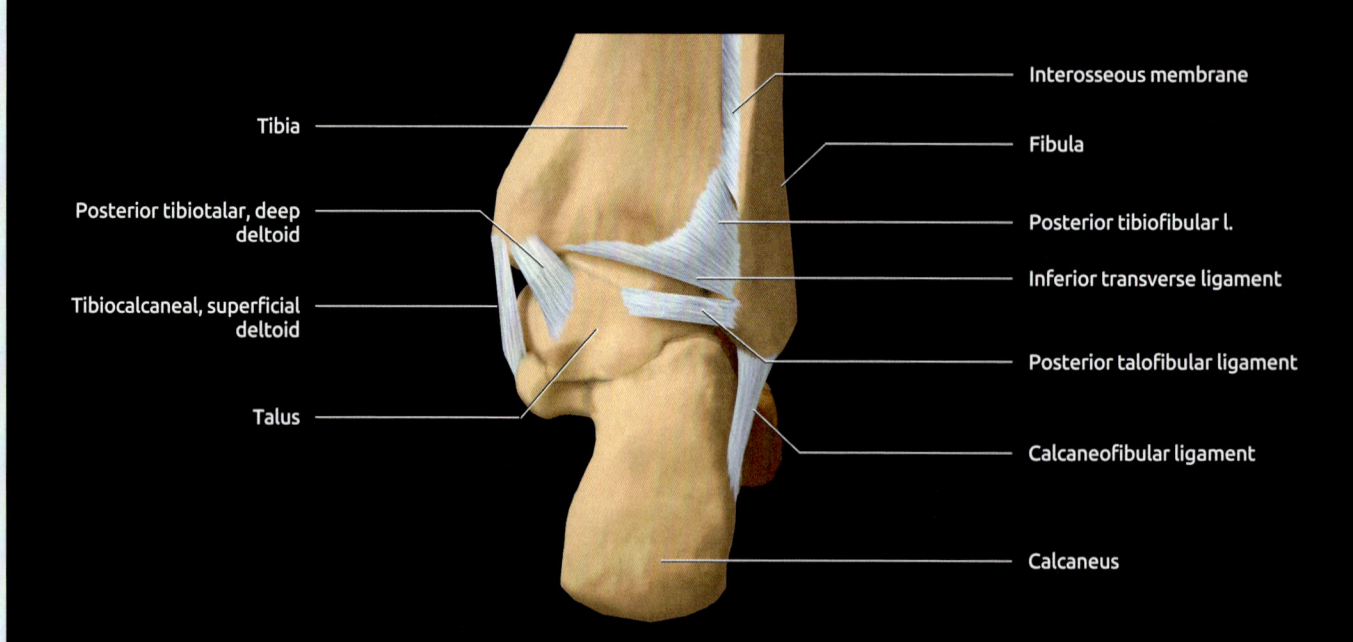

Labels (bottom, posterior view): Tibia, Posterior tibiotalar, deep deltoid, Tibiocalcaneal, superficial deltoid, Talus, Interosseous membrane, Fibula, Posterior tibiofibular l., Inferior transverse ligament, Posterior talofibular ligament, Calcaneofibular ligament, Calcaneus.

(**Top**) *Lateral view of the ankle is shown. Two groups of lateral ligaments support the ankle: 1) the syndesmotic ligaments, including the anterior tibiofibular, posterior tibiofibular, and syndesmotic ligaments, and 2) the lateral collateral ligaments including the anterior talofibular, posterior talofibular, and calcaneofibular ligaments. Other ligaments that bind the lateral hindfoot include the talocalcaneal ligaments, talocalcaneal interosseous ligament and cervical ligament in the sinus tarsi. Note the bifurcate ligament which extends from the calcaneus to the navicular and cuboid.* (**Bottom**) *Posterior view of the ankle is shown. The tibiofibular ligaments are obliquely oriented and their fibular origin is above the fibular fossa. The inferior transverse ligament, which is the inferior aspect of the posterior tibiofibular ligament, extends distal to the tibial posterior surface.*

Ankle Overview

GRAPHICS: HINDFOOT LIGAMENTS

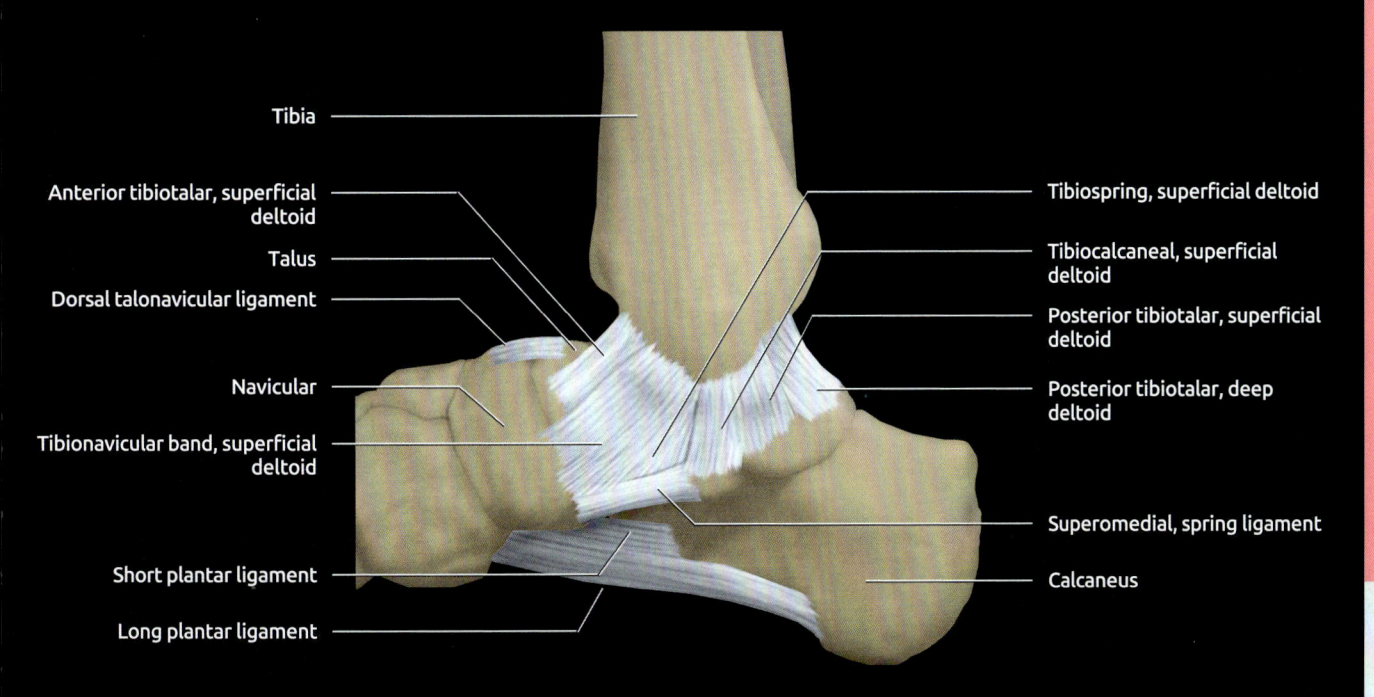

Labels (top, medial view):
- Tibia
- Anterior tibiotalar, superficial deltoid
- Talus
- Dorsal talonavicular ligament
- Navicular
- Tibionavicular band, superficial deltoid
- Short plantar ligament
- Long plantar ligament
- Tibiospring, superficial deltoid
- Tibiocalcaneal, superficial deltoid
- Posterior tibiotalar, superficial deltoid
- Posterior tibiotalar, deep deltoid
- Superomedial, spring ligament
- Calcaneus

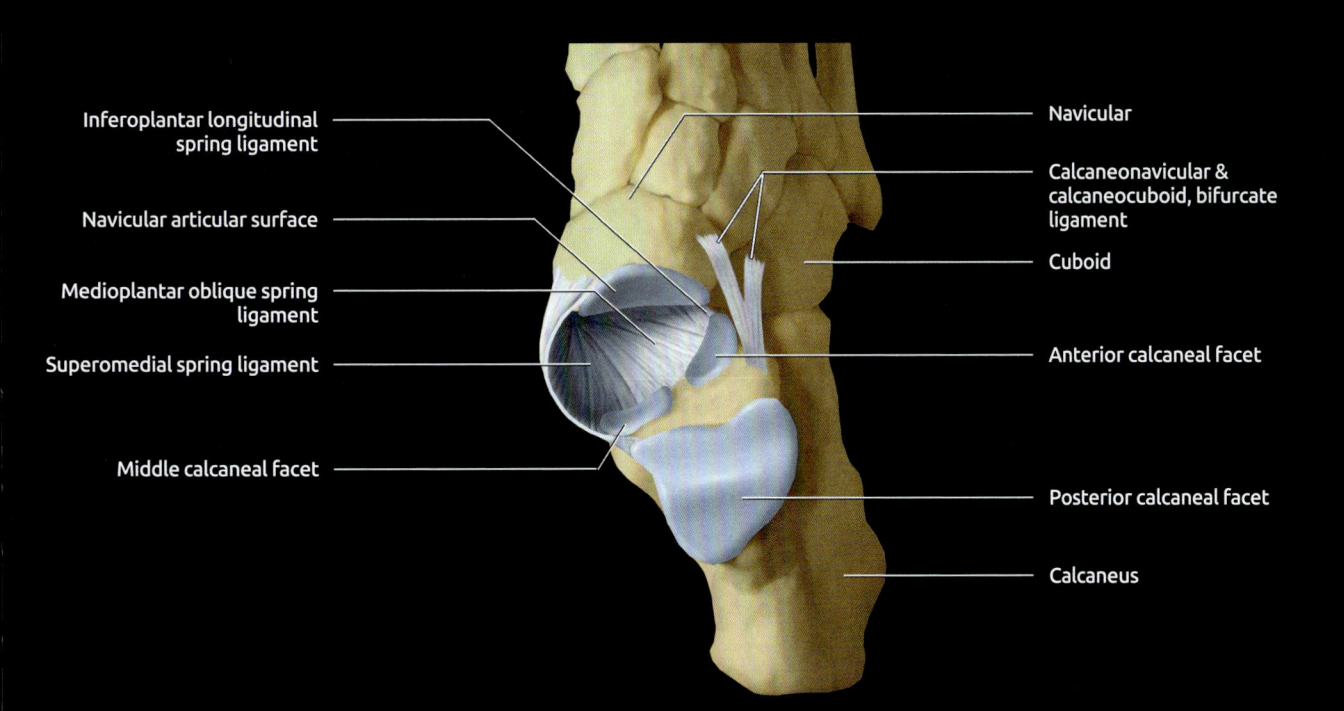

Labels (bottom):
- Inferoplantar longitudinal spring ligament
- Navicular articular surface
- Medioplantar oblique spring ligament
- Superomedial spring ligament
- Middle calcaneal facet
- Navicular
- Calcaneonavicular & calcaneocuboid, bifurcate ligament
- Cuboid
- Anterior calcaneal facet
- Posterior calcaneal facet
- Calcaneus

(Top) *Medial view of the ankle is shown. The deltoid ligament is the major supporter of the ankle. It has many variable components but a commonly accepted division includes the deep anterior and posterior tibiotalar and superficial anterior and posterior tibiotalar, tibiocalcaneal, tibiospring and tibionavicular bands. Note that the superficial deltoid is band-like and distinction between its various components relies on the sites of origins and insertions.* **(Bottom)** *Spring ligament is shown from above with the talus removed. The ligament forms a sling supporting the talar head and is composed of the superomedial, medioplantar oblique, and inferoplantar longitudinal bands. It originates from the sustentaculum tali, tibiospring and coronoid fossa and inserts onto the plantar navicular. The bifurcate ligament originates on the anterosuperior corner of the calcaneus and inserts onto the navicular and cuboid.*

Ankle Overview

GRAPHICS: RETINACULA

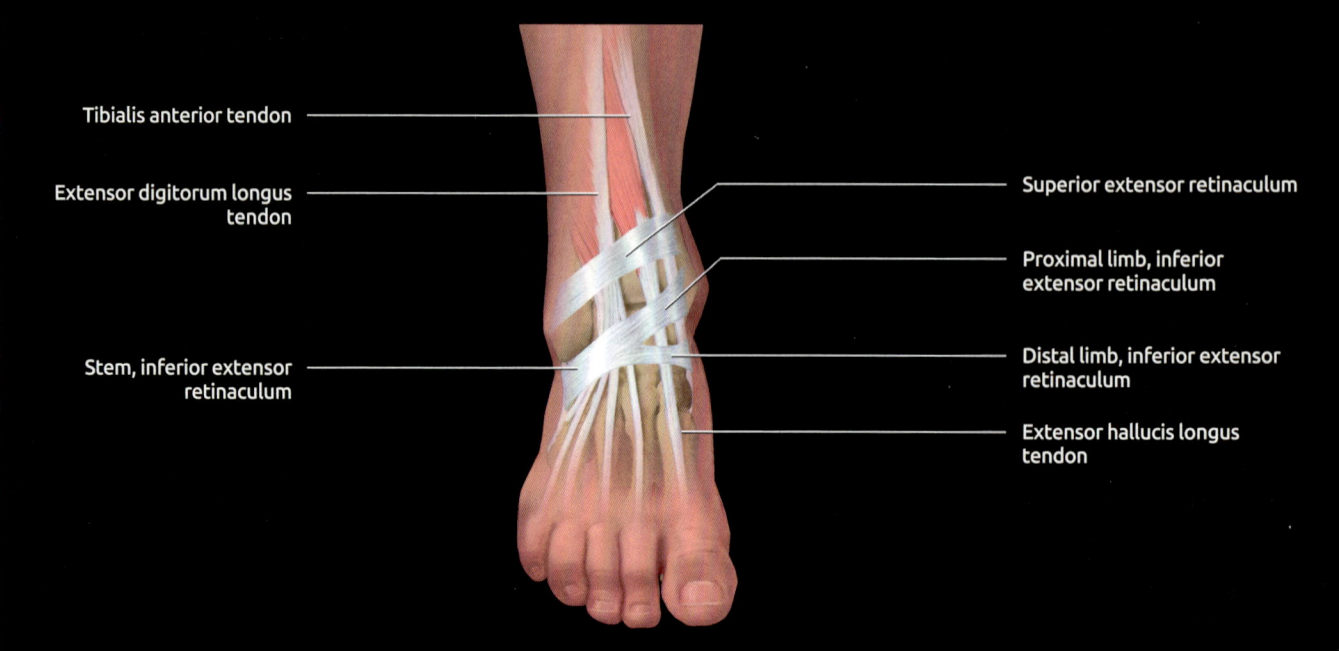

Labels (top image):
- Tibialis anterior tendon
- Extensor digitorum longus tendon
- Stem, inferior extensor retinaculum
- Superior extensor retinaculum
- Proximal limb, inferior extensor retinaculum
- Distal limb, inferior extensor retinaculum
- Extensor hallucis longus tendon

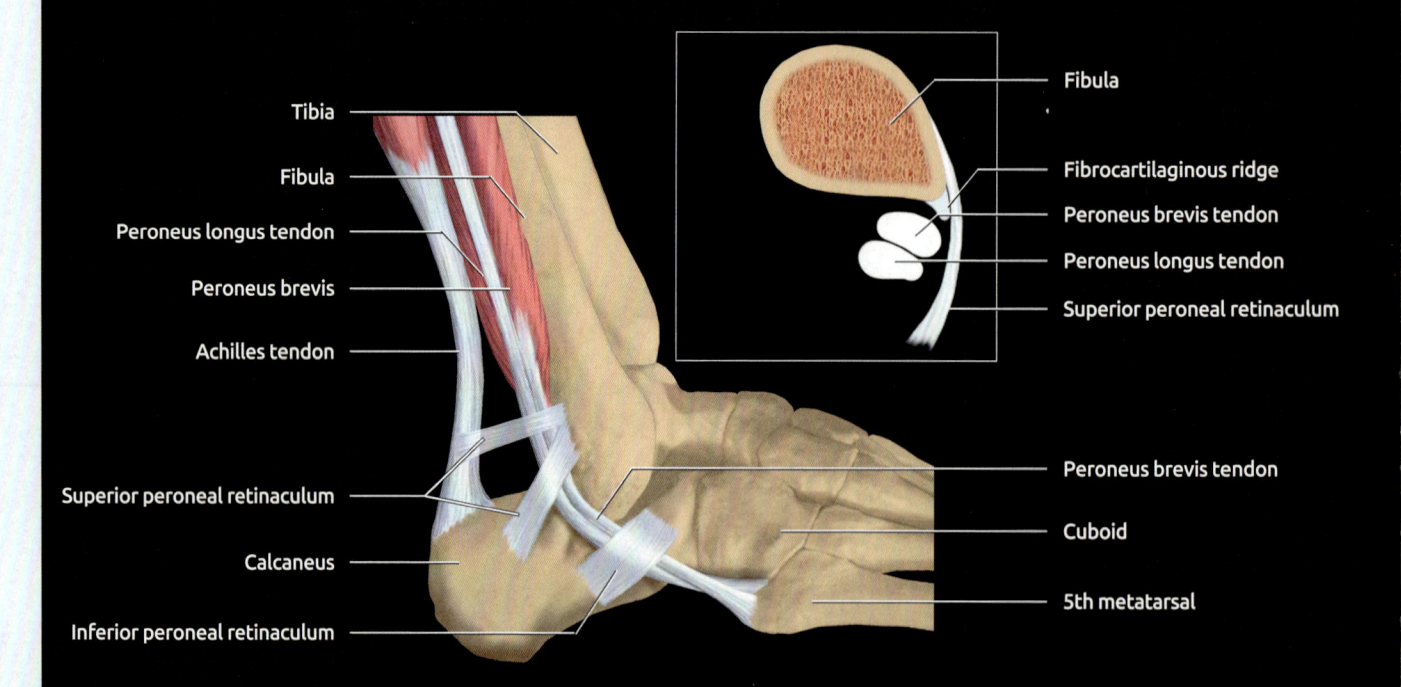

Labels (bottom image):
- Tibia
- Fibula
- Peroneus longus tendon
- Peroneus brevis
- Achilles tendon
- Superior peroneal retinaculum
- Calcaneus
- Inferior peroneal retinaculum
- Fibula
- Fibrocartilaginous ridge
- Peroneus brevis tendon
- Peroneus longus tendon
- Superior peroneal retinaculum
- Peroneus brevis tendon
- Cuboid
- 5th metatarsal

(Top) Extensor retinacula is shown. The superior and inferior extensor retinacula loop over and bind the anterior compartment tendons. The superior extensor retinaculum is above the ankle joint. The inferior extensor retinaculum is Y-shaped and is composed of lateral stem and 2 medial limbs. The stem originates at the calcaneus and the medial limbs attach to the medial malleolus and plantar aponeurosis. (Bottom) Peroneal retinacula is shown. The superior peroneal retinaculum holds the peroneal tendons in the retrofibular groove. The retinaculum has variable insertions but typically inserts on the deep fascia of leg and on the calcaneus. The inferior peroneal retinaculum holds the peroneal tendons against the calcaneus.

Ankle Overview

GRAPHICS: ANKLE TENDONS

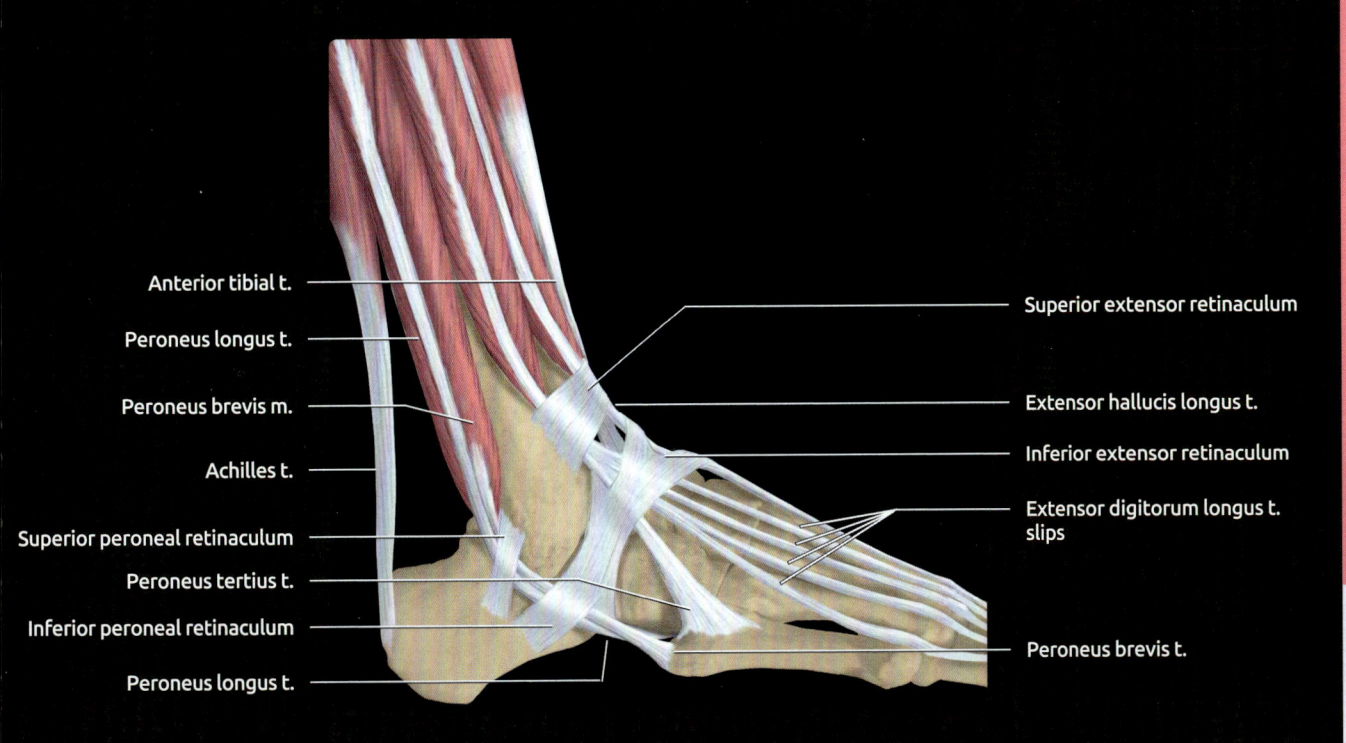

Labels (top, lateral view):
- Anterior tibial t.
- Peroneus longus t.
- Peroneus brevis m.
- Achilles t.
- Superior peroneal retinaculum
- Peroneus tertius t.
- Inferior peroneal retinaculum
- Peroneus longus t.
- Superior extensor retinaculum
- Extensor hallucis longus t.
- Inferior extensor retinaculum
- Extensor digitorum longus t. slips
- Peroneus brevis t.

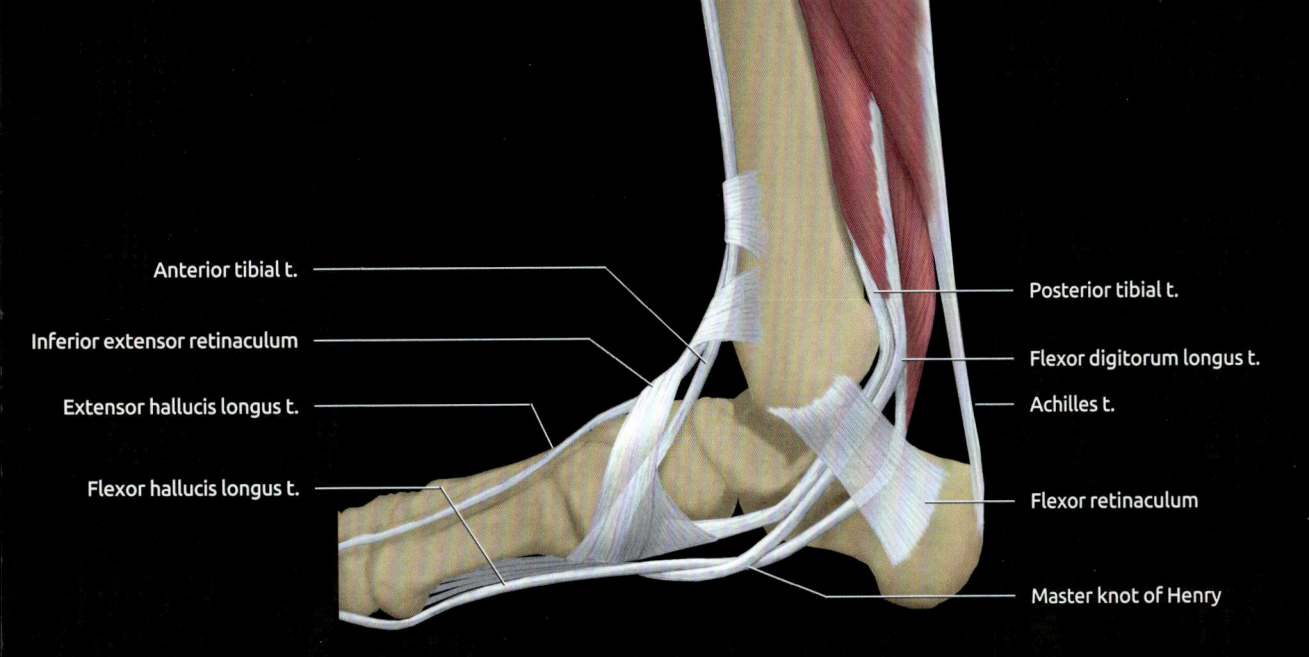

Labels (bottom, medial view):
- Anterior tibial t.
- Inferior extensor retinaculum
- Extensor hallucis longus t.
- Flexor hallucis longus t.
- Posterior tibial t.
- Flexor digitorum longus t.
- Achilles t.
- Flexor retinaculum
- Master knot of Henry

(**Top**) *Lateral view shows how the peroneus brevis & peroneus longus tendons descend posterior to the fibula, maintained within the retromalleolar groove by the superior peroneal retinaculum, and continue along the lateral wall of calcaneus, held in place by the inferior peroneal retinaculum. Fibers of the inferior peroneal retinaculum insert and separate the two tendons. The peroneus longus tendon curves around the cuboid to enter the sole of the foot. Both the peroneus brevis and peroneus tertius tendons insert on the 5th metatarsal base.* (**Bottom**) *Medial view shows the posterior tibial, flexor digitorum longus & flexor hallucis longus tendons traversing under the flexor retinaculum within the tarsal tunnel. The flexor digitorum longus & flexor hallucis longus tendons cross each other under the navicular. The extensor tendons descend deep to the extensor retinacula.*

Ankle Overview

GRAPHICS: ANKLE NERVES

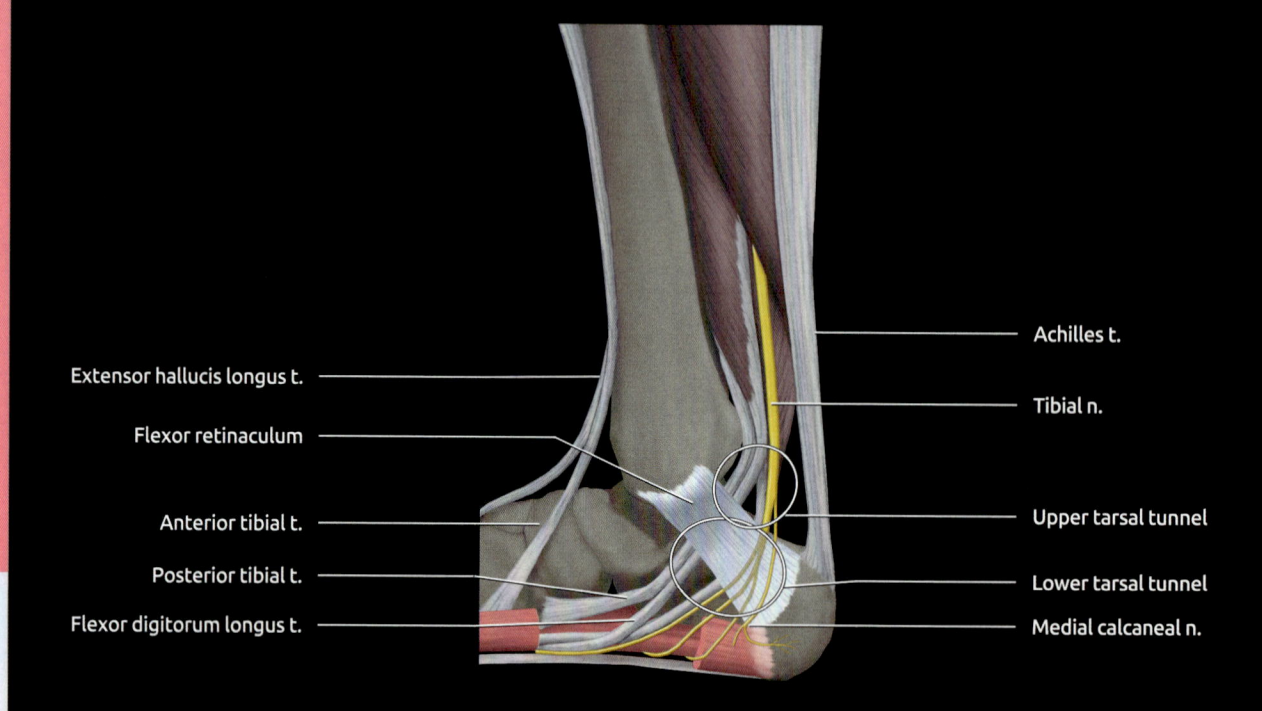

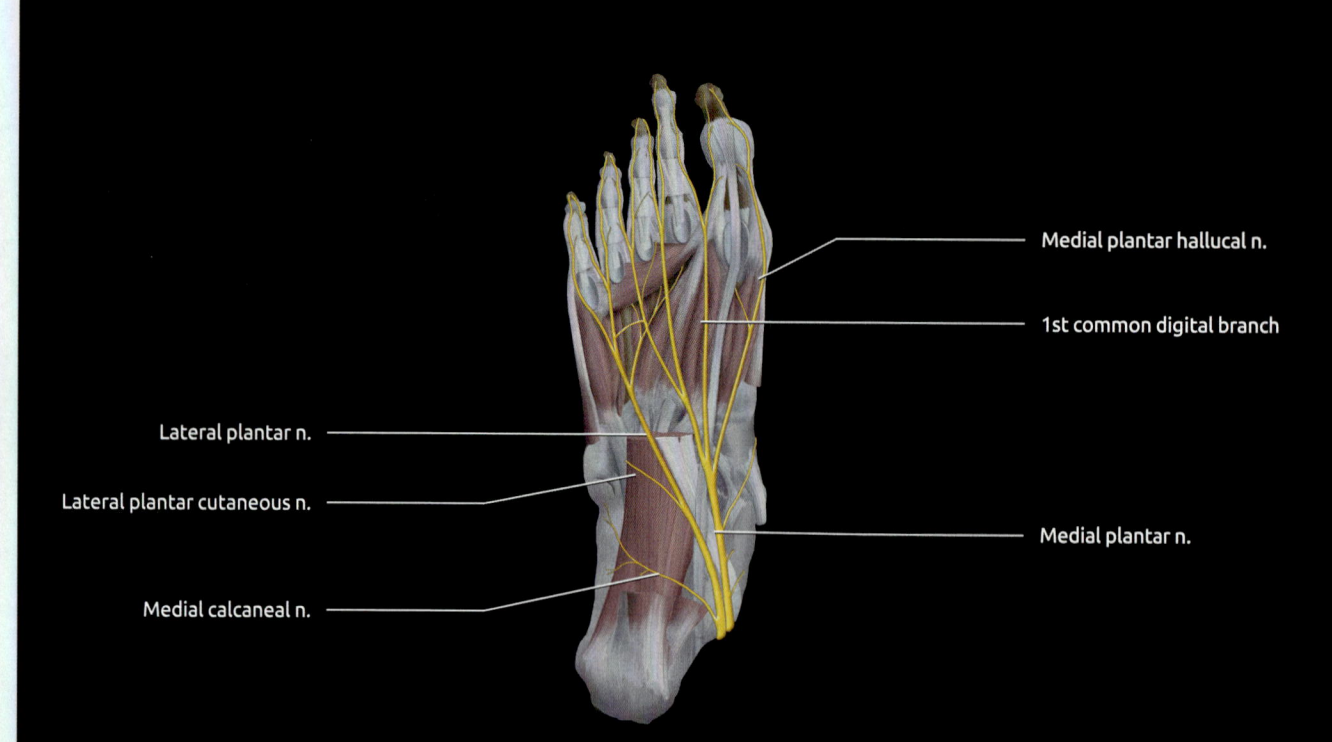

Extensor hallucis longus t.
Flexor retinaculum
Anterior tibial t.
Posterior tibial t.
Flexor digitorum longus t.

Achilles t.
Tibial n.
Upper tarsal tunnel
Lower tarsal tunnel
Medial calcaneal n.

Lateral plantar n.
Lateral plantar cutaneous n.
Medial calcaneal n.

Medial plantar hallucal n.
1st common digital branch
Medial plantar n.

(Top) *The tarsal tunnel is traversed by the posterior tibial, flexor digitorum longus, and flexor hallucis longus tendons, tibial nerve and branches, and posterior tibial vessels (not shown). The roof of the tunnel is the flexor retinaculum, and the floor is the subjacent bones.*
(Bottom) *The medial plantar nerve passes between the abductor hallucis and flexor digitorum brevis (removed) and supplies the abductor hallucis, flexor digitorum brevis, flexor hallucis brevis & 1st lumbrical & provides sensation to medial 2/3 of foot. The lateral plantar nerve passes between the flexor digitorum brevis & quadratus plantae & divides into the superficial branch (divides into 2 common digital nerves) & deep branch (runs deep to flexor tendons). The latter sends a communicating branch to the 3rd digital nerve. The lateral plantar nerve supplies the quadratus plantae, abductor digiti minimi, flexor digiti minimi, adductor hallucis, 2-4 lumbricals, interossei & skin of lateral sole, 5th toe, & lateral 1/2 of 4th toe.*

Ankle Overview

GRAPHICS: ANKLE NERVES

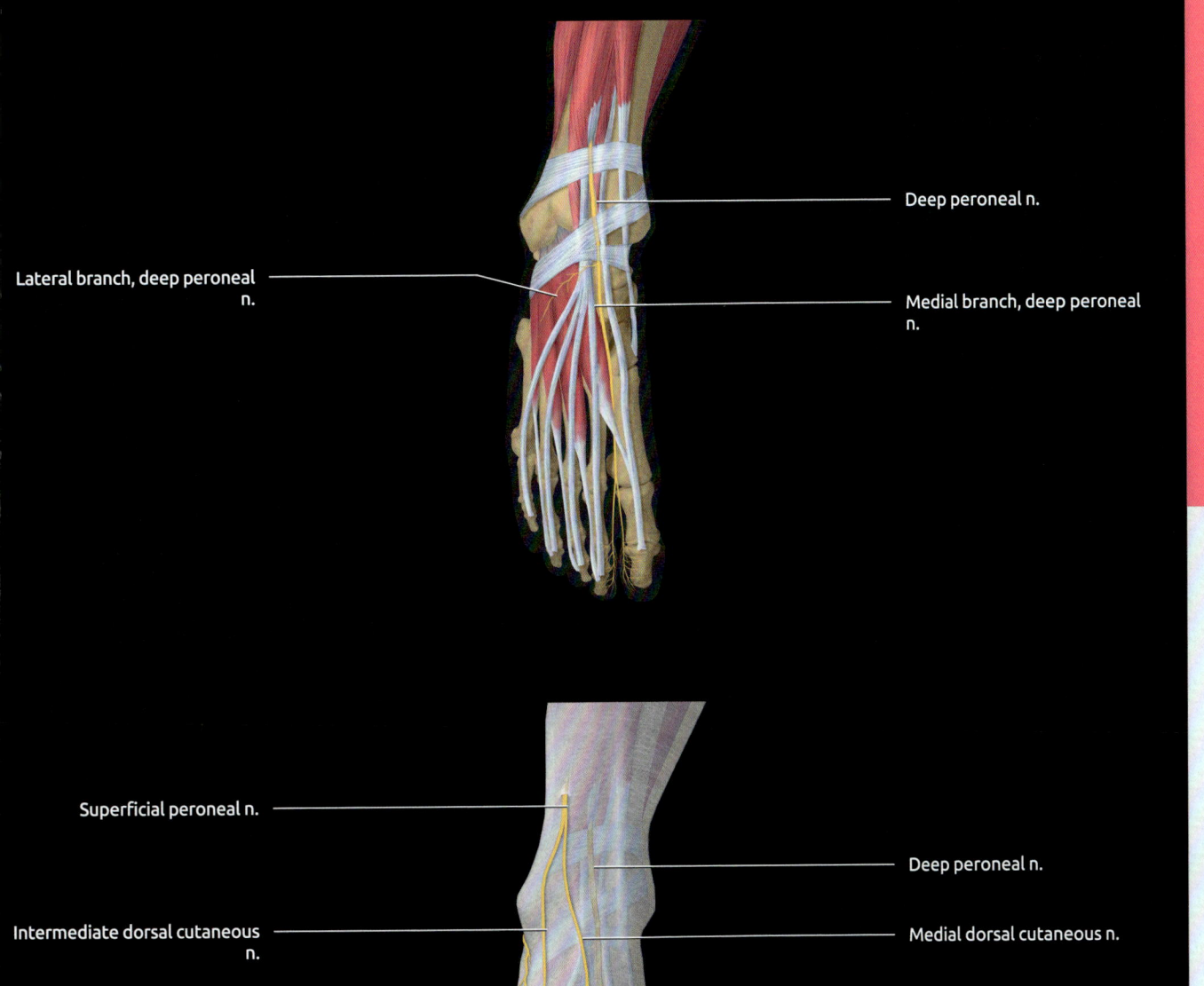

- Deep peroneal n.
- Lateral branch, deep peroneal n.
- Medial branch, deep peroneal n.
- Superficial peroneal n.
- Deep peroneal n.
- Intermediate dorsal cutaneous n.
- Medial dorsal cutaneous n.

(Top) The deep peroneal nerve travels deep to the extensor retinacula and terminates in 2 branches. The lateral branch innervates the extensor digitorum brevis muscle. It sends 3 tiny interosseous branches (not shown) which supply the tarsal and tarsometatarsal joints of the middle 3 toes; the 1st branch also supplies the 2nd dorsal interosseous. The medial branch continues dorsal to talonavicular joint, middle cuneiform and in between the 1st & 2nd metatarsals to provide mostly sensory but some motor supply to the 1st web space. (Bottom) In the distal leg, the superficial peroneal nerve bifurcates to the medial and intermediate dorsal cutaneous nerves. The medial dorsal cutaneous nerve, via 2 dorsal digital nerves, supplies the 1st-3rd toes and communicates with the saphenous and deep peroneal nerve. The intermediate dorsal cutaneous nerve, also via digital branches, supplies 3rd-5th toes and skin of the lateral ankle and communicates with the sural nerve (not shown).

Ankle Overview

GRAPHICS: CUTANEOUS INNERVATION

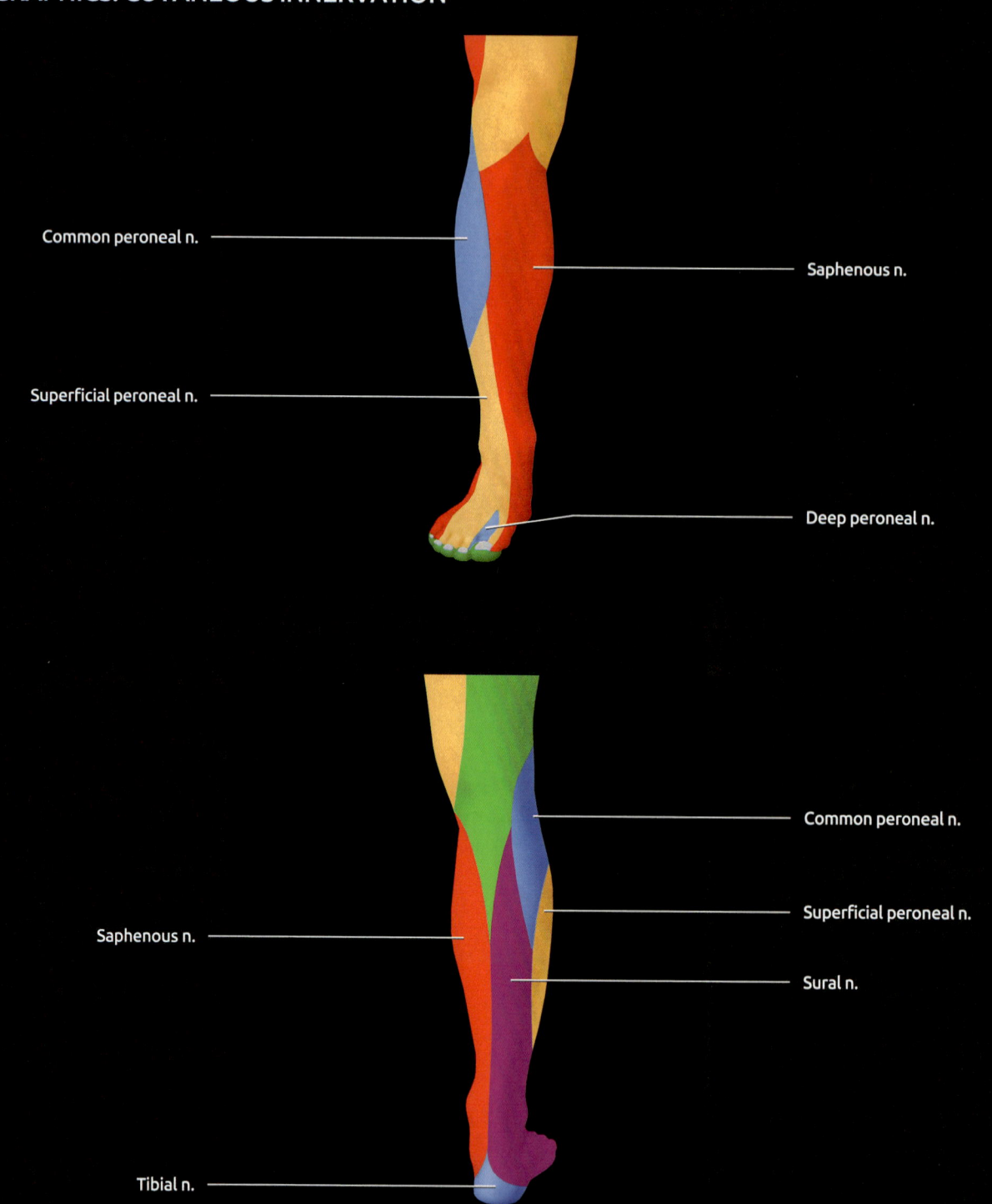

Common peroneal n.
Saphenous n.
Superficial peroneal n.
Deep peroneal n.

Common peroneal n.
Superficial peroneal n.
Saphenous n.
Sural n.
Tibial n.

(Top) Cutaneous innervation of the ventral (anterior) leg is shown. The upper 1/3 and lower 2/3 of the lateral anterior leg are innervated by the common and superficial peroneal nerves respectively. The anterior medial leg is supplied by the saphenous nerve (femoral nerve branch). Most dorsal foot innervation is supplied by the superficial peroneal nerve except for the 1st web space (deep peroneal nerve), medial ankle and foot (saphenous nerve), lateral ankle and foot (sural nerve), and tips of toes (medial and lateral plantar nerves). Variations and overlap in innervation are common. *(Bottom)* Cutaneous innervation of the dorsal (posterior) leg is shown. The medial 1/2 of the posterior leg is supplied by the saphenous nerve (branch of femoral nerve) while the lateral 1/2 is supplied by the sural nerve (formed by a merger of branches of the tibial and common peroneal nerve). The heel is supplied by the tibial nerve. Variations and overlap in innervation are frequent phenomena.

Ankle Overview

GRAPHICS: CUTANEOUS INNERVATION

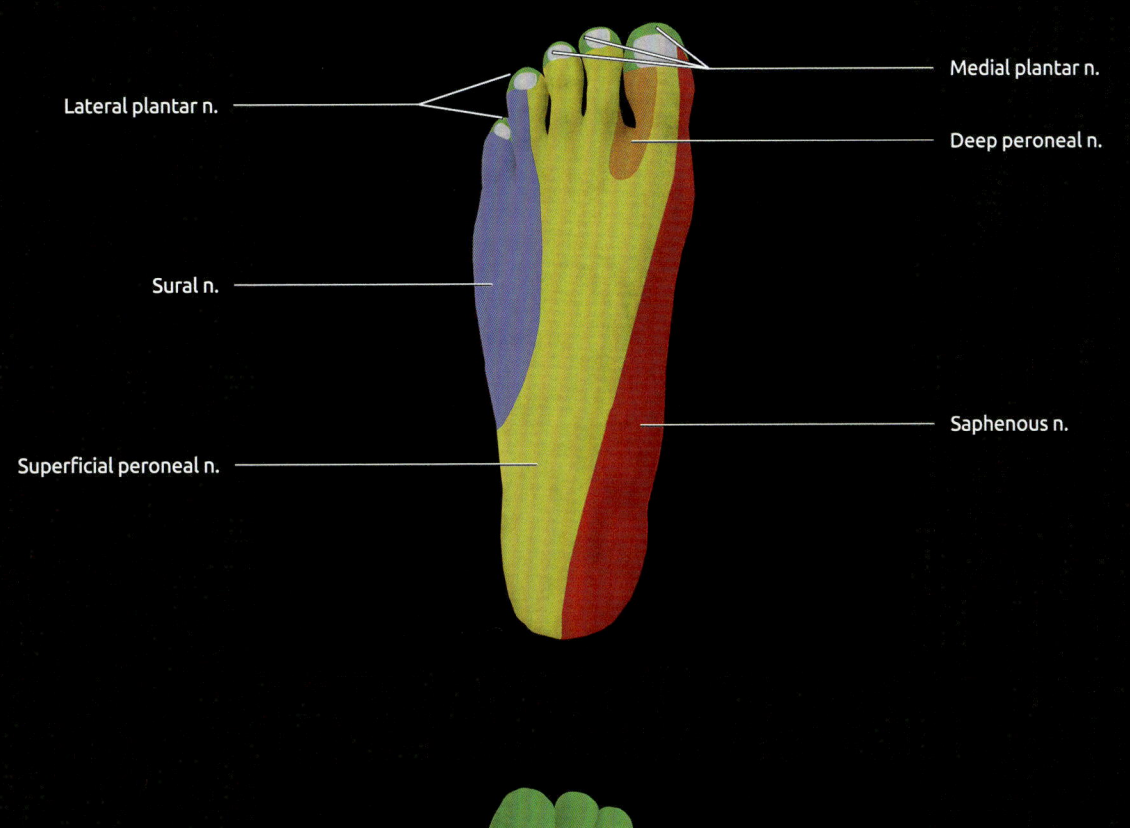

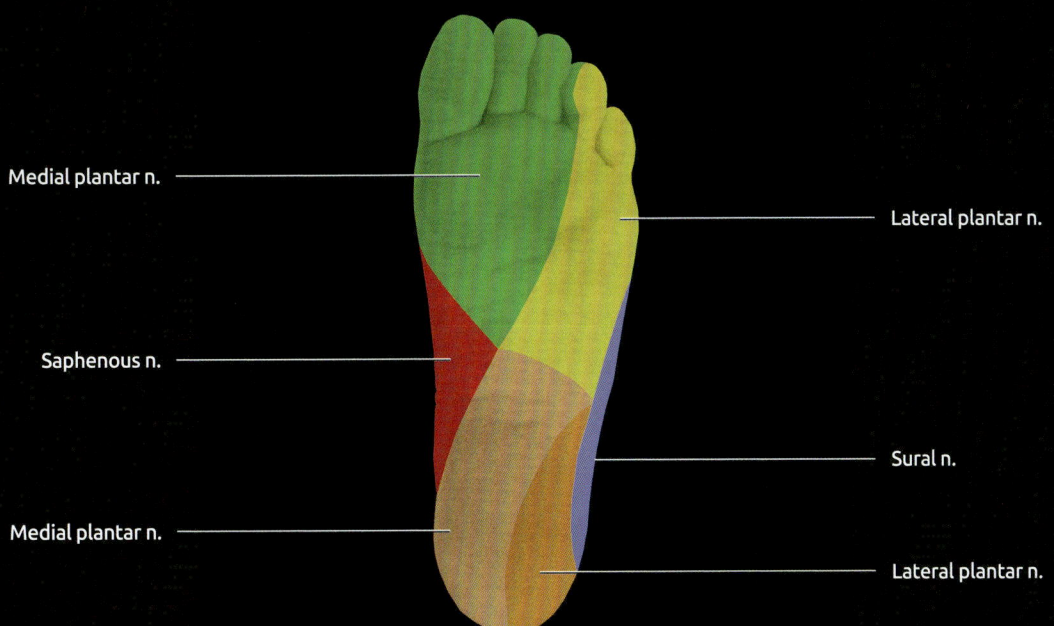

(Top) The dorsal cutaneous innervation is provided mainly by the superficial peroneal nerve, with contributions by the deep peroneal nerve, sural nerve, and saphenous nerve. The medial and lateral plantar nerves provide dorsal innervation to nail beds and tips of toes. (Bottom) The medial plantar nerve supplies the plantar skin of the medial 3 and 1/2 toes. The lateral plantar nerve supplies the lateral 1 and 1/2 toes. There is typically communication between the medial and lateral plantar nerves at the level of the 3rd and 4th common digital nerves. There is also plantar innervation by the sural nerve laterally and saphenous nerve medially. The skin of the heel is innervated medially by the medial calcaneal nerve (a branch of the posterior tibial nerve) and laterally by the lateral calcaneal nerve (branch of sural nerve). The lateral plantar nerve may also give rise to small branches, which pierce the plantar fascia and supply the lateral skin of the heel.

Ankle Radiographic and Arthrographic Anatomy

IMAGING ANATOMY

Overview

- Anteroposterior (AP) view of ankle
  - Obtained in same plane as AP of knee
  - Since ankle is externally rotated relative to knee, this view does not show mortise joint of ankle in profile
  - Imaging finding of correct positioning: Fovea of talus seen in profile
  - Anterior colliculus projects inferior to posterior colliculus
    - Inferior cortex of posterior colliculus seen through anterior colliculus should not be mistaken for fracture
- Mortise view of ankle
  - Ankle internally rotated 15-20°; malleoli should be same distance from film
  - Foot is dorsiflexed
    - Brings larger, anterior portion of talar trochlea into view
  - Imaging finding of correct positioning: Mortise seen in profile
  - Medial, superior, and lateral joint spaces should be equal
- Lateral view of ankle
  - Oriented to axis of hindfoot
  - Imaging findings of correct positioning
    - Medial malleolus not anterior to tibial plafond
    - Fibula at posterior 1/3 of tibial plafond
    - 2 sides of talar trochlea superimposed
- Inversion stress view
  - Talar trochlea may tilt into 5° of varus normally
  - Bilateral symmetry useful
- Eversion or external rotation stress view
  - Loss of congruity of medial ankle gutter is abnormal
- Gravity stress view
  - Patient lies in lateral decubitus position, affected side down
  - Pillow under knee, leg beyond end of table
  - Imaging cassette placed posterior to ankle
  - Image obtained from anterior to posterior (cross-table AP)
  - Reportedly equal in accuracy to manual stress view
- Lateral stress view
  - Lateral view with anterior stress applied
  - Evaluates for anterior subluxation of talus (anterior drawer sign)
- Broden view
  - Evaluation of posterior subtalar joint
  - Ankle in 45° internal rotation
- Os calcis (tangential calcaneal) views
  - May be obtained supine or standing
  - Standing: Patient stands on cassette, leg bent forward, beam angled 45° anteriorly to plantar surface of foot
  - Supine: Cassette posterior to ankle, patient dorsiflexes foot, beam angled 45° cephalad from plantar surface of foot
- Hindfoot alignment view
  - Patient standing, foot straight forward, toes at imaging cassette
  - Imaging cassette 20° from vertical, top margin away from patient's toes
  - X-ray tube parallel to imaging cassette
  - Lead strip at back of heel, perpendicular to axis of foot
  - Normal: Axis of tibia falls within 8 mm of most inferior point on calcaneus

ANATOMY IMAGING ISSUES

Imaging Pitfalls

- Poorly positioned mortise view may mimic syndesmotic injury
  - Useful guideline: If medial body of talus overlaps medial malleolus of tibia, exam is overly rotated and cannot accurately measure overlap of tibia and fibula
- Stress views are often false-negative for instability unless performed under anesthesia

Arthrography

- Anterior approach to ankle
- Patient may be in supine or lateral decubitus position
  - Lateral decubitus position aids in visualization of anterior lip of tibia
  - Useful if lacking a C-arm to allow cross-table lateral imaging
- Needle between anterior tibial tendon and extensor hallucis longus tendons
- Start needle trajectory slightly distal to ankle join line, angle cephalad
  - Allows needle to extend under dorsal lip of tibia
- Contrast should flow away from needle, fill anterior and posterior joint spaces
- Air can be used as contrast agent for therapeutic injections
- MR arthrogram: Gadolinium contrast diluted 1:200 with lidocaine, bupivacaine, iodinated contrast, and normal saline
- 15% of patients have communication with posterior subtalar joint
- Flexor hallucis longus normally communicates with ankle joint, may or may not fill with contrast
- Abnormal extension of contrast used as sign of ligament tear
  - Contrast around peroneal tendons indicates calcaneofibular ligament tear
  - Contrast along lateral talar neck indicates anterior talofibular ligament tear
  - Contrast along posterior tibial tendon sheath indicates superficial deltoid ligament detachment and detachment of medial periosteum

SELECTED REFERENCES

1. Golanó P et al: Ankle anatomy for the arthroscopist. Part II: Role of the ankle ligaments in soft tissue impingement. Foot Ankle Clin. 11(2):275-96, v-vi, 2006
2. Oh CS et al: Anatomic variations and MRI of the intermalleolar ligament. AJR Am J Roentgenol. 186(4):943-7, 2006
3. Bartoníček J: Anatomy of the tibiofibular syndesmosis and its clinical relevance. Surg Radiol Anat. 25(5-6):379-86, 2003
4. Lee SH et al: Ligaments of the ankle: normal anatomy with MR arthrography. J Comput Assist Tomogr. 22(5):807-13, 1998
5. Burks RT et al: Anatomy of the lateral ankle ligaments. Am J Sports Med. 22(1):72-7, 1994

Ankle Radiographic and Arthrographic Anatomy

RADIOGRAPHS

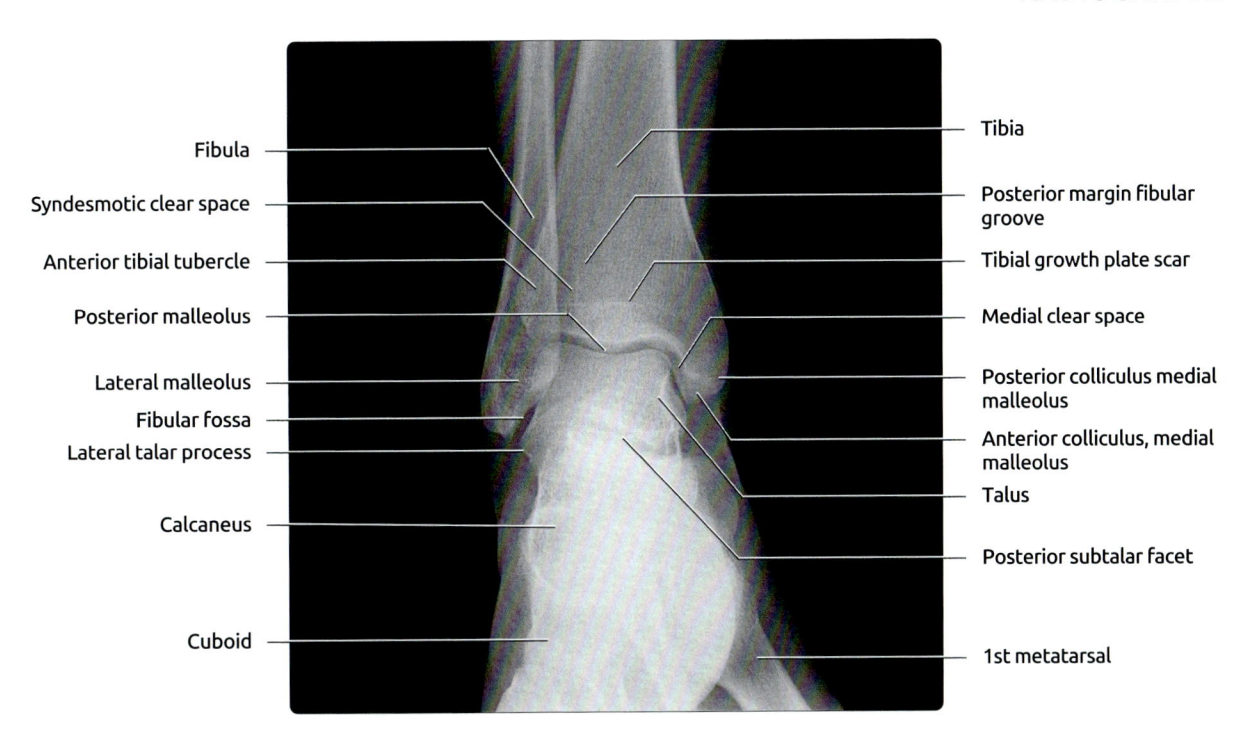

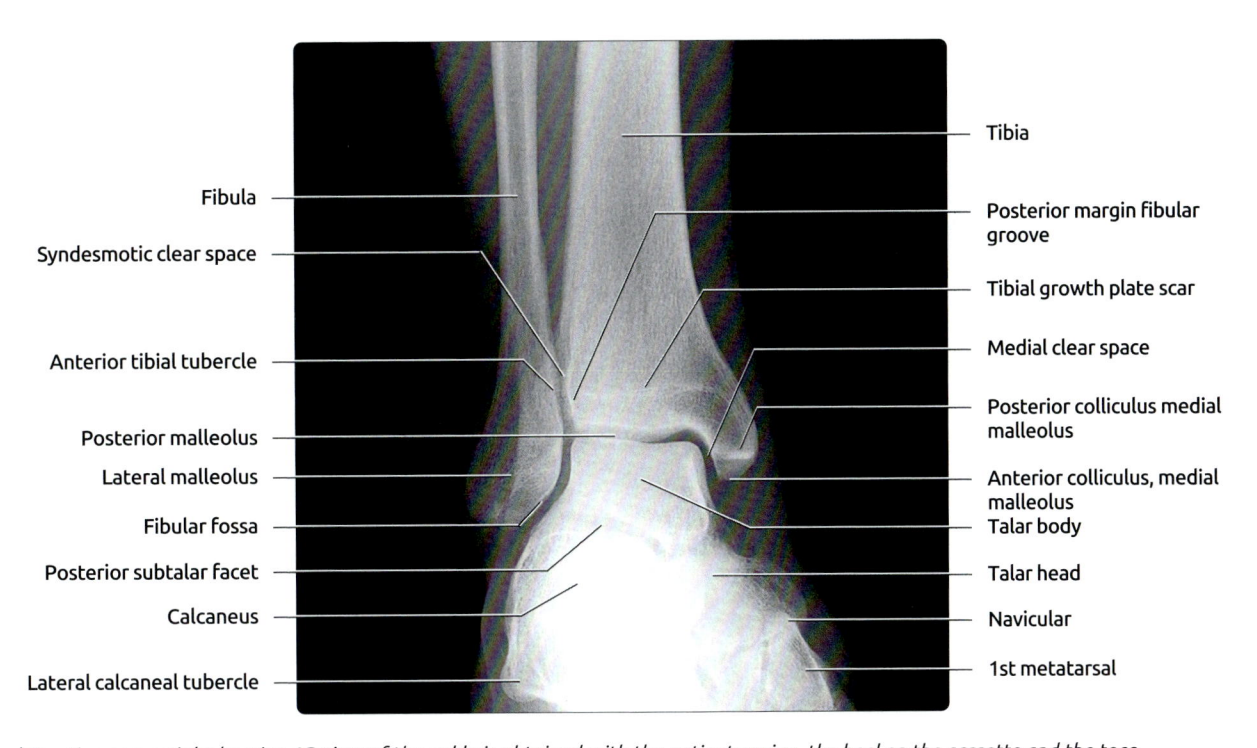

(Top) Routine non-weight-bearing AP view of the ankle is obtained with the patient supine, the heel on the cassette and the toes pointed upward. The x-ray beam is directed at the center of the ankle joint. The talus overlaps the distal fibula obscuring the lateral ankle mortise. Note that the anterior margin of the fibular groove extends further laterally compared to the posterior margin. Similarly, the anterior colliculus of the medial malleolus extends more distally than the posterior colliculus. (Bottom) Non-weight-bearing ankle mortise view (oblique) is obtained with the patient supine and the foot internally rotated until the medial and lateral malleoli are equidistant from the cassette. The lateral ankle mortise is now visualized. The talus should be equidistant from the tibial plafond on both the AP and ankle mortise views.

Ankle Radiographic and Arthrographic Anatomy

RADIOGRAPHS

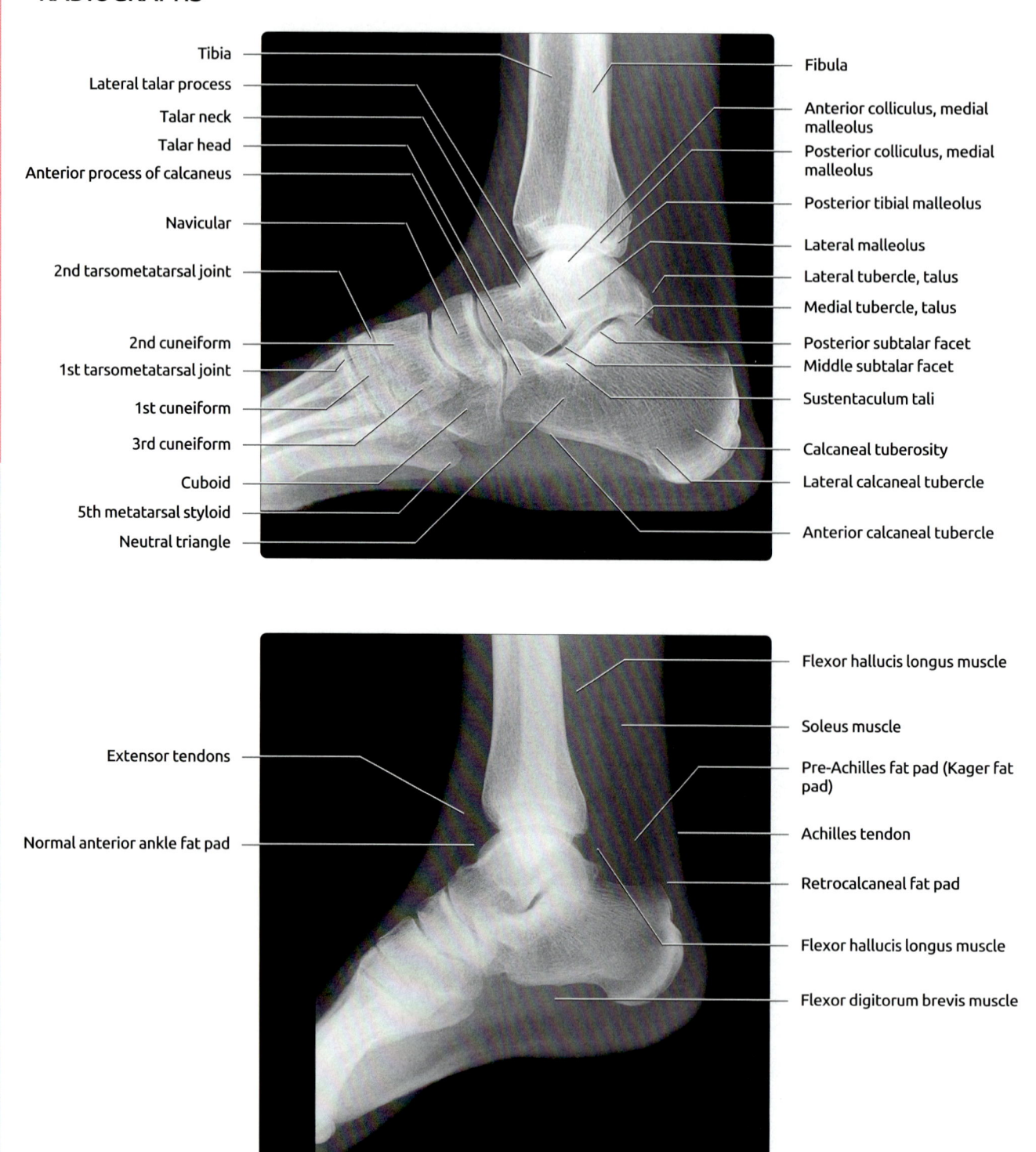

Labels (top image):
- Tibia
- Lateral talar process
- Talar neck
- Talar head
- Anterior process of calcaneus
- Navicular
- 2nd tarsometatarsal joint
- 2nd cuneiform
- 1st tarsometatarsal joint
- 1st cuneiform
- 3rd cuneiform
- Cuboid
- 5th metatarsal styloid
- Neutral triangle
- Fibula
- Anterior colliculus, medial malleolus
- Posterior colliculus, medial malleolus
- Posterior tibial malleolus
- Lateral malleolus
- Lateral tubercle, talus
- Medial tubercle, talus
- Posterior subtalar facet
- Middle subtalar facet
- Sustentaculum tali
- Calcaneal tuberosity
- Lateral calcaneal tubercle
- Anterior calcaneal tubercle

Labels (bottom image):
- Extensor tendons
- Normal anterior ankle fat pad
- Flexor hallucis longus muscle
- Soleus muscle
- Pre-Achilles fat pad (Kager fat pad)
- Achilles tendon
- Retrocalcaneal fat pad
- Flexor hallucis longus muscle
- Flexor digitorum brevis muscle

(Top) Non-weight-bearing lateral view of the ankle depicts both the calcaneus and talus in profile. The posterior, medial, and lateral malleoli are superimposed over one another and over the talus, potentially obscuring fractures at those locations. The lateral view should include the base of the 5th metatarsal. The middle subtalar facet should be seen in tangent on any view which also shows the posterior subtalar facet in tangent. **(Bottom)** The soft tissues of the ankle are emphasized on this lateral view. The Achilles tendon should be uniform in diameter and sharply demarcated. It is separated from the deep flexors by the pre-Achilles fat pad. A small retrocalcaneal fat pad, location of retrocalcaneal bursa, is found between the tendon & calcaneus. Anterior displacement of the small fat pad anterior to the anterior joint line is consistent with joint effusion. Flexor hallucis longus muscle posterior to the ankle should not be mistaken for a joint effusion.

Ankle Radiographic and Arthrographic Anatomy

RADIOGRAPHS

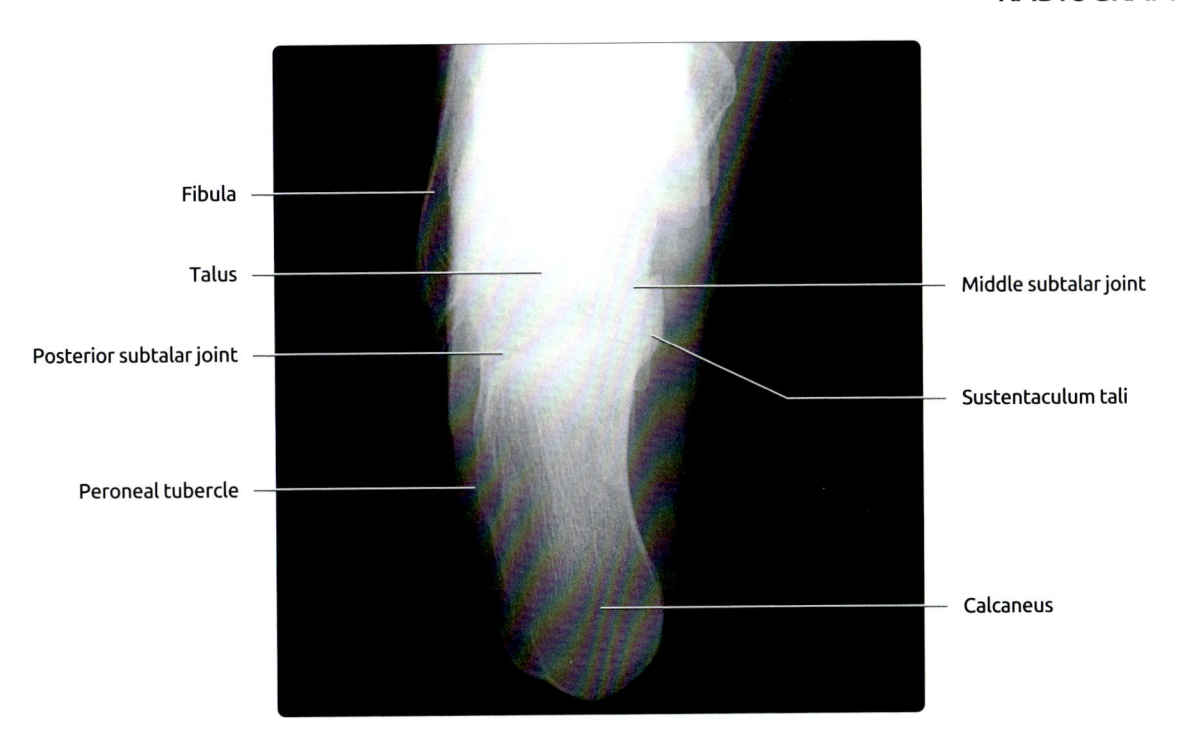

Labels (top image): Fibula; Talus; Posterior subtalar joint; Peroneal tubercle; Middle subtalar joint; Sustentaculum tali; Calcaneus

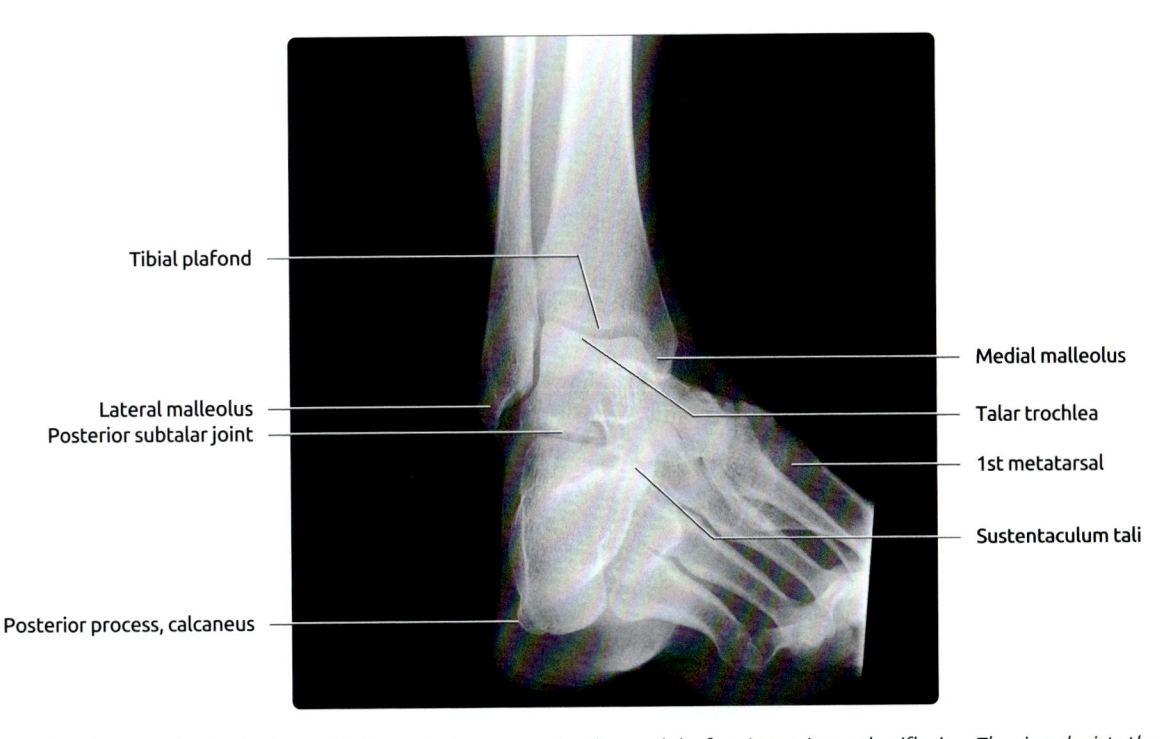

Labels (bottom image): Tibial plafond; Lateral malleolus; Posterior subtalar joint; Posterior process, calcaneus; Medial malleolus; Talar trochlea; 1st metatarsal; Sustentaculum tali

(Top) The calcaneus view is obtained with the patient supine or standing and the foot in maximum dorsiflexion. The view depicts the middle and posterior subtalar joints. **(Bottom)** Broden views are obtained with the patient supine, foot in 45° of internal rotation and 10°, 20°, 30°, and 40° of tube angulation. The views afford visualization of the posterior subtalar joint but have become somewhat obsolete as computed tomography is used more frequently for problem solving in the ankle.

Ankle Radiographic and Arthrographic Anatomy

ARTHROGRAM

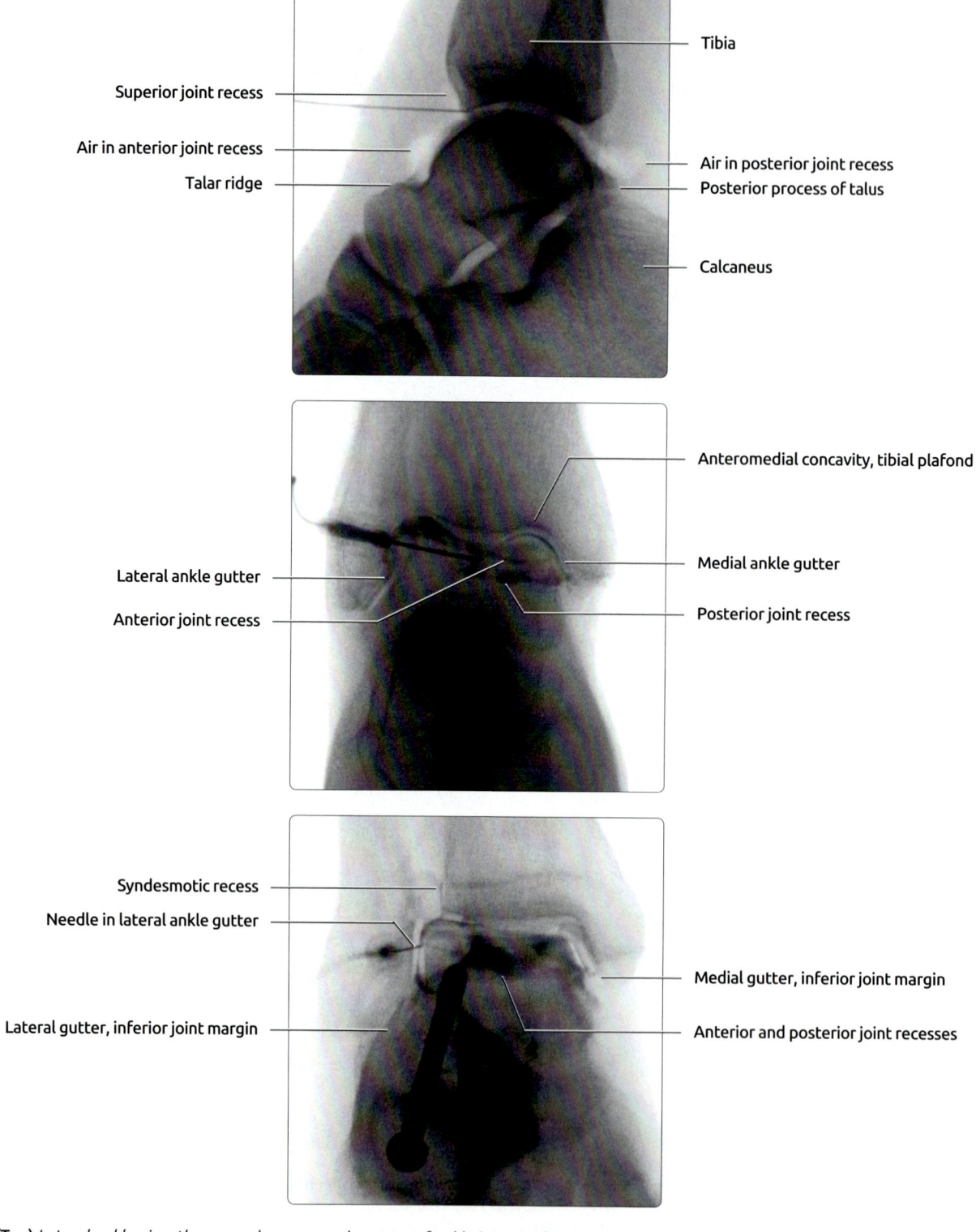

Tibia
Superior joint recess
Air in anterior joint recess
Talar ridge
Air in posterior joint recess
Posterior process of talus
Calcaneus

Anteromedial concavity, tibial plafond
Lateral ankle gutter
Anterior joint recess
Medial ankle gutter
Posterior joint recess

Syndesmotic recess
Needle in lateral ankle gutter
Medial gutter, inferior joint margin
Lateral gutter, inferior joint margin
Anterior and posterior joint recesses

(**Top**) Lateral ankle air arthrogram shows normal contour of ankle joint, with anterior recess extending to talar ridge and posterior recess extending posterior to posterior process of talus. Anteriorly, a superior recess extends slightly above the joint line. Air is useful for therapeutic arthrograms as it avoids the joint irritation and allergic reaction which can be seen with use of iodinated contrast. (**Middle**) AP ankle arthrogram shows the normal extent of filling of medial and lateral joint gutters. The medial gutter does not fill completely due to the presence of the deep deltoid ligament. (**Bottom**) Mortise view Arthrogram shows a normal ankle joint in a patient who had prior subtalar fusion. Approach in this case was via the lateral ankle gutter.

Ankle Radiographic and Arthrographic Anatomy

AXIAL MR ARTHROGRAM

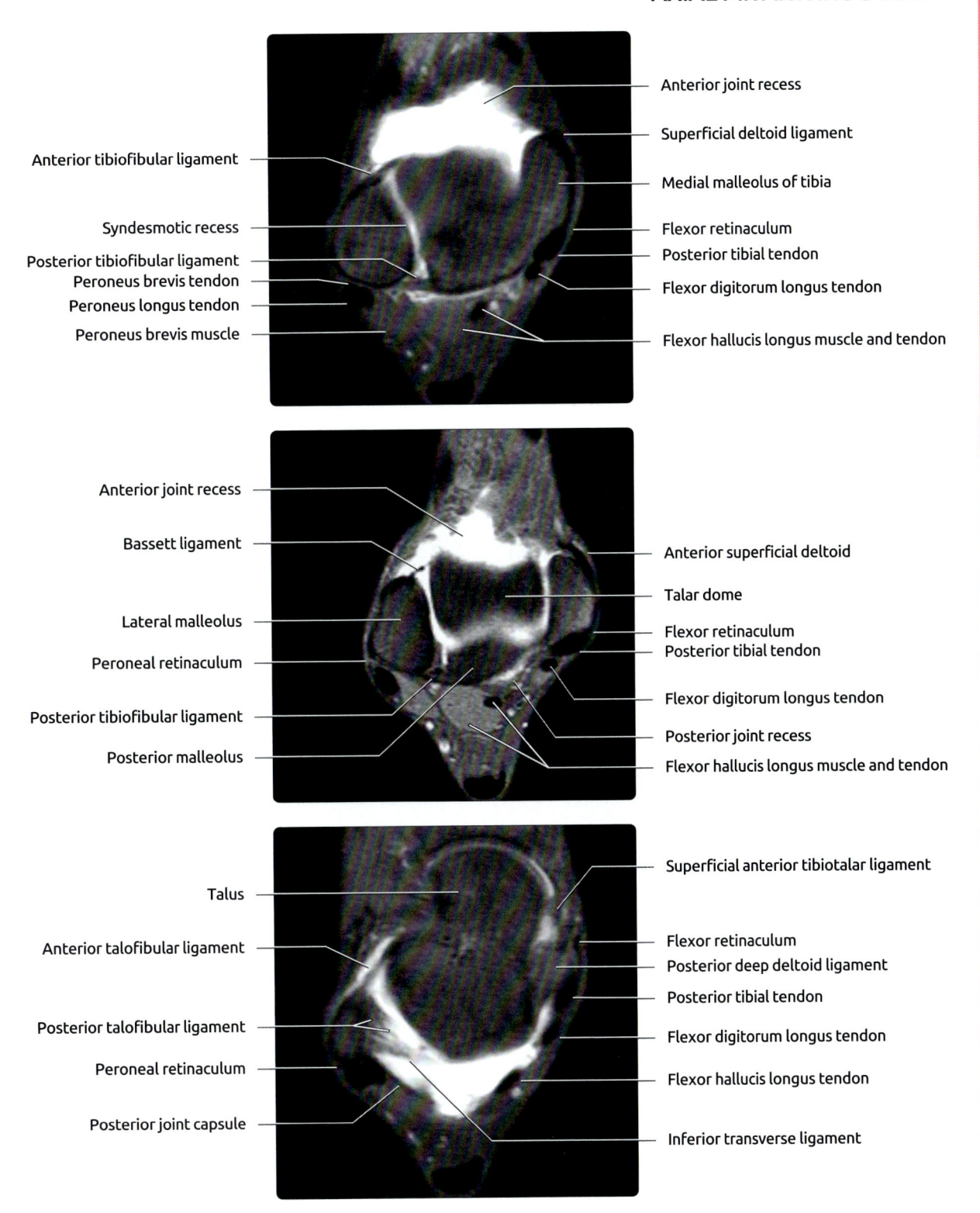

(Top) Selected axial T1 FS MR arthrogram images from different patients through ankle joint are arranged from superior to inferior. At the level of the tibial plafond, axial image shows anterior and posterior ligaments. Fluid extends between tibia and fibula ~ 1 cm cephalad to the plafond in normal syndesmotic recess. Note the rounded anterior joint recess, which extends ~ 5-10 mm above the plafond. (Middle) At the level of the talar dome the accessory tibiotalar ligament (Bassett ligament) is seen arising from the fibula. It courses superiorly and medially and inserts on the anterolateral corner of the tibial plafond. (Bottom) At the superior margin of the talar neck, the anterior talofibular ligament is seen attaching to the anterolateral corner of the talar body. The posterior talofibular ligament is much broader and thicker than the anterior talofibular ligament. It has a fan-shaped appearance with striations similar to those seen in the anterior cruciate ligament.

Ankle Radiographic and Arthrographic Anatomy

AXIAL MR ARTHROGRAM

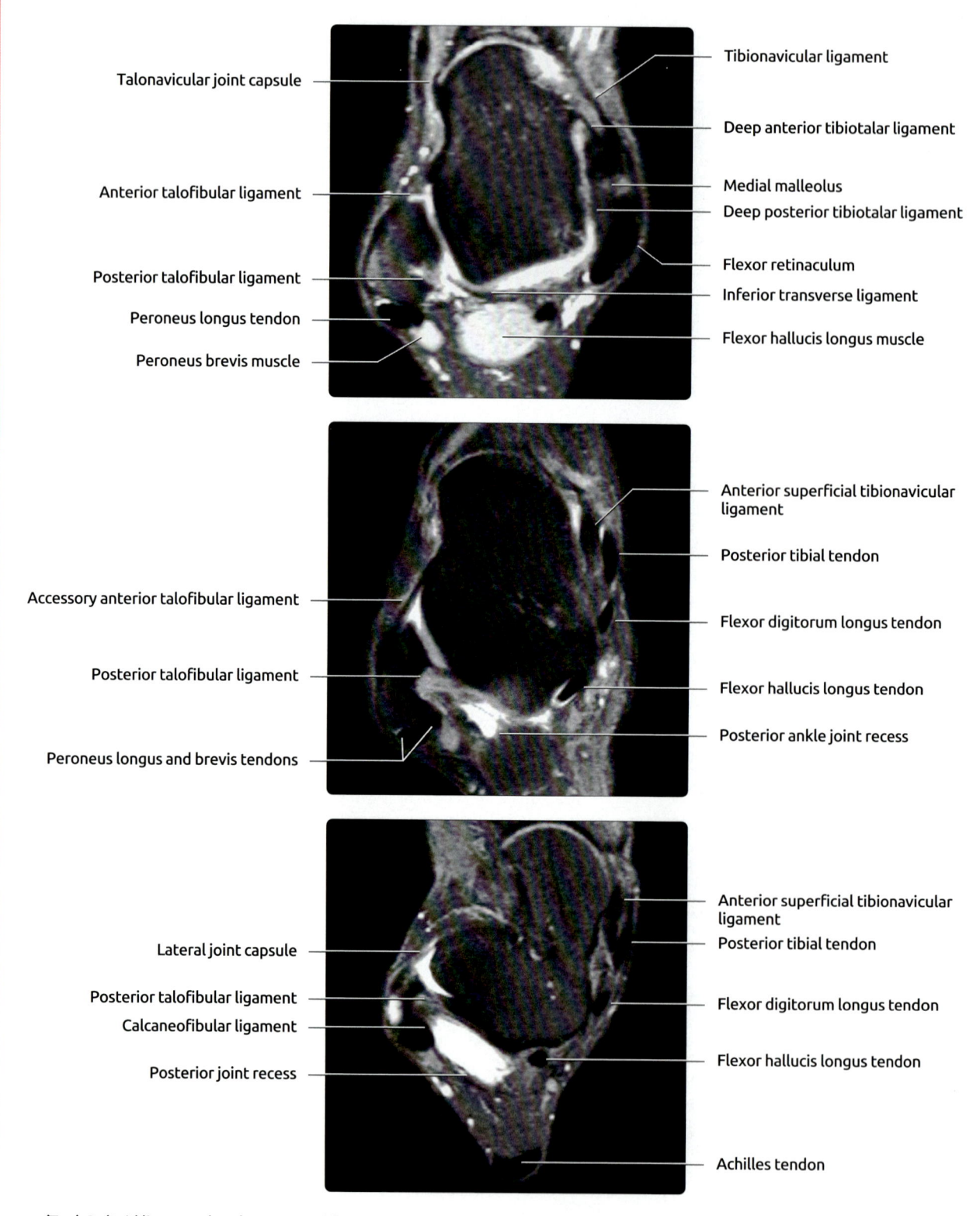

Labels (top image):
- Talonavicular joint capsule
- Anterior talofibular ligament
- Posterior talofibular ligament
- Peroneus longus tendon
- Peroneus brevis muscle
- Tibionavicular ligament
- Deep anterior tibiotalar ligament
- Medial malleolus
- Deep posterior tibiotalar ligament
- Flexor retinaculum
- Inferior transverse ligament
- Flexor hallucis longus muscle

Labels (middle image):
- Accessory anterior talofibular ligament
- Posterior talofibular ligament
- Peroneus longus and brevis tendons
- Anterior superficial tibionavicular ligament
- Posterior tibial tendon
- Flexor digitorum longus tendon
- Flexor hallucis longus tendon
- Posterior ankle joint recess

Labels (bottom image):
- Lateral joint capsule
- Posterior talofibular ligament
- Calcaneofibular ligament
- Posterior joint recess
- Anterior superficial tibionavicular ligament
- Posterior tibial tendon
- Flexor digitorum longus tendon
- Flexor hallucis longus tendon
- Achilles tendon

(**Top**) Deltoid ligament bands are named for attachments. Deep anterior tibiotalar ligament attaches to the small bony prominence at the mid-talar neck. The tibionavicular ligament attaches to the medial eminence of the navicular. Note that the anterior talofibular ligament in this patient is thin and redundant, consistent with prior injury. (**Middle**) The accessory anterior talofibular ligament is inferior to the main portion of the ligament and appears continuous with it on MR. Anterior deltoid fibers course deep to the posterior tibial tendon. (**Bottom**) At the level of the fibular tip, the calcaneofibular ligament is seen extending posteriorly and inferiorly deep to the peroneal tendons. In this patient, the posterior joint recess was continuous with the subtalar joint.

Ankle Radiographic and Arthrographic Anatomy

SAGITTAL MR ARTHROGRAM

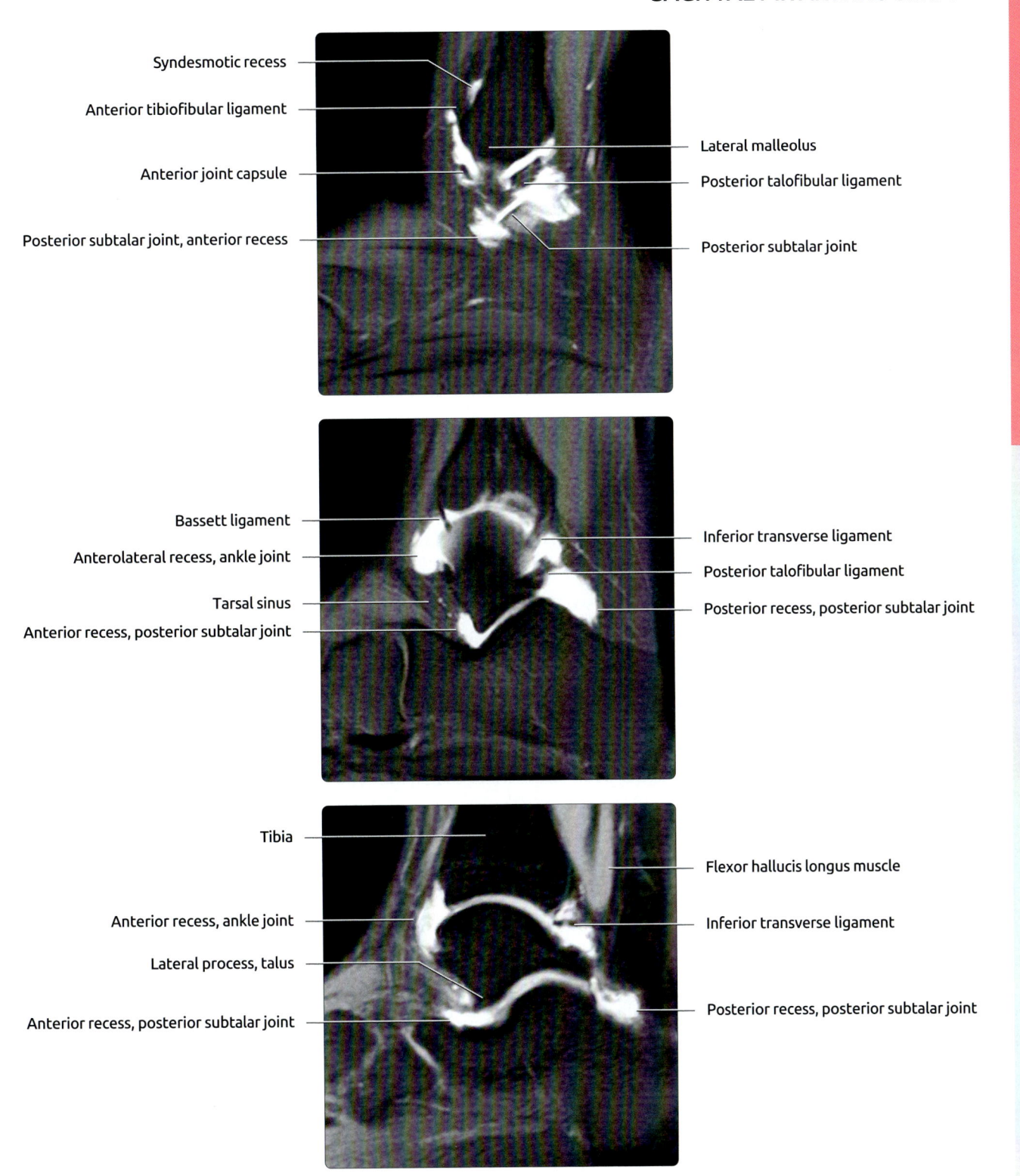

Labels (top image):
- Syndesmotic recess
- Anterior tibiofibular ligament
- Anterior joint capsule
- Posterior subtalar joint, anterior recess
- Lateral malleolus
- Posterior talofibular ligament
- Posterior subtalar joint

Labels (middle image):
- Bassett ligament
- Anterolateral recess, ankle joint
- Tarsal sinus
- Anterior recess, posterior subtalar joint
- Inferior transverse ligament
- Posterior talofibular ligament
- Posterior recess, posterior subtalar joint

Labels (bottom image):
- Tibia
- Anterior recess, ankle joint
- Lateral process, talus
- Anterior recess, posterior subtalar joint
- Flexor hallucis longus muscle
- Inferior transverse ligament
- Posterior recess, posterior subtalar joint

(**Top**) *Selected sagittal T1WI FS MR arthrogram images from different patients were taken through the ankle joint from lateral to medial. On the far lateral image, collateral ligaments are outlined by distended joint recesses. Subtalar joint filling is a normal variant.* (**Middle**) *The oblique course of the Bassett ligament, the accessory anterior tibiofibular ligament inferior to main anterior tibiofibular ligament, is well seen on this image. Note also the oblique course of the inferior transverse or intermalleolar ligament.* (**Bottom**) *Inferior transverse (intermalleolar) ligament forms meniscoid structure; in cross section, it may mimic a loose body.*

Ankle Radiographic and Arthrographic Anatomy

SAGITTAL MR ARTHROGRAM

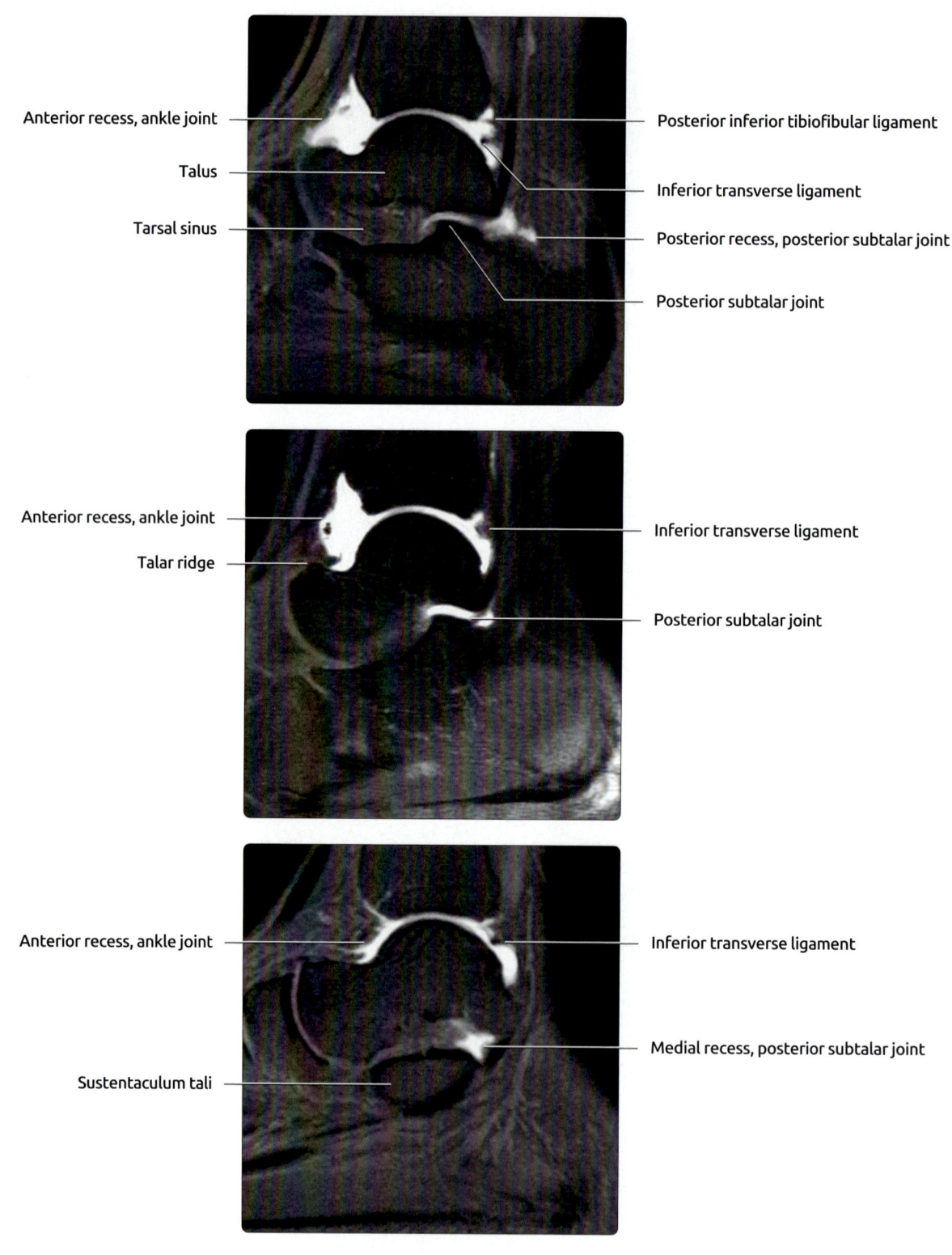

(Top) Labels: Anterior recess, ankle joint; Talus; Tarsal sinus; Posterior inferior tibiofibular ligament; Inferior transverse ligament; Posterior recess, posterior subtalar joint; Posterior subtalar joint.

(Middle) Labels: Anterior recess, ankle joint; Talar ridge; Inferior transverse ligament; Posterior subtalar joint.

(Bottom) Labels: Anterior recess, ankle joint; Sustentaculum tali; Inferior transverse ligament; Medial recess, posterior subtalar joint.

(Top) *Anterior joint recess is large, allowing for a wide range of motion.* **(Middle)** *The anterior tibial attachment of the joint capsule in this patient is slightly high compared to average; some variability should be expected. Distally, the joint capsule attaches to the talar ridge at the junction of the talar neck and head.* **(Bottom)** *At the medial aspect of the ankle joint, the inferior transverse ligament is approaching the tibia. The posterior inferior tibiofibular ligament has already inserted and is no longer visible.*

Ankle Radiographic and Arthrographic Anatomy

CORONAL MR ARTHROGRAM

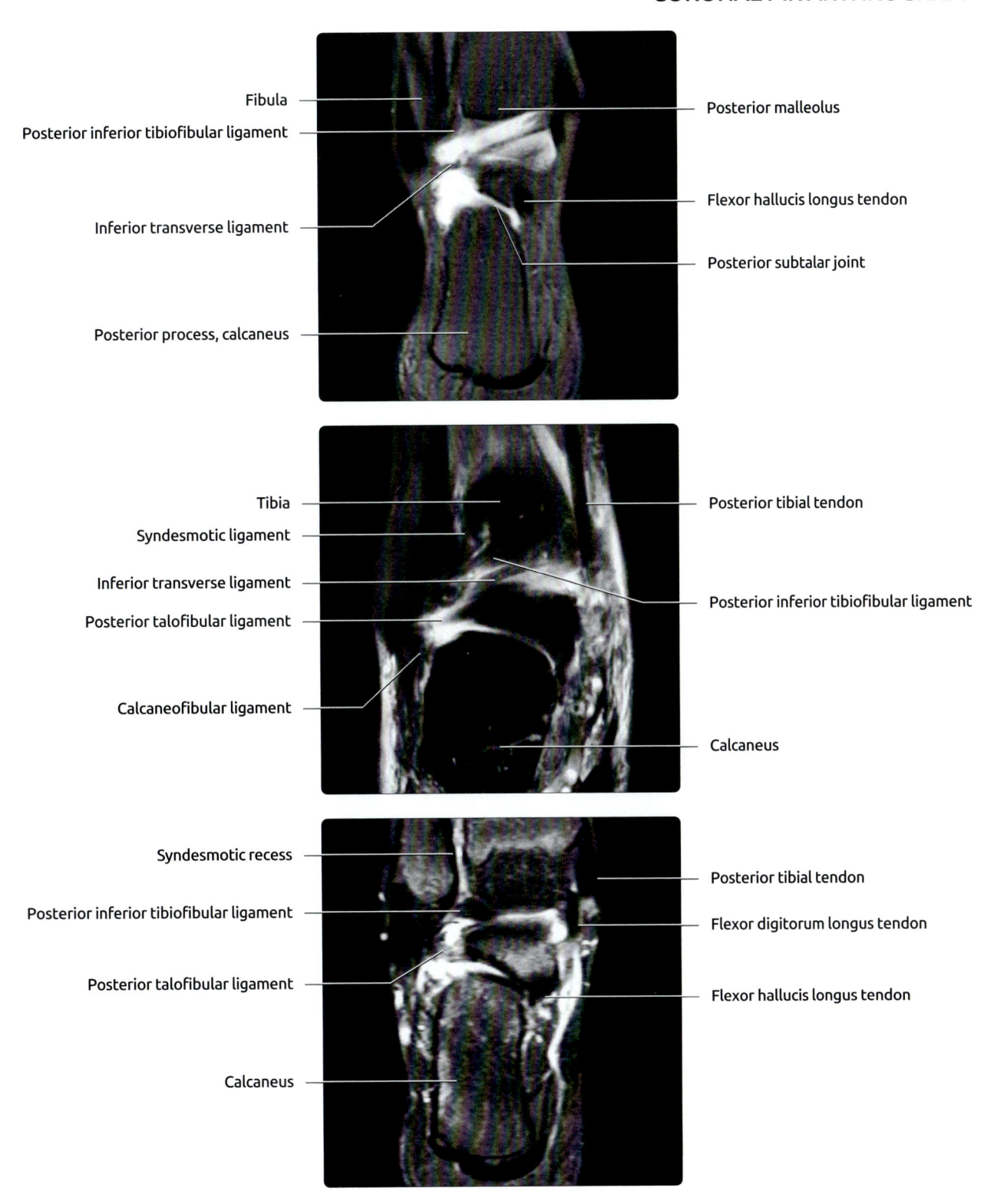

(Top) *Selected coronal T1WI FS MR arthrogram images from different patients show the ankle joint from posterior to anterior. The posterior inferior tibiofibular ligament extends from the posterior malleolus and lateral aspect of the tibia to the fibula, at the level of the plafond. The inferior transverse (intermalleolar) ligament is more inferior and extends from the medial margin of the posterior tibia to the fibula, forming a labrum-like structure across the joint.* **(Middle)** *Slightly more anteriorly, portions of the posterior tibiofibular ligament are visible, and the posterior talofibular ligament comes into view inferior to tibiofibular ligaments.* **(Bottom)** *This young soccer player has an unusually large syndesmotic recess, which may reflect old trauma, but was asymptomatic at time of examination. Although anatomy books usually state the recess is < 1 cm in superoinferior dimension, greater extension proximally is common.*

Ankle Radiographic and Arthrographic Anatomy

CORONAL MR ARTHROGRAM

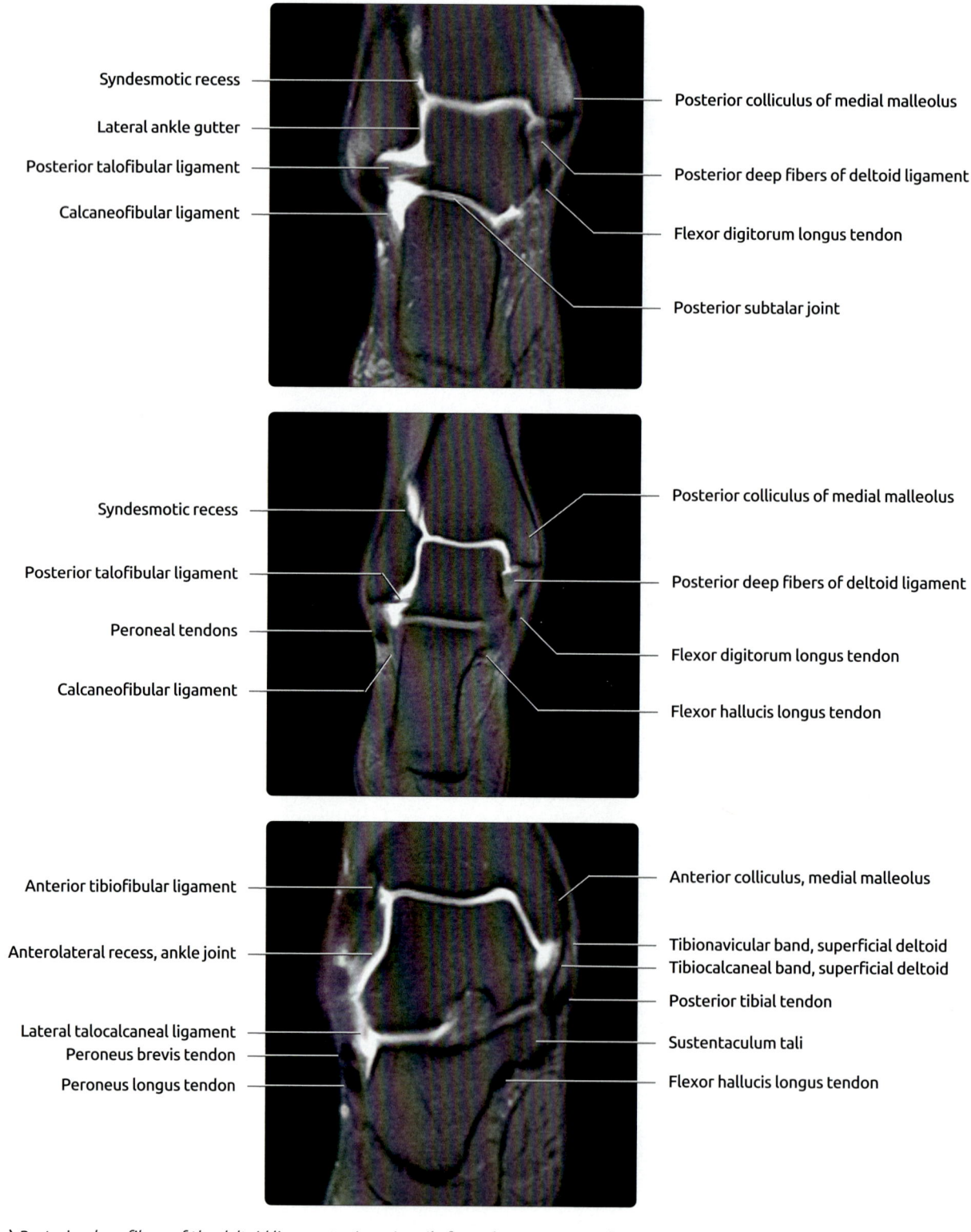

(Top) Posterior deep fibers of the deltoid ligament arise primarily from the posterior surface of the anterior colliculus of the medial malleolus and also from the posterior colliculus. The fibers travel slightly inferiorly to insert on the concavity at the medial aspect of the body of the talus. Contrast deep to calcaneofibular ligament has extended from the subtalar joint. **(Middle)** Note normal contrast filling of the medial and lateral ankle gutters. This outlines the full extent of hyaline cartilage investing articular surfaces. **(Bottom)** Anterior bands of superficial deltoid ligament start to be distinguishable at the level of the anterior colliculus of the medial malleolus.

Ankle Radiographic and Arthrographic Anatomy

CORONAL MR ARTHROGRAM

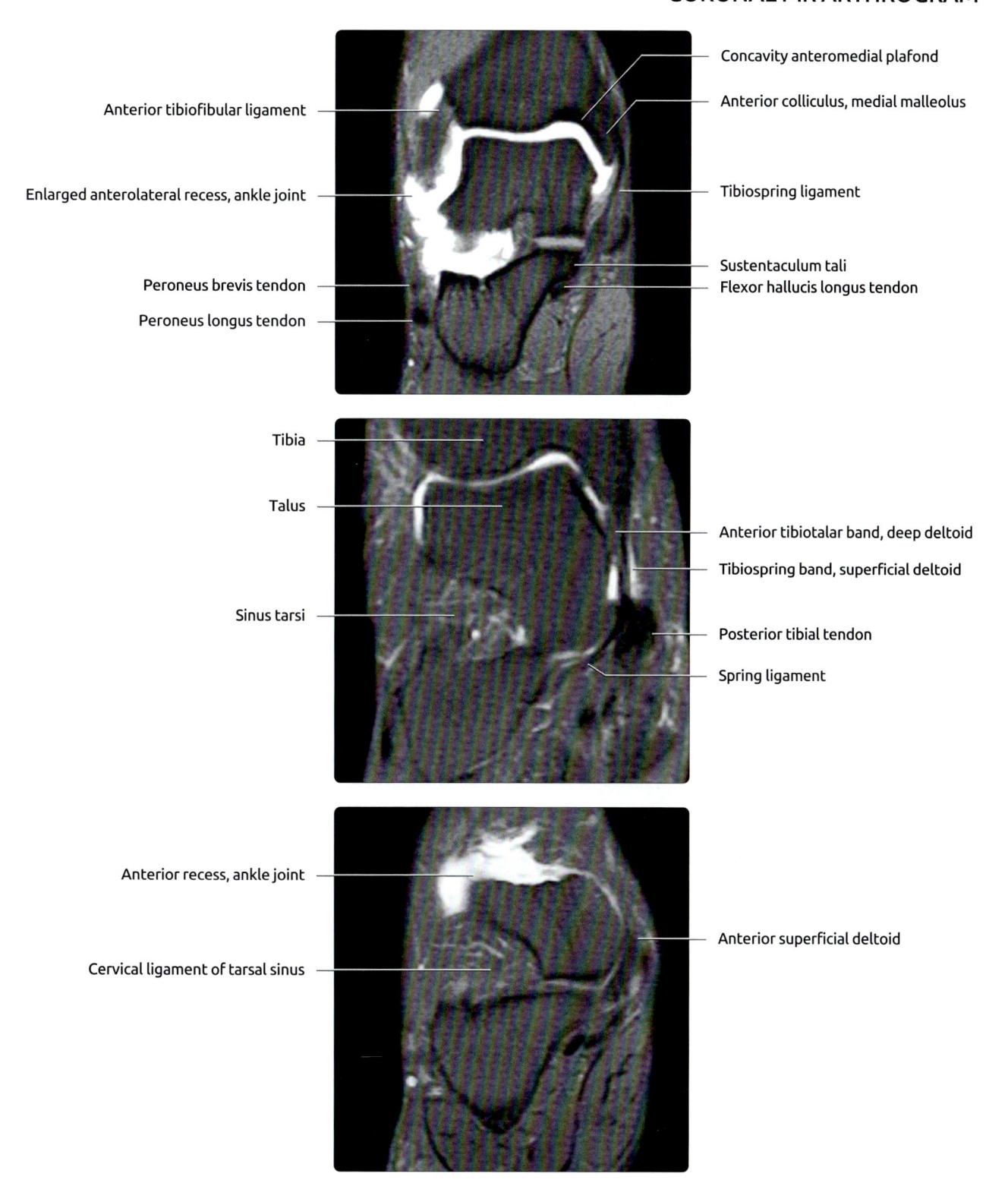

Labels (top image):
- Anterior tibiofibular ligament
- Enlarged anterolateral recess, ankle joint
- Peroneus brevis tendon
- Peroneus longus tendon
- Concavity anteromedial plafond
- Anterior colliculus, medial malleolus
- Tibiospring ligament
- Sustentaculum tali
- Flexor hallucis longus tendon

Labels (middle image):
- Tibia
- Talus
- Sinus tarsi
- Anterior tibiotalar band, deep deltoid
- Tibiospring band, superficial deltoid
- Posterior tibial tendon
- Spring ligament

Labels (bottom image):
- Anterior recess, ankle joint
- Cervical ligament of tarsal sinus
- Anterior superficial deltoid

(**Top**) *The entire oblique course of the anterior tibiofibular ligament is unusually well seen in this patient. The anterolateral joint recess is larger than normal, reflecting an old anterior talofibular ligament (ATFL) injury. The anteromedial portion of the tibial plafond forms a bowl-shaped concavity, which is covered with cartilage.* (**Middle**) *The anterior deep tibiotalar ligament inserts on the proximal talar neck, while the tibiospring ligament superficial to it is continuous with the spring ligament.* (**Bottom**) *The anterior recess of the talar joint ends at the talar neck. The anterior superficial deltoid fibers continue anteriorly to insert on the spring ligament, talar neck, and median eminence of the navicular.*

Ankle MR Atlas

IMAGING ANATOMY

Anatomy Relationships

- Anatomy of joint capsules
  - Ankle joint capsule communicates with flexor hallucis longus tendon sheath
  - Posterior subtalar joint has separate joint capsule
    - 10-15% of cases show continuity with ankle joint capsule
  - Middle, anterior subtalar joint share joint capsule with talonavicular joint
    - Sometimes called talocalcaneonavicular joint
- Deep and superficial deltoid components have different functions
  - Deep deltoid ligament protects against eversion
  - Superficial deltoid ligament protects against twisting injury

Patient Positioning

- Axial imaging may be performed in straight axial position (continuation of plane of leg)
  - Foot is usually plantar flexed when patient is lying comfortably in MR scanner
  - Straight axial imaging results in oblique images through hindfoot
- May angle axial images along axis of talus
  - Same orientation as for axial MR of foot
  - Distal tibia and fibula will be seen at slightly oblique angle
- Choose angle of slices based on area of concern
  - Straight axial: To evaluate distal tibia or Achilles tendon
  - Angled axial: To evaluate remainder of hindfoot
- Coronal imaging has similar issues
  - Usually best to angle perpendicular to axis of talus

Structures Optimally Seen in Axial Plane

- Anterior talofibular ligament reliably evaluated only in this plane
  - Fibular attachment: 1 cm above fibular tip
  - Talar attachment: Most superior image (or next image), which includes talar neck
- Calcaneofibular ligament
  - Majority of ligament well seen
  - Fibular attachment to inferior border of fibular tip is not visible in axial plane
- Extrinsic tendons of ankle and foot
  - Achilles tendon should have concave margin anteriorly
  - Posterior tibial tendon should be 2x size of flexor digitorum longus
- Ankle retinacula
  - Flexor retinaculum
    - Thin sheet of fibrous tissue
    - Attaches medially to pointed prominence at posteromedial margin of tibia
    - Merges laterally with fascia overlying flexor hallucis longus muscle
    - Extends inferiorly to form roof of tarsal tunnel (this portion better seen on coronal images)
  - Peroneal retinaculum
    - Thin sheet of fibrous tissue
    - Attaches laterally to posterolateral border of fibula
    - Attaches medially to lateral margin of calcaneus and Achilles aponeurosis
- Syndesmotic ligaments
  - Obliquely oriented
  - Must evaluate on multiple slices
- Posterior margin of fibula
  - Should be concave
  - Convex posterior margin is associated with peroneal tendon dysfunction
    - Due to increased stress on peroneal retinaculum
- Posterior talofibular ligament
  - Thick, striated appearance
  - Often appears lax in axial plane

Structures Optimally Seen in Sagittal Plane

- Talar dome
  - Small osteochondral lesions may be masked by partial volume artifact on axial, coronal images
- Achilles tendon and pre-Achilles space
- Subtalar joint
- Chopart joint
- Plantar fascia

Structures Optimally Seen in Coronal Plane

- Tarsal sinus ligaments
  - Cervical ligament & extensor retinaculum bands may be confused on sagittal images
  - Cervical ligament anterior to extensor retinaculum
- Hindfoot portions of flexor and peroneal tendons
- Deltoid ligament

ANATOMY IMAGING ISSUES

Imaging Recommendations

- Always include T1 sequence in axial plane in every ankle MR
  - Improves visualization of accessory muscles
  - Helpful in confirming ligament integrity

Imaging Pitfalls

- Anterior inferior tibiofibular ligament
  - Axial images slice obliquely through ligament + accessory Bassett ligament
    - May mimic ligament discontinuity
    - Correlate with coronal images
- Anterior talofibular ligament (ATFL)
  - Joint capsule inferior to ligament often thickens after ATFL tear
  - Do not mistake thickened inferior capsule for intact ATFL
- Accessory muscles
  - Easily overlooked on MR because normal muscle signal intensity
  - Can be symptomatic
  - Clinically can be mistaken for mass
- Posterior tibial tendon dislocation
  - Tendon displaced medially, anteriorly
  - Often overlooked because tendon is normal in signal intensity
- Tarsal sinus
  - Difficult to distinguish cervical ligament from bands of extensor retinaculum in tarsal sinus

Ankle MR Atlas

GRAPHICS OF MUSCLE AND TENDONS OF ANKLE

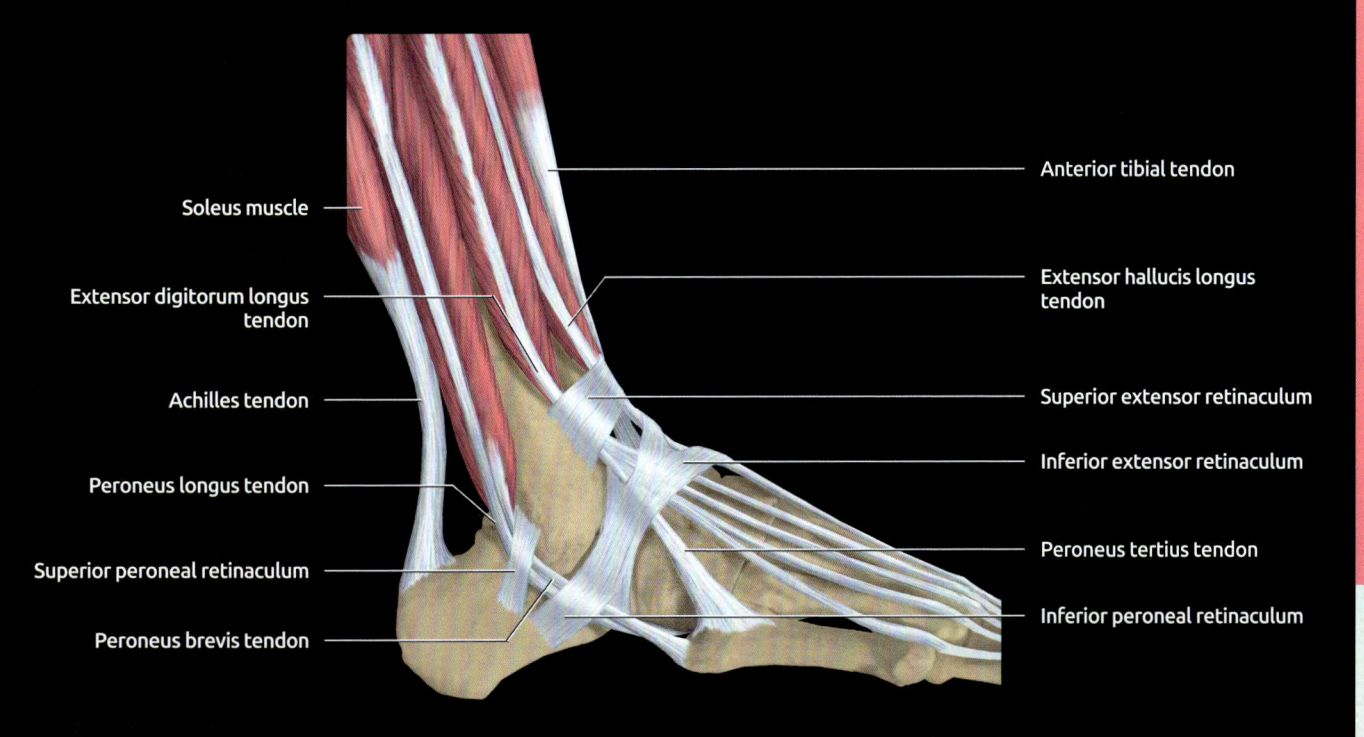

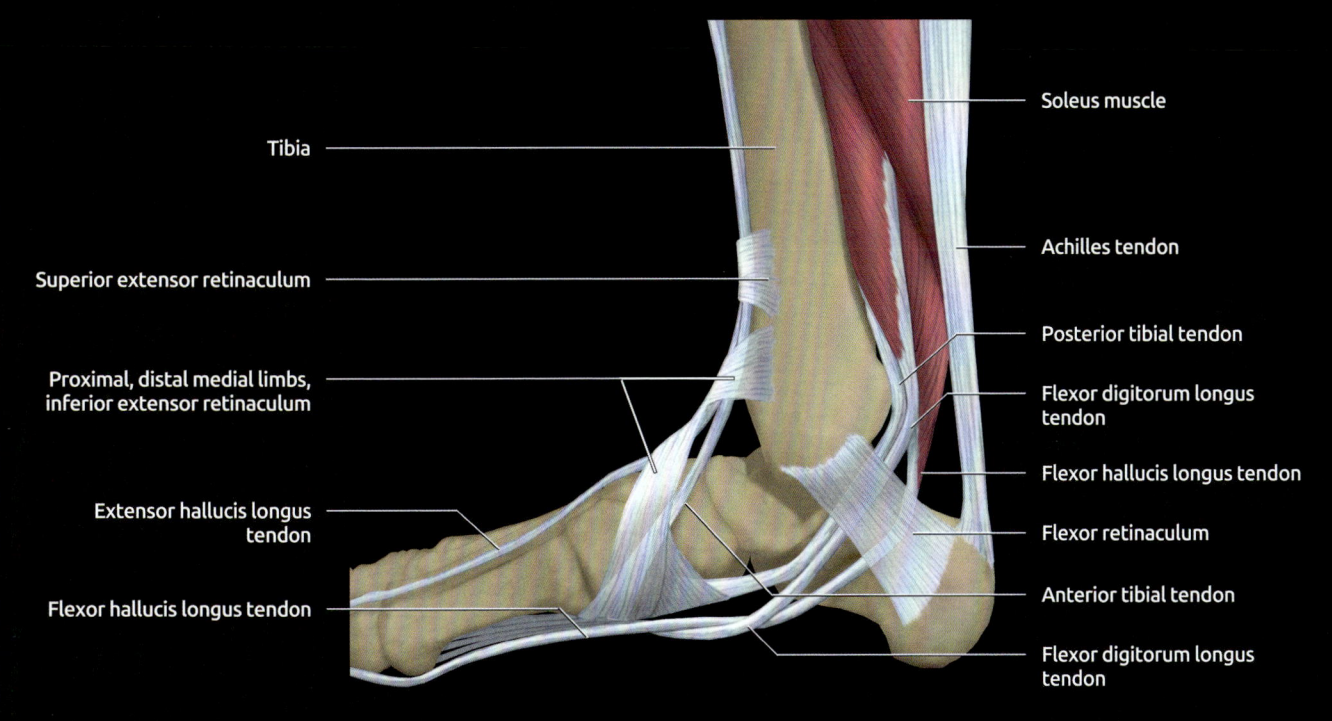

(Top) Lateral view shows the tendons of the ankle. The peroneus brevis & peroneus longus tendons occupy the lateral compartment. They descend posterior to the fibula, held by the superior peroneal retinaculum, & continue along the lateral wall of calcaneus, held by the inferior peroneal retinaculum. Fibers of the inferior peroneal retinaculum insert either into the peroneal tubercle or calcaneal wall and separate the 2 tendons. The peroneus longus tendon curves around the cuboid to enter the sole of the foot. Both the peroneus brevis and peroneus tertius insert on the 5th metatarsal base. (Bottom) Flexor retinaculum is shown. The retinaculum extends from the medial malleolus to the plantar aponeurosis. It binds the posterior compartment tendons & forms the lateral border of tarsal tunnel.

Ankle MR Atlas

AXIAL T1 MR, RIGHT ANKLE

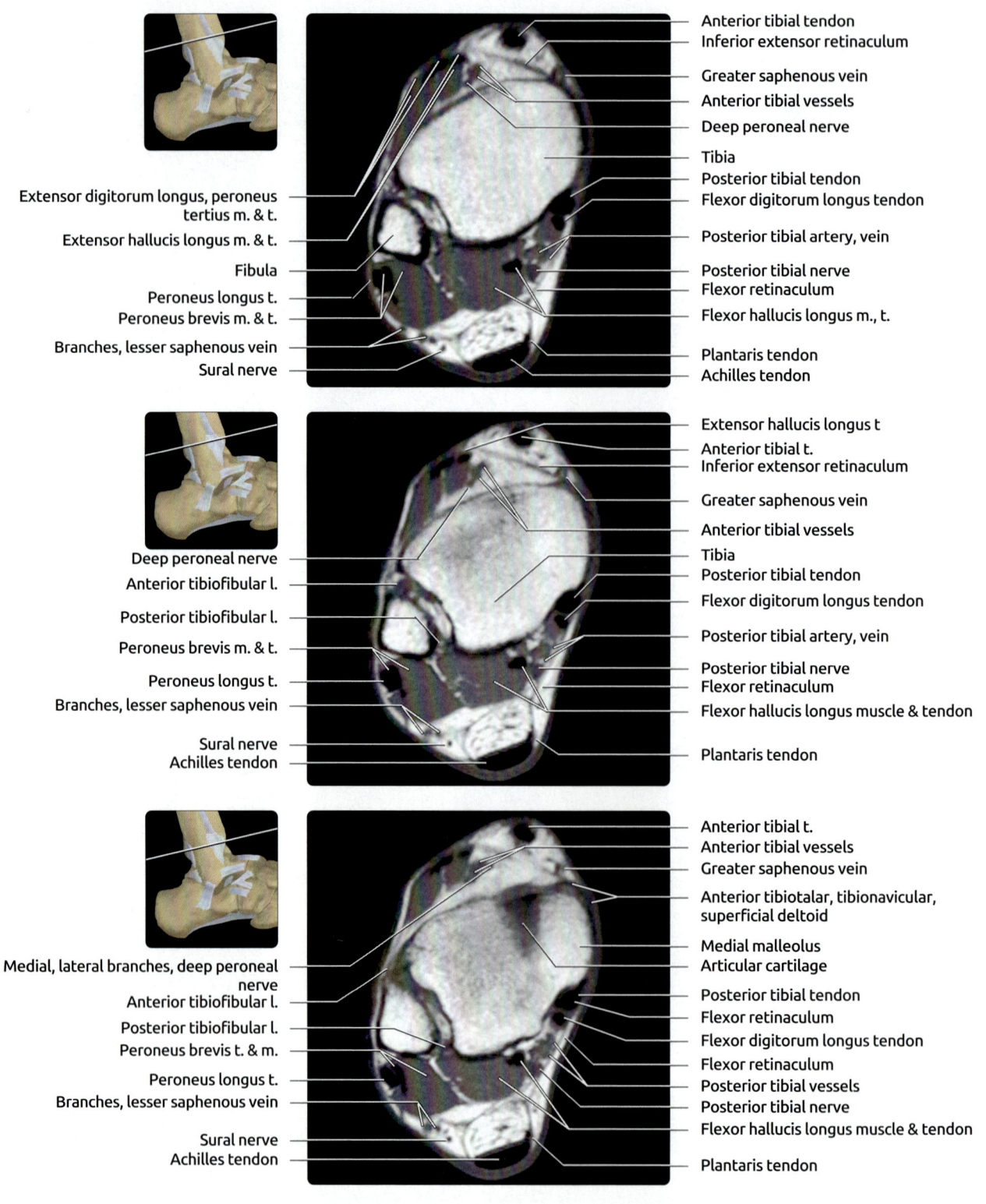

Top image labels (left side):
- Extensor digitorum longus, peroneus tertius m. & t.
- Extensor hallucis longus m. & t.
- Fibula
- Peroneus longus t.
- Peroneus brevis m. & t.
- Branches, lesser saphenous vein
- Sural nerve

Top image labels (right side):
- Anterior tibial tendon
- Inferior extensor retinaculum
- Greater saphenous vein
- Anterior tibial vessels
- Deep peroneal nerve
- Tibia
- Posterior tibial tendon
- Flexor digitorum longus tendon
- Posterior tibial artery, vein
- Posterior tibial nerve
- Flexor retinaculum
- Flexor hallucis longus m., t.
- Plantaris tendon
- Achilles tendon

Middle image labels (left side):
- Deep peroneal nerve
- Anterior tibiofibular l.
- Posterior tibiofibular l.
- Peroneus brevis m. & t.
- Peroneus longus t.
- Branches, lesser saphenous vein
- Sural nerve
- Achilles tendon

Middle image labels (right side):
- Extensor hallucis longus t
- Anterior tibial t.
- Inferior extensor retinaculum
- Greater saphenous vein
- Anterior tibial vessels
- Tibia
- Posterior tibial tendon
- Flexor digitorum longus tendon
- Posterior tibial artery, vein
- Posterior tibial nerve
- Flexor retinaculum
- Flexor hallucis longus muscle & tendon
- Plantaris tendon

Bottom image labels (left side):
- Medial, lateral branches, deep peroneal nerve
- Anterior tibiofibular l.
- Posterior tibiofibular l.
- Peroneus brevis t. & m.
- Peroneus longus t.
- Branches, lesser saphenous vein
- Sural nerve
- Achilles tendon

Bottom image labels (right side):
- Anterior tibial t.
- Anterior tibial vessels
- Greater saphenous vein
- Anterior tibiotalar, tibionavicular, superficial deltoid
- Medial malleolus
- Articular cartilage
- Posterior tibial tendon
- Flexor retinaculum
- Flexor digitorum longus tendon
- Flexor retinaculum
- Posterior tibial vessels
- Posterior tibial nerve
- Flexor hallucis longus muscle & tendon
- Plantaris tendon

(Top) First in series of 18 axial T1 MR images of the right ankle is shown. The cut is just above the tibial plafond and is perpendicular to the long axis of the tibia. **(Middle)** The anterior and posterior tibiofibular ligaments extend from the distal tibia to the fibula and, along with the interosseus ligament, support the distal tibiofibular joint. The anterior surface of the Achilles tendon is flat. The tendon is partially surrounded by a paratenon. The plantaris tendon is found just medial to the Achilles tendon. **(Bottom)** Posterior tibial and flexor digitorum longus tendons lie in a groove posterior to the medial malleolus. They are held in place by the overlying flexor retinaculum. The posterior tibial tendon is 2x the diameter of the flexor digitorum longus tendon.

Ankle MR Atlas

AXIAL T1 MR, LEFT ANKLE

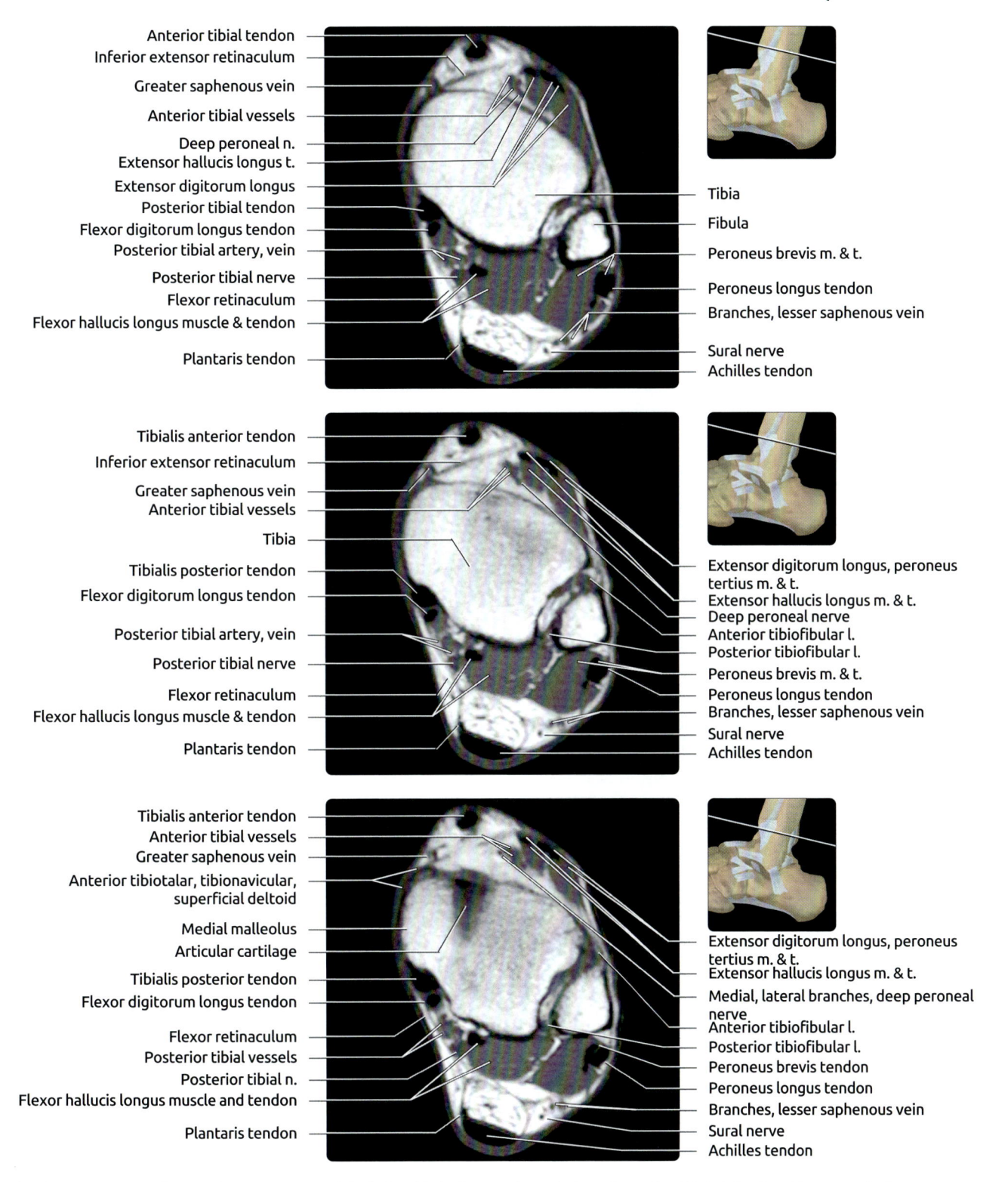

(Top) First in series of 18 axial T1 MR images of the left ankle is shown. The cut is just above the tibial plafond and is perpendicular to the long axis of the tibia. **(Middle)** The anterior and posterior tibiofibular ligaments extend from the distal tibia to the fibula and, along with the interosseous ligament, support the distal fibrous tibiofibular joint. The anterior surface of the Achilles tendon is flat. The tendon is partially surrounded by a paratenon. The plantaris tendon is found just medial to the Achilles tendon. **(Bottom)** Posterior tibial and flexor digitorum longus tendons lie in a groove posterior to the medial malleolus. They are held in place by the overlying flexor retinaculum. The posterior tibial tendon is 2x the diameter of the flexor digitorum longus tendon.

Ankle MR Atlas

AXIAL T1 MR, RIGHT ANKLE

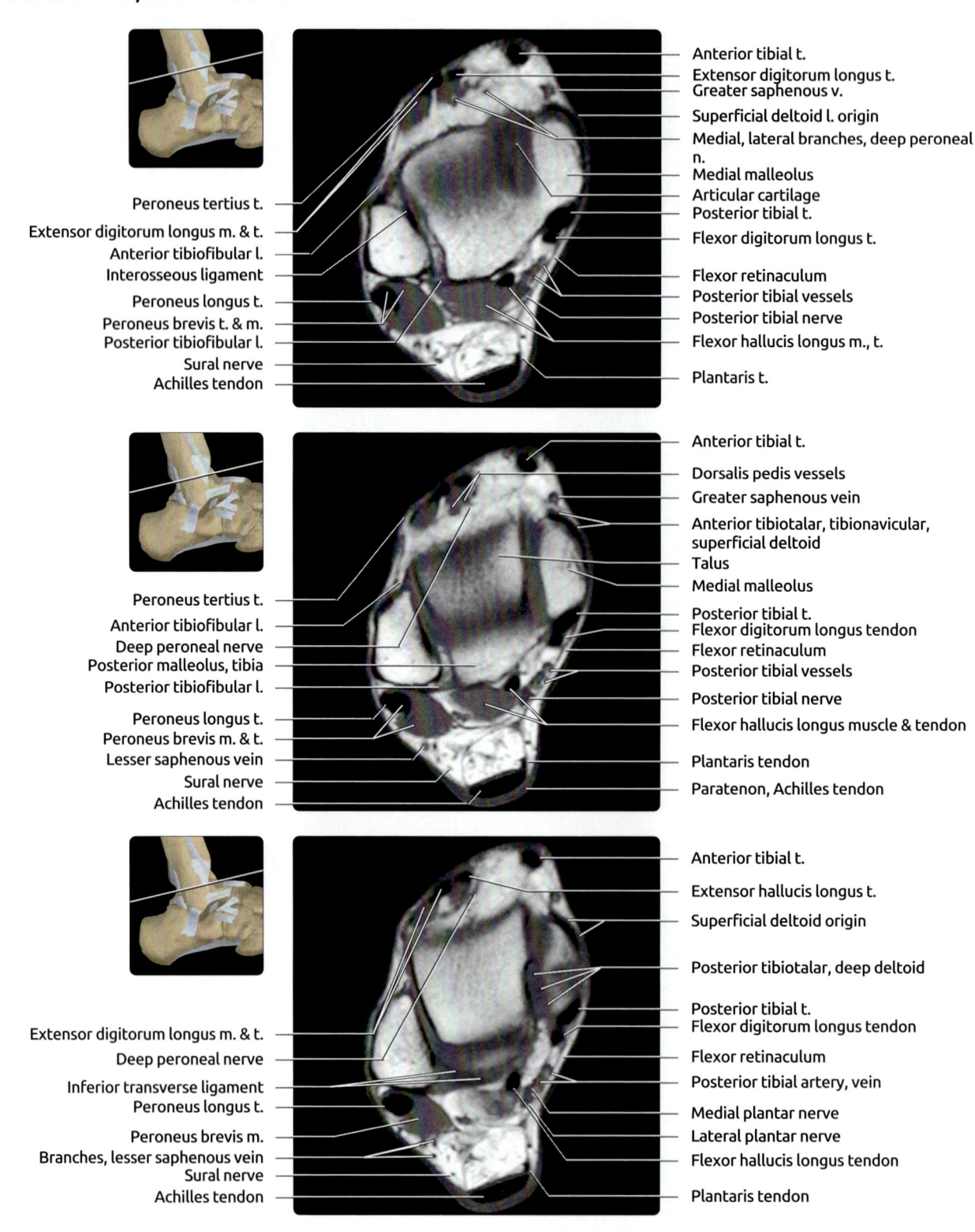

Image 1 labels (left side):
- Peroneus tertius t.
- Extensor digitorum longus m. & t.
- Anterior tibiofibular l.
- Interosseous ligament
- Peroneus longus t.
- Peroneus brevis t. & m.
- Posterior tibiofibular l.
- Sural nerve
- Achilles tendon

Image 1 labels (right side):
- Anterior tibial t.
- Extensor digitorum longus t.
- Greater saphenous v.
- Superficial deltoid l. origin
- Medial, lateral branches, deep peroneal n.
- Medial malleolus
- Articular cartilage
- Posterior tibial t.
- Flexor digitorum longus t.
- Flexor retinaculum
- Posterior tibial vessels
- Posterior tibial nerve
- Flexor hallucis longus m., t.
- Plantaris t.

Image 2 labels (left side):
- Peroneus tertius t.
- Anterior tibiofibular l.
- Deep peroneal nerve
- Posterior malleolus, tibia
- Posterior tibiofibular l.
- Peroneus longus t.
- Peroneus brevis m. & t.
- Lesser saphenous vein
- Sural nerve
- Achilles tendon

Image 2 labels (right side):
- Anterior tibial t.
- Dorsalis pedis vessels
- Greater saphenous vein
- Anterior tibiotalar, tibionavicular, superficial deltoid
- Talus
- Medial malleolus
- Posterior tibial t.
- Flexor digitorum longus tendon
- Flexor retinaculum
- Posterior tibial vessels
- Posterior tibial nerve
- Flexor hallucis longus muscle & tendon
- Plantaris tendon
- Paratenon, Achilles tendon

Image 3 labels (left side):
- Extensor digitorum longus m. & t.
- Deep peroneal nerve
- Inferior transverse ligament
- Peroneus longus t.
- Peroneus brevis m.
- Branches, lesser saphenous vein
- Sural nerve
- Achilles tendon

Image 3 labels (right side):
- Anterior tibial t.
- Extensor hallucis longus t.
- Superficial deltoid origin
- Posterior tibiotalar, deep deltoid
- Posterior tibial t.
- Flexor digitorum longus tendon
- Flexor retinaculum
- Posterior tibial artery, vein
- Medial plantar nerve
- Lateral plantar nerve
- Flexor hallucis longus tendon
- Plantaris tendon

(**Top**) The interosseous ligament is visualized in between the tibia and fibula. This ligament, a thickening of the interosseous membrane, is variable and may be perforated or absent. (**Middle**) The relative position of soft tissue structures posterior to the medial malleolus can be remembered by the mnemonic Tom, Dick, and a very nervous Harry. These signify the posterior tibial tendon, the flexor digitorum tendon, artery, vein, nerve and flexor hallucis longus tendon. (**Bottom**) The deep posterior tibiotalar component of the deltoid ligament originates from the posterior colliculus and is typically striated. The inferior transverse ligament, the very inferior aspect of the posterior tibiofibular ligament, extends distal to the tibial posterior surface.

Ankle MR Atlas

AXIAL T1 MR, LEFT ANKLE

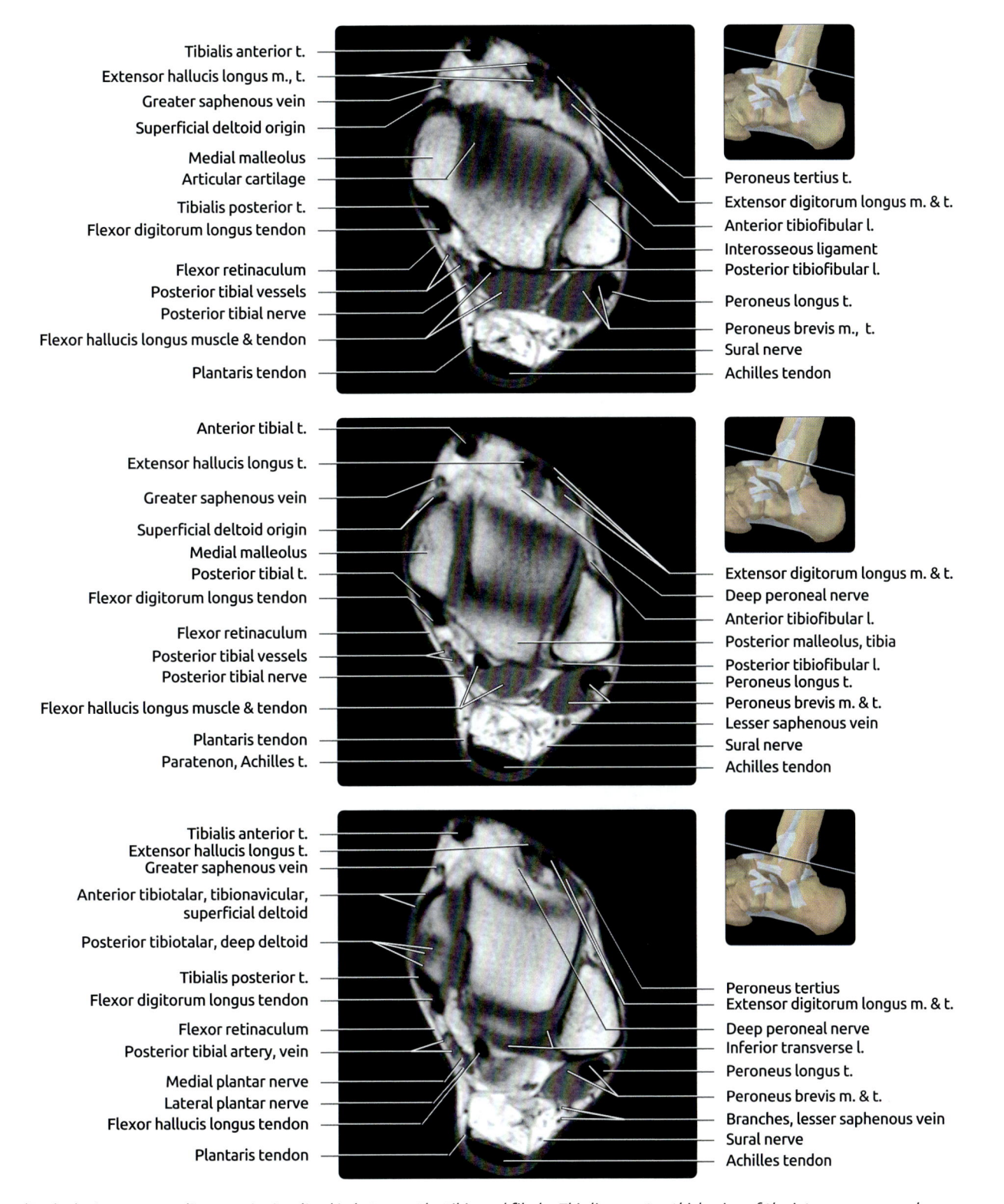

Top image labels (left): Tibialis anterior t.; Extensor hallucis longus m., t.; Greater saphenous vein; Superficial deltoid origin; Medial malleolus; Articular cartilage; Tibialis posterior t.; Flexor digitorum longus tendon; Flexor retinaculum; Posterior tibial vessels; Posterior tibial nerve; Flexor hallucis longus muscle & tendon; Plantaris tendon

Top image labels (right): Peroneus tertius t.; Extensor digitorum longus m. & t.; Anterior tibiofibular l.; Interosseous ligament; Posterior tibiofibular l.; Peroneus longus t.; Peroneus brevis m., t.; Sural nerve; Achilles tendon

Middle image labels (left): Anterior tibial t.; Extensor hallucis longus t.; Greater saphenous vein; Superficial deltoid origin; Medial malleolus; Posterior tibial t.; Flexor digitorum longus tendon; Flexor retinaculum; Posterior tibial vessels; Posterior tibial nerve; Flexor hallucis longus muscle & tendon; Plantaris tendon; Paratenon, Achilles t.

Middle image labels (right): Extensor digitorum longus m. & t.; Deep peroneal nerve; Anterior tibiofibular l.; Posterior malleolus, tibia; Posterior tibiofibular l.; Peroneus longus t.; Peroneus brevis m. & t.; Lesser saphenous vein; Sural nerve; Achilles tendon

Bottom image labels (left): Tibialis anterior t.; Extensor hallucis longus t.; Greater saphenous vein; Anterior tibiotalar, tibionavicular, superficial deltoid; Posterior tibiotalar, deep deltoid; Tibialis posterior t.; Flexor digitorum longus tendon; Flexor retinaculum; Posterior tibial artery, vein; Medial plantar nerve; Lateral plantar nerve; Flexor hallucis longus tendon; Plantaris tendon

Bottom image labels (right): Peroneus tertius; Extensor digitorum longus m. & t.; Deep peroneal nerve; Inferior transverse l.; Peroneus longus t.; Peroneus brevis m. & t.; Branches, lesser saphenous vein; Sural nerve; Achilles tendon

(**Top**) The interosseous ligament is visualized in between the tibia and fibula. This ligament, a thickening of the interosseous membrane, is variable and may be perforated or absent. (**Middle**) The relative position of soft tissue structures posterior to the medial malleolus can be remembered by the mnemonic Tom, Dick and a very nervous Harry. These signify the posterior tibial tendon, the flexor digitorum tenon, artery, vein, nerve and flexor hallucis longus tendon. (**Bottom**) The deep posterior tibiotalar component of the deltoid ligament originates from the posterior colliculus and is typically striated. The inferior transverse ligament, the very inferior aspect of the posterior tibiofibular ligament, extends distal to the tibial posterior surface.

Ankle MR Atlas

AXIAL T1 MR, RIGHT HINDFOOT AXIS

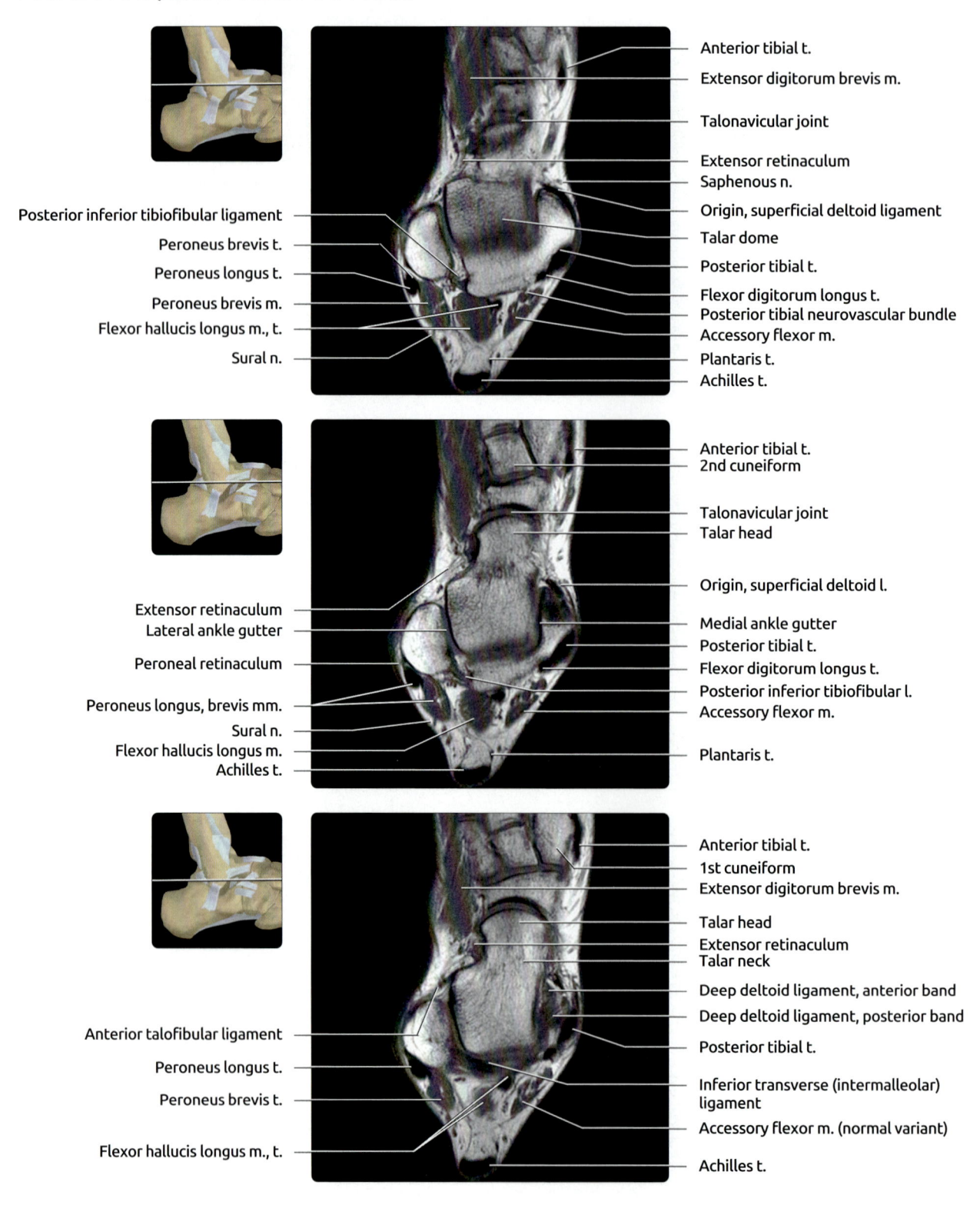

Labels (top image, left side): Posterior inferior tibiofibular ligament; Peroneus brevis t.; Peroneus longus t.; Peroneus brevis m.; Flexor hallucis longus m., t.; Sural n.

Labels (top image, right side): Anterior tibial t.; Extensor digitorum brevis m.; Talonavicular joint; Extensor retinaculum; Saphenous n.; Origin, superficial deltoid ligament; Talar dome; Posterior tibial t.; Flexor digitorum longus t.; Posterior tibial neurovascular bundle; Accessory flexor m.; Plantaris t.; Achilles t.

Labels (middle image, left side): Extensor retinaculum; Lateral ankle gutter; Peroneal retinaculum; Peroneus longus, brevis mm.; Sural n.; Flexor hallucis longus m.; Achilles t.

Labels (middle image, right side): Anterior tibial t.; 2nd cuneiform; Talonavicular joint; Talar head; Origin, superficial deltoid l.; Medial ankle gutter; Posterior tibial t.; Flexor digitorum longus t.; Posterior inferior tibiofibular l.; Accessory flexor m.; Plantaris t.

Labels (bottom image, left side): Anterior talofibular ligament; Peroneus longus t.; Peroneus brevis t.; Flexor hallucis longus m., t.

Labels (bottom image, right side): Anterior tibial t.; 1st cuneiform; Extensor digitorum brevis m.; Talar head; Extensor retinaculum; Talar neck; Deep deltoid ligament, anterior band; Deep deltoid ligament, posterior band; Posterior tibial t.; Inferior transverse (intermalleolar) ligament; Accessory flexor m. (normal variant); Achilles t.

(Top) The axial images from this point inferiorly are angled along the axis of the talus to optimize visualization of hindfoot structures. Note this patient has an accessory flexor muscle. **(Middle)** The malleoli cup the talus creates vertically oriented portions of the ankle joint, which are called the medial and lateral gutters. Both are lined in hyaline cartilage and continuous with the horizontally oriented portion of the joint. **(Bottom)** The deep deltoid ligament has 2 bands. The larger band occupies part of the medial ankle gutter, extending from deep surface of anterior colliculus of medial malleolus to fovea of talus. This band is usually referred to as the deep deltoid ligament, disregarding the anterior band. The small anterior band is variably present; it extends from medial malleolus to talar neck. Anterior talofibular ligament inserts on a squared prominence at the lateral junction of the talar body and neck.

Ankle MR Atlas

AXIAL T1 MR, LEFT HINDFOOT AXIS

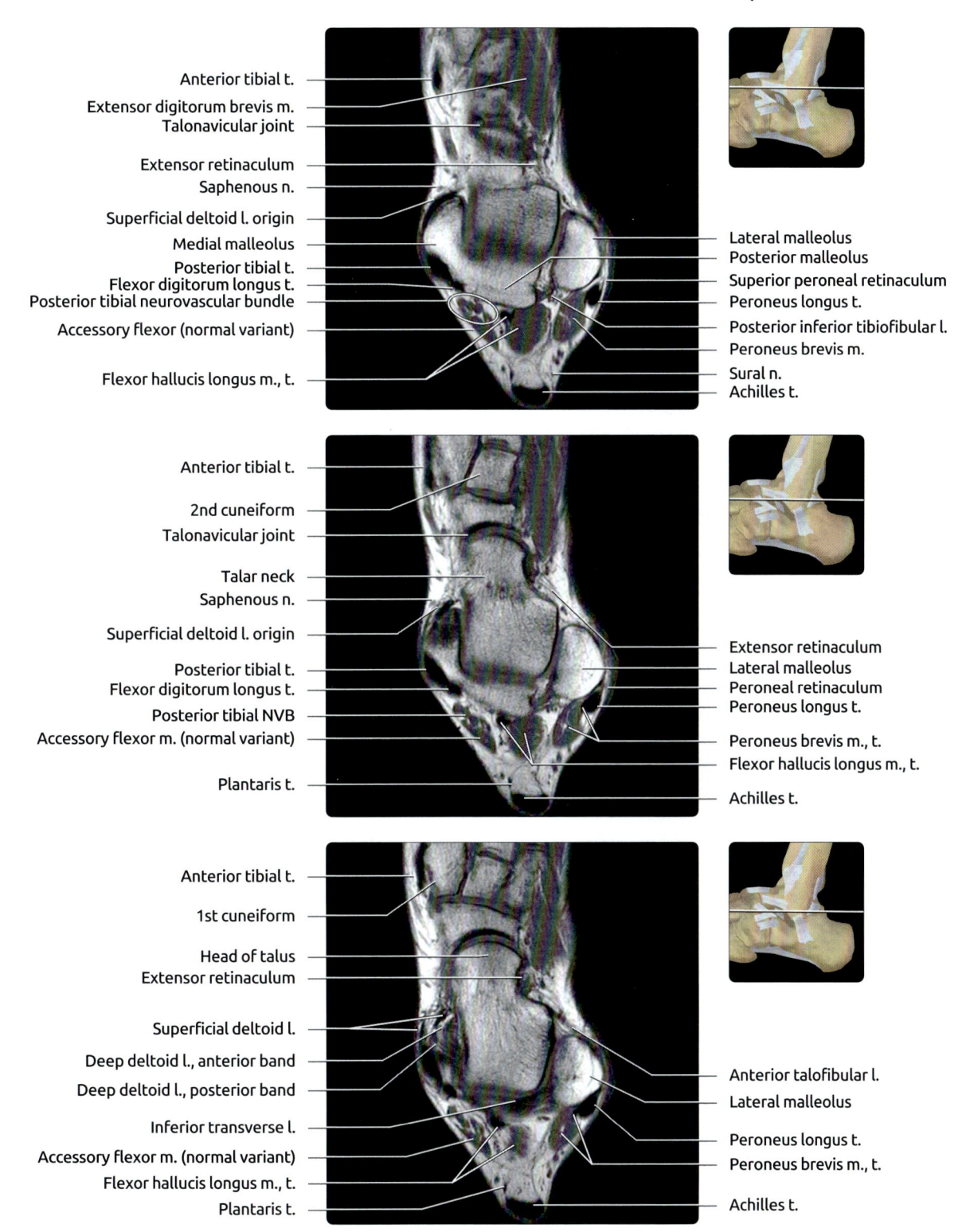

Labels (top image):
- Anterior tibial t.
- Extensor digitorum brevis m.
- Talonavicular joint
- Extensor retinaculum
- Saphenous n.
- Superficial deltoid l. origin
- Medial malleolus
- Posterior tibial t.
- Flexor digitorum longus t.
- Posterior tibial neurovascular bundle
- Accessory flexor (normal variant)
- Flexor hallucis longus m., t.
- Lateral malleolus
- Posterior malleolus
- Superior peroneal retinaculum
- Peroneus longus t.
- Posterior inferior tibiofibular l.
- Peroneus brevis m.
- Sural n.
- Achilles t.

Labels (middle image):
- Anterior tibial t.
- 2nd cuneiform
- Talonavicular joint
- Talar neck
- Saphenous n.
- Superficial deltoid l. origin
- Posterior tibial t.
- Flexor digitorum longus t.
- Posterior tibial NVB
- Accessory flexor m. (normal variant)
- Plantaris t.
- Extensor retinaculum
- Lateral malleolus
- Peroneal retinaculum
- Peroneus longus t.
- Peroneus brevis m., t.
- Flexor hallucis longus m., t.
- Achilles t.

Labels (bottom image):
- Anterior tibial t.
- 1st cuneiform
- Head of talus
- Extensor retinaculum
- Superficial deltoid l.
- Deep deltoid l., anterior band
- Deep deltoid l., posterior band
- Inferior transverse l.
- Accessory flexor m. (normal variant)
- Flexor hallucis longus m., t.
- Plantaris t.
- Anterior talofibular l.
- Lateral malleolus
- Peroneus longus t.
- Peroneus brevis m., t.
- Achilles t.

(**Top**) The axial images from this point inferiorly are angled along the axis of the talus to optimize visualization of hindfoot structures. Note this patient has an accessory flexor muscle. (**Middle**) The malleoli cup the talus creates vertically oriented portions of the ankle joint, which are called the medial and lateral gutters. Both are lined in hyaline cartilage and continuous with the horizontally oriented portion of the joint. (**Bottom**) The deep deltoid ligament has 2 bands. The larger band occupies part of the medial ankle gutter, extending from the deep surface of anterior colliculus of medial malleolus to fovea of talus. This band is usually referred to as the deep deltoid ligament, disregarding the anterior band. The small anterior band is variably present; it extends from medial malleolus to talar neck. Anterior talofibular ligament inserts on a squared prominence at the lateral junction of the talar body and neck.

Ankle MR Atlas

AXIAL T1 MR, RIGHT HINDFOOT AXIS

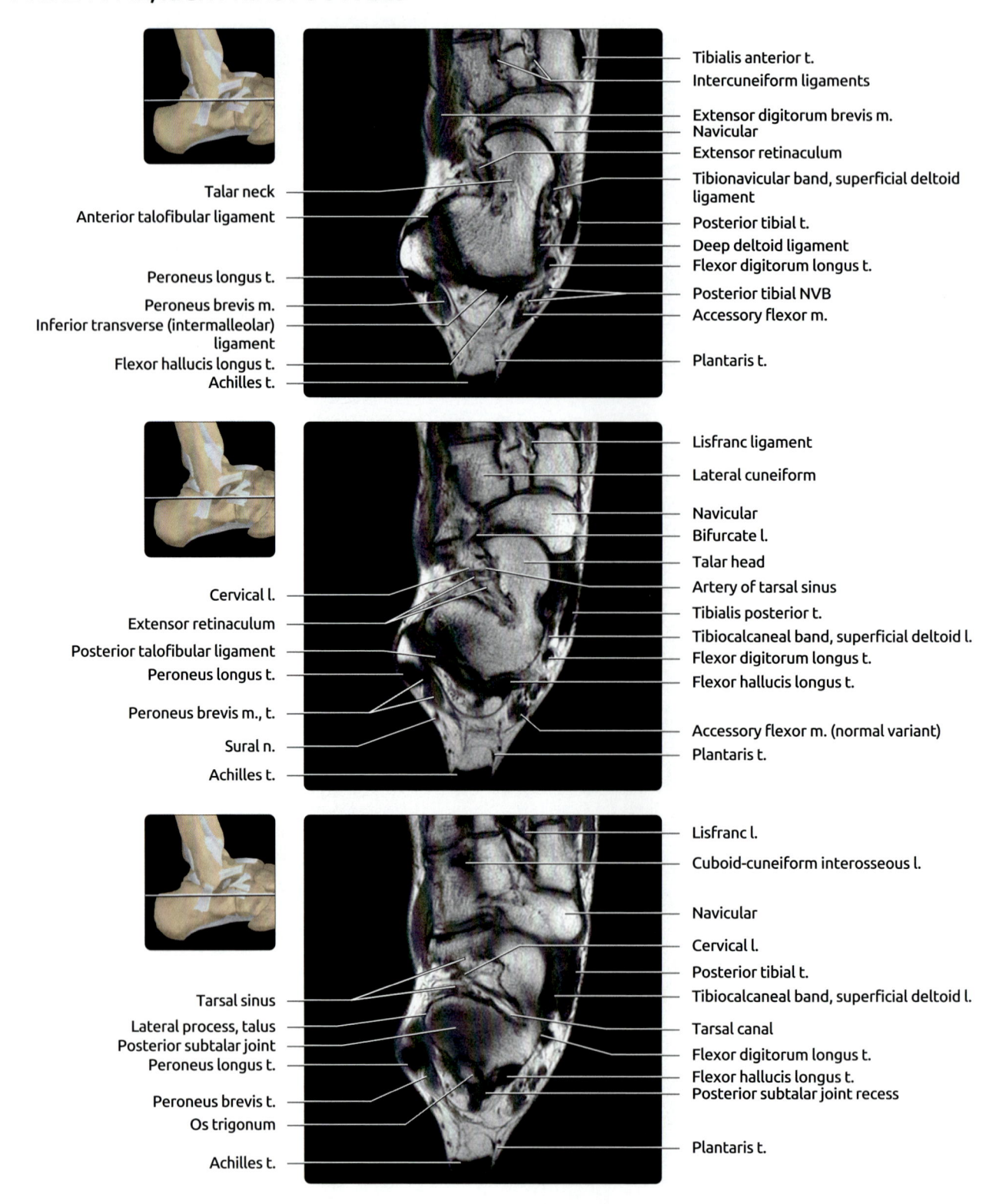

Top image labels (left): Talar neck; Anterior talofibular ligament; Peroneus longus t.; Peroneus brevis m.; Inferior transverse (intermalleolar) ligament; Flexor hallucis longus t.; Achilles t.

Top image labels (right): Tibialis anterior t.; Intercuneiform ligaments; Extensor digitorum brevis m.; Navicular; Extensor retinaculum; Tibionavicular band, superficial deltoid ligament; Posterior tibial t.; Deep deltoid ligament; Flexor digitorum longus t.; Posterior tibial NVB; Accessory flexor m.; Plantaris t.

Middle image labels (left): Cervical l.; Extensor retinaculum; Posterior talofibular ligament; Peroneus longus t.; Peroneus brevis m., t.; Sural n.; Achilles t.

Middle image labels (right): Lisfranc ligament; Lateral cuneiform; Navicular; Bifurcate l.; Talar head; Artery of tarsal sinus; Tibialis posterior t.; Tibiocalcaneal band, superficial deltoid l.; Flexor digitorum longus t.; Flexor hallucis longus t.; Accessory flexor m. (normal variant); Plantaris t.

Bottom image labels (left): Tarsal sinus; Lateral process, talus; Posterior subtalar joint; Peroneus longus t.; Peroneus brevis t.; Os trigonum; Achilles t.

Bottom image labels (right): Lisfranc l.; Cuboid-cuneiform interosseous l.; Navicular; Cervical l.; Posterior tibial t.; Tibiocalcaneal band, superficial deltoid l.; Tarsal canal; Flexor digitorum longus t.; Flexor hallucis longus t.; Posterior subtalar joint recess; Plantaris t.

(**Top**) Inferior transverse ligament, also known as intermalleolar ligament, extends from the posterior surface of medial malleolus to tip of fibula and courses posterior to the talar body. (**Middle**) The extensor retinaculum has 3 bands: Lateral, middle, and medial. They traverse the tarsal sinus and insert on the dorsal surface of the calcaneus, posterior to the cervical l. (**Bottom**) The funnel shape of the tarsal sinus is well seen on this image. It lies between the talus and calcaneus, lateral to the sustentaculum tali. It is primarily filled with fat, through which pass ligaments and the artery of the tarsal sinus. Posteromedially it flows into a narrow space, the tarsal canal, which contains the tibiocalcaneal interosseous ligament.

Ankle MR Atlas

AXIAL T1 MR, LEFT HINDFOOT AXIS

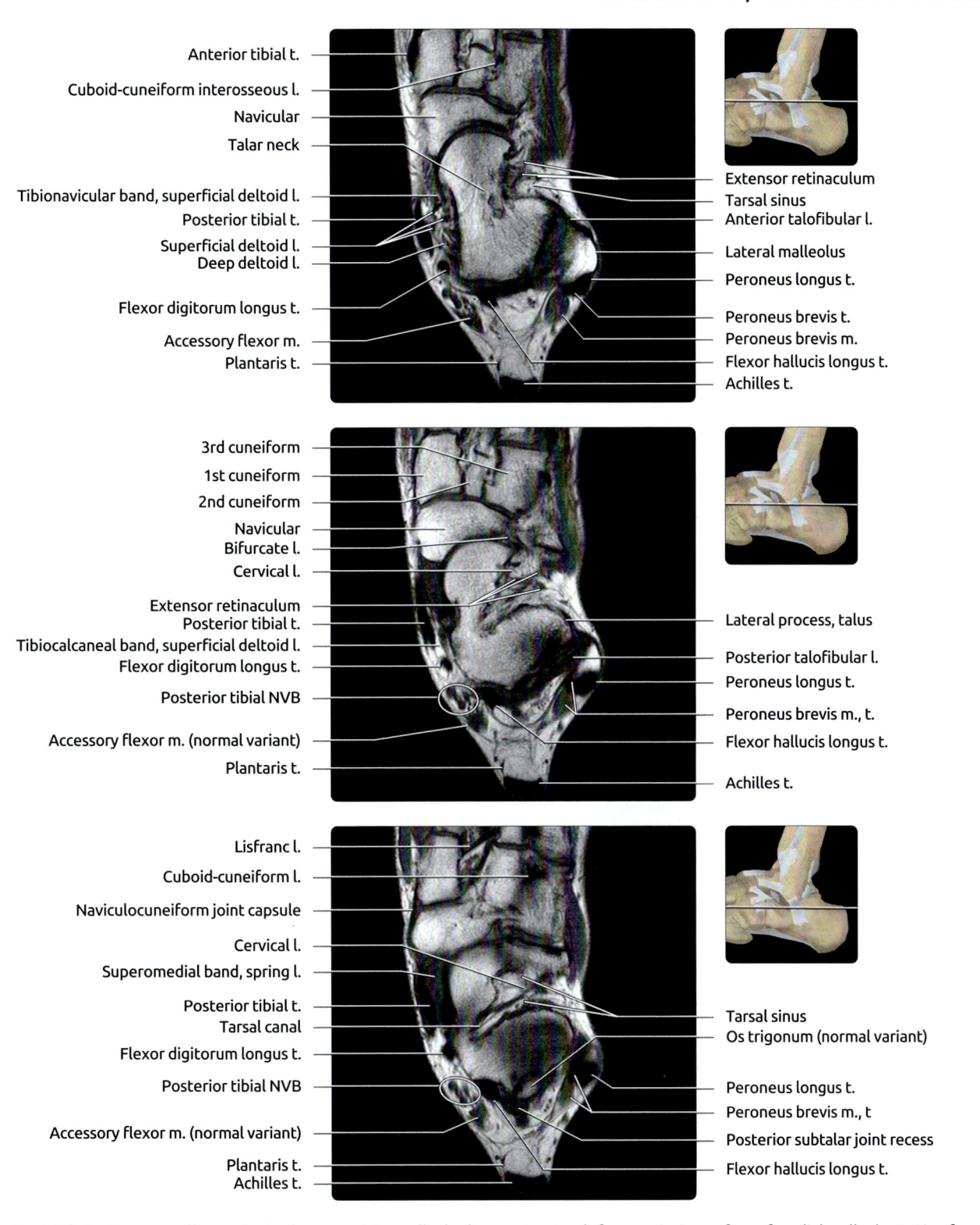

Labels (top image):
- Anterior tibial t.
- Cuboid-cuneiform interosseous l.
- Navicular
- Talar neck
- Tibionavicular band, superficial deltoid l.
- Posterior tibial t.
- Superficial deltoid l.
- Deep deltoid l.
- Flexor digitorum longus t.
- Accessory flexor m.
- Plantaris t.
- Extensor retinaculum
- Tarsal sinus
- Anterior talofibular l.
- Lateral malleolus
- Peroneus longus t.
- Peroneus brevis t.
- Peroneus brevis m.
- Flexor hallucis longus t.
- Achilles t.

Labels (middle image):
- 3rd cuneiform
- 1st cuneiform
- 2nd cuneiform
- Navicular
- Bifurcate l.
- Cervical l.
- Extensor retinaculum
- Posterior tibial t.
- Tibiocalcaneal band, superficial deltoid l.
- Flexor digitorum longus t.
- Posterior tibial NVB
- Accessory flexor m. (normal variant)
- Plantaris t.
- Lateral process, talus
- Posterior talofibular l.
- Peroneus longus t.
- Peroneus brevis m., t.
- Flexor hallucis longus t.
- Achilles t.

Labels (bottom image):
- Lisfranc l.
- Cuboid-cuneiform l.
- Naviculocuneiform joint capsule
- Cervical l.
- Superomedial band, spring l.
- Posterior tibial t.
- Tarsal canal
- Flexor digitorum longus t.
- Posterior tibial NVB
- Accessory flexor m. (normal variant)
- Plantaris t.
- Achilles t.
- Tarsal sinus
- Os trigonum (normal variant)
- Peroneus longus t.
- Peroneus brevis m., t
- Posterior subtalar joint recess
- Flexor hallucis longus t.

(**Top**) *Inferior transverse ligament, also known as intermalleolar ligament, extends from posterior surface of medial malleolus to tip of fibula and courses posterior to the talar body.* (**Middle**) *The extensor retinaculum has 3 bands: Lateral, middle, and medial. They traverse the tarsal sinus and insert on the dorsal surface of the calcaneus, posterior to the cervical l.* (**Bottom**) *The funnel shape of the tarsal sinus is well seen on this image. It lies between the talus and calcaneus, lateral to the sustentaculum tali. It is primarily filled with fat, through which pass ligaments and the artery of the tarsal sinus. Posteromedially it flows into a narrow space, the tarsal canal, which contains the tibiocalcaneal interosseous ligament.*

Ankle MR Atlas

AXIAL T1 MR, RIGHT HINDFOOT AXIS

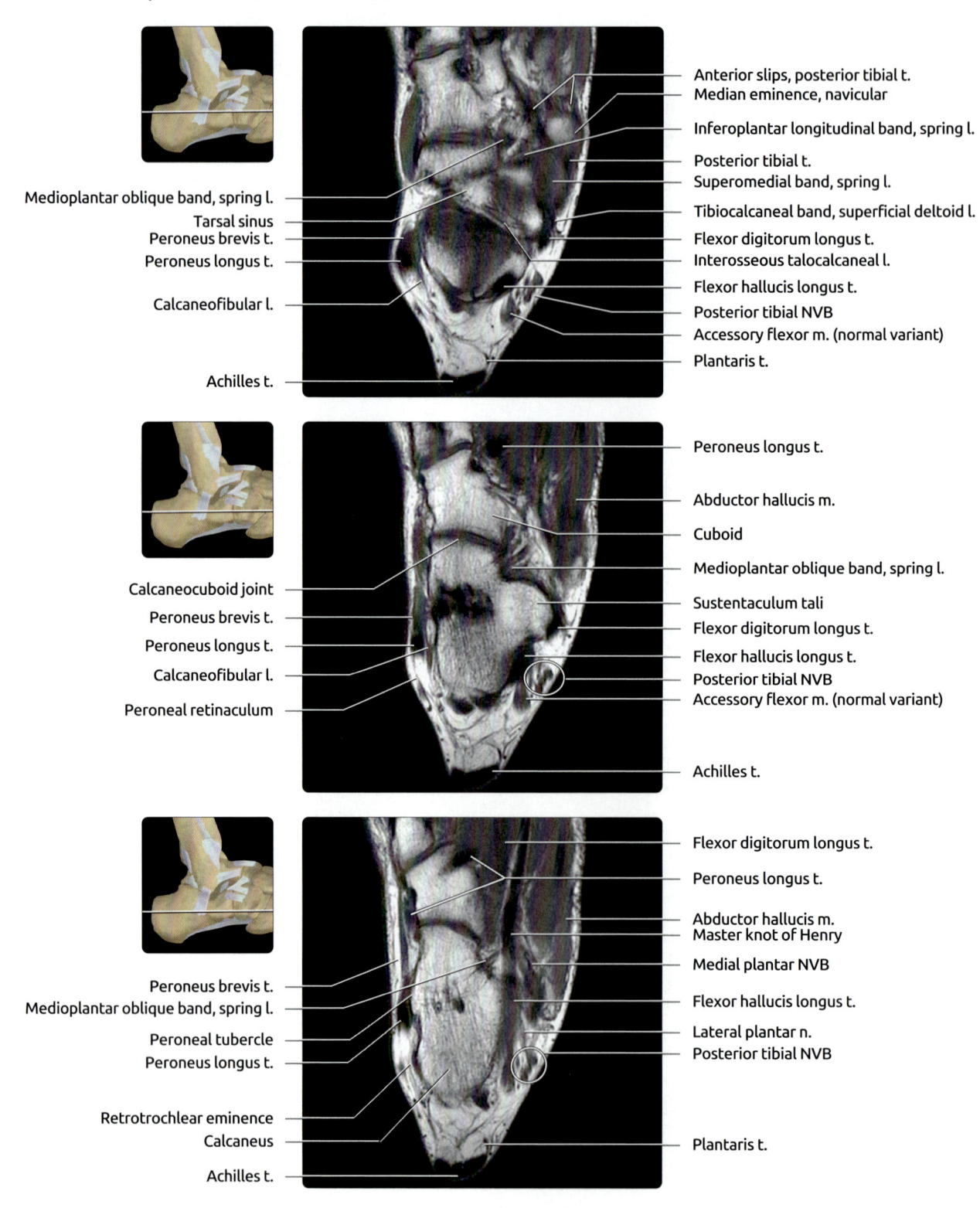

Top image labels (left): Medioplantar oblique band, spring l.; Tarsal sinus; Peroneus brevis t.; Peroneus longus t.; Calcaneofibular l.; Achilles t.

Top image labels (right): Anterior slips, posterior tibial t.; Median eminence, navicular; Inferoplantar longitudinal band, spring l.; Posterior tibial t.; Superomedial band, spring l.; Tibiocalcaneal band, superficial deltoid l.; Flexor digitorum longus t.; Interosseous talocalcaneal l.; Flexor hallucis longus t.; Posterior tibial NVB; Accessory flexor m. (normal variant); Plantaris t.

Middle image labels (left): Calcaneocuboid joint; Peroneus brevis t.; Peroneus longus t.; Calcaneofibular l.; Peroneal retinaculum

Middle image labels (right): Peroneus longus t.; Abductor hallucis m.; Cuboid; Medioplantar oblique band, spring l.; Sustentaculum tali; Flexor digitorum longus t.; Flexor hallucis longus t.; Posterior tibial NVB; Accessory flexor m. (normal variant); Achilles t.

Bottom image labels (left): Peroneus brevis t.; Medioplantar oblique band, spring l.; Peroneal tubercle; Peroneus longus t.; Retrotrochlear eminence; Calcaneus; Achilles t.

Bottom image labels (right): Flexor digitorum longus t.; Peroneus longus t.; Abductor hallucis m.; Master knot of Henry; Medial plantar NVB; Flexor hallucis longus t.; Lateral plantar n.; Posterior tibial NVB; Plantaris t.

(Top) Medioplantar oblique band of spring ligament arises from the coronoid fossa, a portion of the calcaneus just anterior to the sustentaculum tali. (Middle) On this image, the patient's normal variant accessory flexor m. is seen inserting on the flexor hallucis longus t., and so it can be designated as an accessory flexor hallucis longus. Accessory flexor muscles are fairly common, and they can be named according to the muscle they most closely follow or according to their site of insertion. The important points are to recognize them as normal muscles rather than masses and to realize they may result in ankle impingement or even exertional compartment syndromes. (Bottom) The tibial nerve divides in the tarsal tunnel, giving rise to calcaneal branches as well as medial and lateral plantar branches. The lateral plantar n. moves laterally and inferiorly as it extends to the lateral side of the foot. Baxter nerve is its 1st branch, innervating the abductor digiti minimi.

Ankle MR Atlas

AXIAL T1 MR, LEFT HINDFOOT AXIS

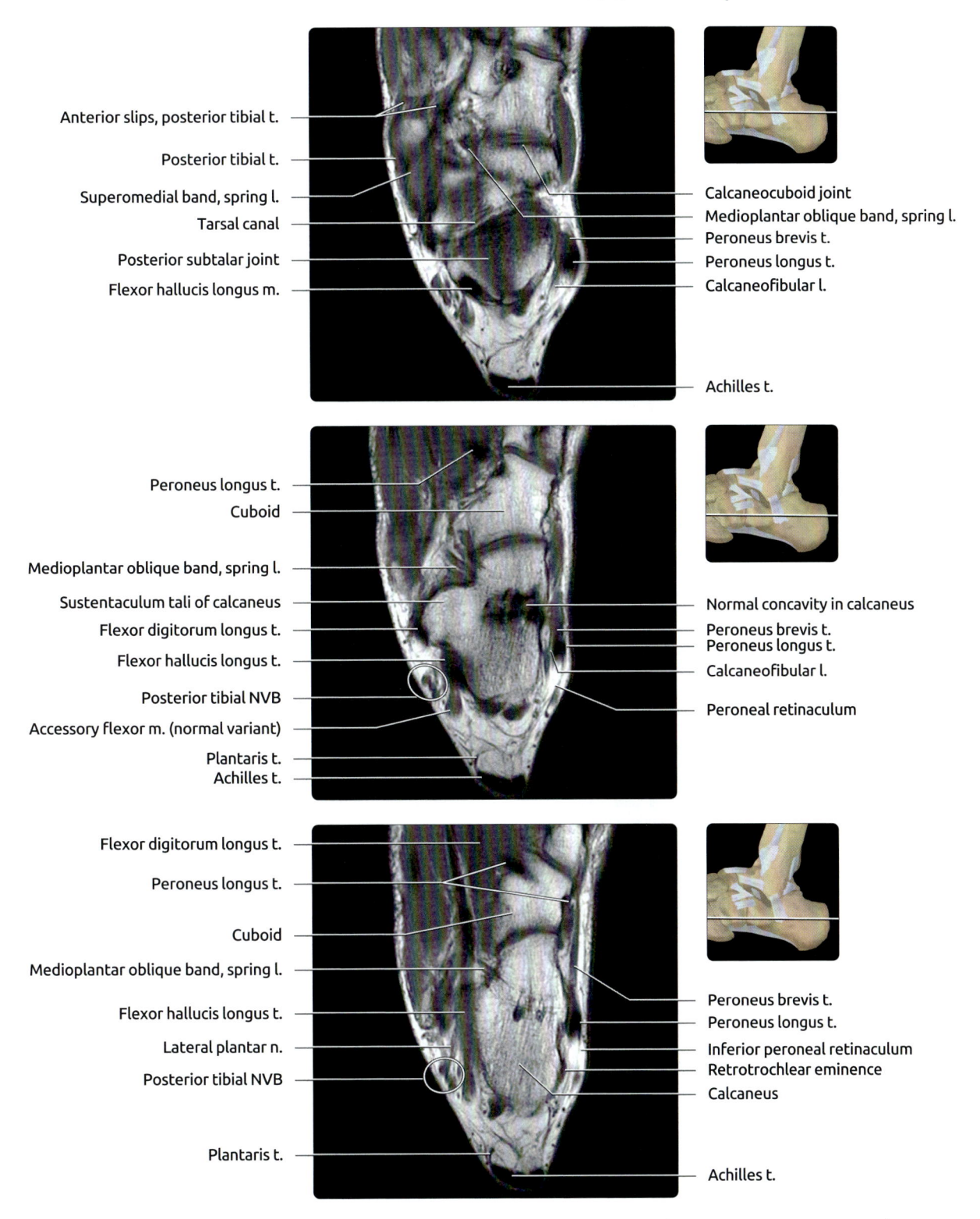

Labels (top image):
- Anterior slips, posterior tibial t.
- Posterior tibial t.
- Superomedial band, spring l.
- Tarsal canal
- Posterior subtalar joint
- Flexor hallucis longus m.
- Calcaneocuboid joint
- Medioplantar oblique band, spring l.
- Peroneus brevis t.
- Peroneus longus t.
- Calcaneofibular l.
- Achilles t.

Labels (middle image):
- Peroneus longus t.
- Cuboid
- Medioplantar oblique band, spring l.
- Sustentaculum tali of calcaneus
- Flexor digitorum longus t.
- Flexor hallucis longus t.
- Posterior tibial NVB
- Accessory flexor m. (normal variant)
- Plantaris t.
- Achilles t.
- Normal concavity in calcaneus
- Peroneus brevis t.
- Peroneus longus t.
- Calcaneofibular l.
- Peroneal retinaculum

Labels (bottom image):
- Flexor digitorum longus t.
- Peroneus longus t.
- Cuboid
- Medioplantar oblique band, spring l.
- Flexor hallucis longus t.
- Lateral plantar n.
- Posterior tibial NVB
- Plantaris t.
- Peroneus brevis t.
- Peroneus longus t.
- Inferior peroneal retinaculum
- Retrotrochlear eminence
- Calcaneus
- Achilles t.

(Top) Medioplantar oblique band of spring ligament arises from the coronoid fossa, a portion of the calcaneus just anterior to the sustentaculum tali. (Middle) On this image, the patient's normal variant accessory flexor m. is seen inserting on the flexor hallucis longus t., and so it can be designated as an accessory flexor hallucis longus. Accessory flexor muscles are fairly common, and they can be named according to the muscle they most closely follow or according to their site of insertion. The important points are to recognize them as normal muscles rather than masses and to realize they may result in ankle impingement or even exertional compartment syndromes. (Bottom) The tibial nerve divides in the tarsal tunnel, giving rise to calcaneal branches as well as medial and lateral plantar branches. The lateral plantar n. moves laterally and inferiorly as it extends to the lateral side of the foot. Baxter nerve is its 1st branch, innervating the abductor digiti minimi.

Ankle MR Atlas

AXIAL T1 MR, RIGHT HINDFOOT AXIS

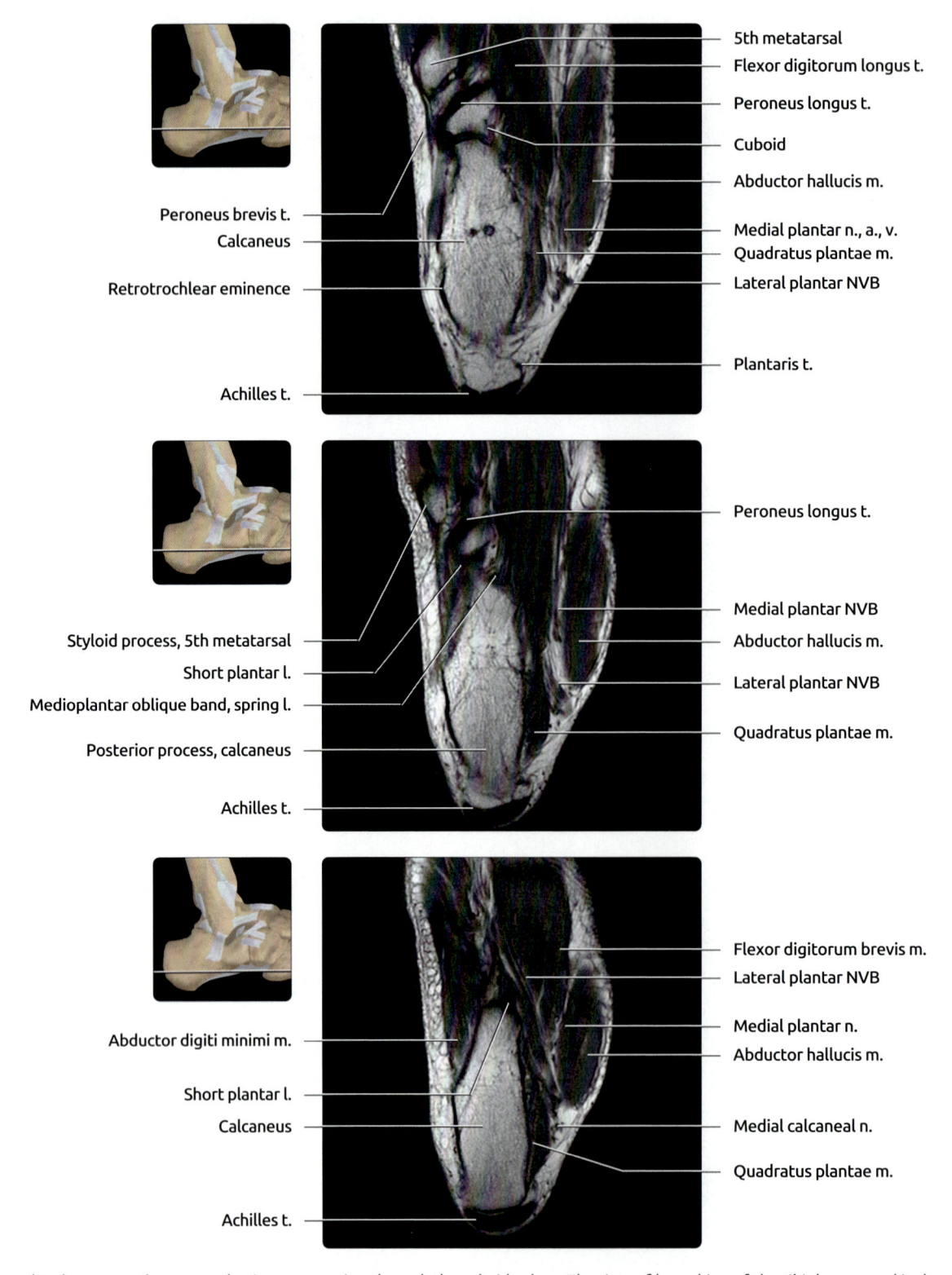

Labels (top image):
- 5th metatarsal
- Flexor digitorum longus t.
- Peroneus longus t.
- Cuboid
- Abductor hallucis m.
- Peroneus brevis t.
- Calcaneus
- Medial plantar n., a., v.
- Quadratus plantae m.
- Retrotrochlear eminence
- Lateral plantar NVB
- Plantaris t.
- Achilles t.

Labels (middle image):
- Peroneus longus t.
- Medial plantar NVB
- Abductor hallucis m.
- Styloid process, 5th metatarsal
- Lateral plantar NVB
- Short plantar l.
- Medioplantar oblique band, spring l.
- Quadratus plantae m.
- Posterior process, calcaneus
- Achilles t.

Labels (bottom image):
- Flexor digitorum brevis m.
- Lateral plantar NVB
- Medial plantar n.
- Abductor digiti minimi m.
- Abductor hallucis m.
- Short plantar l.
- Medial calcaneal n.
- Calcaneus
- Quadratus plantae m.
- Achilles t.

(**Top**) *Peroneus longus tendon is seen coursing through the cuboid sulcus. The sites of branching of the tibial nerve and its branches are fairly variable. Quadratus plantae muscle inserts on flexor digitorum longus tendon, and lumbrical muscles originates on the tendon.* (**Middle**) *The short plantar ligament, also known as the plantar calcaneocuboid ligament, ends at the proximal margin of the cuboid. The long plantar ligament, superficial to it, forms the floor of the cuboid tunnel in which the peroneus longus tendon lies. It is best seen on sagittal images. The roof of the tunnel is the cuboid sulcus.* (**Bottom**) *The lateral plantar nerve lies between the quadratus plantae and flexor digitorum brevis muscles. It divides into deep and superficial branches. The medial plantar nerve lies between the abductor hallucis and flexor digitorum brevis muscles.*

Ankle MR Atlas

AXIAL T1 MR, LEFT HINDFOOT AXIS

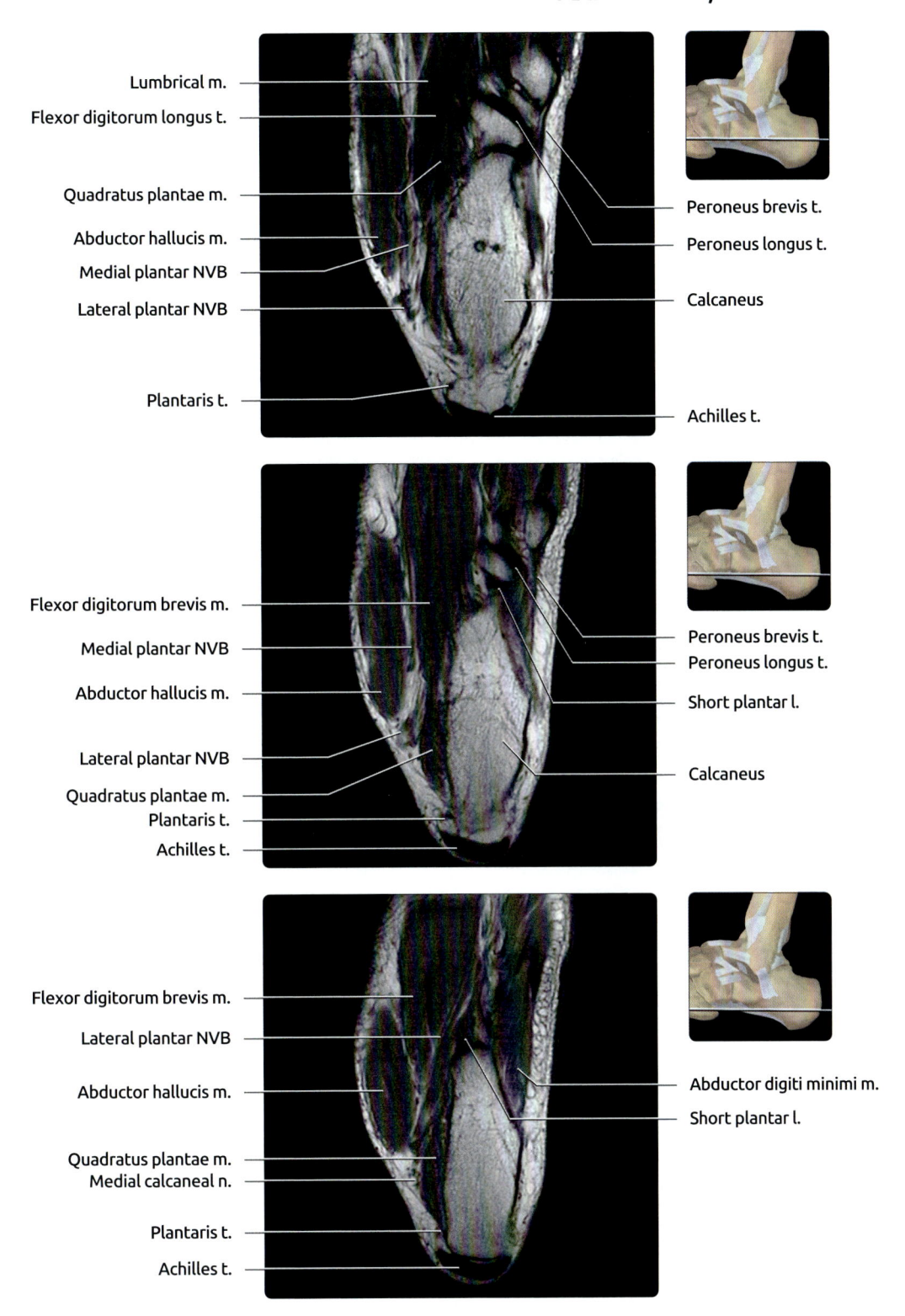

(Top) Peroneus longus tendon is seen coursing through the cuboid sulcus. The sites of branching of the tibial nerve and its branches are fairly variable. Quadratus plantae muscle inserts on flexor digitorum longus tendon, and lumbrical muscles originates on the tendon. (Middle) The short plantar ligament, also known as the plantar calcaneocuboid ligament, ends at the proximal margin of the cuboid. The long plantar ligament, superficial to it, forms the floor of the cuboid tunnel in which the peroneus longus tendon lies. It is best seen on sagittal images. The roof of the tunnel is the cuboid sulcus. (Bottom) The lateral plantar nerve lies between the quadratus plantae and flexor digitorum brevis muscles. It divides into deep and superficial branches. The medial plantar nerve lies between the abductor hallucis and flexor digitorum brevis muscles.

Ankle MR Atlas

CORONAL T1 MR, RIGHT ANKLE

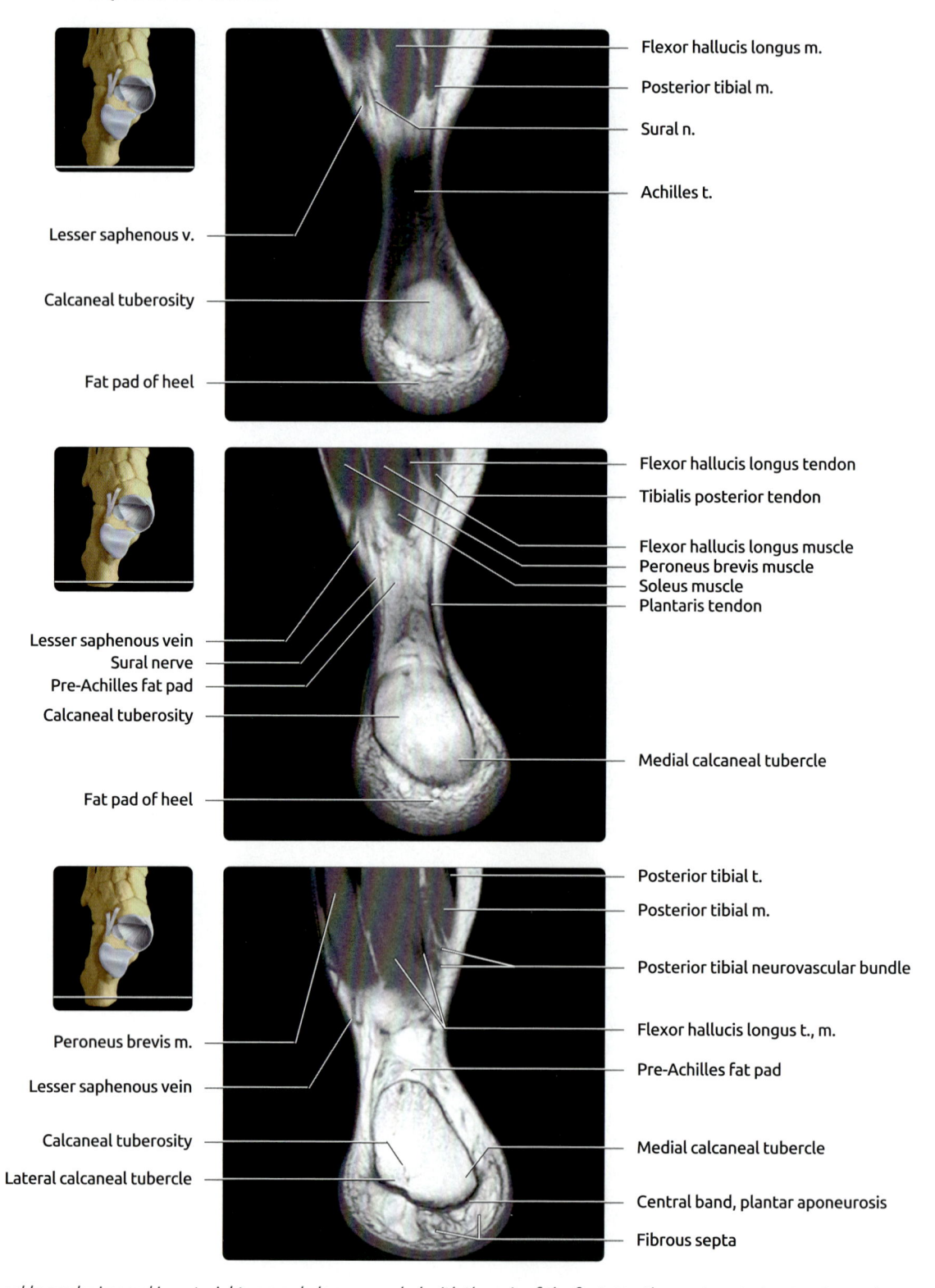

Flexor hallucis longus m.
Posterior tibial m.
Sural n.
Achilles t.

Lesser saphenous v.
Calcaneal tuberosity
Fat pad of heel

Flexor hallucis longus tendon
Tibialis posterior tendon
Flexor hallucis longus muscle
Peroneus brevis muscle
Soleus muscle
Plantaris tendon

Lesser saphenous vein
Sural nerve
Pre-Achilles fat pad
Calcaneal tuberosity

Medial calcaneal tubercle

Fat pad of heel

Posterior tibial t.
Posterior tibial m.
Posterior tibial neurovascular bundle
Flexor hallucis longus t., m.
Pre-Achilles fat pad

Peroneus brevis m.
Lesser saphenous vein
Calcaneal tuberosity
Lateral calcaneal tubercle

Medial calcaneal tubercle
Central band, plantar aponeurosis
Fibrous septa

(Top) The ankle can be imaged in a straight coronal plane or angled with the axis of the foot. For the most posterior structures, the straight coronal is optimal, as shown here. More anterior images in this series will be angled perpendicular to the talus, as shown on accompanying scout images. This improves visualization of the subtalar joint and other hindfoot structures. (Middle) The Achilles tendon is the largest tendon in the body. It inserts into the posterior margin of the calcaneal tuberosity slightly below its superior apex. The plantaris tendon runs along the medial margin of the Achilles tendon, and inserts separately along the medial border of the calcaneus. (Bottom) The flexor hallucis longus muscle is broad and remains muscular more distally than the other muscles of the posterior compartment of the leg; it may be seen down to the ankle joint. The peroneus brevis muscle also descends down to the ankle joint whereas the peroneus longus muscle is no longer visualized at that level.

Ankle MR Atlas

CORONAL T1 MR, LEFT ANKLE

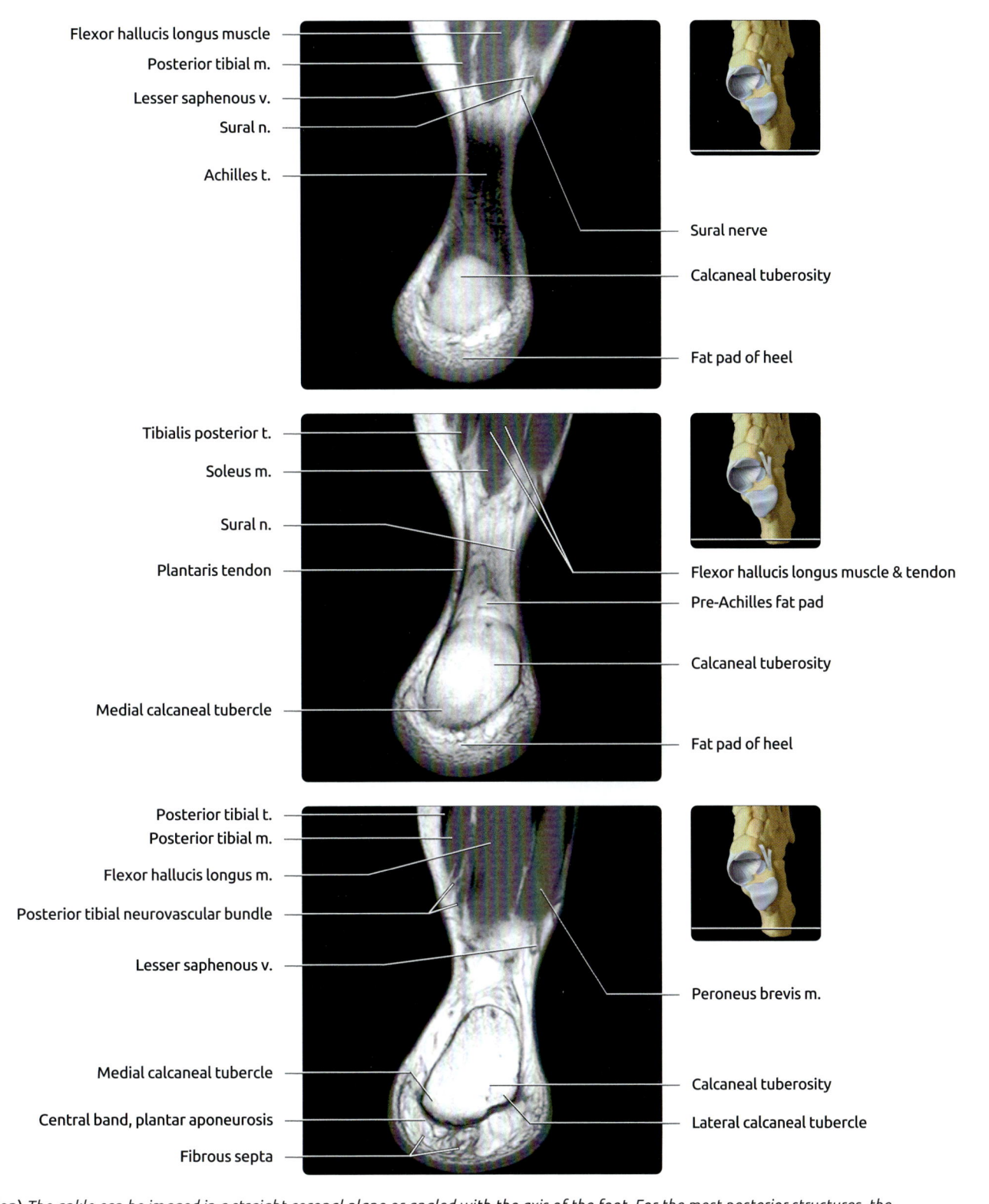

(Top) The ankle can be imaged in a straight coronal plane or angled with the axis of the foot. For the most posterior structures, the straight coronal is optimal, as shown here. More anterior images in this series will be angled perpendicular to the talus, as shown on accompanying scout images. This improves visualization of the subtalar joint and other hindfoot structures. **(Middle)** The Achilles tendon is the largest tendon in the body. It inserts into the posterior margin of the calcaneal tuberosity slightly below its superior apex. The plantaris tendon runs along the medial margin of the Achilles tendon, and inserts separately along the medial border of the calcaneus. **(Bottom)** The flexor hallucis longus muscle is broad and remains muscular more distally than the other muscles of the posterior compartment of the leg; it may be seen down to the ankle joint. The peroneus brevis muscle also descends down to the ankle joint whereas the peroneus longus muscle is no longer visualized at that level.

Ankle MR Atlas

CORONAL T1 MR, RIGHT ANKLE

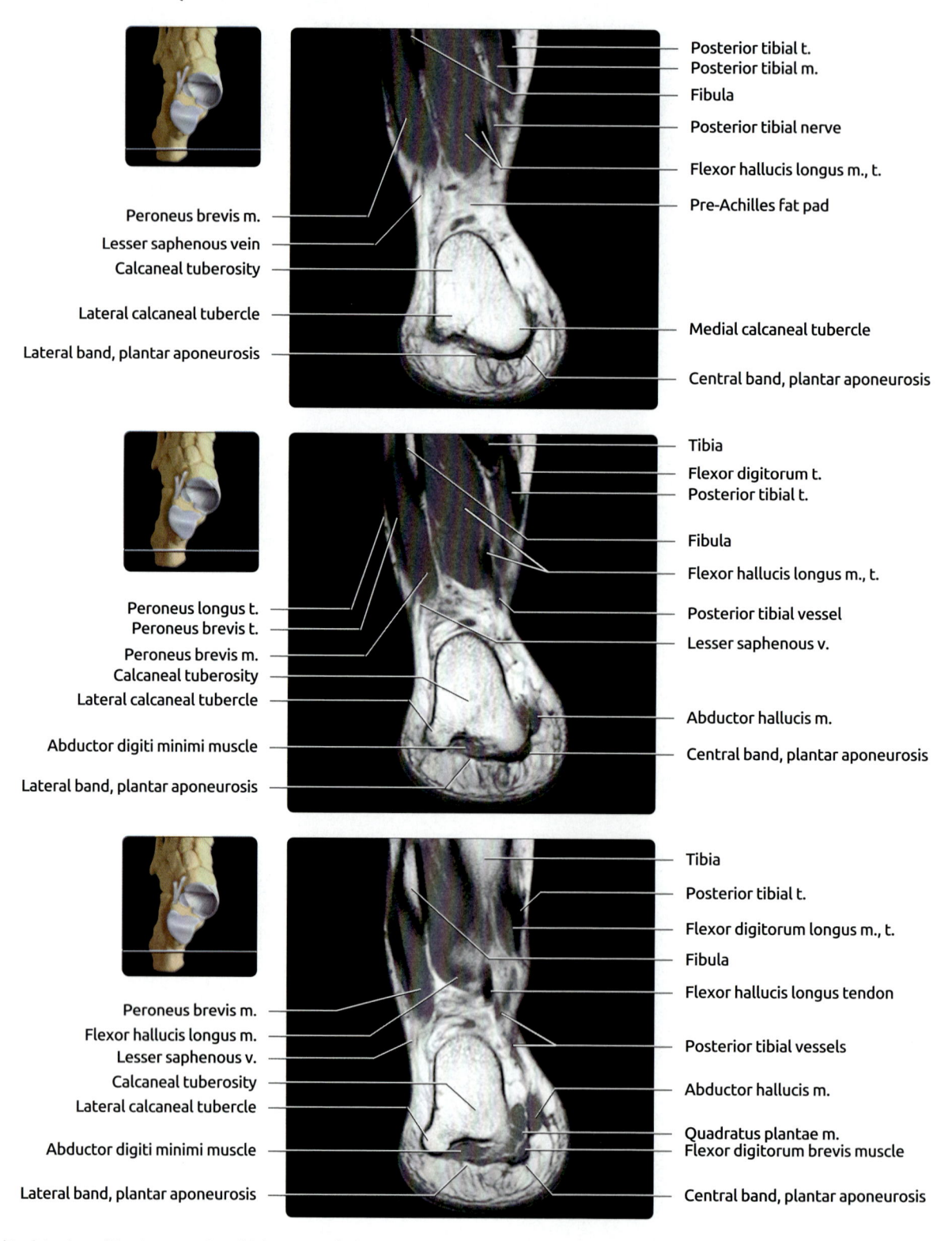

Top image labels (left): Peroneus brevis m.; Lesser saphenous vein; Calcaneal tuberosity; Lateral calcaneal tubercle; Lateral band, plantar aponeurosis

Top image labels (right): Posterior tibial t.; Posterior tibial m.; Fibula; Posterior tibial nerve; Flexor hallucis longus m., t.; Pre-Achilles fat pad; Medial calcaneal tubercle; Central band, plantar aponeurosis

Middle image labels (left): Peroneus longus t.; Peroneus brevis t.; Peroneus brevis m.; Calcaneal tuberosity; Lateral calcaneal tubercle; Abductor digiti minimi muscle; Lateral band, plantar aponeurosis

Middle image labels (right): Tibia; Flexor digitorum t.; Posterior tibial t.; Fibula; Flexor hallucis longus m., t.; Posterior tibial vessel; Lesser saphenous v.; Abductor hallucis m.; Central band, plantar aponeurosis

Bottom image labels (left): Peroneus brevis m.; Flexor hallucis longus m.; Lesser saphenous v.; Calcaneal tuberosity; Lateral calcaneal tubercle; Abductor digiti minimi muscle; Lateral band, plantar aponeurosis

Bottom image labels (right): Tibia; Posterior tibial t.; Flexor digitorum longus m., t.; Fibula; Flexor hallucis longus tendon; Posterior tibial vessels; Abductor hallucis m.; Quadratus plantae m.; Flexor digitorum brevis muscle; Central band, plantar aponeurosis

(**Top**) In the ankle, the posterior tibial nerve and its accompanying vessels descend within a fat plane between the flexor digitorum longus and flexor hallucis longus. The nerve is lateral to the artery and veins. (**Middle**) The medial and lateral tubercles of the calcaneus give origin to the 1st layer of intrinsic muscles of the foot & to the plantar aponeurosis. The abductor digiti minimi muscle originates from the lateral tubercle & the flexor digitorum brevis; abductor hallucis & abductor digiti minimi muscles originate from the medial tubercle. (**Bottom**) The plantar fascia (aponeurosis) is now coming into view. It has 3 proximal parts: A strong, broad, and thick central band covering the flexor digitorum brevis muscle, a lateral band covering the abductor digiti minimi and a thin band covering the abductor hallucis muscle, and continuous with the flexor retinaculum.

Ankle MR Atlas

CORONAL T1 MR, LEFT ANKLE

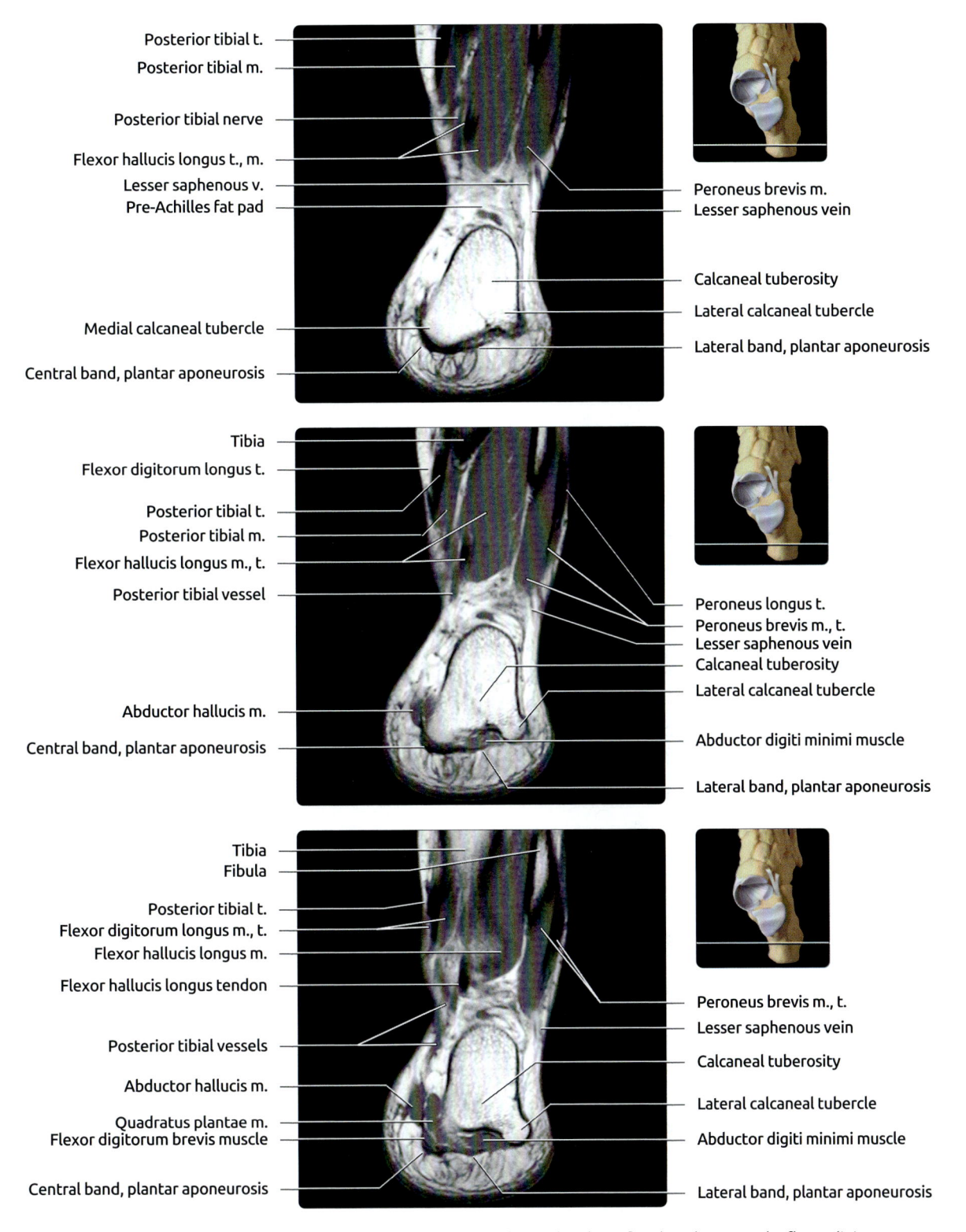

Top image labels (left): Posterior tibial t.; Posterior tibial m.; Posterior tibial nerve; Flexor hallucis longus t., m.; Lesser saphenous v.; Pre-Achilles fat pad; Medial calcaneal tubercle; Central band, plantar aponeurosis

Top image labels (right): Peroneus brevis m.; Lesser saphenous vein; Calcaneal tuberosity; Lateral calcaneal tubercle; Lateral band, plantar aponeurosis

Middle image labels (left): Tibia; Flexor digitorum longus t.; Posterior tibial t.; Posterior tibial m.; Flexor hallucis longus m., t.; Posterior tibial vessel; Abductor hallucis m.; Central band, plantar aponeurosis

Middle image labels (right): Peroneus longus t.; Peroneus brevis m., t.; Lesser saphenous vein; Calcaneal tuberosity; Lateral calcaneal tubercle; Abductor digiti minimi muscle; Lateral band, plantar aponeurosis

Bottom image labels (left): Tibia; Fibula; Posterior tibial t.; Flexor digitorum longus m., t.; Flexor hallucis longus m.; Flexor hallucis longus tendon; Posterior tibial vessels; Abductor hallucis m.; Quadratus plantae m.; Flexor digitorum brevis muscle; Central band, plantar aponeurosis

Bottom image labels (right): Peroneus brevis m., t.; Lesser saphenous vein; Calcaneal tuberosity; Lateral calcaneal tubercle; Abductor digiti minimi muscle; Lateral band, plantar aponeurosis

(**Top**) *In the ankle, the posterior tibial nerve and its accompanying vessels descend within a fat plane between the flexor digitorum longus and flexor hallucis longus muscles. The nerve is lateral to the artery and veins.* (**Middle**) *The medial and lateral tubercles of the calcaneus give origin to the 1st layer of intrinsic muscles of the foot and to the plantar aponeurosis. The abductor digiti minimi muscle originates from the lateral tubercle and the flexor digitorum brevis; abductor hallucis and abductor digiti minimi muscles originate from the medial tubercle.* (**Bottom**) *The plantar fascia (aponeurosis) is now coming into view. It has 3 bands: A strong, broad, and thick central band covering the flexor digitorum brevis muscle, a lateral band covering the abductor digiti minimi, and a thin band covering the abductor hallucis muscle, and continuous with the flexor retinaculum.*

Ankle MR Atlas

CORONAL T1 MR, RIGHT ANKLE

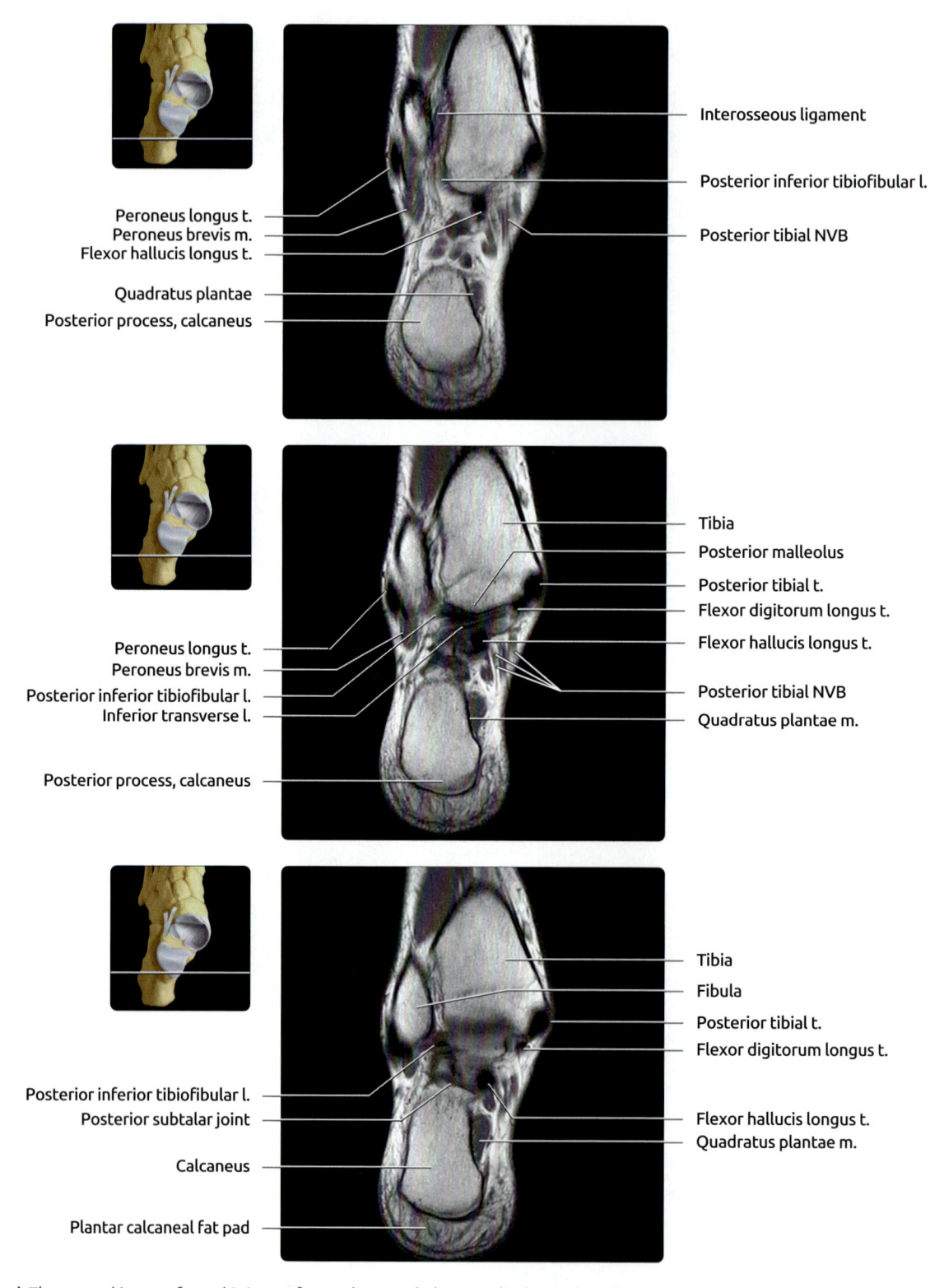

Peroneus longus t.
Peroneus brevis m.
Flexor hallucis longus t.
Quadratus plantae
Posterior process, calcaneus

Interosseous ligament
Posterior inferior tibiofibular l.
Posterior tibial NVB

Peroneus longus t.
Peroneus brevis m.
Posterior inferior tibiofibular l.
Inferior transverse l.
Posterior process, calcaneus

Tibia
Posterior malleolus
Posterior tibial t.
Flexor digitorum longus t.
Flexor hallucis longus t.
Posterior tibial NVB
Quadratus plantae m.

Posterior inferior tibiofibular l.
Posterior subtalar joint
Calcaneus
Plantar calcaneal fat pad

Tibia
Fibula
Posterior tibial t.
Flexor digitorum longus t.
Flexor hallucis longus t.
Quadratus plantae m.

(**Top**) The coronal images from this image forward are angled perpendicular to the talus, which improves visualization of hindfoot structures. For that reason, the calcaneus is seen at a more posterior portion than on the previous images. (**Middle**) The posterior inferior tibiofibular ligament originates from the posterior malleolus and inserts into the fibula above the malleolar fossa. The inferior transverse ligament extends distal to the tibial posterior surface and inserts quite far medially close to the medial malleolus. (**Bottom**) The posterior subtalar joint is broad and curved. Inversion, eversion, and gliding motion occur at this joint.

Ankle MR Atlas

CORONAL T1 MR, LEFT ANKLE

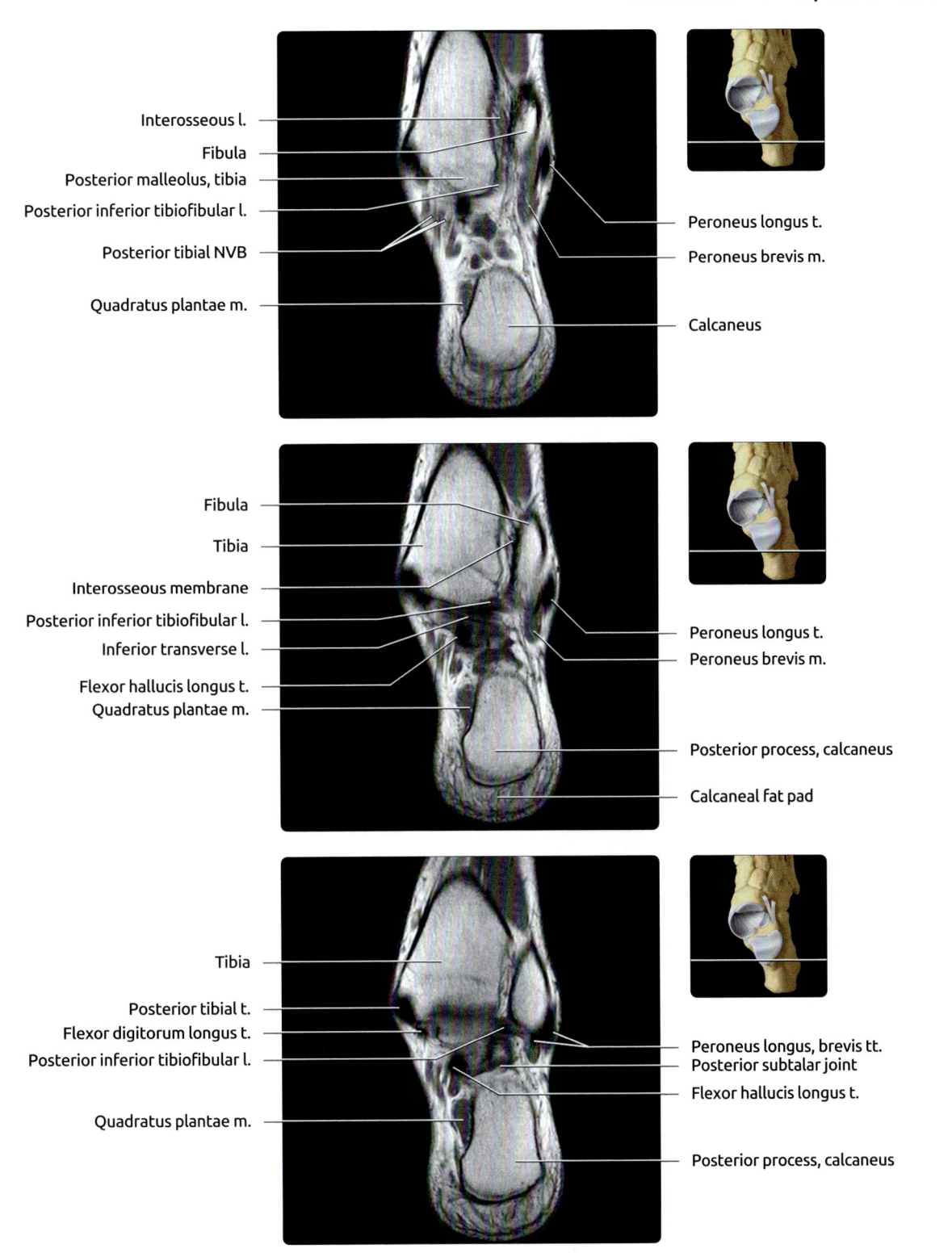

Labels (Top image):
- Interosseous l.
- Fibula
- Posterior malleolus, tibia
- Posterior inferior tibiofibular l.
- Posterior tibial NVB
- Quadratus plantae m.
- Peroneus longus t.
- Peroneus brevis m.
- Calcaneus

Labels (Middle image):
- Fibula
- Tibia
- Interosseous membrane
- Posterior inferior tibiofibular l.
- Inferior transverse l.
- Flexor hallucis longus t.
- Quadratus plantae m.
- Peroneus longus t.
- Peroneus brevis m.
- Posterior process, calcaneus
- Calcaneal fat pad

Labels (Bottom image):
- Tibia
- Posterior tibial t.
- Flexor digitorum longus t.
- Posterior inferior tibiofibular l.
- Quadratus plantae m.
- Peroneus longus, brevis tt.
- Posterior subtalar joint
- Flexor hallucis longus t.
- Posterior process, calcaneus

(Top) The coronal images from this image forward are angled perpendicular to the talus, which improves visualization of hindfoot structures. For that reason, the calcaneus is seen at a more posterior portion than on the previous images. **(Middle)** The posterior inferior tibiofibular ligament originates from the posterior malleolus and inserts into the fibula above the malleolar fossa. The inferior transverse ligament extends distal to the tibial posterior surface and inserts quite far medially close to the medial malleolus. **(Bottom)** The posterior subtalar joint is broad and curved. Inversion, eversion, and gliding motion occur at this joint.

CORONAL T1 MR, RIGHT ANKLE

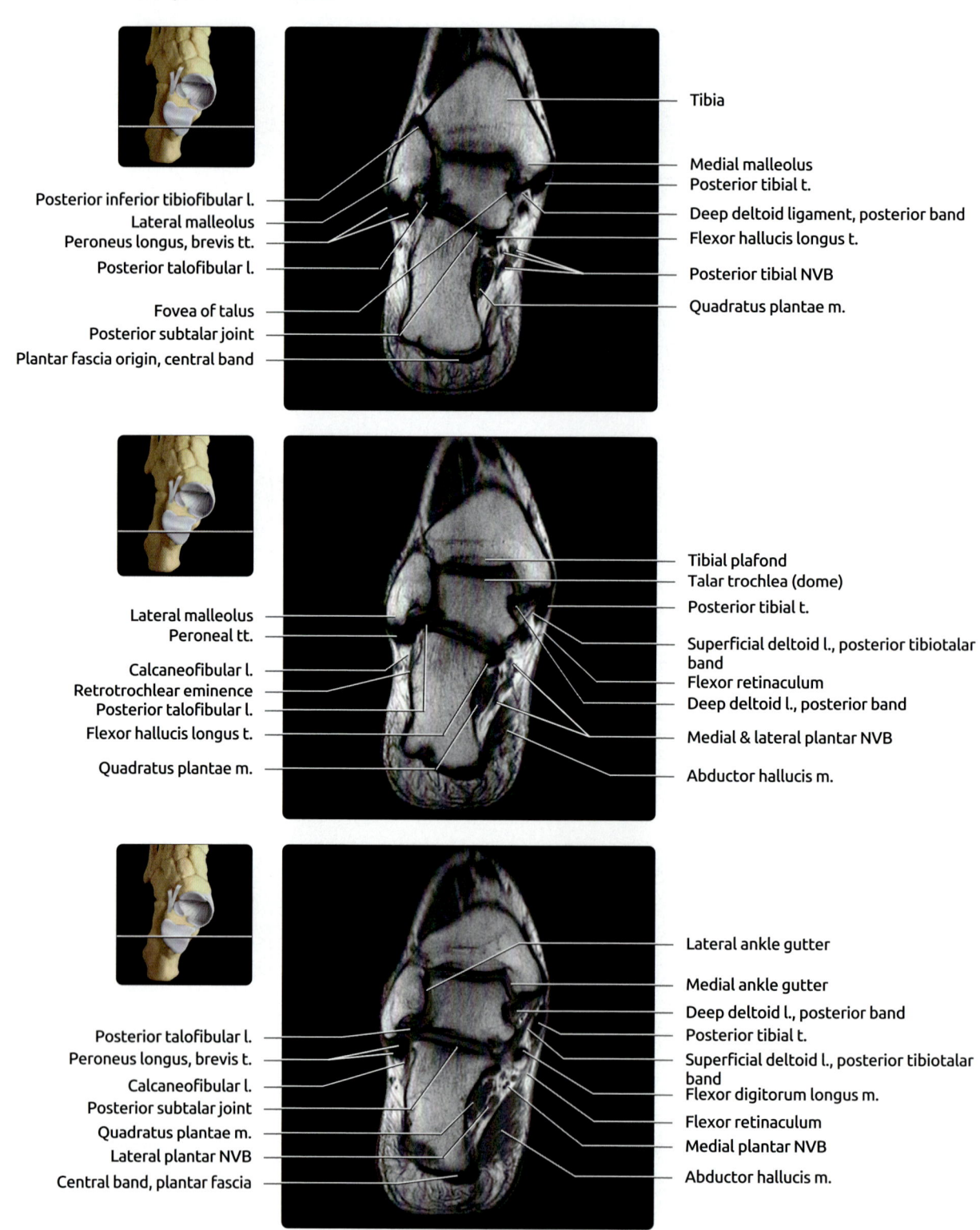

Top image labels:
- Tibia
- Medial malleolus
- Posterior tibial t.
- Deep deltoid ligament, posterior band
- Flexor hallucis longus t.
- Posterior tibial NVB
- Quadratus plantae m.
- Posterior inferior tibiofibular l.
- Lateral malleolus
- Peroneus longus, brevis tt.
- Posterior talofibular l.
- Fovea of talus
- Posterior subtalar joint
- Plantar fascia origin, central band

Middle image labels:
- Tibial plafond
- Talar trochlea (dome)
- Posterior tibial t.
- Superficial deltoid l., posterior tibiotalar band
- Flexor retinaculum
- Deep deltoid l., posterior band
- Medial & lateral plantar NVB
- Abductor hallucis m.
- Lateral malleolus
- Peroneal tt.
- Calcaneofibular l.
- Retrotrochlear eminence
- Posterior talofibular l.
- Flexor hallucis longus t.
- Quadratus plantae m.

Bottom image labels:
- Lateral ankle gutter
- Medial ankle gutter
- Deep deltoid l., posterior band
- Posterior tibial t.
- Superficial deltoid l., posterior tibiotalar band
- Flexor digitorum longus m.
- Flexor retinaculum
- Medial plantar NVB
- Abductor hallucis m.
- Posterior talofibular l.
- Peroneus longus, brevis t.
- Calcaneofibular l.
- Posterior subtalar joint
- Quadratus plantae m.
- Lateral plantar NVB
- Central band, plantar fascia

(Top) The deep deltoid ligament is now coming into view. It has 2 bands. The posterior band is the constant and strong portion and is often referred to simply as deep deltoid ligament. It arises from the posterior border of the anterior colliculus, as well as a small portion of the posterior colliculus of the medial malleolus, and inserts on the fovea at the medial margin of the talar body. **(Middle)** The calcaneofibular ligament is consistently seen on coronal images of the hindfoot deep to the peroneal tendons. It arises from the tip of the lateral malleolus and courses posteriorly, inferiorly, and medially to insert on the retrotrochlear eminence of the calcaneus. **(Bottom)** The contents of the tarsal tunnel, deep extrinsic flexor tendons and posterior tibial neurovascular bundle with its branches, are held beneath the flexor retinaculum. The medial osseous structures provide the floor of the tunnel.

Ankle MR Atlas

CORONAL T1 MR, LEFT ANKLE

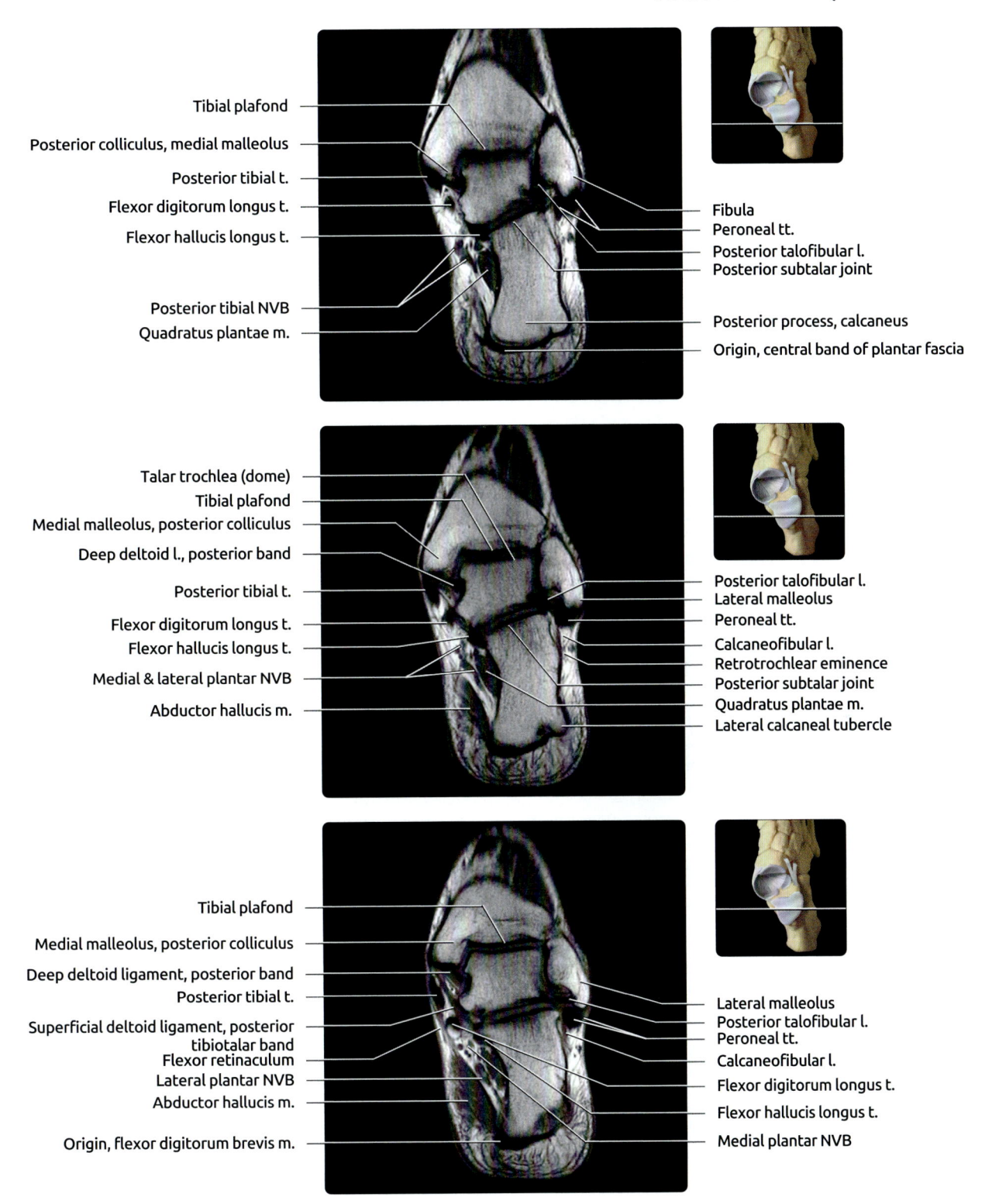

Top image labels (left): Tibial plafond; Posterior colliculus, medial malleolus; Posterior tibial t.; Flexor digitorum longus t.; Flexor hallucis longus t.; Posterior tibial NVB; Quadratus plantae m.

Top image labels (right): Fibula; Peroneal tt.; Posterior talofibular l.; Posterior subtalar joint; Posterior process, calcaneus; Origin, central band of plantar fascia

Middle image labels (left): Talar trochlea (dome); Tibial plafond; Medial malleolus, posterior colliculus; Deep deltoid l., posterior band; Posterior tibial t.; Flexor digitorum longus t.; Flexor hallucis longus t.; Medial & lateral plantar NVB; Abductor hallucis m.

Middle image labels (right): Posterior talofibular l.; Lateral malleolus; Peroneal tt.; Calcaneofibular l.; Retrotrochlear eminence; Posterior subtalar joint; Quadratus plantae m.; Lateral calcaneal tubercle

Bottom image labels (left): Tibial plafond; Medial malleolus, posterior colliculus; Deep deltoid ligament, posterior band; Posterior tibial t.; Superficial deltoid ligament, posterior tibiotalar band; Flexor retinaculum; Lateral plantar NVB; Abductor hallucis m.; Origin, flexor digitorum brevis m.

Bottom image labels (right): Lateral malleolus; Posterior talofibular l.; Peroneal tt.; Calcaneofibular l.; Flexor digitorum longus t.; Flexor hallucis longus t.; Medial plantar NVB

(Top) The deep deltoid ligament is now coming into view. It has 2 bands. The posterior band is the constant and strong portion and is often referred to simply as deep deltoid ligament. It arises from the posterior border of the anterior colliculus, as well as a small portion of the posterior colliculus of the medial malleolus, and inserts on the fovea at the medial margin of the talar body. **(Middle)** The calcaneofibular ligament is consistently seen on coronal images of the hindfoot deep to the peroneal tendons. It arises from the tip of the lateral malleolus and courses posteriorly, inferiorly, and medially to insert on the retrotrochlear eminence of the calcaneus. **(Bottom)** The contents of the tarsal tunnel, deep extrinsic flexor tendons and posterior tibial neurovascular bundle with its branches, are held beneath the flexor retinaculum. The medial osseous structures provide the floor of the tunnel.

Ankle MR Atlas

CORONAL T1 MR, RIGHT ANKLE

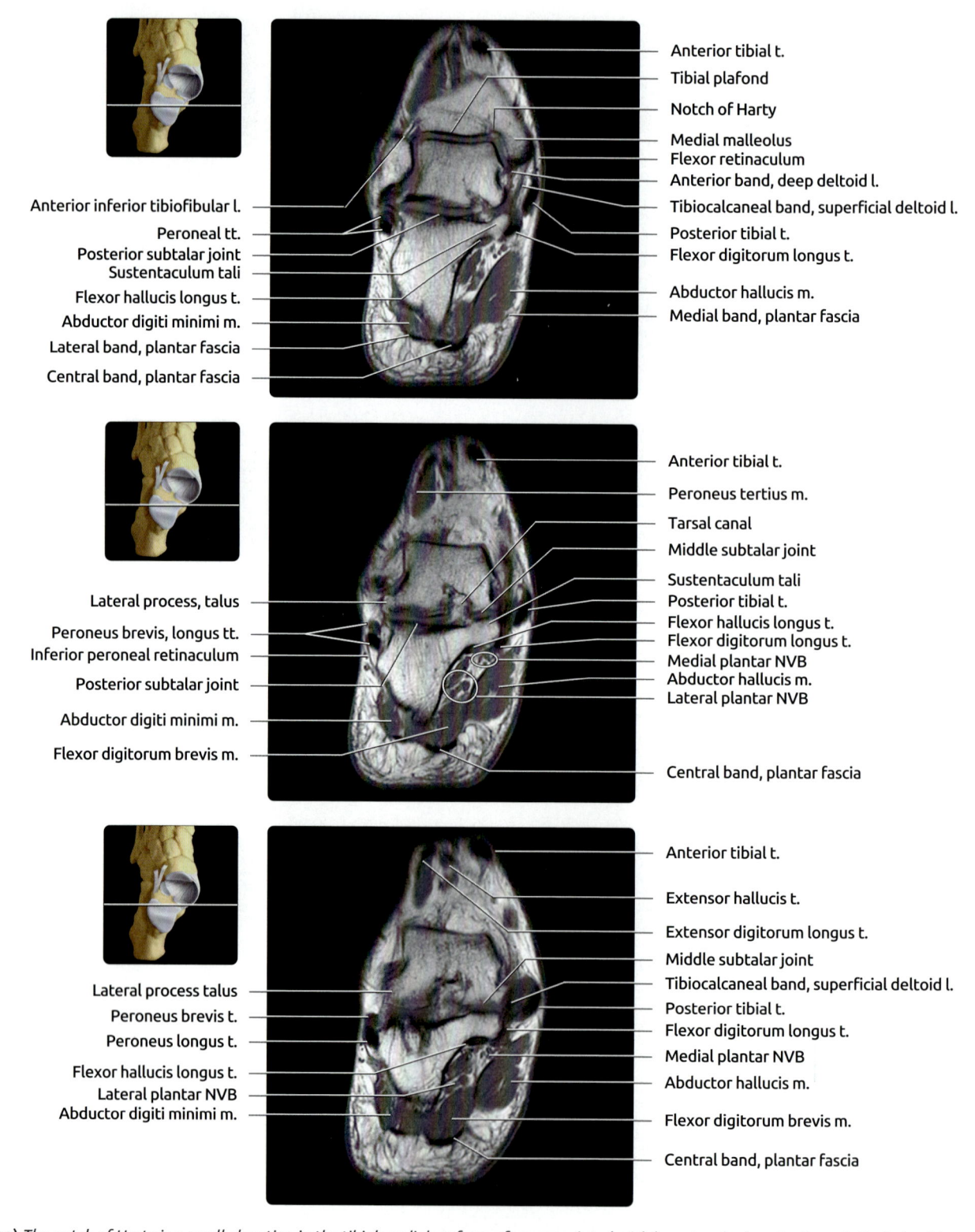

Top image labels:
- Anterior tibial t.
- Tibial plafond
- Notch of Harty
- Medial malleolus
- Flexor retinaculum
- Anterior band, deep deltoid l.
- Tibiocalcaneal band, superficial deltoid l.
- Posterior tibial t.
- Flexor digitorum longus t.
- Abductor hallucis m.
- Medial band, plantar fascia
- Anterior inferior tibiofibular l.
- Peroneal tt.
- Posterior subtalar joint
- Sustentaculum tali
- Flexor hallucis longus t.
- Abductor digiti minimi m.
- Lateral band, plantar fascia
- Central band, plantar fascia

Middle image labels:
- Anterior tibial t.
- Peroneus tertius m.
- Tarsal canal
- Middle subtalar joint
- Sustentaculum tali
- Posterior tibial t.
- Flexor hallucis longus t.
- Flexor digitorum longus t.
- Medial plantar NVB
- Abductor hallucis m.
- Lateral plantar NVB
- Central band, plantar fascia
- Lateral process, talus
- Peroneus brevis, longus tt.
- Inferior peroneal retinaculum
- Posterior subtalar joint
- Abductor digiti minimi m.
- Flexor digitorum brevis m.

Bottom image labels:
- Anterior tibial t.
- Extensor hallucis t.
- Extensor digitorum longus t.
- Middle subtalar joint
- Tibiocalcaneal band, superficial deltoid l.
- Posterior tibial t.
- Flexor digitorum longus t.
- Medial plantar NVB
- Abductor hallucis m.
- Flexor digitorum brevis m.
- Central band, plantar fascia
- Lateral process talus
- Peroneus brevis t.
- Peroneus longus t.
- Flexor hallucis longus t.
- Lateral plantar NVB
- Abductor digiti minimi m.

(Top) The notch of Harty is a small elevation in the tibial medial surface, often associated with low signal sclerosis above it, that should not be mistaken for tibial osteochondral lesion. The sustentaculum tali is a medial protuberance of the calcaneus; its most posterior portion, seen here, is nonarticular. More anteriorly it forms the inferior margin of the middle subtalar joint. **(Middle)** The majority of the sustentaculum tali articulates with a medial projection of the talus. The flexor hallucis longus tendon is seen coursing beneath the sustentaculum tali. Both it and the peroneus brevis show slightly increased signal intensity due to magic angle artifact. **(Bottom)** The tibialis anterior tendon is the largest extensor tendon. It can be followed on sequential coronal images and inserts on the 1st cuneiform and base of 1st metatarsal. The posterior tibial nerve has split into the medial and lateral plantar nerves. The medial plantar nerve travels superior to the lateral plantar nerve and close to the flexor hallucis longus tendon.

Ankle MR Atlas

CORONAL T1 MR, LEFT ANKLE

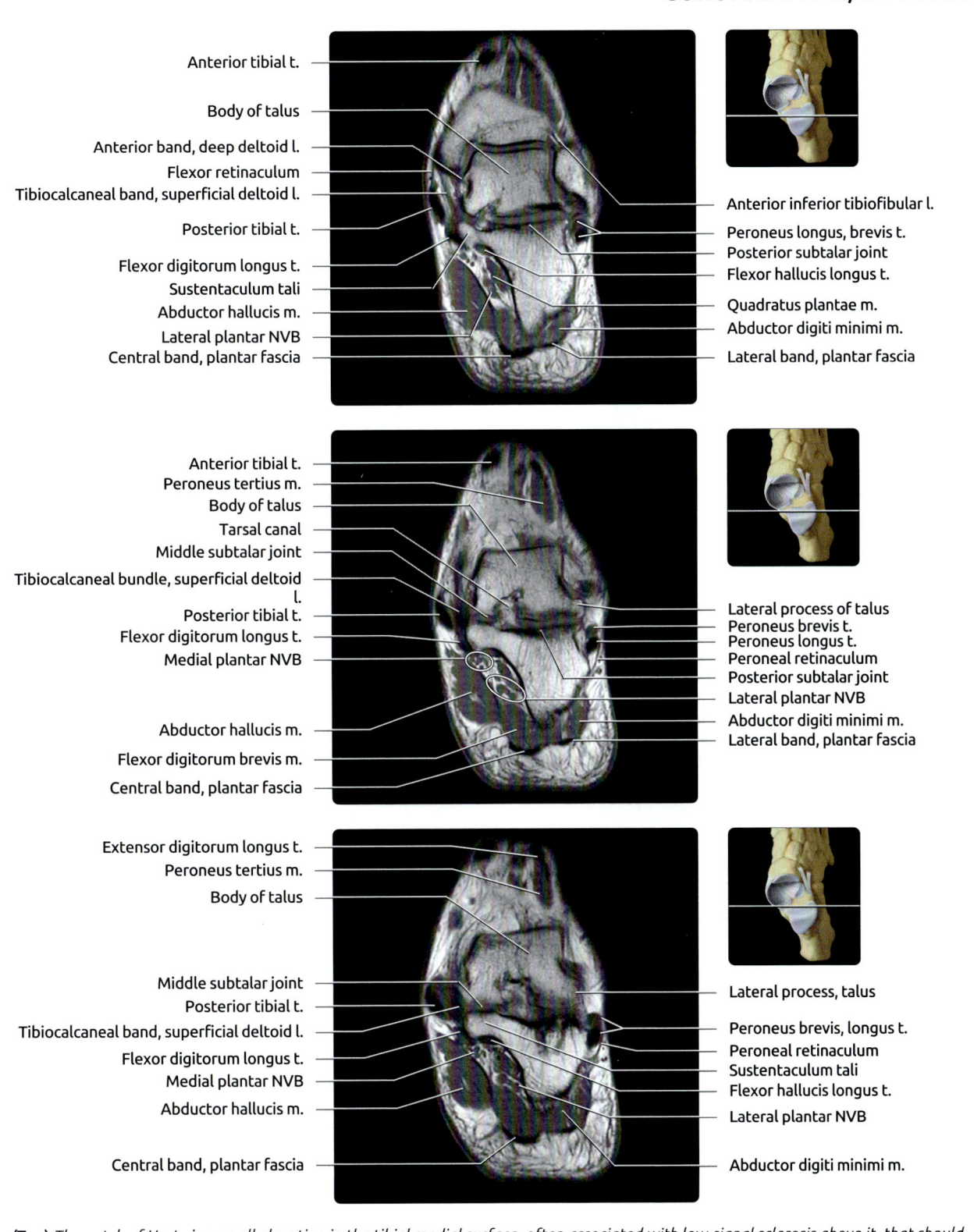

Top image labels (left):
- Anterior tibial t.
- Body of talus
- Anterior band, deep deltoid l.
- Flexor retinaculum
- Tibiocalcaneal band, superficial deltoid l.
- Posterior tibial t.
- Flexor digitorum longus t.
- Sustentaculum tali
- Abductor hallucis m.
- Lateral plantar NVB
- Central band, plantar fascia

Top image labels (right):
- Anterior inferior tibiofibular l.
- Peroneus longus, brevis t.
- Posterior subtalar joint
- Flexor hallucis longus t.
- Quadratus plantae m.
- Abductor digiti minimi m.
- Lateral band, plantar fascia

Middle image labels (left):
- Anterior tibial t.
- Peroneus tertius m.
- Body of talus
- Tarsal canal
- Middle subtalar joint
- Tibiocalcaneal bundle, superficial deltoid l.
- Posterior tibial t.
- Flexor digitorum longus t.
- Medial plantar NVB
- Abductor hallucis m.
- Flexor digitorum brevis m.
- Central band, plantar fascia

Middle image labels (right):
- Lateral process of talus
- Peroneus brevis t.
- Peroneus longus t.
- Peroneal retinaculum
- Posterior subtalar joint
- Lateral plantar NVB
- Abductor digiti minimi m.
- Lateral band, plantar fascia

Bottom image labels (left):
- Extensor digitorum longus t.
- Peroneus tertius m.
- Body of talus
- Middle subtalar joint
- Posterior tibial t.
- Tibiocalcaneal band, superficial deltoid l.
- Flexor digitorum longus t.
- Medial plantar NVB
- Abductor hallucis m.
- Central band, plantar fascia

Bottom image labels (right):
- Lateral process, talus
- Peroneus brevis, longus t.
- Peroneal retinaculum
- Sustentaculum tali
- Flexor hallucis longus t.
- Lateral plantar NVB
- Abductor digiti minimi m.

(**Top**) The notch of Harty is a small elevation in the tibial medial surface, often associated with low-signal sclerosis above it, that should not be mistaken for tibial osteochondral lesion. The sustentaculum tali is a medial protuberance of the calcaneus; its most posterior portion, seen here, is nonarticular. More anteriorly it forms the inferior margin of the middle subtalar joint. (**Middle**) The majority of the sustentaculum tali articulates with a medial projection of the talus. The flexor hallucis longus tendon is seen coursing beneath the sustentaculum tali. Both it and the peroneus brevis show slightly increased signal intensity due to magic angle artifact. (**Bottom**) The tibialis anterior tendon is the largest extensor tendon. It can be followed on sequential coronal images and inserts on the 1st cuneiform and base of 1st metatarsal. The posterior tibial nerve has split into the medial and lateral plantar nerves. The medial plantar nerve travels superior to the lateral plantar nerve and close to the flexor hallucis longus tendon.

Ankle MR Atlas

CORONAL T1 MR, RIGHT ANKLE

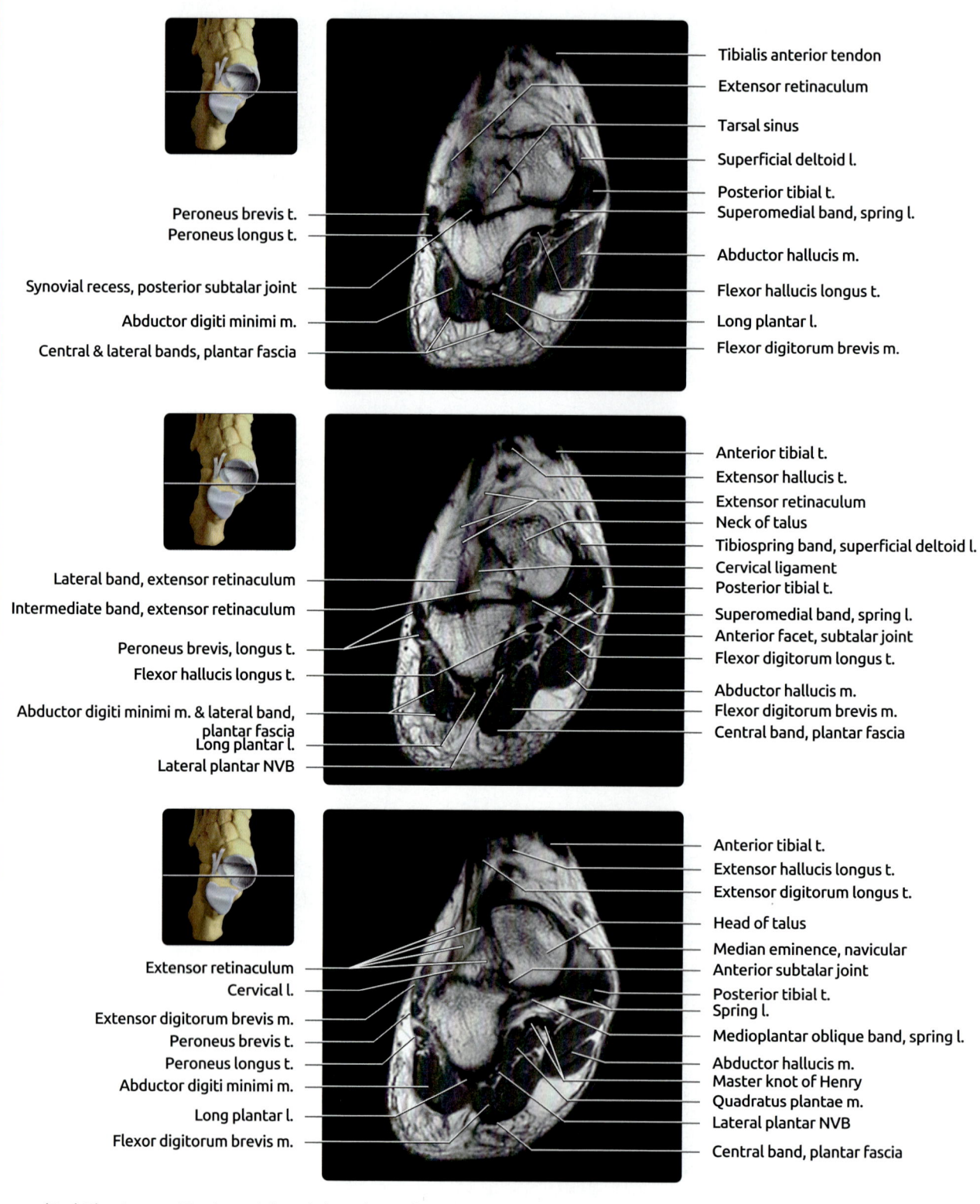

Top image labels:
- Tibialis anterior tendon
- Extensor retinaculum
- Tarsal sinus
- Superficial deltoid l.
- Posterior tibial t.
- Superomedial band, spring l.
- Abductor hallucis m.
- Flexor hallucis longus t.
- Long plantar l.
- Flexor digitorum brevis m.
- Peroneus brevis t.
- Peroneus longus t.
- Synovial recess, posterior subtalar joint
- Abductor digiti minimi m.
- Central & lateral bands, plantar fascia

Middle image labels:
- Anterior tibial t.
- Extensor hallucis t.
- Extensor retinaculum
- Neck of talus
- Tibiospring band, superficial deltoid l.
- Cervical ligament
- Posterior tibial t.
- Superomedial band, spring l.
- Anterior facet, subtalar joint
- Flexor digitorum longus t.
- Abductor hallucis m.
- Flexor digitorum brevis m.
- Central band, plantar fascia
- Lateral band, extensor retinaculum
- Intermediate band, extensor retinaculum
- Peroneus brevis, longus t.
- Flexor hallucis longus t.
- Abductor digiti minimi m. & lateral band, plantar fascia
- Long plantar l.
- Lateral plantar NVB

Bottom image labels:
- Anterior tibial t.
- Extensor hallucis longus t.
- Extensor digitorum longus t.
- Head of talus
- Median eminence, navicular
- Anterior subtalar joint
- Posterior tibial t.
- Spring l.
- Medioplantar oblique band, spring l.
- Abductor hallucis m.
- Master knot of Henry
- Quadratus plantae m.
- Lateral plantar NVB
- Central band, plantar fascia
- Extensor retinaculum
- Cervical l.
- Extensor digitorum brevis m.
- Peroneus brevis t.
- Peroneus longus t.
- Abductor digiti minimi m.
- Long plantar l.
- Flexor digitorum brevis m.

(Top) *The sinus tarsi is a lateral, funnel-shaped space between the talus and calcaneus, which is continuous with the tarsal canal located posteromedial to it. A joint recess from the posterior subtalar joint extends into the posteroinferior portion of the tarsal sinus.*
(Middle) *Three bands of extensor retinaculum extend into tarsal sinus, crossing the cervical ligament. The subcutaneous fat between the abductor hallucis and flexor digitorum brevis muscle is typically not traversed by septa and therefore can be mistaken for a lipoma.*
(Bottom) *The flexor digitorum longus and flexor hallucis longus tendon approximate & then cross each other under the navicular, at the knot of Henry. The cervical ligament crosses the insertions of the extensor retinaculum in the tarsal sinus. Medioplantar oblique band of spring ligament originates from calcaneus immediately anterior to sustentaculum tali. Medioplantar oblique and superomedial bands arise from the sustentaculum.*

Ankle MR Atlas

CORONAL T1 MR, LEFT ANKLE

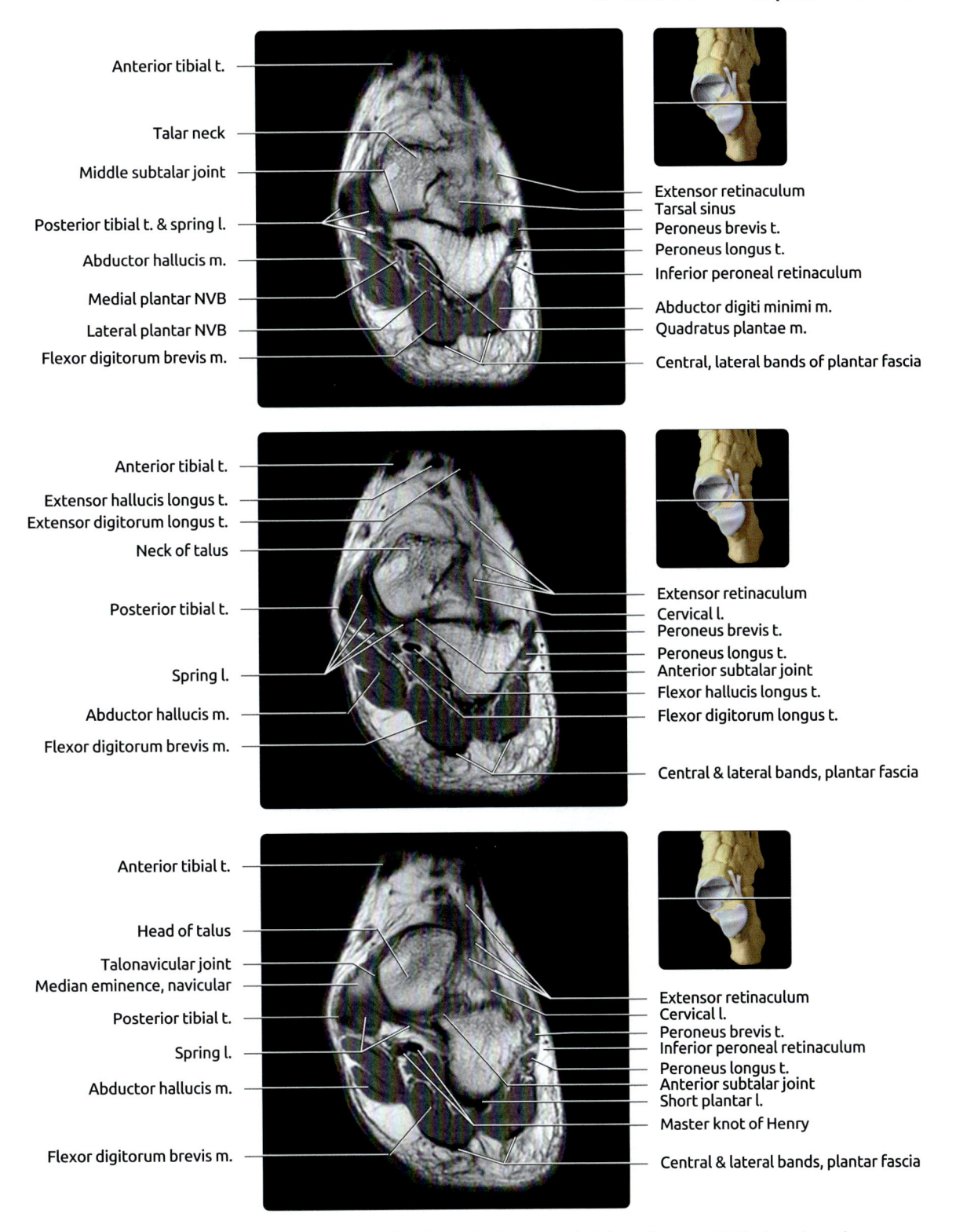

Labels (Top image):
- Anterior tibial t.
- Talar neck
- Middle subtalar joint
- Posterior tibial t. & spring l.
- Abductor hallucis m.
- Medial plantar NVB
- Lateral plantar NVB
- Flexor digitorum brevis m.
- Extensor retinaculum
- Tarsal sinus
- Peroneus brevis t.
- Peroneus longus t.
- Inferior peroneal retinaculum
- Abductor digiti minimi m.
- Quadratus plantae m.
- Central, lateral bands of plantar fascia

Labels (Middle image):
- Anterior tibial t.
- Extensor hallucis longus t.
- Extensor digitorum longus t.
- Neck of talus
- Posterior tibial t.
- Spring l.
- Abductor hallucis m.
- Flexor digitorum brevis m.
- Extensor retinaculum
- Cervical l.
- Peroneus brevis t.
- Peroneus longus t.
- Anterior subtalar joint
- Flexor hallucis longus t.
- Flexor digitorum longus t.
- Central & lateral bands, plantar fascia

Labels (Bottom image):
- Anterior tibial t.
- Head of talus
- Talonavicular joint
- Median eminence, navicular
- Posterior tibial t.
- Spring l.
- Abductor hallucis m.
- Flexor digitorum brevis m.
- Extensor retinaculum
- Cervical l.
- Peroneus brevis t.
- Inferior peroneal retinaculum
- Peroneus longus t.
- Anterior subtalar joint
- Short plantar l.
- Master knot of Henry
- Central & lateral bands, plantar fascia

(Top) The sinus tarsi is a lateral, funnel-shaped space between the talus and calcaneus, which is continuous with the tarsal canal located posteromedial to it. A joint recess from the posterior subtalar joint extends into the posteroinferior portion of the tarsal sinus. (Middle) Three bands of extensor retinaculum extend into tarsal sinus, crossing the cervical ligament. The subcutaneous fat between the abductor hallucis and flexor digitorum brevis muscle is typically not traversed by septa and therefore can be mistaken for a lipoma. (Bottom) The flexor digitorum longus and flexor hallucis longus tendon approximate & then cross each other under the navicular, at the knot of Henry. The cervical ligament crosses the insertions of the extensor retinaculum in the tarsal sinus. Medioplantar oblique band of spring ligament originates from calcaneus immediately anterior to sustentaculum tali. Medioplantar oblique and superomedial bands arise from the sustentaculum.

CORONAL T1 MR, RIGHT ANKLE

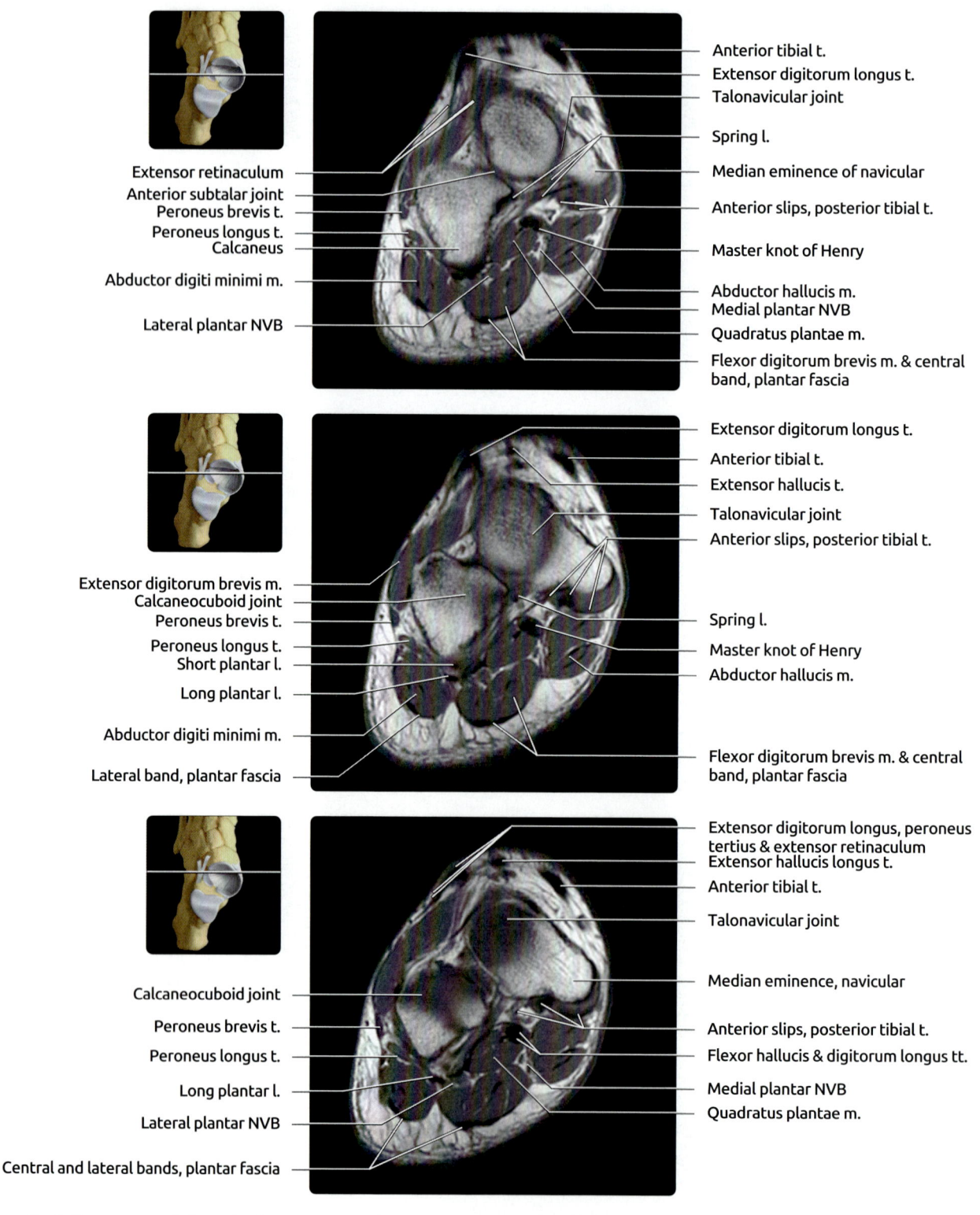

Image 1 labels (Top):
- Anterior tibial t.
- Extensor digitorum longus t.
- Talonavicular joint
- Spring l.
- Median eminence of navicular
- Anterior slips, posterior tibial t.
- Master knot of Henry
- Abductor hallucis m.
- Medial plantar NVB
- Quadratus plantae m.
- Flexor digitorum brevis m. & central band, plantar fascia
- Extensor retinaculum
- Anterior subtalar joint
- Peroneus brevis t.
- Peroneus longus t.
- Calcaneus
- Abductor digiti minimi m.
- Lateral plantar NVB

Image 2 labels (Middle):
- Extensor digitorum longus t.
- Anterior tibial t.
- Extensor hallucis t.
- Talonavicular joint
- Anterior slips, posterior tibial t.
- Spring l.
- Master knot of Henry
- Abductor hallucis m.
- Flexor digitorum brevis m. & central band, plantar fascia
- Extensor digitorum brevis m.
- Calcaneocuboid joint
- Peroneus brevis t.
- Peroneus longus t.
- Short plantar l.
- Long plantar l.
- Abductor digiti minimi m.
- Lateral band, plantar fascia

Image 3 labels (Bottom):
- Extensor digitorum longus, peroneus tertius & extensor retinaculum
- Extensor hallucis longus t.
- Anterior tibial t.
- Talonavicular joint
- Median eminence, navicular
- Anterior slips, posterior tibial t.
- Flexor hallucis & digitorum longus tt.
- Medial plantar NVB
- Quadratus plantae m.
- Calcaneocuboid joint
- Peroneus brevis t.
- Peroneus longus t.
- Long plantar l.
- Lateral plantar NVB
- Central and lateral bands, plantar fascia

(**Top**) *The anatomy of the spring ligament is complex. Fortunately for practical reading of MR, tears are usually attritional, chronic, and involve all components.* (**Middle**) *Portions of the calcaneocuboid and talonavicular joints are seen en face. Peroneal tendons are diverging. Peroneus brevis tendon will become a thin ribbon as it inserts on the 5th metatarsal base. Peroneus longus is coursing medially and inferiorly toward the cuboid tunnel.* (**Bottom**) *Flexor hallucis and digitorum longus tendons have crossed. Quadratus plantae will insert on flexor digitorum longus. Anterior tibial tendon is starting to wrap around the medial side of the foot to its insertions on 1st cuneiform and 1st metatarsal.*

Ankle MR Atlas

CORONAL T1 MR, LEFT ANKLE

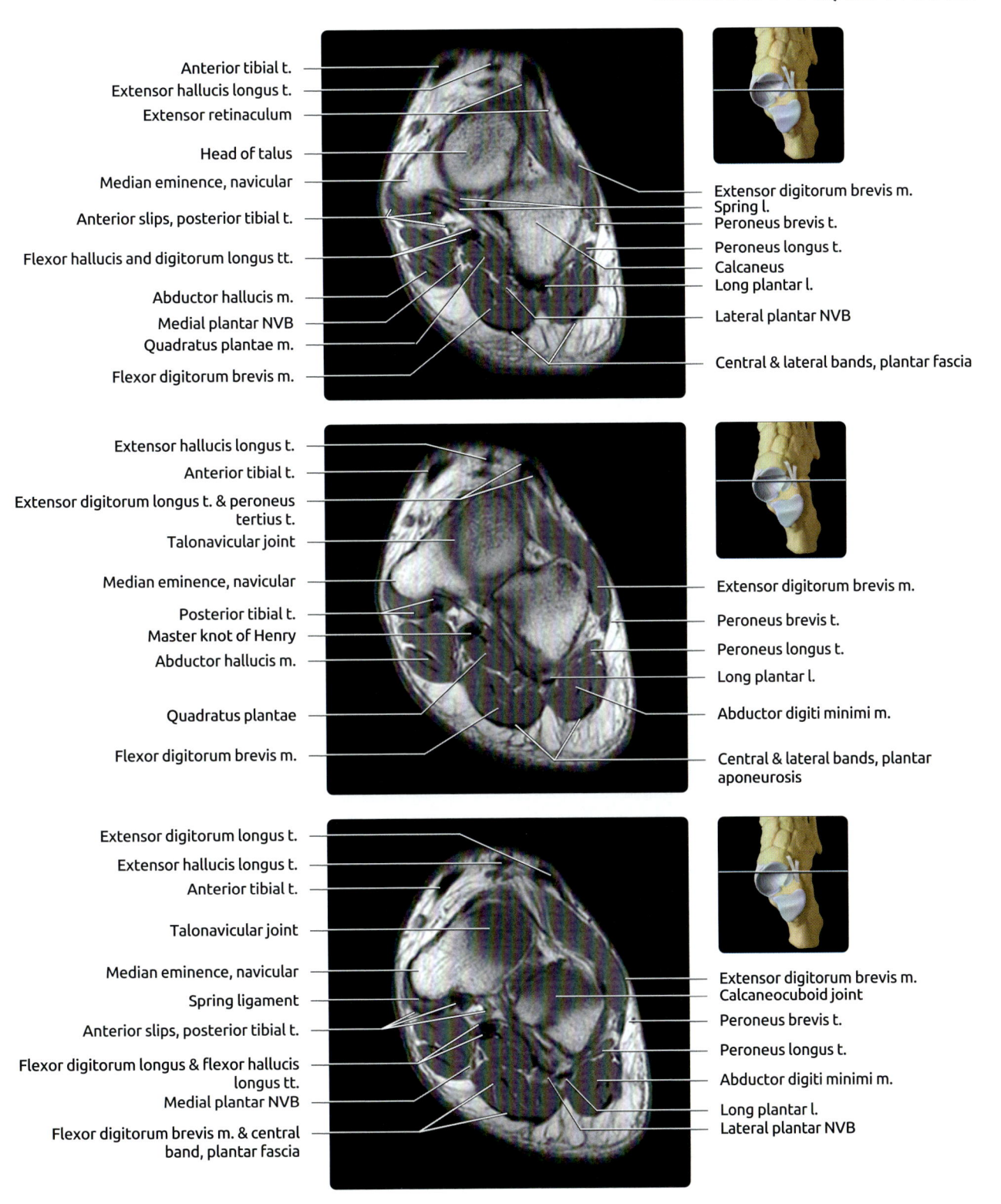

Top image labels (left):
- Anterior tibial t.
- Extensor hallucis longus t.
- Extensor retinaculum
- Head of talus
- Median eminence, navicular
- Anterior slips, posterior tibial t.
- Flexor hallucis and digitorum longus tt.
- Abductor hallucis m.
- Medial plantar NVB
- Quadratus plantae m.
- Flexor digitorum brevis m.

Top image labels (right):
- Extensor digitorum brevis m.
- Spring l.
- Peroneus brevis t.
- Peroneus longus t.
- Calcaneus
- Long plantar l.
- Lateral plantar NVB
- Central & lateral bands, plantar fascia

Middle image labels (left):
- Extensor hallucis longus t.
- Anterior tibial t.
- Extensor digitorum longus t. & peroneus tertius t.
- Talonavicular joint
- Median eminence, navicular
- Posterior tibial t.
- Master knot of Henry
- Abductor hallucis m.
- Quadratus plantae
- Flexor digitorum brevis m.

Middle image labels (right):
- Extensor digitorum brevis m.
- Peroneus brevis t.
- Peroneus longus t.
- Long plantar l.
- Abductor digiti minimi m.
- Central & lateral bands, plantar aponeurosis

Bottom image labels (left):
- Extensor digitorum longus t.
- Extensor hallucis longus t.
- Anterior tibial t.
- Talonavicular joint
- Median eminence, navicular
- Spring ligament
- Anterior slips, posterior tibial t.
- Flexor digitorum longus & flexor hallucis longus tt.
- Medial plantar NVB
- Flexor digitorum brevis m. & central band, plantar fascia

Bottom image labels (right):
- Extensor digitorum brevis m.
- Calcaneocuboid joint
- Peroneus brevis t.
- Peroneus longus t.
- Abductor digiti minimi m.
- Long plantar l.
- Lateral plantar NVB

(Top) The anatomy of the spring ligament is complex. Fortunately for practical reading of MR, tears are usually attritional, chronic, and involve all components. (Middle) Portions of the calcaneocuboid and talonavicular joints are seen en face. Peroneal tendons are diverging. Peroneus brevis tendon will become a thin ribbon as it inserts on the 5th metatarsal base. Peroneus longus is coursing medially and inferiorly toward the cuboid tunnel. (Bottom) Flexor hallucis and digitorum longus tendons have crossed. Quadratus plantae will insert on flexor digitorum longus. Anterior tibial tendon is starting to wrap around medial side of foot to its insertions on 1st cuneiform and 1st metatarsal.

Ankle MR Atlas

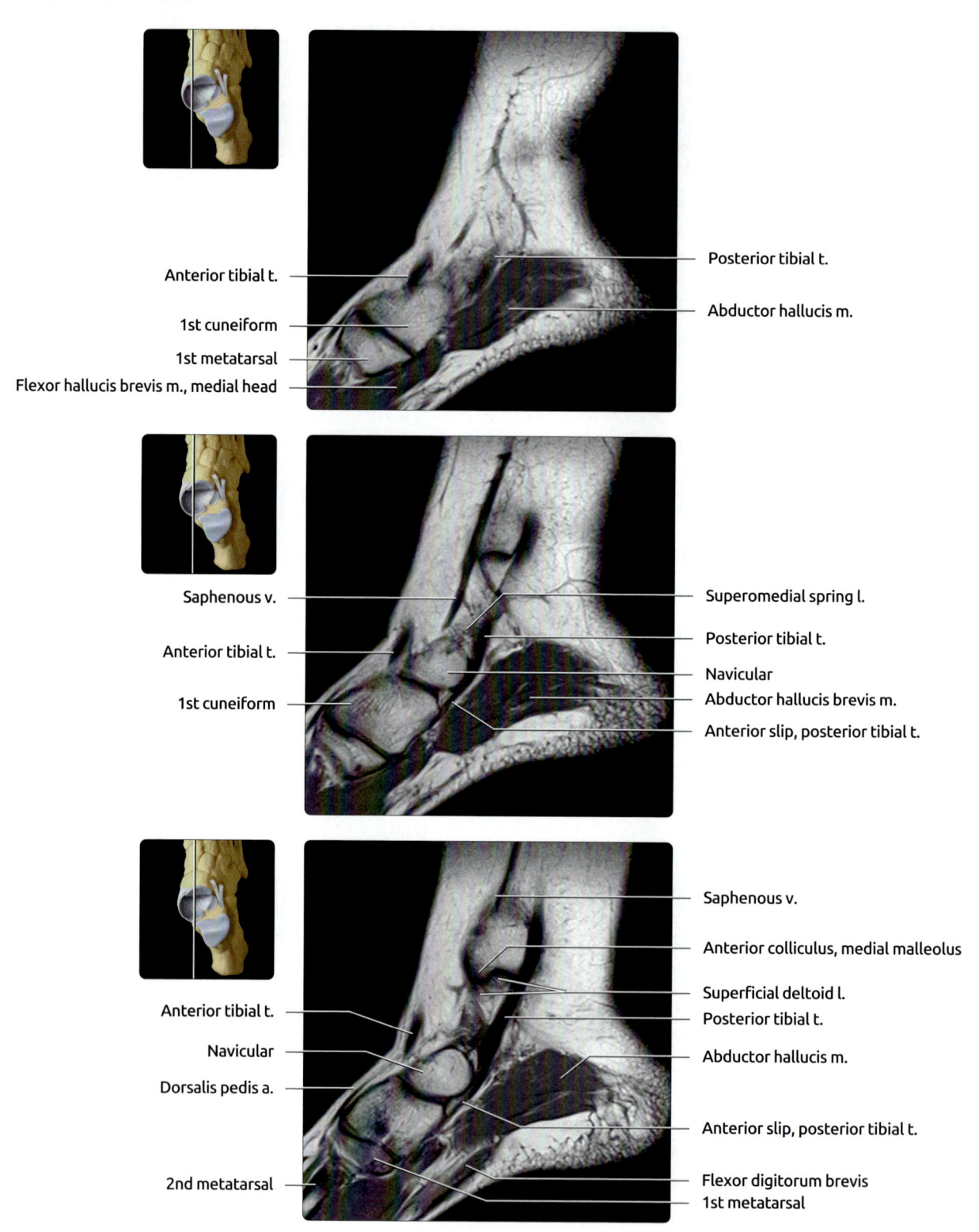

SAGITTAL T1 MR

Anterior tibial t.
1st cuneiform
1st metatarsal
Flexor hallucis brevis m., medial head
Posterior tibial t.
Abductor hallucis m.

Saphenous v.
Anterior tibial t.
1st cuneiform
Superomedial spring l.
Posterior tibial t.
Navicular
Abductor hallucis brevis m.
Anterior slip, posterior tibial t.

Anterior tibial t.
Navicular
Dorsalis pedis a.
2nd metatarsal
Saphenous v.
Anterior colliculus, medial malleolus
Superficial deltoid l.
Posterior tibial t.
Abductor hallucis m.
Anterior slip, posterior tibial t.
Flexor digitorum brevis
1st metatarsal

(**Top**) *Serial sagittal T1 MR images show the ankle from medial to lateral. On this furthest medial image, the anterior tibial tendon is seen wrapping around the medial margin of the 1st cuneiform. It will insert on the plantar-medial margin of the 1st cuneiform and metatarsal.* (**Middle**) *There is a sturdy slip of posterior tibial tendon extending from the navicular to the 1st cuneiform. Superomedial band of spring ligament is partly visible.* (**Bottom**) *A few fibers of the anterior portions of the superficial deltoid ligament are visible arising from the medial surface of the medial malleolus. The bands are named for their attachments: Anterior and posterior tibiotalar, tibiocalcaneal, tibiospring, and tibionavicular.*

Ankle MR Atlas

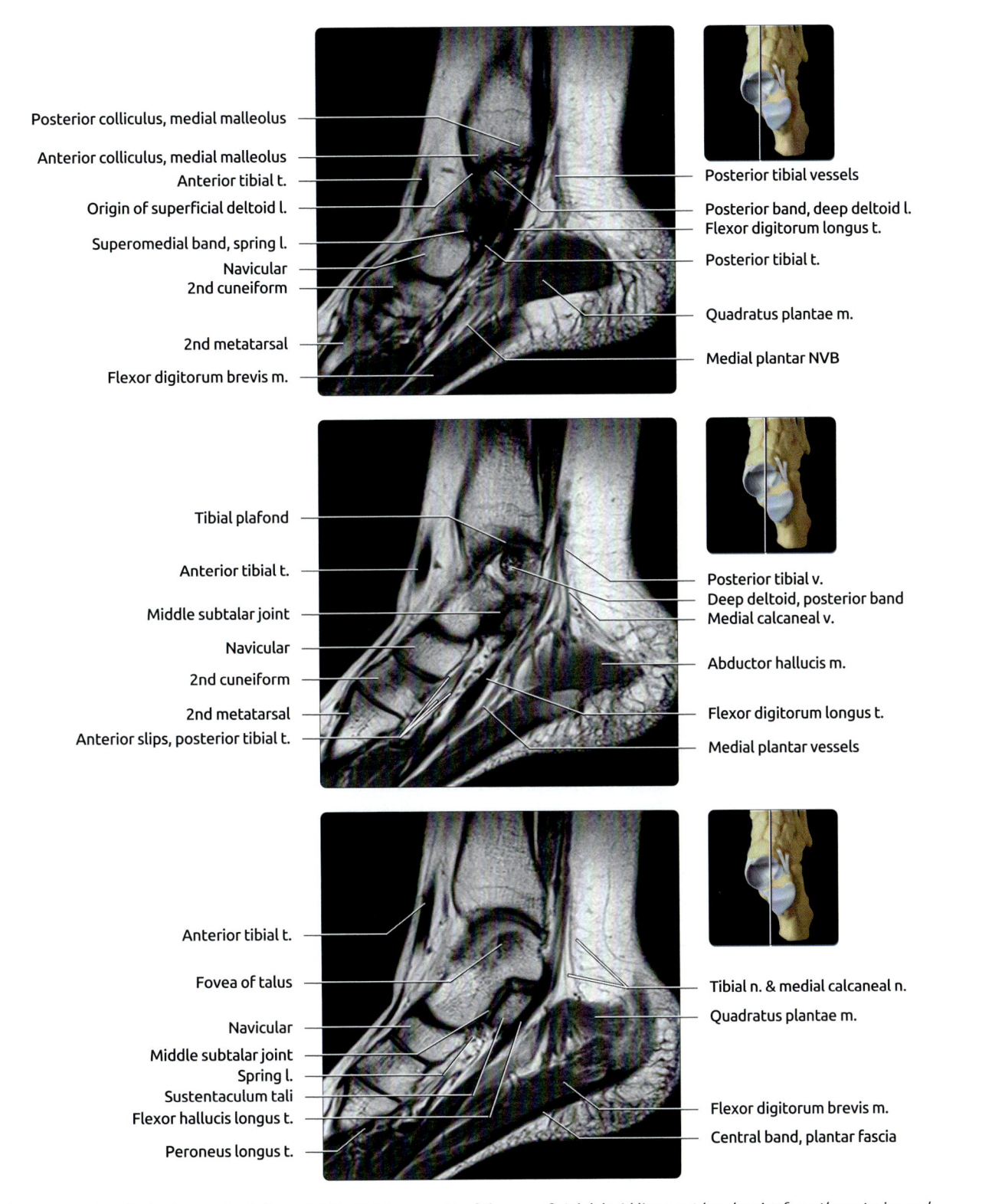

SAGITTAL T1 MR

Top image labels (left):
- Posterior colliculus, medial malleolus
- Anterior colliculus, medial malleolus
- Anterior tibial t.
- Origin of superficial deltoid l.
- Superomedial band, spring l.
- Navicular
- 2nd cuneiform
- 2nd metatarsal
- Flexor digitorum brevis m.

Top image labels (right):
- Posterior tibial vessels
- Posterior band, deep deltoid l.
- Flexor digitorum longus t.
- Posterior tibial t.
- Quadratus plantae m.
- Medial plantar NVB

Middle image labels (left):
- Tibial plafond
- Anterior tibial t.
- Middle subtalar joint
- Navicular
- 2nd cuneiform
- 2nd metatarsal
- Anterior slips, posterior tibial t.

Middle image labels (right):
- Posterior tibial v.
- Deep deltoid, posterior band
- Medial calcaneal v.
- Abductor hallucis m.
- Flexor digitorum longus t.
- Medial plantar vessels

Bottom image labels (left):
- Anterior tibial t.
- Fovea of talus
- Navicular
- Middle subtalar joint
- Spring l.
- Sustentaculum tali
- Flexor hallucis longus t.
- Peroneus longus t.

Bottom image labels (right):
- Tibial n. & medial calcaneal n.
- Quadratus plantae m.
- Flexor digitorum brevis m.
- Central band, plantar fascia

(**Top**) *Posterior tibial artery and vein lie medial to tibial nerve. All of the superficial deltoid ligament bands arise from the anterior and superficial surface of the medial malleolus.* (**Middle**) *The bulbous valves on veins help to distinguish them from arteries and nerves. The distinction is more readily apparent on fluid-sensitive sequences, as the vessels are usually higher signal intensity than the nerves.* (**Bottom**) *The fovea of the talus, inferior to the cartilaginous portion of the joint, is the site of insertion of the posterior band of the deep deltoid ligament.*

Ankle MR Atlas

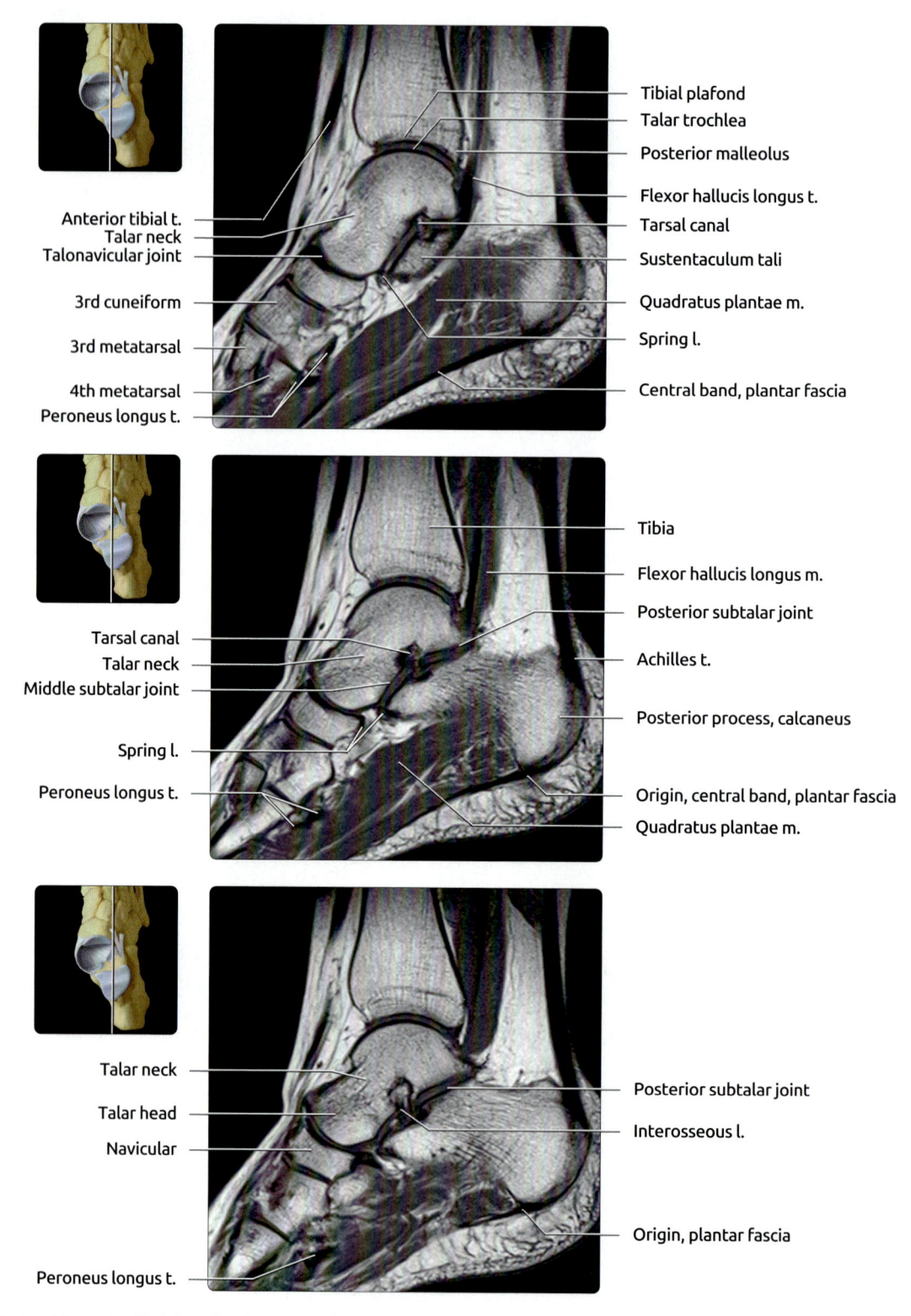

SAGITTAL T1 MR

Labels (top image):
- Tibial plafond
- Talar trochlea
- Posterior malleolus
- Flexor hallucis longus t.
- Tarsal canal
- Sustentaculum tali
- Quadratus plantae m.
- Spring l.
- Central band, plantar fascia
- Anterior tibial t.
- Talar neck
- Talonavicular joint
- 3rd cuneiform
- 3rd metatarsal
- 4th metatarsal
- Peroneus longus t.

Labels (middle image):
- Tibia
- Flexor hallucis longus m.
- Posterior subtalar joint
- Achilles t.
- Posterior process, calcaneus
- Origin, central band, plantar fascia
- Quadratus plantae m.
- Tarsal canal
- Talar neck
- Middle subtalar joint
- Spring l.
- Peroneus longus t.

Labels (bottom image):
- Posterior subtalar joint
- Interosseous l.
- Origin, plantar fascia
- Talar neck
- Talar head
- Navicular
- Peroneus longus t.

(Top) The talar trochlea, miscalled the talar dome, articulates with the tibial plafond. The plafond extends further inferiorly in its posterior portion, a broad expansion of the tibia called the posterior malleolus. **(Middle)** The posterior subtalar joint is shorter in anteroposterior dimension medially than it is laterally. The middle subtalar joint lies anterior to it and also extends further medially. **(Bottom)** The interosseous talocalcaneal l. lies in the tarsal canal, the narrow posteromedial extension of the tarsal sinus.

Ankle MR Atlas

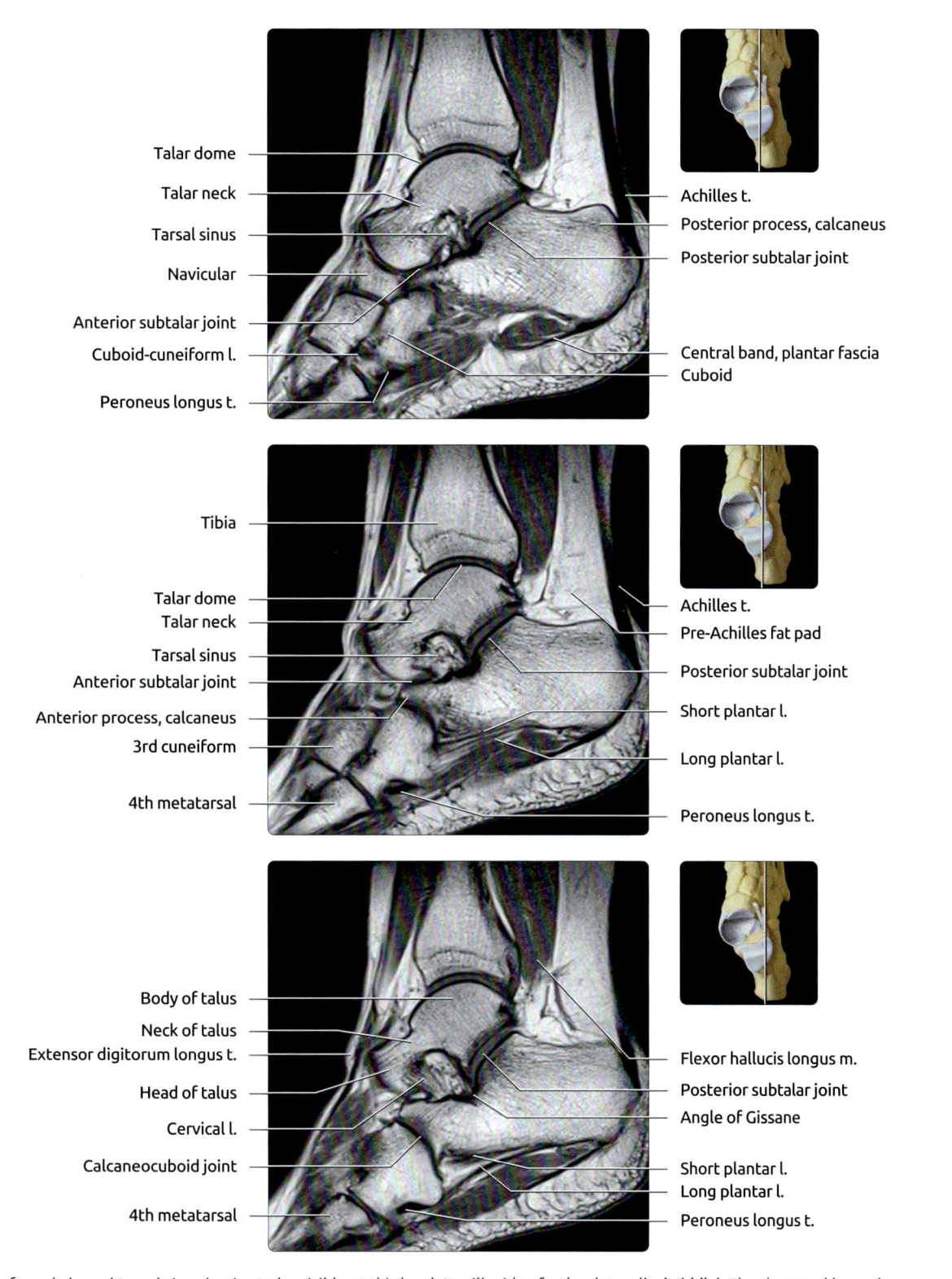

SAGITTAL T1 MR

- Talar dome
- Talar neck
- Tarsal sinus
- Navicular
- Anterior subtalar joint
- Cuboid-cuneiform l.
- Peroneus longus t.
- Achilles t.
- Posterior process, calcaneus
- Posterior subtalar joint
- Central band, plantar fascia
- Cuboid

- Tibia
- Talar dome
- Talar neck
- Tarsal sinus
- Anterior subtalar joint
- Anterior process, calcaneus
- 3rd cuneiform
- 4th metatarsal
- Achilles t.
- Pre-Achilles fat pad
- Posterior subtalar joint
- Short plantar l.
- Long plantar l.
- Peroneus longus t.

- Body of talus
- Neck of talus
- Extensor digitorum longus t.
- Head of talus
- Cervical l.
- Calcaneocuboid joint
- 4th metatarsal
- Flexor hallucis longus m.
- Posterior subtalar joint
- Angle of Gissane
- Short plantar l.
- Long plantar l.
- Peroneus longus t.

(Top) *The funnel-shaped tarsal sinus begins to be visible at this level. It will widen farther laterally.* (Middle) *The short and long plantar ligaments are coming into view.* (Bottom) *Note that when the foot is not weight bearing, the calcaneocuboid joint normally appears subluxated. The joint has a sinusoidal contour. The calcaneus moves inferiorly relative to the cuboid when a person stands.*

Ankle MR Atlas

SAGITTAL T1 MR, ANKLE

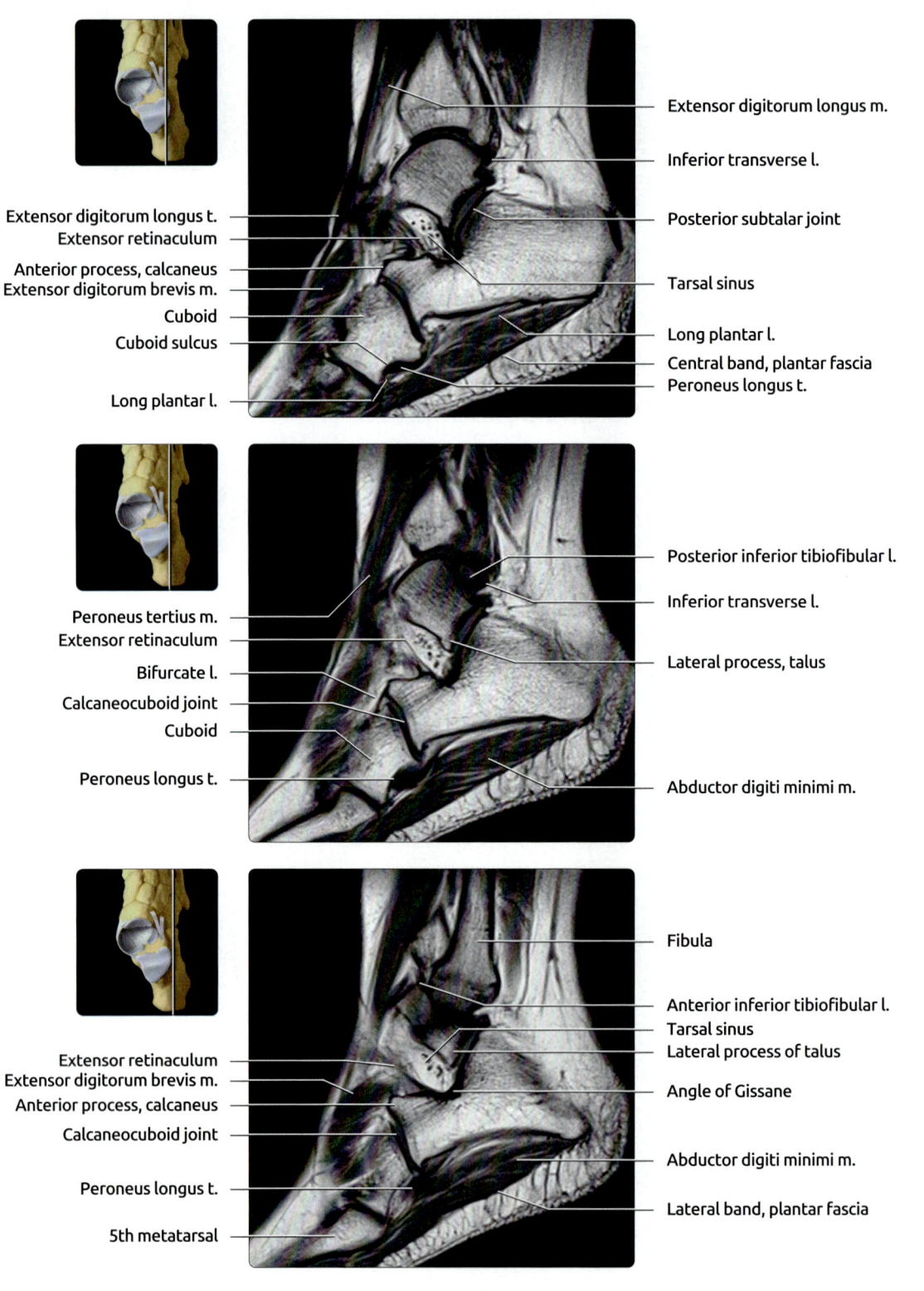

Labels (top image):
- Extensor digitorum longus t.
- Extensor retinaculum
- Anterior process, calcaneus
- Extensor digitorum brevis m.
- Cuboid
- Cuboid sulcus
- Long plantar l.
- Extensor digitorum longus m.
- Inferior transverse l.
- Posterior subtalar joint
- Tarsal sinus
- Long plantar l.
- Central band, plantar fascia
- Peroneus longus t.

Labels (middle image):
- Peroneus tertius m.
- Extensor retinaculum
- Bifurcate l.
- Calcaneocuboid joint
- Cuboid
- Peroneus longus t.
- Posterior inferior tibiofibular l.
- Inferior transverse l.
- Lateral process, talus
- Abductor digiti minimi m.

Labels (bottom image):
- Extensor retinaculum
- Extensor digitorum brevis m.
- Anterior process, calcaneus
- Calcaneocuboid joint
- Peroneus longus t.
- 5th metatarsal
- Fibula
- Anterior inferior tibiofibular l.
- Tarsal sinus
- Lateral process of talus
- Angle of Gissane
- Abductor digiti minimi m.
- Lateral band, plantar fascia

(**Top**) *The long plantar ligament converts the cuboid sulcus into a tunnel through which passes the peroneus longus t.* (**Middle**) *The inferior transverse ligament can mimic a loose body. It extends from the posteromedial tibia to the tip of the fibula. The calcaneocuboid limb of the bifurcate ligament is also well seen on this image.* (**Bottom**) *Extensor retinaculum is seen coursing over the dorsum of the hindfoot. It sends 3 limbs into the tarsal sinus.*

Ankle MR Atlas

SAGITTAL T1 MR, ANKLE

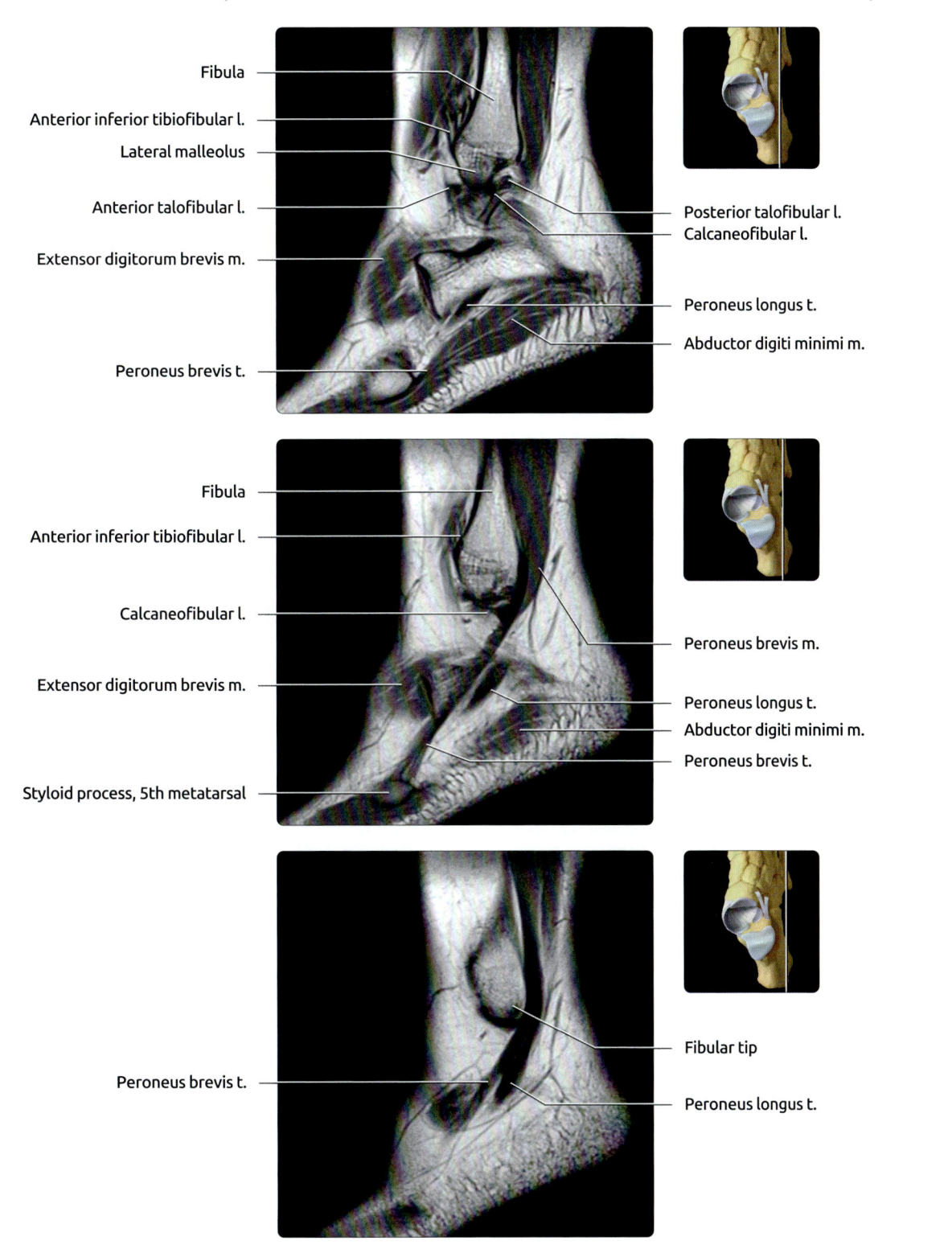

Top image labels:
- Fibula
- Anterior inferior tibiofibular l.
- Lateral malleolus
- Anterior talofibular l.
- Extensor digitorum brevis m.
- Peroneus brevis t.
- Posterior talofibular l.
- Calcaneofibular l.
- Peroneus longus t.
- Abductor digiti minimi m.

Middle image labels:
- Fibula
- Anterior inferior tibiofibular l.
- Calcaneofibular l.
- Extensor digitorum brevis m.
- Styloid process, 5th metatarsal
- Peroneus brevis m.
- Peroneus longus t.
- Abductor digiti minimi m.
- Peroneus brevis t.

Bottom image labels:
- Peroneus brevis t.
- Fibular tip
- Peroneus longus t.

(Top) The striated appearance of the anterior inferior tibiofibular ligament is well shown. The most inferior fascicle, the Bassett ligament, is reportedly a normal variant but is almost always visible on MR. (Middle) The peroneus brevis tendon is anterior to the longus in the foot. It is seen attaching to the styloid process of the 5th metatarsal. (Bottom) The farthest lateral image in this sequence shows the divergence of the peroneus brevis and longus tendons.

Ankle Tendons

GROSS ANATOMY

Organizing Anatomy
- Muscles originate at knee or leg, become tendinous around ankle, tendons insert in foot
- 3 compartments: Anterior, lateral, and posterior
- Anterior compartment from medial to lateral contains anterior tibial, extensor hallucis longus, extensor digitorum longus, and peroneus tertius (variably present) tendons
- Posterior compartment has deep and superficial compartments
  - Superficial: Achilles and plantaris tendons
  - Deep from medial to lateral contains posterior tibial, flexor digitorum longus, and flexor hallucis longus tendons
- Lateral compartment contains peroneus longus and brevis tendons

Transition From Leg to Foot
- Tendons (except Achilles) all dramatically change course from leg to foot
- Positions are maintained by retinacula, fibrous bands, which hold tendons close to underlying bones and joints
  - Extensor retinaculum
    - Bursa usually present deep to inferior extensor retinaculum
  - Flexor retinaculum
  - Peroneal retinaculum

Tendon Sheaths
- All tendons of ankle except Achilles have sheaths
- Achilles surrounded by loose tissue called paratenon
- Flexor hallucis longus tendon sheath communicates with ankle joint

Anterior Compartment: Innervation by Deep Peroneal Nerve (N.)
- Anterior tibial
  - Largest tendon of anterior compartment
  - Origin: Upper 2/3 lateral tibia, interosseous membrane, intermuscular septum
  - Insertion: Medial margin of 1st cuneiform and 1st metatarsal
  - Action: Dorsiflexion, inversion
  - Variant: Tendon may be bifid; may have small accessory muscle (of Gruber)
  - Variant: May insert on navicular or more distally on 1st digit
- Extensor hallucis longus
  - Origin: Proximal fibula and interosseous membrane
  - Insertion: Distal phalanx, 1st toe (sometimes to proximal phalanx)
  - Action: Dorsiflexion of 1st toe and foot
- Extensor digitorum longus
  - Origin: Lateral tibial condyle, upper 3/4 fibula, upper interosseous membrane
  - Insertion: 2nd-5th toes, join extensor digitorum brevis
  - Action: Dorsiflexion of toes
- Peroneus tertius
  - Origin: Distal fibula and interosseous membrane
  - Insertion: Dorsal margin of 5th metatarsal base
  - Variably present

Lateral Compartment: Innervation by Peroneal N.
- Peroneus longus
  - Origin: Proximal fibula
  - Insertion: 1st cuneiform and 1st metatarsal base
  - Action: Plantar flexion and eversion
  - Travels from lateral to medial plantar surface of foot through cuboid sulcus
- Peroneus brevis
  - Origin: Lower 2/3 fibula, deep to peroneus longus
  - Insertion: 5th metatarsal styloid process (also called tuberosity)
  - Action: Plantar flexion and eversion
  - Muscle normally terminates at tip of fibula, but muscle belly may be low-lying
- Peroneus quartus (variably present)
  - Origin: Distal, lateral fibula
  - Insertion: Variable, usually on peroneus brevis or calcaneus

Superficial Posterior Compartment: Innervation by Tibial N.
- Achilles tendon
  - Conjoined tendon of gastrocnemius and soleus muscles
  - Insertion: Posterior tuberosity of calcaneus
  - Action: Plantar flexion of foot
  - Anterior margin is concave; AP diameter < 6 mm on axial images
  - Soleus muscle may be low-lying and extend nearly to calcaneus
- Plantaris
  - Origin: Posterior margin of lateral femoral condyle
  - Insertion: Posterior process calcaneus, medial to Achilles
  - Action: Plantar flexion of foot

Deep Posterior Compartment: Innervation by Tibial N.
- Posterior tibial
  - Origin: Posterior tibia, fibula, and interosseous membrane
  - Insertion: Median eminence of navicular
    - Small slips extend anteriorly to 1st-3rd cuneiforms, cuboid, 2nd-4th metatarsals (± 5th metatarsal)
  - Action: Inversion, plantar flexion of foot
- Flexor digitorum longus
  - Origin: Posterior tibia and intermuscular septum with posterior tibial muscle
  - Note: Crosses lateral to posterior tibial muscle above ankle
  - Insertion: 2nd-5th toes
  - Quadratus plantae inserts onto it, flexor digitorum brevis slips arise from it
- Flexor hallucis longus
  - Origin: Posterior fibula and interosseous membrane
  - Insertion: Distal phalanx of 1st toe
  - Action: Plantar flexion of 1st toe
  - Note: Communicates with ankle joint; fluid in tendon sheath is normal
  - Note: Intersects with flexor digitorum longus tendon at master knot of Henry, in midfoot

Ankle Tendons

GRAPHICS: LATERAL ANKLE TENDONS AND SHEATHS

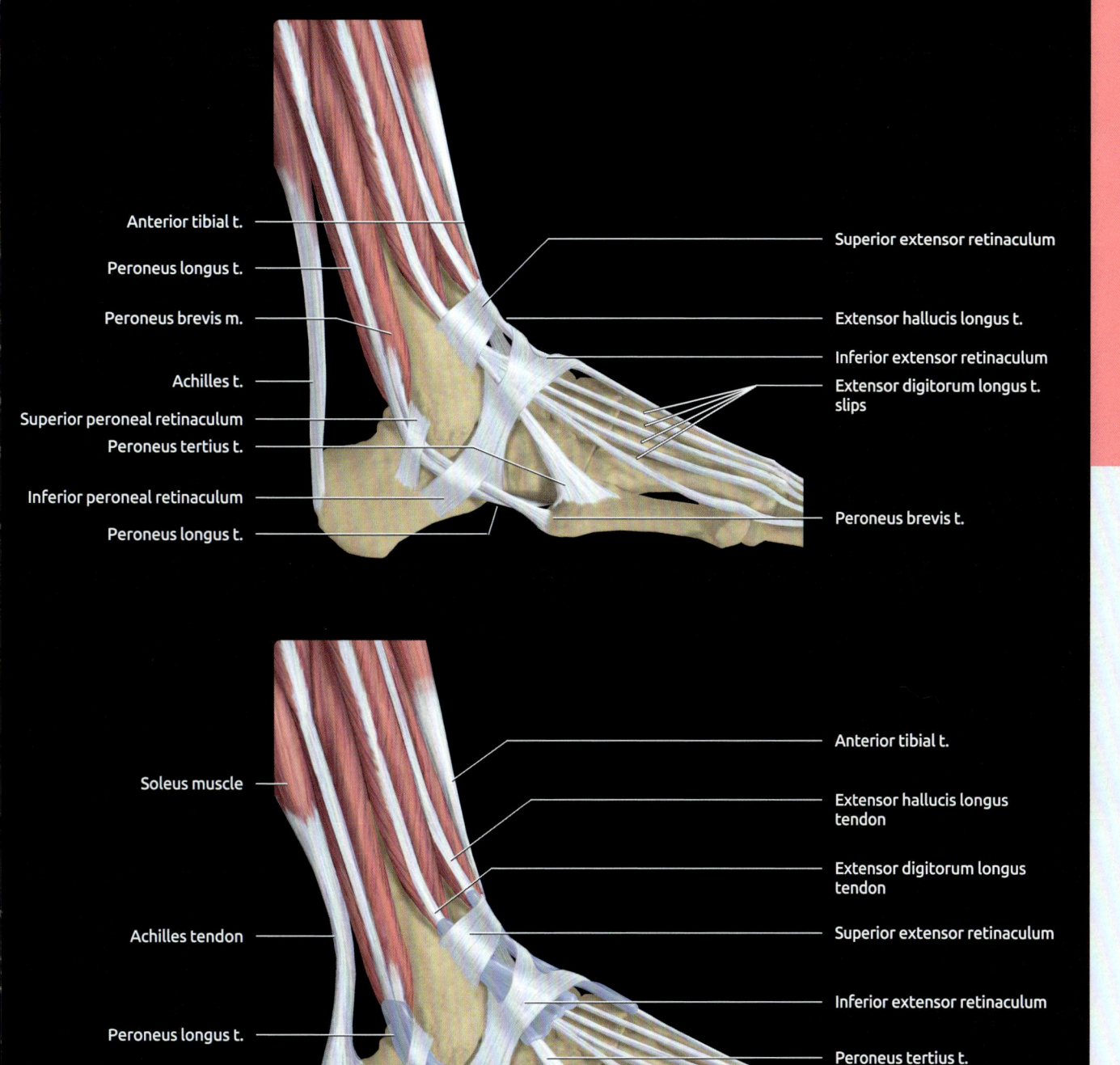

Top image labels:
- Anterior tibial t.
- Peroneus longus t.
- Peroneus brevis m.
- Achilles t.
- Superior peroneal retinaculum
- Peroneus tertius t.
- Inferior peroneal retinaculum
- Peroneus longus t.
- Superior extensor retinaculum
- Extensor hallucis longus t.
- Inferior extensor retinaculum
- Extensor digitorum longus t. slips
- Peroneus brevis t.

Bottom image labels:
- Soleus muscle
- Achilles tendon
- Peroneus longus t.
- Superior peroneal retinaculum
- Peroneus brevis t.
- Anterior tibial t.
- Extensor hallucis longus tendon
- Extensor digitorum longus tendon
- Superior extensor retinaculum
- Inferior extensor retinaculum
- Peroneus tertius t.
- Inferior peroneal retinaculum

(**Top**) *Lateral view shows how the peroneus brevis and peroneus longus tendons descend posterior to the fibula, maintained within the retromalleolar groove by the superior peroneal retinaculum and continue along the lateral wall of calcaneus, held in place by the inferior peroneal retinaculum. Fibers of the inferior peroneal retinaculum insert and separate the 2 tendons. The peroneus longus tendon curves around the cuboid to enter the sole of the foot. Both the peroneus brevis and peroneus tertius tendons insert on the 5th metatarsal base.* (**Bottom**) *Lateral view shows the tendon sheaths, which provide tendons with vascularity, smooth gliding, and greater freedom of movement. The Achilles tendon is the only ankle tendon without a tendon sheath; it is surrounded by paratenon. The peroneal tendons share a common sheath above the inferior peroneal retinaculum. More distally each tendon is enveloped by its own sheath. The peroneus longus tendon has a 2nd sheath under the sole of the foot.*

Ankle Tendons

GRAPHICS: TENDONS OF ANKLE

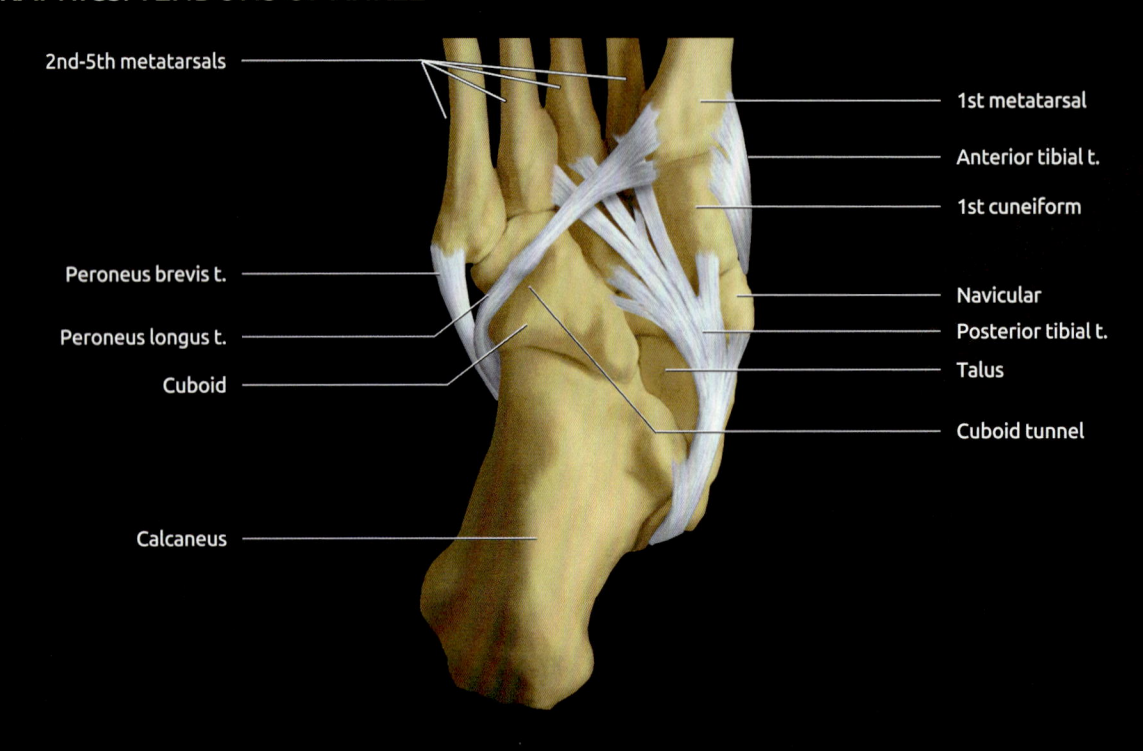

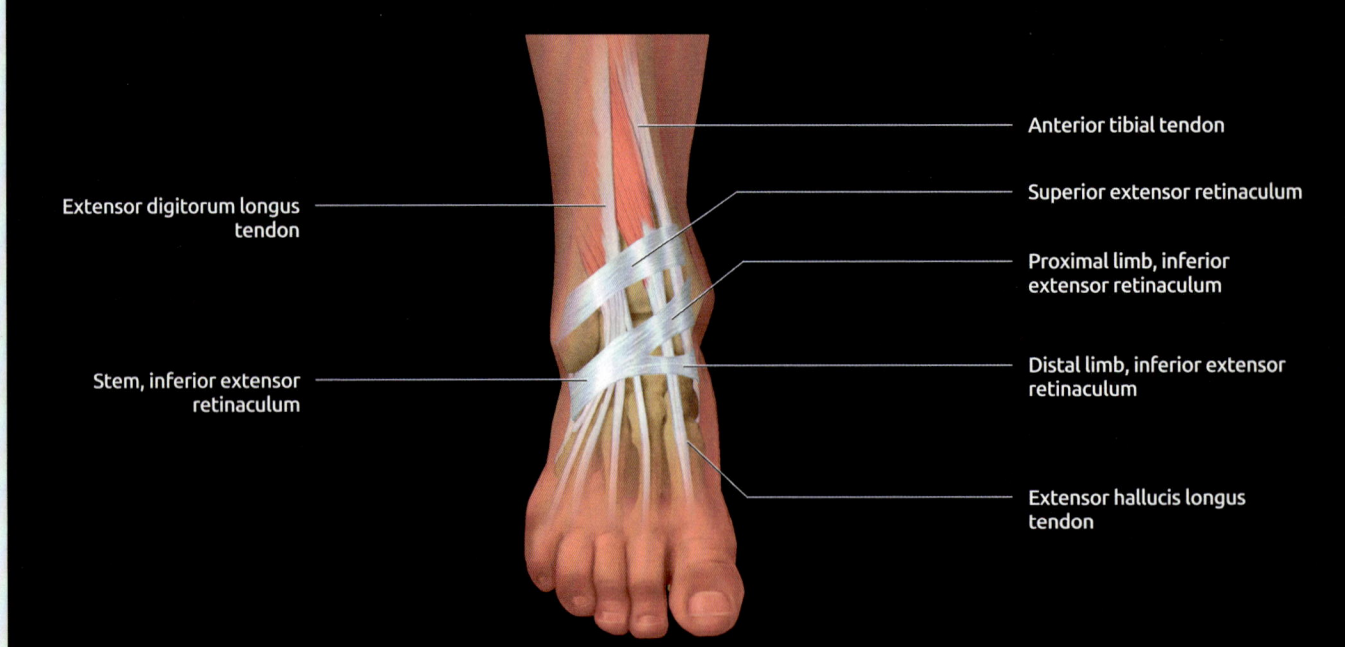

(Top) Graphic shows the insertions of long tendons on the plantar foot. The posterior tibial tendon inserts on all the tarsal bones (excluding talus) and on 2nd-4th metatarsal bases. The posterior and anterior tibial tendons and peroneus longus tendon insertions together form a sling supporting the medial longitudinal arch. (Bottom) Anterior view shows the extrinsic tendons held by the superior and inferior extensor retinacula and extending to their insertions.

Ankle Tendons

GRAPHICS: TENDONS AND SHEATHS

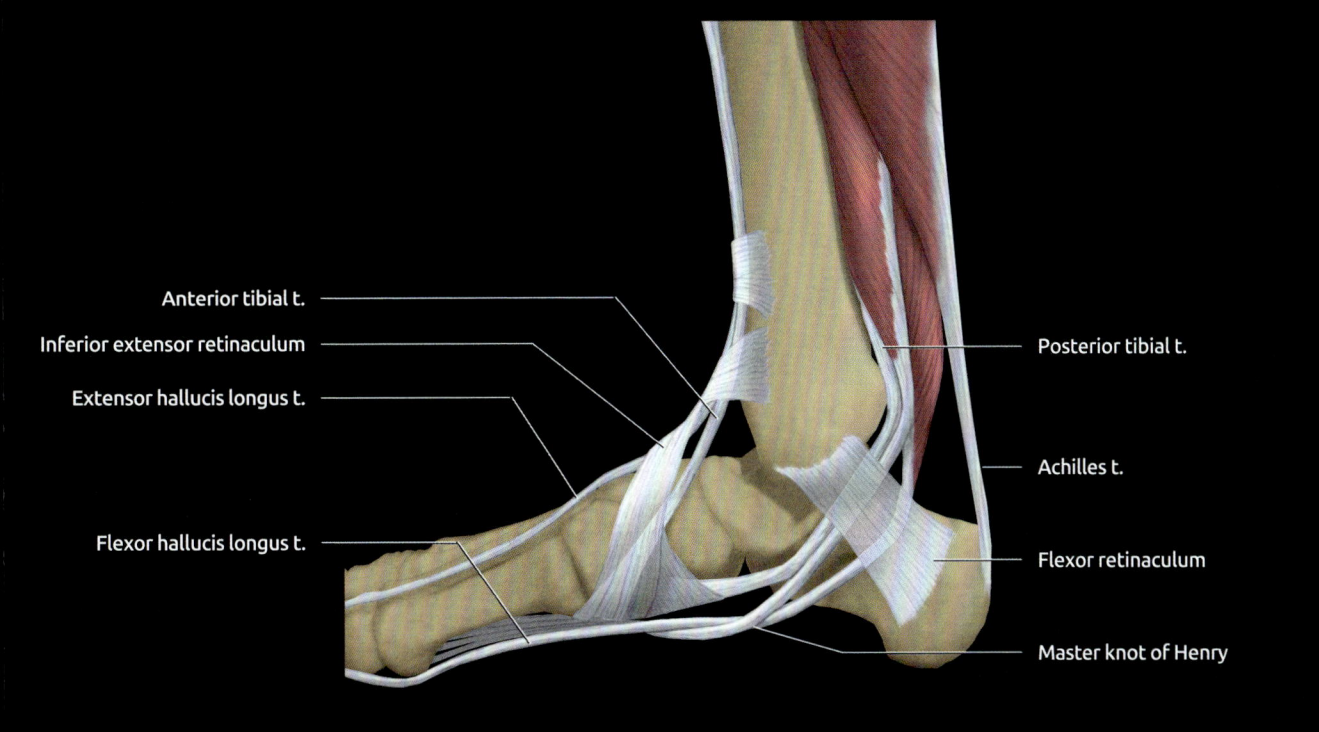

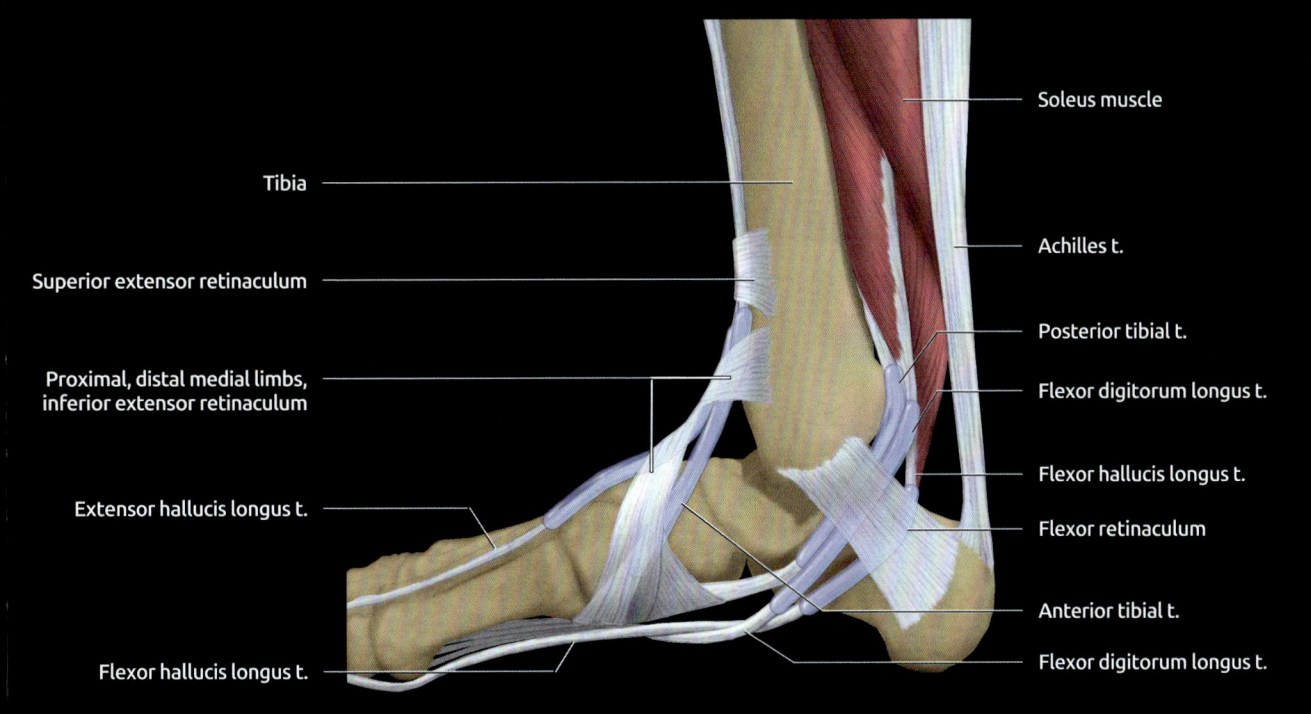

(Top) Medial view shows the posterior tibial, flexor digitorum longus, and flexor hallucis longus tendons traversing under the flexor retinaculum within the tarsal tunnel. The flexor digitorum longus and flexor hallucis longus tendons cross each other under the navicular. The extensor tendons descend deep to the extensor retinacula. (Bottom) The sheath of posterior tibial tendon ends ~ 1-2 cm proximal to its navicular insertion. Minimal tendon sheath fluid is normal except in flexor hallucis longus sheath where a large amount of fluid is common due to normal communication with ankle joint.

Ankle Tendons

ACHILLES TENDON, AXIAL MR

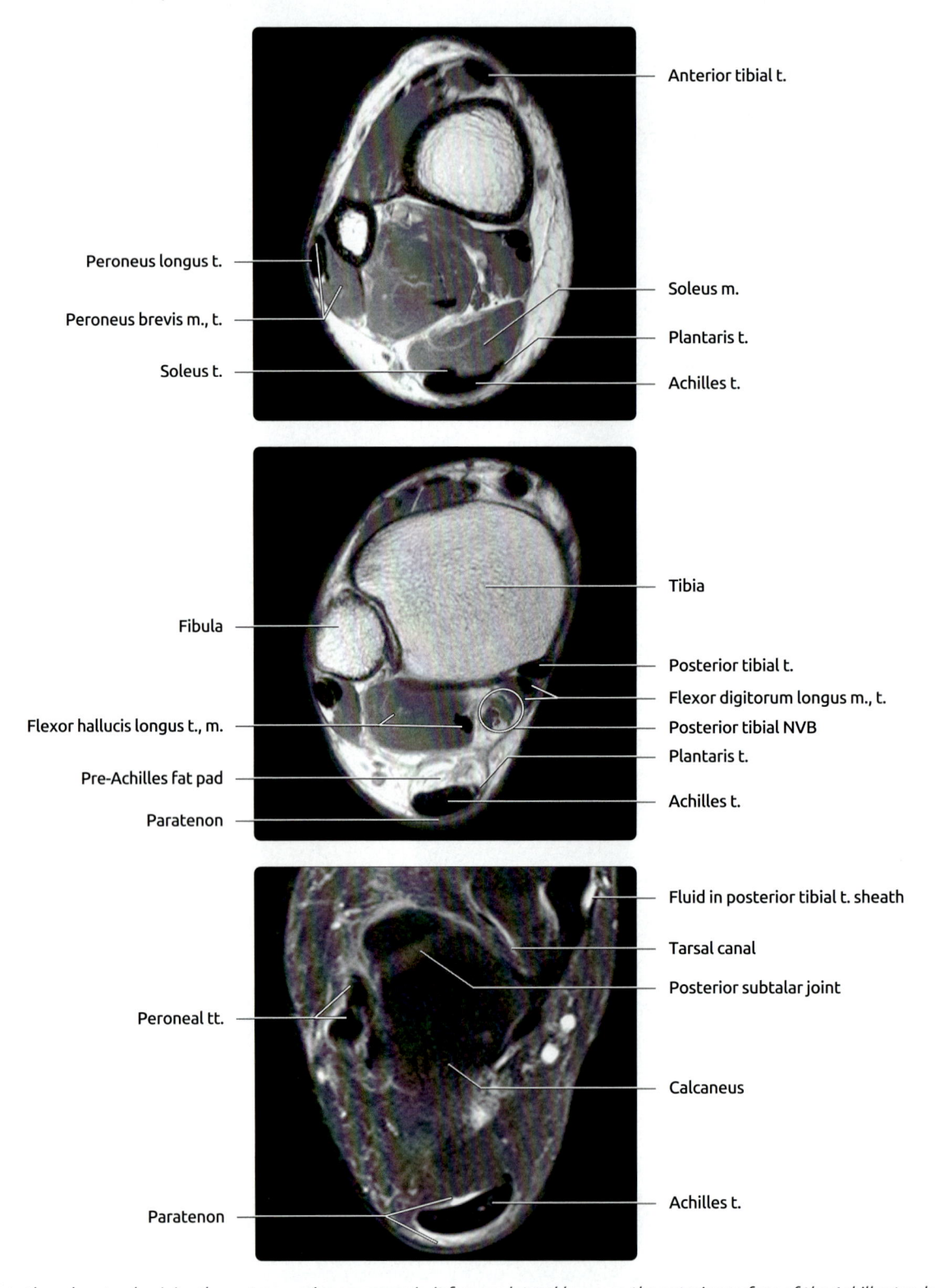

Labels (top image): Peroneus longus t.; Peroneus brevis m., t.; Soleus t.; Anterior tibial t.; Soleus m.; Plantaris t.; Achilles t.

Labels (middle image): Fibula; Flexor hallucis longus t., m.; Pre-Achilles fat pad; Paratenon; Tibia; Posterior tibial t.; Flexor digitorum longus m., t.; Posterior tibial NVB; Plantaris t.; Achilles t.

Labels (bottom image): Peroneal tt.; Paratenon; Fluid in posterior tibial t. sheath; Tarsal canal; Posterior subtalar joint; Calcaneus; Achilles t.

(**Top**) As the soleus tendon joins the gastrocnemius aponeurosis, it forms a lateral bump on the anterior surface of the Achilles tendon, as seen on this axial image. The Achilles tendon spirals as it descends down the calf so that the gastrocnemius contribution is mainly on the lateral and posterior surface of the tendon. (**Middle**) The anterior surface of the Achilles tendon is now flat to slightly concave. Note the subtle normal heterogeneity of the tendon. The large pre-Achilles (Kager) fat pad separates the Achilles tendon from the deep posterior compartment tendons. This fat pad is typically traversed by fine, low-signal vessels and septa. Note the plantaris tendon descending along the medial aspect of the Achilles tendon. (**Bottom**) Axial PD FS MR shows the paratenon, the tissue surrounding the Achilles tendon in lieu of a tendon sheath. Note that the tendon has a normal, concave anterior contour and thickness (< 6 mm). There is also a small amount of fluid in the posterior tibial tendon sheath, an incidental finding.

Ankle Tendons

ACHILLES TENDON, AXIAL MR

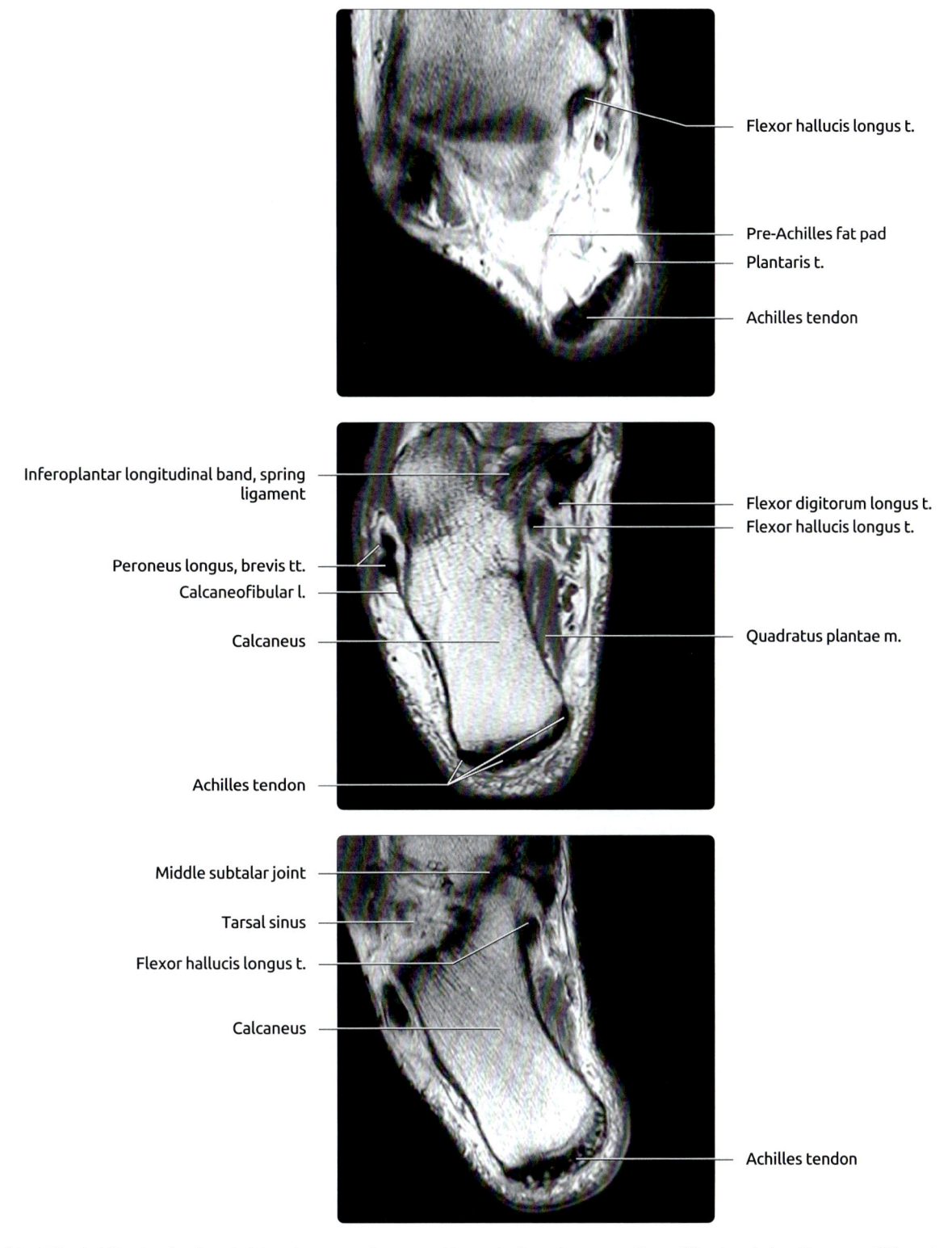

(Top) The Achilles tendon inserts into a large rough area on the posterior calcaneus, a few millimeters below the apex of the calcaneal tuberosity. The tendon develops a flat contour ~ 4 cm above its insertion as seen in this image. Note normal heterogeneity of the tendon. The tendon may be cartilaginous at its very distal aspect. *(Middle)* Note the broad insertion of the Achilles tendon to the calcaneus. *(Bottom)* Note the interdigitation of the bone and tendon at the insertion of the Achilles tendon to the calcaneus.

of the Ankle Tendons

ACHILLES TENDON, SAGITTAL MR

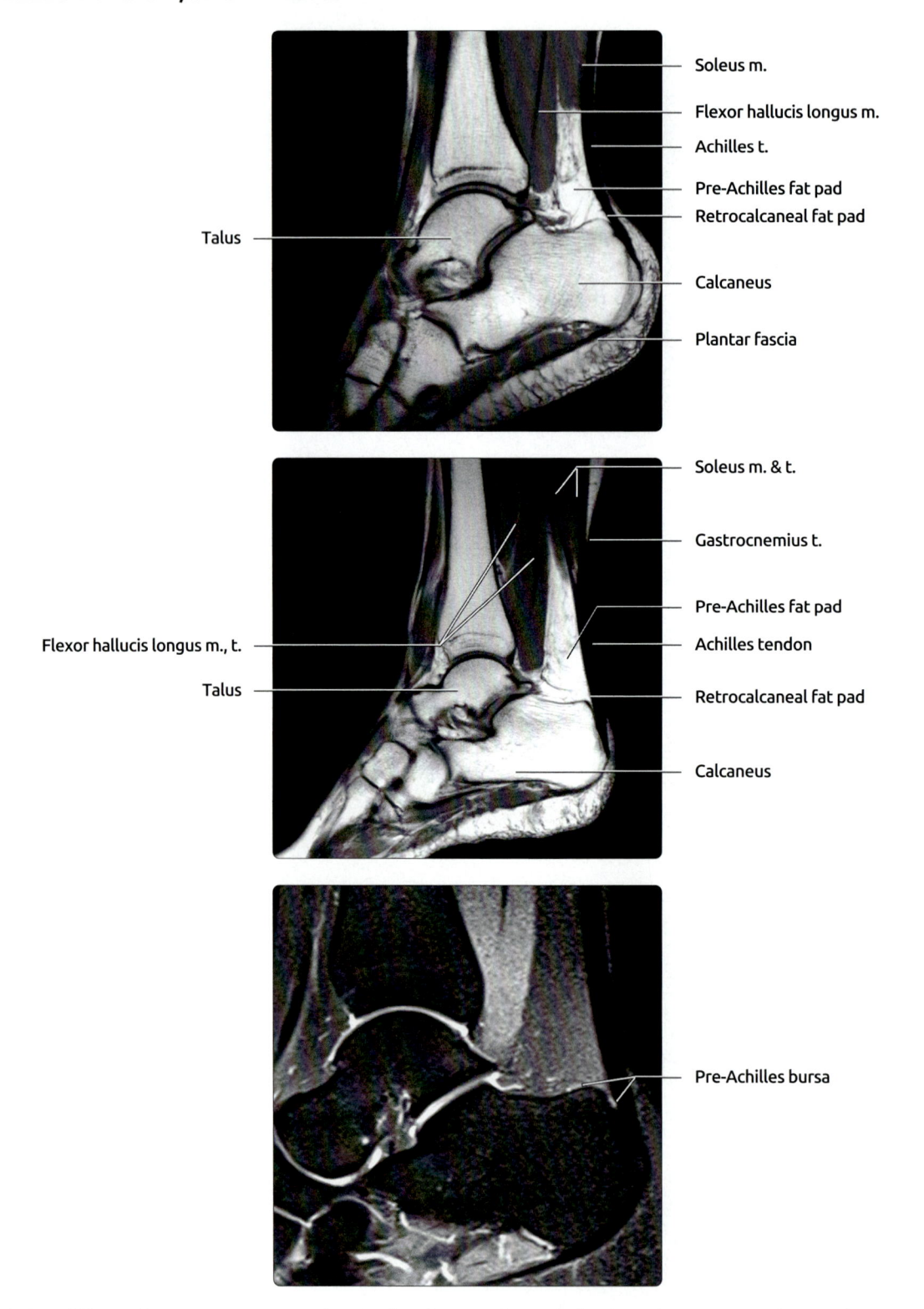

Labels (Top): Talus; Soleus m.; Flexor hallucis longus m.; Achilles t.; Pre-Achilles fat pad; Retrocalcaneal fat pad; Calcaneus; Plantar fascia

Labels (Middle): Flexor hallucis longus m., t.; Talus; Soleus m. & t.; Gastrocnemius t.; Pre-Achilles fat pad; Achilles tendon; Retrocalcaneal fat pad; Calcaneus

Labels (Bottom): Pre-Achilles bursa

(Top) The Achilles tendon measures ~ 15 cm in length. The soleus muscle may be low-lying, however, extending nearly to the tendon insertion on the calcaneus (not seen in this case). (Middle) Note the merger of the soleus tendon with the gastrocnemius tendon/aponeurosis. Tears of the Achilles tendon typically occur 2-6 cm above the insertion of the Achilles tendon, an area that is well seen on routine sagittal ankle images. Tears of the Achilles musculotendinous junction, however, may require imaging more proximally. (Bottom) The pre-Achilles bursa is also known as the retrocalcaneal bursa. It is normal to see a small amount of fluid in the bursa, as shown here. The retro-Achilles bursa is an adventitious bursa due to impingement of the heel, usually related to shoes.

Ankle Tendons

POSTERIOR TIBIAL TENDON, AXIAL MR

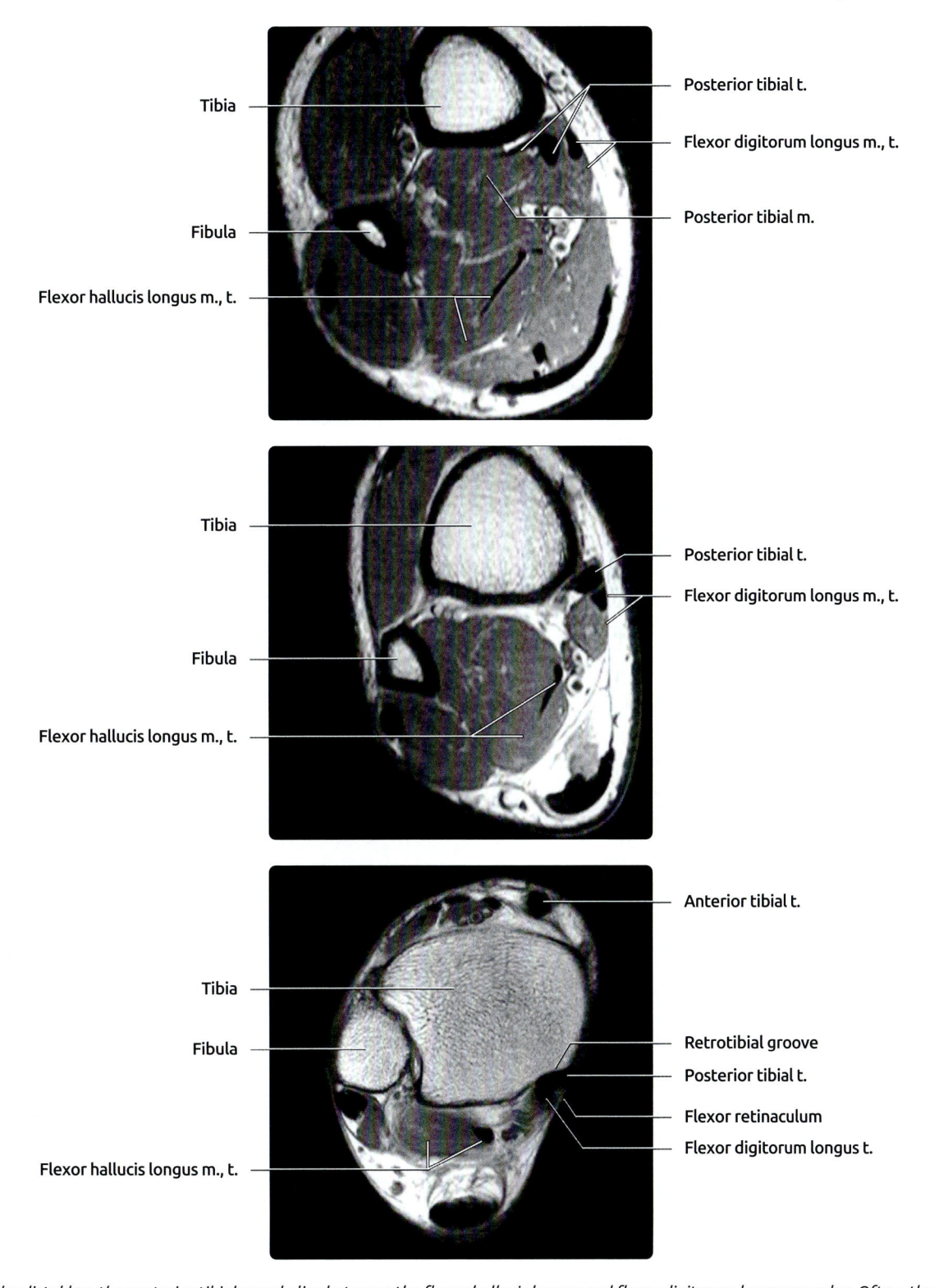

Top image labels: Tibia; Fibula; Flexor hallucis longus m., t.; Posterior tibial t.; Flexor digitorum longus m., t.; Posterior tibial m.

Middle image labels: Tibia; Fibula; Flexor hallucis longus m., t.; Posterior tibial t.; Flexor digitorum longus m., t.

Bottom image labels: Tibia; Fibula; Flexor hallucis longus m., t.; Anterior tibial t.; Retrotibial groove; Posterior tibial t.; Flexor retinaculum; Flexor digitorum longus t.

(Top) In the distal leg, the posterior tibial muscle lies between the flexor hallucis longus and flexor digitorum longus muscles. Often, the muscle has 2 tendinous slips (as seen here), which typically fuse into 1 slip by the time the tendon reaches the ankle joint. Occasionally, the 2 tendon slips are still seen at the ankle joint and should not be mistaken for a torn tendon. (Middle) A few cm above ankle joint, the posterior tibial tendon crosses deep to the flexor digitorum longus tendon to become the most medial tendon of the deep posterior compartment. (Bottom) Just above the ankle joint, the posterior tibial and flexor digitorum longus tendon lie deep to the flexor retinaculum, within a common retrotibial groove, posterior to the tibia and medial malleolus. Each tendon, however, is enclosed within its own separate tendon sheath. The flexor retinaculum holds the tendons in place within the retrotibial groove. Posterior tibial tendon is 2x the size of the flexor digitorum longus tendon.

Ankle Tendons

POSTERIOR TIBIAL TENDON, CORONAL MR

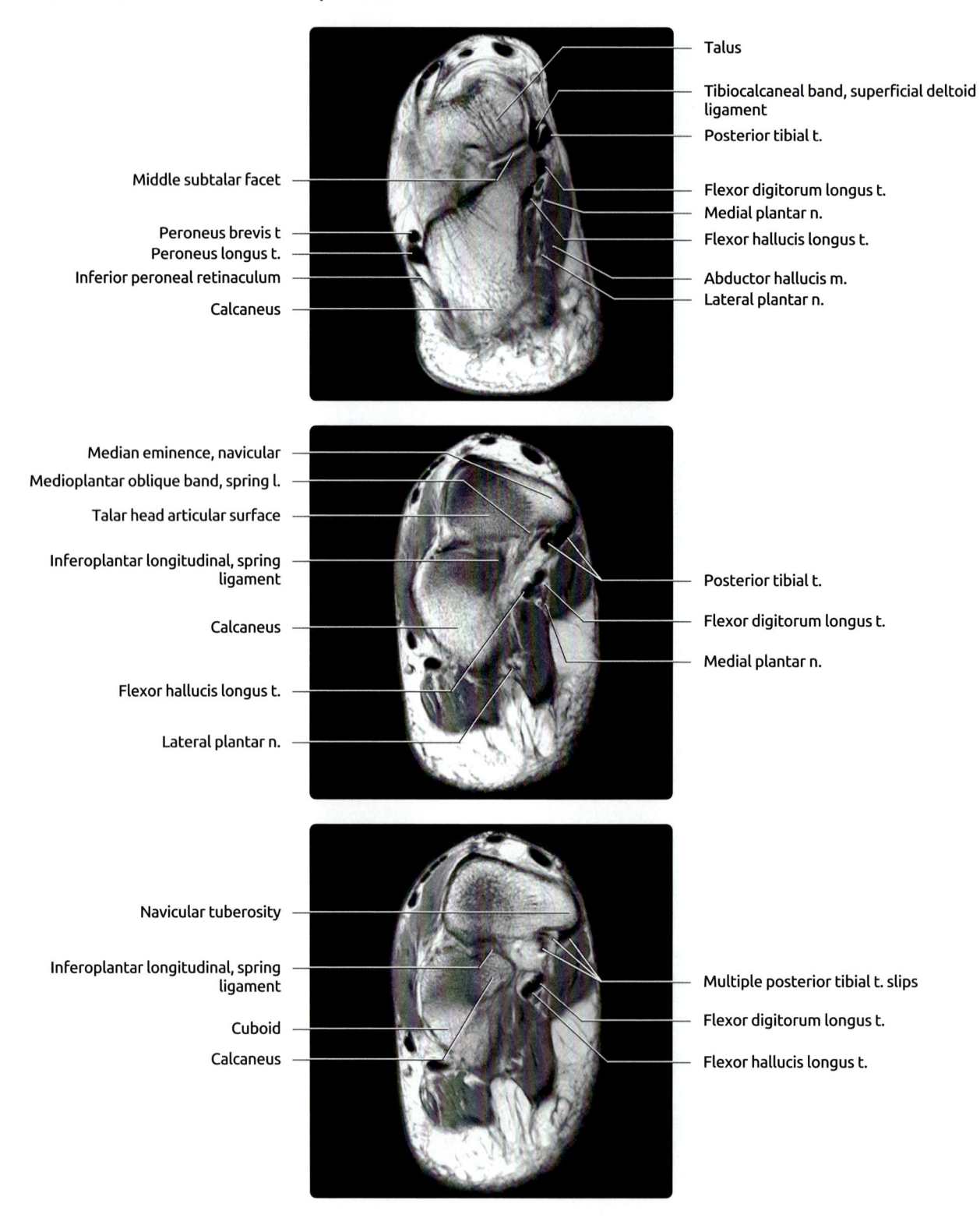

Labels (top image):
- Talus
- Tibiocalcaneal band, superficial deltoid ligament
- Posterior tibial t.
- Flexor digitorum longus t.
- Medial plantar n.
- Flexor hallucis longus t.
- Abductor hallucis m.
- Lateral plantar n.
- Middle subtalar facet
- Peroneus brevis t
- Peroneus longus t.
- Inferior peroneal retinaculum
- Calcaneus

Labels (middle image):
- Median eminence, navicular
- Medioplantar oblique band, spring l.
- Talar head articular surface
- Inferoplantar longitudinal, spring ligament
- Calcaneus
- Flexor hallucis longus t.
- Lateral plantar n.
- Posterior tibial t.
- Flexor digitorum longus t.
- Medial plantar n.

Labels (bottom image):
- Navicular tuberosity
- Inferoplantar longitudinal, spring ligament
- Cuboid
- Calcaneus
- Multiple posterior tibial t. slips
- Flexor digitorum longus t.
- Flexor hallucis longus t.

(**Top**) *Coronal image through the hindfoot shows that as the posterior tibial tendon courses anteriorly, medial to the talar head, it lies superficial to the deltoid ligament.* (**Middle**) *In the foot, the posterior tibial tendon divides into 2 major components, as seen in this image: 1) larger, more medial division inserts directly into the navicular tuberosity and 2) lateral, smaller division inserts to all other tarsal bones (excluding talus), and 2nd-4th metatarsal bases. The posterior tibial tendon may appear heterogeneous at its navicular insertion due to magic angle phenomenon or partial volume averaging of tendon slips.* (**Bottom**) *Coronal T1WI MR is anterior to the main portion of the posterior tibial tendon onto the navicular. Several small slips are seen extending anteriorly.*

Ankle Tendons

POSTERIOR TIBIAL TENDON DISTAL SLIPS, MR

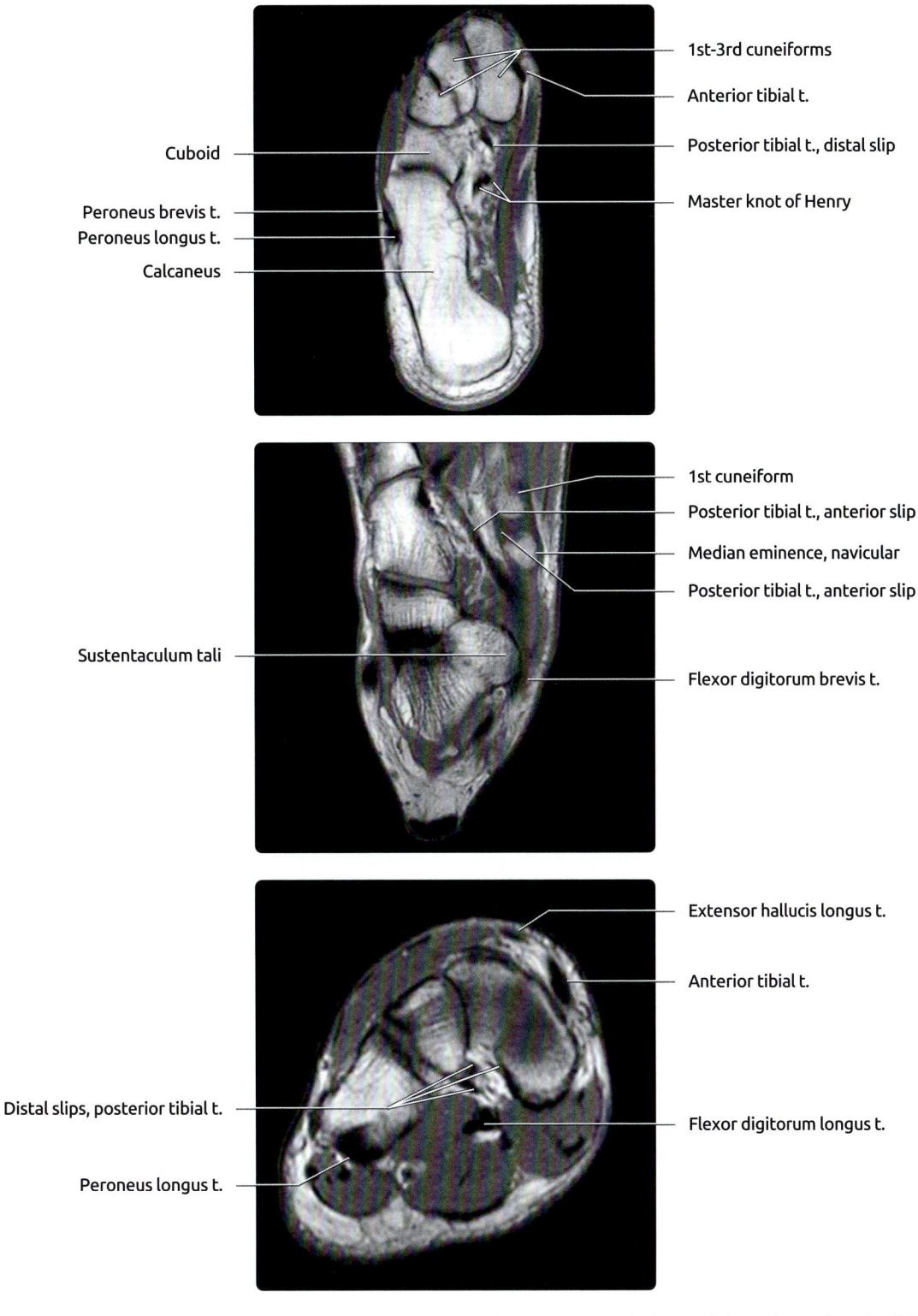

(Top) Oblique axial T1 MR shows one of the distal tibialis posterior tendon slips approaching the bases of the 2nd cuneiform. (Middle) Axial T1 MR shows that the lateral anterior slip of the posterior tibial tendon diverges from the main tendon insertion slightly before its insertion on the plantar margin of the median eminence of the navicular. A medial slip extends directly anterior from the plantar margin of the navicular, inserting on the 1st cuneiform. The role of these slips in maintaining the arch of the foot is evident on this image. (Bottom) Coronal T1 MR in the same patient shows 3 slips of tibial tendon attaching to 1st and 3rd cuneiforms. Anterior slips are variable in size.

Ankle Tendons

DISTAL POSTERIOR TIBIAL TENDON

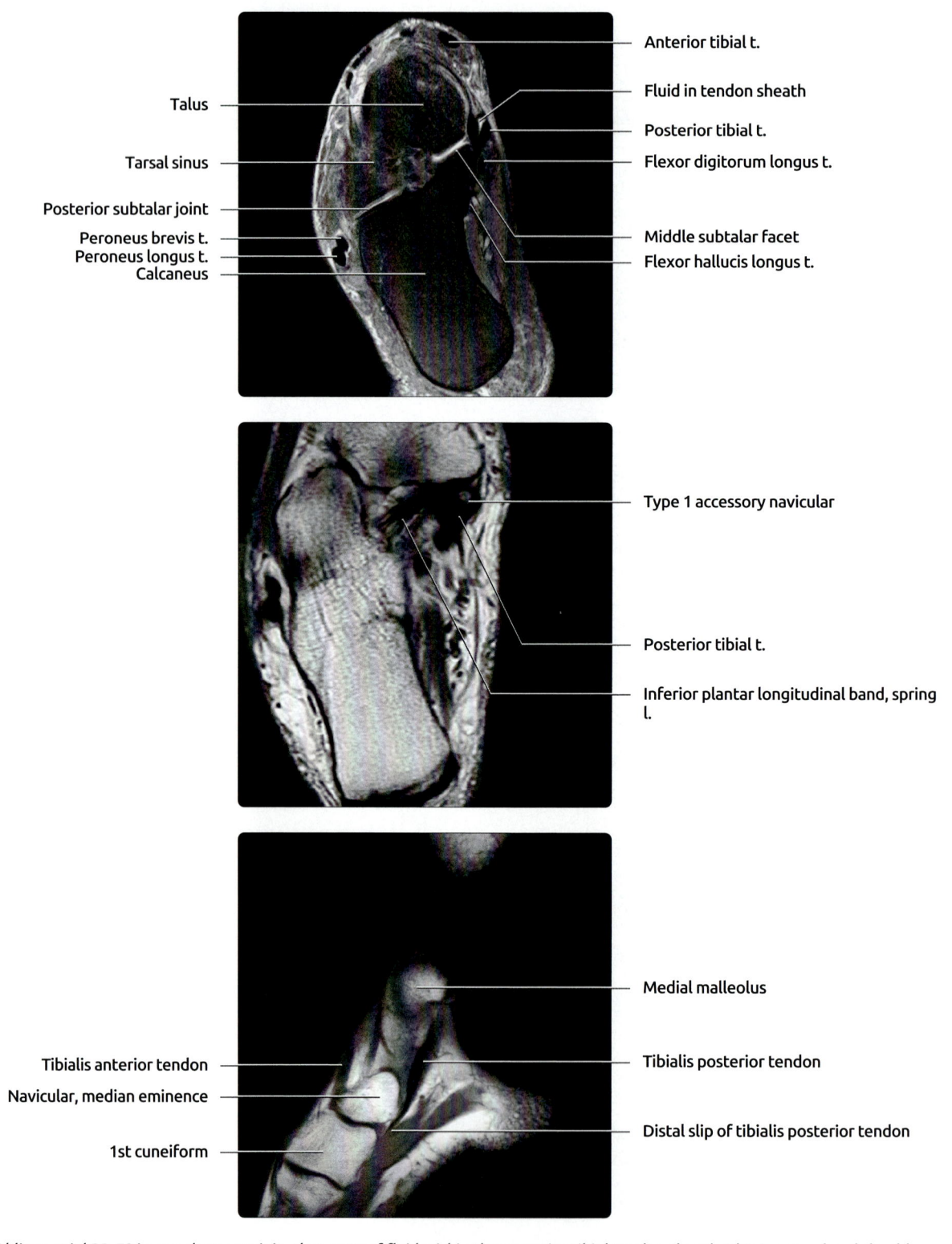

Talus
Tarsal sinus
Posterior subtalar joint
Peroneus brevis t.
Peroneus longus t.
Calcaneus

Anterior tibial t.
Fluid in tendon sheath
Posterior tibial t.
Flexor digitorum longus t.
Middle subtalar facet
Flexor hallucis longus t.

Type 1 accessory navicular

Posterior tibial t.

Inferior plantar longitudinal band, spring l.

Tibialis anterior tendon
Navicular, median eminence
1st cuneiform

Medial malleolus

Tibialis posterior tendon

Distal slip of tibialis posterior tendon

(Top) Oblique axial PD FS image shows a minimal amount of fluid within the posterior tibial tendon sheath. This is normal and should not be misinterpreted as tenosynovitis. (Middle) Heterogeneity at the insertion of the posterior tibial tendon may be related to the presence of type 1 accessory navicular. Three types of ossifications can occur at the navicular tuberosity (median eminence). Type 1 is a small sesamoid bone embedded in the posterior tibial tendon. Type 2 is a large triangular ossification representing a nonfused accessory ossification of the navicular. A synchondrosis is present between the ossification and the navicular. Most of the fibers of the posterior tibial tendon insert into the accessory ossification center rather than to the navicular; this weakens the tendon's actions and causes stress on the synchondrosis. Type 3 is a fused accessory ossification producing a cornuate navicular. (Bottom) Sagittal T1WI MR shows the posterior tibial tendon inserting on the inferior surface of the median eminence of the navicular.

Ankle Tendons

FLEXOR HALLUCIS LONGUS TENDON, AXIAL MR

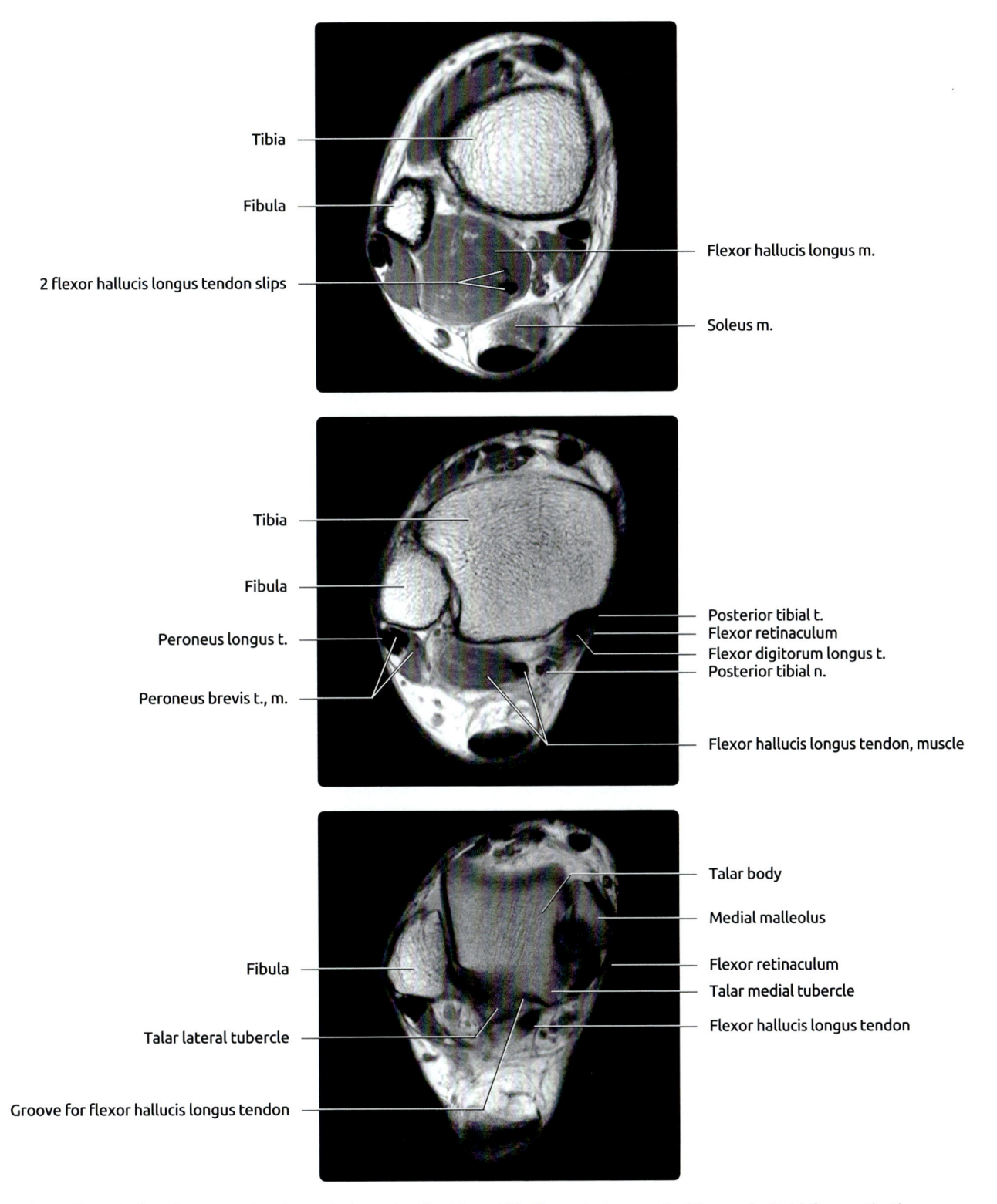

Labels (Top image): Tibia; Fibula; 2 flexor hallucis longus tendon slips; Flexor hallucis longus m.; Soleus m.

Labels (Middle image): Tibia; Fibula; Peroneus longus t.; Peroneus brevis t., m.; Posterior tibial t.; Flexor retinaculum; Flexor digitorum longus t.; Posterior tibial n.; Flexor hallucis longus tendon, muscle

Labels (Bottom image): Fibula; Talar lateral tubercle; Groove for flexor hallucis longus tendon; Talar body; Medial malleolus; Flexor retinaculum; Talar medial tubercle; Flexor hallucis longus tendon

(**Top**) *The flexor hallucis longus tendon descends down the distal leg within the posterior aspect of its muscle. Not infrequently, the tendon is formed by 2 major tendon slips, which usually merge into a single tendon above the ankle joint but sometimes remain separate quite far distally. The secondary irregularity and heterogeneity of the tendon should not be misinterpreted for disease.* (**Middle**) *The flexor hallucis longus tendon and muscle are seen just above the tibial plafond. The posterior tibial and flexor digitorum are purely tendinous at this level.* (**Bottom**) *The flexor hallucis longus tendon traverses 2 major tunnels in the ankle and hindfoot. The 1st tunnel is between the medial and lateral tubercles of the talus. A fibrous band converts the groove into a tunnel. The 2nd tunnel is under the sustentaculum tali of the calcaneus.*

Ankle Tendons

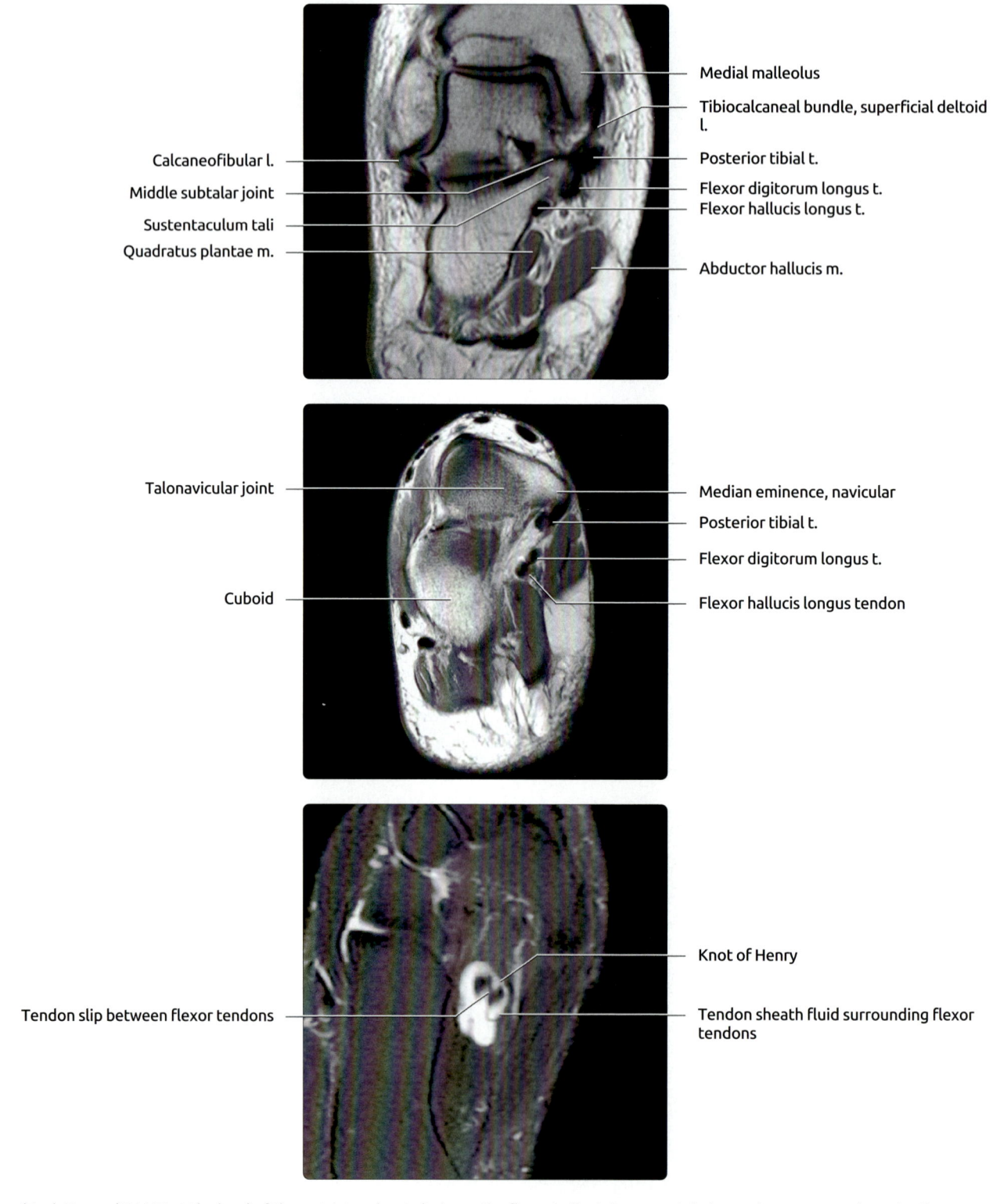

FLEXOR HALLUCIS LONGUS TENDON

Labels (Top image):
- Medial malleolus
- Tibiocalcaneal bundle, superficial deltoid l.
- Posterior tibial t.
- Flexor digitorum longus t.
- Flexor hallucis longus t.
- Abductor hallucis m.
- Calcaneofibular l.
- Middle subtalar joint
- Sustentaculum tali
- Quadratus plantae m.

Labels (Middle image):
- Talonavicular joint
- Cuboid
- Median eminence, navicular
- Posterior tibial t.
- Flexor digitorum longus t.
- Flexor hallucis longus tendon

Labels (Bottom image):
- Tendon slip between flexor tendons
- Knot of Henry
- Tendon sheath fluid surrounding flexor tendons

(Top) *Coronal T1 MR at the level of the sustentaculum tali shows the flexor hallucis longus t. inferior to the sustentaculum, the flexor digitorum longus at the medial margin of the sustentaculum, and the posterior tibial tendon the most superior of the tendons.* (Middle) *Plantar to the navicular tuberosity (median eminence), the flexor hallucis longus tendon 1st approaches and then crosses the flexor digitorum longus tendon at the master knot of Henry.* (Bottom) *Fluid within the flexor hallucis longus tendon sheath may extend quite far distally into the knot of Henry. This is typically an incidental finding and of no clinical significance. Isolated fluid in this area, however, without fluid proximal to it, may indicate tenosynovitis. The medial plantar nerve follows the flexor hallucis longus tendon and may be impinged upon by the fluid.*

Ankle Tendons

FLEXOR HALLUCIS LONGUS TENDON, CORONAL MR

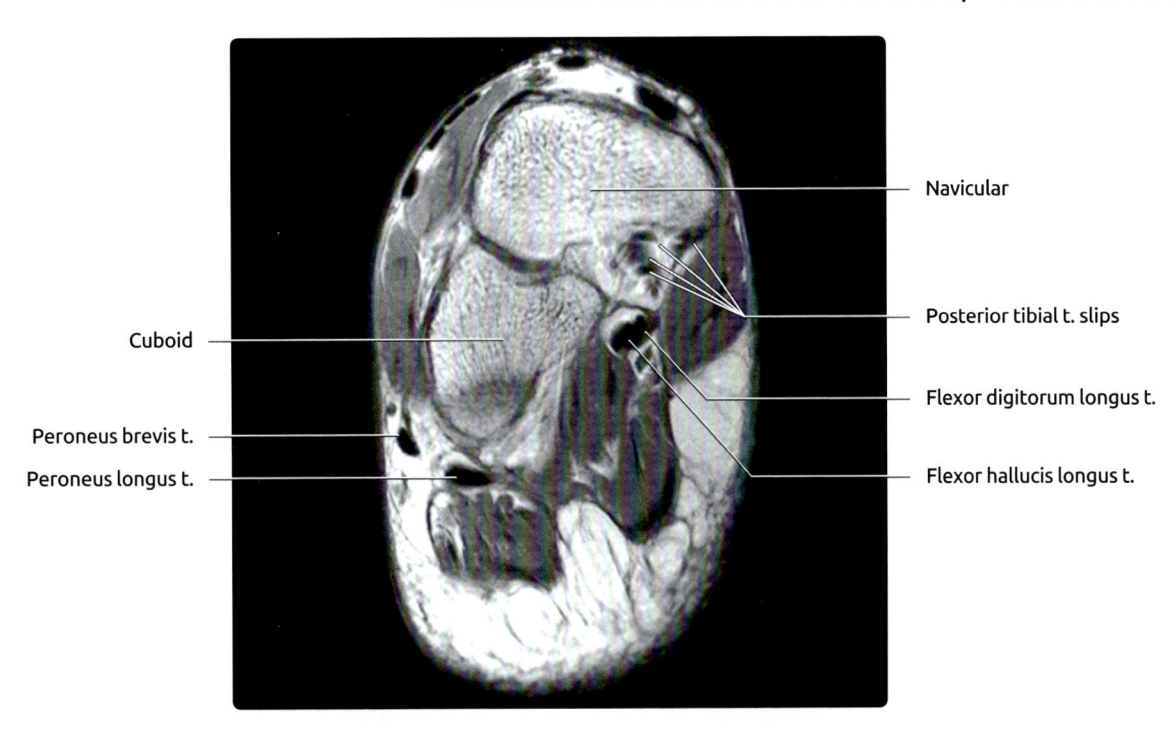

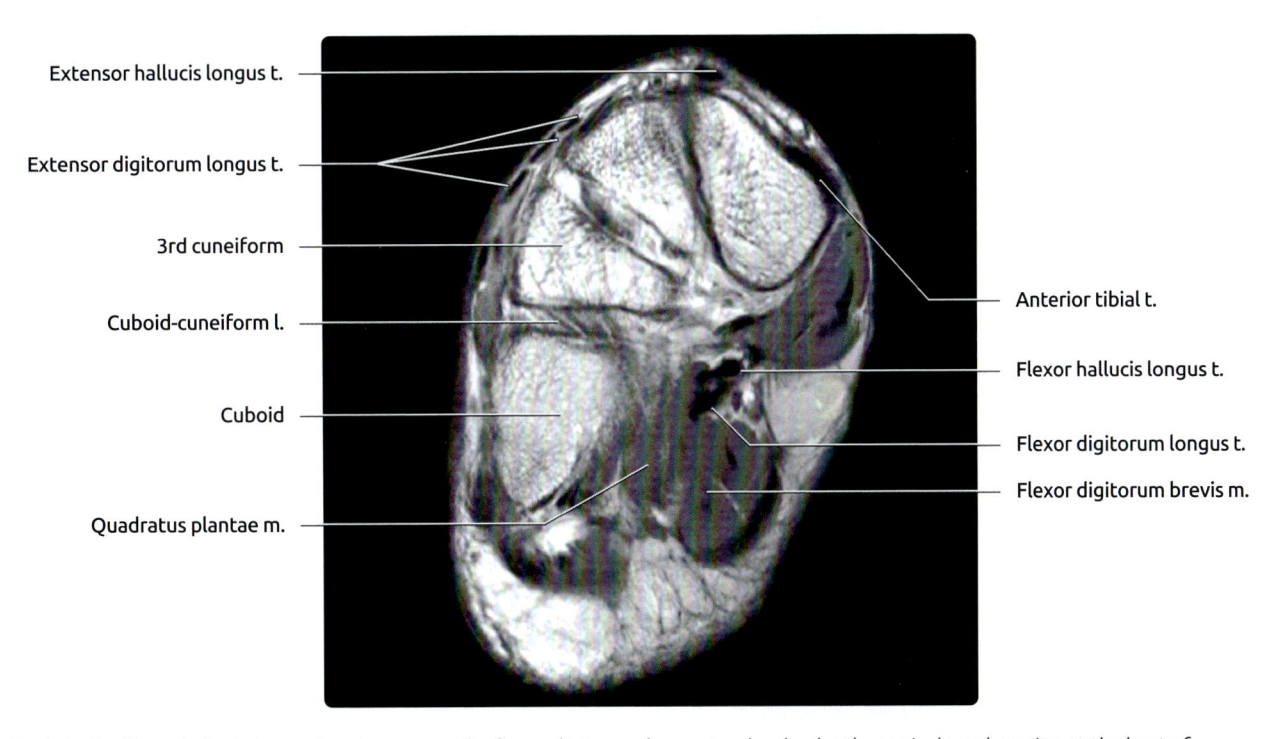

- Navicular
- Posterior tibial t. slips
- Cuboid
- Flexor digitorum longus t.
- Peroneus brevis t.
- Peroneus longus t.
- Flexor hallucis longus t.

- Extensor hallucis longus t.
- Extensor digitorum longus t.
- 3rd cuneiform
- Cuboid-cuneiform l.
- Anterior tibial t.
- Cuboid
- Flexor hallucis longus t.
- Flexor digitorum longus t.
- Flexor digitorum brevis m.
- Quadratus plantae m.

(Top) As the flexor hallucis longus tendon crosses the flexor digitorum longus tendon (under the navicular tuberosity, at the knot of Henry), it sends a fibrous slip to the latter tendon. This slip prevents the flexor hallucis longus tendon from significant proximal retraction if it tears distal to the knot of Henry. (Bottom) Distal to the knot of Henry, the flexor hallucis longus tendon is located superiorly and medially to the flexor digitorum longus tendon.

Ankle Tendons

FLEXOR HALLUCIS LONGUS TENDON

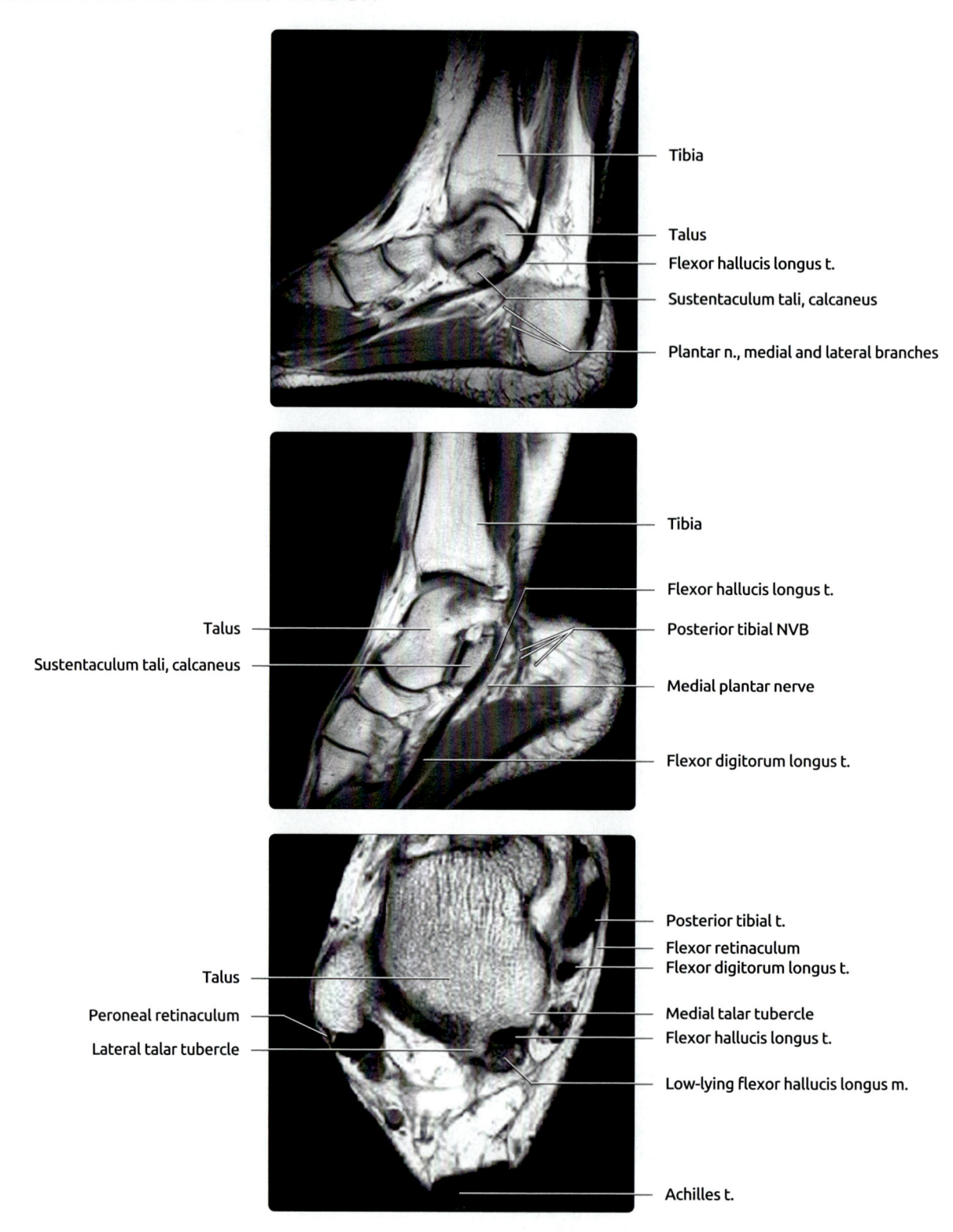

Tibia
Talus
Flexor hallucis longus t.
Sustentaculum tali, calcaneus
Plantar n., medial and lateral branches

Talus
Sustentaculum tali, calcaneus

Tibia
Flexor hallucis longus t.
Posterior tibial NVB
Medial plantar nerve
Flexor digitorum longus t.

Talus
Peroneal retinaculum
Lateral talar tubercle

Posterior tibial t.
Flexor retinaculum
Flexor digitorum longus t.
Medial talar tubercle
Flexor hallucis longus t.
Low-lying flexor hallucis longus m.
Achilles t.

(Top) The flexor hallucis longus tendon is well seen on sagittal images of the ankle as it descends under the sustentaculum tali. (Middle) Note that the distal flexor digitorum longus tendon is typically seen on the same sagittal image in which the flexor hallucis longus tendon is noted to descend under the sustentaculum tali. This is due to the crossing over of the tendons in the knot of Henry under the navicular tuberosity. Note also the medial plantar nerve's proximity to the flexor hallucis longus tendon. (Bottom) Typically, the muscle of the flexor hallucis longus extends to the ankle joint and is not seen at the level of the talar groove. In a low-lying flexor hallucis longus muscle, as in this patient, muscle tissue extends into the groove and may produce impingement symptoms.

Ankle Tendons

PERONEAL TENDONS, AXIAL MR

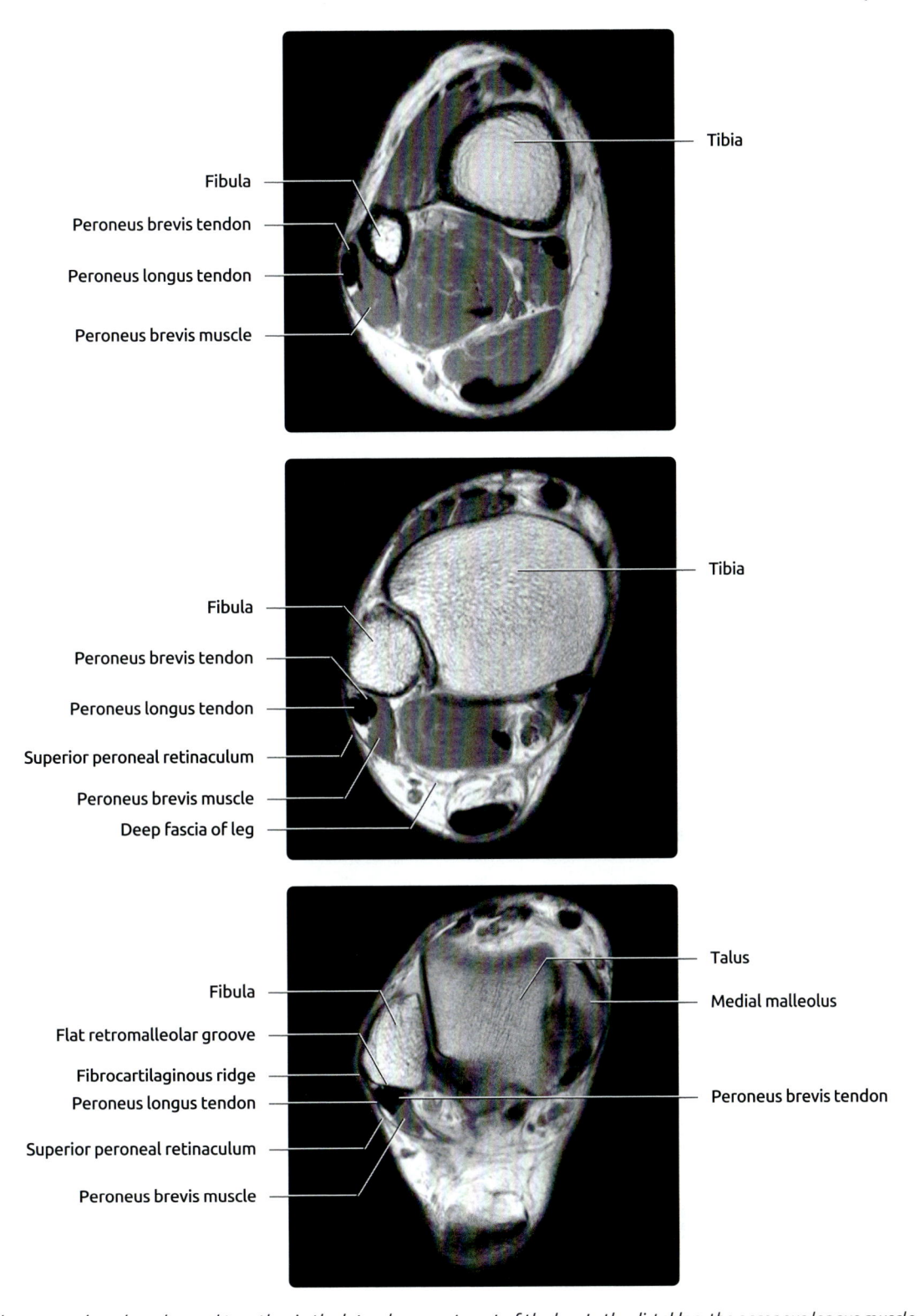

(Top) The peroneal tendons descend together in the lateral compartment of the leg. In the distal leg, the peroneus longus muscle has become entirely tendinous, while both muscle and tendon of the peroneus brevis are visualized. Note that in the distal leg, the peroneal tendons are lateral rather than posterior to the fibula; this should not be misinterpreted as subluxation of the tendons. (Middle) More distally, peroneal tendons lie directly posterior to the distal fibula. The peroneus brevis tendon is typically crescentic in shape and is located anteromedial to the peroneus longus tendon. The superior peroneal retinaculum extends from the distal fibula to calcaneus and deep leg fascia and maintains the peroneal tendons within the retromalleolar groove. (Bottom) The superior peroneal retinaculum is a reinforcement of the leg aponeurosis. It is seen as a low-signal band originating from the lateral distal fibula, at the retromalleolar groove, ~ 1 cm above the fibular tip. It can be followed to its insertion to the deep fascia of the leg.

Ankle Tendons

PERONEAL TENDONS, AXIAL MR

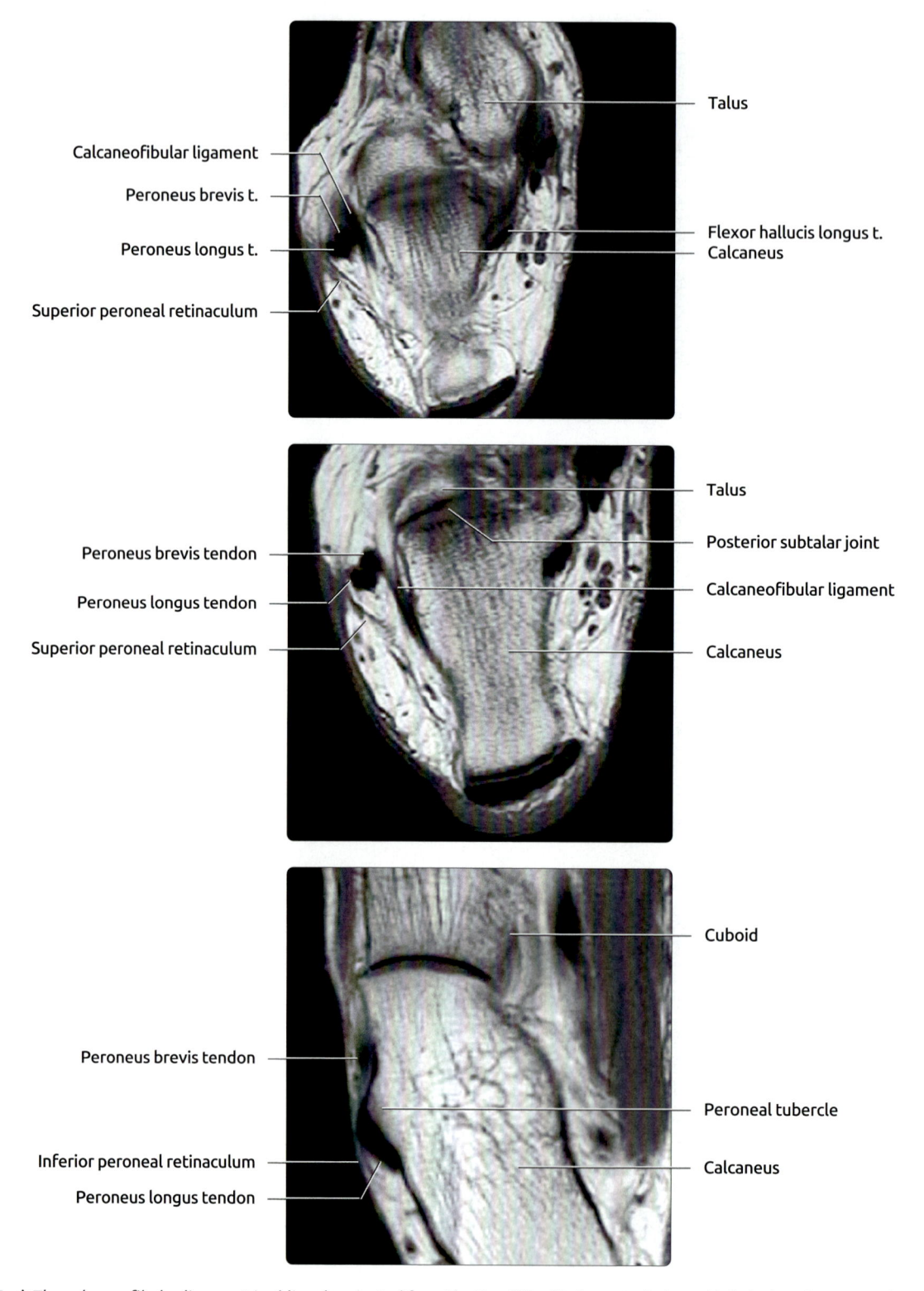

Calcaneofibular ligament
Peroneus brevis t.
Peroneus longus t.
Superior peroneal retinaculum

Talus
Flexor hallucis longus t.
Calcaneus

Peroneus brevis tendon
Peroneus longus tendon
Superior peroneal retinaculum

Talus
Posterior subtalar joint
Calcaneofibular ligament
Calcaneus

Peroneus brevis tendon
Inferior peroneal retinaculum
Peroneus longus tendon

Cuboid
Peroneal tubercle
Calcaneus

(Top) The calcaneofibular ligament is obliquely oriented from the tip of the fibula posteriorly and inferiorly. It inserts on the calcaneus deep to the peroneal tendons. (Middle) The peroneal retinaculum is superficial to the peroneal tendons, while the calcaneofibular ligament lies deep to the tendons. (Bottom) The peroneal tubercle, a normal variant, is a calcaneal wall protuberance that separates the peroneal tendons. Hypertrophy of the tubercle predisposes to peroneus longus tendon tear.

Ankle Tendons

PERONEAL TENDONS

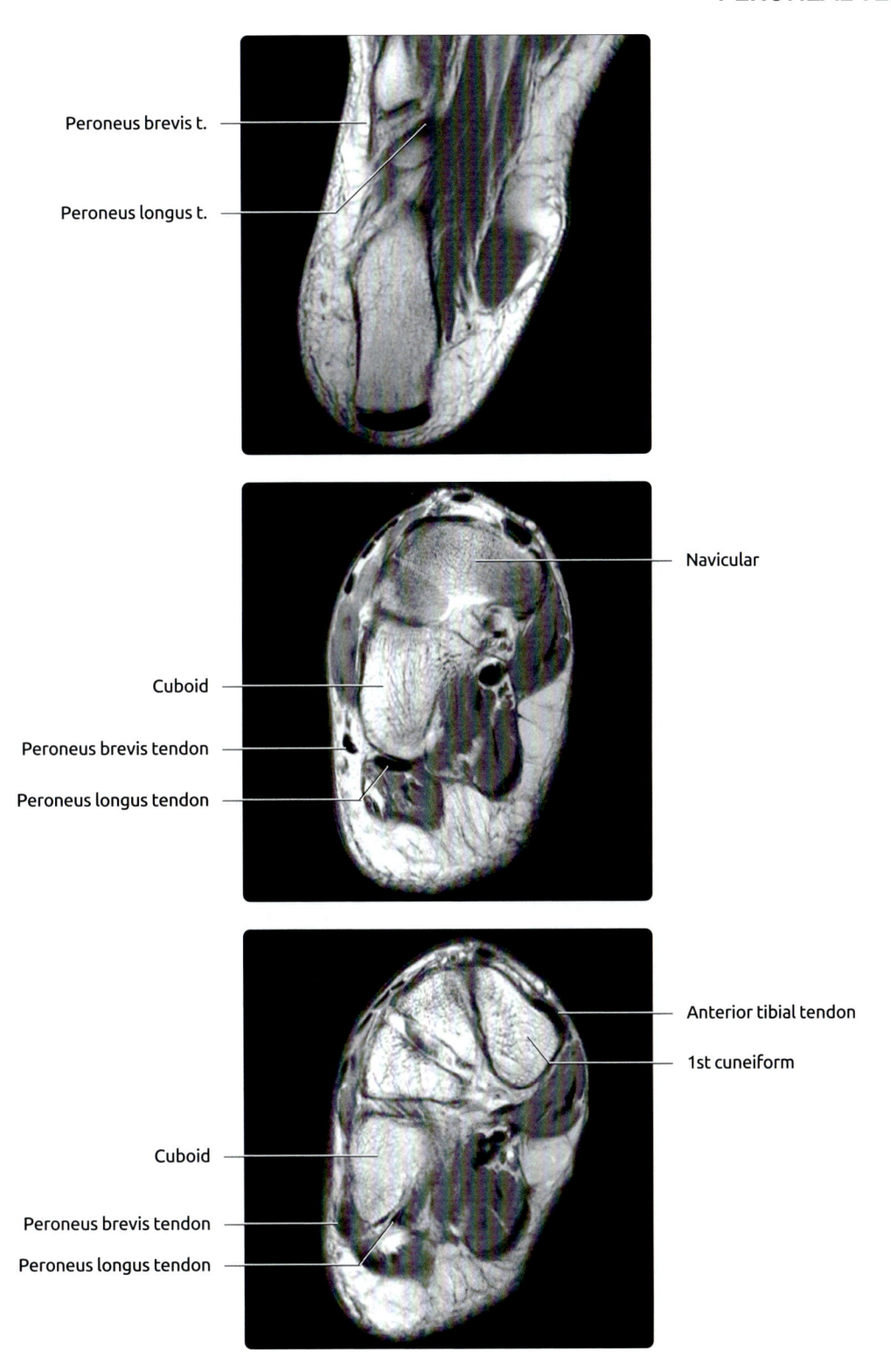

Peroneus brevis t.
Peroneus longus t.

Navicular
Cuboid
Peroneus brevis tendon
Peroneus longus tendon

Anterior tibial tendon
1st cuneiform
Cuboid
Peroneus brevis tendon
Peroneus longus tendon

(Top) Peroneus brevis tendon becomes a thin ribbon as it approaches its insertion on the styloid process of the 5th metatarsal. Peroneus longus tendon is seen coursing anteromedially in the cuboid sulcus toward its attachment on the medial plantar surface of the foot. *(Middle)* Coronal image shows the peroneus brevis tendon continuing toward its insertion on the 5th metatarsal base. The peroneus longus tendon enters the cuboid tunnel, plantar to the cuboid, and continues along the sole of the foot toward its insertion on 1st cuneiform and 1st metatarsal base. *(Bottom)* The distal course of the peroneus longus tendon along the plantar surface of the foot is best seen on short-axis midfoot images but may also be seen on distal axial images of the ankle. The tendon is often suboptimally seen on T1WI due to magic angle effect. Note the insertion of the anterior tibial tendon on the 1st cuneiform.

Ankle Tendons

PERONEAL TENDONS, CORONAL T2WI FS MR

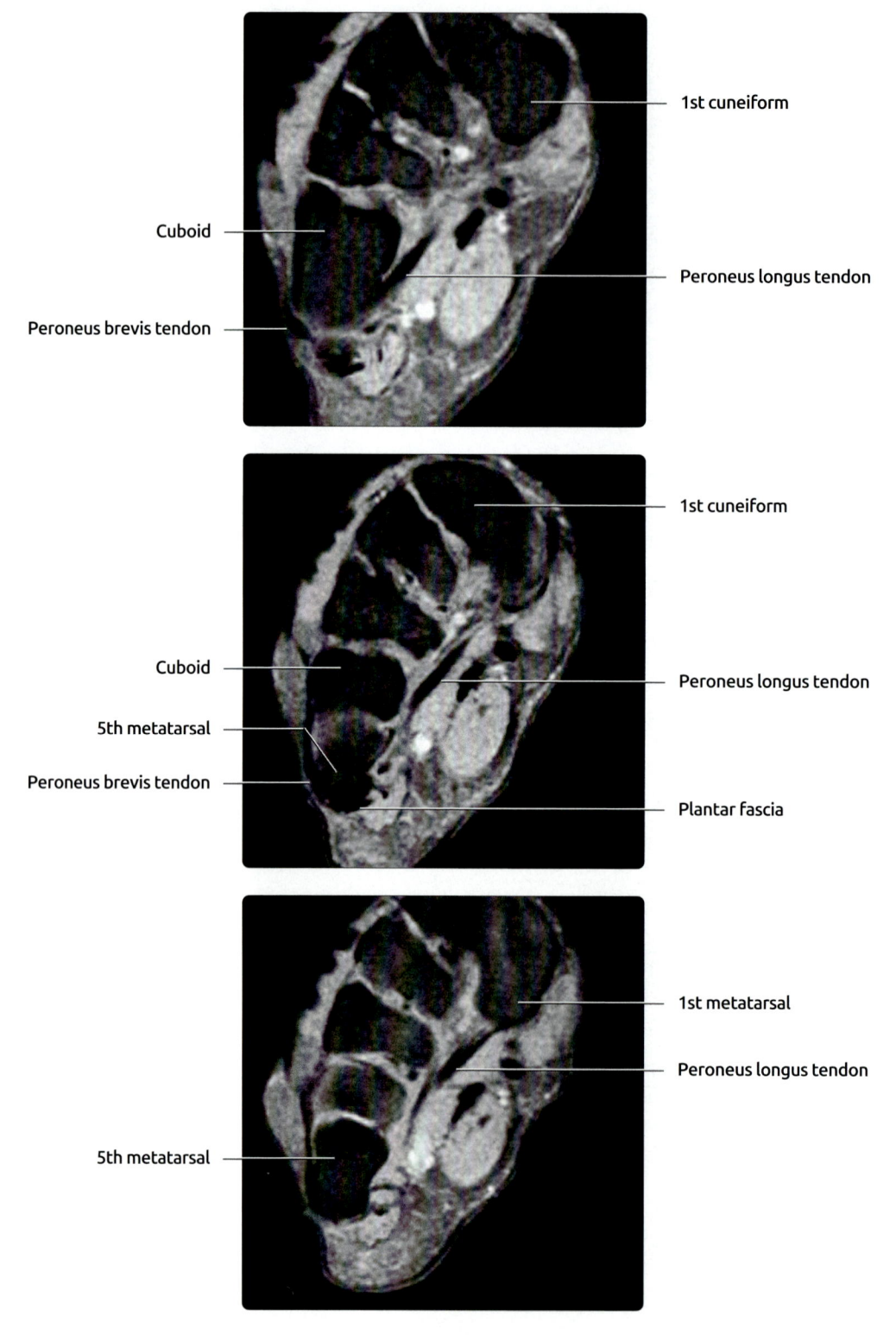

(Top) The course of the peroneus longus tendon along the plantar surface of the foot is frequently better seen on axial FS T2-weighted images due to the relative lack of the magic angle effect. (Middle) On a more distal axial image, the peroneus longus tendon continues deep to the 3rd compartment muscles. Note the insertion of the peroneus brevis tendon on the base of the 5th metatarsal. The peroneus brevis and plantar fascia insert onto the plantar base of the 5th metatarsal, while the peroneus tertius tendon inserts on the dorsal base of the 5th metatarsal. (Bottom) Note the normal striation of the very distal peroneus longus tendon as it divides into slips to several insertion sites.

Ankle Tendons

PERONEAL TENDONS, SAGITTAL MR

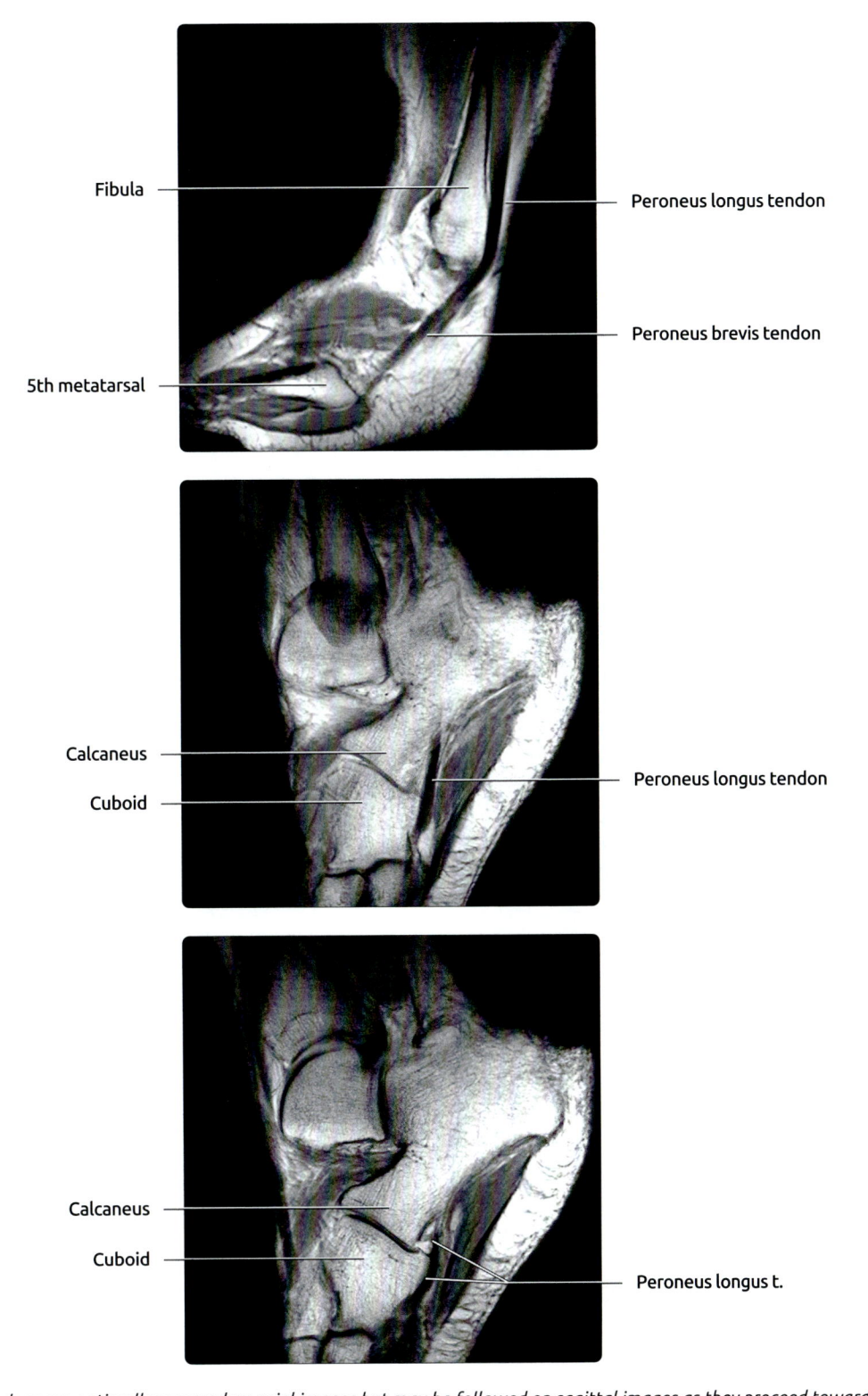

(Top) The peroneal tendons are optimally assessed on axial images but may be followed on sagittal images as they proceed toward their insertion sites. The peroneus brevis tendon is predisposed to friction and tearing as it descends within the fibular retromalleolar groove. **(Middle)** The peroneus longus tendon traverses within 2 fibroosseous tunnels. It 1st shares the retromalleolar groove with the peroneus brevis tendon. It then descends along the lateral wall of the calcaneus where it can undergo friction posterior to the peroneal tubercle. Its final tunnel is plantar to the cuboid within the cuboid tunnel. In this image, the peroneus longus tendon descends along the lateral wall of the calcaneus approaching its cuboid tunnel. **(Bottom)** In this image, the peroneus longus is seen starting to curve under the plantar surface of the cuboid to enter the cuboid tunnel.

Ankle Tendons

PERONEAL TENDONS

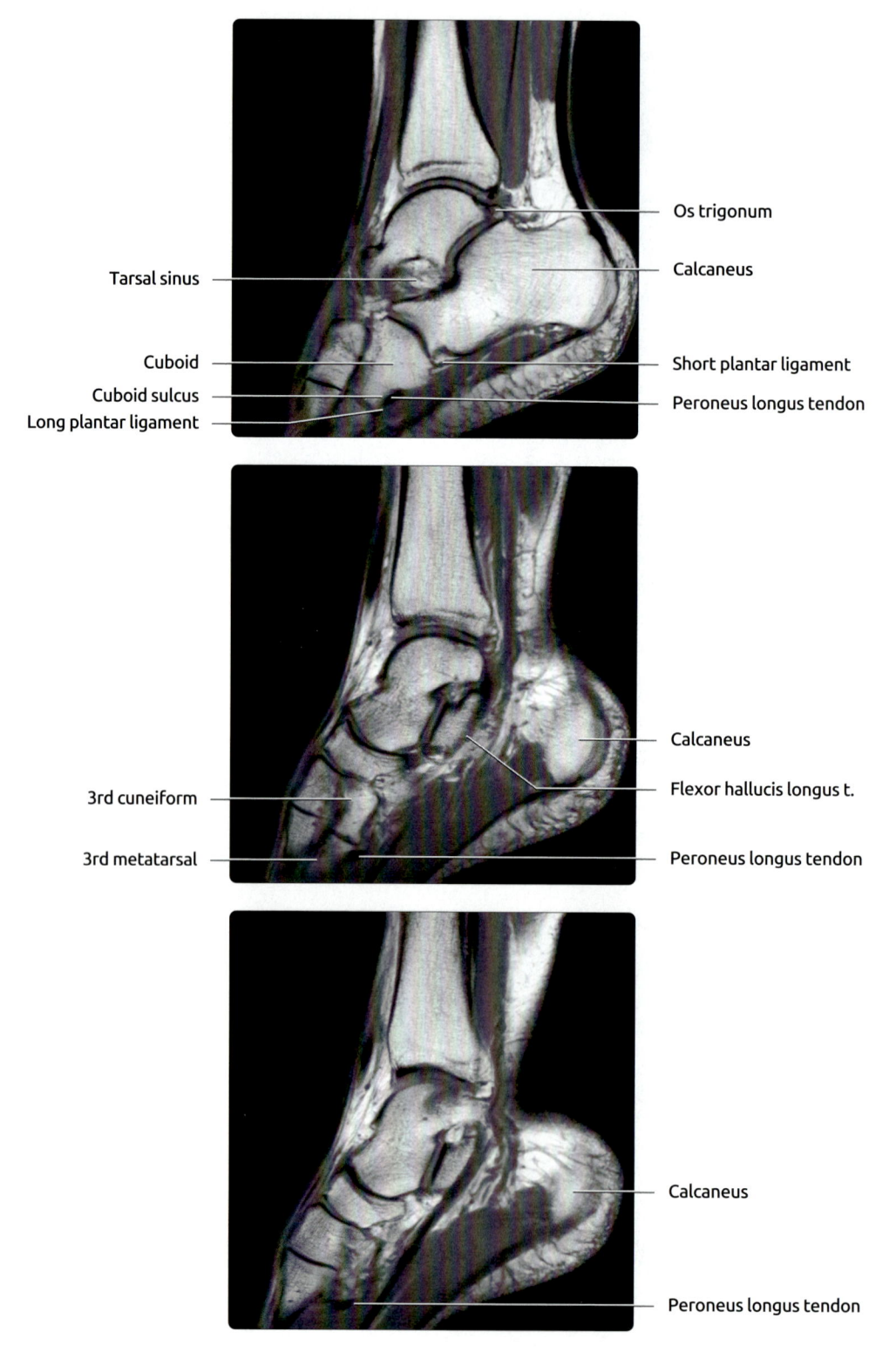

(Top) The peroneus longus tendon has now entered the tunnel under the cuboid. The tendon is held in place by a strong fibrous band derived from the long plantar ligament. Sequential sagittal images allow visualization of the peroneus longus tendon as it obliquely crosses the sole of the foot. The tendon is typically seen in cross section as a small linear, low-signal structure deep to the plantar muscles. *(Middle)* The peroneus longus tendon is seen obliquely traversing the plantar surface of the sole toward its insertion. *(Bottom)* The peroneus longus tendon is now under the 2nd metatarsal base. The insertion to the metatarsal is not always well seen on T1WI due to striation and magic angle effect.

Ankle Tendons

PERONEAL TENDONS

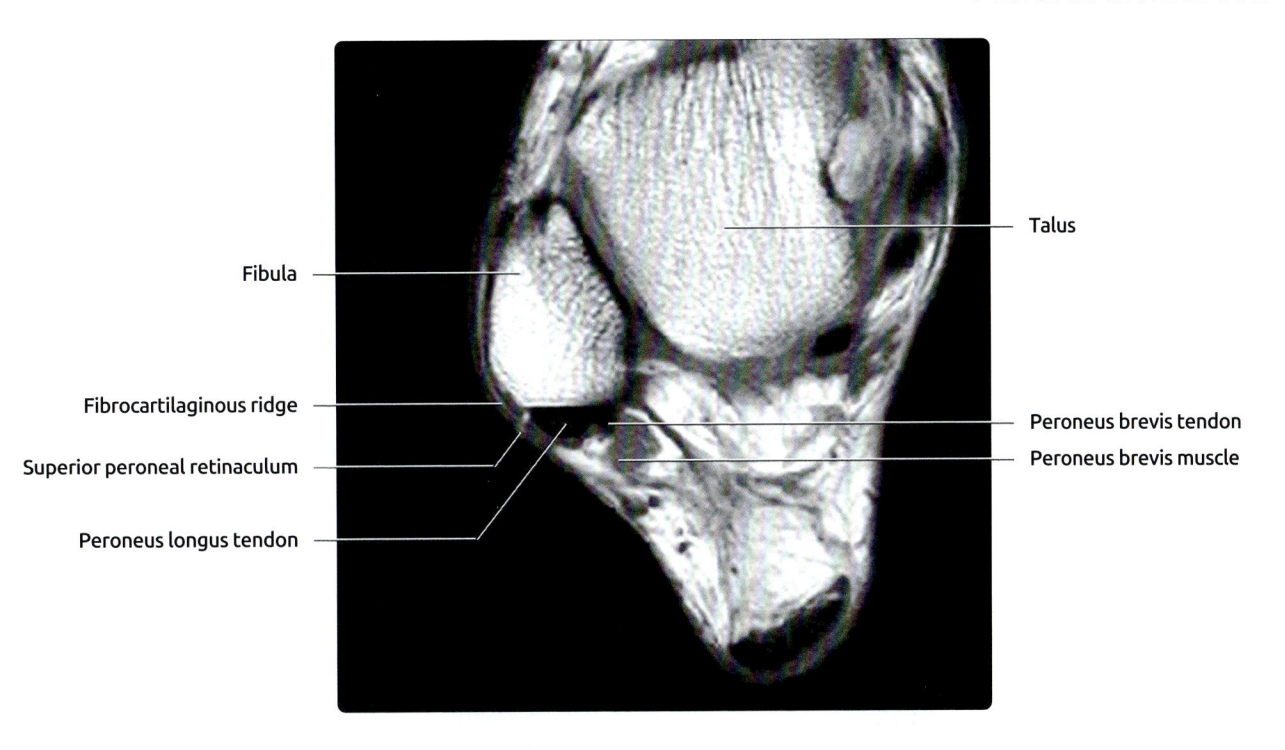

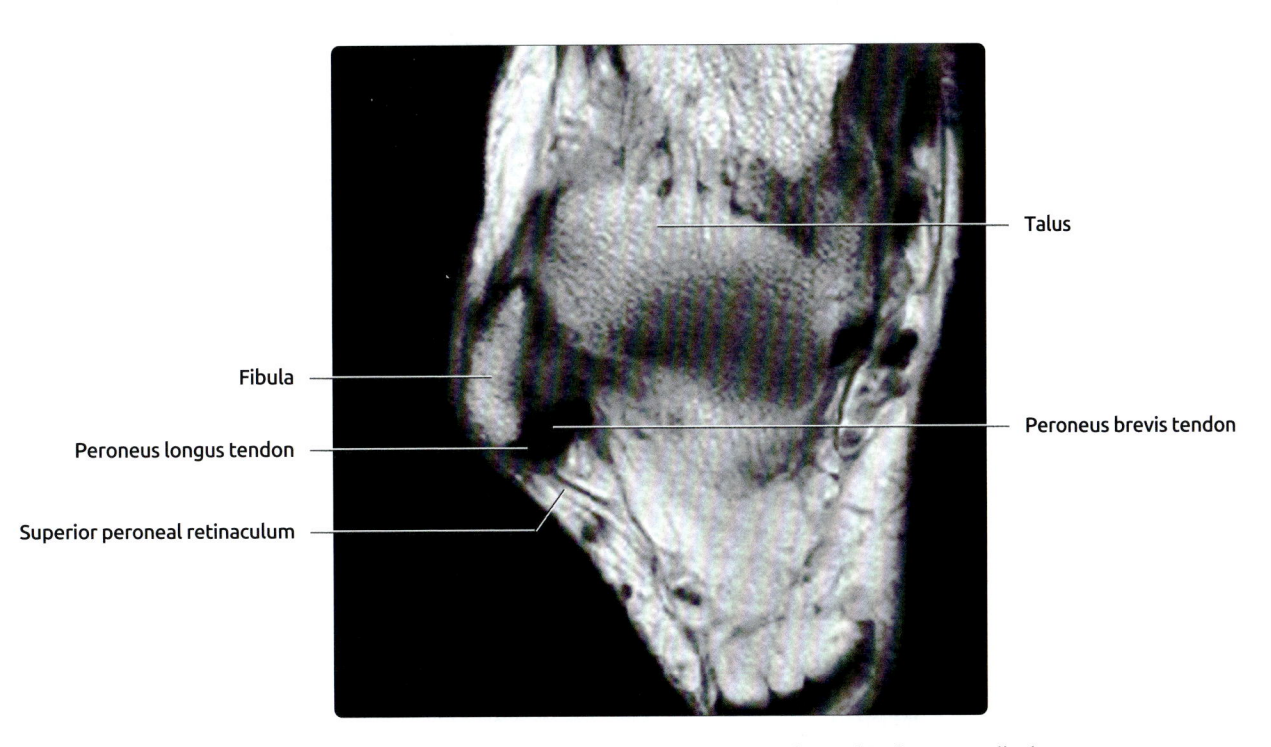

(Top) Usually, the peroneus brevis tendon is anteromedial to the peroneus longus tendon within the retromalleolar groove. Occasionally, however, the peroneus brevis tendon is located medial to the peroneus longus tendon. In those instances, as the tendons descend distally, the peroneus brevis tendon may appear medially subluxed relative to the distal fibular tip. This is a normal finding that should not be misinterpreted for disease. *(Bottom)* Note the pseudosubluxation of the peroneus brevis tendon relative to the distal fibular tip. This is a normal finding.

Ankle Tendons

ANTERIOR TIBIAL TENDON

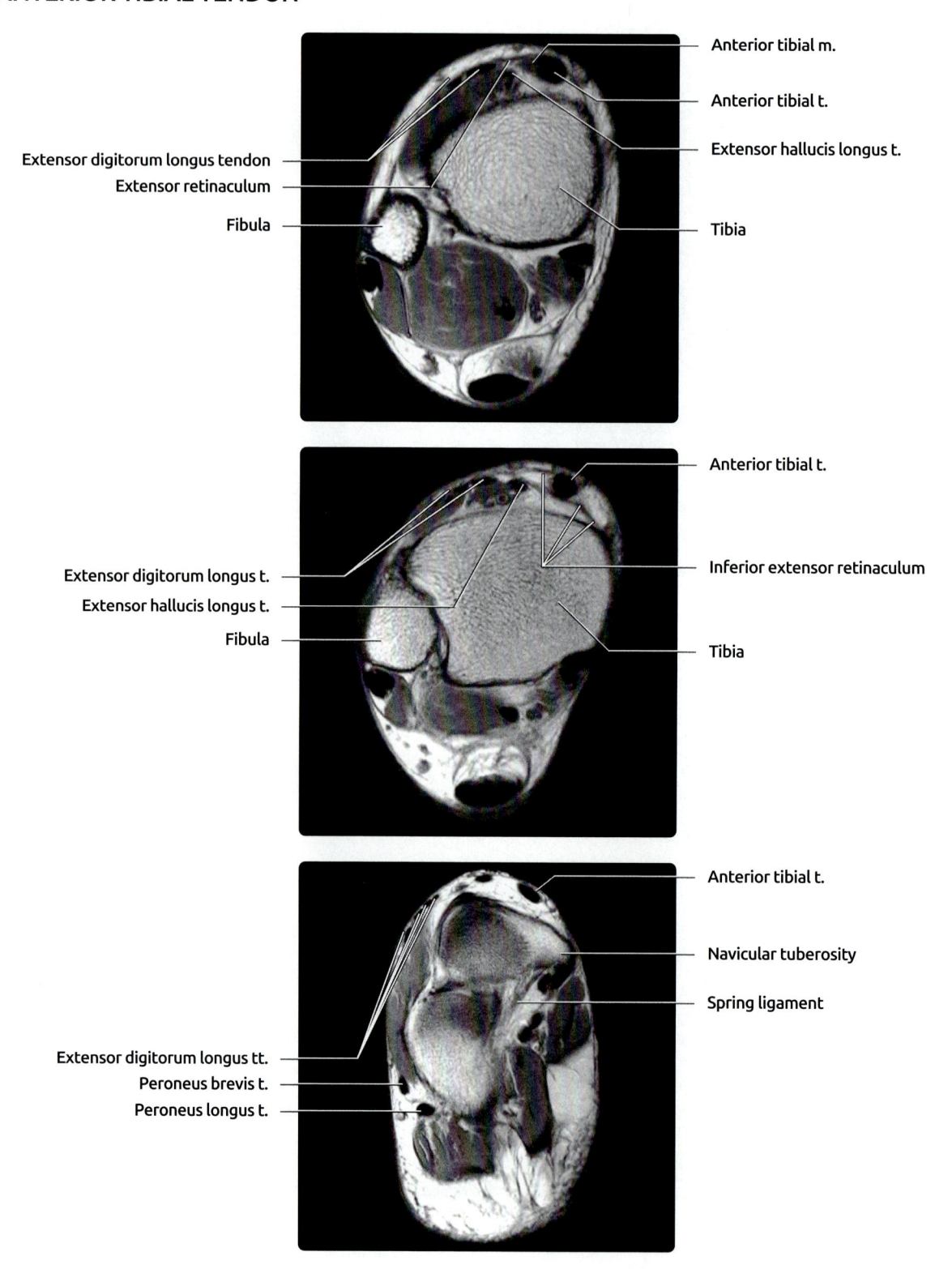

Top image labels:
- Anterior tibial m.
- Anterior tibial t.
- Extensor hallucis longus t.
- Tibia
- Extensor digitorum longus tendon
- Extensor retinaculum
- Fibula

Middle image labels:
- Anterior tibial t.
- Inferior extensor retinaculum
- Tibia
- Extensor digitorum longus t.
- Extensor hallucis longus t.
- Fibula

Bottom image labels:
- Anterior tibial t.
- Navicular tuberosity
- Spring ligament
- Extensor digitorum longus tt.
- Peroneus brevis t.
- Peroneus longus t.

(**Top**) *The anterior tibial muscle becomes completely tendinous at the level of the ankle. At the ankle, the tendon is enveloped by the superior and inferior extensor retinacula. It descends obliquely and medially to insert on the medial and inferior surfaces of the 1st cuneiform and base of the 1st metatarsal.* (**Middle**) *Note the limbs of the inferior extensor retinaculum superficial and deep to the anterior tibial tendon. This tendon is rarely injured, except by direct laceration. Attritional tears are rarely seen, primarily seen in elderly women.* (**Bottom**) *The tibialis anterior tendon is quite superficial and can be easily palpated under the skin in the medial ankle. It is the most commonly injured tendon of the extensor compartment tendons. It usually undergoes chronic degeneration, often related to impingement by the enveloping retinacula or, more commonly, by osteophytes originating from the talonavicular or navicular-cuneiform joints. Bony irregularities of the medial surface of the 1st cuneiform can also predispose the tendon to tears.*

Ankle Tendons

ANTERIOR TIBIAL TENDON

Labels (top image): Extensor hallucis longus t.; Extensor digitorum brevis t.; Cuboid; Peroneus brevis t.; Peroneus longus t.; Anterior tibial t.; 1st cuneiform

Labels (middle image): Anterior tibial tendon; Navicular tuberosity; 1st cuneiform; Medial malleolus; Tibialis posterior tendon; Distal slip of tibialis posterior tendon

Labels (bottom image): 1st metatarsal; 1st cuneiform; Cuboid; Peroneus brevis t.; Peroneus longus t.; Calcaneus; Anterior tibial t.; Anterior slips, posterior tibial t.

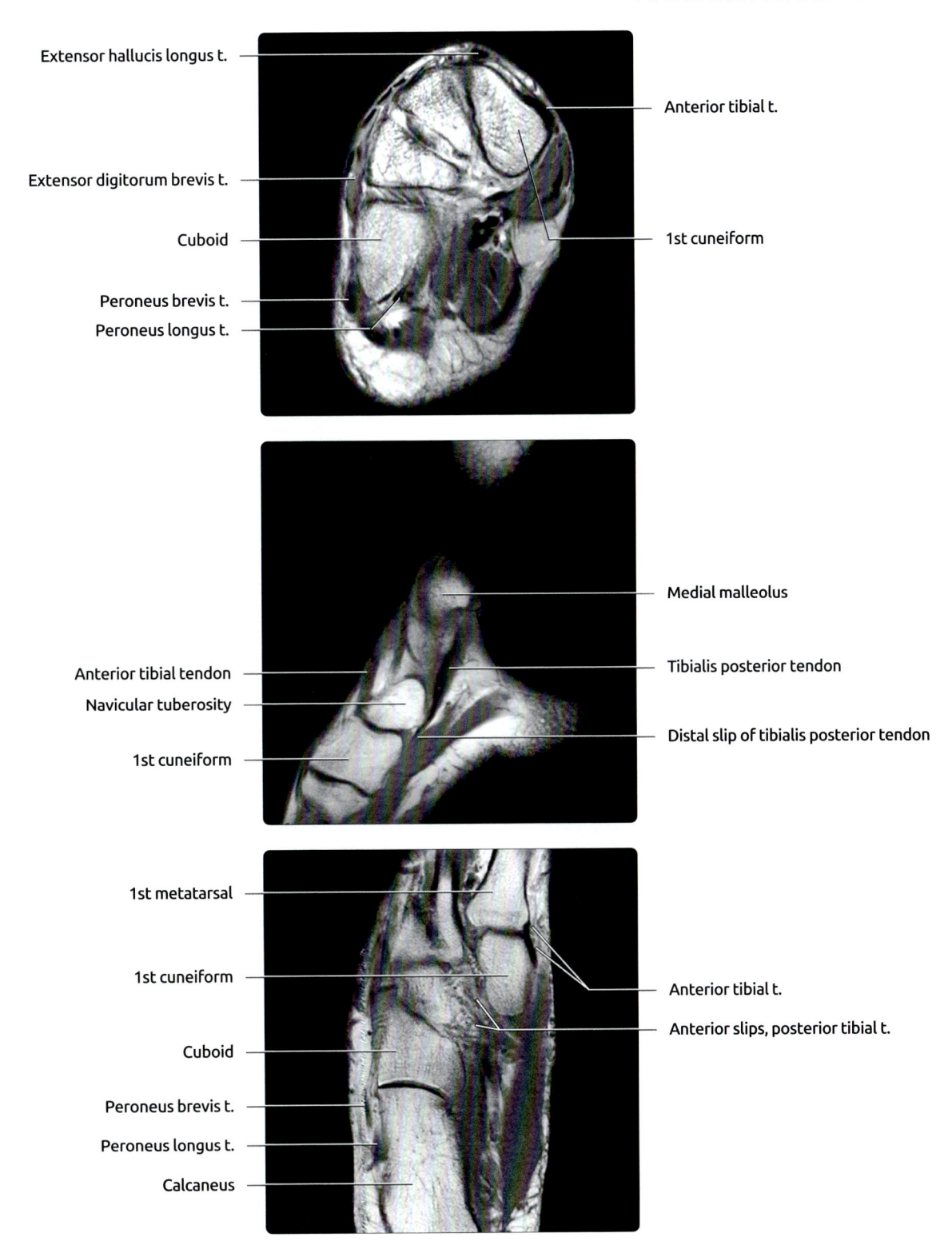

(**Top**) Note the insertion of the anterior tibial tendon to the medial surface of the 1st cuneiform. The insertion to the 1st metatarsal is usually less prominent on MR ankle images and may be better depicted on oblique axial midfoot images. (**Middle**) The anterior tibial tendon is seen wrapping around the navicular toward its insertion on the 1st cuneiform and 1st metatarsal. Careful evaluation of this area sometimes reveals tendinosis of the tibialis anterior, which can be overlooked on routine axial images of the ankle. The tibialis anterior, tibialis posterior, and peroneus longus tendons form a sling around the medial axis of the midfoot supporting the medial longitudinal arch. (**Bottom**) Note the insertion of the anterior tibial tendon to both the 1st cuneiform and 1st metatarsal on this axial ankle view.

Ankle Ligaments

GROSS ANATOMY

Syndesmotic Tibiofibular Ligaments
- Stabilize against eversion
- **Anterior inferior tibiofibular**: Oblique course from anterior lateral corner tibia inferiorly and laterally to fibula
  - Bassett ligament: Separate fascicle, usually present inferior to main band
- **Posterior inferior tibiofibular**
  - Main band oriented horizontally from posterior malleolus to posterior margin of fibula
  - Inferior transverse (or intermalleolar) band: Oblique course from medial, posterior tibia to fibular tip
- **Interosseous ligament**: Thickening of interosseous membrane, which extends length of tibial and fibular shafts
  - Extends to ~ 1 cm above tibial plafond (variable)
  - Synovial recess of ankle joint present inferior to ligament

Lateral Collateral Ligaments
- 3 separate ligaments
- Stabilize against inversion, internal rotation, anterior subluxation
- **Anterior talofibular**: Oblique course from 1 cm above fibular tip to superior margin of talar neck
  - Reliably seen on axial images only
  - Inserts on talus on 1st or 2nd superior axial images, which includes talar neck
- **Calcaneofibular**: Oblique course from fibular tip posteriorly, and inferiorly to lateral margin of calcaneus
  - Deep to peroneal tendons; well seen on axial and coronal images
- **Posterior talofibular**: Horizontal course from lateral talar body to medial margin of fibula
  - Striated appearance should not be mistaken for tear
  - Well seen on coronal and axial images

Deltoid Ligament
- Well seen on axial and coronal images
- **Deep deltoid ligament**
  - Stabilizes against eversion
  - Main (posterior) band
    - Most structural important portion of deltoid
    - Originates primarily from posterior border of anterior colliculus of medial malleolus
    - Courses inferiorly, medially, and anteriorly
    - Inserts on medial fovea of talar body
    - Has striated appearance
  - Anterior band is small, variably present, and of doubtful clinical importance
    - Originates at anterior margin of medial malleolus
    - Inserts on medial talus at junction of body and neck
- **Superficial deltoid ligament**
  - Stabilizes against rotation
  - Multiple bands, named for their attachments
  - Anterior superficial components originate from anterior corner medial malleolus as continuous band; continuous with periosteum and flexor retinaculum
  - Tibiocalcaneal: Inserts at sustentaculum tali; strongest band
  - Tibiospring: Merges with spring ligament
  - Tibionavicular: Inserts on medial border of navicular, deep to posterior tibial tendon
  - Posterior tibiotalar band: Variably present; originates more posteriorly on medial malleolus, inserts posterior talar body

Tarsal Canal and Tarsal Sinus Ligaments
- **Cervical ligament**: Stabilizes subtalar joint
  - Oblique course in tarsal sinus from inferolateral talar neck to superolateral calcaneus
  - Best seen on coronal images
  - On sagittal and axial images, it may be confused with bands of extensor retinaculum
- **Talocalcaneal interosseous ligament**: Stabilizes subtalar joint
  - Short, vertical ligament in tarsal canal
- **Roots, inferior extensor retinaculum**: 3 bands attach in tarsal sinus
  - Medial: Medial calcaneal insertion in posterior tarsal sinus, anterior to talocalcaneal interosseous ligament
  - Intermediate: Mid-dorsal calcaneal insertion adjacent to cervical ligament
  - Lateral: Lateral margin calcaneal insertion lateral to extensor digitorum brevis muscle origin
  - Best seen on coronal images

Spring Ligament
- 3 bands
- From calcaneus to navicular, supports talar head and medial longitudinal arch
- **Superomedial**: Strongest, hammock-shaped, best seen on axial images
  - Origin: Sustentaculum tali and tibiospring band of deltoid
  - Insertion: Superomedial navicular
  - Deep to posterior tibial tendon
- **Medioplantar oblique**
  - Best seen on axial images
  - Origin: Coronoid fossa of calcaneus
  - Insertion: Plantar, medial navicular
  - Striated appearance, oblique course
- **Inferoplantar longitudinal**
  - Best seen on axial and sagittal images
  - Origin: Coronoid fossa; insertion: Navicular beak
  - Short, straight course

Bifurcate Ligament
- Best seen on sagittal images
- Origin: Dorsal margin of calcaneal anterior process; insertion via 2 limbs to navicular and cuboid

Short and Long Plantar Ligaments
- Best seen on sagittal and axial images
- Support longitudinal arch

Short Plantar Ligament (Plantar Calcaneocuboid)
- Origin: Calcaneal anterior tubercle; insertion: Cuboid

Long Plantar Ligament: Superficial to Short Plantar Ligament
- Origin: At and anterior to medial, lateral, anterior tubercles; insertion: Cuboid, bases 2nd-5th metatarsals

Ankle Ligaments

HINDFOOT LIGAMENTS

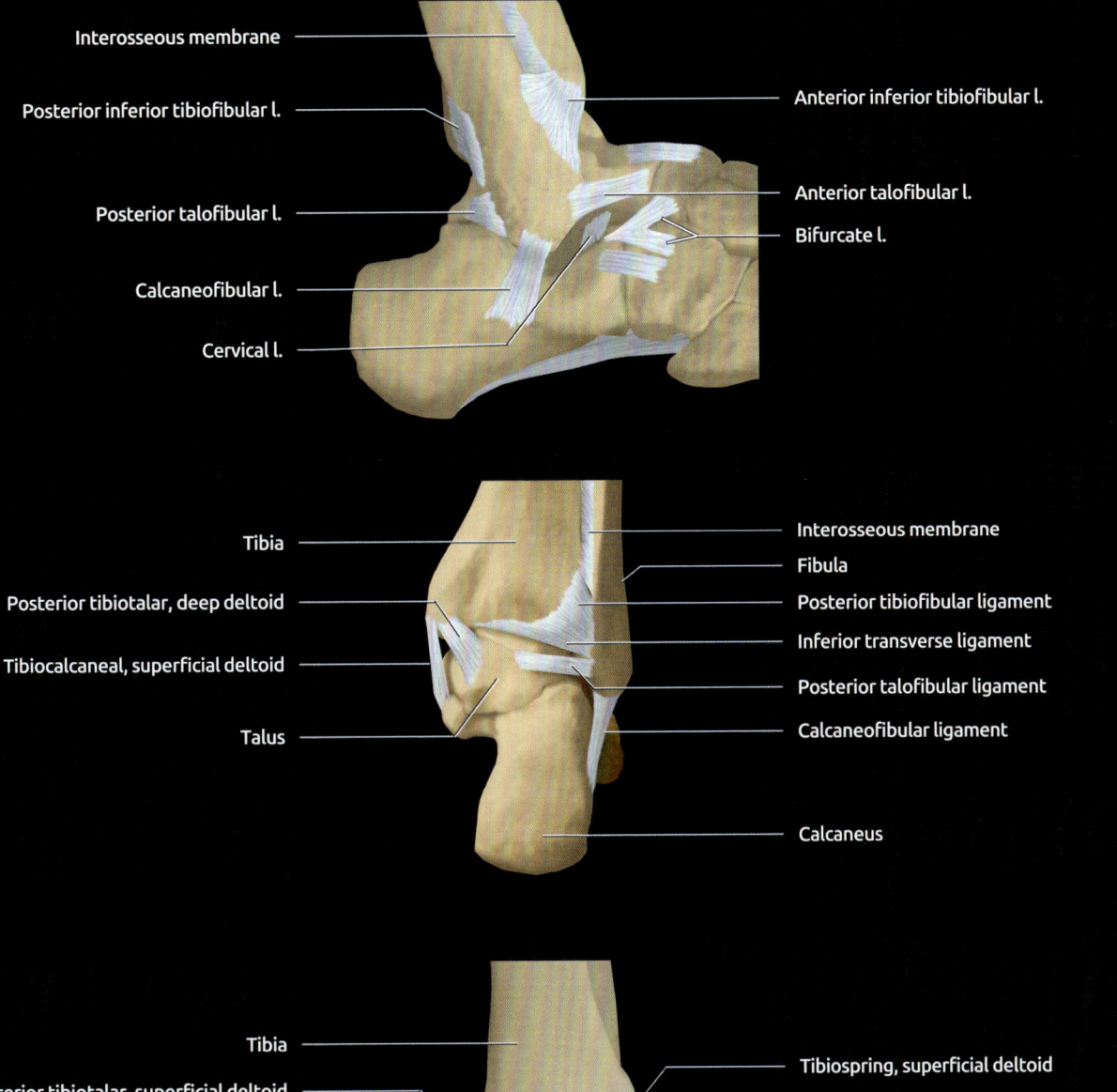

Top image labels:
- Interosseous membrane
- Posterior inferior tibiofibular l.
- Posterior talofibular l.
- Calcaneofibular l.
- Cervical l.
- Anterior inferior tibiofibular l.
- Anterior talofibular l.
- Bifurcate l.

Middle image labels:
- Tibia
- Posterior tibiotalar, deep deltoid
- Tibiocalcaneal, superficial deltoid
- Talus
- Interosseous membrane
- Fibula
- Posterior tibiofibular ligament
- Inferior transverse ligament
- Posterior talofibular ligament
- Calcaneofibular ligament
- Calcaneus

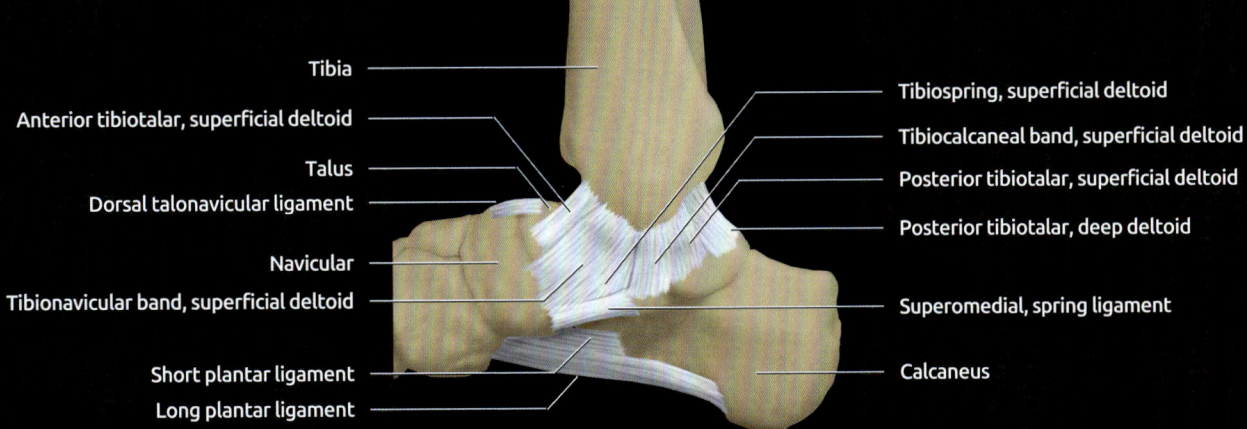

Bottom image labels:
- Tibia
- Anterior tibiotalar, superficial deltoid
- Talus
- Dorsal talonavicular ligament
- Navicular
- Tibionavicular band, superficial deltoid
- Short plantar ligament
- Long plantar ligament
- Tibiospring, superficial deltoid
- Tibiocalcaneal band, superficial deltoid
- Posterior tibiotalar, superficial deltoid
- Posterior tibiotalar, deep deltoid
- Superomedial, spring ligament
- Calcaneus

(**Top**) Lateral view of the ankle is shown. Syndesmotic ligaments, including the anterior inferior tibiofibular, posterior inferior tibiofibular, and interosseous ligaments stabilize against eversion injury. Lateral collateral ligaments, including the anterior talofibular, posterior talofibular, and calcaneofibular ligaments stabilize against inversion and anteroposterior translation. The subtalar joint is stabilized by the cervical ligament and interosseous ligament (not shown). The bifurcate ligament stabilizes against inversion. Plantar ligaments stabilize the longitudinal arch. (**Middle**) Posterior view of the ankle is shown. The tibiofibular ligaments are obliquely oriented and their fibular origin is above the fibular malleolar fossa. The inferior transverse ligament (the inferior portion of the posterior tibiofibular ligament) extends distal to the tibial posterior surface. (**Bottom**) Medial view of ankle is shown. The superficial deltoid originates from the superficial margin of the medial malleolus. The bands are named for their insertions.

Ankle Ligaments

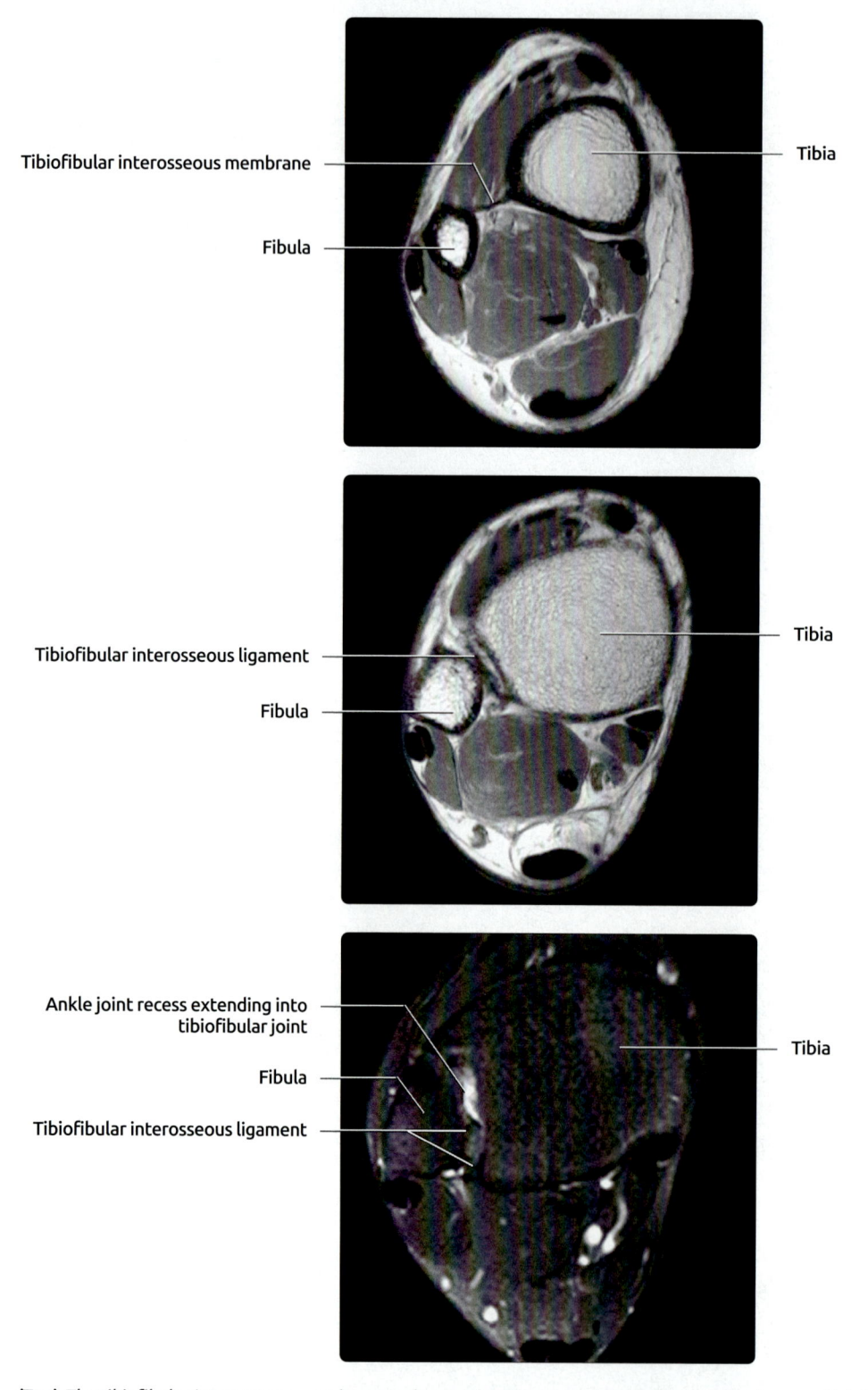

TIBIOFIBULAR SYNDESMOTIC LIGAMENTS

Tibiofibular interosseous membrane — Tibia
Fibula

Tibiofibular interosseous ligament — Tibia
Fibula

Ankle joint recess extending into tibiofibular joint — Tibia
Fibula
Tibiofibular interosseous ligament

(Top) The tibiofibular interosseous membrane is shown. The membrane is typically visualized as a well-defined, low signal structure, binding the tibia and fibula. Its distal thickening is the interosseous ligament. Just above the ankle joint, the membrane becomes less defined and may even be discontinuous. **(Middle)** The tibiofibular interosseous ligament is shown. The ligament is a distal thickening of the tibiofibular membrane. Occasionally, it may be visualized as a distinct structure, as in this image, but often it may be poorly defined, discontinuous, and even absent. **(Bottom)** A fluid-filled recess, measuring between 0.5-1.0 cm, extends from the ankle joint into the tibiofibular fibrous joint. The tibiofibular ligament is frequently present at the superior margin of the recess. In this particular case it extends posterior to the recess.

Ankle Ligaments

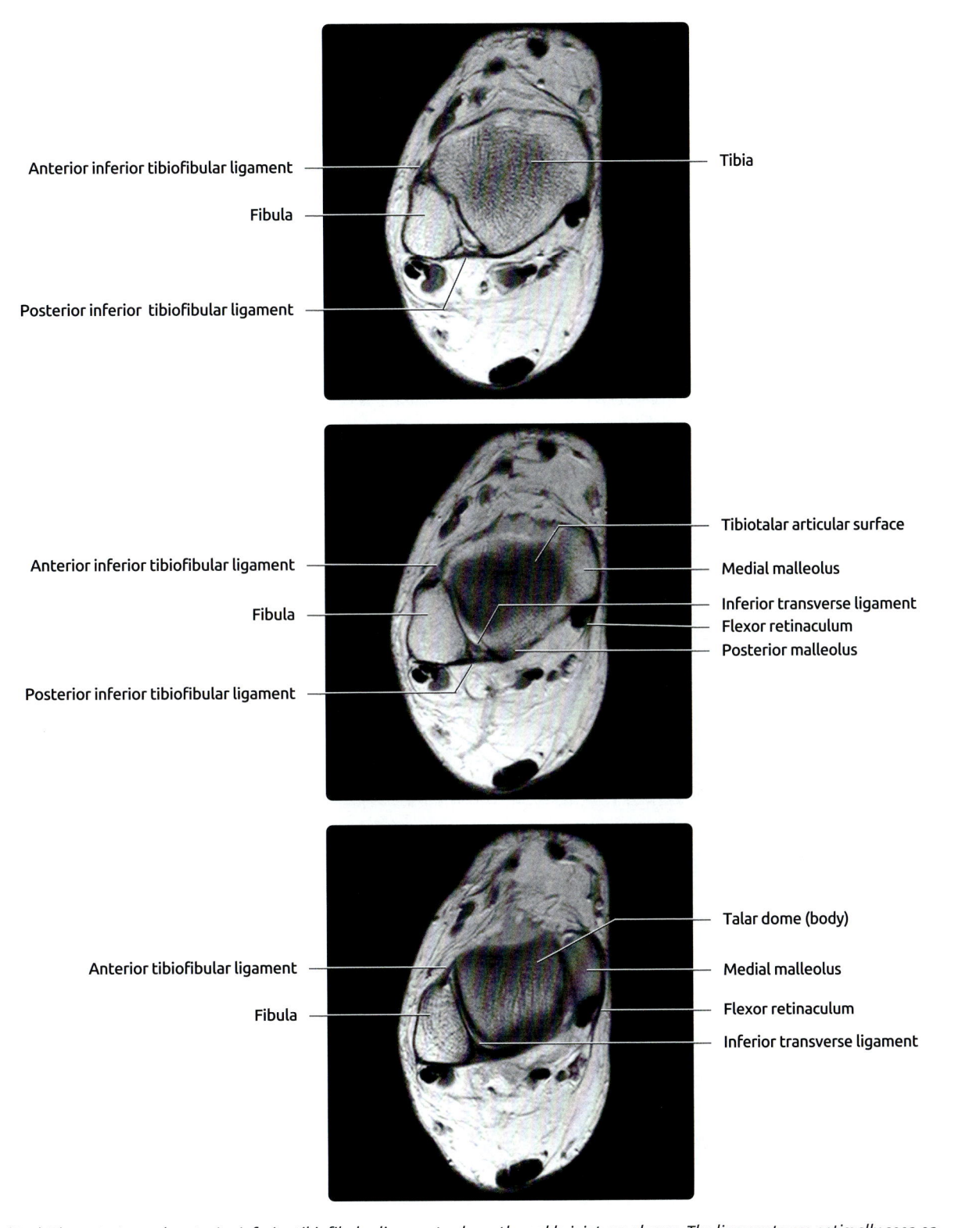

TIBIOFIBULAR SYNDESMOTIC LIGAMENTS

Anterior inferior tibiofibular ligament
Fibula
Posterior inferior tibiofibular ligament
Tibia

Anterior inferior tibiofibular ligament
Fibula
Posterior inferior tibiofibular ligament
Tibiotalar articular surface
Medial malleolus
Inferior transverse ligament
Flexor retinaculum
Posterior malleolus

Anterior tibiofibular ligament
Fibula
Talar dome (body)
Medial malleolus
Flexor retinaculum
Inferior transverse ligament

(Top) The anterior and posterior inferior tibiofibular ligaments above the ankle joint are shown. The ligaments are optimally seen on axial images. The anterior inferior tibiofibular ligament may appear discontinuous due to fat between the ligament and the accessory Bassett ligament. (Middle) Anterior and posterior tibiofibular ligaments at the ankle joint are shown. The ligaments are visualized at, or slightly below, the ankle joint. Note that at this level, the fibula is round, without the more distal medial indentation of the malleolar fossa. (Bottom) The anterior and posterior tibiofibular ligaments at the talar dome (talus is square at this level) are shown. The very inferior aspect of the anterior tibiofibular ligament has been coined the Bassett ligament. The inferior transverse ligament is continuous with the posterior inferior tibiofibular ligament but extends distal to the posterior tibial articular surface.

Ankle Ligaments

Ankle

TIBIOFIBULAR SYNDESMOTIC LIGAMENTS

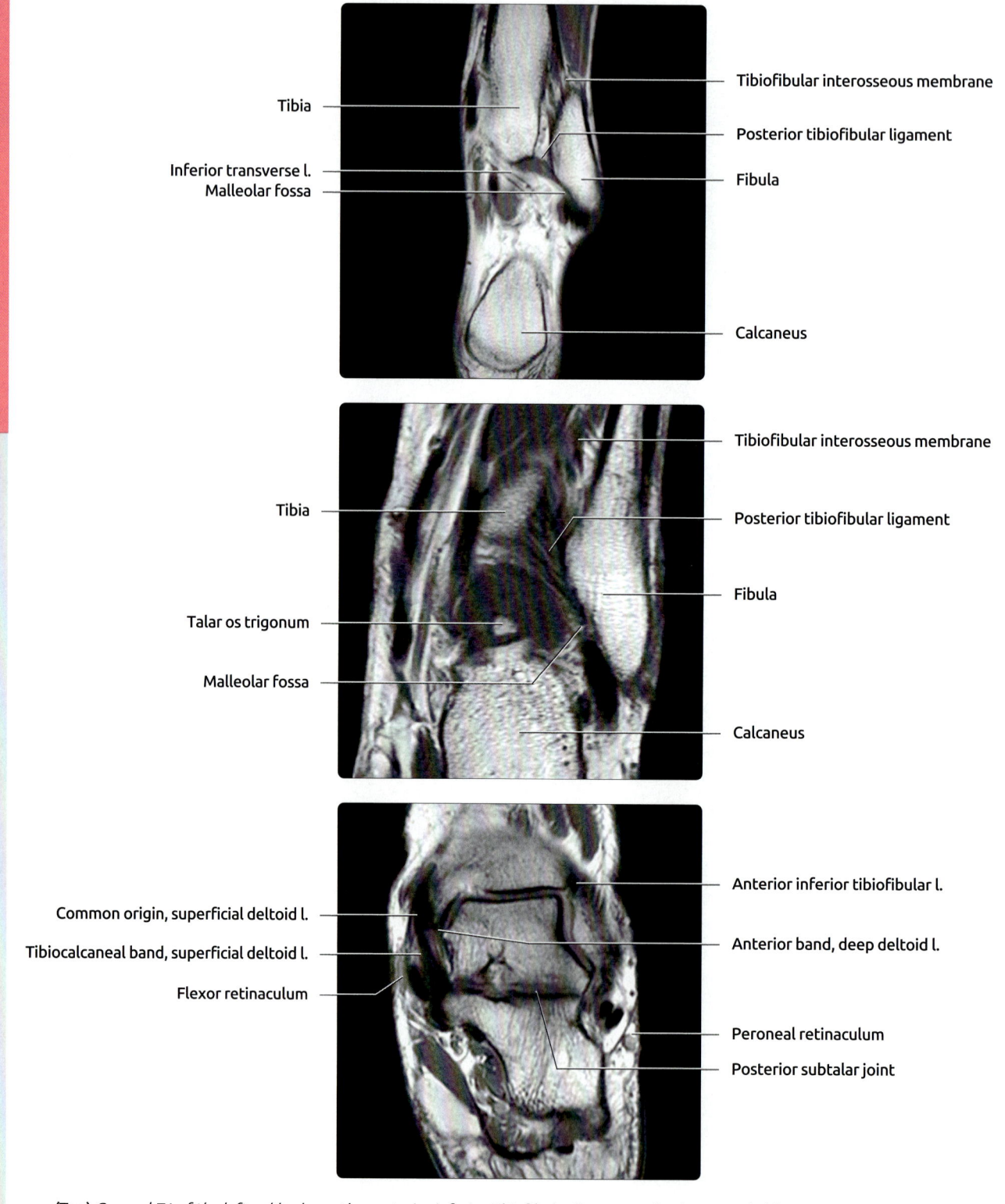

(Top) Coronal T1 of the left ankle shows the posterior inferior tibiofibular ligament. The downward oblique course of the ligament is best appreciated on coronal images. The ligament descends from its superior position on the tibia toward its more inferior fibular insertion. Note that the ligament inserts on the fibula above the malleolar fossa. (Middle) Coronal T1 of the left ankle shows the posterior inferior tibiofibular ligament. The striation of the ligament is due to fat interposed between its fascicles and should not be misinterpreted as a tear on axial images. (Bottom) The anterior inferior tibiofibular ligament has an oblique from the anterior margin of the tibia, inferiorly and laterally to the fibula. The Bassett ligament forms a separate fascicle inferior to the main portion of the ligament.

1008

Ankle Ligaments

TIBIOFIBULAR SYNDESMOTIC LIGAMENTS

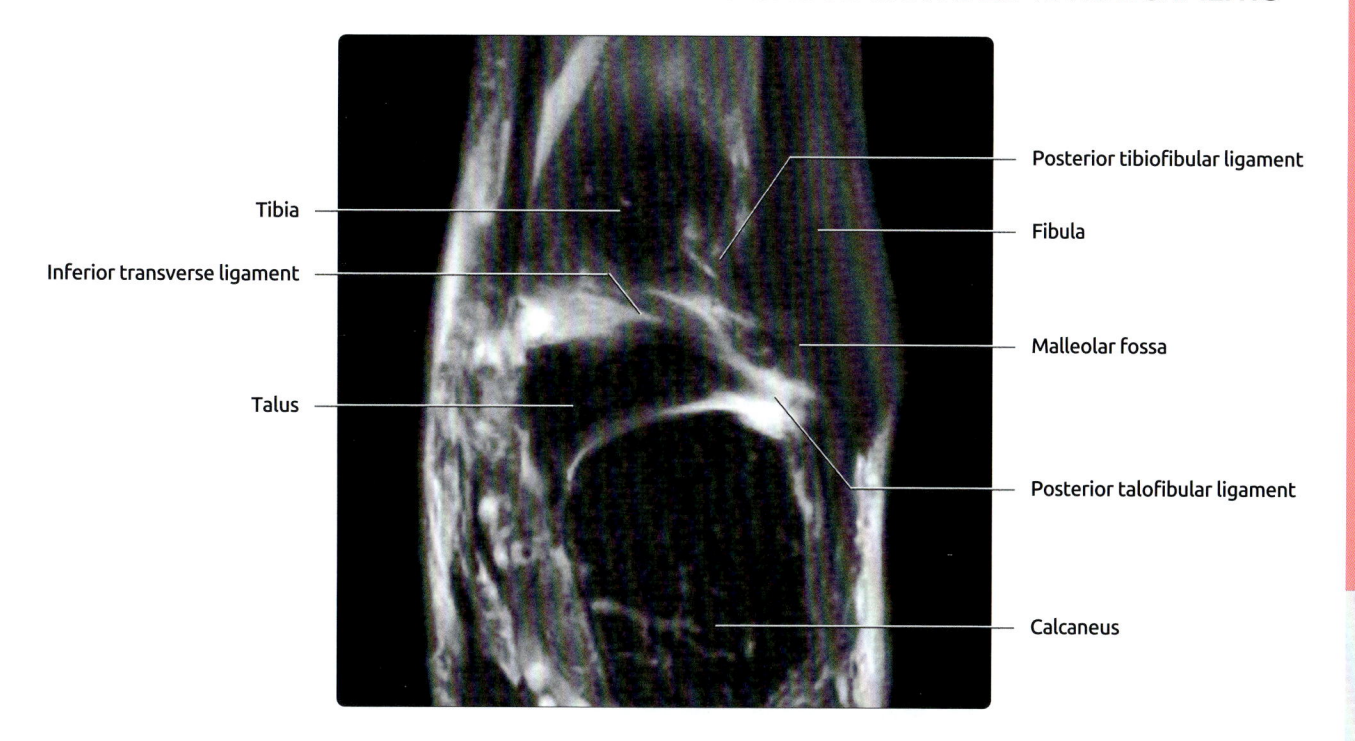

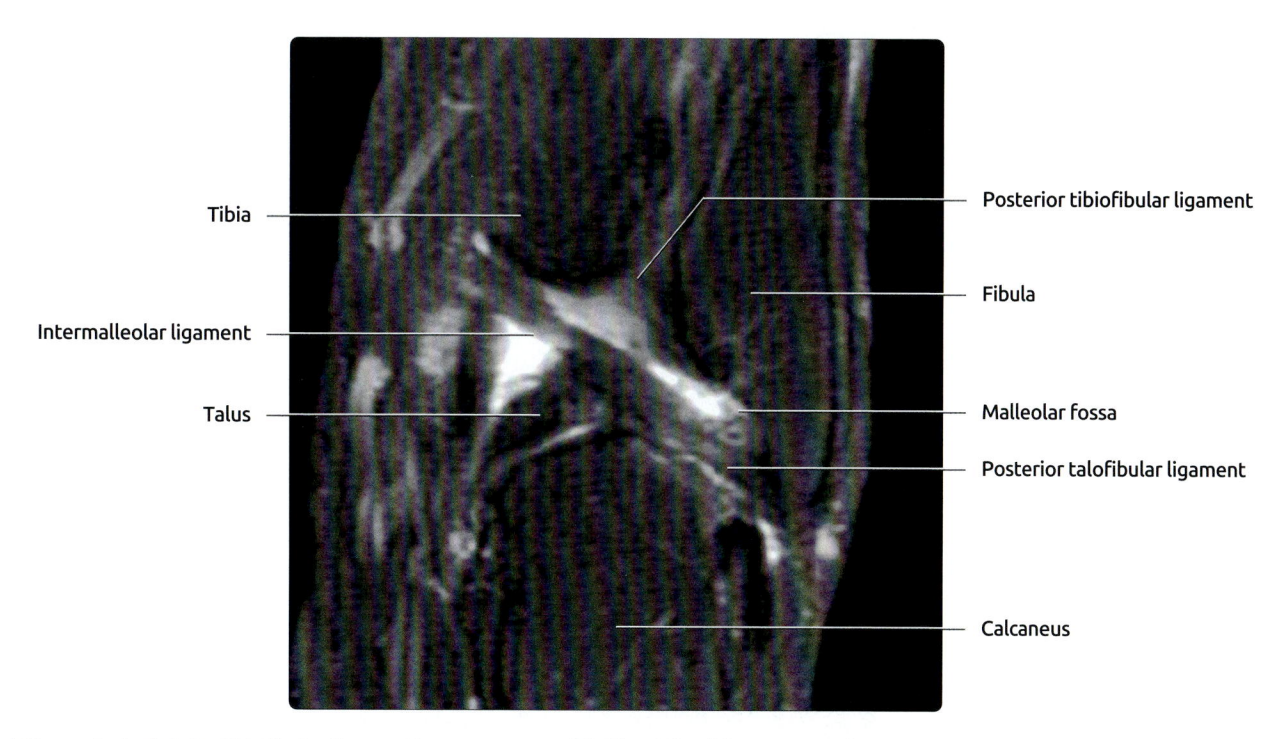

(Top) The posterior inferior tibiofibular ligament is seen on coronal fluid-weighted fat-suppressed image. Note that the inferior transverse ligament extends distal to the posterior tibia, forming a posterior labrum and deepening the posterior ankle joint. Its tibial insertion is quite far medial, almost to the level of the medial malleolus. The tibiofibular ligaments insert onto the fibula above the malleolar fossa, while the talofibular ligaments insert below it. **(Bottom)** The intermalleolar ligament is seen on this coronal fluid-weighted fat-suppressed image. The intermalleolar ligament, also called the tibial slip, is a normal variant that extends from the posterior talofibular ligament almost to the tibial medial malleolus. This ligament is found between the inferior transverse and posterior talofibular ligaments. It may be difficult to distinguish it from the inferior transverse ligament.

Ankle Ligaments

TIBIOFIBULAR SYNDESMOTIC LIGAMENTS

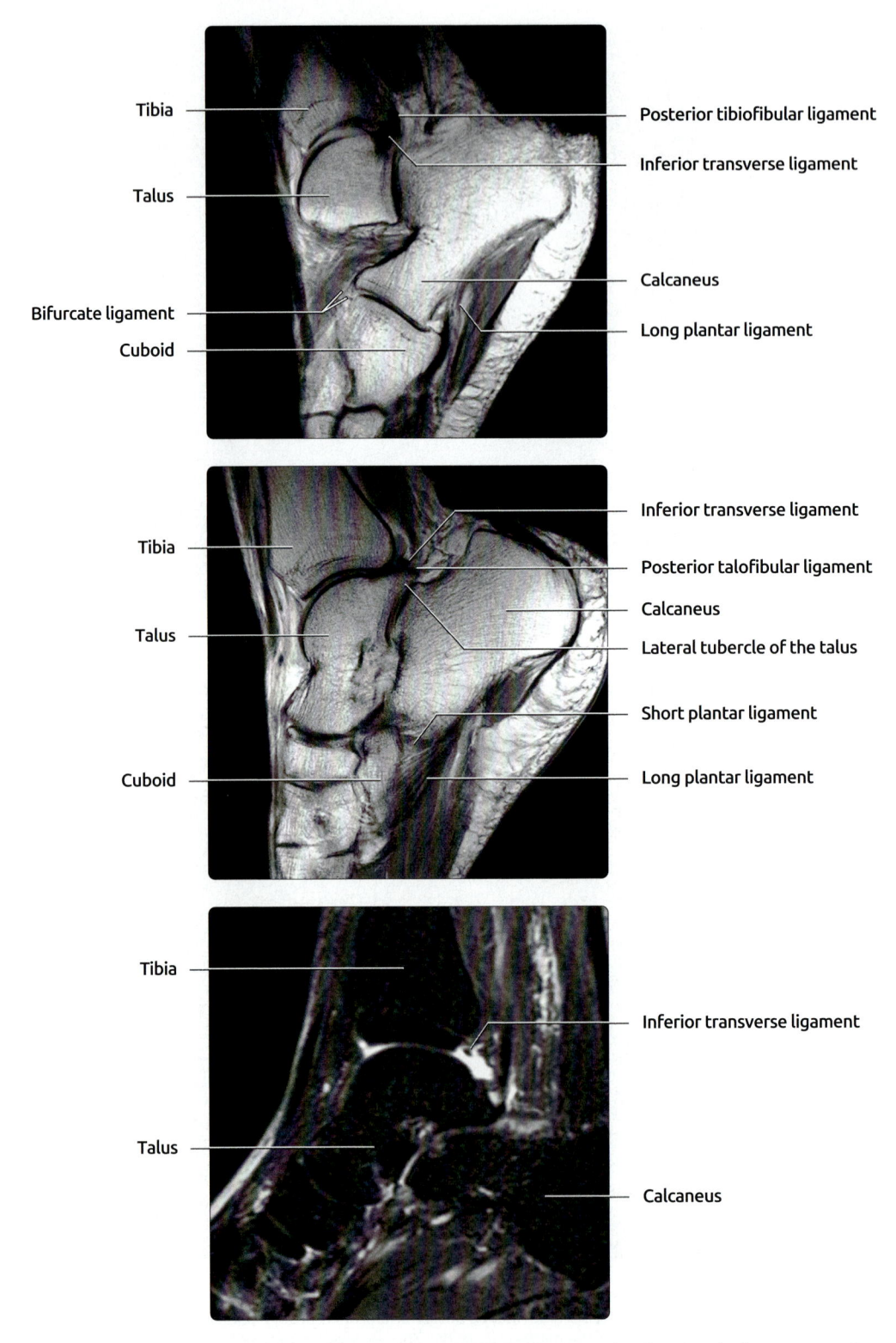

(Top) Sagittal T1-weighted MR image shows the inferior extent of the tibiofibular ligament distal to the tibial posterior surface. The sagittal images are suboptimal for visualizing the tibiofibular and talofibular ligaments. (Middle) On sagittal images, the tibiofibular and talofibular ligaments are typically seen in cross section as small, low signal intensity, oval structures posterior to the talus and should not be misinterpreted as intraarticular bodies. Following the ligaments on sequential images will obviate this problem. Note that the posterior talofibular ligament is barely visualized as it originates from the lateral tubercle of the talus. (Bottom) Sagittal STIR MR image depicts the inferior transverse ligament surrounded by fluid, simulating an intraarticular body.

Ankle Ligaments

TIBIOFIBULAR SYNDESMOTIC LIGAMENTS

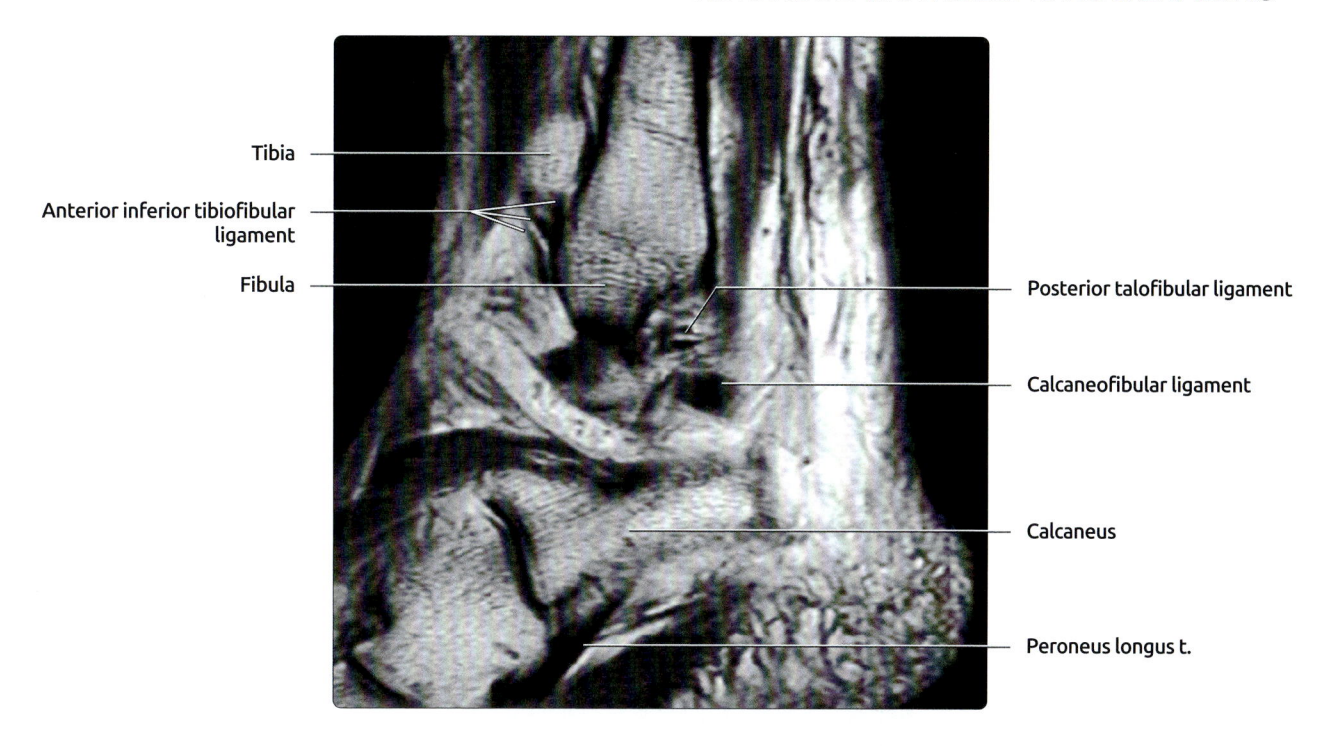

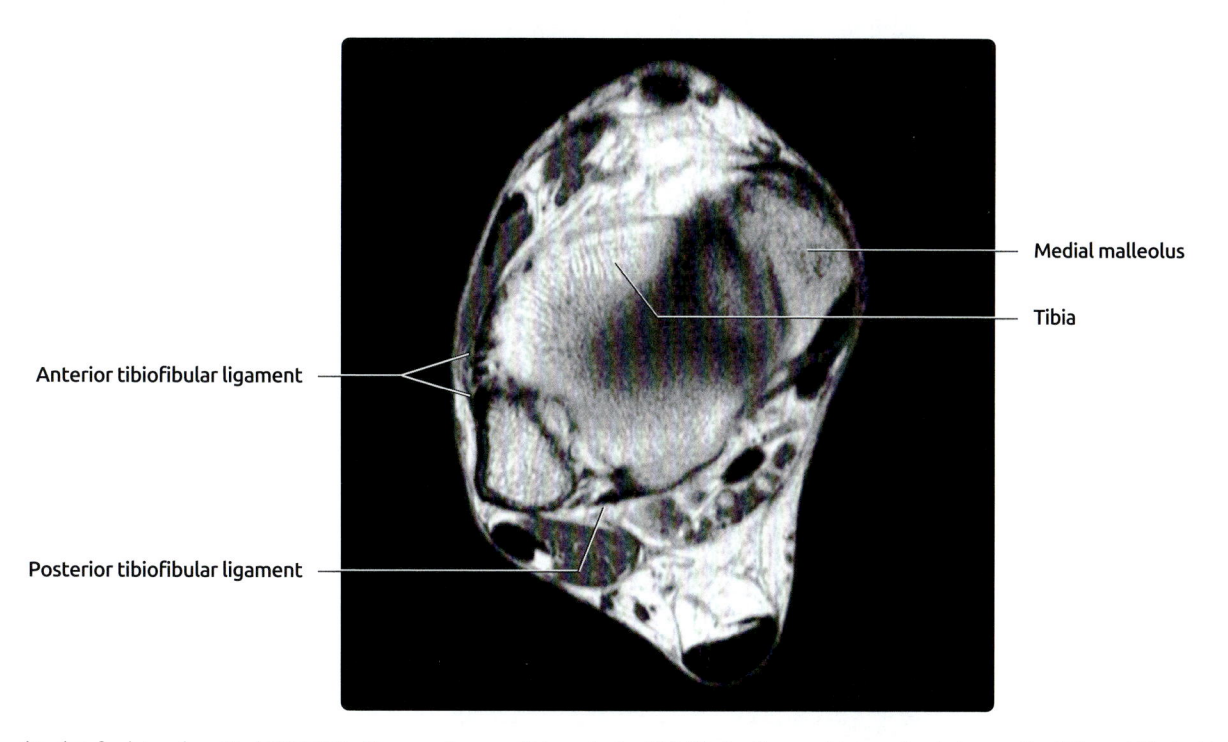

(Top) A far lateral sagittal T1WI MR allows a glimpse of the anterior tibiofibular ligament traversing between the tibia and fibula. Note the striation of the ligament. The calcaneofibular ligament is also visualized. (Bottom) Normal striation of the anterior inferior tibiofibular ligament is seen on this axial T1WI. Because of the oblique descent of the anterior tibiofibular ligament and the fat interposed between its fascicles, it may appear discontinuous. This should not be misinterpreted as a tear.

Ankle Ligaments

DELTOID AND SYNDESMOTIC LIGAMENTS

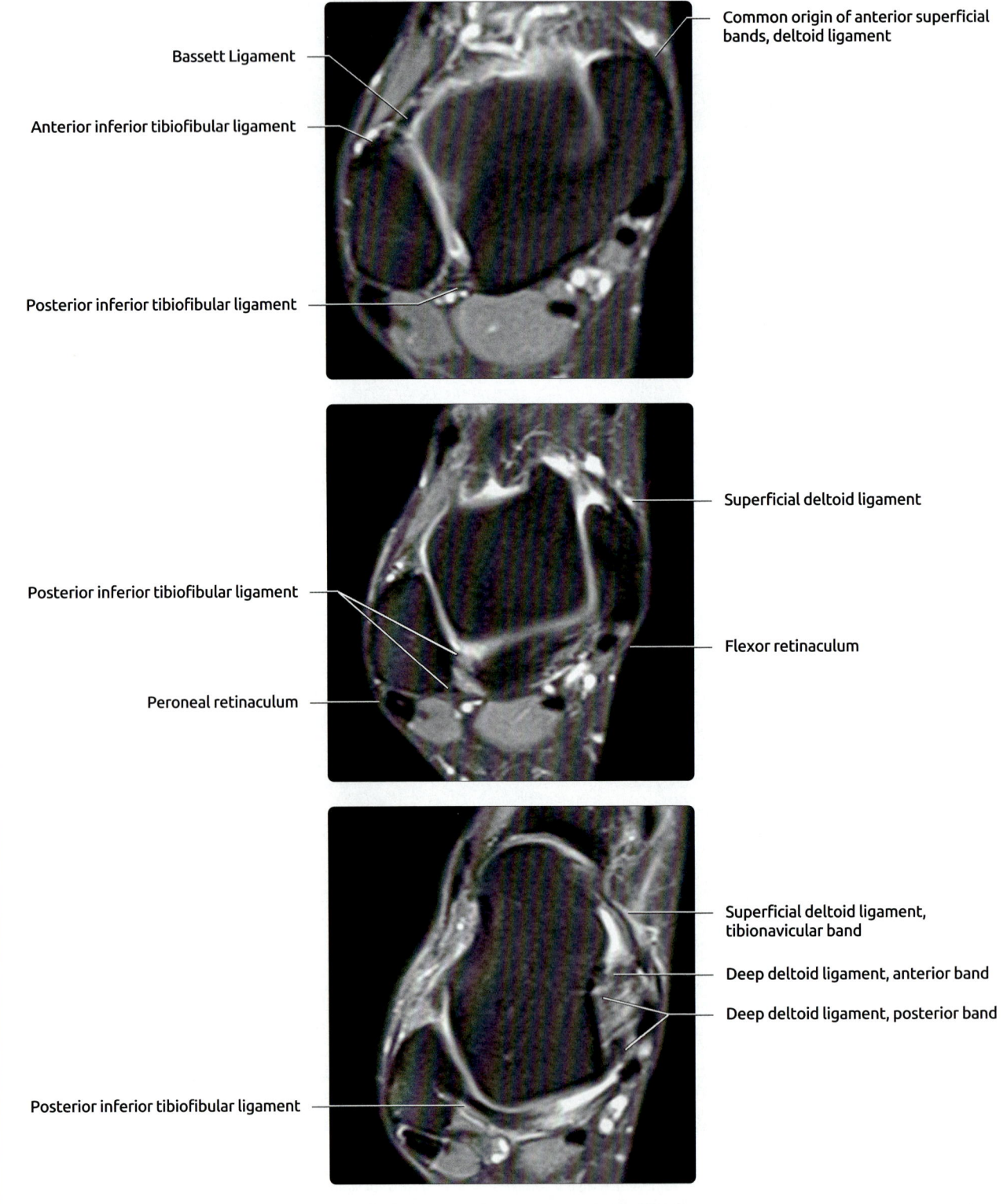

Labels (Top image): Bassett Ligament; Anterior inferior tibiofibular ligament; Posterior inferior tibiofibular ligament; Common origin of anterior superficial bands, deltoid ligament

Labels (Middle image): Posterior inferior tibiofibular ligament; Peroneal retinaculum; Superficial deltoid ligament; Flexor retinaculum

Labels (Bottom image): Posterior inferior tibiofibular ligament; Superficial deltoid ligament, tibionavicular band; Deep deltoid ligament, anterior band; Deep deltoid ligament, posterior band

(**Top**) Axial T2 FS MR shows the common origin of the anterior bands of the superficial ligament from the medial malleolus. Laterally, the image includes portions of the anterior inferior tibiofibular ligament and the Basset ligament. The juxtaposition of the 2 ligamentous bands can be mistaken for a ligament tear. (**Middle**) Axial T2 FS MR shows fibers of the superficial deltoid ligament. The ligament bands are not distinguishable at this point. The posterior inferior tibiofibular ligament is thick and striated. (**Bottom**) Axial T2 FS MR demonstrates the broad extent of the deep deltoid ligament from anterior to posterior. A striated appearance, with taut individual fibers, is normal. The tibionavicular band of superficial deltoid is outlined here by joint effusion.

Ankle Ligaments

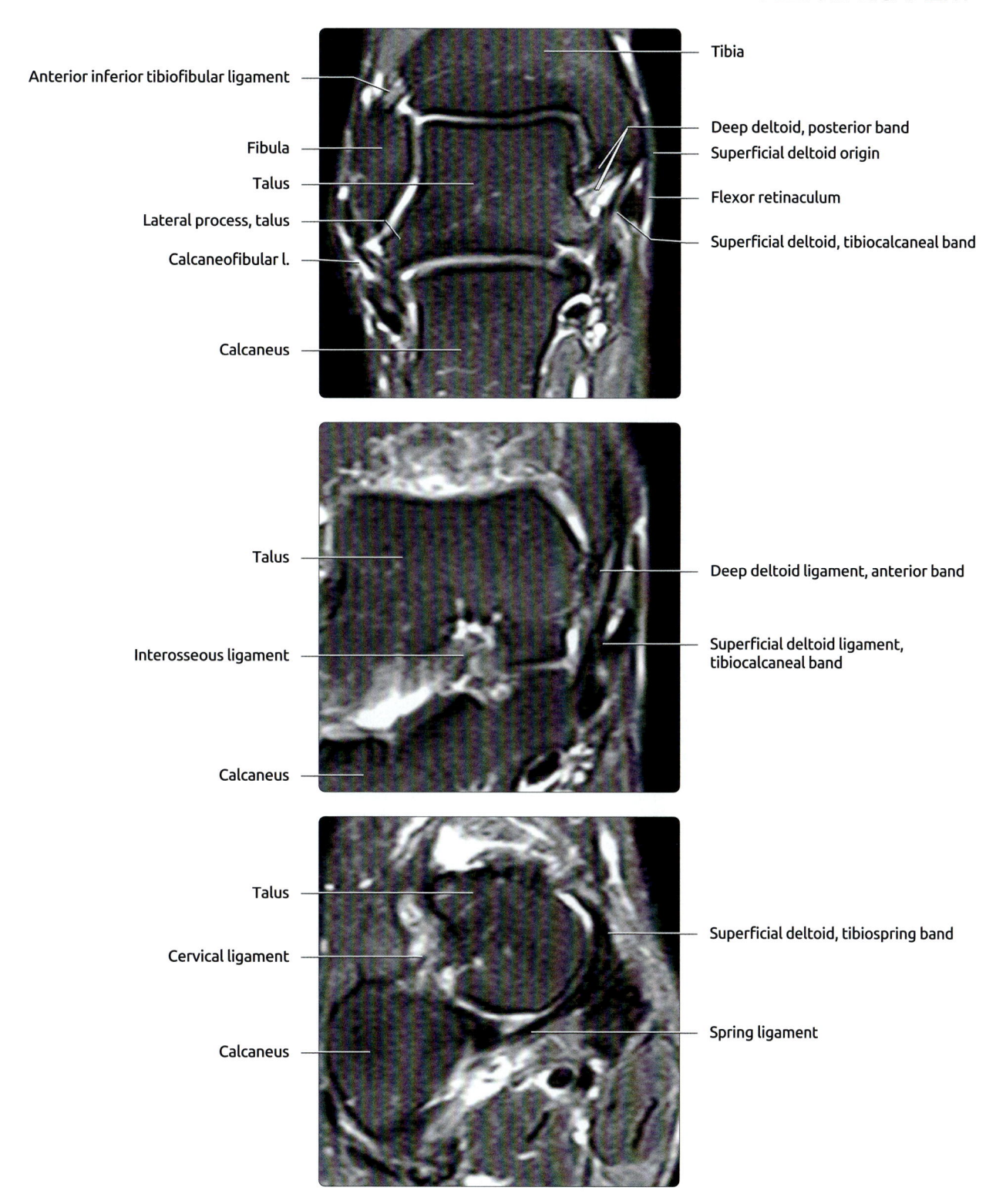

DELTOID LIGAMENT

Labels (top image): Anterior inferior tibiofibular ligament; Fibula; Talus; Lateral process, talus; Calcaneofibular l.; Calcaneus; Tibia; Deep deltoid, posterior band; Superficial deltoid origin; Flexor retinaculum; Superficial deltoid, tibiocalcaneal band

Labels (middle image): Talus; Interosseous ligament; Calcaneus; Deep deltoid ligament, anterior band; Superficial deltoid ligament, tibiocalcaneal band

Labels (bottom image): Talus; Cervical ligament; Calcaneus; Superficial deltoid, tibiospring band; Spring ligament

(**Top**) *Coronal T2 FS MR shows the fan-shaped deep deltoid extending from the medial malleolus to the medial fovea of the talar body. The normal ligament has a striated appearance and does not completely fill the fovea. The posterior band is the primary band of the deep deltoid ligament. The anterior inferior tibiofibular ligament has a short, oblique course.* (**Middle**) *Coronal T2 FS MR shows the anterior band of the deep deltoid ligament. This small band is of doubtful significance, and variably present. The tibiocalcaneal band of the superficial deltoid is the strongest component of the superficial deltoid.* (**Bottom**) *Coronal T2 FS MR at the level of the talar head shows the tibiospring band of the superficial deltoid ligament continuous with the spring ligament.*

Ankle Ligaments

DEEP DELTOID LIGAMENT, CORONAL MR

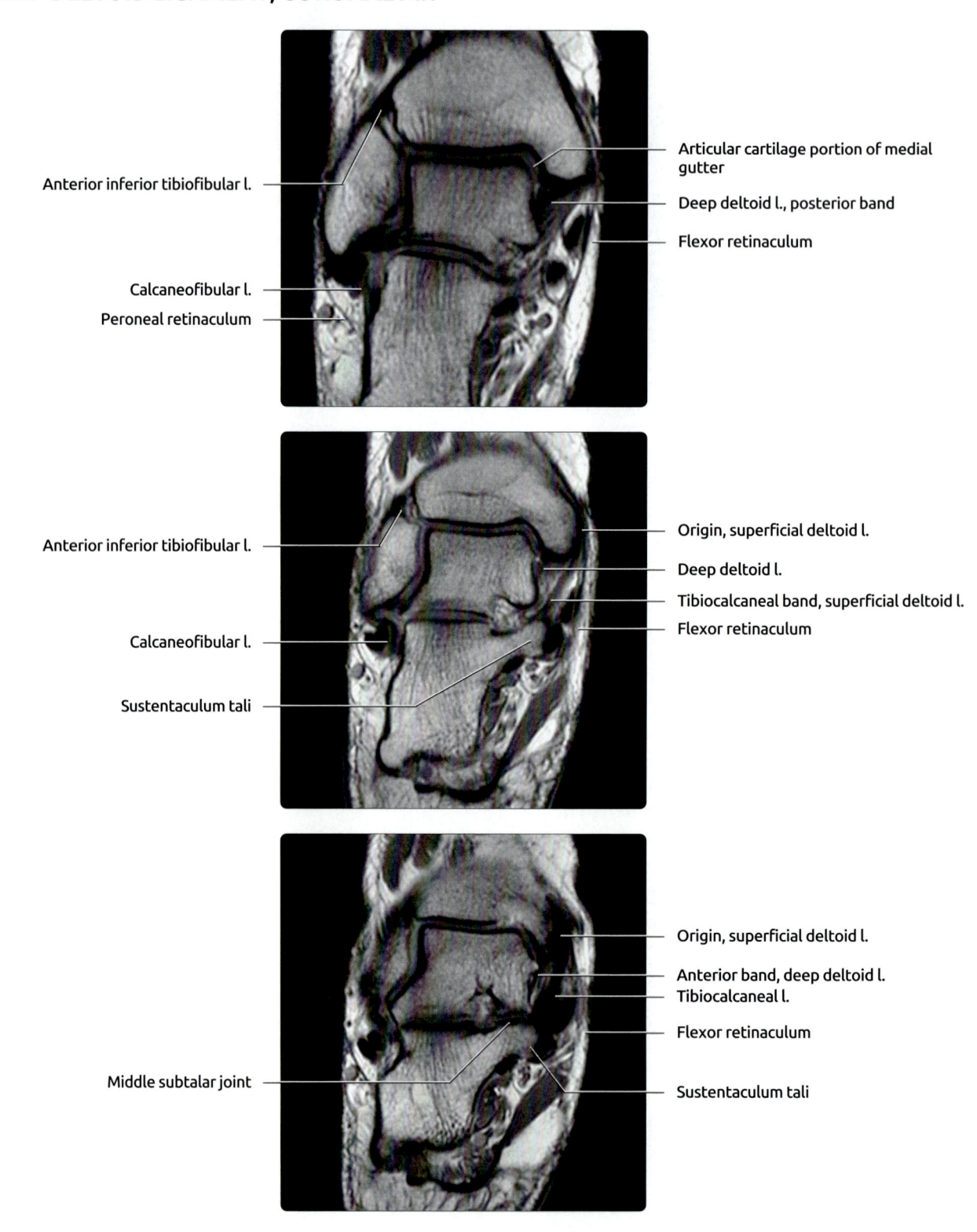

(Top) The posterior band of the deep deltoid ligament is often simply designated as the deep deltoid, disregarding the small, variably present anterior band. It has a striated appearance and an oblique course from the posterior margin of the anterior colliculus of the medial malleolus and the posterior colliculus to the fovea at the medial talus. *(Middle)* The anterior bands of the superficial deltoid have a common origin from the superficial, medial, and anterior margin of the medial malleolus. The tibiocalcaneal band is the strongest band. It inserts on the sustentaculum tali of the calcaneus. *(Bottom)* The tibiocalcaneal band of the superficial deltoid is always present in uninjured patients. In this normal volunteer, it is slightly thicker than is usually seen.

Ankle Ligaments

LATERAL COLLATERAL LIGAMENTS

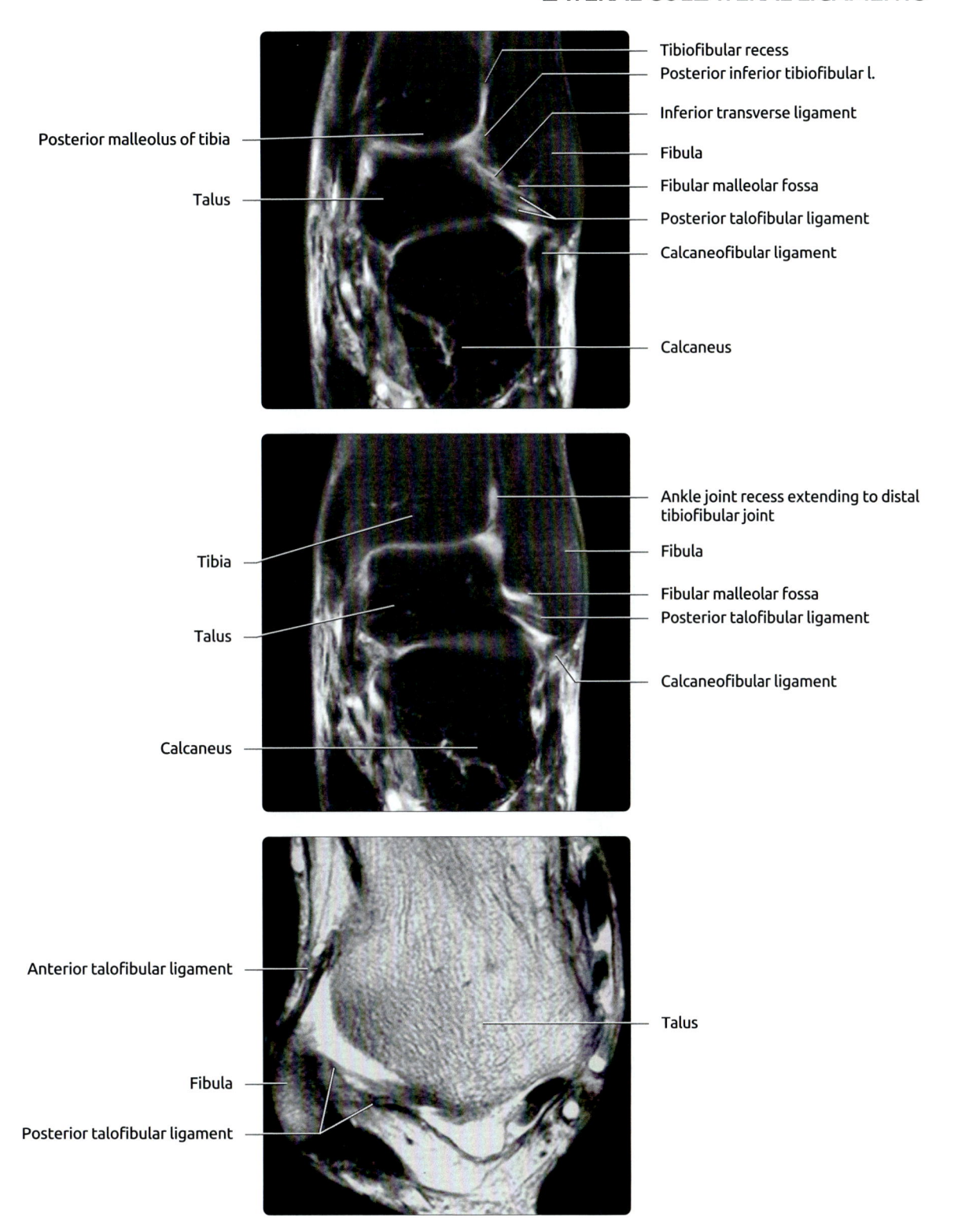

(Top) Coronal T2 fat-suppressed image shows the lateral collateral ligaments. The lateral collateral ligaments consist of anterior and posterior talofibular, as well as calcaneofibular ligaments. Although they are in close proximity to the syndesmotic ligaments, their function, protecting against inversion, internal rotation, and anterior subluxation are very different. (Middle) A slightly more anterior coronal T2 fat-suppressed image is shown. The posterior talofibular ligament is visualized as a distinct structure from the posterior tibiofibular ligament. (Bottom) Lateral collateral ligaments are shown on this T2 axial image. The ligaments are optimally seen on axial images. Since these ligaments are thickening of the capsule, they are highlighted by fluid. Note the fan-shaped and striated fibular insertion of the posterior talofibular ligament, which should not to be mistaken for a tear.

Ankle Ligaments

LATERAL COLLATERAL LIGAMENTS

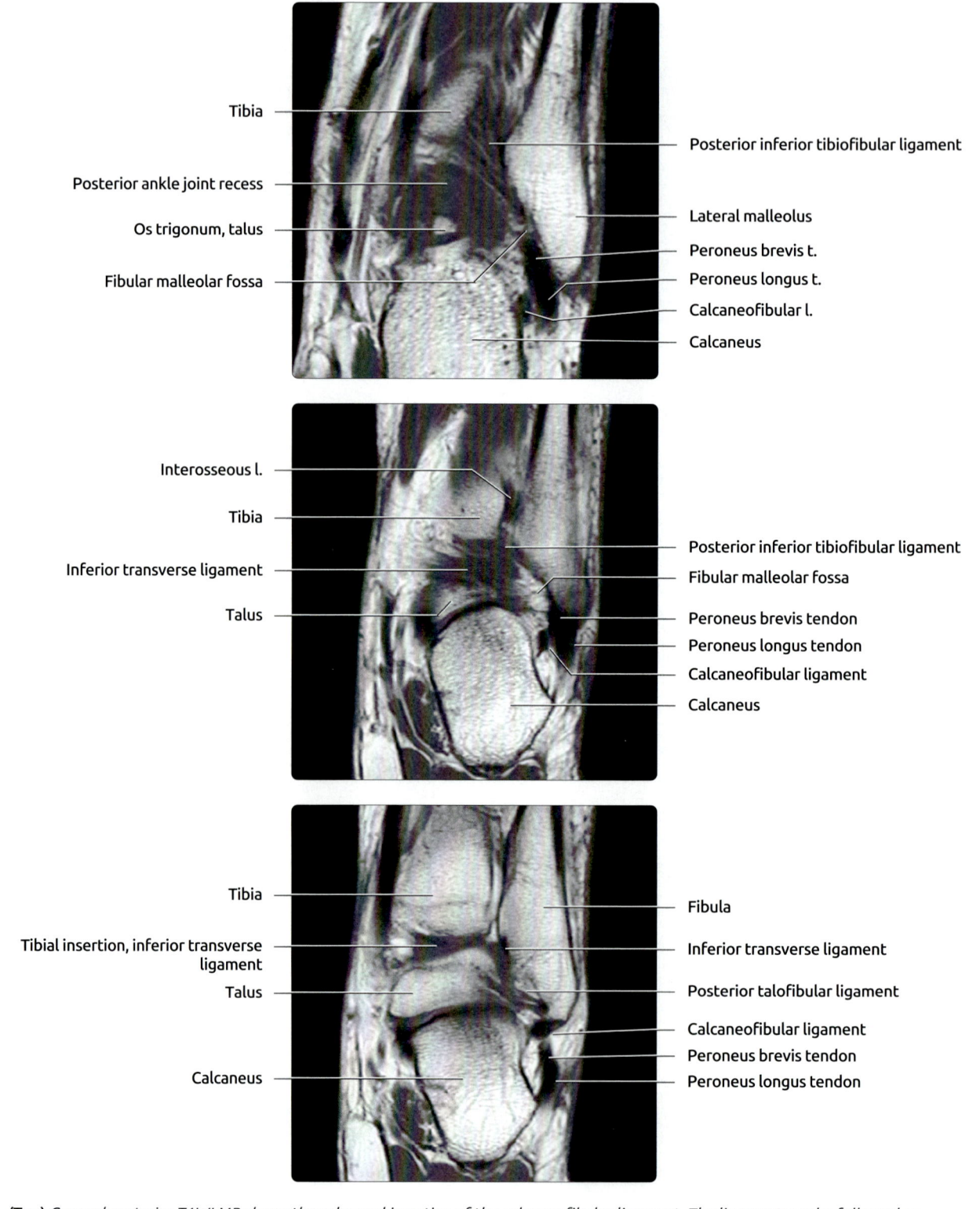

(Top) Coronal posterior T1WI MR shows the calcaneal insertion of the calcaneofibular ligament. The ligament can be followed on sequential coronal images from its fibular origin to its calcaneal insertion. (Middle) The calcaneofibular ligament is seen on a more anterior coronal T1WI. Note proximity of the ligament to peroneal tendons, which can be used to locate the ligament. A tear of the ligament may produce reactive fluid within the common peroneal tendon sheath; this should not to be mistaken for peroneal tenosynovitis. (Bottom) In a more anterior image, the origin of the calcaneofibular ligament from the tip of the fibula is visualized.

Ankle Ligaments

LATERAL COLLATERAL LIGAMENTS

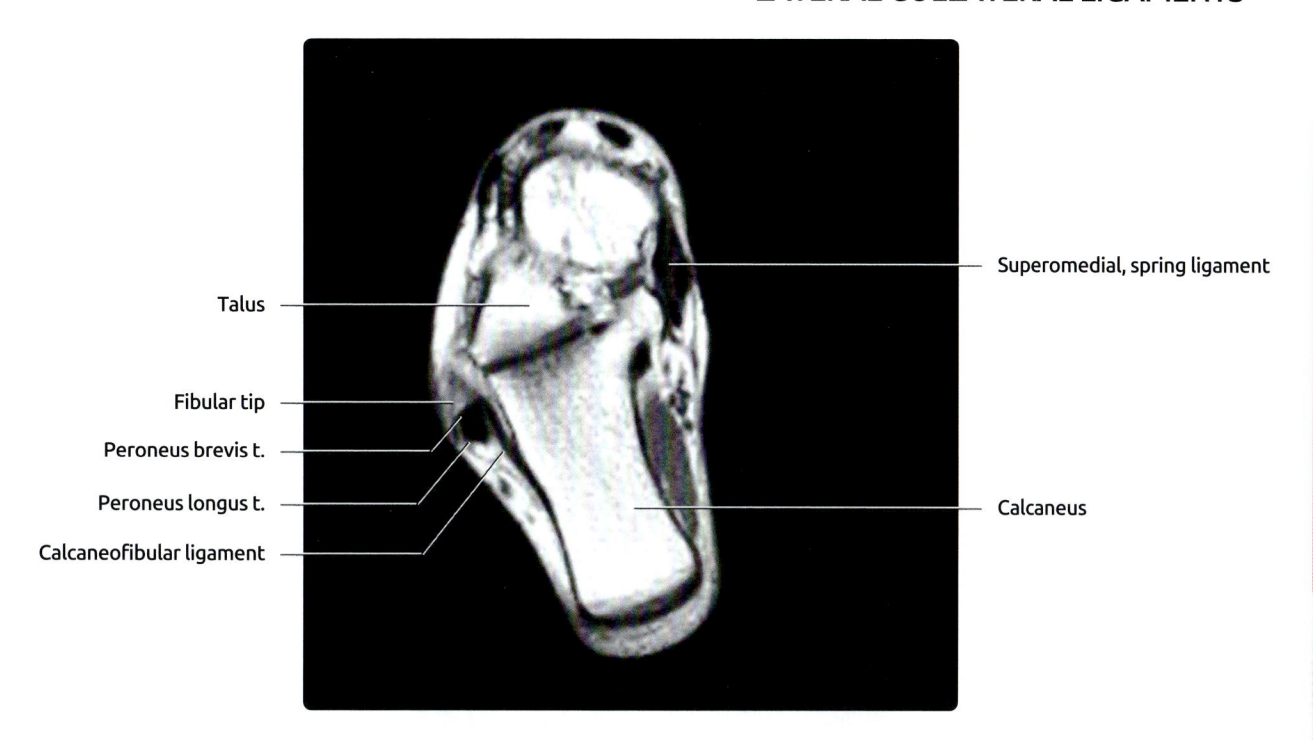

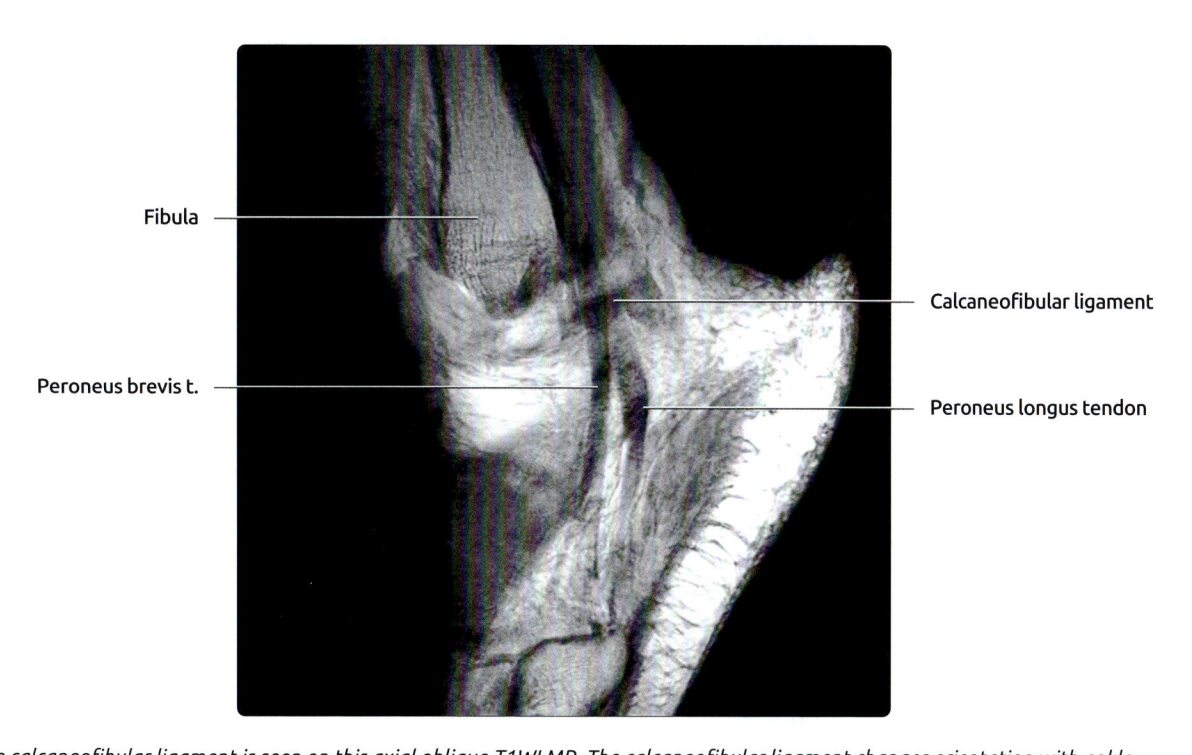

(Top) The calcaneofibular ligament is seen on this axial oblique T1WI MR. The calcaneofibular ligament changes orientation with ankle movements. In mild plantar flexion, the ligament becomes close to horizontal in orientation and may be visualized on axial images as it hugs the calcaneus, deep to the peroneal tendons. Its location deep to the peroneal tendons is a clue in locating this ligament. (Bottom) On this far lateral sagittal MR image, the calcaneofibular ligament may be visualized, due to partial volume averaging, as a low signal shadow superimposed on the peroneal tendons. Note that in this patient, scanned in plantarflexion, the calcaneofibular ligament is relatively horizontal. In general, mild plantar flexion of the ankle aids in detecting the calcaneofibular ligament on axial images.

Ankle Ligaments

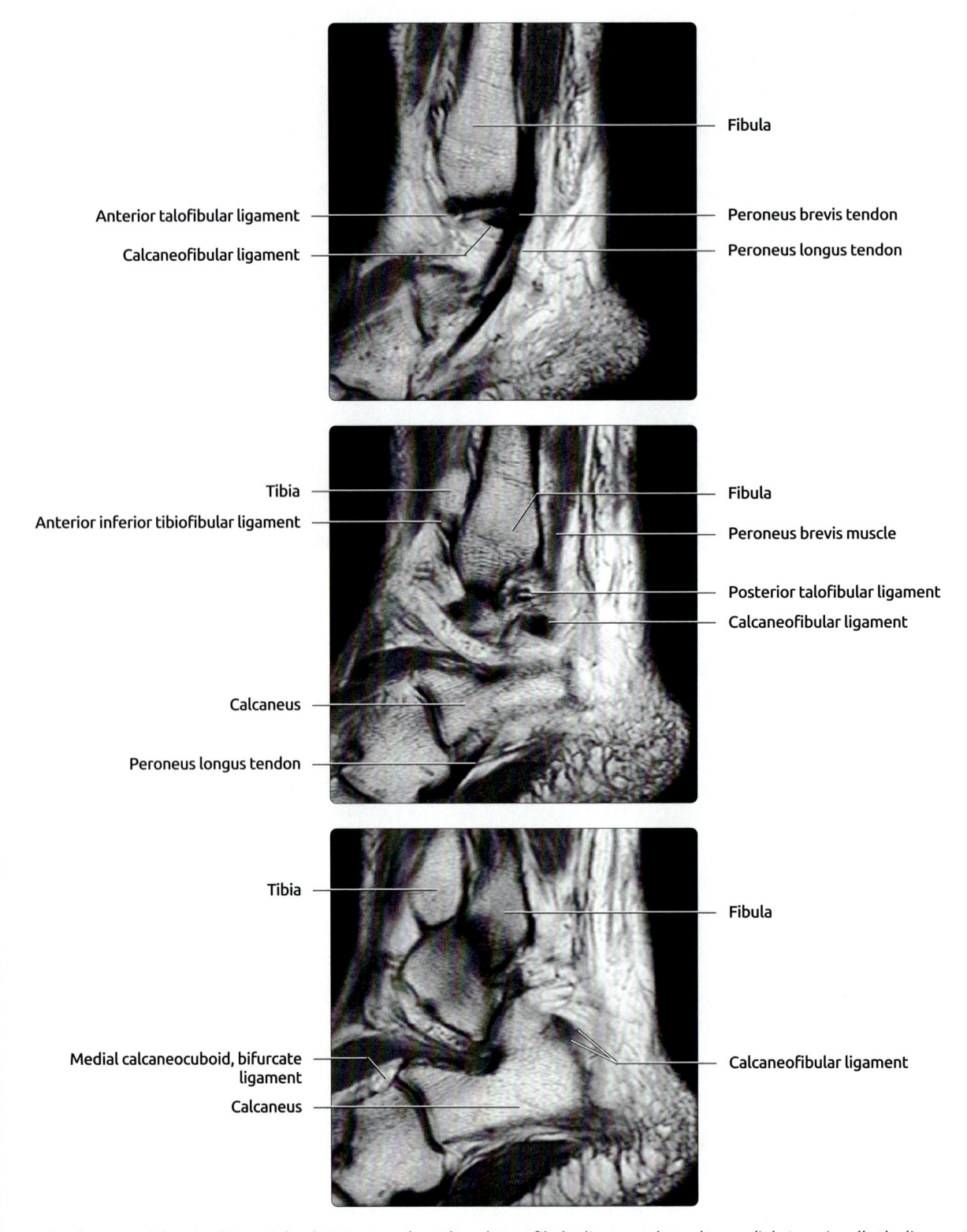

LATERAL COLLATERAL LIGAMENTS

(Top) Sequential sagittal T1-weighted MR images show the calcaneofibular ligament, lateral to medial. Occasionally the ligament may be visualized on sequential sagittal images from its fibular origin to its posterior calcaneal insertion. *(Middle)* The calcaneofibular ligament is now visualized as it is traversing the region deep (medial) to the peroneal tendons (peroneals are not well seen in this image). Note also the striated posterior talofibular ligament behind (posterior to) the fibula. *(Bottom)* Sagittal T1WI shows the calcaneofibular ligament. The calcaneofibular ligament is now seen in cross section as it inserts onto the calcaneus.

Ankle Ligaments

DELTOID LIGAMENT

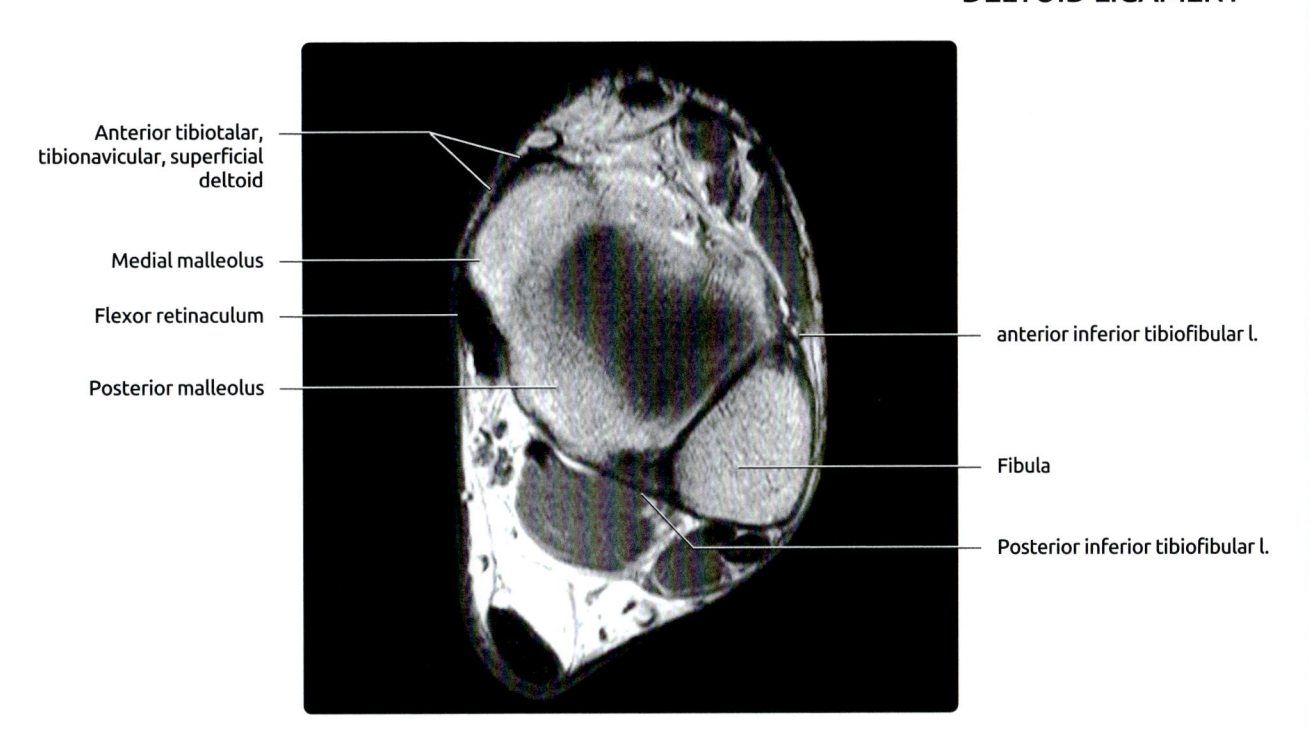

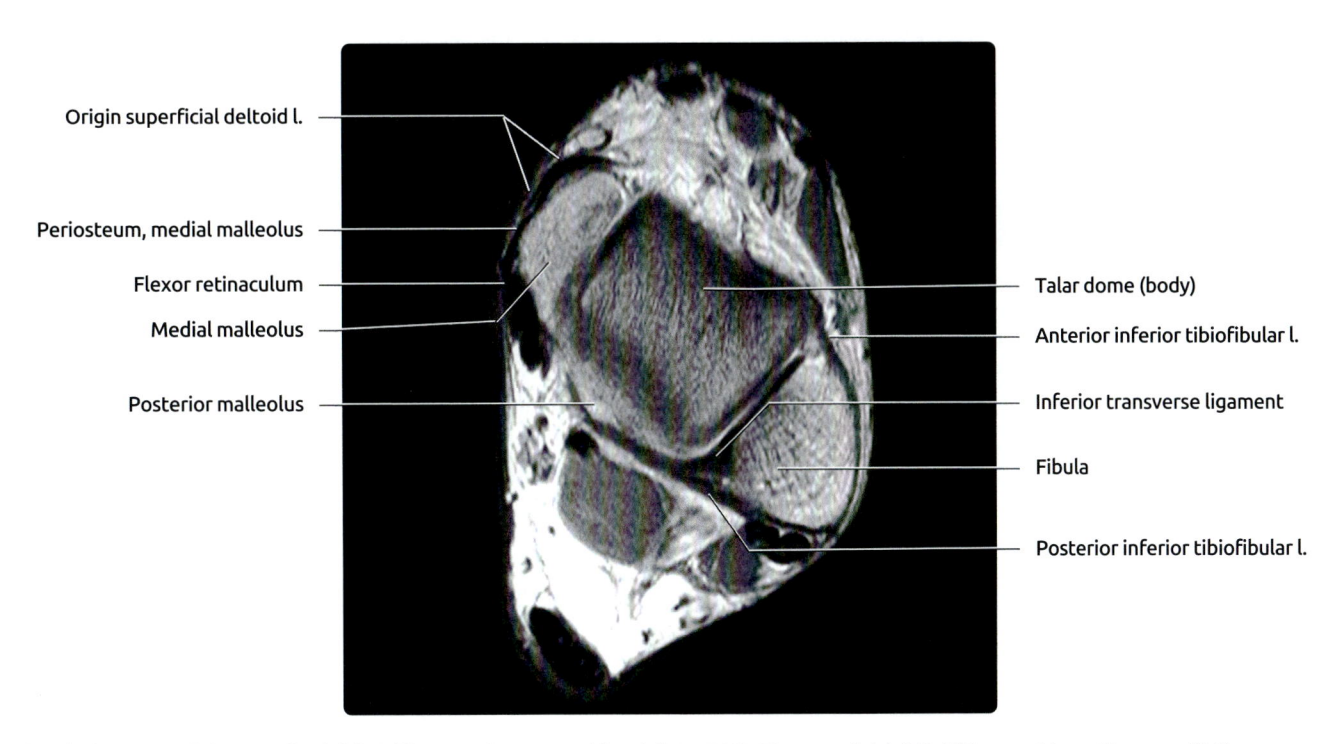

Labels (top image):
- Anterior tibiotalar, tibionavicular, superficial deltoid
- Medial malleolus
- Flexor retinaculum
- Posterior malleolus
- anterior inferior tibiofibular l.
- Fibula
- Posterior inferior tibiofibular l.

Labels (bottom image):
- Origin superficial deltoid l.
- Periosteum, medial malleolus
- Flexor retinaculum
- Medial malleolus
- Posterior malleolus
- Talar dome (body)
- Anterior inferior tibiofibular l.
- Inferior transverse ligament
- Fibula
- Posterior inferior tibiofibular l.

(Top) The origin of the superficial deltoid ligament is seen on this axial T1WI MR. The superficial deltoid ligament is continuous with the periosteum of the medial malleolus, which is continuous with the flexor retinaculum origin. (Bottom) Axial T1WI MR, located slightly more distally, depicts the origin of the superficial deltoid. Its continuity with the periosteum of the medial malleolus, and the flexor retinaculum, is evident. This entire fascial layer may be avulsed from anterior to posterior due to twisting injury.

Ankle Ligaments

DELTOID LIGAMENT

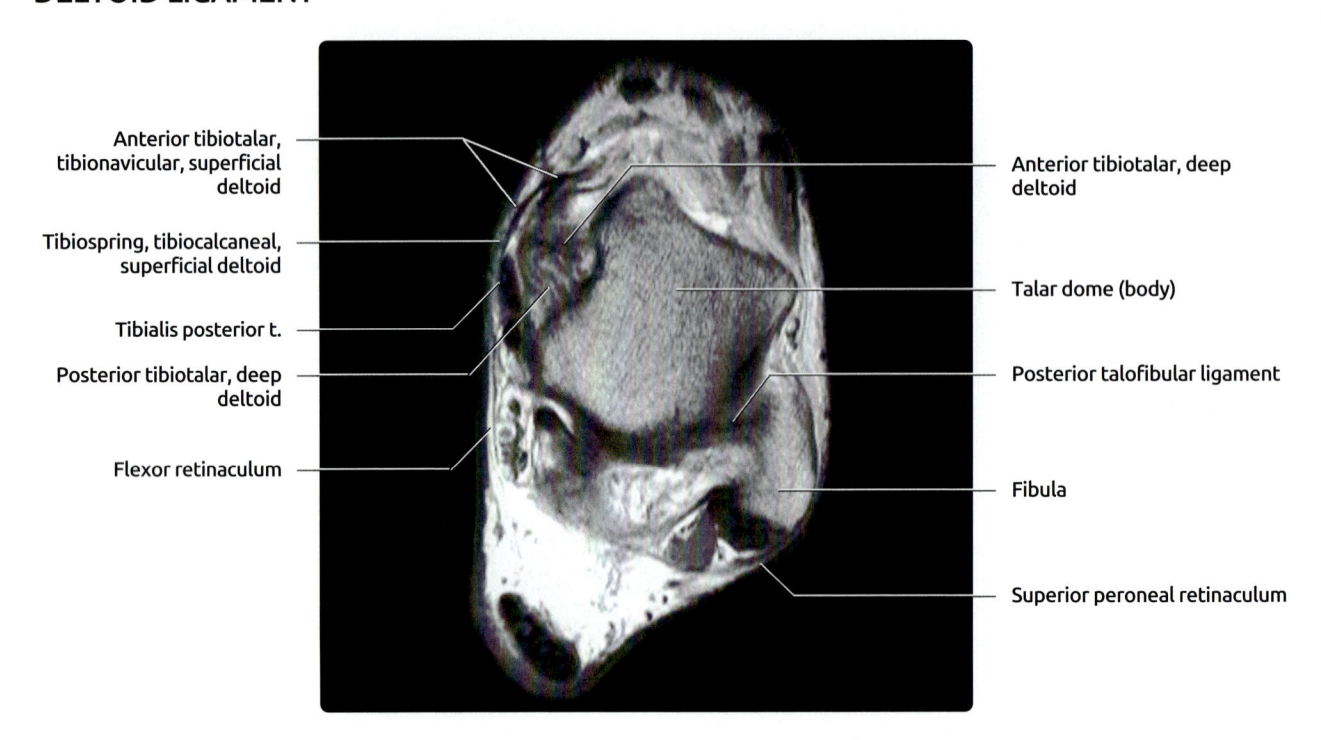

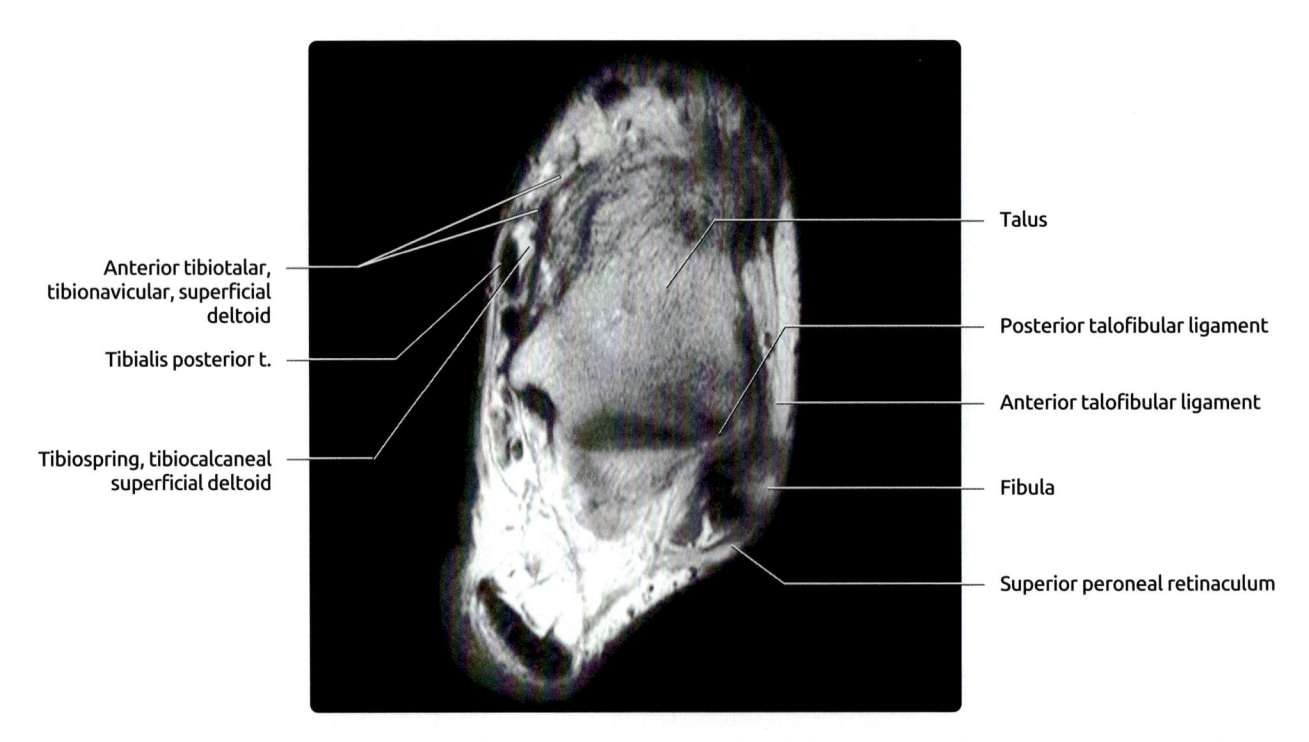

(Top) Axial T2WI MR, at the level of talar dome, depicts the superficial deltoid bands diverging toward their insertions. The striated appearance of the deep deltoid ligament is well seen. (Bottom) Axial T2WI MR, located slightly more distally, depicts the tibiocalcaneal and tibiospring ligaments of the deltoid. The tibiospring ligament is slightly anterior to the tibiocalcaneal band and merges with the spring ligament.

Ankle Ligaments

TARSAL CANAL & SINUS TARSI LIGAMENTS

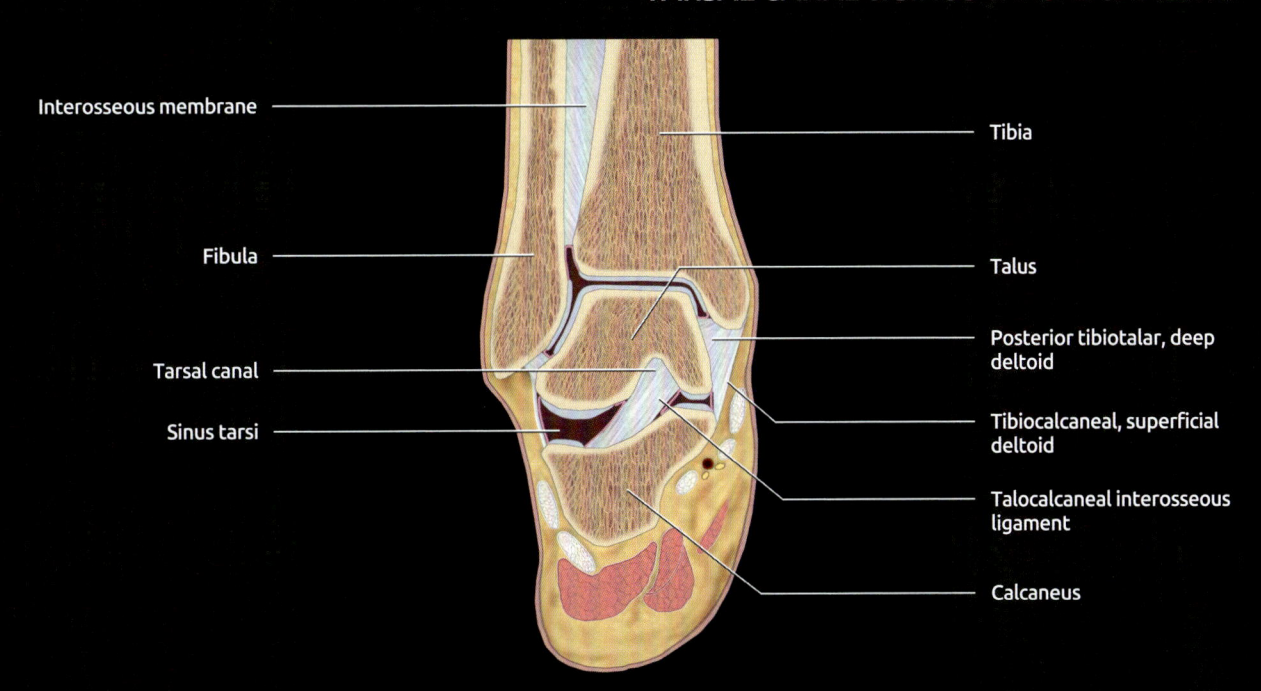

Top image labels:
- Interosseous membrane
- Fibula
- Tarsal canal
- Sinus tarsi
- Tibia
- Talus
- Posterior tibiotalar, deep deltoid
- Tibiocalcaneal, superficial deltoid
- Talocalcaneal interosseous ligament
- Calcaneus

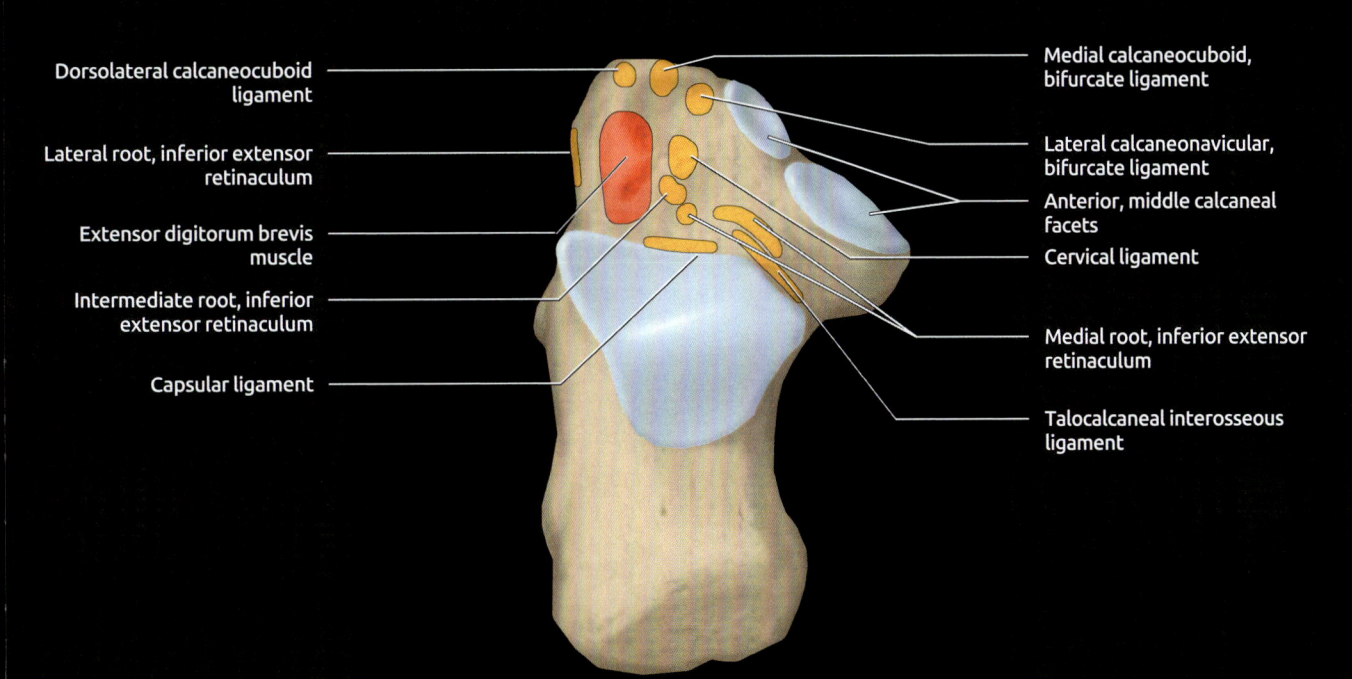

Bottom image labels:
- Dorsolateral calcaneocuboid ligament
- Lateral root, inferior extensor retinaculum
- Extensor digitorum brevis muscle
- Intermediate root, inferior extensor retinaculum
- Capsular ligament
- Medial calcaneocuboid, bifurcate ligament
- Lateral calcaneonavicular, bifurcate ligament
- Anterior, middle calcaneal facets
- Cervical ligament
- Medial root, inferior extensor retinaculum
- Talocalcaneal interosseous ligament

(Top) A drawing of tarsal canal ligaments is shown. The tarsal canal is a space between the posterior subtalar joint and sustentaculum tali, traversed by the talocalcaneal interosseous ligament. The sinus tarsi is a more lateral space between the talus and calcaneus, which is continuous with the tarsal canal. The sinus tarsi is traversed by the roots of the inferior extensor retinaculum and by the cervical ligament. (Bottom) Calcaneal insertions of sinus tarsi ligaments are shown. The talocalcaneal interosseous ligament is most medial and posterior, while the cervical ligament is most anterior. The intermediate root of the inferior extensor retinaculum is immediately posterior to the cervical ligament, while the lateral root is lateral to the origin of the extensor digitorum brevis muscle. The medial root has 2 calcaneal and 1 talar insertions.

Ankle Ligaments

TARSAL CANAL & TARSAL SINUS LIGAMENTS

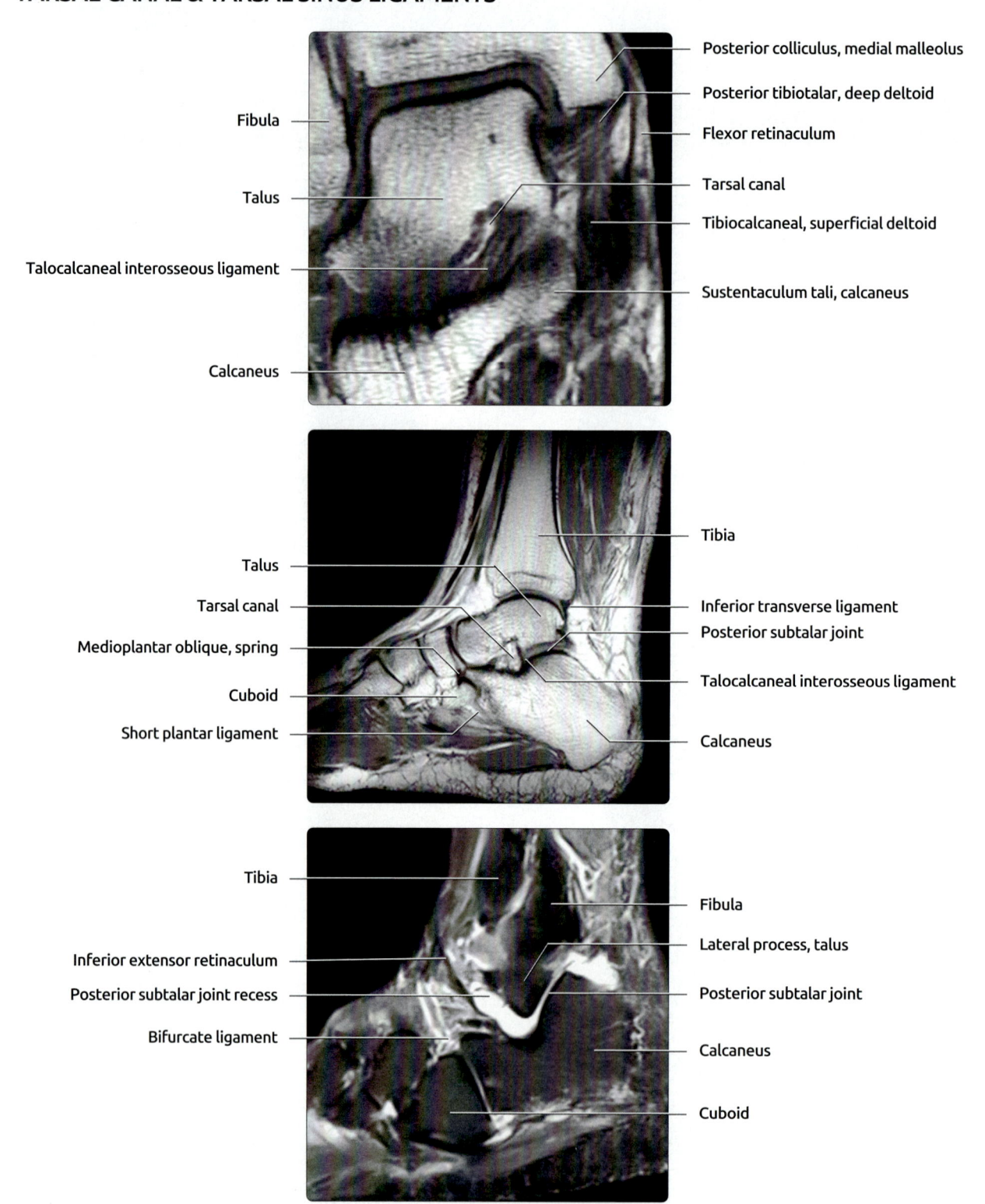

(Top) Coronal MR shows the talocalcaneal interosseous ligament. The ligaments calcaneal insertion is just anterior to the posterior subtalar joint. The ligament then traverses the tarsal canal and ascends obliquely and medially to insert on the talar sulcus. The talocalcaneal interosseous ligament is best identified on coronal and sagittal images as the most posterior and medial of sinus tarsi ligaments. (Middle) Sagittal MR image depicts the interosseous ligament as a band extending from the talus to the calcaneus, found anterior to the posterior subtalar joint. This ligament is typically found on the most medial sagittal images of the sinus tarsi. (Bottom) Tarsal sinus fluid often implies acute or chronic disease. However, a fluid-filled recess may extend from the posterior subtalar joint into the sinus tarsi. This should not be misinterpreted as pathology of the sinus tarsi.

Ankle Ligaments

TARSAL CANAL & TARSAL SINUS LIGAMENTS

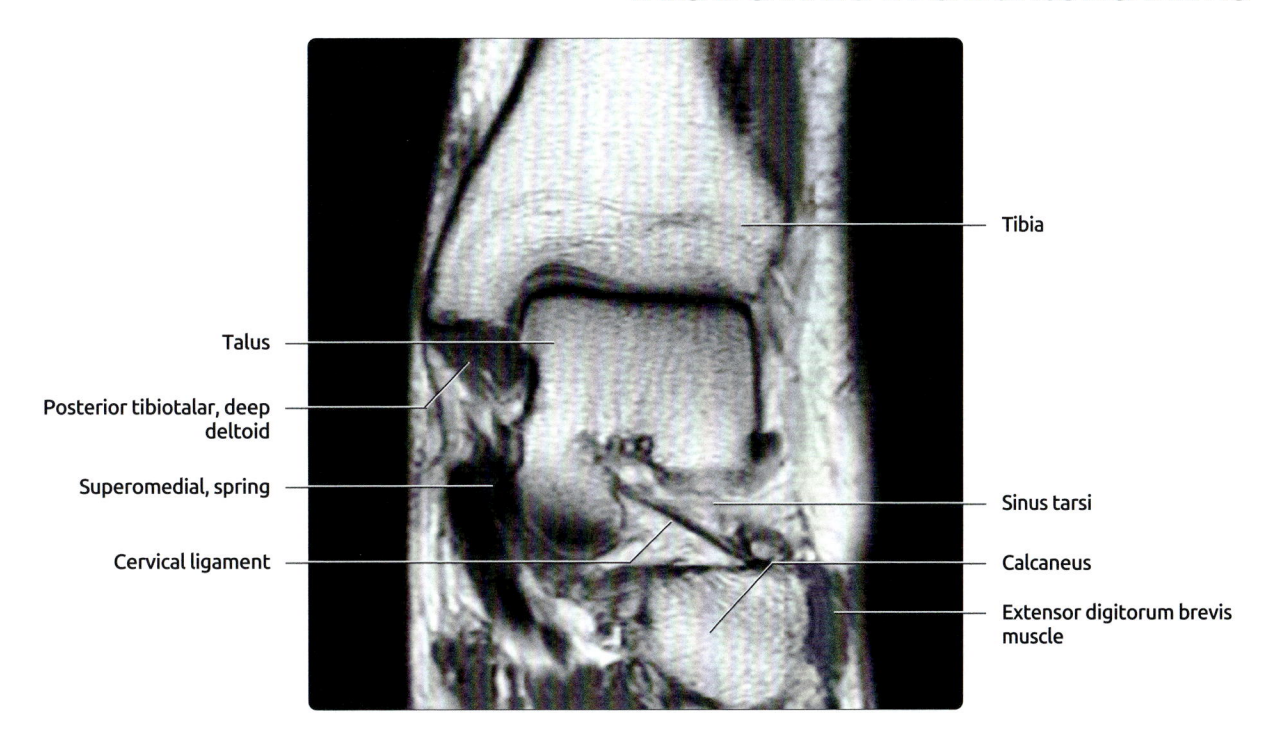

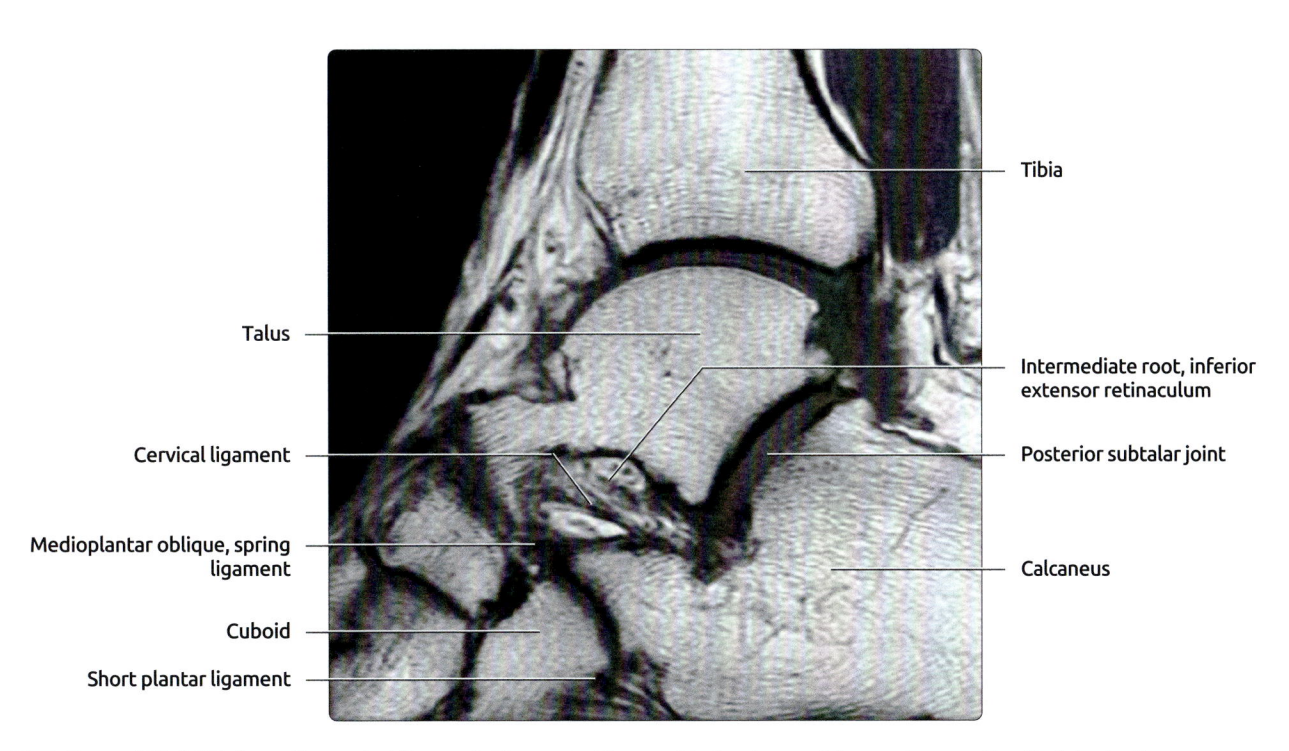

Top image labels:
- Tibia
- Talus
- Posterior tibiotalar, deep deltoid
- Superomedial, spring
- Cervical ligament
- Sinus tarsi
- Calcaneus
- Extensor digitorum brevis muscle

Bottom image labels:
- Tibia
- Talus
- Intermediate root, inferior extensor retinaculum
- Cervical ligament
- Posterior subtalar joint
- Medioplantar oblique, spring ligament
- Calcaneus
- Cuboid
- Short plantar ligament

(**Top**) Coronal T1WI MR shows the cervical ligament. The cervical ligament is the strongest ligament connecting the talus to the calcaneus. It is also the most anterior ligament of the sinus tarsi. Its calcaneal origin is medial to the origin of the extensor digitorum brevis muscle. The ligament ascends upward anteriorly and medially to insert on the inferior aspect of the talar neck. The ligament becomes more horizontal in valgus and more vertical in varus position of the calcaneus. (**Bottom**) Sagittal T1WI MR shows the cervical ligament. The ligaments anterior course from the calcaneus to the talus is better appreciated on sagittal images. Note the intermediate root of the inferior extensor retinaculum located immediately posterior to the cervical ligament.

Ankle Ligaments

TARSAL CANAL & TARSAL SINUS LIGAMENTS

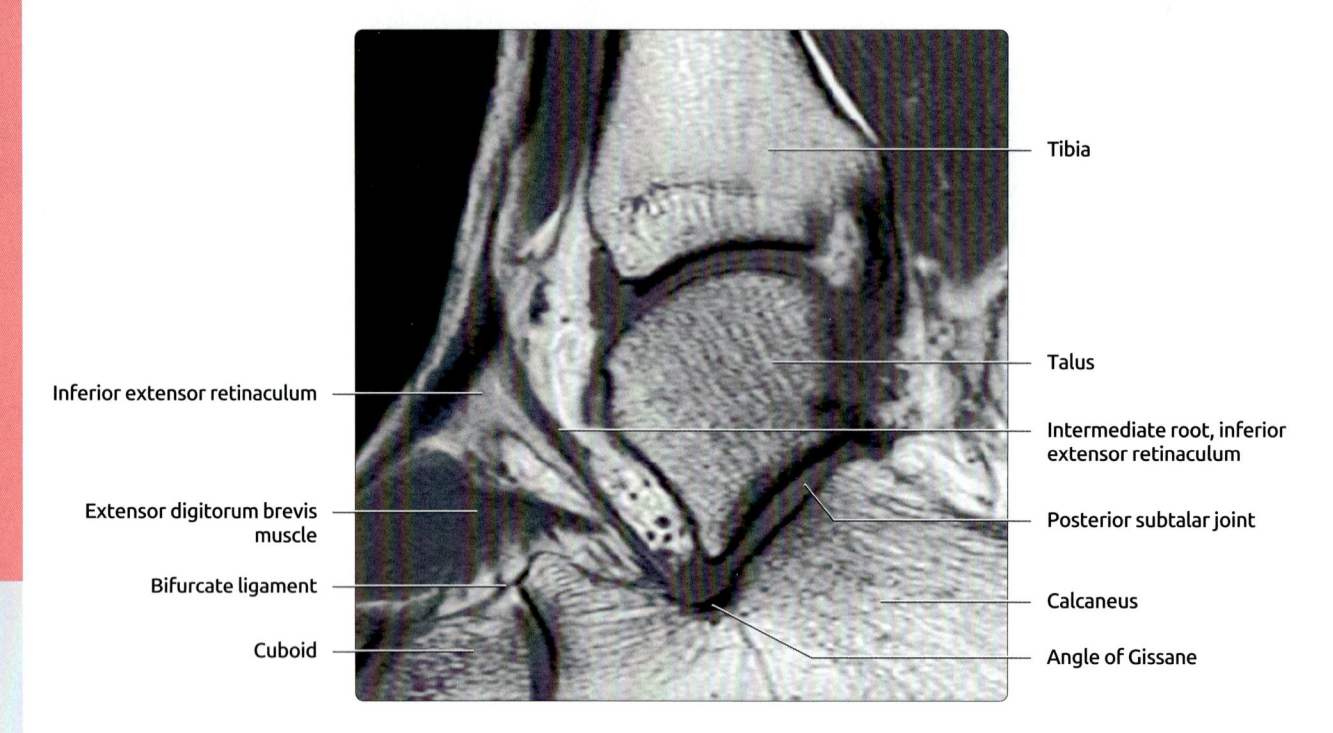

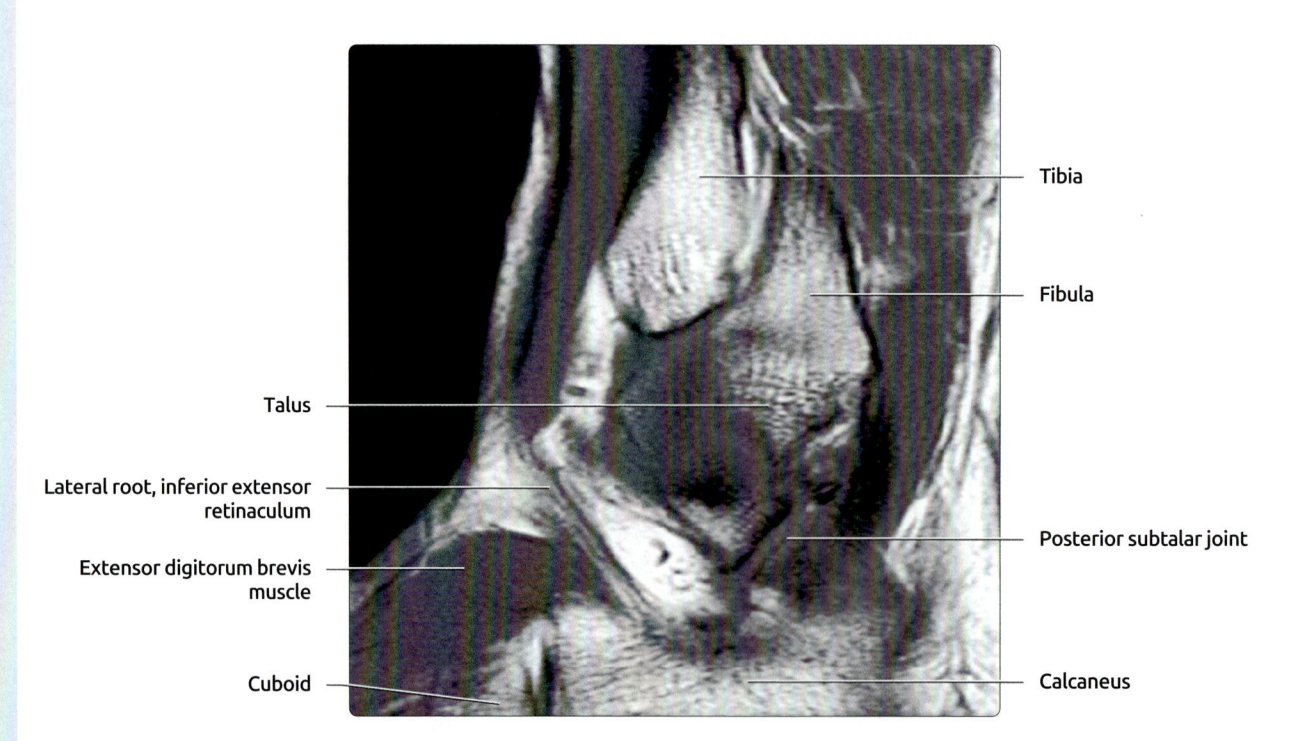

Top image labels:
- Inferior extensor retinaculum
- Extensor digitorum brevis muscle
- Bifurcate ligament
- Cuboid
- Tibia
- Talus
- Intermediate root, inferior extensor retinaculum
- Posterior subtalar joint
- Calcaneus
- Angle of Gissane

Bottom image labels:
- Talus
- Lateral root, inferior extensor retinaculum
- Extensor digitorum brevis muscle
- Cuboid
- Tibia
- Fibula
- Posterior subtalar joint
- Calcaneus

(Top) *Sagittal MR shows roots of the extensor retinaculum. The intermediate root inserts into the calcaneus slightly posterior to the cervical ligament. The medial root has medial and lateral calcaneal insertions and 1 talar insertion. The intermediate root and lateral component of the medial root may insert very close to each other on the calcaneus, but the latter is found closer to the posterior subtalar joint.* (Bottom) *Sagittal T1WI MR shows the lateral root of the inferior extensor retinaculum. The root inserts into the calcaneus lateral to the origin of the extensor digitorum brevis muscle. It is continuous with the inferior peroneal retinaculum and deep fascia. The ligament is found on very far lateral sagittal images of the sinus tarsi.*

Ankle Ligaments

SPRING LIGAMENT

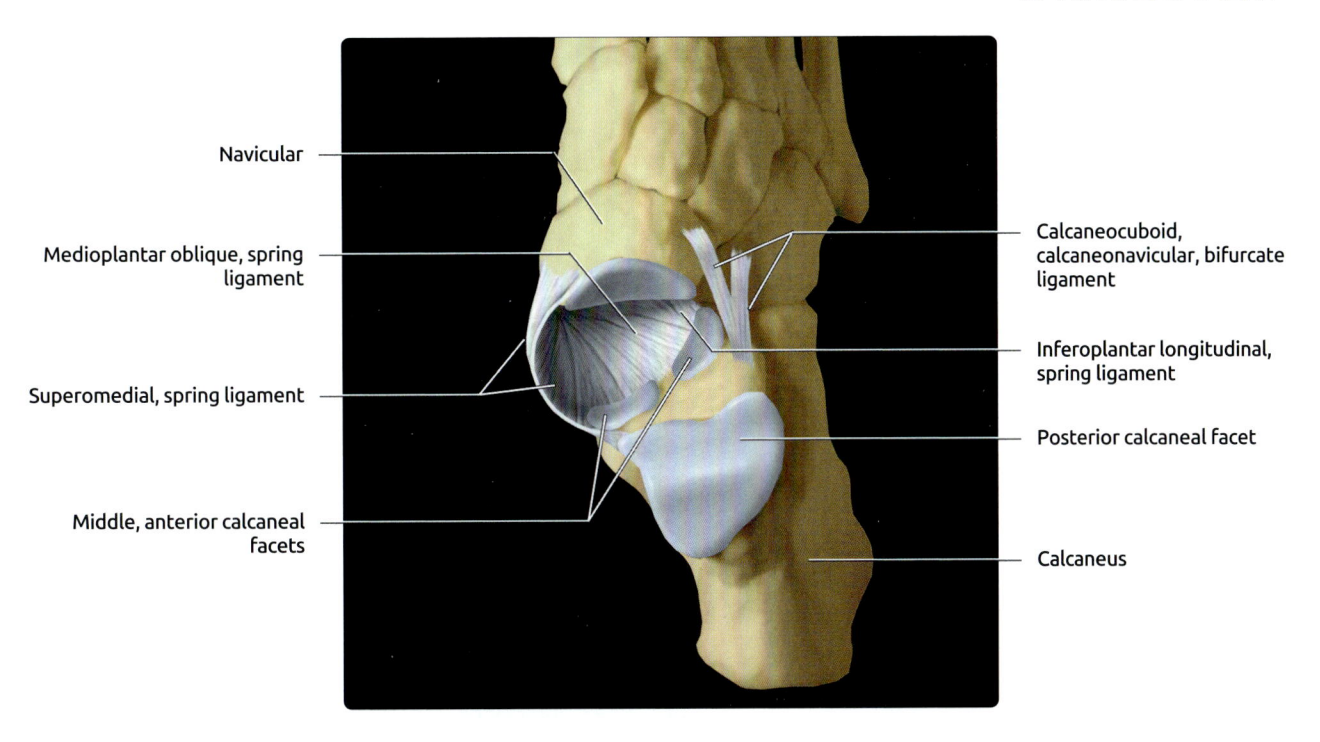

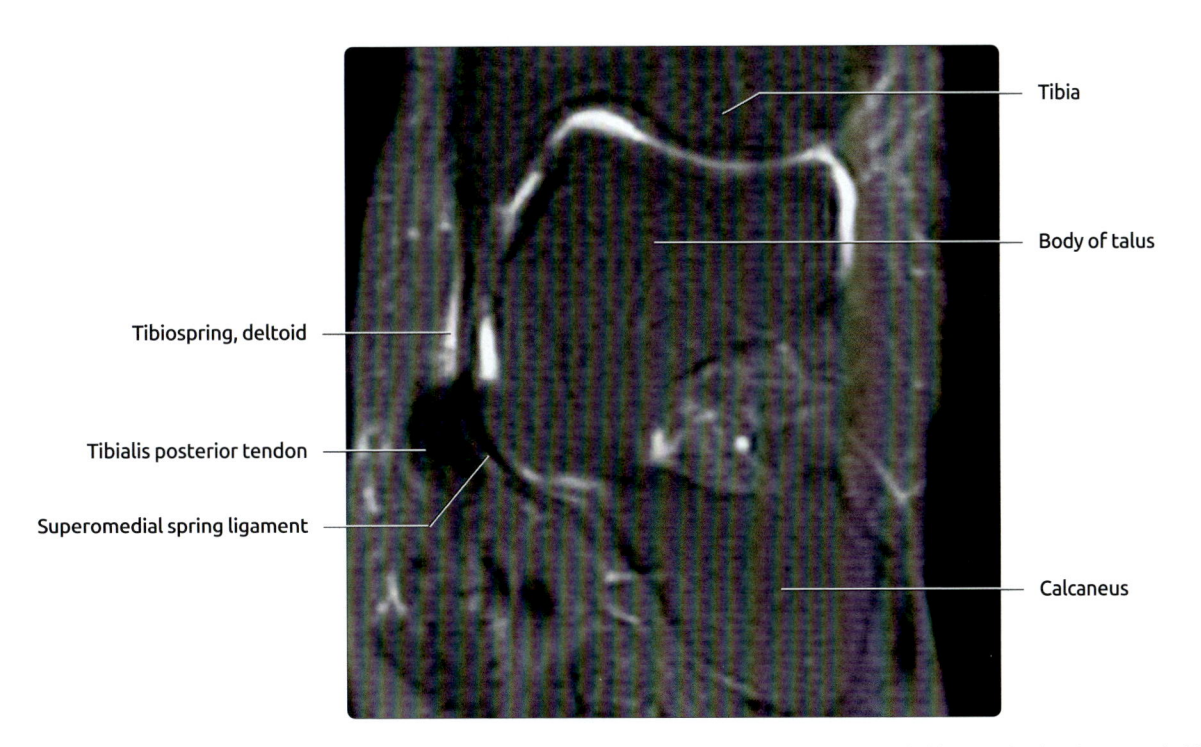

(Top) The spring ligament is a hammock-shaped structure which supports the talar head and medial longitudinal arch. Coronal oblique and sagittal images provide optimal visualization of the components of the spring ligament; however, routine ankle images are also useful. The superomedial component originates from the sustentaculum tali and inserts into superomedial navicular and the tibiospring ligament. It is best seen on coronal and axial images and occasionally on a far medial sagittal image. The medioplantar oblique is best seen on axial images, while the inferoplantar longitudinal is seen on both axial and sagittal images. (Bottom) Coronal fat-suppressed T2WI shows the superomedial spring ligament. The ligament hugs the talar head and is contiguous with the tibiospring component of the deltoid ligament. Note the proximity of the tibialis posterior tendon to the ligament.

Ankle Ligaments

SPRING LIGAMENT

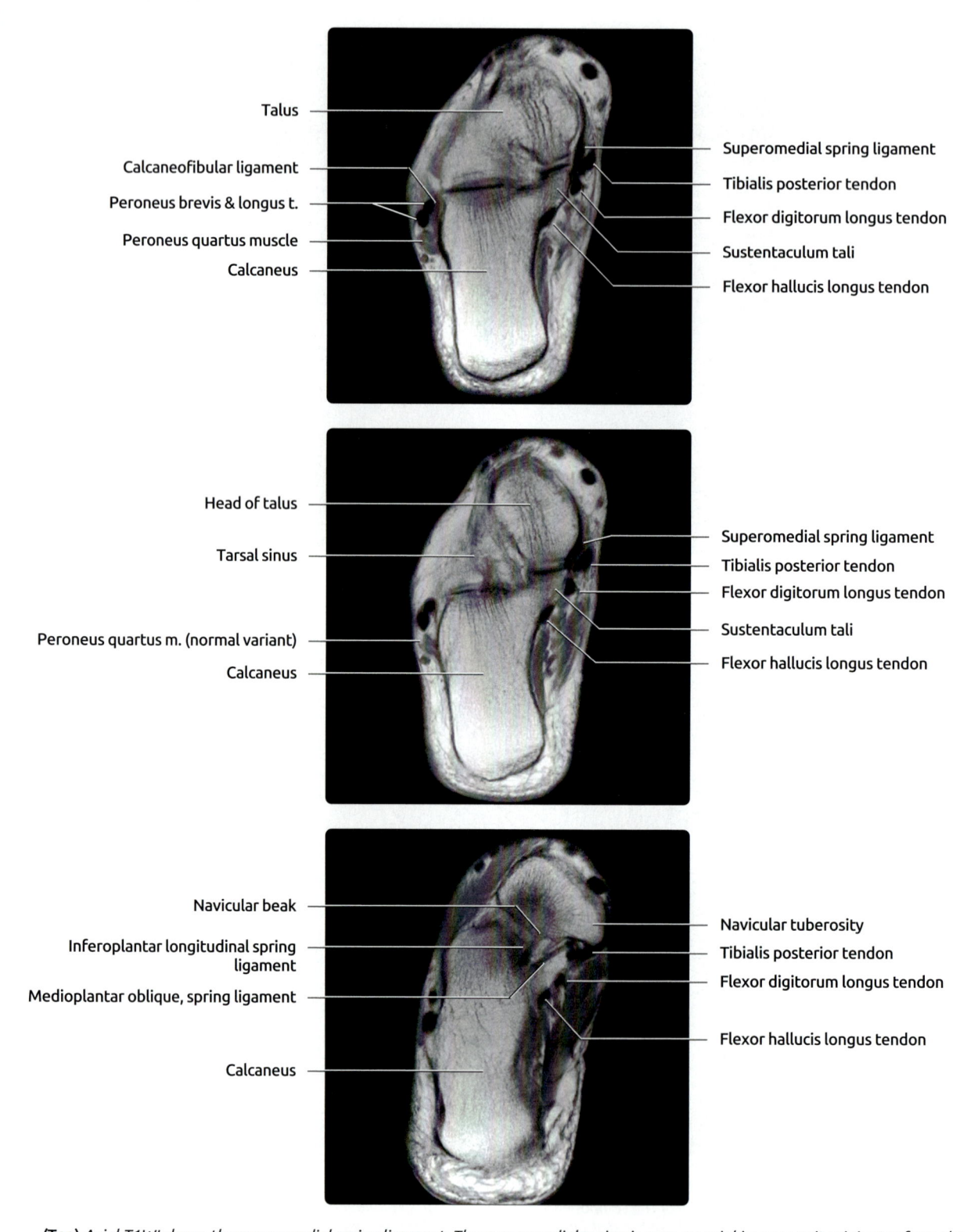

(Top) Axial T1WI shows the superomedial spring ligament. The superomedial spring is seen on axial images as it originates from the sustentaculum tali and curves around the talar head toward its navicular insertion (latter not seen). Notice the proximity of the tibialis posterior tendon. **(Middle)** A more distal axial T1WI shows the superomedial spring ligament. **(Bottom)** A more distal axial T1WI is shown. The medioplantar oblique and inferoplantar longitudinal components of the spring ligament originate from the calcaneus at the coronoid fossa (between the sustentaculum tali and anterior calcaneal process). The medioplantar oblique is consistently seen as it inserts into the plantar navicular, just lateral to the navicular tuberosity and tibialis posterior tendon. The inferoplantar longitudinal inserts on the beak of the navicular.

Ankle Ligaments

SPRING LIGAMENT

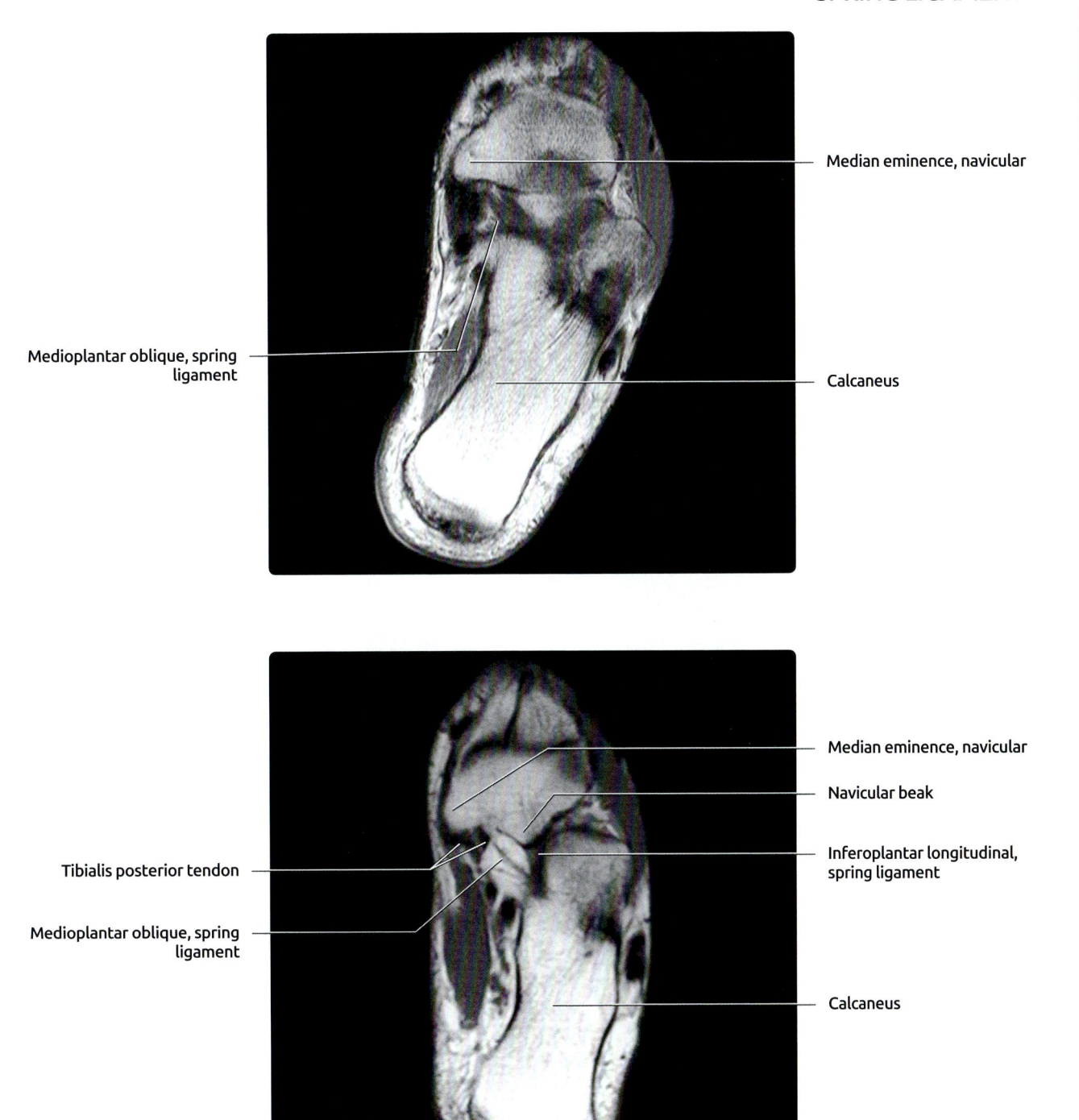

(Top) Axial T1WI image shows the medioplantar oblique component of the spring ligament. The ligament is frequently striated and is often relatively thick. **(Bottom)** A more distal axial T1WI is shown. Note the navicular beak at the insertion of the inferoplantar component of the spring ligament. Because of the straight course of the inferoplantar longitudinal component of the spring ligament, it is often seen on axial and sagittal images.

Ankle Ligaments

SPRING LIGAMENT

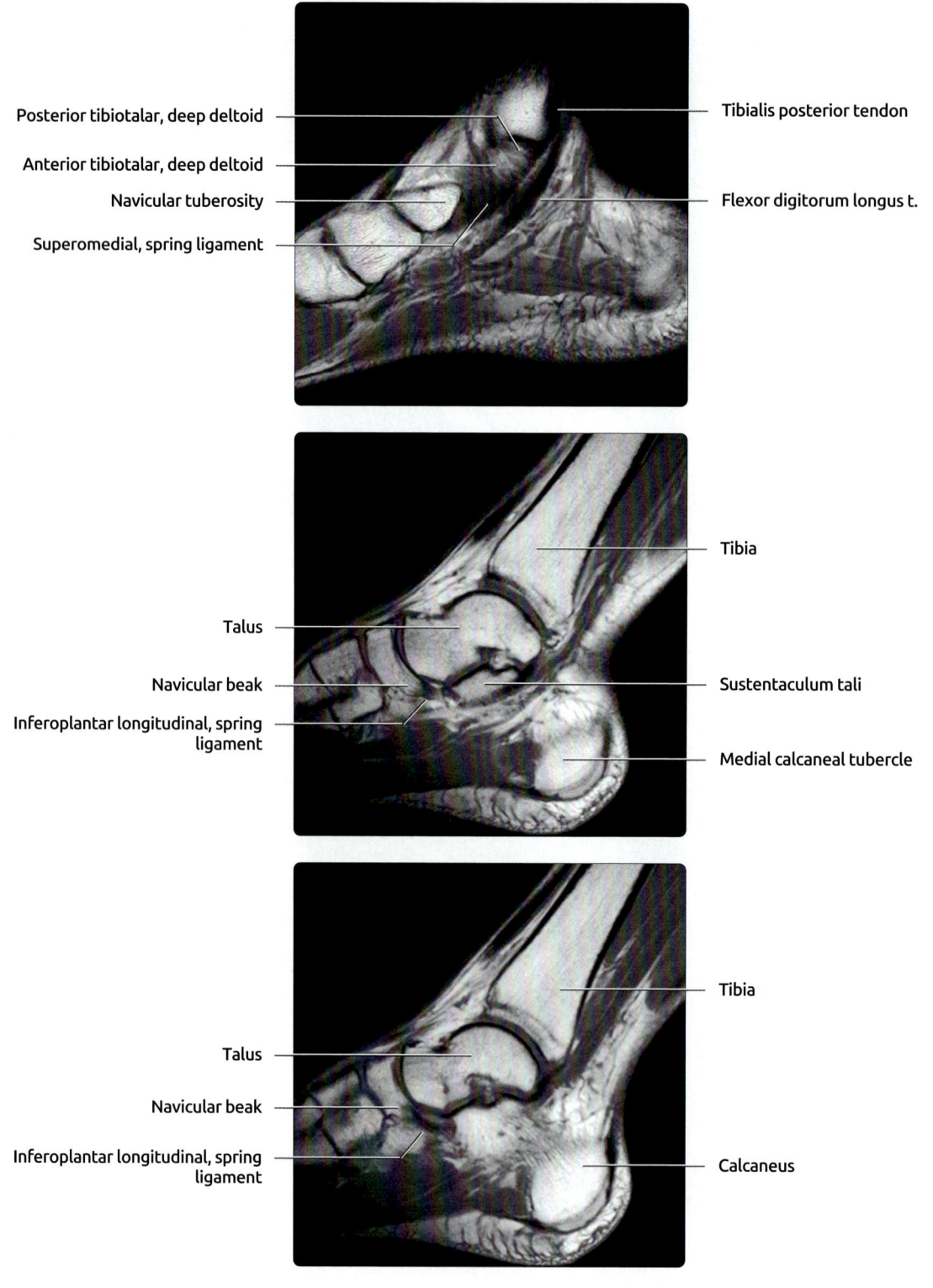

(Top) The superomedial component of the spring ligament is sometimes seen on a far medial image as a low signal band medial to the talar head and lateral to the tibialis posterior tendon. *(Middle)* The inferoplantar longitudinal band of the spring ligament is shown. Because of its oblique course, the medioplantar oblique component of the spring ligament is difficult to identify on routine sagittal images and may been seen on cross section as an oval low signal structure. However, the inferoplantar longitudinal component, because of its straight and short course, is frequently seen on sagittal images. Visualization of the beak of the navicular aids in identifying the ligament. *(Bottom)* Inferoplantar longitudinal ligament is shown. The ligament is a low signal band extending from the navicular beak to the coronoid fossa of the calcaneus.

Ankle Ligaments

BIFURCATE LIGAMENT

Top image labels:
- Talus
- Lateral calcaneonavicular, bifurcate
- Cuboid
- Calcaneus
- Long plantar ligament

Middle image labels:
- Talus
- Lateral root, inferior extensor retinaculum
- Medial calcaneocuboid, bifurcate
- Calcaneus
- Cuboid

Bottom image labels:
- Navicular
- Tibionavicular, superficial deltoid
- Talus
- Cuboid
- Lateral calcaneonavicular component, bifurcate ligament
- Medial calcaneocuboid component, bifurcate ligament
- Anterior process, calcaneus
- Cervical ligament

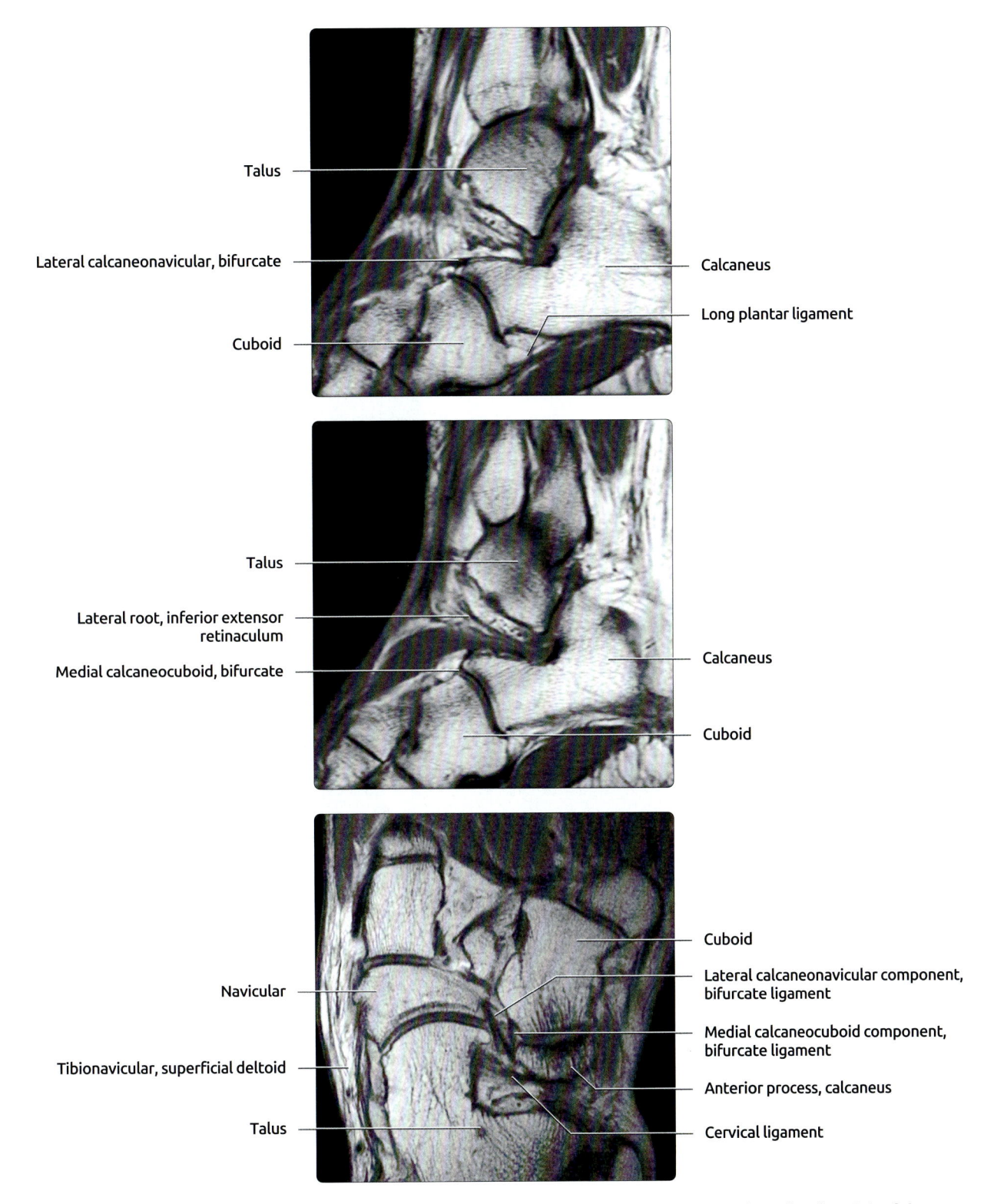

(Top) The lateral calcaneonavicular ligament of the bifurcate ligament is best seen on a sagittal image just lateral to the origin of the inferoplantar longitudinal component of the spring ligament. It is seen as a fine, curved, low signal structure originating from the anterior process of the calcaneus. (Middle) The medial calcaneocuboid component of the bifurcate ligament originates lateral to the lateral calcaneonavicular component. It is often quite a delicate, low signal intensity structure, which may be absent in some individuals. (Bottom) The bifurcate ligament is occasionally seen on axial oblique images of the hindfoot.

Ankle Ligaments

LONG & SHORT PLANTAR LIGAMENTS

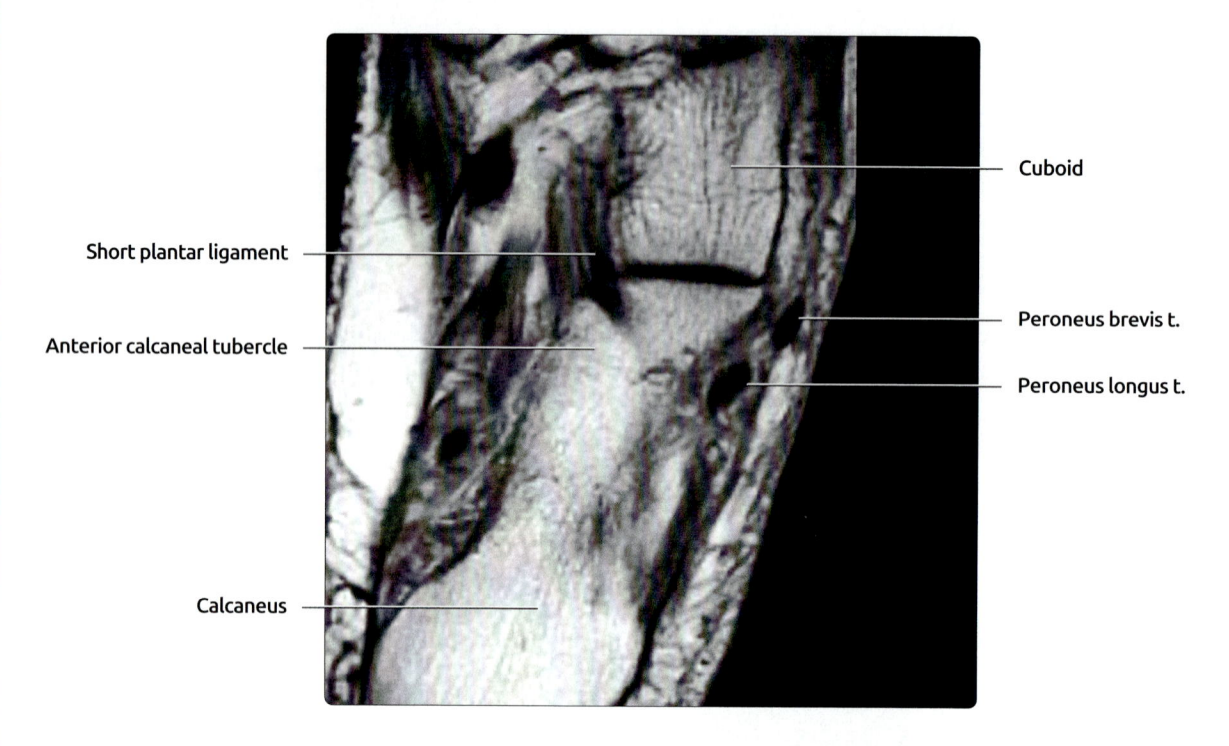

(Top labels): Short plantar ligament; Anterior calcaneal tubercle; Calcaneus; Cuboid; Peroneus brevis t.; Peroneus longus t.

(Bottom labels): Long plantar ligament; Anterior calcaneal tubercle; Long plantar ligament; Cuboid; Peroneus brevis t.; Peroneus longus t.; Calcaneus

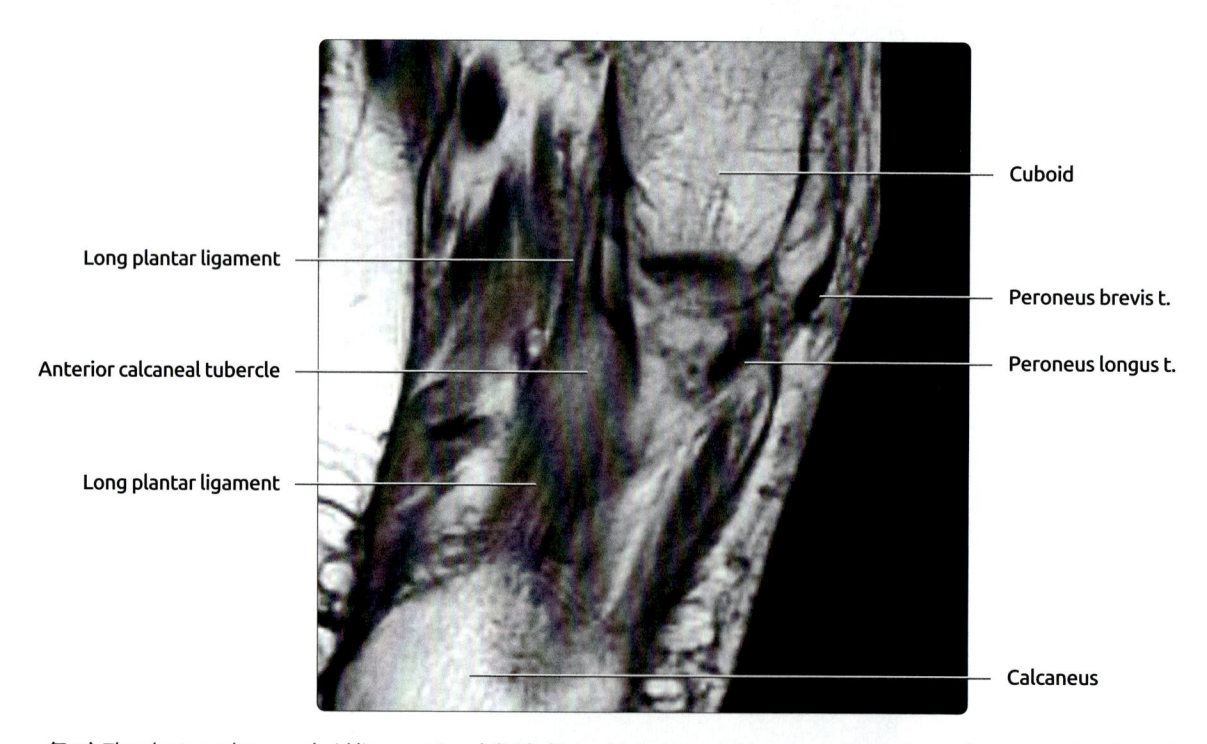

(Top) The plantar calcaneocuboid ligament is subdivided into short, deep, and long superficial plantar ligaments. The short plantar ligament, also called the short plantar calcaneocuboid ligament, is more medial than the long plantar ligament. It originates from the anterior tubercle of the calcaneus and inserts on the entire posterior plantar surface of and on the beak of the cuboid. (Bottom) A more distal (plantar) axial image in the same patient is shown. The long plantar ligament originates from the anterior tubercle and more posteriorly from the anterior aspect and intertubercular segment of the posterior calcaneal tuberosities. Its deeper fibers, representing the bulk of ligament, insert on the cuboid crest and its superficial fibers form a thinner layer, which forms the roof of the cuboid tunnel of the peroneus longus tendon and inserts on the 2nd-5th metatarsal bases.

Ankle Ligaments

LONG & SHORT PLANTAR LIGAMENTS

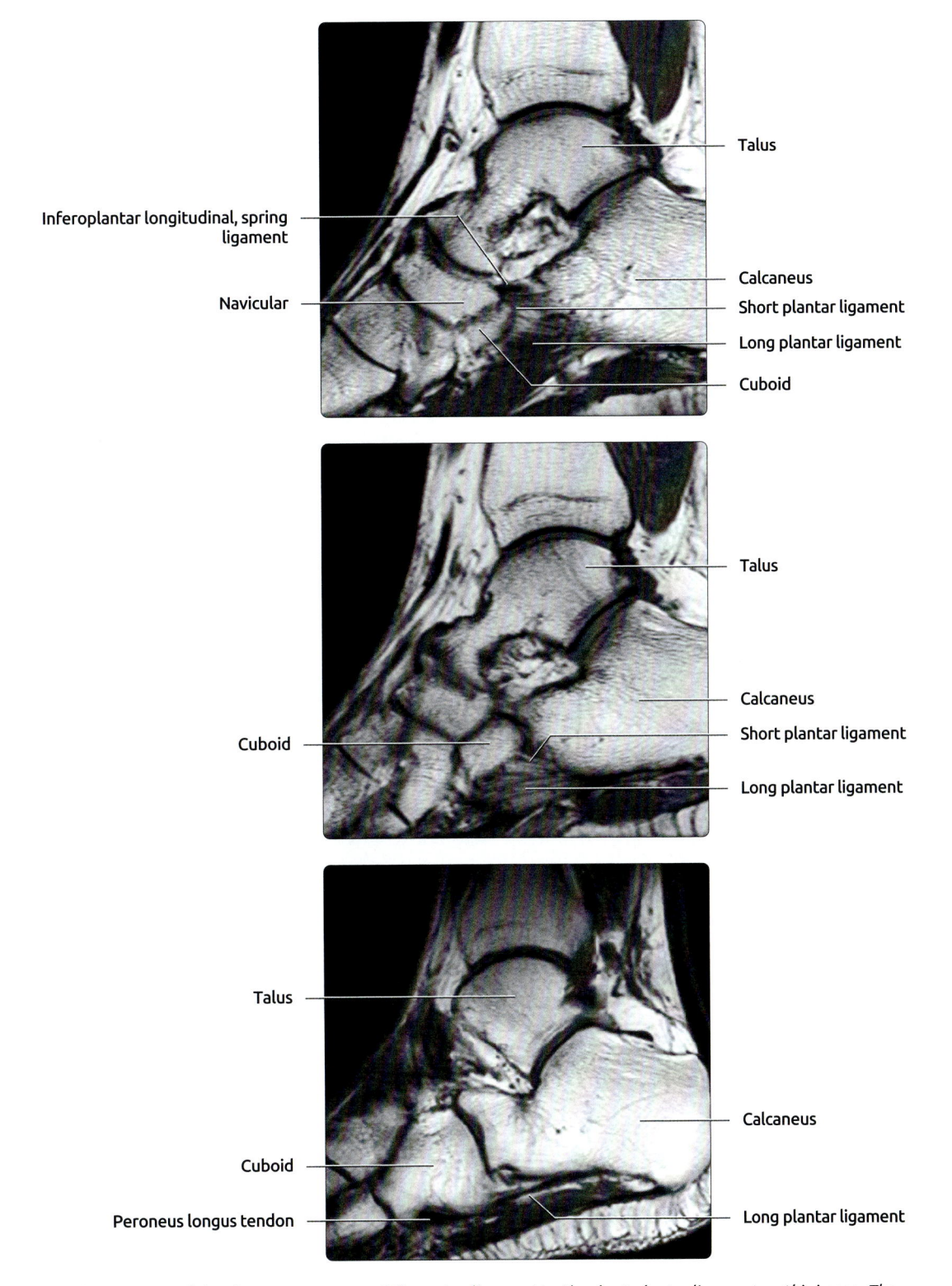

(Top) Note the proximity of the plantar component of the spring ligament to the short plantar ligament on this image. The inferoplantar longitudinal ligament inserts into the beak of the navicular. The short plantar ligament is found more plantarly and is deeper than the long plantar ligament. It inserts on the cuboid. **(Middle)** A more lateral sagittal image in the same patient is shown. Note the marked striation of both the short and long plantar ligaments. **(Bottom)** A more lateral sagittal image in a different patient is shown. The superficial fibers of the long plantar ligament continue distal to the cuboid to insert onto the bases of 2nd-5th metatarsals, and thus form the roof of the peroneus longus tunnel, under the cuboid.

SECTION 12
Foot

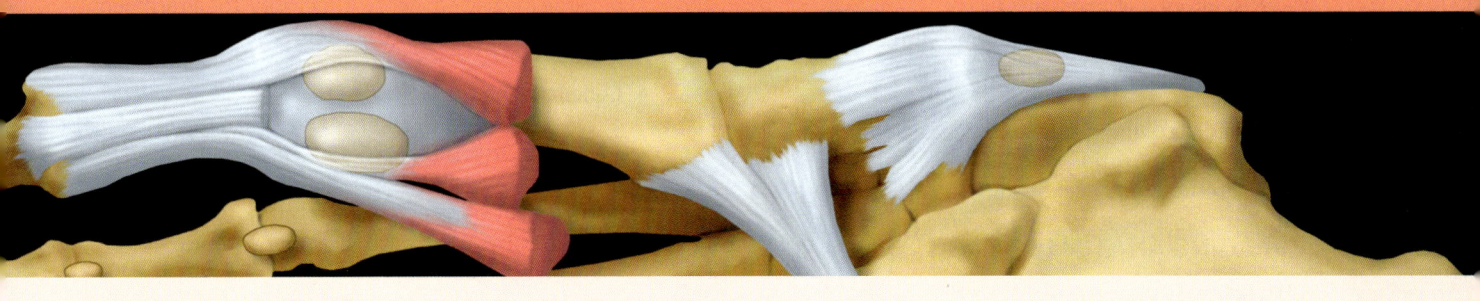

Foot Overview	**1034**
Foot Radiographic and Arthrographic Anatomy	**1042**
Foot MR Atlas	**1054**
Intrinsic Muscles of Foot	**1084**
Tarsometatarsal Joint	**1090**
Metatarsophalangeal Joints	**1096**
Foot and Ankle Normal Variants and Imaging Pitfalls	**1100**
Foot and Ankle Measurements and Lines	**1128**

Foot Overview

TERMINOLOGY

Definitions

- **3 major divisions from proximal to distal**
  - **Hindfoot**: Calcaneus and talus
  - **Midfoot**: Navicular, cuneiforms, and cuboid
  - **Forefoot**: Metatarsals and phalanges
- **2 columns**
  - **Medial column**: Talus, navicular, cuneiforms 1-3, digits 1-3
  - **Lateral column**: Calcaneus, cuboid, digits 4 and 5

IMAGING ANATOMY

Arches of Foot

- Foot is arched from posterior to anterior and from medial to lateral
- **Transverse arch of foot**
  - Triangular cuneiform bones and metatarsal bases form arch
  - Major supporting structures of transverse arch
    - Spring ligament, Lisfranc ligament, intermetatarsal and intertarsal ligaments
- **Longitudinal arch of foot**
  - From posterior process calcaneus to metatarsal heads, apex in midfoot
  - Medial side is higher than lateral
  - Metatarsals slant downward from apex of arch to metatarsophalangeal (MTP) joint
    - This is called inclination angle
    - Inclination angle decreases from 20° at 1st to 5° at 5th metatarsal
  - Major supporting structures of longitudinal arch: Plantar fascia, long and short plantar ligaments, spring ligament, posterior tibial tendon, peroneus longus tendon

Distribution of Weight Bearing

- 50% of weight borne on subtalar joint and calcaneus
- Remainder transmitted to metatarsophalangeal joints, greatest weight on 1st toe

Bony Anatomy

- **Cuboid bone**
  - Roughly cuboidal shape
  - 1 ossification center: Ossifies between 9th fetal month and 6 months age
  - Articulates with calcaneus, navicular, 3rd cuneiform, 4th and 5th metatarsals, rarely head of talus
    - Dorsal ligaments (calcaneocuboid, cubonavicular, cuneocuboid, cubometatarsal) strengthen each of these articulations
    - Short and long plantar ligaments attach to plantar surface
  - Sulcus at lateral margin, under which passes peroneus longus tendon
- **Navicular bone**
  - Curved shape, concave proximally and convex distally
  - 1 ossification center: Ossifies in 3rd year of life
  - Articulates with talus, cuboid, cuneiforms
    - Single facet proximally for articulation with head of talus
    - 3 facets distally for cuneiform articulations
    - 1 facet laterally for articulation with cuboid
    - Connected to anterior process of calcaneus by bifurcate ligament
    - Connected to sustentaculum tali by spring ligament
  - Large median eminence (tuberosity) for attachment of posterior tibial tendon is located plantar to main body of navicular
- **Cuneiform bones**
  - Wedge shaped, with base of wedge at dorsal surface of 2nd and 3rd cuneiforms, dorsomedial surface 1st cuneiform
  - 1st cuneiform (medial cuneiform)
    - Articulates with navicular, 2nd cuneiform, 1st metatarsal
    - 1 or 2 ossification centers: Ossify in 2nd year of life
  - 2nd cuneiform (middle or intermediate cuneiform)
    - Articulates with navicular, 1st and 3rd cuneiforms, 2nd metatarsal
    - 1 ossification center: Ossifies in 3rd year of life
  - 3rd cuneiform (lateral cuneiform)
    - Articulates with navicular, 2nd cuneiform, cuboid, 3rd metatarsal
- **Metatarsal bones**
  - 2 ossification centers: Shaft ossifies in 9th prenatal week, epiphysis in 3rd-4th years of life
    - 1st metatarsal has epiphysis at proximal end, others at distal end
  - 2nd-5th metatarsals have articulations at bases with adjacent metatarsals
  - 1st metatarsal
    - Articulates with 1st cuneiform, 1st proximal phalanx, sesamoids of metatarsal head
    - Variable articulation with 2nd metatarsal base
  - 2nd-3rd metatarsals
    - Articulate with respective cuneiforms and proximal phalanges
    - 2nd metatarsal base recessed relative to 1st and usually 3rd
  - 4th-5th metatarsals
    - Articulate with cuboid and respective proximal phalanges
    - Styloid process of 5th metatarsal extends lateral to cuboid
- **Phalanges**
  - 1st toe is biphalangeal, other toes are triphalangeal
  - 5th toe sometimes has failure of segmentation of middle and distal phalanges
  - 2 ossification centers: Shaft ossifies in 9th-15th prenatal weeks, epiphysis during 2nd-8th years

Musculature

- **Plantar muscles**: 4 layers
  - 1st layer: Abductor hallucis, flexor digitorum brevis, abductor digiti minimi, peroneus brevis
  - 2nd layer: Quadratus plantae (flexor accessorius), flexor digitorum and hallucis longus, lumbricals
  - 3rd layer: Flexor hallucis brevis, adductor hallucis, flexor digiti minimi brevis, tibialis posterior
  - 4th layer: Plantar interossei (3), dorsal interossei (4)
  - Peroneus longus courses across all layers, from superficial plantar laterally to deep plantar medially

Foot Overview

- **Dorsal muscles**: 2 muscle layers
  - Superficial layer: Tibialis anterior, extensor hallucis longus, extensor digitorum longus, peroneus tertius
  - Deep layer: Extensor hallucis brevis, extensor digitorum brevis
  - In forefoot, long and short extensors run side by side in single layer

Compartments

- **4 plantar compartments** divided by fascial layers
- **Medial plantar compartment**
  - Contains abductor hallucis, flexor hallucis longus, and flexor hallucis brevis
- **Central plantar compartment**
  - Superficial subcompartment: Contains flexor digitorum brevis, distal portion of flexor digitorum longus
  - Intermediary subcompartment: Contains proximal plantar portion of flexor digitorum longus, quadratus plantae, lumbricals
  - Deep subcompartment: Limited to forefoot, contains adductor hallucis
- **Lateral plantar compartment**
  - Contains abductor and flexor digiti minimi
- **Interosseous compartment**
  - Contains plantar and dorsal interosseous muscle
- **Dorsal compartment**
  - Superficial layer: Extrinsic extensor tendon
  - Deep layer: Intrinsic extensor muscle

Major Ligaments

- Plantar fascia (aponeurosis): 3 portions extend from tuberosity of calcaneus to transverse metatarsal ligaments of toes
  - Medial band: Thin structure superficial to abductor hallucis muscle
  - Central band: Thick, strong structure superficial to flexor digitorum brevis
    - Divides into separate bands to each toe; these are linked by transverse bands
    - Distally sends septa superficially into subcutaneous fat and deep to MTP joints
  - Lateral band: Thin structure superficial to abductor digiti minimi
  - Medial and lateral bands sometimes terminate at level of mid metatarsals
- Long plantar ligament: Originates calcaneal tuberosity, inserts cuboid and bases 2nd-4th metatarsals
  - Forms tunnel roof for peroneus longus tendon
- Short plantar (plantar calcaneocuboid) ligament: Deep to long ligament, inserts more proximally on cuboid
- Plantar calcaneocuboid (spring) ligament: Originates sustentaculum tali, inserts plantar aspect navicular
- Bifurcate ligament: Originates anterior process of calcaneus dorsally, inserts navicular and cuboid
- Lisfranc ligament: Originates 1st cuneiform, inserts base 2nd metatarsal
- Intermetatarsal ligaments: Dorsal and plantar ligaments between 2nd-5th metatarsal bases
- Transverse metatarsal ligaments: Superficial and deep ligaments between metatarsal heads

Nerves

- **Tibial nerve** divides into medial calcaneal, medial and lateral plantar branches at level of tarsal tunnel
  - **Medial calcaneal nerve**: Sensory to skin of heel, medial hindfoot
  - **Medial plantar nerve**
    - Between 1st and 2nd muscle layers, accompanies medial plantar artery
    - Motor branches: Abductor hallucis, flexor digitorum and hallucis brevis, 1st lumbrical
    - Plantar digital nerves to 1st-3rd toes, medial aspect 4th toe
  - **Lateral plantar nerve**: Has deep and superficial divisions
    - Motor branches: Flexor digiti minimi brevis, lumbricals, interossei, adductor hallucis
    - Superficial lateral plantar nerve: Between 1st and 2nd muscle layers
    - Plantar digital nerves to 5th toe, lateral aspect 4th toe
    - Deep lateral plantar nerve: Between 3rd and 4th muscle layers; accompanies lateral plantar artery
- **Deep peroneal nerve**: Dorsum of foot, between tibialis anterior and extensor hallucis longus
  - Motor branch: Extensor digitorum brevis
- **Superficial peroneal nerve**: Divides into medial and lateral branches at dorsum of foot
  - Sensory branches to dorsal foot
- **Sural nerve**: Lateral, superficial branch of tibial nerve
  - Extends along lateral margin of foot
  - Sensory branches to lateral foot

Arteries

- Posterior tibial artery divides into medial and lateral plantar arteries at level of tarsal tunnel
  - Plantar arteries accompany medial and deep lateral plantar nerves
- Peroneal artery accompanies superficial peroneal nerve down anterolateral aspect ankle
  - May join or replace posterior tibial artery
- Anterior tibial artery continues into foot as dorsalis pedis artery, deep to extensor retinaculum
  - Divides into multiple branches in midfoot, forming arcade

Bursae

- Extensor digitorum brevis: Between muscle and 2nd cuneiform and metatarsal bases
- Extensor hallucis longus: Between tendon and 1st cuneiform and metatarsal bases
- Abductor digiti minimi: Between muscle and tuberosity of 5th metatarsal
- Metatarsophalangeal joints: Bursa located dorsally, between metatarsal heads, and medial to 1st metatarsal head

Foot Motion

- **Supination**: Elevation of medial arch of foot; inversion + adduction
- **Pronation**: Depression of medial arch of foot; eversion + abduction

Foot Overview

GRAPHICS, NERVES & ARTERIES OF FOOT

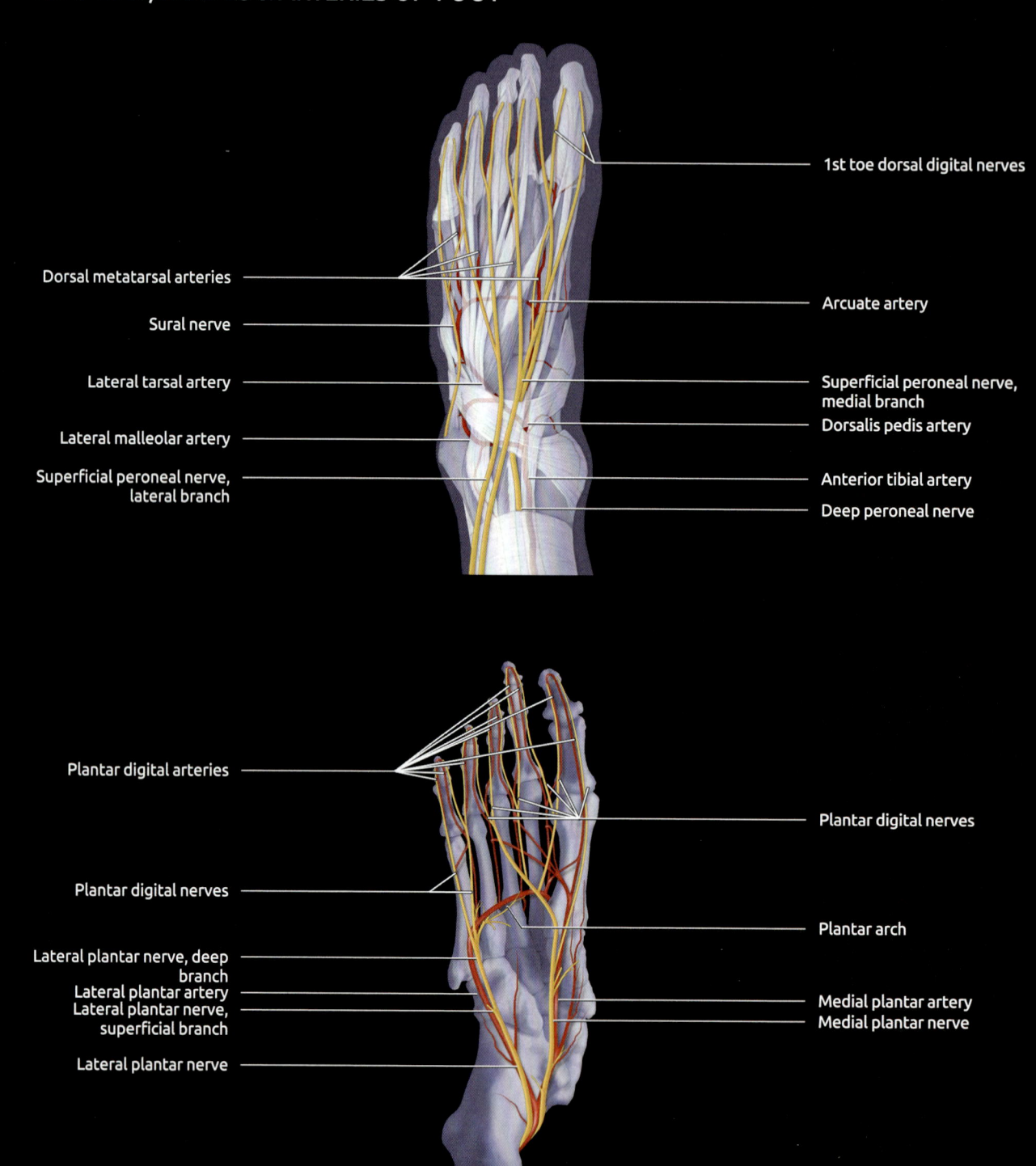

- Dorsal metatarsal arteries
- Sural nerve
- Lateral tarsal artery
- Lateral malleolar artery
- Superficial peroneal nerve, lateral branch
- 1st toe dorsal digital nerves
- Arcuate artery
- Superficial peroneal nerve, medial branch
- Dorsalis pedis artery
- Anterior tibial artery
- Deep peroneal nerve

- Plantar digital arteries
- Plantar digital nerves
- Lateral plantar nerve, deep branch
- Lateral plantar artery
- Lateral plantar nerve, superficial branch
- Lateral plantar nerve
- Plantar digital nerves
- Plantar arch
- Medial plantar artery
- Medial plantar nerve

(Top) *Graphic shows arteries and nerves at the dorsal aspect of foot. The deep peroneal nerve accompanies the anterior tibial artery. The superficial peroneal nerve divides into medial and lateral branches in the distal 1/3 of the leg. The anterior tibial artery is called the dorsalis pedis in foot. It terminates in the arcuate artery, which communicates with the plantar arterial arch and in digital vessels.*
(Bottom) *Graphic shows arteries and nerves at the plantar aspect of foot. The posterior tibial nerve and artery divide into medial and lateral plantar branches. These divide further into digital branches to medial and lateral aspects of each toe. The plantar arch sends vessels dorsally, as well as to plantar aspect of toes.*

Foot Overview

GRAPHICS, LIGAMENTS OF FOOT

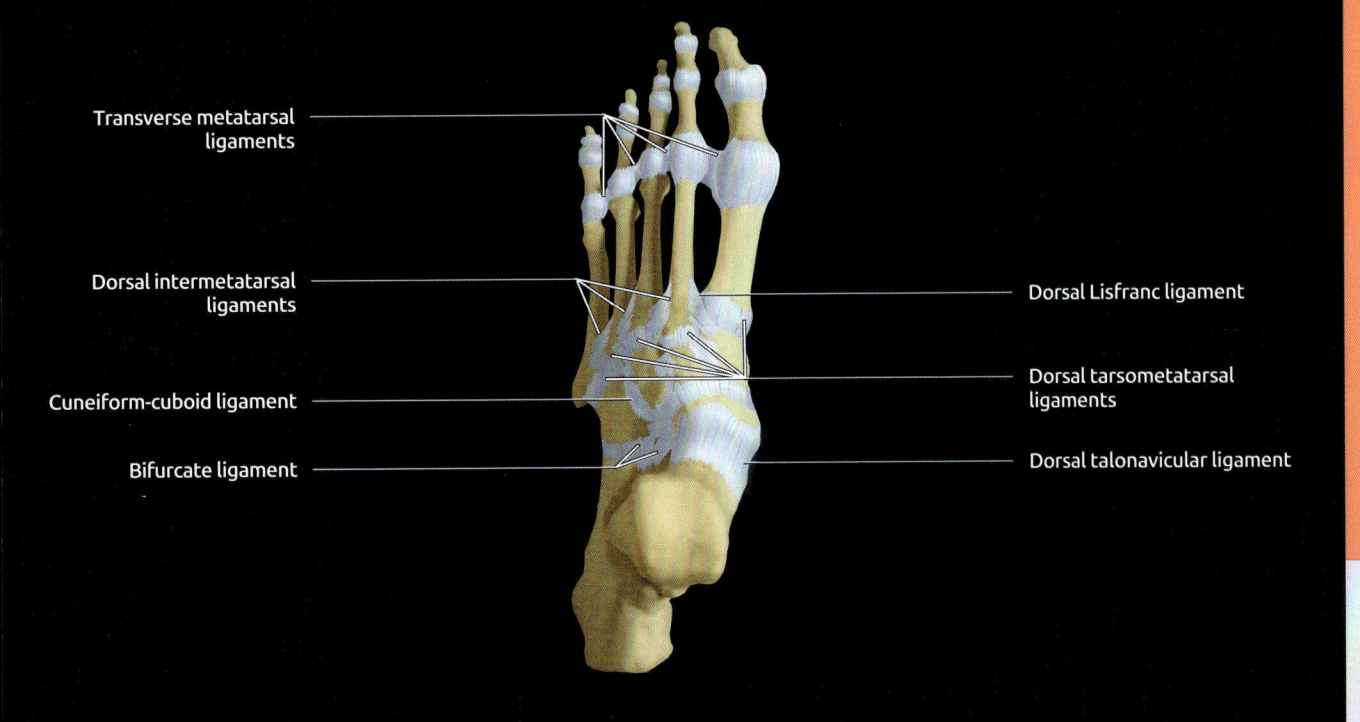

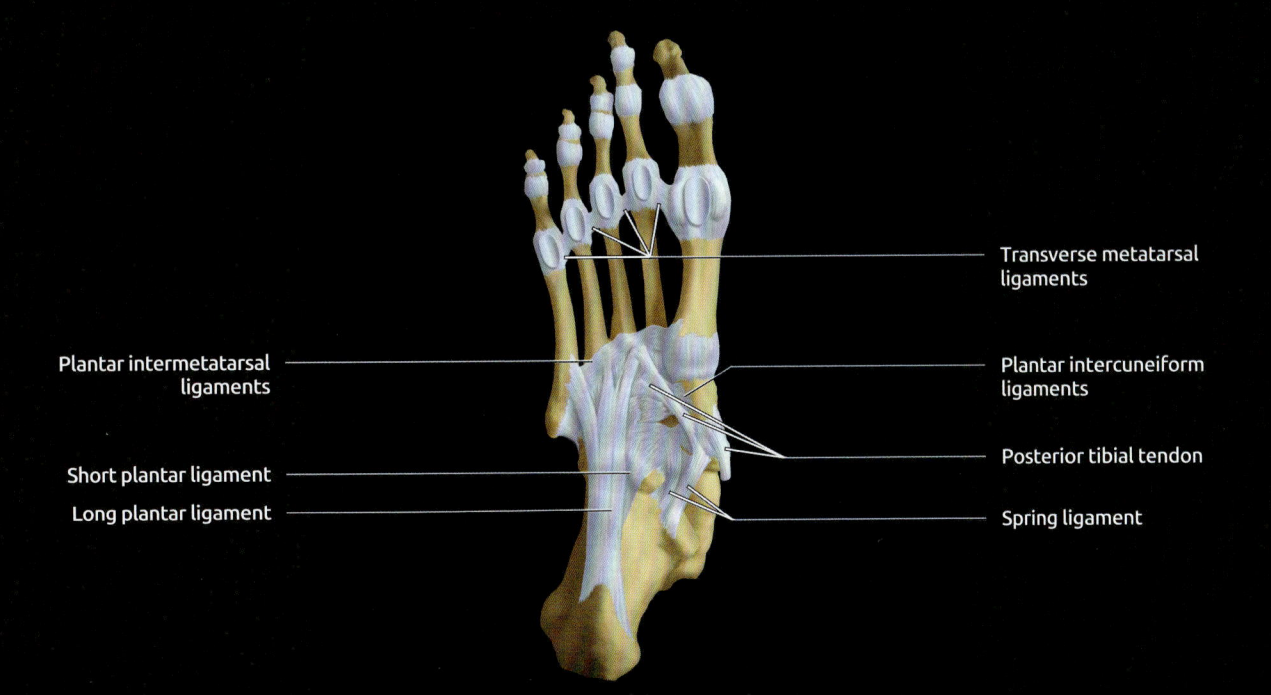

Transverse metatarsal ligaments

Dorsal intermetatarsal ligaments

Cuneiform-cuboid ligament

Bifurcate ligament

Dorsal Lisfranc ligament

Dorsal tarsometatarsal ligaments

Dorsal talonavicular ligament

Plantar intermetatarsal ligaments

Short plantar ligament

Long plantar ligament

Transverse metatarsal ligaments

Plantar intercuneiform ligaments

Posterior tibial tendon

Spring ligament

(Top) Graphic of dorsal ligaments shows dense ligaments between tarsal bones and between tarsals and metatarsals. Ligaments are generally named for the bones they bridge. Exceptions are the bifurcate ligament, which extends from the anterior process calcaneus to the cuboid and navicular, and the dorsal Lisfranc ligament, which extends from the 1st cuneiform to 2nd metatarsal. **(Bottom)** Graphic of plantar ligaments shows ligaments deep to the plantar fascia, as well as the navicular, cuneiform and metatarsal insertions of the posterior tibial tendon. The spring ligament, a.k.a. the plantar calcaneonavicular ligament, originates on the sustentaculum tali and anterior calcaneus and inserts on the navicular. Deep intertarsal ligaments are also shown and are named for bones they bridge.

Foot Overview

GRAPHICS, COLUMNS & LONGITUDINAL ARCH

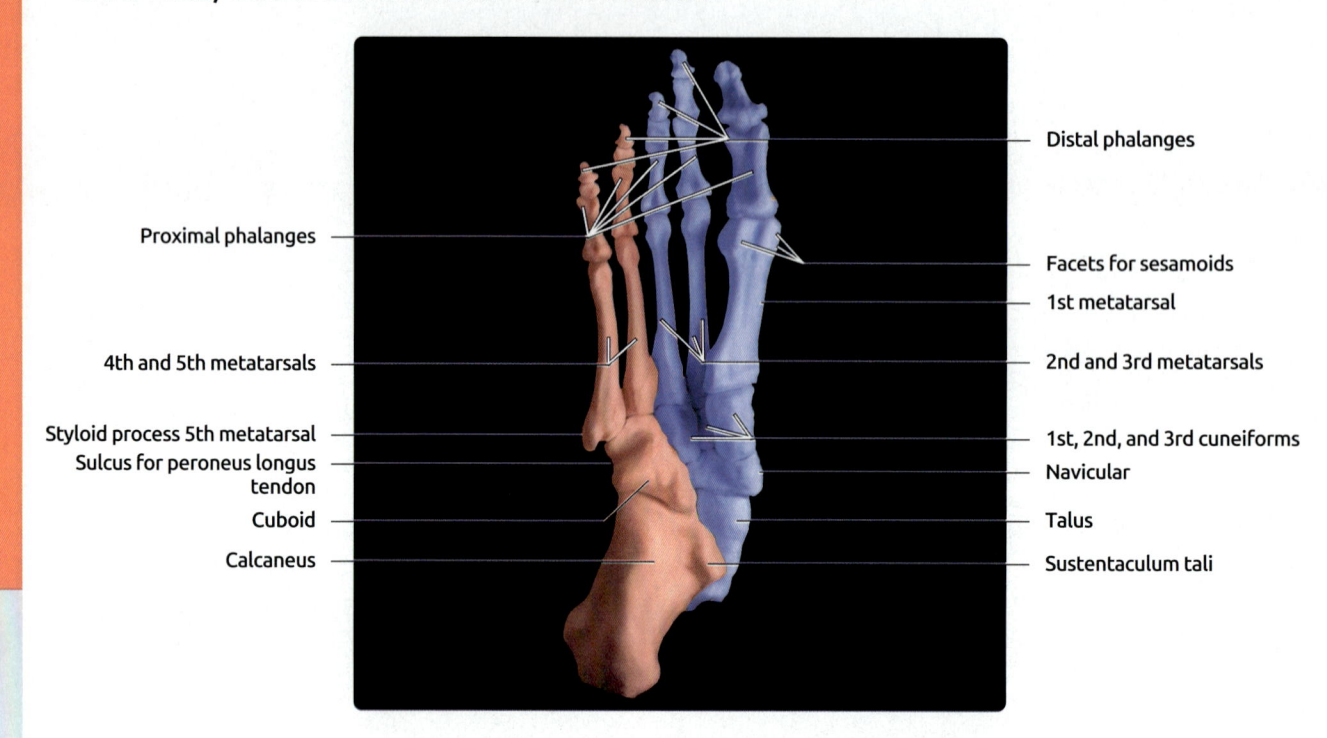

Labels on top image:
- Distal phalanges
- Proximal phalanges
- Facets for sesamoids
- 1st metatarsal
- 4th and 5th metatarsals
- 2nd and 3rd metatarsals
- Styloid process 5th metatarsal
- 1st, 2nd, and 3rd cuneiforms
- Sulcus for peroneus longus tendon
- Navicular
- Cuboid
- Talus
- Calcaneus
- Sustentaculum tali

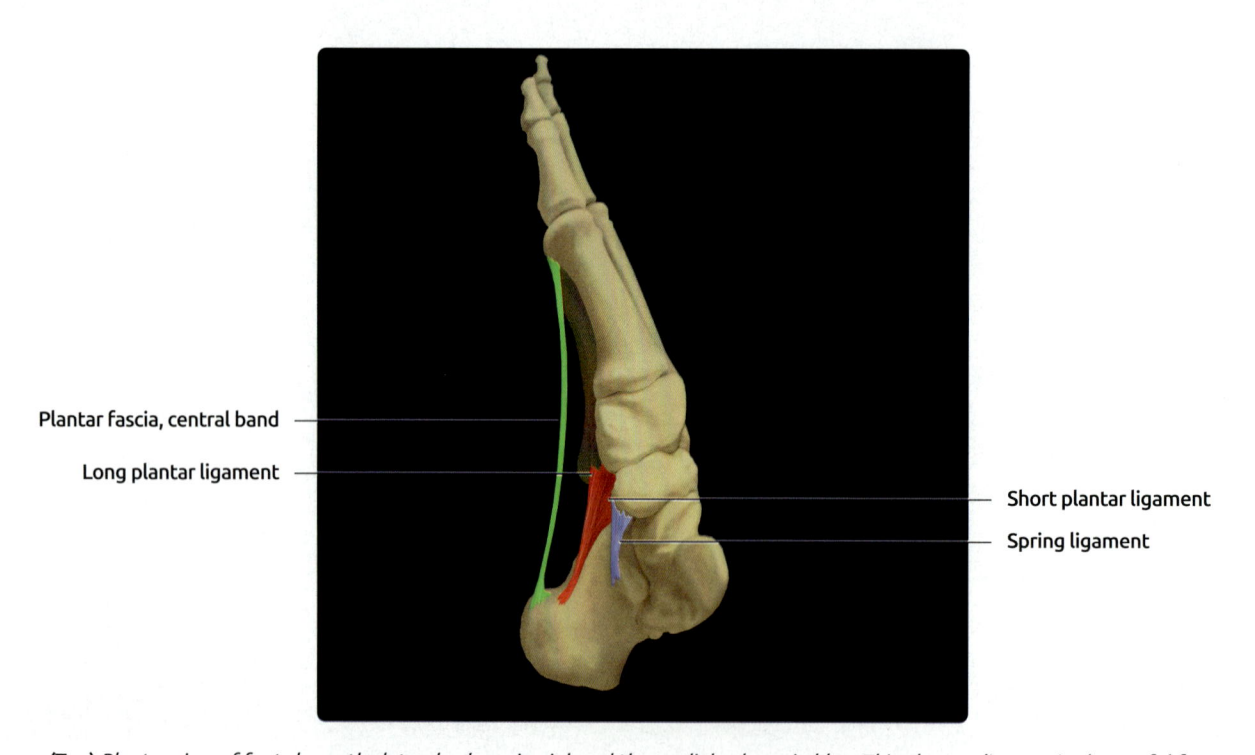

Labels on bottom image:
- Plantar fascia, central band
- Long plantar ligament
- Short plantar ligament
- Spring ligament

(Top) Plantar view of foot shows the lateral column in pink and the medial column in blue. This plantar diagram is also useful for showing the appearance of the transverse arch created by wedge-shaped cuneiform bones. Plantar margins of cuneiforms are closely apposed, and the 2nd cuneiform is recessed. (Bottom) Graphic shows the longitudinal arch of the foot from the medial side together with a schematic representation of major plantar ligaments helping maintain the longitudinal arch. The plantar fascia is the most important structure for maintaining the arch. It acts like a tie beam between the ends of the arch: Calcaneal tuberosity and metatarsal heads. Long and short plantar ligaments originate on the calcaneus, with the short plantar ligament deep to the long plantar ligament. Both insert on the cuboid. The long plantar ligament also sends fibers to metatarsal bases. The spring ligament extends from the sustentaculum tali and adjacent anteromedial calcaneus to the plantar surface of navicular.

Foot Overview

GRAPHICS, TRANSVERSE ARCH

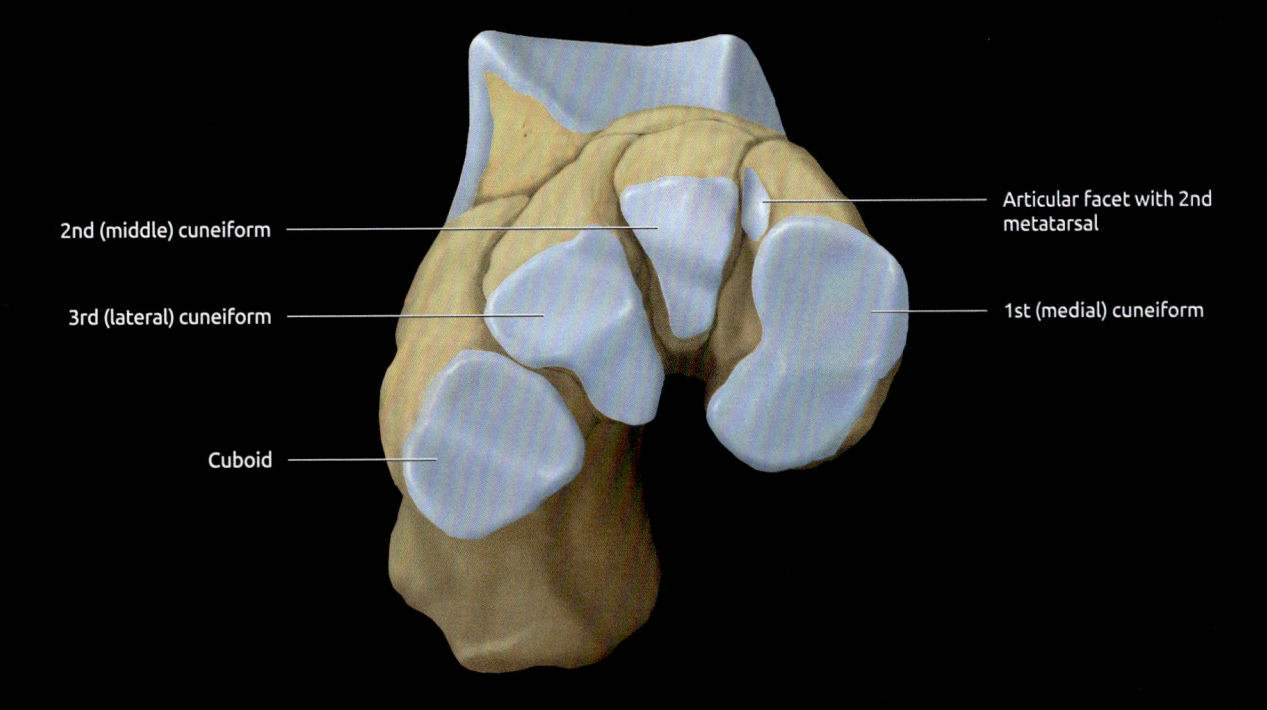

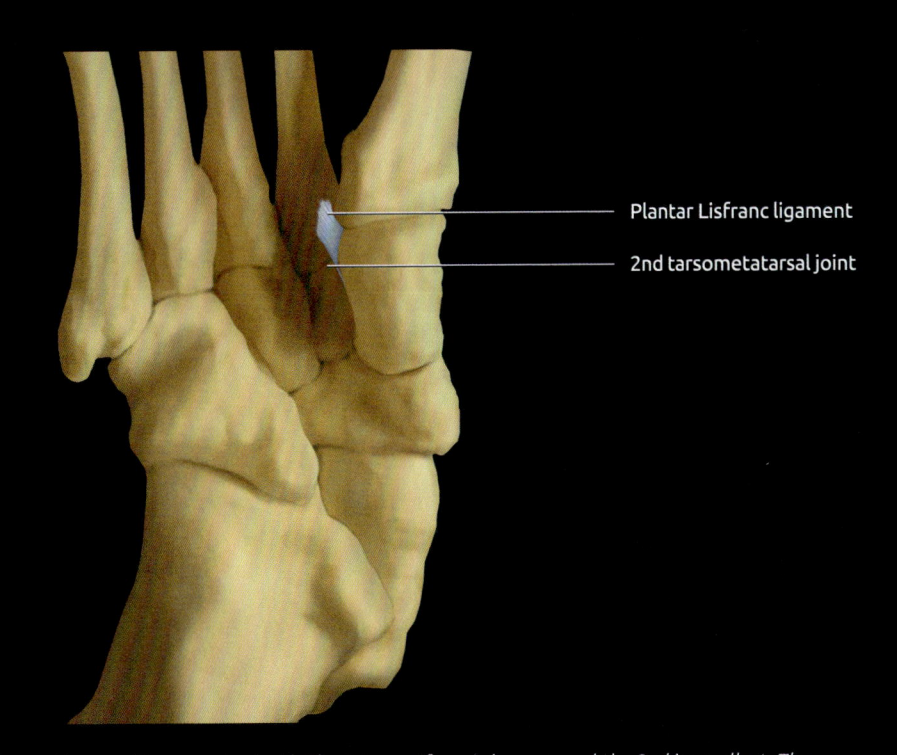

2nd (middle) cuneiform

3rd (lateral) cuneiform

Cuboid

Articular facet with 2nd metatarsal

1st (medial) cuneiform

Plantar Lisfranc ligament

2nd tarsometatarsal joint

(Top) Graphic shows the transverse arch formed by cuneiforms and cuboid. The 1st cuneiform is largest, and the 2nd is smallest. The arch is continued anterior to this image by configuration of proximal portions of metatarsals. Interosseous and intercuneiform ligaments maintain the shape of the arch together with the peroneus longus tendon. Note the multifaceted articular surfaces at the tarsometatarsal joint. *(Bottom)* Graphic shows the transverse arch from the plantar side of the foot. The arch is formed by bones, but stability is dependent on ligaments. Lisfranc ligaments are critically important in maintaining the arch. There are 3 distinct Lisfranc ligaments extending from the 1st cuneiform to the base of 2nd metatarsal: Dorsal, interosseous, and plantar. The interosseous ligament is the strongest of them and is structurally most important.

Foot Overview

GRAPHICS, MUSCULATURE OF FOOT

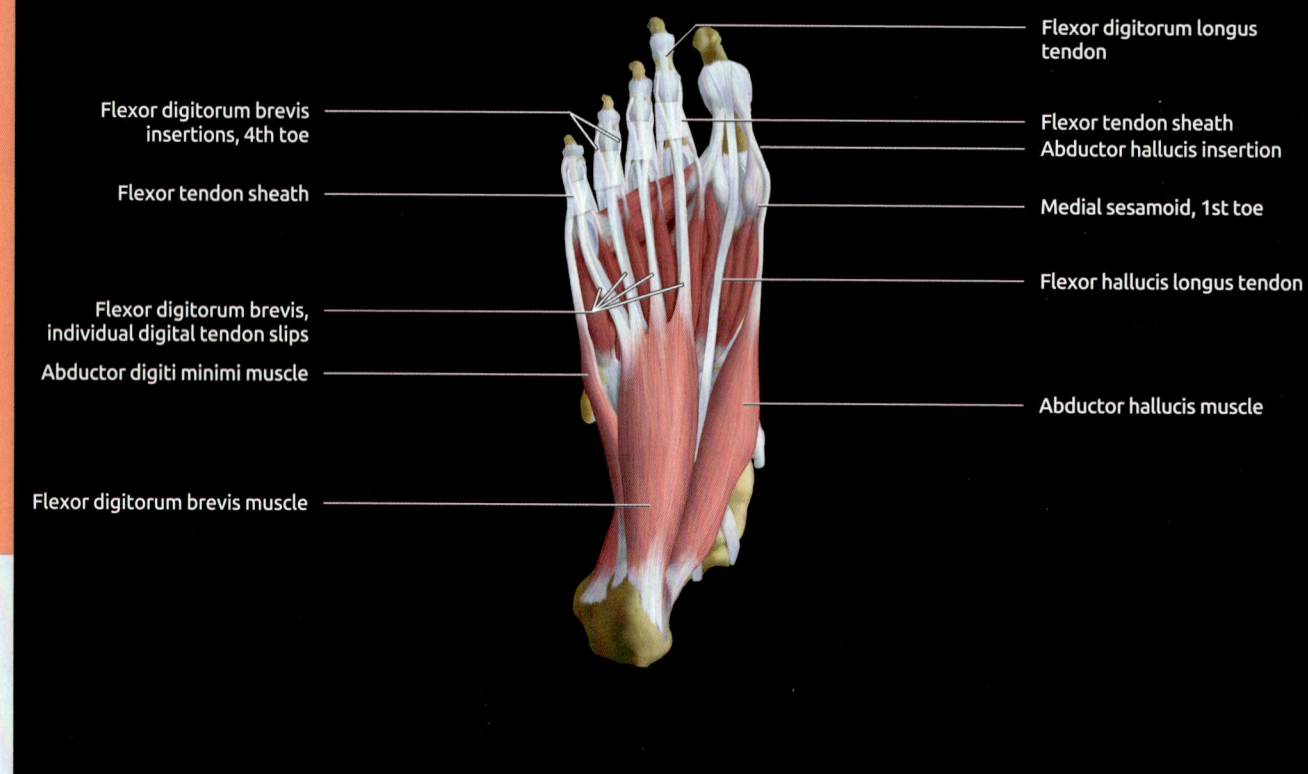

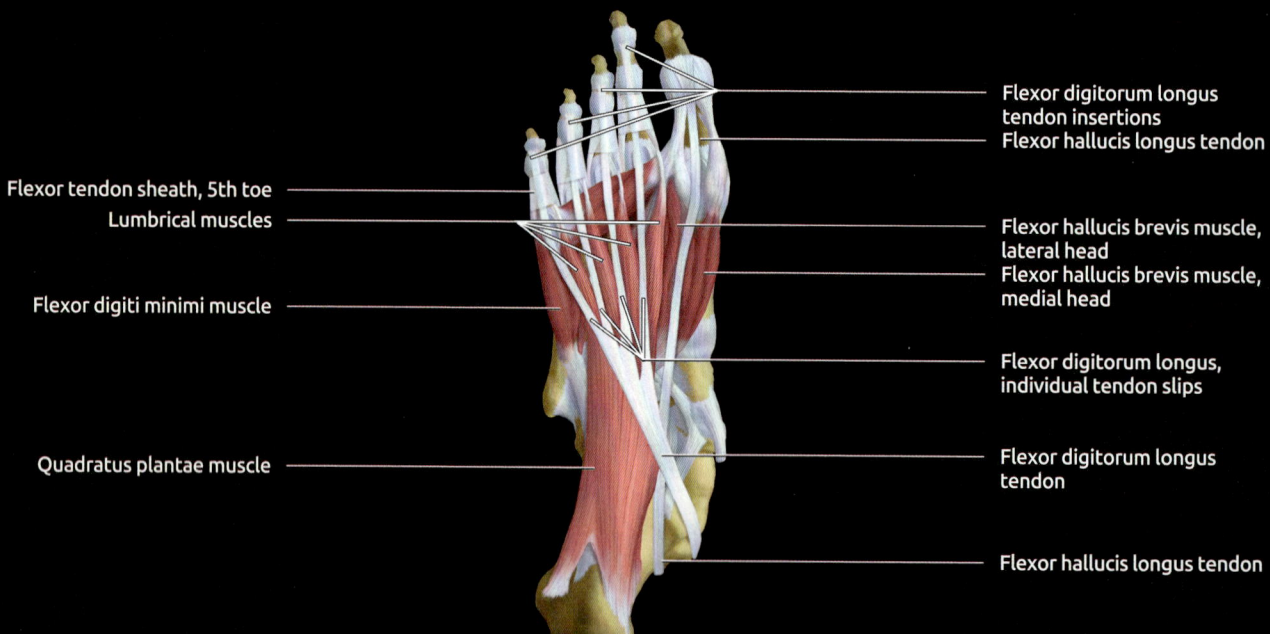

(Top) Graphic shows the superficial layer of plantar foot muscles: Abductor digiti minimi, flexor digitorum brevis, and abductor hallucis. The deep muscles are partially visible deep to the superficial layer. Flexor digitorum brevis tendons split in each digit (4th digit labeled) attaching at the lateral aspects of the middle phalangeal bases. Flexor tendon sheaths hold the flexor mechanism in close proximity to the phalanges. (Bottom) Graphic shows the 2nd layer of plantar muscles. The interesting arrangement of interactions between flexors is well seen: Quadratus plantae inserting on the flexor digitorum longus tendon, and lumbricals arising from individual flexor digitorum longus tendon slips. In the toes, flexor tendons are contained with fibrous tendon sheaths.

Foot Overview

GRAPHICS, MUSCULATURE OF FOOT

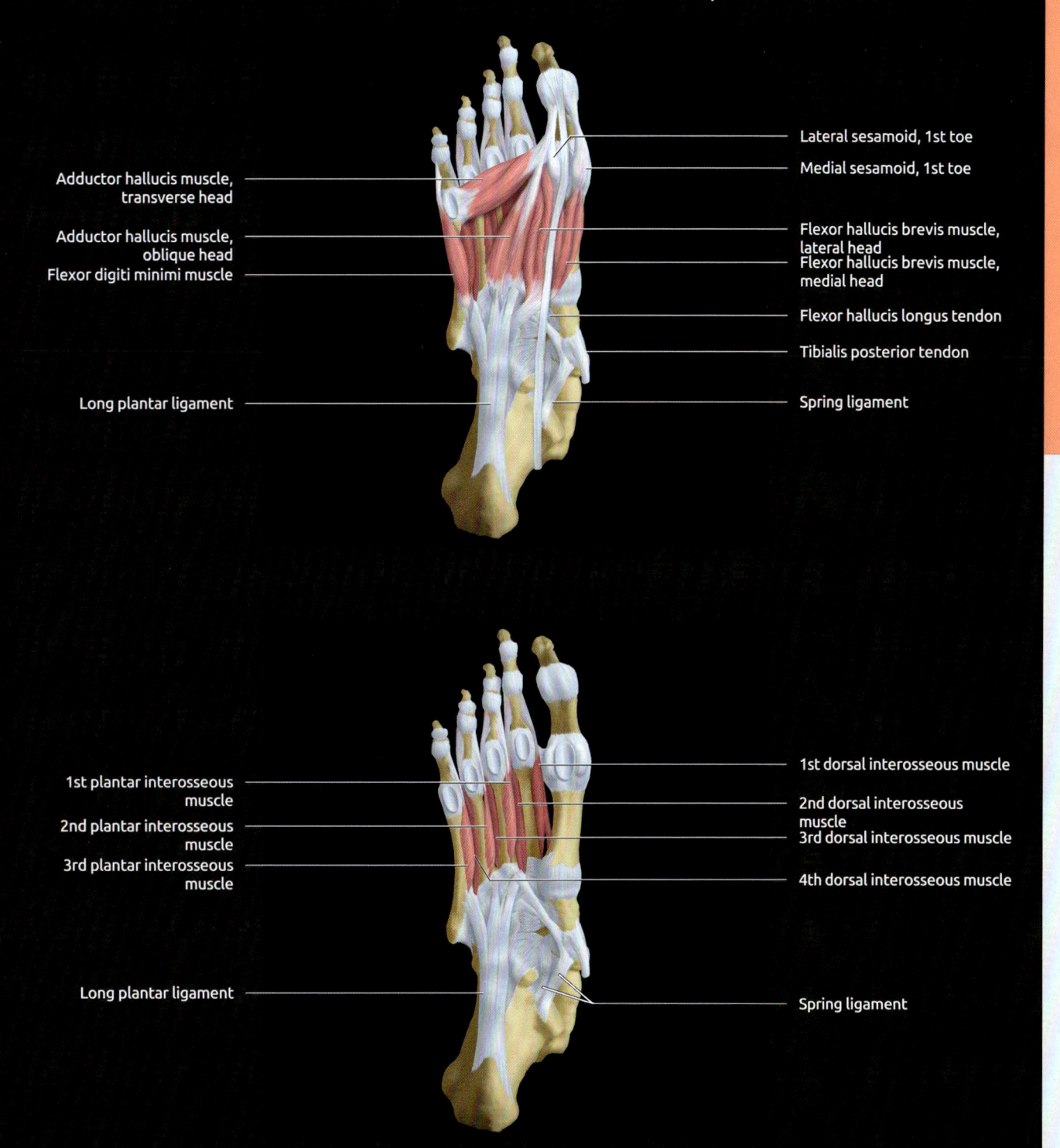

Labels (top image):
- Adductor hallucis muscle, transverse head
- Adductor hallucis muscle, oblique head
- Flexor digiti minimi muscle
- Long plantar ligament
- Lateral sesamoid, 1st toe
- Medial sesamoid, 1st toe
- Flexor hallucis brevis muscle, lateral head
- Flexor hallucis brevis muscle, medial head
- Flexor hallucis longus tendon
- Tibialis posterior tendon
- Spring ligament

Labels (bottom image):
- 1st plantar interosseous muscle
- 2nd plantar interosseous muscle
- 3rd plantar interosseous muscle
- Long plantar ligament
- 1st dorsal interosseous muscle
- 2nd dorsal interosseous muscle
- 3rd dorsal interosseous muscle
- 4th dorsal interosseous muscle
- Spring ligament

(Top) *Graphic shows the 3rd layer of plantar muscles. This layer contains the flexor hallucis brevis and flexor digiti minimi, as well as the adductor hallucis muscle. The oblique head of adductor hallucis is thick and broad, whereas the transverse head is thin and occasionally congenitally absent.* (Bottom) *Graphic shows the 4th layer of plantar muscles, the interosseous muscles. There are 4 dorsal interossei. They have bipennate origins from 2 adjacent metatarsals. The 1st dorsal interosseous inserts on the medial side of the 2nd proximal phalanx. Remaining dorsal interossei insert on the lateral side of the corresponding proximal phalanx. There are 3 plantar interossei. The 1st plantar interosseous muscle originates from medial side of 3rd metatarsal and inserts on medial side of 3rd proximal phalanx. The 2nd and 3rd plantar interossei originate on medial sides of 4th and 5th metatarsals, respectively, and insert on medial side of corresponding proximal phalanx.*

Foot Radiographic and Arthrographic Anatomy

ANATOMY IMAGING ISSUES

Imaging Recommendations
- Foot alignment can only be evaluated accurately on weight-bearing radiographs
  - Calcaneocuboid, talonavicular joints often appear subluxated on non-weight-bearing lateral, but normal on weight-bearing lateral
  - If pes planus is seen on non-weight-bearing view this is a true-positive finding
  - If pes cavus is seen on non-weight-bearing view this may be a false-positive finding
- Care must be taken to have patients stand naturally
- Patients may pronate foot instead of holding natural stance unless both feet are side-by-side
- Standard series consists of AP, lateral, and oblique views of foot
- Helpful to have steps and elevated platform for patients to stand while films obtained
  - Allows x-ray beam to be centered on foot
- Sesamoid view
  - Patient prone, toes dorsiflexed against plate, x-ray beam from posterior to anterior **or**
  - Patient supine, toes dorsiflexed by band holding them in position **or**
  - Patient standing, toes dorsiflexed against plate, x-ray beam angled toward sesamoids from posterior to anterior
- Toe films
  - Helpful to cone down on region of concern
  - Use pencil or other device to move overlapping toes out of view on lateral radiograph

General Arthrographic Technique
- Position foot and angle fluoroscopic beam to place joint of concern in tangent
- 25-gauge 1.5 inch needle used for both anesthesia and joint injection
  - Permits procedure with only 1 needle stick for patient
- Use standard mixture of gadolinium contrast of choice diluted 1:200; diluent is iodinated contrast + bupivicaine + normal saline
- Position patient to show joint in tangent
- Tape helpful to prevent foot from sliding on table
- Observe under fluoroscopy for contrast extravasation
- Do not overdistend the joints; only small amount of fluid needed to fill joint
- Usually feel slight "give" as joint is entered, and anesthetic flows without resistance

Posterior Subtalar Joint Injection
- Patient in decubitus position, contralateral side down
- Position foot so that lateral process of talus is in profile
- Enter joint at angle of Gissane, between calcaneus & lateral process of talus

Middle or Anterior Subtalar Joint or Talonavicular Joint Injection
- These joints communicate
- Access all 3 from dorsal approach to talonavicular joint
- Patient supine, knee bent, foot flat on table
- Midportion of talonavicular is most dorsal and easiest to access
- Can also approach middle subtalar joint from medial approach; patient lateral decubitus, medial side of foot up

Calcaneocuboid Joint Injection
- Patient supine, knee bent, sole of foot on table
- Rotate foot internally to optimally visualize joint in profile
- Access from dorsal approach

Navicular-Cuneiform Joint Injection
- Patient supine, knee bent, foot flat on table
- May need to angle beam or foot slightly to see joint in tangent
- Access from dorsal approach

Tarsometatarsal Joint Injection
- 3 separate joint cavities
- 1st tarsometatarsal joint has separate joint capsule
- 2nd-3rd tarsometatarsal joints share a joint capsule
- 4th-5th tarsometatarsal joints share a joint capsule
- Tarsometatarsal injection usually fills intermetatarsal joints, sometimes fills intercuneiform joints

1st Metatarsophalangeal Joint Injection
- Patient supine
- Knee bent, foot flat against table
- Check lateral view for dorsal osteophytes, which can block access
- Dorsal approach

2nd-5th Metatarsophalangeal Joint Injection
- Dorsal approach through extensor tendon
- Dynamic fluoroscopic evaluation important to look for small ligament tears

Tendon Sheath Injection Technique
- Usually easiest under ultrasound guidance
- Can perform under fluoroscopy utilizing bony landmarks & palpation of tendon
- Use 25-gauge needle
- Since tendons are superficial, best stability for injection is passing needle through tendon and entering tendon sheath deep to tendon
- Contrast (fluoroscopy) or injectate (ultrasound) must flow readily away from needle and follow tendon sheath contour

MR Arthrography
- Helpful for evaluation of ligament tears
- Utilize small FOV, 3 planes of T1 and 2 planes of fluid-sensitive imaging

SELECTED REFERENCES
1. Theumann NH et al: Metatarsophalangeal joint of the great toe: normal MR, MR arthrographic, and MR bursographic findings in cadavers. J Comput Assist Tomogr. 26(5):829-38, 2002
2. Yao L et al: Plantar plate of the foot: findings on conventional arthrography and MR imaging. AJR Am J Roentgenol. 163(3):641-4, 1994
3. Karpman RR et al: Arthrography of the metatarsophalangeal joint. Foot Ankle. 9(3):125-9, 1988

Foot Radiographic and Arthrographic Anatomy

AP & OBLIQUE FOOT RADIOGRAPHS

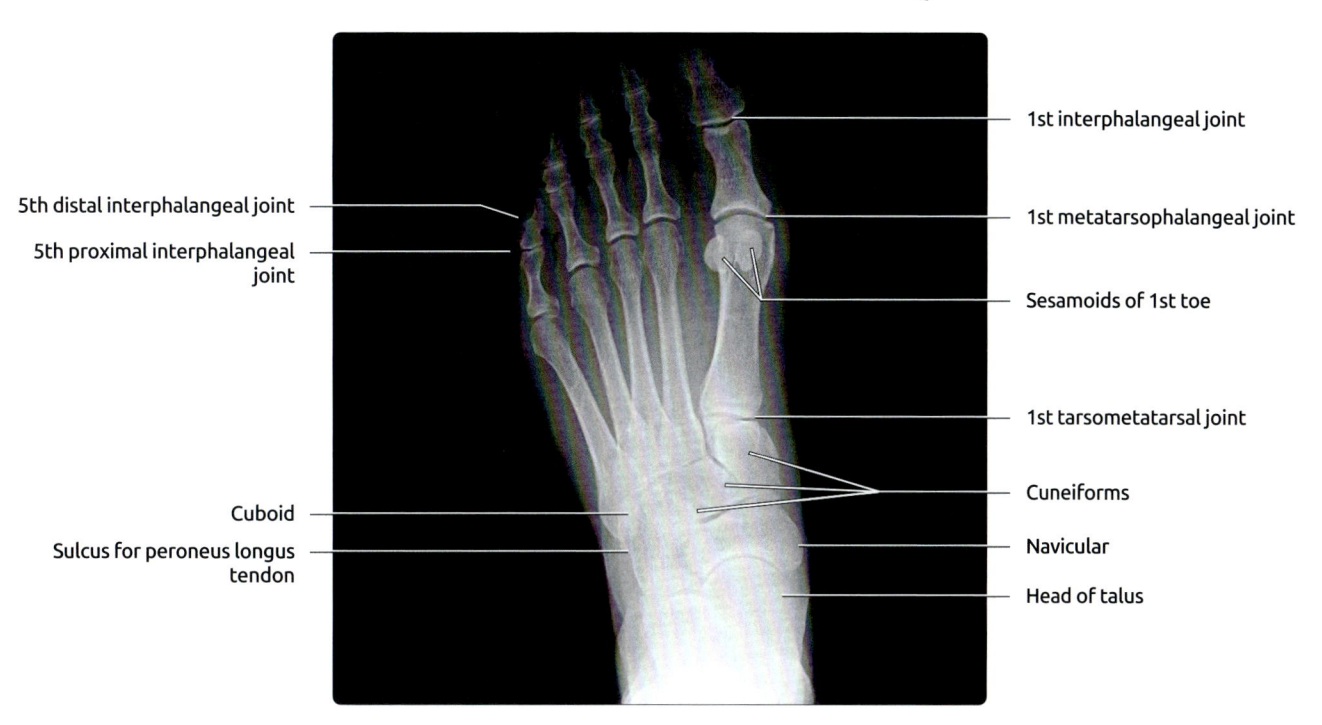

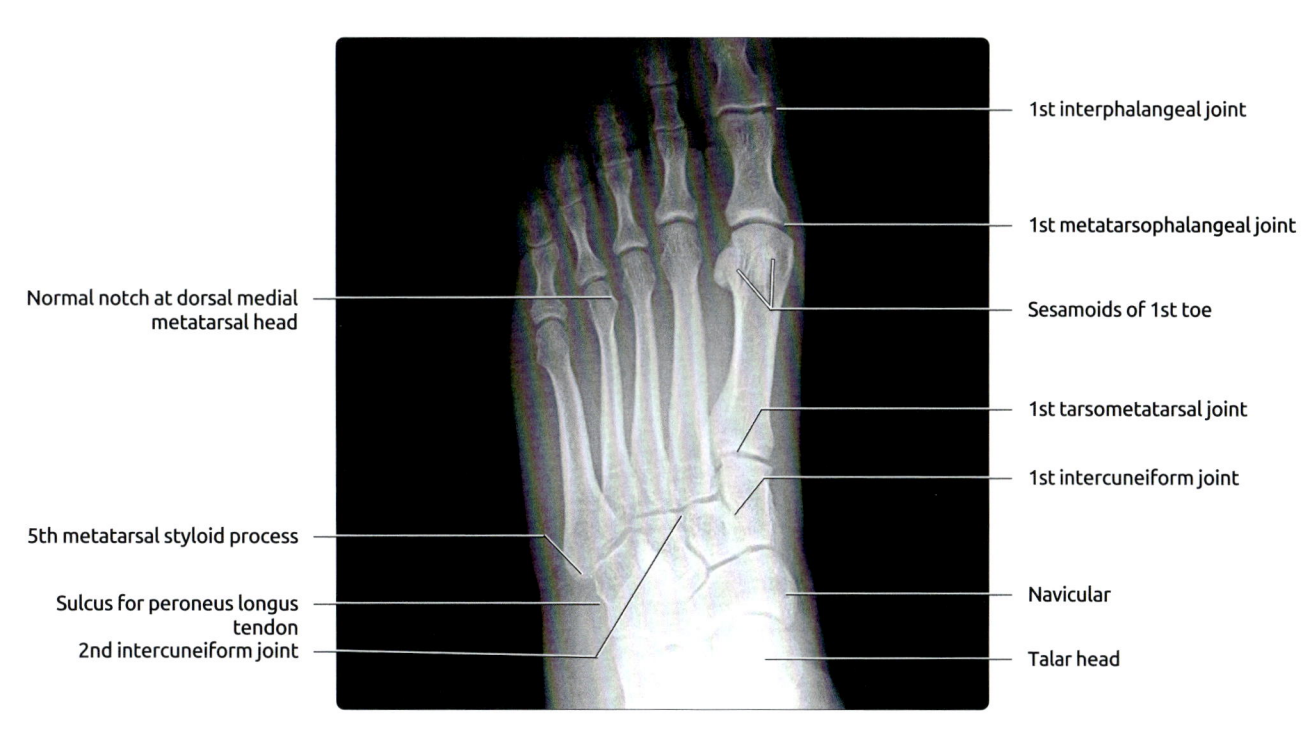

(Top) *Anteroposterior weight-bearing radiograph of the foot shows a normal amount of overlap of the bones of the midfoot. Articulations between cuboid and navicular, between cuneiforms, and between cuboid and lateral cuneiform are not seen in profile. Tarsometatarsal joints are sometimes in profile, but joints may not be visible due to obliquity of joint; this should not be mistaken for joint fusion.* (Bottom) *On oblique view, intercuneiform joints, tarsometatarsal joints, and styloid process (also called tuberosity) at the base of the 5th metatarsal are usually better seen than on anteroposterior view. A normal notch at the medial margin of the metatarsal heads is often thrown into profile on this view and should not be mistaken for erosion.*

Foot Radiographic and Arthrographic Anatomy

LATERAL FOOT: WEIGHT BEARING AND NON-WEIGHT BEARING

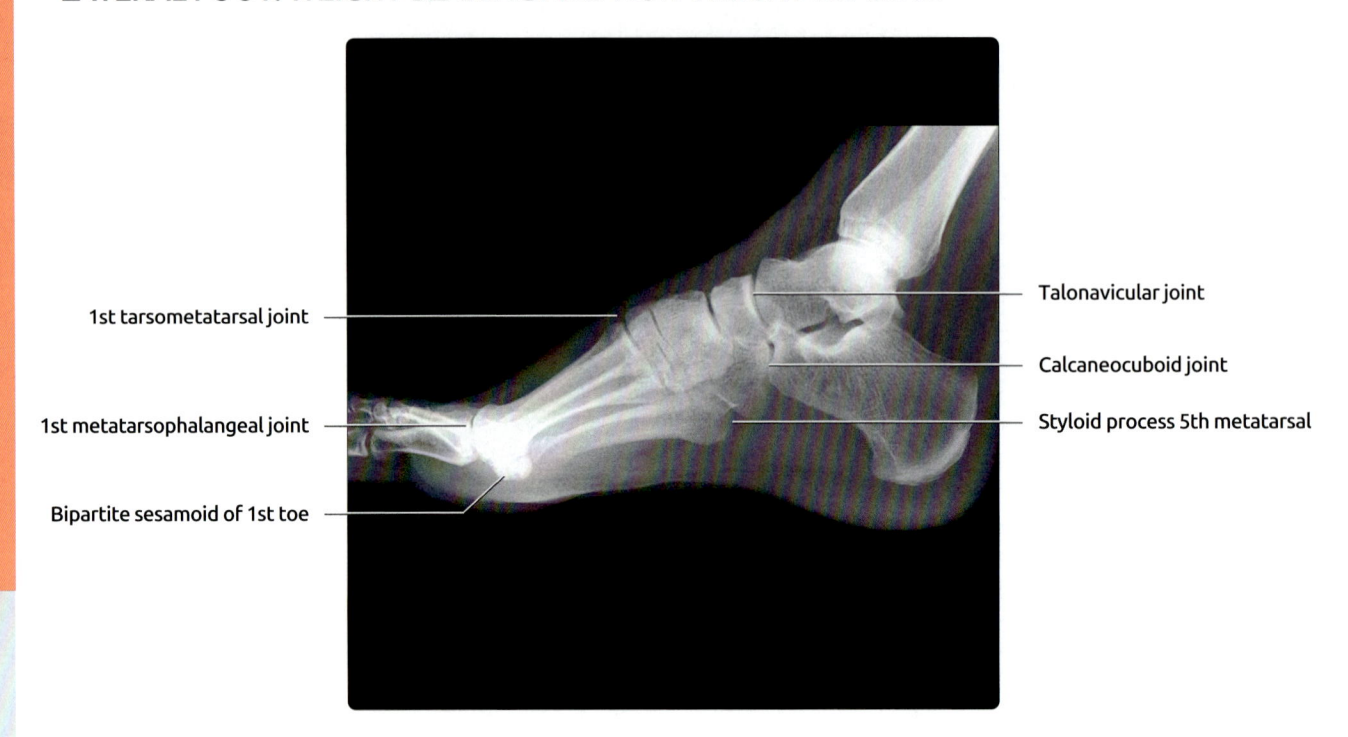

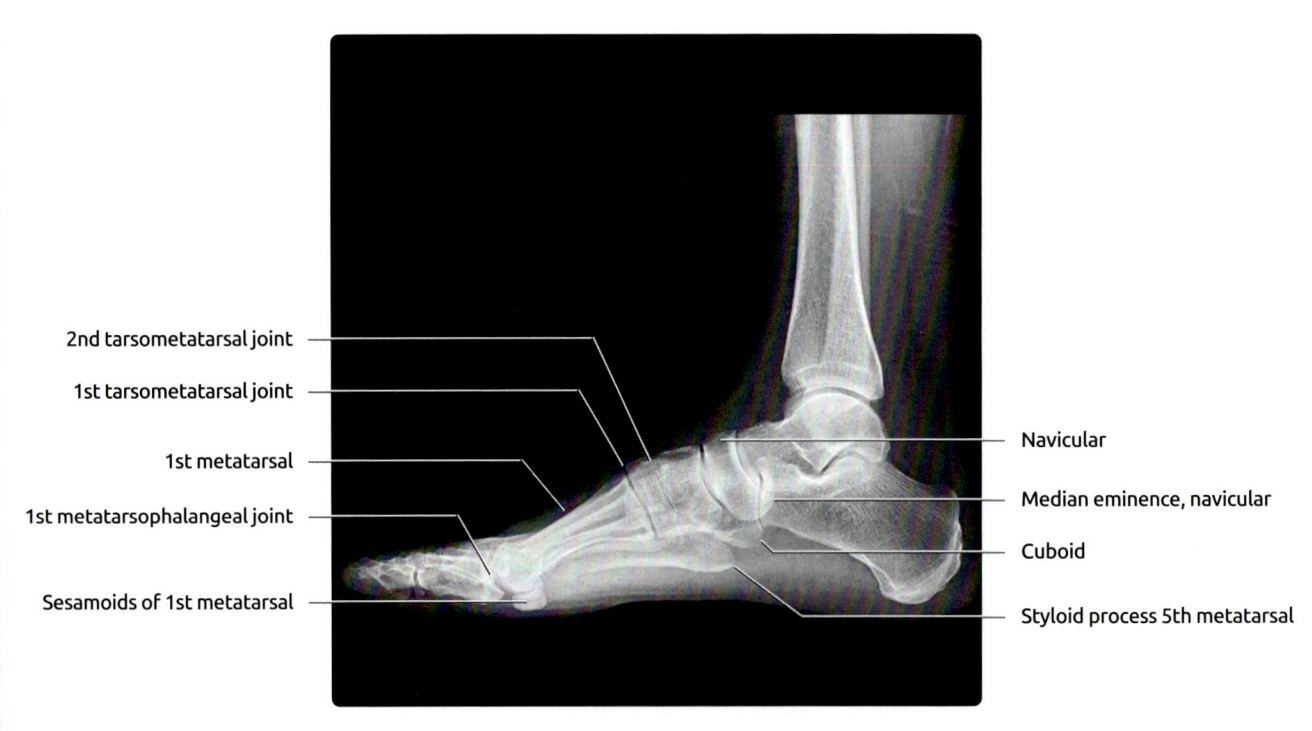

Labels (top image):
- 1st tarsometatarsal joint
- 1st metatarsophalangeal joint
- Bipartite sesamoid of 1st toe
- Talonavicular joint
- Calcaneocuboid joint
- Styloid process 5th metatarsal

Labels (bottom image):
- 2nd tarsometatarsal joint
- 1st tarsometatarsal joint
- 1st metatarsal
- 1st metatarsophalangeal joint
- Sesamoids of 1st metatarsal
- Navicular
- Median eminence, navicular
- Cuboid
- Styloid process 5th metatarsal

(Top) *On this non-weight-bearing lateral radiograph, the longitudinal arch of the foot usually appears higher than on a weight-bearing view. The calcaneocuboid and talonavicular joints appear subluxated inferiorly on this view but that is a normal finding that resolves on weight-bearing radiographs.* **(Bottom)** *Lateral weight-bearing radiograph shows the longitudinal arch of the foot, from the posterior process of calcaneus to the 1st MTP joint. Note the relatively plantar position of the median eminence (tuberosity) of the navicular. The line drawn along the center of the talar axis will continue along the axis of the 1st metatarsal in a normally aligned foot. The 1st and 2nd metatarsal bases are both at the dorsal aspect of the foot; they can be distinguished by the more proximal position of the 2nd metatarsal.*

Foot Radiographic and Arthrographic Anatomy

POSTERIOR SUBTALAR JOINT ARTHROGRAPHY

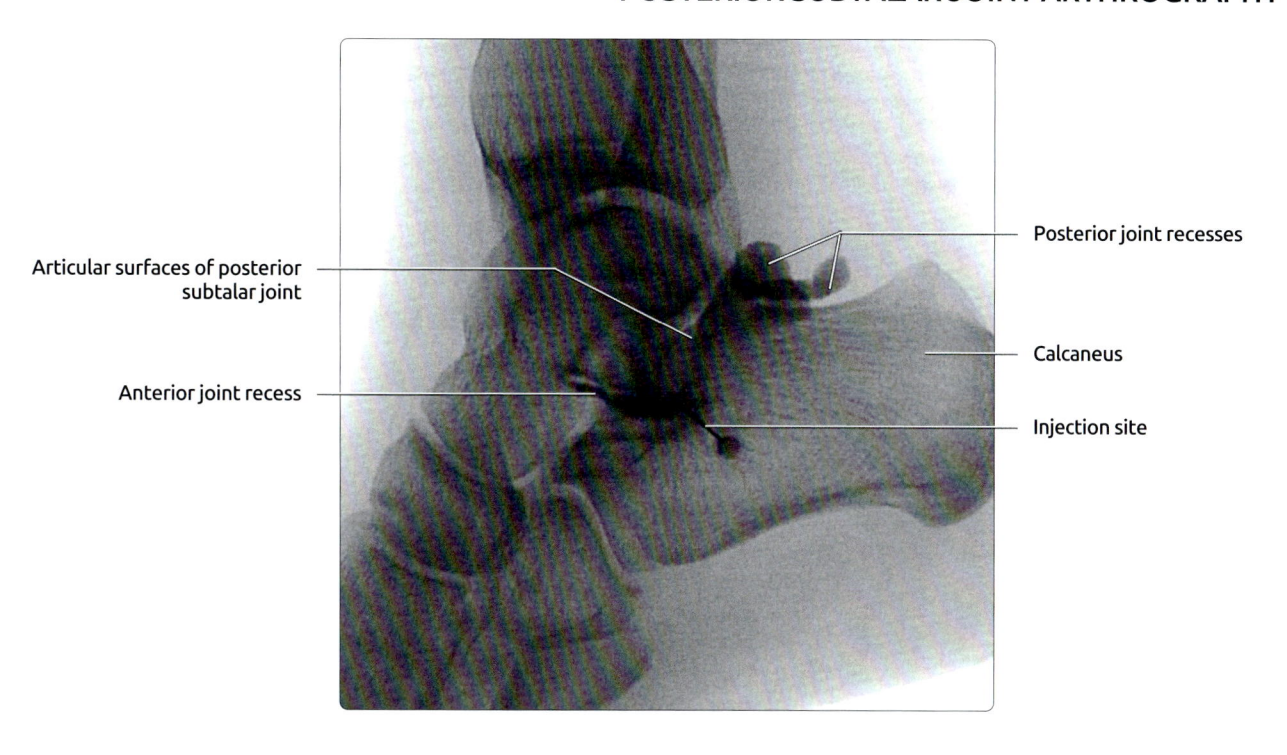

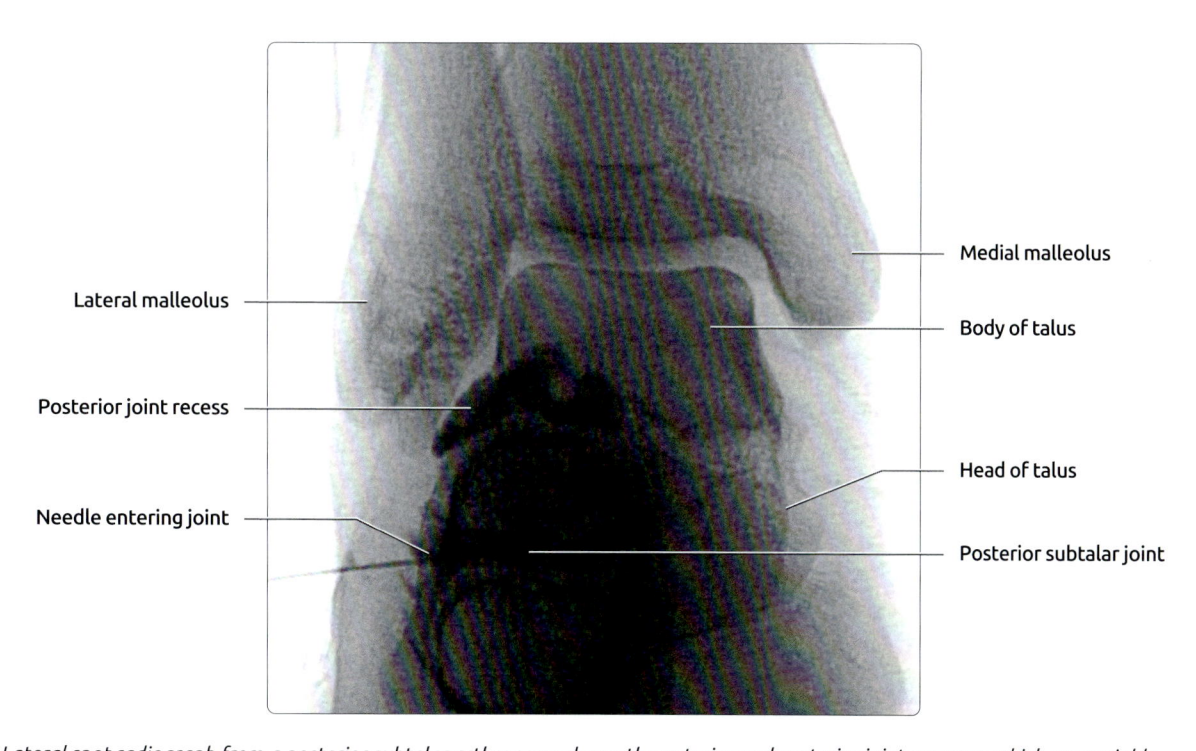

Articular surfaces of posterior subtalar joint

Anterior joint recess

Posterior joint recesses

Calcaneus

Injection site

Lateral malleolus

Posterior joint recess

Needle entering joint

Medial malleolus

Body of talus

Head of talus

Posterior subtalar joint

(Top) *Lateral spot radiograph from a posterior subtalar arthrogram shows the anterior and posterior joint recesses, which are variable in size. The anterior recess normally extends into the posterior portion of the sinus tarsi, as in this case.* (Bottom) *Anteroposterior spot radiograph from the same posterior subtalar joint arthrogram shows the joint recesses superimposed on the talus. The joint is difficult to see on this view, which is useful primarily for confirming needle position. Note that the lateral margin of the joint is well below the level of the fibular tip.*

Foot Radiographic and Arthrographic Anatomy

POSTERIOR SUBTALAR JOINT MR ARTHROGRAPHY

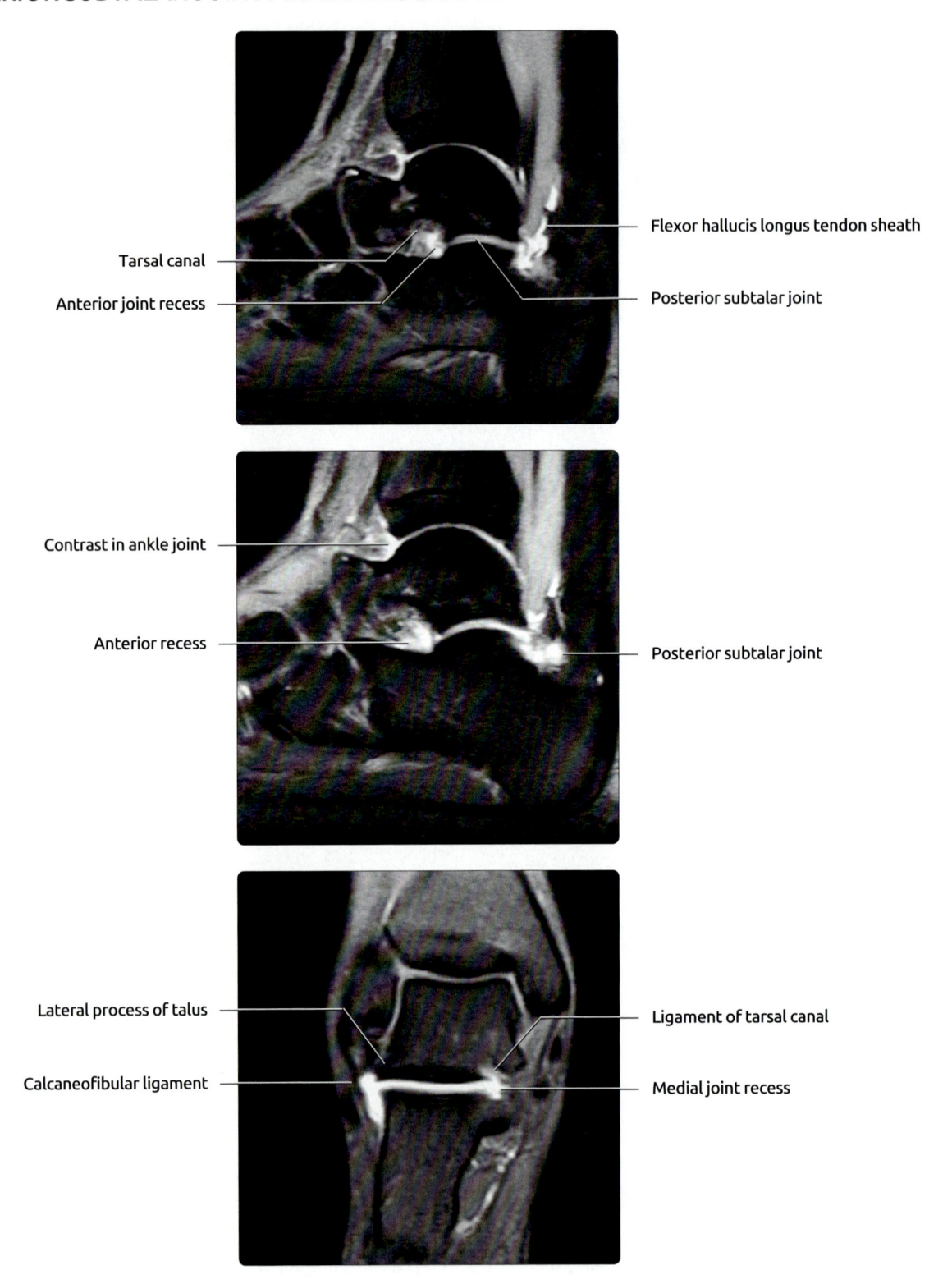

Tarsal canal
Anterior joint recess
Flexor hallucis longus tendon sheath
Posterior subtalar joint

Contrast in ankle joint
Anterior recess
Posterior subtalar joint

Lateral process of talus
Calcaneofibular ligament
Ligament of tarsal canal
Medial joint recess

(Top) Sagittal PD T1WI FS MR at the medial margin of the posterior subtalar joint shows the relatively small size of the joint compared to its size laterally. Contrast in the flexor hallucis longus tendon sheath and tibiotalar joint are normal variants present in 15% of the population. (Middle) Sagittal PD FS MR shows fluid filling the normal anterior and posterior recesses of the posterior subtalar joint. (Bottom) Coronal T1WI FS MR through the posterior subtalar joint shows the normal recess into the tarsal canal. Laterally, contrast often extends to the undersurface of the calcaneofibular ligament. In other patients a well-defined talocalcaneal ligament contains contrast closer to the joint.

Foot Radiographic and Arthrographic Anatomy

TALOCALCANEONAVICULAR JOINT ARTHROGRAPHY

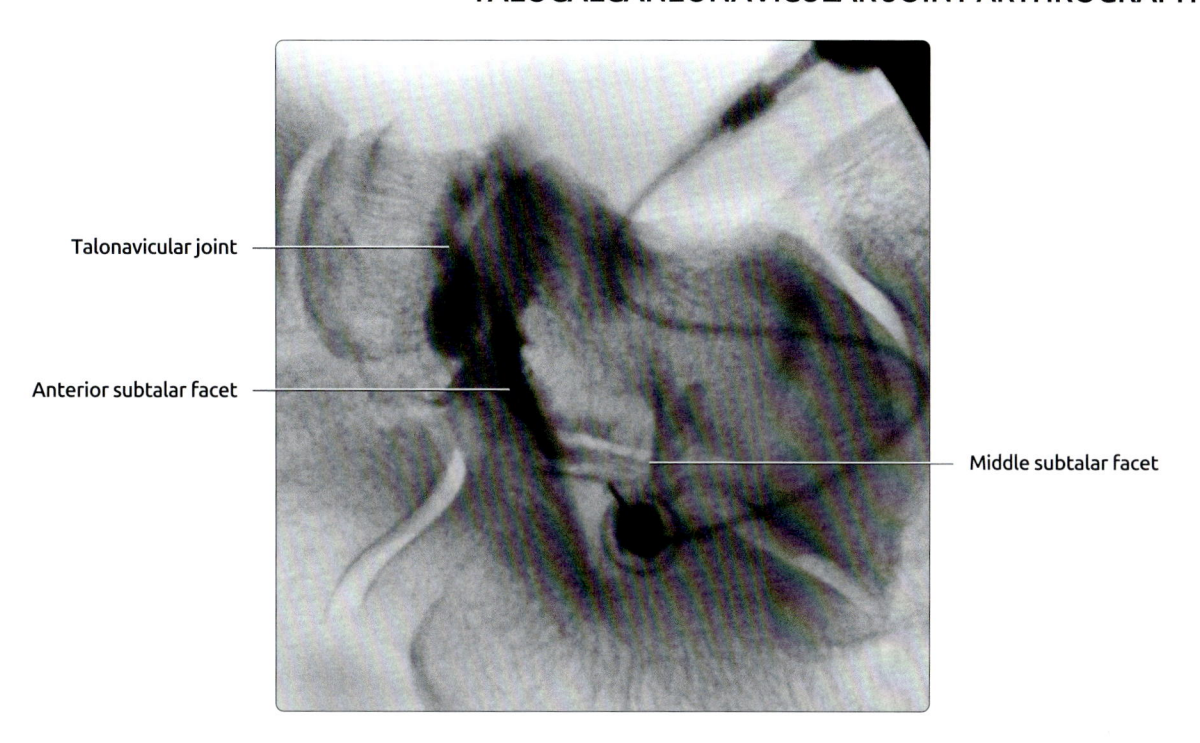

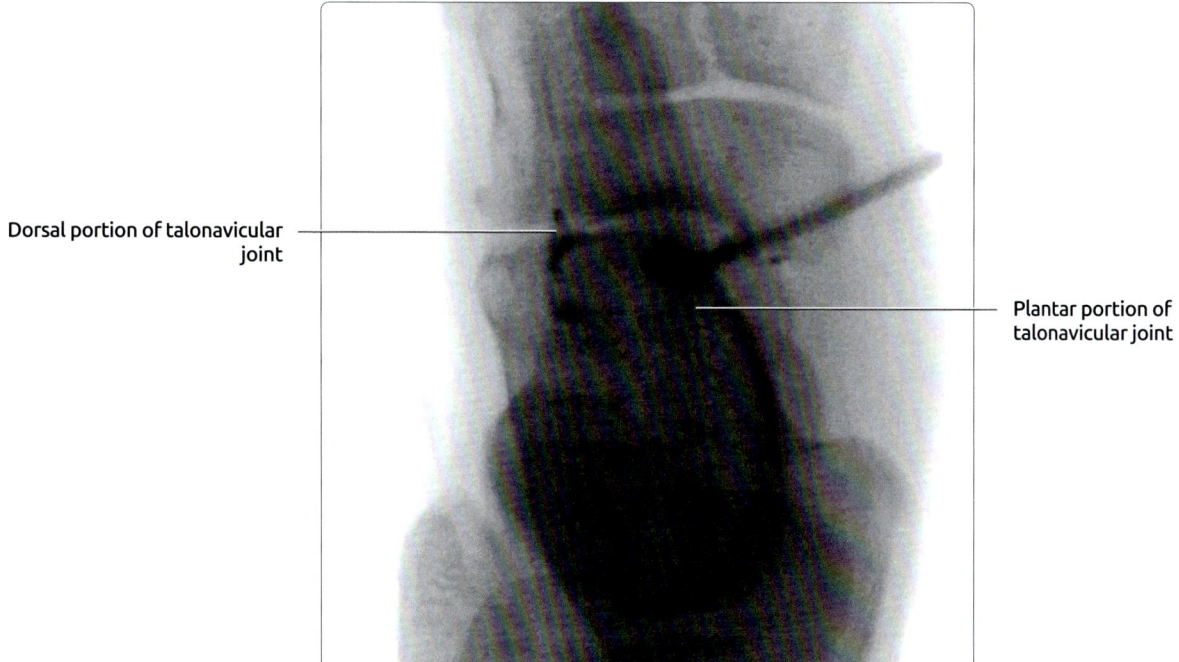

(Top) Lateral spot radiograph obtained after middle subtalar joint injection. The talonavicular joint, anterior subtalar facet, and middle subtalar facet form a common joint cavity. (Bottom) Anteroposterior spot radiograph in a different patient from a talonavicular joint injection shows contrast in joint recesses. The rounded talar head articulates with the disc-shaped navicular.

Foot Radiographic and Arthrographic Anatomy

CALCANEOCUBOID JOINT ARTHROGRAPHY

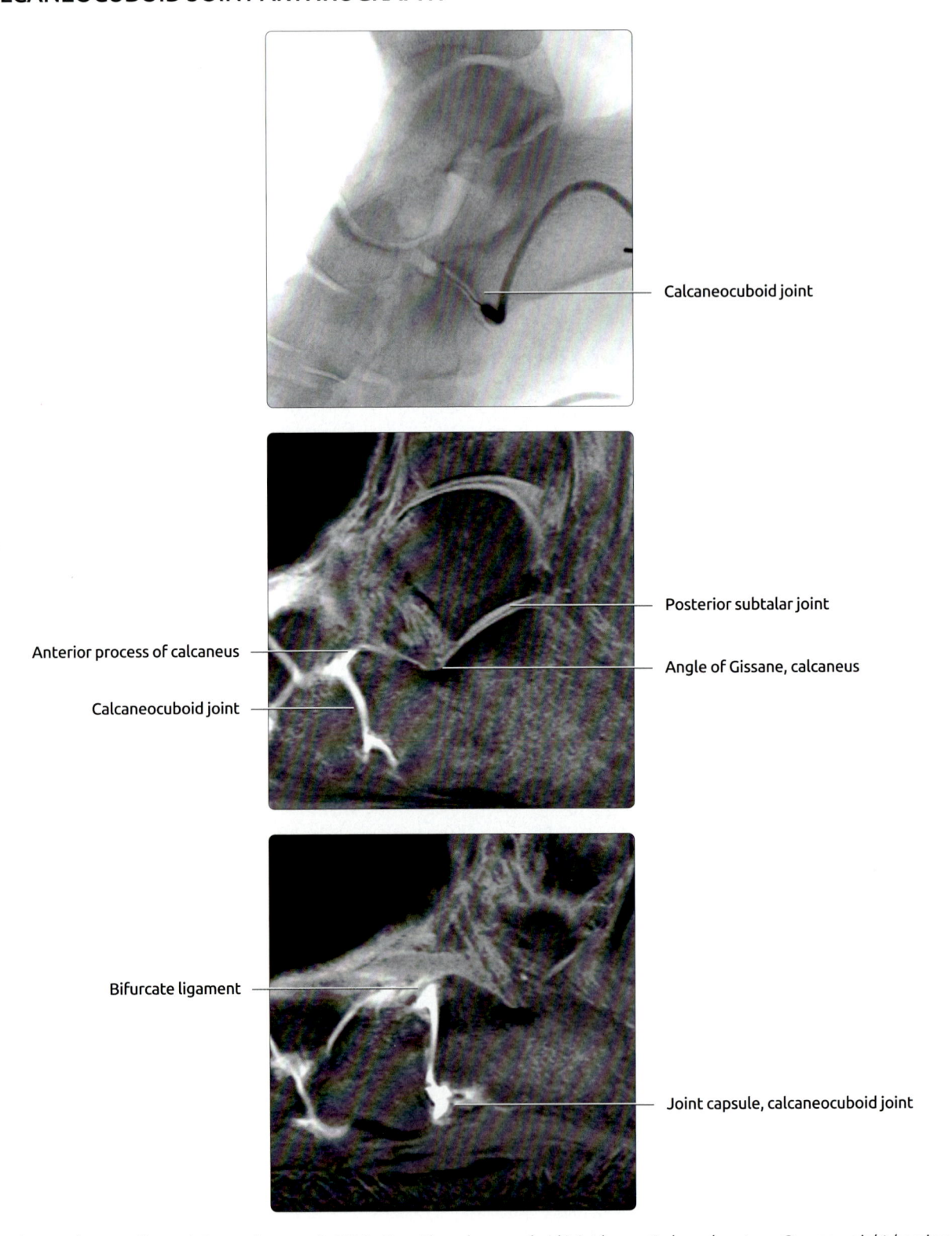

Calcaneocuboid joint

Anterior process of calcaneus

Calcaneocuboid joint

Posterior subtalar joint

Angle of Gissane, calcaneus

Bifurcate ligament

Joint capsule, calcaneocuboid joint

(Top) *Lateral spot radiograph from calcaneocuboid injection. The calcaneocuboid joint has an S-shaped contour. On non-weight-bearing films, the cuboid usually appears to be subluxated slightly inferior to the calcaneus.* **(Middle)** *Sagittal MR arthrography of the calcaneocuboid joint shows contrast outlining joint surfaces and joint recesses. The anterior process of the calcaneus forms a triangular tip and does not articulate with the navicular.* **(Bottom)** *Sagittal MR arthrography lateral to the previous image shows the bifurcate ligament extending from the anterior process of the calcaneus to the cuboid and navicular.*

Foot Radiographic and Arthrographic Anatomy

NAVICULOCUNEIFORM JOINT ARTHROGRAPHY

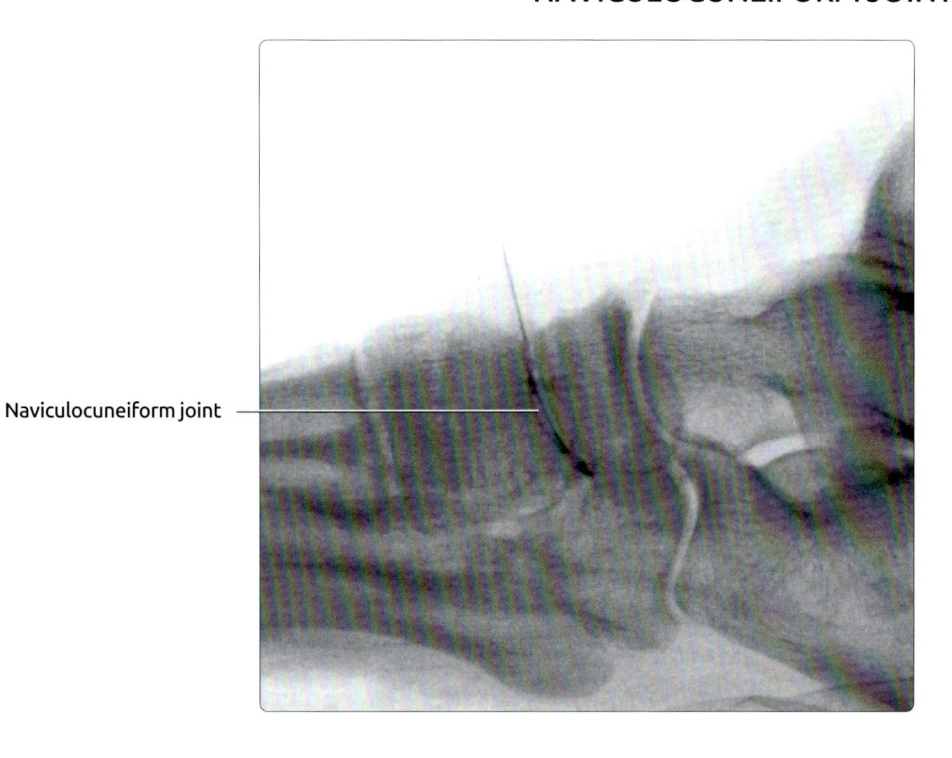

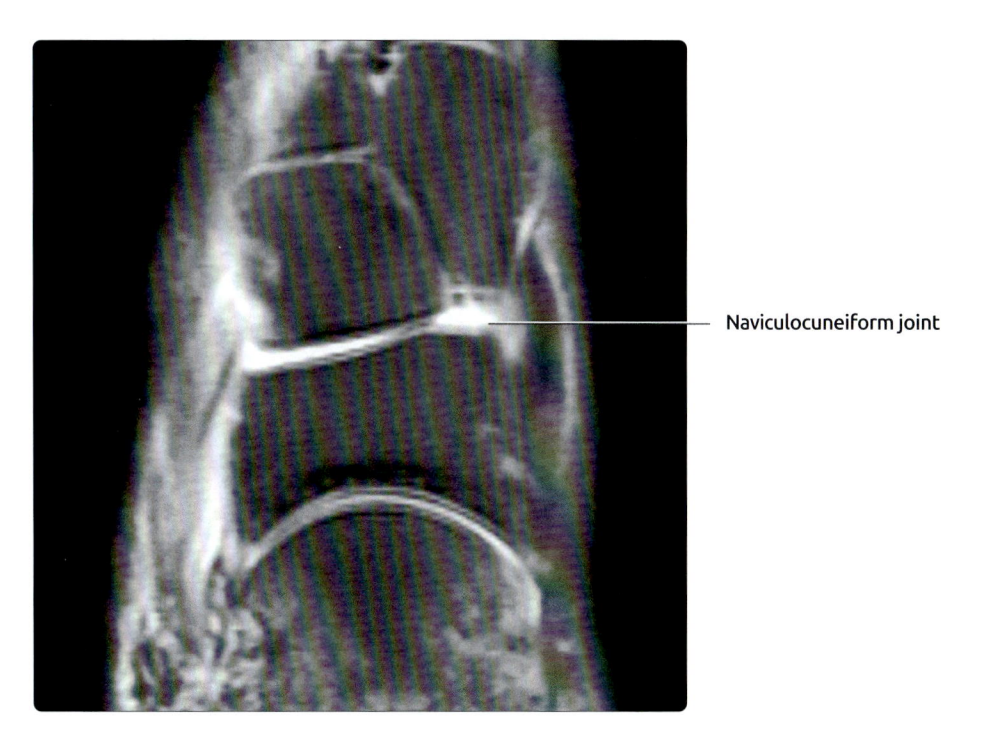

Naviculocuneiform joint

Naviculocuneiform joint

(Top) Lateral spot radiograph of naviculocuneiform arthrogram shows that the naviculocuneiform joint has a contour similar to that of the talonavicular joint. It often communicates with intercuneiform joints. (Bottom) Axial naviculocuneiform MR arthrography shows that the naviculocuneiform joint has 3 contiguous facets for articulation with each of the cuneiforms.

Foot Radiographic and Arthrographic Anatomy

INTERCUNEIFORM & TARSOMETATARSAL JOINTS

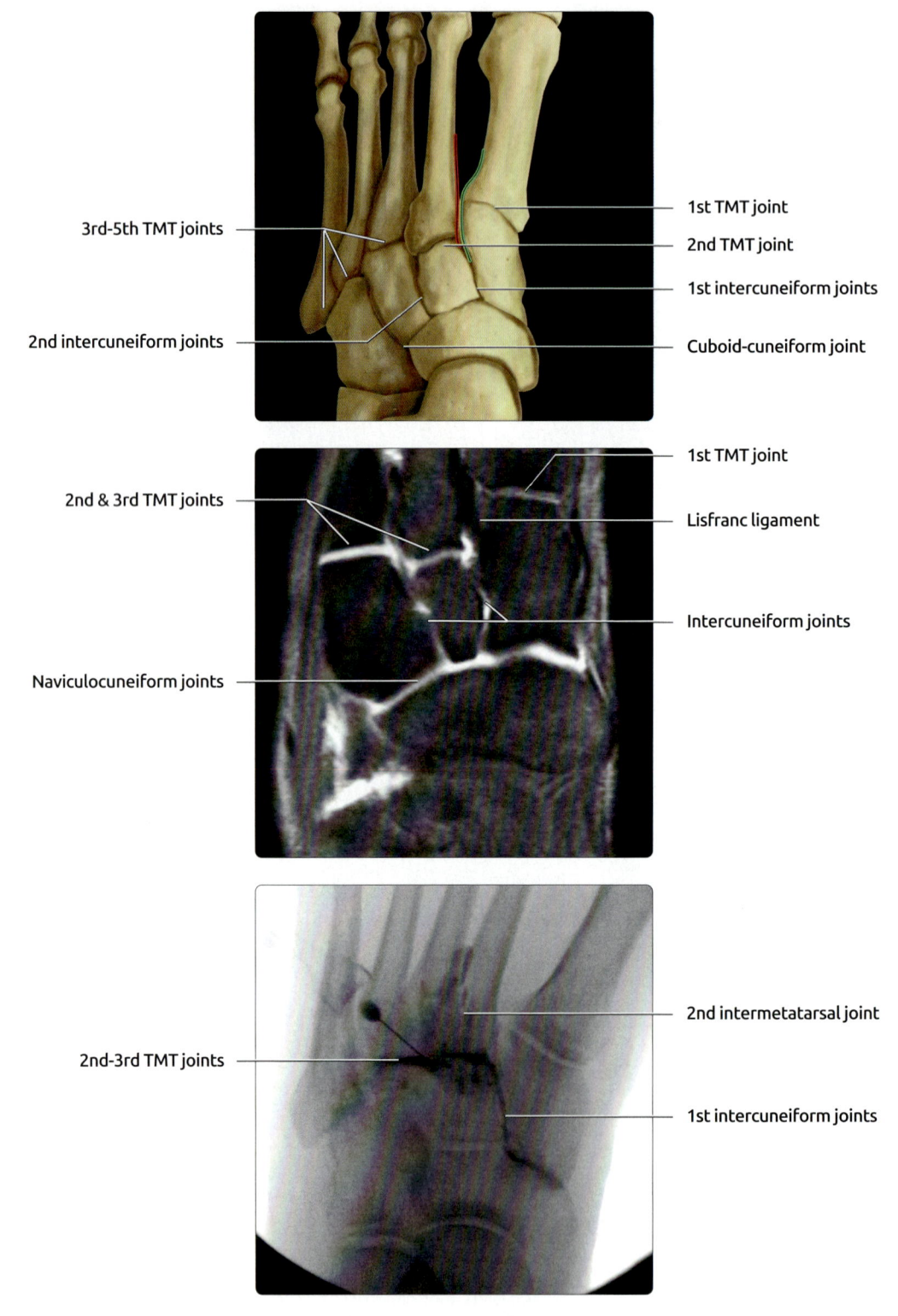

Labels (top graphic): 3rd-5th TMT joints; 2nd intercuneiform joints; 1st TMT joint; 2nd TMT joint; 1st intercuneiform joints; Cuboid-cuneiform joint

Labels (middle): 2nd & 3rd TMT joints; Naviculocuneiform joints; 1st TMT joint; Lisfranc ligament; Intercuneiform joints

Labels (bottom): 2nd-3rd TMT joints; 2nd intermetatarsal joint; 1st intercuneiform joints

(**Top**) *Graphic shows that the TMT joint forms a shallow arc from medial to lateral. It is stabilized by the recessed position of the 2nd TMT and by the Lisfranc ligament between the 1st cuneiform and 2nd metatarsal base. The 1st cuneiform is centered on the 1st metatarsal; the medial margin of the 2nd cuneiform is aligned with the medial margin of the 2nd metatarsal; the 5th metatarsal extends beyond the cuboid.* (**Middle**) *Axial MR arthrography with contrast filling intercuneiform, naviculocuneiform, and 2nd and 3rd tarsometatarsal joints shows variable communications between the Antercuneiform joints, tarsometatarsal joints, and naviculocuneiform joints.* (**Bottom**) *The 2nd and 3rd TMT joints form a single joint cavity, also communicating with the 2nd intermetatarsal joint. The communication seen here, with the 1st intercuneiform joint, is uncommon.*

Foot Radiographic and Arthrographic Anatomy

1ST METATARSOPHALANGEAL JOINT ARTHROGRAPHY

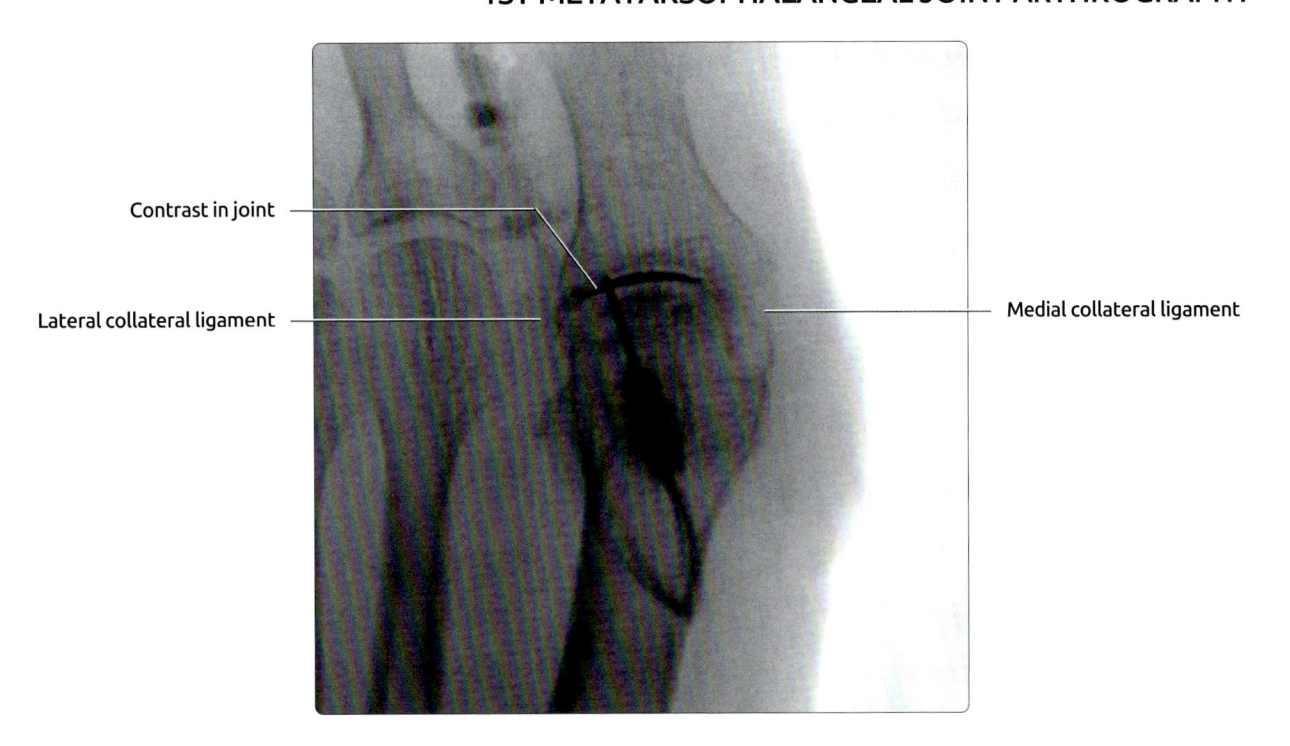

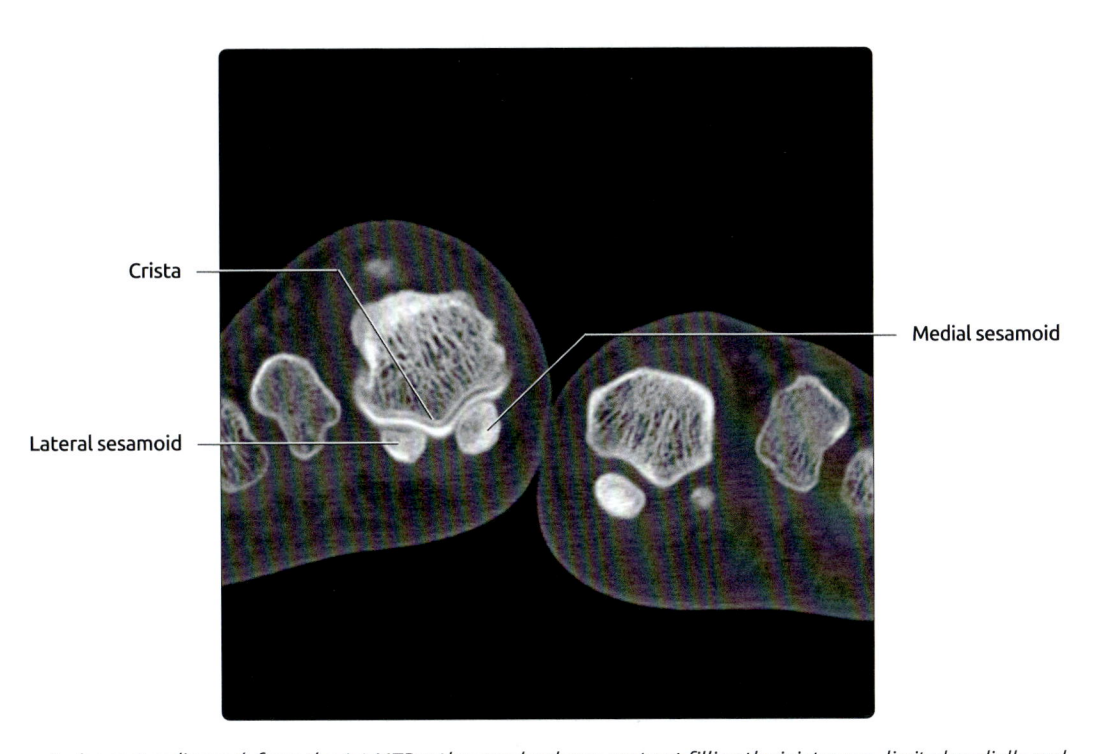

(Top) Anteroposterior spot radiograph from the 1st MTP arthrography shows contrast filling the joint space, limited medially and laterally by collateral ligaments. (Bottom) Coronal CT arthrogram shows the normal synovial articulation between the sesamoids and 1st metatarsal head.

Foot Radiographic and Arthrographic Anatomy

1ST MTP MR ARTHROGRAPHY

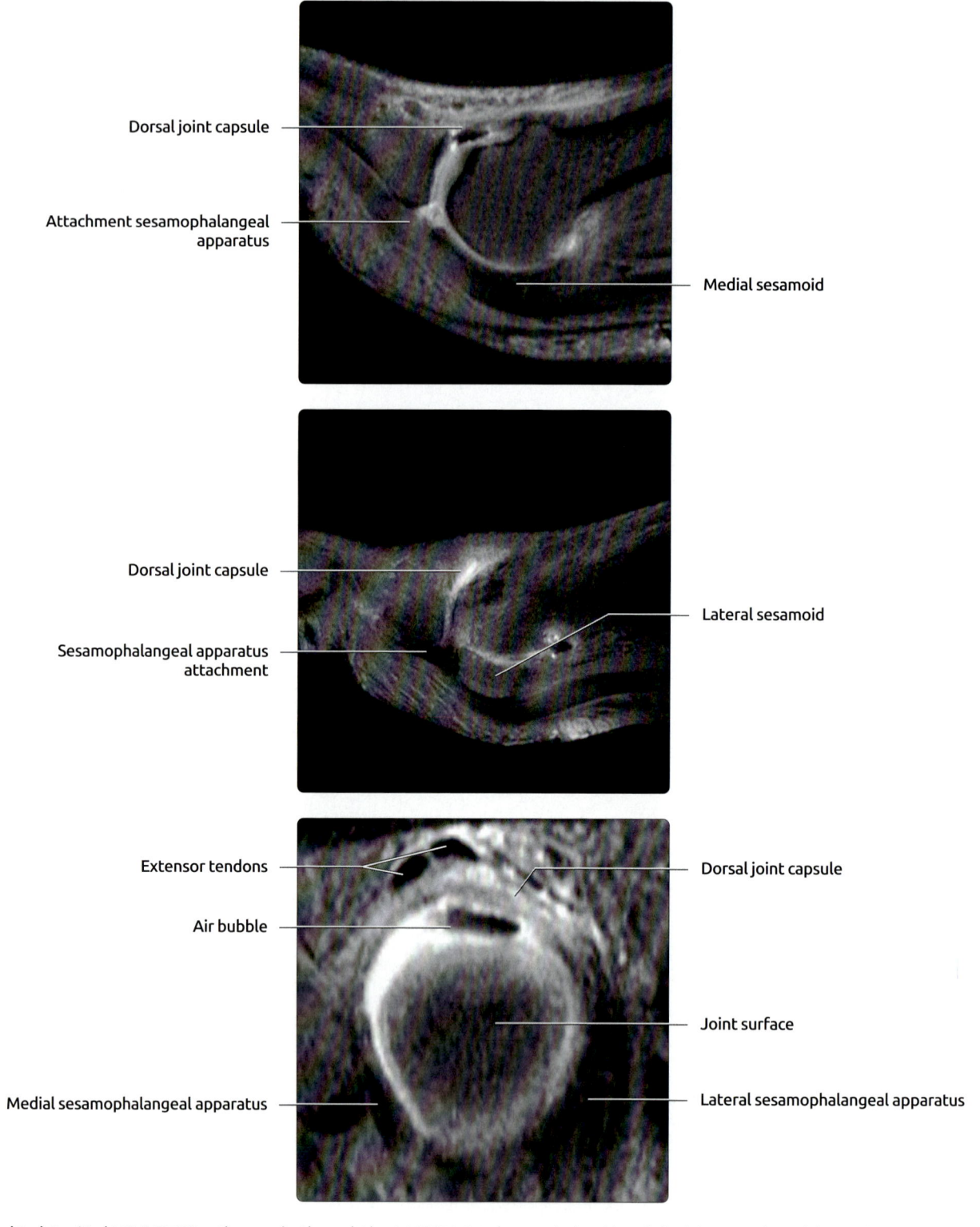

(Top) Sagittal T1WI FS MR arthrography through the 1st MTP joint shows relationships of the joint capsule and the medial sesamoid. The sesamophalangeal apparatus includes the plantar plate, sesamoids, and tendons in which sesamoids sit. It attaches to the base of the proximal phalanx. (Middle) Sagittal T1WI FS MR arthrography through the lateral margin of 1st MTP joint shows relationships of the joint capsule and the lateral sesamoid. Sesamophalangeal apparatus is shown attaching to lateral, plantar margin of 1st proximal phalangeal base. (Bottom) Coronal T1WI FS MR arthrography shows the sesamophalangeal apparatus at the periphery of the plantar aspect of the joint, close to the distal attachments.

Foot Radiographic and Arthrographic Anatomy

2ND MTP JOINT

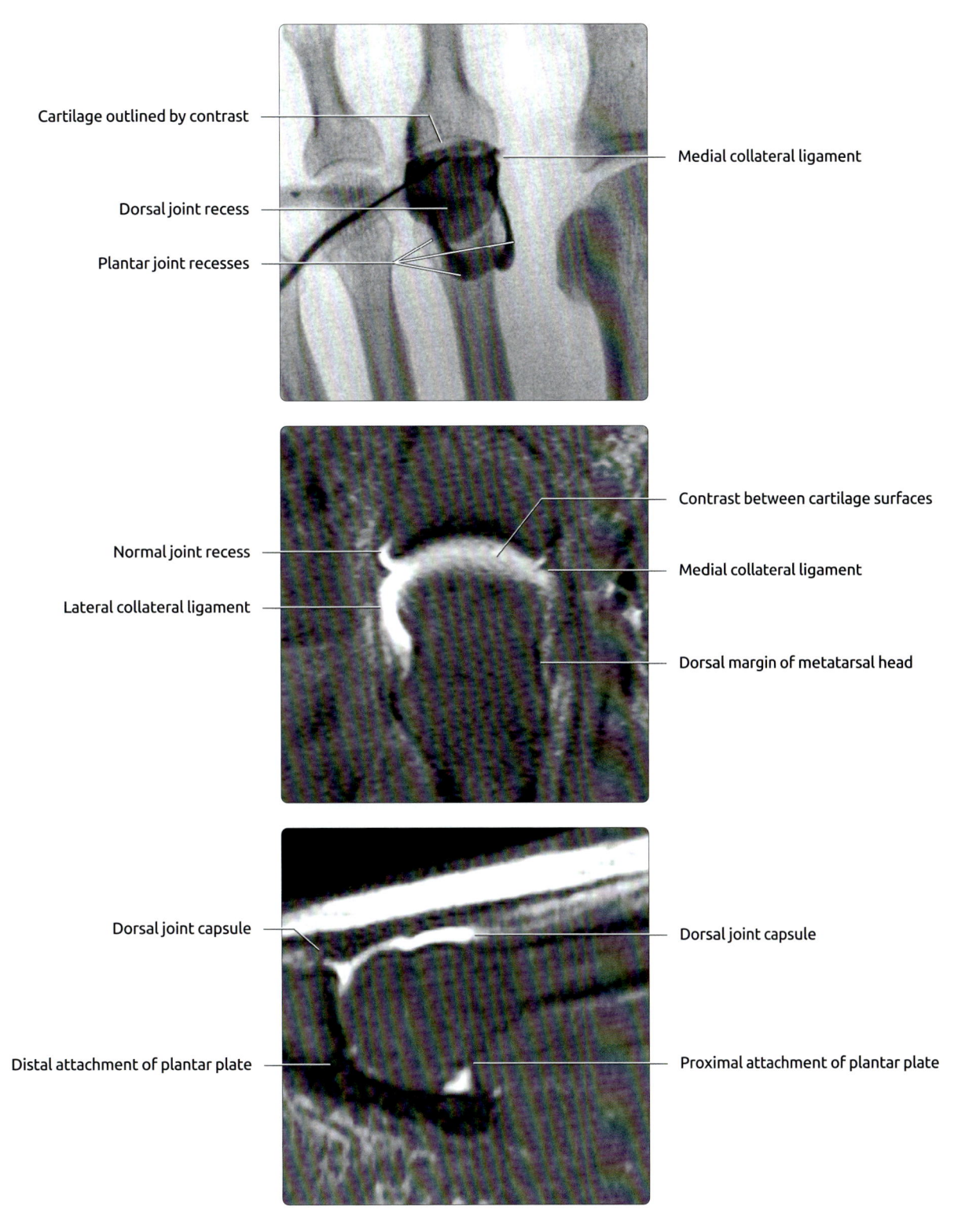

- Cartilage outlined by contrast
- Medial collateral ligament
- Dorsal joint recess
- Plantar joint recesses

- Contrast between cartilage surfaces
- Normal joint recess
- Medial collateral ligament
- Lateral collateral ligament
- Dorsal margin of metatarsal head

- Dorsal joint capsule
- Dorsal joint capsule
- Distal attachment of plantar plate
- Proximal attachment of plantar plate

(Top) Anteroposterior spot radiograph from the 2nd MTP arthrography shows normal filling of the capacious plantar recesses. The joint capsule is tightly adherent at the medial and lateral collateral ligaments. (Middle) Axial T1WI MR arthrography shows the collateral ligaments and articular cartilage outlined by contrast. (Bottom) Sagittal T1WI MR arthrogram through the 2nd MTP joint shows attachment of the plantar plate to the metatarsal neck. The plantar and dorsal joint recesses are normally fairly redundant, unlike the tight attachments at the base of the proximal phalanges.

Foot MR Atlas

TERMINOLOGY

Definitions

- Axial (horizontal) plane of foot
  - Long axis of foot
  - Slightly oblique compared to axial plane in leg
  - Hindfoot: Images angled along long axis of talus
  - Midfoot and forefoot: Images angled along long axis of 2nd metatarsal
- Coronal plane of foot
  - Short axis of foot
  - Hindfoot: Images angled perpendicular to neck of talus
  - Midfoot and forefoot: Images angled perpendicular to long axis of 2nd metatarsal

IMAGING ANATOMY

Structures Best Seen in Axial Plane

- Lisfranc ligament (3 separate bands, from 2nd cuneiform to 1st metatarsal base)
  - Dorsal band: Most superior slice through 2nd cuneiform and 1st metatarsal
  - Interosseous band: Thick band centrally located, must have taut appearance
  - Plantar band: Thinnest band, at plantar margin of 2nd cuneiform
- Spring ligament (plantar bands)
  - From calcaneus to navicular
  - Medioplantar oblique: Originates on coronoid fossa of calcaneus, anterior to sustentaculum tali, inserts on navicular lateral to posterior tibial tendon
  - Inferoplantar longitudinal: Short, straight course from coronoid fossa of calcaneus to navicular beak

Structures Best Seen in Coronal Plane

- Tarsal tunnel
  - Fibroosseous tunnel in medial hindfoot
    - Roof: Flexor retinaculum
    - Floor: Medial margins of talus & calcaneus
  - Contains: Posterior tibial neurovascular bundle and branches, posterior tibial tendon, flexor hallucis longus & flexor digitorum longus tendons
  - Importance: Mass, venous varicocity, cyst, or anomalous muscle may cause impingement on tibial nerve or its branches
    - Results in tarsal tunnel syndrome: Pain, numbness, muscle weakness, and atrophy
- Tarsal sinus
  - Funnel-shaped space between talar neck and dorsal margin of calcaneus
  - Contains: Cervical ligament, limbs of extensor retinaculum, artery of tarsal sinus
  - Importance: Injury may lead to fibrosis, pain at lateral hindfoot, subjective instability
- Tarsal canal
  - Posteromedial extenson of tarsal sinus
  - Contains: Interosseous ligament
  - Significance: Ligament tear can be associated with subtalar instability
- Spring ligament, superomedial band
  - Strongest portion of spring ligament
  - Originates on sustentaculum tali, tibiospring band of superficial deltoid ligament
  - Inserts on medial navicular
- Intrinsic muscles
  - Interrelationships of muscle layers usually best seen on coronal images
- Compartments of foot
  - 4 plantar compartments divided by fascial layers
  - Medial, middle (superficial & deep), lateral
  - Significance: Infection usually limited to 1 compartment unless patient has had prior surgery

Structures Best Seen in Sagittal Plane

- Tarsometatarasal joints
  - Due to obliquity of joints, partial volume averaging may cause interpretative difficulties in other planes
  - Significance: Joint disorders, instability
- Plantar plate of metatarsophalangeal joints
  - Plantar thickening of joint capsule
  - Extends from metatarsal neck to base of proximal phalanx
  - 1st metatarsophalangeal plantar plate incorporates its sesamoids
  - Significance: Injury to plantar plate can result in dorsal subluxation or dislocation at joint
- Phalanges
  - Due to their normally flexed position, difficult to localize abnormalities on axial, coronal images
  - Significance: Osteomyelitis often involves terminal phalanges, best seen on sagittal images

MR Protocol

- Use dedicated foot coil or knee coil
- Usually patient supine, some authors prefer patient prone, foot plantar flexed
  - Prone position results in some distortion of normal anatomy
- Usually angle along 2nd metatarsal axis for sagittal images
  - Modify for other regions of interest
- Coronal should be perpendicular to metatarsals
- Axial should be along plane of 2nd metatarsal
- High-density pad around forefoot often improves image quality
- T1-weighted imaging usually obtained in sagittal, axial planes
- Fluid-sensitive imaging in coronal, sagittal planes
- For osteomyelitis, obtain T1-weighted images in all 3 planes

ANATOMY IMAGING ISSUES

Imaging Pitfalls

- Talonavicular joint recess between plantar bands of spring ligament can be confused with ligament rupture
- Bursae between metatarsal heads may be mistaken for neuromas
- Divergence of metatarsals may create confusion on sagittal images as to exact digit being imaged
- Flexion of toes may mimic abnormality due to partial volume averaging

Foot MR Atlas

GRAPHICS: DORSAL AND PLANTAR FOOT LIGAMENTS

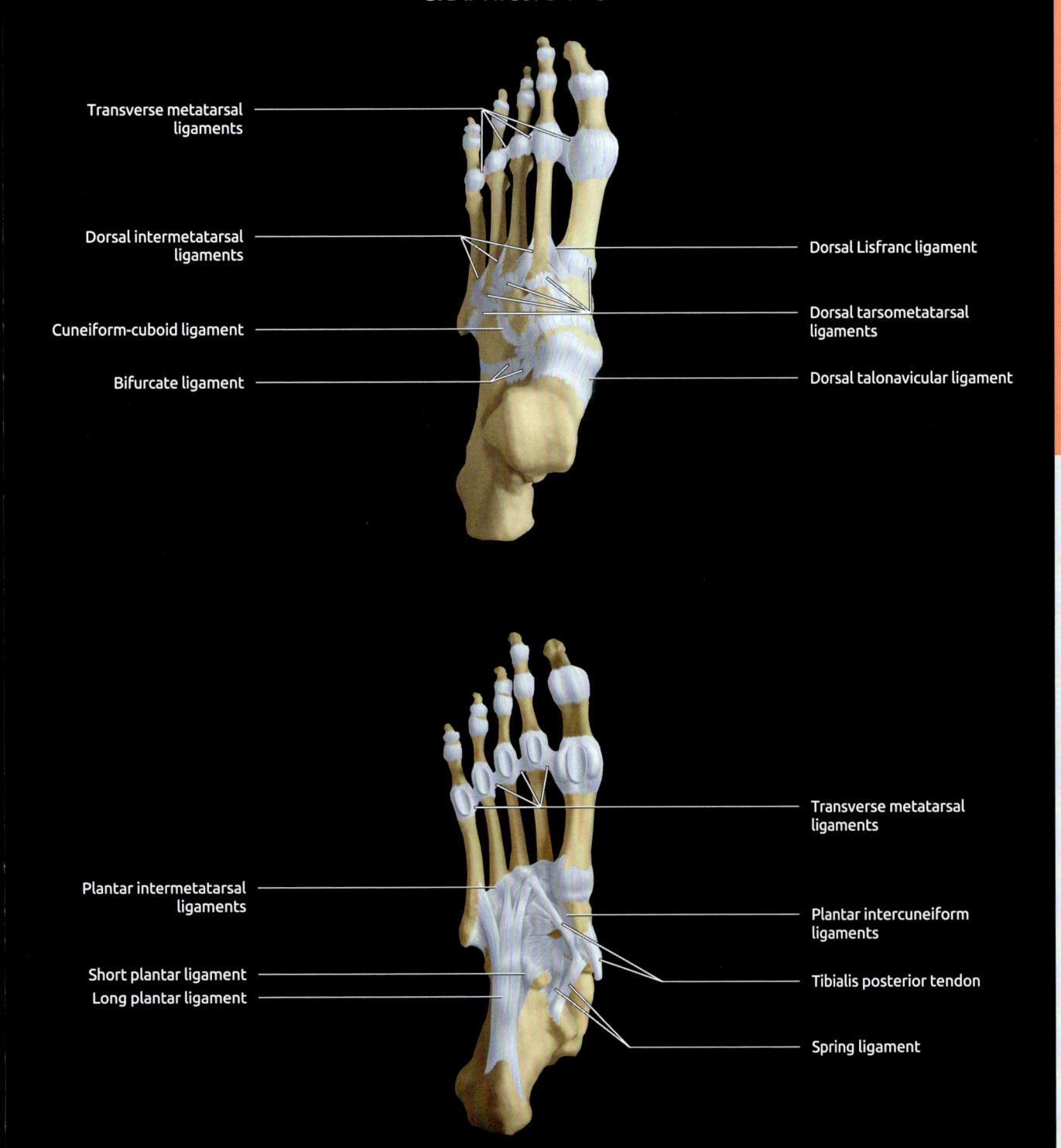

Labels (top, dorsal view): Transverse metatarsal ligaments; Dorsal intermetatarsal ligaments; Cuneiform-cuboid ligament; Bifurcate ligament; Dorsal Lisfranc ligament; Dorsal tarsometatarsal ligaments; Dorsal talonavicular ligament.

Labels (bottom, plantar view): Plantar intermetatarsal ligaments; Short plantar ligament; Long plantar ligament; Transverse metatarsal ligaments; Plantar intercuneiform ligaments; Tibialis posterior tendon; Spring ligament.

(Top) *Graphic of dorsal ligaments shows dense ligaments between tarsal bones, and between tarsals and metatarsals. Ligaments are generally named for the bones they bridge. Exceptions are the bifurcate ligament, which extends from the anterior process calcaneus to the cuboid and navicular, and the dorsal Lisfranc ligament, from the 1st cuneiform to 2nd metatarsal.* (Bottom) *Graphic of plantar ligaments shows ligaments deep to the plantar fascia as well as proximal and distal attachments of the tibialis posterior tendon. The spring ligament, a.k.a. the plantar calcaneonavicular ligament, originates on the sustentaculum tali and anterior calcaneus and inserts on the navicular. Deep intertarsal ligaments are also shown, and are named for bones they bridge.*

Foot MR Atlas

AXIAL (LONG AXIS) T1 MR, RIGHT FOOT

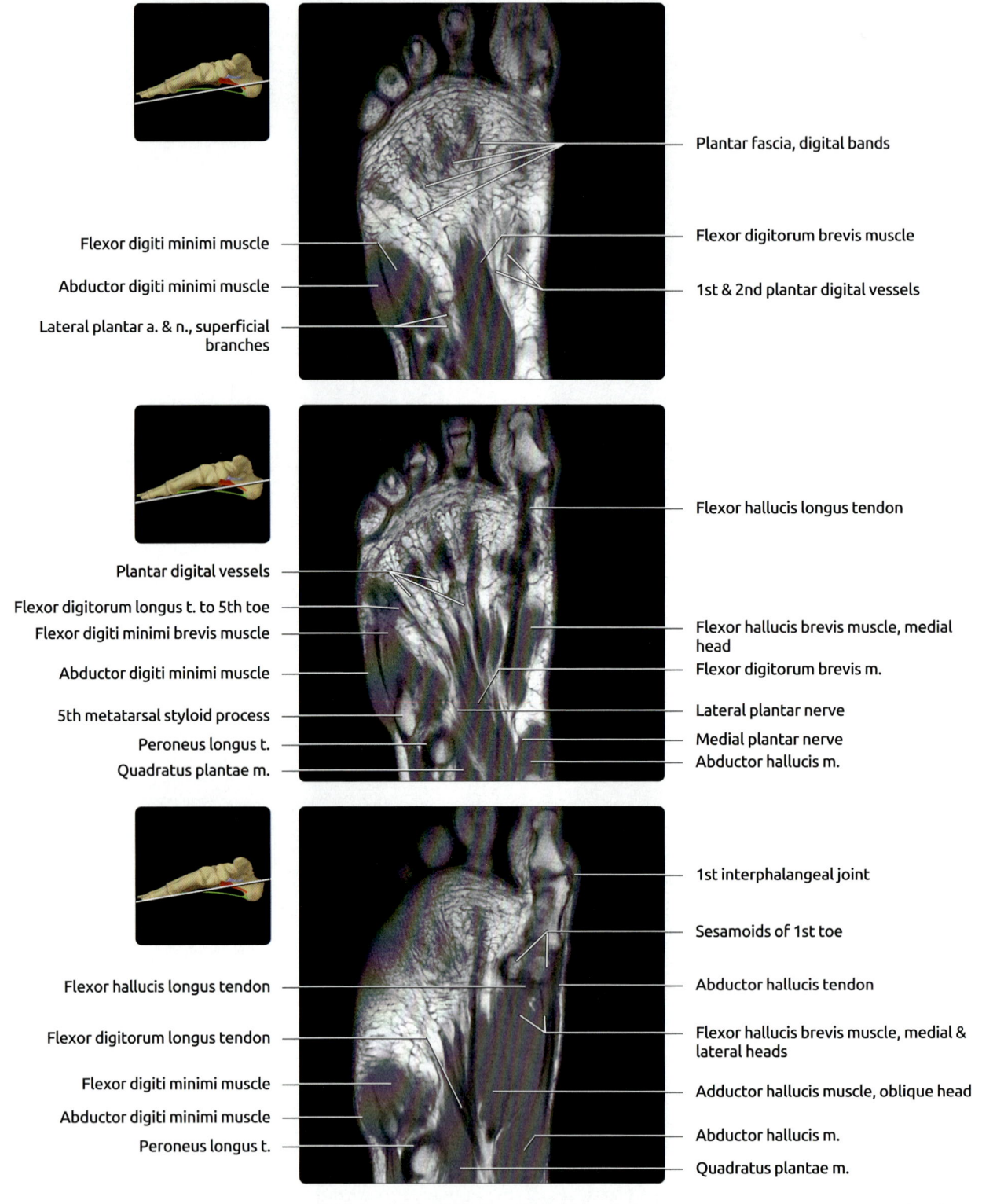

Top image labels:
- Plantar fascia, digital bands
- Flexor digitorum brevis muscle
- 1st & 2nd plantar digital vessels
- Flexor digiti minimi muscle
- Abductor digiti minimi muscle
- Lateral plantar a. & n., superficial branches

Middle image labels:
- Flexor hallucis longus tendon
- Flexor hallucis brevis muscle, medial head
- Flexor digitorum brevis m.
- Lateral plantar nerve
- Medial plantar nerve
- Abductor hallucis m.
- Plantar digital vessels
- Flexor digitorum longus t. to 5th toe
- Flexor digiti minimi brevis muscle
- Abductor digiti minimi muscle
- 5th metatarsal styloid process
- Peroneus longus t.
- Quadratus plantae m.

Bottom image labels:
- 1st interphalangeal joint
- Sesamoids of 1st toe
- Abductor hallucis tendon
- Flexor hallucis brevis muscle, medial & lateral heads
- Adductor hallucis muscle, oblique head
- Abductor hallucis m.
- Quadratus plantae m.
- Flexor hallucis longus tendon
- Flexor digitorum longus tendon
- Flexor digiti minimi muscle
- Abductor digiti minimi muscle
- Peroneus longus t.

(Top) 1st in a series of axial (long axis) T1 MR images of the right foot, shown from plantar to dorsal. Plantar fascia, superficial to the flexor digitorum brevis muscle, is seen dividing into digital bands in the forefoot. **(Middle)** The medial plantar nerve courses lateral to the medial plantar artery, between the abductor hallucis and flexor digitorum brevis. The lateral plantar nerve courses between the flexor digitorum brevis muscle and quadratus plantae muscle and continues laterally, dividing into deep and superficial branches at the level of the 5th metatarsal base, between the flexor digitorum brevis and abductor digiti minimi. **(Bottom)** Medial and lateral heads of flexor digitorum brevis muscle are seen attaching to sesamoids of the 1st toe. Their distal insertion onto the base of the 1st proximal phalanx is not seen on this image.

Foot MR Atlas

AXIAL (LONG AXIS) T1 MR, LEFT FOOT

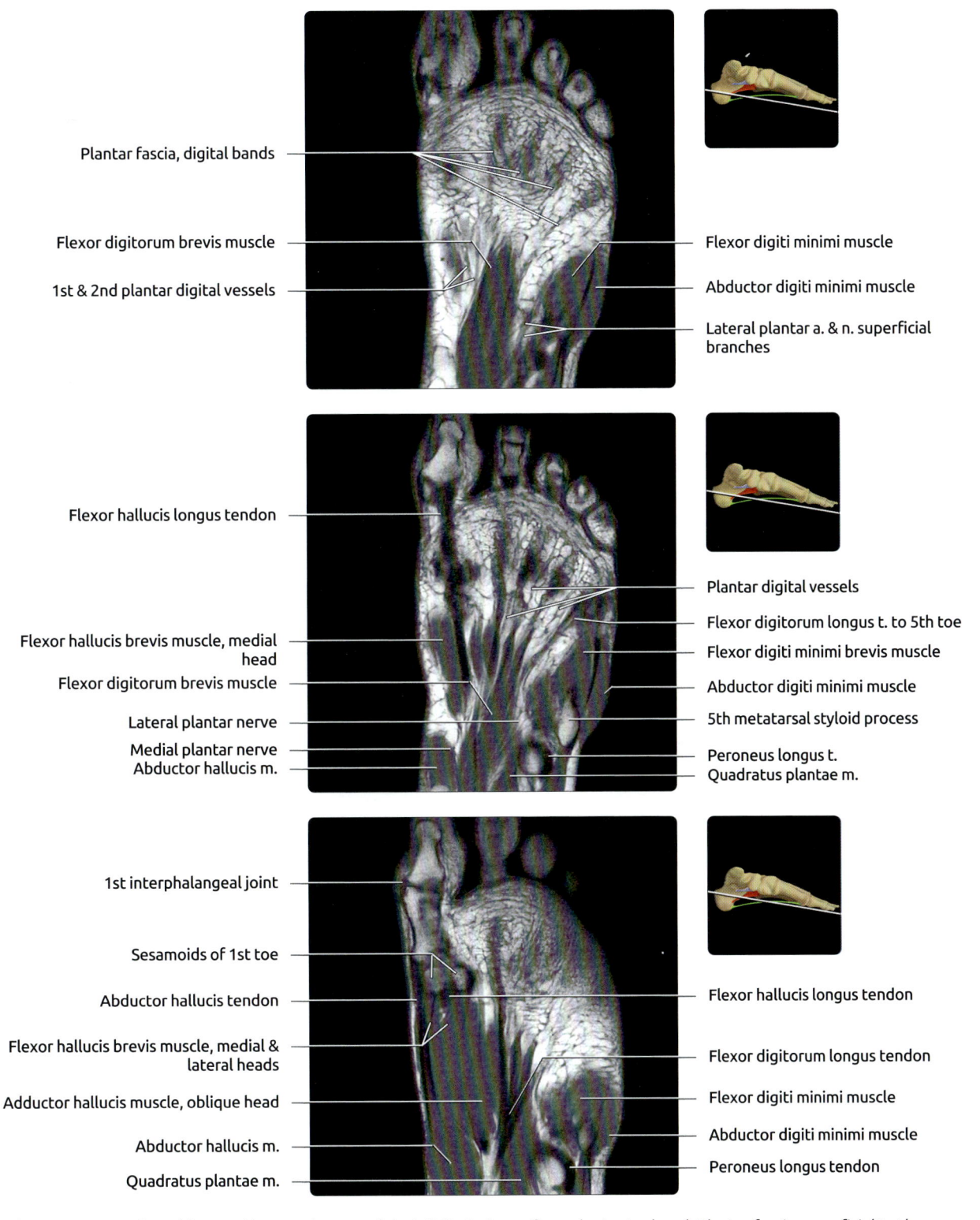

Labels (top image):
- Plantar fascia, digital bands
- Flexor digitorum brevis muscle
- 1st & 2nd plantar digital vessels
- Flexor digiti minimi muscle
- Abductor digiti minimi muscle
- Lateral plantar a. & n. superficial branches

Labels (middle image):
- Flexor hallucis longus tendon
- Flexor hallucis brevis muscle, medial head
- Flexor digitorum brevis muscle
- Lateral plantar nerve
- Medial plantar nerve
- Abductor hallucis m.
- Plantar digital vessels
- Flexor digitorum longus t. to 5th toe
- Flexor digiti minimi brevis muscle
- Abductor digiti minimi muscle
- 5th metatarsal styloid process
- Peroneus longus t.
- Quadratus plantae m.

Labels (bottom image):
- 1st interphalangeal joint
- Sesamoids of 1st toe
- Abductor hallucis tendon
- Flexor hallucis brevis muscle, medial & lateral heads
- Adductor hallucis muscle, oblique head
- Abductor hallucis m.
- Quadratus plantae m.
- Flexor hallucis longus tendon
- Flexor digitorum longus tendon
- Flexor digiti minimi muscle
- Abductor digiti minimi muscle
- Peroneus longus tendon

(**Top**) *1st in a series of axial (long axis) T1 MR images of the left foot, shown from plantar to dorsal. Plantar fascia, superficial to the flexor digitorum brevis muscle, is seen dividing into digital bands in the forefoot.* (**Middle**) *The medial plantar nerve courses lateral to the medial plantar artery, between the abductor hallucis and flexor digitorum brevis. The lateral plantar nerve courses between the flexor digitorum brevis muscle and quadratus plantae muscle and continues laterally, dividing into deep and superficial branches at the level of the 5th metatarsal base, between the flexor digitorum brevis muscle and abductor digiti minimi.* (**Bottom**) *The medial and lateral heads of the flexor digitorum brevis muscle are seen attaching to the sesamoids of the 1st toe. Their distal insertion onto base of 1st proximal phalanx is not seen on this image.*

1057

Foot MR Atlas

AXIAL (LONG AXIS) T1 MR, RIGHT FOOT

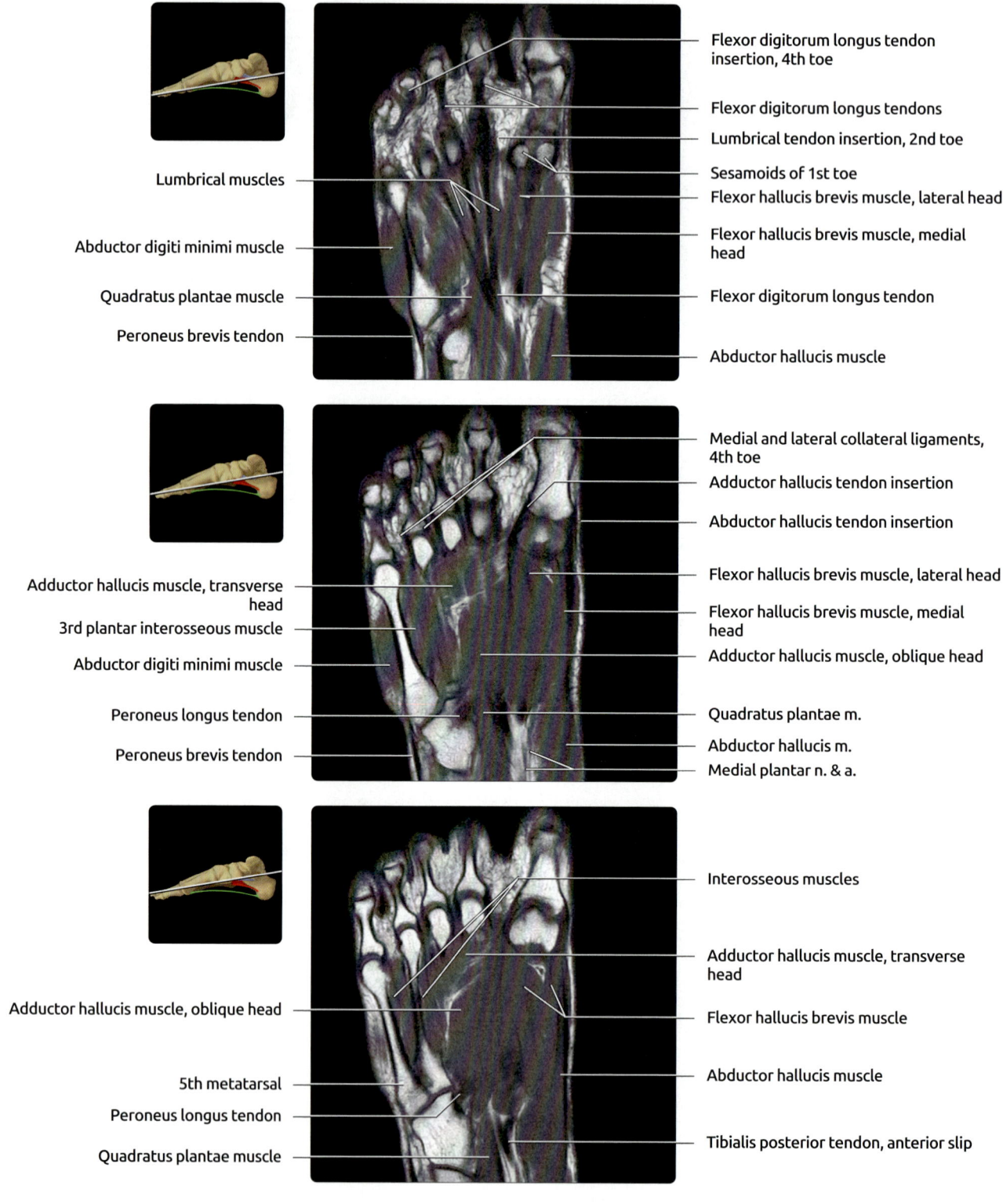

Labels (top image):
- Flexor digitorum longus tendon insertion, 4th toe
- Flexor digitorum longus tendons
- Lumbrical tendon insertion, 2nd toe
- Sesamoids of 1st toe
- Flexor hallucis brevis muscle, lateral head
- Flexor hallucis brevis muscle, medial head
- Flexor digitorum longus tendon
- Abductor hallucis muscle
- Lumbrical muscles
- Abductor digiti minimi muscle
- Quadratus plantae muscle
- Peroneus brevis tendon

Labels (middle image):
- Medial and lateral collateral ligaments, 4th toe
- Adductor hallucis tendon insertion
- Abductor hallucis tendon insertion
- Flexor hallucis brevis muscle, lateral head
- Flexor hallucis brevis muscle, medial head
- Adductor hallucis muscle, oblique head
- Quadratus plantae m.
- Abductor hallucis m.
- Medial plantar n. & a.
- Adductor hallucis muscle, transverse head
- 3rd plantar interosseous muscle
- Abductor digiti minimi muscle
- Peroneus longus tendon
- Peroneus brevis tendon

Labels (bottom image):
- Interosseous muscles
- Adductor hallucis muscle, transverse head
- Flexor hallucis brevis muscle
- Abductor hallucis muscle
- Tibialis posterior tendon, anterior slip
- Adductor hallucis muscle, oblique head
- 5th metatarsal
- Peroneus longus tendon
- Quadratus plantae muscle

(**Top**) Note the insertion of the quadratus plantae muscle into the flexor digitorum longus tendon just proximal to its division into slips to 4 lateral toes. The lumbrical muscles arise from individual slips of the flexor digitorum longus tendon, and insert on the medial aspect of the proximal phalanx. A flexor digitorum longus tendon slip to the 5th digit is variably present. (**Middle**) Terminology for adductor and abductor hallucis muscles becomes clear once it is remembered that abductor pulls 1st toe away from 2nd toe, and adductor pulls it toward 2nd toe (i.e., axis of reference here is the foot, not the entire body). (**Bottom**) The oblique head of the adductor hallucis muscle is thick and broad, while the transverse head is thinner and sometimes congenitally absent.

Foot MR Atlas

AXIAL (LONG AXIS) T1 MR, LEFT FOOT

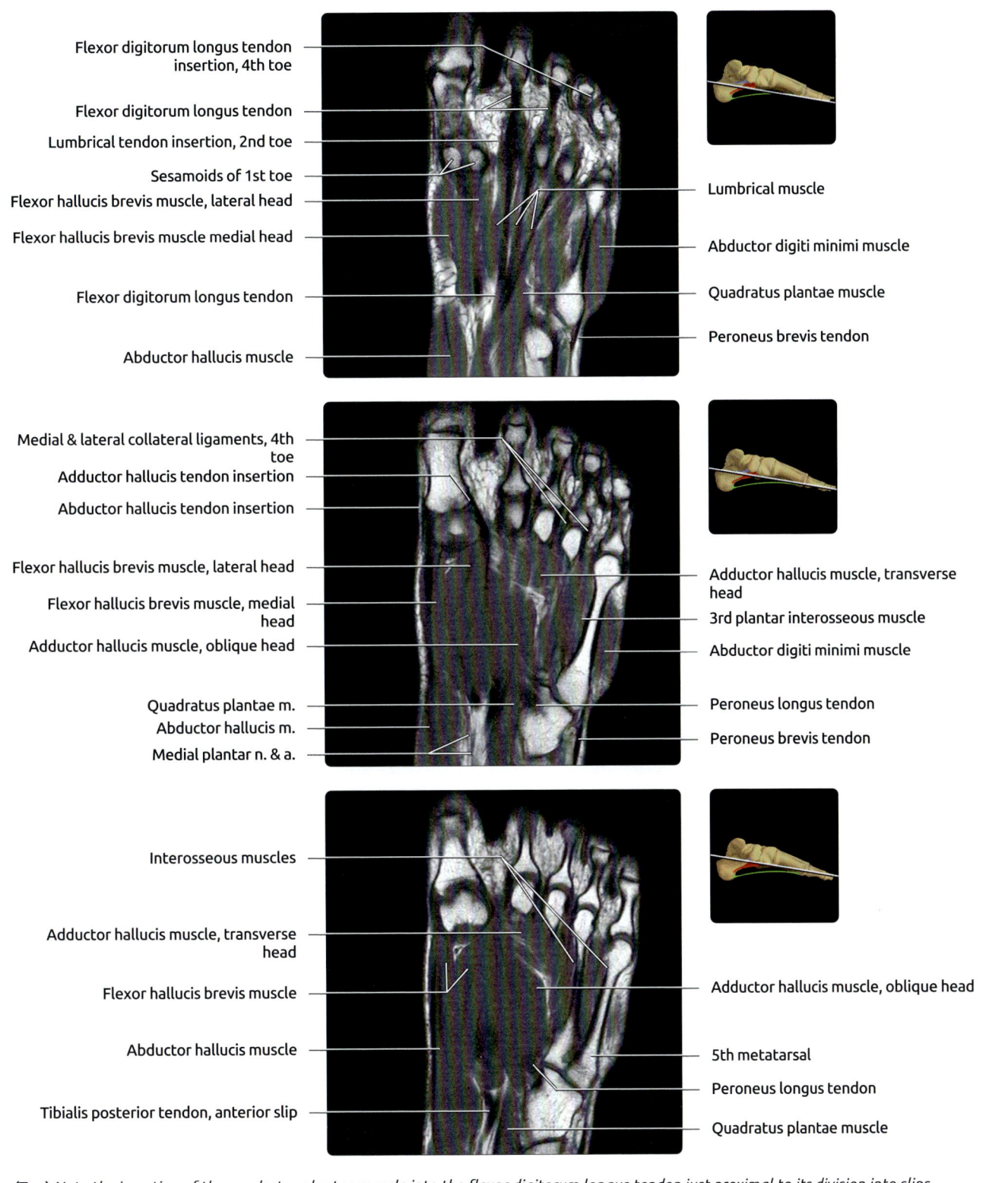

Labels (top image):
- Flexor digitorum longus tendon insertion, 4th toe
- Flexor digitorum longus tendon
- Lumbrical tendon insertion, 2nd toe
- Sesamoids of 1st toe
- Flexor hallucis brevis muscle, lateral head
- Flexor hallucis brevis muscle medial head
- Flexor digitorum longus tendon
- Abductor hallucis muscle
- Lumbrical muscle
- Abductor digiti minimi muscle
- Quadratus plantae muscle
- Peroneus brevis tendon

Labels (middle image):
- Medial & lateral collateral ligaments, 4th toe
- Adductor hallucis tendon insertion
- Abductor hallucis tendon insertion
- Flexor hallucis brevis muscle, lateral head
- Flexor hallucis brevis muscle, medial head
- Adductor hallucis muscle, oblique head
- Quadratus plantae m.
- Abductor hallucis m.
- Medial plantar n. & a.
- Adductor hallucis muscle, transverse head
- 3rd plantar interosseous muscle
- Abductor digiti minimi muscle
- Peroneus longus tendon
- Peroneus brevis tendon

Labels (bottom image):
- Interosseous muscles
- Adductor hallucis muscle, transverse head
- Flexor hallucis brevis muscle
- Abductor hallucis muscle
- Tibialis posterior tendon, anterior slip
- Adductor hallucis muscle, oblique head
- 5th metatarsal
- Peroneus longus tendon
- Quadratus plantae muscle

(Top) Note the insertion of the quadratus plantae muscle into the flexor digitorum longus tendon just proximal to its division into slips to 4 lateral toes. The lumbrical muscles arise from individual slips of the flexor digitorum longus tendon and insert on the medial aspect of the proximal phalanx. A flexor digitorum longus tendon slip to 5th digit is variably present. **(Middle)** Terminology for adductor and abductor hallucis muscles becomes clear once it is remembered that the abductor pulls the 1st toe away from the 2nd toe, and the adductor pulls it toward the 2nd toe (i.e., axis of reference here is foot, not entire body). **(Bottom)** The oblique head of the adductor hallucis muscle is thick and broad, while the transverse head is thinner and sometimes congenitally absent.

Foot MR Atlas

AXIAL (LONG AXIS) T1 MR, RIGHT FOOT

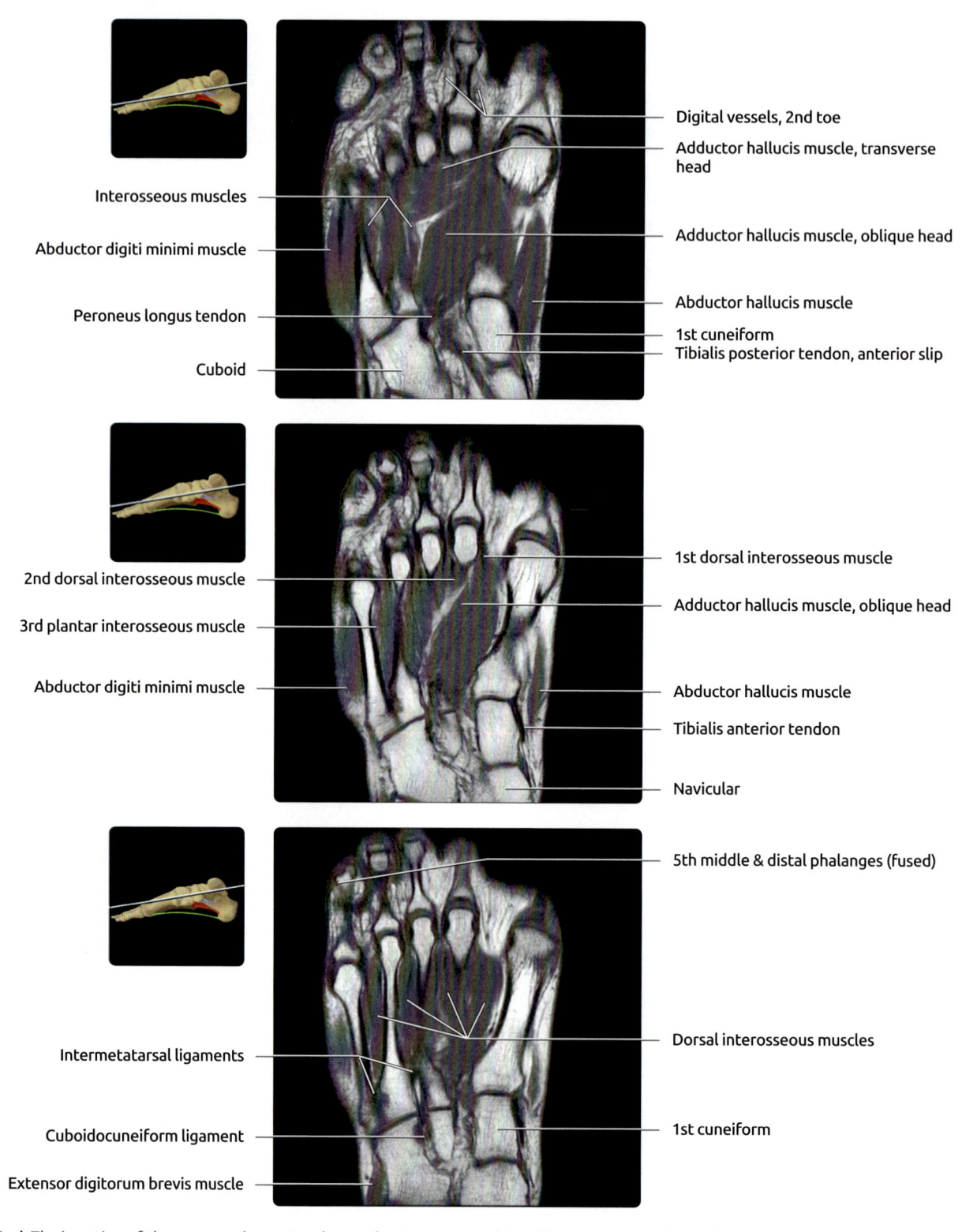

Labels (top image):
- Digital vessels, 2nd toe
- Adductor hallucis muscle, transverse head
- Adductor hallucis muscle, oblique head
- Abductor hallucis muscle
- 1st cuneiform
- Tibialis posterior tendon, anterior slip
- Interosseous muscles
- Abductor digiti minimi muscle
- Peroneus longus tendon
- Cuboid

Labels (middle image):
- 1st dorsal interosseous muscle
- Adductor hallucis muscle, oblique head
- Abductor hallucis muscle
- Tibialis anterior tendon
- Navicular
- 2nd dorsal interosseous muscle
- 3rd plantar interosseous muscle
- Abductor digiti minimi muscle

Labels (bottom image):
- 5th middle & distal phalanges (fused)
- Dorsal interosseous muscles
- 1st cuneiform
- Intermetatarsal ligaments
- Cuboidocuneiform ligament
- Extensor digitorum brevis muscle

(Top) The insertion of the peroneus longus tendon on the 1st metatarsal is well seen. Note the thread-like digital vessels at the medial and lateral margins of the 2nd toe. (Middle) The plantar interossei arise from the medial margin of 3 lateral toes and insert on the medial aspect of the base of their respective proximal phalanges. (Bottom) There are 4 dorsal interosseous muscles, each with 2 heads ("bipennate") arising from the bases of the adjacent metatarsals. The 1st dorsal interosseous inserts on the medial aspect of the 2nd proximal phalanx base, and the 2nd-4th on to the lateral aspect of the base of the 2nd-4th metatarsals.

Foot MR Atlas

AXIAL (LONG AXIS) T1 MR, LEFT FOOT

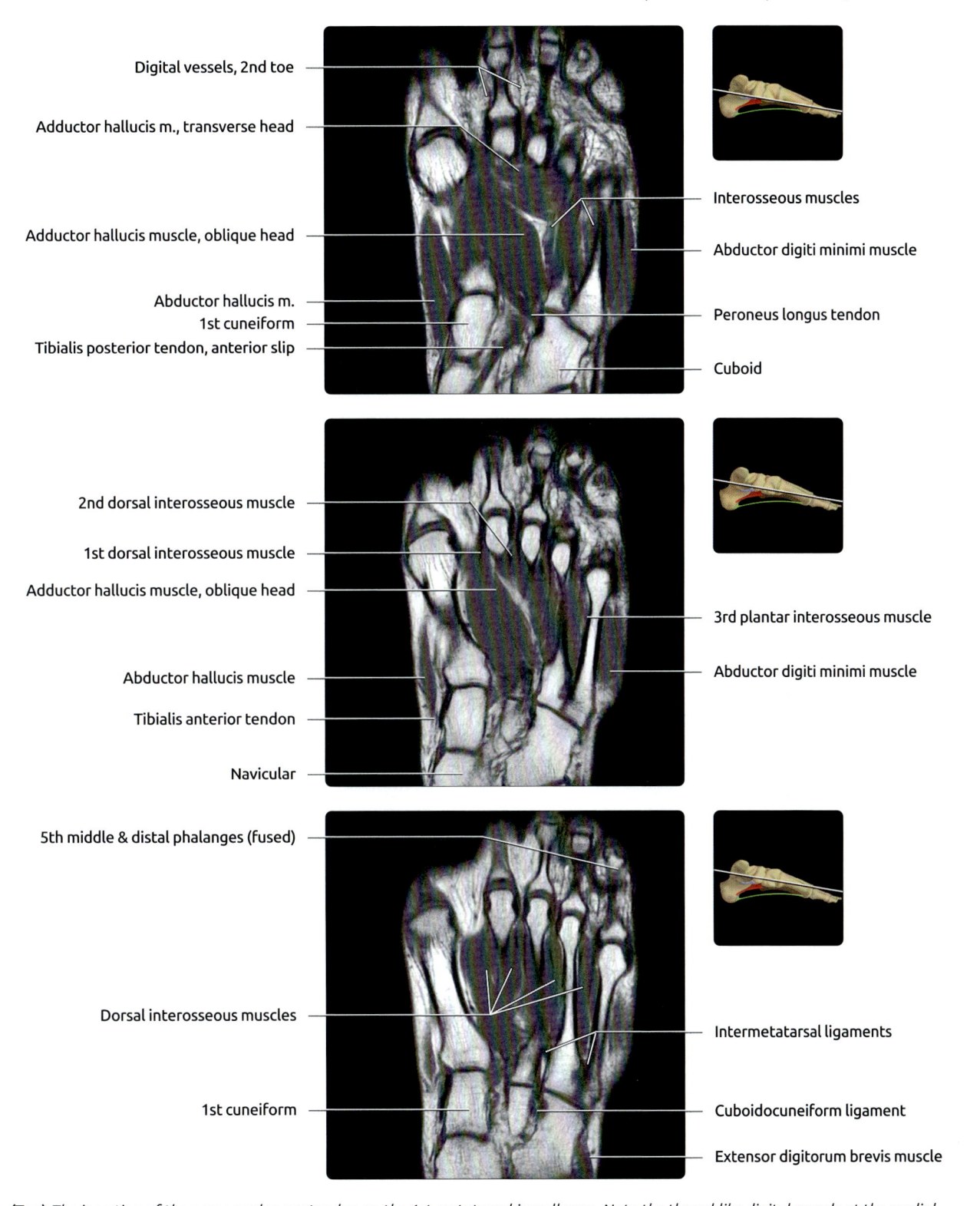

Labels (top image):
- Digital vessels, 2nd toe
- Adductor hallucis m., transverse head
- Adductor hallucis muscle, oblique head
- Abductor hallucis m.
- 1st cuneiform
- Tibialis posterior tendon, anterior slip
- Interosseous muscles
- Abductor digiti minimi muscle
- Peroneus longus tendon
- Cuboid

Labels (middle image):
- 2nd dorsal interosseous muscle
- 1st dorsal interosseous muscle
- Adductor hallucis muscle, oblique head
- Abductor hallucis muscle
- Tibialis anterior tendon
- Navicular
- 3rd plantar interosseous muscle
- Abductor digiti minimi muscle

Labels (bottom image):
- 5th middle & distal phalanges (fused)
- Dorsal interosseous muscles
- 1st cuneiform
- Intermetatarsal ligaments
- Cuboidocuneiform ligament
- Extensor digitorum brevis muscle

(**Top**) The insertion of the peroneus longus tendon on the 1st metatarsal is well seen. Note the thread-like digital vessels at the medial and lateral margins of the 2nd toe. (**Middle**) The plantar interossei arise from the medial margin of the 3 lateral toes, and insert on the medial aspect of the base of their respective proximal phalanges. (**Bottom**) There are 4 dorsal interosseous muscles, each with 2 heads ("bipennate") arising from the bases of the adjacent metatarsals. The 1st dorsal interosseous inserts on the medial aspect of the base of the 2nd proximal phalanx, and the 2nd-4th on to the lateral aspect of the base of the 2nd-4th metatarsals.

Foot MR Atlas

AXIAL (LONG AXIS) T1 MR, RIGHT FOOT

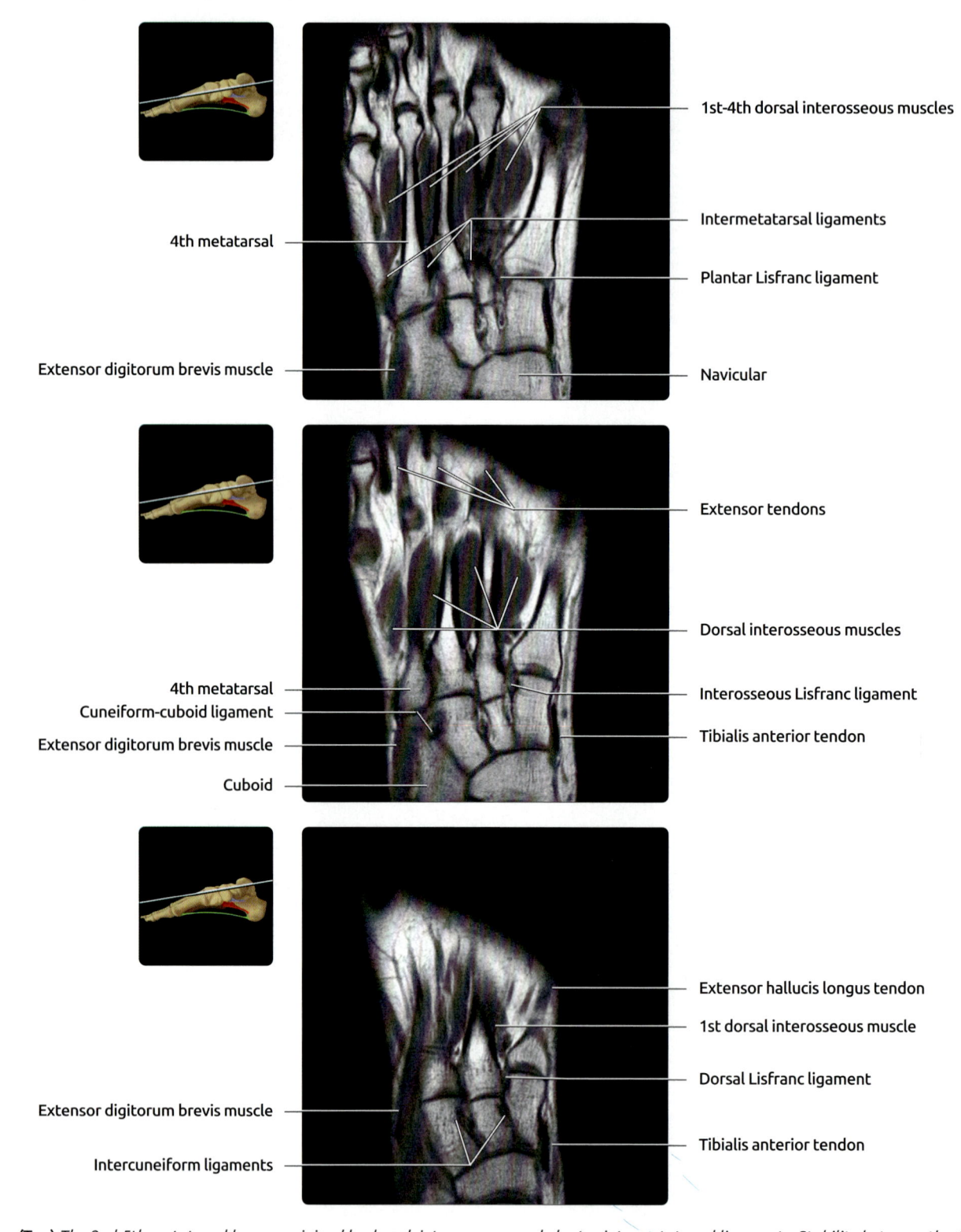

Labels (Top): 4th metatarsal; Extensor digitorum brevis muscle; 1st-4th dorsal interosseous muscles; Intermetatarsal ligaments; Plantar Lisfranc ligament; Navicular

Labels (Middle): 4th metatarsal; Cuneiform-cuboid ligament; Extensor digitorum brevis muscle; Cuboid; Extensor tendons; Dorsal interosseous muscles; Interosseous Lisfranc ligament; Tibialis anterior tendon

Labels (Bottom): Extensor digitorum brevis muscle; Intercuneiform ligaments; Extensor hallucis longus tendon; 1st dorsal interosseous muscle; Dorsal Lisfranc ligament; Tibialis anterior tendon

(Top) The 2nd-5th metatarsal bases are joined by dorsal, interosseous, and plantar intermetatarsal ligaments. Stability between the 1st and 2nd rays is achieved by the 3 ligaments from the 1st cuneiform to the base of the 2nd metatarsal: Dorsal, interosseous, and plantar. The interosseous 1st cuneiform to the 2nd metatarsal ligament is the broadest and strongest and is a true Lisfranc ligament; however, "plantar" and "dorsal Lisfranc ligament" are terms that are commonly and appropriately used. **(Middle)** Note the articulations between the metatarsal bases. These are constant at the lateral toes, but variability is seen in the articulations between the 1st and 2nd metatarsals where an articulation is variably present. **(Bottom)** Extensor digitorum brevis muscle originates at the lateral margin of the calcaneus and fans out to toes. The tibialis anterior tendon wraps around the 1st cuneiform to insert on its plantar surface as well as on the plantar surface of the 1st metatarsal.

Foot MR Atlas

AXIAL (LONG AXIS) T1 MR, LEFT FOOT

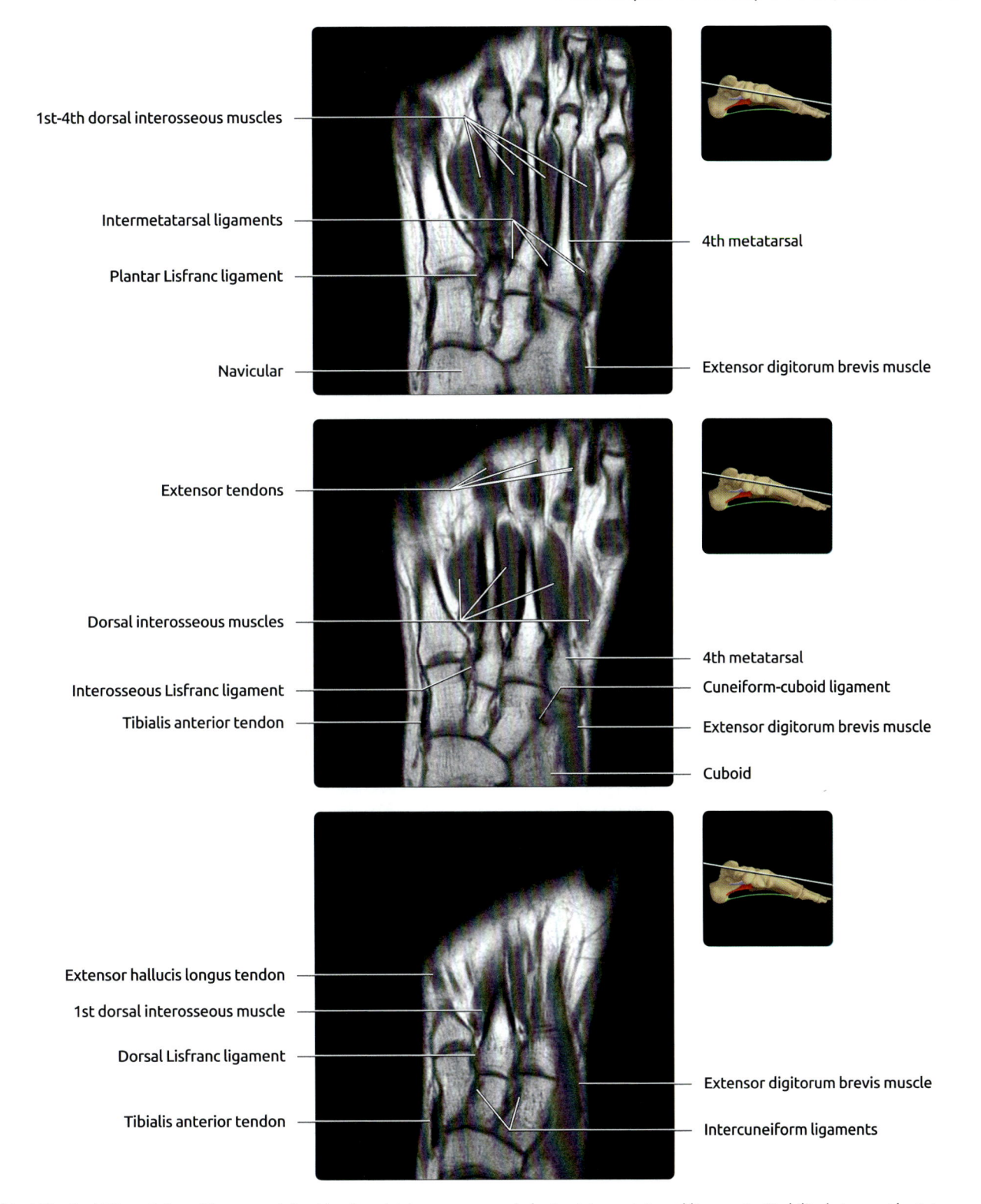

Top image labels:
- 1st-4th dorsal interosseous muscles
- Intermetatarsal ligaments
- Plantar Lisfranc ligament
- Navicular
- 4th metatarsal
- Extensor digitorum brevis muscle

Middle image labels:
- Extensor tendons
- Dorsal interosseous muscles
- Interosseous Lisfranc ligament
- Tibialis anterior tendon
- 4th metatarsal
- Cuneiform-cuboid ligament
- Extensor digitorum brevis muscle
- Cuboid

Bottom image labels:
- Extensor hallucis longus tendon
- 1st dorsal interosseous muscle
- Dorsal Lisfranc ligament
- Tibialis anterior tendon
- Extensor digitorum brevis muscle
- Intercuneiform ligaments

(Top) *The 2nd-5th metatarsal bases are joined by dorsal, interosseous, and plantar intermetatarsal ligaments. Stability between the 1st and 2nd rays is achieved by 3 ligaments from the 1st cuneiform to the base of the 2nd metatarsal: Dorsal, interosseous, and plantar. Interosseous 1st cuneiform to 2nd metatarsal ligament is broadest and strongest and is a true Lisfranc ligament; however, "plantar" and "dorsal Lisfranc ligament" are terms that are commonly and appropriately used.* **(Middle)** *Note the articulations between metatarsal bases. These are constant at the lateral toes, but variability is seen in the articulations between the 1st and 2nd metatarsals, where an articulation is variably present.* **(Bottom)** *The extensor digitorum brevis muscle originates at the lateral margin of the calcaneus and fans out to toes. The tibialis anterior tendon wraps around the 1st cuneiform to insert on its plantar surface as well as on the plantar surface of the 1st metatarsal.*

Foot MR Atlas

CORONAL (SHORT AXIS) T1 MR, RIGHT FOOT

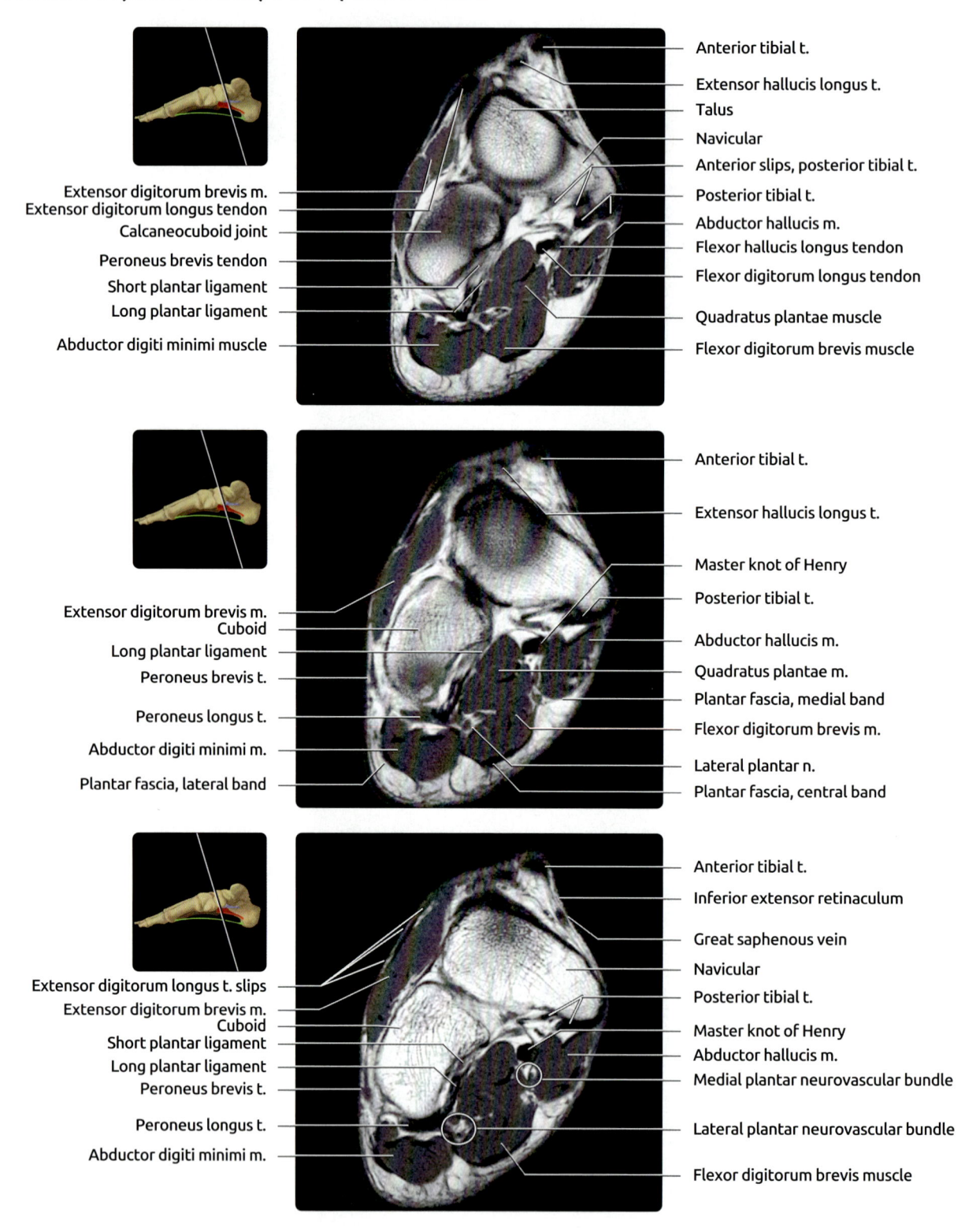

Labels (top image):
- Anterior tibial t.
- Extensor hallucis longus t.
- Talus
- Navicular
- Anterior slips, posterior tibial t.
- Posterior tibial t.
- Abductor hallucis m.
- Flexor hallucis longus tendon
- Flexor digitorum longus tendon
- Quadratus plantae muscle
- Flexor digitorum brevis muscle
- Extensor digitorum brevis m.
- Extensor digitorum longus tendon
- Calcaneocuboid joint
- Peroneus brevis tendon
- Short plantar ligament
- Long plantar ligament
- Abductor digiti minimi muscle

Labels (middle image):
- Anterior tibial t.
- Extensor hallucis longus t.
- Master knot of Henry
- Posterior tibial t.
- Abductor hallucis m.
- Quadratus plantae m.
- Plantar fascia, medial band
- Flexor digitorum brevis m.
- Lateral plantar n.
- Plantar fascia, central band
- Extensor digitorum brevis m.
- Cuboid
- Long plantar ligament
- Peroneus brevis t.
- Peroneus longus t.
- Abductor digiti minimi m.
- Plantar fascia, lateral band

Labels (bottom image):
- Anterior tibial t.
- Inferior extensor retinaculum
- Great saphenous vein
- Navicular
- Posterior tibial t.
- Master knot of Henry
- Abductor hallucis m.
- Medial plantar neurovascular bundle
- Lateral plantar neurovascular bundle
- Flexor digitorum brevis muscle
- Extensor digitorum longus t. slips
- Extensor digitorum brevis m.
- Cuboid
- Short plantar ligament
- Long plantar ligament
- Peroneus brevis t.
- Peroneus longus t.
- Abductor digiti minimi m.

(Top) 1st of 24 sequential coronal T1 MR images show the right foot from the Chopart joint to the phalanges. At the level of the talonavicular and calcaneocuboid joint (together known as the Chopart joint), the flexor digitorum longus and flexor hallucis longus tendons converge, exchanging fibers at the master knot of Henry. (Middle) Plantar fascia (aponeurosis) has 3 divisions: Medial overlies the abductor hallucis, central overlies the flexor digitorum brevis, and lateral overlies the abductor digiti minimi. The central portion is the strongest and functionally most important. (Bottom) The posterior tibial neurovascular bundle bifurcates into medial and lateral plantar divisions at the origin of the abductor hallucis muscle. The medial plantar neurovascular bundle courses between the abductor hallucis and quadratus plantae. The lateral plantar neurovascular bundle diverges laterally between the quadratus plantae and flexor digitorum brevis.

Foot MR Atlas

CORONAL (SHORT AXIS) T1 MR, LEFT FOOT

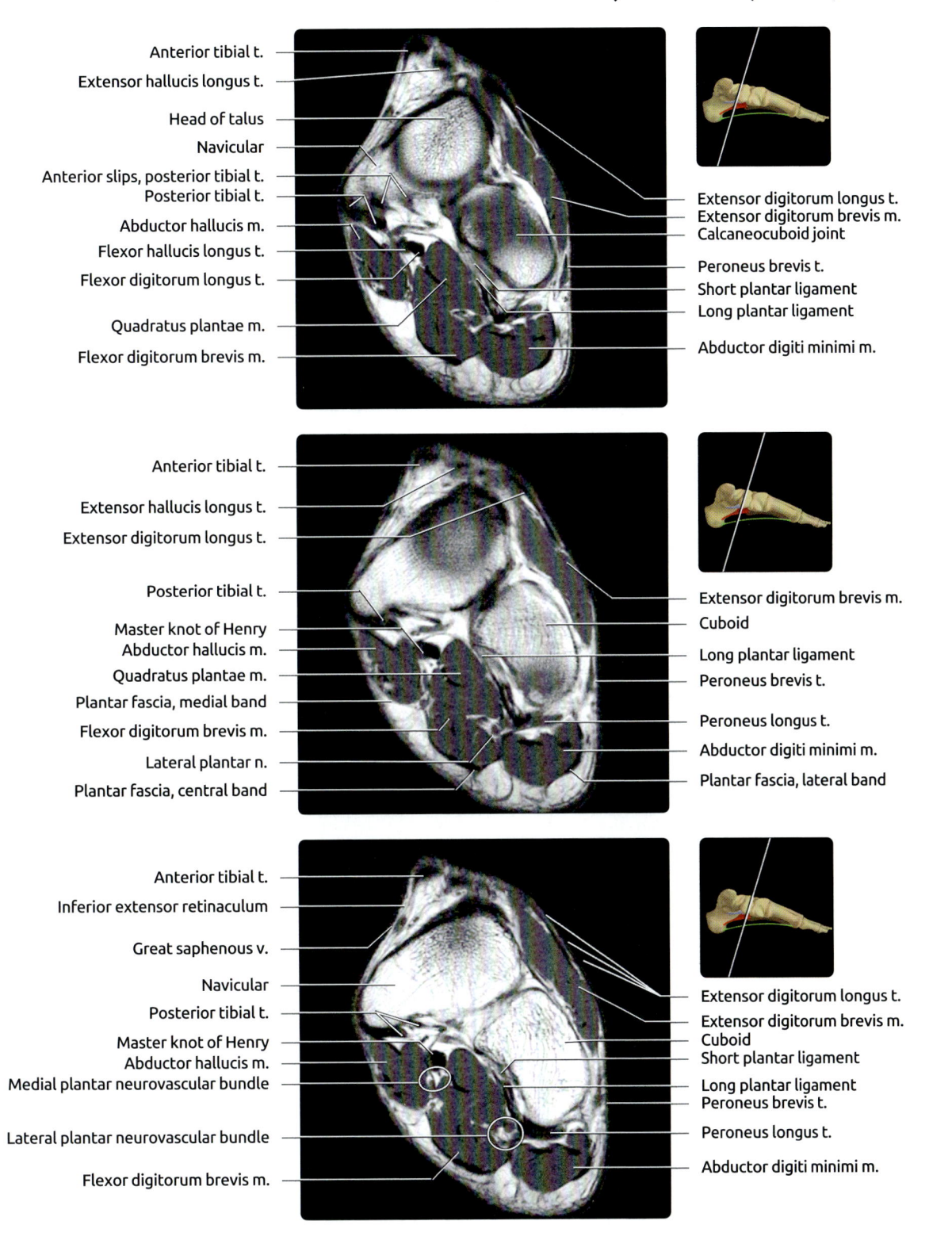

Top image labels (left): Anterior tibial t.; Extensor hallucis longus t.; Head of talus; Navicular; Anterior slips, posterior tibial t.; Posterior tibial t.; Abductor hallucis m.; Flexor hallucis longus t.; Flexor digitorum longus t.; Quadratus plantae m.; Flexor digitorum brevis m.

Top image labels (right): Extensor digitorum longus t.; Extensor digitorum brevis m.; Calcaneocuboid joint; Peroneus brevis t.; Short plantar ligament; Long plantar ligament; Abductor digiti minimi m.

Middle image labels (left): Anterior tibial t.; Extensor hallucis longus t.; Extensor digitorum longus t.; Posterior tibial t.; Master knot of Henry; Abductor hallucis m.; Quadratus plantae m.; Plantar fascia, medial band; Flexor digitorum brevis m.; Lateral plantar n.; Plantar fascia, central band

Middle image labels (right): Extensor digitorum brevis m.; Cuboid; Long plantar ligament; Peroneus brevis t.; Peroneus longus t.; Abductor digiti minimi m.; Plantar fascia, lateral band

Bottom image labels (left): Anterior tibial t.; Inferior extensor retinaculum; Great saphenous v.; Navicular; Posterior tibial t.; Master knot of Henry; Abductor hallucis m.; Medial plantar neurovascular bundle; Lateral plantar neurovascular bundle; Flexor digitorum brevis m.

Bottom image labels (right): Extensor digitorum longus t.; Extensor digitorum brevis m.; Cuboid; Short plantar ligament; Long plantar ligament; Peroneus brevis t.; Peroneus longus t.; Abductor digiti minimi m.

(**Top**) 1st of 24 sequential coronal T1 MR images through the left foot from the Chopart joint to the phalanges. At the level of the talonavicular and calcaneocuboid joint (together known as Chopart joint), the flexor digitorum longus and flexor hallucis longus tendons converge, exchanging fibers at the master knot of Henry. (**Middle**) Plantar fascia (aponeurosis) has 3 divisions: Medial overlies the abductor hallucis, central overlies the flexor digitorum brevis, and lateral overlies the abductor digiti minimi. The central portion is the strongest and functionally most important. (**Bottom**) The posterior tibial neurovascular bundle bifurcates into medial and lateral plantar divisions at the origin of the abductor hallucis muscle. The medial plantar neurovascular bundle courses between the abductor hallucis and quadratus plantae. The lateral plantar neurovascular bundle diverges laterally between the quadratus plantae and flexor digitorum brevis.

Foot MR Atlas

CORONAL (SHORT AXIS) T1 MR, RIGHT FOOT

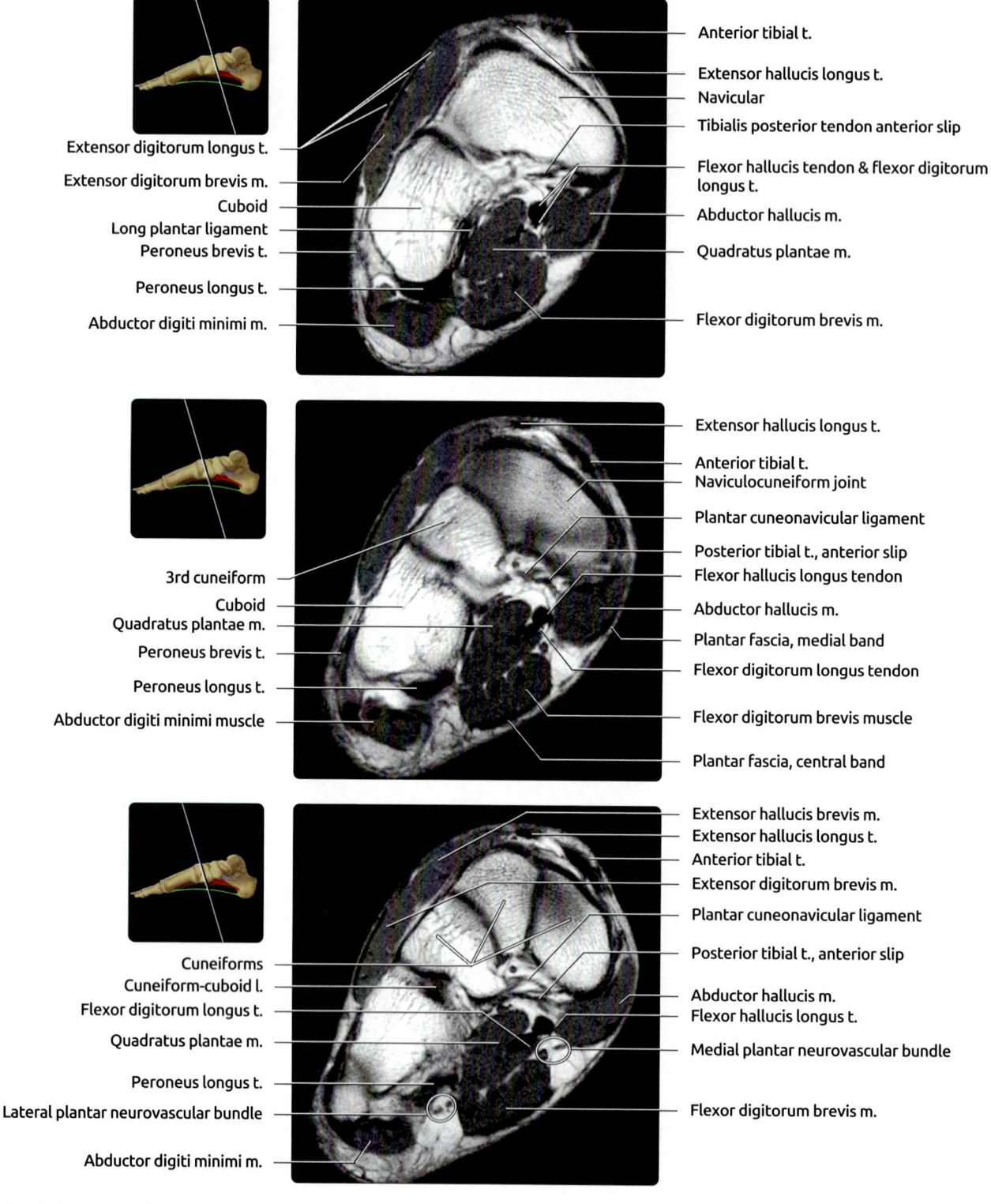

Top image labels (left):
- Extensor digitorum longus t.
- Extensor digitorum brevis m.
- Cuboid
- Long plantar ligament
- Peroneus brevis t.
- Peroneus longus t.
- Abductor digiti minimi m.

Top image labels (right):
- Anterior tibial t.
- Extensor hallucis longus t.
- Navicular
- Tibialis posterior tendon anterior slip
- Flexor hallucis tendon & flexor digitorum longus t.
- Abductor hallucis m.
- Quadratus plantae m.
- Flexor digitorum brevis m.

Middle image labels (left):
- 3rd cuneiform
- Cuboid
- Quadratus plantae m.
- Peroneus brevis t.
- Peroneus longus t.
- Abductor digiti minimi muscle

Middle image labels (right):
- Extensor hallucis longus t.
- Anterior tibial t.
- Naviculocuneiform joint
- Plantar cuneonavicular ligament
- Posterior tibial t., anterior slip
- Flexor hallucis longus tendon
- Abductor hallucis m.
- Plantar fascia, medial band
- Flexor digitorum longus tendon
- Flexor digitorum brevis muscle
- Plantar fascia, central band

Bottom image labels (left):
- Cuneiforms
- Cuneiform-cuboid l.
- Flexor digitorum longus t.
- Quadratus plantae m.
- Peroneus longus t.
- Lateral plantar neurovascular bundle
- Abductor digiti minimi m.

Bottom image labels (right):
- Extensor hallucis brevis m.
- Extensor hallucis longus t.
- Anterior tibial t.
- Extensor digitorum brevis m.
- Plantar cuneonavicular ligament
- Posterior tibial t., anterior slip
- Abductor hallucis m.
- Flexor hallucis longus t.
- Medial plantar neurovascular bundle
- Flexor digitorum brevis m.

(Top) The peroneus longus tendon begins to curve medially beneath the plantar aspect of the cuboid. Long plantar ligament superficial fibers form the roof, and deep fibers form the floor of the tunnel through which it passes. **(Middle)** The navicular and cuneiforms are bridged by plantar cuneonavicular ligaments, which lie deep to the anterior slips of the posterior tibial tendon. **(Bottom)** The quadratus plantae muscle has a broad insertion on the flexor digitorum longus tendon. The anterior tibial tendon is turning medially towards its insertion on the plantar aspect of the 1st cuneiform and 1st metatarsal.

Foot MR Atlas

CORONAL (SHORT AXIS) T1 MR, LEFT FOOT

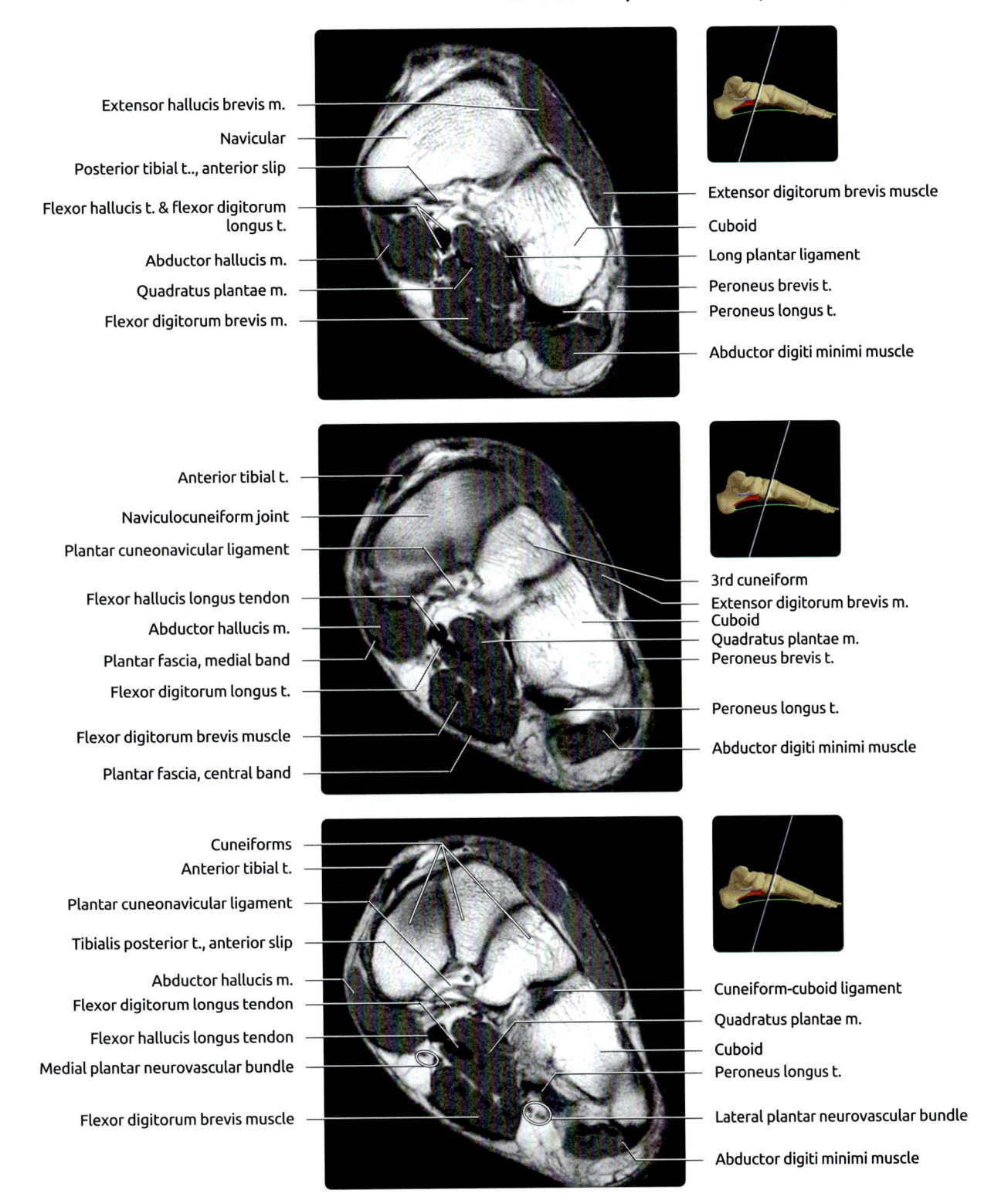

Labels (top image):
- Extensor hallucis brevis m.
- Navicular
- Posterior tibial t., anterior slip
- Flexor hallucis t. & flexor digitorum longus t.
- Abductor hallucis m.
- Quadratus plantae m.
- Flexor digitorum brevis m.
- Extensor digitorum brevis muscle
- Cuboid
- Long plantar ligament
- Peroneus brevis t.
- Peroneus longus t.
- Abductor digiti minimi muscle

Labels (middle image):
- Anterior tibial t.
- Naviculocuneiform joint
- Plantar cuneonavicular ligament
- Flexor hallucis longus tendon
- Abductor hallucis m.
- Plantar fascia, medial band
- Flexor digitorum longus t.
- Flexor digitorum brevis muscle
- Plantar fascia, central band
- 3rd cuneiform
- Extensor digitorum brevis m.
- Cuboid
- Quadratus plantae m.
- Peroneus brevis t.
- Peroneus longus t.
- Abductor digiti minimi muscle

Labels (bottom image):
- Cuneiforms
- Anterior tibial t.
- Plantar cuneonavicular ligament
- Tibialis posterior t., anterior slip
- Abductor hallucis m.
- Flexor digitorum longus tendon
- Flexor hallucis longus tendon
- Medial plantar neurovascular bundle
- Flexor digitorum brevis muscle
- Cuneiform-cuboid ligament
- Quadratus plantae m.
- Cuboid
- Peroneus longus t.
- Lateral plantar neurovascular bundle
- Abductor digiti minimi muscle

(Top) The peroneus longus tendon begins to curve medially beneath the plantar aspect of the cuboid. The long plantar ligament superficial fibers form the roof, and deep fibers form the floor of the tunnel through which it passes. **(Middle)** The navicular and cuneiforms are bridged by plantar cuneonavicular ligaments, which lie deep to the anterior slips of the tibialis posterior tendon. **(Bottom)** The quadratus plantae muscle has a broad insertion on the flexor digitorum longus tendon. The anterior tibial tendon is turning medially towards its insertion on the plantar aspect of the 1st cuneiform and 1st metatarsal.

CORONAL (SHORT AXIS) T1 MR, RIGHT FOOT

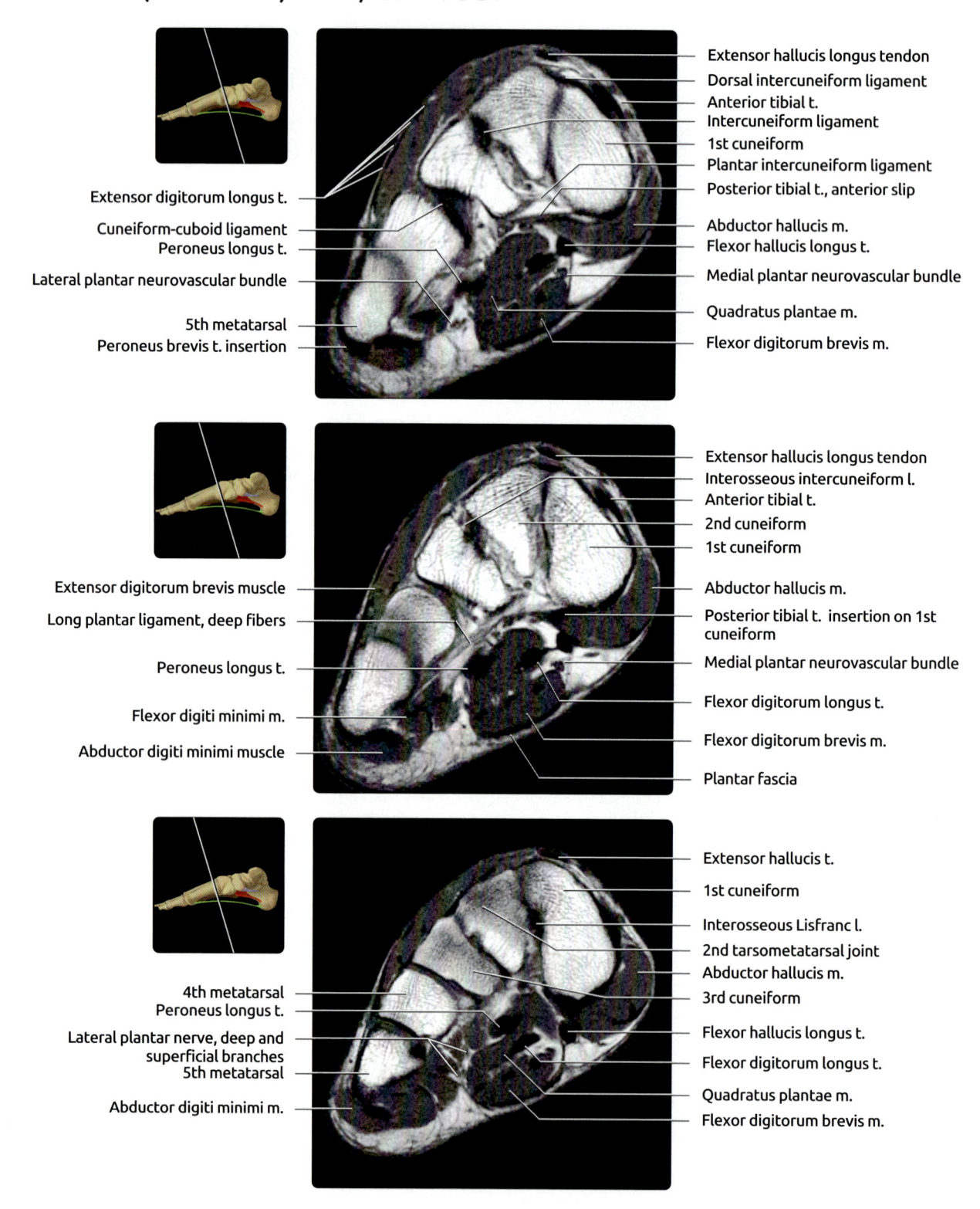

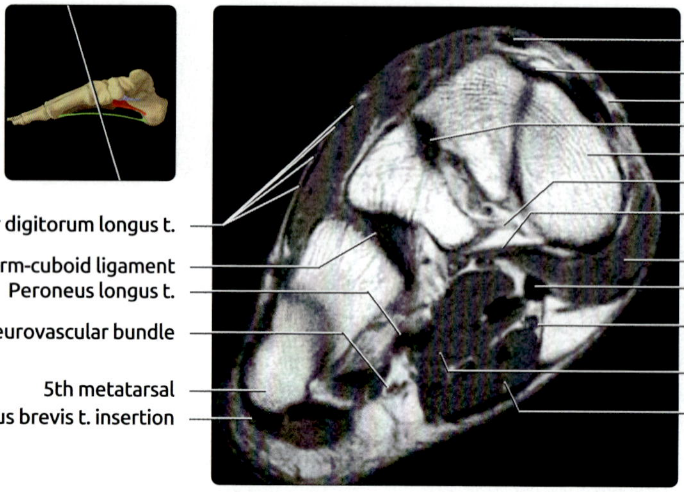
Extensor digitorum longus t.
Cuneiform-cuboid ligament
Peroneus longus t.
Lateral plantar neurovascular bundle
5th metatarsal
Peroneus brevis t. insertion
Extensor hallucis longus tendon
Dorsal intercuneiform ligament
Anterior tibial t.
Intercuneiform ligament
1st cuneiform
Plantar intercuneiform ligament
Posterior tibial t., anterior slip
Abductor hallucis m.
Flexor hallucis longus t.
Medial plantar neurovascular bundle
Quadratus plantae m.
Flexor digitorum brevis m.

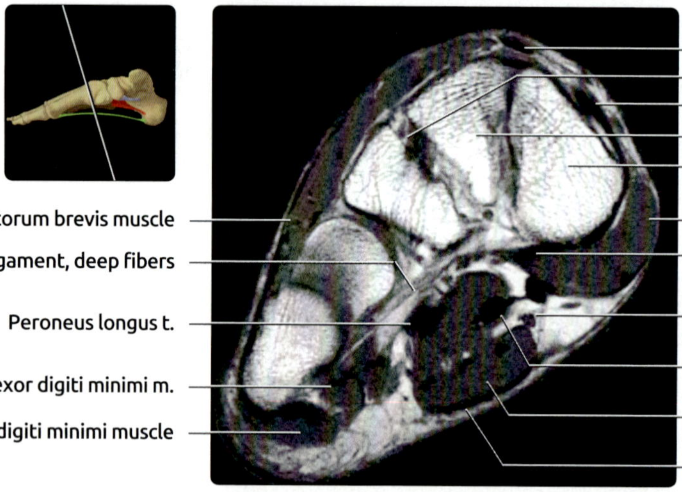
Extensor digitorum brevis muscle
Long plantar ligament, deep fibers
Peroneus longus t.
Flexor digiti minimi m.
Abductor digiti minimi muscle
Extensor hallucis longus tendon
Interosseous intercuneiform l.
Anterior tibial t.
2nd cuneiform
1st cuneiform
Abductor hallucis m.
Posterior tibial t. insertion on 1st cuneiform
Medial plantar neurovascular bundle
Flexor digitorum longus t.
Flexor digitorum brevis m.
Plantar fascia

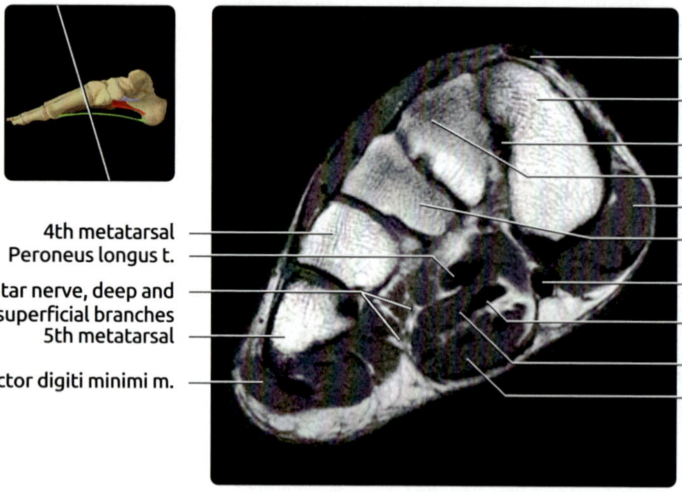
4th metatarsal
Peroneus longus t.
Lateral plantar nerve, deep and superficial branches
5th metatarsal
Abductor digiti minimi m.
Extensor hallucis t.
1st cuneiform
Interosseous Lisfranc l.
2nd tarsometatarsal joint
Abductor hallucis m.
3rd cuneiform
Flexor hallucis longus t.
Flexor digitorum longus t.
Quadratus plantae m.
Flexor digitorum brevis m.

(Top) *The wedge shape of the cuneiform bones create the transverse arch. They are held in position by the dorsal, plantar, and interosseous ligaments.* **(Middle)** *At this level, the 3 major compartmental divisions of the plantar muscles are well seen: The medial compartment beneath the 1st ray, the lateral compartment beneath the 5th ray, and the intermediate compartment beneath the 2nd-4th rays. The compartments are separated by vertically oriented fascial layers.* **(Bottom)** *The interosseous Lisfranc ligament is seen at its origin from the 1st cuneiform.*

Foot MR Atlas

CORONAL (SHORT AXIS) T1 MR, LEFT FOOT

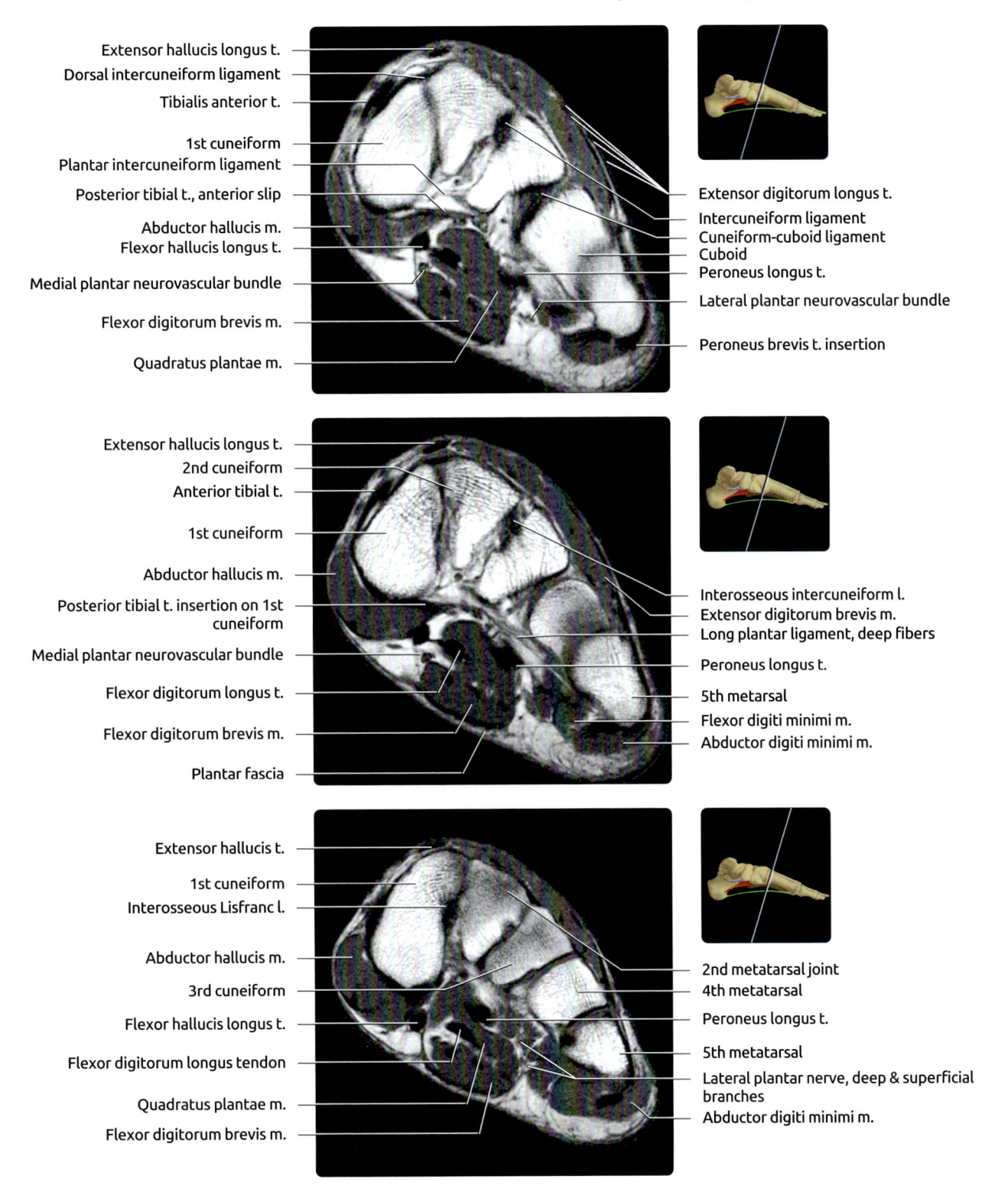

Labels (top image):
- Extensor hallucis longus t.
- Dorsal intercuneiform ligament
- Tibialis anterior t.
- 1st cuneiform
- Plantar intercuneiform ligament
- Posterior tibial t., anterior slip
- Abductor hallucis m.
- Flexor hallucis longus t.
- Medial plantar neurovascular bundle
- Flexor digitorum brevis m.
- Quadratus plantae m.
- Extensor digitorum longus t.
- Intercuneiform ligament
- Cuneiform-cuboid ligament
- Cuboid
- Peroneus longus t.
- Lateral plantar neurovascular bundle
- Peroneus brevis t. insertion

Labels (middle image):
- Extensor hallucis longus t.
- 2nd cuneiform
- Anterior tibial t.
- 1st cuneiform
- Abductor hallucis m.
- Posterior tibial t. insertion on 1st cuneiform
- Medial plantar neurovascular bundle
- Flexor digitorum longus t.
- Flexor digitorum brevis m.
- Plantar fascia
- Interosseous intercuneiform l.
- Extensor digitorum brevis m.
- Long plantar ligament, deep fibers
- Peroneus longus t.
- 5th metarsal
- Flexor digiti minimi m.
- Abductor digiti minimi m.

Labels (bottom image):
- Extensor hallucis t.
- 1st cuneiform
- Interosseous Lisfranc l.
- Abductor hallucis m.
- 3rd cuneiform
- Flexor hallucis longus t.
- Flexor digitorum longus tendon
- Quadratus plantae m.
- Flexor digitorum brevis m.
- 2nd metatarsal joint
- 4th metatarsal
- Peroneus longus t.
- 5th metatarsal
- Lateral plantar nerve, deep & superficial branches
- Abductor digiti minimi m.

(Top) The cuneiform bones form the transverse arch by virtue of their wedge shape. They are held in position by the dorsal, plantar, and interosseous ligaments. (Middle) At this level, the 3 major compartmental divisions of plantar muscles are well seen: The medial compartment beneath the 1st ray, the lateral compartment beneath the 5th ray, and the intermediate compartment beneath the 2nd-4th rays. The compartments are separated by vertically oriented fascial layers. (Bottom) The interosseous Lisfranc ligament is seen at its origin from the 1st cuneiform.

Foot MR Atlas

CORONAL (SHORT AXIS) T1 MR, RIGHT FOOT

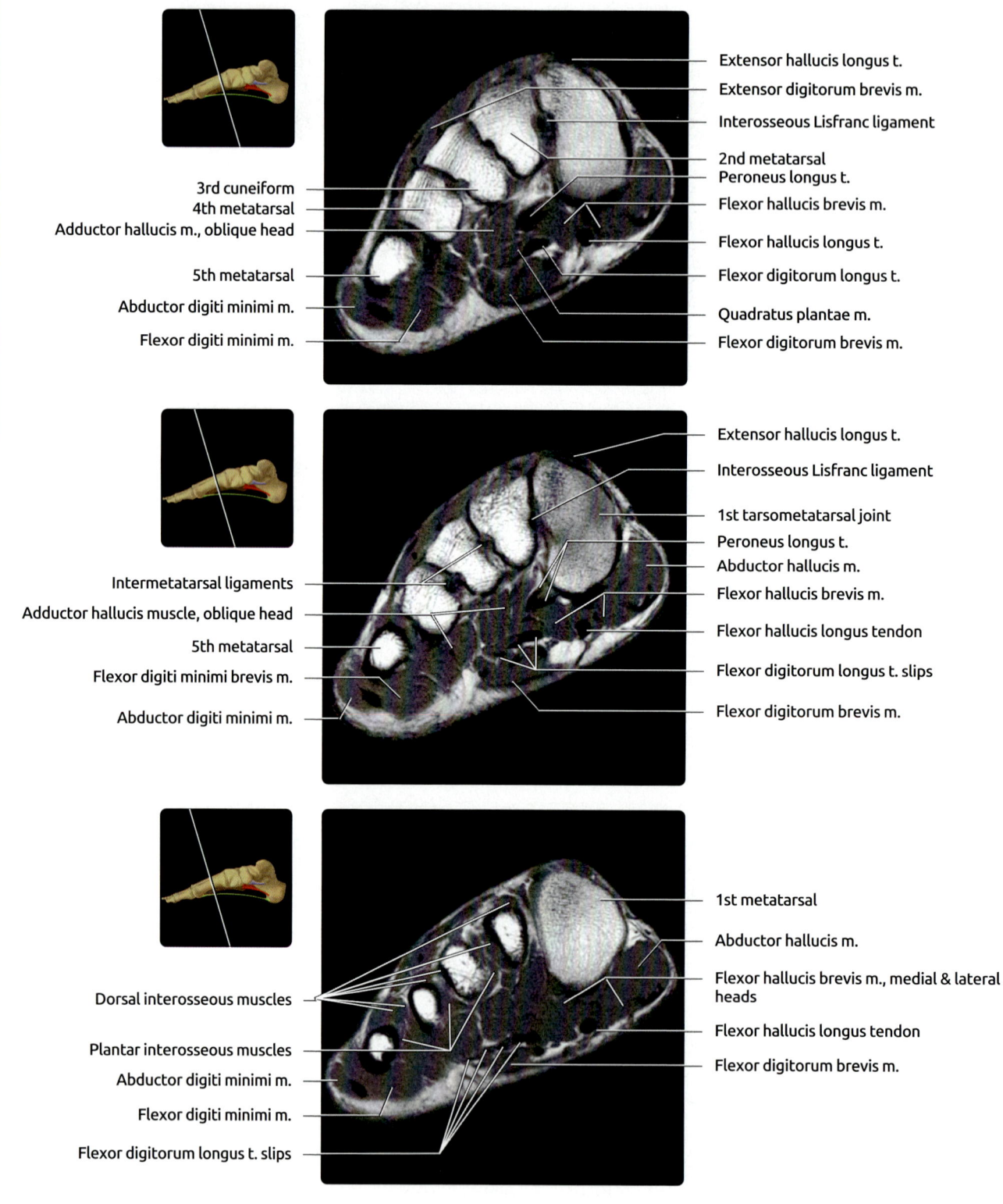

Top image labels:
- 3rd cuneiform
- 4th metatarsal
- Adductor hallucis m., oblique head
- 5th metatarsal
- Abductor digiti minimi m.
- Flexor digiti minimi m.
- Extensor hallucis longus t.
- Extensor digitorum brevis m.
- Interosseous Lisfranc ligament
- 2nd metatarsal
- Peroneus longus t.
- Flexor hallucis brevis m.
- Flexor hallucis longus t.
- Flexor digitorum longus t.
- Quadratus plantae m.
- Flexor digitorum brevis m.

Middle image labels:
- Intermetatarsal ligaments
- Adductor hallucis muscle, oblique head
- 5th metatarsal
- Flexor digiti minimi brevis m.
- Abductor digiti minimi m.
- Extensor hallucis longus t.
- Interosseous Lisfranc ligament
- 1st tarsometatarsal joint
- Peroneus longus t.
- Abductor hallucis m.
- Flexor hallucis brevis m.
- Flexor hallucis longus tendon
- Flexor digitorum longus t. slips
- Flexor digitorum brevis m.

Bottom image labels:
- Dorsal interosseous muscles
- Plantar interosseous muscles
- Abductor digiti minimi m.
- Flexor digiti minimi m.
- Flexor digitorum longus t. slips
- 1st metatarsal
- Abductor hallucis m.
- Flexor hallucis brevis m., medial & lateral heads
- Flexor hallucis longus tendon
- Flexor digitorum brevis m.

(Top) The Lisfranc ligament courses distally between the 1st cuneiform and 2nd cuneiform, attaching to the medial margin of the 2nd metatarsal base. It consists of distinct dorsal, interosseous, and plantar bands. The interosseous band is the strongest portion. **(Middle)** The peroneus longus tendon ends in slips attaching to the base of the 1st metatarsal, the 1st cuneiform, and sometimes, the base of the 2nd metatarsal. The oblique head of the adductor hallucis muscle originates from the bases of the 3rd and 4th metatarsals and from the tendon sheath of the peroneus longus. **(Bottom)** The flexor hallucis brevis muscle has 2 heads, and the flexor hallucis longus tendon is centered between them. The abductor hallucis muscle is closely apposed to the medial head of the flexor hallucis brevis muscle.

Foot MR Atlas

CORONAL (SHORT AXIS) T1 MR, LEFT FOOT

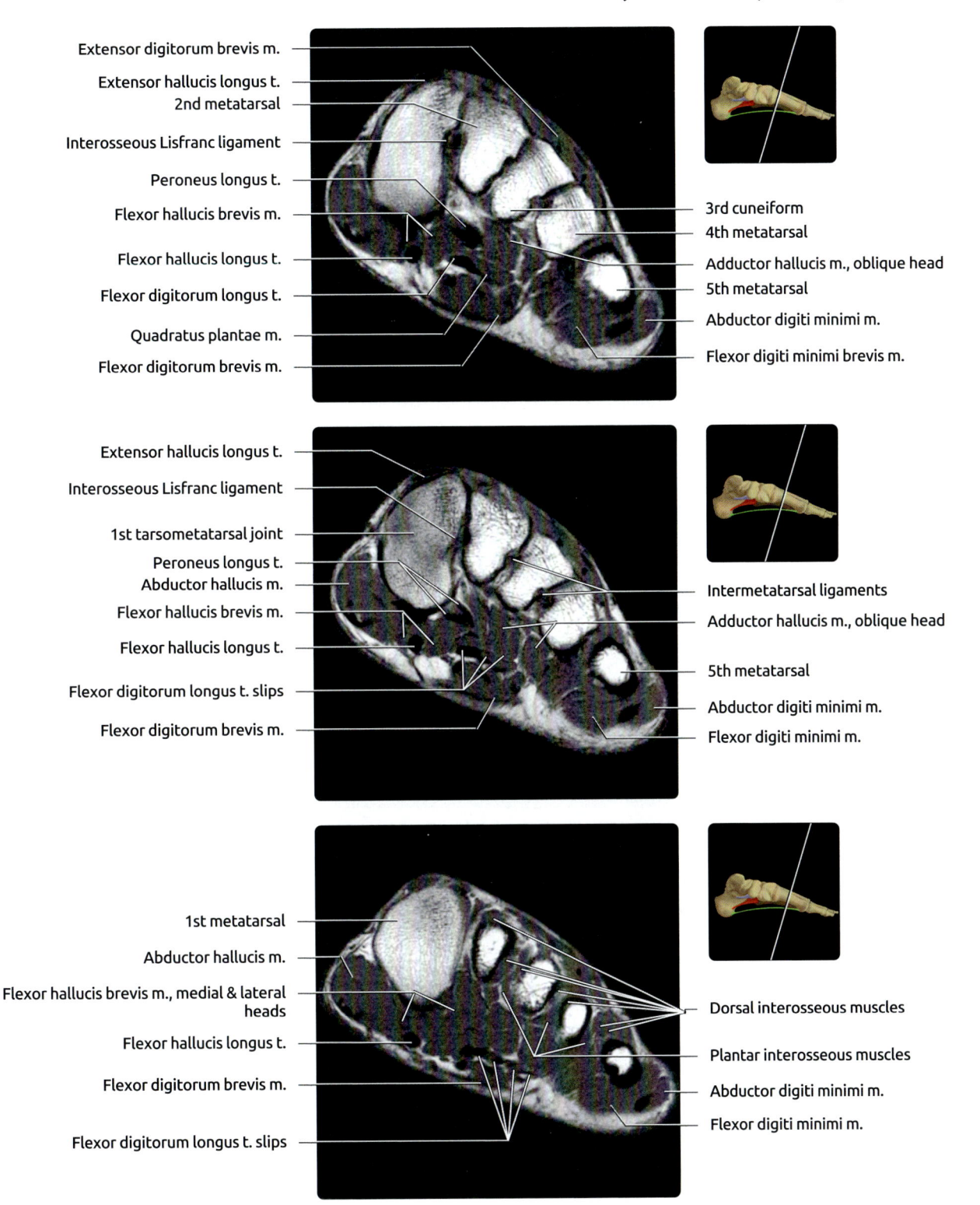

Labels (top image):
- Extensor digitorum brevis m.
- Extensor hallucis longus t.
- 2nd metatarsal
- Interosseous Lisfranc ligament
- Peroneus longus t.
- Flexor hallucis brevis m.
- Flexor hallucis longus t.
- Flexor digitorum longus t.
- Quadratus plantae m.
- Flexor digitorum brevis m.
- 3rd cuneiform
- 4th metatarsal
- Adductor hallucis m., oblique head
- 5th metatarsal
- Abductor digiti minimi m.
- Flexor digiti minimi brevis m.

Labels (middle image):
- Extensor hallucis longus t.
- Interosseous Lisfranc ligament
- 1st tarsometatarsal joint
- Peroneus longus t.
- Abductor hallucis m.
- Flexor hallucis brevis m.
- Flexor hallucis longus t.
- Flexor digitorum longus t. slips
- Flexor digitorum brevis m.
- Intermetatarsal ligaments
- Adductor hallucis m., oblique head
- 5th metatarsal
- Abductor digiti minimi m.
- Flexor digiti minimi m.

Labels (bottom image):
- 1st metatarsal
- Abductor hallucis m.
- Flexor hallucis brevis m., medial & lateral heads
- Flexor hallucis longus t.
- Flexor digitorum brevis m.
- Flexor digitorum longus t. slips
- Dorsal interosseous muscles
- Plantar interosseous muscles
- Abductor digiti minimi m.
- Flexor digiti minimi m.

(Top) The Lisfranc ligament courses distally between the 1st cuneiform and 2nd cuneiform, attaching to the medial margin of the 2nd metatarsal base. It consists of distinct dorsal, interosseous, and plantar bands. The interosseous band is the strongest portion. **(Middle)** The peroneus longus tendon ends in slips attaching to the base of the 1st metatarsal, the 1st cuneiform and sometimes, the base of the 2nd metatarsal. The oblique head of the adductor hallucis muscle originates from the bases of the 3rd and 4th metatarsals and from the tendon sheath of the peroneus longus. **(Bottom)** The flexor hallucis brevis muscle has 2 heads, and the flexor hallucis longus tendon is centered between them. The abductor hallucis muscle is closely apposed to the medial head of the flexor hallucis brevis muscle.

Foot MR Atlas

CORONAL (SHORT AXIS) T1 MR, RIGHT FOOT

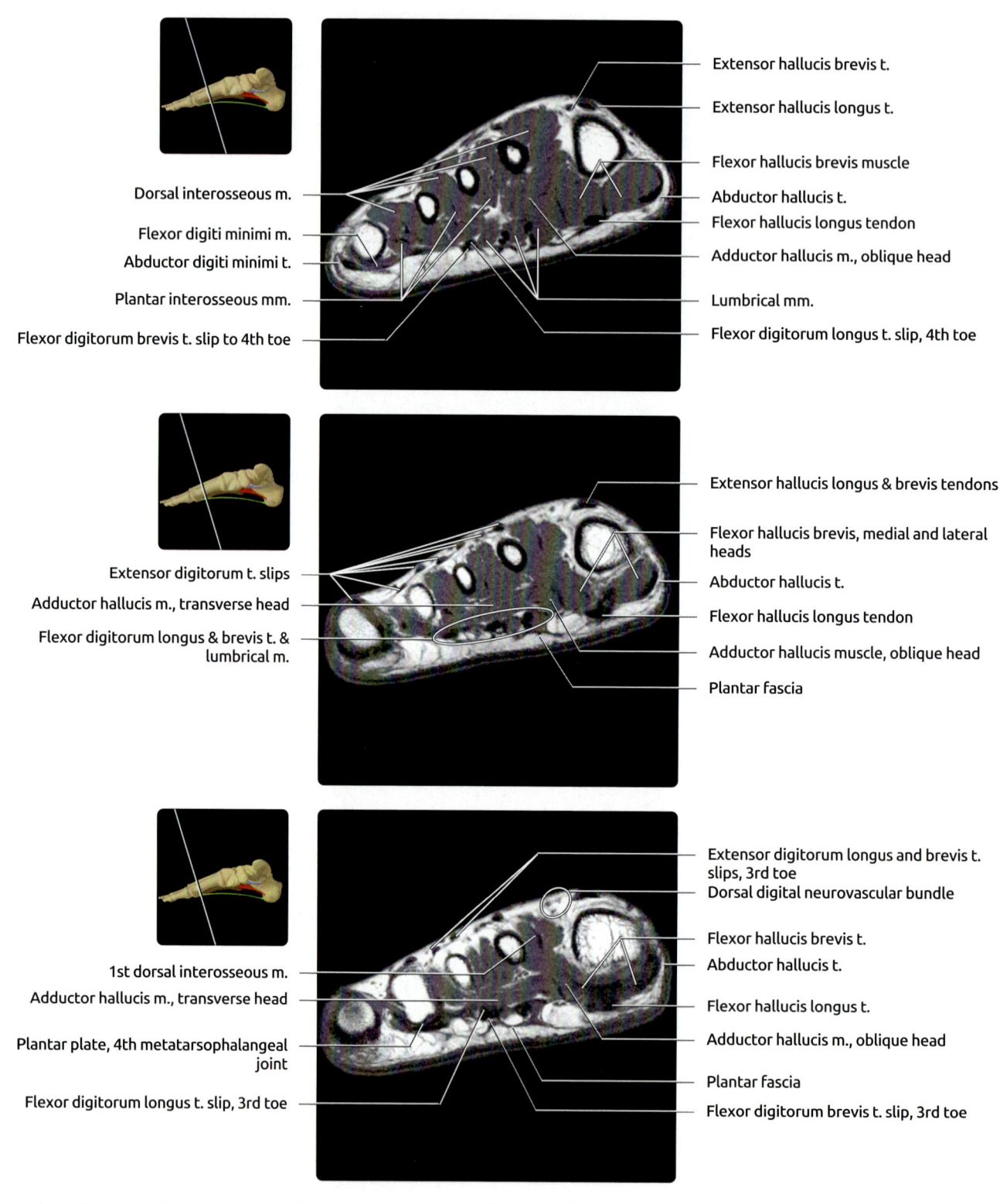

Labels (top image):
- Extensor hallucis brevis t.
- Extensor hallucis longus t.
- Flexor hallucis brevis muscle
- Abductor hallucis t.
- Flexor hallucis longus tendon
- Adductor hallucis m., oblique head
- Lumbrical mm.
- Flexor digitorum longus t. slip, 4th toe
- Dorsal interosseous m.
- Flexor digiti minimi m.
- Abductor digiti minimi t.
- Plantar interosseous mm.
- Flexor digitorum brevis t. slip to 4th toe

Labels (middle image):
- Extensor hallucis longus & brevis tendons
- Flexor hallucis brevis, medial and lateral heads
- Abductor hallucis t.
- Flexor hallucis longus tendon
- Adductor hallucis muscle, oblique head
- Plantar fascia
- Extensor digitorum t. slips
- Adductor hallucis m., transverse head
- Flexor digitorum longus & brevis t. & lumbrical m.

Labels (bottom image):
- Extensor digitorum longus and brevis t. slips, 3rd toe
- Dorsal digital neurovascular bundle
- Flexor hallucis brevis t.
- Abductor hallucis t.
- Flexor hallucis longus t.
- Adductor hallucis m., oblique head
- Plantar fascia
- Flexor digitorum brevis t. slip, 3rd toe
- 1st dorsal interosseous m.
- Adductor hallucis m., transverse head
- Plantar plate, 4th metatarsophalangeal joint
- Flexor digitorum longus t. slip, 3rd toe

(Top) The flexor digitorum brevis and longus tendons have divided into individual slips to the toes. The brevis tendon slips are superficial to those of the longus tendon. The lumbrical muscles are seen adjacent to the flexor digitorum longus tendon slips. **(Middle)** Transverse head of adductor hallucis muscle supports metatarsal heads. It may be congenitally absent. Transverse and oblique heads are shown converging towards their attachment on the lateral sesamoid of the great toe. **(Bottom)** The plantar fascia sends fibers dorsally and superficially in an arborizing pattern.

Foot MR Atlas

CORONAL (SHORT AXIS) T1 MR, LEFT FOOT

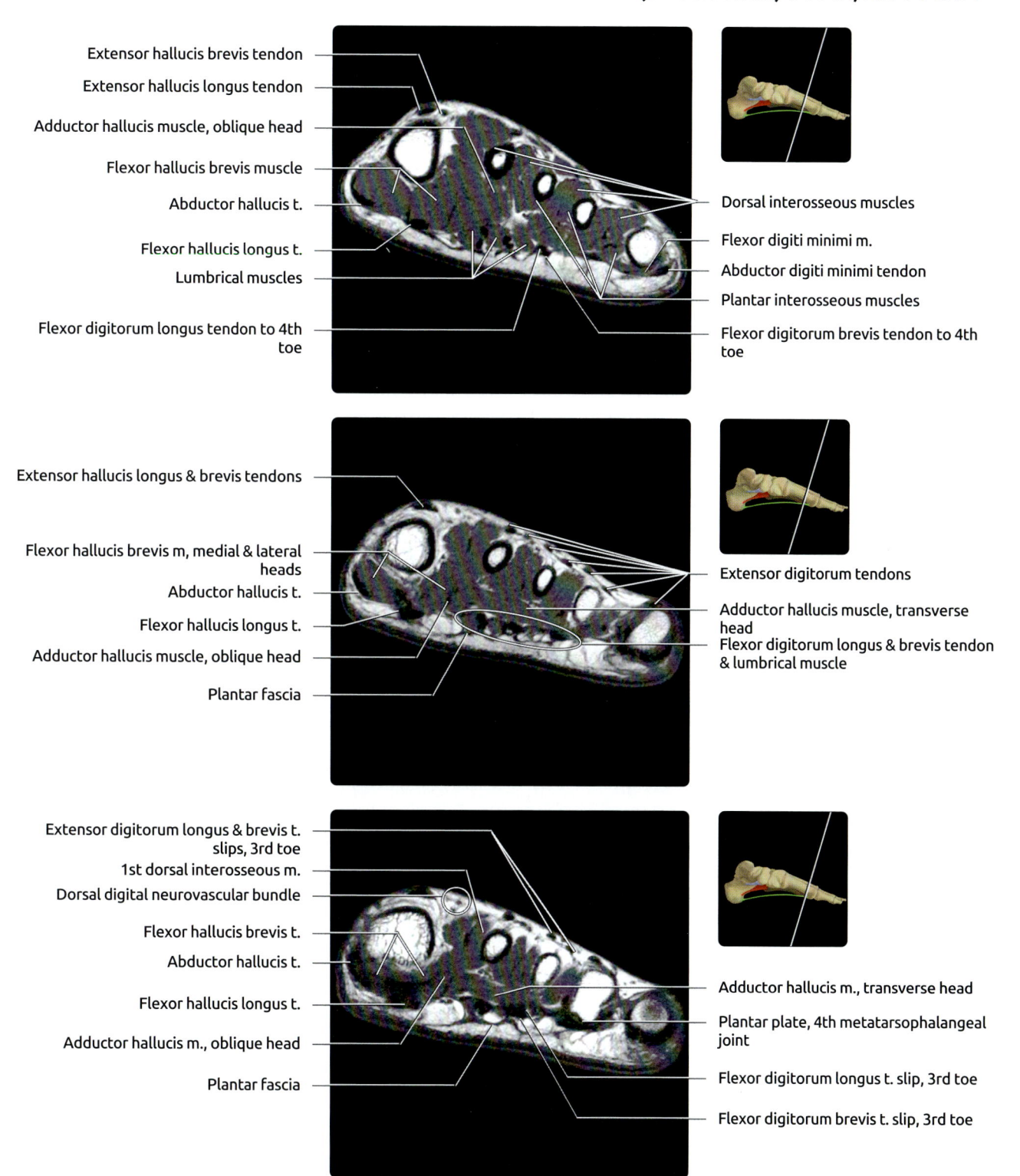

Labels (top image):
- Extensor hallucis brevis tendon
- Extensor hallucis longus tendon
- Adductor hallucis muscle, oblique head
- Flexor hallucis brevis muscle
- Abductor hallucis t.
- Flexor hallucis longus t.
- Lumbrical muscles
- Flexor digitorum longus tendon to 4th toe
- Dorsal interosseous muscles
- Flexor digiti minimi m.
- Abductor digiti minimi tendon
- Plantar interosseous muscles
- Flexor digitorum brevis tendon to 4th toe

Labels (middle image):
- Extensor hallucis longus & brevis tendons
- Flexor hallucis brevis m, medial & lateral heads
- Abductor hallucis t.
- Flexor hallucis longus t.
- Adductor hallucis muscle, oblique head
- Plantar fascia
- Extensor digitorum tendons
- Adductor hallucis muscle, transverse head
- Flexor digitorum longus & brevis tendon & lumbrical muscle

Labels (bottom image):
- Extensor digitorum longus & brevis t. slips, 3rd toe
- 1st dorsal interosseous m.
- Dorsal digital neurovascular bundle
- Flexor hallucis brevis t.
- Abductor hallucis t.
- Flexor hallucis longus t.
- Adductor hallucis m., oblique head
- Plantar fascia
- Adductor hallucis m., transverse head
- Plantar plate, 4th metatarsophalangeal joint
- Flexor digitorum longus t. slip, 3rd toe
- Flexor digitorum brevis t. slip, 3rd toe

(Top) The flexor digitorum brevis and longus tendons have divided into individual slips to the toes. The brevis tendon slips are superficial to those of the longus tendon. The lumbrical muscles are seen adjacent to the flexor digitorum longus tendon slips. **(Middle)** The transverse head of the adductor hallucis muscle supports the metatarsal heads. It may be congenitally absent. The transverse and oblique heads are shown converging towards their attachment on the lateral sesamoid of the great toe. **(Bottom)** The plantar fascia sends fibers dorsally and superficially in an arborizing pattern.

CORONAL (SHORT AXIS) T1 MR, RIGHT FOOT

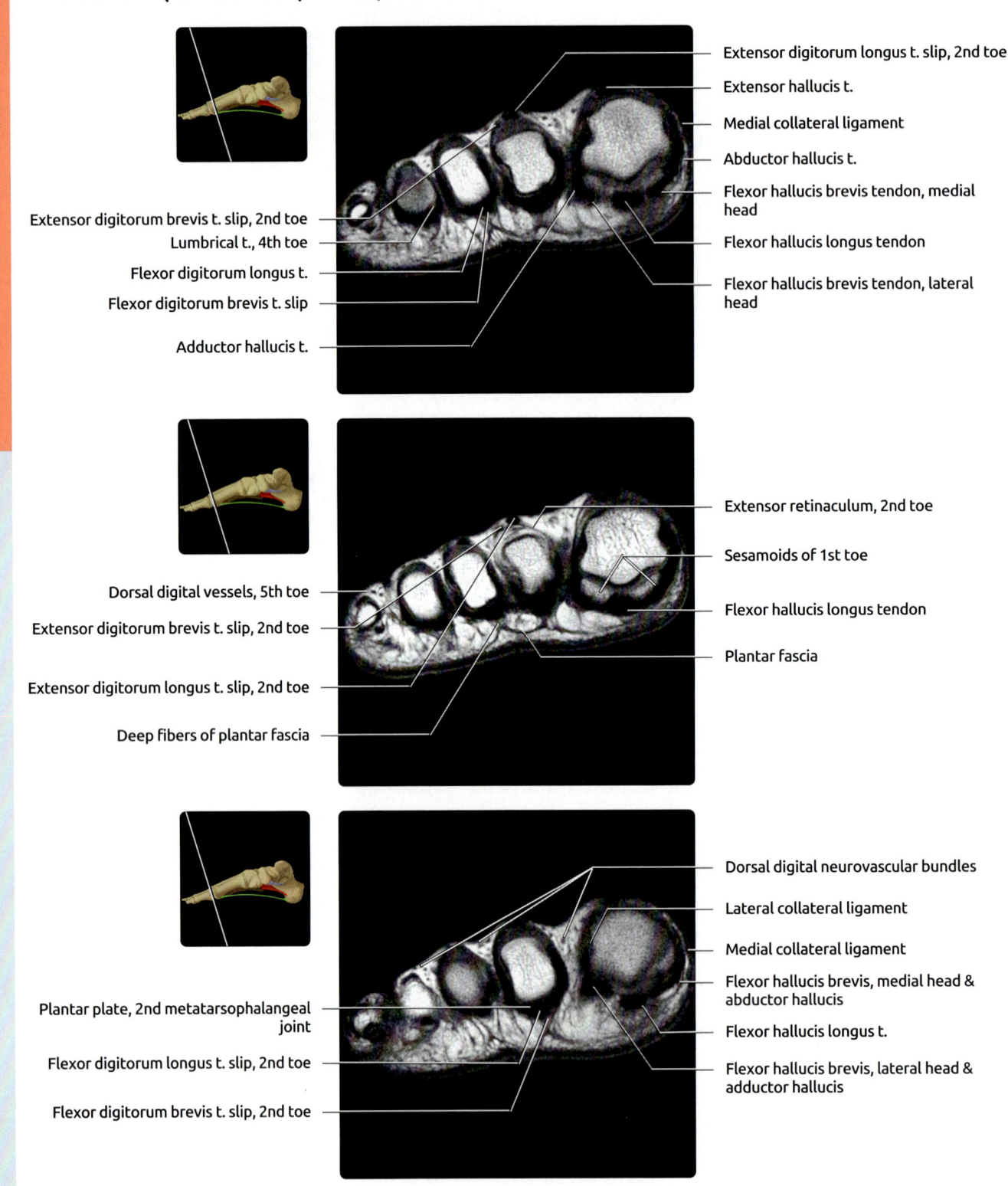

Top image labels:
- Extensor digitorum brevis t. slip, 2nd toe
- Lumbrical t., 4th toe
- Flexor digitorum longus t.
- Flexor digitorum brevis t. slip
- Adductor hallucis t.
- Extensor digitorum longus t. slip, 2nd toe
- Extensor hallucis t.
- Medial collateral ligament
- Abductor hallucis t.
- Flexor hallucis brevis tendon, medial head
- Flexor hallucis longus tendon
- Flexor hallucis brevis tendon, lateral head

Middle image labels:
- Dorsal digital vessels, 5th toe
- Extensor digitorum brevis t. slip, 2nd toe
- Extensor digitorum longus t. slip, 2nd toe
- Deep fibers of plantar fascia
- Extensor retinaculum, 2nd toe
- Sesamoids of 1st toe
- Flexor hallucis longus tendon
- Plantar fascia

Bottom image labels:
- Plantar plate, 2nd metatarsophalangeal joint
- Flexor digitorum longus t. slip, 2nd toe
- Flexor digitorum brevis t. slip, 2nd toe
- Dorsal digital neurovascular bundles
- Lateral collateral ligament
- Medial collateral ligament
- Flexor hallucis brevis, medial head & abductor hallucis
- Flexor hallucis longus t.
- Flexor hallucis brevis, lateral head & adductor hallucis

(Top) The flexor digitorum longus and brevis tendons are centered beneath the metatarsal heads, with the brevis superficial to the longus, in close proximity to the plantar plate of the metatarsophalangeal joints. Lumbrical muscles course medial to the metatarsal heads and will insert on the medial margin of the proximal phalanges. **(Middle)** The medial sesamoid of the 1st toe is in the tendon of the medial head of the flexor hallucis brevis tendon and is also attached to the adductor hallucis tendon. The lateral sesamoid is in the lateral head of the flexor hallucis brevis tendon and is also attached to the abductor hallucis tendon. The flexor hallucis longus tendon courses between the sesamoids. Fibrous septa extending from the main portion of plantar fascia to the metatarsophalangeal (MTP) joints are well seen on this image. **(Bottom)** The plantar plate extends from the metatarsal neck to the base of the proximal phalanx, and is an important stabilizer of the MTP joints.

Foot MR Atlas

CORONAL (SHORT AXIS) T1 MR, LEFT FOOT

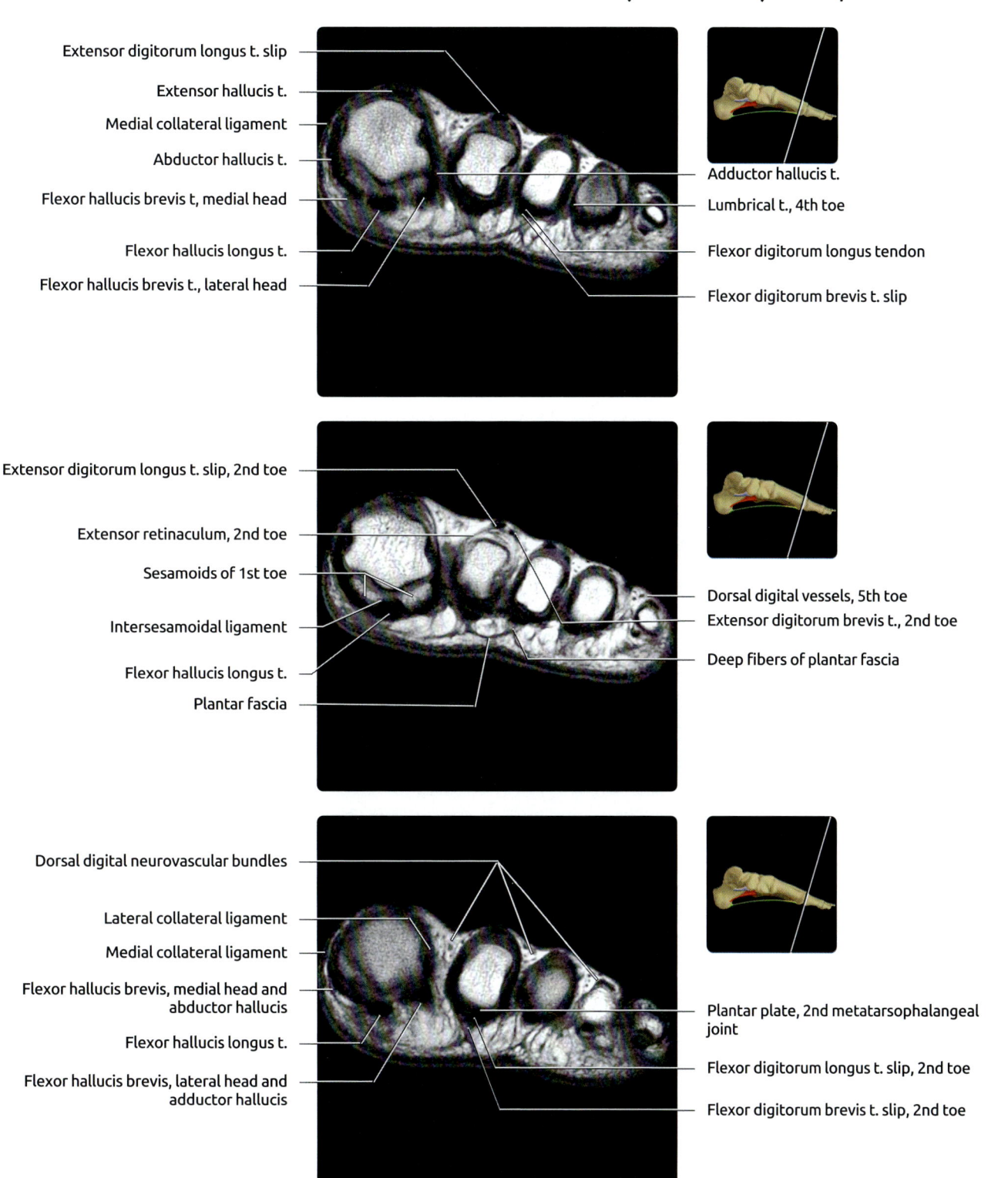

Labels (top image):
- Extensor digitorum longus t. slip
- Extensor hallucis t.
- Medial collateral ligament
- Abductor hallucis t.
- Flexor hallucis brevis t, medial head
- Flexor hallucis longus t.
- Flexor hallucis brevis t., lateral head
- Adductor hallucis t.
- Lumbrical t., 4th toe
- Flexor digitorum longus tendon
- Flexor digitorum brevis t. slip

Labels (middle image):
- Extensor digitorum longus t. slip, 2nd toe
- Extensor retinaculum, 2nd toe
- Sesamoids of 1st toe
- Intersesamoidal ligament
- Flexor hallucis longus t.
- Plantar fascia
- Dorsal digital vessels, 5th toe
- Extensor digitorum brevis t., 2nd toe
- Deep fibers of plantar fascia

Labels (bottom image):
- Dorsal digital neurovascular bundles
- Lateral collateral ligament
- Medial collateral ligament
- Flexor hallucis brevis, medial head and abductor hallucis
- Flexor hallucis longus t.
- Flexor hallucis brevis, lateral head and adductor hallucis
- Plantar plate, 2nd metatarsophalangeal joint
- Flexor digitorum longus t. slip, 2nd toe
- Flexor digitorum brevis t. slip, 2nd toe

(Top) The flexor digitorum longus and brevis tendons are centered beneath metatarsal heads, with brevis superficial to longus, in close proximity to the plantar plate of the metatarsophalangeal joints. The lumbrical muscles course medial to the metatarsal heads and will insert on the medial margin of the proximal phalanges. (Middle) The medial sesamoid of the 1st toe is in the tendon of the medial head flexor hallucis brevis tendon, and is also attached to the adductor hallucis tendon. The lateral sesamoid is in the lateral head flexor hallucis brevis tendon, and is also attached to the abductor hallucis tendon. The flexor hallucis longus tendon courses between the sesamoids. Fibrous septa extending from the main portion of plantar fascia to the MTP joints are well seen on this image. (Bottom) The plantar plate extends from the metatarsal neck to the base of the proximal phalanx and is an important stabilizer of the MTP joints.

Foot MR Atlas

CORONAL (SHORT AXIS) T1 MR, RIGHT FOOT

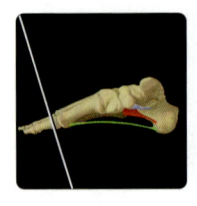

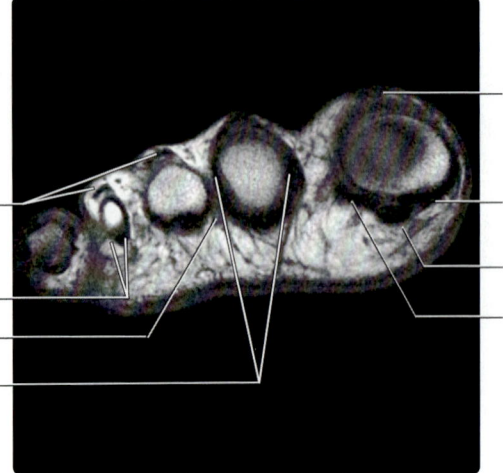

Extensor tendons, 3rd & 4th toes

Flexor digitorum longus & brevis, 4th toe

Plantar digital neurovascular bundle

Medial & lateral collateral ligaments, 2nd toe

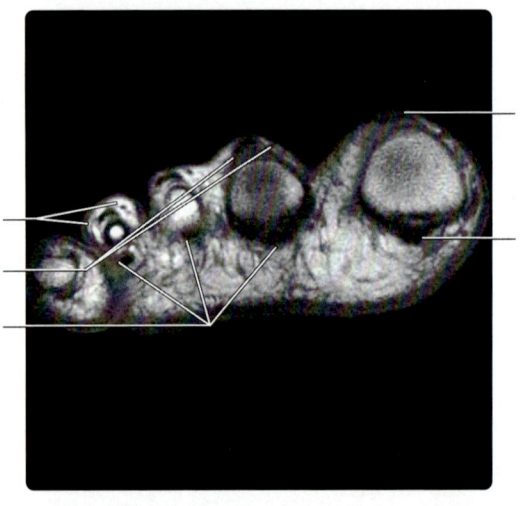

Extensor hallucis longus tendon

Flexor hallucis brevis, medial head & abductor hallucis

Flexor hallucis longus tendon

Flexor hallucis brevis, lateral head & adductor hallucis

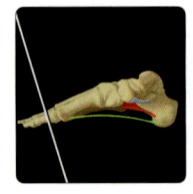

Dorsal digital neurovascular bundles

Extensor retinaculum, 2nd toe

Flexor digitorum tendons

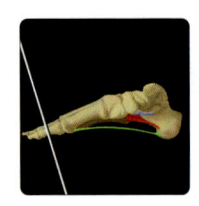

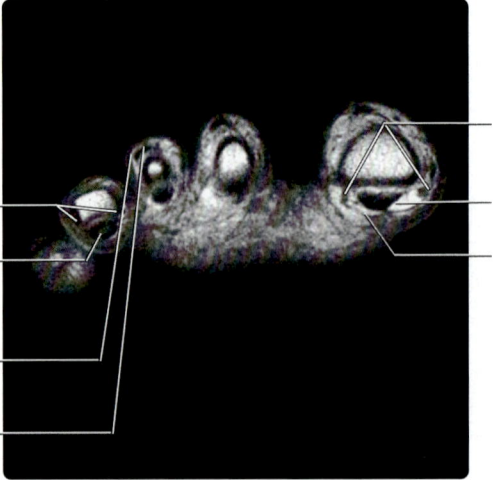

Extensor hallucis longus tendon

Flexor hallucis longus tendon

Flexor retinaculum, 4th toe

Flexor digitorum longus & brevis tendons

Extensor digitorum brevis t. slip, 3rd toe

Extensor digitorum longus t. slip, 3rd toe

Plantar digital neurovascular bundles

Flexor hallucis longus t.

Flexor retinaculum, 1st toe

(Top) The plantar vessels and nerves lie between the metatarsal heads where nerves are susceptible to compression. **(Middle)** The extensor retinacula are seen superficial to the extensor tendons and attaching to the dorsolateral margins of the phalanges. The flexor retinacula are not well seen on this image because of their obliquity to the imaging plane. At the level of the proximal phalanges, the flexor digitorum brevis tendons split into medial and lateral slips, which attach to the middle phalanges. The flexor digitorum longus tendon courses between them. The tiny slips are difficult to distinguish on MR. Dorsal digital neurovascular bundles are present at the medial and lateral aspects of the digits. **(Bottom)** The flexor digitorum brevis divides into 2 tendon slips to each toe, inserting on the middle phalanx. The flexor digitorum longus has a single slip that passes between them to insert on the distal phalanx.

Foot MR Atlas

CORONAL (SHORT AXIS) T1 MR, LEFT FOOT

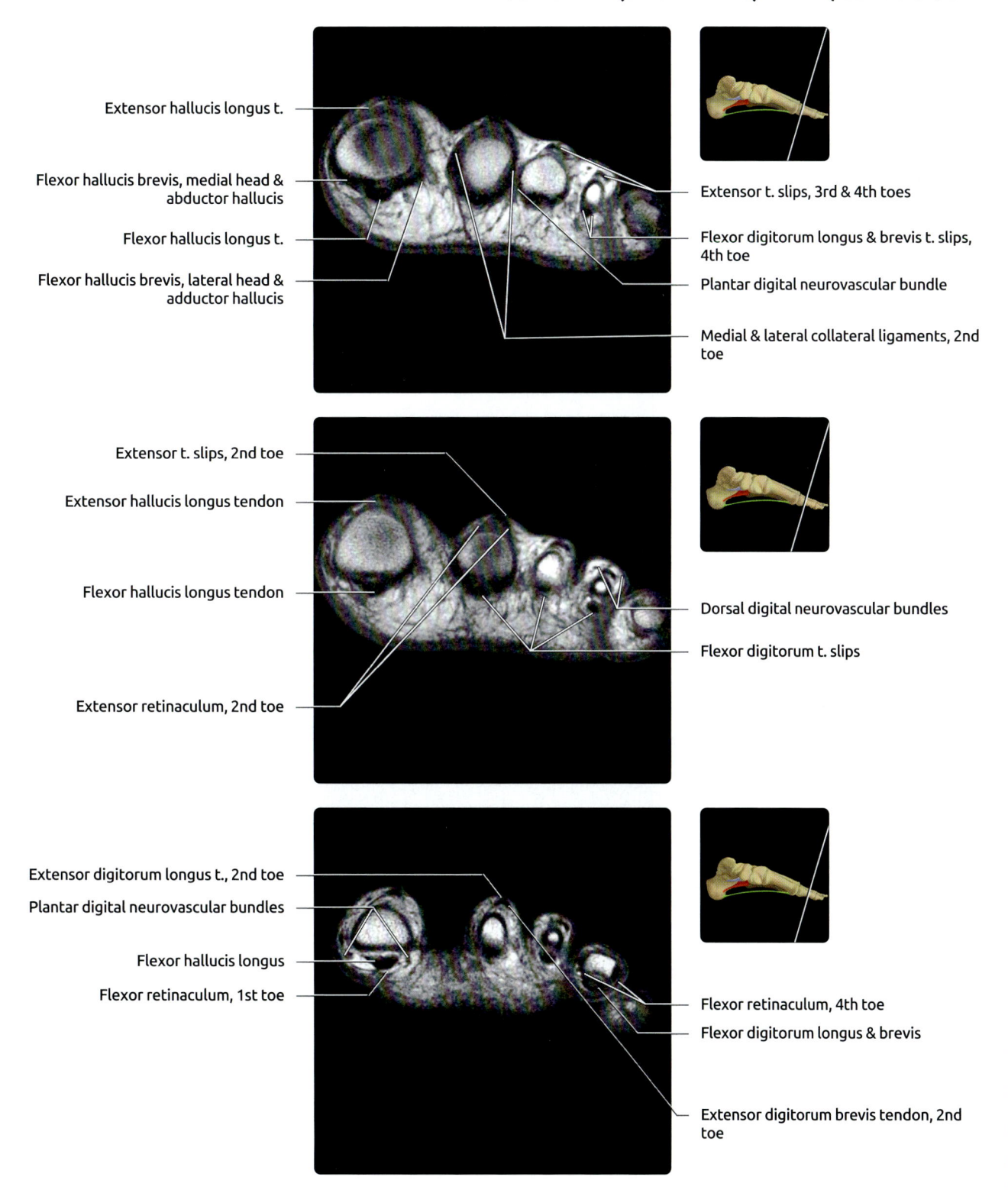

Labels (Top image):
- Extensor hallucis longus t.
- Flexor hallucis brevis, medial head & abductor hallucis
- Flexor hallucis longus t.
- Flexor hallucis brevis, lateral head & adductor hallucis
- Extensor t. slips, 3rd & 4th toes
- Flexor digitorum longus & brevis t. slips, 4th toe
- Plantar digital neurovascular bundle
- Medial & lateral collateral ligaments, 2nd toe

Labels (Middle image):
- Extensor t. slips, 2nd toe
- Extensor hallucis longus tendon
- Flexor hallucis longus tendon
- Extensor retinaculum, 2nd toe
- Dorsal digital neurovascular bundles
- Flexor digitorum t. slips

Labels (Bottom image):
- Extensor digitorum longus t., 2nd toe
- Plantar digital neurovascular bundles
- Flexor hallucis longus
- Flexor retinaculum, 1st toe
- Flexor retinaculum, 4th toe
- Flexor digitorum longus & brevis
- Extensor digitorum brevis tendon, 2nd toe

(Top) The plantar vessels and nerves lie between the metatarsal heads where the nerves are susceptible to compression. (Middle) The extensor retinacula are seen superficial to the extensor tendons and attaching to the dorsolateral margins of the phalanges. The flexor retinacula are not well seen on this image because of their obliquity to the imaging plane. At the level of the proximal phalanges, the flexor digitorum brevis tendons split into medial and lateral slips, which attach to the middle phalanges. The flexor digitorum longus tendon courses between them. The tiny slips are difficult to distinguish on MR. Dorsal digital neurovascular bundles are present at medial and lateral aspects of digits. (Bottom) The flexor digitorum brevis divides into 2 tendon slips to each toe, inserting on the middle phalanx. The flexor digitorum longus has a single slip that passes between them to insert on the distal phalanx.

Foot MR Atlas

SAGITTAL T1 MR, FOOT

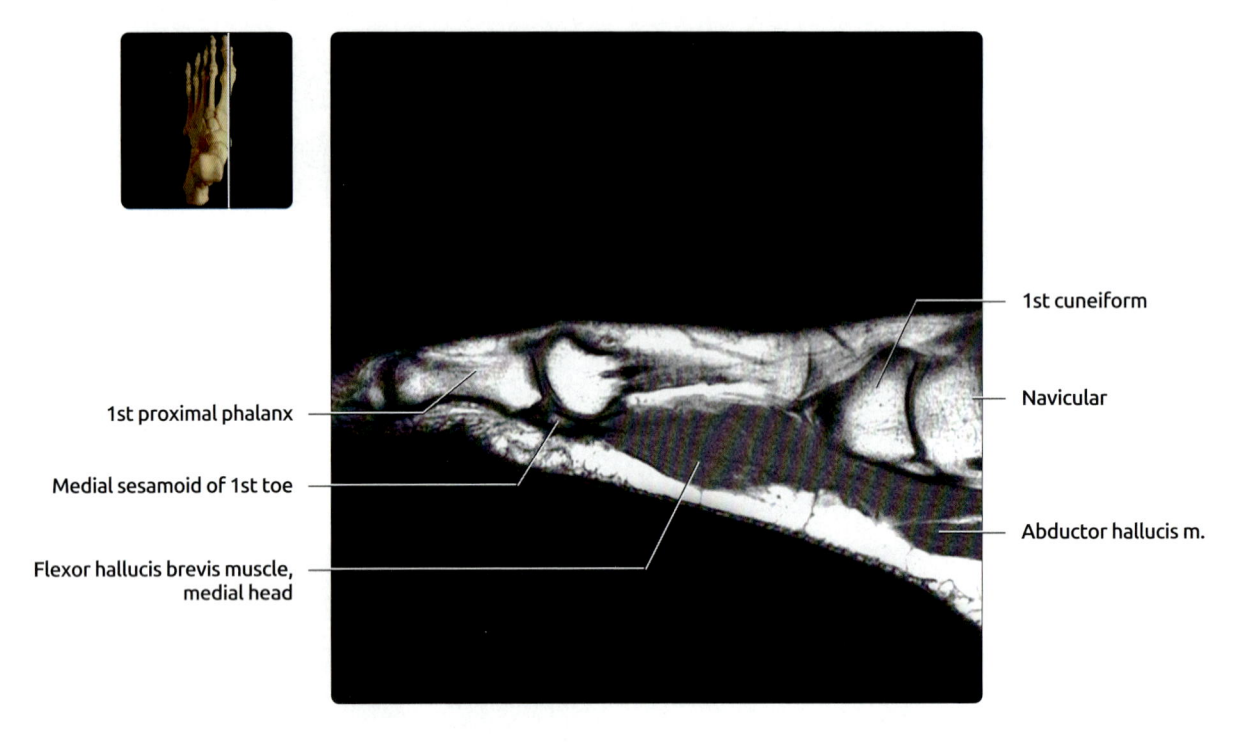

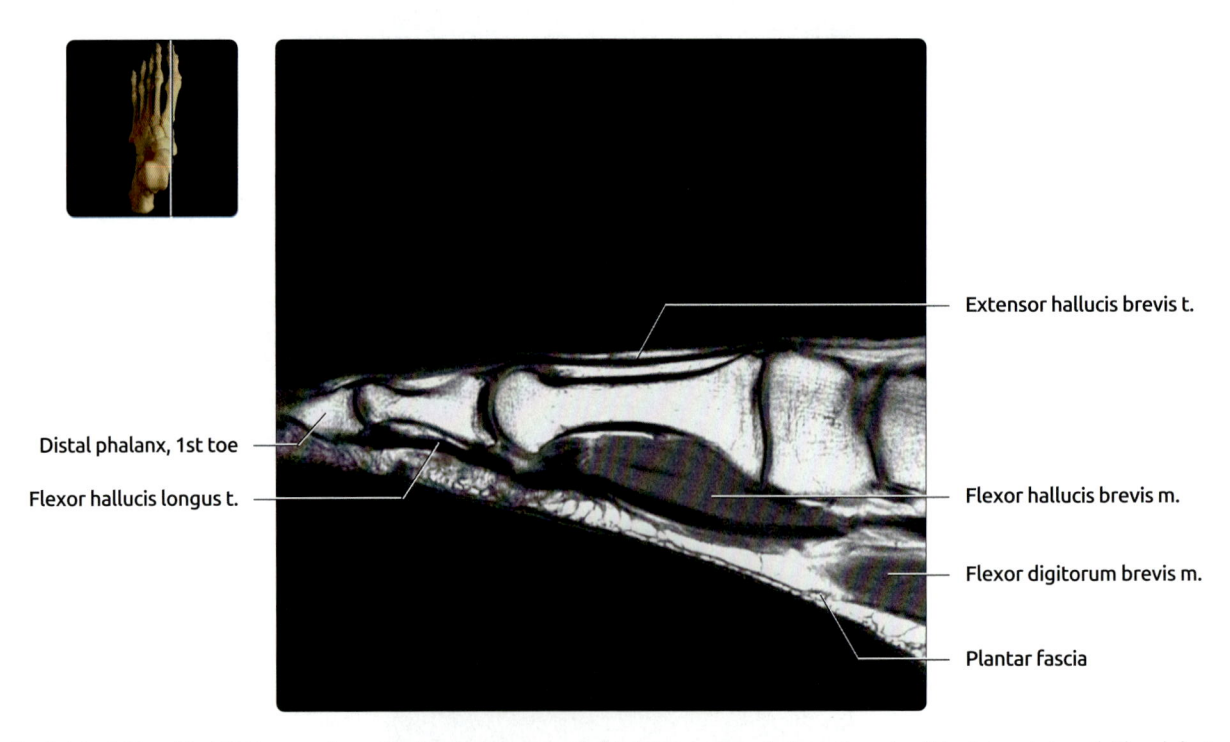

Labels (top image): 1st cuneiform; Navicular; 1st proximal phalanx; Medial sesamoid of 1st toe; Flexor hallucis brevis muscle, medial head; Abductor hallucis m.

Labels (bottom image): Extensor hallucis brevis t.; Distal phalanx, 1st toe; Flexor hallucis longus t.; Flexor hallucis brevis m.; Flexor digitorum brevis m.; Plantar fascia.

(Top) 1st of 15 sagittal MR images shows the forefoot from medial to lateral, aligned along the axis of the 1st metatarsal. The abductor hallucis muscle lies medial to the 1st metatarsal, while the flexor hallucis brevis lies beneath it. **(Bottom)** The flexor hallucis longus tendon courses between the sesamoids of the 1st toe and inserts on the distal phalanx of the 1st toe. The extensor hallucis brevis tendon lies lateral to the longus tendon and inserts on the proximal phalanx of the 1st toe.

Foot MR Atlas

SAGITTAL T1 MR, FOOT

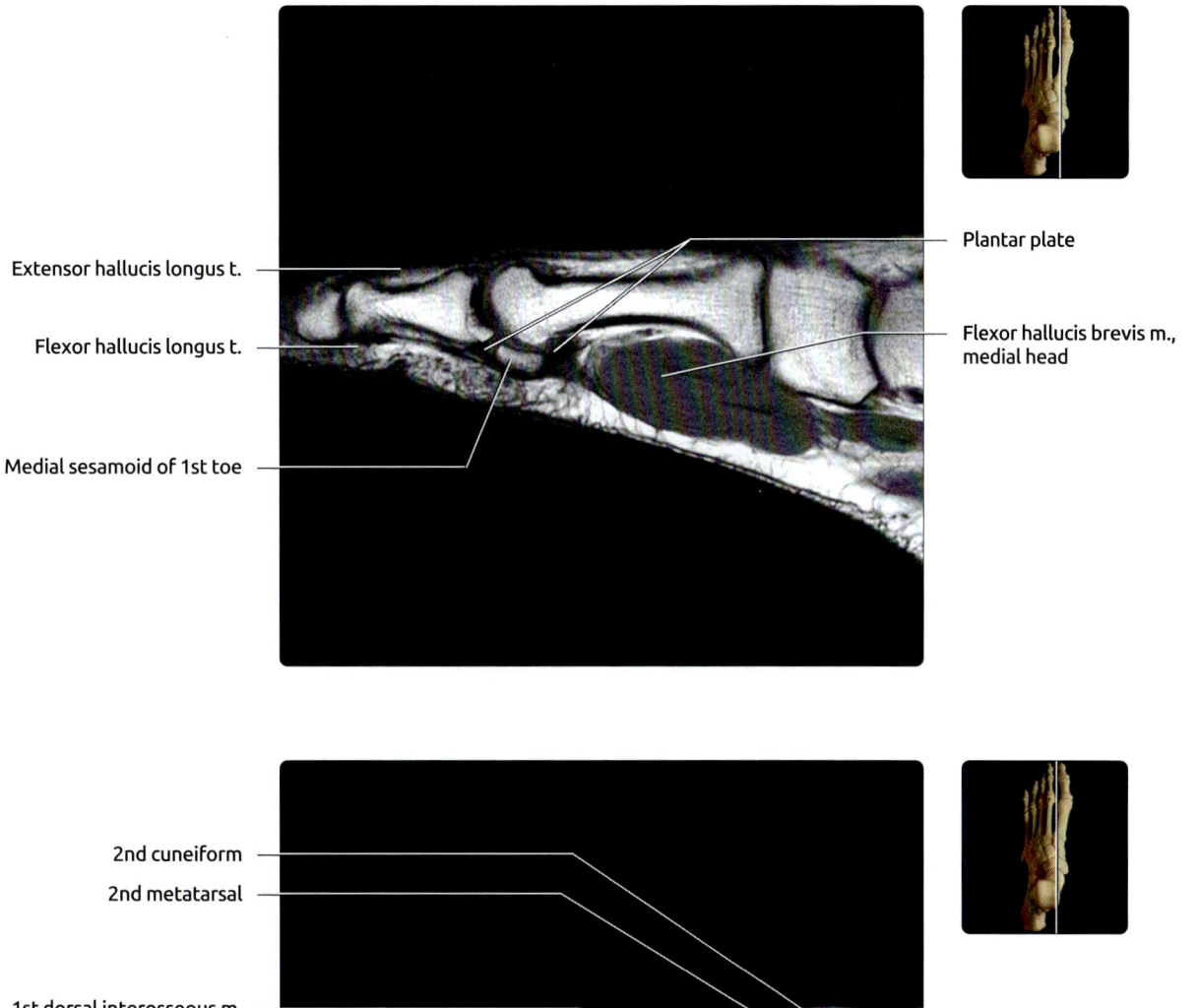

Labels (top image):
- Extensor hallucis longus t.
- Flexor hallucis longus t.
- Medial sesamoid of 1st toe
- Plantar plate
- Flexor hallucis brevis m., medial head

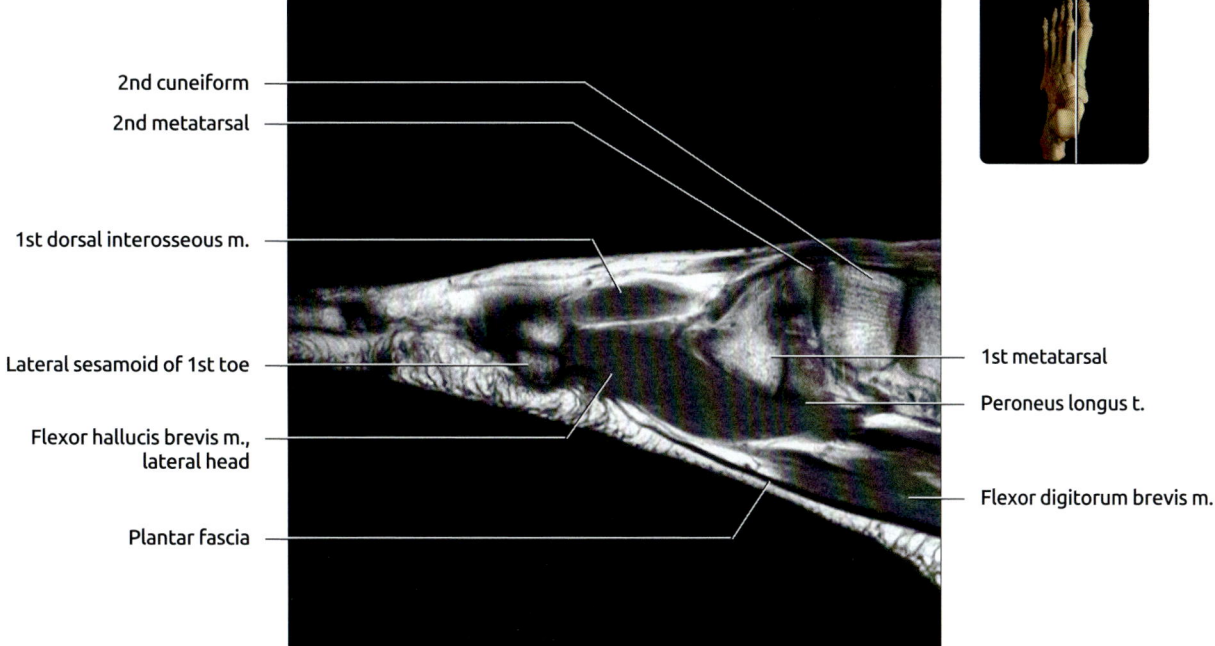

Labels (bottom image):
- 2nd cuneiform
- 2nd metatarsal
- 1st dorsal interosseous m.
- Lateral sesamoid of 1st toe
- Flexor hallucis brevis m., lateral head
- Plantar fascia
- 1st metatarsal
- Peroneus longus t.
- Flexor digitorum brevis m.

(Top) The plantar plate of the 1st metatarsophalangeal joint is a strong fibrocartilaginous thickening of the plantar joint capsule. It is attached to both sesamoids, the metatarsal neck, the medial and lateral collateral ligaments, and the base of the proximal phalanx. (Bottom) The distal portion of the peroneus longus tendon is seen attaching to the 1st metatarsal base.

Foot MR Atlas

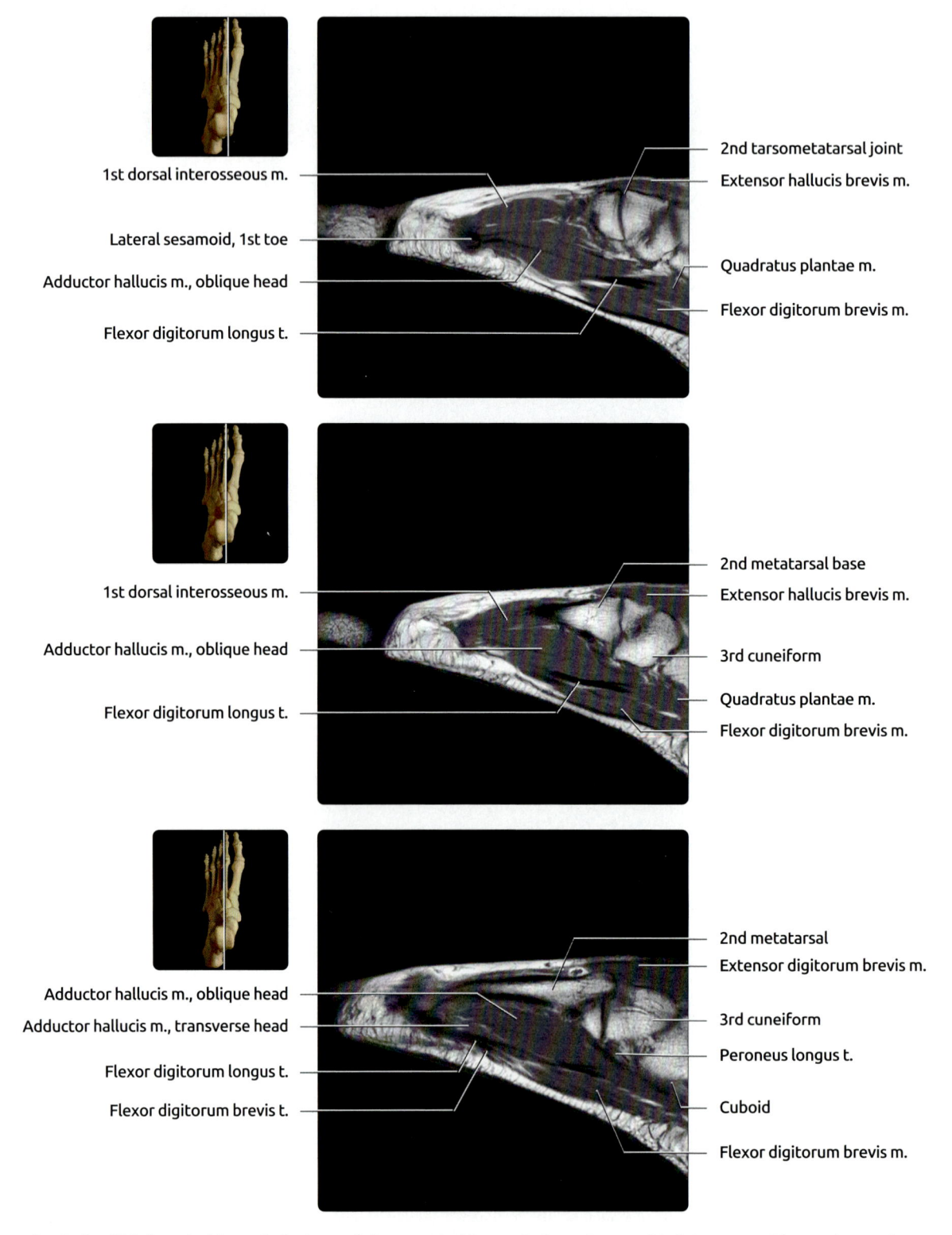

SAGITTAL T1 MR, FOOT

Top image labels:
- 1st dorsal interosseous m.
- Lateral sesamoid, 1st toe
- Adductor hallucis m., oblique head
- Flexor digitorum longus t.
- 2nd tarsometatarsal joint
- Extensor hallucis brevis m.
- Quadratus plantae m.
- Flexor digitorum brevis m.

Middle image labels:
- 1st dorsal interosseous m.
- Adductor hallucis m., oblique head
- Flexor digitorum longus t.
- 2nd metatarsal base
- Extensor hallucis brevis m.
- 3rd cuneiform
- Quadratus plantae m.
- Flexor digitorum brevis m.

Bottom image labels:
- Adductor hallucis m., oblique head
- Adductor hallucis m., transverse head
- Flexor digitorum longus t.
- Flexor digitorum brevis t.
- 2nd metatarsal
- Extensor digitorum brevis m.
- 3rd cuneiform
- Peroneus longus t.
- Cuboid
- Flexor digitorum brevis m.

(Top) The thick, broad adductor hallucis muscle is seen attaching to the lateral sesamoid of the 1st toe. The quadratus plantae muscle is seen attaching to the flexor digitorum longus tendon. **(Middle)** Interspace between the 1st and 2nd metatarsals contains only a dorsal interosseous muscle, attaching to the medial aspect of the 2nd proximal phalanx. The remaining intermetatarsal interspaces contain dorsal and plantar interosseous muscles. The dorsal muscles attach to the lateral aspect of proximal phalangeal bases 2-4, and the plantar muscles attach to the medial aspect of proximal phalangeal bases 3-5. **(Bottom)** The flexor digitorum brevis muscle divides into slips to toes 2-4, and sometimes 5, at the level of the metatarsal shafts. The tendons are superficial to the flexor digitorum longus tendons.

Foot MR Atlas

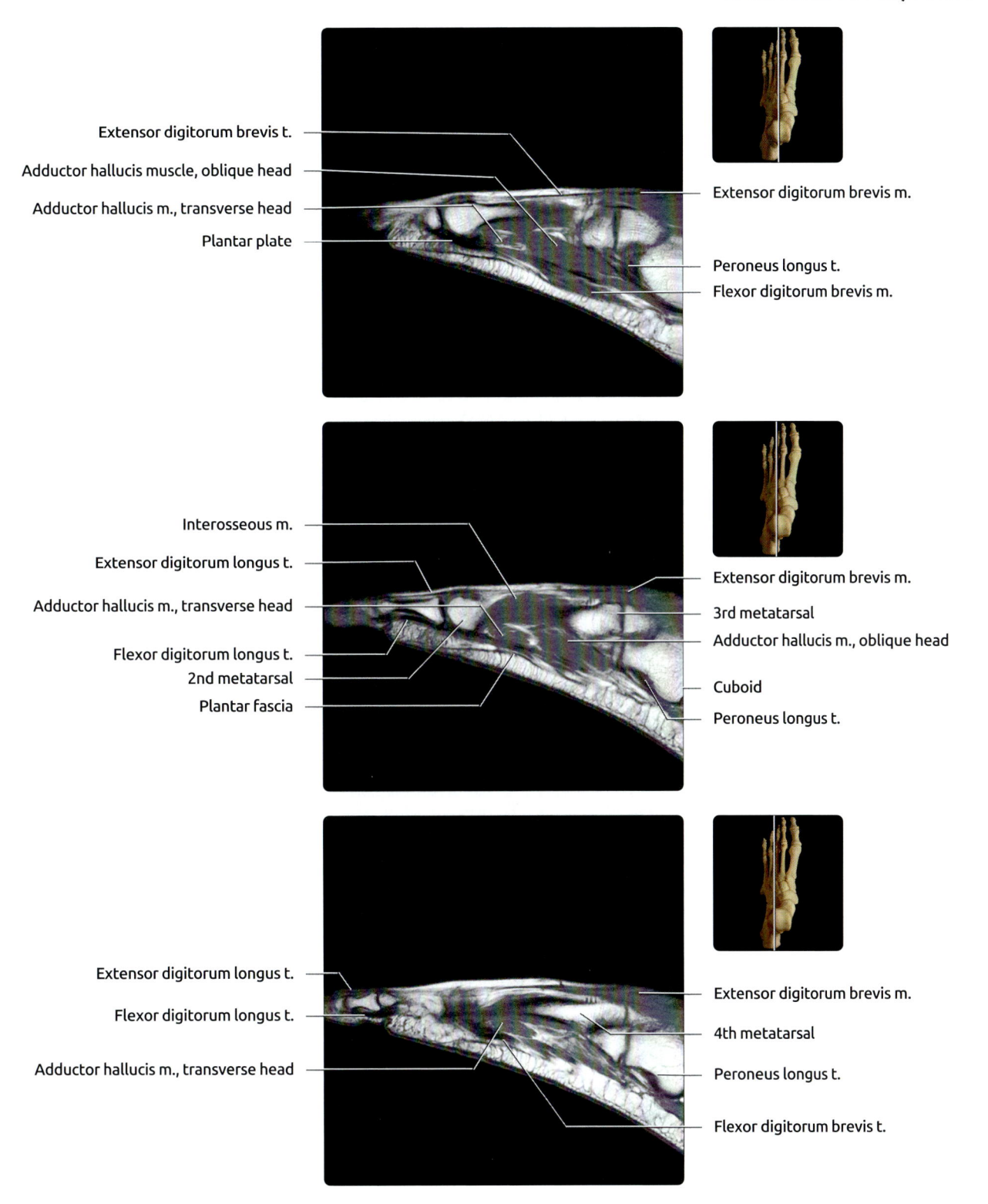

SAGITTAL T1 MR, FOOT

Labels (top image):
- Extensor digitorum brevis t.
- Adductor hallucis muscle, oblique head
- Adductor hallucis m., transverse head
- Plantar plate
- Extensor digitorum brevis m.
- Peroneus longus t.
- Flexor digitorum brevis m.

Labels (middle image):
- Interosseous m.
- Extensor digitorum longus t.
- Adductor hallucis m., transverse head
- Flexor digitorum longus t.
- 2nd metatarsal
- Plantar fascia
- Extensor digitorum brevis m.
- 3rd metatarsal
- Adductor hallucis m., oblique head
- Cuboid
- Peroneus longus t.

Labels (bottom image):
- Extensor digitorum longus t.
- Flexor digitorum longus t.
- Adductor hallucis m., transverse head
- Extensor digitorum brevis m.
- 4th metatarsal
- Peroneus longus t.
- Flexor digitorum brevis t.

(Top) The extensor digitorum longus and brevis tendons run side-by-side in the forefoot, with the brevis lateral to the corresponding longus tendon. The brevis tendon attaches to the lateral margin of the longus tendon. (Middle) In the forefoot, the plantar fascia divides into digital bands. At the level of the metatarsal heads, it arborizes into superficial and deep components. (Bottom) The peroneus longus tendon lies in a groove beneath the cuboid, held in place by the long plantar ligament.

Foot MR Atlas

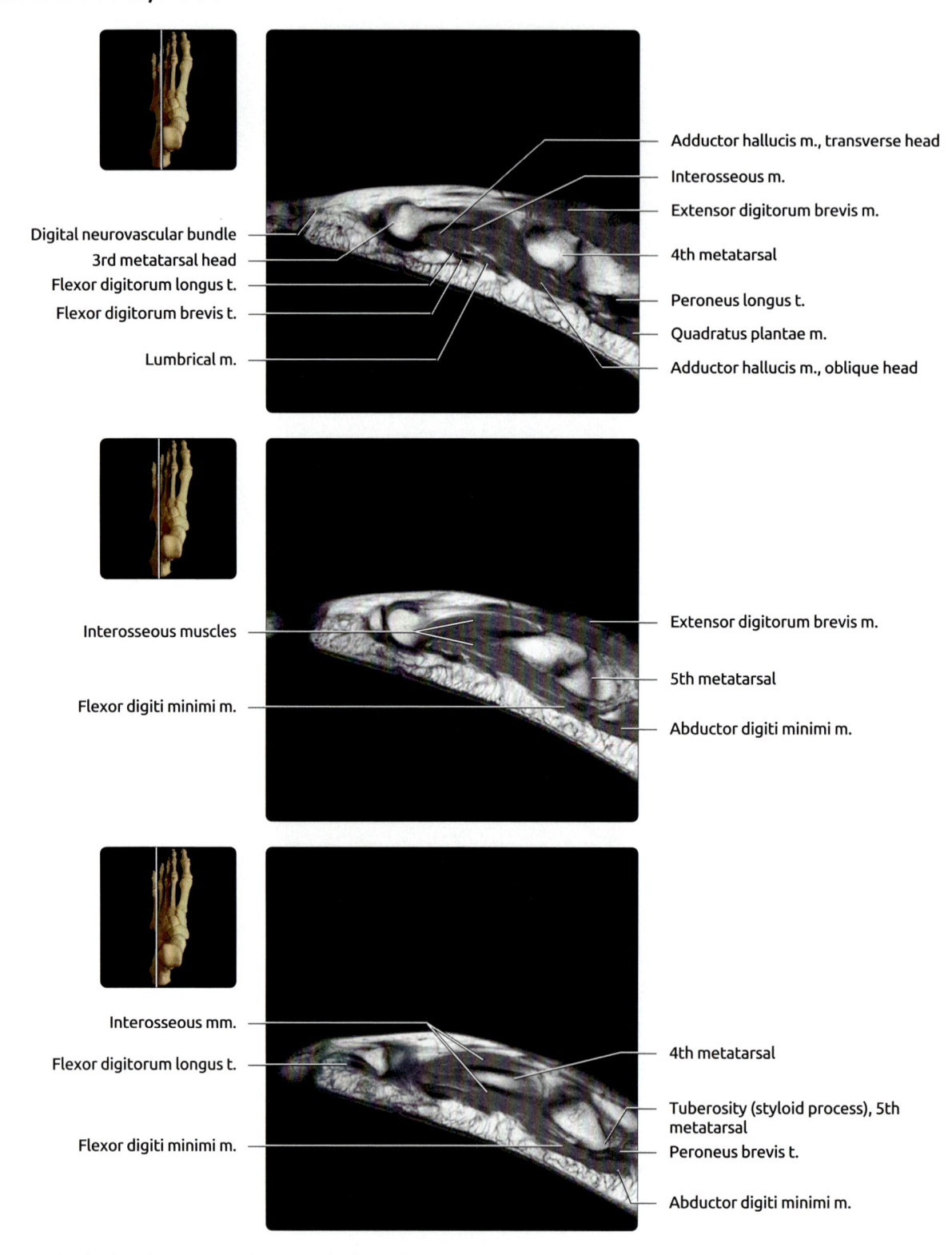

SAGITTAL T1 MR, FOOT

Labels (top image): Digital neurovascular bundle; 3rd metatarsal head; Flexor digitorum longus t.; Flexor digitorum brevis t.; Lumbrical m.; Adductor hallucis m., transverse head; Interosseous m.; Extensor digitorum brevis m.; 4th metatarsal; Peroneus longus t.; Quadratus plantae m.; Adductor hallucis m., oblique head.

Labels (middle image): Interosseous muscles; Flexor digiti minimi m.; Extensor digitorum brevis m.; 5th metatarsal; Abductor digiti minimi m.

Labels (bottom image): Interosseous mm.; Flexor digitorum longus t.; Flexor digiti minimi m.; 4th metatarsal; Tuberosity (styloid process), 5th metatarsal; Peroneus brevis t.; Abductor digiti minimi m.

(Top) The thin lumbrical muscles lie adjacent to the flexor digitorum tendon slips in the 2nd layer of plantar muscles. **(Middle)** Because of the normal fanning of toes, sagittal images angled to the 1st metatarsal will become oblique at the lateral aspect of the foot, as shown on this image. The 3rd metatarsophalangeal joint, as well as the 4th metatarsal and 5th metatarsal base are seen here on a single 3 mm thick slice. In clinical practice, the sagittal axis for imaging the forefoot will be chosen for the metatarsal of concern, or as default along the 1st metatarsal axis. **(Bottom)** The flexor digiti minimi muscle lies at the plantar aspect of the 5th metatarsal, and the abductor digiti minimi muscle lies at its lateral aspect. The peroneus brevis tendon attaches to the tuberosity (styloid process) at the lateral margin of the metatarsal base.

Foot MR Atlas

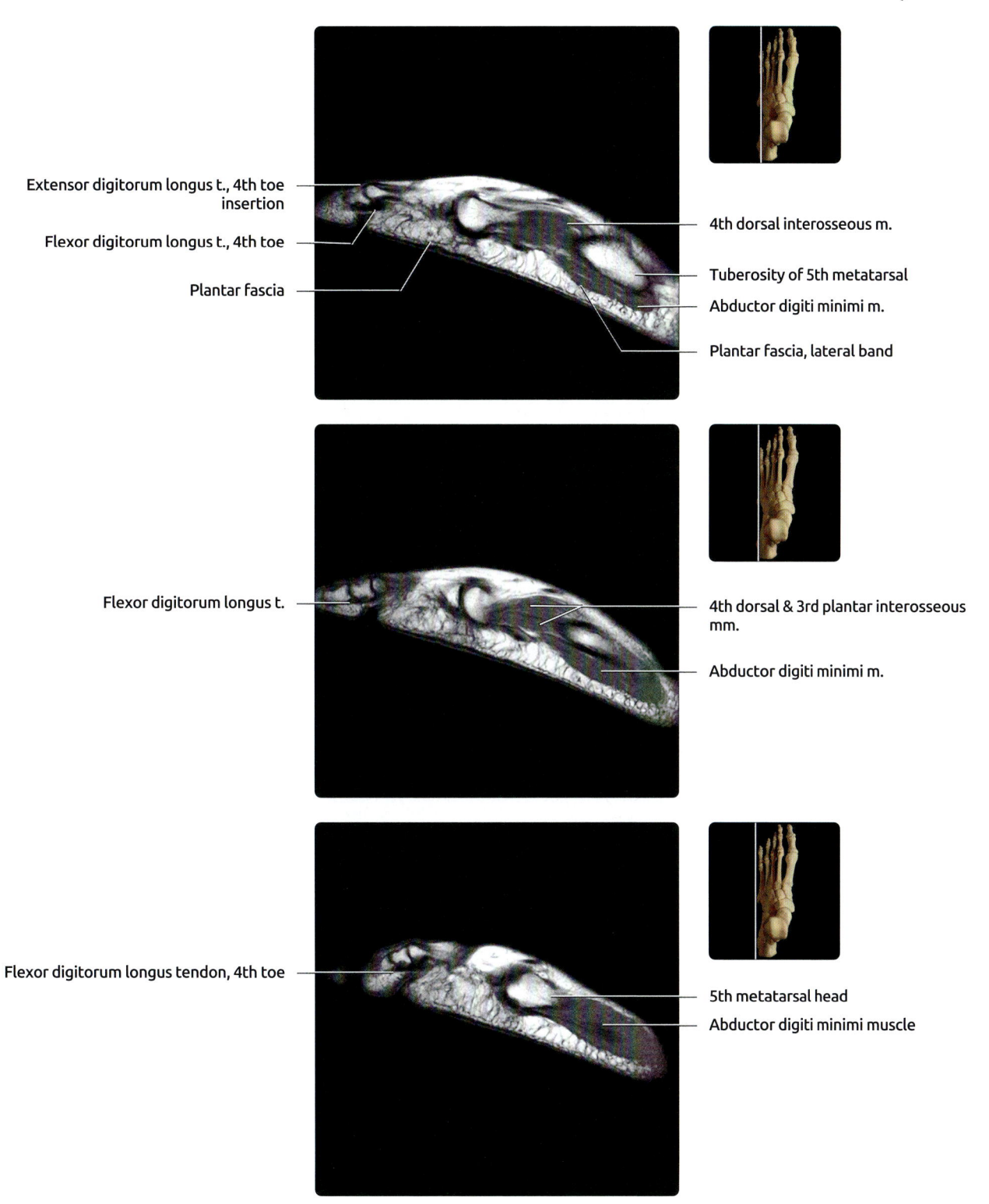

SAGITTAL T1 MR, FOOT

- Extensor digitorum longus t., 4th toe insertion
- Flexor digitorum longus t., 4th toe
- Plantar fascia
- 4th dorsal interosseous m.
- Tuberosity of 5th metatarsal
- Abductor digiti minimi m.
- Plantar fascia, lateral band

- Flexor digitorum longus t.
- 4th dorsal & 3rd plantar interosseous mm.
- Abductor digiti minimi m.

- Flexor digitorum longus tendon, 4th toe
- 5th metatarsal head
- Abductor digiti minimi muscle

(Top) The fine digital fascial network, which is the distal termination of the plantar fascia, is well seen. (Middle) Note that in a resting, non-weight-bearing position, the proximal interphalangeal joint is minimally flexed, and the distal interphalangeal joint is straight. (Bottom) The abductor digiti minimi is the most lateral muscle of the forefoot.

Intrinsic Muscles of Foot

GROSS ANATOMY

Plantar Musculature

- 4 layers of muscles deep to plantar aponeurosis
- Peroneus longus tendon crosses all 4 layers
- **Superficial (1st) muscle layer**
  - Abductor hallucis
    - Origin: Medial aspect posterior process calcaneus, flexor retinaculum, plantar fascia, intermuscular septum
    - Insertion: Medial sesamoid of 1st toe and medial aspect 1st proximal phalangeal base
    - Innervation: Medial plantar nerve
    - Function: Moves 1st toe medially
  - Flexor digitorum brevis
    - Origin: Posterior process calcaneus, plantar fascia, intermuscular septum
    - Divisions: 4 tendon slips split into medial and lateral tendons at metatarsophalangeals (MTPs)
    - Insertion: Medial and lateral margins of bases of middle phalanges
    - Innervation: Medial plantar nerve
    - Function: Flexes proximal interphalangeals (PIPs)
  - Abductor digiti minimi
    - Origin: Posterior process calcaneus
    - Insertion: Base 5th proximal phalanx
    - Innervation: Lateral plantar nerve
    - Function: Moves 5th toe laterally
    - Variant: Abductor ossis metatarsi quinti arises tuberosity 5th metatarsal, merges with abductor digiti minimi
  - Tendon of extrinsic muscle: Peroneus brevis
- **Middle (2nd) muscle layer**
  - Quadratus plantae (also called flexor accessorius)
    - Origin: 2 heads arise from posterior process calcaneus and long plantar ligament
    - Insertion: Tendon of flexor digitorum brevis
    - Innervation: Lateral plantar nerve
    - Function: Flexes lateral 4 toes
  - 4 lumbricals
    - Origin: Tendons of flexor digitorum longus
    - Insertion: Medial side of proximal phalanges of 4 lateral toes, into dorsal hood expansion of extensor tendons
    - Innervation: 1st lumbrical from medial plantar nerve, others by deep branch lateral plantar nerve
    - Function: Maintain extension of interphalangeal joints, flex MTP joints
  - Tendons of 2 extrinsic muscles: Flexor digitorum longus and flexor hallucis longus
    - Fibers from these 2 tendons join at master knot of Henry and exchange fibers
- **Deep (3rd) muscle layer**
  - Flexor hallucis brevis
    - Origin: Lateral head originates from plantar surface cuboid; medial head arises lateral division tibialis posterior and medial intermuscular septum
    - Insertion: Medial and lateral heads insert respectively on medial and lateral aspects base 1st proximal phalanx
    - Contains: Medial and lateral sesamoids of 1st toe
    - Innervation: Medial plantar nerve
    - Function: Flexes proximal phalanx of 1st toe
  - Adductor hallucis
    - Origin: Oblique head originates from bases of 2nd, 3rd, and 4th metatarsals, transverse head originates from 3rd, 4th, and sometimes 5th plantar MTP ligaments
    - Insertion: Lateral sesamoid of 1st toe and base of 1st proximal phalanx
    - Innervation: Deep branch lateral plantar nerve
    - Function: Stabilizes metatarsal heads, flexes proximal phalanx of 1st toe
    - Variant: Transverse head may be absent
  - Flexor digiti minimi brevis
    - Origin: Base of 5th metatarsal and sheath of peroneus longus tendon
    - Insertion: Lateral margin, base of 5th proximal phalanx
    - Innervation: Superficial branch of lateral plantar nerve
    - Function: Flexes MTP joint of 5th toe
  - Tendon of extrinsic muscle: posterior tibial
- **Interosseous (4th) layer**
  - Plantar interossei: 3 muscles, to 3rd, 4th, and 5th toes
    - Origin: Medial bases of 3rd, 4th, and 5th metatarsals
    - Insertion: Medial base of proximal phalanges of same toes
    - Innervation: Deep branch lateral plantar nerve
    - Function: Adduct 3rd-5th toes, flex metatarsophalangeal joints, extend proximal interphalangeal joints
  - Dorsal interossei: 4 muscles, to 2nd, 3rd, 4th, 5th toes
    - Origin: Each has 2 heads, from lateral and medial margins of 2 adjacent metatarsals
    - Insertion: 1st to medial margin 2nd proximal phalanx, 2nd-4th to lateral margin of 2nd-4th proximal phalanges
    - Innervation: Deep branch lateral plantar nerve
    - Function: Deviate toes laterally, flex MTP joints, extend PIP joints

Dorsal Muscles

- Extrinsic muscles: Tendons of anterior tibial, extensor hallucis longus, extensor digitorum brevis, peroneus tertius
- Intrinsic muscles
  - Extensor hallucis brevis: Partially joined to extensor digitorum brevis
    - Origin: Anterior aspect calcaneus
    - Insertion: Base proximal phalanx of 1st toe
    - Innervation: Deep peroneal nerve
    - Function: Extends proximal phalanx
  - Extensor digitorum brevis
    - Origin: Anterolateral aspect calcaneus
    - Insertion: Lateral margins of extensor digitorum longus tendons to 2nd-4th digits and bases middle phalanges
    - Innervation: Deep peroneal nerve
    - Function: Extend phalanges of toes
- In hindfoot, extrinsic tendons superficial to intrinsic tendons
- In forefoot, intrinsic (brevis) tendons lateral to extrinsic (longus) tendons

Intrinsic Muscles of Foot

GRAPHICS, MUSCLE ATTACHMENTS OF FOOT

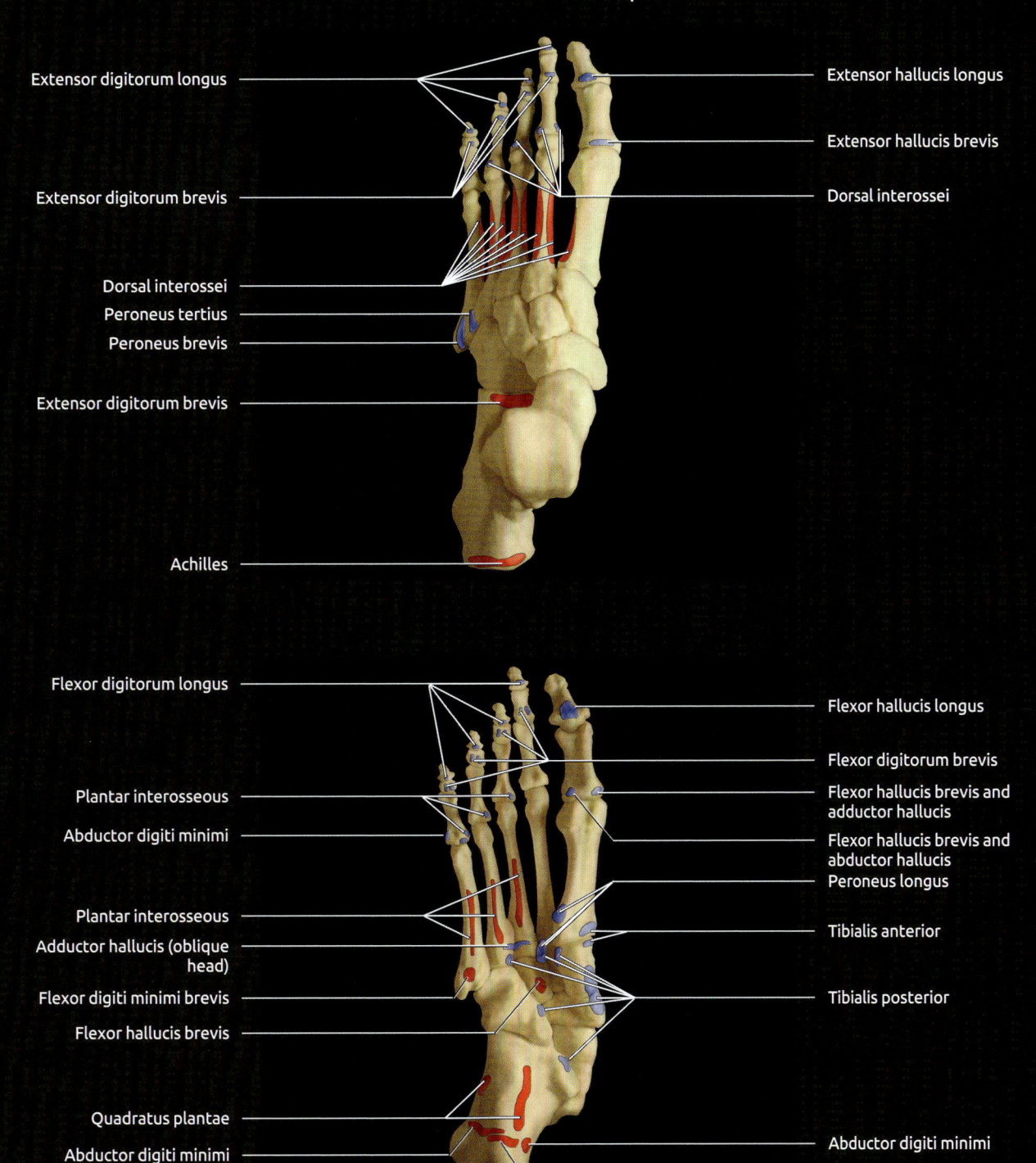

Extensor digitorum longus
Extensor digitorum brevis
Dorsal interossei
Peroneus tertius
Peroneus brevis
Extensor digitorum brevis
Achilles

Extensor hallucis longus
Extensor hallucis brevis
Dorsal interossei

Flexor digitorum longus
Plantar interosseous
Abductor digiti minimi
Plantar interosseous
Adductor hallucis (oblique head)
Flexor digiti minimi brevis
Flexor hallucis brevis
Quadratus plantae
Abductor digiti minimi

Flexor hallucis longus
Flexor digitorum brevis
Flexor hallucis brevis and adductor hallucis
Flexor hallucis brevis and abductor hallucis
Peroneus longus
Tibialis anterior
Tibialis posterior
Abductor digiti minimi
Flexor digitorum brevis

(**Top**) *Graphic shows muscle origins (red) and insertions (blue) at dorsal surface of foot. Note the dorsal interossei insert on proximal phalangeal bases, extensor digitorum brevis on middle phalangeal bases, and extensor digitorum longus on distal interphalangeal bases.* (**Bottom**) *Graphic shows muscle origins (red) and insertions (blue) at plantar surface of foot. Note the multiple attachments of the tibialis posterior tendon. Flexor digitorum brevis tendons to each toe split into 2 slips, attaching at plantar margins of middle phalanges, with the flexor digitorum longus tendon coursing between them to attach at base of distal phalanges.*

Intrinsic Muscles of Foot

GRAPHICS, 1ST & 2ND PLANTAR MUSCLE LAYER

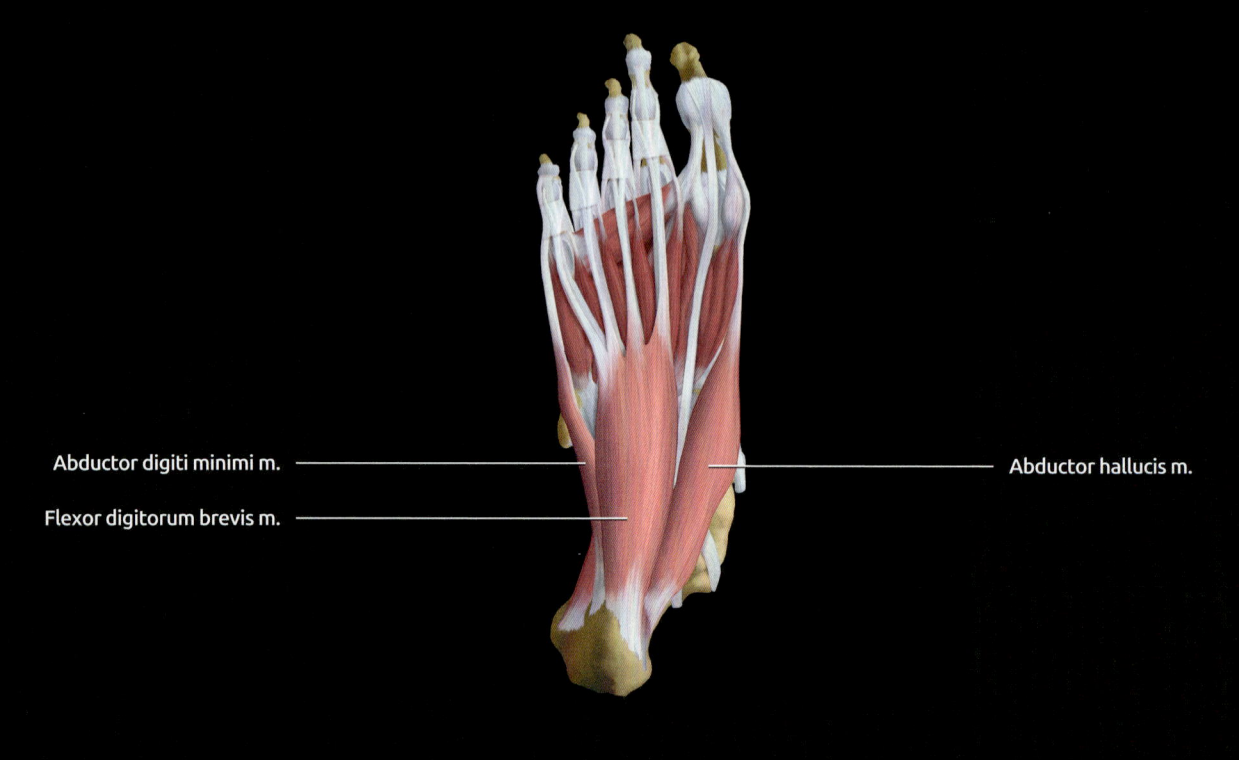

- Abductor digiti minimi m.
- Flexor digitorum brevis m.
- Abductor hallucis m.

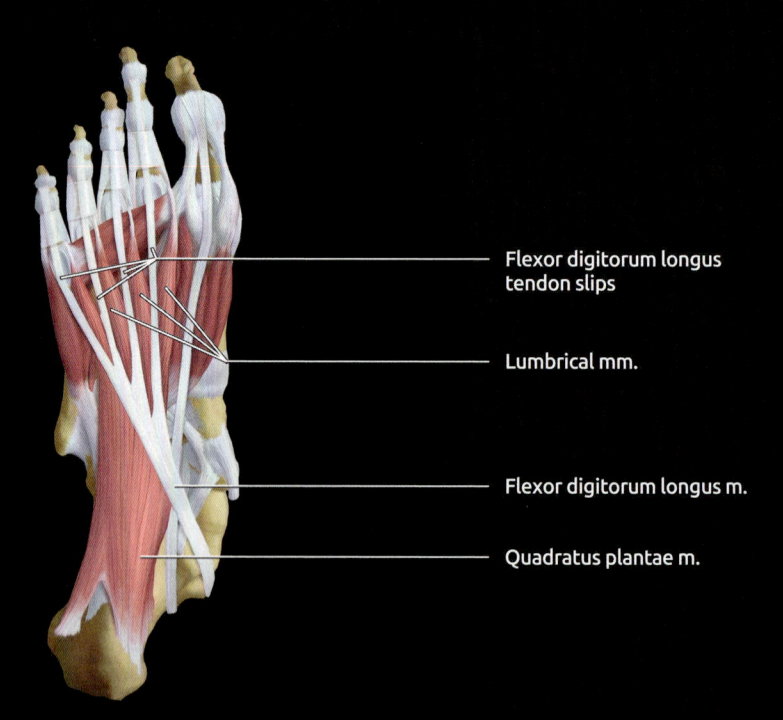

- Flexor digitorum longus tendon slips
- Lumbrical mm.
- Flexor digitorum longus m.
- Quadratus plantae m.

(Top) The 1st, or superficial, layer of plantar muscles is composed of the abductor hallucis, flexor digitorum brevis, and abductor digiti minimi. Abduction in the foot is motion away from the central axis, the 2nd metatarsal. The peroneus brevis (not shown) is the only extrinsic tendon in this layer. (Bottom) The 2nd layer of plantar muscles is composed of the intrinsic muscles, quadratus plantae (also called the flexor accessorius) and the lumbricals, and also the extrinsic tendons of the flexor hallucis longus and flexor digitorum longus. This graphic shows how the lumbricals arise from the tendon slips of the flexor digitorum longus.

Intrinsic Muscles of Foot

GRAPHICS, 3RD & 4TH PLANTAR MUSCLE LAYER

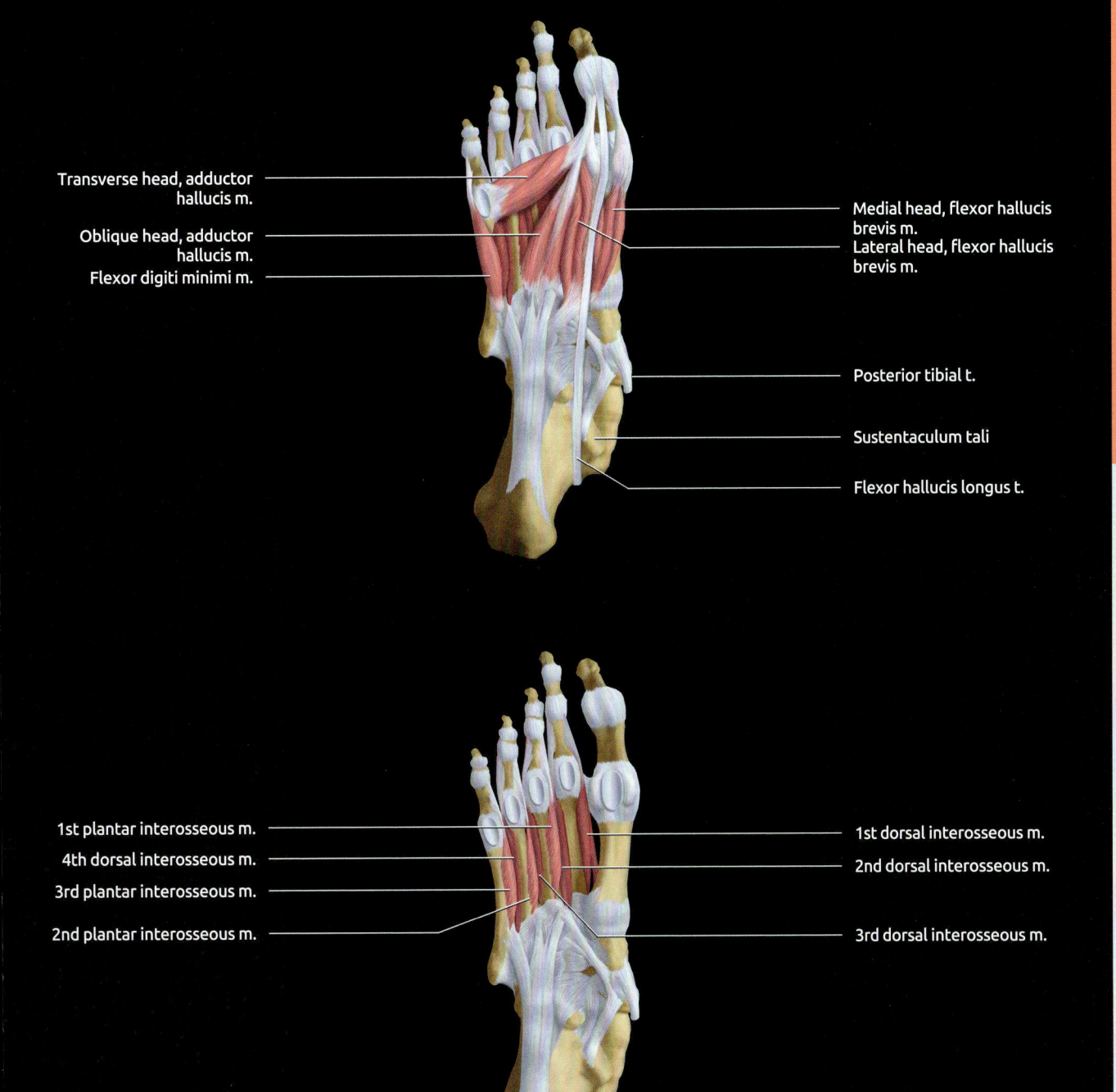

Transverse head, adductor hallucis m.
Oblique head, adductor hallucis m.
Flexor digiti minimi m.

Medial head, flexor hallucis brevis m.
Lateral head, flexor hallucis brevis m.

Posterior tibial t.

Sustentaculum tali

Flexor hallucis longus t.

1st plantar interosseous m.
4th dorsal interosseous m.
3rd plantar interosseous m.
2nd plantar interosseous m.

1st dorsal interosseous m.
2nd dorsal interosseous m.
3rd dorsal interosseous m.

(Top) The 3rd layer consists of 1 extrinsic tendon, the posterior tibial tendon, and 3 intrinsic muscles: Flexor hallucis brevis, (which has medial and lateral heads), the adductor hallucis (which has oblique and transverse heads), and the flexor digiti minimi. *(Bottom)* The 4th layer of plantar muscles contains the interossei. There are 4 dorsal interossei, which have bipennate origins from 2 adjacent metatarsals. The 1st dorsal interosseous inserts on medial side of 2nd proximal phalanx, and the remaining dorsal interossei insert on lateral side of the proximal phalanx corresponding to the metatarsal of origin. There are 3 plantar interossei. They originate from the medial side of the 3rd-5th metatarsals and insert on the medial side of the corresponding proximal phalanges.

Intrinsic Muscles of Foot

CORONAL T1 MR, INTRINSIC FOOT MUSCLES

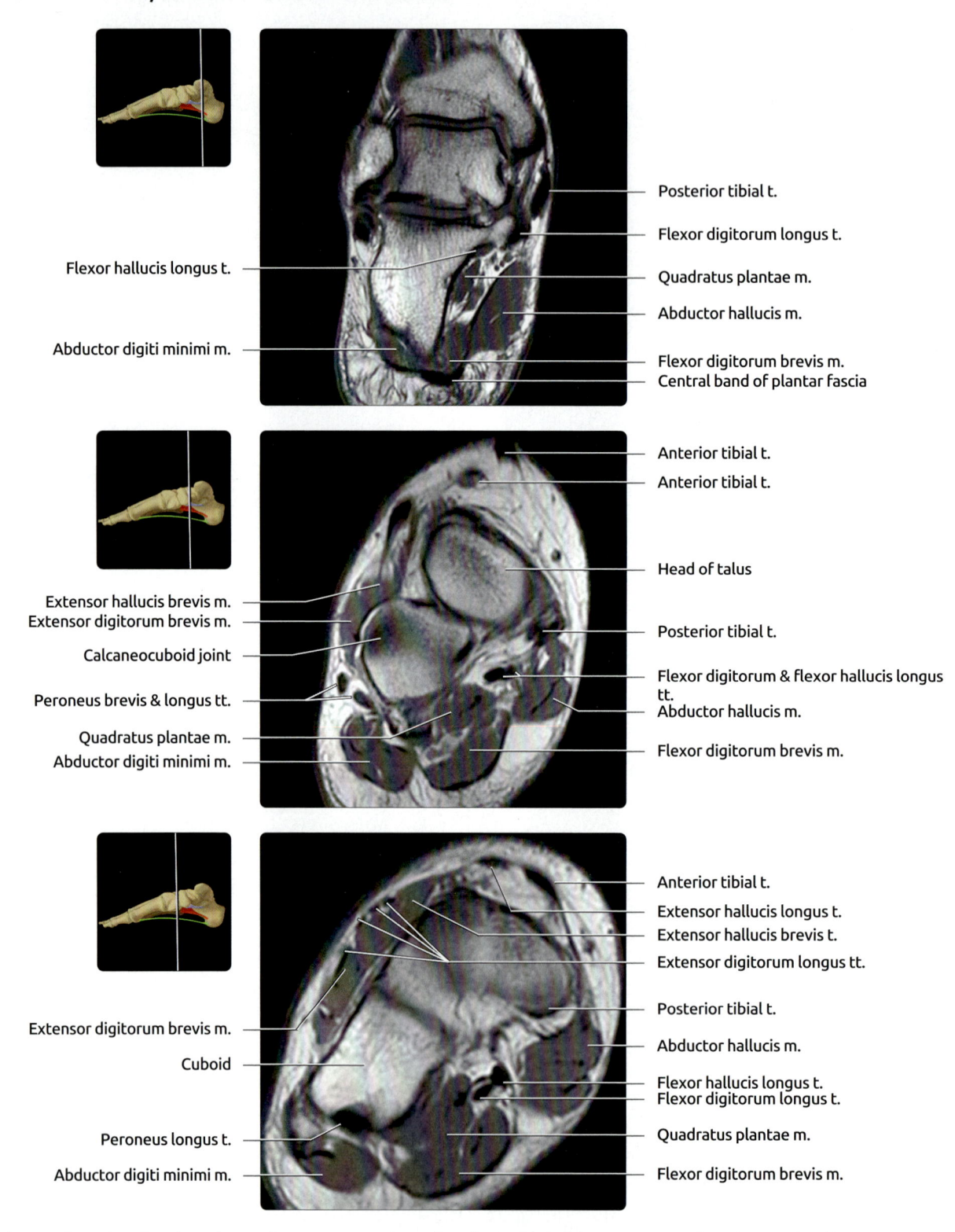

Labels (top image): Flexor hallucis longus t.; Abductor digiti minimi m.; Posterior tibial t.; Flexor digitorum longus t.; Quadratus plantae m.; Abductor hallucis m.; Flexor digitorum brevis m.; Central band of plantar fascia

Labels (middle image): Extensor hallucis brevis m.; Extensor digitorum brevis m.; Calcaneocuboid joint; Peroneus brevis & longus tt.; Quadratus plantae m.; Abductor digiti minimi m.; Anterior tibial t.; Anterior tibial t.; Head of talus; Posterior tibial t.; Flexor digitorum & flexor hallucis longus tt.; Abductor hallucis m.; Flexor digitorum brevis m.

Labels (bottom image): Extensor digitorum brevis m.; Cuboid; Peroneus longus t.; Abductor digiti minimi m.; Anterior tibial t.; Extensor hallucis longus t.; Extensor hallucis brevis t.; Extensor digitorum longus tt.; Posterior tibial t.; Abductor hallucis m.; Flexor hallucis longus t.; Flexor digitorum longus t.; Quadratus plantae m.; Flexor digitorum brevis m.

(**Top**) First of a series of 6 selected coronal T1 MR images shows the relationships of the intrinsic muscles. The superficial layer of plantar muscles includes the abductor hallucis, flexor digitorum brevis, and abductor digiti minimi. In the hindfoot, the quadratus plantae shares the 2nd (middle) level with 2 extrinsic tendons, the flexor hallucis longus and flexor digitorum longus. (**Middle**) This image is at the level of the calcaneocuboid joint. The extensor digitorum brevis and extensor hallucis brevis arise adjacent to each other on the dorsal surface of the calcaneus. (**Bottom**) At the level of the cuboid sulcus, the flexor hallucis and digitorum tendons have crossed. The quadratus plantae muscle is approaching its insertion on the flexor digitorum longus tendon.

Intrinsic Muscles of Foot

CORONAL T1 MR, INTRINSIC FOOT MUSCLES

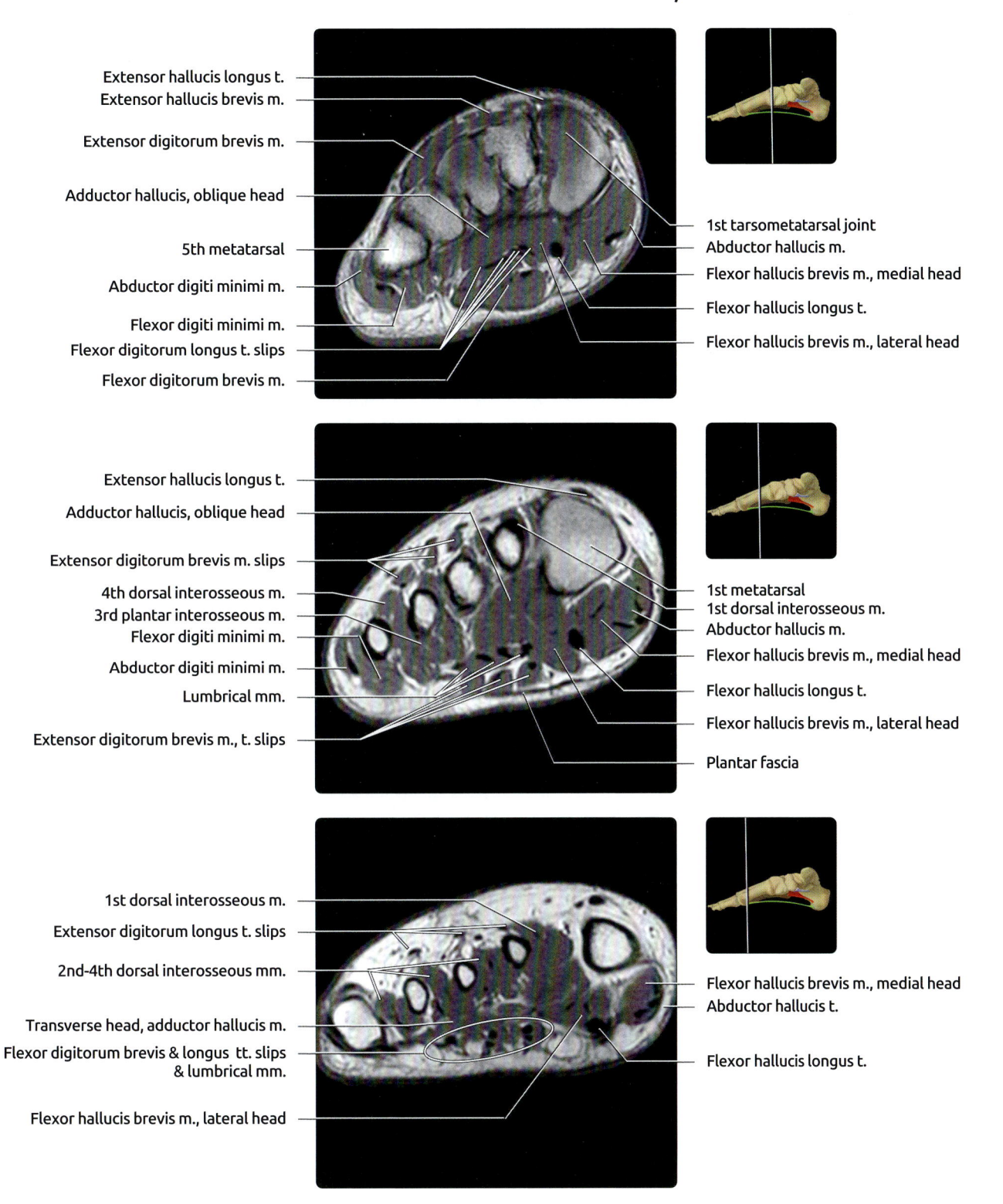

(Top) At the level of the 1st tarsometatarsal joint, the 2 heads of the flexor hallucis brevis muscle are seen flanking the flexor hallucis longus tendon. They lie in the 3rd layer of intrinsic plantar muscles. Flexor digiti minimi muscle, seen here at its origin from the plantar surface of the 5th metatarsal, and adductor hallucis muscle are also part of the deep layer. (Middle) This image is through the proximal metatarsals. The interosseous, or 4th layer of plantar muscles, is composed of the plantar and dorsal interossei. Lumbrical muscles are part of the 2nd plantar layer. The slips of the extensor digitorum brevis muscle are deep and lateral to the corresponding slips of extensor digitorum longus tendon. (Bottom) At the level of the 5th metatarsal head, the abductor digiti minimi and flexor digiti minimi are both tendinous. The transverse head of the adductor hallucis, seen here, is variably present.

Tarsometatarsal Joint

TERMINOLOGY

Synonyms
- Lisfranc joint

IMAGING ANATOMY

Overview
- 1st-5th tarsometatarsal articulations usually considered functionally as 1 joint
- Follows transverse arch configuration established by wedge shape of cuneiforms
  - Bases of 2nd and 3rd metatarsals also have wedge shape
- In coronal plane, joint extends obliquely from anteromedial to posterolateral
  - 2nd metatarsal recessed relative to 1st and 3rd
    - This provides added bony stability ("mortise and tenon" configuration)
    - Some individuals lack recessed position of 2nd metatarsal; they have higher incidence of dislocation
  - Cuboid slightly recessed relative to 3rd cuneiform
    - Creates mortise and tenon configuration in opposite orientation to 2nd tarsometatarsal joint
- Small intermetatarsal joints are present between metatarsal bases 2-5, sometimes bases of 1-2

Motion
- 1st tarsometatarsal joint allows abduction, slight flexion, and extension
- 2nd and 3rd tarsometatarsal joints are relatively immobile
- 4th and 5th tarsometatarsal joints have about 10° of flexion and extension

Synovial Divisions
- 3 separate synovial joint cavities
  - 1st tarsometatarsal joint
  - 2nd-3rd tarsometatarsal joint
    - Usually continuous with joint between 2nd and 3rd cuneiforms, and naviculocuneiform joint
  - 4th-5th tarsometatarsal joint
- Intermetatarsal joints have continuous cavity with tarsometatarsal joints

Ligaments
- **1st tarsometatarsal joint**
  - Dorsal, plantar, and medial and lateral collateral ligaments from 1st cuneiform to 1st metatarsal
- **Tarsometatarsal ligaments 2-5**
  - Dorsal and plantar ligaments at each digit
  - 2nd, 3rd interosseous cuneometatarsal ligaments variably present
- **Lisfranc ligament**
  - Prevents lateral displacement of 2nd cuneiform, helps maintain transverse arch of foot
  - Oblique orientation from 1st cuneiform to 2nd metatarsal
  - 3 separate bands
  - Dorsal bands is most thin
  - Interosseous band is thick, 0.5-1 cm; striated appearance, sometimes 2 separate bands
    - Cuneiform origin is slightly dorsal to metatarsal insertion
  - Interosseous band is a critical stabilizer of Lisfranc joint
  - Plantar band is 2x thickness of dorsal band
    - Attaches to 3rd as well as 2nd metatarsal base, just dorsal to peroneus longus tendon
- **Intermetatarsal ligaments**
  - Dorsal, interosseous, and plantar ligaments between 2nd-5th metatarsal bases
  - No dorsal or plantar ligaments between 1st and 2nd metatarsal bases
    - Weak interosseous ligaments are present in this region
    - Lack of intermetatarsal ligaments between 1st and 2nd metatarsals increases importance of Lisfranc ligament

Bursae
- Bursa between 1st and 2nd metatarsal bases
- Lateral and plantar bursae at base 5th metatarsal, under abductor and flexor muscle origins
- Bursa at plantar 1st tarsometatarsal joint, under origin flexor hallucis brevis
- Bursae at plantar tarsometatarsal joints, under extensor tendons

ANATOMY IMAGING ISSUES

Imaging Recommendations
- Radiographs must be weight bearing to evaluate alignment
  - Abduction stress views may elicit instability
- Axial and coronal MR provide best visualization of Lisfranc ligament
  - Optimize with small flex coil centered at Lisfranc joint

Imaging Pitfalls
- Interosseous Lisfranc ligament structurally most important stabilizer of Lisfranc joint
  - Since obliquely oriented, see on sequential coronal MR images
  - See on axial MR images through midportion of cuneiforms and metatarsal bases

CLINICAL IMPLICATIONS

Clinical Importance
- Injuries of Lisfranc joint commonly missed in emergency department setting
- Isolated tears of Lisfranc ligament occur with plantar flexion, axial load
- Even slight lateral displacement of 2nd metatarsal medial margin relative to medial margin of 2nd cuneiform indicates disruption of Lisfranc ligament
- Flattening of transverse and longitudinal arches of foot and osteoarthritis of Lisfranc joint develop rapidly if ligamentous disruption untreated

SELECTED REFERENCES

1. Castro M et al: Lisfranc joint ligamentous complex: MRI with anatomic correlation in cadavers. AJR Am J Roentgenol. 195(6):W447-55, 2010
2. Johnson A et al: Anatomy of the lisfranc ligament. Foot Ankle Spec. 1(1):19-23, 2008

Tarsometatarsal Joint

RADIOGRAPHS, LISFRANC JOINT

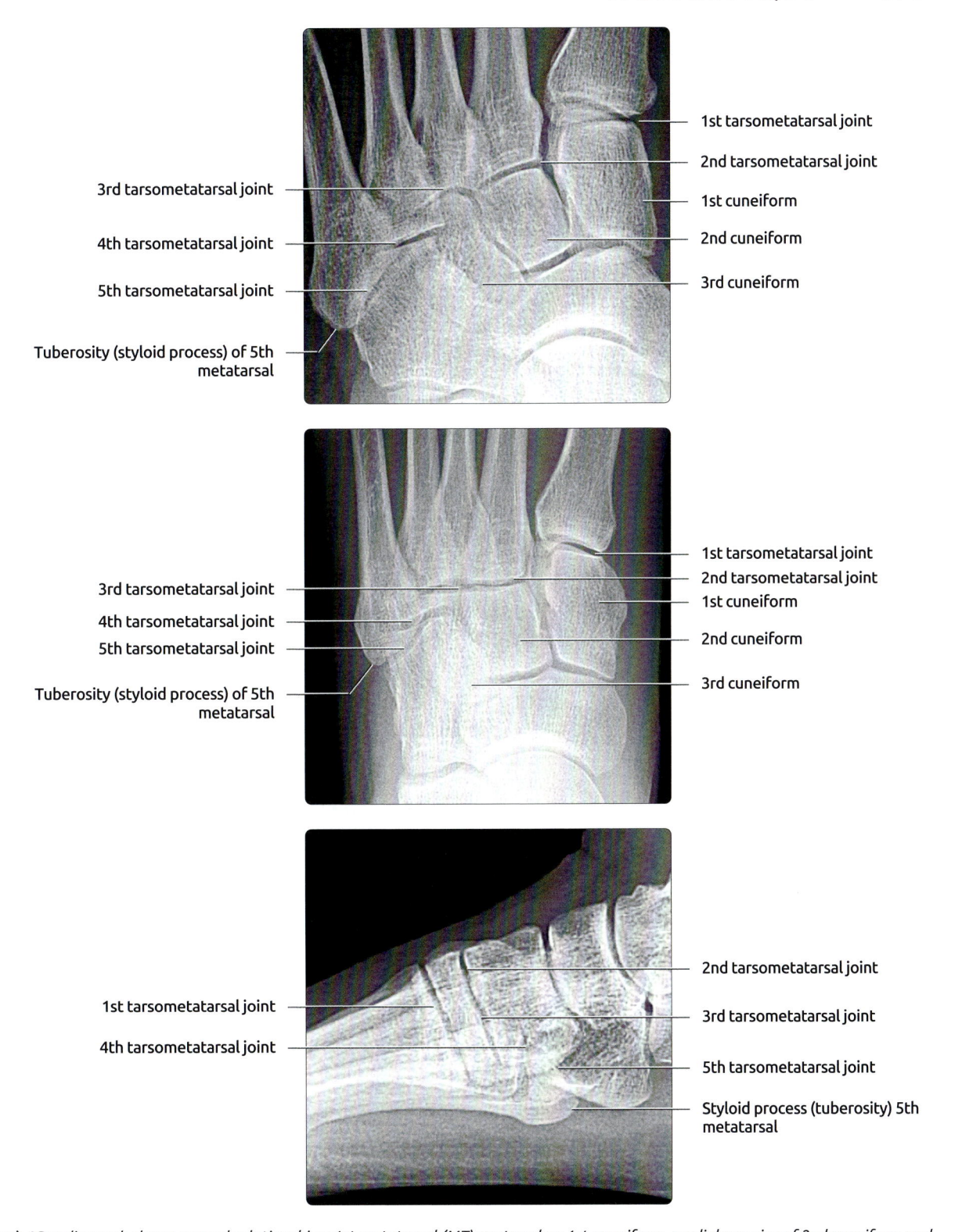

(Top) *AP radiograph shows normal relationships: 1st metatarsal (MT) centered on 1st cuneiform, medial margins of 2nd cuneiform and MT aligned, 5th MT styloid process extending lateral to cuboid.* (Middle) *Anteroposterior radiograph shows that 2nd metatarsal base is not recessed relative to the 3rd, a normal variant which predisposes to dislocation.* (Bottom) *On lateral radiograph, the 1st and 2nd tarsometatarsal joints are at the dorsum of foot, and the 2nd tarsometatarsal joint is located more proximally.*

Tarsometatarsal Joint

SAGITTAL CT, LISFRANC JOINT

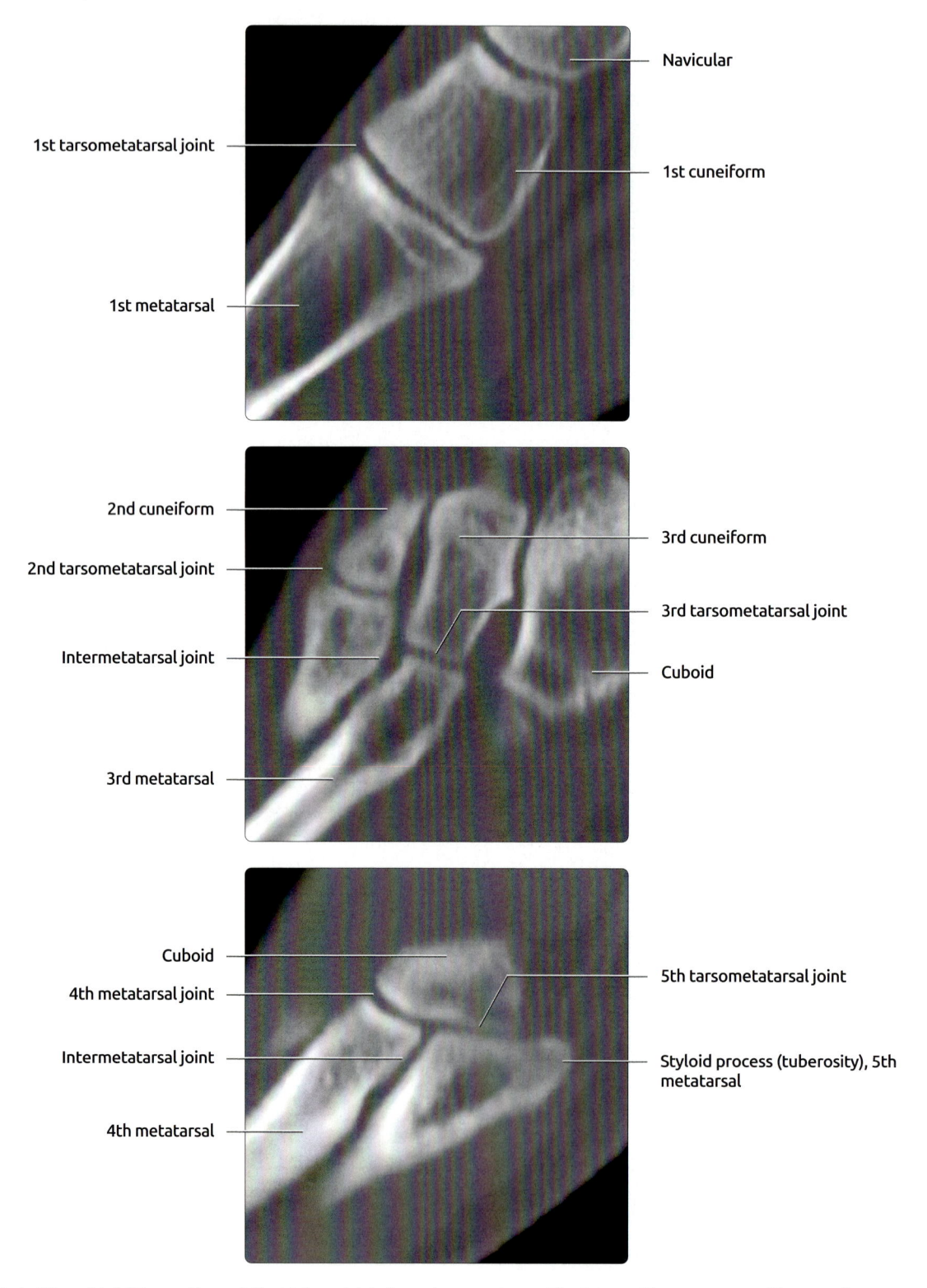

(Top) First of 3 sagittal CT scans through the Lisfranc joint shows bony anatomy. The 1st cuneiform, metatarsal base, and tarsometatarsal joint are much larger than the corresponding bones of the lateral digits. There should be no plantar or dorsal offset of the 1st metatarsal relative to the 1st cuneiform, even on non-weight-bearing studies. (Middle) Sagittal CT through the 2nd and 3rd tarsometatarsal joints shows the recessed position of the 2nd metatarsal base relative to the 3rd. The intermetatarsal joint between the bases of the 2nd and 3rd metatarsals is also well seen. (Bottom) Sagittal CT through the 4th and 5th tarsometatarsal bases shows the articulation of the cuboid with the 4th and 5th metatarsals. The tuberosity (styloid process) of the 5th metatarsal extends beyond the lateral margin of the cuboid.

Tarsometatarsal Joint

GRAPHICS, LISFRANC LIGAMENT

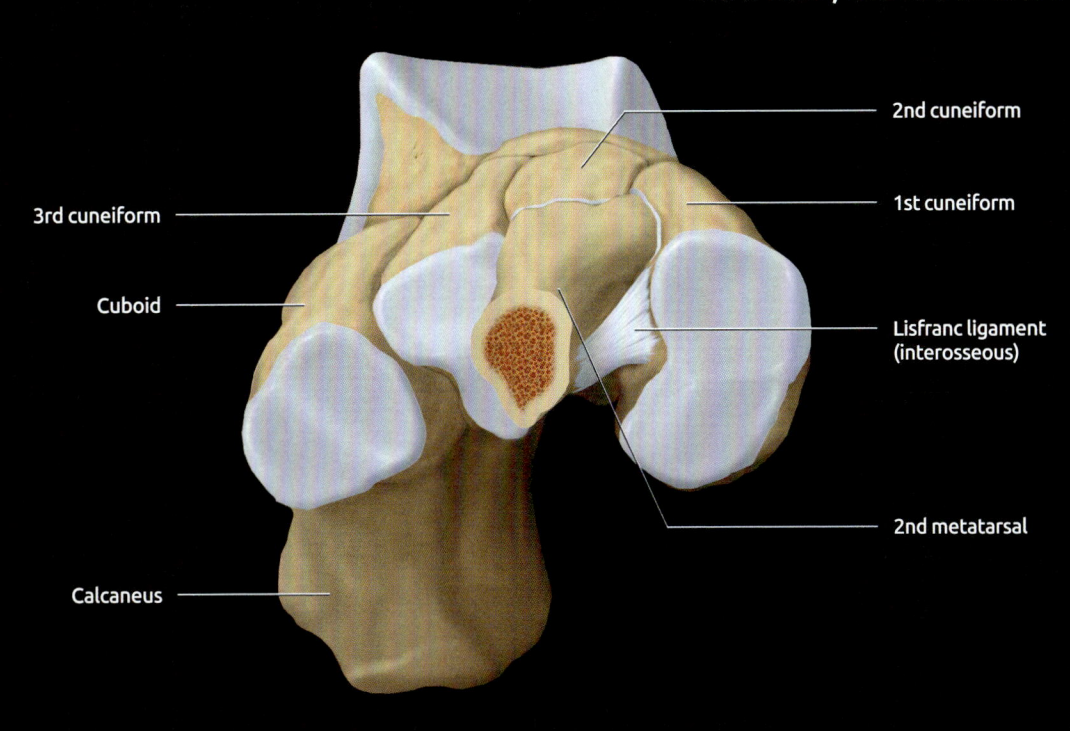

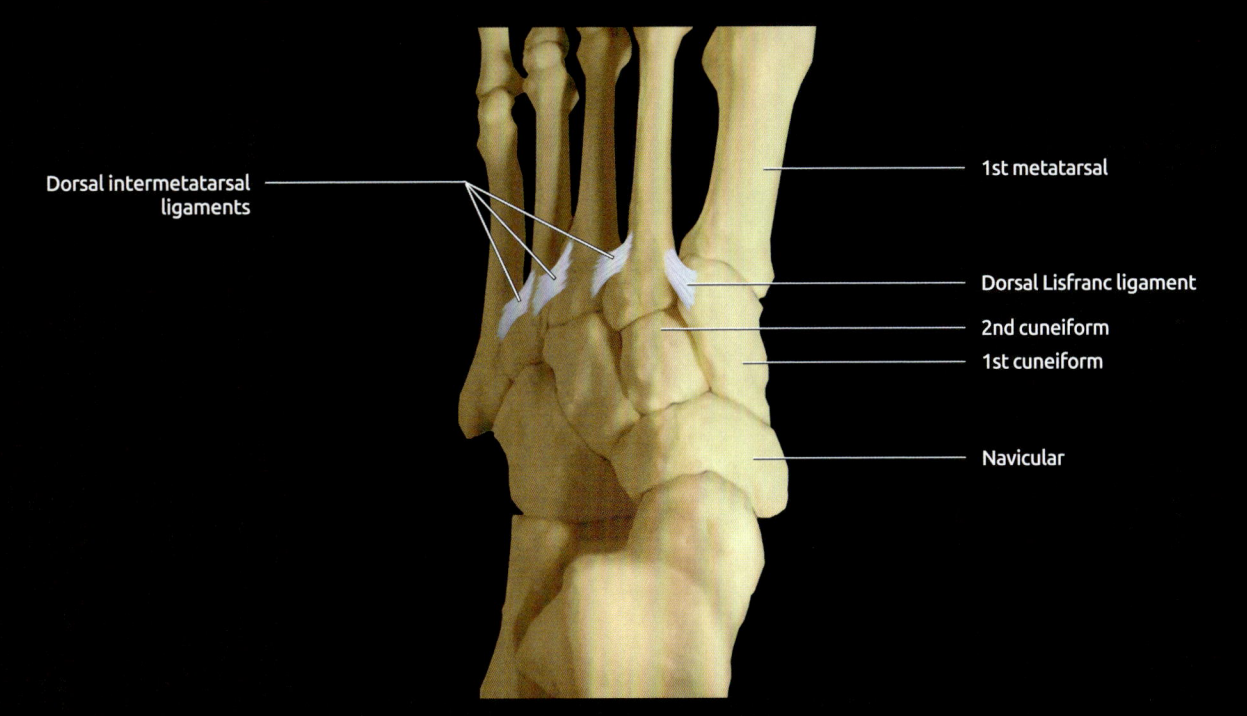

(Top) Three separate ligaments extend from the lateral aspect of the 1st cuneiform to the medial aspect of the 2nd metatarsal: Dorsal, interosseous, and plantar. The interosseous ligament is the strongest of these. The function of all 3 is to prevent lateral displacement of the 2nd metatarsal. (Bottom) Dorsally strong intermetatarsal ligaments are seen between the 2nd-5th metatarsals, but not between the 1st and 2nd metatarsals. The dorsal Lisfranc ligament extends from the 1st cuneiform to the 2nd metatarsal.

Tarsometatarsal Joint

AXIAL T1 MR, LISFRANC LIGAMENT

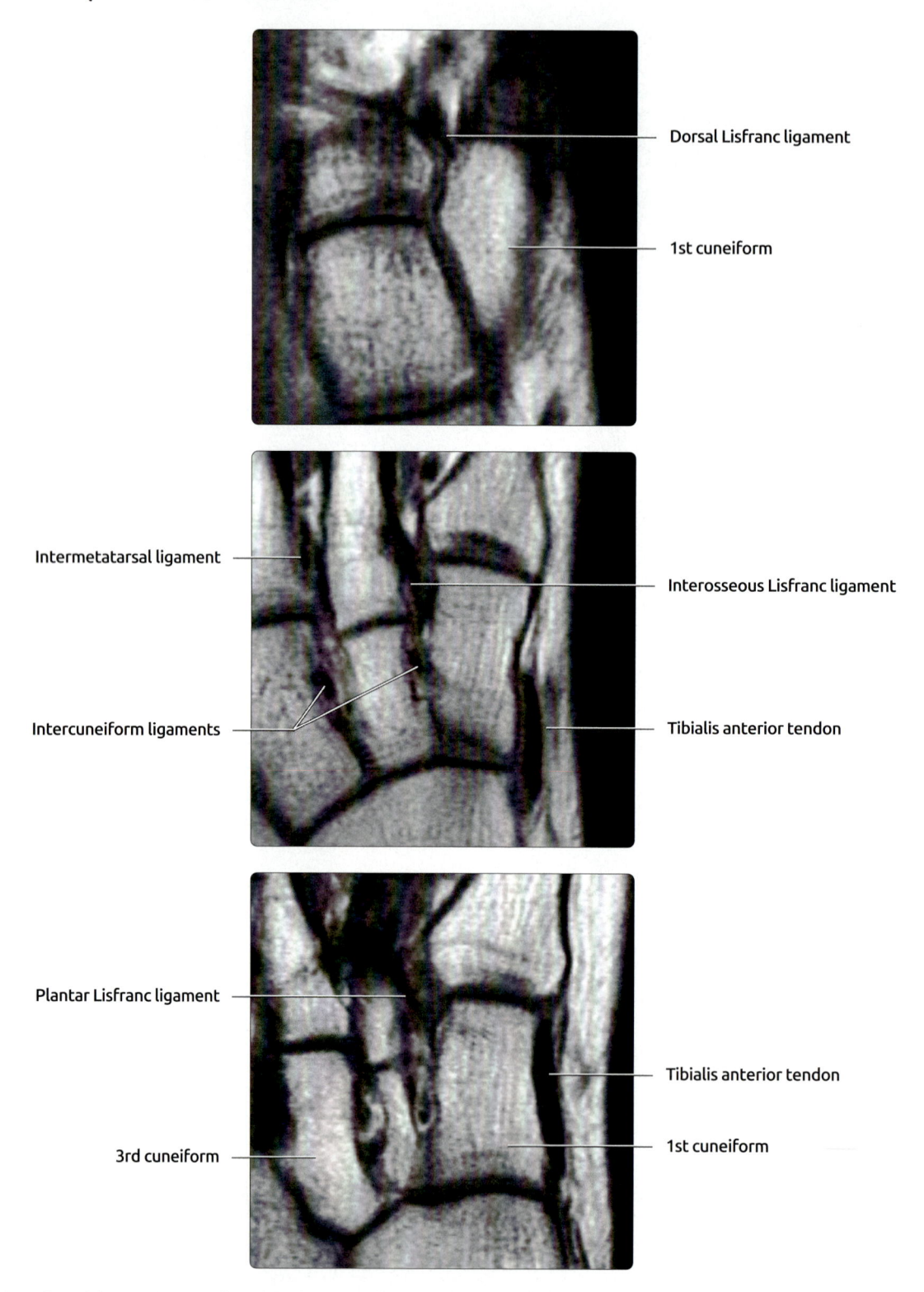

- Dorsal Lisfranc ligament
- 1st cuneiform

- Intermetatarsal ligament
- Interosseous Lisfranc ligament
- Intercuneiform ligaments
- Tibialis anterior tendon

- Plantar Lisfranc ligament
- Tibialis anterior tendon
- 3rd cuneiform
- 1st cuneiform

(Top) First of 3 axial T1 MR images, from dorsal to more plantar positions through the Lisfranc joint. At the dorsal aspect of the tarsometatarsal joint, a thin ligament extends from the 1st cuneiform to the 2nd metatarsal. Isolated injury to Lisfranc ligament occurs with plantarflexion of midfoot, so this ligament is 1st to be injured. (Middle) The interosseous Lisfranc ligament is the primary stabilizer between the 1st and 2nd rays. It is thick and broad when compared to the other interosseous ligaments of the foot. (Bottom) The plantar Lisfranc ligament is a thin structure paralleling the dorsal and interosseous Lisfranc ligaments.

Tarsometatarsal Joint

CORONAL T2 MR, LISFRANC LIGAMENT

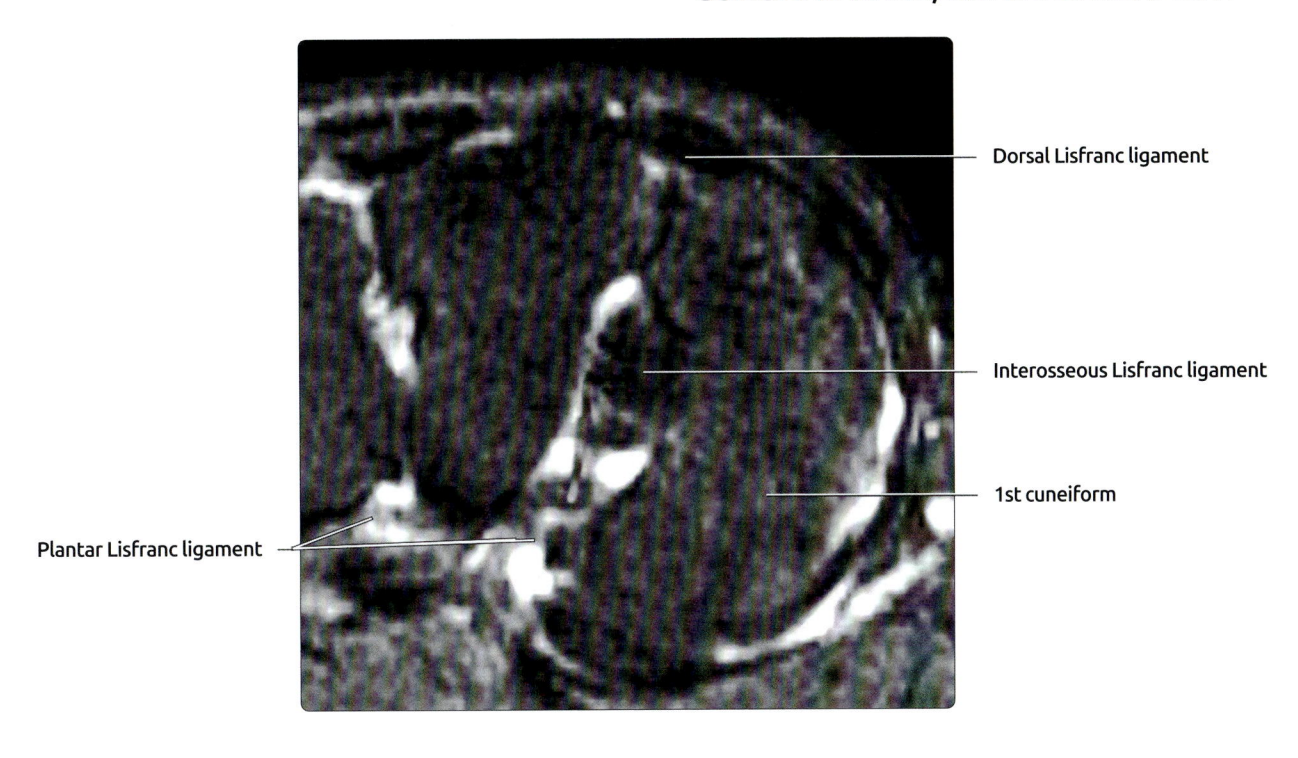

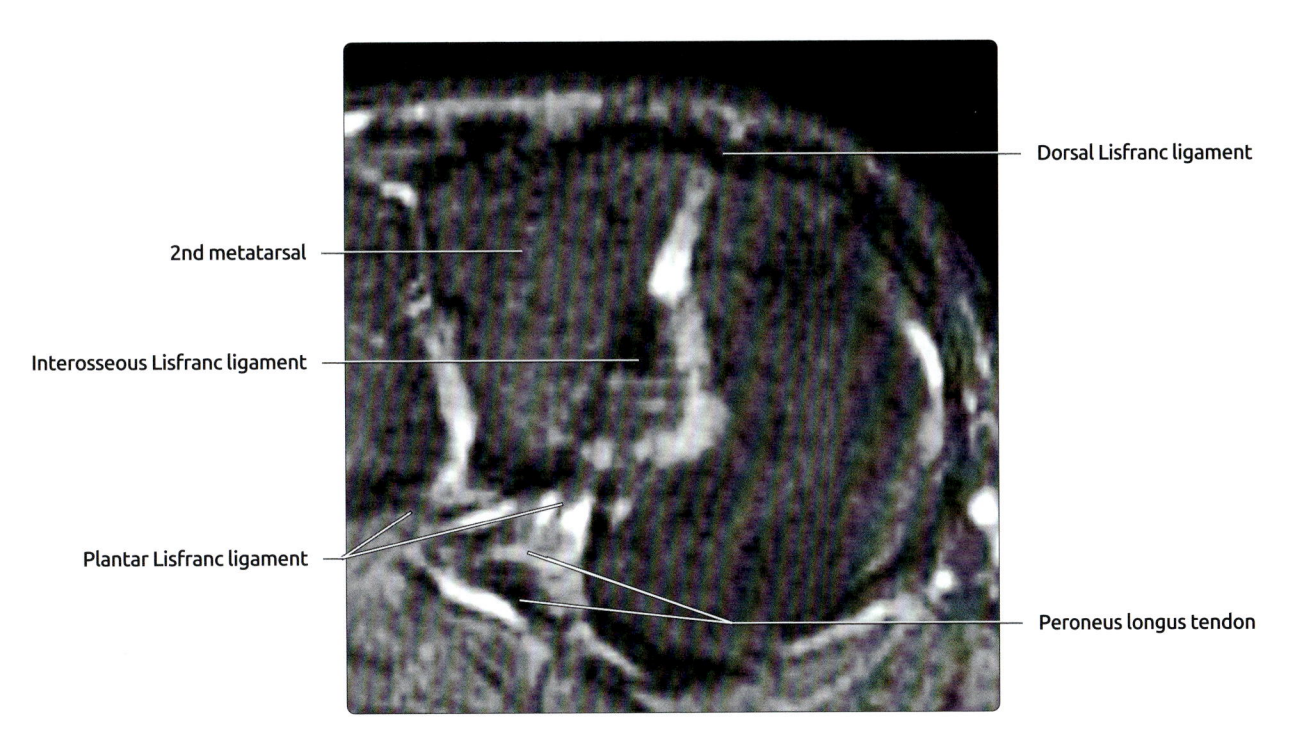

Dorsal Lisfranc ligament

Interosseous Lisfranc ligament

1st cuneiform

Plantar Lisfranc ligament

2nd metatarsal

Interosseous Lisfranc ligament

Plantar Lisfranc ligament

Dorsal Lisfranc ligament

Peroneus longus tendon

(Top) First of 2 coronal T2 MR images of the Lisfranc ligaments. Since the ligaments are obliquely oriented, their entire course will not be seen on a single coronal image. This image shows the origin from the 1st cuneiform. **(Bottom)** This image, adjacent to the previous image, shows the insertion of the interosseous Lisfranc ligament on the 2nd metatarsal base. Note the striated appearance of ligament.

Metatarsophalangeal Joints

IMAGING ANATOMY

Overview
- In normal weight-bearing stance, all of the metatarsal heads are at same level, and all are weight-bearing
  - Metatarsophalangeal (MTP) joints are slightly extended in standing position
- Each metatarsophalangeal joint is a separate synovial cavity

1st Metatarsophalangeal Joint
- Dorsiflexion of toe important in push-off phase of gait
- Metatarsal head has 2 concave facets at plantar surface, 1 for each sesamoid, separated by ridge (crista)
- Distal articular surface of metatarsal head may be flat, rounded, or have central prominence
- Base of proximal phalanx has concave contour
- **Sesamoids**
  - Either sesamoid may be unipartite or bipartite
  - Medial sesamoid in medial head flexor hallucis brevis and abductor hallucis
  - Lateral sesamoid in lateral head flexor hallucis brevis and adductor hallucis and deep metatarsal ligament
  - Medial and lateral sesamoids joined by intersesamoid ligament
    - Intersesamoid ligament is roof of canal in which flexor hallucis longus tendon runs
  - Both are embedded in plantar plate of joint
- **Plantar plate**
  - Fibrocartilaginous plantar capsular thickening extending from metatarsal neck to base proximal phalanx
  - Incorporates sesamoids + tendons distal to sesamoids
- **Sesamophalangeal apparatus**
  - Consists of sesamoids + tendon attachments + plantar plate
  - Inserts on plantar aspect of 1st proximal phalanx
  - Sesamoids fixed in position relative to 1st proximal phalanx, but move relative to 1st metatarsal
  - Therefore displaced laterally in hallux valgus

Lateral Metatarsophalangeal Joints
- Convex metatarsal head articular surface articulates with concave articular surface of proximal phalangeal base
- Plantar aspect of metatarsal head has rounded contour
- Dorsal aspect of metatarsal head is smaller than plantar aspect
  - Has concave or notched contour along medial and lateral margins
- Sesamoids variably present, most commonly at 5th toe
- **Phalangeal apparatus** is combination of plantar plate and proximal phalanx
- **Plantar plate**
  - Fibrocartilaginous plantar capsular thickening extending from metatarsal neck to base proximal phalanx
  - Attached to deep transverse metatarsal ligament, plantar fascia and flexor tendon sheath, medial and lateral collateral ligaments
  - Instability may mimic Morton neuroma symptomatically

Ligaments
- Intermetatarsal ligaments: Between metatarsal heads
- Plantar fascia: Distal attachments to joint capsules
- Medial and lateral collateral ligaments: Well defined at each digit

Bursae
- 1st metatarsophalangeal
  - Dorsal: Variably present separate from tendon sheath of extensor hallucis longus
  - Plantar: Subcutaneous, at plantar and medial aspect of metatarsal head
- Intermetatarsophalangeal
  - Located between metatarsal heads
  - Dorsal to transverse metatarsal ligament
  - Adjacent to plantar digital neurovascular bundle
    - Bursitis may irritate nerve, mimic Morton neuroma
  - Usually absent between 4th and 5th toes
- 5th metatarsophalangeal
  - Plantar: Subcutaneous, at plantar aspect of metatarsal head

Nerves
- Plantar and dorsal nerves course with arterioles along medial and lateral aspects of digits
- Plantar nerves vulnerable to impingement between metatarsal heads

ANATOMY IMAGING ISSUES

Imaging Recommendations
- MTP MR
  - Use wrist or small wrap coil, 10-12 cm FOV
  - 3 mm slices allow excellent visualization of ligaments

CLINICAL IMPLICATIONS

Clinical Importance
- Instability of MTP joints results in pain and deformity of forefoot

Stability of 1st MTP Joint
- Collateral ligaments
- Flexor and extensor hallucis brevis mm
- Flexor and extensor hallucis longus mm have a smaller contribution to stability

Stability of Lateral MTP Joints
- Collateral ligaments
- Plantar plate
  - Rupture of plantar plate results in dorsal subluxation of MTP joint

Short 1st Metatarsal (Morton Foot)
- Normal variant but increases stress on 2nd metatarsal (transfer metatarsalgia)
- Predisposes to
  - Osteonecrosis of 2nd metatarsal head (Freiberg infraction)
  - Stress fracture
  - Dorsal subluxation of 2nd MTP

Metatarsophalangeal Joints

1ST METATARSOPHALANGEAL JOINT

Labels (top figure):
- Adductor hallucis, transverse head
- Adductor hallucis, oblique head
- Flexor hallucis brevis muscle, medial & lateral heads

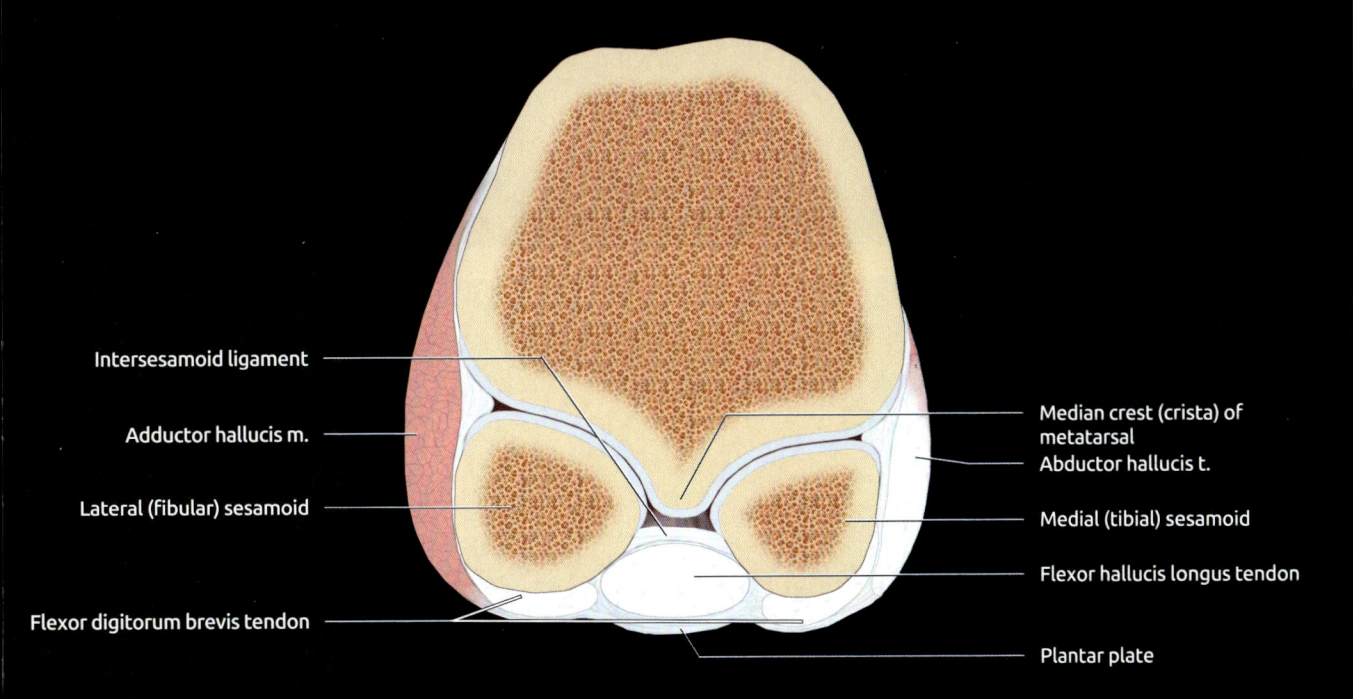

Labels (bottom figure):
- Intersesamoid ligament
- Adductor hallucis m.
- Lateral (fibular) sesamoid
- Flexor digitorum brevis tendon
- Median crest (crista) of metatarsal
- Abductor hallucis t.
- Medial (tibial) sesamoid
- Flexor hallucis longus tendon
- Plantar plate

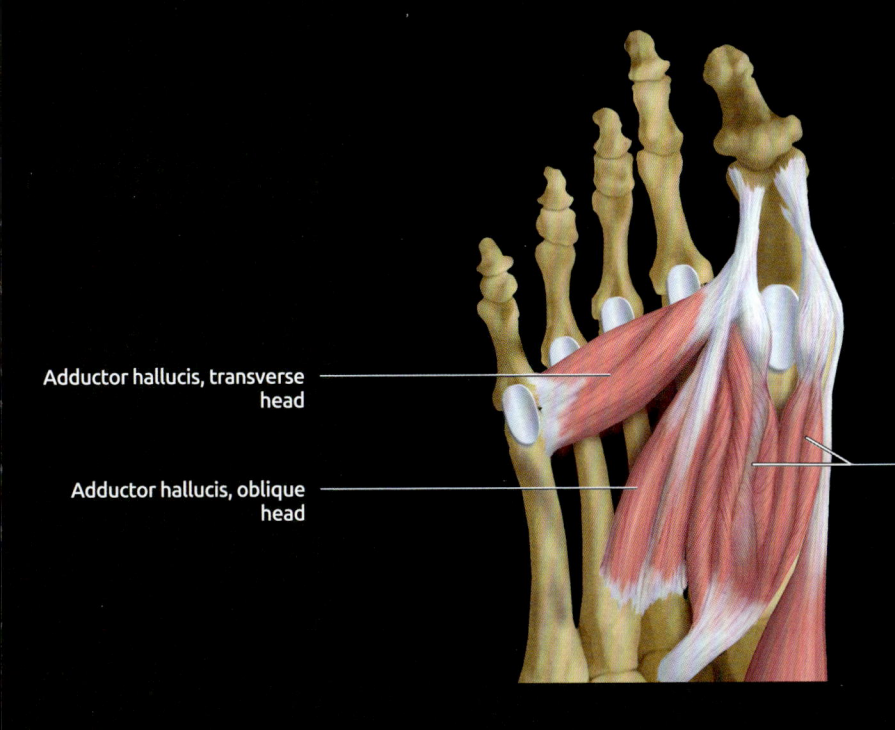

(Top) Axial graphic shows muscle attachments to the sesamoids of the 1st metatarsophalangeal joint. The abductor hallucis and medial head of the flexor hallucis brevis attach to the medial sesamoid. The lateral head of the flexor hallucis brevis and adductor hallucis attach to the lateral sesamoid. *(Bottom)* Coronal graphic shows sesamoids positioned at the plantar surface of the 1st metatarsal head, separated by the median crest of the metatarsal. The sesamoids are united by the intersesamoid ligament. The intersesamoid ligament forms the roof of the groove between the sesamoids, and the flexor hallucis longus tendon runs in this groove.

Metatarsophalangeal Joints

1ST METATARSOPHALANGEAL JOINT

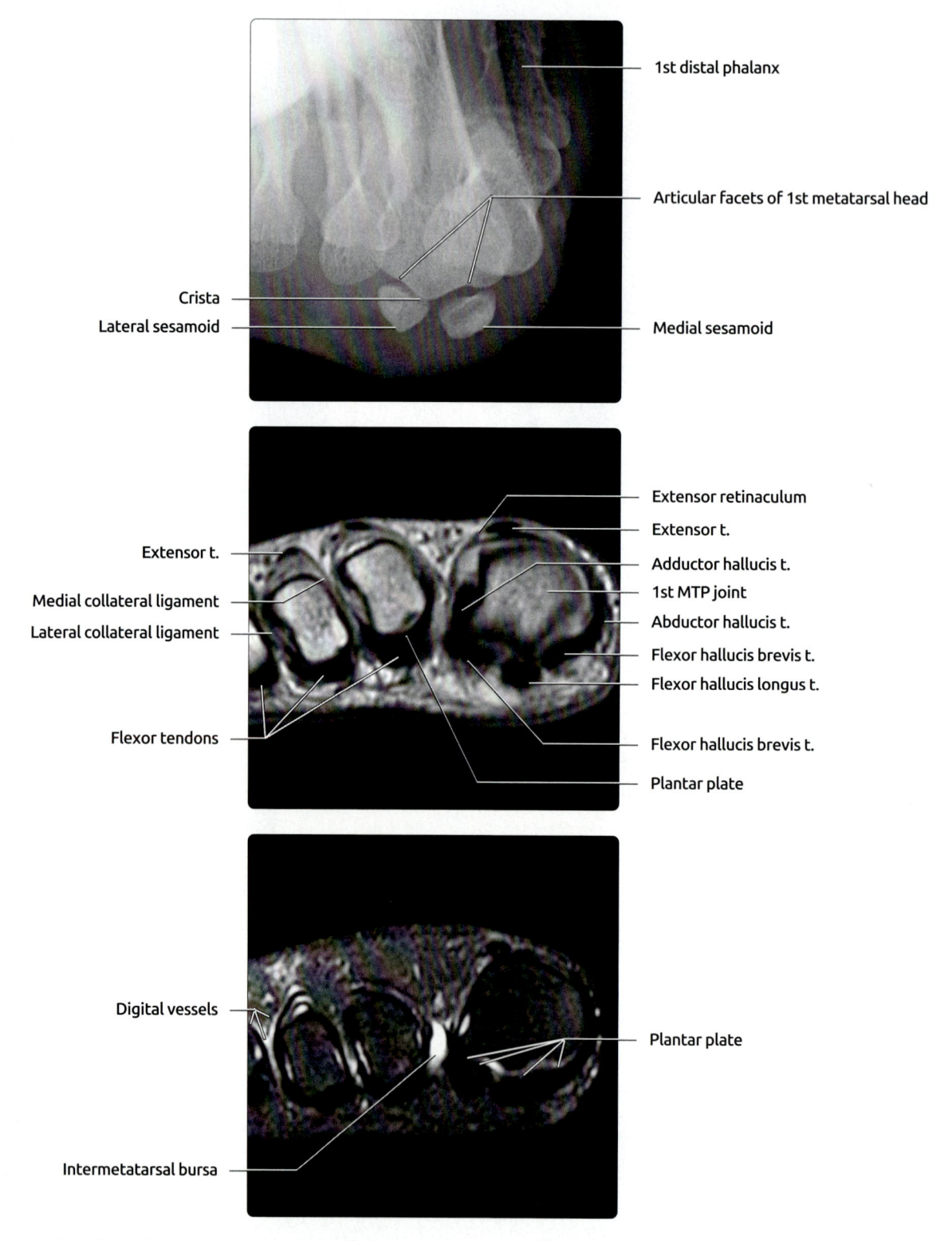

(Top) Sesamoid radiograph obtained tangent to the sesamoids, with the toe dorsiflexed. The sesamoids are centered on articular facets of the metatarsal head. (Middle) Coronal PDWI through the 1st MTP joint and the 2nd-3rd metatarsal heads shows the stabilizing ligaments. Note the plantar plate is much thicker than the dorsal capsule. (Bottom) Coronal T2WI FS shows the normal intermetatarsal bursa between 1st and 2nd metatarsal heads. The digital vessels are also well seen. Both of these normal structures are sometimes mistaken for Morton neuroma.

Metatarsophalangeal Joints

METATARSOPHALANGEAL JOINTS

Labels (top image): Lateral (fibular) sesamoid; Abductor hallucis m.; Lateral head, flexor hallucis brevis m.; Flexor hallucis longus t.; Conjoined tendons forming plantar plate; Medial (tibial) sesamoid; Adductor hallucis t.; Medial head, flexor hallucis brevis m.

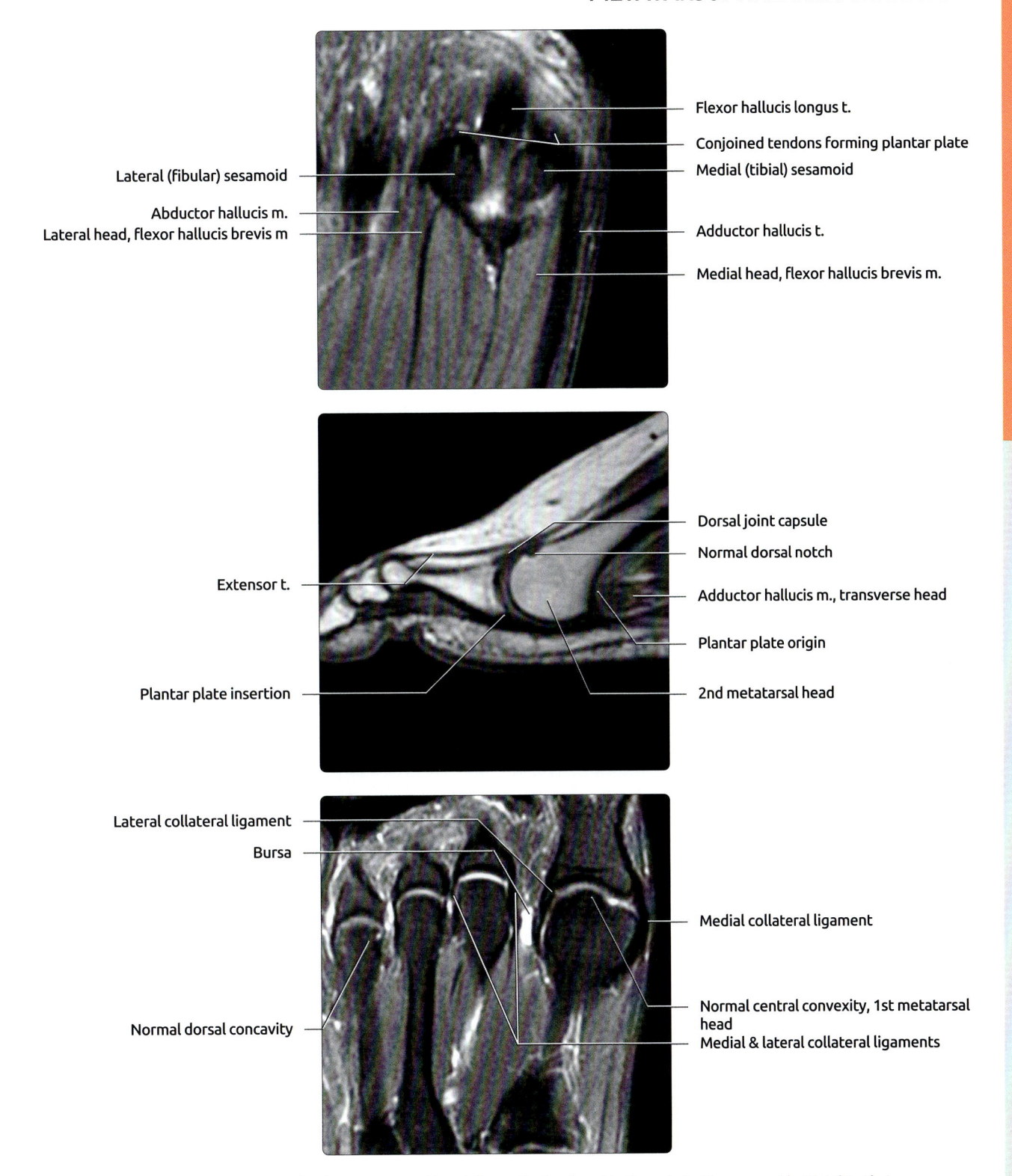

Labels (middle image): Extensor t.; Plantar plate insertion; Dorsal joint capsule; Normal dorsal notch; Adductor hallucis m., transverse head; Plantar plate origin; 2nd metatarsal head

Labels (bottom image): Lateral collateral ligament; Bursa; Normal dorsal concavity; Medial collateral ligament; Normal central convexity, 1st metatarsal head; Medial & lateral collateral ligaments

(Top) Axial PD FS image through sesamoids of 1st metatarsal head shows the tendon attachments to the sesamoids. Distal to their attachment on the sesamoids, the tendons form thickenings in the plantar plate of the 1st metatarsophalangeal joint. (Middle) Sagittal T1WI through the 2nd metatarsophalangeal joint shows the proximal origin of the plantar plate from the metatarsal neck, and its insertion on the base of the proximal phalanx. (Bottom) Axial PD FS shows collateral ligaments of the metatarsophalangeal joints. A small bursa is visible between the 1st and 2nd metatarsophalangeal joints.

Foot and Ankle Normal Variants and Imaging Pitfalls

IMAGING ANATOMY

Overview

- **Distal fibular variants**
  - Absent retromalleolar fibular groove
    - Predisposes to peroneal retinaculum injury, peroneal tendon subluxation
  - Os subfibulare: Accessory center of ossification, anteroinferior margin of fibula
- **Distal tibial variants**
  - Medial malleolus accessory ossification center for anterior colliculus
- **Ankle capsule variants**
  - 10-15% of population have ankle joint capsule communication with subtalar joint
- **Talus variants**
  - Os trigonum: Accessory center of ossification for posterior process talus
  - Stieda process: Enlarged posterior process of talus
- **Calcaneal variants**
  - Peroneal tubercle of calcaneus
    - Variably present at lateral margin, separates peroneus longus and brevis
  - Os calcaneus secondarius: Small ossicle adjacent to anterior process calcaneus
  - Sclerotic ossification center of posterior process
    - May be multipartite, may mimic osteonecrosis (Sever disease)
- **Navicular variants**
  - Accessory navicular (also called os tibiale externum): Ossicle at median eminence of navicular
    - Type 1: Sesamoid in tibialis posterior tendon
    - Type 2: Accessory center of ossification joined to navicular by synchondrosis
    - Type 3: Enlarged median eminence of navicular
  - Os supranaviculare (also called os talonaviculare dorsale or Pirie bone): Dorsal, proximal margin of navicular
  - In childhood navicular may be sclerotic, flat, multipartite
    - May mimic avascular necrosis of navicular (Köhler disease)
- **Cuboid variant: Cuboides secondarium** (rare)
  - Small ossicle at proximal medial aspect of cuboid, between cuboid and navicular
- **Cuneiform variants**
  - Os intercuneiform: Dorsal aspect foot, between 1st and 2nd cuneiforms
  - Medial cuneiform may arise from 2 ossification centers
- **Metatarsal variants**
  - Accessory centers of ossification
    - Pars peronea metatarsalis primi: Between base of 1st metatarsal and 1st cuneiform
    - Os vesalianum: Base of 5th metatarsal
    - Os intermetatarseum: Dorsal, between 1st and 2nd metatarsals
    - Accessory epiphysis: At opposite end of bone from true epiphysis
  - Intermetatarsal joint of 1st and 2nd digits
    - Articular facet between bases of 1st and 2nd metatarsals variably present
  - Morton foot: 1st metatarsal is short relative to 2nd
    - Results in increased stress on 2nd metatarsal
- **Phalangeal variants**
  - Failure of segmentation of middle and distal phalanges
  - Exostosis of 1st distal phalangeal base

Sesamoids

- **Os peroneale**: Sesamoid within peroneus longus muscle, seen adjacent to lateral margin of cuboid
  - May be bipartite or multipartite
- **Sesamoids of great toe**
  - 30% bipartite or multipartite
  - Medial (tibial) sesamoid rarely congenitally absent
  - Interphalangeal sesamoid: At interphalangeal joint, within flexor hallucis longus tendon
- **Sesamoids of 2nd-5th toes**
  - Variably present at metatarsophalangeal or interphalangeal joints

Pediatric Marrow Variation

- May see islands of low T1, high T2 signal in bone marrow in pediatric population
- Residual hematopoietic bone marrow, resolves by age 15

Muscle Variants

- **Accessory soleus**
  - Originates anterior margin soleus, inserts on calcaneus
- **Accessory flexor muscles**
  - Variable origins and insertions, description of course preferred to specific names
- **Peroneus quartus**
  - Originates distal fibula, peroneus brevis, or peroneus longus
  - Variable insertion lateral foot: 5th toe, calcaneus, cuboid, lateral retinaculum
- **Quadratus plantae**: May be absent; may send slip to 5th toe, 2nd-4th toes, or 2nd-3rd toes
- **Opponens digiti minimi**: Variably present muscle slip of flexor digiti minimi, sharing its origin, and inserting on distal 5th metatarsal shaft
- **Peroneus tertius**: Absent in 10% of population

ANATOMY IMAGING ISSUES

Imaging Recommendations

- Use radiographic CT or MR criteria to distinguish normal variants from fracture
  - Fracture: Jagged margins, acute angular contour
  - Accessory ossicle/bipartite ossicle: Smooth, rounded, corticated margins
- Accessory centers may be symptomatic, due to injury of synchondrosis between ossicle and parent bone
  - If symptomatic, edema will be seen on MR, centered on synchondrosis
- Accessory muscles may be symptomatic, should not be mistaken for mass

Foot and Ankle Normal Variants and Imaging Pitfalls

GRAPHIC OF ACCESSORY CENTERS & SESAMOIDS

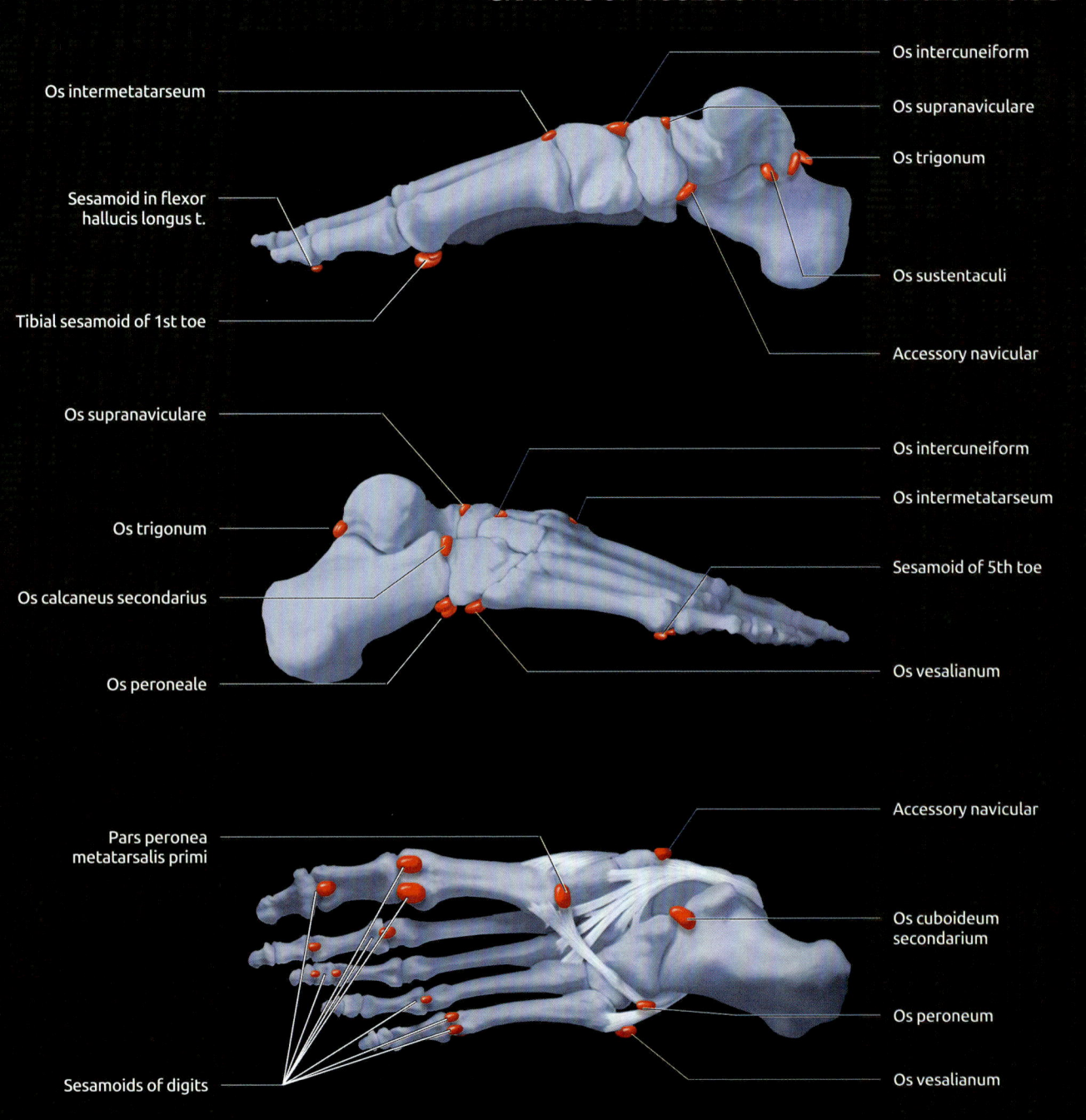

Labels (top view):
- Os intermetatarseum
- Sesamoid in flexor hallucis longus t.
- Tibial sesamoid of 1st toe
- Os intercuneiform
- Os supranaviculare
- Os trigonum
- Os sustentaculi
- Accessory navicular

Labels (medial view):
- Os supranaviculare
- Os trigonum
- Os calcaneus secondarius
- Os peroneale
- Os intercuneiform
- Os intermetatarseum
- Sesamoid of 5th toe
- Os vesalianum

Labels (plantar view):
- Pars peronea metatarsalis primi
- Sesamoids of digits
- Accessory navicular
- Os cuboideum secondarium
- Os peroneum
- Os vesalianum

There are multiple, variably present accessory ossicles of the foot. Os sustentaculi and pars peronea metatarsalis primi are quite uncommon, while the others shown are frequently seen. Ossicles are frequently called by Latin names. Os tibiale externum, however, is usually called by its simple English name, accessory navicular.

Foot and Ankle Normal Variants and Imaging Pitfalls

ANKLE JOINT CAPSULE VARIANTS

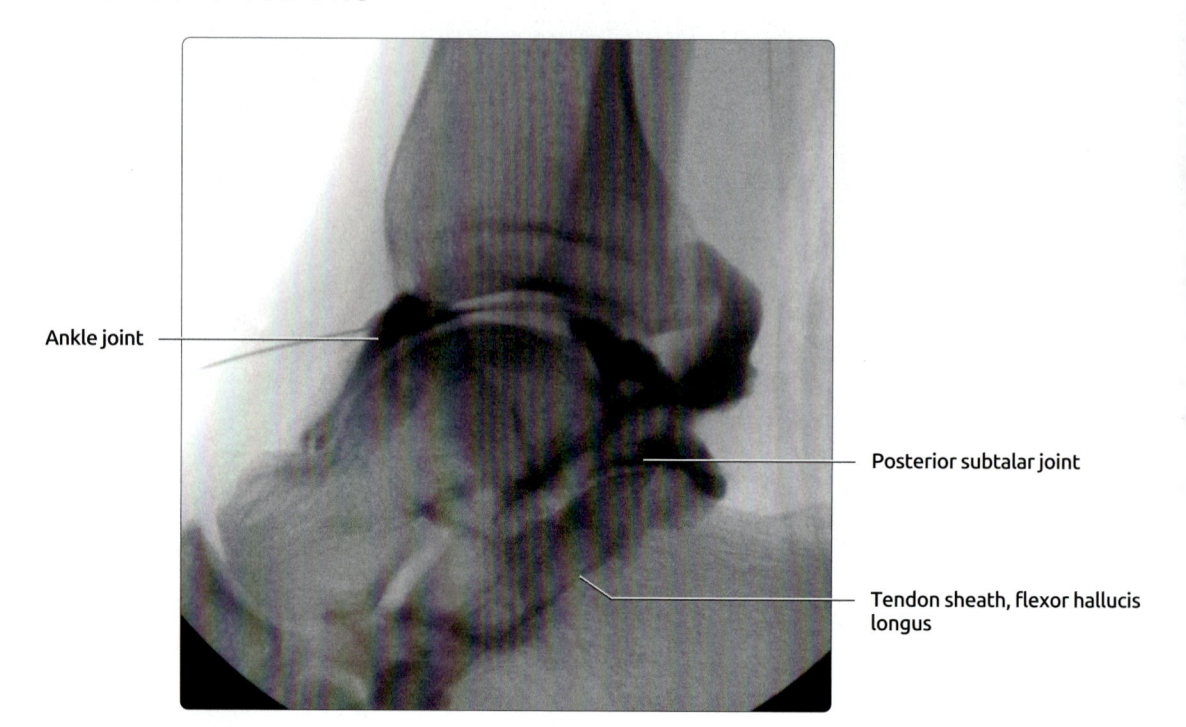

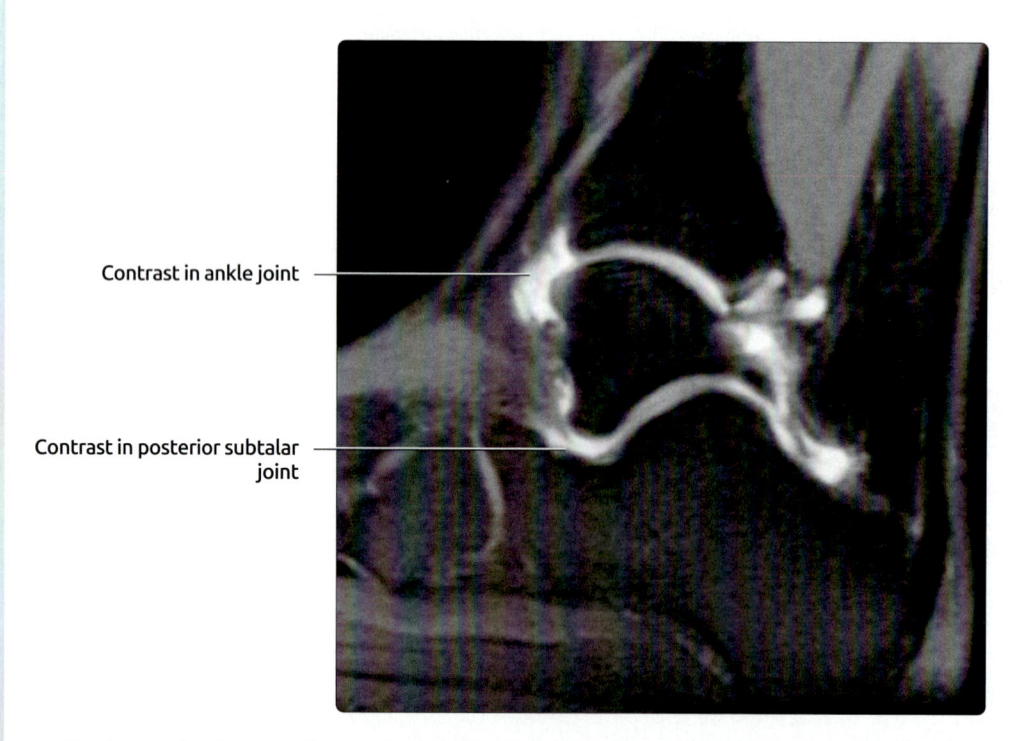

(Top) Lateral arthrogram shows communication of the ankle joint with the flexor hallucis longus tendon sheath and the posterior subtalar joint. Communication to the flexor hallucis longus tendon sheath is always present, but communication with the posterior subtalar joint happens in only 10-15% of the population. (Bottom) Sagittal T1 FS MR arthrogram shows contrast filling ankle and posterior subtalar joints.

ACCESSORY OSSIFICATION CENTER, MEDIAL MALLEOLUS

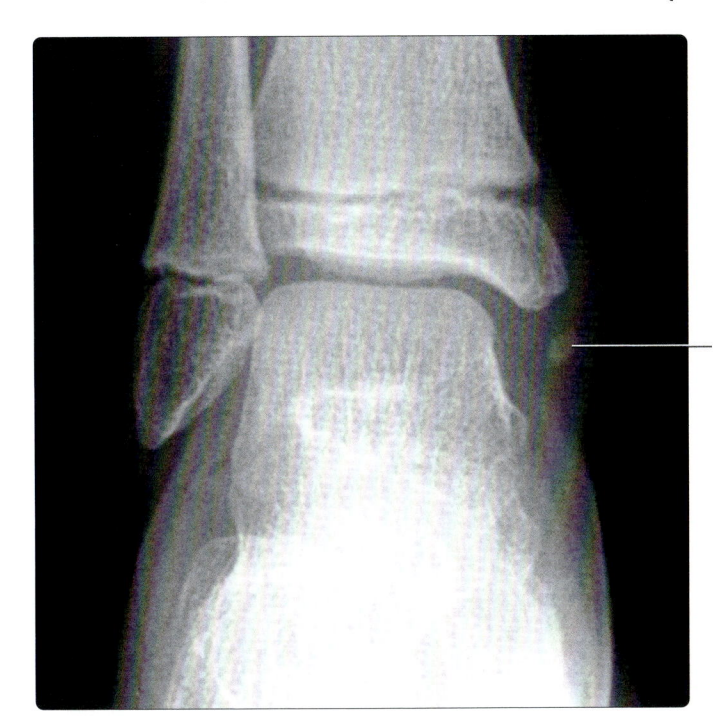

Accessory center of ossification, medial malleolus

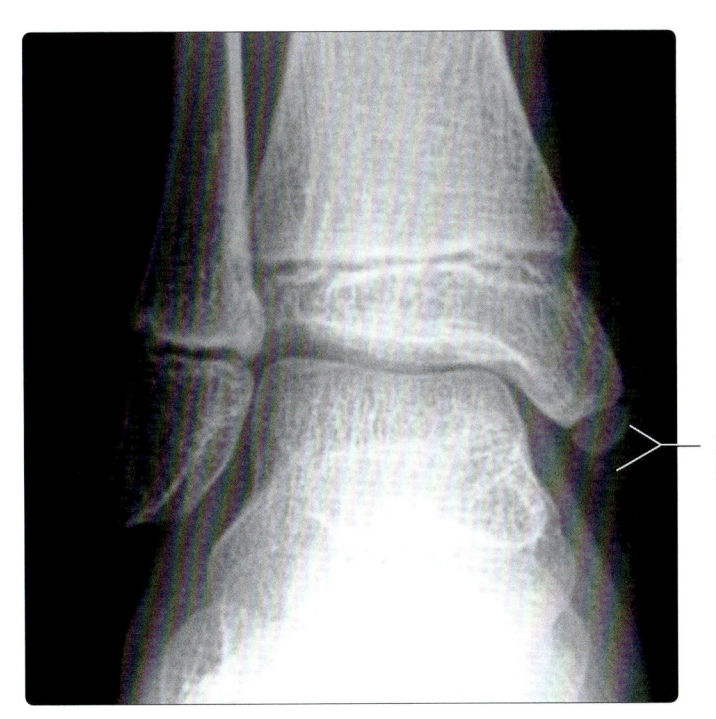

Bipartite accessory of medial malleolus ossification center

(Top) Anteroposterior radiograph shows os subtibiale (accessory medial malleolus center of ossification) in a child. This ossicle occurs in ~ 20% of children, becoming radiographically apparent between 7 and 10 years of age and fusing at skeletal maturity. It may be symptomatic due to injury of synchondrosis, uniting it to the remainder of medial malleolus. (Bottom) Anteroposterior radiograph in a different child shows bipartite os subtibiale (accessory center of ossification of medial malleolus).

Foot and Ankle Normal Variants and Imaging Pitfalls

ACCESSORY OSSIFICATION CENTER, LATERAL MALLEOLUS

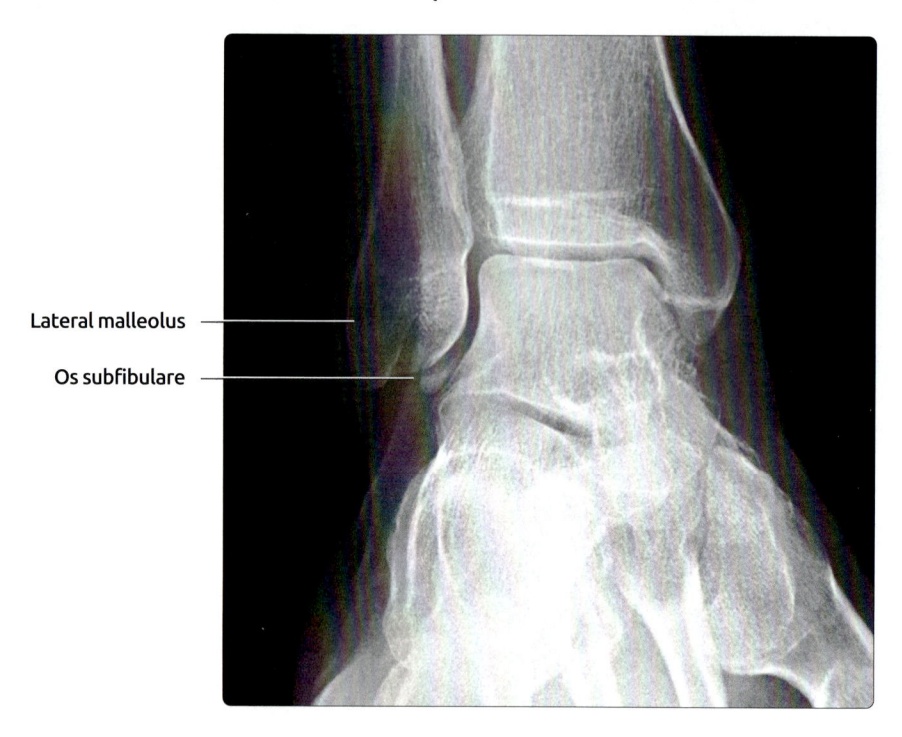

Lateral malleolus
Os subfibulare

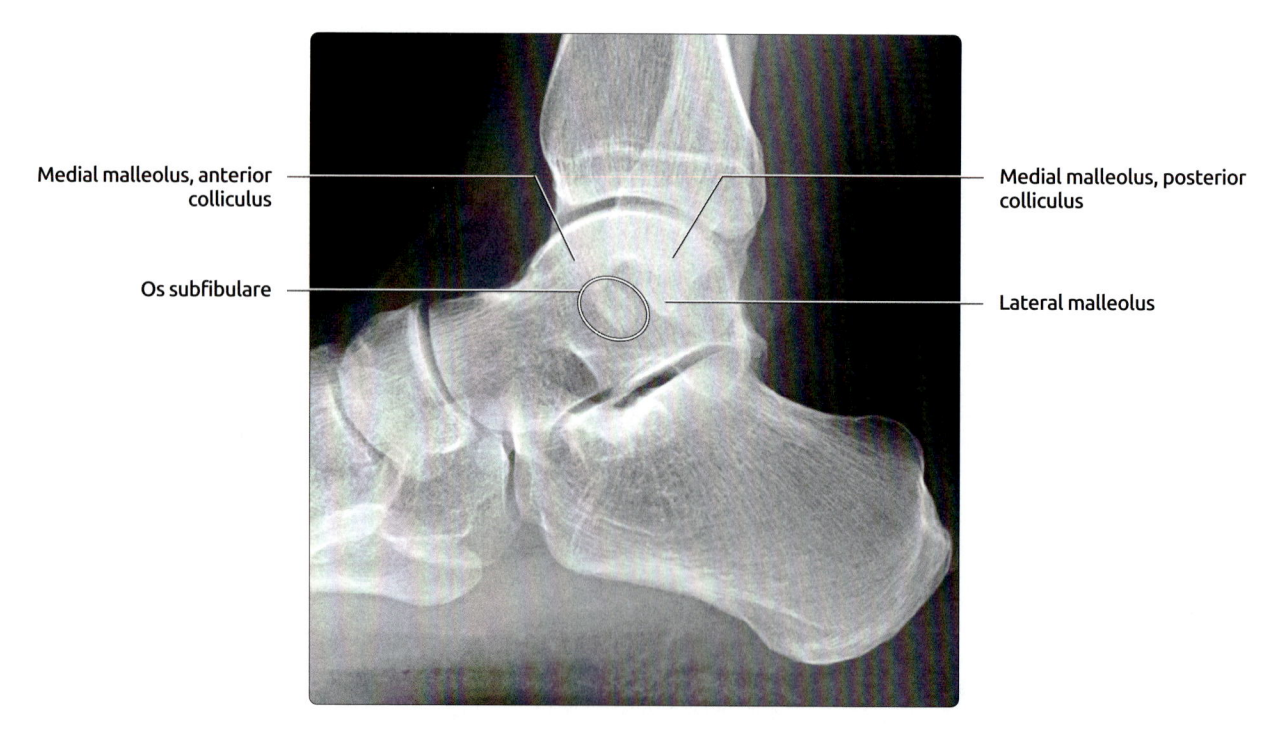

Medial malleolus, anterior colliculus
Os subfibulare
Medial malleolus, posterior colliculus
Lateral malleolus

(Top) Mortise view shows os subfibulare in an adult patient. Os subfibulare occurs in ~ 1% of children but usually fuses by adulthood. Shape of ossicle as well as normal size and configuration of adjacent lateral malleolus help to distinguish ossicle from nonunited fracture. (Bottom) Lateral radiograph in the same patient shows the characteristic location of os subfibulare at the anteroinferior margin of the fibula. Overlap of malleoli may initially be confusing on lateral radiographs, but malleoli and lateral malleolar accessory center of ossification can reliably be identified.

Foot and Ankle Normal Variants and Imaging Pitfalls

OS TRIGONUM AND STIEDA PROCESS

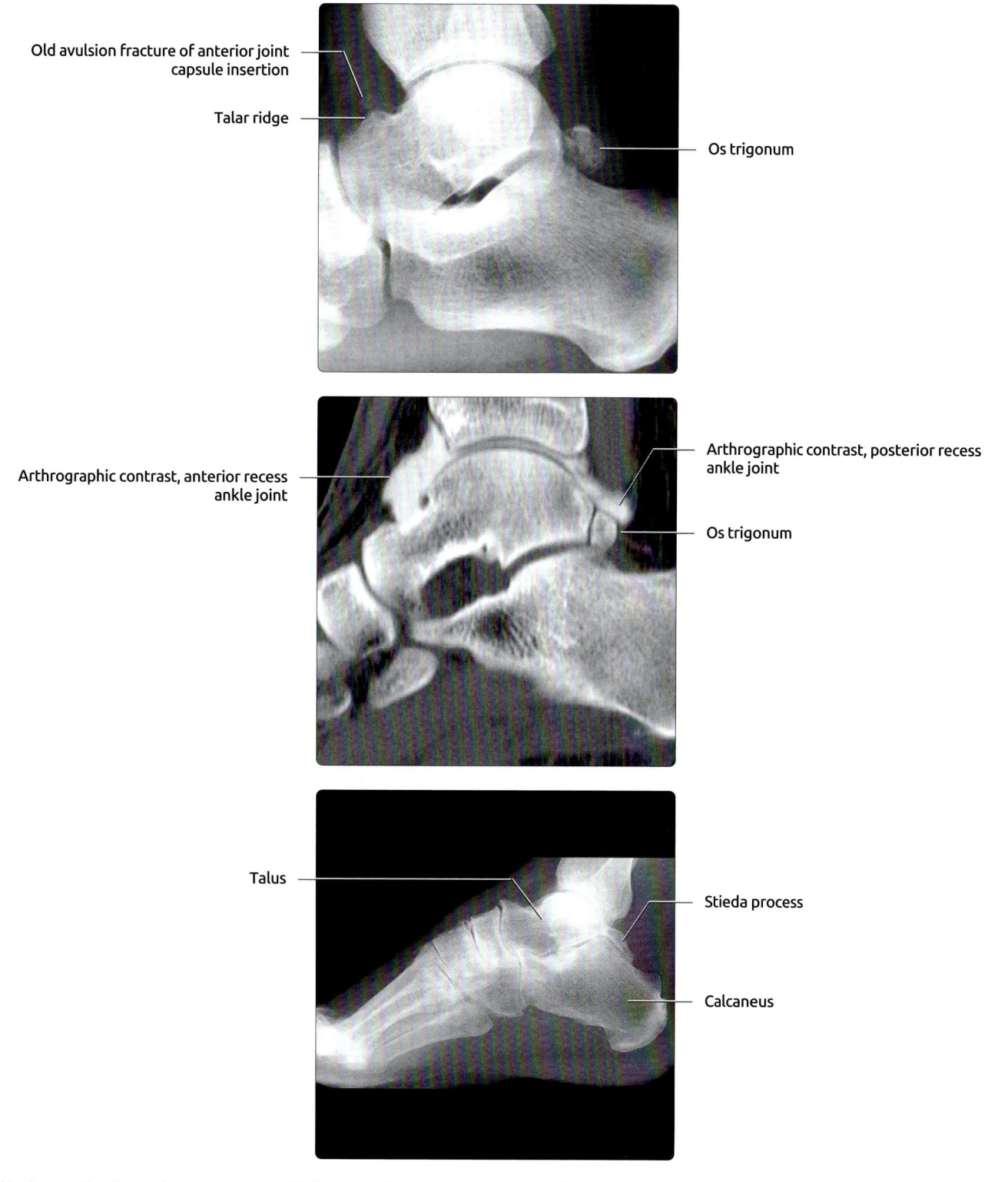

Old avulsion fracture of anterior joint capsule insertion

Talar ridge

Os trigonum

Arthrographic contrast, anterior recess ankle joint

Arthrographic contrast, posterior recess ankle joint

Os trigonum

Talus

Stieda process

Calcaneus

(Top) *Lateral radiograph shows an unusually large os trigonum. Cysts in the ossicle suggest os trigonum syndrome in which there is impingement of the ossicle against talus or flexor hallucis longus. Note that the patient also has a slightly prominent talar ridge, another normal variant. Ossicle adjacent to the talar ridge is an old fracture, not a normal variant.* (Middle) *Sagittal CT arthrogram shows contrast in the ankle joint flowing smoothly over the superior margin of a triangular os trigonum.* (Bottom) *Lateral radiograph shows a Stieda process, an elongated lateral tubercle of the posterior process of the talus. The Stieda process, while a normal variant, can predispose to posterior impingement of the ankle or flexor hallucis longus tendon, especially in plantar flexion.*

Foot and Ankle Normal Variants and Imaging Pitfalls

CALCANEAL VARIANTS

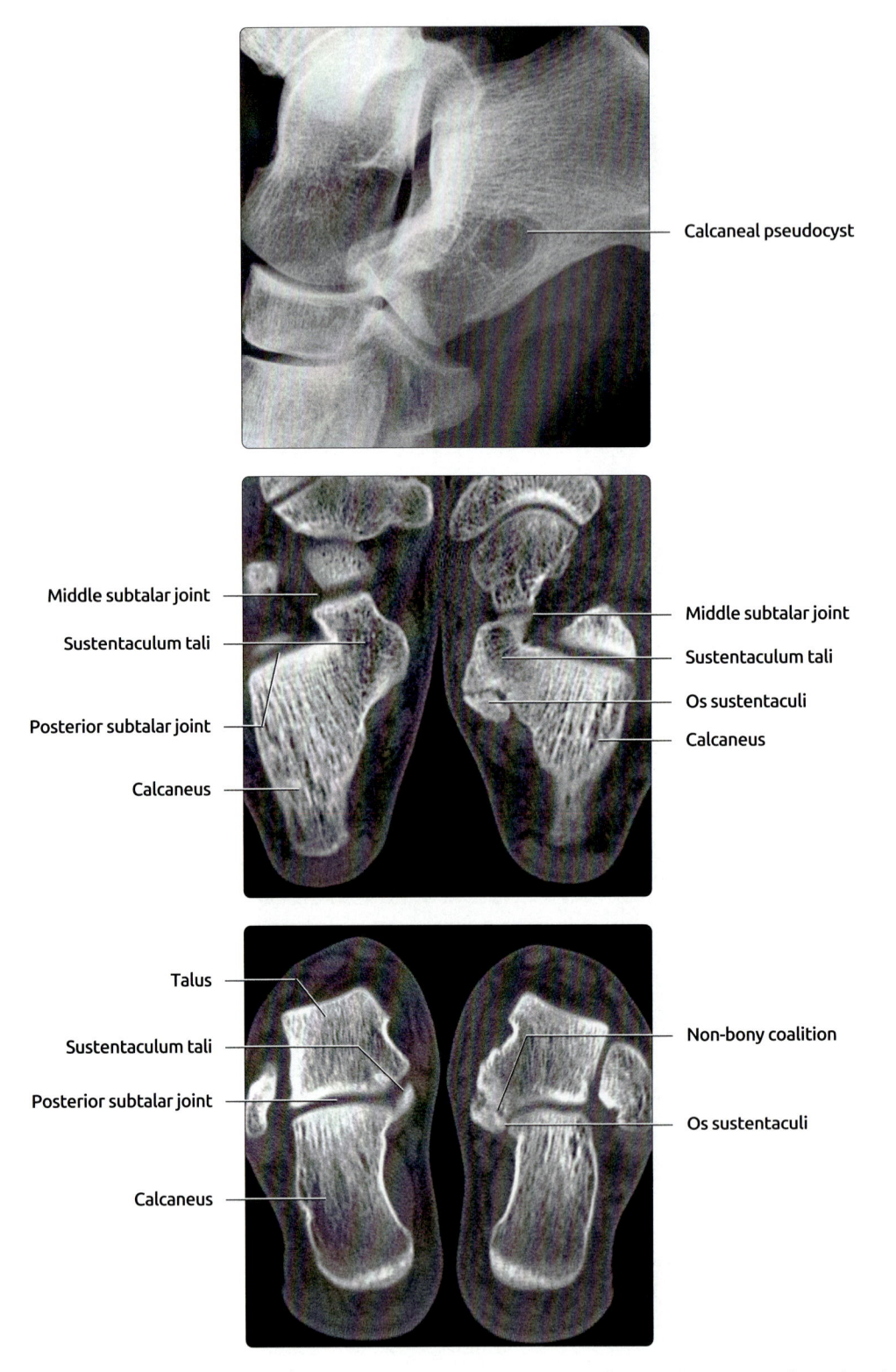

(Top) Lateral radiograph shows a calcaneal pseudocyst. This area of lucency is seen inferior to the sustentaculum tali and reflects the normal paucity of trabeculae in this region. True cysts and lipomas also occur in this region but will show a more well-defined and continuous border. (Middle) Axial oblique CT shows left foot os sustentaculi, a rare ossicle arising from the calcaneus at the posterior margin of sustentaculum tali. The right side is normal. (Bottom) Coronal CT through left-sided os sustentaculi, posterior to sustentaculum tali is shown. Note the non-bony coalition between os sustentaculi and talus, a common finding with this ossicle. Right foot is normal.

Foot and Ankle Normal Variants and Imaging Pitfalls

CALCANEAL VARIANTS

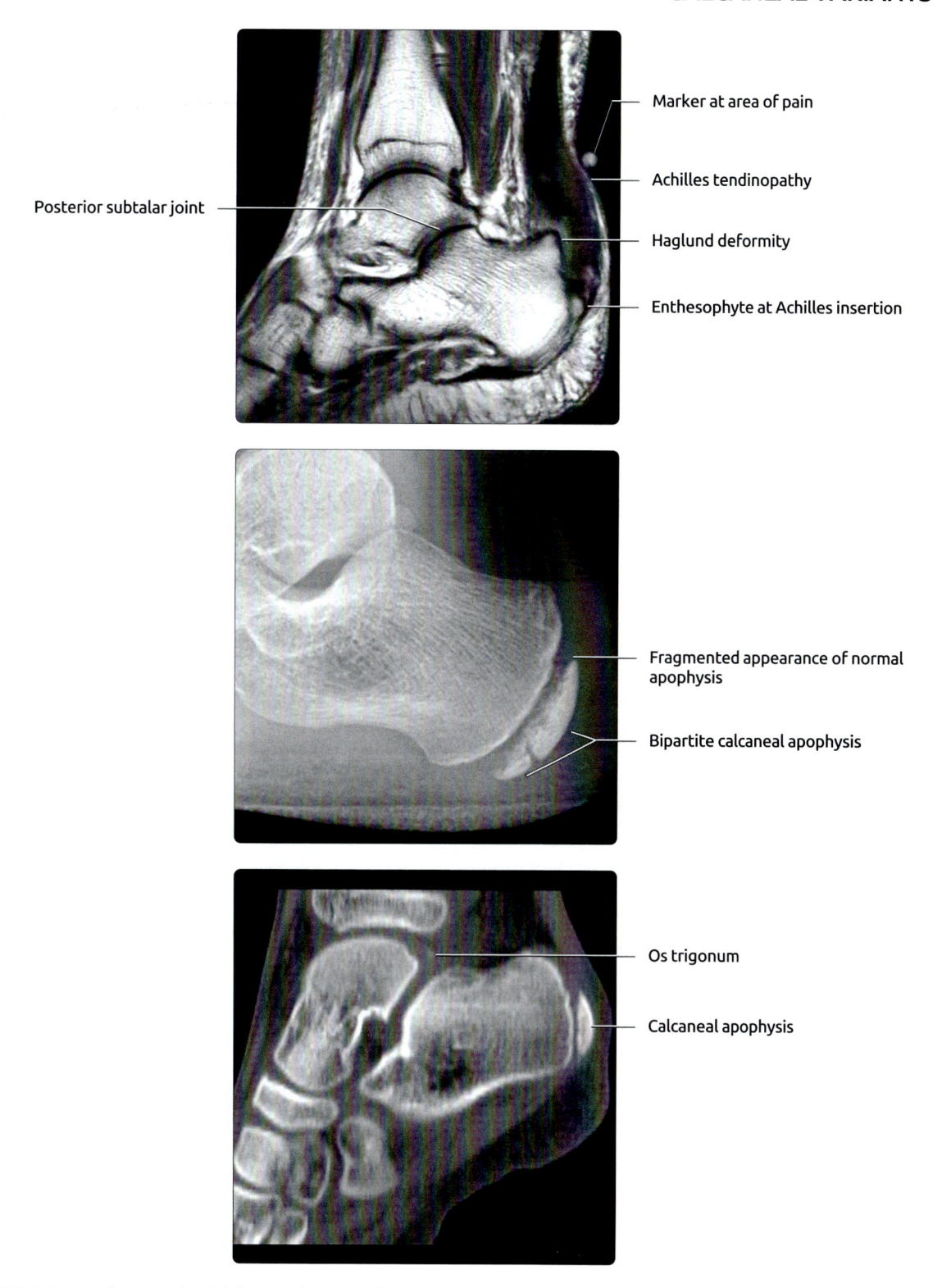

(Top) Sagittal T1WI shows a large Haglund deformity (known as "pump bump"). This is prominence of superior margin of posterior process calcaneus. This normal variant often impinges against high backs of shoes and results in retrocalcaneal bursitis as well as Achilles tendinopathy. (Middle) Lateral radiograph in a child shows bipartite and sclerotic calcaneal apophysis. At the superior margin, apophysis appears to have several tiny fragments, also a normal variant. (Bottom) Sagittal CT shows the normal sclerotic appearance of calcaneal apophysis in a child. Note the undulating contour of adjacent metaphysis, also a normal variant. This patient has also begun to form an os trigonum.

Foot and Ankle Normal Variants and Imaging Pitfalls

CALCANEAL VARIANTS

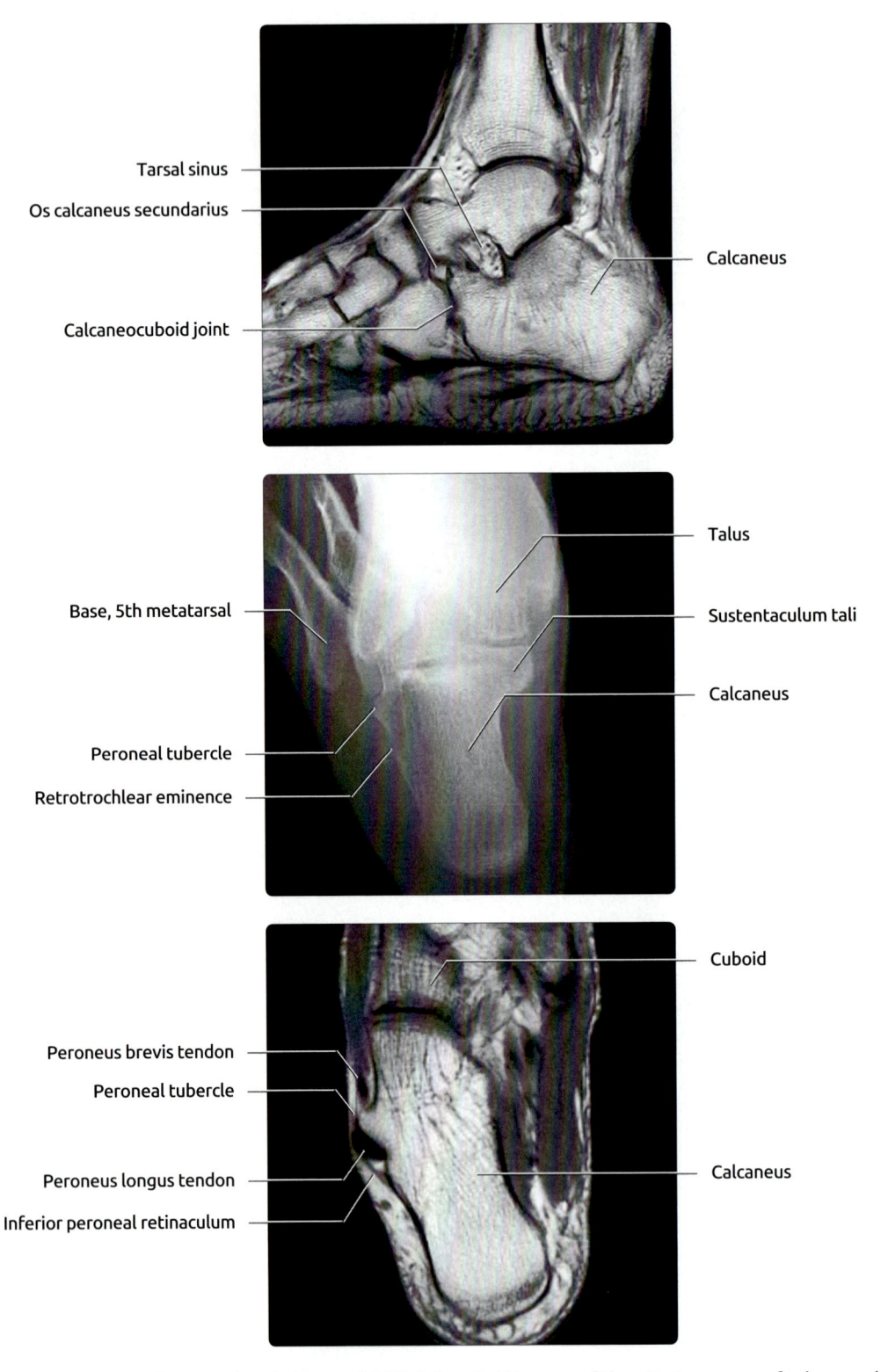

Labels (Top image): Tarsal sinus; Os calcaneus secundarius; Calcaneocuboid joint; Calcaneus

Labels (Middle image): Base, 5th metatarsal; Peroneal tubercle; Retrotrochlear eminence; Talus; Sustentaculum tali; Calcaneus

Labels (Bottom image): Peroneus brevis tendon; Peroneal tubercle; Peroneus longus tendon; Inferior peroneal retinaculum; Cuboid; Calcaneus

(Top) Os calcaneus secundarius, with an incidence of 2-7%, is found at the apex of the anterior process of calcaneus, between the talar head, navicular, and cuboid. The os may be angular or round and may be confused with an old avulsion fracture at the calcaneal origin of the bifurcate ligament. **(Middle)** Calcaneal (a.k.a. axial or Harris) view shows a small peroneal tubercle. The peroneal tubercle, also called trochlear process, is a protuberance of lateral calcaneal wall and is present in ~ 40% of individuals. It separates the peroneus longus and brevis tendons. **(Bottom)** Axial MR of the ankle depicts mildly enlarged peroneal tubercle. The peroneus brevis and peroneus longus tendons are anterior and posterior to the tubercle, respectively. Fibers from the inferior peroneal retinaculum insert on the peroneal tubercle, forming 2 fibroosseous tunnels for each peroneal tendon.

Foot and Ankle Normal Variants and Imaging Pitfalls

MARROW VARIANT, PEDIATRIC

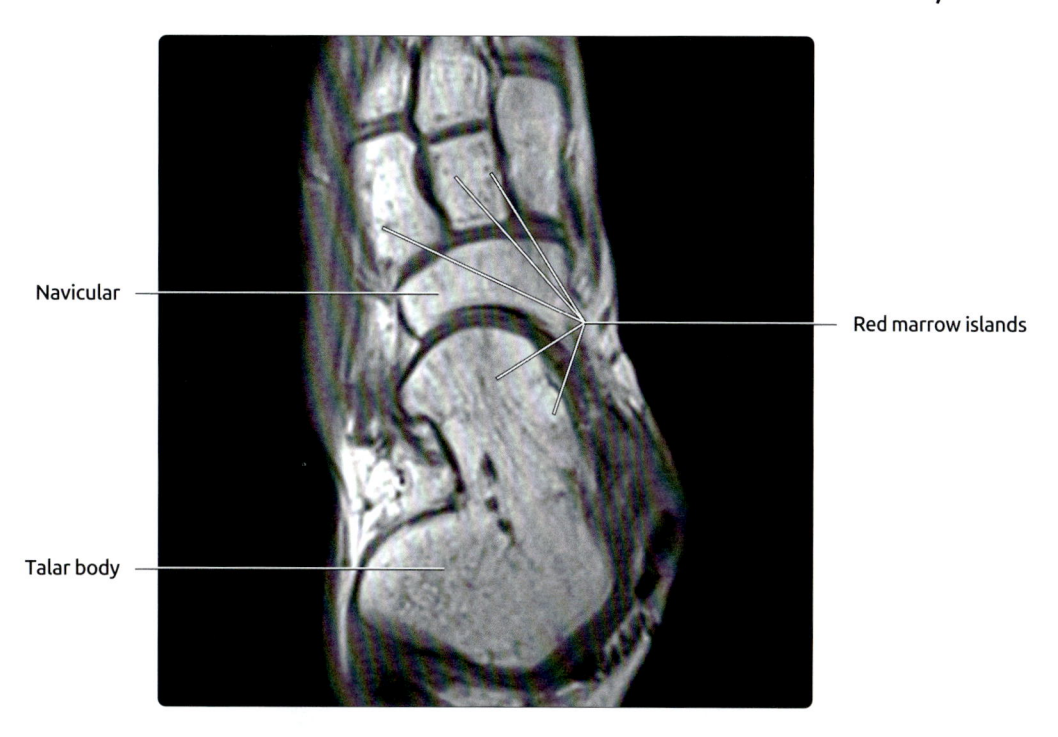

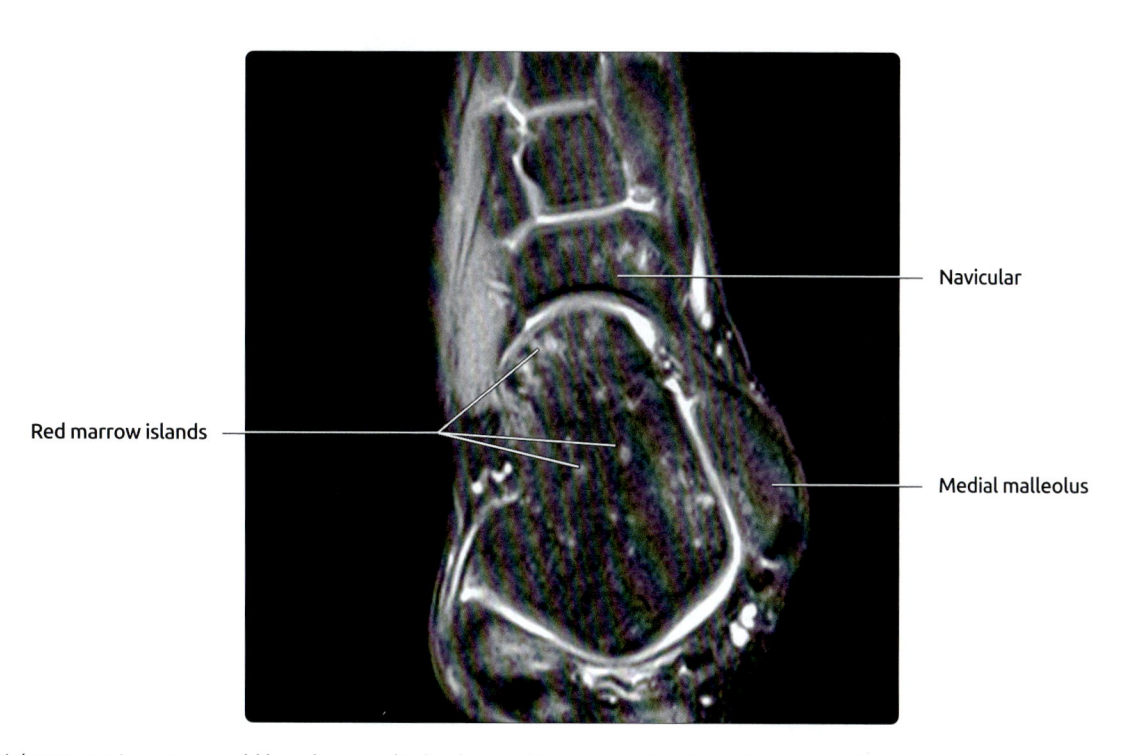

(Top) Axial T1WI MR in a 12-year-old boy shows multiple islands of low signal intensity in the marrow. These are thought to represent residual erythropoietic marrow and resolve by about age 13-14. (Bottom) Axial PD FS MR in the same patient shows the red marrow foci become bright on fluid-sensitive sequences. A few of the foci are labeled. Patient age, the generalized distribution of small foci, and the absence of localizing findings are helpful in making the correct diagnosis of residual erythropoietic marrow.

ACCESSORY NAVICULAR BONE

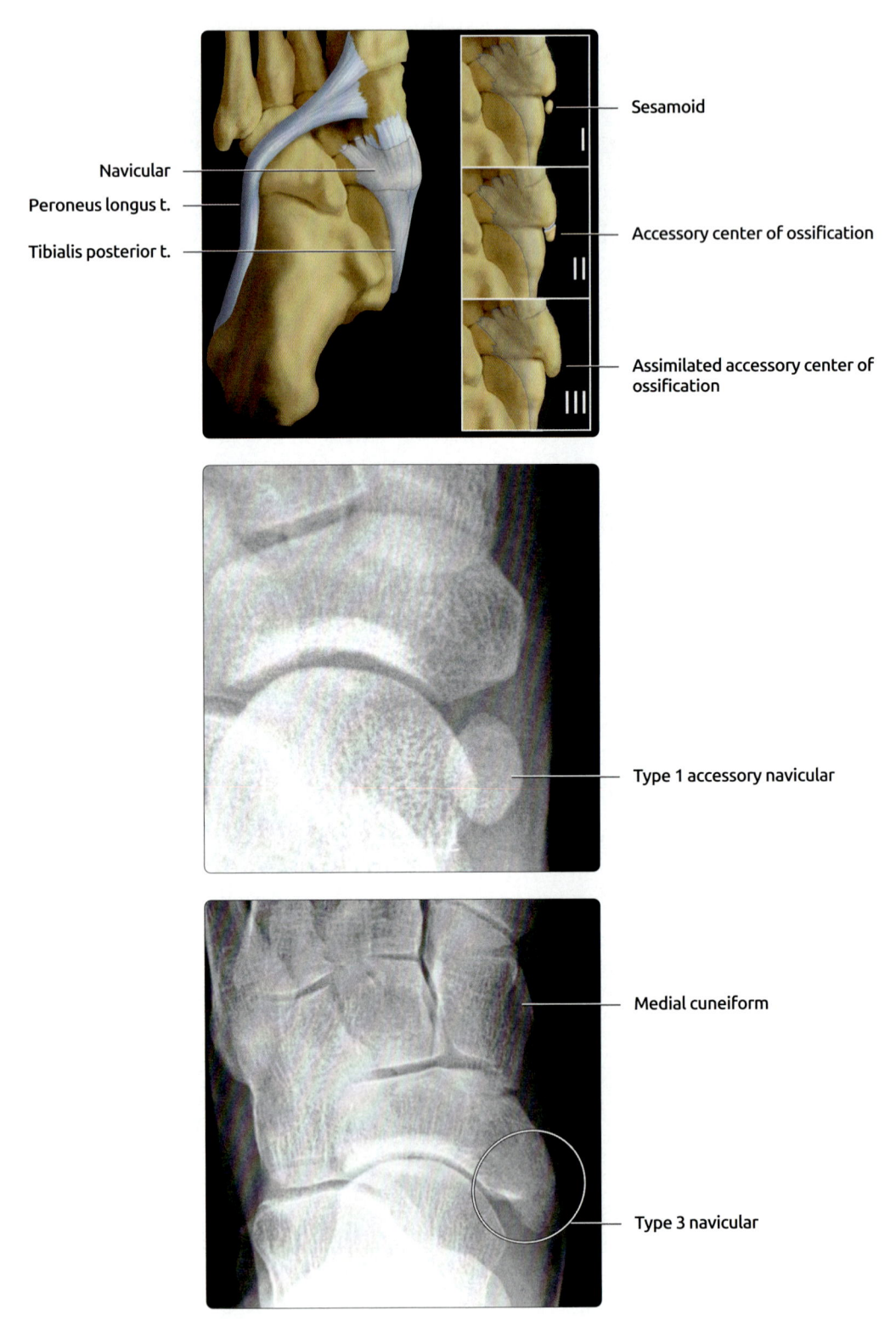

Labels (top graphic): Navicular; Peroneus longus t.; Tibialis posterior t.; Sesamoid (I); Accessory center of ossification (II); Assimilated accessory center of ossification (III)

Labels (middle radiograph): Type 1 accessory navicular

Labels (bottom radiograph): Medial cuneiform; Type 3 navicular

(Top) Graphic shows plantar view of accessory navicular (os tibiale externum) variants. Normally, tibialis posterior tendon attaches to plantar aspect of median eminence of navicular. A type 1 accessory navicular is a sesamoid in posterior tibial tendon. Type 2 is accessory center of ossification. Type 3 is an elongated median eminence ("cornuate navicular"). (Middle) Anteroposterior radiograph shows large type 1 accessory navicular. This ossicle is larger than most type 1 accessory naviculars. It is distinguished from type 2 by the lack of an articular facet with the main navicular body. (Bottom) Anteroposterior radiograph shows a type 3 navicular, also called cornuate or gorilloid. This is an assimilated accessory navicular ossicle, which forms a projection at the medial eminence of the navicular. This configuration may cause impingement on shoes, especially on ski boots.

Foot and Ankle Normal Variants and Imaging Pitfalls

ACCESSORY NAVICULAR BONE

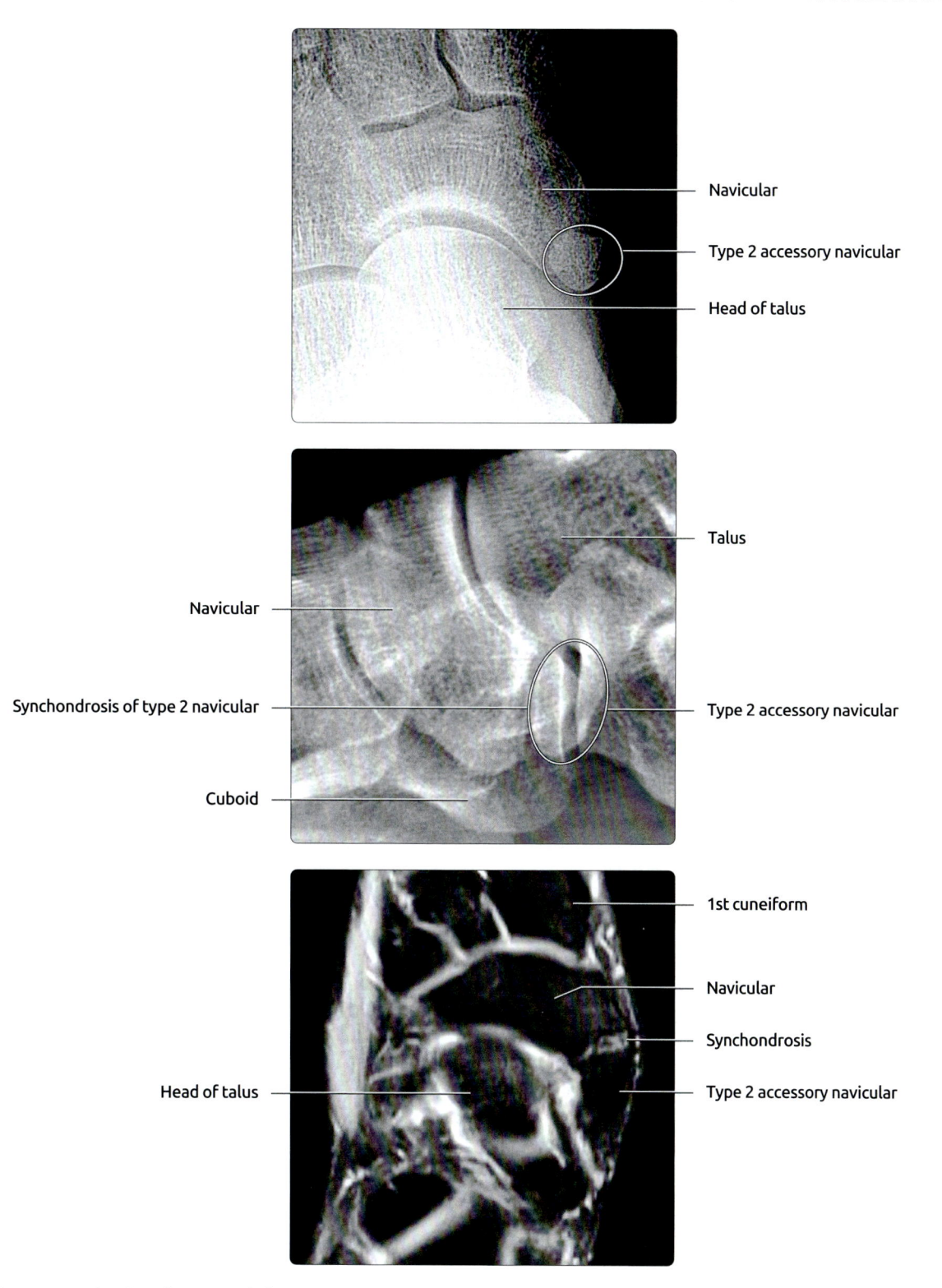

(Top) Anteroposterior view shows rounded type 2 accessory navicular overlying medial eminence of navicular. Synchondrosis with navicular may or may not be seen in the profile on anteroposterior view. (Middle) Lateral radiograph in the same patient shows characteristic, relatively plantar position of accessory navicular. Note its flat anterior facet where it is joined through a synchondrosis to the main navicular. (Bottom) Axial PD MR with FS shows type 2 accessory navicular having a flat facet joined by a synchondrosis to parent navicular.

ACCESSORY NAVICULAR BONE

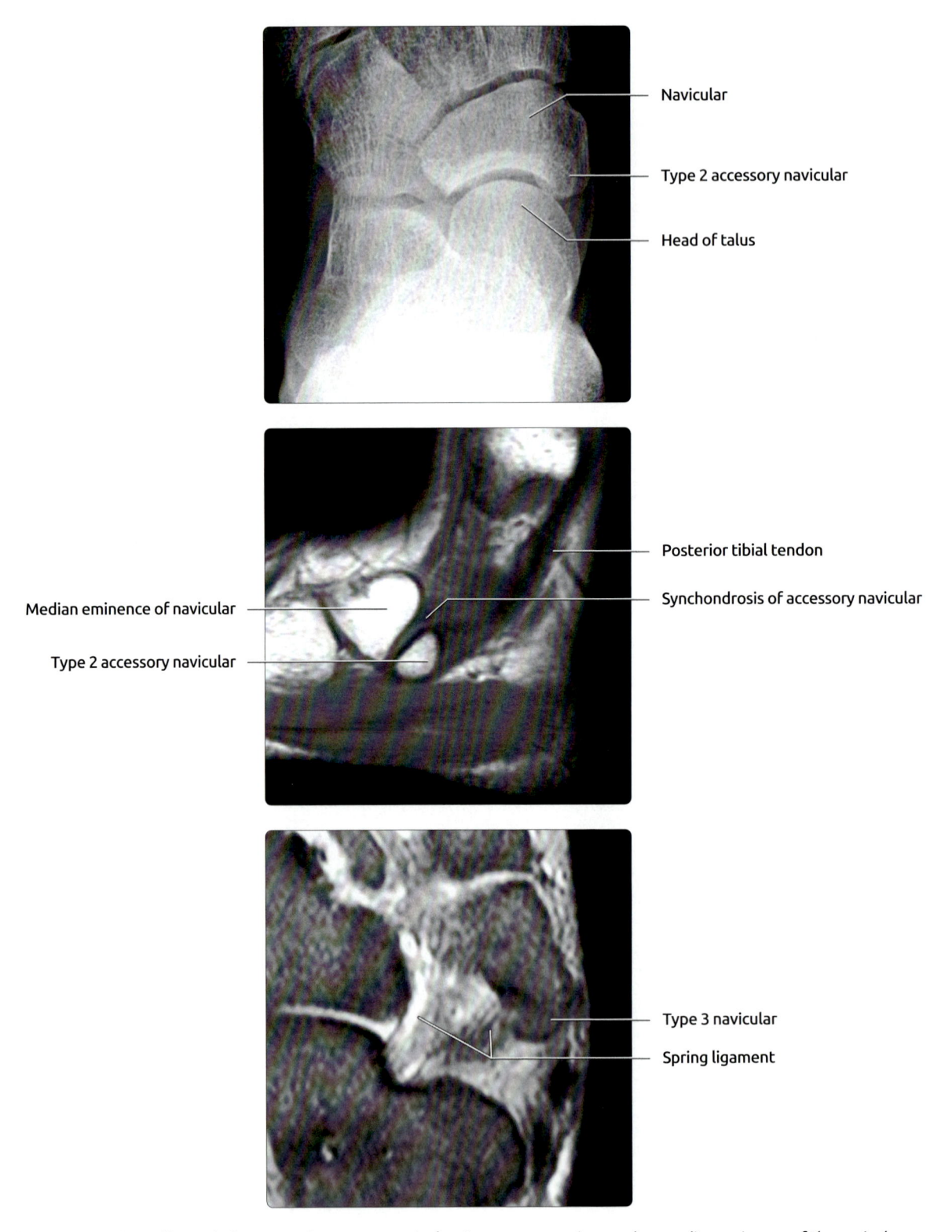

(Top) Anteroposterior radiograph shows type 2 accessory navicular. It appears superimposed on median eminence of the navicular because it is at the plantar margin of navicular. (Middle) Sagittal PD MR in the same patient shows plantar position of type 2 accessory navicular relative to the median eminence of navicular. The accessory ossicle has a flat superior facet and articulates with the navicular via a synchondrosis. Note the attachment of the posterior tibial tendon to accessory navicular, stressing the synchondrosis and predisposing to posterior tibial tendon dysfunction. (Bottom) Axial PD FS MR shows a type 3 accessory navicular. The spring ligament is seen attaching both to the bony prominence and more medially to the main portion of the navicular.

Foot and Ankle Normal Variants and Imaging Pitfalls

NAVICULAR VARIANTS

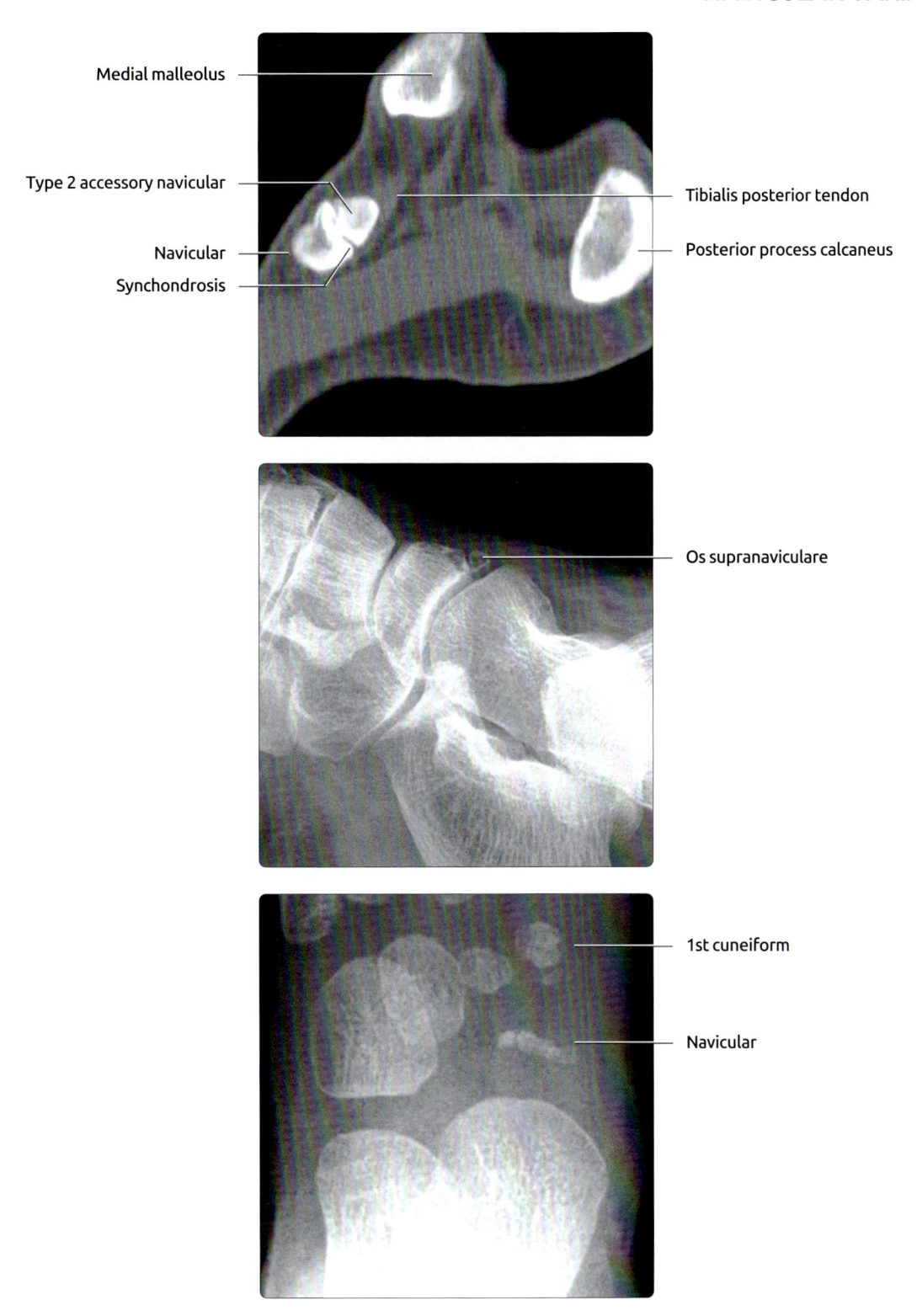

(Top) Sagittal CT shows type 2 accessory navicular and a synchondrosis. (Middle) Lateral radiograph shows a triangular ossicle at the proximal, dorsal margin of the navicular. Os supranaviculare is also known as os talonaviculare dorsale or Pirie bone. Many so-called cases of os supranaviculare probably represent old, nonunited fractures. (Bottom) Anteroposterior radiograph shows an irregular, flattened, sclerotic but asymptomatic navicular. The appearance resolves as the child grows. Note also the dual ossification centers for the 1st cuneiform, also a normal variant. Köhler disease is avascular necrosis of navicular in childhood and has the same appearance.

Foot and Ankle Normal Variants and Imaging Pitfalls

OS CUBOIDES SECONDARIUM

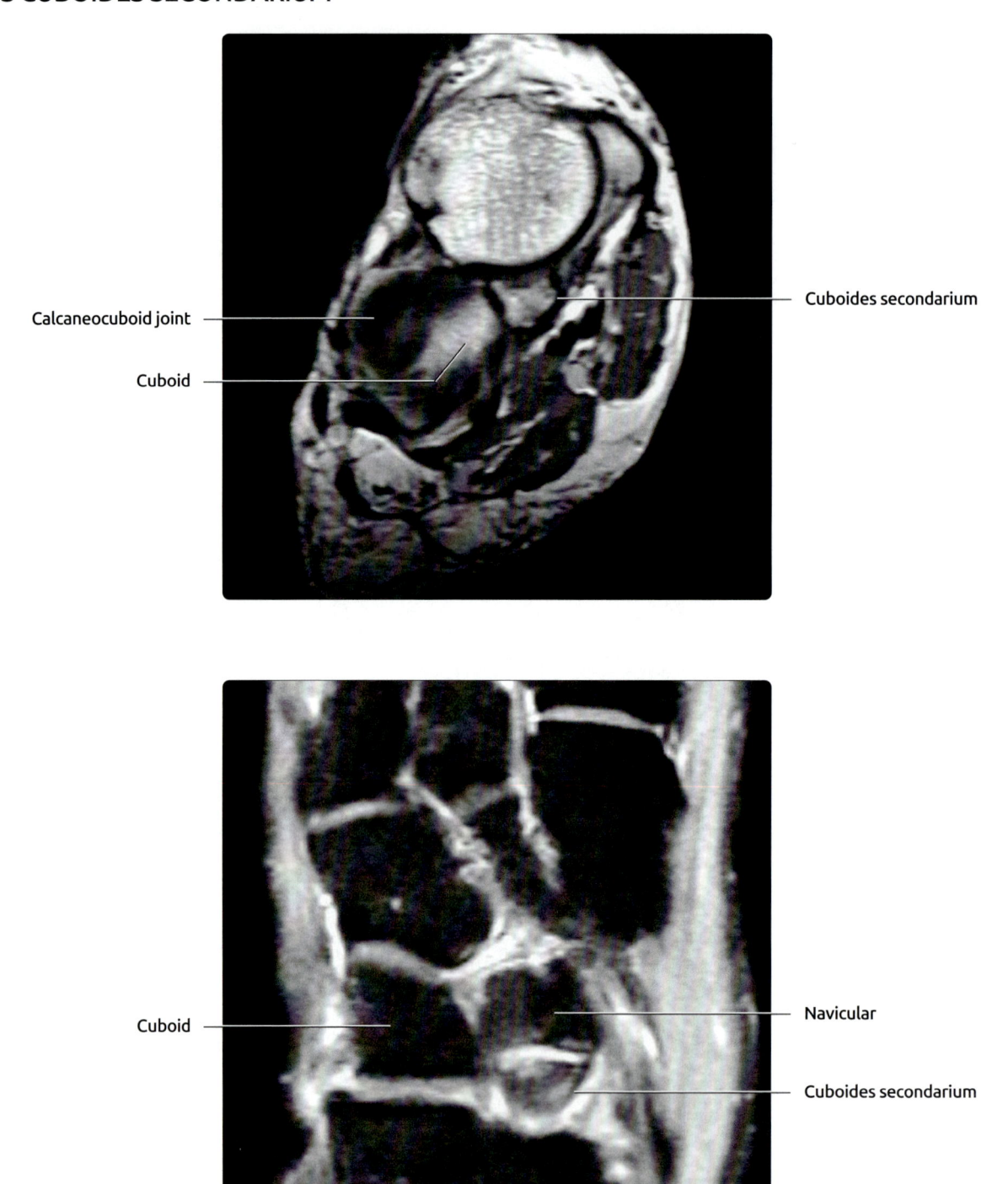

(Top) Coronal T1 MR shows cuboides secondarium ossicle at the proximal, medial, and superior margin of the cuboid between the cuboid and the navicular. This ossicle is rare and difficult to see on radiographs. (Bottom) Axial PD FS MR shows the relationship of the cuboides secondarium ossicle to both the cuboid and navicular.

Foot and Ankle Normal Variants and Imaging Pitfalls

OS PERONEUM

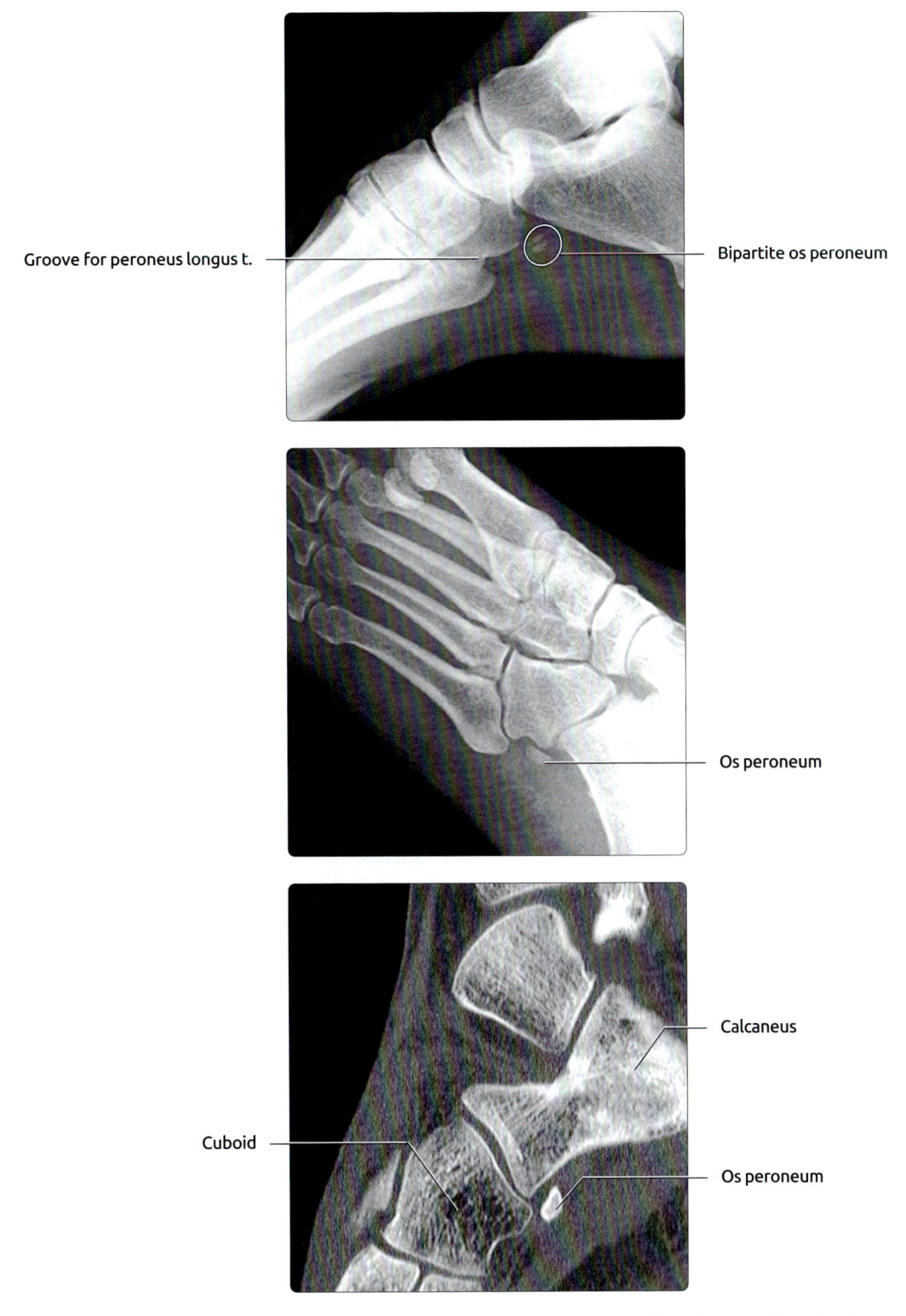

(Top) Lateral radiograph shows bipartite os peroneum. The os peroneum may be unipartite, bipartite, or multipartite. It lies in the peroneus longus tendon, adjacent to the calcaneocuboid joint or cuboid. Proximal displacement of os peroneum can be seen as a radiographic manifestation of a peroneus longus tendon rupture. (Middle) Oblique radiograph shows unipartite os peroneum. The ossicle is just proximal to the point where the peroneus longus courses under the cuboid sulcus. (Bottom) Sagittal CT reformation depicts an os peroneum adjacent to the calcaneocuboid joint.

Foot and Ankle Normal Variants and Imaging Pitfalls

OS VESALIANUM

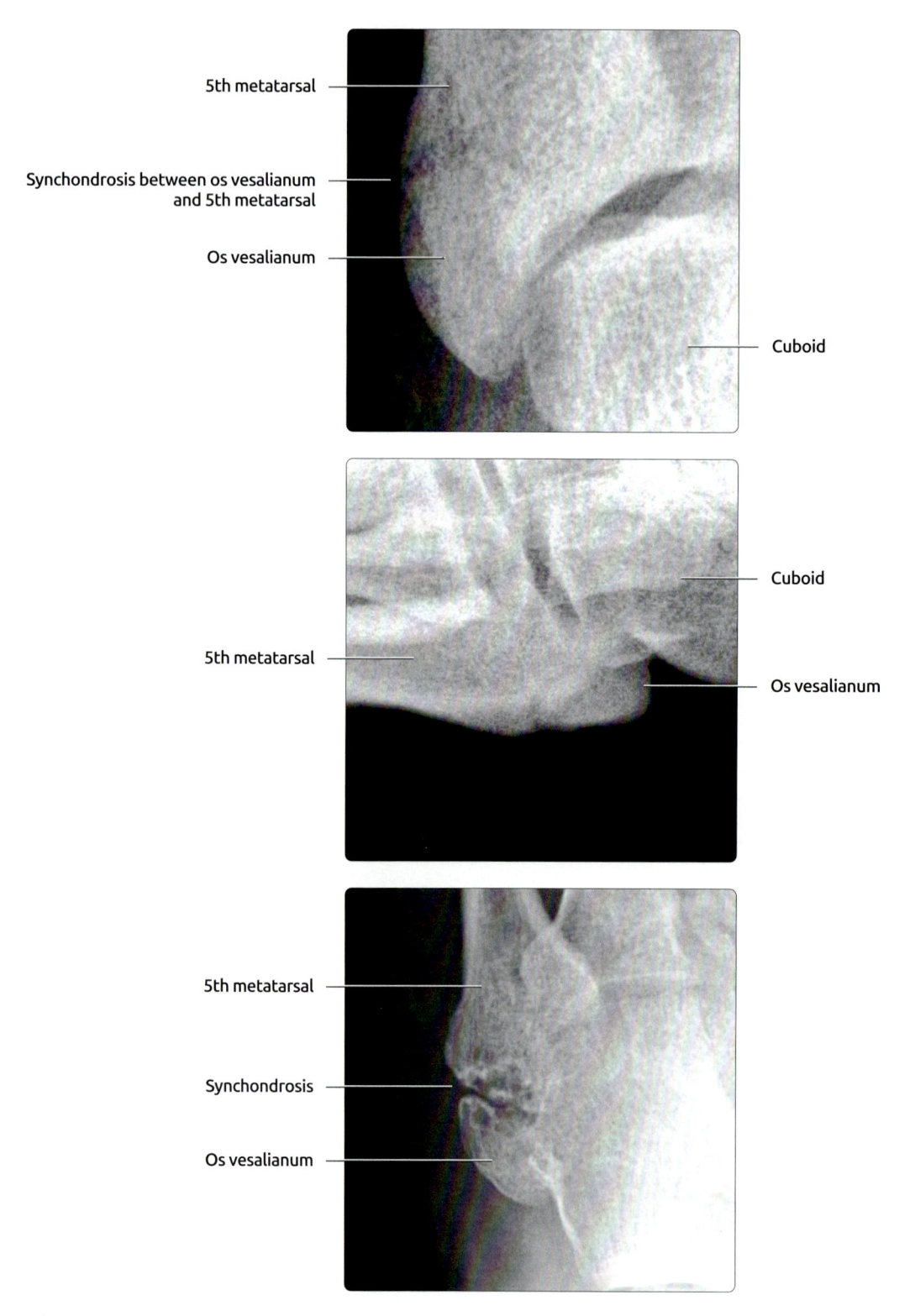

(Top) On anteroposterior radiograph, the os vesalianum overlies the styloid process of the 5th metatarsal, and a synchondrosis may be mistaken for a fracture. (Middle) Lateral radiograph in the same patient shows the rounded contour of the ossicle, consistent with accessory center of ossification rather than a fracture. (Bottom) Anteroposterior radiograph shows a different patient with a large os vesalianum and multiple cysts at the synchondrosis between the os and the 5th metatarsal base. Cysts are most likely stress-related, due to tugging of the peroneus brevis on the os vesalianum and indirectly on the synchondrosis.

Foot and Ankle Normal Variants and Imaging Pitfalls

TARSOMETATARSAL JOINT VARIANTS

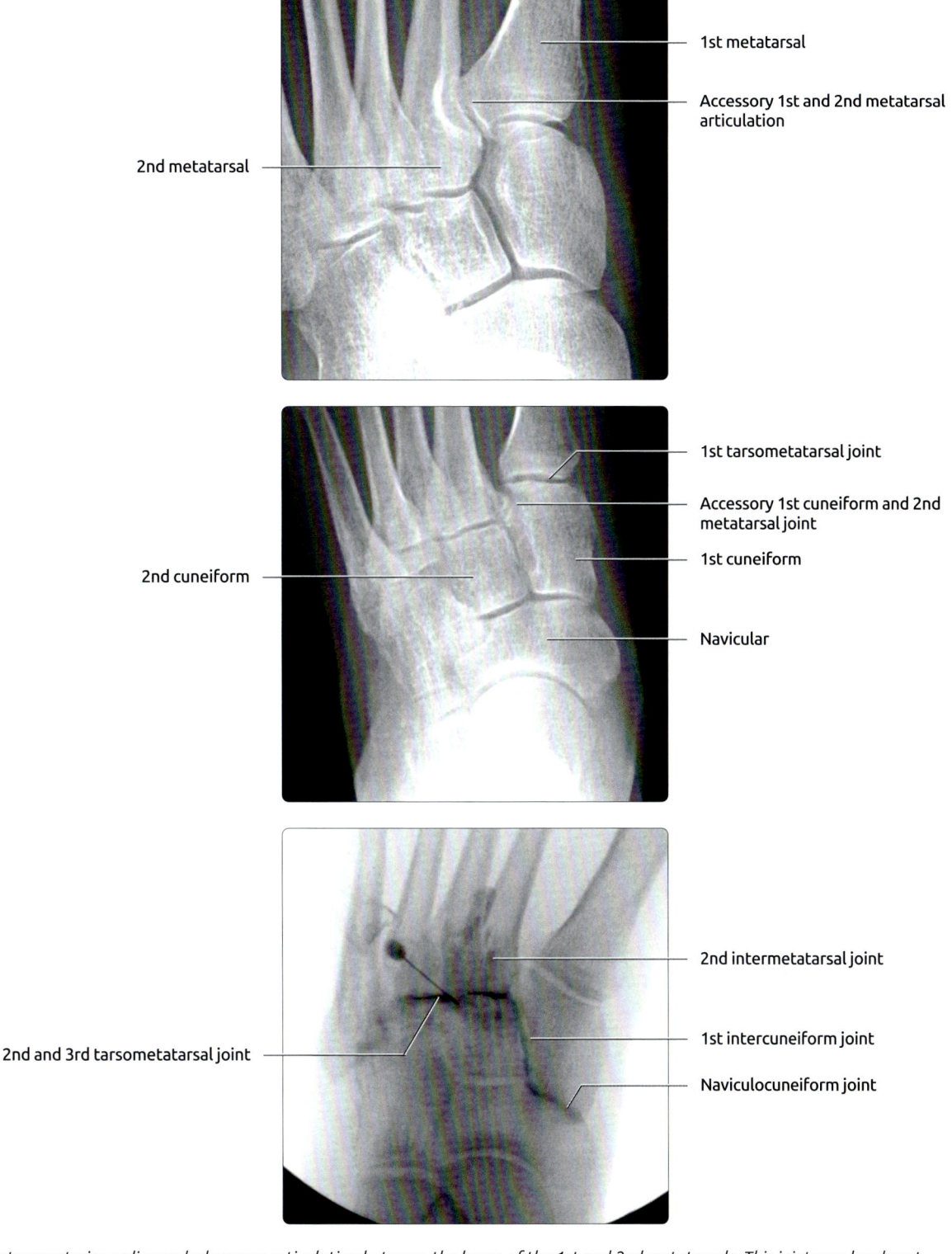

(Top) Anteroposterior radiograph shows an articulation between the bases of the 1st and 2nd metatarsals. This joint may be absent, small, or fairly large, as in this case. (Middle) Anteroposterior radiograph shows an uncommon accessory articulation between the 1st cuneiform and the 2nd metatarsal. (Bottom) Anteroposterior image from the 3rd tarsometatarsal arthrogram shows a normal variant of extension of contrast between 1st and 2nd cuneiforms as well as into naviculocuneiform joint. In most feet, the 2nd and 3rd tarsometatarsal joints form a separate cavity. Extension into the 2nd intermetatarsal joint is usually present, as in this case.

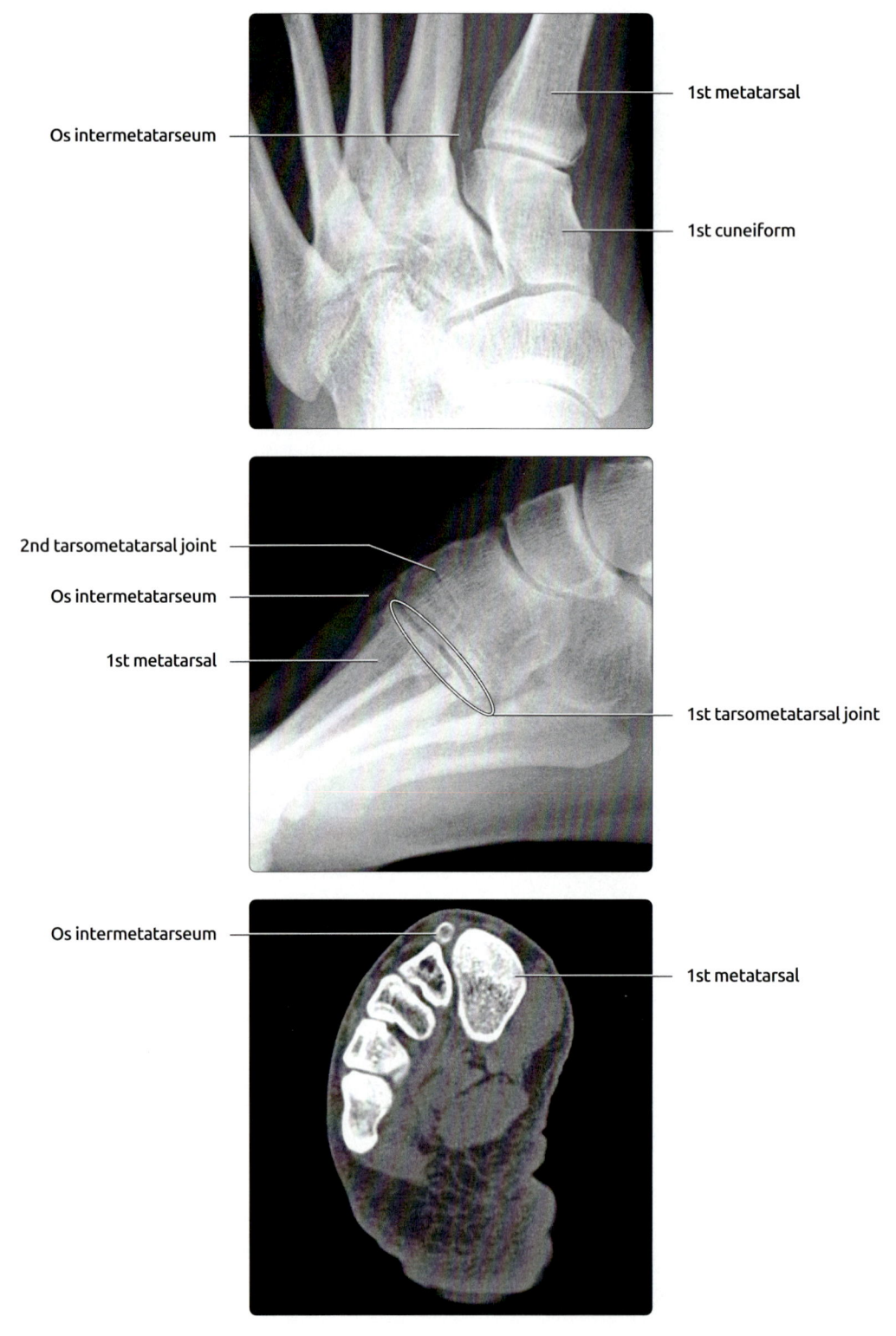

OS INTERMETATARSEUM

Os intermetatarseum — 1st metatarsal — 1st cuneiform

2nd tarsometatarsal joint — Os intermetatarseum — 1st metatarsal — 1st tarsometatarsal joint

Os intermetatarseum — 1st metatarsal

(Top) Anteroposterior radiograph shows a teardrop-shaped os intermetatarseum arising between the 1st and 2nd metatarsal bases. Occasionally, this ossicle will be partially assimilated to the 1st metatarsal base. **(Middle)** On this lateral radiograph, the ossicle is dorsal in position, adjacent to the base of the 1st metatarsal. **(Bottom)** On this coronal CT, the os intermetatarseum is rounded in appearance, and no donor site from adjacent bones is visible. These signs help distinguish it from a fracture fragment.

Foot and Ankle Normal Variants and Imaging Pitfalls

METATARSAL VARIANTS

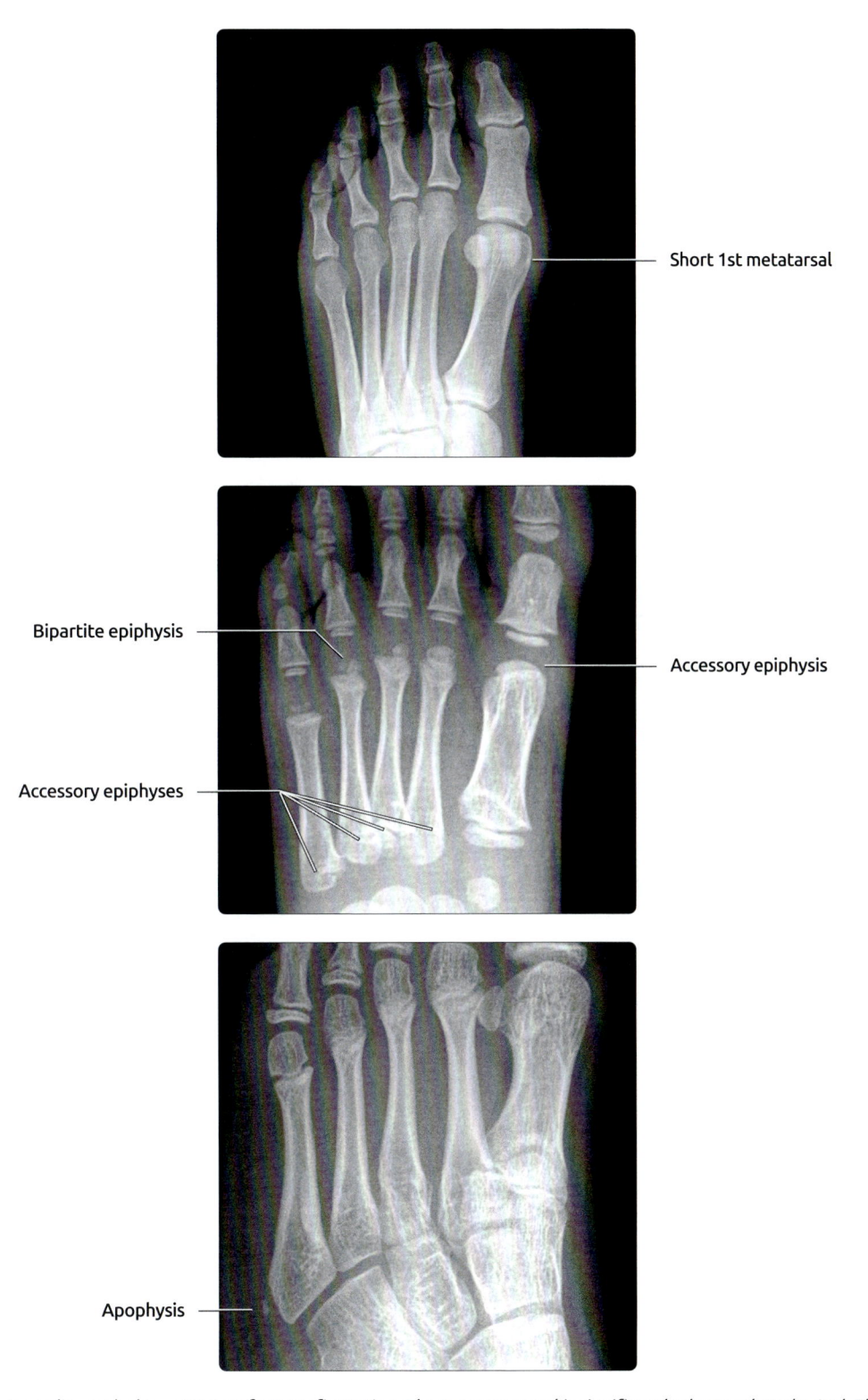

(Top) Anteroposterior radiograph shows Morton foot configuration. The 1st metatarsal is significantly shorter than the 2nd. This is a very common variant that increases stress on the 2nd metatarsal head. (Middle) Anteroposterior radiograph shows multiple accessory epiphyses of the metatarsals. The normal ossification center for the 1st metatarsal is at the proximal end of the bone. The normal ossification centers of the remaining metatarsals are distal. Accessory epiphyses may form at the opposite end of the metatarsal from normal epiphysis. Accessory epiphyses may be complete or incomplete. (Bottom) Normal apophysis at the base of the 5th metatarsal is shown. Fractures in this location tend to be horizontally oriented, while apophysis is longitudinally oriented.

Foot and Ankle Normal Variants and Imaging Pitfalls

1ST METATARSOPHALANGEAL SESAMOID VARIANTS

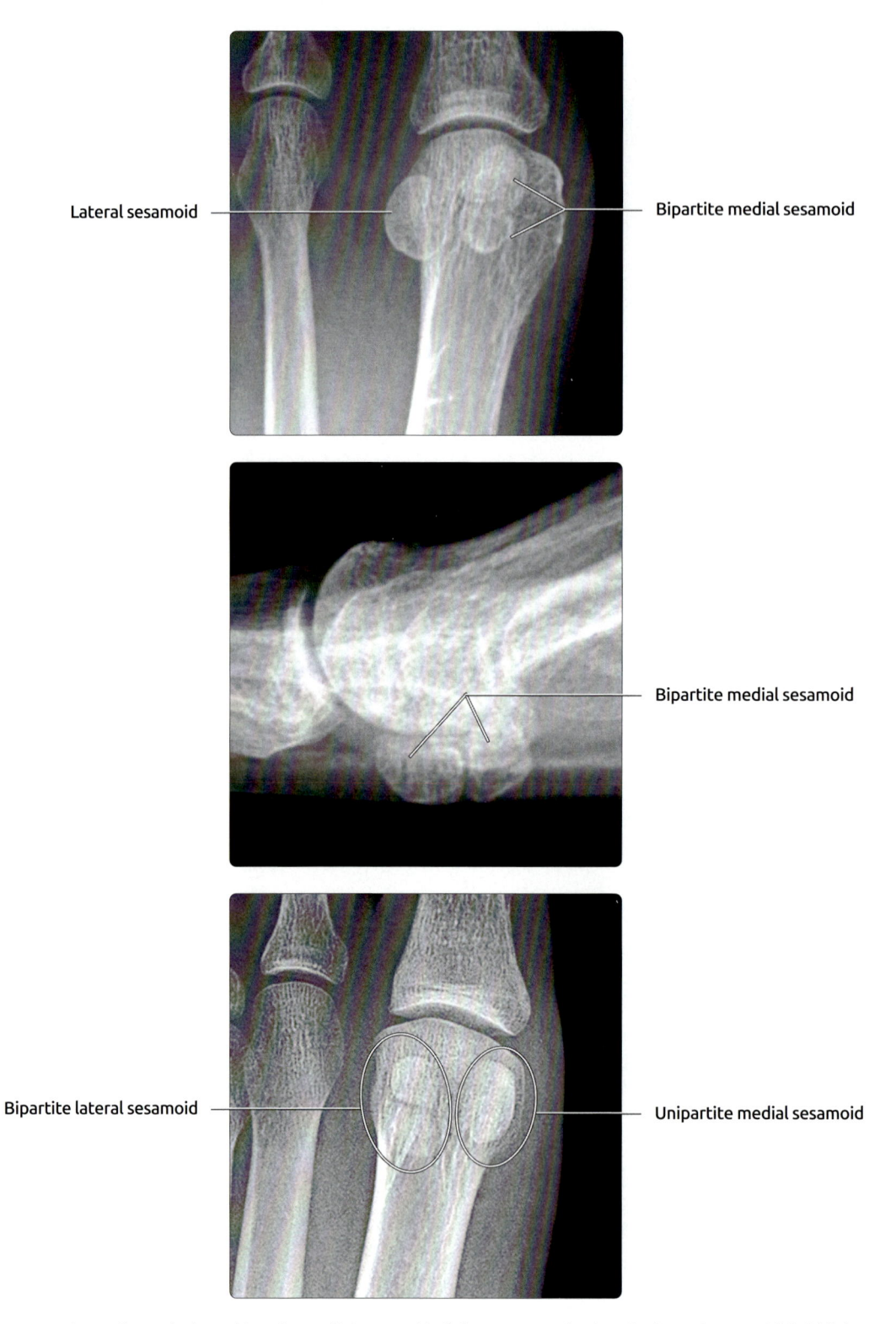

(Top) *Anteroposterior radiograph shows bipartite medial sesamoid of the 1st toe and unipartite lateral sesamoid.* (Middle) *Lateral radiograph shows rounded contour, characteristic of bipartite sesamoids. Fracture fragments, in contrast, will show angular margins.* (Bottom) *Anteroposterior radiograph shows bipartite lateral sesamoid of the 1st toe and unipartite medial sesamoid. Bipartite sesamoids are usually more rounded in contour than fractured sesamoids. Bipartite sesamoids are usually larger than unipartite sesamoids. Bipartite sesamoids may or may not be present on contralateral foot.*

Foot and Ankle Normal Variants and Imaging Pitfalls

SESAMOID VARIANTS

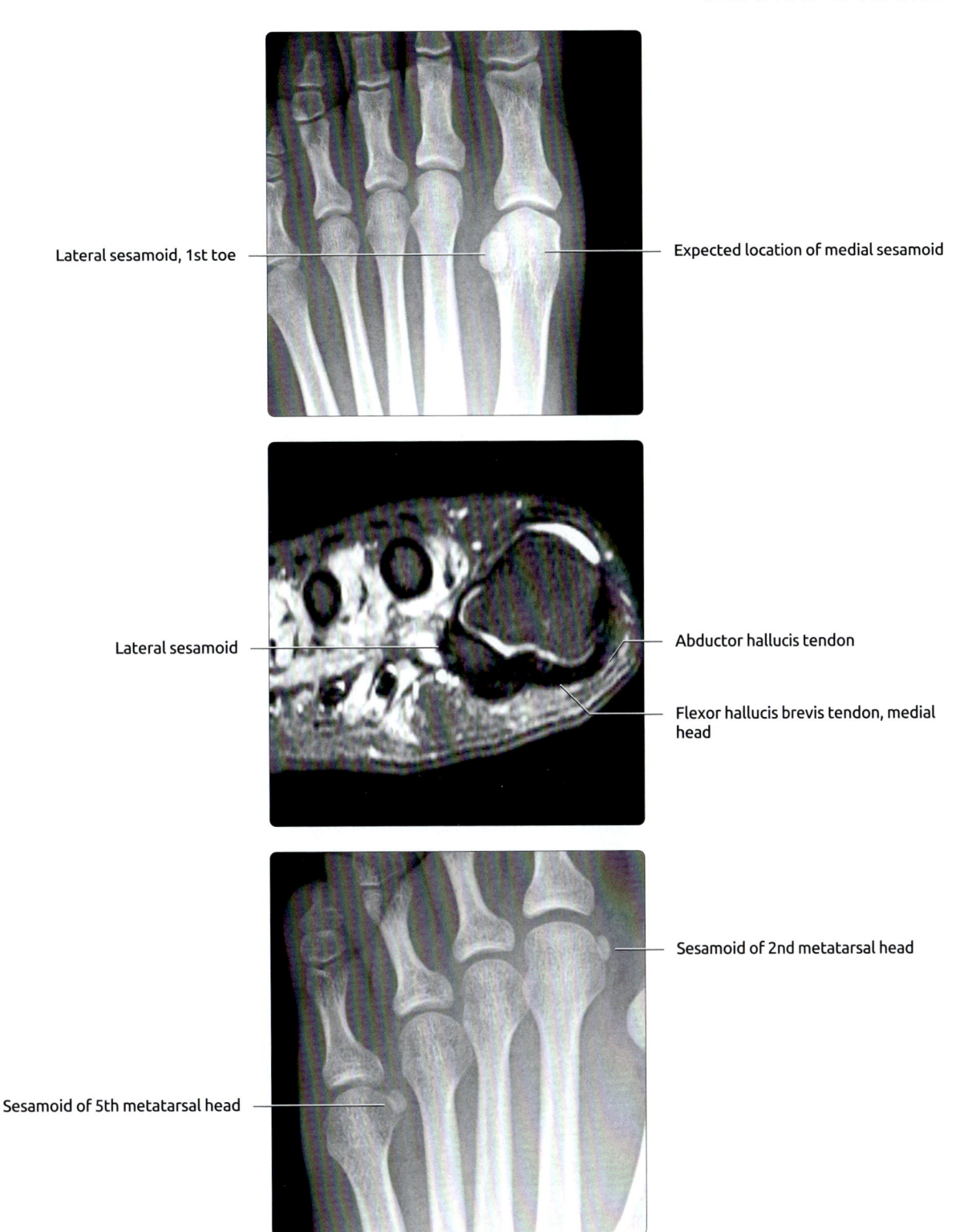

Lateral sesamoid, 1st toe — Expected location of medial sesamoid

Lateral sesamoid — Abductor hallucis tendon / Flexor hallucis brevis tendon, medial head

Sesamoid of 2nd metatarsal head

Sesamoid of 5th metatarsal head

(Top) Anteroposterior radiograph shows absent medial sesamoid in a patient with no history of trauma. This is a very rare normal variant and most cases where the sesamoid is not visible probably reflect resorption of the sesamoid after remote trauma. (Middle) Coronal T2WI FS MR in the same patient confirms absence of the medial sesamoid. (Bottom) Anteroposterior radiograph shows sesamoids of the 2nd and 5th metatarsal heads. Sesamoids of the lateral toes are variably present. They are always small and may be round or oval. The 5th toe may have medial and lateral sesamoids.

TOE VARIANTS

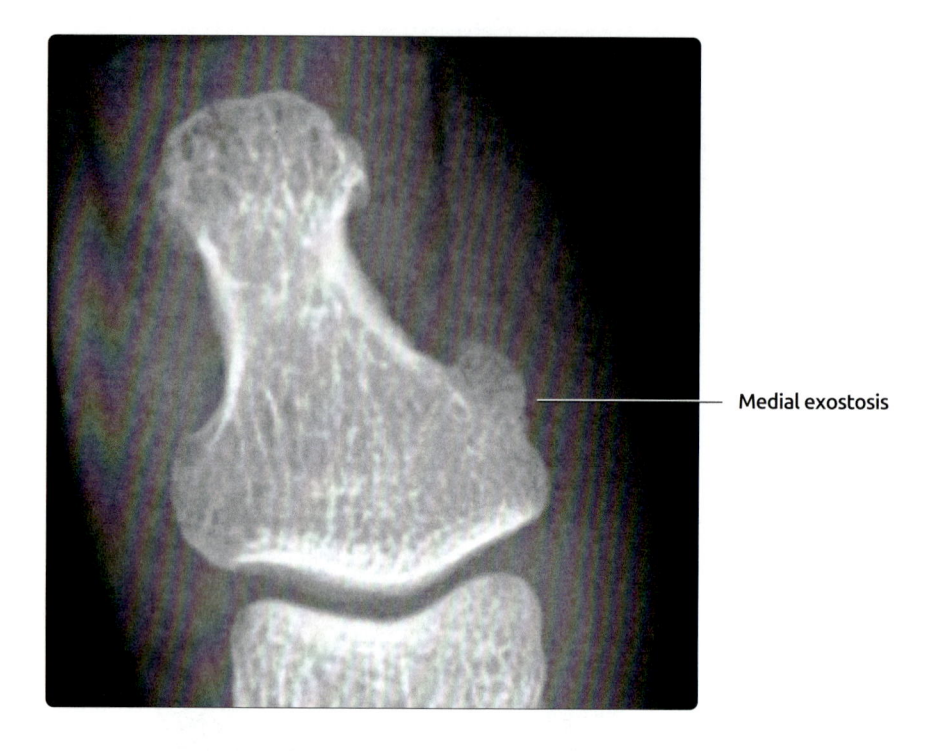

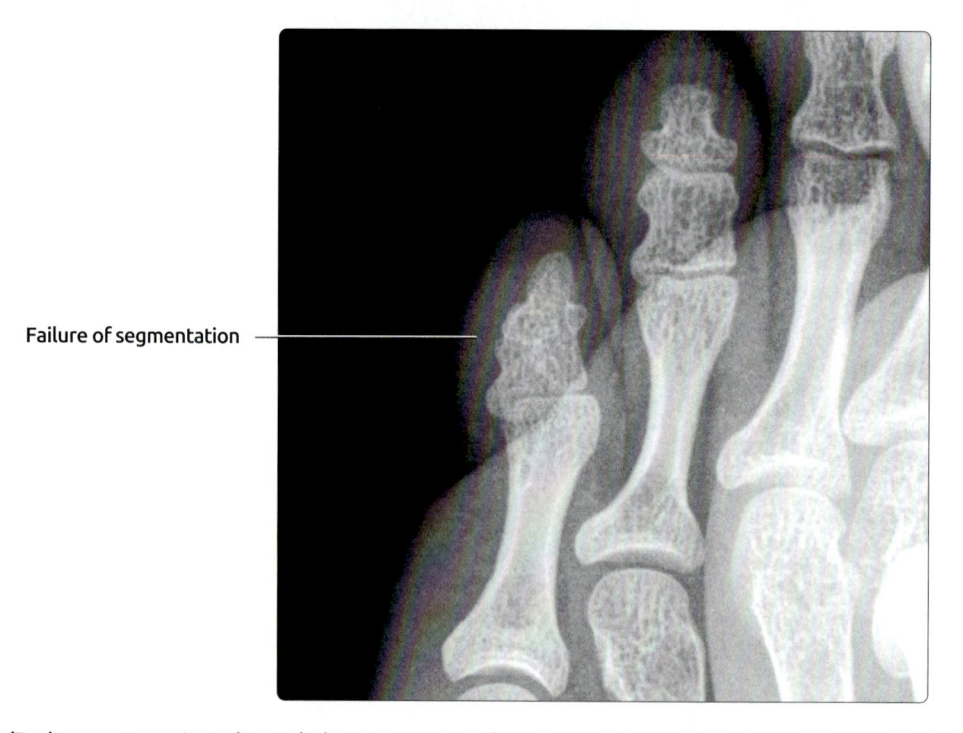

Medial exostosis

Failure of segmentation

(Top) Anteroposterior radiograph shows an exostosis from the medial margin, the base of the 1st distal phalanx. This is commonly seen, often large and asymptomatic. (Bottom) Anteroposterior radiograph shows failure of segmentation of the middle and distal phalanges of the 5th toe. This is a very common normal variant.

Foot and Ankle Normal Variants and Imaging Pitfalls

SOLEUS MUSCLE VARIANTS

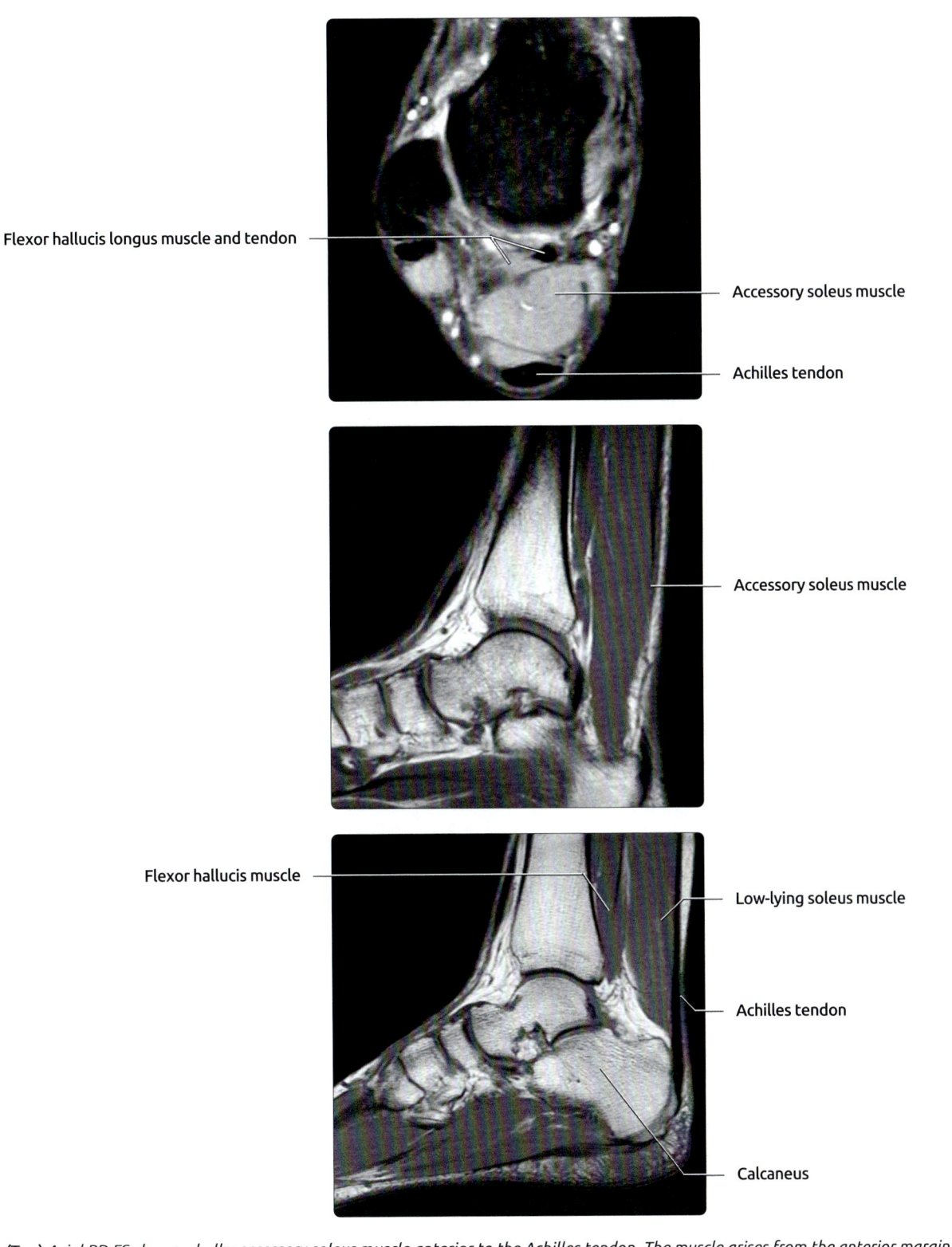

(Top) Axial PD FS shows a bulky accessory soleus muscle anterior to the Achilles tendon. The muscle arises from the anterior margin of soleus and inserts on the medial margin of calcaneus. (Middle) Sagittal T1WI shows a bulky accessory soleus muscle extending to the medial margin of the posterior process of calcaneus. This anomalous muscle may present clinically as a mass, or may cause impingement. (Bottom) Sagittal MR of the low-lying soleus muscle in an asymptomatic patient is shown. In most individuals, the soleus muscle ends between 2.5-7.5 cm above the calcaneus. In ~ 12.5% of individuals, however, the musculotendinous unit is 0-2.5 cm above the calcaneus. A low-lying soleus muscle may presents clinically as calf fullness. (Courtesy J. Bencardino, MD.)

Foot and Ankle Normal Variants and Imaging Pitfalls

ACCESSORY FLEXOR MUSCLES

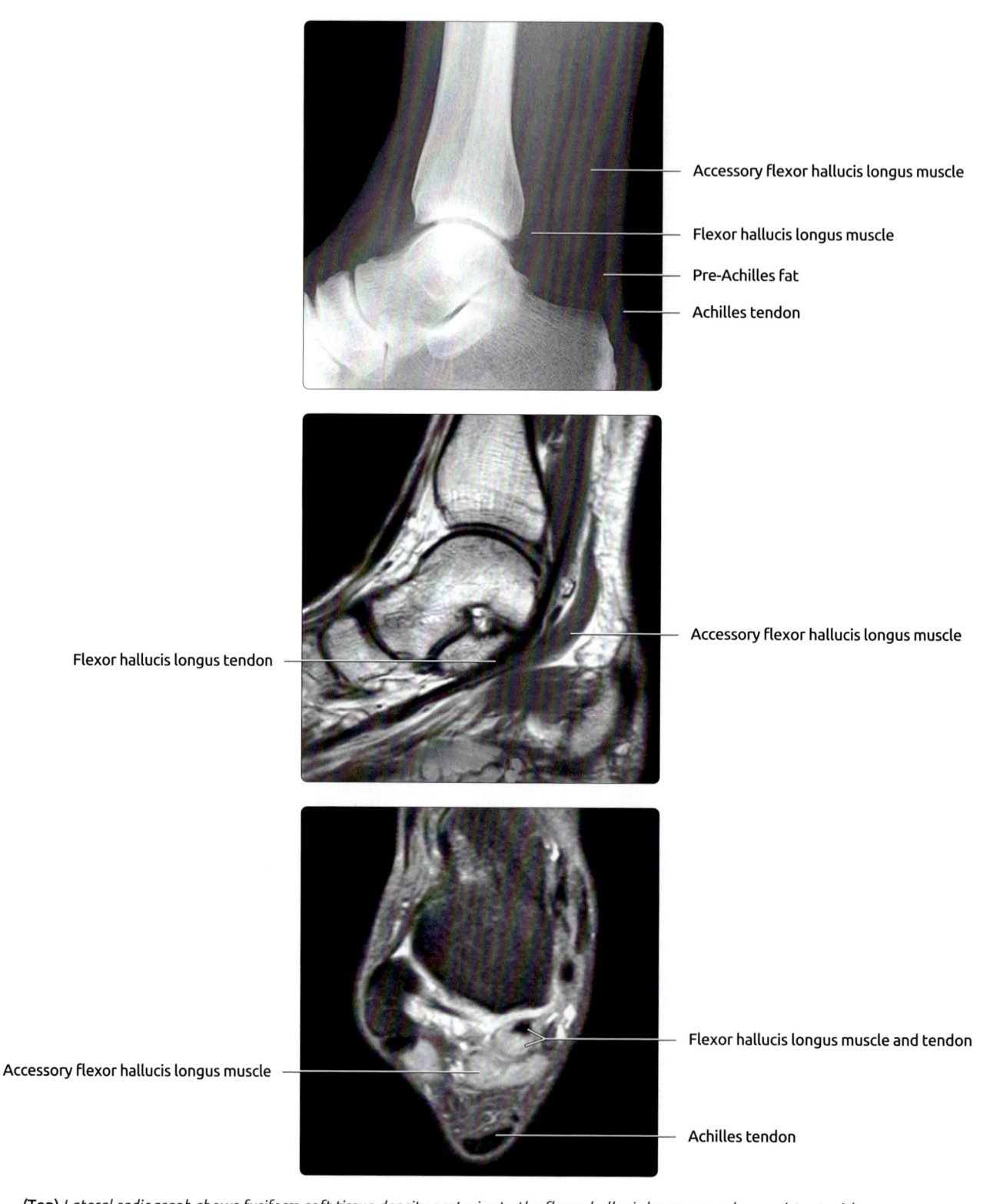

Accessory flexor hallucis longus muscle
Flexor hallucis longus muscle
Pre-Achilles fat
Achilles tendon

Flexor hallucis longus tendon
Accessory flexor hallucis longus muscle

Accessory flexor hallucis longus muscle
Flexor hallucis longus muscle and tendon
Achilles tendon

(Top) Lateral radiograph shows fusiform soft tissue density posterior to the flexor hallucis longus muscle, consistent with an accessory muscle. (Middle) Sagittal T2WI MR in the same patient shows that the muscle travels with and attaches to the flexor hallucis longus tendon. Due to mass effect from the anomalous muscle, patients may present with tarsal tunnel syndrome or with impingement when the foot is plantar flexed. This patient, a ballerina, had limited plantar flexion, which resolved after excision of accessory muscle. (Bottom) Axial PD MR in the same patient shows the accessory flexor hallucis longus muscle posterior to the flexor hallucis longus.

Foot and Ankle Normal Variants and Imaging Pitfalls

ACCESSORY FLEXOR MUSCLES

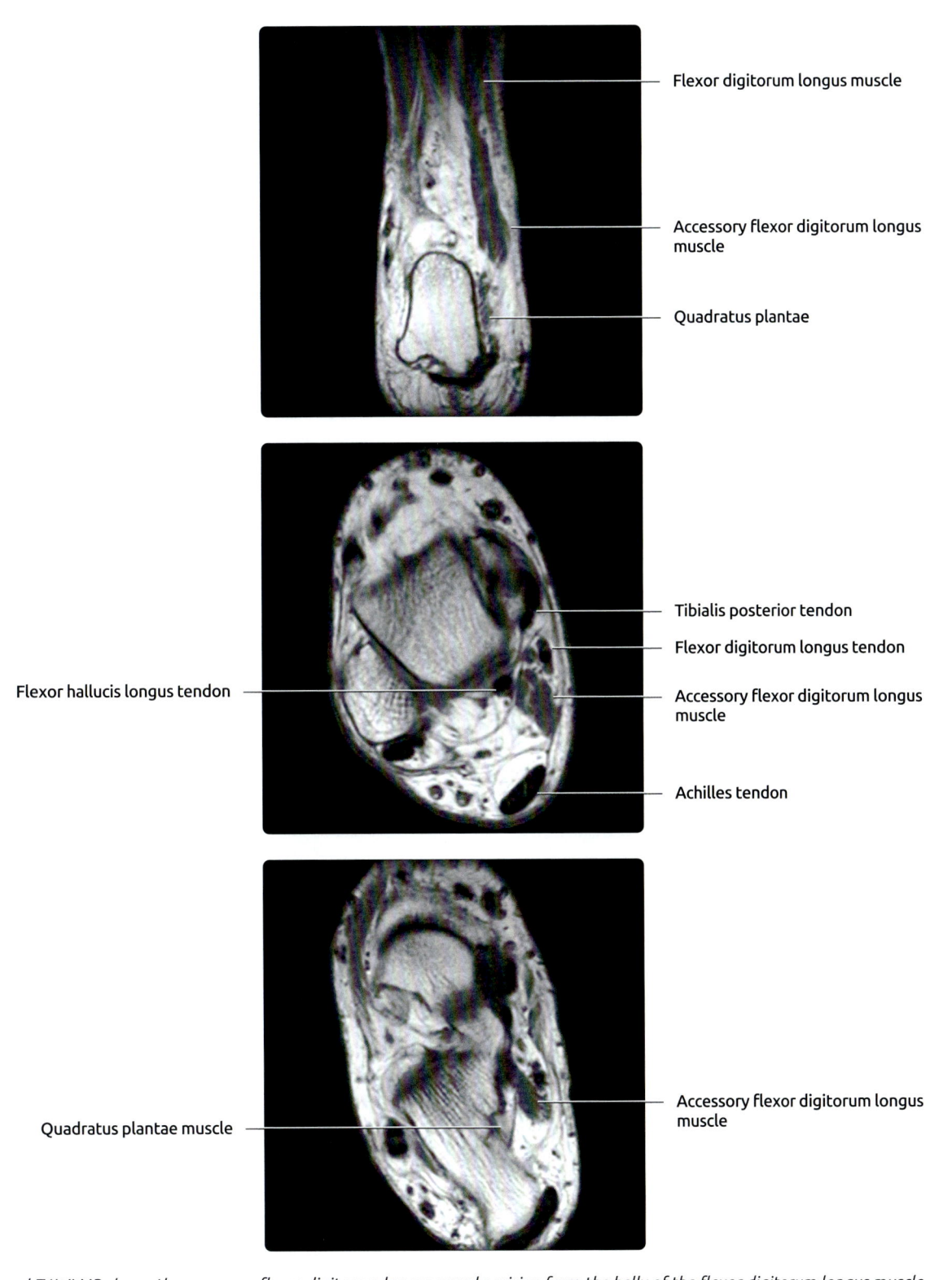

(Top) Coronal T1WI MR shows the accessory flexor digitorum longus muscle arising from the belly of the flexor digitorum longus muscle and inserting on the quadratus plantae muscle. (Middle) Axial PD MR shows the position of the accessory flexor digitorum longus muscle immediately posterior to the flexor digitorum longus tendon and neurovascular bundle. (Bottom) Axial PD MR shows the muscle near its attachment to the atrophic quadratus plantae muscle.

Foot and Ankle Normal Variants and Imaging Pitfalls

FLEXOR MUSCLE VARIANTS

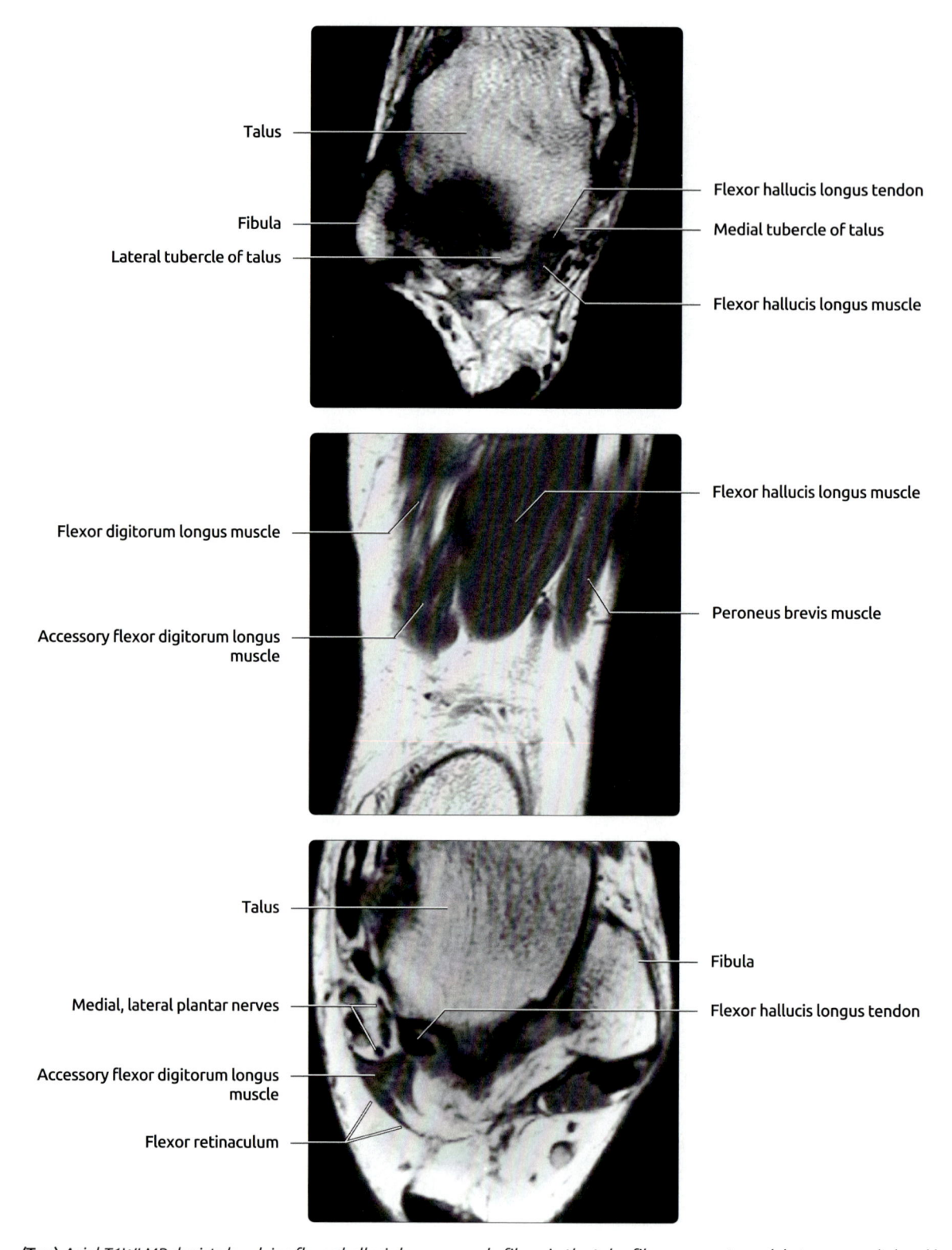

(Top) Axial T1WI MR depicts low-lying flexor hallucis longus muscle fibers in the talar fibroosseous tunnel, between medial and lateral talar tubercles of the posterior talar process. This variant can produce crowding and limit smooth gliding of the tendon in the talar tunnel during foot plantar and dorsiflexion. (Middle) The accessory flexor digitorum longus muscle is optimally visualized on axial images but may be detected on coronal and sagittal images as well. (Bottom) The accessory flexor digitorum longus muscle frequently originates directly from the flexor retinaculum in the ankle region. In those instances, it is typically triangular in shape with the apex pointing toward the talus or tibia and base, abutting against the flexor retinaculum. Because of variable origins and insertions of the accessory flexor digitorum longus and accessory flexor hallucis longus muscles, they are lumped by some authors under the category of "long accessory of long flexors," or "quadratus plantae."

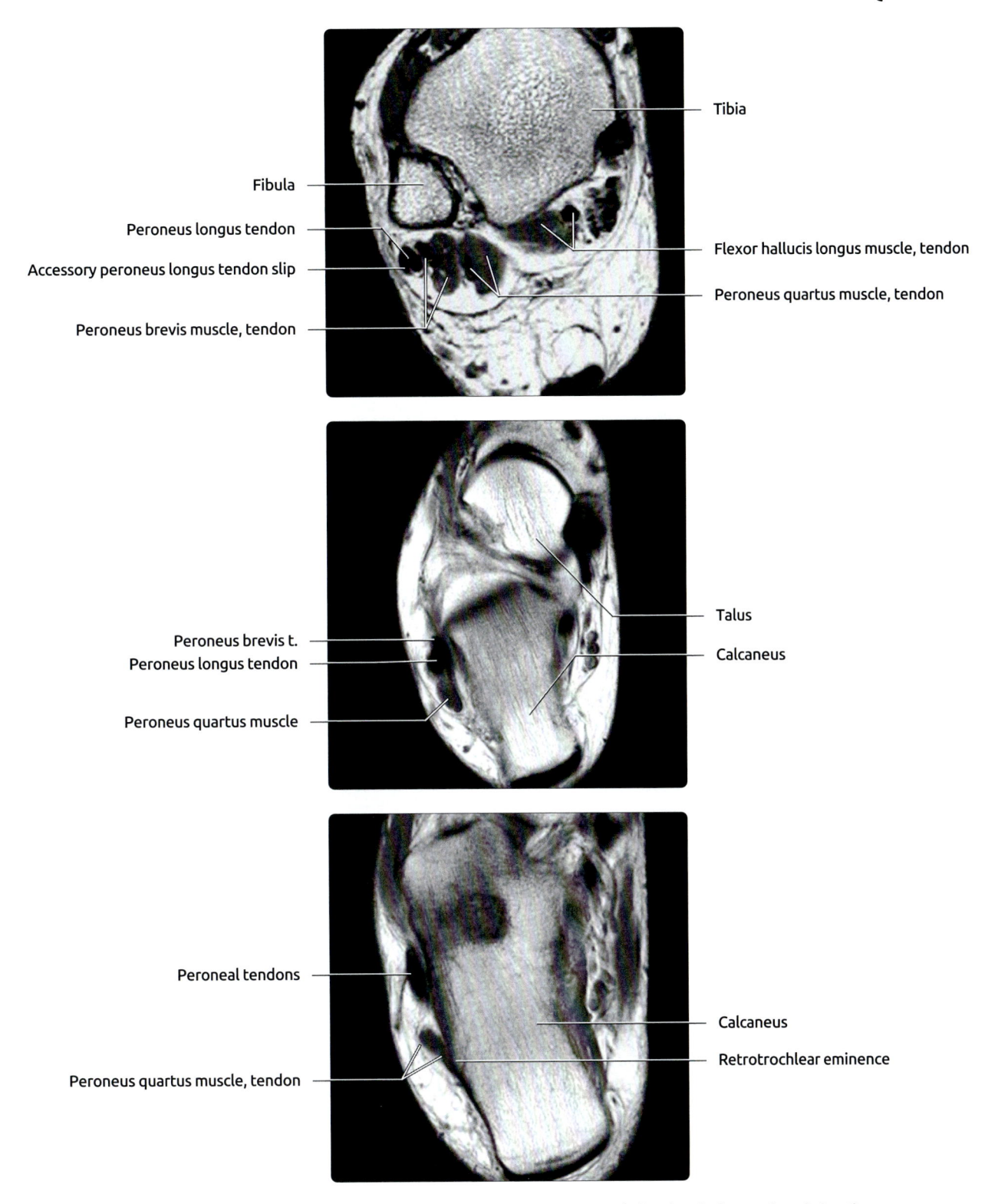

Foot and Ankle Normal Variants and Imaging Pitfalls

PERONEUS QUARTUS

Labels on top image: Fibula; Peroneus longus tendon; Accessory peroneus longus tendon slip; Peroneus brevis muscle, tendon; Tibia; Flexor hallucis longus muscle, tendon; Peroneus quartus muscle, tendon

Labels on middle image: Peroneus brevis t.; Peroneus longus tendon; Peroneus quartus muscle; Talus; Calcaneus

Labels on bottom image: Peroneal tendons; Peroneus quartus muscle, tendon; Calcaneus; Retrotrochlear eminence

(Top) The peroneus quartus is frequently seen on axial MR images as an accessory muscle/tendon distinct and medial to the peroneus brevis muscle. The presence of the peroneus quartus muscle on ankle MR study should prompt the radiologist to search for peroneal tendon tears or dislocation. Note the incidental finding of an accessory slip of the peroneus longus tendon. **(Middle)** The normal peroneus brevis is tendinous by the level of the retromalleolar groove, although significant variations in its distal extent have been described. In this case, a separate peroneus quartus is visible posterior to the peroneus longus and brevis tendons. **(Bottom)** The peroneus quartus inserts into the retrotrochlear eminence and not into, as stated in many reports, the peroneal tubercle. The retrotrochlear eminence is seen in 98% of normal individuals posterior & slightly inferior to the peroneal tubercle. The eminence is typically seen on axial MR images and can be quite small, as seen in this patient.

Foot and Ankle Measurements and Lines

IMAGING ANATOMY

Overview
- Abnormal alignment leads to foot pain and dysfunction

Anatomy Relationships
- Axes of foot are designated on AP radiograph
  - Anatomic axis
    - Line from center of 2nd metatarsal head to midpoint of posterior tuberosity of calcaneus
  - Mechanical axis
    - Line from center of 1st metatarsal head to midpoint posterior calcaneal tuberosity

Longitudinal Arch of Foot
- Flatfoot normally present at birth
- Arch develops in 1st decade of life
- 20% of normal adults have flatfoot deformity

Talometatarsal Angle (Lateral Radiograph)
- Lines drawn along axes of 1st metatarsal and talus
- Normally axes are same
- Pes cavus = talar axis extends dorsal to 1st metatarsal axis
- Pes planus = talar axis extends plantar to 1st metatarsal axis

Talocalcaneal Angles
- Anteroposterior radiograph
  - Lines drawn along central axis of talus and lateral margin of calcaneus
  - 27-56° in newborn
  - 25-45° (mean: 35°) in adult
  - > 45° = hindfoot valgus
  - < 20° = hindfoot varus
- Lateral radiograph
  - Lines drawn along central axis of talus and inferior margin of calcaneus
  - 23-55° in newborn
  - 30-50° (mean: 35°) in adult

Böehler Angle
- Line 1: Anterior process calcaneus to posterior margin posterior facet
- Line 2: Posterior margin posterior facet to superior margin calcaneal tuberosity
- Normal = 20-40°

Gissane Angle
- Line 1: Along superior margin anterior process calcaneus
- Line 2: Along lateral border of posterior subtalar facet
- Normal = 100-130°

Hindfoot Width (AP Radiograph)
- Distance from medial margin head of talus to lateral margin calcaneus
- Normal = 4-5.5 cm

Talonavicular Relationship (AP Radiograph)
- Distance between midpoint articular surfaces talus and navicular at talonavicular joint
- Normal = < 7 mm, > 7 mm indicates hyperpronation

1st-5th Intermetatarsal Angle (AP Radiograph)
- Normal = 14-35°
- Increased in splayfoot

1st Intermetatarsal Angle (AP Radiograph)
- Normal = < 9°
- Increased in metatarsus primus varus

4th-5th Intermetatarsal Angle (AP Radiograph)
- Normal = < 5°
- Increased in bunionette deformity

Forefoot Width (AP Radiograph)
- Distance from medial margin 1st metatarsal head to lateral margin 5th metatarsal head
- Normal = 7-9 cm

Relative Metatarsal Lengths (AP Radiograph)
- 1st metatarsal may be equal, shorter or longer than 2nd
- 2nd-5th metatarsals become progressively shorter
- Can be assessed by metatarsal break angle of Meschan
  - Line 1: Tangential to 1st and 2nd metatarsal head articular surfaces
  - Line 2: Tangential to 2nd and 5th metatarsal head articular surfaces
  - Normal = 140°; < 135° indicates relatively short 1st metatarsal

Hallux-Metatarsophalangeal Angle (AP Radiograph)
- Normal = < 15°; > 15 indicates hallux valgus

Hallux-Interphalangeal Angle (AP Radiograph)
- Normal = 6-14°

Plantar Soft Tissue Measurements
- Thickness increases with weight, decreases with age
- Increased plantar soft tissue thickness: Acromegaly, infection, myxedema
- Calcaneal fat pad: 4-17 mm
- Metatarsal fat pad
  - 1st metatarsal head: 7-25 mm
  - 5th metatarsal head: 1-16 mm

ANATOMY IMAGING ISSUES

Imaging Recommendations
- Assess alignment only on weight-bearing radiographs
- In infants, weight-bearing simulated by pressing the foot gently down on flat surface

SELECTED REFERENCES
1. Jahss M: Disorders of the Foot and Ankle: Medical and Surgical Management. vol 1. 2nd ed. Philadelphia, 1990

Foot and Ankle Measurements and Lines

ANKLE MORTISE ALIGNMENT

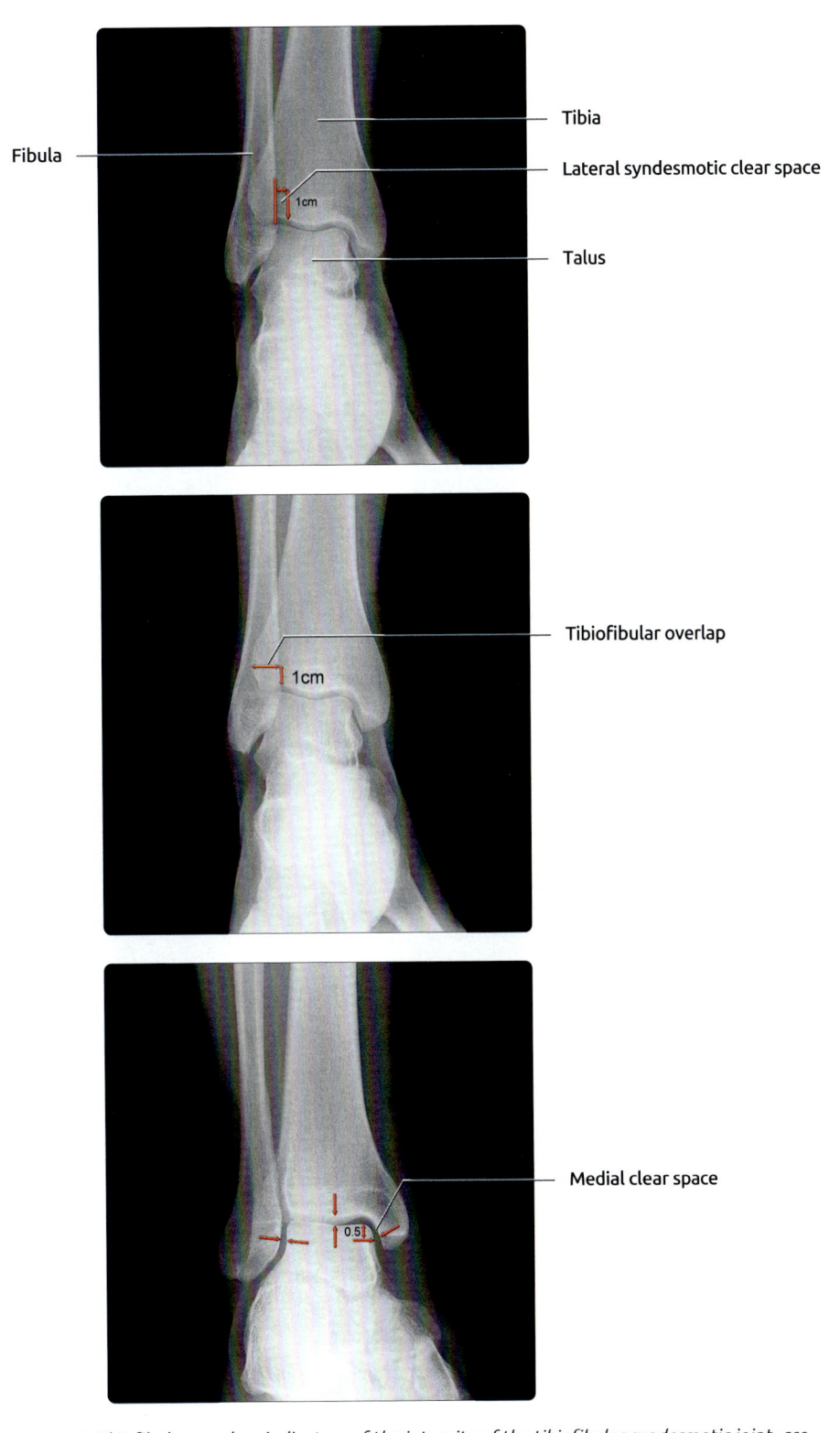

(Top) The lateral syndesmotic clear space & tibiofibular overlap, indicators of the integrity of the tibiofibular syndesmotic joint, are measured approximately 1 cm above the tibial plafond. The lateral syndesmotic clear space is measured from the posterior tibial margin to the medial fibular margin. Normal measurements vary in the literature and range from 4-6 mm on both the AP ankle and ankle mortise views. (Middle) The tibiofibular overlap measurements also vary and range from 6-10 mm in the literature. An overlap of 6 mm, however, on the AP view and 1 mm on the ankle mortise view, are considered normal by most. (Bottom) The talus should be equidistant from the tibial plafond on the AP and ankle mortise views. Minimal tilts are within normal. The normal medial clear space, measured 0.5 cm below the talar articular surface, should be 4 mm in size.

HINDFOOT ALIGNMENT

Talocalcaneal angle (Kite angle)

Axis of tibia

Line drawn perpendicular to tibial axis

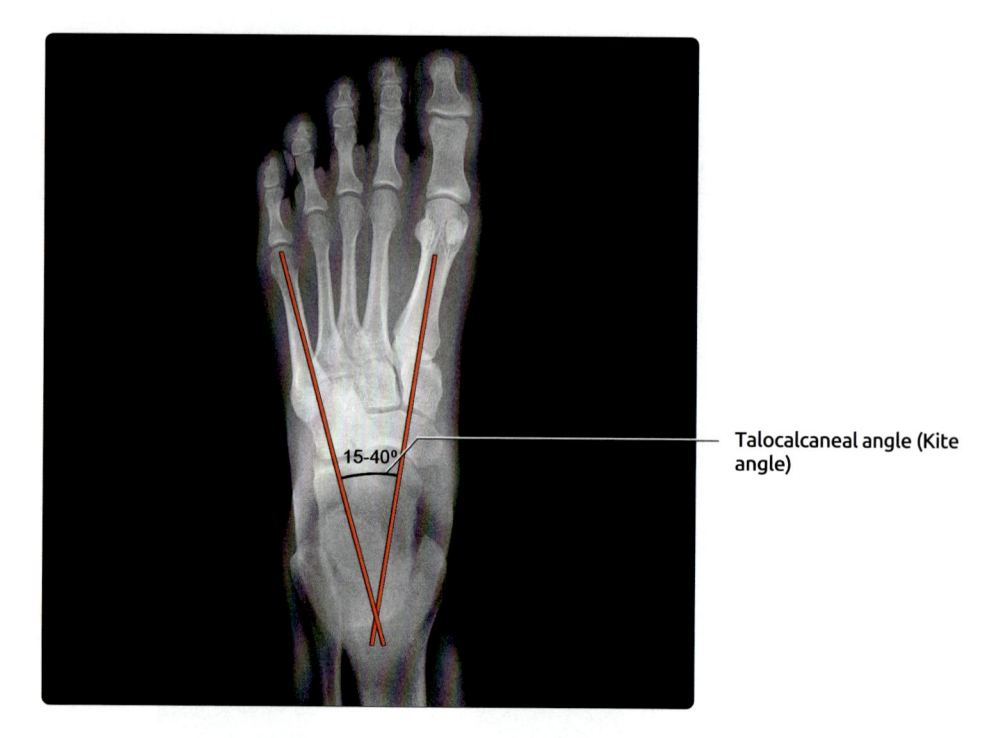

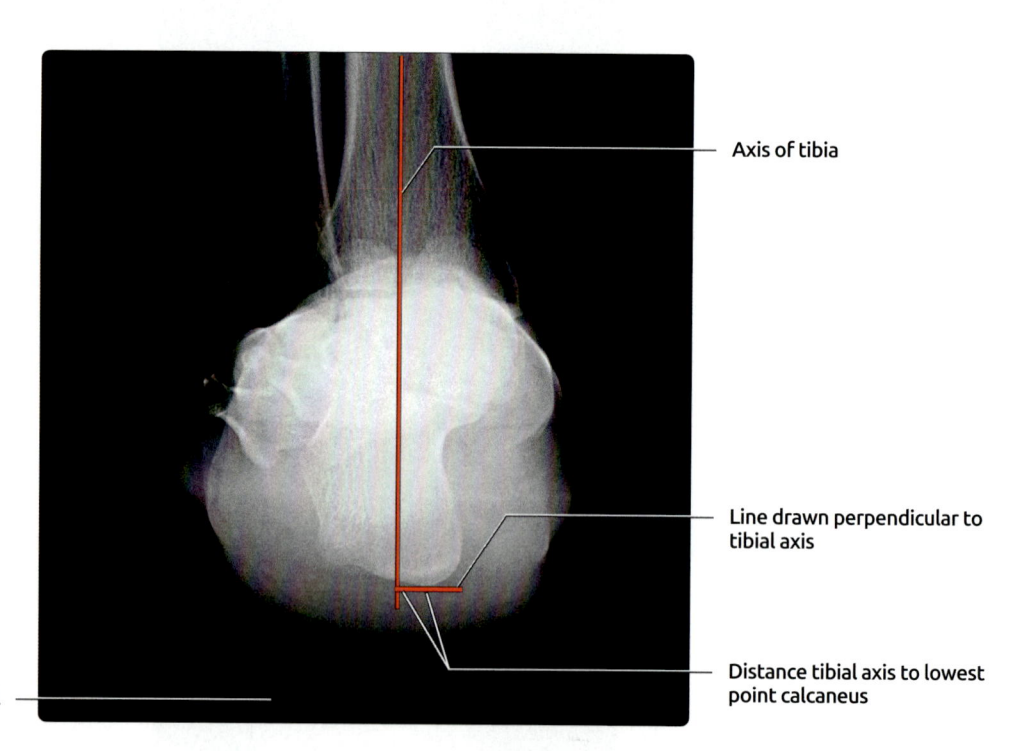

Distance tibial axis to lowest point calcaneus

Marker placed behind heel

(Top) *Normal AP talocalcaneal angle, measured along longitudinal axes of talus & calcaneus is 15-40°. Decrease in AP angle is indicative of varus hindfoot deformity & increase is indicative of valgus hindfoot deformity.* (Bottom) *Hindfoot alignment view obtained with patient standing. Toes are against radiographic cassette which is angled 20° from vertical, with its top edge tilted away from the foot. X-ray beam angled 20° caudal from heel to toes. Distance from the lowest point of the heel to the line bisecting the tibia (""tibial axis"") < 8 mm in normal, asymptomatic subjects. If the distance is > 8 mm, lateral position of the lowest point of the calcaneus indicates hindfoot valgus, medial position indicates varus.*

Foot and Ankle Measurements and Lines

HINDFOOT ALIGNMENT

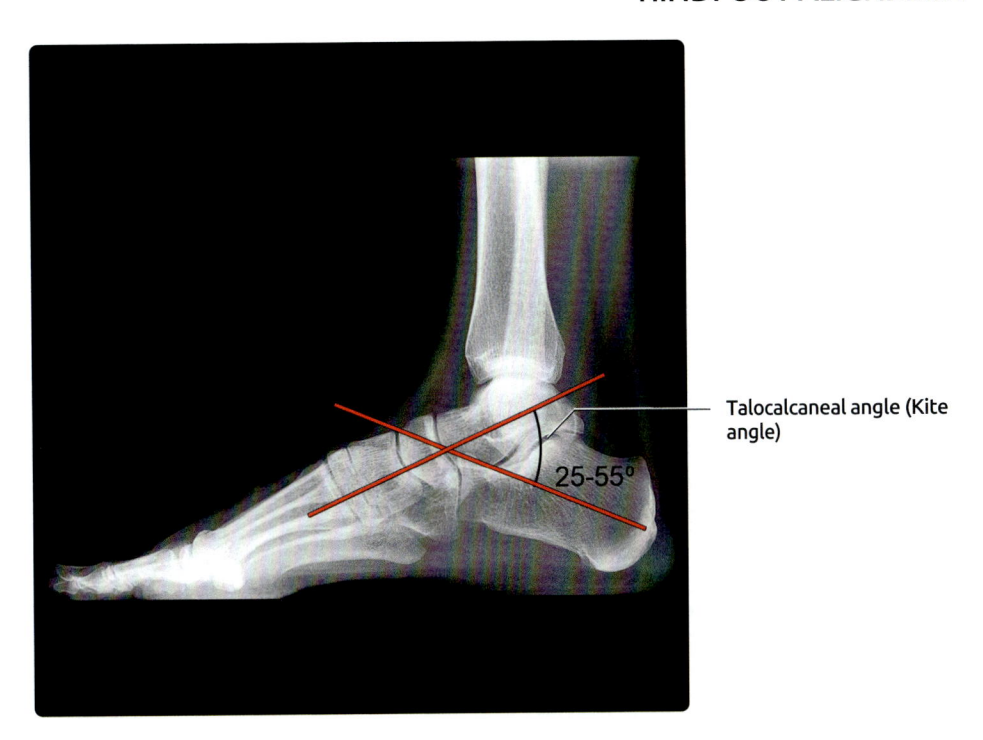

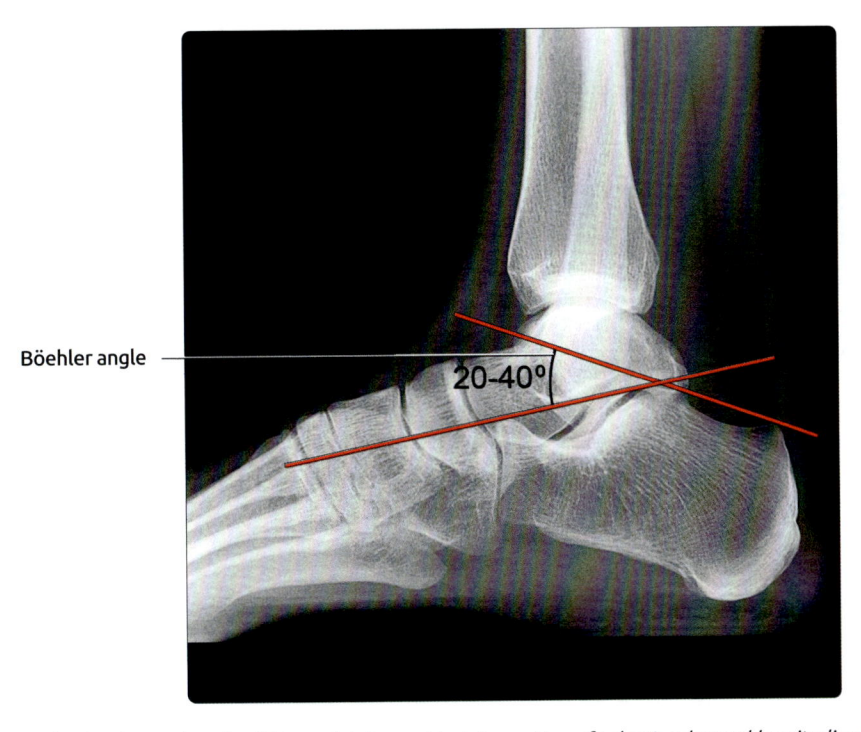

Talocalcaneal angle (Kite angle) — 25-55°

Böehler angle — 20-40°

(Top) Normal lateral talocalcaneal angle, (Kite angle), formed by intersection of talar & calcaneal longitudinal axes, measures 25-55°. Decrease in lateral angle is indicative of varus hindfoot deformity & increase is indicative of valgus hindfoot deformity. **(Bottom)** Böehler angle reflects integrity of the posterior calcaneal facet & calcaneal height. The angle is formed by the intersection of a line drawn along the apices of anterior calcaneal process & posterior calcaneal facet & a line drawn along the apices of posterior calcaneal tuberosity & posterior calcaneal facet. The normal range is 20-40°.

MIDFOOT ALIGNMENT

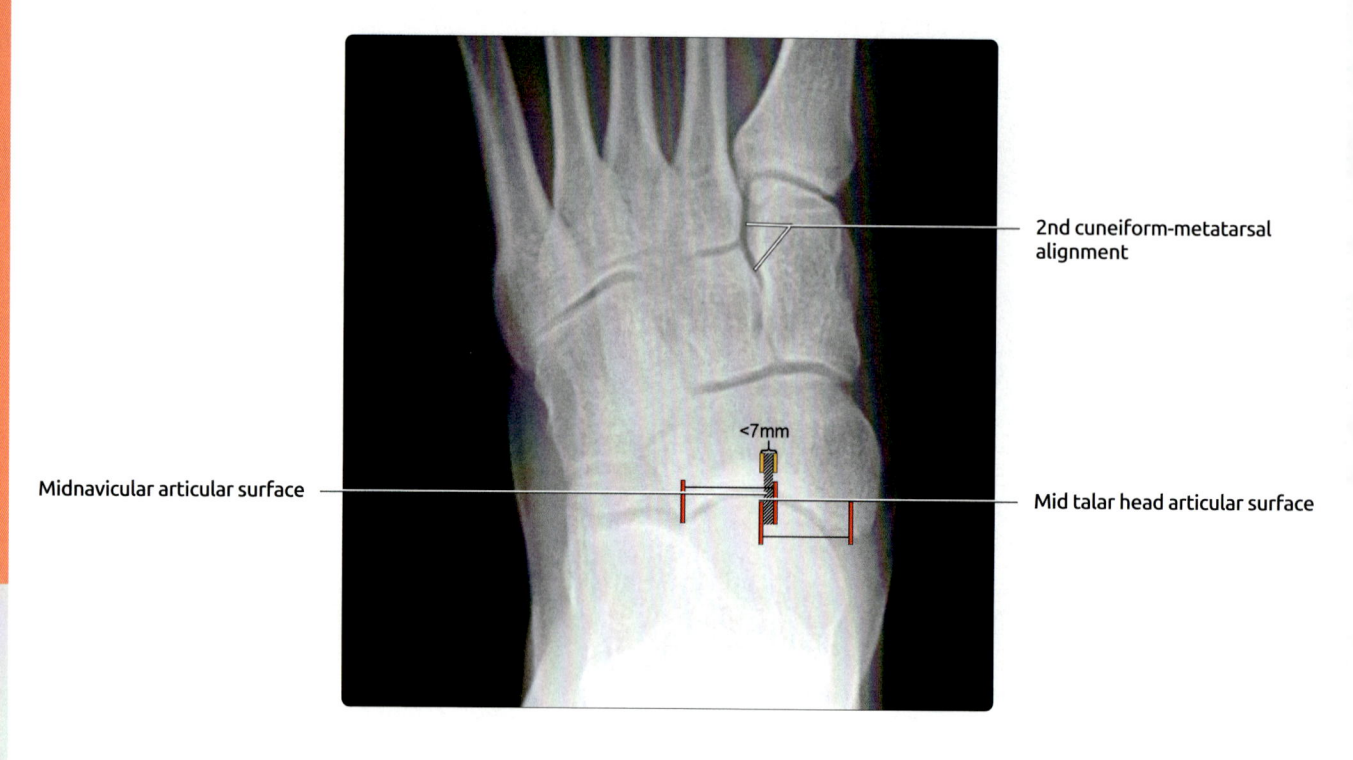

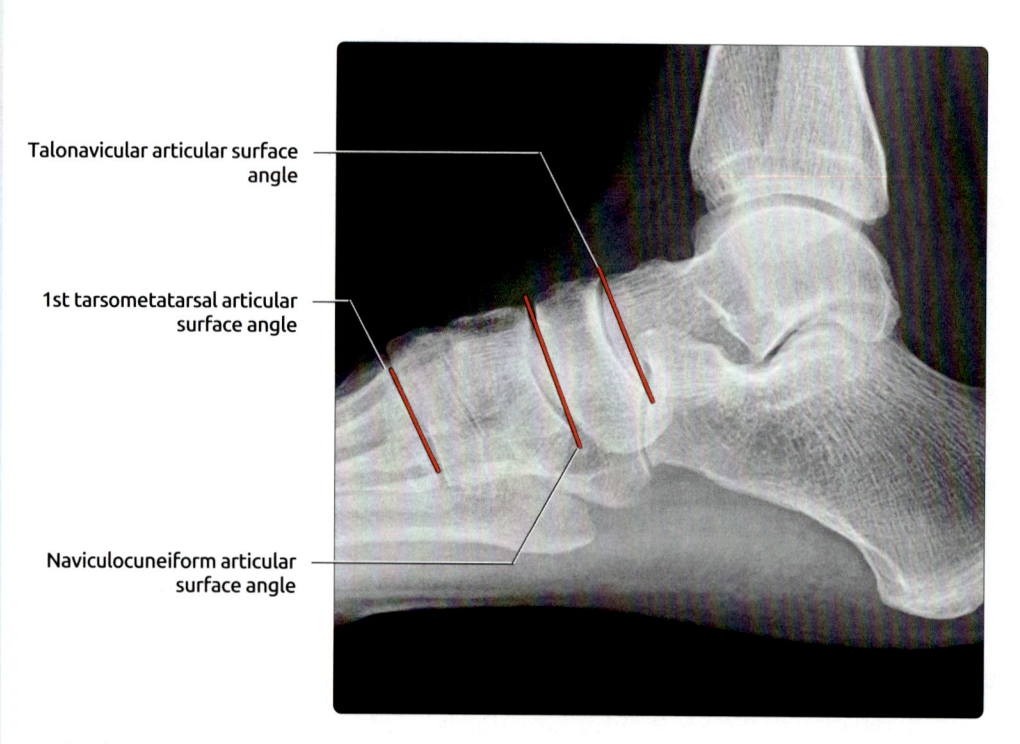

2nd cuneiform-metatarsal alignment

<7mm

Midnavicular articular surface

Mid talar head articular surface

Talonavicular articular surface angle

1st tarsometatarsal articular surface angle

Naviculocuneiform articular surface angle

(Top) Anteroposterior radiograph shows the normal relationship between the talus and navicular. Distance from the midpoint articular surface head of the talus to the midpoint articular surface proximal margin navicular is < 7 mm. The medial margins of 2nd cuneiform and 2nd metatarsal are exactly aligned; lateral displacement indicates Lisfranc ligament rupture. (Bottom) Lateral radiograph shows the normal relationship of the talus, navicular, and cuneiforms. Lateral articular surface angles of talonavicular, naviculocuneiform, and 1st tarsometatarsal joints are approximately parallel.

Foot and Ankle Measurements and Lines

TARSOMETATARSAL JOINT ALIGNMENT

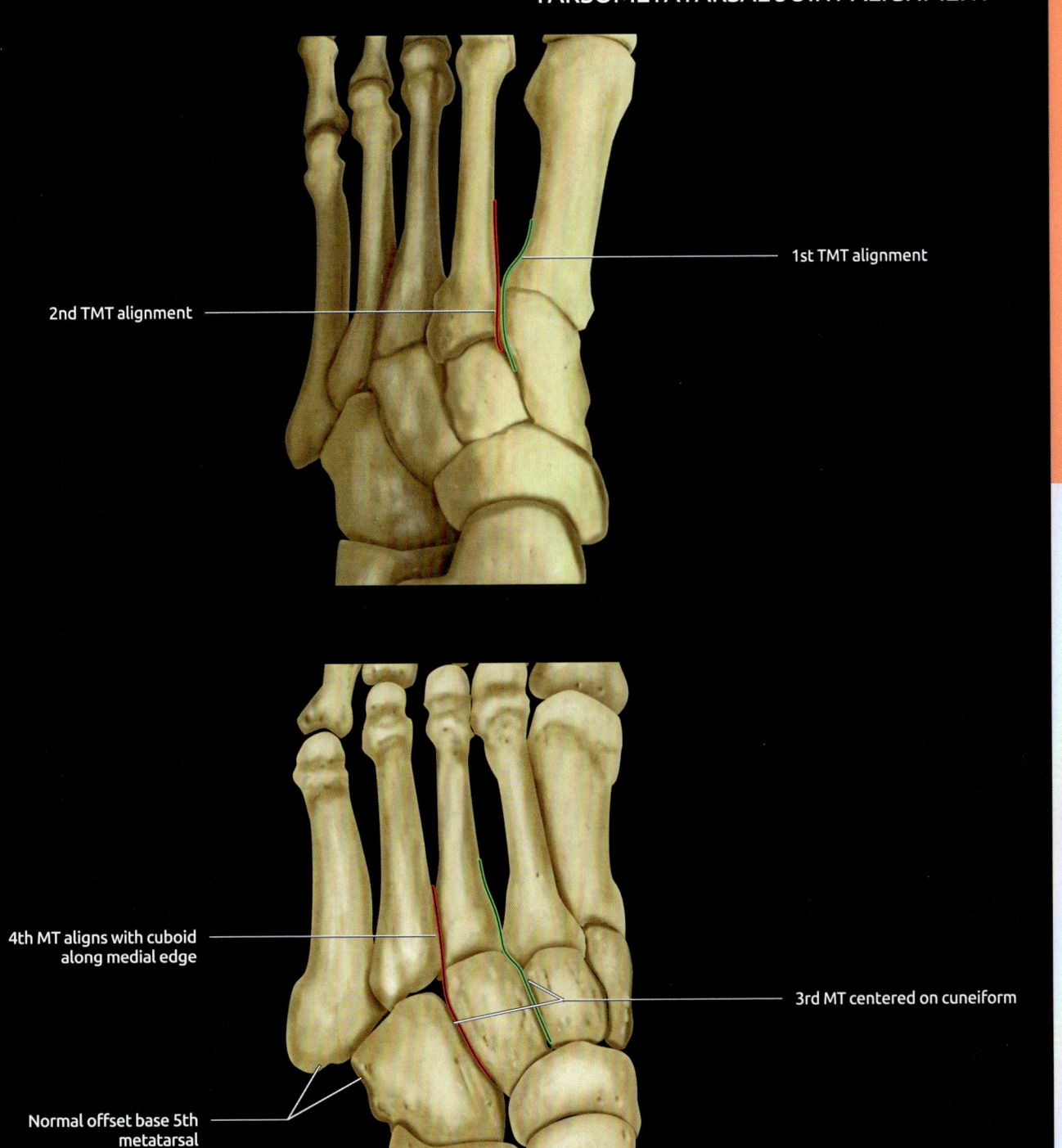

2nd TMT alignment

1st TMT alignment

4th MT aligns with cuboid along medial edge

3rd MT centered on cuneiform

Normal offset base 5th metatarsal

(Top) Anteroposterior graphic shows that the 1st metatarsal is centered on the 1st cuneiform. The line drawn along the lateral margin of the cuneiform and metatarsal is often curved, and there may be focal offset. In contradistinction, the line along medial margins of the 2nd cuneiform and metatarsal should be straight, and any deviation of the line indicates disruption of the Lisfranc ligament. **(Bottom)** Oblique graphic shows the 3rd metatarsal centered on the 3rd cuneiform. The medial margin of the 4th metatarsal is aligned with the medial margin of the cuboid. The 5th metatarsal styloid process extends beyond the lateral margin of the cuboid.

Foot and Ankle Measurements and Lines

LONGITUDINAL ARCH OF FOOT

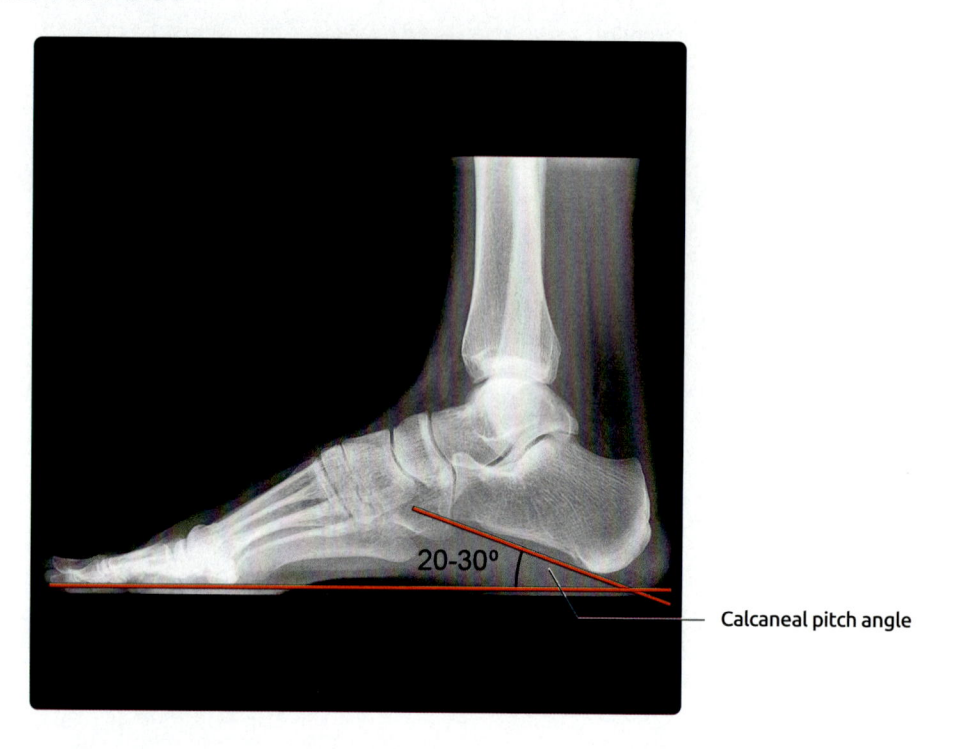

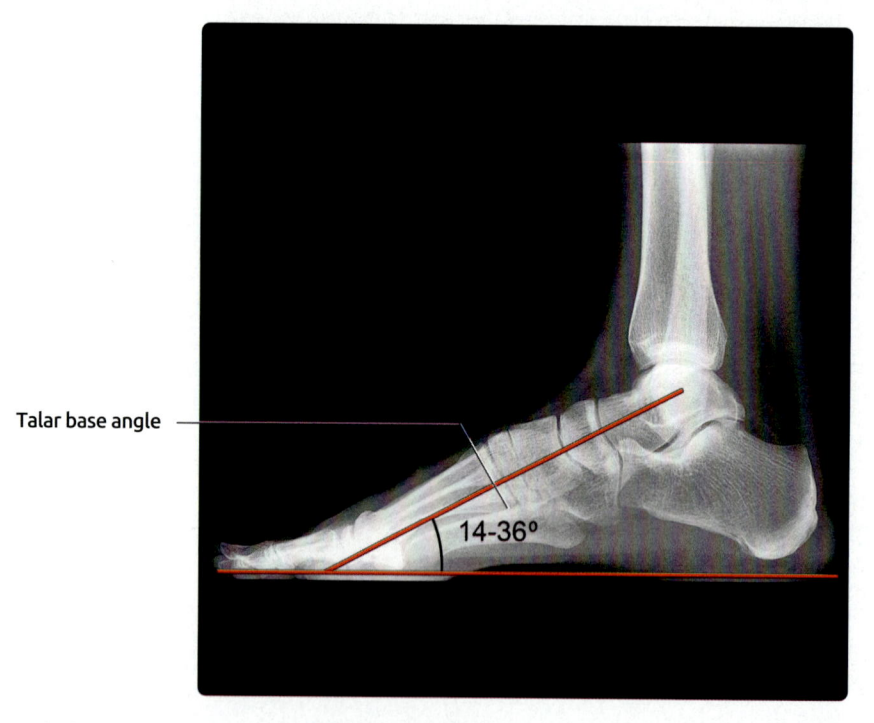

(Top) A weight-bearing lateral view of the foot provides information on the height of the longitudinal arch. The calcaneal pitch is an angle formed by intersection of a line along the plantar aspect of the calcaneus with a line parallel to the floor. It should measure about 20-30°. (Bottom) The normal talar-base angle is formed by the intersection of the longitudinal axis of the talus, with a line parallel to the floor. It normally measures 14-36°.

Foot and Ankle Measurements and Lines

METATARSAL ALIGNMENT LATERAL

Talometatarsal axis

5th metatarsal inclination angle

1st metatarsal inclination angle

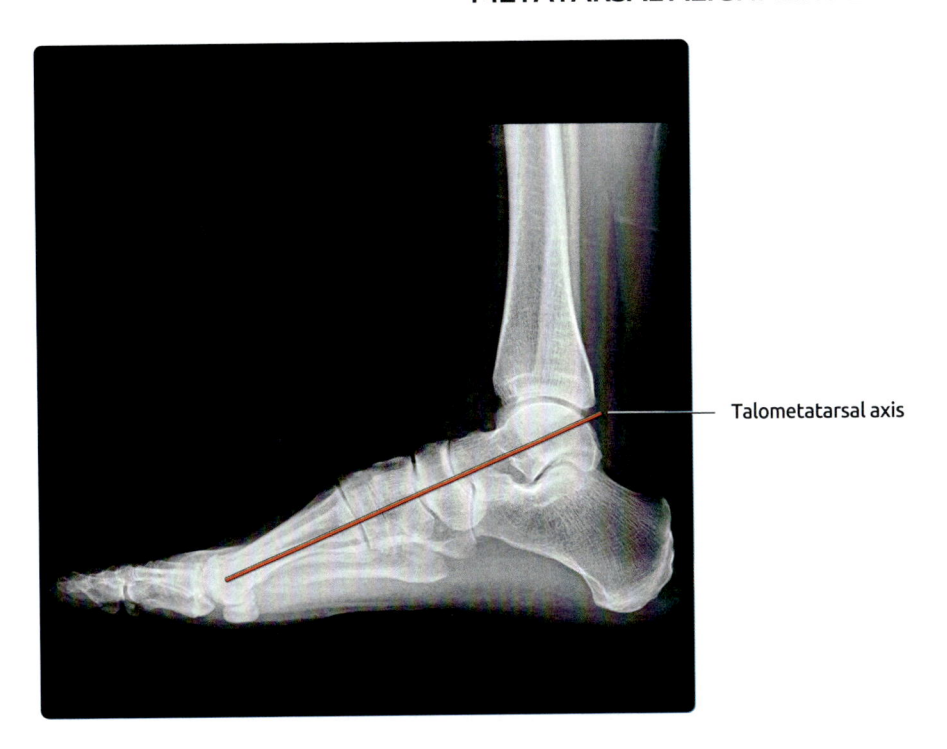

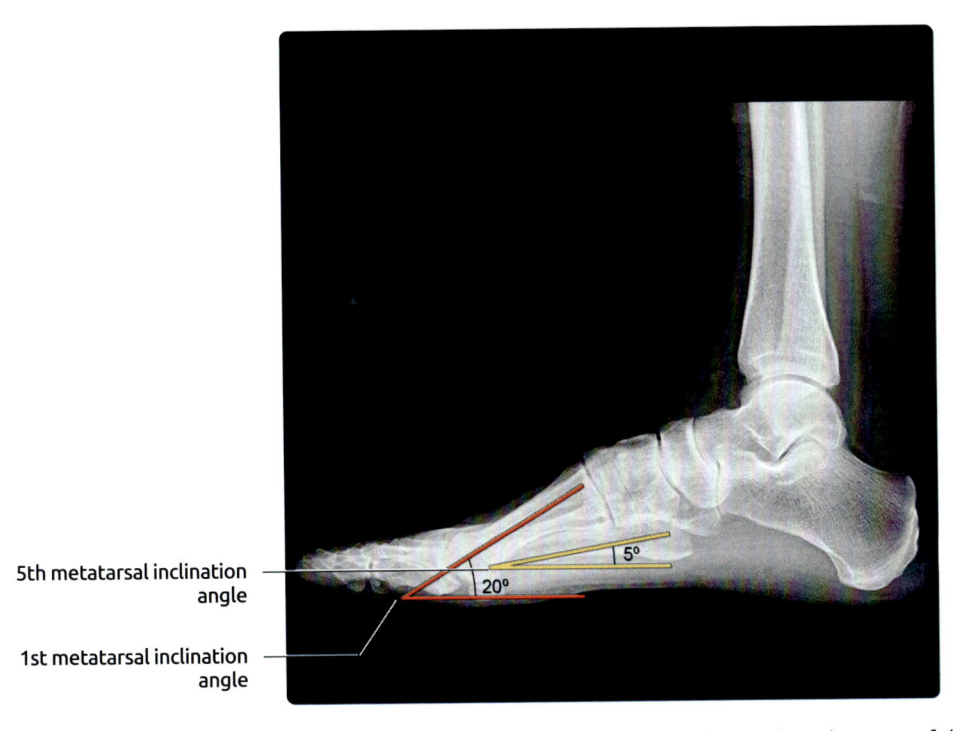

(Top) *Lateral weight-bearing radiograph shows the talometatarsal axis. The line drawn along the center of the talar axis will continue along the axis of the 1st metatarsal in a normally aligned foot. The axis of the talus passes above the 1st metatarsal axis in the pes cavus. It passes below the 1st metatarsal axis in the pes planus.* **(Bottom)** *Lateral weight-bearing radiograph shows the plantigrade inclination of the metatarsals. The inclination angle is the angle between the horizontal and the axis of a metatarsal. It decreases from 20° for the 1st metatarsal to 15° for the 2nd, 10° for the 3rd, 8° for the 4th, and 5° for the 5th.*

METATARSAL ALIGNMENT AP

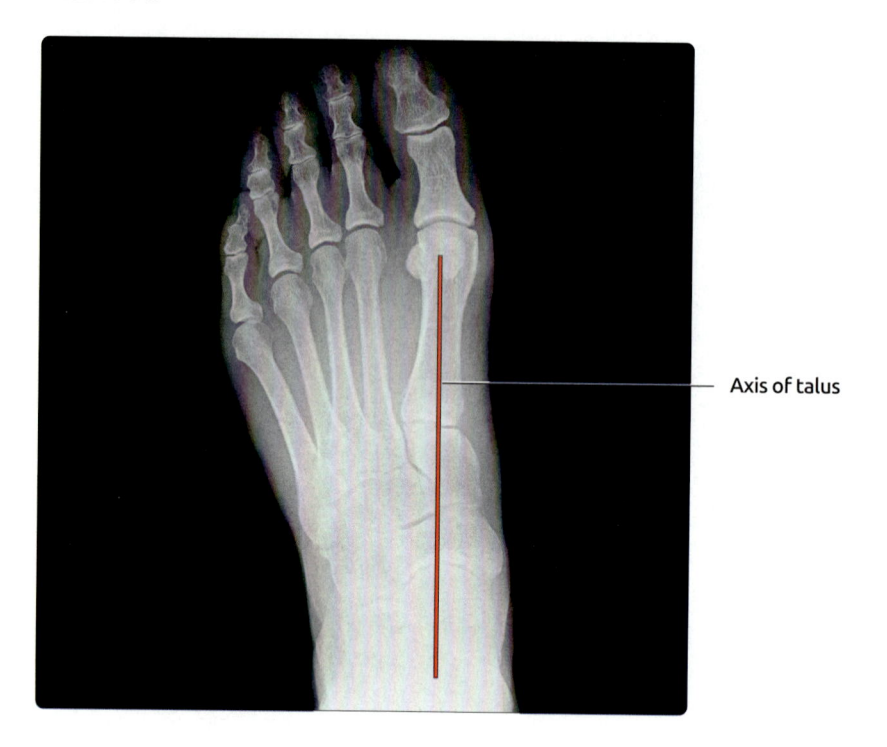

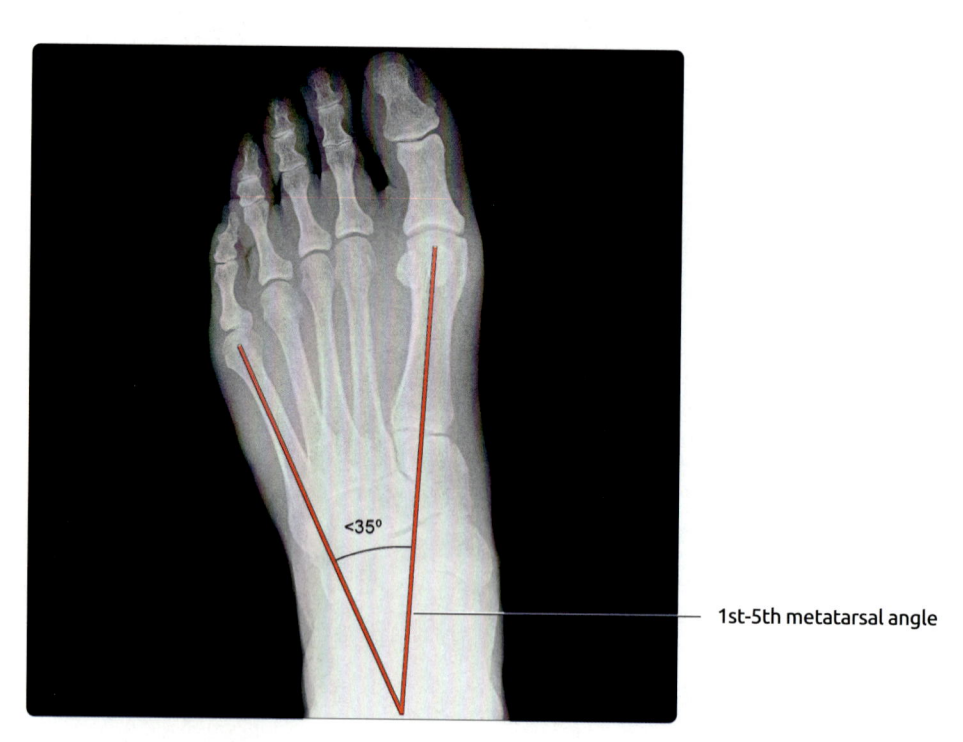

Axis of talus

<35°

1st-5th metatarsal angle

(Top) *Anteroposterior radiograph shows the normal relationship between the axis of the talus and the axis of the 1st metatarsal. The axis of the talus extends along the axis of the 1st metatarsal, or between the 1st and 2nd metatarsal. In the forefoot varus or adductus, the axis of the 1st metatarsal deviates medially from the axis of the talus. In the forefoot valgus or abductus, the 1st metatarsal deviates laterally.* **(Bottom)** *Anteroposterior radiograph shows that metatarsals overlap at the base and fan outward. Splayfoot is present when 1st-5th metatarsal angle is more than 35°. The normal angle between the 1st and 2nd metatarsals is < 9°, and between the 4th and 5th metatarsals is < 5°. An increased 1st-2nd metatarsal angle is termed metatarsus primus varus, and an increased 4th-5th metatarsal angle is termed metatarsus quintus valgus.*

Foot and Ankle Measurements and Lines

METATARSAL LENGTHS

2nd metatarsal length

1st metatarsal length

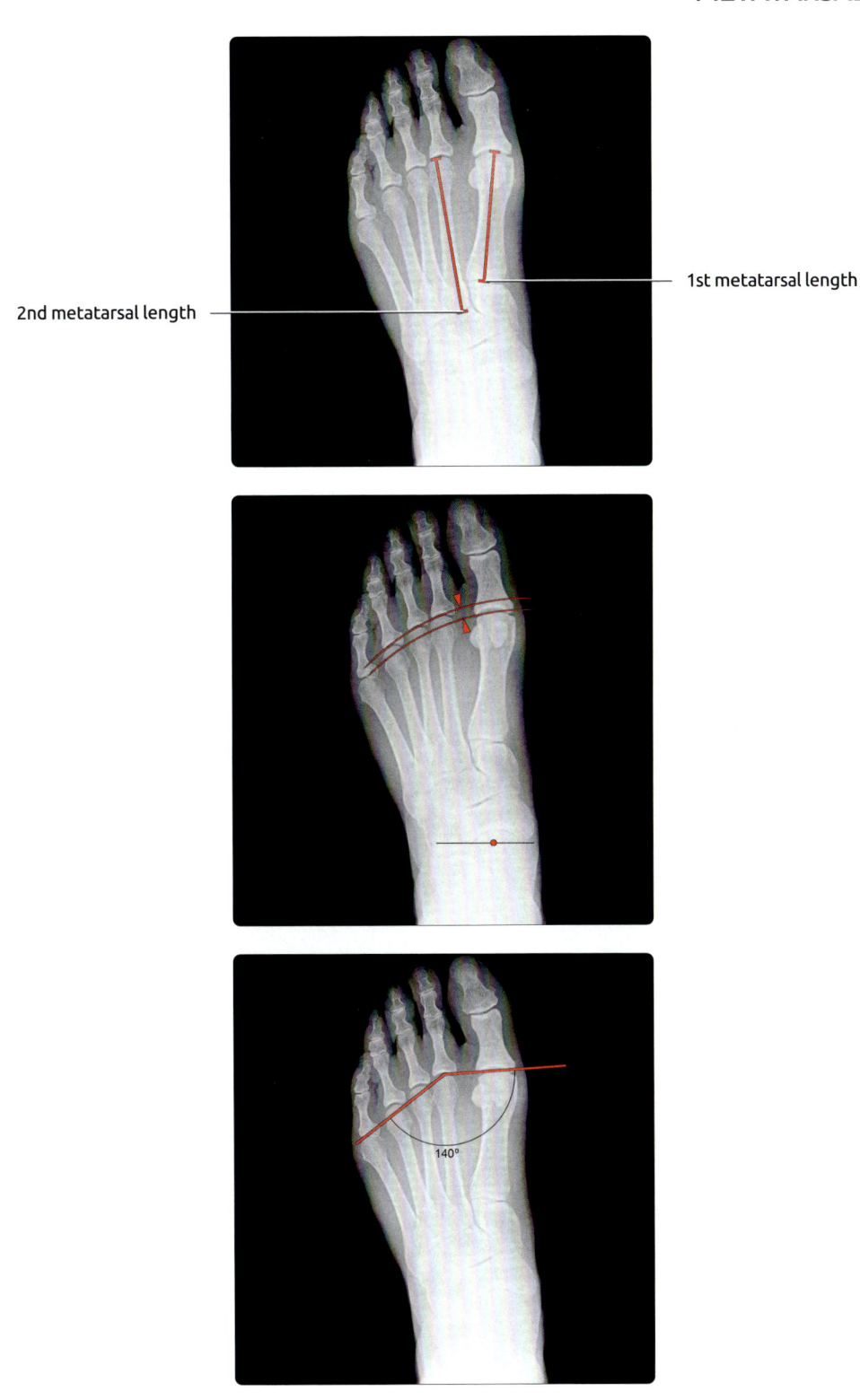

140°

(Top) Anteroposterior radiograph shows the relative metatarsal lengths measured by the method of Stokes. In this method, absolute metatarsal lengths are measured, but overall alignment is not considered. **(Middle)** Anteroposterior radiograph shows relative metatarsal lengths by the method of Hardy and Clapham. An arc is drawn centered on the metatarsal head, with the center of the arc at the center of the talar head. The difference in metatarsal length is measured as the distance between the arcs of the 1st and 2nd metatarsal. **(Bottom)** Anteroposterior radiograph shows the metatarsal break angle of Meschan. This angle is formed between the line tangential to the 1st and 2nd metatarsal head articular surfaces, and the line tangential to the 2nd and 5th metatarsal head articular surfaces. Normal is 140°; < 135° indicates relatively short 1st metatarsal.

Foot and Ankle Measurements and Lines

HALLUX ALIGNMENT

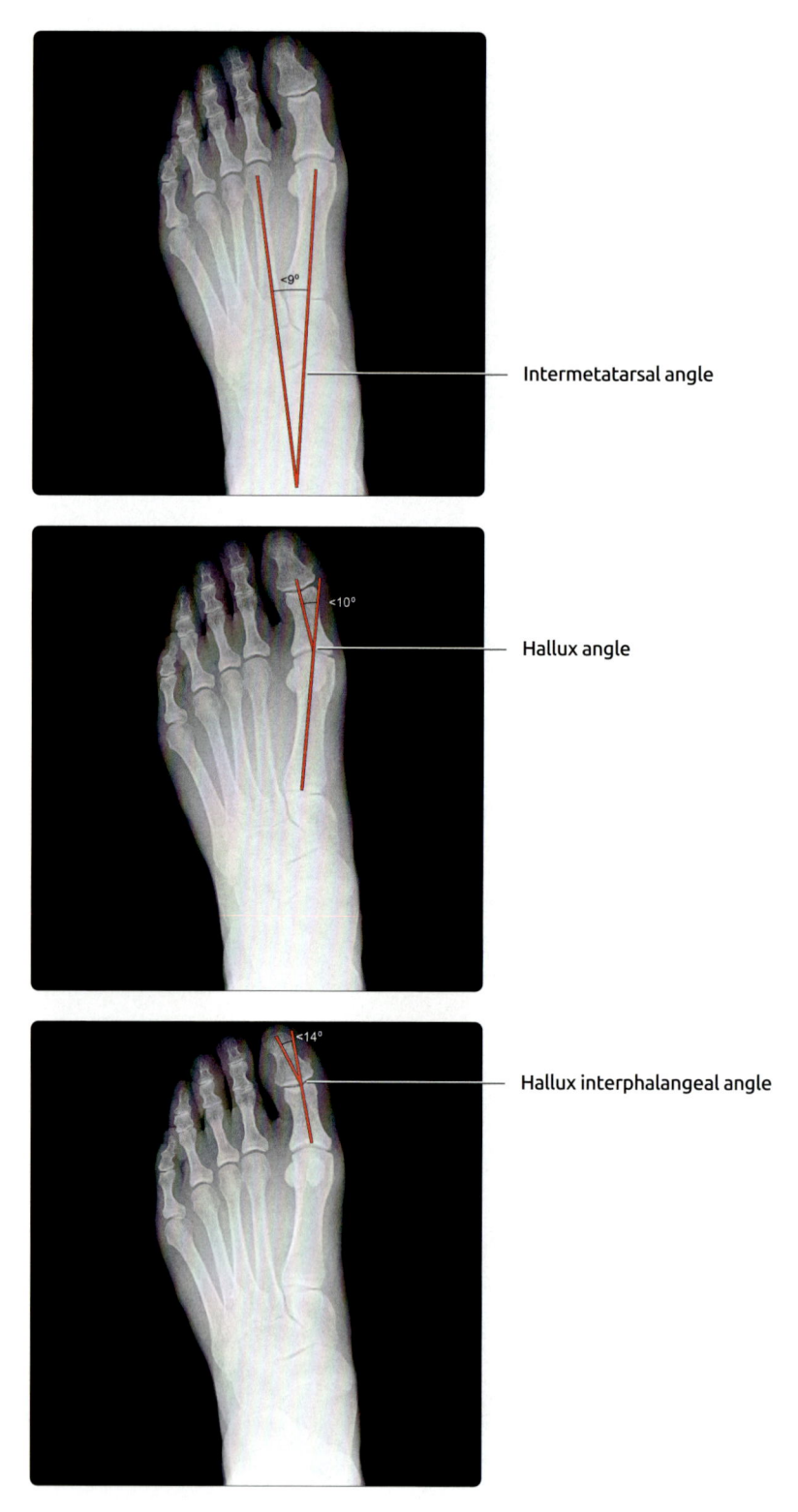

Intermetatarsal angle

Hallux angle

Hallux interphalangeal angle

(Top) Anteroposterior radiograph shows a normal intermetatarsal angle of less than 10°. *(Middle)* Anteroposterior radiograph shows a normal hallux angle of less than 10°. The threshold for definition of hallux valgus varies between 15° and 20°. *(Bottom)* Anteroposterior radiograph shows a hallux interphalangeal angle. Lines are drawn along the axes of the 1st proximal and distal phalanges. Normal angle is 6-14°.

Foot and Ankle Measurements and Lines

SOFT TISSUE MEASUREMENTS

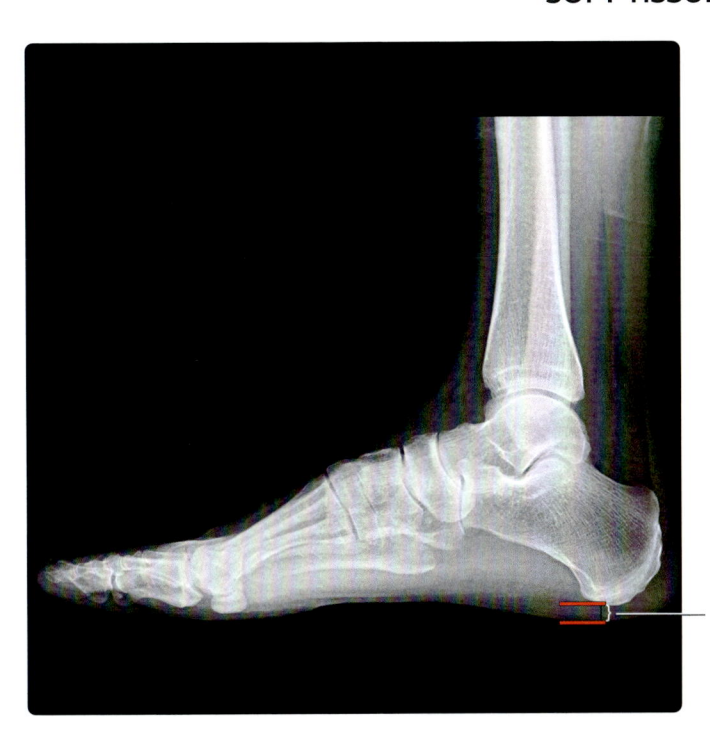

Plantar heel pad thickness

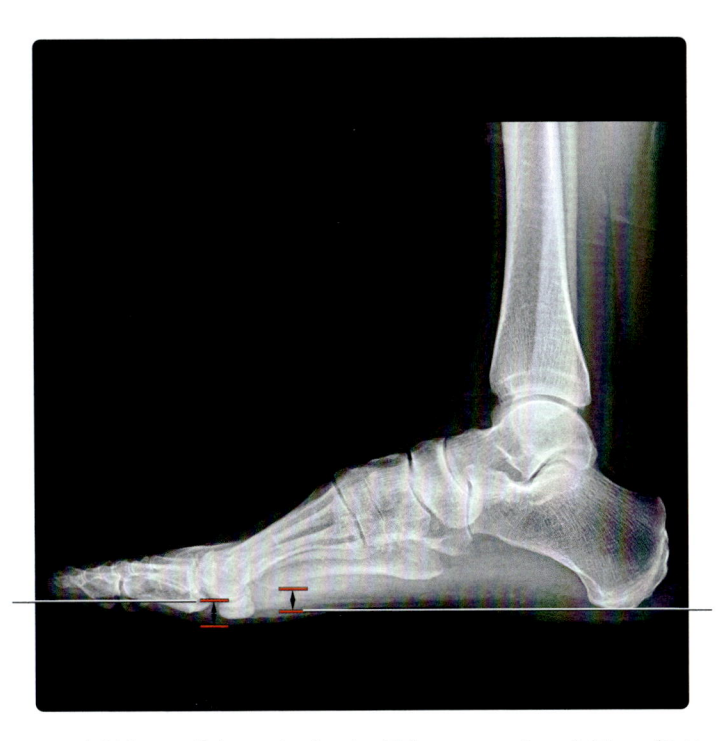

1st metatarsal pad — 5th metatarsal pad

(Top) *Lateral radiograph shows a normal thickness of plantar heel pad, which can range from 4-17 mm.* **(Bottom)** *Lateral weight-bearing radiograph shows a normal thickness of metatarsal soft tissue pads. The 1st measures between 7-25 mm, and the 5th measures between 1-16 mm. Note that it is difficult to discern the soft tissue margin at the lateral aspect of the foot, limiting accuracy of the 5th metatarsal pad measurement.*

INDEX

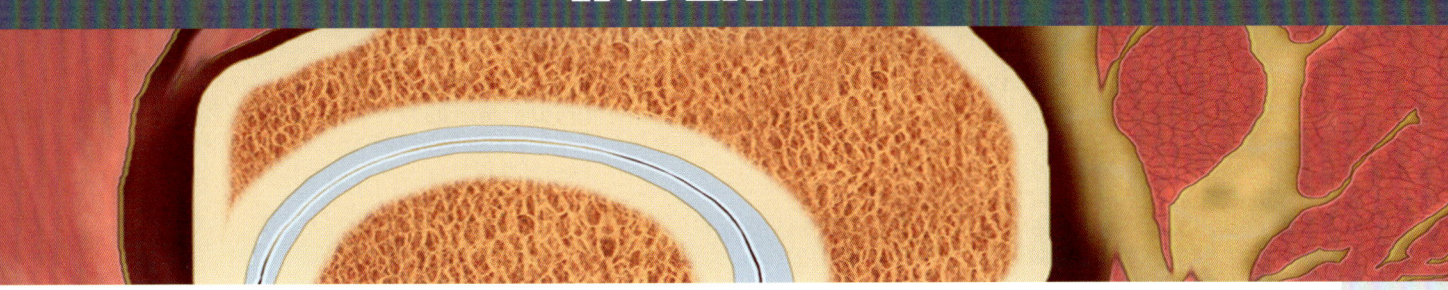

A

A1 pulley, **449, 474–475, 477, 479, 481**
A2 pulley, **464–465, 474–475, 479–481, 483**
A3 pulley, **471, 474–475, 480, 482**
A4 pulley, **474–475, 480, 482–483**
A5 pulley, **474–475**
Abdominal muscle, aponeuroses, **522–525**
Abdominal wall muscle, **515–518**
 - anterior, **528**
Abductor digiti minimi, **352–361, 370–375, 378–379, 400, 402, 405, 407, 412, 414–415, 438, 441, 445, 458–464, 466–467, 470, 474, 476, 925, 958–959, 962–963, 968–973, 978–979, 1035, 1040, 1056–1061, 1064–1073, 1082–1083, 1084–1086, 1088–1089**
 - accessory, **400, 418**
Abductor hallucis, **925, 956, 958–959, 962–963, 966–975, 988, 992, 1040, 1056–1059, 1056–1061, 1064–1071, 1072–1075, 1078, 1084–1086, 1088–1089, 1097–1099, 1121**
Abductor pollicis brevis, **354–361, 368–369, 371, 374–376, 383–385, 399, 402, 411, 414, 438, 445, 447–448, 450–451, 456, 458–461, 466–467, 471, 474**
 - insertion, **449–450**
Abductor pollicis longus, **299, 302, 308–315, 318–319, 321, 331, 344–355, 368–373, 385–386, 399, 401–409, 415, 438, 448, 456, 476**
 - multiple slips, **425**
Abductor pollicis muscle, **448**
ABER (abduction external rotation) plane, shoulder, **86–93**
Aberrant flexor digiti minimi, **425**
Absent retromalleolar fibular groove, **1100**
Accessory abductor digiti minimi, **400, 418**
Accessory anterior talofibular ligament, **940**
Accessory centers, **1100–1101**
Accessory collateral ligaments, **450, 477**
Accessory epiphysis, **426, 1119**
Accessory extensor pollicis longus muscle, **425**
Accessory facet, with hamate, **419**
Accessory flexor digitorum longus muscle, **1125–1126**
Accessory flexor hallucis longus muscle, **1124**
Accessory flexor muscles, **952–957, 1100, 1124–1125**
Accessory muscles, ankle, **946**
Accessory navicular, **990, 1100–1101, 1110–1112**
Accessory ossicle
 - foot, **1101**
 - wrist, **423**
Accessory ossification center, **418, 590, 597, 1100, 1103–1104, 1110**
Accessory palmaris longus, **400, 425**
Accessory peroneus longus tendon slip, **1127**
Accessory radial collateral ligament, **200, 449, 479**
Accessory sacroiliac joint, **591**
Accessory soleus, **1100, 1123**
Accessory ulnar collateral ligament, **449, 479**
Accessory vein, **222–223**
Acetabular angle, **598, 601**
Acetabular cartilage, **587**
Acetabular depth, **598**
Acetabular fossa, **489, 539, 552, 554, 556, 559, 561, 563, 572–573, 580–581, 584–585, 590, 594, 618–619**
 - margins, **584**
 - notch at superior margin, **572**
 - superior margin, **582**
Acetabular index, **598**
Acetabular labrum, **554, 561, 565–568, 573, 594**
 - anterior, **565, 567**
Acetabular notch, **486, 489, 554**
 - superior, **590, 593**
Acetabular overcoverage, **599**
Acetabular rim
 - anterior, **524–525, 603**
 - posterior, **514, 603**
Acetabular roof, **526–527, 560, 564, 566, 576, 587, 596**
 - axis of, **601**
Acetabular undercoverage, **599**
Acetabular version, **598–599**
 - radiographic measurement, **603**
Acetabulum, **508–510, 531–534, 554, 556, 561, 563, 651**
 - anterior wall, **564–565, 576**
 - articular surface, **489**
 - lateral margin, **572**
 - medial wall, **600, 654**
 - posterior column, **565**
 - posterior wall, **576**
Achilles tendinopathy, **1107**
Achilles tendon, **821, 881–882, 884–885, 891, 893, 905–909, 912, 919–920, 925, 928–930, 936, 940, 946, 948–961, 976–977, 980–981, 983, 994, 1123–1124**
 - axial MR, **984–985**
 - distracted ruptured, **820**
 - insertion, **924**
 - sagittal MR, **986**
Acromial plexus, **10**
Acromial process, **87**
Acromial pseudospur, **141**
Acromioclavicular joint, **16–18, 40–41, 72–73, 81–83, 98, 108, 141, 143–146**
Acromioclavicular ligament, **112, 125**
Acromion, **4, 29–30, 66–67, 87–88, 103, 105, 113–114, 124, 134, 141, 143–145, 156–158**
 - base, **145**

INDEX

Acromion process, **8–9, 12–13, 29, 37, 68–73, 81–83, 95, 97–100, 108–110**
 - scapula, **40–43**
Acromion pseudospur, MR pitfalls, **141**
Adductor aponeurosis, **447, 449, 451, 471**
Adductor brevis, **489, 515–517, 520–524, 529, 535–540, 543, 548–551, 553, 557, 562, 572–573, 609–610, 618–631, 650–651, 654–657**
Adductor canal, **608**
Adductor hallucis, **1041, 1084, 1097–1099**
 - oblique head, **1056–1061, 1070–1073, 1080–1082, 1085, 1087, 1089, 1097**
 - transverse head, **1058–1061, 1072–1073, 1080–1082, 1087, 1089, 1097, 1099**
Adductor hiatus, **610, 650, 657**
Adductor longus, **489, 515–523, 529–530, 535–538, 540–544, 546–553, 557, 562, 609–610, 615, 619–635, 650–657**
Adductor magnus, **489, 493, 513–515, 521–526, 529, 539, 550–553, 557, 562, 564–565, 567, 572–573, 609–610, 615, 622–639, 648–652, 654–658, 665–667, 669, 688–691, 730–733, 736**
 - at adductor tubercle, **719**
 - at insertion, **719**
 - ischiocondylar portion, **529, 610, 624–625, 636–647**
Adductor minimus, **529, 541, 557, 566**
Adductor pollicis, **358–361, 370–373, 399, 438, 441, 445, 448–451, 456, 460–461, 466–467, 471, 474**
 - oblique head, **440–441, 445**
 - osseous insertion, **440–441, 445**
 - transverse head, **440–441, 445**
Adductor pollicis brevis, **438**
Adductor pollicis longus tendon, **450**
Adductor tubercle, **617, 672, 719, 736–738**
Air bubble, **29**
Alpha angle, **599, 600–602**
Anatomic axis, **1128**
Anatomic snuffbox, **342, 385–386, 408**
Anconeus, **155, 158, 174–179, 198, 208, 210, 212–213, 216, 224–236, 248, 251, 254–259, 265, 291, 302–309, 321–322**
Anconeus epitrochlearis, **219, 248, 280, 291**
Angle of Gissane, **1024, 1048**
Angle of Wiberg, **598–603**
Ankle
 - arthrogram, **938**
 - articulations, **918**
 - axial T1 MR, **948–959**
 - coronal T1 MR, **960–973**
 - cutaneous innervation, **932–933**
 - graphics, muscles and tendons, **947**
 - ligaments, **918, 1004–1031**
 - measurements, **1128–1139**
 - MR atlas, **946–979**
 - nerves, **920, 930–931**
 - normal variants, **1100–1127**
 - osseous structures, **918**
 - overview, **918–933**
 - radiography, **934–945**
     AP, **935**
     axial MR, **939–940**
     Broden view, **937**
     coronal MR, **943–945**
     lateral, **936**
     mortise view, **938**
     oblique, **935**
     os calcis views, **934**
     sagittal MR, **941–942**
 - retinacula, **919, 928**
 - sagittal T1 MR, **974–979**
 - spaces, **920**
 - tendons, **919, 929, 980–1003**
     axial MR, **984–985, 987, 989, 991, 995–996**
     coronal MR, **988, 993**
     coronal T2WI FS MR, **998**
     graphics, **981–983**
     sagittal MR, **986, 999**
 - vessels, **920**
Ankle gutter
 - lateral, **952**
 - medial, **952**
Ankle joint capsule, **1102**
Ankle joint recess
 - extending into tibiofibular joint, **1006**
 - extending to distal tibiofibular joint, **1015**
 - posterior, **940, 1016**
Ankle mortise, alignment, **1129**
Ankle retinacula, **946**
Ankle (talocrural) joint, **918**
Annular ligament, **198, 200, 204–205, 209–210, 213, 216, 228–229, 270–272, 274, 276–277, 279, 304–305**
 - anterior aspect, **276**
 - insertion, **280**
 - notch, **281**
 - posterior aspect, **276**
Annular pulleys, **472**
Anomalous muscles, wrist, **400, 425**
Antebrachial fascia, **344–345**
Anterior abdominal wall musculature, **528**
Anterior acetabular labrum, **552**
Anterior acetabular rim, **578**
Anterior ankle fat pad, **936**
Anterior calcaneal facet, **927**
Anterior calcaneal tubercle, **936, 1030**
Anterior center-edge angle, **598–603, 602**
Anterior circumflex humeral artery, **10, 37, 82–84, 157**
 - anterolateral branch, **140**
Anterior circumflex humeral vein, anterolateral branch, **140**
Anterior circumflex humeral vessels, **56–57, 72–75, 83, 99–100**
Anterior colliculus, **881, 883, 935**
Anterior column
 - hip, **559, 564**
 - pelvis, **577**
Anterior compartment, thigh, **611**
Anterior cortex humeral shaft, **295**

INDEX

Anterior cruciate ligament (ACL), **664–666, 675–676, 678, 680, 682–685, 692–695, 710–713, 722–723, 729–731, 733, 739–740, 747–750, 756–758, 763–767, 768–769, 771–774, 776–777, 779, 782, 784, 836–840, 842–844, 848**
- angle, relative to femur and tibia, **873**
- anteromedial band, **752, 760, 768, 785, 845**
- anteromedial bundle, **681, 770**
- "foot" attachment, **769**
- insertion on tibia, **837**
- intermediate fibers, **752**
- isometric tunnel locations, **875**
- medial, **841**
- origin, **768, 771**
- posterolateral band, **710–711, 752, 760, 768, 785, 845**
- posterolateral bundle, **681, 770**
- proximal fibers, **841**
- synovium covering, **784**
- tibial attachment, **675**
- 2° signs of tear, **872**

Anterior facet, **570**
Anterior fat pad, **196–197, 215, 222–225, 245–246, 734**
- in coronoid fossa, **264**
- normal, **282**

Anterior glenoid labrum, **30**
Anterior glenoid rim, **16**
Anterior gluteal line, **489**
Anterior humeral line, **292**
Anterior inferior glenoid rim, **18**
Anterior inferior iliac spine, **486, 489–490, 506, 518, 527, 542–543, 556, 560, 563, 566, 575, 577–578, 587, 616**
Anterior inferior labrum, **92**
Anterior interosseous artery, **199, 303, 332**
Anterior interosseous nerve, **195, 199, 217–218, 303**
Anterior joint capsule, **563, 566–567**
- insertion, **4**

Anterior joint recess, **35, 196, 206–207, 209, 211, 586, 588, 938–939, 1045–1046, 1105**
Anterior labrum, **26–27, 31–32, 35, 46–53, 91–92, 117–118, 130–131, 134–135, 559, 563, 565–566, 583–585, 587, 593**
Anterior lateral meniscocruciate ligament, **763, 836**
Anterior lateral trochlear ridge, **716–717**
Anterior leg muscles, **664**
Anterior longitudinal ligament, **488**
Anterior margin, acetabulum, **578**
Anterior medial crural fascia, **791**
Anterior medial trochlear ridge, **716–717**
Anterior meniscal fascicle, **774**
Anterior meniscocruciate ligament, **764, 773, 837–838**
Anterior oblique ligament, **451**
Anterior recess, knee, **677**
Anterior recurrent tibial artery, **893**
Anterior rim, **525, 603**
- acetabulum, **575**

Anterior subtalar facet, **923, 1047**
Anterior subtalar joint, **946**
Anterior superficial deltoid, **939, 945**
Anterior superior iliac spine, **486, 489–490, 500, 519, 527, 556, 575–577, 609, 615**

Anterior superior labrum, **90**
Anterior suprapatellar (quadriceps) fat pad, **736**
Anterior talofibular ligament, **918, 939–940, 941, 946, 952–955, 979, 1004–1005, 1015, 1018, 1020**
Anterior tibial artery, **663, 669, 879, 884–885, 887–893, 896–897, 920, 1035–1036**
Anterior tibial muscle, **1002**
Anterior tibial tendon, **929–930, 947–953, 955, 968–976, 980–984, 987, 989–990, 993, 997, 1002–1003, 1064–1069, 1088**
Anterior tibial tubercle, **935**
Anterior tibial vessels, **898–909**
Anterior tibiofibular ligament, **918, 926–927, 939, 941, 944–945, 948–951, 979, 1007, 1011**
- inferior, **968–969, 978–979, 1004–1005, 1007–1008, 1011–1014, 1018–1019**

Anterior tibiotalar band, deep deltoid, **945**
Anterior tibiotalar ligament, **927, 948–951**
Anterior tubercle, **923–924**
Anterior ulnar recurrent artery, **303**
Anterior wall, **559, 587**
- acetabulum, **578, 588**
- pelvis, **577**

Anterolateral joint recess, **945**
Anterolateral ligament, **694–699**
- insertion, **698–699**

Anteromedial knee, **665, 669**
Anterosuperior labrum, **88–89**
Anterosuperior rim, of acetabulum, **584**
Aponeurosis, **519, 530–531, 533–536, 544, 546–553**
Apophysis, **292, 1119**
Arcade of Frohse, **218**
Arcs of Gilula, **432**
Arcuate artery, **1036**
Arcuate ligament, **388, 542–543, 546, 664, 683, 731–732, 783, 795, 797–803, 805–808, 810, 822**
- lateral, **792, 802–803, 809**
- medial, **761, 792, 802–803, 807, 810**
- origin, **803, 810**
- of Osborne, **197, 224–225, 253, 275**

Arcuate line, **490, 575, 577, 586**
- S1, **579**

Arcuate popliteal ligament and capsule, **724–726**
Arcuate pubic ligament, **528**
Arm. *See also* Elbow; Forearm; Wrist.
- graphics
    anterior, **157**
    axial, **159**
    posterior, **158**
- left
    axial T1 MR, **161, 163, 165, 167, 169, 171, 173, 175, 177, 179**
    coronal T1 MR, **181, 183, 185, 187**
- MR atlas, **154–191**
- radiographic anatomy, **154–191**
- right
    axial T1 MR, **160, 162, 164, 166, 168, 170, 172, 174, 176, 178**
    coronal T1 MR, **180, 182, 184, 186**
    sagittal T1 MR, **188–191**

INDEX

- rotation, **33**
Articular branch, **646–647**
Articular cartilage, **135, 556, 559, 948–951, 1014**
 - glenoid, **135**
 - proximal phalanx, **477**
Articularis genus muscle, **609, 812, 818**
Articulation, with 3rd metacarpal, **422**
Assimilation joint, **591**
Auricular surface, **490**
Av pulley, **474**
Avian spur, **285–286, 289**
 - with ligament of Struthers, **289**
Avian spur seen en face, **286**
Axillary artery, **10, 58–59, 79–80, 80, 82, 97**
 - distal, **58–59**
Axillary fat, **64–65**
Axillary nerve, **9, 11, 56–57, 66–68, 70–71, 76–77, 81, 83–84, 95, 98–100, 110–111, 158, 180–185**
Axillary neurovascular bundle, **12, 131**
Axillary pouch, **22, 29, 127, 131**
Axillary recess, **21, 24, 29–30, 33, 91–92**
Axillary recess en face, **21**
Axillary vein, **79–80, 91, 97**
Axillary vessels, **76–77, 182, 184–185**

B

Baker (popliteal) cyst, **682, 781**
Basicervical region, **616**
Basilic vein, **159, 166–176, 178–179, 184–188, 195, 197, 215, 220–225, 238–241, 244, 252–254, 261, 263, 332, 344–345, 378**
Bassett ligament, **939, 941, 979, 1008, 1012**
Baxter nerve, **956–957**
Biceps, **5, 29, 34, 37, 62–65, 87, 157, 160–179, 186–187, 189–190, 197–198, 211–213, 215–217, 224–233, 238–241, 246, 250–251, 256, 261–262, 267, 269, 302, 316–317, 512, 536–537, 562, 564, 620**
 - attachment, **149**
 - bicipital recess outlining, **21**
 - deep sulcus, **33**
 - distal, **249**
 - entering bicipital groove, **101**
 - long head, **6, 8–9, 12, 14, 20, 22–24, 26–29, 31–33, 35, 37, 46–65, 72–77, 83–84, 87–89, 94, 95, 98–99, 101, 102–104, 106–107, 109–111, 113–114, 116–118, 120–121, 124, 127–137, 139–140, 148, 154, 157, 159, 186–187, 190**
 - short head, **6, 8, 12, 22, 37, 46–51, 54–65, 72–77, 82, 87, 95, 98–100, 105, 108–109, 113, 130, 131, 132, 154, 157, 159, 184–187, 189, 664, 732, 882**
 - transverse ligament overlying, **22**
Biceps anchor, **9, 22, 26, 30, 88–89, 98**
 - normal variants, **33–34**
Biceps aponeurosis, **197, 217–218, 226–231, 245–246, 248, 250–251, 254–256, 264**
Biceps brachii, **212, 220–225, 242–243, 245–247, 248, 250, 252–255, 257, 264–266, 269, 304–307, 316–317, 321–322**

Biceps femoris, **562, 566, 610, 614, 623, 640, 644–649, 657–658, 664, 668–669, 674–676, 681, 683, 688–711, 722–727, 731–732, 737, 738, 754–755, 759, 783–784, 796, 798–801, 804–806, 808–810, 819, 882, 884, 886, 891, 893–895, 915**
 - expansion, **700–701, 896–897**
 - fibrous extension, **676, 799**
 - hypertrophied, **812, 816–817**
 - inserting on fibular head, **891**
 - insertion, **704–705, 796, 808, 811**
 - long head, **489, 493, 512–513, 557, 610, 622–645, 648–649, 657–659, 796–799, 805, 808, 811**
   anterior arm, **798**
   conjoined origin with semitendinosus, **512–513, 526, 655–658**
   direct arm, **798**
   insertion, **805–806, 811**
 - short head, **610, 634–645, 648, 658–659, 796–799, 805**
   anterior arm, **798, 805**
   direct arm, **798**
   insertion, **798**
Biceps groove, **25, 88**
Biceps labral complex (BLC), **114–116, 120, 126–127, 138**
 - normal variants, **33, 136–137**
 - type 1, **33, 136–137**
 - type 2, **33, 136–137**
 - type 3, **33, 136–137**
Biceps recess, joint, **34**
Biceps sling, **14, 25**
Biceps tendon sheath, contrast in, **88**
Bicipital aponeurosis, **176–177**
Bicipital bursa, **267**
Bicipital fascia, **155**
Bicipital groove, **74–75, 114, 132, 137, 140**
Bicipital labral complex, **87**
Bicipital recess, **28**
 - joint, **27**
Bicipital tendon, **35**
Bicipital tubercle, **209**
Bicipitoradial bursa, **194, 249, 267**
Bifid piriformis, **596**
Bifurcate ligament, **926–927, 954–955, 978, 1004–1005, 1010, 1018, 1021–1022, 1024, 1029, 1035, 1037, 1048, 1055**
 - calcaneocuboid, **927, 1018, 1021, 1029**
 - calcaneonavicular, **927, 1025, 1029**
Bigelow ligament, **555**
Bipartite calcaneal apophysis, **1107**
Bipartite epiphysis, **1119**
Bipartite lateral sesamoid, **1120**
Bipartite lunate, wrist, **418**
Bipartite medial sesamoid, **1120**
Bipartite os peroneum, **1115**
Blumensaat line, **672, 678, 745, 873**
Böehler angle, **1128, 1131**
Bone marrow, **4**
Bowed extensor tendon, **423**

INDEX

Brachial artery, **8, 10, 37, 60–65, 155, 157, 159, 188–189, 194–195, 197–199, 215–217, 220–224, 226–229, 245, 252–257, 264, 280, 289, 303–307, 316–317**
- deep, **9–10, 60–65, 159–171, 181–183**
    ascending branch, **10**
- deep branch, **199, 303**
- median nerve traveling with, **289**

Brachial fascia, **155**
Brachial plexus, **79–80, 182, 184–185**
- posterior cord, **11**
- upper trunk, **11**

Brachial veins, **159, 306–307**
Brachial vessels, **160–171, 182–185**
Brachialis, **6–7, 154, 159, 162–179, 184–191, 197–198, 211–213, 215–217, 220–222, 224–231, 237–242, 244–247, 248, 251–256, 261–265, 268–269, 302, 304–307, 316–317, 321–322**
Brachioradialis, **157–158, 170–179, 186–187, 191, 197–198, 209, 212–213, 215–217, 220–233, 236–243, 246–247, 248, 251–258, 261–262, 266, 291, 302–311, 316–321, 327**
Buford complex, **32, 126, 138**
- normal variant, **150–151**

Buford ligament, glenohumeral ligament, MR pitfall, **118**
Bursae, **5, 1090**
- metatarsophalangeal joints, **1096, 1099**

C

C1 pulley, **474–475**
C2 pulley, **474–475**
C3 pulley, **474–475**
C5 spinal nerve, **11**
C6 spinal nerve, **11**
C7 spinal nerve, **11**
C8 spinal nerve, **11**
Calcaneal apophysis, **1107**
Calcaneal facet
- anterior, **927**
- middle, **927**
- posterior, **927, 1025**

Calcaneal nerve, medial, **1035**
Calcaneal pitch angle, **1134**
Calcaneal pseudocyst, **1106**
Calcaneal tubercle
- anterior, **936, 1030**
- lateral, **935–936, 960–963, 967**
- medial, **960–963, 1028**

Calcaneal tuberosity, **923–924, 936, 960–963**
Calcaneocuboid bifurcate ligament, **927**
- medial, **1021, 1029**

Calcaneocuboid joint, **956–957, 972–973, 977–978, 1042, 1048, 1064–1065, 1088, 1108, 1114**
Calcaneocuboid ligament, **1035**
- dorsal, **926**
- dorsolateral, **1021**
- plantar, **958–959**
- short plantar, **1030**

Calcaneofibular ligament, **918, 926, 940, 943–944, 946, 956–957, 966–967, 979, 985, 992, 996, 1004–1005, 1011, 1013–1018, 1026, 1046**
- insertion, **924**

Calcaneonavicular bifurcate ligament, **927, 1029**
- medial, **1021**

Calcaneus, **910, 918, 923–928, 935, 937–938, 943, 956–959, 964–965, 972–973, 982, 984–986, 988–990, 994, 996, 999–1000, 1003, 1005, 1008–1011, 1013, 1015–1018, 1021–1031, 1038, 1045, 1093, 1105–1106, 1108, 1115, 1123, 1127**
- anterior process, **923–924, 936, 977–978, 1048**
- body, **923**
- posterior facet for, **922**
- posterior process, **937, 943, 964, 967, 976–977, 1113**
- sulcus, **923–924**

Calcar, **594**
Capitate, **326, 329, 335–337, 343, 350–357, 364–371, 381–383, 394, 396–397, 423**
- articulating with normal lunate facet, **419**
- cyst with, **423**
- normal cartilage at articulation of, **419**

Capitellar articular cartilage, **207**
Capitellar epiphysis, **280–281**
- irregular ossification, **287**

Capitellum, **202–203, 207–208, 210, 212, 238, 240, 246, 261, 265, 274, 286–287, 290, 294–295, 321–322**
- 1st to ossify, **295**
- fragmentation, **288**
    worsening, **288**
- pseudodefect, **208, 210, 247, 265, 280, 283–284**
- reconstituted, **288**

Capitohamate ligament, **330, 354–355, 391–392, 396–397**
Capitolunate angle, **428**
Capitulum, **174–177, 186, 190**
Capsular insertion, **582**
Capsular junction, **780**
Capsular ligament, **1021**
Capsule, **103**
Capsulolabral complex, **5**
Carpal angle, **428, 432**
Carpal arch, dorsal, **332**
Carpal boss, wrist, **422**
Carpal coalitions, **418, 420**
Carpal height ratio, **428, 433**
Carpal ligament, volar, **342**
Carpal row, proximal, **314–315**
Carpal translation, **428**
Carpal tunnel
- anatomic spaces, **342**
- region, **372–373**
- roof of, **440–441, 443, 445**
- zone III, **478**
- zone IV, **478**

Carpal tunnel view, **334, 337**
Carpometacarpal alignment, **432**
Carpometacarpal compartment
- common, **338**
- 1st, **338**

INDEX

Carpometacarpal joint, **326**
 - 1st, **436, 444, 446–449, 451, 455**
 - 2nd-5th, **436**
 - 3rd, **336**
 - 5th, **335**
 - capsule, **380**
Carpometacarpal ligaments, **330, 389, 391–392**
Cartilaginous loose body, **677**
Caton method, **858–859**
Center-edge angle, **598, 602**
Central cartilage defect, shoulder, **22**
Central convexity, **1099**
Central disc, **589**
Central plantar compartment, foot, **1035**
Cephalic vein, **12, 48–49, 54–65, 74–77, 81–82, 100–101, 109–111, 132, 159–179, 191, 195, 197, 215, 222–227, 242–243, 252–253, 262, 304–307, 321, 332, 344, 348–353, 354–355, 357, 385**
 - deltopectoral groove, **52–53, 83**
 - median, **191**
Cervical artery, transverse, **10**
Cervical ligament, **926, 954–955, 970–971, 977, 1004–1005, 1013, 1021, 1023, 1029**
Chondromalacia hamate, **419**
Chondromalacia lunate, **419**
Circumflex artery
 - lateral, **562, 566–567, 570, 663**
 - medial, **561–562, 564–565, 568**
Circumflex femoral artery
 - lateral, **525–527, 541, 612, 620–621**
 - medial, **525, 527, 565, 612**
Circumflex femoral vein
 - lateral, **525–527, 613, 620–621**
 - medial, **525, 527, 613**
Circumflex iliac artery
 - deep, **612**
 - superficial, **612**
Circumflex scapular artery, **8, 10–11, 37, 157**
Circumflex scapular vessels, **72–73**
Circumflex vein
 - lateral, **562, 566, 570**
 - medial, **561–562, 564–565, 568**
Circumflex vessels, **595**
Clavicle, **4, 16–17, 19–20, 30, 40–43, 72, 74–77, 80–81, 96–98, 114, 156, 186–187**
 - distal, **16, 18, 81, 108, 113, 122–123, 125, 134, 143–144**
Cloquet node, **615**
Coccygeal plexus, **487**
Coccygeus, **490, 522–523, 557**
Coccyx, **486, 492, 508–510, 520, 546**
Collateral ligament
 - accessory, **450, 477**
 - fibular, **675–676, 681, 683, 698–699**
 - lateral, **664, 667, 670, 692–697, 700–701, 706–709, 727, 731–733, 749, 758–759, 797–800, 806, 809, 811, 1004–1005, 1015–1018, 1051, 1053, 1058–1059, 1074–1077, 1096, 1098–1099**
   accessory, **270–271**
   origin, **726**
 - main, **477**

 - medial, **665–666, 669, 670, 675–676, 680–681, 690–693, 696–699, 710–713, 718, 730–731, 733, 738, 749, 756–758, 789, 791, 793–794, 803, 881, 894–897, 1051, 1053, 1058–1059, 1074–1077, 1096, 1098–1099**
   deep, **795**
   longitudinal fibers, **694–697, 712–713**
   oblique, **712–713**
   oblique fibers, **694–697**
   superficial, **731**
   superior, **738**
   ulnar, **270**
 - radial, **197, 204–205, 209–210, 212–213, 215, 226–229, 237, 261, 270–279**
 - ulnar, **204–205, 208, 212–213, 225–227, 236–237, 260, 263, 270–272, 275–276, 278**
   lateral, **198, 216, 236–237, 260, 270–271, 273–274, 277–278**
   radial, **205, 208, 210**
Collateral ligament complex, **456, 464–465, 477**
 - lateral, **270**
 - radial, **271**
Colliculus
 - anterior, **881, 883, 935–936, 944**
 - posterior, **881, 883, 935–936**
Common digital tendon sheath, **474–475**
 - zone II, **478**
Common extensor tendon, **174–179, 186–187, 194, 197, 204, 212–213, 215, 226–230, 231, 236–239, 248–249, 251, 253–255, 260–261, 266, 272, 275–276, 278–279**
Common femoral artery, **510–511, 517–519, 523–525, 533–535, 537–538, 542–544, 552, 612, 615, 618–623, 652–656**
Common femoral nerve, **544, 618–621**
Common femoral vein, **510–511, 517–519, 523–525, 533–535, 537–538, 542–544, 552, 613, 615, 618–624, 652–656**
Common femoral vessels, **620**
Common flexor mass, **250**
Common flexor tendon, **175–177, 194, 197, 204, 208, 215, 217, 219, 225–231, 236–239, 244–245, 249, 251, 254–255, 260–261, 263, 272, 275–276, 279**
Common flexor tendon sheath, **400, 402**
Common iliac artery, **612**
Common iliac vein, **613**
Common interosseous artery, **199**
Common palmar digital arteries, **437, 443, 457**
Common peroneal nerve, **613, 644–647, 658, 663, 668, 674, 676, 688–705, 722–725, 798, 814, 819, 880, 889–890, 892–897, 915, 920, 932**
Concave condyle, **455**
Concave proximal phalangeal head, **454**
Concavity anteromedial plafond, **945**
Conjoined origin, semitendinosus and long head biceps femoris, **512–513, 526, 537, 618–620**
Conjoined tendon, **473, 476–477, 507, 528, 544–545, 683**
 - EDC contribution, **476**
 - short head biceps and coracobrachialis, **130**
Conoid tubercle, clavicle, **42–43**
Contrast outlining superior joint recesses, **580**

INDEX

Coracoacromial arch, **5, 36**
Coracoacromial ligament, **5, 42–45, 72–77, 82–83, 87, 95, 99, 106–107, 110–111, 112–114, 122, 124, 129, 134, 141, 157**
Coracobrachialis, **6, 8, 12, 37, 46–60, 62–65, 72–77, 81–82, 98–100, 105, 108–109, 130–132, 154, 157, 159–161, 184–187, 189**
Coracoclavicular ligament, **5, 44–45, 96, 107, 112**
 - conoid band, **113, 123**
 - conoid component, **76–77, 80**
 - coronoid component, **107**
 - trapezoid band, **113, 122–123**
 - trapezoid component, **76–77, 81, 97**
Coracohumeral ligament (CHL), **5, 14, 22–31, 44–45, 76–77, 82, 102–110, 112–116, 119–124, 127–129, 134, 148**
 - axial, **121**
 - coronal oblique, **122**
 - lateral band, **29**
 - lateral head, **27**
 - medial band, **29**
 - sagittal oblique, **120**
Coracoid ligament, **109**
Coracoid process, **4, 8, 23, 25, 27, 30, 32, 37, 45–47, 76–77, 81, 86–88, 95, 97–98, 104, 108, 113, 116, 120–124, 129–130, 156–157, 182–187**
 - scapula, **16–20**
Coronal oblique, axis for images, **585**
Coronary ligament, **681**
Coronoid, **202–203, 272, 301**
Coronoid fossa, **202–203, 238–239, 923**
 - anterior, **206**
Coronoid process, **202–203, 209, 227–229, 236–239, 245, 264, 278–279, 304–305, 318–319**
 - capsular attachment, **211**
 - ulna, **256**
Cortical defect, **830**
Coxa profunda, **600**
Crista, **1051, 1097–1098**
Crista medialis, **883**
CRITOE mnemonic, **292**
Cruciate ligaments, **670, 686, 749, 768–785**. *See also* Anterior cruciate ligament; Posterior cruciate ligament.
Cruciform pulleys, **472**
Crural fascia, **690–691, 702–703, 710–711, 738, 784, 786, 791, 795**
Cubital retinaculum, **215, 219**
Cuboid, **923–928, 935–936, 982, 988–989, 992–993, 996–1000, 1003, 1010, 1022–1024, 1029–1031, 1034, 1038–1039, 1043–1044, 1060–1067, 1069, 1080–1081, 1092–1093, 1108, 1111, 1114–1116**
Cuboid-cuneiform interosseous ligament, **954–955**
Cuboid-cuneiform joint, **1050**
Cuboid-cuneiform ligament, **993**
Cuboid sulcus, **958–959, 978, 1000**
Cuboid tunnel, **982, 1030**
Cuboides secondarium, **1100, 1114**
Cuboidocuneiform ligament, **1060–1061**

Cuneiform, **925, 1034, 1043**
 - 1st, **925, 936, 952–953, 955, 974, 982, 989–990, 997–998, 1003, 1038–1039, 1060–1061, 1068–1069, 1078, 1091–1095, 1111, 1113, 1117–1118**
 - 2nd, **936, 952–953, 955, 975, 1038–1039, 1068–1069, 1079, 1091–1093, 1117**
 - 3rd, **936, 955, 976–977, 989, 993, 1000, 1038–1039, 1066–1071, 1080, 1091–1094**
 - lateral, **954**
 - medial, **1110**
Cuneiform-cuboid ligament, **1037, 1055, 1062–1063, 1066–1069**
Cuneiform-metatarsal, 2nd, alignment, **1132**
Cutaneous nerve
 - antebrachial, median, **11**
 - brachial, medial, **11**
 - lateral, **303**
 - posterior femoral, **493**

D

Deep anterior tibiotalar ligament, **940**
Deep brachial artery, **95, 303**
Deep circumflex iliac artery, **612**
Deep circumflex iliac vein, **613**
Deep compartment, hip, **580**
Deep deltoid ligament, **919, 926–927, 946, 951–955, 966–967, 1004–1005, 1008, 1012–1014, 1020–1023, 1028**
 - anterior band, **952–953, 968–969**
 - posterior band, **952–953, 966–967, 975**
Deep femoral artery, **514–517, 612, 624–635, 650–652, 656**
Deep femoral vein, **514–517, 613, 624–635, 650–652, 656**
Deep flexor tendon, **480**
Deep inguinal ring, **529**
Deep medial collateral ligament, **795**
Deep palmar arch, **303, 332, 358–359, 443, 460**
Deep peroneal nerve, **814, 880, 889–893, 898–907, 915, 920, 931–933, 948–951, 1035–1036**
 - lateral, **893, 920, 931**
 - medial, **893, 920, 930**
Deep semimembranosus bursa, **780**
Deep transverse metacarpal ligament, **464–465, 474, 479**
Deltoid, **6–7, 9, 12–13, 32, 42–48, 54–66, 68, 70–73, 75–85, 95–101, 106–111, 116–118, 120–125, 127, 129–134, 140–141, 154, 158–163, 180–181, 182, 186–187, 190**
 - anterior belly, **8, 12, 37, 40–43, 46–47, 49–53, 129–130, 186–187**
 - lateral, **85**
 - middle belly, **12, 42–43, 74–75, 85, 129, 134, 184–185, 191**
 - posterior attachment, **182–183**
 - posterior belly, **8, 12, 37, 47, 49–55, 66, 67, 79, 129–131, 180–181**
Deltoid ligament, **918–919, 1012–1013**
 - bands, **940**

INDEX

- deep, **919, 926–927, 945, 946, 951–955, 966–967, 1004–1005, 1008, 1012–1014, 1020–1023, 1028**
- insertion, **922**
- posterior deep, **939, 944**
- superficial, **919, 926–927, 939, 944, 946, 948–953, 970, 974–975, 1004–1005, 1008, 1012–1014, 1019–1020**
- tibiotalar component, **922**

Deltoid tuberosity, **156, 160–163, 182–183**
Deltopectoral groove, **54–55, 187**
Denervation syndromes, knee anatomy, **687**
Descending geniculate artery, **612, 669**
Digastric flexor digitorum superficialis, of 2nd digit, **418**
Digit extensor tendon, 5th, **464**
Digital arteries
- common palmar, **437, 443**
- proper, **437, 443**

Digital neurovascular bundle, **1082**
- dorsal, **1072–1077**
- plantar, **1076–1077**

Digital tendon sheath, common, **474–475**
Digital vessels, **1098**
- 2nd toe, **1060–1061**
- plantar, **1056–1057**

Digits, duplication, **418**
Direct inguinal hernia, **529**
Disc remnant, **492, 520**
Discoid meniscus, **813, 845–847**
- anterior horn, **845**
- body, **845**
- morphology, **846**
- posterior horn, **845**

Distal anterior band of pes, **712–713**
Distal carpal tunnel, **356–357**
Distal interosseous ligament, **389**
Distal interphalangeal joint, **454, 480**
- 2nd, **453**
- 3rd, **453**
- 5th, **1043**
- capsule, **476**
- volar plate, **472**
- zone II, **478**

Distal phalanx, **455, 1038, 1078**
- 1st, **453, 1098**
- 2nd, **453**
- 4th, **480**
- 5th, **480**

Distal pole scaphoid, **335**
Distal radioulnar compartment, **337**
Distal radioulnar joint (DRUJ), **334–335, 337, 367, 429, 433**
Distal radioulnar ligament, **389**
Distal radius, **329, 343**
Distal ulna, **329, 343**
Dorsal bone contour, **454**
Dorsal calcaneocuboid ligament, **926**
Dorsal carpal arch, **332**
Dorsal compartment, foot, **1035**
Dorsal concavity, **1099**
Dorsal cutaneous nerve
- intermediate, **931**
- medial, **931**

Dorsal digital expansion, **479**
Dorsal digital nerves, **1036**
Dorsal digital neurovascular bundles, **1072–1077**
Dorsal hood, **449, 479**
Dorsal intercarpal ligament, **330, 341, 350–353, 364–365, 380–383**
Dorsal intermetatarsal ligaments, **1037, 1055, 1093**
Dorsal interossei, **378–379, 456, 473, 475–477, 1041, 1084–1085, 1087, 1089**
- 1st, **439, 460–463, 466–469, 471, 479**
- 2nd, **439, 460–463**
    musculotendinous junction, **468–469**
- 3rd, **439, 442, 460–463, 468–470**
    contributing to lateral band, **469**
- 4th, **439, 442, 460–463, 468–470, 476**

Dorsal joint recess, **339, 341**
Dorsal Lisfranc ligament, **1037, 1055, 1062–1063, 1093–1095**
Dorsal metacarpal artery, **332**
- 5th, **332**

Dorsal metatarsal arteries, **1036**
Dorsal midcarpal ligament, **388**
Dorsal notch, **1099**
Dorsal radiocarpal ligament, **330, 341, 350–351, 364–365, 380–383, 388, 392, 394, 396–397**
Dorsal radioulnar ligament, **346–349, 364, 366–367, 380, 391, 393**
Dorsal sacral foramen, **492**
Dorsal sacroiliac ligament, **498–500, 502**
Dorsal scaphotriquetral ligament, **330, 348–351, 364–365, 383, 392, 394, 396–397**
Dorsal scapular artery, **10**
- anastomoses with, intercostal arteries, **10**

Dorsal stabilizing ligaments, **392**
Dorsal subcutaneous venous plexus, **468**
Dorsal superior joint recess, **212**
Dorsal talonavicular ligament, **926–927, 1005, 1037, 1055**
Dorsal tarsometatarsal ligaments, **1037, 1055**
Dorsal transverse recess, **390, 394, 397**
Dorsal triangular structure, **470**
Dorsal vein, **362–363**
Dorsal venous plexus tributary, **332**
Dorsalis pedis artery, **893, 974, 1036**
Dorsalis pedis vessels, **950**
Dorsolateral calcaneocuboid ligament, **1021**
Ductus deferens, **505**

E

Elbow. *See also* Forearm.
- arthrography, **200–213**
    anatomy, **207**
    axial MR arthrogram, **212–213**
    coronal MR arthrogram, **208–209**
    needle placement, **206**
    sagittal MR arthrogram, **210–211**
- axial anatomy, **215–216**
- bursae, **194**
- carrying angle of, **292–293**
- cubital fossa, **217**

INDEX

- FABS
    - positioning and image, **268**
    - T1 MR, left elbow, **269**
- graphics
    - arteries and nerves, **199**
    - axial, **197–198**
    - biceps aponeurosis, **250**
    - biceps tendon, **250**
    - collateral ligament complex, **271**
    - collateral ligaments, **272**
    - common extensor, **251**
    - common flexor tendons, **251**
    - coronal cross section, **204**
    - joint capsule, **196, 204**
    - ligament, anatomy, **205**
- joint, **194**
- left
    - axial T1 MR, **221, 223, 225, 227, 229, 231, 233**
    - coronal T1 MR, **235, 237, 239, 241, 243, 259–262, 278–279**
    - sagittal T1 MR, **244–247, 263–266**
- ligaments, **194, 270–279**
    - coronal MR arthrography, **274**
- measurements
    - and lines, **292–295**
    - normal angulation, **292**
- median nerve entrapment, **218**
- MR atlas, **214–247**
- muscles and tendons, **248–269**
- nerves, **195**
- order of ossification
    - anterior humeral line and, **295**
    - epiphyses/apophyses, **292**
- osseous, **280**
- overview, **194–199**
- radial nerve entrapment, **218**
- radiography, **200–213**
    - AP and lateral, **202**
    - external oblique and radial head views, **203**
    - normal variants, **280–291**
- right
    - axial T1 MR, **220, 222, 224, 226, 228, 230, 232, 252–258, 275–277**
    - coronal T1 MR, **234, 236, 238, 240, 242**
- ulnar nerve entrapment, **219**
- veins, **266**
- vessels, **194–195**
Enthesophyte, at Achilles insertion, **1107**
Epicondylar axis, **870**
Epigastric artery
 - inferior, **501, 506, 522, 545, 612**
 - superficial, **612**
Epigastric vein, inferior, **500–501, 506, 522, 545, 613**
Epiphysis, **426**
 - accessory, **426, 1119**
 - capitellar, **280, 281**
 - elbow, **292**
 - radial head, **281**
 - trochlear, **280**
Erector spinae, **490, 495–502, 512, 520–523, 550, 557**
Exostosis, medial, **1122**

Extensor carpi radialis accessory, **400**
Extensor carpi radialis brevis, **198, 204, 209, 216, 232–233, 238–241, 248, 251, 257–258, 262, 266, 274–276, 306–311, 313–315, 318, 320–321, 327, 331, 339–340, 344–359, 364–365, 383–384, 398, 401, 403–407, 409–410, 417, 423, 439**
Extensor carpi radialis intermedius, **400**
Extensor carpi radialis longus, **159, 170–179, 184–185, 191, 197–198, 212, 215–216, 220–233, 236–240, 247, 248, 251–258, 260–262, 266, 278, 302–310, 313–315, 318, 320–321, 327, 331, 344–359, 364–367, 384–385, 398, 401, 403–410, 416–417**
Extensor carpi ulnaris (ECU), **198, 230–231, 233–237, 246–249, 251, 257–260, 265, 276–277, 303, 306–311, 314–315, 318–319, 327, 331, 344–347, 349, 356–357, 366–369, 378–379, 393, 396, 401, 403–407, 413, 415–416, 429–430, 439, 476–477**
 - groove, **329, 343**
Extensor compartment, wrist
 - 1st, **429**
 - 2nd, **429**
 - 3rd, **429**
Extensor digiti minimi (EDM), **248, 251, 308–314, 314–315, 318–319, 321, 322, 327, 331, 344–361, 399, 401, 403–407, 412, 416–417, 429, 462–463, 473, 476**
Extensor digiti tendon, **345**
Extensor digitorum, **198, 210, 216, 228–233, 236–239, 247, 248, 251, 255–258, 260, 266, 277, 303, 304–311, 313–315, 318–321, 327, 331, 345, 347, 349–351, 355–356, 358–363, 378–382, 398, 401, 403, 882, 889–891, 898–899, 902–903**
 - slips, **344, 348, 352–354, 357–361, 404–407, 411–412, 417**
Extensor digitorum brevis, **925, 952–954, 970, 972–973, 978–979, 1003, 1023–1024, 1035, 1060–1071, 1074–1077, 1080–1082, 1084–1085, 1088–1089**
Extensor digitorum communis (EDC), **456, 458–459, 462–465, 468–470, 472–473**
 - to 2nd digit, **476**
 - 4th, contribution to 5th EDC tendon, **476**
 - to 5th digit, **476**
 - central slip, **476**
Extensor digitorum longus, **664, 708–713, 724–725, 731–732, 879, 882, 896–897, 900–902, 904–909, 911, 914, 919, 928–929, 947–951, 968–973, 977–978, 980–982, 993, 1002, 1064–1066, 1068–1069, 1072–1077, 1081, 1083, 1085, 1088–1089**
 - insertion, **890**
 - slips, **929**
Extensor digitorum manus brevis, **400, 418, 425**
Extensor digitorum profundus, central tendon slip of, **439**
Extensor hallucis, **879, 882**
Extensor hallucis brevis, **1084–1085, 1088–1089**
Extensor hallucis longus, **889–891, 900–909, 911, 913–914, 919, 928, 930, 947–951, 951, 970–973, 980–983, 989, 993, 1002–1003, 1035, 1063–1066, 1068–1073, 1076–1077, 1079, 1085, 1088–1089**
 - insertion, **890**
Extensor hood, **441, 464–465, 470–471, 473, 476, 479**

INDEX

Extensor indicis, **299, 302, 312–315, 331, 345–348, 350–354, 355–356, 357, 382–383, 399, 401, 403–407, 411, 462–463, 469, 473, 476**
Extensor mechanism, **670–671**
- hand, **472–483**
- knee, **663, 686, 734–741, 858–861**
- terminal tendon, **439**

Extensor muscles, **217**
Extensor pollicis brevis, **299, 302, 310–315, 318–319, 331, 344–355, 367–371, 385–387, 399, 401–409, 439, 456, 476**
Extensor pollicis longus, **299, 302, 308–315, 322, 327, 331, 344–365, 383, 399, 401, 403–408, 410, 416–417, 439, 448, 456, 468–469, 476**
- accessory, **400**
- course, **408**
- groove, **329, 343**

Extensor retinaculum, **174–175, 328, 331, 342, 344–351, 403, 409, 476, 893, 952–955, 970–973, 978, 1098**
- 2nd toe, **1075–1077**
- distal fibers, **350–351**
- inferior, **878, 889–890, 908–909, 919, 981–983, 1002**
    intermediate root, **1021, 1023–1024**
    lateral root, **1021, 1024, 1029**
    medial root, **1004, 1021, 1024**
- superior, **878, 889–890, 892, 919, 981–983**

Extensor tendons, **346–347, 404, 447, 449, 479, 936, 1062–1063, 1098–1099**
- 3rd & 4th toes, **1076–1077**
- common, **302, 304–305**

External iliac artery, **491, 501, 503–509, 517–518, 522–523, 531–532, 539, 541–543, 560**
External iliac vein, **501, 503–509, 517–518, 522–523, 531–532, 539, 541–543, 560**
External iliac vessels, **502, 506**
External lip, **489**
External marker, **314–315**
External oblique, **489, 495–500, 525–527, 528, 544–545, 557**
- aponeurosis, **495, 500–504, 527**

External pudendal artery, **612**
External rotators, **526–527, 565, 569, 572, 655**
Extraarticular bursae, **671**
Extracapsular fat stripe, **745**
Extrinsic ligaments
- dorsal, **392**
- volar, **391, 397**

Extrinsic muscles, **444**
Extrusion index, **599**

F

Fabella, **617, 683, 802, 804, 812, 822**
Fabellofibular ligament, **664, 683, 732, 797–799, 801–802, 804, 822**
Facet joint, **579**
False pelvis, **494**
Femoral angle of inclination, **599, 600**

Femoral artery, **487, 536, 553, 559, 561, 663**
- common, **510–511, 517–519, 523–525, 533–535, 537–538, 542–544, 552, 612, 615, 618–623, 652–656**
- deep, **514–517, 612, 624–635, 650–652, 656**
- lateral circumflex, **525–527, 541, 612, 620–621**
- medial circumflex, **525, 527, 565, 612**
- superficial, **515–517, 612, 624–639, 650–652, 655–656**

Femoral canal, **615**
Femoral cartilage, **678**
Femoral condylar sulcus, lateral, **672**
Femoral condyle, **649–650**
- irregularity, **828**
- lateral, **617, 657–658, 672, 679, 728–729, 745, 767, 769–771, 776–777, 784, 818, 826, 843, 868**
- medial, **617, 655–656, 672, 677, 684, 745, 749, 766, 769, 771, 776, 780, 785, 789, 794, 842–843, 849**

Femoral cutaneous nerve, posterior, **493**
Femoral diaphysis, **616–617, 650–651**
- long axis, **600**

Femoral head, **508–510, 515–517, 524–527, 531–535, 539–541, 552, 554, 559–561, 564–567, 573, 578, 583–585, 588, 601, 616, 652, 655**
- cartilage, **587, 590**
- center, **600, 602**
- coverage, **599**
- lateral migration, **601**
- line center, **602**

Femoral head-neck offset, **599**
Femoral neck, **511, 563, 567–570, 578, 586–587, 618, 657–658, 870**
- anterior cortex, **601**
- long axis, **600–601**
- normal cutback of, **578**

Femoral nerve, **498, 500–503, 505, 507, 509–511, 516–517, 532–533, 535–537, 540, 559–562, 608, 615, 620, 622–623, 663**
- common, **544, 618–621**

Femoral shaft, **569, 578**
Femoral torsion, **858, 870**
Femoral triangle, **607**
- apex, **615**

Femoral vein, **536, 553, 559, 561**
- common, **510–511, 517–519, 523–525, 533–535, 537–538, 542–544, 552, 613, 615, 618–624, 652–656**
- deep, **514–517, 613, 624–635, 650–652, 656**
- lateral circumflex, **525–527, 613, 620–621**
- medial, **525, 527**
- medial circumflex, **613**
- superficial, **515–517, 613, 624–639, 650–652, 655–656**

Femoral version, **599**
Femoral vessels, **608**
Femur, **515–516, 567, 570, 625–636, 638–641, 644–645, 651, 818**
- bony anatomy, **606**
- cam morphology, **590**
- distal, **686**
- supracondylar, **650–651**

Fibro-osseous connection, **423**
Fibrocartilaginous ridge, **995, 1001**
Fibrous septa, **960–961**

INDEX

Fibula, **676, 683, 878, 918, 926, 928, 935–937, 943, 948–949, 962–965, 967, 978–979, 984, 987, 991, 995, 999, 1001–1002, 1005–1009, 1011, 1013, 1015–1022, 1024, 1126–1127, 1129**
- head, **727**
- posterior margin, **946**
- proximal, **686**

Fibular collateral ligament, **675–676, 681, 683, 698–699**
Fibular fossa, **935**
Fibular head, **804, 883, 886, 893**
Fibular malleolar fossa, **1015–1016**
Fibular neck, **883**
Fibular styloid, **810**
Fibular tip, **979, 1017**
Fingernail, **447**
Flexor accessorius muscle, **1084**
Flexor carpi radialis, **157, 178–179, 198, 216, 230–233, 240–241, 245, 249, 251, 256–258, 261–262, 264, 303–317, 321, 327, 331, 344–357, 370–371, 374–377, 383–385, 398, 401–402, 404–407, 410, 429, 438, 458–459**
- insertion, **458–459**

Flexor carpi ulnaris, **158, 197–198, 211, 213, 215–216, 219, 226–237, 249, 251, 255–260, 263, 302–315, 318–319, 322–323, 327, 331, 340, 344–351, 374, 376–377, 379, 398, 401–402, 404–405, 406–407, 413–414, 429, 438**

Flexor digiti minimi, **300, 360, 361, 379, 415, 425, 438, 441, 445, 458, 459–463, 466–467, 470, 474, 1041, 1056–1057, 1087, 1089**
- insertion site, **441, 445**

Flexor digiti minimi brevis, **358–361, 402, 414, 1084–1085**
Flexor digitorum, **298, 310–311, 356–357, 372–373, 412, 470, 820–821, 884–885, 887–888, 902–903, 906–907, 962**

Flexor digitorum brevis, **925, 936, 989, 993, 1040, 1056–1057, 1064–1071, 1072–1075, 1078–1081, 1080–1082, 1084–1086, 1088–1089, 1097**

Flexor digitorum longus, **879, 881, 888, 893, 900–909, 911–913, 920, 929–930, 939–940, 943–944, 947–959, 962–971, 966, 973, 975, 980, 983–985, 987–994, 1026, 1040, 1056–1059, 1064–1077, 1080–1083, 1085–1086, 1088–1089, 1125–1126**

Flexor digitorum profundus, **198, 208, 211, 213, 216, 226–239, 244–245, 255–261, 264, 299, 302–311, 314–315, 318–319, 322–323, 327, 331, 345–348, 350–357, 358–361, 370–373, 379–383, 398, 401–402, 404–407, 411–412, 415, 438, 442, 456, 458–459, 464–467, 470–471, 474–475, 480–483**

Flexor digitorum superficialis, **198, 208, 216, 227–233, 236–239, 244–245, 249, 251, 256–258, 260–261, 263–264, 302–313, 315–317, 322, 327, 331, 343, 345–361, 372–377, 380–382, 398, 401–402, 404–407, 411–412, 414–415, 429, 438, 456, 458–459, 464–465, 471, 472, 474–475, 479–483**
- 2nd digit, **471**
- insertion, **470–471**
- zone I, **478**
- zone II, **478**

Flexor hallucis, **887, 898–899, 1123**

Flexor hallucis brevis, **925, 1041, 1084–1085, 1098**
- lateral head, **1056–1059, 1070–1077, 1079, 1087, 1089, 1097, 1099**
- medial head, **1056–1059, 1070–1079, 1087, 1089, 1097, 1099, 1121**

Flexor hallucis longus, **820, 879, 883, 887, 893, 900–910, 912–913, 920, 929, 936, 939–941, 943–945, 947–957, 960–963, 973, 975–977, 980, 983–988, 990–992, 994, 996, 1000, 1026, 1040–1041, 1056–1057, 1064–1079, 1085, 1087–1089, 1097–1099, 1102, 1123–1127**
- accessory, **821**
- axial MR, **991**
- coronal MR, **993**
- groove for, **921–924**
- origin, **887**

Flexor hallucis longus tendon sheath, **1046**
Flexor mechanism, hand, **472–483**
Flexor muscles, **306–307**
Flexor musculotendinous junctions, **346–347**
Flexor pollicis brevis, **311, 358–361, 370–371, 383–385, 399, 402, 438, 441, 445, 447–448, 460–461, 471**

Flexor pollicis longus, **299, 302, 308–315, 318, 321, 327, 331, 344–361, 372–373, 375, 383–384, 398, 401–402, 404–407, 414–415, 438, 447–449, 451, 458–463, 466–467, 471**
- insertion, **447, 464–465**

Flexor pollicis longus tendon sheath, **402**
Flexor pulleys, **444, 472**
Flexor retinaculum, **328, 331, 342, 350–355, 357–359, 372, 374, 381–382, 391, 402, 405, 407, 414, 421, 440–441, 443, 445, 448, 458–459, 474, 878, 887–888, 919, 929–930, 939–940, 946–951, 966–969, 983, 987, 991, 994, 1007–1008, 1012–1014, 1019–1020, 1022, 1126**
- 1st toe, **1076–1077**
- 4th toe, **1076–1077**
- superficial portion, **405, 407**

Flexor sheath, **464–465**
Flexor tendon, **212, 213, 464–465, 470, 474, 477, 481, 1098**
- common, **302, 316, 323**
- origins of, **275**

Flexor tendon sheath, **1040**
- common, **400**

Focal periphyseal edema (FOPE) zone, **812, 835**
Foot
- arches, **1034**
- arteries, **1035–1036**
- axial T1 MR, long axis, **1056–1063**
- bony anatomy, **1034**
- bursae, **1035**
- columns, **1038**
- compartments, **1035**
- coronal T1 MR, **1064–1077**
- cuboid bone, **1034**
- cuneiform bones, **1034**
- graphics, **1036–1041, 1055, 1085–1087**
- ligaments, **1035, 1037**
- longitudinal arch, **1034, 1038, 1128, 1134**
- measurements, **1128–1139**

INDEX

- metatarsal bones, **1034**
- metatarsophalangeal joints, **1096–1099**
- motion, **1035**
- MR atlas, **1054–1083**
- muscles, **1084–1089**
    - coronal T1 MR, **1088–1089**
    - dorsal, **1035**
    - plantar, **1034, 1040–1041, 1086–1087**
- navicular bone, **1034**
- nerves, **1035–1036**
- normal variants, **1100–1127**
- overview, **1034–1041**
- phalanges, **1034**
- radiography, **1042–1053**
    - AP, **1043**
    - lateral, **1044**
    - oblique, **1043**
- sagittal T1 MR, **1078–1083**
- tarsometatarsal joint, **1090–1095**
- transverse arch, **1034, 1038–1039**

Forearm
- AP and lateral radiographs, **301**
- arteries, **299–300**
- articulations, **298**
- axial T1 MR, **304–315**
- coronal T1 MR, **316–319**
- graphics, axial view, **303**
- interosseous fibrous attachments, **298–299**
- muscles, **299**
- nerves, **300**
- origins and insertions, **302**
- radiographic anatomy and MR atlas, **298–323**
- sagittal T1 MR, **320–323**
- supine, **268**

Forefoot, **1034**
- width, **1128**

Fovea capitis, **209, 213, 539, 552, 554, 563–564, 573, 575, 582, 584, 594, 616**

Foveal strut, **393**

G

Gastrocnemius, **666, 730, 745, 878, 902–903, 986**
- aponeurosis, **884**
- lateral, **668, 702–705, 710–711, 723–724, 754–755, 771, 783–784, 882, 884, 891**
- lateral head, **610, 657–658, 664, 667–668, 675, 679, 681, 683, 690–701, 704–707, 723–727, 731–733, 759, 804–807, 814–816, 819, 886, 894–899, 913–915**
    - aberrant origin, **816–817**
- medial, **668, 702–711, 718–722, 736, 771, 780–781, 784, 803, 884, 889**
- medial head, **610, 656–657, 666–668, 675, 677, 681–682, 685, 688–701, 706–711, 719, 732–733, 744, 746, 804, 815–817, 884, 886, 894–903, 910–912**
- 3rd head, **815**

Gemellus, **561, 564, 567–569, 572, 614**
- inferior, **489, 493, 511, 535, 555, 562, 566–568, 610**
- superior, **489, 493, 510, 533, 555, 566–568, 610**

Genicular branches, **708–709**

Geniculate artery
- descending, **669**
- inferior lateral, **612, 669, 714–715**
- inferior medial, **669, 710–713, 716–717, 721**
- superior lateral, **612, 644–647, 669, 688–689, 712–715, 726–727**
- superior medial, **642–645, 669, 688–689, 714–715, 718, 721**

Geniculate vein
- lateral superior, **644–647, 714–715**
- medial superior, **642–645, 714–715**

Genitofemoral nerve, **495, 497, 500, 505**

Gerdy tubercle, **680, 698–701, 714–715, 727, 757, 798, 883**

Gilula arcs, **428**

Gissane angle, **1128**

Glenohumeral joint, **98**
- conventional arthrography, **20**

Glenohumeral joint space, **4**

Glenohumeral ligament, **14, 81, 108, 112**
- anterior, **107**
- anterior band, **127–128, 131, 133–134**
- arthrogram, **115**
- inferior, **5, 14, 98, 127, 131–134**
    - anterior band, **9, 22, 24–25, 27, 29–30, 32, 34**
    - axillary pouch, **9, 32**
    - posterior band, **9, 22, 24, 27, 29–30, 32**
- middle, **5, 9, 14, 22, 25–27, 30–32, 35, 98, 108–109, 127–128, 130–131, 133–134, 148, 150–151**
- MR ligament, Buford ligament, **118**
- posterior band, **127**
- size/presence, **138**
    - MR variant, **148**
- superior, **5, 9, 14, 22–23, 25–26, 29–30, 32, 102–111, 127–129, 133–134, 148**

Glenoid, **4, 9, 14, 27, 30, 32, 46–53, 70–75, 106, 117–118, 125, 130–133, 135, 139–141, 150–151, 181**
- anterior, **146–147**
- articular cartilage, **33**
- articular surface, **31**
- bony cortex, **27**
- cartilage, **151**
- deep sulcus, **33**
- hypoplastic, **138, 146**
    - inferior, **146**
    - posterior, **146–147**
    - variant, **146–147**
- mid, **32, 134**
- posterior margin, **24**

Glenoid fossa, **16, 18–20, 22, 114, 127**
- anterior rim, **17**
- inferior rim, **17**
- posterior rim, **17**
- scapula, **81**

Glenoid labrum, **9, 14, 24, 32**
- anterior, **30**
- inferior, **9, 30**
- posterior, **22, 30**
- superior, **20, 24, 26, 33, 106**

Glenoid rim
- anterior, **16**

INDEX

- anterior inferior, **18**
- posterior, **16**

Gluteal artery
- inferior, **487, 512, 524–525, 527, 560, 562, 565, 612**
- superior, **487, 503–505, 515, 524–525, 612**

Gluteal line
- anterior, **489**
- inferior, **489**
- posterior, **486, 489–490**

Gluteal muscles, **555**

Gluteal vein
- inferior, **512, 524–525, 527, 560, 562, 613**
- superior, **503–505, 515, 524–525, 560, 613**

Gluteus maximus, **489, 493, 497–515, 521–527, 531–538, 549–551, 555, 557, 560–561, 563–571, 610, 615, 618–629, 648–649, 654–659**

Gluteus medius, **489, 491, 493, 495–511, 514–517, 525–527, 555, 557, 560–572, 592, 610, 618–619, 621, 650–651, 656–659**

Gluteus minimus, **489, 493, 500–510, 514–518, 526–527, 555, 557, 560–563, 565–573, 609–610, 618, 650–652, 657–659**

Gonadal artery, **505**
Gonadal vein, **505**
Gonadal vessel, **497**

Gracilis, **489, 493, 513–516, 520–521, 529, 539–541, 549–550, 557, 609–610, 615, 622–652, 654–655, 665–666, 668–669, 674–675, 681, 688–711, 718–719, 730–731, 759, 786, 788–791, 795, 819, 881–882, 884–885, 894–897**

Greater arc, **432**

Greater saphenous vein, **515–518, 522–523, 543–544, 613, 620–627, 629–655, 668, 692–695, 698–705, 708–711, 880, 894–897, 949–951, 1064–1065**

Greater sciatic foramen, **488, 491**
Greater sciatic notch, **489–490, 494, 552, 564, 577, 588**
Greater trochanter, **509–511, 515–516, 556, 559, 562–563, 570–572, 575, 578, 585, 616, 650, 657–659**
Greater trochanteric bursa, **555, 558**
Greater tuberosity, **4, 24, 27, 47–51, 70–73, 87–88, 114, 130, 156–157**
- humerus, **16–20, 158**
- osteophyte, **143**

Guyon canal, **342, 350–353, 372–373**

H

Haglund deformity, **1107**
Hallux alignment, **1138**
Hallux angle, **1138**
Hallux-interphalangeal angle, **1128, 1138**
Hallux-metatarsophalangeal angle, **1128**

Hamate, **329, 335, 343, 352–357, 364–369, 379–381, 397, 419, 421**
- body, **337, 380, 424**
- hook, **329, 335, 337, 343, 354–357, 370–373, 380, 421, 448, 454–455, 466–467, 470**
- normal cartilage at articulation of, **419**

Hamate-pisiform coalition, **421**

Hamstring, **592, 657**
- origins, **536, 538, 588**

Hand
- additional view, **454**
- extensor mechanism, **472–483**
- extensor tendons, **277**
- flexor mechanism, **472–483**
- imaging pitfalls, **456**
- joints, **436**
- left
    - axial T1 MR, **458, 460, 462, 479–480**
    - coronal T1 MR, **466, 468**
- MR atlas, **456–471**
- muscles, **437, 456**
- nerves, **437, 443**
- normal variants and imaging pitfalls, **418–427**
- overview, **436–443**
- radiographic anatomy, **452–455**
    - lateral, **453**
    - PA, **453**
    - posteroanterior, **455**
- right
    - axial PD FS MR, **481–482**
    - axial T1 MR, **459, 461**
    - coronal T1 MR, **467**
    - sagittal PD FS MR, **483**
    - sagittal T1 MR, **470–471**
- tendon injury zones, **478**
- vessels, **437**
- volar, **438**

Hilgenreiner line, **598, 601–602**

Hindfoot, **918, 1034**
- alignment, **1130–1131**
- ligaments, **926–927, 1005**
- muscle attachment, **925**
- retinacula, **928**
- width, **1128**

Hip. *See also* Pelvis; Thigh.
- acetabular labral variants, **590**
- arthrographic technique, **580**
- axial T1 MR, **560–562**
- bony variants, **590, 591–592**
- bursae, **558**
- coronal T1 MR, **572–573**
- glenoid labrum variants, **595**
- graphics, **559**
- ligaments, **556**
- measurements and lines, **598–603**
- MR anatomy, **558–573**
- muscles, **555**
    - attachments, innominate bone, **557**
    - and nerve variants, **590**
- normal variants and imaging pitfalls, **590–597**
- oblique angled axial T1 MR, **563**
- overview, **554–557**
- pediatric variants, **597**
- pelvis and
    - AP, **575**
    - axial MR arthrogram, **584**
    - coronal MR arthrogram, **581–583**
    - inlet and outlet, **576**

INDEX

radiographic and arthrographic anatomy, **574–589**
sacroiliac and pubic symphysis arthrography, **589**
sagittal MR arthrogram, **586–588**
- sagittal T1 MR, **564–571**
Hip anteversion, **870**
Hip flexors, **607**
Hip joint
- contrast in, **580, 589**
- ligaments, **555**
- posterior portion of, **577**
Hoffa fat pad, **672, 676–678, 694–695, 714–717, 722, 724–726, 734, 747, 754, 757, 761, 772**
- apex, **764, 837, 844**
Humeral angle, **292**
Humeral artery
- anterior circumflex, **8, 10**
- posterior circumflex, **9–11**
Humeral ligament, transverse, **8**
Humeroradial joint, articulation, **194**
Humeroulnar joint, **202**
- articulation, **194**
Humerus, **4, 52–53, 159, 162–163, 166–167, 169, 189–191**
- anatomic head, **17**
- anatomic neck, **16, 20, 33, 70–71, 136**
- capitellum, **254–255**
- distal, **197, 215, 252**
- head, **12, 16–19, 26, 44–45, 69, 82, 85, 89–93, 98–99, 116, 121, 123–124, 142**
    articular surface, **16**
    cartilage, **87**
    posterior, normal flattening, radiographic pitfall, **142**
    posterolateral, **18**
- intercondylar ridge, **208, 211**
- lateral epicondyle, **253–254**
- medial epicondyle, **253–254**
- mid, **159**
- proximal, **114**
- proximal diaphysis, **54–59**
- shaft, **19, 82, 99–100, 145, 156, 159**
- surgical neck, **16, 20, 54–55, 70–71**
- trochlea, **254–255, 261**
Humphrey, meniscofemoral ligament of, **677, 684–685, 742, 745–747, 752, 768–769, 776–779, 795, 799, 812–813**
Hunter canal, **608**
Hyaline cartilage, **24, 27, 34, 671, 677**
- glenoid, **24**
- humeral head, **24**
- radius, **395**
Hypothenar eminence, **331**
Hypothenar muscles, **358–359, 379, 400, 437, 473**

I

Iliac apophysis, **597**
Iliac artery, **491, 495–499**
- common, **612**
- deep circumflex, **612**
- external, **491, 501, 503–509, 517–518, 522–523, 531–532, 539, 541–543, 560**
- internal, **491, 501, 503–505, 513–516, 521–522, 612**
- superficial circumflex, **612**
Iliac crest, **486, 489–490, 493, 519, 568–569, 575–577, 615–616**
- tubercle, **486, 489**
Iliac fossa, **486, 490**
Iliac spine
- anterior inferior, **486, 489–490, 506, 518, 527, 542–543, 556, 560, 563, 566, 616**
- anterior superior, **486, 489–490, 500, 519, 527, 556, 609, 615**
- posterior inferior, **486, 489–490, 504, 524**
- posterior superior, **486, 489–490, 493, 524**
Iliac vein, **495–499**
- common, **613**
- deep circumflex, **613**
- external, **501, 503–509, 517–518, 522–523, 531–532, 539, 541–543, 560**
- internal, **501, 503–505, 513–516, 521–522, 613**
Iliac vessels, **500**
Iliac wing, **491, 542, 566, 578, 616**
Iliacus, **490, 496–502, 515–519, 524–525, 527, 539–541, 543, 557, 560, 563–565, 609, 615**
Iliofemoral ligament, **489, 527, 555, 556–557, 559, 561–562, 565, 567–569, 581, 586–587**
Iliohypogastric nerve, **528**
Ilioinguinal nerve, **528**
Ilioischial line, **530, 575, 598, 600**
Iliolumbar ligament, **488, 490, 514, 557, 591**
Iliopectineal fold, **590**
Iliopectineal junction, **490, 523–524, 542**
Iliopectineal line, **530, 575, 578**
Iliopsoas, **503–511, 516–519, 523–527, 531–538, 540–544, 552, 559–568, 572–573, 609–610, 618–623, 650–652, 654–657**
- bursa, **555, 558–559**
Iliopubic tract, **528**
Iliotibial band, **514–517, 560–562, 607, 609–610, 618–628, 642, 650, 659, 664–665, 676, 680, 684, 690–697, 731–732, 757, 894–895**
Iliotibial tract, **607, 642–647, 688–691, 698–701, 710–715, 727, 737, 738, 796, 799, 801, 891, 893**
Ilium, **486, 491, 495–502, 504–506, 512–518, 523, 525–527, 539–540, 559, 565, 572, 578**
Indirect inguinal hernia, **529**
Inferior acromioclavicular ligament, **113–114, 125**
Inferior epigastric artery, **501, 506, 522, 545, 612**
Inferior epigastric vein, **500–501, 506, 522, 545, 613**
Inferior extensor retinaculum, **878, 889–890, 908–909, 919, 929, 947–949, 981–983, 1002**
- intermediate root, **1021, 1024**
- lateral root, **1004, 1021, 1024**
- medial root, **1004, 1021, 1024**
- stem, **928**
Inferior fascicle, **761, 802**
Inferior gemellus, **489, 493, 511, 535, 562, 566–568, 610**
Inferior geniculate artery
- lateral, **612, 669, 714–715**
- medial, **612, 669, 710–713, 716–717, 721**

INDEX

Inferior glenohumeral ligament, **14, 86, 98, 112, 127**
 - anterior band, **22, 24, 25, 27, 29–30, 32, 34, 74–75, 90–91, 108, 127–128, 131–134**
 - axillary pouch, **32, 81, 98–99**
 - posterior band, **22, 24, 27, 29–30, 32, 72–73, 127, 131, 133**
Inferior glenohumeral ligament complex, **114, 119**
 - anterior band, **114–115**
 - axillary pouch, **108, 114, 119, 133**
 - posterior band, **114, 119**
Inferior glenoid labrum, **30, 33**
Inferior glenoid rim, anterior, **18**
Inferior gluteal artery, **487, 493, 512, 524–525, 527, 560, 562, 565, 612**
Inferior gluteal nerve, **493**
Inferior gluteal vein, **493, 512, 524–525, 527, 560, 562, 613**
Inferior iliac spine
 - anterior, **486, 489–490, 506, 518, 527, 542–543, 556, 560, 563, 566, 616**
 - posterior, **486, 489–490, 504, 524**
Inferior (ischiopubic) ramus, **556**
Inferior joint capsular attachments, **582**
Inferior joint recess, **207–210, 213, 580**
Inferior labrum, **27, 30, 34, 72–73, 92–93, 120**
Inferior patellar tendon, **664–666, 672, 696–701, 714–717, 723–726, 730–732, 734, 735–736, 746–747, 753–755, 760, 788, 881–882, 889, 891, 893–895, 913**
Inferior patellotibial ligament, **665, 692–695, 716–717, 722, 730**
Inferior peroneal retinaculum, **892, 919, 928–929, 947, 957, 968, 971, 981, 988, 996, 1108**
Inferior popliteomeniscal fascicle, **679, 742, 750–751, 754–755, 759, 761, 802**
Inferior pubic ligament, **528**
Inferior pubic ramus, **489–490, 530, 538–540, 550–551, 575, 579, 586, 620–621**
Inferior ramus, **515–516, 522–523, 528, 616, 621, 651**
Inferior tibiofibular joint, **918**
Inferior transverse ligament, **564, 566, 918, 926, 939–943, 950–954, 964–965, 978, 1005, 1007–1010, 1015–1016, 1019, 1022**
 - facet for, **921**
 - scapular, **112**
Inferior ulnar collateral artery, **303**
Inferomedial joint recess, **581, 583**
Inferoplantar longitudinal spring ligament, **927, 1004, 1025–1028, 1031**
Infraglenoid tubercle, **54–55, 81, 97, 180–181**
Infraglenoid tuberosity, **132**
Infrapatellar (Hoffa) fat pad, **675–676, 678, 694–695, 714–717, 722, 724–726, 734, 735, 747, 754, 757, 761**
Infrapatellar plica, **685, 739, 772, 818, 844**
Infraspinatus, **7–8, 9, 12–13, 14, 24, 26, 28–30, 32, 35, 37, 44–71, 78–85, 91–101, 103, 105–106, 108–111, 115, 117–121, 127–135, 141, 148, 158, 180–183**
 - anterior fibers, **70–71**
Infraspinatus bursa, **5**
Inguinal canal, **494, 529**
Inguinal hernias, **529**

Inguinal ligament, **489, 508–509, 519, 522–524, 528, 531–534, 544–545, 550–551, 557, 615, 653**
 - proximal, **507**
 - reflected, **528**
Inguinal lymph nodes, **653**
Innominate bone, **557**
Insall-Salvati methods, **858–859**
Intercarpal joint, 2nd, **366**
Intercarpal ligament, dorsal, **341, 392, 396–397**
Intercondylar area, fat within, **771**
Intercondylar notch, **649–650, 672, 678, 684, 745, 752**
Intercondylar ridge, **209**
Intercondylar roof, **657**
Intercostobrachial nerve, **11**
Intercruciate recess, **680, 768, 782, 784–785**
Intercrural fibers, **529**
Intercuneiform joint, **1050**
 - 1st, **1117**
Intercuneiform ligament, **954, 1039, 1062–1063, 1069, 1094**
 - dorsal, **1068–1069**
 - interosseous, **1068–1069**
 - plantar, **1037, 1055, 1068–1069**
Interligamentous recess, **396**
Interligamentous sulcus, **390–391**
Intermalleolar ligament, **941, 943, 954–955, 1009**
Intermediate dorsal cutaneous nerve, **931**
Intermediate sacral crest, **492**
Intermetacarpal ligament, **358–359**
Intermetatarsal angle, **1128, 1138**
Intermetatarsal bursa, **1098**
Intermetatarsal joint, **1092**
 - 2nd, **1050, 1117**
Intermetatarsal ligaments, **1035, 1060–1063, 1070–1071, 1090, 1094, 1096**
 - dorsal, **1037, 1055, 1093**
 - plantar, **1037, 1055**
Intermuscular septum, **898–899**
Internal iliac artery, **491, 501, 503–505, 513–516, 521–522, 612**
Internal iliac vein, **501, 503–505, 513–516, 521–522, 613**
Internal iliac vessels, **502**
Internal oblique, **489, 495–506, 523–527, 528, 544–545, 550–551, 557**
Internal oblique/transversus aponeurosis, **495**
Internal pudendal artery, **493, 507, 559**
Internal pudendal nerve, **493**
Internal pudendal vein, **493, 507, 559**
Interossei, **360–361, 441, 1058–1063, 1070–1073, 1079–1083**
 - compartment, **1035**
 - dorsal, **456, 473, 476, 1041, 1084–1085, 1087, 1089**
   1st, **448–450**
 - palmar, **456**
 - plantar, **1041, 1084–1085, 1087, 1089**
Interosseous artery
 - anterior, **303, 310–311**
 - common, **303**
 - posterior, **303, 308–309**
 - recurrent, **199, 303**
Interosseous borders, leg, **883**

INDEX

Interosseous ligament, **490, 512–513, 523, 557, 918, 950–951, 964, 1004–1005, 1013, 1016, 1039**
- distal, **389**
- proximal, **389**
- small, **397**
- talocalcaneal, **956, 1004, 1021–1022**
- tibiofibular, **1006**

Interosseous Lisfranc ligament, **1062–1063, 1070–1071, 1094–1095**

Interosseous membrane, **298, 302, 308–311, 318–319, 321–322, 878, 889–890, 892–893, 926, 1005, 1021**
- tibiofibular, **1006, 1008**

Interosseous nerve, posterior, **308, 327**

Interphalangeal joint, **436, 446–447, 1043**
- 1st, **444, 447, 450, 1043, 1056–1057**
- 5th, **1043**
- distal
    5th, **1043**
    capsule, **476**
    volar plate, **472, 483**
- proximal, 5th, **1043**

Intersesamoid ligament, **1075, 1097**

Intertrochanteric crest, **556, 616**

Intertrochanteric line, **556, 575, 580, 594**

Intertrochanteric ridge, **572**

Intertubercular groove, **16, 20, 156**

Intracapsular fatty tissue, **747**

Intraosseous ligament, **512–513**

Intrinsic ligaments, **391**

Intrinsic muscles, **444**
- thenar, **444**
- thumb, graphics, **445**

Ischial apophysis, **597**

Ischial ramus, **486, 489–490**

Ischial spine, **486, 489–491, 510, 530, 576–577, 579, 586, 615, 655**

Ischial tuberosity, **486, 489–491, 493, 512–514, 524–525, 530, 535–538, 557, 559, 564–566, 575–578, 616, 618–621, 649–650, 654, 656**

Ischiocavernosus, **490, 557**

Ischiofemoral ligament, **555, 556, 581**

Ischiopubic synchondrosis, **597**

Ischium, **486, 514–515, 524–525, 562, 618–619, 649, 654–655**

J

Joint capsule, **9, 12, 14, 22, 84, 99–100, 107, 114, 194, 200, 581, 585, 671, 799**. *See also* Posterior capsule.
- ankle, **946**
- anterior, **196**
- calcaneocuboid joint, **1048**
- dorsal, **1052–1053, 1099**
- humeral attachment, **21**
- posterior, **196, 939**

Junctura tendinum, **462–463, 476**

K

Kager fat pad. *See* Pre-Achilles fat pad.
Kite angle, **1130–1131**
Knee, **600**. *See also* Leg.
- angulation, mechanical axis, **860**
- arthroscopic photographs, **728–729**
- articular capsule, **686**
- axial anatomy, **674–675**
- coronal, **680–681**
- cruciate ligaments/posterior capsule, **768–785**
- 3D CT, **664–667**
- 3D reconstruction CT, origins and insertions, **730–733**
- extensor mechanism, **663, 686, 734–741**
- graphics
    axial, **676**
    posterior superficial and deep muscles and nerves, **668**
    vessels and anastomotic network, **669**
- imaging pitfalls, **813**
- internal structures, **663, 686**
- lateral supporting structures, **663, 687, 796–811**
- left
    axial T1 MR, **689, 691, 693, 695, 697, 699, 701**
    coronal T1 MR, **703, 705, 707, 709, 711, 713, 715, 717**
- ligamentous variants, **812–813**
- measurements and lines, **858–875**
- medial supporting structures, **663, 686–687, 786–795**
- menisci, **686, 742–767, 813**
- motion, **662**
- MR atlas, **686–733**
- muscles, **662–663**
    variants, **812**
- needle placement for arthrography or injection, **673**
- nerves, **663**
- osseous variants, **812**
- overview, **662–669**
- plica variant, **813**
- posterolateral corner structures, **683**
- radiographic and arthrographic anatomy, **670–685**
- retinacula, **734–741**
- right
    axial T1 MR, **688, 690, 692, 694, 696, 698, 700**
    coronal, **702, 704, 706, 708, 710, 712, 714, 716**
- sagittal
    lateral, **678–679**
    medial, **677**
    T1 MR, **718–727**
- standard radiographs, **672**
- vessels, **663**
Knot of Henry, **992**

L

L4
- nerve root, **493, 495**
- vertebral body, **495**

INDEX

L4/L5, facet joint, **495**
L5
- enlarged transverse process, **591**
- nerve root, **493, 497–501, 503–504**
- normal lateral process, **591**
- vertebral body, **496–498**

L5/S1, facet joint, **497**
Labral degeneration, **590**
Labrocapsular recess, **580, 582, 584, 590**
Labrocapsular sulcus, **586, 595**
Labrocartilaginous cleft, **554**
Labroligamentous sulci, **554**
Labrum, **5, 71–72, 81, 97–98, 108, 126–137, 149, 556, 582**
- anterior, **12, 147, 150–151, 559, 563, 565–566, 593**
    inferior, **151**
- anterosuperior, **150**
- attachment types, **126, 138**
- deep sulcus, **33**
- inferior, **149**
- normal, sagittal, **128**
    axial PD FS MR, **129–132**
- posterior, **146–147, 149, 150–151, 559, 563**
- posterior inferior portion, **54–55**
- sagittal graphic, **127**
- superior, **149–150, 559**
- variants, **133**
    attachment, **135**
    Buford complex, **134**

Lacertus fibrosus. *See* Biceps aponeurosis.
Lacunar ligament, **528**
Lateral ankle gutter, **938, 944, 952, 966**
Lateral antebrachial cutaneous nerve, **157, 159, 344**
Lateral arm arcuate ligament, **802–803, 809**
Lateral bands, **442, 464–465, 468–469, 473, 475, 477, 480**
- contribution to central slip, **476**
- interosseous tendons beginning, **464**

Lateral calcaneal tubercle, **935–936, 960–963, 967**
Lateral calcaneonavicular, bifurcate ligament, **1029**
Lateral center-edge angle, **598–603**
Lateral circumflex artery, **562, 566–567, 570, 663**
Lateral circumflex femoral artery, **525–527, 541, 612, 620–621**
Lateral circumflex femoral vein, **525–527, 562, 566, 570, 613, 620–621**
Lateral collateral ligament, **664, 667, 670, 692–697, 700–701, 706–709, 727, 731–733, 749, 758–759, 797–802, 805–806, 809, 811, 1051, 1053, 1058–1059, 1074–1077, 1096, 1098–1099**
- bursa deep to, **803**
- insertion, **798, 805**
- origin, **726, 755, 809, 811**

Lateral collateral ligaments, **1004–1005, 1015–1018**
Lateral condyle, **454**
Lateral cord, **11**
Lateral crural extension of retinaculum, **738**
Lateral crus, **529**
Lateral cutaneous nerve, **303**
- forearm, **199**

Lateral epicondyle, **156, 174–175, 197, 202, 204, 208, 212, 215, 222–225, 272, 275, 278, 287, 304–305, 672**
- apophysis, **280**

Lateral femoral condylar peak, **672**
Lateral femoral condylar sulcus, **672**
Lateral femoral condyle, **617, 657–658, 672, 679, 728–729, 745, 767, 769–771, 776–777, 784, 818, 826, 843, 868**
- "defect," **832**
- developmental variation, **828–832**

Lateral femoral recess, **679**
Lateral femoral sulcus, **874**
Lateral gastrocnemius, **668, 702–705, 710–711, 723–724, 771, 783–784, 884, 891**
Lateral geniculate nerve, **810**
Lateral geniculate vein, **810**
Lateral inferior geniculate artery, **612, 669, 714–715**
Lateral intermuscular septum, **166–167, 191**
Lateral joint capsule, **572**
Lateral joint recesses, **679**
Lateral leg muscles, **664**
Lateral malleolar artery, **1036**
Lateral malleolus, **883, 885, 892, 935–937, 939, 941, 953, 955, 966–967, 979, 1016, 1045, 1104**
- facet for, **921–922**

Lateral meniscocruciate ligament, anterior, **763**
Lateral meniscus, **675–676, 681–684, 696–697, 728, 742, 750, 753, 759**
- anterior horn, **676, 678–680, 712–713, 723–726, 748–751, 753–758, 763, 765, 772–774, 836–838, 844, 847, 849**
- anterior root, **675–676**
- body, **679–680, 708–711, 748–751, 755–756, 758, 760, 809, 847, 849, 855**
- "bow tie," **727**
- coverage, **874**
- discoid, **760, 813, 845**
- fascicle, **765, 839**
- junction of body/anterior horn, **765, 839**
- posterior, **874**
- posterior horn, **678–679, 681, 683, 706–709, 722–726, 748–750, 752–753, 756, 759, 762, 766, 770, 775–777, 779, 783, 802, 804, 806–807, 809, 811, 842, 847**
- posterior roots, **676**
- roots, **723, 742, 750–753, 756–757, 774**

Lateral patellar cartilage, **674**
Lateral patellar facet, **672, 674**
Lateral patellar retinaculum, **609, 690–691**
Lateral patellofemoral recess, **674, 679–680**
Lateral plantar artery, **1056–1057**
Lateral plantar compartment, foot, **1035**
Lateral plantar nerve, **930, 933, 950–951, 956–957, 988, 994, 1035, 1064–1065, 1126**
- cutaneous, **930**
- superficial branch, **1056–1057, 1068–1069**

Lateral plantar neurovascular bundle, **1064–1069**
Lateral recesses, **680**
Lateral retinaculum, **664, 692–693, 696–697, 714–717, 727, 731, 734, 735, 737, 738, 889, 891, 894–895**
Lateral sacral crest, **486, 492**
Lateral sesamoid, **1051**
- 1st toe, **1041**

xvii

INDEX

Lateral superior geniculate artery, **612, 644–647, 669, 688–689, 712–715, 726–727**
Lateral superior geniculate nerve, **714–715**
Lateral superior geniculate vein, **644–647, 714–715**
Lateral supporting structures, knee, **687, 796–811**
 - layer 1 (superficial), **796**
 - layer 2 (middle), **796**
 - layer 3 (deep), **796**
Lateral supracondylar line, **617**
Lateral supracondylar region, **197**
Lateral supracondylar ridge, **168–173**
Lateral syndesmotic clear space, **1129**
Lateral talar process, **935–936**
Lateral talocalcaneal ligament, **944**
Lateral tarsal artery, **893, 1036**
Lateral tibial plateau, **678, 728**
Lateral tibial spine, **672, 680–681**
Lateral trochlea, **864**
 - cartilage, **675**
Lateral trochlear ridge, anterior, **716–717**
Lateral tubercle, **923, 925**
Lateral ulnar collateral ligament (LUCL), **194, 198, 200**
Latissimus dorsi, **6–9, 12–13, 37, 60–75, 78–82, 87, 95–99, 100, 108, 113, 154, 157–158, 159, 180–187, 489, 557**
Leg, **812–857**
 - axial T1 MR
    left, **895, 897, 901, 903, 905, 907, 909**
    right, **894, 896, 900, 902, 904, 906, 908**
 - coronal T1 MR, **910–911**
 - deep fascia, **995**
 - imaging pitfalls, **813**
 - ligamentous variants, **812–813**
 - meniscal variant, **813**
 - muscles, **878–879**
    attachments, **881–882**
    variants, **812**
 - nerves of, **880, 893**
 - osseous variants, **812**
 - plica variant, **813**
 - radiographic anatomy and MR atlas, **878–915**
 - radiographs, **883**
 - retinacula, **878**
 - sagittal T1 MR, **912–914**
 - vessels, **879–880**
Lesser arc, **432**
Lesser saphenous vein, **692–693, 702–703, 721, 896–897, 904–909, 948–951, 960, 962–963**
Lesser sciatic foramen, **491**
Lesser sciatic notch, **489–490, 494**
Lesser trochanter, **515, 526–527, 556, 562, 567–568, 572, 575, 577, 578, 581, 609, 616, 620–621, 650, 657**
Lesser tuberosity, **4, 24–25, 27, 49–51, 74–75, 84, 88–89, 114, 122, 131, 151**
 - humerus, **16–20**
Levator ani, **490–491, 513–514, 557**
Levator scapulae, **7**
Ligament of Struthers, **280**
Ligamentum teres, **555, 556, 559, 582, 584–585, 588, 590, 593, 595**
Limbus labrum, **595**
Linea alba, **495–496, 519, 545**

Linea aspera, **616–617, 622, 624, 628–631, 633–637, 639, 658**
Linea terminalis, **592**
Lisfranc joint. *See* Tarsometatarsal joint.
Lisfranc ligament, **954–955, 1035, 1039, 1050, 1090**
 - dorsal, **1037, 1055, 1062–1063, 1093–1095**
 - interosseous, **1062–1063, 1070–1071, 1094–1095**
 - plantar, **1039, 1062–1063, 1094–1095**
Lister tubercle, **298, 302, 314, 326, 329, 331, 336, 343–347, 362–365, 383, 404, 406, 417, 429–430**
Liver, **186–187**
Long dorsal sacroiliac ligament, **488, 520–521**
Long plantar ligament, **926, 927, 970, 972–973, 977–978, 1000, 1004–1005, 1010, 1029–1031, 1035, 1037–1038, 1041, 1055, 1064–1069**
Long radiolunate ligament, **327, 348–349, 371, 383**
Longitudinal arch, foot, **1034, 1038, 1128, 1134**
Longitudinal fibers medial collateral ligament, **694–697, 712–713**
Lower trunk, **11**
Lumbar plexus, **487**
Lumbosacral trunk, **493**
Lumbosacral vertebra, transitional, **590**
Lumbrical, **425, 441, 456, 462–463, 473, 475, 477, 959, 1086, 1089**
 - 1st, **442, 466–467**
 - 2nd, **442, 467**
 - 3rd, **442, 466– 467, 470, 476**
 - 4th, **442, 466–467**
 - anomalous origin, **400**
 - insertion, **1058–1059**
 - proximal origin, **418**
Lunate, **326, 329, 335–337, 341, 343, 346–351, 366–371, 380–383, 394, 396, 420, 424, 453–454**
 - bipartite, **418**
 - cartilage, **395**
 - extra facet of, **419**
 - fossa, **301, 326, 329, 343, 393**
 - overhang, **431**
 - type II, **418–419**
 - volar lip of, **397**
Lunatocapitate angle, **433**
Lunatotriquetral ligament, **337, 339, 341, 368–369, 395**
 - dorsal band, **341**
Lung, **78–79, 96–97**
Lunotriquetral angle, **428, 433**
Lunotriquetral ligament, **330, 368–369, 391, 393–395**
 - dorsal, **395**
 - proximal, **395**
Lymph node, **79, 519**
Lymphatics, **519, 544–545**

M

Magic angle phenomenon, **456**
Main collateral ligament, **477**
Malleolar fossa, **1008–1009**
 - fibular, **1015–1016**

INDEX

Malleolus
- lateral, **883, 885, 892, 935–937, 939, 941, 953, 955, 966–967, 979, 1016, 1045, 1104**
- medial, **881, 883, 935–936, 944, 948–951, 953, 966–968, 974–975, 990–992, 995, 1003, 1007, 1011, 1019, 1022, 1045, 1103–1104, 1109, 1113**
- posterior, **935, 939, 943, 976, 1007, 1015, 1019**

Master knot of Henry, **929, 956, 970–971, 970–973, 983, 989, 1064–1065**
Mechanical axis, **599, 600, 1128**
Medial ankle gutter, **938, 952, 966**
Medial arm arcuate ligament, **802–803, 807, 810**
Medial calcaneal nerve, **930, 958–959, 975, 1035**
Medial calcaneal tubercle, **960–963, 1028**
Medial calcaneocuboid, bifurcate ligament, **1018, 1021, 1029**
Medial capsuloligamentous complex, **786, 794–795**
- deep layer (layer 3), **786**
- middle layer (layer 2), **786, 795**
- superficial layer (layer 1), **786, 788, 795**

Medial circumflex, ascending and descending branches, **612**
Medial circumflex artery, **561–562, 564–565, 568, 585–586**
Medial circumflex femoral artery, **525, 527, 565, 612**
Medial circumflex femoral vein, **525, 527, 613**
Medial circumflex vein, **561–562, 564–565, 568, 585, 613**
Medial circumflex vessels, **563**
Medial clear space, **935, 1129**
Medial collateral ligament, **194, 665–666, 669, 670, 675–676, 680–681, 690–693, 696–699, 710–713, 718, 730–731, 733, 738, 749, 756–758, 789, 791, 793–794, 803, 881, 894–897, 918–919, 1051, 1053, 1058–1059, 1074–1077, 1096, 1098–1099**
- bursa, **758, 794**
- deep, **795**
- fat between superficial and deep fibers, **794**
- insertion, **911**
- longitudinal fibers, **694–697, 712–713**
- oblique, **712–713, 758–759, 791, 803**
- oblique fibers, **694–697**
- origin, **791**
- superficial, **731, 756–758, 794–795**
- superior, **738**
- two arms, **792**

Medial compartment, thigh, **611**
Medial condyle, **454, 719**
Medial cord, **11**
Medial crus, **529**
Medial cubital vein, **172–179**
Medial cuneiform, **1110**
Medial cutaneous nerve
- brachial, **159, 166–169**
- forearm, **195, 199**

Medial dorsal cutaneous nerve, **931**
Medial epicondyle, **156, 174–177, 186–187, 197, 199, 202–204, 212, 215, 222–225, 244, 263, 272, 274–275, 278, 286, 289, 291, 292, 295, 302, 316–317, 323, 672**
Medial exostosis, **1122**
Medial facet signal abnormality, **741**

Medial femoral circumflex artery, **612**
Medial femoral circumflex vessels, **587**
Medial femoral condylar notch, **762**
Medial femoral condylar peak, **672**
Medial femoral condyle, **617, 655–656, 672, 677, 684, 714–715, 718, 729, 745, 749, 766–767, 769, 771, 776, 780, 785, 789, 794, 842–843, 849**
Medial gastrocnemius, **668, 702–711, 718–722, 736, 771, 780–781, 784, 803, 884, 889**
Medial inferior geniculate artery, **669, 710–713, 716–717, 721**
Medial intermuscular septum, **158, 188**
Medial joint recess, **1046**
Medial malleolus, **881, 883, 935–937, 944, 948–951, 953, 966–968, 974–975, 990–992, 995, 1003, 1007, 1011, 1019, 1022, 1045, 1103–1104, 1109, 1113**
- anterior colliculus, **935–936, 944–945**
- facet for, **921–922**
- posterior colliculus, **935–936, 944, 967, 975**

Medial meniscomeniscal ligament, **766, 767, 843**
Medial meniscus, **676, 681, 684, 696–697, 729, 742–746, 748, 757**
- anterior horn, **675, 677, 680, 682, 684, 714–715, 719–722, 743–746, 748–749, 757, 761, 764, 773, 837, 841, 849, 854**
    originating from tibial plateau, **848–849**
- body, **675–676, 680, 710–713, 743–744, 748–750, 756–758, 794, 849**
- junction anterior horn/body, **714–715**
- junction body/posterior horn, **708–709**
- posterior horn, **676–677, 682, 685, 706–707, 709, 719–721, 743–746, 748–749, 756, 758–759, 761, 770, 780–781, 852**
    superior recess, **761**
- posterior root, **675–676**
- roots, **722, 742, 746, 756–757**

Medial oblique meniscomeniscal ligament, **766**
Medial patella, **723**
Medial patellar facet, **672, 674**
Medial patellar retinaculum, **609, 615, 665, 730–731**
Medial patellofemoral ligament, **665–666, 690–691, 730, 733, 734–738, 757, 787–788, 791**
Medial patellofemoral recess, **674, 677**
Medial patellofibular ligament, **731**
Medial patellomeniscal ligament, **736, 737, 787**
Medial plantar artery, **1036, 1058–1059**
Medial plantar compartment, foot, **1035**
Medial plantar hallucal nerve, **930**
Medial plantar nerve, **930, 933, 950–951, 958–959, 966–969, 988, 992, 994, 1035, 1036, 1056–1057, 1126**
Medial plantar neurovascular bundle, **1064–1069**
Medial plica, **685, 728, 741**
Medial retinacular complex, **787, 795**
Medial retinaculum, **692–693, 696–697, 712–717, 719–720, 722–723, 791, 795, 889, 894–895**
Medial retinaculum complex, **734, 736–738**
Medial sesamoid, 1st toe, **1040–1041**
Medial superior geniculate artery, **642–645, 669, 688–689, 714–715, 718, 721**
Medial superior geniculate nerve, **714–715**

INDEX

Medial superior geniculate vein, **642–645, 714–715**
Medial supporting structures, knee, **686–687, 786–795**
Medial supracondylar line, **617**
Medial supracondylar region, **197**
Medial supracondylar ridge, **168–173**
Medial tibial plateau cartilage, **729, 799**
Medial tibial spine, **672, 680–681, 770**
Medial trochlea, **728**
  - cartilage, **675**
Medial tubercle, **923–925**
Medial wall, **559**
Median artery, **332**
Median crest
  - metatarsal, **1097**
  - sacral, **492**
Median eminence, **1027, 1044**
Median eminence, navicular, **956, 970–973, 988–990, 992, 1112**
Median nerve, **8, 11, 37, 155, 157, 159–179, 182–183, 188–189, 195, 197–199, 212, 214–218, 217, 220–233, 240–241, 244, 252–258, 261–262, 264, 289, 303–315, 327, 333, 344, 346–355, 357–359, 361, 374–375, 383, 404–407, 411, 414, 429, 437, 443**
  - recurrent branch of, **443**
  - variants, **418**
Median sacral crest, **503**
Medioplantar oblique band, spring ligament, **956–957, 970–971**
Medioplantar oblique spring ligament, **927, 1004, 1022–1023, 1025–1028**
Meniscal fascicle, anterior, **774**
Meniscal homologue, **339, 393**
Meniscal ligaments, **684**
Meniscal ossicle, **813, 850–854**
  - fat saturated, **853**
  - unusual location, **855**
Menisci, knee, **670, 686, 742–767**. *See also* Lateral meniscus; Medial meniscus.
Meniscocapsular junction, **743, 795**
Meniscocruciate ligament, **763–764, 773, 813, 838**
  - mimicking meniscal tear, **840**
  - mimicking partial ACL tear, **841**
  - from transverse ligament, **836–837**
Meniscofemoral ligament, **670, 680–681, 684, 742, 746–747, 752, 756–758, 762, 786, 794–795**
  - of Humphrey, **677, 684–685, 742, 745–747, 752, 768–769, 776–779, 795, 799, 812–813**
  - of Wrisberg, **721–722, 742, 762, 768, 775, 795, 799, 812–813**
Meniscomeniscal ligaments, **772, 838**
  - medial, **767**
  - oblique, **742, 766**
Meniscopopliteal ligament. *See* Superior fascicle.
Meniscotibial ligament, **665–666, 669, 730–731, 733, 756–758, 786, 794, 881**
Metacarpal, **436, 452, 477**
  - 1st, **337, 361, 453**
       hypoplastic, **420**
  - 2nd, **453**
  - 3rd, **335–336, 366, 381**
  - 4th, **366–367**
  - 5th, **337, 361, 368, 378, 453**
Metacarpal base, **358**
  - 1st, **329, 343, 356–361, 368–373, 385, 467**
  - 2nd, **329, 343, 358–361, 364–369, 383–385**
  - 3rd, **329, 343, 358–365, 367–369, 382–383, 423**
       edema, **423**
  - 4th, **329, 343, 358–361, 364–365, 367–369, 379–381**
  - 5th, **329, 343, 356–361, 369, 371, 378–379**
Metacarpal head, **452**
  - 1st, **447–448, 450**
  - 2nd, **450, 453, 479**
  - 3rd, **453**
  - 4th, radial aspect, **470**
  - articular cartilage, **477**
  - dorsal concavity of, **450**
  - dorsal contour of, **454**
Metacarpal joint, 5th, **370**
Metacarpophalangeal joint, **436**
  - 1st, **444, 446–447, 450, 455**
  - 4th, **479**
  - 5th, **464**
  - zone IV, **478**
  - zone VI, **478**
Metaphyseal beak, **601**
Metaphyseal notch, **280–281**
Metatarsal, **1034**
  - 1st, **935, 937, 974, 982, 998, 1003, 1038, 1044, 1089, 1092–1093, 1118–1119**
       inclination angle, **1135**
       length, **1137**
       pad, **1139**
  - 1st-5th angle, **1136**
  - 2nd, **974–975, 982, 1038–1039, 1093, 1095, 1117, 1121**
       length, **1137**
  - 3rd, **976, 1000, 1038, 1092**
  - 4th, **976–977, 1038, 1062–1063, 1068–1071, 1081–1082, 1092**
  - 5th, **928, 958, 978–979, 982, 998–999, 1038, 1058–1059, 1068–1071, 1082–1083, 1089, 1108, 1116, 1121**
       inclination angle, **1135**
       pad, **1139**
       styloid, **936**
       tuberosity, **1082–1083, 1091–1092**
  - alignment
       AP, **1136**
       lateral, **1135**
  - lengths, **1137**
       relative, **1128**
  - median crest, **1097**
Metatarsal articulation, accessory, **1117**
Metatarsal head
  - 1st, articular facets, **1098**
  - 2nd, **1099**
Metatarsal head, dorsal medial, notch at, **1043**
Metatarsal ligaments, transverse, **1055**
Metatarsophalangeal joint, **1035, 1096–1099**
  - 1st, **1042–1044, 1051–1052, 1096–1098**

INDEX

- 2nd, **1053**
    - plantar plate, **1074–1075**
- 2nd-5th injection, **1042**
- 4th, plantar plate, **1072–1073**
- lateral, **1096**

Mid talar head articular surface, **1132**
Midcarpal compartment, **338**
Midcarpal joint, **334**
Midcarpal ligament
- dorsal, **388**
- volar, **388**

Middle calcaneal facet, **927**
Middle collateral artery, **158–159**
Middle glenohumeral ligament (MGHL), **14, 21–22, 25–27, 30–32, 35, 49–51, 89–90, 98, 112, 114–115, 117–119, 127, 149–151**
- arthrogram, **117**

Middle phalangeal base, biconcave contour of, **454**
Middle phalanx
- 2nd, **453**
- 3rd, **482**
    - head of, **480**
    - midshaft, **482**
- 4th, **482**
    - base, **482**
- 5th, **453, 480**

Middle subtalar facet, **936, 988, 990, 1047**
Middle subtalar joint, **937, 968–969, 971, 975–976, 985, 992, 1014, 1106**
Middle trunk, **11**
Midfoot, **1034**
- alignment, **1132**

Midnavicular articular surface, **1132**
Morton foot, **1096, 1100**
Motion artifacts, **857**
Multipartite patella, **823**
Muscular branches, **612**
Musculocutaneous nerve, **8, 11, 37, 157, 159, 195, 199, 217, 303**

N

Navicular, **925–927, 935–936, 955, 974–977, 982, 993, 997, 1005, 1025, 1027, 1031, 1034, 1038, 1043–1044, 1060–1067, 1078, 1092–1093, 1109–1114**
- articular surface, **921, 927**
- beak, **1026–1028**
- facet for, **921–922**
- tuberosity, **988, 1002–1003, 1026, 1028**

Naviculocuneiform articular surface angle, **1132**
Naviculocuneiform joint, **1042, 1049–1050, 1066–1067, 1117**
Neck cutback, **578**
Neck junction, **567**
Needle, **580, 589**
Neural foramen, **576–577, 579, 586**
Neurovascular bundle, **50, 54–61, 98, 132**
- axillary, **52–53**
- brachial, deep, **66–67**
- of deep palmar arch, **470**
- digital. *See* Digital neurovascular bundle.
- plantar. *See* Plantar neurovascular bundle.
- posterior tibial, **952–953, 960–961**
- proper digital, **465, 482**

Neutral triangle, **936**
Nonbony coalition, **421**
Normal concave lunate facet, **419**
Normal joint recess, wrist, **339**
Notch of Harty, **968**
Notches, **427**
Nutrient canal, **634**
Nutrient foramen, **455**
Nutrient groove, **454, 617**

O

Oblique cord, **270–271, 318–319**
Oblique fibers medial collateral ligament, **694–697**
Oblique ligament, posterior, **677, 694–697, 719**
Oblique medial collateral ligament, **791**
Oblique meniscomeniscal ligament, **742, 766, 772, 813, 842–844**
Oblique muscle
- external, **495–500, 525–527, 528, 544–545, 557**
    - aponeurosis, **495, 500–504**
- internal, **495–506, 523–527, 528, 544–545, 550–551, 557**

Oblique popliteal ligament, **694–697, 720–721, 723, 744, 781–782, 786, 793, 797, 799–803, 806, 894–895**
Oblique pulley, **449, 474**
- zone I, **478**
- zone II, **478**

Obturator artery, **487, 510, 560–561, 612**
Obturator canal, **539**
- and vessels, **511**

Obturator externus, **489, 514–517, 520–527, 536–542, 548–551, 553, 555, 562–569, 572–573, 609–610, 618–621, 650–652, 654–656**
- bursa, **555, 556, 558, 581, 586**

Obturator foramen, **486, 488, 490–491, 530, 534, 556, 616**
Obturator groove, **490**
Obturator internus, **490–491, 493, 506–516, 521–526, 531–537, 539–540, 549–553, 555, 557, 560–562, 564–569, 572, 610, 614, 618–621, 649, 651, 654**
- nerve to, **493**

Obturator membrane, **536, 553, 615**
Obturator nerve, **491, 496–498, 503–507, 510, 533, 560–561, 564, 608, 663**
Obturator ring, **577**
Obturator ring/foramen, **494**
Obturator vein, **510, 613**
Olecranon, **202, 219, 234–235, 237, 275–276, 276, 280, 285, 301–302, 304–305, 322–323**
- pseudoeffect and avian spur, **285**

Olecranon articular cartilage, **207**
Olecranon bursa, **196**
- subcutaneous, **194**

Olecranon foramen, **202**

INDEX

Olecranon fossa, **172–173, 189, 202–203, 208, 212, 224–225, 236–239, 260, 274**
 - ulna, **211**
Olecranon process, **174–177, 197, 202–204, 208, 212–213, 215, 224–227, 253–255, 259, 264, 304–305**
Olecranon recess, **207, 211**
Omohyoid, **79**
Opponens digiti minimi, **356–361, 378–380, 402, 412, 438, 440–441, 445, 456, 460–461, 466–467, 470, 474, 1100**
Opponens pollicis, **354–361, 382–385, 399, 414, 438, 445, 447–448, 450–451, 456, 458–461, 471**
Opponens pollicis brevis, **466–467**
Os acetabuli, **590, 594**
Os acromiale, **4, 138, 143–144**
 - 3D CT, **145**
 - MR, **144–145**
 - radiographs, **143–144**
Os calcaneus secondarius, **1100–1101, 1108**
Os calcis views, **934**
Os cuboides secondarium, **1114**
Os cuboideum secondarium, **1101**
Os hamuli, **424**
Os intercuneiform, **1100–1101**
Os intermetatarseum, **1100–1101, 1118**
Os peroneale, **1100–1101**
Os peroneum, **1101, 1115**
Os styloideum, **422–423**
Os subfibulare, **1100, 1104**
Os supranaviculare, **1100–1101, 1113**
Os sustentaculi, **1101, 1106**
Os talonaviculare dorsale, **1100**
Os tibiale externum, **1100**
Os trigonum, **954–955, 1000, 1008, 1016, 1100–1101, 1105, 1107**
Os vesalianum, **1100–1101, 1116**
Osseous defect, **285**
Ossicle, accessory
 - foot, **1101**
 - wrist, **423**
Osteitis condensans ilii, **590–591**
Osteitis pubis, **529**

P

Palmar aponeurosis, **352–353, 356–361, 460–461**
Palmar arch
 - deep, **387, 457**
    neurovascular bundle, **470**
 - superficial, **457**
Palmar brevis, **458**
Palmar carpal arch, **332**
Palmar carpal ligament, **458–459**
Palmar cutaneous branch, **303, 333**
Palmar digital arteries, common, **437, 443, 460**
Palmar interossei, **379, 438–439, 456, 473, 475, 477, 479**
 - 1st, **442, 460–463**
    musculotendinous junction, **468–469**
 - 2nd, **442, 460–463, 470, 479**
 - 3rd, **442, 460–463, 470**
Palmar intrinsic muscles, **440**

Palmar plate, **480**
Palmaris brevis, **379–380, 459–461**
Palmaris longus, **178–179, 198, 213, 216, 228–233, 236–241, 249, 251, 256–258, 260–263, 303–309, 311–317, 321, 327, 398, 404, 406, 429**
 - accessory, **400**
 - insertion, **460–461**
 - variants, **418**
Palmaris muscle, **310**
Panner disease, **280, 288**
Pannus, margin of, **580**
Paraglenoid fossa, **590**
Paraglenoid sulcus, **591–592**
Parasymphysis, **519**
Paratenon, **950–951, 984**
Pars peronea metatarsalis primi, **1100–1101**
Patella, **617, 652, 656–658, 664–665, 676, 683, 685, 686, 728, 740, 784**
 - apex, pathologic cartilage thinning, **674**
 - bipartite, **812, 823–824**
 - cartilage, **677–678**
 - congruence
    dynamic assessment, **858, 869**
    to trochlea, **858, 868**
 - dorsal defect, **812, 825–827**
 - equator, **673**
 - height, measurement, **858–859**
 - lateral facet, **867**
 - medial, **723**
 - medial facet, **867**
 - multipartite, **823**
 - stabilizers, **736–738**
    medial, **786–787**
 - superior, **738**
 - tilt, measurement, **858, 867**
 - translational force exerted on, measurement, **858, 861**
Patella cubiti, **280**
Patellar ligament, **609**
Patellar median ridge, **674**
Patellar retinaculum, **799**
 - lateral, **609, 690–691**
 - medial, **609, 615, 665, 730–731**
Patellar tendon, **675, 678, 685, 734**
 - inferior, **664–666, 672, 696–701, 714–717, 723–726, 730–732, 734–736**
Patellofemoral ligament, medial, **665–666, 690–691, 730, 733, 787**
Patellomeniscal ligament, medial, **736–737, 787**
Patellotibial ligament, **734–738, 787, 788**
 - inferior, **665, 692–695, 716–717, 722, 730**
Pecten, **487, 489, 528, 530, 542**
Pectineal ligament, **528**
Pectineofoveal fold, **587, 593**
Pectineus, **489–490, 510–511, 515–518, 521–526, 529–530, 533–544, 549–553, 557, 561–562, 564–567, 573, 609–610, 615, 618–625, 651–657**
Pectinofoveal fold, **582, 593**
Pectoral nerve
 - lateral, **11**
 - medial, **11**

INDEX

Pectoralis major, **6, 12, 52–65, 82–83, 99–100, 109–110, 132, 154, 159, 187**
Pectoralis minor, **6, 12, 46–64, 130–132, 186–187**
Pelvic splanchnic nerves, **493**
Pelvis. *See also* Hip; Thigh.
- acetabular labral variants, **590**
- anterior
  - axial T1 MR, **531–538**
  - coronal T1 MR, **517–519, 539–545**
  - oblique axial T1MR, **552–553**
  - osseous anatomy, **528**
  - sagittal T1 MR, **546–551**
- bones and ligaments, **488**
  - external surface, **489**
  - internal surface, **490**
- bony variants, **590, 591–592**
- cartilage defect, **593**
- glenoid labrum variants, **595**
- and hip
  - AP, **575**
  - axial MR arthrogram, **584**
  - coronal MR arthrogram, **581–583**
  - inlet and outlet, **576**
  - radiographic and arthrographic anatomy, **574–589**
  - sacroiliac and pubic symphysis arthrography, **589**
  - sagittal MR arthrogram, **586–588**
- horizontal axis, **603**
- lateral, sagittal T1 MR, **524–527**
- lower, axial T1 MR, **507–511**
- measurements and lines, **598–603**
- mid
  - axial T1 MR, **501–506**
  - coronal T1 MR, **515–516**
  - sagittal T1, **520–523**
- MR atlas, **494–527**
- muscle and nerve variants, **590**
- normal variants and imaging pitfalls, **590–597**
- overview, **486–493**
- pediatric variants, **597**
- perpendicular to horizontal, **603**
- posterior, **493**
  - coronal T1 MR, **512–514**
- upper, axial T1 MR, **495–500**
- wall, internal surface, **491**
Perforating arteries, **612**
Perforating peroneal artery, **893**
Perforating veins, **613**
Perforating vessels, **612, 624–625, 632–633, 782, 784**
Perforation, in disc, **589**
Perilabral sulcus, **586**
Periosteum, **1019**
Perkin line, **599, 601**
Peroneal artery, **884–885, 887–888, 893, 1035**
- perforating, **893**
Peroneal nerve, **640, 814, 818, 915**
- common, **493, 613, 644–647, 658, 663, 668, 674, 676, 688–705, 722–725, 798, 814, 819, 880, 889–890, 892–897, 915, 920, 932**
- deep, **814, 880, 889–893, 898–907, 915, 920, 931–932, 948–951, 1035–1036**
  - lateral, **920, 931**
  - medial, **920, 930**
- recurrent, **915**
- superficial, **814, 880, 889–890, 892–893, 915, 920, 931–933, 1035–1036**
Peroneal retinaculum, **939, 946, 952–953, 956–957, 969, 994, 1008, 1012, 1014**
- inferior, **892, 919, 928, 947, 957, 968, 971, 981, 988, 996, 1108**
- superior, **878, 919, 928, 947, 953, 981, 995–996, 1001, 1020**
Peroneal tendons, **944, 972–973, 984, 997, 1000–1001, 1127**
- axial MR, **995–996**
- coronal MR, **998**
- sagittal MR, **999**
Peroneal trochlea, **923**
Peroneal tubercle, **923–924, 937, 956, 996, 1108**
- calcaneus, **1100**
Peroneal tunnel, **893, 915**
Peroneal vessels, **898–907, 910**
Peroneus brevis, **879, 881–882, 891–892, 898–910, 914, 919, 928–929, 939–940, 944–945, 947–959, 960–965, 968–973, 979, 980, 981–982, 984–985, 988–991, 993, 995–999, 1001–1003, 1016–1018, 1026, 1030, 1058–1059, 1064–1069, 1082, 1085, 1088, 1108, 1126–1127**
Peroneus digiti minimi, **879**
Peroneus longus, **664, 704–711, 727, 731–732, 879, 882, 889, 891–893, 896–910, 914–915, 919, 928–929, 939–940, 944–945, 947–959, 962–965, 968–973, 975–979, 981–982, 984, 988–991, 993, 995–1003, 1011, 1016–1018, 1026, 1030–1031, 1056–1061, 1064–1071, 1079–1082, 1085, 1088, 1095, 1108, 1110, 1115, 1127**
- groove for, **924–925**
- origin, **892, 915**
- sulcus, **1038, 1043**
- tunnel, **1031**
Peroneus quartus, **879, 980, 1026, 1100, 1127**
Peroneus tertius, **879, 891, 919, 929, 947–951, 948–949, 968–969, 972–973, 978, 980–981, 1085, 1100**
Persistent median artery, **418**
Pes anserinus, **609, 615, 712–715, 786, 788–791, 795, 896–897**
Phalangeal apparatus, **1096**
Phalanges, **436, 442, 452**. *See also* Middle phalanx; Proximal phalanx.
- 5th middle & distal (fused), **1060–1061**
- foot, **1034**
Pirie bone, **1100**
Piriformis, **489, 491, 493, 503–509, 512–514, 521–526, 551–553, 555, 557, 560, 563–570, 572, 610, 614, 650, 655–656**
- duplicated, **596**
- nerve to, **493**
Piriformis fossa, **594**
Pisiform, **326, 329, 331, 335–337, 339–340, 343, 350–353, 370–375, 378–380, 394, 396–397, 413–414, 421, 424, 453–454, 466–467**
Pisiform-5th metacarpal ligament, **413**

INDEX

Pisiform-triquetral joint, **337**
Pisiform-triquetral recess, **337, 340, 454**
Pisohamate ligament, **351, 372–375, 378–380, 415**
Pisometacarpal ligament, **378, 413**
Pisotriquetral joint, **379, 397**
Pisotriquetral recess, **337**
Plantar aponeurosis, **962**
 - central band, **960–963**
 - lateral band, **962–963**
Plantar arch, **1036, 1038**
Plantar calcaneocuboid ligament, **958–959**
Plantar cuneonavicular ligament, **1066–1067**
Plantar digital arteries, **1036**
Plantar digital nerves, **1036**
Plantar digital neurovascular bundles, **1076–1077**
Plantar digital vessels, **1056–1057**
Plantar fascia, **962–963, 986, 998, 1035, 1037, 1068–1069, 1072–1075, 1078–1079, 1081, 1083, 1096**
 - central band, **966–970, 972–973, 975–978, 1038, 1065–1067, 1088–1089**
 - deep fibers, **1074–1075**
 - digital bands, **1056–1057**
 - lateral band, **968–970, 972, 978, 1064–1065, 1083**
 - medial band, **1064–1067**
Plantar heel pad, thickness, **1139**
Plantar intercuneiform ligaments, **1037, 1055**
Plantar intermetatarsal ligaments, **1037, 1055**
Plantar interossei, **1041, 1084, 1085, 1087, 1089**
Plantar joint recess, **1053**
Plantar ligament
 - long, **926–927, 970, 972–973, 977–978, 1004–1005, 1010, 1029–1031, 1035, 1037–1038, 1041, 1055, 1064–1069**
 - short, **926–927, 958–959, 971–972, 977, 1004–1005, 1010, 1022–1023, 1030–1031, 1035, 1037–1038, 1055, 1064–1065**
Plantar Lisfranc ligament, **1039, 1062–1063, 1094–1095**
Plantar muscles, foot, **1034, 1040–1041**
Plantar nerve
 - lateral, **930, 933, 950–951, 956–957, 988, 994, 1035–1036, 1064–1065, 1126**
    cutaneous, **930**
    superficial branch, **1056–1057, 1068–1069**
 - medial, **930, 933, 950–951, 958–959, 966–969, 988, 994, 1035–1036, 1056–1057, 1126**
Plantar neurovascular bundle, **821**
 - lateral, **1064–1069**
 - medial, **1064–1069**
Plantar plate, **1053, 1096–1099**
Plantar soft tissue, measurements, **1128**
Plantaris, **610, 664, 666–668, 690–695, 698–711, 723–726, 732–733, 753–754, 783, 793, 810, 814–815, 819, 878, 884–886, 894–903, 906–907, 910, 912, 920, 948–961, 980, 984–985**
 - musculotendinous junction, **885**
Plica, **593, 685, 734**
 - inferior, **734**
 - infrapatellar, **685, 739, 772, 813, 818, 844**
 - lateral, **734**
 - medial, **685, 728, 734, 741**
 - superior, **734**
 - suprapatellar, **739–740**
 - variant, **813**
Popliteal artery, **612, 640–650, 657–658, 663, 669, 688–701, 708–711, 721–722, 747, 782, 812, 879, 884–885, 887–888, 892–893**
Popliteal fascicles, **683**
Popliteal-fibular ligament, **683**
Popliteal fossa, **610, 649**
Popliteal hiatus, **679, 728, 749–751, 754–756, 759, 761, 783, 796, 800, 806–807, 822, 846**
 - fluid in, **809, 811**
Popliteal ligament, oblique, **694–697, 720–721, 723, 744, 781, 786, 793, 797, 799–800, 802, 894–895**
Popliteal sulcus, **672, 758, 796**
Popliteal tendon, **664, 727, 732, 748–751, 754–756, 758–759, 761, 783**
Popliteal vein, **613, 640–650, 657–658, 688–689, 704–709, 722, 782**
Popliteal vessels, **643, 645, 649, 704–705, 720**
Popliteofibular ligament, **761, 783, 796–802, 804–807, 809–810, 822, 886**
Popliteomeniscal fascicle
 - inferior, **679, 742, 750–751, 754–755, 759, 761, 802**
 - superior, **678–679, 683, 742, 750–751, 754–755, 761, 796, 801, 804, 806**
Popliteomeniscal ligament, **761**
Popliteus, **610, 666–669, 675–676, 678–679, 681, 683–684, 692–701, 706–711, 720–726, 728, 731–733, 742, 746–756, 758, 761–762, 771, 783–784, 792, 796, 799–811, 822, 846, 878–879, 881, 885–886, 893–899, 910–914**
 - insertion, **886**
 - musculotendinous junction, **753, 760, 801–802, 807–808, 810, 845, 886**
 - origin, **726, 749, 755, 799, 806, 809–811**
Posterior acetabular rim, **578**
Posterior antebrachial cutaneous nerve, **158–159**
Posterior calcaneal facet, **927, 1025**
Posterior capsule, **676–677, 692–693, 719–721, 723, 743–747, 752–753, 761, 768–769, 771, 780–784, 792, 795, 799–803, 805, 807**
 - incomplete, **768**
 - perforations, **782**
 - and posterior cruciate ligament, fat interposed between, **782**
 - spaces within, **768**
Posterior circumflex humeral artery, **82–84, 95, 98–100, 110–111, 158, 516**
 - branches, **101**
Posterior circumflex humeral vessels, **56–59, 66–68, 70–71, 81, 180–185**
Posterior colliculus, **881, 883, 935, 1022**
Posterior column
 - hip, **559**
 - pelvis, **577**
Posterior compartment
 - arm, **164–165**
 - thigh, **611**
Posterior condylar cartilage, **675**

INDEX

Posterior cord, **11**
Posterior cruciate ligament, **664, 666–667, 675–678, 680–685, 692–697, 706–713, 720–722, 729, 731–733, 740, 745–746, 748–750, 756, 758–759, 766, 768–772, 775–779, 784–785, 794–795, 841–842, 844, 912**
 - anterolateral bundle, **768**
 - insertion, **684, 747, 759, 768–769, 849**
 - isometric tunnel locations, **875**
 - origin, **675, 720, 768–771, 777, 785**
 - posteromedial (oblique) bundle, **768**
 - ratio/angle, **872**
 - synovium covering, **784**
Posterior cruciate recess, **771, 784–785**
Posterior crural fascia, **706–707**
Posterior deep fibers, of deltoid ligament, **944**
Posterior epicondyle, **736**
Posterior fat, **769**
Posterior fat pad, **172–173, 189, 196–197, 215, 222–223, 245–246, 264**
Posterior femoral condyle cartilage, **677**
Posterior femoral cutaneous nerve, **493**
Posterior glenoid labrum, **22, 30, 114**
Posterior glenoid rim, **16**
Posterior gluteal line, **486, 489–490**
Posterior humeral cortex, **109**
Posterior inferior iliac spine, **504, 524**
Posterior inferior labrum, **92–93**
Posterior interosseous artery, **199, 303, 332**
Posterior interosseous nerve, **216, 327**
Posterior joint capsule, **563, 566, 584, 587, 679, 720**
Posterior joint recess, **27, 30, 35, 196, 208, 581, 588, 681, 769, 938, 1045**
Posterior labrum, **26–27, 30–31, 35, 47–53, 91–93, 117–118, 128, 130–132, 134–135, 559, 563, 581, 584–585, 587**
Posterior lateral femoral condyle cartilage, **674**
Posterior malleolus, **935, 939, 943, 976, 1007, 1015, 1019**
Posterior margin fibular groove, **935**
Posterior medial femoral condyle cartilage, **674**
Posterior medial meniscal root, **685**
Posterior medial recesses, **677**
Posterior oblique ligament, **677, 694–697, 719, 780, 786, 791–792, 795, 803**
Posterior recess, **677–678**
Posterior recess ankle joint, **1105**
Posterior rim, **526, 532, 603**
 - acetabulum, **575**
Posterior rotator interval, **14, 30**
Posterior subtalar facet, **923, 935–936**
Posterior subtalar joint, **937, 941–944, 946, 954–955, 957, 964–970, 976–978, 984, 990, 996, 1008, 1022–1024, 1042, 1045–1046, 1102, 1106–1107**
Posterior superior iliac spine, **486, 489–490, 493, 524, 575, 576**
Posterior superior labrum, **89–90**
Posterior suprapatellar (prefemoral) fat pad, **735, 761**
Posterior talofibular ligament, **918, 926, 939–941, 943–944, 946, 954, 1004–1005, 1009–1011, 1015–1016, 1018, 1020**
Posterior tibial artery, **669, 879–880, 884–885, 887, 893, 896–897, 920, 948–951, 1035–1036**
Posterior tibial cortex, **911**
Posterior tibial malleolus, **936**
Posterior tibial muscle, **960–963, 987**
Posterior tibial nerve, **898, 902–903, 948–951, 962–963**
Posterior tibial neurovascular bundle, **952–953, 960–961**
Posterior tibial tendon, **929–930, 939–940, 943–945, 948–957, 960–975, 980, 982–984, 991–994, 1003, 1037, 1064–1069, 1087–1088**
 - axial MR, **987**
 - coronal MR, **988**
 - dislocation, **946**
 - distal, **990**
 - distal slips, **989**
Posterior tibial vein, **948–951**
Posterior tibial vessels, **898–910, 948–951, 962–963, 975**
Posterior tibiofibular ligament, **926, 939, 948–951, 1005, 1008–1011**
 - inferior, **942–943, 952, 964–966, 1005, 1007–1012, 1015–1016, 1019**
Posterior tibiotalar ligament, **926–927, 950–951, 1005, 1020–1023, 1028**
Posterior ulnar recurrent artery, **174–177, 198, 303**
Posterior wall, **559, 587**
 - acetabulum, **578, 581**
 - pelvis, **577**
Posterolateral capsule, **796**
Posterolateral corner, **798–799**
Posterolateral structures, **800–810**
Posteromedial capsule, **787**
Posteromedial distal femoral metaphyseal cortical defect, **812, 833–834**
Posteromedial oblique ligament, **682**
Posteromedial structures, knee, **792–793**
Posteromedial tibia, **666**
Posterosuperior labrum, **87, 581**
Posterosuperior rim of acetabulum, **584**
Pre-Achilles bursa, **986**
Pre-Achilles fat, **1124**
Pre-Achilles fat pad, **821, 891, 936, 960–963, 977, 984–986**
Precruciate joint recess, **769**
Prefemoral fat pad, **672, 674, 678, 688–689, 716–717, 735, 761**
Pregastrocnemius recess, **678**
Prestyloid recess, **390, 393–394, 397**
Princeps pollicis artery, **303, 443, 457**
Processus vaginalis, **529**
Pronator quadratus, **299, 302, 312–315, 318–319, 327, 331, 344–345, 368–373, 381–383, 398, 402**
Pronator teres, **157, 178–179, 198, 209, 212–213, 215–218, 222–233, 238–241, 244–246, 251, 253–258, 261–265, 280, 302–309, 316–317, 321–323**
Proper digital arteries, **437, 443, 460**
Proper digital neurovascular bundles, **464**
Proximal carpal row, **315**
Proximal humeral diaphysis, **120**
Proximal interosseous ligament, **389**

INDEX

Proximal interphalangeal joint, **454**
- 2nd, **454, 468–469**
- 3rd, **453**
- 5th, **453, 1043**

Proximal phalanx, **442, 449, 454–455, 471, 1038**
- 1st, **446, 450, 453, 479, 1078**
    - duplicated, **427**
- 2nd, **451, 453**
- 3rd
    - base, **481**
    - diaphysis, **481**
    - proximal aspect, **481**
- 4th, **481**
    - diaphysis, **481**
- 5th, **479, 481**
- articular cartilage, **477**
- base, **455**
- capsule, **476**
- head, volar aspect, condyles of, **482**

Proximal radioulnar joint, **194, 202–204, 208–209, 213, 265, 272**
- ligaments of, **194**

Proximal row carpal ligaments, **394**
Proximal tibiofibular joint, **672, 679, 683, 878, 883**
Proximal tibiofibular ligament, **802–803**
Pseudoepiphyses, **426**
Pseudoerosions, wrist, **418**
Pseudospur, **592**
- acromion, MR pitfalls, **141**

Psoas, **495–502, 515–517, 525, 540–541, 560, 562, 564–565, 609, 615**
Psoas minor, **490, 557**
Pubic angle, **528**
Pubic arch, **528**
Pubic body, **486, 521, 530, 535, 537, 542–543, 547, 616**
Pubic bone, **519, 528, 530, 536–537, 547, 654**
Pubic crest, **528, 530, 543–544, 546–547**
Pubic ramus, **576**
- inferior, **489–490, 530, 538–540, 550–551, 620–621**
- superior, **486–487, 489–490, 517, 530, 540–543, 550–552, 556, 616, 652**

Pubic spine, **592**
Pubic symphysis, **488, 530, 542, 552–553, 575–576, 579, 586, 597, 652**
Pubic tubercle, **487, 489, 528, 530, 535, 544, 548–549, 556, 575, 592, 615–616**
Pubis, **486–487, 491, 556**
- body, **490**

Pubofemoral ligament, **555, 556**
Pudendal artery
- external, **612**
- internal, **507, 559**

Pudendal nerve, **514**
Pudendal vein, internal, **507, 559**
Pulley system, **474**
Pulvinar, **554, 556, 559, 564, 582, 593, 595**

Q

Q-angle, **858, 861**
Quadrangular space, **5, 36**
Quadrate ligament, **270**
Quadratus femoris, **489, 493, 513–514, 526–527, 555, 557, 562, 565–572, 609–610, 614, 618–623, 650, 657–659**
Quadratus lumborum, **490, 557**
Quadratus plantae, **925, 958–959, 962–967, 969–973, 975, 985, 992–993, 1040, 1056–1059, 1064–1071, 1080, 1082, 1084–1086, 1088, 1100, 1125**
Quadriceps, **617, 644–647, 652, 657–658, 664, 666, 669, 672, 688–689, 716–717, 724, 726–727, 732, 734–735, 889, 891**
- aponeurosis, **730**
- fat pad, **736**
- insertion, **730**
- tendon, **734, 736**

Quadrilateral plate, **532, 561, 563, 572–573**
- of acetabulum, **584**

Quadrilateral space, **5, 13, 36, 56–57**
- graphics, **13**

R

Radial artery, **198–199, 216, 230, 232–233, 258, 265, 303, 308–309, 316–317, 332–333, 344, 346–353, 357, 372–375, 385, 437, 440, 443, 448, 457–461**
Radial articular cartilage, **207**
Radial bursa, **400, 402, 474**
Radial collateral artery, **158–159, 190**
Radial collateral ligament (RCL), **194, 197, 200, 204–205, 209–210, 212–213, 215, 229, 238–239, 247, 270–279, 330, 384–385, 391, 396, 449–450, 464–465, 468–469, 479**
- accessory, **200, 449, 479**

Radial deviation (PA), **334**
Radial height, **428**
Radial inclination, **428, 431**
Radial nerve, **9, 11, 58–65, 95, 155, 158–173, 181–183, 189–190, 195, 197–198, 214–218, 217, 220–227, 238–240, 247, 253, 261, 266, 303, 306–311, 327, 333, 344, 346–353, 354–355, 437**
- branches, **166–167, 174–179**
- deep branch, **195, 198–199, 216–218, 228–233, 240–241, 254–258**
- superficial branch, **195, 198–199, 216–218, 228–231, 240–241, 254–257, 265, 327**

Radial notch, **301**
Radial recurrent artery, **199, 303**
Radial sesamoid, **447**
Radial styloid, **301–302, 326, 329, 331, 341, 343, 367–369, 384–385, 396, 410, 429**
Radial styloid base, **346–347**
Radial styloid process, **348–349, 366–367**
Radial tilt, **431**

INDEX

Radial tuberosity, **202–203, 230–233, 238–239, 250, 261, 267–269, 282, 285, 301**
- lucency, **280**
    mimicking lesion, **282**
Radial vein, **230, 232–233, 346–347, 351**
Radial vessel, **310–311**
Radial volar (palmar) tilt, **428**
Radialis indicis artery, **303, 443, 457**
Radiocapitellar joint, **202–203, 206**
Radiocapitellar joint space, **290**
Radiocapitellar line, **292**
- elbow, **293**
Radiocarpal compartment, **338, 396**
Radiocarpal joint (RCJ), **334, 338–339**
Radiocarpal joint recess, dorsal, **341**
Radiocarpal ligament
- dorsal, **327, 341, 388, 392, 394, 396–397**
- volar, **327, 388**
Radiolunate angle, **433**
Radiolunate ligament
- long, **327, 388, 396**
- short, **388, 394, 396**
Radiolunotriquetral ligament, **340**
- dorsal, **340**
Radioscaphocapitate ligament, **327, 330, 339–341, 348–353, 381–384, 388, 391, 394, 396–397**
- long, **391**
Radioscapholunate ligament, **327, 396**
Radioulnar angle, **428, 433**
Radioulnar bursa, **194**
Radioulnar joint, **326, 329, 343**
- distal, **429–430**
- proximal, **246, 265**
Radioulnar ligament
- distal, **389**
- dorsal, **327, 348–349, 366–367, 380, 391–392, 396**
- volar, **348–349, 380**
Radioulnar ratio, **428–429**
Radius, **190, 198, 216, 257–258, 269, 302–303, 306–315, 318–321, 320–321, 335–336, 364–373, 380–383, 430**
- distal, **321, 326, 340**
- head, **156, 178–179, 191, 198, 202–203, 206–211, 216, 228–229, 236–237, 240, 246–247, 255, 260–261, 265, 272, 278, 287, 289, 292, 295, 301–302, 304–305, 321–322**
    epiphysis, **281**
    posterior aspect, **273**
- neck, **202–204, 228–231, 238–239, 256, 281–282, 301, 306–307**
- shaft, **266, 294, 301**
Rectus abdominis, **495–510, 519–523, 528, 530–536, 544–549, 552–553, 564, 619, 654**
Rectus femoris, **489, 507–511, 517–519, 524–527, 534, 537–538, 541–543, 557, 560–563, 565–569, 571, 573, 609–610, 615, 618–645, 652–653, 655–658, 723–726, 734, 735, 889, 891**
- reflected head, **583**
Recurrent peroneal nerve, **915**
Red marrow islands, **1109**
Retro-Achilles bursa, **986**
Retrocalcaneal bursa, **986**
Retrocalcaneal fat pad, **936, 986**
Retrocondylar bursa, **780–781**
Retromalleolar groove, **995**
Retrotibial groove, **987**
Retrotrochlear eminence, **956–958, 966–967, 1108, 1127**
Rhomboideus major, **7**
Rhomboideus minor, **7**
Rib, **79, 96, 156**
Rotator cuff, **5, 14, 94–101**
- graphics, **9, 95**
- right, sagittal T2 FS MR, **96–101**
Rotator interval, **5, 14, 22, 36, 82, 102–111**
- anatomy, **104**
- axial T2 MR arthrogram, **106**
- coronal T2 MR arthrogram, **107**
- graphics, **23, 103**
- lower, **102**
- posterior, **14, 30**
- sagittal PD FS arthrogram, **105**
- sagittal T1 FS MR arthrogram, **108–111**
Rotators, external, **526–527, 565, 569, 572, 655**

S

S1
- nerve root, **498–504, 513, 521–522**
- neural foramen, **550, 592**
- segment, **491–492**
S2
- nerve, **549**
- nerve root, **500–504, 522**
- segment, **492**
S3
- nerve root, **503**
- segment, **492**
S4 segment, **492**
S5 segment, **492**
Sacral ala, **486, 492**
Sacral arc, **492, 616**
Sacral crest, median, **486, 492**
Sacral foramen anterior, **492**
Sacral hiatus, **486, 492, 506, 520**
Sacral plexus, **487, 491, 493, 505**
Sacral promontory, **486, 492**
Sacral tuberosity, **492**
Sacrococcygeal junction, **492**
Sacroiliac joint, **493, 499–503, 512–513, 575–576, 579, 586, 589, 616**
- accessory, **590, 591**
- anterior margin, **577**
- posterior, **576**
- synovial portion, **500, 512–514**
- views, **579**
Sacroiliac ligament
- long dorsal, **488, 520–521**
- short dorsal, **488**
- ventral, **488**
Sacrospinous ligament, **488, 490–491, 508–510, 522–523, 531–532, 557, 615**

INDEX

Sacrotuberous ligament, **488, 490–491, 493, 508–511, 522–525, 531–535, 557, 562, 610, 615**
Sacrum, **486, 491–492, 498–507, 512–515, 520–523, 546–550, 616**
- base, **492**
- graphics, **492**

Sagittal band, **464–465, 476–477, 479**
Saphenous nerve, **628, 643–644, 646, 668, 880, 920, 931, 933, 952–953**
Saphenous vein
- greater, **515–518, 522–523, 543–544, 613, 620–627, 629–655, 668, 692–695, 698–705, 708–711, 880, 894–897, 949–951, 1064–1065**
- lesser, **692–693, 702–703, 721, 896–897, 904–909, 948–951, 960–963**
- small, **668, 880**

Sartorius, **489, 506–511, 517–519, 523–527, 531–538, 544–545, 557, 560–567, 609, 611, 615, 618–656, 665–666, 668–669, 674–675, 688–713, 718–719, 730–731, 758–759, 774, 784, 786, 788–791, 793, 795, 817, 819, 881–882, 884–885, 889, 894–897, 910**

Scaphocapitate ligament, deep portion, **396–397**
Scaphoid, **326, 329, 335–337, 341, 343, 348–355, 366–373, 383, 385, 394, 396–397, 420, 424, 446, 453–454**
- cartilage, **395**
- distal pole, **334, 336, 340, 384, 397**
- fossa, **301, 329, 343, 393**
- proximal pole, **337, 340, 396**
- tubercle, **335, 337, 339**
- waist, **329, 343**

Scapholunate angle, **428, 433**
Scapholunate distance, **428**
Scapholunate joint, **340**
Scapholunate ligament, **330, 338–341, 348–349, 367–371, 391, 393–395**
- dorsal, **393–396**
- proximal, **394–395**
- volar, **394**

Scaphotrapeziotrapezoid articulation, **354–355**
Scaphotrapeziotrapezoid ligament, **330**
Scaphotrapezium-trapezoid ligament, **391**
Scaphotriquetral ligament, dorsal, **339–341, 392, 394, 396–397**

Scapula, **4, 32, 54–56, 58–63, 65, 70–71, 79, 96, 114, 130, 132, 134, 156**
- acromion, **16–20**
- blade, **24, 30**
- body, **16–17, 19–20, 50–53, 80, 97, 130–132**
- glenoid fossa, **97**
- inferior angle, **19**
- lateral border, **19**
- medial border, **19**
- spine, **13, 17–18, 37, 42–47, 68–69, 71–73, 78–80, 89–93, 96–97, 106, 108, 116, 121, 124, 129, 134**
- surgical neck, **17**

Scapular artery, dorsal, **10**
Scapular ligament, superior transverse, **12, 95**
Scapular nerve, dorsal, **11**
Sciatic buttress, **576**

Sciatic foramen, greater, **488**
Sciatic nerve, **493, 506–511, 513, 523–527, 531–534, 552–553, 560–562, 564–565, 567, 596, 608, 614, 618–643, 658, 668**
Sciatic notch
- greater, **489–490, 552, 564**
- lesser, **489–490**

Semimembranosus, **489, 493, 512–513, 526, 536–537, 557, 562, 566–567, 610, 615, 618–649, 655–658, 665–669, 674–675, 677, 681–682, 685, 688–697, 702–711, 718–722, 730–733, 736, 759, 771, 780–781, 786, 789–791, 792–793, 795, 803–804, 816–817, 819, 881, 886, 894–895**
- anterior branch, **803**
- branch to oblique popliteal ligament, **696–697**
- capsular expansion, **719**
- direct and capsular parts, **696–697**
- direct branch, **698–699**
- expansion, **704–705**
- insertion, **677, 706–709, 780, 789–790**
- posteromedial tibial insertion, **789**
- slip to medial collateral ligament, **792–793, 803**
- slip to oblique popliteal, **793**
- tibial attachment, **792–793, 803**

Semitendinosus, **489, 493, 512, 527, 536–537, 557, 562, 564, 566–567, 610, 615, 620, 622–649, 655–658, 665–666, 668–669, 674–675, 682, 688–703, 705–709, 718–719, 721, 730–731, 771, 786, 788–789, 791, 795, 816–817, 819, 881, 882, 884, 894–897**
- conjoined origin long head biceps femoris, **512–513, 526, 655–658**

Serratus anterior, **6, 61–65, 78–79, 131–132, 180–187**
Sesamoid, **418, 427, 446, 454–455, 471, 1096, 1100–1101, 1110**
- 1st toe, **1043–1044, 1056–1059, 1074–1075, 1078–1080**
- 2nd-5th toes, **1100**
- 5th toe, **1101**
- of digits, **1101**
- facets, **1038**
- in flexor hallucis longus tendon, **1101**
- great toe, **1100**
- lateral, **1051–1052, 1097–1099, 1120–1121**
  1st toe, **1041**
- medial, **1051–1052, 1097–1099, 1121**
  1st toe, **1040–1041**

Sesamophalangeal apparatus, **1096**
- attachment, **1052**
- lateral, **1052**
- medial, **1052**

Shenton line, **599, 601**
Short head biceps, **664**
Short plantar ligament, **927, 958–959, 971–972, 977, 1000, 1004–1005, 1010, 1022–1023, 1030–1031, 1035, 1037–1038, 1055, 1064–1065**
Short radiolunate ligament, **330, 381–382**
Shoulder. *See also* Arm.
- 3D CT reconstruction, muscle origins and insertions, **6–7**
- ABER (abduction external rotation) plane, **86–93**
  anterior and superior views, **87**

INDEX

T1 FS MR arthrogram, **88–93**
- anterior, **113–114**
- arthrography, **14–35**
  - conventional, **20**
  - normal, **21**
- axial, superior to inferior, **26–27**
- contrast outlines cartilage surface, **21**
- graphics, **22**
  - anterior, **8**
  - neural structures, **11**
  - neurovascular structures, **9**
  - posterior, **8**
  - quadrilateral space, **13**
  - rotator cuff, **9**
  - shoulder musculature, **8**
  - spinoglenoid notch, **12**
  - superficial dissection, **37**
  - suprascapular notch, **12**
  - vascular structures, **10**
- imaging pitfalls, **138–151**
- labrum, **126–137**
- left
  - axial T1 MR, **39, 41, 43, 45, 47, 49, 51, 53, 55, 57, 59, 61, 63, 65**
  - coronal oblique T1 MR, **67, 69, 71, 73, 75, 77**
  - sagittal oblique T1 MR, **79, 81, 83, 85**
- ligaments, **5, 112–125**
- MR atlas, **36–85**
- normal variants, **138–151**
  - bicipital groove, vessels lateral, **140**
  - distal supraspinatus tendon, hyperintensity, **139**
- oblique coronal, posterior to anterior, **24, 25**
- overview, **4–13**
- radiography, **14–35**
  - AP external and internal rotation, **16**
  - axillary view, **18**
  - Garth view, **17**
  - Grashey view, **17**
  - scapular Y and AP scapula views, **19**
  - Stryker notch view, **18**
  - supraspinatus outlet view, **19**
  - West Point view, **18**
- right
  - axial T1 MR, **38, 40, 42, 44, 46, 48, 50, 52, 54, 56, 58, 60, 62, 64**
  - coronal oblique T1 MR, **66, 68, 70, 72, 74, 76**
  - sagittal oblique T1 MR, **78, 80, 82, 84**
- rotator cuff and biceps tendon, **94–101**
- rotator interval, **102–111**
- sagittal, **114**
  - lateral to medial, **28–30**
- sublabral window, **31**
Sigmoid notch, **276, 326, 329, 343, 346–347, 393, 430**
Sinus tarsi, **920, 944, 970–971, 1021, 1023**
Slight dorsal displacement, **430**
Small saphenous vein, **668, 880**
Soft tissue, measurements, **1139**
Soleal line, **708–709, 886**

Soleus, **610, 666–669, 709, 721–726, 732–733, 878, 881, 884–885, 891, 893, 896–905, 910–914, 936, 947, 960–961, 981, 983–984, 986, 991**
- accessory, **820, 1100, 1123**
- tibial origin, **708**
Sourcil, **572, 575**
Space of Poirier, **390–391**
Spermatic cord, **506**
Sphincter urethra, **557**
Sphincter urethra muscle, **490**
Spinoglenoid notch, **9, 36, 48, 92, 134**
- graphics, **12**
Spinous process, **579, 586**
Sports hernia, **529**
Spring ligament, **919, 945, 972–973, 1002, 1004, 1013, 1026–1028, 1037–1038, 1041, 1055, 1112**
- facet for, **921–922**
- inferoplantar longitudinal, **927, 1004, 1025–1028, 1031**
  band, **956, 985, 988**
- medioplantar oblique, **927, 1004, 1022–1023, 1025–1028**
  band, **956–958, 970, 988**
- superomedial, **927, 1004–1005, 1017, 1023, 1025, 1028**
  band, **955–957, 970, 974–975**
Stellate crease/lesion, **590, 593**
Stieda process, **1105**
Styloid process, **340, 958, 979, 1038, 1044, 1056–1057, 1082**
Styloid strut, **393**
Subacromial-subdeltoid bursa, **5, 9, 32, 72–73, 127, 133**
- contrast in, **20**
Subcapital region, **616**
Subchondral cysts, **28, 31**
Subclavian artery, **10**
Subclavius, **80**
Subcoracoid bursa, **5**
Subcutaneous fat, **38–39, 85**
Subdeltoid bursa, conventional arthrography, **20**
Subgastrocnemius bursa, **744, 780–781, 784**
Subgluteus medius bursa, **558–559**
Subgluteus minimus bursa, **558**
Subinguinal space, **494**
Sublabral cleft, **138**
Sublabral foramen, **106, 126, 133, 138, 149**
- normal variant, **149**
Sublabral recess, **34, 135, 590, 595**
Sublabral sulcus, **33, 130, 584–585, 595**
Sublabral window, **31**
- contrast in, **31**
Sublime tubercle, **274**
Subsartorial canal, **608**
Subscapular nerve, **11**
Subscapular recess, **4–5, 89–90, 105, 108**
Subscapularis, **6, 8–9, 12, 14, 22, 25, 27, 29–30, 32, 35, 37, 44–65, 72–84, 87–91, 94–101, 103, 105–111, 113, 115, 117–120, 122–125, 127–137, 139–140, 148, 150–151, 157, 180–182, 184–185**
- insertion at lesser tuberosity, **87**
- superficial fibers, **118**
Subscapularis recess, **21, 25, 30, 35**

INDEX

Subtalar facet
- anterior, **923–924, 1047**
- middle, **923–924, 936, 1047**
- posterior, **923–924, 935–936**

Subtalar joint, **918**
- anterior, **921, 946**
- middle, **921, 937, 968–969, 971, 975–976, 985, 992, 1014, 1106**
- posterior, **921, 937, 941–944, 946, 954–955, 957, 964–970, 976–978, 984, 990, 996, 1008, 1022–1024, 1042, 1045–1046, 1048, 1106–1107**

Superficial anterior tibiotalar ligament, **939**
Superficial circumflex iliac artery, **612**
Superficial deltoid fibers, anterior, **945**
Superficial deltoid ligament, **919, 926–927, 939, 946, 948–953, 970, 974–975, 1004–1005, 1008, 1012–1014, 1019–1020**
- tibiocalcaneal band, **944, 954–956, 968–969, 988, 992**
- tibionavicular band, **944, 954–955**
- tibiospring band, **945, 970**

Superficial epigastric artery, **612**
Superficial fascia, **784**
Superficial femoral artery, **515–517, 612, 624–639, 650–652, 655–656**
Superficial femoral vein, **515–517, 613, 624–639, 650–652, 655–656**
Superficial inguinal ring, **529**
Superficial medial collateral ligament, **756–758, 794–795**
Superficial palmar arch, **303, 332, 418, 443, 460**
- radial artery contribution, **443, 460**

Superficial peroneal nerve, **814, 880, 889–890, 892–893, 915, 931–933, 1035–1036**
Superficial semimembranosus bursa, **780**
Superficial veins, **376–377**
Superior acetabular labrum, **560, 567**
Superior acetabular notch, **593**
Superior acromioclavicular ligament, **113–114, 125**
Superior articular facet, **492**
Superior articular process, **492**
Superior extensor retinaculum, **878, 889–890, 892, 919, 928–929, 947, 981–983**
Superior fascicle, **754–788, 761, 783, 802, 806–807**
Superior gemellus, **489, 493, 510, 533, 566–568, 610**
Superior geniculate artery
- lateral, **612, 644–647, 669, 688–689, 712–715, 726–727**
- medial, **612, 642–645, 669, 688–689, 714–715, 718, 721**

Superior geniculate vein
- lateral, **644–647, 714–715**
- medial, **642–645, 714–715**

Superior glenohumeral ligament (SGHL), **14, 22–23, 25–26, 29–30, 32, 99, 102–111, 112, 114–116, 120–121, 127–130**
- arthrogram, **116**

Superior glenoid, **88–89, 134**
Superior glenoid labrum, **24, 26, 33, 136**
- meniscoid, **33**

Superior gluteal artery, **487, 493, 503–505, 515, 524–525, 612**
Superior gluteal nerve, **493**
Superior gluteal vein, **493, 503–505, 515, 524–525, 560, 613**
Superior gluteal vessels, **566**
Superior iliac spine
- anterior, **486, 489–490, 500, 519, 527, 556, 609, 615**
- posterior, **486, 489–490, 493, 524**

Superior joint recess, **584–585, 938**
Superior labrum, **34, 72–73, 89, 107, 116, 121, 125, 128–129, 559, 582–584**
- anterior, **32**

Superior medial collateral ligament, **738**
Superior patella, **738**
Superior peroneal retinaculum, **878, 919, 928–929, 947, 953, 981, 995–996, 1001, 1020**
Superior popliteomeniscal fascicle, **678–679, 683, 742, 750–751, 754–755, 761, 796, 801, 804, 806**
Superior pubic ligament, **528, 543**
Superior pubic ramus, **486–487, 489–490, 517, 530, 540–543, 550–552, 556, 575, 579, 586, 616, 652**
Superior pubic root, **573**
Superior ramus, **517–519, 522–523, 528**
Superior sublabral recess, **126**
Superior transverse scapular ligament, **95, 112, 114**
Superior ulnar collateral artery, **159, 303**
Superior ulnar collateral vessels, **166–167**
Superolateral joint recess, **580–581**
Superomedial joint recess, **580–581, 583**
Superomedial spring ligament, **927, 974, 1004–1005, 1017, 1023, 1025, 1028**
Supinator, **198, 208–210, 213, 216, 218, 228–233, 236–240, 246–247, 249, 256–258, 260–261, 265–266, 268, 302–303, 306–311, 316–319, 321–322**
- crest, **274, 277**
- fossa, **301**

Supra-acetabular ilium, **507**
Supracondylar femur, **650–651**
Supracondylar spur, **280, 285–286, 289**
Supraglenoid tubercle, **9, 46–47, 73**
Suprapatellar bursa, **672, 735, 761**
Suprapatellar fat pad, **672, 735**
Suprapatellar joint recess, **818**
Suprapatellar plica, **677–678, 685, 739–740**
Suprapatellar recess, **677–678, 690–691**
Suprascapular artery, **9–10, 46–49, 72–75, 129–130**
- infraspinatus branch, **10**

Suprascapular branch vessels, **79, 96**
Suprascapular nerve, **9, 11, 46–47, 49, 72–75, 130**
- infraspinatus branch, **12**
    in splenoid notch, **12**
- in suprascapular notch, **12**

Suprascapular neurovascular bundle, **80, 97**
Suprascapular notch, **36, 134**
Suprascapular vessels, **12, 40–41, 44–45, 78**
Supraspinatus, **6–9, 12–13, 14, 22, 24–29, 29–30, 32, 37, 40–47, 70–80, 82, 84–85, 87, 90–91, 94–101, 103, 105–111, 113, 116, 119–121, 124–125, 127–130, 133–134, 137, 139, 148, 151, 158, 180, 184–185**
- anterior direct, **42–43, 83, 100**
- direct component, **46–47, 83**
- footprint, **21**

INDEX

- leading edge, **28**
- oblique, **42–43, 46–47, 100**
- posterior oblique component, **129**
- posterior oblique fibers, **70–71, 83**

Supraspinatus fossa, **79, 96**
Sural nerve, **668, 721, 880, 896–901, 904–909, 920, 932–933, 948–953, 960–961, 1035–1036**
Sustentaculum tali, **923–925, 936–937, 942, 944–945, 956–957, 968–969, 975–976, 989, 992, 994, 1014, 1022, 1026, 1028, 1038, 1087, 1106, 1108**
Symphyseal surface, **490**
Symphysis pubis, **511, 518, 528, 530, 615–616**
- axial T1 MR, **531–538**
- coronal T1 MR, **539–545**
- oblique axial T1MR, **552–553**
- sagittal T1 MR, **546–551**

Synchondrosis, **1111–1113, 1116**
Syndesmotic clear space, **935**
- lateral, **1129**

Syndesmotic ligaments, **946**
Syndesmotic portion of joint, **579**
Syndesmotic recess, **938–939, 941, 943–944**
Synovial fold, **200**
Synovial fringe, **200, 204, 208–210, 246, 265, 274, 283**
- hyperplastic, **280, 290**

Synovial joint capsule, **554–555**
Synovium, **103, 784**

T

T1 spinal nerve, **11**
Talar base angle, **1134**
Talar head articular surface, **988**
Talar os trigonum, **1008**
Talar ridge, **938**
Talocalcaneal angle, **1128, 1130–1131**
Talocalcaneal interosseous ligament, **1004, 1021–1022**
Talocalcaneal ligament, lateral, **944**
Talocalcaneonavicular joint, **946, 1047**
Talofibular ligament
- anterior, **918, 926, 939–940, 941, 946, 952–955, 979, 1004–1005, 1015, 1018, 1020**
- posterior, **918, 926, 939–941, 943–944, 946, 954, 1004–1005, 1009–1011, 1015–1016, 1018, 1020**

Talometatarsal angle, **1128**
Talometatarsal axis, **1135**
Talonavicular articular surface angle, **1132**
Talonavicular joint, **952–953, 971–973, 976, 992, 1042, 1044, 1047**
Talonavicular joint capsule, **940**
Talonavicular ligament, dorsal, **926–927, 1005, 1037, 1055**
Talonavicular relationship, **1128**
Talus, **884–885, 918, 921–922, 925–927, 935, 937, 939, 942, 945, 982, 986, 988, 990, 994–996, 1001, 1005, 1009–1010, 1013, 1015–1017, 1020–1024, 1026, 1028–1029, 1031, 1038, 1105–1106, 1108, 1126–1127, 1129**
- anterior facet, **922**
- axis, **1136**
- body, **921, 969, 977, 991, 1025, 1045, 1109**
- dome, **939, 946, 952, 977, 1007, 1019–1020**
- fovea, **966, 975**
- head, **918, 921–922, 935–936, 952–954, 970–971, 973, 976–977, 1026, 1045, 1088, 1111–1112**
- lateral process, **918, 921–922, 935, 936, 941, 954–955, 968–969, 978, 1013, 1022, 1046**
- lateral tubercle, **921–922, 936, 991, 994, 1126**
- medial tubercle, **921–922, 936, 991, 994**
- neck, **918, 921–922, 936, 952–955, 970–971, 976–977**
- posterior process, **918, 922, 938**
- ridge, **938, 942, 1105**
- sulcus, **921–922**
- trochlea, **922, 937, 966–967, 976**

Tarsal artery, lateral, **893**
Tarsal canal, **920, 954–955, 957, 968–969, 976, 984, 1004, 1021–1024, 1046**
Tarsal sinus, **941–942, 945, 954–956, 970–971, 977–978, 985, 990, 1000, 1004, 1021–1024, 1026, 1108**
- ligaments, **946**

Tarsal tunnel, **920, 930**
Tarsometatarsal articular surface angle, 1st, **1132**
Tarsometatarsal joint, **1042, 1050, 1090–1095**
- 1st, **936, 1043–1044, 1050, 1070–1071, 1089, 1090–1092, 1117–1118**
- 2nd, **936, 1039, 1044, 1050, 1068, 1080, 1117–1118**
- 3rd, **1091–1092, 1117**
- 3rd-5th, **1050**
- 4th, **1091**
- 5th, **1091–1092**
- alignment, **1133**
- axial T1 MR, **1094**
- coronal T2 MR, **1095**
- graphics, **1093**
- radiographs, **1091**
- sagittal CT, **1092**

Tarsometatarsal ligaments, **1090**
- dorsal, **1037, 1055**

Teardrop, **554, 575, 616**
Tendon injury zones, hand, **478**
Tendon sheaths, **94, 481, 980–981, 1042, 1102**
- flexor, **472, 481**
- fluid in, **456**
- wrist, **340, 400**

Tensor fascia lata, **489, 504–511, 518–519, 557, 560–563, 568–571, 573, 609, 615, 618–625, 652–653, 657–659**
Tensor fascia suralis, **819**
Teres major, **6–9, 12–13, 37, 58–65, 67–73, 78–82, 87, 95–99, 108, 113, 154, 157–159, 180–185**
Teres minor, **7–9, 12–13, 14, 27–30, 32, 37, 50–55, 68–71, 78–84, 82, 85, 93, 94–99, 98–101, 103, 105, 108–111, 115, 118–120, 127–128, 130–134, 131–134, 140, 158, 180–181**
Terminal sulcus, **679**
Terminal tendon, **439, 476–477**
Terminal tuft, **447, 452, 454–455**
- 4th, **453**

Thenar, **358–359, 399–400, 437**
Thenar eminence, **331**

xxxi

INDEX

Thigh
- adductor muscles, **529**
- anterior, **609**
    coronal T1 MR, **652–653**
- arterial anatomy, **612**
- central, sagittal T1 MR, **656–658**
- compartments, **606, 611**
- fascia, **608**
- femoral triangle, **615**
- femur radiographs
    distal, **617**
    proximal, **616**
- lateral, sagittal T1 MR, **659**
- left distal, axial T1 MR, **643, 645, 647**
- left mid, axial T1 MR, **627, 629, 631, 633, 635, 637, 639, 641**
- medial, sagittal T1 MR, **654–655**
- mid, coronal T1 MR, **650–651**
- muscles
    anterior, **606–607**
    medial, **606, 615**
    posterior, **607**
- posterior, **610**
    coronal T1 MR, **648–649**
- posterior cutaneous nerve of, **668**
- radiographic anatomy and MR atlas, **607–659**
- right distal, axial T1 MR, **642, 644, 646**
- right mid, axial T1 MR, **626, 628, 630, 632, 634, 636, 638, 640**
- sciatic nerve and dermatomes, **614**
- upper left, axial T1 MR, **619, 621, 623, 625**
- upper right, axial T1 MR, **618, 620, 622, 624**
- venous anatomy, **613**

Thoracic artery
- internal, **10**
- lateral, **10**
- superior, **10**

Thoracic nerve, long, **11**
Thoracoacromial artery, **10**
- acromial branch, **10, 70–71**
- branches, **42–43, 81, 98**
- clavicular branch, **10**
- deltoid branch, **10**
- posterior branch, **10**

Thoracoacromial vessels, **97**
Thoracodorsal artery, **10**
Thoracodorsal nerve, **11**
Thoracolumbar fascia, **495**

Thumb
- anatomy, **444–451**
    axial, **448**
    features, **444**
- coronal MR, **450**
- orientation, **452**
- proximal phalanx, **479**
- radiographs, **446, 455**
- sagittal MR, **447**
- tip of, **480**

Thyrocervical trunk, **10**
Thyroid artery, inferior, **10**

Tibia, **918, 926–928, 935–936, 938, 941, 943, 945, 947–951, 962–966, 976–977, 983–984, 987, 991, 994–995, 1002, 1005–1011, 1013, 1015–1016, 1018, 1021–1025, 1028, 1127, 1129**
- anterior, **1002**
- anteromedial bare area, **889**
- axis, **1130**
- distal, transverse axis, **871**
- insertion of anterior cruciate ligament on, **764**
- insertion of posterior cruciate ligament on, **746–747**
- posterior, **987**
- proximal, **686**

Tibial apophysis, **883**
Tibial artery, **888**
- anterior, **879, 884–885, 887–893, 896–897, 1035–1036**
- posterior, **669, 879–880, 884–885, 887, 896–897, 948–951, 1035–1036**

Tibial growth plate scar, **935**
Tibial nerve, **493, 614, 640, 644–647, 663, 668, 674, 688–695, 698–705, 720, 722–723, 818, 880, 884–886, 888, 893, 896–909, 920, 930, 932, 1035**
- posterior, **898, 902–903, 948–951, 962–963**

Tibial plafond, **600, 937–938, 966–968, 975**
Tibial plateau, **745, 749**
- anterior horn medial meniscus originating from, **848–849**
- lateral, **678, 728**
- medial, **849**

Tibial sesamoid, 1st toe, **1101**
Tibial slip, **1009**
Tibial spine, **770**
Tibial tendon
- anterior, **947–949, 980, 982, 1002–1003, 1064–1069**
- posterior, **948–957, 960–975, 980, 982–983, 987–988, 991–992, 1037, 1064–1069**
    axial MR, **987**
    coronal MR, **988**
    distal, **990**
    distal slips, **989**

Tibial torsion, **858, 871**
Tibial tubercle, **672, 862, 935**
Tibial tubercle trochlear groove method (TT-TG), **858, 862–863**
Tibial vein, posterior, **975**
Tibial vessels
- anterior, **898–909, 948–949**
- posterior, **898–910, 948–951, 962–963, 975**

Tibialis anterior, **664, 726–727, 731–732, 879, 881–882, 889, 891, 896–909, 911–914, 919, 925, 928, 949, 951, 954, 970, 990, 1060–1063, 1085, 1094**
Tibialis posterior, **667, 669, 708–709, 732–733, 820–821, 879, 884–888, 893, 896–909, 911, 913, 920, 925, 951, 954, 961, 990, 1003, 1020, 1025–1028, 1041, 1055, 1085, 1110, 1113, 1125**
- anterior slip, **1058–1061, 1066–1067**
- fibular origin, **666, 733**
- tibial origin, **666, 733, 887**

Tibiocalcaneal band, **1004–1005, 1008, 1013–1014, 1020–1022**
Tibiocalcaneal ligament, **926–927**

INDEX

Tibiofibular interosseous membrane, **1006, 1008**
Tibiofibular joint, **686**
 - inferior, **918**
 - proximal, **672, 679, 683, 878**
Tibiofibular ligament, **811**
 - anterior, **918, 926–927, 939, 941, 944–945, 948–951, 979**
   inferior, **1004–1005, 1007–1008, 1011–1014, 1018–1019**
 - posterior, **918, 926, 948–951**
   inferior, **1004–1005, 1007, 1012, 1015–1016, 1019**
Tibiofibular overlap, **1129**
Tibiofibular syndesmotic ligaments, **1004–1011**
Tibionavicular band, **927, 1004–1005, 1012, 1019–1020, 1029**
Tibionavicular ligament, **940, 948–951**
Tibiospring band, **1004–1005, 1013, 1020, 1025**
Tibiospring ligament, **927, 945**
Tibiotalar articular surface, **1007**
Tibiotalar ligament, deep, anterior, **940**
Transcondylar line, **863, 870–871**
 - posterior, **864**
Transverse arch, foot, **1034, 1038–1039**
Transverse humeral ligament, **14, 37, 112–113, 113**
Transverse intermeniscal ligament, **676**
Transverse ligament, **9, 27, 32, 35, 49, 95, 134, 157, 555, 556, 559, 564–565, 581–582, 585, 588, 595, 684–685, 696–697, 714–715, 722–726, 742, 746–750, 752–754, 757, 763–765, 773, 813, 837–838, 848–849**
 - inferior, **564, 566, 918, 921, 926, 939–943, 1005, 1007–1008, 1010, 1015–1016, 1019, 1022**
 - meniscocruciate ligament arising from, **836–837**
Transverse meniscal ligament, **748–749**
Transverse metatarsal ligaments, **1035, 1037, 1055**
Transverse recess, dorsal, **390, 394, 397**
Transverse scapular ligament, superior, **95**
Transversus abdominis, **490, 495–505, 523–527, 528, 544–545, 549–551, 557**
Trapeziocapitate ligament, **330, 354–355, 391–392**
Trapeziotrapezoid ligament, **327, 330, 392**
Trapezium, **326, 329, 335–337, 343, 354–357, 368–375, 384–385, 424, 446–447, 453, 466–467**
 - articulation, **451**
 - hook, **337, 424**
 - tubercle, **448**
Trapezius, **6–7, 38–43, 66–67, 70–81, 96–97**
 - anterior fibers, **40–41**
Trapezoid, **326, 329, 335–337, 340, 343, 354–357, 365, 367–371, 383–384, 420, 446, 451**
Triangular fibrocartilage, **338–339, 366–369, 379–380, 391, 393, 395**
 - articular disc, **366–367**
 - attachment, normal cartilage underlying, **339**
 - distal margin, **338**
Triangular fibrocartilage complex (TFCC), **338, 429**
Triangular ligament, **476**
Triangular space, **13**

Triceps, **9, 12–13, 37, 56–57, 95, 158, 163–168, 171–175, 180–183, 188–189, 196–197, 211–212, 215, 219, 221–225, 234–235, 245–249, 252–253, 259, 264, 302, 322**
 - lateral head, **7–9, 12–13, 58–69, 82–83, 95, 99–101, 108–109, 154, 158–169, 180–183, 190–191, 220–223, 234–237, 246–247, 260, 265–266**
 - long head, **7–9, 12–13, 37, 54–57, 56, 58–59, 61–69, 78–82, 95–99, 108, 132, 154, 158–173, 180–185, 189–190, 220–223, 234–239, 244–245, 260, 263–264**
 - medial head, **7, 154–155, 159, 162–171, 180–183, 189–190, 219–221, 234–237, 245–246, 260, 264**
 - snapping, **249**
Tricipital aponeurosis, **174–175**
Triquetrocapitate ligament (TC), **370–371, 391**
Triquetrohamate ligament, **330, 391–392, 396–397**
Triquetrum, **326, 329, 335–337, 341, 343, 348–353, 366–371, 378–380, 392, 394, 396–397, 420, 424, 453**
Triradiate cartilage, **597**
Trochanter
 - greater, **509–511, 515–516, 556, 559, 562–563, 570–572, 616, 650, 657–659**
 - lesser, **515, 526–527, 556, 562, 567–568, 572, 609, 616, 620–621, 650, 657**
Trochanteric bursa, **559**
Trochlea, **174–176, 186, 188–189, 196, 202–203, 207, 209, 211–212, 226–227, 238–241, 244–245, 264, 285, 287, 295, 304–305, 316–317, 322**
 - depth, **858, 865**
 - facet
   asymmetry, **858, 865**
   lateral, **865**
   medial, **865–866**
 - fragmented, **286**
 - inclination, measurement, **858, 864**
 - irregular ossification of, **285–287**
 - lateral, **864, 866–869**
 - sulcus angle, **858, 866**
Trochlear cartilage, **677–678**
Trochlear cleft, **196**
Trochlear groove, **280, 672**
Trochlear groove line, **863**
Trochlear notch, **285**
Trochlear ridge, **280**
True pelvis, **494**
Truncation artifact, **856**

U

Ulna, **178–179, 198, 211, 213, 216, 228–231, 233, 246, 257–258, 267, 269, 276, 303, 306–313, 314–315, 318–319, 322, 366–371, 378–380, 453**
 - distal, **322, 326**
 - head, **302, 318–319, 329, 343, 364–365, 379**
   inclination, **428, 433**
 - olecranon process, **156, 182–185**
 - radial notch, **198, 216**
 - shaft, **301**
 - sublime tubercle, **204, 208–209, 274**

INDEX

- trochlear head, **260**
- trochlear notch, **211, 245, 264**

Ulnar angle, **292**

Ulnar artery, **198–199, 230–233, 240–241, 258, 261–262, 303, 308–309, 316–317, 332, 344–359, 372–375, 380, 421, 437, 443, 457–459**

Ulnar bursa, **400, 402, 474**

Ulnar collateral ligament (UCL), **197, 200, 204–205, 208–209, 212–213, 238–239, 251, 260, 263, 270–272, 275–276, 278, 449–450, 464–465, 468–469, 471, 479**
- accessory, **449, 479**
- anterior, **199**
- anterior band, **205, 272, 274, 275–276**
- insertion, **449**
- lateral, **198, 216, 228, 236–237, 260, 270–271, 273–274, 277–278**
- posterior band, **205, 211, 251, 272, 275**
- radial, **205, 208–210**
- superior, **199**
- transverse band, **205, 251, 272**

Ulnar deviation (PA), **334**

Ulnar fossa, **329, 343**

Ulnar minus, **431**

Ulnar nerve, **11, 155, 159–179, 182–183, 188, 195, 197–199, 205, 208, 212–213, 214–216, 219–233, 236–237, 244–245, 253–258, 260, 275, 291, 303–311, 314–315, 327, 333, 344–361, 372–374, 380, 404–407, 413–415, 421, 437, 443, 458–459**
- superficial branch, **356–358**

Ulnar neutral, **431**

Ulnar notch, **202, 281**

Ulnar plus, **431**

Ulnar recess, **390, 397**

Ulnar recurrent artery, **197, 215, 224–225**
- posterior, **199, 216, 219**

Ulnar sagittal band, **479**

Ulnar sesamoid, thumb, **447, 449, 451**

Ulnar shaft, **202**

Ulnar styloid, **301–302, 329, 335–336, 343, 346–347, 362–363, 368–369, 413, 428, 429, 430**

Ulnar styloid process, **346–347, 378**

Ulnar tuberosity, **203, 245, 256, 268–269, 301**

Ulnar variance, **428**

Ulnar vein, **344–345, 348–353, 356–357, 372–375**

Ulnocapitate ligament, **348–349, 352–353, 370–371, 391, 393–394, 396–397**

Ulnocarpal structures, **389–390**

Ulnolunate ligament, **327, 330, 348–349, 370–371, 391, 393, 396**

Ulnotriquetral ligament (UT), **348–349, 379, 391, 393–395**

Unipartite medial sesamoid, **1120**

Upper trunk, **11**

Ureter, **497, 500, 503, 505, 507**

Urinary bladder, **553**

V

Valgus/varus, standing AP view, **858**

Vastus intermedius, **562–563, 568–569, 609–610, 620, 622, 624, 626–647, 650–652, 657–659, 724–726, 735, 818**

Vastus lateralis, **513–518, 527, 562–563, 569–573, 609–610, 618–647, 649–653, 657–659, 688–689, 712–717, 724–727, 735, 737–738, 889, 891**

Vastus medialis, **515–516, 527, 540, 609–610, 615, 620, 622–647, 649–652, 655–657, 669, 680, 688–689, 712–726, 788–789, 818, 889**
- aponeurosis, **716–717**

Vastus medialis obliquus (VMO), **646–647, 651, 688–691, 734–738, 787–788, 791**

Ventral S1 foramen, **502**

Ventral sacroiliac ligaments, **488**

Vertebral artery, **10**

Vinculum breve, **472, 475**

Vinculum longum, **475**

Volar carpal ligament, **342, 351**

Volar joint recess, normal, **341**

Volar midcarpal ligament, **388**

Volar plate, **449, 466–467, 470–471, 479, 482**
- DIP joint, **483**
- MCP joint, **483**
- membranous portion, **477**
- PIP
    membranous portion, **483**
    portion of 3rd, **482**
- thick portion, **477**

Volar radiocarpal ligament, **327, 330**

Volar radioulnar ligament (VRU), **346–349, 368–369, 380, 391, 393, 396**

Volar recess, **340**

Volar superior joint recess, **212**

Volar tilt, **433**

Volume artifacts, **857**

W

Wrisberg, meniscofemoral ligament of, **721–722, 742, 762, 768, 775, 795, 799, 812–813**

Wrist
- anatomic spaces, **328**
- anteroposterior arthrogram, **338**
- central axis, **428**
- compartments, **338, 344**
- extensor tendons, **277**
- graphics, **330**
    arteries, **332**
    ligaments, **330**
    lunate axis, **433**
    nerves, **333**
    tendons, **331**
    veins, **332**
- joints, **326**

INDEX

- left
    - axial T1 MR, **345, 347, 349, 351, 353, 355, 357, 359, 361**
    - coronal T1 MR, **363, 365, 367, 369, 371, 373, 375, 377**
- ligaments, **327, 388–397**
    - axial GRE MR, **396**
    - graphics, **330**
- measurements and lines, **428–433**
    - carpal relationships, **432**
    - distal radius and ulna, **431**
- miscellaneous bony variants, **427**
- motion, **326–327**
- MR arthrogram findings, **334, 339**
    - axial T1, **341**
- MR atlas, **342–387**
- multiple joint recesses, **340**
- muscles and tendons, **327–328, 398–417**
    - graphics, **331**
    - variants, **418**
- nerves, **327**
- neurovascular variants, **418**
- normal variants and imaging pitfalls, **418–427**
- osseous structures, **326**
- overview, **326–333**
- pronated
    - 3D CT anatomy, **343**
    - 3D reconstruction CT, **329**
- radiographic and arthrographic anatomy, **334–341**
    - carpal tunnel view, **334**
    - clenched fist view, **334**
    - imaging pitfalls, **334**
    - PA, **334–335**
    - radial and ulnar deviation, **335**
    - semisupinated view, **334, 337**
- recesses, **390**
- retinacula, **328**
- right
    - axial T1 MR, **344, 346, 348, 350, 352, 354, 356, 358, 360**
    - coronal T1 MR, **362, 364, 366, 368, 370, 372, 374, 376**
- tendons
    - 3D reconstruction CT, **408**
    - axial T1 MR, **406–407**
    - coronal GRE MR, **414–417**
    - graphics, **402–405**
    - sagittal T1 MR, **410–412**
- vessels, **327**

Z

Zona orbicularis, **555, 559, 563, 568–569, 572, 580–582, 585, 587, 595**
Zones of vulnerability, wrist, **432**